Brief Contents for Volume 2

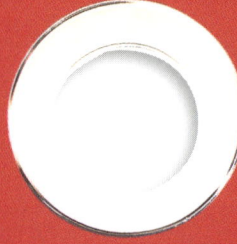

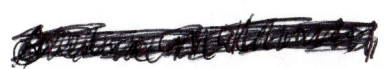

VOLUME **1**

PARAMEDIC PRACTICE TODAY ABOVE AND BEYOND

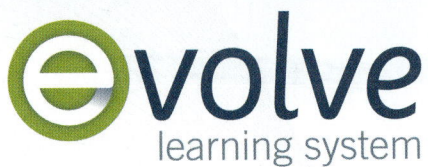

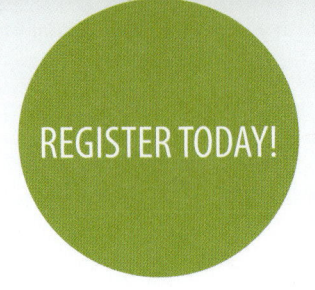

REGISTER TODAY!

To access your Student Resources, visit:

http://evolve.elsevier.com/Aehlert/paramedic

Instructor Resources

- Chapter Pretest
- Detailed Lesson Plan
- Classroom Activities
- PowerPoint Presentation with Speaker Notes
- ExamView Test Bank

Student Resources

- Learning Objectives
- Chapter Summary
- PowerPoint Lecture Notes
- Anatomy Challenges
- Body Spectrum Electronic Anatomy Coloring Book
- Drug Calculators
- Fluid and Electrolytes Presentation
- Heart and Lung Sounds
- Link to the National Registry Skill Sheets
- Medical Terminology Review
- Mosby's Essential Drug List
- Study Tips
- English/Spanish Audio Glossary
- Weblinks
- And more

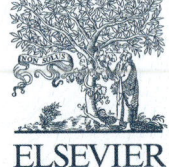

ELSEVIER

VOLUME **1**

PARAMEDIC PRACTICE TODAY ABOVE AND BEYOND

Editor

BARBARA AEHLERT, RN, BSPA

Associate Editor

ROBERT VROMAN, BS, NREMT-P

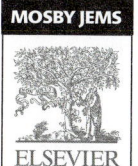

MOSBY JEMS
ELSEVIER

11830 Westline Industrial Drive
St. Louis, Missouri 63146

PARAMEDIC PRACTICE TODAY: ABOVE AND BEYOND
Volume 1
Two-Volume Set

ISBN: 978-0-323-04374-8
ISBN: 978-0-323-04389-2

Notice

Knowledge and best practice in this field are constantly changing. As new research and experience broaden our knowledge, changes in practice, treatment and drug therapy may become necessary or appropriate. Readers are advised to check the most current information provided (i) on procedures featured or (ii) by the manufacturer of each product to be administered, to verify the recommended dose or formula, the method and duration of administration, and contraindications. It is the responsibility of the practitioner, relying on their own experience and knowledge of the patient, to make diagnoses, to determine dosages and the best treatment for each individual patient, and to take all appropriate safety precautions. To the fullest extent of the law, neither the Publisher nor the Editor assumes any liability for any injury and/or damage to persons or property arising out of or related to any use of the material contained in this book.

The Publisher

Library of Congress Cataloging-in-Publication Data

Aehlert, Barbara.
  Paramedic practice today : above and beyond / Barbara Aehlert.--lst ed.
    p. cm.
  Includes bibliographical references and index.
  ISBN 978-0-323-04374-8 (vol. 1, hardcover : alk paper)--ISBN 978-0-323-04375-5 (vol. 2, hardcover : alk paper)--ISBN 978-0-323-04389-2 (two volume set, hardcover : alk. paper) 1. Emergency medicine. 2. Emergency medical technicians. I. Title.
  RC86.7.A355 2010
  616.02'5--dc22

2008041746

Executive Editor: Linda Honeycutt
Senior Developmental Editor: Laura Bayless
Publishing Services Manager: Patricia Tannian
Project Manager: Jonathan M. Taylor
Designer: Amy Buxton

Working together to grow
libraries in developing countries

www.elsevier.com | www.bookaid.org | www.sabre.org

ELSEVIER | BOOK AID International | Sabre Foundation

Printed in Canada

Last digit is the print number: 9 8 7 6 5 4 3 2

For our paramedic students and instructors (past, present, and future) who make a personal commitment every shift to provide optimal emergency care to each patient—as if that patient were a member of their own family.

Contributors

Barbara Aehlert, RN, BSPA
Southwest EMS Education, Inc.
Phoenix, Arizona
Pursley, Texas

Imoigele P. Aisiku, MD, MSCR, MBA
Assistant Professor
Department of Anesthesia/Critical Care &
   Emergency Medicine
Virginia Commonwealth University
Richmond, Virginia

Deanna Aftab Guy, MD
Assistant Professor of Pediatrics
Division of Pediatric Endocrinology
Vanderbilt University Medical Center
Children's Hospital at Vanderbilt
Nashville, Tennessee

David K. Anderson, BS, EMT-P
Director of EMS Education
NW Regional Training Center
Vancouver, Washington

Augie Bamonti III, EMT-P, FF
EMS Training Officer
Chicago Heights Fire Department
Chicago Heights, Illinois

Jeffrey K. Benes, BS, NREMT-P
EMS Coordinator
Aurora Medical Centre
Kenosha, Wisconsin

Scott Bourn, PhD, RN, NREMT-P
National Director of Clinical Programs
American Medical Response National Resource Center
Greatwood Village, Colorado

Jennie A. Buchanan, MD
Chief Resident in Emergency Medicine
Denver Health
Denver, Colorado

Chris Cebollero, NREMT-P
Clinical Services Manager
MedStar
Fort Worth, Texas

Jo Ann Cobble, EdD, NREMT-P, RN
Dean, Division of Health Professions
Oklahoma City Community College
Oklahoma City, Oklahoma

Kevin T. Collopy, BA, NREMT-P, WEMT
Lead Instructor, Wilderness Medical Associates
Bell Ambulance, Inc.
Milwaukee, Wisconsin

Peter Connick, EMT-P, EMT I/C
Captain
Chatham Fire-Rescue
Chatham, Massachusetts
Adjunct Faculty
Cape Cod Community College EMS Program
Emergency Medical Teaching Services Inc
Dennis, Massachusetts

Elizabeth Criss, RN, MEd, CEN, CCRN
Clinical Educator
University Medical Center
Tucson, Arizona

Phil Currance, EMT-P, RHSP
Deputy Commander, National Medical Response
   Team—Central Task Force
U.S. Department of Homeland Security
Denver, Colorado

Randy D. Danielsen, PhD, PA-C
Dean and Professor
Arizona School of Health Sciences
A.T. Still University
Mesa, Arizona

Roy Danks, DO
Kansas Surgical Consultants
Wichita, Kansas

Thom Dick, BA
Quality Care Coordinator
Platte Valley EMS
Brighton, Colorado

Steven Dralle, LP, BA
Director of Operations
American Medical Response–South Texas
San Antonio, Texas

Marc Eckstein, MD, FACEP
Medical Director
Los Angeles Fire Department
Associate Professor of Emergency Medicine
Keck School of Medicine of the University of
    Southern California
Director of Prehospital Care
Los Angeles County/University of Southern
    California Medical Center
Los Angeles, California

Dennis Edgerly, EMT-P
Program Coordinator
HealthONE EMS
Englewood, Colorado

John Elder, EMT-P, CCEMT-P
Forth Worth, Texas

Hunter Elliott, CCEMT-P
Adjunct Faculty
The Center for Emergency Health Services
Williamsburg, Virginia

Jay Fitch, PhD
Fitch & Associates, LLC
Platte City, Missouri

Jeffery S. Force, BA, NREMT-P
EMS Program Director
Pikes Peak Community College
Colorado Springs, Colorado

Greg Frailey, DO
Williamsport Hospital
Williamsport, Pennsylvania

Mark Goldstein, RN, BSN, EMT-P I/C
EMS Coordinator
William Beaumont Hospital–Royal Oak
Royal Oak, Michigan

John B. Gosford, EMT-P
Adjunct Faculty
North Florida Community College
Madison, Florida
CE Broker
Jacksonville, Florida

Keith Griffiths
President
The Red Flash Group
Encinitas, California

Seth C. Hawkins, MD, FACEP
Assistant Medical Director of Special Operations
Burke County EMS
Attending Physician
Blue Ridge HealthCare
Morganton, North Carolina

John C. Hopkins, Paramedic
Retired
Lexington, South Carolina

Davis E. Hill, EMT-P
Program Director
Managing Agricultural Emergencies
The Pennsylvania State University
University Park, Pennsylvania

Lorri Johnston, EMT-P
Owner and Instructor
Emergency Medical Instructor Services
New Carlisle, Indiana
Instructor
LaPorte Hospital
LaPorte, Indiana

Rodger J. Kelley, RN-CEN, EMT-P, I/C
Emergency Department
Ingham Regional Medical Center/Lansing
    Community College
Lansing, Michigan

Josh Krimston, Firefighter/Paramedic
Director of Operations
EPIC Medics
La Mesa, California

Douglas F. Kupas, MD, EMT-P
Clinical Professor of Emergency Medicine
Department of Emergency Medicine
Geisinger Health System
Danville, Pennsylvania

David T. Lake, BS, MS, EMT-D
Vice President of Academic Affairs
Wichita Area Technical College
Director, State of Kansas Board of EMS, Retired
Wichita, Kansas

Andrea Legamaro, RN
Emergency Room RN
McKinney, Texas

Paul Maxwell, Paramedic
President/Founder
EPIC Medics
San Diego, California

Joanne McCall, RN, MA, CEN, CFN, SANE-A
Senior Education Specialist
St. John Providence Park Hospital
Novi, Michigan

Christine C. McEachin, BSN, CEN, MBA, Paramedic/IC
Clinical Nurse Specialist
Emergency Service Line
William Beaumont Hospital–Troy
Troy, Michigan

Michelle M. McLean, MD, EMT-P
Clinical Faculty
Emergency Medicine Residency
Michigan State University
Covenant Emergency Care Center
Saginaw, Michigan

Michael Meoli, FF/EMTP-TEMS
SEAL Team 17
San Diego Fire Department Special Weapons and Tactics
San Diego Fire Department
San Diego, California

Michael G. Miller, BS, RN, NREMT-P
Coordinator EMS Education
Creighton University EMS Education
Omaha, Nebraska

Joseph B. Mittelman II, BS, NREMTP
Murray City Fire Department
Murray, Utah

Kirk E. Mittelman, BS, NREMTP
Mt. Nebo Training Association
Payson, Utah

Margaret A. Mittelman, BS
Utah Valley State College
Provo, Utah

Ron Moore, Battalion Chief
McKinney Fire Department
McKinney, Texas

Earl H. Neal, BS, EMT-P
Executive Director
Johnson County Ambulance District
Warrensburg, Missouri

Robert G. Nixon, MBA, EMT-P
Manager, Clinical and Educational Services
American Medical Response
New Haven, Connecticutt

William Northington, MD, NREMT-P
Instructor, Department of Emergency Medicine
University of Pittsburgh
Pittsburgh, Pennsylvania

Roger Parvin, Jr, NREMT-P
Field Training Officer
Louisville Metro EMS
Louisville, Kentucky

Mary Jane Pavlick, RN, BA
Program Manager, Emergency Management
Hillcrest Hospital, A Cleveland Clinic Hospital
Mayfield Heights, Ohio

Thomas F. Payton, MD, MBA, EMT-P
Staff Physician, Emergency Medicine
Geisinger Health System
Danville, Pennsylvania

Randall G. Perkins, EMT-P
Paramedic Program Director
Scottsdale Community College
Scottsdale, Arizona

Warren J. Porter, MS, BA, LP, PNCCT
EMS Programs Manager
Garland Fire Department
Garland, Texas

Roy Ramos, NREMT-P
Director Education/Training
Thompson Valley EMS
Loveland, Colorado

William Raynovich, EdD, MPH, NREMTP
Assistant Professor and Director
Creighton University EMS Education
Omaha, Nebraska

Howard Rodenberg, MD, MPH
Director, Division of Health
State Health Officer
Kansas Department of Health and Environment
Topeka, Kansas
Clinical Associate Professor
Department of Preventive Medicine
University of Kansas School of Medicine–Wichita
Wichita, Kansas

Gregory Scott, MBA
EMD QA Instructor
EMD Consultant
Priority Dispatch Corporation
EMD Consultant
National Academies of Emergency Dispatch
Salt Lake City, Utah

Everett Stephens, MD, FAAEM
Assistant Clinical Professor
Department of Emergency Medicine
University of Louisville
Louisville, Kentucky

Rod Thompson, CEP
Deputy Fire Chief
Scottsdale Fire Department
Scottsdale, Arizona

Chris Tilden, PhD
Director, Office of Local and Rural Health
Kansas Department of Health and Environment
Topeka, Kansas
Adjunct Instructor
Department of Health Policy and Management
University of Kansas Medical School
Kansas City, Kansas

Tom Vines
Training Officer
Carbon County Sheriff's Search and Rescue
Red Lodge, Montana

Robert Vroman, BS, NREMT-P
HealthONE EMS
Englewood, Colorado

Richard A. Walker, MD
Associate Professor
Section of Emergency Medicine
University of Nebraska Medical Center
Clinical Director
Nebraska Medical Center Emergency Services
Omaha, Nebraska

Chris Weber, PhD
President
Dr. Hazmat, Inc.
Ann Arbor, Michigan

Elizabeth M. Wertz, RN, BSN, MPM, EMT-P, PHRN,
   FACMPE
Chief Executive Officer
Pediatric Alliance, PC
Chairperson, EMSC Advisory Committee
Pennsylvania Emergency Health Services Council
Pittsburgh, Pennsylvania

Stephen R. Wirth, JD, BA, MS, EMT-P
Partner, Attorney at Law
Page, Wolfberg & Wirth, LLC
Mechanicsburg, Pennsylvania

Christopher M. Woleben, MD, FAAP
Assistant Professor, Emergency Medicine
Pediatric Division
Virginia Commonwealth University Medical Center
Richmond, Virginia

Douglas M. Wolfberg, JD
Partner, Attorney at Law
Page, Wolfberg & Wirth, LLC
Mechanicsburg, Pennsylvania

Lynn Yancey, MD
Department of Emergency Medicine
University of Colorado Health Sciences Center
Denver, Colorado

Jesse Yarbrough, EMT-P
Operations Paramedic
Louisville Metro EMS
Louisville, Kentucky

Adam M. Yates, MD
Emergency Medicine Attending Physician
Mercy Hospital of Pittsburgh
Pittsburgh, Pennsylvania

Brian S. Zachariah, MD, MBA, FACEP
Associate Professor
Director, Division of Emergency Medicine
University of Texas Medical Branch–Galveston
Galveston, Texas

Reviewers

Michael Armacost, MA, NREMT-P
Owner, Athena Learning Services
Frederick, Colorado
Instructor/Simulation Faculty
Exempla Healthcare
Wheatridge, Colorado

Kathleen A. Ballman, RN, MSN, ACNP, CEN, NREMT-P
Paramedic Training Program
Bethesda North Hospital
Cincinnati, Ohio

Mark Barrier, AAS, NREMT-P, CCEMT-P, EMD
Burke County Emergency Services
Morganton, North Carolina

Rhonda Beck, NREMT-P
Houston Healthcare EMS
Warner Robins, Georgia

Daniel Benard, BS, EMTP-IC
EMS Program Director
Kalamazoo Valley Community College
Kalamazoo, Michigan

Jeffrey K Benes, BS, NREMT-P
EMS Coordinator
Aurora Medical Centre
Kenosha, Wisconsin

Michael Berg, Flight Paramedic
Berklyn Medical Solutions
Gilbert, Arizona

James Blivin, NREMT-P, RRT
F.D. Paramedic/Instructor
Chambersburg, Pennsylvania

Chip Boehm, RN, EMT-P, FF, EMS I/C III
Portland Fire Department
Portland, Maine

Kristen Borchelt, NREMT-P
Cincinnati Children's Hospital
Cincinnati, Ohio

Rob Bozicevich, Paramedic
Instructor
Woodstock, Georgia

Joyce S. Bradley, NREMT-P, AAS, BHCS
Dona Ana Community College
Las Cruces, New Mexico

Bob Breese, CCEMT-P, FP-C
Monroe Community College
Rochester, New York

Brady Breon, AAS, BS, MS, NREMT-P
EMS Operations Chief
Jersey Shore Area EMS
Faculty
Pennsylvania College of Technology
Williamsport, Pennsylvania

Richard Britz, NREMT-P
EMS Captain
Bulverde Spring Branch EMS
Spring Branch, Texas

Rod Brouhard, AA, EMT-P
Former EMS Program Director
Modesto Junior College
Modesto, California

Robert J. Carter, NREMT-P
Flight Paramedic/Instructor
STAT MedEvac
West Mifflin, Pennsylvania
Centre for Emergency Medicine
Pittsburgh, Pennsylvania

Robert Clark, EMT-P, EMSI
Fire Fighter, Paramedic
Warrensville Heights Fire Department
Warrensville Heights, Ohio
Instructor
Cuyahoga Community College
Highland Hill, Ohio

Jo Ann Cobble, EdD, NREMT-P, RN
Dean, Division of Health Professions
Oklahoma City Community College
Oklahoma City, Oklahoma

Kevin T. Collopy, BA, NREMT-P, WEMT
Lead Instructor, Wilderness Medical Associates
Bell Ambulance, Inc.
Milwaukee, Wisconsin

Peter Connick, EMT-P, EMT I/C
Captain
Chatham Fire-Rescue
Chatham, Massachusetts
Adjunct Faculty
Cape Cod Community College EMS Program
Emergency Medical Teaching Services, Inc.
Dennis, Massachusetts

Jon Cooper, NREMT-P
Baltimore City Fire and EMS Academy
Baltimore, Maryland

Ken H. Davis, AS, NREMT-P, CCEMT-P
Eastern New Mexico University
Roswell, New Mexico

John A. DeArmond, NREMT-P
Emergency Management Resources
Half Moon Bay, California

Janice Dorey, RN, BS
EMS Education Coordinator
Advocate Christ Medical Center EMS Academy
Oak Lawn, Illinois

Steven Dralle, LP, BA
Director of Operations
American Medical Response–South Texas
San Antonio, Texas

Kelly J. Drennan, EMT-P
Capital Region EMS
Jefferson City, Missouri

John Dudte, MPA, MICT I/C
Assistant Medical Director
District of Columbia Fire and EMS Department
Washington, D.C.

Cindy Edwards, AAS, NREMT-P, LP
Course Coordinator
Bulverde Spring Branch EMS Training Institute
Spring Branch, Texas

Steven Ernest, NREMT-P
EMS Operations Coordinator/Paramedic Program
    Coordinator
Kish Health System
Flight Medic
OSF Lifeline Helicopter
DeKalb, Illinois

Thomas E. Ezell III, NREMT-P, CCEMT-P
James City County Fire Department
Williamsburg, Virginia

Mark Fair, BS, NREMT-P, PI, CTM
Director
Fayette Regional Health System School of Paramedic
    Science
Connersville, Indiana

Joe Ferrell, MS, NREMT-P
EMS Regulation Manager
Iowa Department of Public Health
Des Moines, Iowa

Janet Fitts, RN, BSN, CEN, TNS, EMT-P
Educational Consultant
Prehospital Emergency Medical Education
Pacific, Missouri

**Joyce Foresman-Capuzzi, RN, BSN, CEN, CPN, CTRN,
    PHRN, EMT-P**
Business Development Representative
Temple Health System Transport Team, Temple
    University Health System
Philadelphia, Pennsylvania

Jason Foth, Firefighter/Paramedic
Marshfield Fire and Rescue Department
Marshfield, Wisconsin

Gregory T. Friese, MS, NREMT-P, WEMT
President
Emergency Preparedness Systems, LLC
Plover, Wisconsin

Fidel O. Garcia, EMT-P
President
Professional EMS Education
Mesa State College
Grand Junction, Colorado

Rudy Garrett, AS, NREMT-P, CCEMT-P
Flight Paramedic
Lifenet Kentucky
Lexington, Kentucky

Maylyn Geissler, NREMT-P
Education Coordinator
National EMS Academy
Covington, Louisiana

**Lisa Gilmore, MSN/Ed, RN, CEN, CFRN, CC/NREMT-P,
    FP-C**
STC Education Coordinator/Flight Nurse
St. John's Emergency Trauma Center
Springfield, Missouri

Chuck Gipson, AAS, NREMT-P, CCP
Medic, EMS
Des Moines, Iowa

Lynn Goldstein, PharmD
Emergency Medicine Specialist
William Beaumont Hospital–Royal Oak
Royal Oak, Michigan

Mark Goldstein, RN, BSN, EMT-P I/C
EMS Coordinator
William Beaumont Hospital–Royal Oak
Royal Oak, Michigan

James Goss, BS, BA, MHS, MICP
Lead Paramedic Instructor
Northern California Training Institute
Roseville, California
Faculty
Loma Linda University
Loma Linda, California

Thomas G. Gottschalk, Critical Care Paramedic
Educator
Platinum Educational Group, LLC
Jenison, Michigan

Danna S. Hatley, PharmD
Clinical Phramacist
East Alabama Medical Center
Opelika, Alabama

Robert M. Hawkes, MS, PA-C, NREMT-P
EMS Program Director
Southern Maine Community College
South Portland, Maine

Agustin Hernandez, AAS, NREMT-P, I/C
United States Army
Fort Detrick, Maryland

Jon Hibbard, AS, EMT-P, EMS-I
President
Connecticut Medical Training Academy
Windsor Locks, Connecticut

Stephen Hines, BSc, Dip IMC RCS Ed
London Ambulance Service NHS Trust
London, United Kingdom

John C. Hopkins, Paramedic
Retired
Lexington, South Carolina

Mark Hornshuh, BS, EMT-P
Portland Community College
Portland, Oregon

David Hostler, PhD, CSCS
Emergency Responder
Human Performance Lab
Department of Emergency Medicine
University of Pittsburgh
Pittsburgh, Pennsylvania

Eric Howard, NREMT-P, CCEMT-P, FP-C
Senior Flight Crew Member, Flight Paramedic
St. John's Life Line, St. John's Regional Health Center
Springfield, Missouri

Bill Hufford, REMT-P, PI, CTM
Director
Tri-County Training Academy
Connersville, Indiana

Stephen J Huisman, NREMT-P
President/Owner
Great Lakes EMS Academy
Grand Rapids, Michigan

Robert L. Jackson, Jr., EMT-P, CCEMTP, NREMT-P, MAR, MAPS
University of Missouri Health Care
Columbia, Missouri

Captain Thomas Jarman, NREMT-P, AAS
Prince William County Department of Fire and Rescue
Prince William, Virginia

Lorri Johnston, EMT-P
Owner and Instructor
Emergency Medical Instructor Services
New Carlisle, Indiana
Instructor
LaPorte Hospital
LaPorte, Indiana

Scott Jones, MBA, EMT-P
Director, Paramedic Academy
Chairperson, Allied Health
Victor Valley College
Victorville, California

Chad S. Kim, NREMT-P, BA, I/C
Eastern New Mexico University
Roswell, New Mexico

Don Kimlicka, NREMT-P, CCEMT-P
EMS Coordinator
Saint Clare's Hospital
Weston, Wisconsin

Gregory R. LaMay, AS, NREMT-P
Associate Training Specialist
Texas Engineering Extension Service
College Station, Texas

Jane L. LaMay, BSN
Somerville, Texas

Robert W. Lamey, MSIT, NREMT-P
Retired
Baltimore, Maryland

Chris Parker, MSN/ED, RN, LICP
Office of the Medical Director, Austin County
    EMS System
Adjunct Faculty
Austin Community College
South Austin Hospital
Austin, Texas

Dennis Parker, MA, EMT-P, I/C
Tennessee Tech University
Cookeville, Tennessee

Richard Patterson, NR/CCEMT-P, MICP, FP-C
Director of Operations, Flight Paramedic, ALS Instructor
Critical Care Concepts, Inc.
Suffolk, Virginia

Captain Tim Peebles, AAS, NREMT-P
EMS Coordinator
Hall County Fire Services
Gainesville, Georgia

Tim Penic, NREMT-P
Field Operations Supervisor
Medstar EMS
Fort Worth, Texas

Warren J. Porter, MS, BA, LP, PNCCT
EMS Programs Manager
Garland Fire Department
Garland, Texas

Merle Potter, NREMT-P
Paramedic/EMS Educator
Wyoming Life Flight
Wyoming Medical Center
Casper, Wyoming

Gregg D. Ramirez, BS, EMT-P
Student Services Director
Northwest Regional Training Center
Vancouver, Washington

Kathleen Rankin, MICT I/C, NREMT-P, AAS
Paramedic, Adjunct Faculty
Johnson County MED-ACT
Johnson County, Kansas

John Rasmussen, REMT-P, PhD
Captain, Support Services
Greenville County EMS
Greenville, South Carolina

David Rathbun, EMT-P, AA
Chairperson
Tactical Emergency Medical Services
LaCanada, California

Kenneth J. Reardon
Flight Paramedic
LifeNet
Valhalla, New York

Lori Reeves, BA, PS/CCP
Program Director
Rural Health Education Partnership, Indiana Hills
    College
Ottumwa, Iowa

Mark Register, BS, NREMT-P
Lead Paramedic Instructor
Aiken Technical College
Low Country Regional Council EMS
Aiken, South Carolina

William E. Rich, AAS-EMT, EMT-P, CEM
Center for Disease Control and Prevention
Atlanta, Georgia

Larry Richmond, AS, NREMT-P, CCEMT-P
EMS Education Manager
Mountain Plains Health Consortium
Fort Meade, South Dakota

Becky Ridenhour, PharmD
The Medicine Shoppe
Troy, Missouri

Michael W. Robinson, MA, CFO, NREMT-P
Division Chief
Baltimore County Fire Department
Baltimore, Maryland

George Schulp, EMT-P/PI
Director, Education Services
EMS Coordinator
Superior Air-Ground Ambulance Services
Highland, Indiana

Stephen M. Setter, PharmD, CDE, CGP, DVM
Associate Professor of Pharmacotherapy
Washington State University-Spokane
Spokane, Washington

Maureen Shanahan, RN, BSN, MN
EMT Program Coordinator
City College of San Francisco
San Francisco, California

Judson Smith, BSBA, NREMT-P, CCEMT-P
Overland Park Fire Department
Overland Park, Kansas

Derek Sobelman, MPA, NREMT-P
EMS Training Captain
Olathe Fire Department
Olathe, Kansas

Andrew E. Spain, MA, EMT-P
Assistant Manager, Emergency Centers
University of Missouri Health Care
Columbia, Missouri

Randolph Scott Spies, AS, NREMT-P
Emergency Services Program Coordinator
Blue Ridge Community and Technical College
Martinsburg, West Virginia

Robert Spranger, LP
Methodist Dallas Medical Center
Dallas, Texas

David Stamey, CCEMT-P
EMS Training Administrator
District of Columbia Fire and EMS Department
Washington, D.C.

Nerina J. Stepanovsky, PhD, RN, NREMT-P
Chief Flight Nurse
U.S. Air Force Reserve
MacDill Air Force Base, Florida
EMS Program Director
St. Petersburg College
St. Petersburg, Florida

Michael A. Stern, NREMT-P, CCEMT-P
Deputy Chief
Grand County EMS
Granby, Colorado

David L. Sullivan, MA, NREMT-P
EMS/CME Program Director
Critical Care Transport Paramedic and SWAT (Tactical
    Paramedic)
St. Petersburg College, Pinellas County EMS Sunstar
    Paramedics
Pinellas Park, Florida
Largo, Florida

Christopher T. Sweeney, NREMT-P, FFI, FFII
Covington Fire Department
Covington, Kentucky

John Tartt, MPH, EMT-P, DHA(c)
Director, Emergency Medical Science
Carolinas College of Health Sciences
Carolinas HealthCare System
Charlotte, North Carolina

Dave M. Tauber, NREMT-P, CCEMT-P, FP-C, I/C
Advanced Life Support Institute
Conway, New Hampshire

Chet Thorne, NREMT-P, I/C, BSN, PALS ACLS
Albuquerque Fire Department
Albuquerque, New Mexico

Donna G. Tidwell, BS, RN, EMT-P
Tennessee Department of Health EMS Division
Nashville, Tennessee

William F. Toon, MeD, NREMT-P
Battalion Chief, Training
Olathe, Kansas

Mark Trueman, BS, NREMT-P
Pennsylvania College of Technology
Williamsport, Pennsylvania

Larry Vandegriff, BS, NREMT-P
Paramedic Instructor, Flight Paramedic
Lifenet Georgia
Griffin, Georgia

Susan Van Egghen, EMT-P
New York State Course Instructor Coordinator and
    Regional Faculty
Albany, New York

Lisa Vargas, EMT-P, BS
Primary Paramedic Instructor
National College of Technical Instruction
Buellton, California

Jimmy Walker, NREMT-P
Training Coordinator/EMT, EMT-I, Paramedic
    Instructor
South Carolina Midlands EMS
West Columbia, South Carolina

Laura L. Walker, DM, NREMT-P
Center Director
Weber Simulation Center
Norfolk, Virginia

Michael J. Ward
Assistant Professor of Emergency Medicine
The George Washington University
Washington, D.C.

John J. Watts, MPH, MEP, NREMT-P
Regional Emergency Response and Recovery
    Coordinator, Region 7
Carolinas HealthCare System
Charlotte, North Carolina

Michael Whitehurst, EMT-P
Albemarle Hospital
Elizabeth City, North Carolina

Marc Yeston, NREMT-P
Canyon District Ranger
National Park Sevice
Grand Canyon, Arizona

Acknowledgments

We would like to thank Jeff Sargent, Cathy Thanner, Roy Ryals, and the employees of Southwest Ambulance for making their staff, facility, vehicles, and equipment available to us for many of the photographs used in this text.

Moulage make-up provided by Graftobian Make-up Company, makers of the EMS Makeup/Severe Trauma Kit. For more information, please visit www.graftobian.com.

Because being "good enough" isn't good enough for you . . .

Congratulations on your choice to pursue a career in paramedicine. Whether you are just starting out, looking for a refresher, or seeking to perfect your skills, your success in this dynamic field depends on preparation that goes **above and beyond** the standard.

You need the best.

The most clinically comprehensive foundation for practice, **Paramedic Practice Today: Above and Beyond** is designed to help you achieve complete success on the National Registry examination and prepare you for *any* challenge you may encounter in practice.

Paramedic Practice Today: Above and Beyond is more than just a paramedic textbook; it is part of a complete learning system composed of innovative tools that work together to give you the most effective learning experience:

- Textbook
- Companion DVD-ROMs
- Student Workbook
- Virtual Patient Encounters
- Evolve Resources for Students

HOW TO USE THIS TEXTBOOK

The best possible preparation for the National Registry examination and professional success begins with a solid foundation in the principles and skills of paramedic practice. A conversational, easy-to-read style simplifies topics and helps you master National Standard Curriculum objectives and the new National Education Standards. In addition, content corresponding directly to the National Registry of EMTs National EMS Practice Analysis provides unparalleled preparation for the National Registry examination.

Streamlined division and chapter openers help you to navigate each volume with ease and learn more efficiently. *Chapter Objectives* identify learning goals, and the *Chapter Outlines* present a brief overview of each chapter.

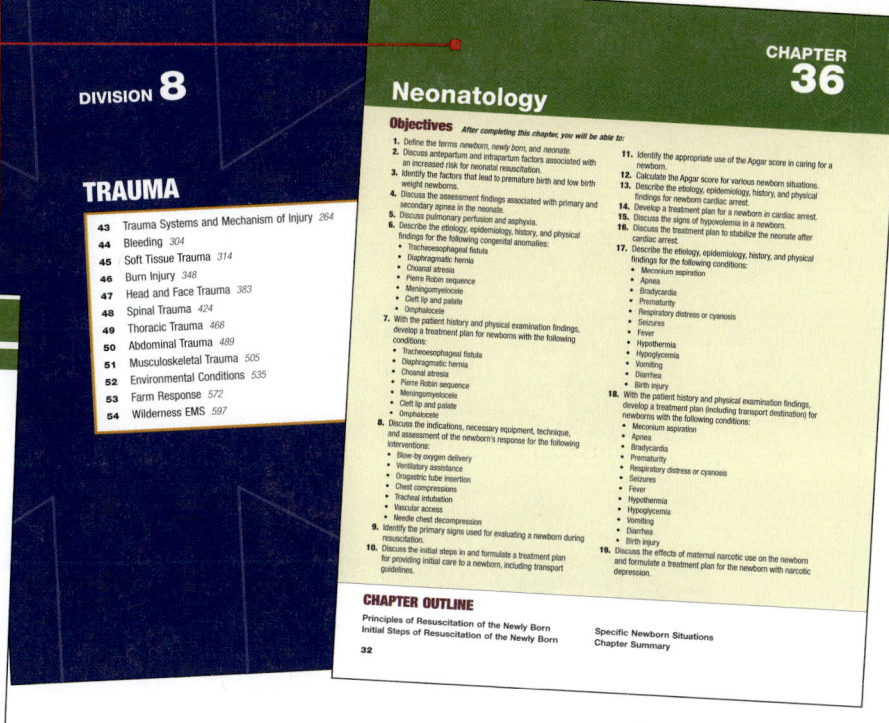

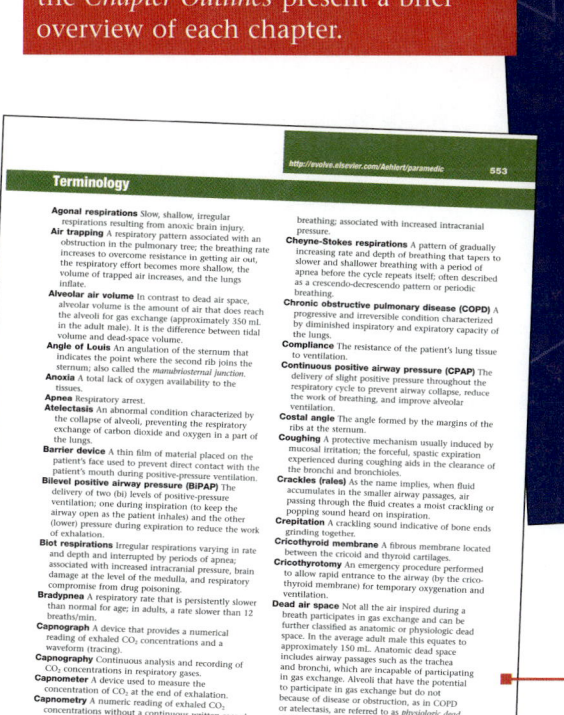

Key terms are bolded in each chapter for easy identification. These terms are discussed in the text and are defined for quick reference in the Terminology section at the end of each chapter.

Four-part case scenarios put material into context, enabling you to follow each case from presentation to conclusion. Questions throughout each scenario test your knowledge of each step and are followed by complete answers and expert insight at the end of each scenario.

Forty-nine illustrated, step-by-step skill sequences in this two-volume package guide you through each action to help you review important skills before performing them in class.

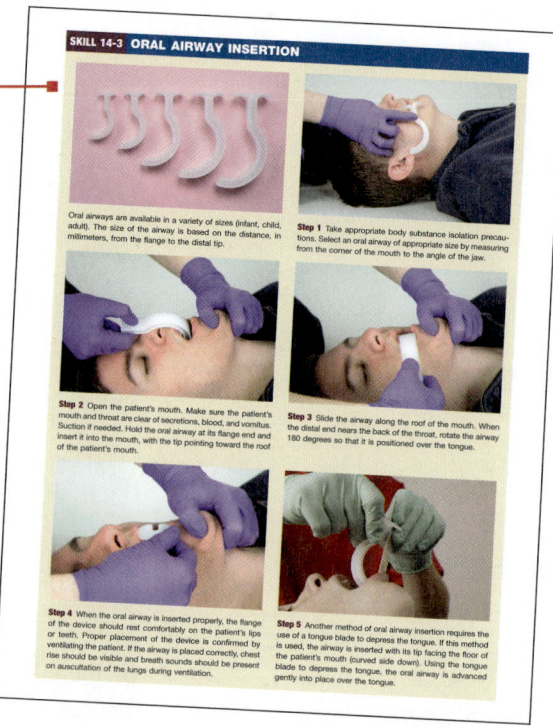

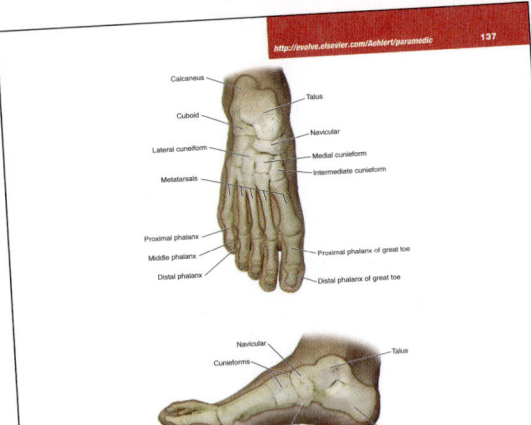

Figure 7-24 The foot consists of seven tarsal bones.

the functional system should at least be mentioned. Functionally, joints fall into three categories. Synarthroses are immovable and include joints such as the suture, gomphosis, and synchondrosis. Amphiarthroses are slightly movable and include joints such as the syndesmosis and symphysis. Diarthroses are movable and include the synovial joints.

Fibrous Joints

Fibrous joints consist of two bones united by fibrous tissue that have little or no movement (Figure 7-25). The joints are further divided on the basis of structure into sutures, syndesmoses, or gomphoses. **Sutures** (seams between flat bones) are located in the skull bones. These may be completely immobile in adults. In the newly born, the sutures have gaps called **fontanels**. These gaps allow the skull to expand or contract during birth. They also allow growth of the head during development. A

syndesmosis is a type of joint in which the bones are united by fibrous connective tissue, forming an intraosseous membrane or ligament. It is a temporary joint in which the cartilage is replaced by bone later in life. The ligaments may provide some movement of the joint. An example is the radioulnar syndesmosis that binds the radius and ulna together (Figure 7-26). **Gomphoses** consist of a peg that fits into a socket. The peg is held in place by fine bundles of collagenous connective tissue. The joints between the teeth and the sockets along the processes of the mandible and maxilla are examples of gomphoses (see Figure 7-26).

Cartilaginous Joints

Cartilaginous joints unite two bones with hyaline cartilage (synchondroses) or fibrocartilage (symphyses). This is a slightly movable joint in which the bones are connected by a fibrocartilage disk or ligaments.

Extensive illustrations clarify key concepts and reinforce your understanding.

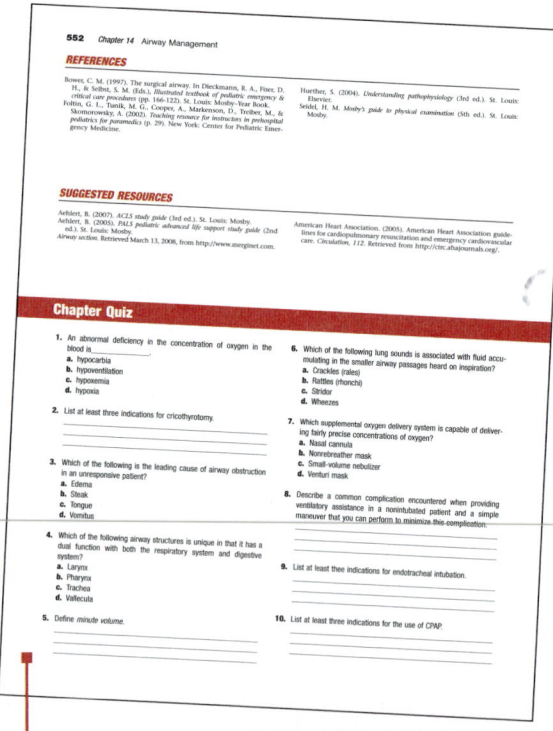

Bulleted summaries at the conclusion of each chapter help you review essential information quickly and easily.

Chapter quizzes included at the end of each chapter test your understanding of chapter content with a variety of multiple-choice, true/false, short-answer, and matching questions. Answers and rationales at the end of each volume provide instant feedback and help you identify areas requiring additional study and review.

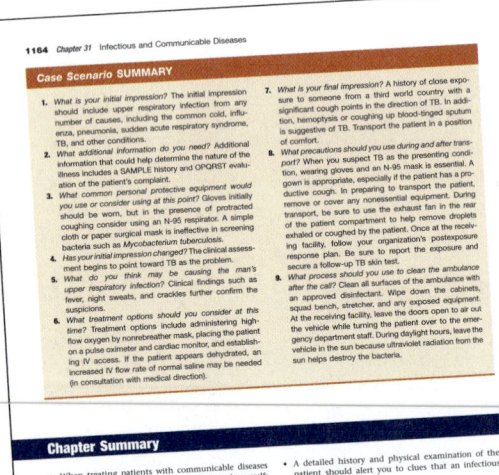

***Pediatric Pearl* boxes** identify important distinctions for managing pediatric patients.

PEDIATRIC*Pearl*

Maintaining appropriate temperature is particularly important in the pediatric patient because children have a large body surface area/weight ratio, providing a greater area for heat loss.

***Cultural Considerations* boxes** provide helpful information for interacting with people of various cultures.

CULTURAL*Considerations*

When talking with patients, try to avoid using medical terms. Ask the patient questions and explain what you are going to do to help by using words that are easy to understand. This is important when communicating with any patient, but it is particularly important when speaking with patients for whom English is a second language.

***Geriatric Considerations* boxes** alert you to special considerations for elderly patients.

GERIATRIC*Considerations*

Urinary retention in the elderly may lead to delirium. Carefully question the recent urinary history and bladder habits for any older adult who has a sudden onset of delirium.

***Paramedic Pearl* boxes** highlight important information in the text.

PARAMEDIC*Pearl*

Remember to communicate with the patient throughout your assessment. Make him or her feel a part of your team, not just an object of your work.

A comprehensive, timesaving index presented at the end of each volume spans *both* volumes of the textbook, enabling you to find topics of interest from both volumes in one place.

Drugs and herbal supplements are indexed at the back of the applicable volumes, providing essential dosage information on 50 herbal supplements and approximately 100 drugs.

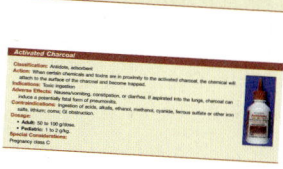

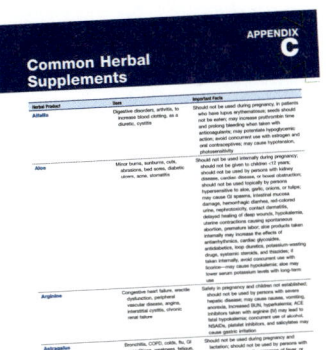

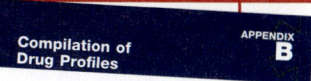

The comprehensive glossary presented at the end of each volume provides clear definitions for more than 2200 key terms.

The heart rate ruler included in *Volume 1* is a quick, easy tool for use in ECG interpretation, as outlined in *Basic Dysrhythmias: Interpretation & Management* by Robert J. Huszar, MD.

A 12-lead placement card accompanying *Volume 1* details placement and purpose for both anterior and posterior leads.

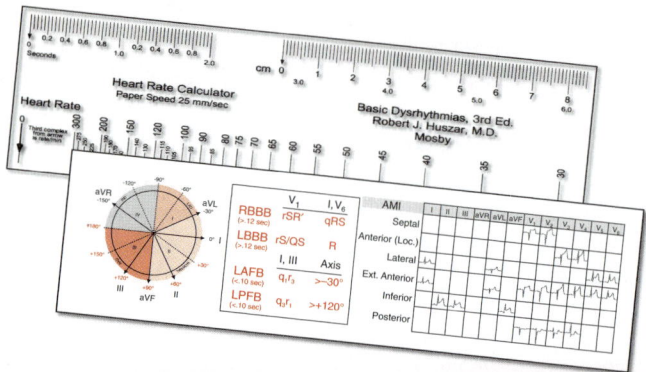

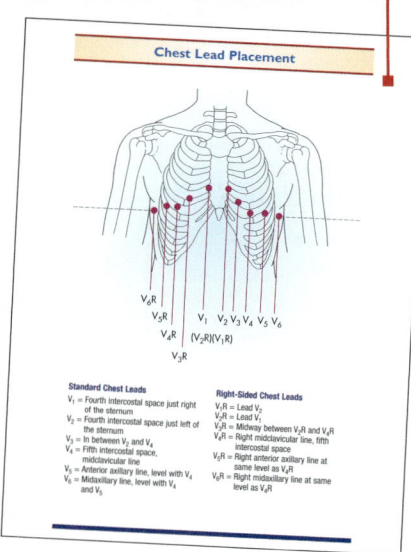

A complete *Pediatric Quick Reference* **foldout card,** packaged in *Volume 2*, presents key information from *Mosby's Comprehensive Pediatric Emergency Care* in a concise, pocket-sized format for fast reference wherever you go.

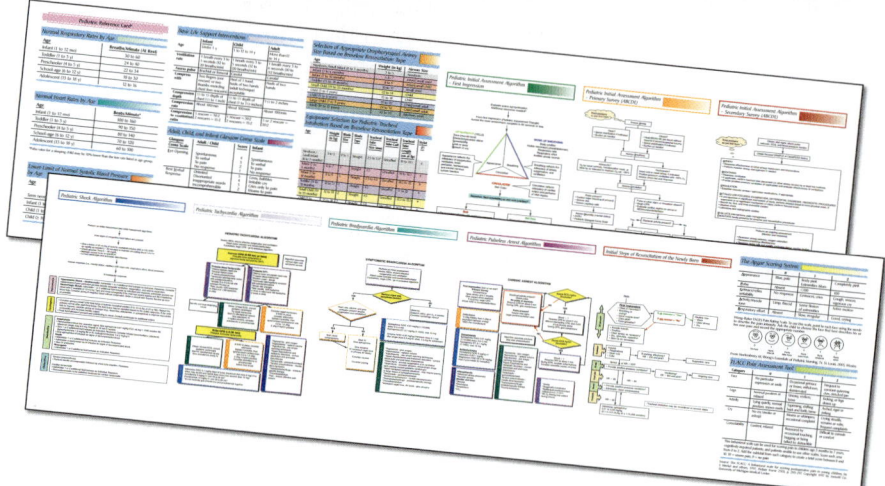

Go *beyond* the textbook for greater understanding . . .

COMPANION DVD-ROMS

Load the companion DVD-ROMs included with each volume on your computer to access video footage produced exclusively for **Paramedic Practice Today: Above and Beyond.** These detailed videos guide you through the performance of key skills, while medical animations, lecture videos, and skill clips from other Elsevier resources broaden your understanding of core concepts.

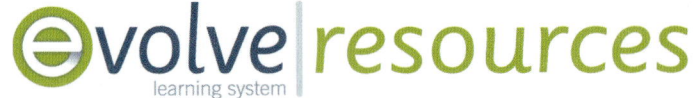

Enhance your knowledge with FREE online access to additional classroom resources, reference materials, and interactive games and activities on a companion Evolve website.
http://evolve.elsevier.com/Aehlert/paramedic

CLASSROOM RESOURCES

- **Lecture notes** drawn from instructor PowerPoint presentations provide printable outlines for each slide.

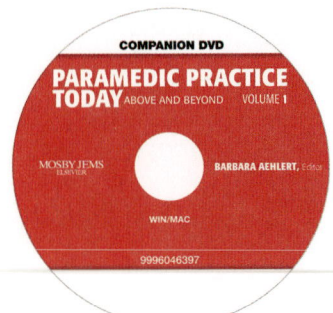

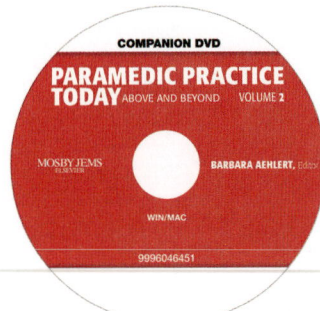

- **Study tips** help you prepare for in-class examinations, the National Registry examination, and skills stations testing.

ADDITIONAL REFERENCE MATERIALS

- **An *English-Spanish Talking Glossary*** strengthens your medical vocabulary with glossary terms and definitions in both English and Spanish, accompanied by English and Spanish audio pronunciations to help you confidently use key words in practice.

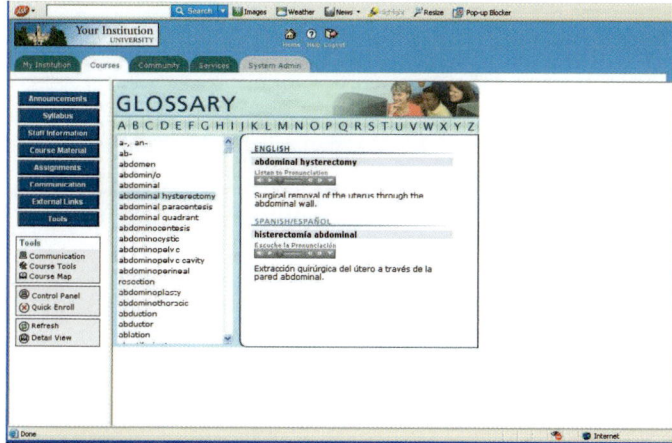

- **Twenty-seven heart and lung audio files** help you learn to recognize conditions based on common sounds.
- **A presentation on *Fluids and Electrolytes*** expands your knowledge of these key areas.

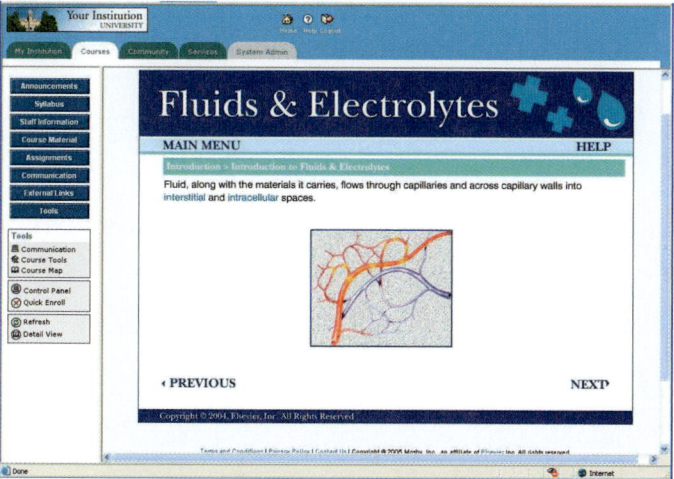

- **Dosage calculators, a *Medication Identification Guide*, and *Mosby's Essential Drug List*** familiarize you with medications common to paramedic practice and help you identify appropriate dosage amounts.

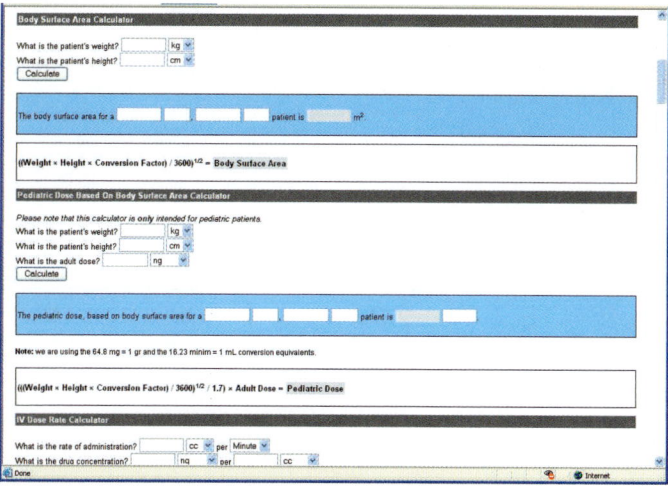

CHAPTER GAMES AND ACTIVITIES

- ***Drug Calculation Exercises*** offer valuable practice determining proper drug dosages.

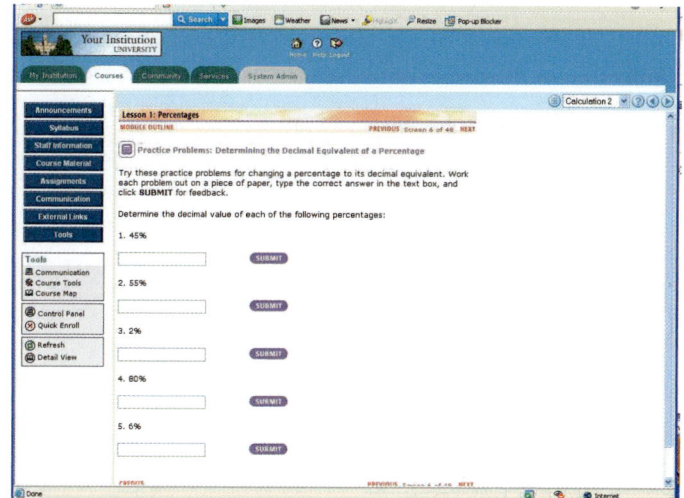

- *A Medical Terminology Review* and a variety of **vocabulary games** reinforce your understanding of key terms and definitions through fun, engaging exercises.
- **Approximately 200 interactive *Anatomy Challenges*** help you master important anatomy and physiology concepts presented in the textbook.

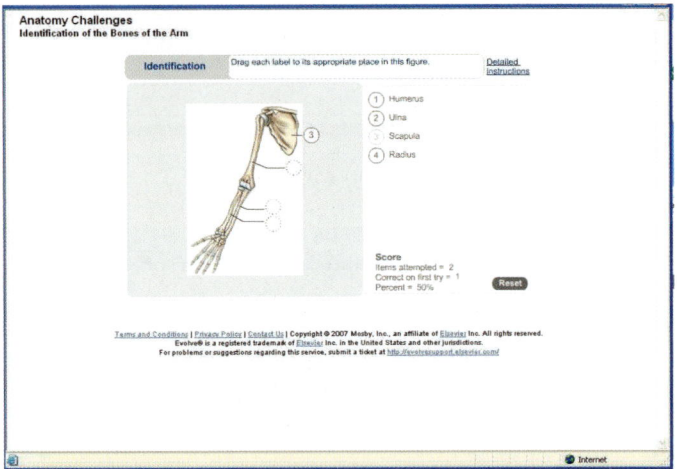

- *A Body Spectrum* **interactive coloring book** tests your knowledge of anatomy and physiology with 80 illustrations that challenge you to identify anatomic components and complete related quizzes.

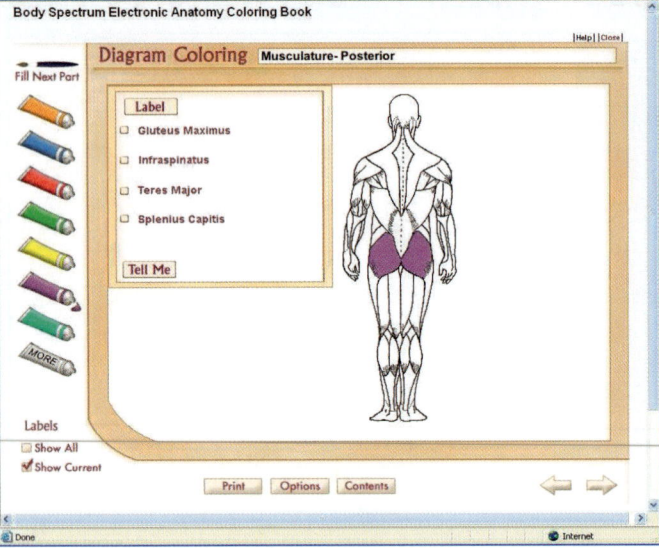

WORKBOOKS

Practice your skills and prepare for your examinations with detailed, chapter-by-chapter review opportunities in two workbook volumes that correspond directly to the two volumes of the text.
Sold separately.

Volume 1

2009 • Approx. 448 pp., illustd. • ISBN: 978-0-323-04377-9

Volume 2

2009 • Approx. 352 pp., illustd. • ISBN: 978-0-323-04378-6

2-Volume Set

2009 • Approx. 800 pp., illustd. • ISBN: 978-0-323-04390-8

- **Multiple question formats** include matching, short-answer, multiple-choice, true/false, labeling, and case studies to test your knowledge in a variety of different ways.

- **Chapter objectives** identify learning goals and guide you through your review.

- **Chapter summaries** outline the most important points from each corresponding textbook chapter.

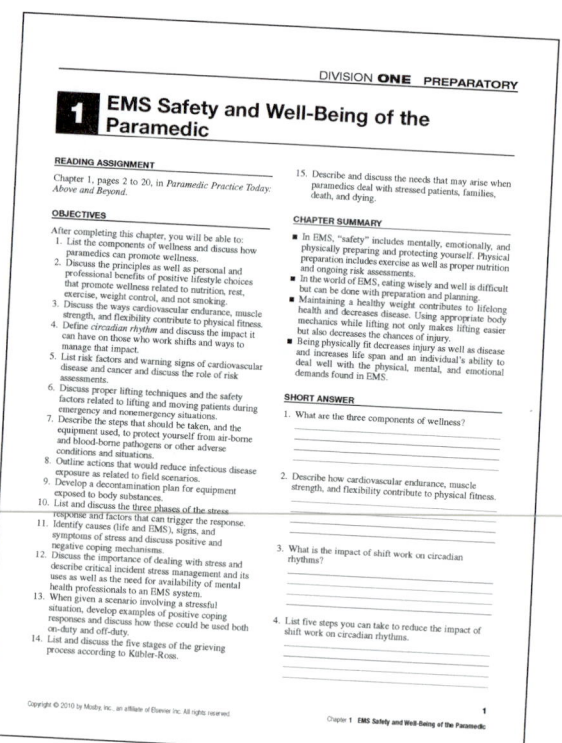

VIRTUAL PATIENT ENCOUNTERS

Obtain realistic patient care experience without leaving the classroom! This workbook/software combination creates a virtual environment in which you can interact with patients and gain experience in critical thinking and decision-making.

Sold separately.

2009 • Approx. 320 pp., illustd. • ISBN: 978-0-323-04920-7

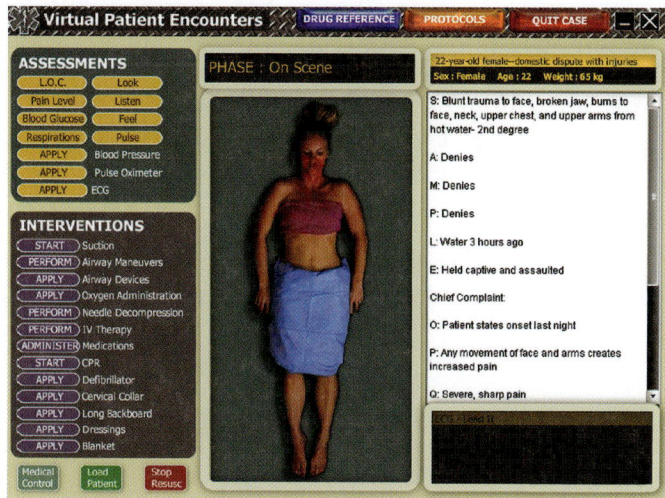

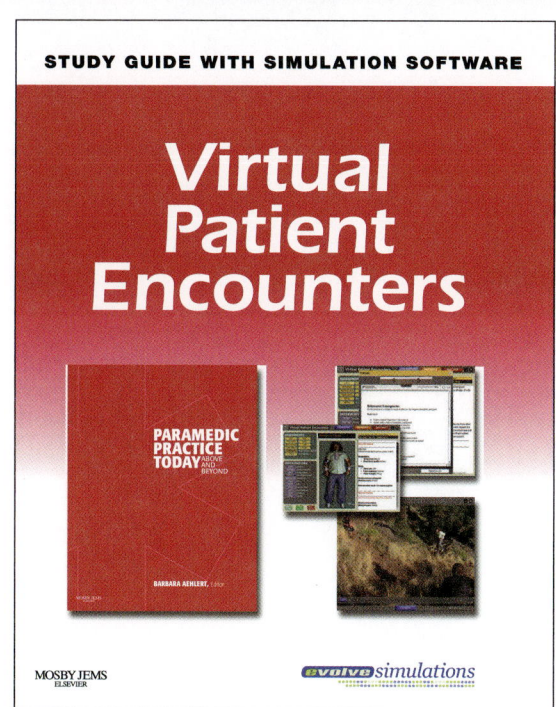

RAPID PARAMEDIC

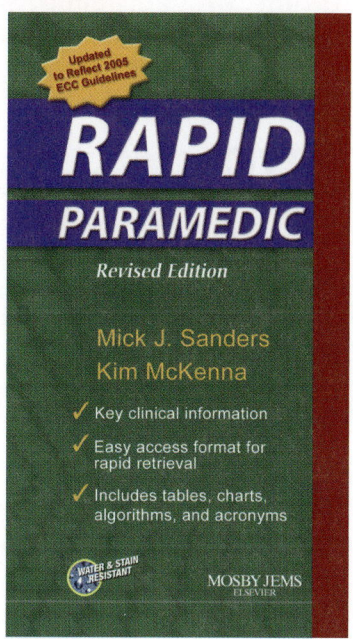

Respond quickly and confidently with this full-color paramedic field guide. Useful both as a classroom resource and as a field reference, **RAPID Paramedic** distills the essentials of paramedic practice into a pocket-sized, spiral-bound, fluid-resistant quick reference to provide the fastest, most convenient access to the information you need in paramedic practice.

Sold separately.

2007 • 172 pp., illustd. • ISBN: 978-0-323-04762-2

Take learning to a new level . . .

Paramedic Practice Today is supported by extensive **instructor resources** that provide everything needed for easy, efficient class preparation.

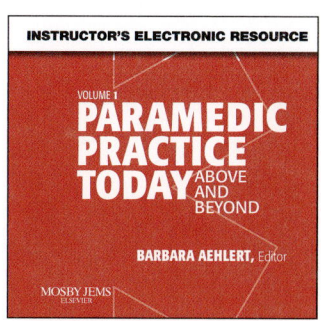

The extensive **Instructor's Electronic Resource** includes everything needed to make preparing for class quick and easy: detailed lesson plans, lecture outlines, PowerPoint presentations with *Speaker Notes* and embedded skills video clips, and even tables that correlate content to the National EMS Practice Analysis (on which the National Registry examination is based), NSC objectives, and National Education Standards.

Customizable lesson plans, lecture outlines, and PowerPoint presentations with *Speaker Notes* **and embedded skills videos** streamline course preparation.

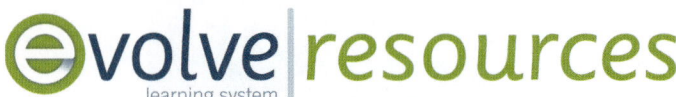

Evolve Resources save preparation time and help instructors teach more effectively with online access to all of the instructor electronic resources and valuable course management tools:

- **Chapter quizzes** can be assigned to students and completed directly through the website.
- **Helpful tables** correlate content to the **NREMT National EMS Practice Analysis, NSC objectives,** and **National Education Standards.**

Paramedic Practice Today: Above and Beyond is intended to be the most effective paramedic learning resource and provide the best preparation for paramedic practice and the National Registry examination. If you have any questions about the components of this learning system, if you would like to place an order, or if you have suggestions about how **Paramedic Practice Today** could go even further **above and beyond,** please contact Elsevier at 1-800-545-2522 or visit http://www.mosbyjems.com.

Barbara Aehlert, RN, BSPA

Contents

**DIVISION 3 AIRWAY MANAGEMENT
AND VENTILATION**

DIVISION 6 SHOCK

Appendices

Contents for Volume 2

Strategies for Successfully Studying and Taking Examinations

Studying is a skill and, like any skill, it has certain steps or procedures that lead to success. In the academic arena, there are four distinct time frames that require study skills: before class, during class, after class, and while taking examinations. The most successful students have developed study skills in each of these areas. Each of us is an individual; therefore we each have a unique learning style that works best for us. We learn in different ways, and many effective study techniques can be used, based on our learning styles. However, some study techniques are essential and common across all learning styles and will therefore be useful to most students.

STUDYING BEFORE CLASS

Some of the essential and common study techniques that should be used before class are:

- Plan on attending class regularly and being actively involved in classroom activities.
  - Although some subjects may seem boring, simply reading the assignments and taking tests does not promote the best learning. One of the best ways to improve learning is developing knowledge and understanding through classroom discussion and interaction with your instructor. Both listening and participating in class discussions are critical to understanding the subject matter.
- Set a regular time for studying each day.
  - Schedule study time for the time of day you are most alert. For example, if your attention is more focused in the morning, try to schedule your study time for that period.
- Study in a consistent and quiet place.
  - Study produces the best results when distractions are kept to a minimum and the surroundings are familiar. Avoid distractions such as noise, music, television, and radio. Ensure that there is adequate lighting to avoid unnecessary eyestrain. Studying on a bed should be avoided to reduce the possibility of overrelaxation, inattentiveness, and sleepiness.
- Study in half-hour intervals with 10-minute breaks.
  - This format will provide reasonable study time and allow relaxation breaks. The mind will only process so much information without a break. A tired mind is not a good study tool.
- Have everything you need available before you start.
  - This includes textbooks, notebooks, pencils, pens, highlighters, calculators, and anything else that will be required for completion of the assignment.

- Know how to use your textbook.
- Learn to use reference materials.
- Read and pay careful attention to assigned materials.
  - This requires reading class assignments and preparing homework assignments before the start of class. Trying to read the assignment while the instructor is presenting the lesson or during classroom discussions causes your hearing and sight to compete for attention, resulting in memory confusion. Plan to read the assignment at least twice. The first reading should be approached as though reading a novel or newspaper (conversational reading). This will allow you to capture the main points in your short-term memory. The second reading should be accomplished while outlining the assignment to allow the prominent points to be recorded into long-term memory.
- Read the assignment again and use outlines to emphasize critical points.
  - Outlining allows you to organize information into useful patterns, which improves recall, application, and problem-solving skills. Use the chapter and section headings as the major points in the outline and then use the following questions to add subpoints.
    - What is the main point of the section?
    - What are the major anatomic, physiologic, and pathophysiologic concepts?
    - Who is most affected by this information or these concepts?
    - When is this important to me, my EMS partner, and/or my patient?
    - Why is this important to me, my EMS partner, and/or my patient?
    - How is this important to me, my EMS partner, and/or my patient?
    - Where will this information be most useful to me?
- Develop your own examples or case studies of information in the assignment.
  - As you develop your own examples and case studies, ask yourself why the author put this information in the reading and what it teaches you about similar situations that you might see in the day-to-day operations as a paramedic. By putting key concepts or illustrations into your own words instead of simply memorizing the words of the author of the assignment, it is easier to understand and remember your own examples

and case studies because they are a product of your learning style and method of processing new information.

STUDYING DURING CLASS

There is no substitute for attending class. Using notes taken by a classmate with a different learning style may not prove beneficial to you.

Some of the essential and common study techniques that should be used during class are:

- Get involved by asking questions on topics that are confusing to you.
  - Remember, your classmates bring a wide variety of perspective and experience to the class discussion and may use a phrase or example that will help your understanding of a concept or principle. In addition, providing your thoughts and insights on topics that you have mastered and actively participating in discussion groups will allow you to hear your own words and explanations of concepts and principles. This may help you to find flaws in your logic or reinforce your understanding of a topic.
- Ask the "stupid" question.
  - Every student at some time has failed to ask a question because he or she thought it might sound stupid or that everybody else already understood the concept being taught. The old adage "the only stupid question is the one that isn't asked" has a lot of validity. You are attending class to learn a topic. If you don't ask, you won't learn.
- Take effective notes.
  - Notes should be focused on critical concepts and principles. Use the outline you developed before class to identify the important points. Write down "additional information" gained during the lecture or classroom discussion that enhances your outline. Take notes in your own words rather than trying to write verbatim what the instructor or classmate said. It is easier to understand and remember your own words, because they are a product of your learning style and method of processing new information.

STUDYING AFTER CLASS

Some of the essential and common study techniques that should be used after class are:

- Study in half-hour intervals with 10-minute breaks.
  - This format will provide reasonable study time and allow relaxation breaks. The mind will only process so much information without a break. A tired mind is not a good study tool.
- Have everything you need available before you start.

- This includes textbooks, notebooks, pencils, pens, highlighters, calculators, and anything else that will be required for completion of the assignment.
  - Know how to use your textbook.
  - Use additional study materials, such as your workbook, *Virtual Patient Encounters,* and Evolve Resources, to reinforce learning.
  - Learn to use reference materials.
- Develop and use flashcards, acronyms, and memory mnemonics for recall topics.
  - Flashcards and mnemonics are useful for memorizing information at a recall level. They are useful for recall of medical terminology, normal laboratory values, normal age-specific vital signs, rhythm strip recognition, and medication dosages.
- Be selective of the materials to study.
  - There is entirely too much information in any lecture or textbook to be included on an examination or to be added to your memory. While studying, anticipate possible questions that might be included on a test. Use your outline and class notes to highlight areas that have a high potential for inclusion on a test. Concepts and principles that are critical to life and limb or have critical ethical or legal implications are most likely to appear on comprehensive examinations.
- Get involved with study groups.
  - As mentioned earlier, classmates bring a wide variety of perspective and experience to the study groups and may help your understanding of a concept or principle. Remember to take notes in your words so that they match your learning style. Ask the members of the study group to confirm your list of important topics that may appear on a test.
- Set a regular time for studying each day.
  - Schedule study time for the time of day you are most alert. For example, if your attention is more focused in the morning, try to schedule your study time for that period.
- Study in a consistent and quiet place.
  - Study produces the best results when distractions are kept to a minimum and the surroundings a familiar. Avoid distractions such as noise, music, television and radio. Ensure there is adequate lighting to avoid unnecessary eyestrain. Studying on a bed should be avoided to reduce the possibility of overrelaxation, inattentiveness, and sleepiness.
- Study each day for upcoming tests.
  - Consistent study, spread out over a period of time, has been proven to be far more effective in retention of knowledge than "cramming" or massing study the day before class or hours before an examination. Start your study far enough in advance of a class or a test so that you can read and practice the critical information several times over a period of days, not hours.

TAKING EXAMINATIONS

Like studying, there are specific strategies that enhance student success when preparing to take a high-stakes certification examination.

- Course examinations help you determine how well you have managed the topics presented and help you identify whether your study materials and habits are effective.
- There is no substitute for good study habits when preparing for an examination.
  - It is important to remember that using any examination preparation strategy is ineffective if you have not spent time studying effectively. Effective study habits, as outlined earlier, are the single most effective method of improving examination scores. Remember to study consistently over a period of days, not hours. "Cramming" for a test is usually not effective. Focus your study on the critical items most likely to be included on the test. There is too much information in any lecture or textbook to be added to your memory.
- Eat a nutritious meal the night before an examination.
  - Avoid stimulants and depressants.
- Get plenty of rest the night before the examination.
  - Arriving at the examination site well rested will help to reduce anxiety and improve focus and mental acuity necessary for the critical thinking associated with high-stakes certification examinations.
- Take steps to avoid hunger and other physical distraction during the examination.
  - Be sure to eat before arriving at the examination to avoid hunger pains during the examination. Ensure that you empty your bladder before entering the examination room to avoid the distraction of a full bladder during the examination.
- Find out as much information about the test as possible.
  - If you are taking the National Registry of Emergency Medical Technicians test, visit their website at http://www.nremt.org/about/CBT_Home.asp to learn about the examination and take a visual tour of the testing facility. If you are taking a state certification examination, ask your instructor to describe what you should expect when you take the examination. Ensure that you know where and when the examination will be administered and what materials you will need to bring to the examination site.
- Arrive early at the examination site.
  - To reduce any last minute pressure and to allow for unavoidable delays in travel, plan on arriving at the examination site 15 to 20 minutes earlier than the scheduled time.
- Layer clothing to accommodate for variable room temperatures. It is better to be a bit cooler than too warm while taking an examination.
- Expect to experience some stress and anxiety.
  - It is natural to feel stress and anxiety. Do not become focused on the stress or anxiety and do not become overly concerned. A small amount of stress and anxiousness will help you do your best on the examination.
- Stay away from other individuals who are extremely nervous or worried.
  - You have enough stress of your own and do not need to multiply your level of stress by "buying" into others' emotions. Remember, stress is contagious and increasing stress will not help improve test performance.
- Take steps to reduce unproductive stress.
  - Keep a positive and upbeat attitude by deciding to do your best on things you know and understand, and refusing to dwell on those things that you do not know. It is too late to learn new material; simply make sure that you do well on the things that you know and understand.
  - Focus on the task of taking the examination. Answer one question at a time to the best of your ability. Avoid thinking about the remaining questions and do not worry about what others are doing.
  - Try to slow down and focus by taking several deep breaths before reading the first question. If you feel anxiety returning, repeat the deep breathing sequence.

PREPARING FOR EXAMINATIONS

Depending on the developer of the examination, you may be presented with a traditional pen and paper multiple-choice examination or a computer-adaptive multiple-choice examination. Although some of the strategies are similar, it is important to be aware of the type of examination you will be taking and apply the appropriate test-taking strategies to meet the examination format.

Pen and Paper Multiple-Choice Examination

The following are general test-taking strategies for pen and paper examinations that contain multiple-choice questions. Many of these strategies are appropriate for computer-adaptive testing as well.

- Read the examination instructions carefully or listen carefully to the examination proctor if he or she is required to read the instructions to you. If you do not understand any of the instructions or require clarification, ask the proctor for more detailed explanation before you begin reading the examination questions.

- Be sure that you know how much time you have to complete the examination and then plan your time for each part of the test. Allow a few minutes to review your answers before turning in your examination material.
- Read the stem of each question carefully and completely before considering an appropriate response.
- Answer examination items in the order presented and avoid the urge to skip questions. Identify any answer of which you are not completely certain by making a mark in the margin of the answer sheet next to the suspect answer. Once you have completed the test, review the examination question and answers that you marked in the margin. Correct any absolute errors that you identify, but do not change any answers unless you are extremely confident that you have made a mistake.
- Do not stay too long on any single question. If you find a question that appears to be difficult, rule out any answer that does not make sense and then make your best guess among the remaining answer choices. Mark the question for review at the end of the examination and continue with the rest of the examination.
- When confronted with a question that appears to have more than one correct answer, be alert for two or more concepts in the answer phrase. Some test developers will make the first concept of an answer choice correct and the second incorrect. Remember, all parts of the answer must be correct or the entire answer choice is incorrect.
- Reread all questions that contain the words *not, least, except* in the stem. These words have a negative connotation and can be confusing. If they appear on the examination, rereading the stem two or three times will help ensure a better understanding of the question and related answers.
- Be aware of qualifying words in the stem or the answer choices, such as *always, never, all, most, largest, smallest, best,* and *worst*. These words help to identify the correct answer choice, but are easily missed when reading a question. Sometimes test developers use a bold font to make the words more apparent. If you see this on a test, it is a clue that the word has serious implications for understanding the questions and related answers.
- Look for grammar and syntax agreement between the stem of the question and the related answers.

Any answer that has a grammatical or syntactical mismatch with the stem of the question must be considered incorrect.

Computer-Adaptive Examination

In addition to the test-taking strategies listed in the previous section, the following are strategies that are unique to computer-adaptive testing:

- If a difficult question is presented to you, use the strategies listed in the section outlining multiple-choice pen and paper examination strategies to select the correct answer.
  - In computer-adaptive testing, you are not permitted to skip questions or review answers as the end of the examination. You are presented only one question at a time and must answer the question before another question is presented to you.
- Avoid random guessing at the correct answer.
  - Random guessing can significantly reduce your overall examination scores. If you are unsure of an answer to a question, ignore any answer choice that is absolutely incorrect, and then use the strategies outlined in the pen and paper multiple-choice examination section to help choose the best answer.
- Expect to get tougher questions.
  - Don't panic—computer-adaptive tests are designed to present you with questions that you will have about a 50/50 probability of answering correctly. This type of test is designed to test you at your maximum ability level; therefore you should not be surprised when you get difficult questions. Once again, don't panic. Take a deep breath and use your test-taking strategies to make the best guess about the correct answer.
- Regardless of the question, always make your best guess at the correct answer.
  - Every examination will contain pilot questions. You will not be able to identify these questions and they may appear anywhere during the examination. You should simply answer every question to the best of your ability even though pilot questions do not count toward your official examination score.

VOLUME **1**

PARAMEDIC PRACTICE TODAY ABOVE AND BEYOND

DIVISION 1

PREPARATORY

EMS Safety and Well-Being of the Paramedic

Objectives *After completing this chapter, you will be able to:*

1. List the components of wellness and discuss how paramedics can promote wellness.
2. Discuss the principles as well as personal and professional benefits of positive lifestyle choices that promote wellness related to nutrition, rest, exercise, weight control, and not smoking.
3. Discuss the ways cardiovascular endurance, muscle strength, and flexibility contribute to physical fitness.
4. Define circadian rhythm and discuss the impact it can have on those who work shifts and ways to manage that impact.
5. List risk factors and warning signs of cardiovascular disease and cancer and discuss the role of risk assessments.
6. Discuss proper lifting techniques and the safety factors related to lifting and moving patients during emergency and nonemergency situations.
7. Describe the steps that should be taken, and the equipment used, to protect yourself from airborne and bloodborne pathogens or other adverse conditions and situations.
8. Outline actions that would reduce infectious disease exposure as related to field scenarios.
9. Develop a decontamination plan for equipment exposed to body substances.
10. List and discuss the three phases of the stress response and factors that can trigger the response.
11. Identify causes (life and EMS), signs, and symptoms of stress and discuss positive and negative coping mechanisms.
12. Discuss the importance of dealing with stress.
13. When given a scenario involving a stressful situation, develop examples of positive coping responses and how these could be used both on and off duty.
14. List and discuss Kübler-Ross' five stages of the grieving process.
15. Describe and discuss the needs that may arise when paramedics deal with stressed patients, families, death, and dying.

Chapter Outline

Wellness
Consequences of Poor Health Habits
Injury Prevention
Preventing the Spread of Disease

Stress
Death and Dying
Chapter Summary

Case Scenario

You and your partner are called to a private residence for a "man having difficulty breathing." You arrive before the police or fire responders. Because of the potentially urgent nature of the call, you ascend the two flights of stairs that lead up to the front door. After ringing the doorbell, you hear a woman's voice urgently requesting you to enter the house. She sounds frightened. You cannot hear or see any other approaching emergency vehicles.

Questions

1. Should you enter the home? Why or why not?

In the early days of EMS, many individuals had a sense that part of the job included putting themselves on the line to save lives and help patients. Little or no caution on the part of responders resulted in personnel entering unsecured scenes and often unnecessarily placing their lives at risk. Gloves were reserved for special circumstances such as childbirth, and little, if any, protective equipment was available.

EMS has matured and the world has changed. Today, one of the first rules of being a good EMT is to protect yourself. Some years ago, "protecting yourself" meant waiting a safe distance away until the scene was secure. With the advent of HIV/AIDS and increases in infectious diseases such as hepatitis and tuberculosis, the idea of protecting yourself has broadened to include concepts such as standard precautions and immunizations. Concerns about physical, mental, and emotional well-being has also become a part of protecting yourself and your peers. After the events of September 11, 2001, respirators became more important, as did varying levels of personal protective equipment (PPE). Use of such equipment may have prevented or reduced some of the health problems, particularly those affecting the pulmonary system, suffered by responders who worked at or near ground zero.

Today, scene safety, requests for lifting assistance when needed, use of PPE, fitness, and nutrition are all part of "protecting yourself." A paramedic who is injured cannot help others. One who becomes infected with a communicable disease may have to leave the profession.

This chapter focuses on the concepts of wellness, which include wellness itself, injury prevention, prevention of disease transmission, and stress management.

WELLNESS

[OBJECTIVE 1]

Each person lives somewhere on the continuum between wellness and illness. Good choices and positive lifestyle habits such as good nutrition, fitness, and sufficient rest provide the foundation for health as well as the prevention of disease and injury.

Physical, mental, and emotional well-being are the three components of wellness (Figure 1-1). Paramedics can promote wellness in their communities by assisting with health screenings and educating the public about wellness and injury prevention. As a community role model, you should set a positive example by obtaining all appropriate immunizations and boosters and undergoing regular tuberculosis screenings and other pertinent risk assessments such as colonoscopies and mammograms.

Physical Well-Being

Where an individual "lives" on the wellness continuum depends to a great extent on his or her lifestyle, habits,

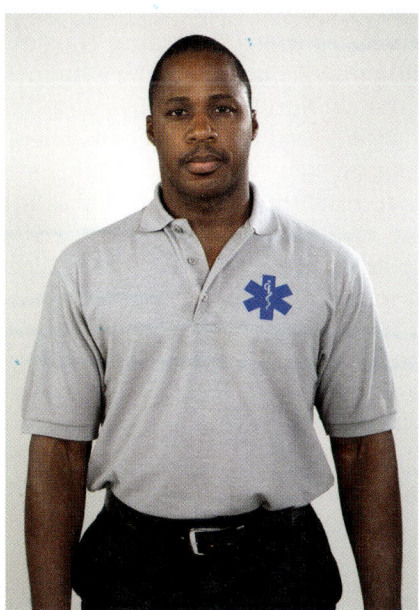

Figure 1-1 Physical, mental, and emotional well-being are the three components of wellness.

and choices. Many of the components affecting physical well-being are discussed below.

Nutrition

[OBJECTIVE 2]

Many EMS personnel live on fast food from drive-through establishments and high-calorie snacks from the corner market. Eating in a healthy manner may be more difficult while on the run (literally) than in many jobs, but it can be done. Planning ahead and carrying a small cooler with healthy foods is a good solution.

To enhance understanding of nutritional components, each is briefly discussed. Carbohydrates are primarily found in plant foods and are commonly referred to as *starches* and *sugars*. Milk sugar (lactose) is one example from an animal source. Carbohydrates are the primary source of energy for the body.

Fats add a lot of flavor to foods but should be eaten sparingly. Saturated fats usually are found in meat and dairy products and can raise cholesterol levels, which can increase the risk of heart disease. Unsaturated fats are divided into two categories. Polyunsaturated fats, the first category, are found in plant oils such as corn, soybean, and sunflower. Omega-3 fatty acids (a type of polyunsaturated fat) are primarily found in cold-water fish such as mackerel, salmon, and tuna but also are found in flax oil. Polyunsaturated fats are considered healthy for human beings because they help decrease blood cholesterol levels. Monounsaturated fats, the second category, are liquid and include healthy vegetable oils such as canola and olive oil. Trans fats are unsaturated fats that may be monounsaturated or polyunsaturated. They are considered a negative dietary addition because they seem to have the same effect on blood cholesterol as saturated fats. Trans fats are formed when vegetable oils are processed to make solids or to make them more stable so they will have a longer shelf life. They are found in a variety of packaged foods, including cookies and crackers. Legislation now requires that the amount of fat (saturated, unsaturated, and trans) be listed on the nutrition label of every food product to help consumers make well-informed choices.

Proteins are sometimes called the building blocks of life. They are needed for tissue growth, rebuilding, and repair. As proteins are processed during digestion, they break down into amino acids. Essential amino acids are required for cells and for body growth. They are not produced by the body, so they must be ingested. Nonessential amino acids are not needed for cell growth, but they are produced by the body. Protein is found in meat, fowl, fish, dairy products, and in some plant foods such as legumes and beans. Protein can be used for energy for the body, but carbohydrates should be the primary energy source.

Minerals such as calcium, iron, magnesium, and zinc, to name a few, are inorganic elements that naturally occur in the earth. They must come from the diet and play an important role in biochemical reactions in the body. All good multivitamins contain a number of needed minerals.

The word *vitamin* is defined as any one of a group of substances, other than proteins, carbohydrates, fats, and organic salts, that is needed for normal growth, development, and metabolism. Vitamins are important for metabolism, and intake can be by food or supplements. Vitamins are either water soluble or fat soluble. Water soluble vitamins cannot be stored in the body, so they must be obtained through diet or supplements on a daily basis. Vitamins A, D, E, and K are fat soluble.

Many people do not think of water as a nutrient, but it is a critical element needed for health. Cellular function depends on an adequate fluid environment. Total body weight for adults is approximately 60% water. Maintaining adequate hydration is an extremely important health issue. A common recommendation is to drink at least six to eight 8-oz glasses of water per day, but this requirement may change based on factors such as environmental conditions, altitude, and activity level.

One additional component that should be included in any discussion of nutrition is fiber, which comes from plant foods or fiber supplements. Soluble fiber can be found in legumes, barley, and some fruits and vegetables. It helps control blood sugar levels and may help lower blood cholesterol levels. Whole grains and some vegetables contain insoluble fiber, which helps retain water in the colon and can reduce or prevent constipation. Fiber is thought to help prevent some intestinal diseases such as diverticulosis, hemorrhoids, and perhaps some kinds of cancer. Figure 1-2 shows the Food Pyramid developed by the United States Department of Agriculture. Portion sizes are listed for each category based on a diet of 2000 calories per day. The stick figure climbing up the side of the pyramid represents the need for daily exercise and physical activity.

Good nutrition is important to maintain a healthy weight or to lose weight. A healthy diet includes consuming at least five servings of fruits and vegetables a day, a small amount of lean protein (5 to 6 ounces), low-fat dairy (3 cups), and whole grains (3 servings). Sugars, fats, and non–whole grain starches should be eaten in moderation. Being at a normal weight reduces the risk of injury and usually results in an increased energy level. A commonly used method of assessing body weight in relation to body height is the body mass index (BMI) (Table 1-1).

The key to reducing weight is to consume fewer calories than are expended in the course of a day. Magic diets do not exist. Healthy food choices and appropriate-sized portions, combined with exercise, is still the right choice. Set realistic goals, document or chart your success, get an exercise buddy, or meet with a group of like-minded people to make progress toward your goal.

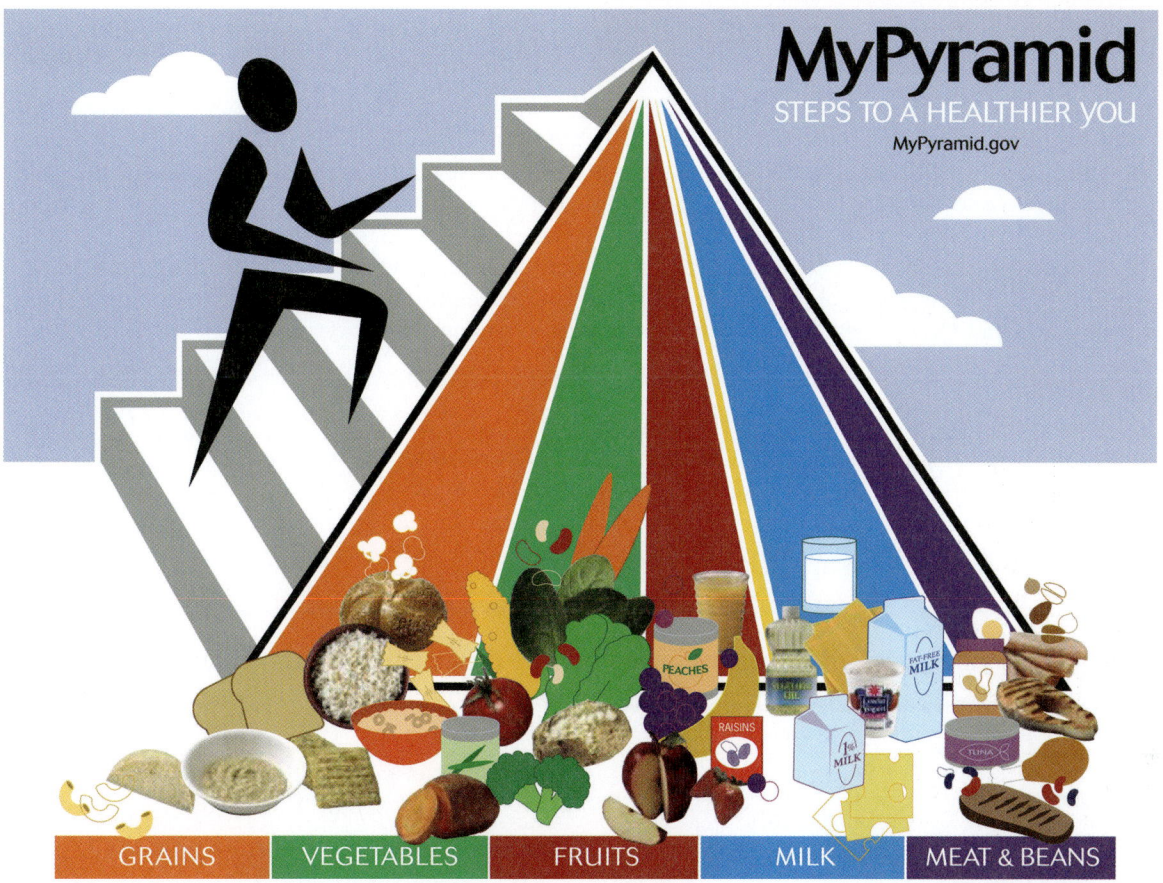

MyPyramid
STEPS TO A HEALTHIER YOU
MyPyramid.gov

GRAINS	VEGETABLES	FRUITS	MILK	MEAT & BEANS

GRAINS Make half your grains whole	**VEGETABLES** Vary your veggies	**FRUITS** Focus on fruits	**MILK** Get your calcium-rich foods	**MEAT & BEANS** Go lean with protein
Eat at least 3 oz. of whole-grain cereals, breads, crackers, rice, or pasta every day 1 oz. is about 1 slice of bread, about 1 cup of breakfast cereal, or ½ cup of cooked rice, cereal, or pasta	Eat more dark-green veggies like broccoli, spinach, and other dark leafy greens Eat more orange vegetables like carrots and sweetpotatoes Eat more dry beans and peas like pinto beans, kidney beans, and lentils	Eat a variety of fruit Choose fresh, frozen, canned, or dried fruit Go easy on fruit juices	Go low-fat or fat-free when you choose milk, yogurt, and other milk products If you don't or can't consume milk, choose lactose-free products or other calcium sources such as fortified foods and beverages	Choose low-fat or lean meats and poultry Bake it, broil it, or grill it Vary your protein routine — choose more fish, beans, peas, nuts, and seeds

For a 2,000-calorie diet, you need the amounts below from each food group. To find the amounts that are right for you, go to MyPyramid.gov.

Eat 6 oz. every day	Eat 2½ cups every day	Eat 2 cups every day	Get 3 cups every day; for kids aged 2 to 8, it's 2	Eat 5½ oz. every day

Find your balance between food and physical activity
- Be sure to stay within your daily calorie needs.
- Be physically active for at least 30 minutes most days of the week.
- About 60 minutes a day of physical activity may be needed to prevent weight gain.
- For sustaining weight loss, at least 60 to 90 minutes a day of physical activity may be required.
- Children and teenagers should be physically active for 60 minutes every day, or most days.

Know the limits on fats, sugars, and salt (sodium)
- Make most of your fat sources from fish, nuts, and vegetable oils.
- Limit solid fats like butter, stick margarine, shortening, and lard, as well as foods that contain these.
- Check the Nutrition Facts label to keep saturated fats, *trans* fats, and sodium low.
- Choose food and beverages low in added sugars. Added sugars contribute calories with few, if any, nutrients.

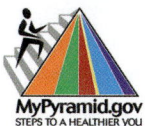
MyPyramid.gov
STEPS TO A HEALTHIER YOU

U.S. Department of Agriculture
Center for Nutrition Policy and Promotion
April 2005
CNPP-15

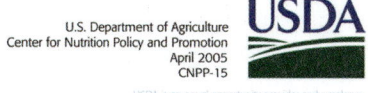
USDA

USDA is an equal opportunity provider and employer

Figure 1-2 The U.S. Department of Agriculture Food Pyramid emphasizes the daily intake of fruits, vegetables, and whole grains. It recommends a smaller daily intake of protein and stresses the need for consistent, daily activity to maintain normal weight and health.

Case Scenario—continued

You tentatively enter the home and see a middle-aged woman across the room urgently motioning you to a very large man seated on the couch. You estimate the patient weighs 350 to 400 pounds. From across the room you can see that his skin is pale, his lips are blue, and he is laboring to breathe. Several metered-dose inhalers are on the table by the couch, and a nasal cannula connects the man to an oxygen tank sitting beside him. His eyelids are fluttering as if he is falling asleep. The man's wife urges you to "help him," stating that "this episode of his congestive heart failure is worse than the time they put a breathing tube in and kept him in ICU for a week." Your partner completes her assessment just as two police officers arrive, informing you that the fire crew was diverted to a cardiac arrest several blocks away.

Questions

2. *What is your general impression of this patient?*
3. *What additional assessment will be important in the evaluation of this patient?*
4. *What intervention will be most useful for the patient at this time?*
5. *The patient is unable to ambulate, even with assistance. Should you attempt to transfer him to the stretcher and remove him from the home, or wait until additional help arrives?*

TABLE 1-1	Body Mass Index
Category	**Value**
Underweight	<18.5
Normal weight	18.5-24.9
Overweight	25-29.9
Obese	30 or greater

Body mass index is the body weight (in kilograms) divided by height squared (meters squared).

Physical Fitness

[OBJECTIVES 2, 3, 4]

An individual's level of physical fitness has a great impact on well-being, wellness, enhanced quality of life, and risk for injury. Benefits of physical fitness include the following:

- Decreased resting heart rate and blood pressure
- Increased oxygen-carrying capacity
- Increased muscle mass and metabolism
- Improved personal appearance and self-image
- Motor skill maintenance throughout life.

Recommendations for physical activity and exercise range from 30 minutes three to four times per week to 30 minutes six to seven times per week. There is no "right" amount of exercise. Age, fitness level, medications, and underlying medical problems can all have an impact on what is the right amount of exercise for an individual. For weight loss, 60 minutes of exercise six to seven times per week is recommended. Before beginning any new fitness effort, undergo a physical examination by your healthcare provider. It provides a baseline for comparing future improvements and may identify areas of concern. One measure used to identify levels of exertion is the target zone for heart rate. One recommenda-

tion is to maintain heart rate in the target zone for at least 20 minutes during an exercise session. To figure your target zone:

- Subtract your age from 220
- Multiple the result by 70%

For example, if you are 20 years old:

- 220 − 20 = 200
- 200 × 70% (0.70) = a target zone of 140 beats/min

When beginning an exercise program, start slowly both in terms of time and level of activity. Work up to more strenuous exercises continued for a longer period. Overdoing exercise at the beginning can cause sore muscles and lead to discomfort or injury. In some people this may result in a loss of motivation.

One goal of exercise and fitness is to increase muscle strength and flexibility. EMS requires significant lifting, so muscle strength is mandatory. Flexibility helps prevent injuries when lifting, particularly in less-than-ideal circumstances, such as on water beds, in overturned vehicles, and so forth.

Several possible approaches can be helpful when working to increase strength. Isometric exercise does not result in joint movement. Examples of isometric exercise include pushing or pulling against an immovable object or contracting the abdominal muscles (Figure 1-3). Although the muscle is strengthened, little if any bulk is added. Isotonic exercise moves the joints and therefore flexes and extends muscles (Figure 1-4). The amount of weight moved or lifted during isotonic exercise is referred to as resistance. A repetition describes the isotonic movement from the beginning position through the range of motion and back to the starting position. The number of repetitions done together (one or more times during a workout) is called a set. Increasing the resistance and/or repetitions or sets results in increased strength and some increase in muscle bulk.

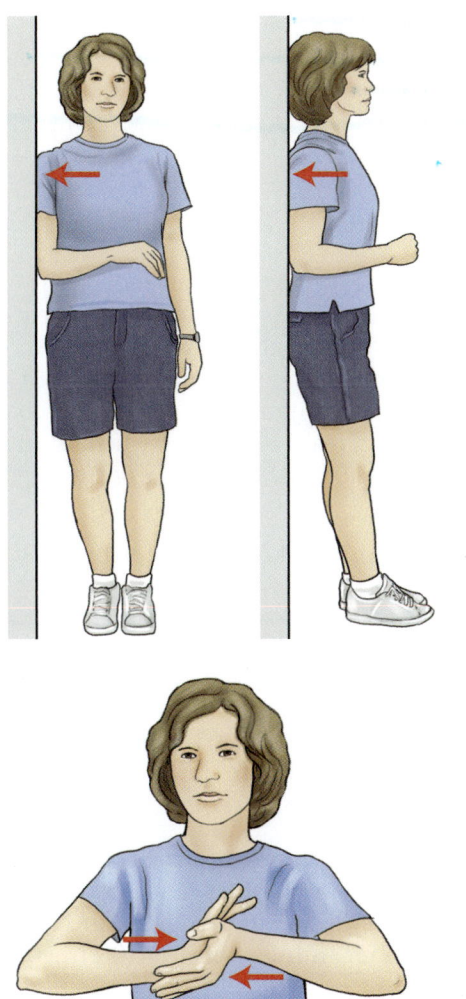

Figure 1-3 Isometric exercises increase muscle strength but do not result in joint movement.

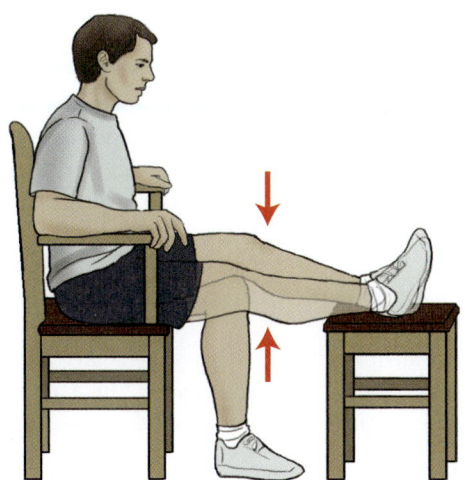

Figure 1-4 Isotonic exercises strengthen muscles by moving joints.

Muscle flexibility helps decrease injuries; strain is less likely when the individual has full range of motion. Flexibility can be developed and improved by smooth, slow stretching exercises—no bouncing! Muscles should be stretched *after* a warm-up. Stretching cold muscles, like bouncing, can increase the likelihood of injury.

Back pain and injuries are common in EMS. Lifting properly is critical and is discussed later in this chapter. Keeping muscles fit and flexible is also part of the equation for injury prevention. Any sudden onset of back pain while lifting should be evaluated as soon as possible. Sore or tired muscles after a busy shift should be treated gently, allowed to rest and, if severe enough, treated with ice and antiinflammatory medications per physician recommendation.

Rest

The importance of sleep is seldom emphasized in today's world, although many articles have been published on this topic. People commonly get by on 5 hours of sleep or less per night. Fatigue has been shown to increase skill response times and affect judgment. The amount of sleep recommended is 7 to 8 hours per day. In EMS, where 24-hour shifts are common and the majority of paramedics regularly work extra shifts or a second job, getting needed sleep can be a challenge.

Most human beings tend to have a relatively normal **circadian rhythm,** which means a daytime work schedule and nighttime sleep schedule. **Circadian** refers to a daily rhythmic activity cycle based on 24-hour intervals. Shift workers from all walks of life have documented difficulty with sleep patterns when their schedules deviate from the norm.

Sleep deprivation can lead to irritability, problems with relationships, illness, decreased job performance, and even depression. Some actions that can enhance the ability to sleep include the following:

- Avoid drinking caffeine or exercising during the last few hours before the desired sleep time.
- Give yourself a little break after the end of a shift to unwind before heading to bed.
- Eat carbohydrates that may help induce sleep.
- As much as possible, maintain the same kind of sleep schedule whether you are on or off duty.

Mental and Emotional Well-Being

Physical fitness, good nutrition, and sufficient rest contribute to both mental and emotional well-being. Identifying and managing stress also is an important component discussed later in this chapter. Each of these contributes to increased quality of life, general good health, and wellness.

Substance misuse and abuse can be detrimental to mental, emotional, and physical health. **Addictive behaviors** can involve something generally considered "safe," such as caffeine, but can lead to health problems for some people. Many people who are involved in high-stress jobs have "crutches" such as nicotine or alcohol that have become addictions for them. Unfortunately, those habits can lead to problems with health, relationships, job performance, and disease. Problems may be psychological or psychosocial. Problems may also be physiologic, true physical **addiction,** in which the individual develops withdrawal symptoms when the substance is withheld.

Many organizations and programs, as well as new medications, can help individuals control addictive behaviors. Most employers have employee or peer assistance programs designed to provide resources. Assistance for smokers, for example, may include nicotine patches or gum, counseling, behavior modification programs including hypnosis, or support groups. Smoking leads to cardiovascular and pulmonary disease as well as cancer. The first step to change is to admit a problem exists; the second step is to seek help.

CONSEQUENCES OF POOR HEALTH HABITS

[OBJECTIVES 5, 6]
Poor health habits eventually move an individual away from health and wellness and toward illness and disease. For example, obesity, smoking, a sedentary lifestyle, lack of appropriate health care and health screenings, and an unhealthy diet are examples of poor health habits that can increase the incidence of cancer, cardiovascular disease, and stroke.

> **PARAMEDIC*Pearl***
>
> Although not all disease is preventable, as a paramedic you have a responsibility to yourself and the patients you serve to take action to prevent and control those diseases that can be affected by lifestyle changes and medical management.

Cardiovascular Disease

Cardiovascular disease is a common cause of death in the United States. Such disease shortens life and has a significant impact on the quality of life. Warning signs of heart disease may include chest discomfort; pain that spreads to shoulders, neck, arms, or jaw; nausea or vomiting; indigestion; shortness of breath; back pain; dizziness; and unexplained fatigue. Maintaining fitness through a regular exercise routine, sound diet, stress management, and the avoidance of smoking are the keys to avoiding or preventing cardiovascular diseases and disorders. Other factors that have an effect include the following:

- Controlling high blood pressure
- Maintaining normal weight
- Keeping cholesterol and triglyceride levels within current guidelines

- Controlling diabetes
- Getting regular physicals, including risk assessments
- Making sure women use estrogen with caution, if at all

Cancer

Certain actions as well as diet can reduce the chances of developing certain cancers. Foods such a broccoli, blueberries, and high-fiber grains are thought to minimize the risk of certain cancers. Sun exposure, a diet high in fat, and a diet containing a lot of charcoaled foods are thought to increase the risk. Wear hats and use sunscreen when possible. Be alert for warning signs such as the following:

- A change in bowel or bladder habits
- A sore throat that will not heal
- Unusual bleeding or discharge
- A thickening or lump in the breast or elsewhere
- Indigestion or difficulty swallowing
- An obvious change in a wart or mole
- A nagging cough or hoarseness

If any of these signs or symptoms develops, see your physician.

Risk assessment screenings such as mammograms, prostate exams, colonoscopies, and monthly breast self-checks should be done regularly per current guidelines. Being proactive regarding your health is to your benefit.

Obesity

Obesity has been labeled an epidemic in the United States. It leads to many health risks and problems, including cardiovascular disease, arthritis, certain cancers, hypertension, and diabetes, to name a few. Maintain a normal weight to prevent obesity and protect yourself from its associated health problems.

INJURY PREVENTION

Many injuries can be prevented by using appropriate body mechanics when lifting and moving patients. As much as possible, clear the path that will be used as the patient is moved. Although one person should be in charge of the move, anyone involved must be able to stop the action when needed for safety.

> **PARAMEDIC*Pearl***
>
> Never hesitate to call for lifting assistance when needed because of patient size or location. Make good choices because back injuries can be career enders.

General guidelines for proper lifting and moving techniques include the following:

- Move a load only if you can safely handle it.
- Ask for help when you need it for any reason.
- Keep your palms up whenever possible.
- Take the time to establish good footing and balance.
- Keep a wide base of support by separating your feet by a comfortable distance, usually shoulder width apart.
- When lifting, bend your knees and lift with your legs. Do not bend forward and lift with your back. Flatten your lower back and tighten your abdominal muscles.
- Do not hold your breath; exhale during a lift.
- Avoid twisting and turning.
- Move or walk forward whenever possible. This gives you better line of sight and more control. Because of logistics, however, especially in confined or narrow spaces such as hallways in manufactured homes, one rescuer must often walk backward while weight bearing. Move slowly, deliberately, and with small steps. If possible, have a spotter behind the individual moving backward to help maintain stability.
- If trauma is present or suspected, move the patient in the direction of the length (the long axis) of the body.
- When moving a patient down an incline or stairs, have two rescuers on the lower, heavier end of the stretcher or board.
- When a team is lifting a load, only one person should give commands.
- Communicate frequently with your partner or other rescuers involved in the move to evaluate how things are going and make necessary adjustments.
- Keep the weight to be lifted as close to your body and center of gravity as possible. Extending the

arms to move weight away from your body puts more stress on the back and torso. Individuals who are overweight have more difficulty safely lifting because keeping the weight close to the body core is more difficult.
- When possible, push; do not pull.
- Staying alert and conscientiously practicing good lifting technique are key. Even when no spinal injury is suspected, the patient will feel more secure when normal body alignment is maintained during moving (Figure 1-5).

PREVENTING THE SPREAD OF DISEASE

[OBJECTIVE 7]

Many of the topics discussed in this chapter can help you stay healthy and even boost your immune system. Be alert for changes such as chapped hands, lacerations, or fatigue and deal with them properly and quickly.

Infectious diseases are caused by pathogens (viruses and bacteria) that can be spread from one person to another. The time between exposure to a disease pathogen and the appearance of the first signs or symptoms is called the **incubation period**. The most important method you can use to prevent the spread of an infectious disease is handwashing. Make handwashing a habit before and after contact with a patient, after removing your gloves, and between patients.

Entry points for pathogens include needle sticks, skin breaks, inhalation, absorption, ingestion, or through mucus membranes. Because not all infected persons are aware that they have a disease, and some who know will not share the information, treat the blood and body fluids of every patient you deal with as if the fluids are infectious. **Standard precautions** should be practiced during *every* patient encounter. Obtain all appropriate, available immu-

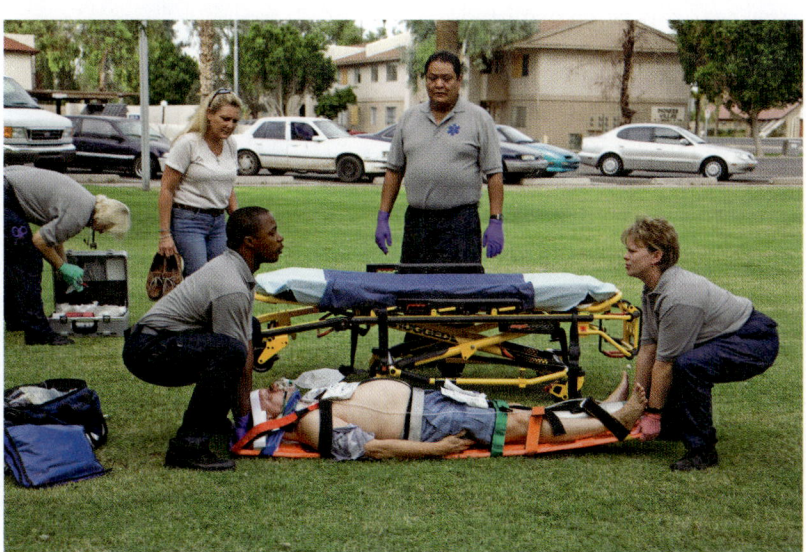

Figure 1-5 Proper lifting technique prevents injuries and prolongs careers.

nizations, get boosters as needed, and have regular routine screenings for tuberculosis.

Personal Protective Equipment

[OBJECTIVE 8]

The equipment used to protect personnel is called **personal protective equipment (PPE):**

- *Gloves.* Don disposable gloves before every patient encounter. Ideally, gloves should be changed between patients. Damaged or discarded gloves should be properly disposed of as soon as possible. If latex gloves are used, they should be nonpowdered to help reduce the chance of developing a latex allergy. Hands should always be washed or cleaned after glove removal.
- *Protective eyewear.* Appropriate eyewear helps protect the mucous membranes of the eyes from blood and fluid spatter as well as from pathogens introduced by coughing or sneezing.
- *Masks.* Don masks when splashes or spatter is possible and when giving nebulized medications, suctioning, inserting airway management devices, and cleaning contaminated equipment. A barrier, even a standard paper face mask, can help contain fluids and particulate matter and decrease contamination.
- *Respirators.* High-efficiency particulate air (HEPA) and N-95 respirators are designed to protect you from patients who have diseases that can be transmitted through respiratory secretions, such as tuberculosis. Fit testing is needed. Per Occupational Health and Safety Administration (OSHA) standards, employers must provide respirators when employee protection is needed. When a patient has a disease such as tuberculosis, you should wear gloves and a HEPA or N-95 (or higher level) respirator and the patient should wear a surgical mask. During transport the ambulance ventilation system should be operated in nonrecirculating mode and a rear exhaust fan should be used, if present (Centers for Disease Control and Prevention, 2005).
- *Gowns.* Disposable gowns can protect clothing from splashes. If uniforms are contaminated, remove them and shower as soon as possible. Contaminated clothing should not be taken home or to a laundromat to launder. OSHA requires that the employer have facilities available for this purpose.

- *Resuscitation equipment.* The primary equipment used in resuscitation should be disposable to prevent disease transmission.

Several levels of PPE are designed for different levels of threat. The levels of protection described for use in the event of a weapons of mass destruction (WMD) event are briefly discussed below as they pertain to biologic agents. Only level D protection does not require specialized training.

- *Level D:* [*Protect from some heat & water*] This level of protection essentially is clothing, a uniform, standard issue turnout gear, or structural firefighting gear. It is appropriate when no respiratory or skin hazard is present but provides no protection from WMD agents (Figure 1-6).
- *Level C:* This level includes chemical-resistant clothing with a hood and an air-purifying respirator. Cloth provides protection only when little chance of splash is present, and the air respirator can provide adequate protection against airborne biologic agents.
- *Level B:* This level consists of a chemical splash-resistant suit with hood and self-contained breathing

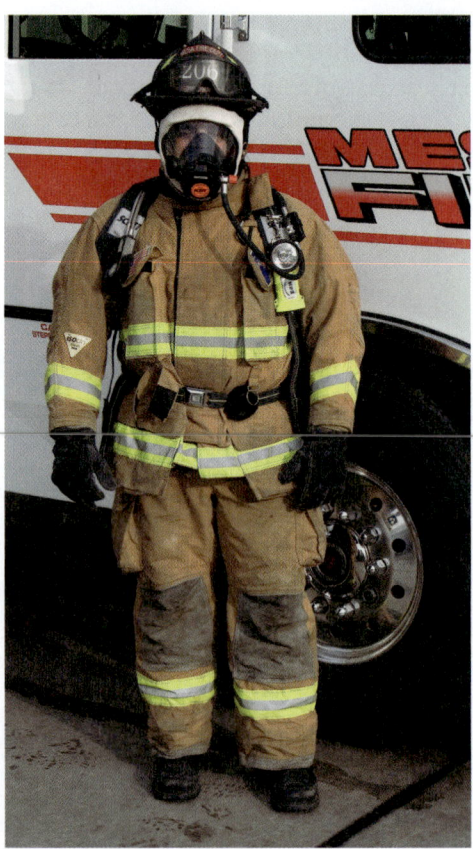

Figure 1-6 Uniforms provided at level D of protection.

apparatus (SCBA). It provides the maximum respiratory protection but less skin protection than level A. It can be used in low-oxygen environments (Figure 1-7).

- Level A: A completely encapsulated chemical-resistant suit with SCBA or other supplied air with escape device. It provides maximum respiratory and skin protection (Figure 1-8). *Very hot!*

Even with all the high-technology gadgets available, frequent handwashing remains one of the most important infection control deterrents. Use soap and water, lather vigorously for up to 1 minute, then rinse and dry. If soap and water are not available, an antimicrobial hand-washing solution or alcohol-based cleaner may be used until washing can occur.

exposure vs contamination

Exposure Management

contamination - skin intact - something on top or vomit on pants

An **exposure** occurs when blood or body fluids come in contact with eyes, mucous membranes, broken or intact skin, or through a needlestick. It also can occur through inhalation or ingestion. If that occurs certain actions must be taken in the time frames required by the employer or facility policy.

- Immediately wash the affected area(s) with soap and water.

- Document the incident. Turn a copy in to the employer or facility and retain one for your records.
- Obtain a medical evaluation and needed screenings or baselines.
- Get any recommended immunization boosters, immune system boosters, or medications.
- Continue follow-up care and evaluation as needed.

Equipment and Unit Maintenance

[OBJECTIVE 9]

PPE and many patient care items are designed for a single use and should be properly disposed of as soon as possible. Nondisposable equipment, including the ambulance, must be cleaned, disinfected, or sterilized:

- **Clean:** Wash the object with soap and water and use approved soaps to clean work areas.
- **Disinfect:** clean with an agent that should kill many of, or most, surface organisms. Equipment that has been in direct contact with a patient, such as a long spine board or splint, should be disinfected. *Bleach 1:10 w/water*
- **Sterilize:** The purpose of sterilization is to kill all microorganisms. Items that enter the body, such

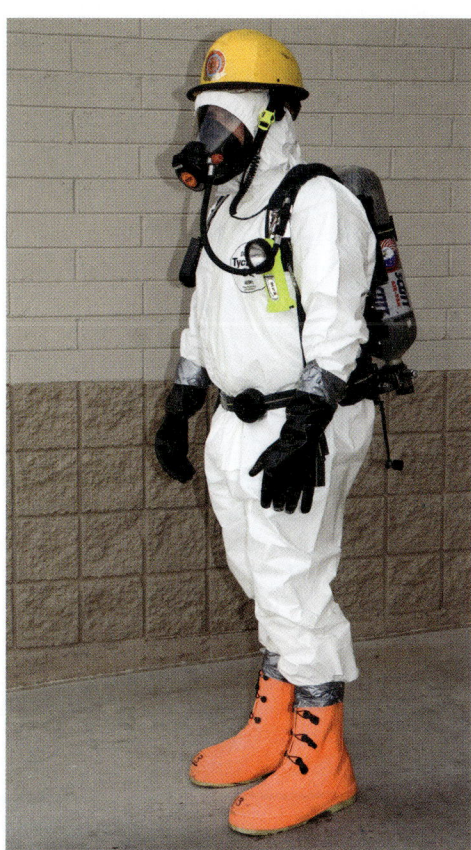

Figure 1-7 Maximum respiratory and pulmonary protection is provided by level B personal protective equipment (PPE).

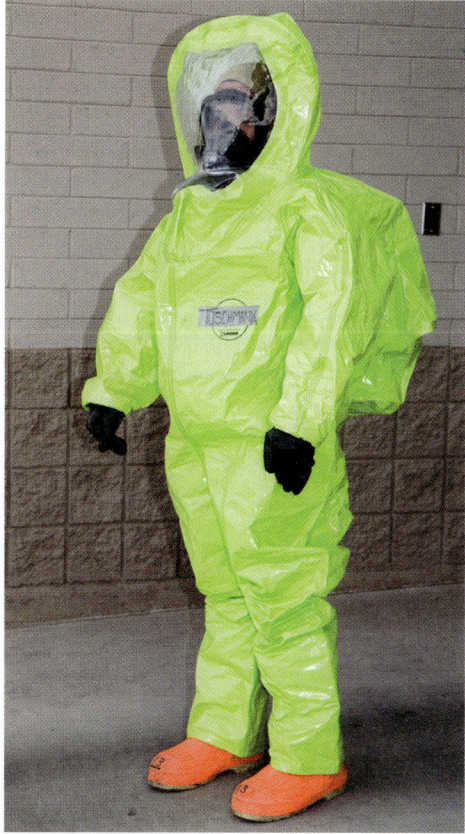

Figure 1-8 Level A personal protective equipment (PPE) provides maximal protection for the rescuer for both the skin and pulmonary system.

as laryngoscope blades, should be sterilized. This can be done by heat, steam, radiation, or an Environmental Protection Agency approved solution.

STRESS

[OBJECTIVES 10, 11, 12, 13, 15]

Stress is a part of everyone's existence and comes in many forms. It can help or hurt performance and relationships. The level of stress is not as important as how it is managed. Part of managing health and wellness is to be aware of your stress level and how well you are dealing with it. **Stress** can be mental, emotional, or physical and is often referred to as pressure, strain, or tension resulting from stimuli. Those stimuli are termed **stressors** and vary widely from individual to individual. Working in extreme heat or cold is a physical stressor. Attempting to resuscitate a child in cardiac arrest is often a mental as well as an emotional stressor. EMS calls provide ample opportunity for stressors of all kinds, as does life itself.

Dr. Hans Selye of the University of Montreal published a book titled *The Stress of Life* and was the first researcher to bring the term into medical usage (Selye, 1956). Selye identified three stages of the stress response.

1. The **alarm reaction** stage is essentially the response of the sympathetic division of the autonomic nervous system to stimuli. The response is designed to prepare the individual to fight or for flight (Box 1-1).
2. If a specific stressor or a build-up of stress lasts long enough, the individual's reaction changes. In the **resistance stage**, the body seems to have developed a tolerance to the stimuli and the autonomic nervous system's response to it. The specific stimulus no longer elicits an alarm reaction.
3. The final stage is **exhaustion**. In the exhaustion stage, the individual's physical performance, judgment, and critical thinking are affected. When **resistance** and the ability to adapt fail and exhaustion begins, the individual's reservoir of resources may be affected. The ability to respond appropriately to other stressors may then fail. The immune system can be affected and the individual may be at risk physically or emotionally. People may reach the **exhaustion stage** during one prolonged or especially challenging response, or it may come as a result of many accumulated stressors that have not been worked through appropriately.

Types of Stress

Getting a new job or promotion, starting school, and getting married are usually considered positive events in a person's life. Are they stressful? Absolutely! Good or positive stress is called **eustress.** Things considered to cause negative stress, or the accumulation of stress, can lead to **distress.** Distress can lead to anxiety and stress-related health problems and disorders (Table 1-2).

Causes and Effects of Stress

Factors that can trigger stress include fatigue, sleep deprivation, loss of something valued by the individual, poor health, nutritional challenges, injury or fear of injury, frustration, poor coping skills or inability to cope, and so forth. Individuals may experience the following:

- Be stressed by different things than are their peers.
- React differently than another individual when both are exposed to the same stressor.
- React differently to the same stressor at different times or days based on the level of stress they are experiencing as well as their nutritional, fatigue, or health status at that time.
- Be affected by previous exposure to a specific stressor, past experience, and their perception of the event.

A list of common signs and symptoms that may be experienced as a result of stress are found in Box 1-2. **Anxiety** may occur in many situations and can be described as a feeling of apprehension, agitation, uneasiness, or fear.

Life is stressful and individuals learn to adapt and cope to survive. Defense mechanisms are one way of adapting or responding to stress. Individuals may become accustomed to, or depend on, a particular mechanism such as denial or blaming others. This helps the individual adjust to the stress-causing situations that confront them.

Coping mechanisms also may be used by the individual to deal with stress and stressful situations. Negative coping could include increased smoking, drinking, or use of other substances. Acting out in anger may vent some emotion but has many negative ramifications. Such actions or activities do not address the issue or solve or alleviate the problem. They simply mask it temporarily.

BOX 1-1 The Alarm Reaction

The responses below are mediated by the autonomic nervous system and coordinated by the hypothalamus. The pituitary gland releases adrenocorticotropic hormone, which leads to the release of adrenaline (epinephrine) and noradrenaline (norepinephrine).

- Pupil dilation
- Increased heart rate
- Increased blood pressure
- Increased glucose production
- Bronchodilation
- Decreased gastrointestinal tract function and motility
- Increased blood flow to large muscles

TABLE 1-2 Holmes and Ray Social Readjustment Scale

SCORE	LIFE EVENT	SCORE	LIFE EVENT
100 ☐	Death of spouse	29 ☐	Son or daughter leaving home
73 ☐	Divorce	29 ☐	Trouble with in-laws
65 ☐	Marital separation from mate	28 ☐	Outstanding personal achievement
63 ☐	Detention in jail or other institution	26 ☐	Spouse beginning or ceasing to work outside the home
63 ☐	Death of a close family member	26 ☐	Beginning or ending formal schooling
53 ☐	Major personal injury or illness	25 ☐	Major change in living conditions
50 ☐	Marriage	24 ☐	Revision of personal habits (dress, manners)
47 ☐	Fired from work	23 ☐	Trouble with boss
45 ☐	Marital reconciliation	20 ☐	Major change in working hours or conditions
45 ☐	Retirement	20 ☐	Change in residence
44 ☐	Major change in the health or behavior of a family member	20 ☐	Change in schools
40 ☐	Pregnancy	19 ☐	Major change in usual type and/or amount of recreation
39 ☐	Sexual difficulties	19 ☐	Major change in church activities
39 ☐	Gain of a new family member	18 ☐	Major change in social activities
39 ☐	Major business readjustment (reorganization, bankruptcy)	17 ☐	Loan less than $50,000
38 ☐	Major change in financial status	16 ☐	Major change in sleeping habits
37 ☐	Death of close friend	15 ☐	Major change in the number of family get-togethers
36 ☐	Change to different line of work	15 ☐	Major change in eating habits
35 ☐	Major change in the number of arguments with spouse	13 ☐	Vacation
31 ☐	Mortgage greater than $50,000	12 ☐	Christmas season
30 ☐	Foreclosure on a mortgage or loan	11 ☐	Minor violations of the law (such as a traffic ticket)
29 ☐	Major change in responsibilities at work	Total: _____	

For each item, mark an "x" in the box to the left if you have experienced such an event in the past 12 months.
Greater than 300 life change units = 80% chance of developing a stress-related illness in the near future; 150 to 299 life change units = 50% chance of illness; and less than 150 life change units = 30% chance of illness.
Reprinted from Holmes, T. H., & Rahe, R. H. (1967). The social readjustment rating scale. *Journal of Psychosomatic Research*, 11, 213-218.

Positive coping mechanisms should be actively developed and used. In this context these methods can involve the following steps used in problem solving.

1. Identify the problem
2. Gather information, look at alternatives
3. Select an action and solution, make a choice
4. Implement the action
5. Evaluate the success of the action, adjust as needed

Being able to see multiple options or solutions to problems comes with time and practice in similar situations. Mastery of this skill is of great benefit in many situations, including on the job.

Examples of positive coping mechanism include the following.

- Exercising to reduce stress, clear the mind, and do something healthy.

- Talking with friends or peers who understand what is causing the stress, which provides support and a safe place to vent.
- Using time management techniques is a solid way to decrease stress, prevent overload, and practice learning to say "no" to extra shifts, new assignments, and so forth.
- Getting plenty of rest because fatigue and sleep deprivation can significantly decrease the ability to manage stress well.
- Following good nutrition, a foundation block for staying healthy and giving your body what it needs to recover and rebuild.
- Scheduling time for fun activities, events, or hobbies that bring pleasure (e.g., music, concerts, sports, reading).
- Reframing an event, situation, or attitude to lay out the facts and examine them from different

| BOX 1-2 | Signs and Symptoms of Stress |

Signs and symptoms of stress vary by individual and by stimulus. Note the "opposite" reactions listed (e.g., diarrhea and constipation), which demonstrate the variety of reactions individuals may have.

Emotional

- Panic reactions or attacks
- Easily startled
- Increased irritability
- Easily angered
- Fear
- Denial
- Responses out of line with stimulus
- Feeling overwhelmed

Physiologic

- Cardiac rhythm disturbances: rapid, irregular
- Chest tightness or pain
- Palpitations
- Dyspnea
- Increased respiratory rate
- Nausea and/or vomiting
- Gastrointestinal problems: diarrhea, constipation
- Sleep disturbances: insomnia, nightmares, sleep all the time
- Sweating
- Headaches
- Increased blood pressure
- Aching muscles and joints

Cognitive

- Difficulty making decisions
- Critical thinking slow or impaired
- Decreased level of awareness (others, self, scene)
- Difficulty concentrating or focusing
- Memory problems
- Strange dreams or nightmares
- Confusion or disorientation

Behavioral

- Hyperactive
- Withdrawn
- Sullen
- Short fuse
- Increased smoking
- Increased use of alcohol or medication
- Change in eating habits, not eating, excessive eating

- Taking deep, slow, controlled breaths to decrease feelings of stress and increase the feeling of calmness or serenity.
- Following guided imagery to take short "mental vacations" or breaks from the current stress by thinking of a favorite spot (e.g., waterfall, mountain, garden) and dwelling briefly on how being there makes you feel.
- Performing relaxation exercises to relax the body progressively by focusing on individual muscle groups one at a time.

Stress in EMS

People who work in EMS and other front-line emergency response groups such as law enforcement and the fire service are subjected to a number of stressors with which most individuals never have to deal. As a paramedic, you may experience environmental, psychosocial, or personality stress as well. The sights, sounds, smells, and emotions of calls can all have an impact. Sirens, screams, fear, anger, inclement weather, abusive patients or families, difficult work spaces, and danger can all cause or lead to feelings of stress.

Everyone, including paramedics, arrives at work and starts the shift with a certain amount of emotional baggage that contributes to the stress load. Problems in the family or with relationships, conflicts with coworkers or supervisors, and financial strain can all lead to stress. The need to perform skills expertly, the need to be liked, guilt over behaviors or perceived failures, or the need to achieve can also add to the burden of stress. Learning what positive coping mechanisms work best for you, and making the practice of them a priority, can help you stay healthy, fit, and successful.

DEATH AND DYING

[OBJECTIVES 14, 15]

Although the primary goals of prehospital professionals deal with saving lives, protecting patients, and preventing future injuries, paramedics must also deal with death and dying. This section deals with those patients with a terminal diagnosis that allows them some time for adjustment.

These situations are often difficult and uncomfortable. Keep in mind that individuals who care deeply about a patient, and patients themselves, may have quite different reactions and behaviors concerning end-of-life issues. Some will be quiet and withdrawn as death approaches or at the time of death, and others will be loud or hysterical. Some are dry eyed, others cry profusely. Remember that grieving is personal, and that reactions may vary based on gender and age as well as the cultural or religious background of the individual. EMS has the difficult job of providing comfort and professional support to the patient and significant others during emotional times. A key objective is to maintain a nonjudgmental attitude at all times on the scene and be open to cultural differences.

viewpoints to get the right perspective (e.g., how big will this problem seem when you look back at it in 6 months or a year? How do you think it would be seen from a patient, hospital, or supervisor's perspective?).

Stages in the Grief Process

The original work in the area of death and dying was published by Elizabeth Kübler-Ross (1969). Her work with terminal patients led her to identify five stages in the grief process. Family members and significant others may also experience some of these phases, as may emergency responders.

1. **Denial** presents with feelings of disbelief, such as "no, that can't be right" when a life-threatening or terminal diagnosis is received.
   It is a common defense mechanism.
2. **Anger** may be evident anywhere along the continuum of frustration to rage. The individual may demonstrate anger toward the medical community, family, friends, God, or any living person. "Why me?" is a frequent thought or question. This can be a very difficult stage for those who deal with or care for the patient.
3. The **bargaining** stage is often characterized by an attempt to "cut a deal" with a higher power. "OK, I'm sick, but just let me live long enough to see my child graduate from high school" is an example of the thinking involved at this stage. Denial is no longer a prime response, and it confirms that the patient has admitted the condition.
4. **Depression** is difficult to deal with at any time, but when it occurs for a terminal patient it means he is looking at his own mortality and his life (accomplishments, mistakes, how he has treated the people that he loves). This "looking back" can lead to great sadness, regret, or despair. These feelings should be respected while providing support to the patient as he works through saying goodbye to everything in his life or supporting the family as they say goodbye to a loved one.
5. **Acceptance** of impending death can lead to peace and a feeling of calm or serenity. A patient in this stage often makes those around him or her uncomfortable or uneasy. Sometimes this leads to the patient comforting the family and friends, which can make others even more uncomfortable. Dying patients need to be as comfortable as possible. Pain control is a priority, as is the patient's need not to die alone.

Not all patients or family members will transition through each stage or go through the stages in the same order. In part, this may be caused by the length of time between diagnosis and death. Not everyone gets to acceptance. An individual may move back and forth through stages such as anger or bargaining.

Dealing with the Dying Patient

Patients with a life-threatening or terminal diagnosis may refuse treatment or choose treatment to give themselves more time. Family may or may not agree with the choices the patient has made. EMS may interact with a patient and family multiple times over the course of an illness or only at the very end. If a terminal patient is to be transported to a hospital or other facility, EMS should ensure that all legal paperwork regarding end-of-life care is transported as well. See Chapter 4 regarding legal issues involved with this matter. This paperwork makes clear what actions are appropriate en route.

Showing care and concern for the dying patient is important for everyone. Facial expressions, words, tone of voice, and gentleness of touch can provide comfort to the patient and the family.

In some cases the patient may be enrolled in hospice. Hospice originated in England in the early 1960s and came to the United States in 1963 through courses taught at Yale University. Hospice is designed for patients who are no longer being treated to cure their disease or condition. Patients are usually enrolled in hospice when they appear to have 6 months or less to live. The goals of hospice organizations include patient comfort, pain relief, and provision of a "good death." In addition, they provide support and assistance for the patient and the family. Family support, including grief counseling, can continue after the death, often up to several months. Hospice may serve the patient at home, in a nursing home, or in a free-standing hospice center. Hospice teams are multidisciplinary based on patient history and needs. The teams include a physician medical director, registered nurse, counselor or social worker, chaplain, pharmacists, and specialists such as respiratory therapists.

Death with Family and Friends

Even though time has been available for adjustment between diagnosis and death, family and friends may not be accepting of the loss of a loved one. Do not take negative statements personally; maintain a calm, professional, appropriate manner at the scene. These individuals often feel guilt or anger toward the situation and may vent emotions such as anger on anyone in their path.

When a death has occurred before the arrival of EMS and nothing can be done, you should be honest and concrete in communications with those at the scene to prevent misunderstandings. For example, use the words "died" or "dead" to achieve this goal. If hospice has been involved, the family was taught *not* to call 9-1-1. The reaction of dialing 9-1-1 in an emergency is deeply ingrained, however, so EMS may be called when no care, treatment, or resuscitation is desired. Following the laws of the state while providing support for grieving families can be hard to balance. Your compassion and professionalism can have a positive impact on the way family and friends deal with the situation.

Case Scenario CONCLUSION

You and your partner decide to initiate treatment and transport. As your partner initiates continuous positive airway pressure and starts an IV, you and the police officers get the stretcher. You load the patient onto the stretcher and roll him out the front door with one person on each corner of the stretcher. Leaving the stretcher in the raised position, you awkwardly lower/bump the patient down the first flight of steps. While negotiating the second set of steps in the same fashion, the stretcher begins to tip sideways. In your effort to stabilize it, you feel a sharp pain in your lower back. After releasing the patient (who is much improved) to the emergency department physician, you contact a supervisor to take your unit out of service because of your severe back pain. Ultimately you are off work for 6 weeks and require surgery for a herniated lumbar disk. You are never able to return to the field.

Looking Back

6. The patient was much improved when delivered to the emergency department and ultimately did well. Given the outcome, do you think you made the right choice when you decided to carry him out of the home without additional assistance? Why or why not?

7. When during this situation could you have called for additional lift assistance? Why didn't you?

8. Had you chosen to initiate treatment but delay transfer from the home until additional assistance arrived, what would you have told the wife?

Age Considerations

In the emotional environment surrounding a death, children are often left out of conversations or shunted to the background or another area in an attempt to shield them. Even the youngest child knows something has happened. Being aware of their needs is important, as are the needs of older adults. Families should be made aware of the need to be alert for any significant changes in habits, patterns of behavior or sleep, irritability, or eating changes of affected children and to seek appropriate help if needed.

From infancy to the age of 3 years, children sense emotions and may respond in a variety of ways to the sadness and tears they feel, see, or hear. For their sake, maintain the familiar, consistent routines they are accustomed to as much as possible. It also helps if the remaining significant people in the child's life make themselves available to the child.

Children 3 to 6 years old do not usually understand the concept of death, but previous experience with loss may have had an impact. They do not understand that the deceased is not coming back and may continue to ask about the person, or when they pass the hospital ask if the deceased is still there. They may feel a sense of responsibility because they have been "bad" or they fear other loved ones also will go away. Caregivers should give the child support and the opportunity to talk about perceptions and feelings. If the child was not responsible for the event, it is important to reinforce that the child was not to blame.

Those in the age range of 6 to 9 years have a more complete understanding of the finality of death. They may need to talk about the death repeatedly and may want specific details of how it occurred. The fear of other significant people in their life dying continues in this age group, and denial is a relatively common coping mechanism.

Children in the 9 to 12-year age range often hold in their emotions and try to act "adult." They, too, want to know the details of the event and may ask some questions repeatedly. They are old enough to feel and show anger toward the deceased or others they believe are somehow responsible, and they often feel guilt. Regression is a possibility for any age child.

Elderly adults may try to take on the role of providing comfort and care to others in the family. Keeping busy is a common method of coping. At times it is used to ignore the reality of the death or postpone grieving. Death can also cause them to look at their own mortality and consider their lives. A family member's death may also bring additional stressors related to financial concerns or their ability to remain independent. Remaining professional and supportive on the scene can help provide some structure and stability in an emotionally charged situation.

Death and EMS

Dealing with death can be emotionally and physically challenging for prehospital personnel. Dying patients can bring back difficult personal memories of friends or loved ones who are deceased or previous difficult ambulance calls. Special challenges exist when the dying patient is close to the age of the responder or one of his or her children, or if the responder knows the patient.

Being professional and appropriate on the scene always is the goal. When a call is over, however, each responder should deal with emotions and concerns in a way that fits his or her needs. Talking to other EMS personnel and working through difficult calls are critical for future health and well-being. Being a paramedic does not make you immune to grief. Recognize it and deal with it, and do so sooner rather than later. Suppressed emotions do not go away; they ferment. Stress from a critical incident or accumulated over a span of time that is not dealt with can lead to **burnout.** Burnout is exhaustion to the point of not being able to effectively perform one's job. It can affect

performance, attitude, relationships, and all other parts of life. Gaining closure after difficult calls is just as important to your well-being as protecting yourself by wearing gloves, using a higher level of PPE, or protecting your patients by keeping the equipment and unit clean. Keep yourself healthy in every sense of the word. Your partner, your patients, and your professional future all depend on it.

Case Scenario SUMMARY

1. *Should you enter the home? Why or why not?* This is one of the most difficult decisions for new paramedics to make. In many cases, entering a home without police accompaniment is safe and without any risk. Unfortunately, when the situation is not safe, the paramedic entering a house alone is completely exposed and often unable to escape without injury. The best practice is to enter with accompaniment. If you do choose to enter without the police, wait for someone inside the house to open the door and lead you to the patient. Doing so gives you an opportunity to spot suspicious situations before you are completely in the home.

2. *What is your general impression of this patient?* This is a high-priority patient. His visible respiratory distress, pallor, cyanosis, and declining mental status all suggest a severe condition. His wife's assessment that this episode is worse than the time he was intubated and in the intensive care unit also is significant. Families of chronically ill patients are often very accurate in their assessments. This patient requires rapid intervention and transport to an appropriate facility.

3. *What additional assessment will be important in the evaluation of this patient?* Vital signs, pulse oximetry, capnography, breath sounds, and additional history of the episode could all be useful but should not cause delays in treatment or transport.

4. *What intervention will be most useful for the patient at this time?* Given the available information, this patient requires high-flow oxygen, potentially assisted ventilation and/or continuous positive airway pressure, and intravenous access. Rapid-sequence intubation is another consideration if permitted by your medical director and local protocols. En route, a 12-lead ECG should be obtained and provided to the staff at the receiving facility. Transport is also critical because he requires physician-level evaluation, a chest radiograph, possible laboratory work, and probable admission to the intensive care unit. Depending on the remainder of the examination (and local protocols), he may also require nitroglycerin, furosemide, and/or morphine during transport.

5. *The patient is unable to ambulate, even with assistance. Should you attempt to transfer him to the stretcher and*

remove him from the home, or wait until additional help arrives? The answer to this question is easy but hard to implement. It is not safe for two trained lifters (you and your partner) and two untrained assistants (the police officers) to place a 350- to 400-pound patient on a 75-pound stretcher with 15 to 20 pounds of equipment and lift/roll/bump him down two flights of stairs. Doing so places the patient at risk of being dropped and the crew at risk of injury.

6. *The patient was much improved when delivered to the emergency department and ultimately did well. Given the outcome, do you think you made the right choice when you decided to carry him out of the home without additional assistance? Why or why not?* Sacrificing yourself for the health of a patient sometimes sounds noble. But is it? Was this patient worth the loss of your career as a paramedic? And can you say with certainty that the patient would not have had as good an outcome if you had waited a short period for lift assistance? Probably not. In addition, moving the stretcher in the raised position was a poor choice for two reasons. First, when dealing with an extremely heavy patient, raising the stretcher is unwise in the first place—it is an unnecessary lift. Second, moving the stretcher in the raised position on an uneven or sloped surface with *any* patient is dangerous because the high center of gravity makes it prone to tipping (as occurred in this case). Once adequate help is available, the best plan would be rolling the patient to the door with the stretcher in the lowered position, carrying him down the steps, rolling him to the ambulance, and *then* raising the stretcher for loading.

7. *When during this situation could you have called for additional lift assistance? Why didn't you?* This is the potentially preventable part of the situation. A call for assistance could have been placed when you first saw the two flights of steps to the home or, at the latest, when you saw the size of the patient. When calls for additional assistance are made early in a call, you can often avoid having to choose between rapid patient care and transport and safety. A key part of scene size-up is recognizing the need for additional assistance early and calling for it.

Continued

Case Scenario SUMMARY—continued

8. *Had you chosen to initiate treatment but delay transfer from the home until additional assistance arrived, what would you have told the wife?* Many paramedics hesitate to start a conversation with family members about decisions to wait for additional help for fear that it will make them appear weak or helpless or anger the family. This fear typically is unwarranted. Explain the need for the delay in terms of the *patient's safety*. In this situation, the patient was in greater danger than the paramedics because he was restrained on the stretcher and unable to protect himself. Had the stretcher tipped over, the patient would likely have been severely injured. Explain that the patient's safety is your highest priority and that temporarily delaying his move from the home until additional assistance arrives will ensure a safe and uneventful transfer.

Chapter Summary

- In EMS, "safety" includes mentally, emotionally, and physically preparing and protecting yourself. Physical preparation includes exercise as well as proper nutrition and ongoing risk assessments.
- In the world of EMS, eating wisely and well is difficult but can be done with preparation and planning.
- Maintaining a healthy weight contributes to lifelong health and decreases disease, but it also makes lifting easier by using appropriate body mechanics and decreases the chances of injury.
- Being physically fit decreases injury as well as disease and increases life span and an individual's ability to deal well with the physical, mental, and emotional demands found in EMS.
- Cardiovascular fitness, muscle strength, and flexibility should all be maintained; they enhance health and help prevent disease.
- Regular medical check-ups and risk assessments increase longevity.
- Rest and sleep are physical requirements and should not be considered luxuries.
- A wide variety of addictive behaviors is possible; identification is the first step to better health, and seeking assistance or treatment is the second.

- Stress management is an important component of remaining healthy in EMS; deal with emotions or they will deal with you; develop and practice positive coping mechanisms.
- One of the areas of self-protection that has become increasingly important is PPE; proper use can save your life.
- Paramedics work to save lives, but all have to deal with death and dying; be prepared through self-assessment of stress levels and by developing healthy coping strategies.
- Dealing with stressed individuals, those who are in pain, or those who have just experienced loss is challenging; keep your cool and remain professional and appropriate.
- Difficult calls and critical incidents bring special stress to the paramedic during and after the event; be alert and aware of your own emotions, feelings, and needs and deal with them in the most positive way possible; get professional help if needed.
- Be prepared for age-related differences found when death affects individuals of different ages, ethnicities, or cultural backgrounds; be supportive and nonjudgmental.

REFERENCES

Centers for Disease Control and Prevention (2005). Guidelines for preventing the transmission of *Mycobacterium tuberculosis* in health-care settings. *Morbidity and Mortality Weekly Report, 54* (RR-17), 1-141.

Kübler-Ross, E. (1997). *On death and dying*, New York: Simon and Schuster.

Selye, H. (1978). *The stress of life* (2nd ed.), New York: McGraw Hill.

SUGGESTED RESOURCES

Benson, H. (1976). *The relaxation response* (9th ed.), New York: Avon Books.

Covey, S. R. (2004). *Seven habits of highly effective people*, New York: Free Press.

Johnson, S. (1999). *Who moved my cheese* (8th ed.), New York: G.P. Putnam's Sons.

National Highway Traffic Safety Administration. (1998). *EMT-Paramedic national standard curriculum*, Washington, DC: U.S. Department of Transportation.

Sternberg, E. (2001). *The science connecting health and emotions*, New York: W. H. Freeman and Co.

Chapter Quiz

1. List the three components of wellness and assess your personal level of well-being in regard to each.

   _____
   _____
   _____
   _____
   _____
   _____

2. In what ways have you seen paramedics promote wellness in your community? What other ways do you think paramedics should consider to have an effect in your community?

   _____
   _____
   _____
   _____
   _____
   _____

3. Evaluate your current lifestyle choices related to nutrition, rest, exercise, weight control, and smoking. What changes should you make to maximize your well-being?

   _____
   _____
   _____
   _____
   _____
   _____

4. List risk factors for cardiovascular disease.

   _____
   _____
   _____
   _____

5. Why are risk assessments such as colonoscopies, mammograms, and prostate exams considered so important?

   _____
   _____

6. What impact can irregular sleep patterns have on performance? How can you decrease the impact?

   _____
   _____
   _____
   _____

7. You inserted an endotracheal tube on the scene. What would you do to the laryngoscope blade before using it on another patient?

   _____

8. What PPE should be used when dealing with the following?
   a. A patient with active tuberculosis

   _____

   b. An elderly patient who has fallen and has hip pain

   _____

   c. A patient from an incoming flight at the airport who is hemorrhaging from his nose and ears

   _____
   _____

9. What would indicate that your partner has reached the third phase of the stress response and action or intervention is needed?

   _____
   _____

10. List as many signs and symptoms of stress as you can remember.

    _____
    _____
    _____
    _____

11. List Kübler-Ross' five stages of the grieving process. Discuss the variation that may be found in how or what order patients or families may experience these stages.

    _____
    _____
    _____
    _____
    _____

12. Why is stress management considered so important for those who work in EMS? Can individuals always handle stress by themselves? What might indicate mental health professionals could be helpful?

    _____
    _____
    _____
    _____
    _____

13. What positive coping mechanisms work best for you? Which ones could be easily used when you are on duty?

    _____
    _____
    _____

Terminology

Acceptance A grief stage in which the individual has come to terms with the reality of his or her (or a loved one's) imminent death.

Addiction The involvement in a repetitive behavior (gambling, substances, etc.). In physical addiction the individual has become dependent on an external substance and develops physical withdrawal symptoms if the substance is unavailable.

Addictive behavior The involvement in repetitive behavior such as gambling or substance abuse.

Alarm reaction The body's autonomic, sympathetic nervous system response to stimuli designed to prepare the individual to fight or flee.

Anger A stage in the grieving process in which the individual is upset by the stated future loss of life.

Anxiety The sometimes vague feeling of apprehension, uneasiness, dread, or worry that often occurs without a specific source or cause identified. It is also a normal response to a perceived threat.

Bargaining A stage of the grieving process. The individual may attempt to "cut a deal" with a higher power to accomplish a specific goal or task.

Burnout Exhaustion to the point of not being able to perform one's job effectively.

Circadian A daily rhythmic activity cycle based on 24-hour intervals or events that occur at approximately 24-hour intervals, such as certain physiologic occurrences.

Circadian rhythm The 24-hour cycle that relates to work and rest time.

Clean To wash with soap and water.

Denial A common defense mechanism that presents with feelings of disbelief, such as "no, that can't be right" when a life-threatening or terminal diagnosis is received; one of the stages of the grief response.

Depression A stage in the grieving process characterized by sorrow and lack of interest in the things that produce pleasure and other signs and symptoms seen in depression from other causes.

Disinfect To clean with an agent that should kill many of, or most, surface organisms.

Distress Stress that is perceived as negative; it may be seen as physical or mental pain or suffering.

Eustress Stress that occurs from events, people, or influences that are perceived as good or positive. Eustress can increase productivity and performance.

Exhaustion The last stage of the stress response and the body's inability to respond appropriately to subsequent stressors.

Exhaustion stage Occurs when the body's resistance to a stressor (decreased reaction to the stress, tolerance) and the ability to adapt fail; the ability to respond appropriately to other stressors may then fail; the immune system can be affected, and the individual may be at risk physically or emotionally.

Exposure When blood or body fluids come in contact with eyes, mucous membranes, nonintact skin, or through a needle stick; it also can occur through inhalation and ingestion.

Incubation period The time between exposure to a disease pathogen and the appearance of the first signs or symptoms

Personal protective equipment (PPE) Equipment used to protect personnel and includes items such as gloves, eyewear, masks, respirators, and gowns.

Resistance The amount of weight moved or lifted during isotonic exercise.

Resistance stage The stage of the stress response in which the specific stimulus no longer elicits an alarm reaction.

Standard precautions Infection control practices in health care designed to be observed with every patient and procedure and prevent the exposure to bloodborne pathogens.

Sterilize To kill all microorganisms.

Stress Mental, emotional, or physical pressure, strain, or tension resulting from stimuli.

Stressor A stimulus that produces stress.

Paramedic Roles and Responsibilities

Objectives *After completing this chapter, you will be able to:*

1. Define the following terms:
   - EMS systems
   - Licensure
   - Certification
   - Profession
   - Professionalism
   - Health care professional
   - Ethics
   - Medical direction
   - Protocols
2. Describe key historical events that influenced the development of national EMS systems.
3. Discuss the role of a national registry and how national groups are important to the development, education, and implementation of EMS.
4. Identify the standards (components) of an EMS system, as defined by the National Highway Traffic Safety Administration.
5. Distinguish between the local and nationally recognized levels of EMS training and education, leading to licensure, certification, and/or registration.
6. Explain paramedic licensure and/or certification, recertification, and reciprocity requirements.
7. Evaluate the importance of maintaining your license and/or certification.
8. Describe the benefits of continuing education for paramedics.
9. Describe how professionalism applies to paramedics while on and off duty.
10. Describe the attributes of a paramedic as a healthcare professional.
11. Give examples of professional behavior in the areas of integrity, empathy, self-motivation, appearance and personal hygiene, self-confidence, communication, time management, teamwork and diplomacy, respect, patient advocacy, and careful delivery of service.
12. List the primary and additional responsibilities of paramedics.
13. Discuss the benefits of paramedics teaching in their community.
14. Analyze how the paramedic can benefit the healthcare system by providing primary care to patients in the prehospital setting.
15. Discuss citizen involvement in the EMS system.
16. Describe the role of the EMS physician, and discuss the benefits of online and offline medical direction.
17. Describe the process for the development of local policies and protocols.
18. Describe the components of continuous quality improvement and its role regarding continuing medical education and research.
19. Explain the basic principles of research, the EMS provider's role in data collection, and the process of evaluating and interpreting research.
20. Describe the importance of quality EMS research to the future of EMS.

Chapter Outline

EMS Systems
EMS Education and Training
Professionalism in EMS
Attributes and Responsibilities of a Paramedic

Medical Direction
Improving System Quality
EMS Research
Chapter Summary

Case Scenario

A local emergency physician shares an article on chest pain management with you and your partner. The article documents a significant reduction in cardiac chest pain in 15 patients who received fentanyl compared with 15 patients who received morphine. The study was performed in a cardiac specialty hospital.

Questions

1. *Based on this information, what are the strengths of this study?*
2. *What are the weaknesses of this study?*

From the beginning, the field of **emergency medical services (EMS)** has been dynamic. It offers opportunities and challenges for anyone who is willing to answer a calling to the profession. This chapter covers the essential roles and responsibilities of a paramedic. A **professional** is a person who has special knowledge and skills. As an EMS professional, the paramedic must conform to high standards of conduct and performance and understand how fulfilling your roles and responsibilities will help EMS continue to grow and advance as a profession.

EMS SYSTEMS

[OBJECTIVE 1]

An **EMS system** is a network of resources that provides emergency care and transportation to victims of sudden illness or injury. The key parts of the EMS system we know today have developed and changed over the last 40 years. These changes have helped identify the essential parts of a functioning EMS system; however, compared with other health professions, EMS is still in its infancy. As a result the EMS profession is still developing its identity and role in healthcare, resulting in an ever-changing view of the role of EMS and the paramedic. The paramedic today is no longer a healthcare technician, but a healthcare professional, and as such requires comprehensive knowledge and education of body systems, functions, treatments and their effects, and knowledge of the chronic conditions encountered in the prehospital setting.

EMS is no longer considered simply a ride to the hospital. The EMS systems of today are an integral part of the medical community. Today's EMS systems are complex and composed of a network of services that provide care and transportation to sick and injured patients. These components include the EMS system as well as emergency departments, surgical treatment, intensive care units, rehabilitation, and long-term care. The EMS system has become the first line of access to medical care and the healthcare network for many people around the country. Paramedics are an integral part of the continuum of medical care, and their actions, or inactions, can have a dramatic impact on others in the system and patient outcome. Because EMS now plays such a critical role in the medical system, it must be continually updated and modified to meet the ever-changing and growing demands of medical care in the community.

Emergency medical technicians (EMTs) and paramedics are the core of most EMS systems. They are responsible for the care of patients until arrival at the hospital. Paramedics today perform interventions that are far more advanced than those performed by early EMS providers, including advanced procedures in the field that were previously performed only in an emergency department. EMS systems today bring the emergency department into the patient's living room or the street, providing immediate initial treatment.

In fact, prehospital professionals provide thorough assessments, aggressive treatments, and patient transport to the appropriate destinations. These actions allow the patient to receive definitive care at the hospital more quickly.

PARAMEDIC*Pearl*

The evolution of EMS is continuing. Of note, EMS has a history of only approximately 40 years, whereas other healthcare professions have a much longer history. This important fact may help you understand why EMS is in such a state of turmoil right now and undergoing an identity crisis. For example, are paramedics professionals or technicians? Members of the healthcare team or a transport service? Is a degree required to be a paramedic?

History of EMS

[OBJECTIVES 2, 3, 4]

Documentation of resuscitation attempts can be found dating back to the first and second centuries AD. However, not until the early eighteenth century were successful mouth-to-mouth ventilation attempts documented.

Baron Dominique-Jean Larrey, chief physician in Napoleon's army, is credited with establishing the first prehospital system for triaging and transporting patients in 1797.

In the United States, civilian ambulance services began in Cincinnati in 1865 and in New York City in 1869. In New York City, ambulances (horse-drawn carriages) were dispatched by telegraph from Bellevue Hospital's Centre Street branch. In the first year alone, the ambulances responded to more than 1800 calls for help throughout the city.

In 1928 the first volunteer rescue squad (Roanoke Life Saving Crew) was organized in Roanoke, Va. Additional volunteer rescue squads were then organized along the New Jersey coast. During World Wars I and II, with the development of the battlefield corps, systems for field treatment and transport were developed. During the 1950s and 1960s, transport of the sick and injured became a needed and expected service in America. At that time, hospitals and funeral homes provided most ambulance transport. However, most transport services had only a driver who possessed no medical training. In time, volunteer fire departments became involved with the development of EMS systems and began to establish rescue operations; some even provided transports. The Miami Fire Department was the first agency to use defibrillators on rescue units.

In the early 1950s mobile army surgical hospital (MASH) units used helicopters for evacuation in the Korean War. The rapid evacuation of patients increased survival rates. In fact, soldiers injured on the battlefields of Korea had a better chance of survival than civilians injured in the United States. This important fact was pointed out in 1966, when The National Academy of Sciences, National Research Council published the report *Accidental Death and Disability: The Neglected Disease of Modern Society.* This report is commonly referred to in the profession as the "white paper." It reported that in 1965, 52 million accidental injuries occurred in the United States, resulting in 107,000 deaths and 10.4 million persons temporarily or permanently disabled. Of these, 49,000 deaths were on highways and resulted from motor vehicle accidents. The remainder of the deaths occurred in homes and offices. This important paper exposed the inadequacies of providing emergency care in the United States and made 29 recommendations for improving care for injured victims, including the creation of trauma committees and trauma registries for collecting data about types of injuries. Eleven of the recommendations were directly related to prehospital EMS.

In response to the findings of the white paper, the U.S. Congress passed the Highway Safety Act of 1966. This act created the U.S. Department of Transportation (DOT) and the **National Highway Traffic Safety Administration (NHTSA)**. The DOT was created as a cabinet-level position and initiated the development of EMS systems across the country. The 1966 act created NHTSA as an agency within the DOT and provided the authority for the development of EMS systems, including the development of curriculum. For the first time the federal government provided funding to help get EMS systems started. In fact, the Highway Safety Act of 1966 required states to develop effective EMS systems or risk losing federal highway construction funds. Over the next 11 years, more than $142 million was set aside for the

development of EMS systems. This led to the beginning of advanced life support (ALS) educational programs, which are key components in EMS paramedic systems today.

In 1973 Congress began funding EMS systems nationwide. The Emergency Medical Services Systems Act of that year established that states would receive federal funding for EMS system development. The Emergency Medical Services Systems Act defined 15 required components of an EMS system. In addition, each state was required to have a lead agency for the regulation of EMS systems (Box 2-1).

The definition of these required components was a good start for the development of EMS systems. However, two key pieces were missing: medical direction and system finance. This was also the beginning of trauma systems and a regionalized approach to trauma care.

In 1981 the Omnibus Budget Reconciliation Act ended the federal funding of EMS system development because these funds were intended to be startup money and not long-term financing. As EMS systems began to grow and trauma systems were integrated, tracking the rates of trauma patient survival became important. As a result, regional EMS councils began to collaborate with the hospitals. In 1988 NHTSA developed a technical assistance program that permitted states to use highway safety funds to support the technical evaluation of existing and proposed EMS programs. Recognizing the deficiencies in the original EMS components, the technical assistance program developed 10 essential elements of an EMS system (Box 2-2). NHTSA also developed guidelines for how states were to implement these elements within a state EMS system. Because they were *guidelines*, individual states could choose what recommendations to adopt and how to implement them. This approach resulted in inconsistencies in the delivery of EMS, a wide variety of

---

BOX 2-1　Required Components of the EMS Act of 1973

1. Manpower
2. Training
3. Communications
4. Transportation
5. Facilities
6. Critical care units
7. Public safety agencies
8. Consumer participation
9. Access to care
10. Patient transfer
11. Coordinated patient record keeping
12. Public information and education
13. Review and evaluation
14. Disaster plan
15. Mutual aid

BOX 2-2 NHTSA's Essential EMS Elements (1988)

1. Regulation and policy
2. Resource management
3. Human resources and training
4. Transportation
5. Facilities
6. Communications
7. Public information and education
8. Medical direction
9. Trauma systems
10. Evaluation

NHTSA, National Highway Traffic Safety Administration.

BOX 2-3 System Attributes from the EMS Agenda for the Future (1996)

1. Integration of health services
2. EMS research
3. Legislation and regulation
4. System finance
5. Human resources
6. Medical direction
7. Education systems
8. Public education
9. Prevention
10. Public access
11. Communication systems
12. Clinical care
13. Information systems
14. Evaluation

Reprinted from National Highway Traffic Safety Administration: *EMS agenda for the future*. Retrieved October 6, 2006, from http://www.nhtsa.dot.gov/people/injury/ems/agenda/apenc.html.

---

certification levels, and many state-to-state differences that do not appear in other areas of health care.

PARAMEDIC*Pearl*

As federal funding was reduced, NHTSA began giving the responsibility for EMS system development back to the states, including the continued funding of the EMS system. States have laws and rules to guide the development and oversight of their EMS systems. State laws are put in place by the state legislatures and carry heavy penalties for not abiding by them. State rules are put in place by state offices with input from the public in further defining or clarifying the laws. These rules are enforceable by the state.

BOX 2-4 Components of the EMS Education System of the Future

- National EMS core content
- National EMS scope of practice
- National EMS education standards
- National EMS education program accreditation
- National EMS certification

In 1991 the National EMS Education and Practice Blueprint identified four levels of EMS professionals: First Responder, EMT-Basic, EMT-Intermediate, and EMT-Paramedic. According to NHTSA, in 1996 at least 44 different levels of EMS personnel certification existed in the United States because of state variations. In 2005 a survey of U.S. states and territories revealed 39 different licensure levels between the EMT and paramedic levels. The existence of so many different levels of EMS professionals has created problems. Some of these problems include public confusion as well as limited professional mobility for EMS personnel.

In 1996, NHTSA created the EMS Agenda for the Future to refocus the goals of EMS systems, including defining 14 essential attributes of an EMS system and developing the EMS Education Agenda for the Future: A Systems Approach (Box 2-3). The education agenda outlines five components necessary for the development of the EMS education system of the future (Box 2-4).

EMS Organizational Relationships

[OBJECTIVE 3]

National organizations are composed of people who share a common interest in promoting the evolution, goals, and/or direction of a particular topic. Many national EMS organizations focus on specific topics in EMS and work to develop the EMS systems of tomorrow. Such organizations include EMS field personnel, directors or chiefs, educators, and data personnel, to name a few. More information about the organizations available in your area can be obtained from your local EMS agency or state office. National organizations work to enhance a specific area of the EMS system while promoting what has already been accomplished. These organizations provide a stronger voice to other organizations or governments by providing information backed by evidence from across the country or a region.

An example of such a national organization is the Committee on Accreditation of Educational Programs for the EMS Professions (CoAEMSP). This organization focuses on ensuring potential students that a school is a sound institution and that it has met certain minimum standards in terms of administration, resources, faculty, and facilities.

The **National Registry of Emergency Medical Technicians (NREMT)** is a national organization that measures the readiness of program graduates to provide safe and effective patient care in the prehospital setting. The NREMT does this by measuring competency through a uniform testing process (Box 2-5). This agency strives

BOX 2-5 National Registry of Emergency Medical Technicians

- Contributes to the development of professional standards
- Verifies competency by preparing and conducting examinations
- Vehicle for simplifying the process of state-to-state mobility (reciprocity)
- Spreads costs of examination development and validation across a large user base

BOX 2-6 Important Events in the Development of EMS National Standard Curricula

1966: The report "Accidental Death and Disability: The Neglected Disease of Modern Society" published
1966: DOT established
1966: DOT established EMT-A curriculum
1971: First version of EMT-A curriculum published
1977: First EMT-P curriculum published
1977: EMT-A curriculum updated
1985: EMT-A was renamed EMT-B and EMT-I was created
1994: EMT-B curriculum updated
1998: EMT-P curriculum updated
1999: EMT-I curriculum updated
2005: National Scope of Practice Model submitted to NHTSA
2005: National EMS Core Content document published by NHTSA
2007: National EMS Scope of Practice Model published by NHTSA
2007: National EMS Education standards drafted

DOT, Department of Transportation; *EMT-A*, Emergency Medical Technician-Ambulance; *EMT-P*, Emergency Medical Technician-Paramedic; *EMT-B*, Emergency Medical Technician-Basic; *EMT-I*, Emergency Medical Technician-Intermediate; *NHTSA*, National Highway Traffic Safety Administration.

to keep testing current and equal across the country. Such standardized testing has helped establish **reciprocity** between states. Reciprocity is what enables EMS professionals to move from one state to another and receive credit for their previous credentialing.

In addition to national organizations, all states have other organizations that represent the personnel and providers involved in the EMS system within that state. These organizations may be advisory councils or boards that govern and regulate the EMS of that state. Advisory councils are usually composed of representatives of the various EMS functions and agencies. These councils provide expert insight to the state offices concerning specific EMS topics. EMS boards are typically composed of individuals who assist in the regulation of EMS. The boards regulate EMS by monitoring agencies, personnel, and training. The boards also determine punishments and sanctions for personnel who have acted outside their scope of practice. A **scope of practice** is a predefined set of skills, interventions, or other activities that the paramedic is legally authorized to perform. Boards also may play a key role in developing the rules and regulations that personnel must follow in that state.

Locally, many regions and districts have additional organizations working to ensure that the EMS system is meeting the demands of the public within a specific community. These local organizations usually include the local medical director, administration of the agency or agencies within the area, local EMS professionals, and citizens from the community.

EMS EDUCATION AND TRAINING

In 1971, NHTSA published the first version of a **National Standard Curriculum (NSC).** This document provided information on course planning and structure, objectives, and detailed lesson plans. It also suggested hours of instruction for the EMT-Ambulance (EMT-A).

In 1977 the first EMT-Paramedic (EMT-P or paramedic) NSC was developed by NHTSA. The curriculum included 15 modules of instruction. In the same year, the EMT-A curriculum was updated to meet the changing and growing needs of that time. In 1985, NHTSA approved

the EMT-Intermediate (EMT-I) curriculum and EMT-A was renamed EMT-Basic (EMT-B). The NSC for the EMT-B was again updated in 1994. The NSC for the EMT-I and EMT-P was updated in 1998.

PARAMEDIC*Pearl*

As is evident from the need for past changes to paramedic education, medicine is dynamic. EMS professionals are responsible for staying current with changes in medical care and not relying on information gained in initial education for their entire career. What was once taught as the standard of care may one day be inappropriate care.

In 2005 the National Association of State EMS Directors (NASEMSD) and the National Council of State EMS Training Coordinators (NCSEMSTC) completed a national project to develop the National EMS Scope of Practice Model for all levels of EMS professionals. This document was published by NHTSA in February 2007 (Box 2-6). It defines the minimal level of knowledge and skills for each level of EMS professional and is intended as a model that will help ensure consistency of state EMS licensure and promote reciprocity.

The NSC outlines the information to be delivered, or taught, at each level of EMS education. EMS professionals must have certain knowledge, be able to perform skills, and be professional in their practice. The NSC is divided into four sections to ensure that all students acquire the necessary competencies:

1. *Didactic*. The didactic portion of the program allows the student to demonstrate his or her acquisition of knowledge. This portion is traditionally done in the classroom. Written examinations are used to assess the information that has been learned (Figure 2-1).

2. *Laboratory*. The laboratory portion of the program allows the student to begin applying his or her knowledge while developing psychomotor skills. This allows the student to practice skills, such as starting intravenous lines, inserting endotracheal tubes on manikins, and using other training equipment without the risk of incorrect performance on patients. Check-off sheets are used to assess the information and skills learned (Figure 2-2).

3. *Clinical*. The clinical portion of the program allows the student to begin using learned skills on patients while being guided and coached by a preceptor. Students in this phase of the program are generally assigned to specific patient types. Then they are given specific skills to practice until they begin to master the associated techniques and knowledge. Evaluation sheets with set criteria are used to assess the clinical portion of the program.

4. *Field internship*. The field internship is the final portion of a paramedic program. This portion of the program allows the student the opportunity to put all the skills together. During this phase, the student can begin functioning as an independent EMS professional. All care provided by the student is monitored by a preceptor (Figure 2-3). The preceptor and student have a "master and apprentice" relationship. During this phase of the program, whether the student can apply the knowledge and skills acquired during the other portions of the program to assess and care for patients appropriately will be determined. Field

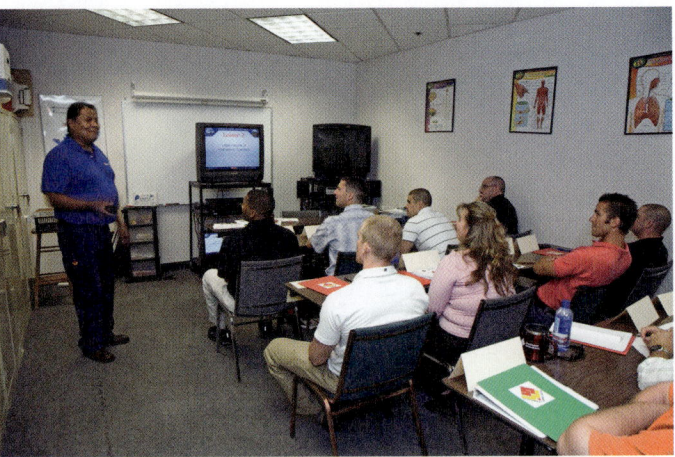

Figure 2-1 The didactic portion of a paramedic program is usually held in a classroom.

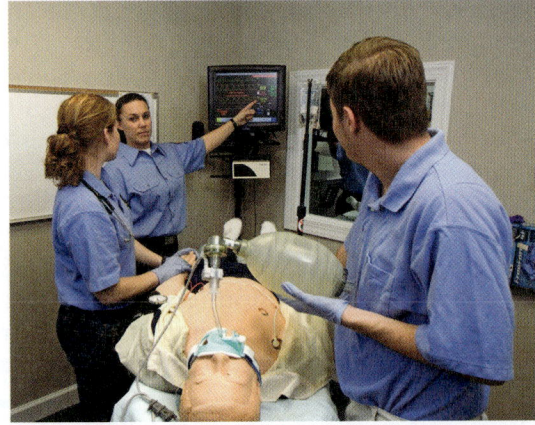

Figure 2-2 The laboratory portion of a paramedic program allows the student to practice skills.

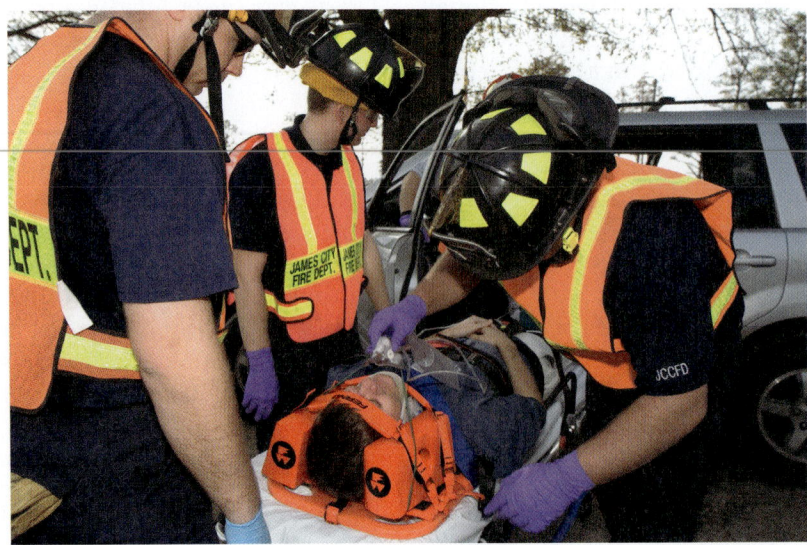

Figure 2-3 During the field internship portion of a paramedic program, all care provided by the student is monitored by a preceptor.

internships are assessed by using evaluation sheets that assess competency on the basis of determined benchmarks. At the end of this phase, the student should be able to function independently as an entry-level paramedic.

The final draft of the National EMS Education Standards is being reviewed by EMS educators and stakeholders while this textbook is in production. This document is an important step toward implementing the vision outlined in the EMS Education Agenda for the Future: a systems approach and will eventually replace the current DOT National Standard Curricula. The National EMS Education Standards outline the minimal terminal objectives to be achieved by entry-level EMS personnel within the parameters outlined in the National EMS Scope of Practice Model.

PARAMEDIC*Pearl*

Because national standards take years to develop, review, and implement, paramedics, as healthcare professionals, should never limit themselves to a static document, but should continue to learn and expand their knowledge.

Levels of EMS Professionals

[OBJECTIVE 5]

The National EMS Scope of Practice Model defines and describes four levels of EMS professionals: emergency medical responder (EMR), EMT, advanced EMT (AEMT), and paramedic. Each level of EMS professional differs in knowledge, skills, and judgment, critical thinking, and decision making. Not every state recognizes all levels of EMS professionals. Although the various levels of EMS professionals may differ from state to state, all EMS professionals work to provide the best patient care at their level of training and expertise.

Each level of EMS professional has its own scope of practice. For example, the scope of practice for an EMT is not the same as the scope of practice for an AEMT or a paramedic. Scope of practice is regulated by the state where the individual works and by the medical director. As new technology or research appears, an EMS professional's scope of practice should change. These changes will reflect the new norms or expectations. An EMS professional can be legally liable if he or she functions outside his or her scope of practice.

Emergency Medical Responder

An **emergency medical responder (EMR)** is an EMS professional who provides initial basic life support care to patients who access the EMS system. EMRs were formerly called *first responders*. An EMR must work with an EMT or higher level personnel during the transport of emergency patients.

Emergency Medical Technician

An **emergency medical technician (EMT)** is the minimal level of training required to transport a patient to an acute care facility. This level of EMS professional can provide noninvasive emergency care, including performing assessments, administering oxygen, and immobilizing a patient. An EMT can assist patients in taking their own prescribed medications. An EMT can also administer specific over-the-counter medications (such as aspirin and oral glucose) with appropriate medical oversight.

Advanced Emergency Medical Technician

An **advanced emergency medical technician (AEMT)** is an EMS professional who provides basic and limited advanced skills to patients who access the EMS system. An AEMT was formerly called an EMT-Intermediate. This level of EMS professional varies drastically from state to state. In some states AEMT skills include giving 50% dextrose to patients who have a low blood sugar and starting intravenous lines. In other states, AEMTs can perform advanced airway skills (including endotracheal intubation), apply cardiac monitoring, and give cardiac and respiratory medications. Many states do not recognize this level of EMS professional.

Paramedic

A paramedic is the highest level of EMS professional in the prehospital setting. This level of EMS professional performs advanced assessments, advanced procedures, and medication administration. A paramedic is competent in all the skills of the EMR, EMT, and AEMT and also can perform a broader range of advanced procedures that the other levels cannot.

Specialized Levels

More specialized levels are specific to individual states. Generally, specialized levels are not replacements for the standard four levels, but rather additional training one can take after receiving the initial EMT or Paramedic credential. For example, a wilderness EMT course is available for EMS personnel who work in remote areas. This course focuses on the long-term stabilization of patients within limited resources.

A critical care paramedic course teaches paramedics additional pharmacology and skills, such as the use of balloon pumps, to help with the care of critically ill patients who depend on equipment. Critical care paramedics commonly work on critical care transport ambulances, which are used to move patients between health care facilities. Other examples of expanding and emerging roles for paramedics include primary care, industrial medicine, sports medicine, and tactical medicine.

Licensure, Certification, and Registration

[OBJECTIVES 1, 6, 7]

To ensure the competence of EMS personnel, all personnel in an EMS system must be certified or licensed by the state in which they provide patient care. Although certification and licensure are terms that often are used interchangeably in EMS, their EMS meanings differ from other healthcare disciplines. This has caused confusion and inconsistency at the national level. The National EMS Scope of Practice Model defines and explains education, certification, licensing, and credentialing as follows:

The National EMS Scope of Practice Model establishes a framework that ultimately determines the range of skills and roles that an individual possessing a State EMS license is authorized to do on a given day, in a given EMS system. It is based on the notion that education, certification, licensure, and credentialing represent four separate but related activities.

- **Education** includes all of the cognitive, psychomotor, and affective learning that individuals have undergone throughout their lives. This includes entry-level and continuing professional education, as well as other formal and informal learning. Clearly, many individuals have extensive education that, in some cases, exceeds their EMS skills or roles.
- **Certification** is an external verification of the competencies that an individual has achieved and typically involves an examination process. While certification exams can be set to any level of proficiency, in health care they are typically designed to verify that an individual has achieved minimum competency to assure safe and effective patient care.
- **Licensure** represents permission granted to an individual by the state to perform certain restricted activities. Scope of practice represents the legal limits of the licensed individual's performance. States have a variety of mechanisms to define the margins of what an individual is legally permitted to perform.
- **Credentialing** is a local process by which an individual is permitted by a specific entity (medical director) to practice in a specific setting (EMS agency). Credentialing processes vary in sophistication and formality.

For every individual, these four domains are of slightly different relative sizes. However, one concept remains constant: an individual may only perform a skill or role for which that person is:

- Educated (has been trained to do the skill or role), and
- Certified (has demonstrated competence in the skill or role), and
- Licensed (has legal authority issued by the state to perform the skill or role), and
- Credentialed (has been authorized by medical director to perform the skill or role). (NHTSA, 2007)

All state certifications and licenses have set dates for when they must be renewed. To renew your license or certification, you must participate in a set amount of continuing education. Continuing education is covered in more detail later in this chapter. If your license or certification expires, your ability to practice prehospital medicine is suspended.

Reciprocity is the ability of an EMS professional to use his or her certification or license to practice in a different state. States have different rules and guidelines for reciprocity. One of the goals outlined in the *EMS Agenda for the Future* is to have a nationally accepted certification process. Such a process would allow EMS professionals to transfer from one state to another easily. **Registration** is the process of entering an individual's name and essential information into a record. NREMT offers examinations for each level of EMS professional. If an individual passes the NREMT examination, his or her name is placed on a registry of EMTs. Currently, many states grant an EMS professional the ability to practice in his or her state through certification or licensure, if the individual is nationally registered.

Lifelong Learning

[OBJECTIVE 8]

The paramedics educated today receive more knowledge and a different set of skills than many of their preceptors did. This is not to say that their preceptors are not as skilled or educated, but rather that the profession is continually changing. The information needed to become a paramedic today is different from what was required in the past. This is largely attributable to new technologies and information that have become available.

Your initial paramedic program is just the beginning of your education. To stay current with trends, technology, and research, you will need to continue your education through smaller courses and enhancements. All states have set minimal criteria that a paramedic must meet through additional training and education to remain certified or licensed.

PARAMEDIC*Pearl*

Lifelong learning is an essential part of a paramedic's job. Through the advancement of knowledge and maintenance of core knowledge and skills, a paramedic is able to provide safe and efficient patient care.

The educational requirements for EMS professionals fall into two categories: refresher education and continuing education. **Refresher education** is the process of updating what you have already learned, including your knowledge and skills. Because a paramedic does not use all the information learned in the classroom every day, refreshing that base of knowledge is important. This also holds true for skills; skills learned during an initial paramedic program must be maintained. Returning to a classroom laboratory or a clinical site helps the paramedic maintain skills competency. For instance, performing an endotracheal intubation is a skill that must be maintained.

Continuing education (CE) is lifelong learning. CE helps ensure that an individual who is certified or licensed continues to keep up with current information and trends (Box 2-7). Again, this applies to knowledge and skills. As EMS advances, drugs will change, skills will change, equipment will change, and knowledge will need to be advanced. The expansion of skills and knowledge is clearly beneficial. This will be guided by the state government, the local EMS system, and medical director. Be sure to research and learn the requirements to maintain a paramedic certificate or license in your area.

BOX 2-7	Benefits of Continuing Education

- Maintenance of core level of knowledge
- Maintenance of fundamental technical and professional skills
- Expansion of skills and knowledge
- Awareness of advances in the profession

PROFESSIONALISM IN EMS

[OBJECTIVES 1, 9]

Paramedicine is a profession. A **profession** is a group of similar jobs or fields of interest that involve a responsibility to serve the public and require mastery of specific knowledge and specialized skills. **Professionalism** is following the standards of conduct and performance for a profession. Professionalism includes attributes such as integrity, empathy, courtesy, honesty, and observance of the highest ethical standards. **Ethics** are expectations established by the community at large reflecting their views of the conduct of a profession. In other words, they are society's expectations of you. **Healthcare** is a business associated with the provision of medical care to individuals. A **healthcare professional** is an individual who has special skills and knowledge in medicine. This person also adheres to the standards of conduct and performance of the medical profession (Box 2-8). As a healthcare professional, a paramedic is expected to uphold the standards associated with medicine.

As a paramedic, you are entrusted with the lives of your patients. Every paramedic must strive to provide the best quality patient care possible to each patient. Paramedics provide quality patient care, instill pride in the profession, strive for high standards, earn the respect of others, and show respect and empathy for all patients.

Paramedics represent a variety of persons, including themselves, their EMS agency, the local EMS office, and

BOX 2-8	Standards of Conduct and Performance of the Medical Profession

A Paramedic:

- Conforms to and upholds the standards associated with the medical profession
- Looks, speaks, acts, and dresses like a professional
- Maintains knowledge and skills
- Provides high-quality patient care
- Treats every patient with respect and empathy
- Serves as a patient advocate
- Earns (and is deserving of) the public's trust
- Instills pride in the profession
- Strives for high standards
- Earns respect of others
- Demonstrates excellence on and off duty

their peers. Unprofessional conduct and/or an unprofessional appearance hurts the image of the profession.

PARAMEDIC *Pearl*

Every EMS professional should have a daily commitment to excellence on and off duty.

Because EMS personnel are highly visible role models and occupy positions of public trust, an EMS professional should respect the profession and act in a professional manner when on and off duty. A professional appearance and professional conduct are vital to establishing credibility and instilling confidence.

PARAMEDIC *Pearl*

By developing standards for education, establishing a scope of practice, and identifying the attributes of a paramedic, expectations of all paramedics are set—regardless of where or when they receive their training.

Case Scenario—continued

On further examination, you discover that the dose ranges used for both fentanyl and morphine in the study are comparable to those in your local protocols. However, in your protocols, fentanyl is indicated only for orthopedic pain, and morphine is indicated for cardiac pain. As you and your partner discuss the study, which was published in a medical journal the previous month, you wonder whether your local protocols are based on outdated research. Later in the shift you are called to treat a 54-year-old man with crushing substernal, cardiac chest pain. He is virtually identical to the patients described in the study.

Questions

3. *Would it be appropriate to "test" fentanyl for management of your patient and compare the patient's response to the response of previous patients who have received morphine? Why or why not?*
4. *Would any additional patient education or discussion be required if you chose to administer the fentanyl?*
5. *If you chose to administer the morphine per your usual protocol, would you have any liability for not choosing to use an alternative therapy that has been proven more effective? Why or why not?*

ATTRIBUTES AND RESPONSIBILITIES OF A PARAMEDIC

Attributes

[OBJECTIVES 10, 11]

As a paramedic, you are entrusted with the care and safety of members of the community. To be effective in this role, you must possess several important **attributes**, which are qualities or characteristics of a person.

Integrity

The single most important attribute a paramedic must possess has been said to be integrity. **Integrity** has been defined as doing the right thing even when no one is looking. The public assumes that paramedics are honest. As a paramedic, you must demonstrate honesty in all actions. Examples of such behavior include telling the truth and keeping complete and accurate documentation.

Empathy

As a paramedic, you must have **empathy** for the patient and his or her situation. Empathy is not the same as sympathy. Sympathy is sharing the feelings of another, but empathy is showing a person care and compassion with an appreciation for the person's situation without sharing the same feelings. No matter how trivial a patient's condition may seem, you must show that you care about the patient and that the patient is your most important concern at that time. You must also extend empathy to the patient's family and friends as well as to other health-care professionals. Some examples of behavior that demonstrates empathy include the following:

- Showing care and compassion for others
- Demonstrating an understanding of patient and family feelings
- Demonstrating respect for others
- Exhibiting a calm, compassionate, and helpful demeanor toward those in need
- Being supportive and reassuring of others

Self-Motivation

As a paramedic, you must be self-motivated. This requires an internal drive to excel. You must also be self-directed, meaning that you are able to complete tasks without being guided each step of the way (Figure 2-4). Some examples of behavior that demonstrates self-motivation include the following:

- Taking initiative to complete assignments
- Taking initiative to improve and/or correct behavior
- Taking on and following through on tasks without needing constant supervision
- Showing enthusiasm for learning and improvement
- Demonstrating a commitment to continuous quality improvement

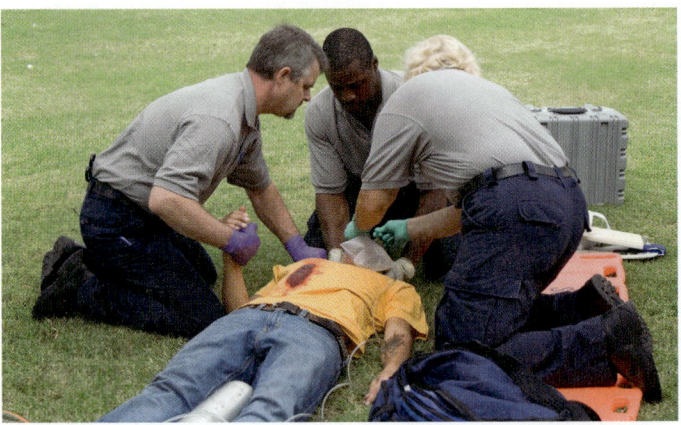

Figure 2-4 A paramedic must be self-motivated and self-directed.

- Accepting constructive feedback in a positive manner
- Taking advantage of learning opportunities

Respect

As a paramedic, you must show respect, consideration, and appreciation to others. Some examples of behavior that demonstrates respect include the following:

- Being polite to others
- Not using derogatory or demeaning terms
- Behaving in a manner that brings credit to you, your employer and peers, and your profession

Appearance and Personal Hygiene

As a paramedic, your appearance and personal hygiene reflect how much you care about yourself. A patient will see you and form an initial opinion on the basis of your appearance before you say your first word. Some examples of behavior that demonstrates good appearance and personal hygiene include the following:

- Keeping clothing and uniform neat, clean, and in good condition
- Having good personal grooming (shaven or neatly trimmed; hair combed and pulled back if long)
- Avoiding the use of overbearing fragrances
- Avoiding wearing jewelry that dangles

PARAMEDIC Pearl

Your personal grooming should demonstrate professionalism.

Self-Confidence

As a paramedic, you must have self-confidence. **Self-confidence** is trust or reliance on oneself. To be self-confident, you must candidly assess and know your personal and professional strengths and limitations. Some examples of behavior that demonstrates self-confidence include the following:

- Demonstrating the ability to trust your personal judgment
- Demonstrating an awareness of your strengths and limitations

Communication Skills

As a paramedic, you must have good communication skills. **Communication** is the exchange of thoughts, messages, and information. Communication is a two-way street. You must be able to convey messages and information accurately and completely to patients and other healthcare professionals. You must also be able to listen to, interpret, and comprehend verbal and written messages. Communication is covered in more detail in Chapters 8 and 18. Your written communication (documentation) must be clear, precise, and thorough. Misinterpreting or misrepresenting information can compromise patient care and lead to mistakes. Documentation is also covered more thoroughly in Chapter 19.

Some examples of behavior that demonstrates good communication include the following:

- Speaking clearly
- Writing legibly
- Listening actively
- Adjusting communication to fit various situations

Time Management

As a paramedic, you must be able to manage your time and maximize the time available. You must prioritize tasks while providing patient care, allowing the patient to receive needed interventions while you transport him or her into the healthcare system as quickly as possible. Some examples of behavior that demonstrates good time management include the following:

- Being punctual
- Completing tasks on time

Teamwork and Diplomacy

Teamwork and diplomacy are important professional attributes. **Teamwork** is the ability to work with others to achieve a common goal. **Diplomacy** is tact and skill in dealing with people. As a paramedic, you work with other healthcare professionals and public safety personnel. On a scene, you direct the care that other EMS professionals provide. Once at the hospital, you need to have a strong working relationship with the nurses and physicians. You should show consideration and appreciation to the patient and members of the healthcare team; this will help provide safe and efficient patient care. Some examples of behavior that demonstrates teamwork and diplomacy include the following:

- Placing the success of the team above your own interests
- Not undermining the team

- Helping and supporting other team members
- Showing respect for all team members
- Remaining flexible and open to change
- Communicating with coworkers in an effort to resolve problems

PARAMEDIC*Pearl*
Having respect for others is important. Earning the respect of others is just as important.

Patient Advocacy

As a paramedic, you are a patient advocate. When a patient enters the EMS system, the patient has, directly or indirectly, requested and trusted you to help make his or her situation better. To the patient, his or her illness or injury is the most important concern. Therefore always act in the best interests of the patient. Respect the patient's rights and beliefs, even if they differ from your own. As a patient advocate, you are responsible for protecting the patient's confidentiality. Patient confidentiality is covered in more detail in Chapter 4. Some examples of behavior that demonstrates patient advocacy include the following:

- Not allowing personal (religious, ethical, political, social, or legal) biases to affect patient care
- Placing the needs of patients above your own self-interest (except when it relates to safety)
- Protecting patient confidentiality

PARAMEDIC*Pearl*
Some patients have special needs that require special equipment or transport units. You must know about the available resources in your area and how to contact these resources when they are needed.

Careful Delivery of Service

As a paramedic, you must demonstrate careful delivery of service, including delivering high-quality patient care with careful attention to detail. It also involves critically evaluating your performance and attitude. Some examples of behavior that demonstrates a careful delivery of service include the following:

- Mastering and refreshing skills
- Performing complete equipment checks
- Operating the ambulance carefully and safely
- Following policies, procedures, and protocols
- Following orders of superiors

Responsibilities

Primary Responsibilities

[OBJECTIVE 12]
Responsibilities are duties that have been entrusted to you. In some instances, responsibility is assumed appropriate with one's duties. This holds true for the paramedic. Many of the things you are responsible for are not written

in a policy or operations manual. If they are written, they may not be detail specific. Nevertheless, you may be held accountable for their successful completion.

Preparation and Safety. As previously covered, one of the paramedic's key attributes is the careful delivery of service. This includes most aspects of your job as it pertains to patient care. The careful delivery of service begins with preparation and safety. Preparation includes being physically, mentally, and emotionally ready to respond to a call. Being unprepared physically can lead to patient injury. If you are unprepared mentally or emotionally, you may initiate an incorrect skill or procedure or calculate a medication dosage incorrectly, causing harm to the patient. Being prepared also requires having the appropriate equipment and supplies ready as well as adequate knowledge and updated skills. The appropriate equipment and supplies, as identified by your agency's policies, help you provide the standard of care in your area. When you are up to date with knowledge and skills, you can provide the appropriate care and respond more quickly to the needs of the patient.

A paramedic must *always* be safety conscious. Personal safety is the first priority. The safety of your crew is next, then that of the patient and, finally, the safety of any bystanders. First and foremost, never place yourself or your crew in danger. You must then look to the safety of the patient, removing him or her from a dangerous environment, keeping him or her secured during transport, and delivering him or her safely to the closest appropriate facility.

Response. You must be ready to respond to a call or request for service at any time. Providing a safe and timely response is part of providing patient care. Learning the most efficient route to a call usually comes with experience.

Scene Assessment. On arrival at a scene, you must immediately size up the scene and determine the number of patients. This must be accomplished safely and quickly because more resources may be needed. You must be able to recognize the mechanism of injury or nature of the patient's illness and prioritize the treatment and management needed for the patient.

Patient Assessment. After making sure that the scene is safe to enter, you will perform an advanced patient assessment and obtain a pertinent medical history. Next you will analyze this information, form a field impression, and then formulate a treatment plan.

Emergency Care. The emergency care you provide may include basic and advanced life-support skills. You must be able to follow local protocols while providing patient care and interacting with the medical director as needed. You must always give the best quality patient care possible, paying careful attention to details. This can be accomplished by maintaining your knowledge and mastering the necessary skills; performing complete equipment checks; providing careful and safe operation of the emergency vehicle; and following policies, procedures, protocols, and orders from the medical director or supervisor.

> **PARAMEDIC*Pearl***
>
> Paying attention to details can make the difference between a patient living and dying.

Destination. After establishing patient care, you will determine the most appropriate destination for the patient. This decision depends on the patient's injury or illness as well as available destinations. You must be able to decide quickly whether to transport the patient by air or ground transportation. If air transport is needed, it should be requested within the first 90 seconds after arriving at the patient.

To select the proper receiving facility, you must possess knowledge of the receiving facilities in your area. Your decision about the destination should be based on hospital resource capabilities and local protocols regarding optimal patient care. Some illnesses or injuries may warrant transport to a specialty center. These conditions include burn patients, stroke patients, obstetrics or high-risk deliveries, spinal cord injuries, and trauma patients.

> **PARAMEDIC*Pearl***
>
> If the patient has an illness or injury that warrants transport to a specialized facility, the paramedic must make the decision using local protocols and/or medical direction to transfer the patient to the most appropriate destination.

Transfer of Care. After transporting the patient to the appropriate destination, you must safely and efficiently transfer him or her to the receiving staff and facility. This includes a brief, courteous report of the emergency care that has been provided thus far. Be sure to transfer the patient's belongings, document what was transferred to whom, and obtain a signature indicating receipt of the items from a staff person at the receiving facility.

Documentation. Documentation is equally as important as patient care. Your documentation must be thorough and accurate and be completed in a timely manner. Moreover, a copy of the prehospital care report should be left with the receiving facility staff.

Returning to Service. On completion of a call, you will prepare the unit to return to service. This may involve restocking supplies or equipment and specialized cleaning of the unit. This should be done as quickly and safely as possible so that the unit is ready to respond to another call.

Additional Responsibilities
[OBJECTIVE 13]

Community Involvement. Your involvement with teaching in the community can have many benefits. These include enhancing the visibility and positive image of EMS professionals. Participating in illness and injury prevention courses also helps improve the overall health of the community. Teaching cardiopulmonary resuscitation and first-aid courses establishes your role as a resource in your community. Cooperative public education efforts (such as a cardiopulmonary resuscitation program jointly offered by a local fire department, the police department, and an ambulance service) improve the integration of EMS with other healthcare and public safety agencies.

Case Scenario CONCLUSION

You and your partner choose to administer morphine according to your local protocol. However, at your next meeting with your medical director, you discuss the article. He appreciates your eagerness to stay current in your profession but points out a number of significant problems with the study.

Looking Back

6. Do you think you did the right thing by following protocol rather that choosing a "new" therapy that might be more effective?
7. How does your relationship with your medical director relate to this situation?
8. What do you think your medical director discussed as the significant problems with the study?

Supporting Primary Care Efforts

[OBJECTIVE 14]

An EMS system is part of a larger healthcare system. Integrating paramedics into the healthcare system can help improve the health of the community, prevent injuries and illnesses, enhance patient compliance with treatment regimens, and ensure a more appropriate use of resources through public education. For example, assisting with health assessments and wellness checkups can enhance patient compliance with treatment regimens. You can help educate the public about when, where, and how to properly use EMS. You can also educate the public about alternatives to ambulance transport, how to locate healthcare professionals outside the emergency department, and where to find local resources, such as freestanding emergency clinics.

Citizen Involvement in EMS

[OBJECTIVE 15]

Paramedics encourage the involvement of citizens in the EMS system. Citizen involvement improves the EMS system in the following ways:

- Including citizens in establishing the needs and limits for EMS use in the community
- Providing an outside, objective view into quality improvement and problem resolution
- Creating informed, independent supporters of the EMS system

Personal Professional Development. As a paramedic, you are responsible for your own personal professional development. Some examples of ways in which this development may occur include the following:

- Exploring alternative career paths in EMS
- Continuing education
- Mentoring
- Getting involved in professional organizations
- Getting involved in work-related issues that affect career growth
- Conducting and supporting research initiatives

MEDICAL DIRECTION

[OBJECTIVES 1, 16, 17]

A **medical director** (also called a **physician advisor**) is a physician who authorizes EMS professionals to perform skills and treatments (Figure 2-5). The medical director plays an integral role in the EMS system. With the use of a medical director, paramedics can extend the services of a physician to their patients when providing care to them. The medical director must approve the skills, procedures, and medications used by paramedics. This approval is outlined under set guidelines called **protocols**. Protocols are written guidelines that outline specific assessments, interventions, and treatments for specific types of illnesses or injuries. These guidelines include what drugs should be used, when skills are appropriate, when to call the hospital for physician consultation, and the patient destination guidelines. **Standing orders** are written instructions that authorize EMS personnel to perform certain medical interventions before establishing direct communication with a physician. Protocols differ from policies. Policies are guidelines for behavior and actions not related to patient care. Some examples of policies include uniform codes and disciplinary procedures. The creation of protocols requires an evaluation of the EMS system and community. The medical director consults with EMS personnel, the state EMS office, and the local hospital or hospitals. He or she then determines what procedures and treatment guidelines would best suit the community. The paramedic must work within the scope of the protocols approved by his or her medical director. Additionally, all protocols must fall within what is allowed by the state scope of practice.

PARAMEDIC Pearl

No treatment protocol will fit all patients. Thus protocols are guidelines. They are not designed to replace common sense or logical thinking.

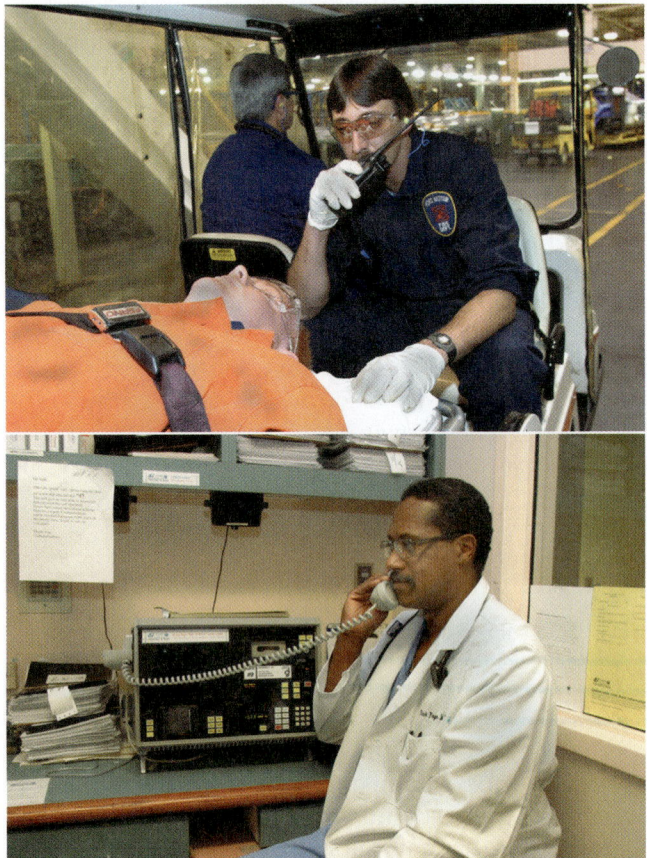

Figure 2-5 A medical director is an essential part of an EMS system.

A medical director's involvement in the development of protocols is an example of **prospective medical direction**. This type of medical direction occurs without direct voice contact between the paramedic and the medical director during patient management. It is considered **offline medical direction**. Prospective medical direction also includes a medical director's participation in training programs and selection of equipment, supplies, and personnel (Box 2-9).

Medical directors are an excellent resource for the paramedic. The paramedic can discuss any questions about medications, disease processes, and even the well-being of the paramedic with the medical director. When a paramedic is on a scene caring for a patient, the medical director may provide online medical direction. **Online medical direction** (also called *direct medical direction*) occurs when a physician gives advice or orders about patient care over the phone or radio (or face-to-face at a scene) while the paramedic attends to the patient. In this scenario, the paramedic provides a summary of the situation and physical findings to the medical director. Then the medical director can offer guidance on how the paramedic should proceed with patient care.

If a physician arrives on scene but is not the paramedic's medical director, the paramedic is obligated to follow the preestablished protocols of his or her medical director. The physician who has arrived on the scene may wish to contact the paramedic's medical director to see how the physician can best assist the EMS crew if he or she desires to help the patient. Physicians are considered the medical conscience of the EMS community. Therefore they should be involved in all aspects of establishing an EMS system.

IMPROVING SYSTEM QUALITY

[OBJECTIVE 18]

Medical directors are directly or indirectly involved in **quality assurance (QA)** and **continuous quality improvement (CQI)**. QA is a retrospective process and CQI is a prospective process. QA reviews the patients transported to ensure that they received the best care possible and that the protocols were followed. If existing protocols were deviated from, the paramedic may be able to defend his or her actions with a logical, medically sound explanation. A medical director's review of the prehospital care reports and participation in the QA process is called **retrospective medical direction.** Retrospective medical direction may include remedial education and/or limitation of patient care functions, if needed.

QA and CQI evaluate many areas of the EMS system, including helping to ensure system efficiency (Box 2-10). A QA or CQI evaluation focuses on the EMS *system*, not the individuals. For example, if studies suggest new or different treatment modalities and offer better patient outcomes, then EMS protocols are amended to reflect those changes. Similarly, EMS agencies evaluate new equipment and update it as appropriate to offer the best care possible consistently.

EMS RESEARCH

[OBJECTIVES 19, 20]

EMS professionals can provide valuable information to help determine how well interventions and treatment work. EMS is a young, growing, and dynamic profession.

BOX 2-10   Quality Improvement

Quality improvement is used to evaluate:
- Medical direction
- Financing
- Training
- Communications
- Prehospital treatment and transport
- Interfacility transports
- Receiving facilities
- Specialty care units
- Dispatch
- Public information and education
- Audit and quality assurance
- Disaster planning
- Mutual aid

For continued growth, information about what works and what does not must be continually evaluated. The paramedic should carefully document the prehospital care report; this is one way EMS professionals can provide information to the EMS system and assist in research.

Research is important for several reasons: (1) it validates existing treatments and protocols, (2) it helps provide better patient care, and (3) it can improve the EMS system. Without data, scientific research would not exist and new technologies would not be available. Research is important to verify that what is being done today does not cause further harm to patients tomorrow. Research is also important to verify whether changes in protocols or patient care are helpful or harmful. Research helps find ways to improve the devices used by paramedics, improve the response to the patient, and provide better equipped paramedics to treat all patients. Paramedics participate in research on many levels; they may be asked to participate in a study or to try a new drug, procedure, or piece of equipment.

After being gathered, data must be carefully analyzed. Data can be used to look continually for ways to improve the EMS system. System areas that need to be evaluated are medical direction, financing, training, communications, prehospital treatment and transport, interfacility transports, receiving facilities, specialty care units, dispatch, public information and education, audit and quality assurance, disaster planning, and mutual aid. This evaluation process must be ongoing and always focused on looking at the bigger picture instead of each component. The process must be dynamic and change as the information or system changes.

Evaluating Research

As previously stated, research data must be analyzed to be useful to the EMS professional. Imagine, for example, an EMS service that would like to introduce a new pro-

cedure. Before the procedure could be included in the local protocols, it would need to be approved by the agency's medical director. The days of introducing new procedures and techniques simply because they are new are gone. These decisions are now being made on the basis of evidence-based medicine. In other words, the medical director will need to know the efficacy of the proposed item: does it have a positive effect on patient outcome? This information is found in the medical literature by evaluating research on the topic at hand, known as a literature review.

Performing a literature review of existing medical research involves several steps. The first is to identify where the information will likely be found. Scientific journals, or those that report original research, should be the source of this information rather than trade journals. In the case of the latter, authors typically write about research articles they have read. Although these articles are generally accurate, they may still be subject to the personal opinions and views of the author. Instead of depending on the opinion of others, you should read the original research yourself and make your own decisions of its value and applicability to your specific situation. Original research is found in publications such as the *Journal of Trauma, New England Journal of Medicine, Journal of the American Medical Association, Prehospital Emergency Care, Annals of Emergency Medicine*, and other such scientific journals. To narrow the focus of which journals to search, begin by looking for those that are specific to the topic you are interested in. Also include those that are likely to address the topic. For example, if your topic lies in the realm of trauma, the *Journal of Trauma* would be appropriate, as would the *Annals of Emergency Medicine* and *Prehospital Emergency Care*.

Once you select the journals you believe will meet your needs, you must ensure they are peer reviewed and the research they contain has been peer reviewed. This means that each item submitted to the journal (other than editorial comments) has been reviewed by an independent panel of experts to ensure it meets all fundamental principles of sound research. If the panel finds it does not, then the article is not accepted for publication. Most scientific journals are peer reviewed; however, if you are in doubt, you can usually determine this by reading the instructions for submission. These generally outline the acceptance process, including the need for review.

With your peer-reviewed journals in hand, begin by reviewing the table of contents to identify which articles are likely to address the topic of your literature review. This process often can be simplified by visiting the Web site of the journal and searching for key words in your topic. To further determine if the article addresses your needs you can read the abstract, which is a summary of the focus of the research project, the methods used, and results and conclusions. The abstract is the first item presented in a research report and generally is available free of charge on the journal's Web site.

Once you select an article that addresses your topic, you must determine the strength of the study. In other words, what was the original hypothesis or aspect of care in question? How was it conducted, and what methods were used? Was it approved by an institutional review board and conducted ethically? Was there author bias in the study? Have the authors disclosed any financial associations with what was being studied? Were the results appropriately analyzed? You should avoid studies and results based on observation or anecdotal evidence. This type of evidence is based on a person's experience rather than scientific principles. The weaknesses of this type of evidence are that reproducibility of the results and whether the study was limited to one experience cannot be determined. The study was likely uncontrolled and subject to personal conjecture. Unfortunately, many of the decisions regarding treatment regimens in EMS in the past have been based on this type of evidence.

Following are some of the types of study designs found in medical literature.

Prospective studies are specifically designed and the participants are followed forward in time. These types of studies are well controlled, are generally randomized, and tend to focus on one variable to determine its effect on patient outcome. They incorporate means to filter all out all other variables that may affect outcome to isolate the one variable in question. These studies often involve the completion of written forms after treating a patient so all appropriate data can be recorded. This ensures consistency among all patients involved in the study.

Retrospective studies occur after the event has taken place. An example is a review of call reports of all chest pain patients to determine the effect of a specific medication that was administered. Although these types of studies can provide valuable information, they also have weaknesses. The largest weakness is that no control over the patient population or other variables is possible, they cannot be randomized, and the data gathered are not designed for the specific study. Needed data to ensure consistency among patients enrolled in the study may not be available to those conducting the study. Advantages of these types of studies are that data are easily accessible and can be quickly gathered.

Cohort studies involve groups of people with common characteristics. These may be age, living conditions, personal habits, or other commonality among the participants of the study. Epidemiologists begin this type of study with a group of people who are disease free and have not been exposed to the agent being studied. For example, if the researchers are trying to determine the association of smoking with lung cancer, the original group will not have anyone who currently has lung cancer or a history of smoking. Over time this group will divide itself into two groups: those who have been exposed to smoking and those who have not. At set intervals these groups will be further divided into those who develop lung cancer and those who do not. Similarities among those who do and do not develop lung cancer will be identified (such as smoking), and conclusions can be drawn regarding risk factors for disease. One of the most famous cohort studies is the Framingham Study, in which 5127 residents of Framingham, Mass., have been followed since 1948 to determine risk factors for heart disease. In the emergency setting cohort studies may differ slightly because following patients for a long period often is not the focus of studies involving emergency medicine. In these situations the cohorts may involve patients who have a similar injury or illness. Each group of patients receives a different treatment, often standard therapy and the therapy being evaluated, to determine the effectiveness of one. These generally are prospective studies because the study is designed to evaluate one facet of treatment and is controlled as described in the section on prospective studies.

Case-control studies start with two groups of individuals, one with the disease or injury in question and one without. Characteristics of both groups are then evaluated in an attempt to identify the causative factors of the condition being studied. These types of studies are observational studies because the researchers do not control any aspects of the study. The difficulty in these studies is ensuring similarities between the two groups so the disease or injury is the only variable studied. Another example of a case-control study is two groups of patients with the same injury yet different outcomes. Researchers could then attempt to determine why the outcome was different in each group. Again, the patients in each group would have to be similar (e.g., age, injury, health status) so the only variable was the aspect of treatment in each group. The major disadvantage of this type of study is the number of variables that could be involved between each patient.

In addition to the design of the study, other factors involved in the study must be considered. These include how patients were divided into groups, how many groups were involved, whether the practitioner or patient knew which group the patient was in, or whether any variables outside the one being studied could have affected the outcome.

Randomized studies are divided into control and study groups at random, with no predetermination of which patient will go into which group. True randomized studies often involve a computer program that determines to which group a patient is assigned. This ensures true randomization and no bias of the researcher in selecting control or study participants. In the EMS setting, this type of system often is impractical because of the emergent nature of prehospital medicine. However, some randomization of patients can be achieved in the prehospital setting. This may be done by reaching into a bag that contains several green and red marbles. The patient can then be assigned to a group based on the color of marble the paramedic pulls out. The disadvantage of this type of system is that each color has a finite number; therefore, as the marbles are depleted from the bag, the chance of one color being selected over another may be increased and true randomization is not achieved. A computer program, on the other hand, can provide an infinite number of possibilities. Other methods that have been used in the prehospital setting include alternating patients in each group and alternating patient assignment based on an even- and odd-day system. Again, these are not true randomization methods, and they often result in the paramedic not being blinded (described below); however, they do avoid researcher bias in determining which patients are assigned to each group.

In *blinded studies* the patient, the practitioner, or both do not know if the standard therapy or therapy being studied is being administered. In a single-blinded study only one party (the patient or the practitioner) is blinded, whereas a double-blinded study has both the patient and practitioner unaware of which treatment is being administered. This avoids any bias of any participants involved. Double-blinded studies are not always possible; however, they do provide the best evidence regarding the effectiveness of the treatment in question. This is because the Hawthorne effect—when a person thinks something should happen, a chance exists that they could be affected by that perception—is avoided in these studies. This may be the patient perceiving an effect that does not exist, or it may be the researcher seeing an effect that does not exist. In addition, when only the patient is blinded the practitioner may subconsciously treat the patient differently or unknowingly question the patient in a way that directs the patient toward reporting effects that should be associated with the therapy being studied. Often in double-blinded studies no one is aware which patients were assigned to which group until the seal on the data is broken. This may be months or even years after the patient was treated and is generally done by statisticians rather than those involved in the patient's care. Sometimes the person evaluating the data is also blinded to the treatment administered. They may simply know the patient was given medication Y or Z but not know which was the standard therapy (or placebo) and which was the study therapy. This further avoids any researcher bias.

Medical research can be divided into the following three distinct categories based on the strength of the study (PHTLS, 2007):

- Class I evidence is the strongest evidence regarding a treatment. It is derived from prospective, controlled, randomized, double-blinded studies.
- Class II evidence comes from literature reviews, nonrandomized or unblinded studies, retrospective studies, case-control series, and cohort studies.
- Class III evidence is derived from case studies, case reports, consensus documents, textbooks, and medical opinion.

Once the type of study, its methods, and its strengths have been determined, it is time to evaluate the study itself. First determine what the hypothesis of the study is. All valid studies should have a clearly stated hypothesis and clearly defined outcome measurements. Studies with a vague hypothesis or vague outcome measurements are subject to manipulation of the data until some effect is found. Results or outcomes that were not part of the original hypothesis also are suspect because they indicate the possibility of data manipulation to achieve an outcome when in reality one may not exist.

Review the patient selection criteria. What was the population being studied? How were they determined and were they randomized? What inclusion criteria existed for entry into the study? All patients should be accounted for, even those who were not included in the final outcome. Additionally, an explanation should be provided for patients who were dropped from the study and not included in the final results. The total number of patients entered in the study should be equal to the total number of patients included in the final results plus those who were dropped. If this is not the case, then the study is suspect of data manipulation. Finally, any discrepancies or unintended occurrences during the study should be reported. For example, if a control patient receives the studied therapy, or if a patient in the study group receives additional treatments, this should be reported.

In addition to selection criteria, the size of the patient population must be evaluated. Small patient samples do not provide a wide range of data to determine if the results would be the same among a large group. Large patient populations have greater applicability and significance compared with small ones. You should also compare the study population to the population you are considering. To determine if the results of the study will apply to your local EMS system, the patients in the study must be similar to the patients in your service area.

Determine how the data were analyzed. Although a complete review of the statistical analysis may not be necessary, you should at least ensure the methods of analysis are appropriate for what was being studied.

Analyze the results of the study. Are the authors' conclusions and results logical compared with the analysis of the data? Be sure to avoid the temptation to simply read the results and make a decision based on them without comparing the results to the actual data from the study. Although this may be an easier method of reading research, you will not have evaluated the research and are taking the authors' conclusions for granted without determining if the data support that conclusion. Finally, determine whether the outcome and results are significant, both statistically and clinically. Statistical significance determines how often the results of the study would happen simply by chance compared with the studied therapy causing the result. In general, 5% is used as the indicator of statistical significance. This means that if the result could occur 5% of the time or less by chance, the study results are considered statistically significant; however, if the result could occur 5% of the time or more by chance, then the results of the study are considered statistically insignificant. Just as important, if not more so, than statistical significance is clinical significance. In other words, is the therapy effective in enough patients to make it a useful treatment for the majority? For example, a medication may cause a statistically significant result, but it may occur in only one of every 100 patients. Would that be worth the addition of the therapy to your treatment options? What if that same medication had a shelf life of 30 days and cost $5000 per dose? On the other hand, suppose a medication could reduce mortality rate by 40%, but the same effect could happen by chance 10% of the time. In this case it is statistically insignificant but is likely clinically significant.

Questions regarding clinical significance and changes in practice cannot be answered in a textbook. These decisions must be made after a critical evaluation of the available medical literature, discussion with your medical director, and evaluation of your patient population. For example, prehospital administration of fibrinolytics would not be appropriate for an EMS service that is never more than 30 minutes from a hospital with 24-hour cardiac catheterization capability, but it may be reasonable for a service that is 5 hours from the nearest medical facility. Your practice as an EMS professional must be based on class I medical evidence whenever possible after a critical evaluation of the available literature and application of that knowledge to your patient population.

Case Scenario SUMMARY

1. *Based on this information, what are the strengths of this study?* The primary strengths are that it was done on human beings (as opposed to animals) and that it compared two groups of patients rather than simply documenting the impact of fentanyl on one group of patients.

2. *What are the weaknesses of this study?* This study has several limitations. First, the sample size is small. Given the information presented, the reader cannot tell whether the patient sample was randomly selected or the patients were chosen by the researchers to receive one drug or the other. The study was also performed in a cardiac specialty hospital—an environment much different than the prehospital setting.

3. *Would "testing" fentanyl for management of your patient and comparing the patient's response to the response of previous patients who have received morphine be appropriate? Why or why not?* No. First and foremost, testing a medication on a patient is unethical. Ethics must take precedence over protocol in this situation. This is, of course, not to say that violating protocol is not also a large issue, but the ethical issue is larger than the protocol issue. Your job and even licensure could be in jeopardy. In addition, for the reasons already discussed, this study is weak. Finally, "testing" must be done in a highly controlled way to ensure patient safety.

4. *Would any additional patient education or discussion be required if you chose to administer the fentanyl?* Yes. When studies involving patients are performed, a highly structured process of research method approval occurs through an institutional review board (IRB). The IRB's role is to ensure that the study will not jeopardize patient health or safety. In addition, the IRB requires researchers to obtain consent from patients, essentially informing them that the treatment is experimental and giving them the option of not participating. In most cases patients will need to sign the consent in the presence of a witness to ensure that they have understood the implications of their choice. However, rules and regulations governing human testing procedures have provisions for providing information to a community in advance of a study, and signed consent may or may not be required.

5. *If you chose to administer the morphine per your usual protocol, would you have any liability for not choosing to use an alternative therapy that has been proven more effective? Why or why not?* You would have no liability if you followed protocols because they define the standard of care for your community (assuming the protocols are correct). On the other hand, you might have *significant* liability if you chose to violate that standard, even if you believed it would be beneficial to the patient. You must understand that you are ultimately responsible for what you do. If you make a medical error that you should have recognized, you will be liable regardless of what is written in protocol or verbal orders received from a physician.

6. *Do you think you did the right thing by following protocol rather that choosing a "new" therapy that might be more effective?* Yes, for all the reasons stated above. Local EMS protocols are created on the basis of the medical standards of care for a particular community and are typically based on reputable scientific research. If you learn of a new medical discovery that you believe is applicable to EMS, your best course of action is to discuss it with your medical director. If it is appropriate for your system, your medical director will initiate a process to have it become a part of the local protocol.

7. *How does your relationship with your medical director relate to this situation?* The provision of prehospital care, especially at the advanced life-support level, requires high-level patient assessment, provisional diagnoses, and intervention. EMTs and paramedics are granted the privilege of performing these activities through their relationship with a licensed physician—their medical director. EMS protocols define the medical activities that the medical director will authorize for the EMS personnel who practice under his or her authority.

Violation of these protocols may have consequences, including termination of privileges by the medical director and potential loss of paramedic certification or licensure.

8. *What do you think your medical director discussed as the significant problems with the study?* Small sample size, nonrandomized patient selection, in-hospital setting.

Chapter Summary

- EMS is a dynamic field with a young but proud history and exciting future.
- EMS systems are an integral part of the medical community.
- Primary education is the beginning of a paramedic's education. Paramedics need to be committed to life-long learning.
- Paramedics need to be licensed or certified to practice. If their credentials expire, they will be unable to practice.

- National, state, and local EMS organizations work to build EMS. Paramedics should participate with these organizations.
- Professionalism is a daily commitment for the paramedic, on and off duty.
- Medical directors function as the medical conscience for EMS systems. They should be consulted in all aspects of an EMS system's development and growth.
- Research is critical if EMS is to grow and expand.

REFERENCE

National Highway Traffic Safety Administration. (2007). *National EMS scope of practice model*, Washington, DC: U.S. Department of Transportation.

SUGGESTED RESOURCES

The Committee on Accreditation of Educational Programs for the EMS Professions: http://www.coaemsp.org/accreditatedprograms.htm.
Genell, L. N. (2001). *Legal concepts and issues in emergency care*, Philadelphia: W. B. Saunders.
McPherson, T. A. (1973). *American funeral cars & ambulances since 1900*, Glen Ellyn, IL: Crestline Publishing.
National Highway Traffic Safety Administration. (2007). *EMS agenda for the future*. Retrieved September 24, 2007, from http://www.nhtsa.dot.gov.

National Registry of Emergency Medical Technicians. (2007). *NREMT news*. Retrieved September 24, 2007, from http://www.nremt.org.
Pons, P., & Cason, D. (Eds.). (1997). *Paramedic field care: a complaint based approach*, St. Louis: Mosby.
Walz, B. (2002). *Introduction to EMS systems*, Albany, NY: Delmar.

Chapter Quiz

1. In what year was EMS created and funded by the U.S. Congress?
   _____

2. What is the name of the bill that ended federal funding to EMS systems?
   _____

3. What does *scope of practice* mean?
   _____

4. What is the first level of EMS professional who is able to offer care and transport to the sick and injured?
   _____

5. The legal ability granted by a state to practice as a paramedic is known as _____.

6. What is the training in which an EMS professional reviews information and skills that he or she previously learned?
   _____

7. To stay current and up to date with new information, should the paramedic attend refresher education or CE courses?
   _____

8. Should the paramedic be able to follow direction as well as be self-directed?
   _____

9. What must be done immediately on arriving at a scene?
   _____

10. What must be done immediately after transferring the patient to a facility?

_____

11. What are the treatment instructions or guidelines given to the paramedic by his or her medical director?

_____

12. Provide three reasons why performing research is important.

_____

_____

_____

Terminology

Advanced emergency medical technician (AEMT) An EMS professional who provides basic and limited advanced skills to patients who access the EMS system.

Attributes Qualities or characteristics of a person.

Certification An external verification of the competencies that an individual has achieved and typically involves an examination process; in healthcare these processes are typically designed to verify that an individual has achieved minimum competency to ensure safe and effective patient care.

Communication The exchange of thoughts, messages, and information.

Continuing education (CE) Lifelong learning.

Continuous quality improvement (CQI) Programs designed to improve the level of care; commonly driven by quality assurance.

Credentialing A local process by which an individual is permitted by a specific entity (medical director) to practice in a specific setting (EMS agency).

Diplomacy Tact and skill in dealing with people.

Emergency medical responder (EMR) An EMS professional who provides initial basic life-support care to patients who access the EMS system; formerly called first responder.

Empathy Showing a person care and compassion with an appreciation for his or her situation without feeling the same emotions.

EMS system A network of resources that provides emergency care and transportation to victims of sudden illness or injury.

Ethics Expectations established by the community at large reflecting their views of the conduct of a profession.

Healthcare A business associated with the provision of medical care to individuals.

Healthcare professional An individual who has special skills and knowledge in medicine and adheres to the standards of conduct and performance of that medical profession.

Integrity Doing the right thing even when no one is looking.

Licensure Permission granted to an individual by a governmental authority, such as a state, to perform certain restricted activities.

Medical director A physician responsible for the oversight of the EMS system and the actions of the paramedics; also known as a physician advisor.

National Registry of Emergency Medical Technicians (NREMT) A national organization developed to ensure that graduates of EMS training programs have met minimal standards by measuring competency through a uniform testing process.

NHTSA National Highway Traffic Safety Administration.

NSC National Standard Curriculum.

Offline medical direction Prospective and retrospective medical direction (e.g., protocols and standard operating procedures).

Online medical direction Direct voice communication by a medical director (or designee) to a prehospital professional while he or she is attending to the patient; also called *direct medical direction*.

Physician advisor A physician responsible for the oversight of the EMS system and the actions of the paramedics; also known as a *medical director*.

Profession A group of similar jobs or fields of interest that involve a responsibility to serve the public and require mastery of specific knowledge and specialized skills.

Professional A person who has special knowledge and skills and conforms to high standards of conduct and performance.

Professionalism Following the standards of conduct and performance for a profession.

Prospective medical direction Physician participation in the development of EMS protocols, procedures, and participation in the education and testing of EMS professionals; a type of offline medical direction.

Protocols A set of treatment guidelines written for the paramedic to follow.

Quality assurance (QA) Programs designed to achieve a desired level of care.

Reciprocity The ability for an EMS professional to use his or her certification or license to be able to practice in a different state.

Refresher education The process of refreshing information and skills previously learned.

Registration The process of entering an individual's name and essential information into a record as a means of verifying initial certification and monitoring recertification.

Retrospective medical direction Physician review of prehospital care reports and participation in the quality improvement process; a type of offline medical direction.

Scope of practice A predefined set of skills, interventions, or other activities that the paramedic is legally authorized to perform when necessary; usually set by state law or regulation and local medical direction.

Standing orders Written instructions that authorize EMS personnel to perform certain medical interventions before establishing direct communication with a physician.

Teamwork The ability to work with others to achieve a common goal.

Illness and Injury Prevention

Objectives *After completing this chapter, you will be able to:*

1. Describe the incidence, morbidity, and mortality of unintentional and alleged unintentional events.
2. Identify the human, environmental, and socioeconomic impact of unintentional and alleged unintentional events.
3. Identify the role of EMS in local municipal and community prevention programs.
4. Identify situations in which you can intervene in a preventive manner.
5. Document primary and secondary injury prevention opportunities.
6. Recognize the ways in which culture plays a role in injury patterns.
7. Identify national resources available for injury prevention data, strategies, and activities.

Chapter Outline

An Essential Activity
An Extensive Problem
The Science of Injury Prevention
The Cost of Injuries
Reasons for EMS Involvement
Epidemiologic Triad
Haddon Matrix

The "EP5" Matrix
The Teachable Moment
A Successful Drowning Prevention Program
Drawing from Personal Experience: SAFE
Examples of Successful EMS-Conceived Programs
Chapter Summary

Case Scenario

You and your first-response engine company respond to a new residential neighborhood for a "child who fell out of a window." On arrival, you find a police officer maintaining manual cervical spine stabilization for a 4-year-old girl. According to the child's father, they were playing in his daughter's bedroom when she fell backward, popping the screen out of the window, and falling 20 to 25 feet onto the concrete driveway. She was unconscious for a brief period. She is awake and alert, her skin is pale, and she appears quite frightened.

Questions

1. *What is your general impression of this patient?*
2. *What physical assessment findings are most pertinent at this time?*
3. *What treatment should be immediately initiated?*

Paramedics are in a perfect position to decrease the rate of injuries and make a difference in communities. This chapter provides a broad overview of the science of injury prevention, specifically as it relates to patients. The following anecdote illustrates the conflicting nature of injury prevention.

A small, mountaintop community was experiencing a major problem. The narrow and winding road that led up to the town had been plagued by deadly motor vehicle accidents. In fact, at one hairpin turn nearly one vehicle "went over the side" each week, resulting in numerous serious injuries

and deaths. So many accidents had occurred that the local towing company could barely keep up. The town council held an emergency meeting to determine a plan to deal with the crisis. The town civil engineer had suggested reinforcement of the guardrails to prevent cars from going over the side. The police chief thought they should reduce the speed limit and post more traffic officers on the road for enforcement. The local trauma surgeon wanted to see a community education program, targeted at the high-risk population to alert them of potential hazards. The town council, however, mulled over all these suggestions before it came to its own conclusion: purchasing more tow trucks!

AN ESSENTIAL ACTIVITY

Several years have passed since the publication of "The Consensus Statement on the EMS Role in Primary Injury Prevention" (National Highway Traffic Safety Administration [NHTSA], 1996). The authors of the statement, representing every possible EMS constituency, make it clear that **primary injury prevention**, or keeping an injury from occurring (Figure 3-1), is an "essential" activity. Moreover, it is an activity that must be undertaken by the leaders, decision makers, and providers of every EMS system. The old adage "an ounce of prevention is worth a pound of cure" is essential to modern EMS. From a medical standpoint, avoiding an injury has a much greater effect on a (potential) patient's life than any treatment the medical community can provide after the fact. Looking at the problem from a financial view, prevention is much less expensive than treatment and any associated rehabilitation. Of course, avoiding the impact of traumatic incidents on the victim and family is incalculable. Traditionally, however, EMS providers have focused on **secondary injury prevention**, or preventing further injury from an event that has already occurred (e.g., providing spinal immobilization to motor vehicle accident victims). Fortunately, over the last several years this view of EMS has been changing and more departments are involved in injury prevention activities. A perfect example of this model involves fire departments and the decrease in fires as a result of prevention activities. The EMS profession must similarly continue to increase its efforts in injury prevention.

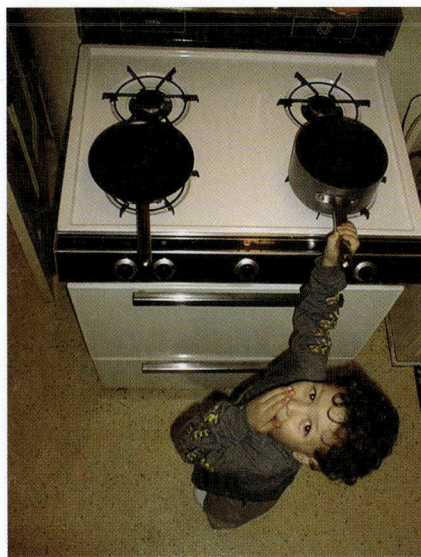

Figure 3-1 More lives can be saved by preventing injuries from occurring.

AN EXTENSIVE PROBLEM

[OBJECTIVE 1]

To many health experts, unintentional injuries are the largest public health problem currently facing the country. In fact, unintentional injuries historically are the leading killer of Americans aged 1 to 44 years, according to data collected by the National Center for Health Statistics (Figure 3-2). Two exceptions to this were in 1999 and 2001, when unintentional injury was the leading cause of death in Americans aged 1 to 34 years and the second leading cause of death in Americans aged 35 to 44 years. In the 35- to 44-year-old age group, **unintentional injury** was only slightly behind malignant neoplasms, the leading cause of death in this age group. However, even during these years, if unintentional and intentional injuries (homicide and suicide) are combined, injury was by far the leading cause of death in people aged 35 to 44 years as well as those aged 1 to 34 years. For all ages unintentional injuries are the fifth leading killer, behind heart disease, cancer, cerebrovascular events (stroke), and the effects of chronic lower airway disease. When unintentional and intentional injuries are combined, traumatic injury becomes the fourth leading cause of death for all age groups (Centers for Disease Control and Prevention [CDC], 2004).

More than 150,000 people die from unintentional injuries in the United States each year. When an additional 33 million visits to the emergency department for unintentional injuries are added to this figure, the results are staggering (Figure 3-3). The "costs of trauma" are far reaching. They include the loss of years of productive life for the trauma patient, financial impact on both families and the healthcare system, the emotional effect on patients and their families, and the financial impact on the community in terms of increased costs of governmental programs and increased insurance costs to pay for trauma care.

The director of the Center for Injury Prevention Policy and Practice at San Diego State University, David Lawrence, explains that people simply get accustomed to these numbers. He adds, "When you look at the number of people who are injured and killed in motor vehicle crashes [alone], we have the equivalent of a medium-size plane crash every day" (Krimston & Griffiths, 2003). When the numbers are spread across 50 states, however, they become so common as to be almost invisible to the national media (Figure 3-4).

THE SCIENCE OF INJURY PREVENTION

To prevent injuries, the nature of these injuries must be understood. An **injury** is defined as intentional or unintentional damage to a person that results from acute exposure to thermal, mechanical, electrical, or chemical energy or from the absence of essentials such as heat or oxygen. **Unintentional injuries** occur without intent to harm. In contrast, **intentional injuries** include all

10 Leading Causes of Death by Age Group, United States – 2003

Rank	<1	1-4	5-9	10-14	15-24	25-34	35-44	45-54	55-64	65+	Total
				Age Groups							
1	Congenital Anomalies 5,621	Unintentional Injury 1,717	Unintentional Injury 1,096	Unintentional Injury 1,522	Unintentional Injury 15,272	Unintentional Injury 12,541	Unintentional Injury 16,766	Malignant Neoplasms 49,843	Malignant Neoplasms 95,692	Heart Disease 563,390	Heart Disease 685,089
2	Short Gestation 4,849	Congenital Anomalies 541	Malignant Neoplasms 516	Malignant Neoplasms 560	Homicide 5,368	Suicide 5,065	Malignant Neoplasms 15,509	Heart Disease 37,732	Heart Disease 65,060	Malignant Neoplasms 388,911	Malignant Neoplasms 556,902
3	SIDS 2,162	Malignant Neoplasms 392	Congenital Anomalies 180	Suicide 244	Suicide 3,988	Homicide 4,516	Heart Disease 13,600	Unintentional Injury 15,837	Chronic Low. Respiratory Disease 12,077	Cerebro-vascular 138,134	Cerebro-vascular 157,689
4	Maternal Pregnancy Comp. 1,710	Homicide 376	Homicide 122	Congenital Anomalies 206	Malignant Neoplasms 1,651	Malignant Neoplasms 3,741	Suicide 6,602	Liver Disease 7,466	Diabetes Mellitus 10,731	Chronic Low. Respiratory Disease 109,139	Chronic Low. Respiratory Disease 126,382
5	Placenta Cord Membranes 1,099	Heart Disease 186	Heart Disease 104	Homicide 202	Heart Disease 1,133	Heart Disease 3,250	HIV 5,340	Suicide 6,481	Cerebro-vascular 9,946	Alzheimer's Disease 62,814	Unintentional Injury 109,277
6	Unintentional Injury 945	Influenza & Pneumonia 163	Influenza & Pneumonia 75	Heart Disease 160	Congenital Anomalies 451	HIV 1,588	Homicide 3,110	Cerebro-vascular 6,127	Unintentional Injury 9,170	Influenza & Pneumonia 57,670	Diabetes Mellitus 74,219
7	Respiratory Distress 831	Septicemia 85	Septicemia 39	Chronic Low. Respiratory Disease 81	Influenza & Pneumonia 224	Diabetes Mellitus 657	Liver Disease 3,020	Diabetes Mellitus 5,658	Liver Disease 6,428	Diabetes Mellitus 54,919	Influenza & Pneumonia 65,163
8	Bacterial Sepsis 772	Perinatal Period 79	Benign Neoplasms 38	Influenza & Pneumonia 72	Cerebro-vascular 221	Cerebro-vascular 583	Cerebro-vascular 2,460	HIV 4,442	Suicide 3,843	Nephritis 35,254	Alzheimer's Disease 63,457
9	Neonatal Hemorrhage 649	Chronic Low. Respiratory Disease 55	Chronic Low. Respiratory Disease 37	Benign Neoplasms 41	Chronic Low. Respiratory Disease 191	Congenital Anomalies 426	Diabetes Mellitus 2,049	Chronic Low. Respiratory 3,537	Nephritis 3,806	Unintentional Injury 34,335	Nephritis 42,453
10	Circulatory System Disease 591	Benign Neoplasms 51	Cerebro-vascular 29	Cerebro-vascular 40	HIV 178	Influenza & Pneumonia 373	Influenza & Pneumonia 992	Viral Hepatitis 2,259	Septicemia 3,651	Septicemia 26,445	Septicemia 34,069

Source: National Vital Statistics System, National Center for Health Statistics, CDC.
Produced by: Office of Statistics and Programming, National Center for Injury Prevention and Control, CDC.

Figure 3-2 Unintentional injuries are the leading cause of death in the United States for ages 1 to 44 years.

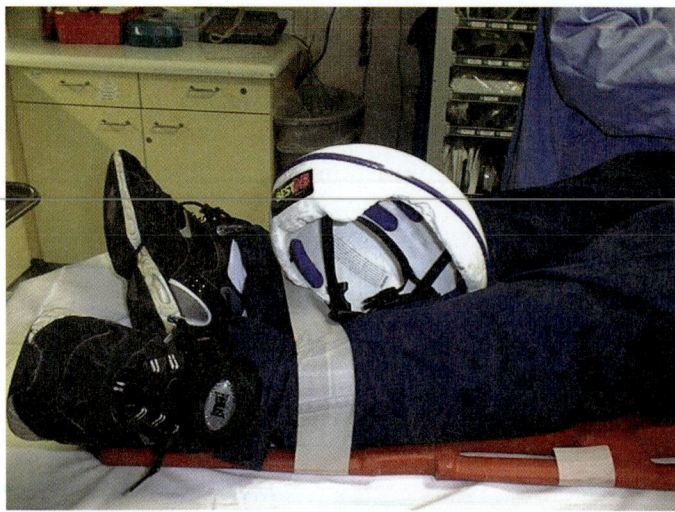

Figure 3-3 More children die from unintentional injuries than from childhood illnesses.

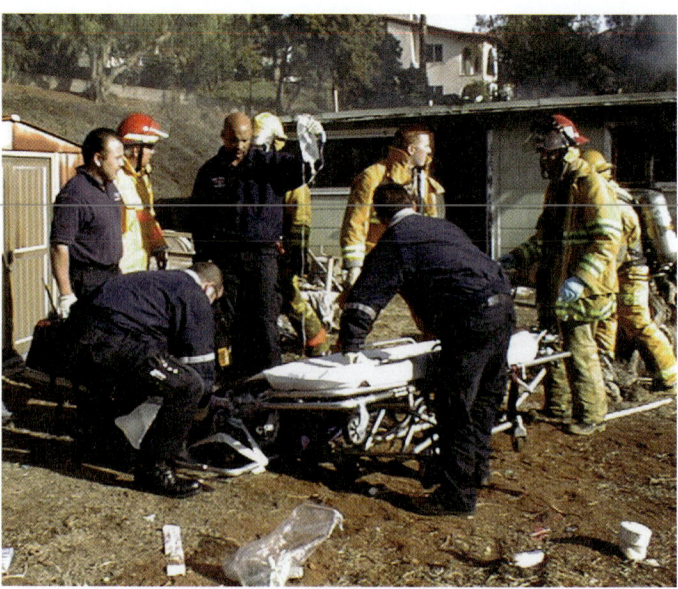

Figure 3-4 More than 150,000 people die in the United States each year from unintentional injuries.

injuries and deaths that are self-inflicted or perpetrated by another person, usually involving some type of violence.

Some people are more prone to injuries because of their actions or the actions of those around them. In general, these persons are at risk for injury. An **injury risk** is defined as a real or potentially hazardous situation that puts individuals at risk for sustaining an injury. Recently, injury risk has escalated because of an increased perceived need for "pushing the envelope" and the development of extreme sports (e.g., human catapulting) and related products (e.g., small motorcycles known as *pocket bikes*).

To track these potential hazards and create prevention programs, **injury surveillance** is conducted. Injury surveillance is an ongoing systematic collection, analysis, and interpretation of injury data essential to the planning, implementation, and evaluation of public health practice, closely integrated with the timely dissemination of the data to those who need to know. **Epidemiology** is the study of the causes, patterns, prevalence, and control of disease in groups of people. The run reports that paramedics are required to write after each call are read and analyzed by **epidemiologists**. These epidemiologists then pass their findings to injury prevention specialists. The specialists create programs and campaigns to prevent the injury from occurring.

In most cases, measuring death **(mortality)** rates is much easier than measuring nonfatal injury **(morbidity)** rates. Nearly all reported deaths involve some type of tracking, either through the medical examiner's office, the police department, or a personal physician. However, nonfatal injuries are difficult to track because reporting systems are not in place or are not well developed for clinics, physicians' offices, school nurses' offices, and even the home medicine cabinet. Great strides have been taken to glean important injury data from places such as emergency departments and trauma centers, yet these figures are only a small part of the big picture.

THE COST OF INJURIES

[OBJECTIVE 2]
Roxanne Hoffman, coordinator for the San Diego Safe Kids Coalition and strong proponent of using EMS personnel in injury-prevention activities, believes that changing the way society views unintentional injuries requires eliminating the word *accident* from society's vocabulary. Hoffman explains, "People still tend to dismiss them [unintentional injuries] as accidents"—as though they were destined to happen. "These are not accidents; they can be prevented." She adds, "People don't realize how many lives are affected by unintentional injuries—physically, emotionally, and economically" (Krimston & Griffiths, 2003).

The cost of these injuries to society, beyond personal suffering, must be considered as well as how it compares with the cost of other major diseases or conditions.

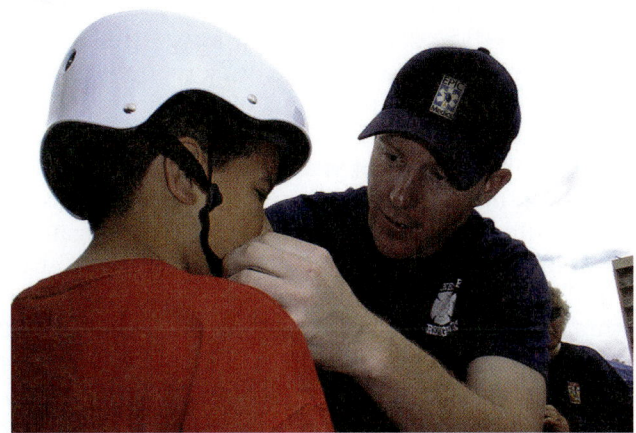

Figure 3-5 Only 20% to 25% of cyclists currently wear helmets.

According to the National Safety Council's 2005 U.S. injury statistics, "Accidents also accounted for more than 24 million nonfatal injuries in 2005, putting major stress on our nation's health care system. The economic cost of all fatal and nonfatal injuries amounted to $625.5 billion nationally, or $5,500 per household" (National Safety Council, 2007).

For instance, consider the case of the bicycle helmet (Figure 3-5). According to NHTSA, the estimated cost of bicycle-related injuries and deaths for all ages is approximately $8 billion (NHTSA, 2004). For every $10 bicycle helmet, this country saves approximately $30 in direct health costs and an additional $365 in associated societal costs. The NHTSA estimates that if 85% of all child cyclists wore helmets every time they rode a bicycle for only 1 year, the lifetime medical cost savings would total between $109 and $142 million. Unfortunately, only 20% to 25% of cyclists currently wear helmets.

Who pays for these costs? Unfortunately, everyone pays through either higher taxes (public sources such as federal, state, and local government pay approximately one fourth of associated injury costs) or higher insurance premiums (private sources such as insurance companies pick up nearly three fourths of all injury-related costs) (CDC, 2001).

Full societal costs of injuries can be measured by using **years of potential life lost (YPLL)** to calculate the costs. This method assumes that, on average, most people live a productive life until the age of 65 years. For example, if a 22 year old is killed in a bicycle accident, 43 years of potential life are lost (YPLL = 65 − Age at death). The YPLL associated with injuries is far greater than the YPLL linked with cancer or heart disease. Several reasons exist for this. First, younger people typically participate in more risk-taking activities than do older generations and as a result are more susceptible to fatal injuries. Older people do die from injuries, but when they do fewer YPLL are lost than in a younger patient. In the example above, the 22-year-old patient had 43 YPLL. Suppose that the patient was 64 years old when he was struck on the bicycle; in this case only 1 year was lost.

Because medical conditions such as heart disease and cancer cause death at a later age, they typically result in a lower YPLL than trauma. However, in some instances, such as congenital heart disease, a medical condition can cause a significant loss of years of potential life. Finally, years of life lost are associated with death secondary to injury or illness as well as disability. Consider again the 22-year-old in a bicycle crash. If the patient did not die, but rather remained in a comatose state for the rest of his life, the term YPLL could still be applied. Although the patient did not lose potential life, he did lose years in which he would be earning income, paying taxes, and making other contributions to society.

EMS leaders at national and state levels have initiated a movement to introduce science to injury prevention and make it a more important part of the EMS mission. Most persons involved with EMS readily admit that many of the providers in the field who were to implement these programs originally were not enthusiastic. Many still are not, but attitudes are changing. A study conducted by Herb Garrison, MD, Director of the East Carolina Injury Prevention Program, used the National Registry of EMTs to measure provider attitudes toward injury prevention (Griffiths, 1999). The results clearly showed a positive attitude by EMS providers. A survey that included questions about injury prevention was mailed to EMTs, EMT-intermediates, and paramedics scheduled for recertification. Approximately 19,000 of 29,000 who applied for recertification returned the survey, a return rate of nearly 66%. Of those polled, 58% believed that EMS should be involved in conducting community-oriented injury prevention programs. Thirty-five percent said EMS involvement in injury prevention programs should be limited to programs and training focused on preventing injuries to the EMS provider. Only 5% thought that EMS should have no involvement in injury prevention (Griffiths, 1999).

REASONS FOR EMS INVOLVEMENT

[OBJECTIVE 3]

Unlike any other medical professional, EMS providers are unique in that they see citizens in their own homes and environments and during activities of daily life. As a result, EMS providers have ample opportunities for prevention education that other health care professionals do not have. Additional advantages of EMS involvement in prevention education are listed below. As previously stated, more benefits exist for both the community and the healthcare system from preventing injuries and illness than from trying to treat them after they have already occurred.

- *EMS providers are widely distributed among the population.* Nearly every community in the United States is covered by some form of emergency medical services, from Maine's seaside town of Lubec (Lubec 55) to the California border town of San Ysidro (Medic 30).
- *EMS providers reflect the makeup of the community.* From its earliest days in Pittsburgh, EMS has often tapped the local populace to care for its own.
- *In a rural setting, EMS providers may be the most medically educated individuals available.* EMS providers may be the only source of help, whether they are an hour drive down the mountain to the nearest emergency department or 200 miles offshore on an oil platform.
- *The United States has more than 840,000 EMS providers.* Even a fraction of these providers would create a formidable injury prevention army.
- *EMS providers are high-profile role models.* Since the early days of Johnny Gage and Roy DeSoto (from the television show *Emergency!*), EMS providers have always been looked upon as mentors.
- *EMS providers are considered a champion of the healthcare consumer.* EMS providers work in concert with their patients and their patients' families.
- *EMS providers are welcome in the schools and other environments.* In today's climate of standardized testing and assessments, cuts in programs, and diminishing funding, EMS providers are still offered unparalleled access to students (Figure 3-6).
- *EMS providers are considered authorities on injury and prevention.* Because they see the results of injury

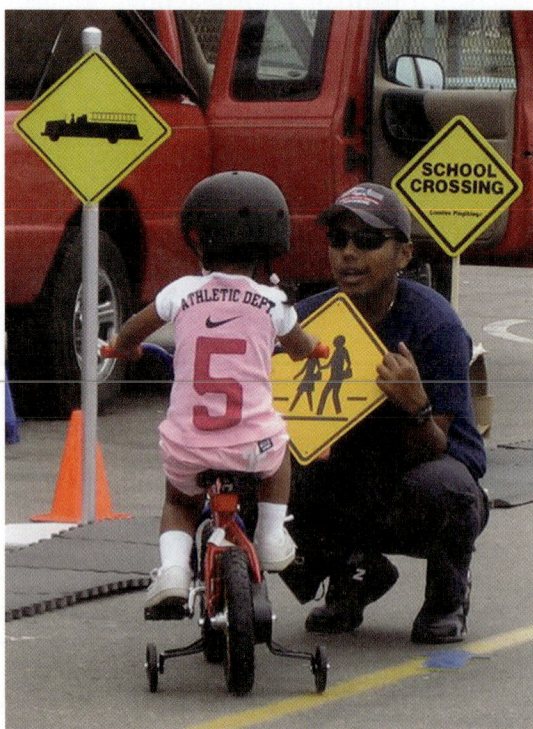

Figure 3-6 In today's climate of standardized testing and assessments, cuts in programs, and diminishing funding, EMS providers are still offered unparalleled access to students.

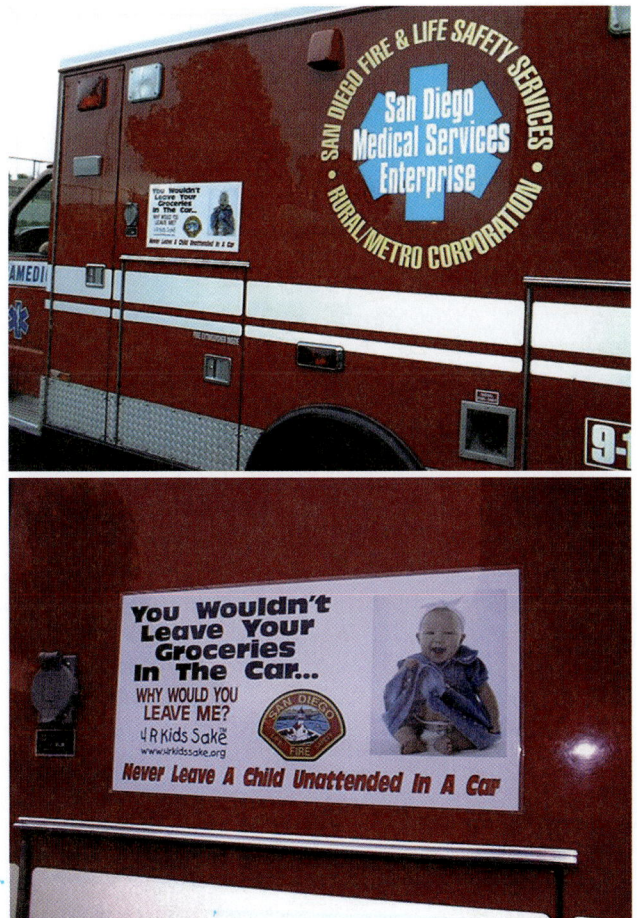

Figure 3-7 Because they see the results of injury every day, EMS providers are in a unique position to discuss the facts and consequences of injuries and prevention.

every day, EMS providers are in a unique position to discuss the facts and consequences of injuries and prevention (Figure 3-7).

If paramedics have the duty to respond to injuries and illness, then they have the duty to prevent injuries and illness. The fire service has successfully incorporated fire prevention into its profession. In fact, the prevention activities of fire departments have saved more lives than has pulling victims out of burning buildings. In fact, fire-related deaths have steadily decreased since President Calvin Coolidge proclaimed the first National Fire Prevention Week in October 1925. Since that call for action, the number of fire-related deaths has dropped from approximately 1 in 8000 Americans to 1 in 95,000 (United States Fire Administration, 2006).

Essential Leadership Activities

Injury and illness prevention for the public is obviously important, but so is injury and illness prevention for EMS providers. This responsibility lies with both the individual EMS professional and the management and leadership of EMS departments. Currently, all employers are required to have policies and procedures in place that address workplace safety. These include the use of personal protective equipment on calls and safe driving strategies. One in every five emergency responders is estimated to be injured each year (Dailey, 2006). Because the job is physically demanding and inherently dangerous, both employer and employee should take responsibility for provider safety.

One good example of an employer-led program designed to reduce worker injury was developed by the Rural Metro Corporation, Scottsdale, Ariz. The company studied the leading causes of job-related injury and illness and used the findings to develop new policies and procedures to reduce those causes (Box 3-1). Next, it developed a comprehensive six-part training program to be implemented companywide. Finally, it created and distributed a 20-minute awareness video to more than 6000 field employees.

EMS leadership must identify and support employees interested in participating in primary injury prevention activities within the community. This may be accomplished with budgetary support providing salary for off-duty personnel involved in injury-prevention activities or by allowing personnel to conduct activities while on duty, in uniform, and with the full sanction of their host agency.

Essential Provider Activities

EMS personnel can contribute to injury prevention efforts in their communities in many ways. Contribution is possible whether you work on an ambulance that responds to only a few calls per shift or a unit that runs nonstop from start to finish. Possible injury prevention activities include car seat safety checks, safe railroad crossing checks, bicycle safety fairs, fall prevention in the elderly, and drowning prevention activities, among countless other opportunities. The format in which the EMS professional provides education also has many possibilities. It

---

BOX 3-1　Causes of Job-Related Injury and Illness at Rural Metro Corporation

- Loading and unloading patients into an ambulance
- Patient transfer (bed to gurney, gurney to chair, scene to gurney)
- Transferring patient down stairs
- Gurney operations on uneven ground (gurney in pothole, gurney through grass)
- Compensating for patient movement on gurney
- Not using partner correctly
- Moving or transferring equipment (drug box, oxygen cylinder, monitor)
- Transporting obese patients
- Entering or exiting the vehicle

may be a prepared program, a program developed by an individual, a formal education event, or education of citizens during your daily interaction with them.

Regardless of what the topic is or how the education is delivered, the first step in any injury prevention program is to determine what education is needed in the community and where to target this education. This information can be gained in a variety of ways. Often personnel will notice they are responding to several of the same types of calls and begin to wonder if a pattern to these incidents exists. A review of run reports or hospital records might then indicate that many calls of a specific type do occur.

For example, if a community were to recognize an increase in injuries and fatalities from motor vehicle collisions, residents would likely want to reduce the number of these accidents. Rather than using a shotgun approach to the problem, which may not be effective, the problem should be studied to determine the most effective strategy for that particular community. In one case, a review of EMS and hospital records revealed that the highest number of injuries and fatalities were among 16- to 24-year-old males involved in street racing. It also was noted that all the individuals were wearing their seatbelts at the time of the crash. Had the community chosen to fund a seat belt campaign, few results would have occurred from their efforts. However, by realizing that street racing in young men was the issue, their education efforts could be more closely focused, potentially yielding a better result.

Injury prevention activities do not always have to be directly focused on the patient. An EMS service in one community responded to several calls in a 2-month period for children age 3 years and younger falling out of second- and third-story windows. Working directly with this patient group obviously would have little effect on the problem. However, by working with local builders and contractors to develop prevention strategies for both new and existing construction, these types of incidents were dramatically reduced.

Once a problem is identified, an injury prevention program must be developed that provides the greatest benefit for the resources available. Several tools can be used to identify how best to approach the problem, such as in the preceeding examples in which education about the dangers of street racing and collaboration with housing contractors were the best prevention approaches.

EPIDEMIOLOGIC TRIAD

One tool for injury prevention is the epidemiologic triad (Figure 3-8). This model of injury prevention has been in use for decades and examines the three main factors of injury and illness: the host, agent, and environment. When using this tool, the interrelations of each element are examined. Injury prevention is then targeted at disrupting one of the "legs" and breaking the triad.

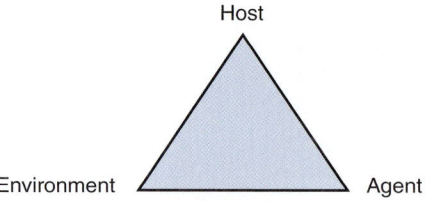

Figure 3-8 The epidemiologic triad.

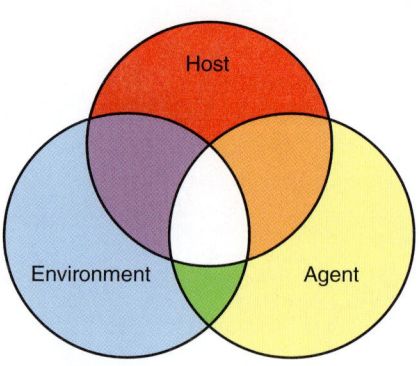

Figure 3-9 An alternate view of the epidemiologic triad.

Host factors can include age, risk-taking activity, gender, psychological profile, judgment, and other items that determine an individual's risk of injury.

In the classic view of this triad (for illness prevention), agent factors typically refer to a disease-causing microorganism or behavior (e.g., smoking). In injury prevention, agent factors typically refer to the amount of energy exchange causing injury to the body. Factors that affect these primarily are speed, distance, time, and other factors that increase the amount of available energy to destroy body tissues.

Environment factors include the environment in which the injury occurred, such as icy roads, distracted drivers, paths too close to a cliff edge, and trip hazards in the home.

An alternative view of this triad has been developed over the years in which each element is seen as a circle that has a certain amount of overlap with the other two circles (Figure 3-9). This model is preferred by many because it recognizes the fact that although all injuries and illnesses have several factors, some factors are unique to each element and cannot be changed. Targeting prevention activities as close as possible to the point at which all three circles overlap achieves the greatest outcome.

To put this model into action, take the example of reducing injuries and fatalities among teenage drivers. The host factors include the age of the drivers, risk-taking activity, and judgment compromise based on the lack of driving experience. Agent factors may include increased speed. Environmental factors may include distractions in the vehicle from friends or electronic devices.

Addressing each factor individually may cause a slight decrease in teen-involved accidents; however, addressing all three factors will have a much greater effect. In fact, many states have done this by increasing the driving age (host factor), restricting who can be in the car with a teenage driver (environmental factor), and increasing education regarding the dangers of speed (agent factor).

HADDON MATRIX

In the early 1960s, Dr. William Haddon expanded on the principles of the epidemiologic triad. Through his work, Haddon determined that all injuries have three time phases. He called these the pre-event, event, and post-event phases. By combining these time phases with the epidemiologic triad, he developed what is now known as the Haddon Matrix (Figure 3-10). By further evaluating all the components of an injury before it occurs, during the injury process, and after it occurs, better and more effective prevention strategies can be performed because each square of the matrix represents a possible intervention point. With this tool the EMS provider can determine which point(s) will have the greatest effect on injury prevention.

EMS traditionally has only participated in the post-event phase, the "you crash, we dash" model. As the EMS profession has developed, however, more agencies are using this matrix to take a proactive approach in their communities. An example of this is a community that noticed an increase in pediatric head trauma resulting from bicycle collisions. A review of the data showed that helmet use was minimal in these patients. The local EMS agency targeted the pre-event phase in both the host and agent. They stocked their ambulances with bicycle helmets, and whenever they saw a child riding without a helmet they took the opportunity to educate the child about bicycle safety (host) and gave the child a helmet (agent). As a result, these types of injuries were significantly reduced. A completed Haddon Matrix for a motor vehicle crash is depicted in Figure 3-11.

	Host	Agent	Environment
Pre-event			
Event			
Post event			

Figure 3-10 The Haddon Matrix.

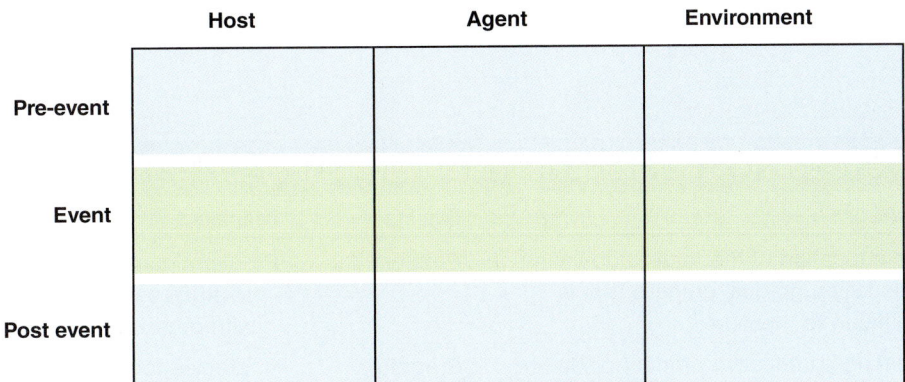

	Host	Agent	Environment
Pre-event	Driver's: Age Judgment Physical condition Tired Impaired Experience	Condition of car Safety features	Road hazards Road conditions Distractions in car
Event	Safety device use Physical condition	Speed Objects in car Type of collision Interior surfaces struck	Other vehicles Object struck "Landing" surface
Postevent	Age General health status Type of injury	Time until found Continued injury	EMS response time Trauma system access

Figure 3-11 A completed Haddon Matrix for a motor vehicle crash.

In the early 1970s Haddon developed what he called his "10 countermeasures for injury prevention." Each countermeasure provides a point at which the EMS professional can target injury prevention activities, as follows:

1. Prevent the initial creation of the hazard.
2. Reduce the hazard being produced.
3. Prevent the release of the hazard.
4. Slow the rate of the release of the hazard.
5. Separate the hazard in terms of time and space.
6. Provide protection from the hazard with a barrier.
7. Modify the hazard.
8. Increase strength or resistance against the hazard.
9. Minimize the damage done by the hazard.
10. Stabilize and repair or rehabilitate what is damaged by the hazard.

THE "EP5" MATRIX

Successful injury prevention programs must be based on how well they integrate the critical elements of injury prevention into the program or intervention. Once the EMS professional knows what the problem is and where to target prevention activities, a prevention program can be developed. Prevention efforts are commonly based on the "Five E's" of injury prevention (Table 3-1). Many times addressing one of these alone will be unsuccessful in reducing injury, requiring programs to address several items. The use of this plan along with the methods in the preceding paragraphs will ensure a strong injury prevention program. In addition to the five E's listed, many experts also add *e*conomic incentives and *e*valuation to their programs. An injury prevention programs components, the "Five P's," are explained in Table 3-1.

Education

Education was long considered the mainstay of injury prevention and is still often the first strategy chosen when considering a new program. Education alone, however, has been shown to not be an effective method of preventing injury. This is because education only affects the host in the epidemiologic triad and does nothing to affect the agent or environment. Add to that the fact that most educational programs are short in duration compared with the time necessary to modify an individual's behavior. As a result, although education is

TABLE 3-1	Specific Interventions (*E*'s) and Overall Program Components (*P*'s)			
Five *E*'s	**Definitions**	**Five *P*'s**	**Definitions**	
Education	The education of the target population. Usually a gradual process that is difficult to measure.	Problem	Problem identification through the use of data or studies. Compare problem magnitude with other injuries that affect the community.	
Engineering	Creating an effective product or device that requires minimal effort on the part of the user or offers automatic or passive protection without thought on the part of the user. Examples include air bags in cars, smoke detectors in homes, and ground fault interrupter outlets in bathrooms and kitchens.	Program	Strategies for implementing a variety of interventions with an evaluation component that creates continuous feedback on effectiveness.	
Enforcement	Legislation, regulations, or litigation that modifies behavior and ensures compliance. Examples include blood alcohol level limits and laws requiring children to wear bicycle helmets.	Partnership	Collaboration with other organizations or public or private agencies.	
Environment	A change in the physical environment or culture of the environment that creates or enhances effectiveness of a program, product, or device.	Preparation	Readying for implementation with training of participants, data collection, identification of resources, analysis of similar interventions cited in the literature, and follow-up with community partners.	
EMS	Engaging EMS personnel into participating in the program.	Policy	Advocacy or actual public or private policy change or law that addresses an identified issue.	

an important piece of any injury prevention program, it rarely works when used alone.

Engineering

Engineering interventions are built into the agent or the environment and are most effective when they do not require any interaction by the host. Examples include airbags in a motor vehicle, the emergency stopping devices in the event of an elevator failure, and other automatic safety devices. Other engineering interventions depend on interaction from the host, which makes them vulnerable to not being used. Fall protection devices for window washers, seatbelts, and helmets all require host interaction to be effective.

Enforcement

Enforcement activities are based on the ability of a governmental agency to mandate or disallow certain activities or the production of certain items deemed to be dangerous. Enforcement is only effective, however, if the public chooses to obey the regulations. In short, the answer to the question "Is the penalty for being caught so low that the activity is worth it?" must be "no." When choosing this strategy the penalty for the infraction must be a deterrent. Although in general the populace tends to follow enforcement actions, they generally do not work alone. People are much more likely to follow rules and regulations if they understand why they are in place; as a result, enforcement should always be paired with education.

Environment

As previously discussed, one factor of the epidemiologic triad is the environment. Activities that change the environment or remove the environmental factor will "break" the triangle, thereby reducing injury. Other environmental factors may include changing the view of the community in a way that increases their receptiveness of an injury prevention program or increases their compliance with existing enforcement activities.

Emergency Medical Services

These activities are specific to the EMS profession in injury prevention. As previously discussed, EMS professionals can play a large role in injury prevention based on numbers of providers, knowledge and experience, and public visibility.

Economic Incentives

The treatment of trauma is expensive, and all members of the community must pay for this treatment in one way or another. Highlighting the cost savings of avoiding injury can be an effective prevention method. These strategies also are common in the business and manufacturing sectors. Products that lead to injury often result in litigation against the companies that produced them. As a result, companies make great efforts to produce safe products in an effort to avoid injuries to consumers.

Evaluation

Evaluation is crucial to any injury prevention program. The question "Is this working?" must be asked. If a program is not effective, then valuable resources are being used with no outcome and a new strategy must be implemented. Although evaluation should begin early in any prevention program, EMS providers must also realize that reduction in injury may not be immediate. Just as a review of data is needed to identify a problem, enough data must be available to review to determine if the program had an effect. Always evaluate, but be sure not to dismiss the program in the absence of overnight success.

In short, an effective injury prevention program begins with identifying the problem (research available data), determining which intervention points will be the most effective (Haddon Matrix), and developing a plan that will best address these intervention points (the five *E*'s). If any component is missing, injuries are unlikely to be reduced. Table 3-1 summarizes these components using the EP5 matrix.

THE TEACHABLE MOMENT

[OBJECTIVE 4]

Not all educational events take place through formal injury prevention programs. EMS personnel are in a unique position to educate their patients and their family members as well as bystanders. One way to impart this education is through the **teachable moment**. This is the time immediately after an injury has occurred when the patient and observers remain acutely aware of what has happened and may be more receptive to learning how the event or illness could have been prevented (U.S. Department of Transportation/NHTSA, 1998). Speaking with patients or bystanders immediately after they have experienced a crisis may be the best way to deliver effective injury prevention messages.

Teachable moments can also be preemptive, or take place before an injury happens. If you happen to be at an elderly patient's home for a medical call and notice a trip hazard in the home, educating the patient at that time may avoid an injury from a fall later. These moments can also be unrelated to trauma. You may find a patient who has difficulty understanding his or her prescription instructions. By taking the time to clarify them, you could prevent that patient from succumbing to the effects of an overdose or underdose of medication.

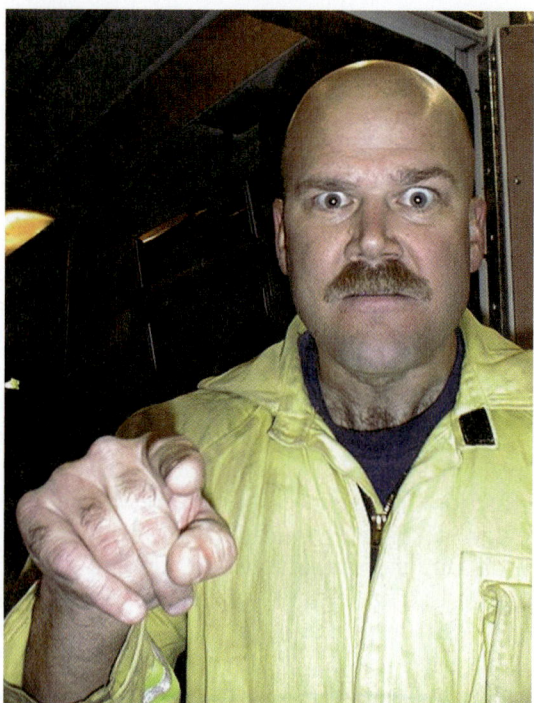

Figure 3-12 The prevention message can be delivered the right way or the wrong way. Avoid being accusatory or judgmental during the teachable moment.

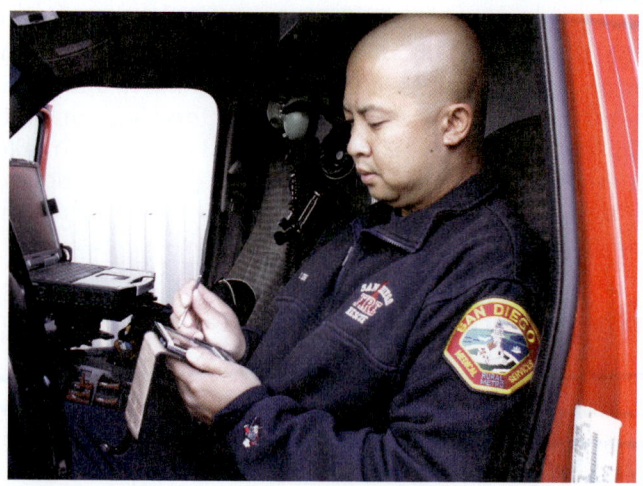

Figure 3-13 Be sure to completely fill out all the required fields in an EMS report no matter how minute the details may seem.

Of course, these teachable moments take a back seat to patient care. However, when the situation stabilizes, you can then proceed with prevention education, which may include discussing seatbelts, helmets, unsafe driving, or driving under the influence. You should remain calm and positive and project a caring and supportive demeanor. Humiliating a patient or yelling will most likely result in the opposite effect (Figure 3-12).

Teachable moments may occur on the scene or in the back of the ambulance. They can involve family members, friends, caregivers, or strangers. The teachable moment also can be an emotional outlet for experienced EMS providers who have responded to the same preventable injuries time and time again.

Paramedics are often able to draw from their previous experiences in dealing with tragedies and effectively communicate their concerns to diverse audiences.

Documentation

[OBJECTIVE 5]

The first way EMS professionals can help is by properly documenting calls involving injuries. These data are imperative for local injury-prevention efforts as well as state and national monitoring. **Epidemiologists**, people who study the causes, distribution, and control of disease in populations, have identified leading causes of injury and how to correct them by sifting through EMS paper-

work. To guarantee "clean" data, you must completely fill out all the required fields in an EMS report no matter how minute the details may seem (Figure 3-13). Information such as a patient's gender or whether he or she was restrained during a motor vehicle crash is imperative for accurate analysis. Your narrative section is equally important. Be as accurate and detailed as possible when reporting the circumstances behind an injury. Although you may have checked the appropriate box on your prehospital care report for the presence of a car seat after a crash, do not forget to describe where the car seat was found, whether it was forward or rear facing, if it was properly installed, and where the child was on your arrival. Narratives are used to paint a picture of what happened from the paramedic's point of view and from the viewpoint of the patient and bystanders. According to the NHTSA Public Information, Education, and Relations in EMS (PIER) curriculum, "Only a narrative can fully portray the physical and emotional characteristics at a scene, detail the **chronology** [the arrangement of events in time] of events, picture the conditions of a road or other features, and depict the conditions, actions, and reactions of the people involved in an injury event." This firsthand information is often "lost" in hospital and police reports that rely on third- and fourth-hand information hours or days later.

The analyzed data are used to develop focused prevention activities, acquire public support, and justify funding.

Case Scenario—continued

Shortly after you begin treatment, the ambulance arrives and you transfer patient care to the paramedic on the ambulance. While speaking with the girl's parents, they angrily comment that this is the second child who has fallen out of a window in their neighborhood. The child's father takes you upstairs to the bedroom, where you see that the window's location in the room and height on the wall make it highly likely that it will be immediately adjacent to a child sitting on the bed. When the father shows you the screen construction, you see that the clips that hold it in place could be easily bent or broken with minimal pressure.

After returning to your station, you mention the conversation to your battalion chief. Together you search the department's records and find three similar calls in the neighborhood during the previous year. After further investigation, you discover that all three calls involved the same model of home.

Questions

4. Should you and your department share this injury trend with anyone? Why or why not? If you chose to communicate the information, whom should you contact?
5. What organization in your community is responsible for injury prevention?
6. Should EMS organizations interact with organizations responsible for injury prevention? How?

A SUCCESSFUL DROWNING PREVENTION PROGRAM

In 1994 drowning was the second leading cause of accidental death for children and youths younger than 20 years old in Alaska. From the period of 1991 to 1994, 37 fatalities occurred, an average of nine per year. This rate was more than twice the national average. Most of the fatalities occurred in open skiffs or canoes, more than half occurred in lakes and rivers, and 22% of boating fatalities occurred among those younger than 19 years old. Of critical importance, more than 90% of those who died had not been wearing a life jacket.

Bob Painter, assistant fire chief of the Homer, Ala., Fire Department, knew two children who had drowned in his jurisdiction. For a population of approximately 4000, two is both very personal and statistically significant. Painter proposed a project that he called "Kids Don't Float" (KDF). It was named after a successful program in New York City called "Kids Can't Fly," aimed at preventing children from falling out of windows. KDF zeroed in on the fact that 90% of victims had not used flotation devices (determination of problem). So KDF combined a life jacket loaner program at the harbors with a water safety education program (educate). Painter's project was developed through collaboration with local groups: the Homer Fire Department, Homer Safe Kids, the Coast Guard Auxiliary, and the Homer School District (develop a plan).

Beginning in spring 1996, these groups erected 15 signboards on which to hang the loaner life jackets in communities around Katchemak Bay, where the town of Homer is situated. The concept was simple—make it easy for people to grab a life jacket on their way to a boat and return it when they are done. The signboards also provided an opportunity for an effective educational message. In 1997 and 1998, Painter evaluated the effec-

tiveness of the life jacket loaner board program in promoting life jacket use. The observed wear rate went from 16% to 35%—an increase of 119%—in the target community after the signboards were erected compared with no increase in the control community (evaluate).

Now, 12 years later, 268 KDF life jacket loaner boards are located by lakes, rivers, and bays in nearly every region of the state (Figure 3-14). The success of this project can also be measured in lives saved in Alaska. A 10-year-old Kotzebue boy was playing near the sound when his friend got swept into deeper water by the current. Neither child could swim, but the boy bravely grabbed a KDF life jacket, dog paddled out to his friend, and pulled her to shore. Three other likely saves have been reported. Two children wearing KDF jackets survived a boating accident on the

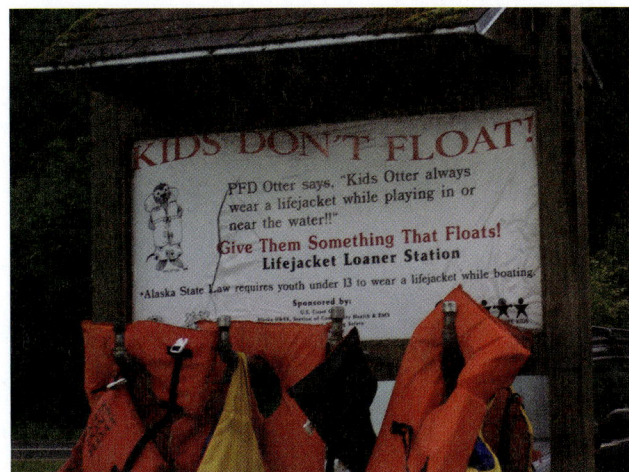

Figure 3-14 Personal flotation device loaner boards are a key component of the "Kids Don't Float" program and have helped increase the wear rate by 119%.

Kenai River. A child fell off the dock in Klawock, and his friends acted quickly by throwing him a KDF life jacket until he could be rescued.

KDF has truly been a collaborative effort both at the state level and in the communities where each of these loaner boards was built and is maintained. The KDF program became a prominent component of the Alaska Boating Safety Bill and was frequently mentioned in testimony by those supporting the bill. The law was passed by the Alaska legislature in May 2000. Along with the legislation came funding for more boards and more life jackets (enforcement). The National Safe Boating Council and National Safe Kids have adopted this program for national promotion.

National recognition is gratifying, but the real reward, Painter will tell you, is seeing kids don life jackets whenever they go out on the water (Griffiths & Maxwell, 2002).

DRAWING FROM PERSONAL EXPERIENCE: SAFE

In Vince Easevoli's 20 years as a firefighter/paramedic for Miami-Dade Fire Rescue, he has responded to nearly every imaginable call for help. However, he noticed a disproportionate number of calls involving teenagers and tragic car accidents, which seemed to have a common denominator: the teens were not wearing seatbelts.

In 1987, Easevoli decided to stop the cycle of preventable injuries and deaths. With the help of fellow firefighter/paramedic Ralph Jiminez and others, he started Stay Alive From Education (SAFE).

Much work was necessary; unintentional injuries continued to be the leading cause of death for Floridians ages 1 to 34 years. Seatbelt use statewide was only 58%, well below the national average. The goal of the SAFE program is to offer young adults information that allows them to make educated and rational decisions concerning their safety and well-being in an effort to reduce injuries and fatalities and give them the opportunity to become responsible and healthy adults.

SAFE program instructors, all experienced paramedics, use a hands-on approach to teach students about the consequences of irresponsible actions. Students learn about crash dynamics and participate in dramatic demonstrations of what happens to trauma patients.

Since the program's start in Dade County, it has grown to include teams in six other counties in Florida as well as teams in California and New Jersey. On average, more than 55,000 students attend the SAFE program each year. The University of Miami recently conducted a study on Florida SAFE's effectiveness and documented a dramatic increase in seatbelt use by SAFE graduates (Krimston & Griffiths, 2003).

Case Scenario CONCLUSION

The patient whom you originally treated was admitted to the hospital with a skull fracture, a small subdural hematoma, and a fractured humerus. Your battalion chief decided to contact the company that built the homes to inform them of what you learned. The builder was quite interested in the information and immediately changed the window height for future projects. The builder also provided alternative clips to existing homeowners to improve the security of the screen. Your department has not responded to any further calls related to this problem.

Looking Back

7. *Was contacting the builder appropriate? Should you have contacted the family instead? What about a public health entity?*

8. *Bringing this injury trend to the attention of the builder or family may have resulted in legal action by the family. You and/or your department may have been called to testify. Does this reality affect the decision to follow up on the trend? How?*

9. *Had the girl not had severe injuries, would following up on the injury trend not have been as appropriate? Why or why not?*

CULTURAL*Considerations*

[OBJECTIVE 6]

Motor vehicle crashes are the leading cause of death for Latinos ages 1 to 34 years and the third leading cause of death for all ages, surpassed only by heart disease and cancer, according to new statistics released by the Centers for Disease Control and Prevention. The death rate from motor vehicle crashes for Hispanic children between the ages of 5 and

12 years is 72% higher than the rate for non-Hispanic children, according to NHTSA. Furthermore, young Latinos drive half as many miles as their non-Hispanic white counterparts, but they are twice as likely to die in a traffic fatality (NHTSA, 2008)

"The biggest problem is that the Latino community has not received information about car seats and seat belt use in a way that resonates with them," said Rebéca Barrera, president of the National Latino Children's Institute (NLCI). Barrera added, "Many Latinos think that they can keep their children safe by hugging them tightly on their laps in the front seat of the car. And although this is one sign of love, in today's fast-paced world a more effective way to keep your child safe is in a car seat or a booster seat."

Corazón de mi Vida, which was developed by NLCI, in partnership with NHTSA and Nationwide Insurance, uses the cultural strengths of the Latino community as the foundation for passenger restraint education, emphasizing the valuable role children play in the lives of their families and society. Cultural values, traditions, and spirituality are incorporated into the program to help change behavior.

"The words 'corazón de mi vida' mean 'you are the center of my life.' This phrase captures the essence of child passenger safety for Latinos. The belief in this message is so powerful that it will change the behaviors of Latinos who may not know how urgent it is for their children to ride in the back seat, buckled up in a safety seat," Barrera explains.

NLCI found that more than half of the parents attending Corazón de mi Vida events around the country did not own safety seats until they participated in the program. In addition, almost every child safety seat checked at Corazón de mi Vida events failed inspection.

"By taking into account Latino cultural traditions and lifestyles, NLCI outreach strategies recognize the good things parents are already doing for their children. Corazón de mi Vida builds on parents' love for their children and invites them to become partners in keeping their children safe—all with a distinct Latino sabor [flavor]," Barrera added.

NLCI also found that the Latino extended family structure, coupled with poverty, can create difficult situations when it comes to using child safety seats.

"Safety seats are expensive, and they take up space," explained Conrad Gonzales, NLCI's director of safety programs. He continued, "Many Latino families are large, and some work in businesses that require trucks, and this may be the only family vehicle. Accommodating the whole family in a small car or truck poses problems.

"Only the most expensive trucks can accommodate more than two persons in seats, and because elders ride in the most comfortable seats, some children ride in the bed of the truck. Frequently, mothers hold the youngest child in their lap, thinking this is the safest place for them."

In addition to space and economic considerations, religious and cultural views can be misinterpreted when it comes to passenger restraints. "Phrases handed down through the centuries," Barrera said, "such as 'lo que Dios quiera' [whatever God wills], might suggest, 'What's the point? I have no control over my destiny.' Instead of ignoring or blaming the concept of fatalism, Corazón de mi Vida incorporates spiritual beliefs by holding car seat blessings and encouraging people to 'help God keep them safe.'"

Tested in 12 cities with diverse Latino populations, Corazón de mi Vida has proven that Latinos will respond to messages and buckle up their children when the message speaks to their hearts.

The program uses appealing culture-based materials combined with four unique community activities. At parent pláticas, often hosted at child care centers, churches, clinics, and community centers, parents discuss child passenger safety and common attitudes. Culturally based materials are distributed and participants watch a demonstration of the correct installation of a safety seat. At safety seat blessings, a religious leader blesses the car seats to be distributed and reminds parents that they have been entrusted with their child's well-being.

EXAMPLES OF SUCCESSFUL EMS-CONCEIVED PROGRAMS

Safety Corridor

Lt. John Creel, a 20-year veteran EMT and firefighter from Hoodland (Oregon) Fire District 74, has the rare gift of bringing people together toward a common goal. The ability to build coalitions among diverse interests to obtain cooperation is critically important for injury prevention challenges that cross agencies and geographic boundaries. In the early 1990s motor vehicle accidents on a stretch of highway through Oregon's Cascade Range near Mount Hood claimed eight to 10 lives per year (Figure 3-15). One mountainous stretch of U.S. Highway 26 from Sandy, Ore., to the Highway 35 junction had the worst record, with Hoodland Fire responding to an average of nearly 200 accidents per year in that segment.

Creel initially wanted to find a way to reduce the number of crashes occurring near Hoodland. He began a local effort to raise awareness of the problem. In a short time, his efforts mushroomed into a regional and statewide effort to reduce motor vehicle crashes throughout the 25 miles of the Mount Hood corridor. Creel successfully enlisted the help of other fire agencies, the Oregon Department of Transportation, the state police, and the county sheriff and organized a local community group to apply the necessary political pressure.

Creel developed an important tool in his safety efforts: a map. This map showed where crashes occurred as well as displayed the hidden dangers of the route. He released statistics in community flyers and wrote columns for local newspapers. Through public education, stepped-up traffic enforcement (fines were doubled in the "safety corridor"), and highway engineering, motor vehicle accidents have declined by 60% (Griffiths &

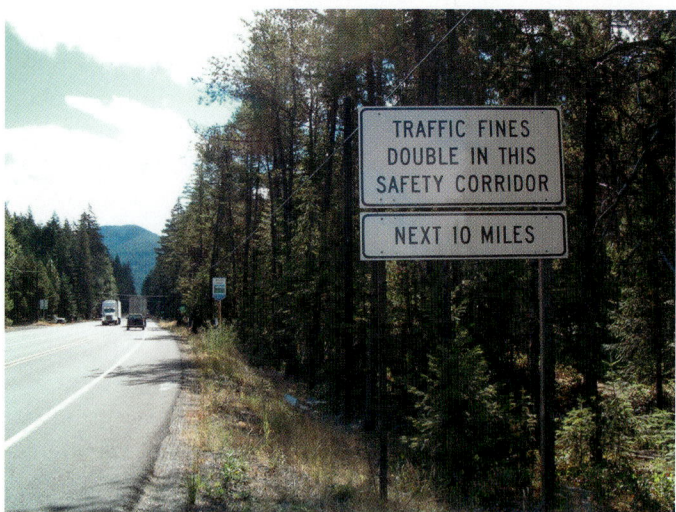

Figure 3-15 Increases in traffic fines, redesigned roads, increased signage and striping, and reduced speed limits are all part of the Mount Hood safety corridor.

Maxwell, 2002). An EP5 breakdown of the plan is shown in Table 3-2.

The next time you are called to the scene of a car accident, fall, drowning, or other injury, think about how the incident could have been prevented. Consider ways that you could have helped prevent it. The time is always right to do something about unintentional injuries.

TABLE 3-2	EP5 Breakdown of Safety Corridor
Five *E*'s	**Application**
Education	Distributed maps showing locations of crashes on Highway 26 corridor; placed crashed vehicle in front of fire station to serve as a reminder to passing motorists
Engineering	Redesigned road to include rumble strips and turnouts for disabled vehicles
Enforcement	Reduced speed limit in corridor, doubled traffic fines, and added signs to warn drivers of increased fines
Environment	Added chain-up areas, increased signage, improved striping, increased winter maintenance, and de-icers
EMS	Hoodland Fire District
Five *P*'s	**Application**
Problem	Increased number of vehicle crashes on 25-mile stretch of highway
Program	Six months of meeting and planning, enforcement help from Oregon State Police, engineering assistance from Oregon Department of Transportation, education provided by Hoodland Fire District
Partnership	Citizens Advisory Committee, Oregon Department of Transportation, United States Forest Service, Federal Highway Administration, U.S. Army Corps of Engineers
Preparation	Conducted Mount Hood corridor study, analyzed data, trained and educated partners
Policy	Lowered speed limit for corridor, increased traffic fines

EPIC Medics

On May 8, 1996, a San Diego County paramedic unit responded to a call to assist a 2-year-old boy named Nicholas Rosecrans who had wandered away from a daycare center and into the unfenced pool of the house next door. The paramedics' resuscitative efforts were successful only to the point of return of a pulse; 12 hours later, Nicholas was released from life support and pronounced dead. A few days later, the paramedics who responded to the accident received a heartbreaking letter from Nicholas' mother Lynn, thanking the paramedics for their efforts and for the time they had given her to say goodbye to her son.

This incident and its aftermath so touched paramedic Paul Maxwell that he vowed to do everything in his power to try to end the rash of preventable child drownings occurring in his district and to make Nicholas' death the last child drowning he would have to answer.

Maxwell contacted the San Diego Safe Kids Coalition, which welcomed him with open arms. The coordinator of the coalition immediately recognized the value of using a paramedic as a spokesperson to influence public policy and deliver the prevention messages. "Our paramedic should know . . . he sees it everyday," she would say to the press. Together they used EMS data, the media, and many other strategies to help influence the passage of Bill AB3305, which requires barriers surrounding all new pool construction in California.

Fellow paramedic Josh Krimston joined Maxwell in organizing other paramedics to use their professional experience to turn this tragedy into action. Together they founded Eliminate Preventable Injuries of Children (EPIC) Medics.

Members of EPIC Medics have received numerous awards, including State of California Paramedic of the Year, Emergency Medical Services for Children (EMS-C) National Heroes Award, and other leadership awards.

Case Scenario SUMMARY

1. *What is your general impression of this patient?* This patient is high priority. Her mechanism of injury, loss of consciousness, and pallor demonstrate high potential for a neurologic injury and shock.

2. *What physical assessment findings are most pertinent at this time?* Assessment should focus on signs of shock and neurologic injury. Skin color, temperature, level of orientation and mental status examination, sensory/motor examination, and vital signs are all important. She should also be checked for other injuries.

3. *What treatment should be immediately initiated?* High-flow oxygen and spinal stabilization.

4. *Should you and your department share this injury trend with anyone? Why or why not? If you chose to communicate the information, whom should you contact?* You should communicate information about community injury risks immediately. Injury prevention is a part of the stated mission of many EMS organizations and is a community responsibly for all healthcare professionals. In some communities, failing to report such information places liability on the organization. Depending on the community, information should be reported to public health officials, local injury prevention organizations, or EMS regulatory agencies. If in doubt, begin by informing your medical director.

5. *What organization in your community is responsible for injury prevention?* As previously noted, all healthcare organizations and professionals share responsibility for injury prevention. In most communities, the public health department has oversight of injury prevention, although specific injury prevention organizations may also exist.

6. *Should EMS organizations interact with organizations responsible for injury prevention? How?* Yes. Because EMS organizations are in a good position to monitor injury patterns (as this case demonstrates), they should become active in local prevention activities such as bicycle helmet, seatbelt, and child safety programs. Because they are trusted by the citizens, EMS organizations have an opportunity to communicate prevention plans to the public and collaborate with other organizations to reduce injury frequency rates.

7. *Was contacting the builder appropriate? Should you have contacted the family instead? What about a public health entity?* The outcome of this case makes it hard to fault the battalion chief for contacting the builder. However, in most cases contacting the builder may be a more appropriate action for public health or other injury prevention organizations. However, one thing is certain: contacting *someone* is better than hesitating because you are not sure whom to contact. Again, if in doubt, start by communicating the information to your medical director.

8. *Bringing this injury trend to the attention of the builder or family may have resulted in legal action by the family. You and/or your department may have been called to testify. Does this reality affect the decision to follow up on the trend? How?* Injury prevention involves identifying injury patterns, looking for the root causes behind patterns, and applying interventions that reduce those causes. None of these activities is specifically focused on assessing blame. Nevertheless, because people or organizations are sometimes related to root causes, a risk that blame will be assigned is always present, along with accusations of liability. As true advocates for patient health and safety, EMS cannot avoid injury prevention activities because of fear of causing anger or getting too involved in a situation. If our actions result in genuine reductions in death and injury, the efforts are worthwhile.

9. *Had the girl not had severe injuries, would following up on the injury trend have been as appropriate? Why or why not?* Studies in injury-causing behavior demonstrate that risky activities may be repeated hundreds of times before they cause any significant injury. Our job in injury prevention is to identify and reduce root causes *before* significant injuries occur. The fact that three children incurred the same preventable injury is adequate justification to investigate a root cause, regardless of whether any of the injuries was severe.

Chapter Summary

- Paramedics are in a perfect position to decrease injuries and make a difference in communities.
- Primary injury prevention, or keeping an injury from occurring, is an essential activity. It must be undertaken by the leaders, decision makers, and providers of every EMS system. Traditionally, EMS providers have focused on secondary injury prevention, or preventing further injury from an event that has already occurred.
- In the United States, unintentional injuries are the leading cause of death for individuals aged 1 to 34 years.
- An injury is defined as intentional or unintentional damage to a person that results from acute exposure to thermal, mechanical, electrical, or chemical energy or the absence of essentials such as heat or oxygen.

Chapter Summary—continued

- Unintentional injuries occur without intent to harm. In contrast, intentional injuries include all injuries and deaths that are self-inflicted or perpetrated by another person, usually involving some type of violence.
- Some people are more prone to injuries as a result of their actions or the actions of those around them. An injury risk is defined as a real or potentially hazardous situation that puts individuals at risk for sustaining an injury.
- Injury surveillance is the ongoing systematic collection, analysis, and interpretation of injury data essential to the planning, implementation, and evaluation of public health practice. Your run reports contribute to this collection of data.
- Measuring death (mortality) rates is much easier than measuring nonfatal injury (morbidity) rates. Nearly all reported deaths involve some type of tracking, whereas nonfatal injuries are quite difficult to track because reporting systems generally exclude clinics, physicians' offices, school nurses' offices, and the home medicine cabinet.
- Unintentional injuries are predictable and therefore are preventable.
- EMS personnel are well suited to injury prevention education for the following reasons:
  - They are widely distributed among the population
  - More than 600,000 are in the United States
  - They are high-profile role models
  - They are welcome in schools and other environments
  - They are champions of the healthcare consumer
- They reflect the composition of the community
- They may be the most medically educated individuals in a rural setting
- They are considered authorities on injury and prevention
- If paramedics have the duty to respond to injuries and illness, then they have the duty to prevent injuries and illness.
- Because the job is physically demanding and inherently dangerous, both employer and employee should take responsibility for EMS provider safety.
- All employers are required to have policies and procedures in place that address workplace safety, including topics such as the use of personal protective equipment on calls and safe driving strategies.
- A teachable moment is the time immediately after an injury has occurred when the patient and observers remain acutely aware of what has happened and may be more receptive to learning how the event or illness could have been prevented. Speaking with patients or bystanders after they have experienced a crisis may be the best way to deliver effective injury prevention messages.
- KDF, SAFE, and EPIC Medics are examples of provider-driven community injury prevention programs.
- To start your own local injury prevention program, first evaluate the five *E*'s (*e*ducation, *e*nforcement, *e*ngineering, *e*nvironment, and *E*MS). Components of an injury prevention program include the five *P*'s (*p*roblem, *p*rogram, *p*artnership, *p*reparation, and *p*olicy).

REFERENCES

Centers for Disease Control and Prevention. (2001). *CDC injury fact book, 2001-2002*. Retrieved October 7, 2006, from http://http://www.cdc.gov.

Centers for Disease Control and Prevention. (2003). *10 Leading causes of death by age group, United States, 2003*. Retrieved April 5, 2007, from ftp://ftp.cdc.gov.

Dailey, B. (2006). Musculoskeletal injury prevention. Protect your personnel from on-the-job injury. *Journal of Emergency Medical Services*, *31*, 60-64, 66.

Griffiths, K. (1999). Injury prevention takes root. EMS evolves to assume expanded mission. *Journal of Emergency Medical Services*, *24*, 56-60, 62-64, 66-67.

Griffiths, K., & Maxwell, P. (2002). Best practices in injury prevention: National award highlights programs across the nation. *Journal of Emergency Medical Services*, *27*, 60-74.

Krimston, J., & Griffiths, K. (2003). Best practices in injury prevention: The Nicholas Rosecrans Award. *Journal of Emergency Medical Services*, *28*, 66-83.

National Highway Traffic Safety Administration. (1996). *Consensus statement: The role of out-of-hospital emergency medical services in primary injury prevention*. Retrieved April 26, 2008, from http://http://www.nhtsa.dot.gov.

National Highway Traffic Safety Administration. (2004). *Traffic safety facts*. Retrieved April 5, 2007, from http://www.nhtsa.dot.gov.

National Highway Traffic Safety Administration. (2008). *Latino/Hispanic American outreach*. Retrieved January 4, 2008, from http://http://www.nhtsa.dot.gov.

National Latino Children's Institute. (2006). *Corazon de mi vida*. Retrieved April 5, 2007, from http://http://www.nlci.org.

National Safety Council. (2007). *Injury facts, 2005-2006*. Retrieved April 16, 2007, from http://http://www.nsc.org.

United States Department of Transportation/National Highway Traffic Safety Administration. (1998). *Paramedic: National standard curriculum*. Retrieved April 5, 2007, from http://http://www.nhtsa.dot.gov.

United States Fire Administration. (2006). *Fire statistics*. Retrieved January 4, 2008, from http://http://www.usfa.dhs.gov/statistics.

SUGGESTED RESOURCES

[OBJECTIVE 7]

4 R Kids Sake
   PO Box 77693
   Corona, CA 92877-0123
   (951) 278-1820
   http://www.4rkidssake.org
AAA Traffic Safety
   607 14th Street NW
   Suite 201
   Washington, DC 20005
   (202) 638-5944
   http://www.aaafoundation.org
American Association of Poison Control Centers
   (800) 222-1222
   http://www.aapcc.org
American Trauma Society
   8903 Presidential Parkway, Suite 512
   Upper Marlboro, MD 20772
   (800) 556-7890
   http://www.amtrauma.org
Bicycle Helmet Safety Institute
   4611 Seventh Street South
   Arlington, VA 22204-1419
   (703) 486-0100
   http://www.bhsi.org
Centers for Disease Control and Prevention
   1600 Clifton Road
   Atlanta, GA 30333
   (800) CDC-INFO
   http://www.cdc.gov
Children's Safety Network
   (619) 594-1995
   http://www.injuryprevention.org
Designated Drivers Association
   PO Box 81362
   San Diego, CA 92138-1362
   (866) 373-SAFE
   http://www.ddasd.org
Emergency Medical Services for Children
   Health Resources and Services Administration
   Maternal and Child Health Bureau
   Parklawn Building, Room 18-05
   5600 Fishers Lane
   Rockville, MD 20857
   (202) 884-4927
   http://www.ems-c.org
EPIC Medics
   4775 Maple Avenue
   La Mesa, CA 91941
   (619) 303-4228
   http://www.epicmedics.org
Every 15 Minutes
   PO Box 20034
   Lehigh Valley, PA 18002-0034
   (610) 814-6418
   http://www.every15minutes.com
Farm Safety 4 Just Kids
   PO Box 458
   Earlham, IA 50072
   (800) 423-5437
   http://www.fs4jk.org
Foundation Center
   (800) 424-9836
   http://www.fdncenter.org
Governor's Highway Safety Association
   750 First Street NE, Suite 720
   Washington, DC 20002
   (202) 789-0942
   http://www.ghsa.org
The Grantsmanship Center
   PO Box 17220
   Los Angeles, CA 90017
   (213) 482-9860
   http://www.tgci.com

Harborview Injury Prevention & Research Center
   325 Ninth Avenue, Box 359960
   Seattle, WA 98104
   (206) 744-9430
   http://depts.washington.edu/hiprc
Home Safety Council
   1250 Eye Street, NW, Suite 1000
   Washington, DC 20005
   (202) 330-4900
   http://www.homesafetycouncil.org
Injury Free Coalition
   http://www.injuryfree.org
International Child Abuse Network
   4024 N. Durfee Avenue
   El Monte, CA 91732
   (626) 455-4585
   http://www.ican-ncfr.org
International Play Equipment Manufacturers Association
   4305 North Sixth Street, Suite A
   Harrisburg, PA 17110
   (888) 944-7362
   http://www.ipema.org
Kids and Cars
   2913 West 113th Street
   Leawood, KS 66211
   (913) 327-0013
   http://www.kidsandcars.org
Kids in Cars
   918 Glenn Avenue
   Washington, MO 63090
   (636) 390-8268
   http://www.kidsincars.org
Kids in Danger
   116 West Illinois Street, Suite 5E
   Chicago, IL 60610-4532
   (312) 595-0649
   http://www.kidsindanger.org
Mothers Against Drunk Driving
   511 E. John Carpenter Freeway, Suite 700
   Irving, TX 75062
   (800) GET-MADD
   http://www.madd.org
National Fire Academy
   16825 South Seton Avenue
   Emmitsburg, MD 21727
   (301) 447-1000
   http://www.usfa.fema.gov/training/nfa
National Fire Protection Agency
   1 Batterymarch Park
   Quincy, MA 02169-7471
   (800) 344-3555
   http://www.nfpa.org
National Institute on Alcohol Abuse and Alcoholism
   5635 Fishers Lane, MSC 9304
   Bethesda, MD 20892-9304
   http://www.collegedrinkingprevention.gov
National Safety Council
   1121 Spring Lake Drive
   Itasca, IL 60143-3201
   (800) 621-7619
   http://www.nsc.org
National Highway Traffic Safety Administration
   400 Seventh Street, SW
   Washington, DC 20590
   (888) 327-4236
   http://www.nhtsa.gov
No Dog Bites
   2100 L Street, NW
   Washington, DC 20037
   (202) 452-1100
   http://www.hsus.org/pets/pet_care/dog_care/stay_dog_bite_free/index.html

Safe Kids Worldwide
   1301 Pennsylvania Avenue NW, Suite 1000
   Washington, DC 20004-1707
   (202) 662-0600
   http://www.safekids.org
Safe Routes to School
   730 Martin Luther King, Jr. Blvd, Suite 300
   Campus Box 3430
   Chapel Hill, NC 27599-3430
   (919) 962-7419
   http://www.walktoschool-usa.org
SafeUSA
   624 North Broadway
   Baltimore, MD 21205
   (410) 955-2397
   http://www.safeusa.org
Stay Alive From Education (SAFE)
   71 Jean Lafitte Drive
   Key Largo, FL 33037
   (305) 852-2651
   http://www.safeprogram.com

Think First
   26 South La Grange Road, Suite 103
   La Grange, IL 60525
   (800) 844-6556
   http://www.thinkfirst.org
U.S. Consumer Product Safety Commission
   4330 East West Highway
   Bethesda, MD 20814
   (800) 638-2772
   http://www.cpsc.gov
Water Awareness in Residential Neighborhoods
   5351 East Thompson, #138
   Indianapolis, IN 46237
   (317) 536-1874
   http://www.warnonline.org

Chapter Quiz

1. Unintentional injuries are the leading cause of death for what age group(s) in the United States?

2. True or False: Most injuries have predictable and preventable components.

3. List five reasons why EMS providers should be involved in injury prevention.

4. Why are data imperative for injury prevention efforts? Who looks at the data?

5. Give an example of a teachable moment unique to the paramedic profession.

6. The five *E*'s of injury prevention are:

7. Give an example of a grassroots community group and what role it might play in a community prevention effort.

Questions 8 to 18 describe different situations that result in injuries to children. A list of injury prevention strategies is provided. Next to each question, write the letter(s) of the strategy(ies) that could prevent the injury from occurring or reduce the severity of the injury. Each question may have more than one answer.

Injury Prevention Strategies

A. Mandatory flame-retardant sleepwear for children
B. Separate bike trails and road traffic with cement medians
C. A low-cost child car seat program for newborns and toddlers
D. Media campaign to promote safe storage of firearms
E. Enforcement of bicycle helmet law for riders younger than 14 years
F. Required fencing around private pools
G. Required window railings on upper-story windows
H. Stop! Drop! Roll! School education programs
I. Firearm and hunter safety program
J. Required safety helmets during youth equestrian events
K. Education and public awareness campaign about childhood pedestrian safety

8. _____ A 13-year-old unhelmeted bicycle passenger is killed in a crash.

9. _____ A child on a bike falls from a curb into traffic.

10. _____ A 7-year-old boy darts out from parked cars onto a busy street and is hit by a moving car.

11. _____ An unsupervised toddler falls from a second-story apartment window.

12. _____ A 7-year-old boy plays with his dad's loaded, unsecured gun and shoots a friend.

13. _____ A 2-year-old is unrestrained and killed in a motor vehicle crash.

14. _____ An unsupervised 2-year-old drowns in a neighbor's backyard pool.

15. _____ A newborn is ejected from a vehicle during an accident and dies.

16. _____ A 10-year-old is cooking breakfast and her pajamas catch on fire.

17. _____ A 12-year-old sustains a head injury from a fall while riding a horse.

18. _____ An 8-year-old shoots a pellet gun at his younger brother, causing an eye injury.

Terminology

Chronology The arrangement of events in time.

Epidemiology The study of the causes, patterns, prevalence, and control of disease in groups of people.

Epidemiologist Medical professional who studies the causes, distribution, and control of disease in populations.

Injury Intentional or unintentional damage to a person that resulted from acute exposure to thermal, mechanical, electrical, or chemical energy or from the absence of such essentials as heat or oxygen.

Injury risk A real or potential hazardous situation that puts individuals at risk for sustaining an injury.

Injury surveillance An ongoing systematic collection, analysis, and interpretation of injury data essential to the planning, implementation, and evaluation of public health practice, closely integrated with the timely dissemination of the data to those who need to know.

Intentional injury Injuries and deaths self-inflicted or perpetrated by another person, usually involving some type of violence.

Morbidity Nonfatal injury rates.

Mortality Death rate.

Primary injury prevention Keeping an injury from occurring.

Secondary injury prevention Preventing further injury from an event that has already occurred.

Teachable moment The time just after an injury has occurred when the patient and observers remain acutely aware of what has happened and may be more receptive to learning how the event or illness could have been prevented.

Unintentional injury Injuries and deaths not self-inflicted or perpetrated by another person (accidents).

Years of potential life lost (YPLL) A method that assumes that, on average, most people will live a productive life until the age of 65 years.

Legal and Regulatory Issues

Objectives *After completing this chapter, you will be able to:*

1. Distinguish legal from ethical responsibilities.
2. Describe the basic structure of the legal system in the United States.
3. Distinguish administrative, civil, and criminal law as they pertain to the paramedic.
4. Identify and explain the importance of laws relevant to the paramedic.
5. Define the following terms:
   - Abandonment
   - Advance directives
   - Assault
   - Battery
   - Breach of duty
   - Causation
   - Confidentiality
   - Consent (expressed, implied, informed, involuntary)
   - Damages
   - Defamation
   - Do not resuscitate orders
   - Duty to act
   - Emancipated minor
   - False imprisonment
   - Immunity
   - Invasion of privacy
   - Liability
   - Libel
   - Medical practice act
   - Minor
   - Negligence
   - Scope of practice
   - Slander
   - Standard of care
   - Tort (intentional, unintentional)
6. Distinguish the scope of practice from the standard of care for paramedic practice.
7. Discuss the concept of medical direction, including offline and online medical direction, and its relation to the standard of care of a paramedic.
8. Distinguish licensure from certification as they apply to the paramedic.
9. Explain the concept of liability as applied to paramedic practice, including physicians providing medical direction and paramedics supervising other care providers.
10. List the specific problems or conditions that paramedics are required to report. Identify in each instance to whom the report is made.
11. Describe the four elements that must be present to prove negligence.
12. Given a scenario in which a patient is injured while a paramedic is providing care, determine whether the four components of negligence are present.
13. Given a scenario, identify patient care behaviors that would protect the paramedic from claims of negligence.
14. Discuss the legal concept of immunity, including Good Samaritan statutes and governmental immunity, as it applies to the paramedic.
15. Distinguish assault from battery and describe how to avoid each.
16. Describe the differences between expressed, informed, implied, and involuntary consent.
17. Given a scenario in which a paramedic is presented with a conscious patient in need of care, describe the process used to obtain consent.
18. Identify the steps to take if a patient refuses care.
19. Given a refusal of care scenario, demonstrate appropriate patient management and care techniques.
20. Describe what constitutes abandonment.
21. Identify the legal issues involved in the decision to reduce the level of care being provided during transportation.
22. Explain the importance and necessity of patient confidentiality and the standards for maintaining patient confidentiality that apply to the paramedic.
23. Describe the conditions under which the use of force, including restraint, is acceptable.
24. Identify the legal issues involved in the decision not to transport a patient.
25. Describe how hospitals are selected to receive patients based on patient need and hospital capability as well as the paramedic's role in such selection.
26. Explain the purpose of advance directives as they relate to patient care and how paramedics should care for a patient who is covered by an advance directive.
27. Discuss your responsibilities regarding resuscitation efforts for patients who are potential organ donors.
28. Describe the actions you should take to preserve evidence at a crime or accident scene.
29. Describe the importance of providing accurate documentation (oral and written) in substantiating an incident.
30. Describe the required characteristics of a prehospital care report for it to be considered an effective legal document.
31. Given a scenario, prepare a prehospital care report, including an appropriately detailed narrative.

Chapter Outline

Case Scenario

You are an advanced life support fire department first-response paramedic. You and your engine company respond to a "rollover accident with injuries." When you arrive you find a new-looking Ford Mustang in a dry creek bed approximately 100 feet off the highway down a 35-foot embankment. The vehicle's roof appears caved in and the car has significant damage down the entire side. A man who appears to be in his early twenties is leaning against the driver's side of the car picking glass out of a large abrasion on his left forearm. As you approach you see that he is somewhat pale and appears to be breathing hard. He informs you that he took the corner too fast and rolled the car down the embankment. He states that he is the only person involved in the car accident.

Questions

1. What is your general impression of this patient?
2. What additional assessment will be important in the evaluation of this patient?
3. What intervention should you initiate at this time?

[handwritten: federal law > state law > local law]

[handwritten: Statutory law = established by groups. administrative law = changes to established law]

[OBJECTIVE 1]

Jurisprudence is the theory and philosophy of law. Paramedics have legal duties and ethical responsibilities. Your legal duties are defined by **statutes** and regulations and are based on generally accepted standards. You have legal duties to the patient, medical director, and public. Paramedics also must uphold many ethical responsibilities (see Chapter 5). Ethics are moral principles based on societal standards that identify desirable conduct. The ethical responsibilities of paramedics are identified in Box 4-1.

BOX 4-1   Ethical Responsibilities of a Paramedic

- Being dedicated to the profession of paramedicine
- Treating patients with dignity and respect
- Being obliged to care for the physical and emotional needs of patients
- Maintaining and mastering clinical skills
- Participating in continuing education and refresher training
- Critically reviewing your performance and continuously seeking to improve your care
- Reporting honestly
- Respecting privacy and confidentiality of patients
- Working cooperatively and with respect for other emergency professionals
- Respecting the wishes and desires of patients

THE LEGAL SYSTEM

[OBJECTIVE 2]

Paramedics, like other healthcare providers, must operate within the legal system. This system is composed of many levels—local, state, and federal. Different types of law also exist, such as criminal, civil, and administrative.

In addition, paramedics must abide by operational policies, clinical protocols, and other state and/or local requirements that govern their practice. EMS law comes from the three branches of government. The legislative branch includes, for example, Congress and the state legislatures. This branch is the source of **statutory law**. The judicial branch includes state and federal courts. This branch is the source of **case law**. Finally, the executive branch includes the state governors and the administrative agencies that make regulations. This branch is the source of **administrative law**.

[handwritten: common law]

PARAMEDIC Pearl

In the legal process, a trial court determines the outcome of individual cases. Cases may be decided by a judge or jury. An appellate court has the power to review the decisions by trial courts or other appeals courts. Decisions made by an appellate court may set precedent for later cases based on similar legal issues and facts.

Local, State, and Federal Regulation of Paramedic Practice

The regulation of paramedic practice at the local level generally consists of ordinances, rules, regulations, or protocols. These items concern issues such as response times, clinical practice, and patient destination. The requirements for paramedic performance and EMS system operations may also be defined by contracts between ambulance services and local governmental agencies.

At the state level, paramedic practice is typically regulated by laws and regulations that deal with the certification or licensing of providers, ambulance service licensing, provider scope of practice, handling and storage of controlled substances, disciplinary enforcement, and related issues. Most regulation regarding advance directives and do not resuscitate (DNR) issues occur at the state level.

At the federal level, regulation of paramedic practice and EMS includes highly technical and complex laws and regulations. These laws and regulations pertain to reimbursement for ambulance services (Medicare), as well as patient privacy and confidentiality, including the security of electronic information (the Health Insurance Portability and Accountability Act [HIPPA]). Federal law also addresses issues of patient destination and hospital diversion (the Emergency Medical Treatment and Active Labor Act [**EMTALA**]).

Administrative, Civil, and Criminal Law

[OBJECTIVE 3]

Laws and regulations generally fall under the headings of administrative, civil, or criminal.

Administrative Law

Administrative law consists of rules and regulations that come from governmental agencies, such as a state EMS office, or a federal agency, such as the Centers for Medicare and Medicaid Services (CMS). CMS establishes reimbursement policy and regulations. The right of the governmental agency to create rules and regulations results when a legislative body passes a statutory law that gives an agency the right to create rules and regulations (administrative law) that govern a particular activity. In the case of EMS, this often is the state EMS act. This act often outlines the goals and objectives of the state but charges an agency with putting it into practice. Administrative agencies, usually state EMS offices, typically hold the authority to impose disciplinary sanctions. These may include revoking or suspending a provider's certification for unprofessional conduct or the violation of applicable laws or regulations pertaining to paramedic practice.

One key concept of administrative law is the idea of **due process**. Administrative agencies seeking to

discipline a licensed or certified provider must do so by giving him or her, at a minimum, notice of the charges and/or proposed disciplinary action and a chance to be heard regarding those charges. This usually occurs through a written complaint or similar document followed by an opportunity for a hearing. State law then typically affords certain appeal rights to providers who disagree with the disciplinary decision of the administrative agency.

Civil Law

Civil law is an area of law that deals with private complaints brought by a **plaintiff** (typically an injured party seeking redress) against a **defendant** (the party against whom liability is sought) for wrongdoing (tort). **Tort** is the legal word for a "wrong" under the law. Torts can be either unintentional or intentional and are explained in more detail later in this chapter. Civil law concerns itself with issues such as professional malpractice. It is typically enforced through the court system, most often at the state level. Penalties generally include fines.

Criminal Law

Criminal law is an area of law in which an individual is prosecuted on behalf of society for violating laws designed to safeguard society. Criminal laws are enforced by the local, state, or federal government. Penalties can include fines and imprisonment. Criminal law plays an increasingly common role in EMS. It may be relevant in issues of vehicle operations and drug diversion.

> **PARAMEDIC*Pearl***
>
> Most civil and criminal cases are heard in state courts. The case is first heard by a state trial court. An appeal may be reviewed by state courts of appeal and, finally, the supreme court of the state.

Paramedic Scope of Practice

[OBJECTIVES 4, 5, 6]

Paramedics operate under a **scope of practice.** A scope of practice is a predefined set of skills, interventions, or other activities that the paramedic is authorized to perform. The paramedic scope of practice is typically defined at the state level. However, in many states local EMS systems and physician medical directors are given substantial control over the clinical practice of paramedics.

The paramedic scope of practice is typically determined by many documents at many levels. For instance, the National Highway Traffic Safety Administration (NHTSA) publishes the National Standard Curriculum for paramedic training (NHTSA, 1998). States then typically adopt their own standards and paramedic scope of practice. The scope of practice often is defined in state laws, regulations, or protocols.

The paramedic's scope of practice should be distinguished from the concept of the **standard of care.** The standard of care relates to professional malpractice claims and is covered in more detail later in this chapter. In brief, the standard of care in a malpractice or negligence case is the conduct that is expected of a reasonably prudent paramedic under similar circumstances.

PARAMEDIC*Pearl*

The concepts of scope of practice and standard of care often are confused. Think of scope of practice as a description of what you *legally* can and cannot do as a paramedic. The difference between the general public, other healthcare professionals, and you is your paramedic scope of practice. Doing something outside your scope of practice is illegal, and you can face criminal prosecution. On the other hand, the standard of care addresses your competency and professional judgment as a paramedic. Failing to do the right thing or doing the right thing but failing to do it properly can result in civil prosecution.

Medical Direction

[OBJECTIVE 7]

Medical direction, or physician oversight of paramedic practice, is a vital and longstanding part of the EMS system. Medical direction and physician oversight of paramedics typically occur prospectively (before care), concurrently (during care), or retrospectively (after care). Medical direction can occur both online and offline. It may even be practiced as a combination of these approaches (see Chapter 2).

Prospective medical direction includes the development of clinical practice standards. These standards include items such as training curricula and protocols. These standards establish, in advance, the parameters in which paramedics can practice. They also define the expectations that EMS providers must satisfy in the delivery of patient care. Often these documents also define the paramedic scope of practice. In some parts of the country, medical directors have the authority to discipline a paramedic for violations of clinical standards or remove a paramedic from clinical practice.

Concurrent medical direction occurs when a paramedic consults a physician or other advanced healthcare professional by telephone, radio, or other electronic means during the delivery of patient care or transport. Such consultation permits the physician and paramedic to work together to decide on the best patient care. Technologic advances continually affect the delivery of concurrent medical direction. For example, the ability to transmit real-time video and clinical information in digital form will improve the accuracy and timeliness of clinical decision making.

Retrospective medical direction occurs after the fact, or after patient care has been delivered. This type of medical direction is typically achieved through quality improvement programs, case reviews, and similar approaches. Retrospective medical direction allows paramedics and their medical directors to evaluate the effectiveness of the care given. It also allows them to discover ways to improve skills, protocols, or other aspects of patient care.

Licensure and Certification

[OBJECTIVES 8, 9]

Paramedics are typically licensed or certified at the state level. However, additional qualifications or credentials may be required at the local level. In the past, much has been made of the difference between licensure and certification. However, licensure and certification have few differences from a practical perspective. Both typically involve some minimal training or educational requirements (such as completing a set number of hours of training in an accredited training or educational program). Both also typically involve a minimal level of demonstrated proficiency (such as achieving a minimal score on a written test or practical skills evaluation).

One broad difference between licensure and certification is that **licensure** often is thought of as recognition of minimal competency and the completion of prescribed education or training. **Certification** is often viewed as evidence of competency in certain skills or tasks. Some also believe licensure holds more professional esteem than certification, but this is largely subjective. Generally little difference in salary, scope of practice, or other aspects of paramedicine exists between the provider who is licensed and the one who is certified.

Although this varies by state, paramedics are periodically required to recertify or renew their licenses. In some states, this is done by attaining a minimal number of hours of continuing education. In other states, paramedics can renew their credentials through testing or some other evaluation method.

State laws vary on this subject, but saying that paramedics practice "under" a physician's license is generally inaccurate. This concept of the paramedic's authority being derived from a physician was popular in the early days of paramedicine. However, this concept is outdated and inaccurate today for the most part. Paramedic certification or licensure brings with it a discrete scope of practice and legal authority to provide care. This, of course, is subject to individual state laws that grant physicians the authority to approve or oversee paramedic practice. Paramedics are independently licensed or certified professionals. They are subject to the physician direction or oversight granted to medical directors under the law.

In a similar vein, paramedics cannot generally confer (grant) a higher scope of practice to basic life support providers. For instance, a paramedic cannot permit an emergency medical technician (EMT) to intubate a patient under the paramedic's direction if the action exceeds the EMT's scope of practice. The EMT may certainly assist the

[Handwritten notes top margin: Child, elder, sexual — Document which nurse you told. Also call hotline]

paramedic as long as it is within the EMT's scope of practice. However, the EMT cannot violate his or her own scope of practice.

Medical Practice Acts

[Handwritten note: 47 states require national registry (not IL yet)]

State **medical practice acts** regulate the practice of medicine by physicians. Such laws vary from state to state. These laws may address the ability of physicians to delegate certain tasks to nonphysician practitioners, including paramedics. State EMS laws and regulations generally provide more detail in this area. You should be familiar with any limits or restrictions placed on physicians in your jurisdiction and their power to delegate certain tasks.

Motor Vehicle Laws

Paramedics who work in the prehospital setting are typically involved in operating emergency vehicles. These vehicles include ambulances, fire engines, paramedic response vehicles, and bicycles. States typically regulate emergency vehicle operations, usually as part of the state's motor vehicle code. Additional laws may be found in the state's EMS act or similar law.

The laws pertaining to the operation of emergency vehicles vary widely by state. Some states permit emergency vehicles to exceed the posted speed limits; some do not. Some states grant other special privileges to emergency vehicles. Most state laws also affect the drivers of other motor vehicles overtaken by an emergency vehicle using its flashing lights and/or audible warning devices. For example, drivers are typically required to yield to emergency vehicles, grant them the right of way, slow down, and pull to the right side of the road.

Regardless of what special privileges may or may not exist for emergency vehicles under state law or regulations, operators of emergency vehicles must drive with due regard for the safety of their crew, the patient, and the public at large. Several emergency vehicle operators have been charged with criminal violations of state vehicle laws, including vehicular manslaughter, negligent homicide, and reckless driving. Lights and sirens do not excuse emergency vehicle operators from their responsibilities to drive safely and within the law.

PARAMEDIC Pearl

State laws and regulations may address the use of flashing lights and audible warning devices. In general, lights and sirens are overused and do not usually save time in any clinically significant fashion in EMS. When weighed against the hazards and liability they create, lights and sirens should be used sparingly and with caution. In addition, emergency vehicle operators should be appropriately trained and experienced in proper driving techniques, which is required in some states.

Mandatory Reporting Requirements

[OBJECTIVE 10]

As mandated by state laws, paramedics in many parts of the country must report certain injuries or conditions to the appropriate authorities. For instance, many states require that paramedics and other healthcare professionals report instances of suspected child abuse to law enforcement or other designated child protection agencies. Some states also require the reporting of suspected elder abuse, animal bites, injuries inflicted with firearms, and burns.

The laws regarding mandatory reporting requirements vary by state. Be sure to learn the applicable laws of your state regarding mandatory reporting. Where state laws require certain injuries or illnesses to be reported, HIPAA (the federal law and regulations dealing with patient privacy) permits those disclosures to be made. HIPAA is covered in more detail later in this chapter.

LEGAL ACCOUNTABILITY FOR THE PARAMEDIC
Liability and Malpractice

[OBJECTIVES 11, 12, 13]

[Handwritten note: Negligence 1. Have duty to act 2. Breached duty 3. Injury occurred 4. you caused injury (proximate cause)]

Liability is the legal responsibility of a party for the consequences of his or her acts or omissions. **Professional malpractice** actions are among the most common types of legal actions in which paramedics and other EMS providers may become involved. Professional malpractice is a type of tort case that addresses whether the paramedic was negligent. **Negligence** is defined as the failure to act as a reasonably prudent and careful person would act under similar circumstances. If a paramedic is sued in a malpractice case, he or she is referred to as the defendant. The injured party who brings the lawsuit is the plaintiff. An injured plaintiff typically has a limit to the amount of time in which he or she can initiate a lawsuit seeking damages for an injury. That period is the **statute of limitations** and varies by state.

A negligence lawsuit alleging medical malpractice by a paramedic falls under the heading of an **unintentional tort.** An unintentional tort is one that the defendant did not mean to commit; it is simply a case in which a bad outcome occurred as a result of the failure to use reasonable care. In addition, negligence also can be found on the part of the injured plaintiff. This is called **contributory negligence.** In some states, contributory negligence can reduce the amount of monetary damages awarded to a plaintiff who prevails in a tort case.

Regardless of the level of training, certification, or licensure held by the healthcare provider, a plaintiff must prove four elements to impose malpractice liability on a healthcare provider in a negligence case (Box 4-2).

BOX 4-2   Components of Negligence

1. Duty
2. Breach of duty
3. Damages
4. Causation

Duty

The first element that must be established in a malpractice case is the existence of a legal duty, also referred to as a **duty to act**. The plaintiff must establish that the defendant had a legal obligation to the plaintiff. Having a legal duty typically means that the paramedic must act with due regard for the patient and uphold the applicable standard of care.

Ordinarily, a paramedic who is part of an ambulance service or other EMS crew dispatched or called to assist a person in need has formed a legal relationship with that person. That, in turn, gives rise to a legal duty under the law of negligence. To the contrary, a healthcare provider who happens on the scene of an accident as a passerby and who was not summoned to the scene as part of his or her job duties typically does not have a legal duty to act. Of course, whether the provider is compelled to act out of a sense of *moral* duty is an entirely different matter.

Breach of Duty

The second element of negligence in a malpractice case is a **breach of duty**. A breach of duty means that the paramedic must be found to have violated the standard of care applicable to the circumstances. The standard of care is, generally speaking, what the reasonably prudent paramedic would do under similar circumstances. Therefore the standard of care is measured objectively, rather than subjectively, in a malpractice case. Courts and juries are not permitted to use "20-20 hindsight" in evaluating whether a paramedic acted reasonably. They must judge whether the paramedic acted reasonably under the circumstances as they were presented at the time and not after the fact.

A breach of duty can occur by **malfeasance** (performing a wrongful act), **misfeasance** (performing a legal act in a harmful manner), or **nonfeasance** (failure to perform a required act or duty).

Evidence of the standard of care can come from many sources (Box 4-3). Violation of an applicable law or regulation by the paramedic can constitute **negligence per se.** In general, this means that the plaintiff can establish negligence without needing to prove what would be reasonable and prudent under similar circumstances. The law also recognizes the principle of **res ipsa loquitur,** which means "the thing speaks for itself." This type of liability can be imposed when an injury could only have been caused by a negligent act. A classic example is a surgical sponge being left inside a patient after surgery. An EMS example might involve a patient who is strapped to a stretcher and completely under the paramedic's

BOX 4-3   How Is a Paramedic's Standard of Care Determined?

- Scope of practice
- EMS protocols
- Applicable EMS policies or procedures
- National standard curriculum
- Literature (journals, EMS textbooks)
- Expert witnesses
- Juries

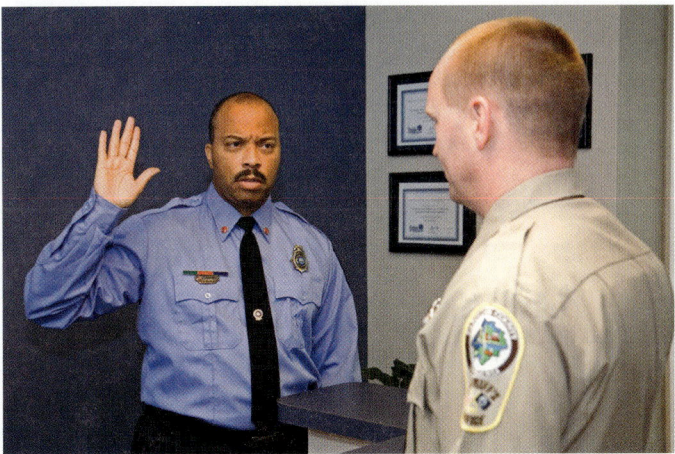

Figure 4-1 Paramedics are sworn in to give testimony, just as any witness.

control. The stretcher is overturned, resulting in facial injuries to the patient. Such acts do not occur without negligence.

Other sources of the standard of care can be protocols or applicable policies or procedures. Documents such as the national standard curriculum or EMS textbooks such as this one can also be used to establish evidence of the standard of care. In most cases, evidence of the standard of care, and its violation by a paramedic or other healthcare provider, is established in court through the testimony of one or more expert witnesses (Figure 4-1).

Damages

The third element that a plaintiff must prove in a malpractice case against a paramedic is **damages,** which refers to compensable harm or other losses incurred by the plaintiff because of the negligence of the defendant. The remedy for damages in a malpractice case is money—financial compensation to the injured party. Many types of damages can be awarded in a malpractice case, including pain and suffering, medical expenses, funeral expenses, and wage loss. In extreme cases, courts can award punitive (punishing) damages against a defendant. Punitive damages can be awarded in some states to punish gross negligence or willful and wanton misconduct. Most insurance policies will not cover punitive damage awards. They will, however, cover damages arising from ordinary negligence up to the coverage limits of the policy.

Causation

The fourth element a plaintiff must prove to bring a successful malpractice case against a paramedic is **causation** (also known as *proximate cause*). Simply put, *causation* means that the defendant's negligence must have caused or created the harm to the plaintiff. To be a legal cause of a plaintiff's harm, a defendant's negligent conduct must ordinarily be a substantial factor in causing that type of harm.

A plaintiff's harm can have more than one legal cause. Moreover, one defendant's actions do not excuse the negligence of another defendant. For instance, a patient who is first injured in an assault by another person, and then is the victim of medical malpractice by the responding paramedics, would have a viable tort claim against the person who assaulted him as well as a viable negligence claim against the paramedics.

Defenses and Immunity Laws

[OBJECTIVE 14]

Paramedics and other EMS providers can be sued for malpractice or any number of other types of cases, but most states have laws that offer some defense in cases of ordinary negligence. Many state EMS laws contain **immunity** provisions. These provisions protect paramedics for acts of ordinary negligence or acts or omissions done in good faith. Immunity is the protection from legal liability in accordance with applicable laws. Good Samaritan laws also may offer protection in some cases, though these laws ordinarily exist for the benefit of individuals who aided an injured person but otherwise had no legal duty to do so. These laws may apply to volunteer paramedics.

willful & wanton added to a Good Sam law

Paramedics who work for public agencies also may have a form of local government immunity when acting within the course and scope of their official duties.

Regardless of whether your state has immunity laws on the books, most such laws offer protection only when the paramedic acts in good faith and only for acts of ordinary negligence. These laws do not usually offer protection for acts of gross negligence.

Although relatively few cases against paramedics go to trial, an individual paramedic is certainly entitled to put up a vigorous defense in a malpractice case. Most often this defense involves attacking the elements of breach of duty or causation in court (i.e., whether the standard of care was violated and/or whether any breach of a standard of care was the legal cause of the plaintiff's harm). Most EMS organizations carry malpractice insurance (called *professional liability insurance*). Under those policies, the insurer (provided it is given prompt notice of the claim) must provide a defense for the organization's paramedics in malpractice cases. As part of that defense, the insurer must typically hire a lawyer to represent the interests of the paramedic. Some paramedics or EMS organizations still retain their own personal lawyer to oversee these types of cases along with the lawyer hired by the insurer.

PARAMEDIC *Pearl*

The difference between ordinary and gross negligence can be subjective. This is most often decided by a judge relatively early in a court case. Paramedics and other EMS professionals should not think of immunity statutes as a hammock on which they can rest, but as a safety net on which they can rely if necessary.

Case Scenario—continued

The patient states that he was not wearing a seatbelt and that he "found himself" outside the vehicle after the accident. In addition to the left forearm abrasion he has a laceration above the right eye. When you ask a colleague to initiate manual spinal immobilization the patient waves him off and bluntly states "I'm not going to the hospital. Period." The transporting ambulance arrives and you work with the paramedic to complete the survey. The patient has a broad abrasion across the right chest that is tender to palpation, and breath sounds may be diminished in the area. He also reports some pain in his lower back. Vital signs are pulse, 124 beats/min; blood pressure, 128/82 mm Hg; and respirations, 24 breaths/min. No evidence is present of alcohol or drug use. As you and the ambulance paramedic find each of these injuries, you explain their potential severity to the patient. He maintains his wish to not be transported to the hospital.

Questions

4. *What are this patient's potential injuries?*
5. *What additional treatment should be initiated?*
6. *If the patient continues to refuse after your best effort to convince him, should you leave him at the scene or transport him against his will? Why?*
7. *What strategies should be used to attempt to convince the patient to accept treatment and transport?*
8. *What role, if any, does the base hospital physician play in this situation?*

Intentional Torts

[OBJECTIVE 15]

In addition to the unintentional tort of negligence, paramedics also can be subject to intentional torts. **Intentional torts** are wrongs in which the defendant meant to cause the harmful action (Box 4-4).

Battery is touching or making contact with another person without that person's consent. **Assault** is a threat of imminent bodily harm to another person by someone with the obvious ability to carry out the threat. **False imprisonment** is the confinement or restraint of a person against his or her will or without appropriate legal justification. The principles of informed consent, covered later in this chapter, are important for the paramedic because consent is a defense to the torts of battery and false imprisonment.

Invasion of privacy refers to disclosing or publishing personal or private facts about a person to a person or persons not authorized to receive such information. **Libel** and **slander** are torts that fall under the heading of **defamation.** Defamation is the publication of false information about a person that tends to blacken the person's character or injure his or her reputation. Libel occurs in written form, and slander occurs in spoken form.

Special Liability Issues

In addition to liability from both unintentional and intentional torts, paramedics and others in the EMS system can face liability in a host of other situations. Paramedics who work for public agencies (such as city or county EMS systems) may, in addition to incurring tort liability, also face liability under civil rights laws. For instance, federal laws prohibit discriminating against individuals on the basis of race, age, gender, and other protected classifications. You must be sensitive not to discriminate while providing care to any patient based on such protected classifications.

In addition, others in the EMS system can incur "derivative" liability for the acts of a negligent paramedic. For instance, a medical director or online physician can be named in a malpractice lawsuit along with the paramedic. The paramedic's ambulance service or EMS organization can also be named as a defendant under the doctrine of **respondeat superior**. This doctrine holds that the "master" is liable for the acts of his "servant."

BOX 4-4	**Examples of Intentional Torts**

- Assault
- Battery
- False imprisonment
- Invasion of privacy
- Libel
- Slander

PARAMEDIC-PATIENT RELATIONSHIPS

Consent and Refusal of Care

Consent

[OBJECTIVES 16, 17]

A competent patient is entitled to make decisions about the care he or she wishes to receive. However, in some cases patients are unable to make informed decisions about their condition or treatment. Moreover, in some cases the law provides other ways in which emergency medical providers can obtain permission to provide care.

A competent patient, or the patient's legally responsible decision maker, can give **consent**, or informed permission, for care and/or transportation by EMS providers. For consent to be valid, it must be informed (Box 4-5). That is, the patient must be given enough information to make an informed decision on whether to accept a particular course of treatment. The patient must ordinarily be given the information that a reasonable person would find relevant to his or her medical decision making. This also depends on what is reasonable under the circumstances.

The patient or responsible decision maker must also be competent to grant consent for care or refuse it. A person must be legally competent, meaning that he or she is old enough to grant consent (typically aged 18 years). A person also must be mentally competent (i.e., able to understand the information given to him or her and make an informed decision regarding healthcare).

Consent can be expressed or implied. A patient or his or her responsible decision maker can give **expressed consent** either verbally or through some physical expression of consent. Nonverbal expressions of consent may include, for example, a nod of the head or rolling up the sleeve to allow an intravenous line to be started. If the patient's legally responsible decision maker is not present at the scene (e.g., a minor's parents are at work), the legally responsible decision maker can give consent by telephone as long as that person is properly informed of the patient's condition and the risks and benefits, as previously discussed.

BOX 4-5	**Informed Consent**

The patient or responsible decision maker must be properly informed about the following:
- Nature of the illness or injury
- Treatment recommended
- Benefits of treatment
- Risks and dangers of treatment
- Alternative treatment possible and associated risks
- Dangers of refusing treatment (including transport)

In a true emergency, a patient can be given treatment under the doctrine of implied consent. With **implied consent**, you may presume that a patient who is ill or injured and, for any reason (e.g., unconscious, incapacitated, patient is a minor) unable to give consent, would consent to receiving the necessary emergency care for his or her condition.

Involuntary consent may seem to be a contradiction in terms. It describes a situation in which care is provided to a person under specific legal authority, even if the person does not consent to the care. For instance, many states have laws permitting a patient who poses a threat to himself or others to be involuntarily treated or committed for observation for a limited period. In addition, the consent for the emergency care of prisoners or those in custody of law enforcement, prison, or a correctional institution can be given by those with lawful custody of the inmate or prisoner.

A competent patient who gives consent can later withdraw that consent. He or she can do so as long as he or she is properly informed of the risks involved.

PARAMEDIC*Pearl*

The principles of consent and refusal of care are important to understand and apply in your daily activities as a paramedic. Consent for medical care is important because, without it, you can be subjected to claims of battery, false imprisonment, or negligence. For instance, battery (under civil law) is an intentional tort that can arise from a nonconsensual touching of or contact with another person. Because consent—whether expressed or implied—is a defense to a battery action, you must obtain consent and document that consent on the prehospital care report.

When treating a **minor** (who, in most states, is defined as a person younger than 18 years), you must recall that they do not have the authority to consent for medical treatment or refuse care. Although some states do permit certain minors to make medical decisions, state law varies widely on this subject. Be sure to check your state's law regarding the right of minors to consent for medical care.

A term often used in healthcare, sometimes incorrectly, is **emancipated minor**. An emancipated minor is typically a self-supporting minor. Two common factors that apply here are marriage and active duty with the armed forces. Other factors vary widely from state to state. Often the minor must receive an actual court order of emancipation for this status. Research your own state laws regarding emancipation.

Parents or legal guardians typically can give consent for a minor. In some states government agencies having custody of a minor may grant consent for medical care. For instance, school officials may grant consent for emergency healthcare for a minor under the principle of *parens patriae*. Literally translated, this phrase means, "parent of

the country." In more practical terms, this refers to the role of the state as guardian of persons under a legal disability, such as juveniles. The doctrine of *parens patriae* also extends to governmental child services organizations with custody over a minor (e.g., children in foster care).

A competent adult can appoint a legal representative with a document called a power of attorney (also referred to as a healthcare power of attorney or durable power of attorney). The person appointed to act as the patient's legal representative is typically called the *agent*. The agent is, subject to state law, permitted to exercise the powers granted in the power of attorney document. Adults can also have court-appointed legal guardians. These persons are authorized to make medical decisions on the adult's behalf.

Some states have laws that grant other family members the ability to make healthcare decisions for an incompetent or incapacitated patient. For instance, some state laws grant authority to a spouse, son or daughter, sibling, or other relative to make emergency decisions for an incapacitated person in need of healthcare.

Refusal of Care
[OBJECTIVES 18, 19]

Closely related to the idea of patient consent is the concept of "refusal of care." The basic rule is that a competent patient (or legally responsible decision maker) who is properly informed of the risks of not receiving treatment and the benefits of treatment is permitted to refuse medical care and/or transportation. This even includes refusing lifesaving emergency care.

In any refusal situation, you must determine whether the patient is both legally and mentally competent to make an informed refusal decision. In addition, you must determine that the patient understands the risks of refusal. Any patient refusal of care should be carefully documented. The minimal documentation that must be completed for refusals of care is shown in Box 4-6. The patient or legally responsible decision maker also should be asked to sign a refusal of care form that includes a release of liability (Figure 4-2).

BOX 4-6   Minimal Documentation Requirements for Refusals of Care

- A record of the patient's mental status
- Findings of the paramedic's assessment of the patient
- Details about any potential mechanism of injury or present illness
- Specific risks discussed with the patient and the patient's understanding of those risks
- Involvement of any medical direction in the refusal
- Signature of patient or legally responsible decision maker on refusal of care form that includes a release of liability

REFUSAL OF SERVICES

I hereby refuse the emergency medical services and/or transportation offered and advised by the above named service provider and its emergency personnel, _____ hospital, and the emergency medical and nursing personnel from said hospital giving directions to the service provider. I understand that my refusal may jeopardize the health of the patient, and hereby release the above named parties from any and all claims of liability in connection with my refusal.

_____
Signature of Patient or Legally Authorized Representative

_____
Signature of EMT

_____   _____
Witness   Date

Figure 4-2 Patient refusal form.

Abandonment

[OBJECTIVES 20, 21]

In EMS, patient **abandonment** is the withdrawal by a paramedic or other EMS provider from the care of a person who requires emergency medical attention without making arrangements for care to be transferred to another qualified provider. Patient abandonment lawsuits are rare but can occur.

In cases in which the patient does not require medical assistance, the patient terminates the relationship, or patient care is transferred to another medical provider, patient abandonment does not occur. Abandonment is chiefly confined to the situation in which a patient requires care and the provider terminates the relationship with the patient without making proper arrangements for the care to be assumed by another appropriate provider.

PARAMEDIC Pearl

A misconception in EMS exists that transferring care to a provider with less training or certification constitutes abandonment. That is not the case. In many instances in the delivery of healthcare, patients are referred from a "higher" level of care to a "lower" one. For instance, a physician may refer a patient to a physical therapist for further specialized care. A physician may leave the discharge instructions of a patient to a nurse or physician assistant for review with the patient. Similarly, in EMS, a paramedic may transfer care to an EMT or other basic life support–level provider if the patient has been assessed and determined not to need advanced life support interventions. Of course, this assessment and conclusion should be adequately documented on the prehospital care report.

Confidentiality and HIPAA

[OBJECTIVE 22]

Confidentiality is the protection of patient information in any form and the disclosure of that information only as needed for patient care or as otherwise permitted by law. State laws regarding the invasion of privacy and similar issues have long addressed this subject. However,

BOX 4-7	Examples of Individually Identifiable Health Information

- Name
- Address
- Employer
- Relatives' names
- Dates relating to patient
- Phone and fax numbers
- Finger or voice print
- Photograph
- Health plan beneficiary number
- E-mail address/Web site
- Social Security number
- Medical record number
- Employee or account number
- Vehicle or device number
- License numbers
- Any unique identifier or code

federal law now requires that almost every type of healthcare provider in the United States protect the privacy and security of patient information under HIPAA. This law requires that all individually identifiable health information (commonly referred to as *protected health information* [PHI]) be safeguarded and used only for purposes specifically permitted by the regulations (Box 4-7). For instance, HIPAA permits PHI to be used in treatment, payment, and healthcare operations. Providers involved in the care of the patient can freely share information among themselves for treatment purposes. Providers can use a patient's PHI to submit claims and invoices for their services. Providers may also use a patient's PHI—provided they use only the minimal amount of PHI necessary—for operational purposes, such as quality improvement and other management functions.

HIPAA greatly restricts the types of disclosures of PHI that you may make to law enforcement officers. For instance, you can share certain limited information with law enforcement, on their request, to identify or locate a suspect or a fugitive. The HIPAA privacy rule provides very detailed information about the situations in which a release of PHI to law enforcement is permitted. HIPAA also restricts the disclosure of PHI to the media and others.

Every entity or organization subject to HIPAA is required to have an appointed privacy officer. Such entities also are required to provide training to their entire workforce regarding the organization's privacy practices. Healthcare providers also are required, in most circumstances, to give patients a notice of privacy practices. Such a notice describes the organization's privacy policies and informs patients of their healthcare privacy rights.

PARAMEDIC*Pearl*

Protecting the confidentiality of patient information—whether in verbal form, written form, electronic form, or otherwise—is the responsibility of every paramedic and healthcare provider.

Patient Restraints

[OBJECTIVE 23]

As a paramedic, you may encounter violent patients or patients with physical or mental conditions. You may need to use restraints to care for these patients adequately. Restraints should be used only as a last resort when patients pose a threat to themselves or others. Make every verbal attempt to calm the patient before resorting to restraints. Moreover, do your best to avoid physical confrontation or placing yourself in a volatile situation. If the scene is not safe, request appropriate assistance, including law enforcement, so the scene can be made safe. Select the least intrusive type of restraint and restrain the patient no more than is necessary to protect the patient or others. Patient restraint use is defined by the following rules:

- They must be used cautiously.
- They must be used consistently with any applicable protocols.
- They must be used in a way that protects the patient and preserves his or her dignity to the maximal extent possible.

Patient restraints may be physical or chemical. **Physical restraints** include straps, splints, and other devices that prevent movement of all or part of the patient's body. **Chemical** or **pharmacologic restraints** include agents such as sedatives that can suppress a patient's neurologic and/or motor capabilities. The use of chemical restraints can reduce the threat the patient poses to you.

Use of patient restraints should be guided by medical control—either online, offline, or both. Medically valid protocols or other policies on patient restraint should be in place to govern the use of restraints in the field. The use of restraints should be carefully documented on the patient care report. This documentation should

include the reasons that restraints were needed, the efforts aimed at avoiding the use of restraints, the type of restraints used, the duration that the restraints were used, the patient's response to the restraints, and other key factors.

Carefully monitor the patient's condition when restraints are used. Pay extremely careful attention to preventing positional asphyxia and other life-threatening complications that can arise. Patients should never be restrained in a manner that compromises or impairs their respiratory or circulatory functions or that could cause permanent injury. Ensure you have enough personnel whenever patient restraint is required. The literature generally recommends a minimum of four providers (one for each extremity) to restrain a patient safely.

PATIENT DISPOSITION AND DESTINATION ISSUES

Transport

[OBJECTIVE 24]

The majority of EMS responses end in the transport of a patient to a hospital emergency department or similar receiving facility. In such cases, a competent patient should ordinarily be given a choice of facility. However, that choice is, of course, subject to reasonable limitations. For example, a patient ordinarily needs only to be transported to a local hospital or approved receiving facility; if a patient wishes to be transported to a long-distance destination and the transport would deprive a community of valuable emergency resources, the patient should be transported to a local hospital. The patient is then free to make private arrangements for transportation to the facility of his or her choice.

Document the transfer of care on the patient care report. At a minimum, document the destination to which the patient was transported, the time of arrival, and the patient's condition on arrival.

Some EMS systems have adopted protocols or other guidelines regarding the issue of patient destination. For instance, most states have destination protocols for trauma patients. In some cases, these call for a patient who meets the protocol's inclusion criteria to be directed to a more distant trauma center instead of a closer community hospital. In other cases, patients who meet other specialty care criteria, such as burn patients or pediatric patients, also are directed by protocols to specialty centers rather than community hospitals, even if those hospitals are closer.

These types of protocols often place you in a difficult position—choosing between the requirements of a protocol and the clearly expressed wishes of a competent patient. In general, follow applicable system protocols. Any variation from those protocols should be handled only in consultation with your medical control authorities.

EMTALA and Hospital Diversions

[OBJECTIVE 25]

In many areas of the country hospital diversions continue to pose big problems for ambulance services. This issue has different names in different parts of the country. Whether you call it "ER diversion," "hospital bypass," or a "reroute," the problem is the same. Your incoming ambulance is told to go to another destination.

The federal EMTALA governs much of the diversion issue. This law requires that a hospital provide a medical screening examination to anyone who comes to that hospital. It further requires that the hospital provide stabilizing treatment to anyone with an emergency medical condition without regard to the patient's ability to pay.

Under EMTALA regulations, a hospital, with few exceptions, cannot divert an incoming ambulance to another hospital unless the hospital is on "diversionary status," or more simply put, "diversion." That means that the hospital lacks the "staff or facilities to accept any additional emergency patients." However, the regulations also state that if an ambulance disregards a diversionary order and comes to the hospital's emergency department anyway, the hospital's EMTALA obligations still apply. The regulations also consider that ambulances owned and operated by the hospital are considered "hospital property" for EMTALA purposes.

In some cases, hospitals have given diversionary orders to ambulances when the hospital is not in a formal diversionary status as defined by EMTALA regulations. In other cases, ambulances disregard diversionary orders and bring the patient to the hospital anyway. The law is clear. When the ambulance arrives at the hospital's emergency department, the hospital must accept the patient and provide the medical screening examination without undue delay, regardless of any diversionary order it previously gave.

In any diversion situation, thoroughly document all the facts and circumstances surrounding the diversion. Document who gave the diversionary order and the precise nature of the order. Document the specific reason for the diversion and the explanation of the diversion to the patient. If the patient insists on going to the diverted facility, explain the risks to the patient, just as you would in any other informed refusal situation. For instance, if a patient with chest pain insists on going to a facility on diversionary status, you should inform the patient of the risks, including delays in the diagnosis or treatment of his or her condition. Document the patient's understanding of these risks. Also, if in the best interests of the patient, do your best to convince the patient to go to a more appropriate destination.

Nontransport/Against Medical Advice

In some cases patients either refuse transport against medical advice or transport is not warranted based on the circumstances or the patient's condition. All cases that do not end in transport should be documented on the prehospital care report. For instance, if no patient is found, document the address to which you responded, the time of arrival, your survey of the scene or search of the area, and other related details.

In the event that the patient refuses transportation, make sure that the patient is competent to make medical decisions. Clearly document the patient's refusal of transportation.

An increasing number of EMS systems permit paramedics, in consultation with medical direction and in accordance with strictly defined protocols, to make no-transport decisions in the field. EMS systems in many parts of the country are overused as a source of primary care for the indigent and in medically underserved areas. Thus not every person who calls for an ambulance truly needs one. Although the literature reports mixed results on the ability of paramedics to properly and safely identify patients who do not require transport, any such decisions should be made in consultation with medical direction and appropriate medical control.

RESUSCITATION ISSUES

Advance Directives and Do Not Resuscitate Orders

[OBJECTIVE 26]

Not same as DNR

Most, if not all, states have laws that pertain to advance directives for healthcare. An **advance directive** is a document in which a competent person gives instructions to be followed regarding his or her healthcare in the event the person later becomes incapacitated and unable to make or communicate those decisions to others (Figure 4-3). An advance directive typically does not become effective unless it is documented in writing and only when the patient becomes terminally ill and/or enters a permanent vegetative or nonresponsive state. State law varies on the ability of paramedics and other EMS providers to honor advance directives for healthcare.

A majority of states have also adopted specific EMS or out-of-hospital DNR programs (Figure 4-4). These programs vary by state but share common characteristics. For example, most state EMS DNR programs feature EMS-specific means of identifying patients with valid DNR orders. These methods often include a DNR bracelet, necklace, form, or card.

DNR typically means that the paramedic should withhold cardiac compressions, intubation, artificial ventilation, resuscitative drugs, defibrillation, and other invasive resuscitative measures. This definition varies by state. You should still administer other appropriate care to a DNR patient as indicated. Other care includes, when appropriate, supplemental oxygen, pain control, basic airway management, and other basic steps for a patient's physical comfort. "Do not resuscitate" does *not* mean "do not treat."

Jim Doyle
Governor

Helene Nelson
Secretary

State of Wisconsin

Department of Health and Family Services

DIVISION OF PUBLIC HEALTH

1 WEST WILSON STREET
P O BOX 2659
MADISON WI 53701-2659

608-266-1251
FAX: 608-267-2832
www.dhfs.state.wi.us

To Whom It May Concern:

Enclosed is the Declaration to Physicians (Living Will) form you requested. This form makes it possible for adults in Wisconsin to state their preferences for life-sustaining procedures and feeding tubes in the event the person is in a terminal condition or persistent vegetative state.

Be sure to read both sides of the form carefully and understand it before you complete and sign it.

The withholding or withdrawal of any medication, life-sustaining procedure or feeding tube may not be made if the attending physician advises that doing so will cause pain or reduce comfort, and the pain or discomfort cannot be alleviated through pain relief measures.

Two witnesses are required. Witnesses must be at least 18 years of age, not related to you by blood, marriage or adoption, and not directly financially responsible for your health care. Witnesses may not be persons who know they are entitled to or have a claim on any portion of your estate. A witness cannot be a health care provider who is serving you at the time the document is signed, an employee of the health care provider, other than a chaplain or a social worker, or an employee other than a chaplain or social worker of an inpatient health care facility in which you are a patient. Valid witnesses acting in good faith are immune from civil or criminal liability.

You should make relatives and friends aware that you have signed the document and the location where it is kept. A signed form may be kept in a safe, easily accessible place until needed. The document may be filed for safekeeping for a fee with the Register in Probate of your county of residence, but it is not required that it be filed. The fee for filing with the Register in Probate has been set by State Statute at $8.00.

You are responsible for notifying your attending physician of the existence of the Declaration. An attending physician who is notified shall make the Declaration part of your medical records. A Declaration that is in its original form or is a legible photocopy or electronic facsimile copy is presumed to be valid.

If you have both a Declaration to Physicians and a Power of Attorney for Health Care, the provisions of a valid Power of Attorney for Health Care supersede any directly conflicting provisions of a valid Declaration to Physicians.

Up to four copies of the Declaration to Physicians are available free to anyone who sends a stamped, self-addressed, business-size envelope to: Living Will, Division of Public Health, P.O. Box 2659, Madison, Wisconsin 53701-2659. You may make additional copies of the enclosed blank form. The form is also available on the Department of Health and Family Services Web page http://dhfs.wisconsin.gov/forms/DPHnum.asp .

If you have questions about the availability of the Declaration to Physicians (Living Will) form or obtaining larger quantities of the form, you may contact the Division of Public Health at (608) 266-1251.

INSTRUCTIONS FOR DECLARATION TO PHYSICIANS FORM

Definitions

"Declaration" means a written, witnessed document voluntarily executed by the declarant under State Statute 154.03 (1), but is not limited in form or substance to that provided in State Statute 154.03 (2).

"Department" means the Department of Health and Family Services.

"Feeding tube" means a medical tube through which nutrition or hydration is administered into the vein, stomach, nose, mouth or other body opening of a qualified patient.

"Terminal condition" means an incurable condition caused by injury or illness that reasonable medical judgment finds would cause death imminently, so that the application of life-sustaining procedures serves only to postpone the moment of death.

Wisconsin.gov

"Persistent vegetative state" means a condition that reasonable, medical judgment finds constitutes complete and irreversible loss of all the functions of the cerebral cortex and results in a complete, chronic and irreversible cessation of all cognitive functioning and consciousness and a complete lack of behavioral responses that indicate cognitive functioning, although autonomic functions continue.

"Qualified patient" means a declarant who has been diagnosed and certified in writing to be afflicted with a terminal condition or to be in a persistent vegetative state by two physicians, one of whom is the attending physician, who have personally examined the declarant.

"Attending physician" means a physician licensed under State Statute Chapter 448 who has primary responsibility for the treatment and care of the patient.

"Health care professional" means a person licensed, certified or registered under State Statutes Chapters 441, 448 or 455.

"Inpatient health care facility" has the meaning provided under State Statute 50.135 (1) and includes community-based residential facilities as defined in State Statute 50.01 (1g).

"Life-sustaining procedure" means any medical procedure or intervention that, in the judgment of the attending physician, would serve only to prolong the dying process but not avert death when applied to a qualified patient.

"Life-sustaining procedure" includes assistance in respiration, artificial maintenance of blood pressure and heart rate, blood transfusion, kidney dialysis and other similar procedures, but does not include (a) the alleviation of pain by administering medication or by performing an medical procedure; or (b) the provision of nutrition or hydration.

Procedures for signing Declarations

A Declaration must be signed by the declarant in the presence of two witnesses. If the declarant is physically unable to sign a Declaration, the Declaration must be signed in the declarant's name by one of the witnesses or some other person at the declarant's express direction and in his or her presence; such a proxy signing shall either take place or be acknowledged by the declarant in the presence of two witnesses.

Effect of Declaration

The desires of a qualified patient who is competent supersede the effect of the Declaration at all times. If a qualified patient is incompetent at the time of the decision to withhold or withdraw life-sustaining procedures or feeding tubes, a Declaration executed under this chapter is presumed to be valid.

Revocation of Declaration

A Declaration may be revoked at any time by the declarant by any of the following methods:

1) By being canceled, defaced, obliterated, burned, torn or otherwise destroyed by the declarant or by some person who is directed by the declarant and who acts in the presence of the declarant.
2) By a written revocation, signed and dated by the declarant expressing the intent to revoke.
3) By a verbal expression by the declarant of his or her intent to revoke the Declaration, but only if the declarant or a person acting on behalf of the declarant notifies the attending physician of the revocation.
4) By executing a subsequent Declaration.

The attending physician shall record in the declarant's medical records the time, date and place of the revocation and time, date and place, if different, that he or she was notified of the revocation.

Liabilities

No physician, inpatient health care facility or health care professional acting under direction of a physician may be held criminally or civilly liable, or charged with unprofessional conduct of any of the following:

1) Participating in the withholding or withdrawal of life-sustaining procedures or feeding tubes under Chapter 154, subchapter II.
2) Failing to act upon a revocation unless the person or facility has actual knowledge of the revocation.
3) Failing to comply with a Declaration, except that failure by a physician to comply with a Declaration of a qualified patient constitutes unprofessional conduct if the physician refuses or fails to make a good faith attempt to transfer the patient to another physician who will comply with the Declaration.

DPH0060A (Rev. 08/05)

DEPARTMENT OF HEALTH & FAMILY SERVICES
Division of Public Health
DOH 0060 (Rev. 4/96)

Effective Date
April 6, 1996
S. 154.03(1),(2)

PLEASE BE SURE YOU READ THE FORM CAREFULLY AND UNDERSTAND IT BEFORE YOU COMPLETE AND SIGN IT

DECLARATION TO PHYSICIANS
(WISCONSIN LIVING WILL)

I, ______________________________

, being of sound mind, voluntarily state my desire that my dying not be prolonged under the circumstances specified in this document. Under those circumstances, I direct that I be permitted to die naturally. If I am unable to give directions regarding the use of life-sustaining procedures or feeding tubes, I intend that my family and physician honor this document as the final expression of my legal right to refuse medical or surgical treatment.

1. If I have a **TERMINAL CONDITION**, as determined by 2 physicians who have personally examined me, I do not want my dying to be artificially prolonged and I do not want life-sustaining procedures to be used. In addition, the following are my directions regarding the use of feeding tubes:

☐ YES, I want feeding tubes used if I have a terminal condition.

☐ NO, I do not want feeding tubes used if I have a terminal condition.

If you have not checked either box, feeding tubes will be used.

2. If I am in a **PERSISTENT VEGETATIVE STATE**, as determined by 2 physicians who have personally examined me, the following are my directions regarding the use of life-sustaining procedures:

☐ YES, I want life-sustaining procedures used if I am in a persistent vegetative state .

☐ NO, I do not want life-sustaining procedures used if I am in a persistent vegetative state.

If you have not checked either box, life-sustaining procedures will be used.

3. If I am in a **PERSISTENT VEGETATIVE STATE**, as determined by 2 physicians who have personally examined me, the following are my directions regarding the use of feeding tubes:

☐ YES, I want feeding tubes used if I am in a persistent vegetative state.

☐ NO, I do not want feeding tubes used if I am in a persistent vegetative state.

If you have not checked either box, feeding tubes will be used.

If you are interested in more information about the significant terms used in this document, see section 154.01 of the Wisconsin Statutes or the information accompanying this document.

ATTENTION: You and the 2 witnesses must sign the document at the same time.

Signed ______________________ **Date** __________

Address ______________________ **Date of Birth** __________

I believe that the person signing this document is of sound mind. I am an adult and am not related to the person signing this document by blood, marriage or adoption. I am not entitled to and do not have a claim on any portion of the person's estate and am not otherwise restricted by law from being a witness.

Witness Signature ______________________ **Date Signed** __________

Print Name ______________________

Witness Signature ______________________ **Date Signed** __________

Print Name ______________________

DIRECTIVES TO ATTENDING PHYSICIAN

1. This document authorizes the withholding or withdrawal of life-sustaining procedures or of feeding tubes when 2 physicians, one of whom is the attending physician, have personally examined and certified in writing that the patient has a terminal condition or is in a persistent vegetative state.

2. The choices in this document were made by a competent adult. Under the law, the patient's stated desires must be followed unless you believe that withholding or withdrawing life-sustaining procedures or feeding tubes would cause the patient pain or reduced comfort and that the pain or discomfort cannot be alleviated through pain relief measures. If the patient's stated desires are that life-sustaining procedures or feeding tubes be used, this directive must be followed.

3. If you feel that you cannot comply with this document, you must make a good faith attempt to transfer the patient to another physician who will comply. Refusal or failure to make a good faith attempt to do so constitutes unprofessional conduct.

4. If you know that the patient is pregnant, this document has no effect during her pregnancy.

* * * * *

The person making this living will may use the following space to record the names of those individuals and health care providers to whom he or she has given copies of this document:

____

____

____

____

Figure 4-3 Advance directives.

DO NOT RESUSCITATE (DNR) REQUEST

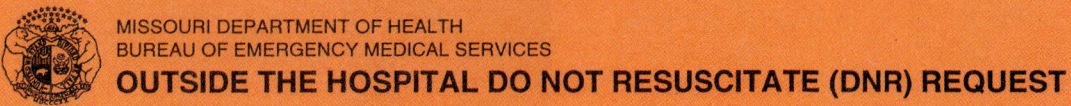

MISSOURI DEPARTMENT OF HEALTH
BUREAU OF EMERGENCY MEDICAL SERVICES

OUTSIDE THE HOSPITAL DO NOT RESUSCITATE (DNR) REQUEST

| | DNR # | 13132 |

I, _____, request limited emergency care as herein described.
  (name)

I understand DNR means that if my heart stops beating or if I stop breathing, no medical procedure to restart breathing or heart functioning will be instituted.

I understand this decision will <u>not</u> prevent me from obtaining other emergency medical care by outside the hospital care providers and/or medical care directed by a physician prior to my death.

I understand I may revoke this directive at any time.

I give permission for this information to be given to the outside the hospital care providers, doctors, nurses, or other health personnel as necessary to implement this directive.

I hereby agree to the "Do Not Resuscitate" (DNR) order.

Patient/Appropriate Surrogate Signature **(Mandatory)**	Date
▶	
Witness **(Mandatory)**	Date
▶	

REVOCATION PROVISION

I hereby revoke the above declaration.

| Signature | Date |
| | |

I AFFIRM THIS DIRECTIVE IS THE EXPRESSED WISH OF THE PATIENT/PATIENT'S APPROPRIATE SURROGATE, IS MEDICALLY APPROPRIATE, AND IS DOCUMENTED IN THE PATIENT'S PERMANENT MEDICAL RECORD.

In the event of a cardiac or respiratory arrest, no cardiopulmonary resuscitation will be initiated.

Physician's Signature **(Mandatory)** ▶	Date
Physician - Printed Name	Physician's Telephone Number
Address	Facility or Agency Name

MO 580-1936 (8-94)   EMS-21

THIS DNR REQUEST FORM SHOULD BE KEPT WITH THE PATIENT IN A VISIBLE LOCATION AT ALL TIMES.
THIS FORM WILL NOT BE ACCEPTED IF IT HAS BEEN AMENDED OR ALTERED IN ANY WAY.

DO NOT RESUSCITATE (DNR) REQUEST

Figure 4-4 Do not resuscitate (DNR) orders.

Withholding or Discontinuing Resuscitation

Apart from the issue of advance directives/DNR orders, many EMS systems permit paramedics to withhold or discontinue resuscitation based on medical direction or other authority. Some states also permit paramedics to make a pronouncement of death. Consult your state law or regulations to determine the extent of paramedic authority in your system.

Organ Donation

[OBJECTIVE 27]

In some cases, EMS providers can play a critical role in the organ donation process. For patients who may be viable organ donors (e.g., unresponsive patients with severe head injuries, gunshot wounds to the head) and who still have a pulse, paramedics can play a critical role in maintaining the viability of the organs until they can be harvested. Paramedics, particularly in states where they are permitted to pronounce death, should be

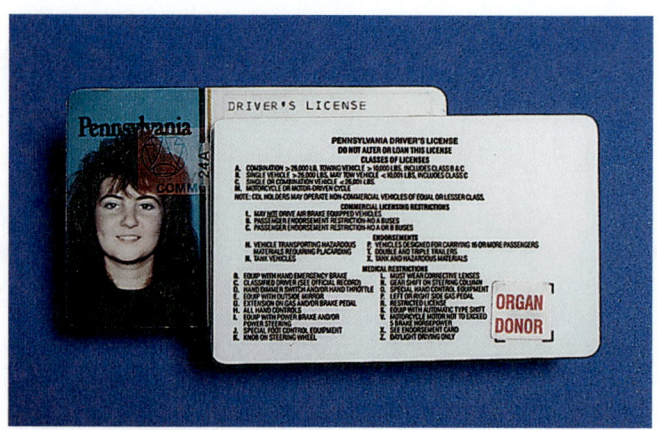

Figure 4-5 Organ donation information.

sensitive to the identification of potential organ donors (Figure 4-5). Work with medical direction and your local organ procurement organization to begin the procedures for maintaining viable transplant organs whenever possible.

Case Scenario CONCLUSION

The situation becomes somewhat more complex because you and the ambulance paramedic disagree about the most appropriate course of action. You believe the patient should be transported against his will, whereas the other paramedic, to whom you have transferred the care of the patient, has initiated the refusal process. Ultimately the patient was released at the scene by the ambulance paramedic.

Looking Back

9. *Who has "control" of this patient? Who decides whether this patient is transported?*
10. *Do you believe this patient has the "right" to refuse? Why or why not?*
11. *What documentation should be performed related to a patient refusal?*
12. *As the fire paramedic, do you have legal responsibility for the refusal decision once you have transferred care to the transporting paramedic?*

10-1 = I need help

CRIME AND ACCIDENT SCENE RESPONSIBILITIES

[OBJECTIVE 28]

As a paramedic, you will often be involved in responses to crime scenes or other locations where a law enforcement investigation or other forensic investigation may occur. Above all, ensure the safety of the scene and the safety of you and your crew when responding to any incident in which a potential crime has occurred.

If the scene is safe, the next priority becomes patient care. Even if insistent law enforcement officials on the scene beg or direct you not to touch the patient for fear of disturbing potential evidence, if a patient is in need of emergency care, then providing that care must be your priority. If assessment and treatment can be provided in a manner that preserves potential evidence, then due care should be taken to preserve that evidence to the maximal extent possible.

For example, if you can avoid cutting or tearing a patient's clothing around the area of a bullet hole, the intact hole may provide valuable forensic evidence to investigators. If you do not need to move items such as tables, chairs, or other furniture at a crime scene to tend to a patient, then take care not to do so. If you must move, displace, or destroy potential evidence while providing patient care, document the previous condition of the scene as much as possible. If time and circumstances permit you to take a photograph, you may do so, though any pictures that contain individually identifiable patient information should be protected in the same manner as prehospital care reports and other protected health information.

DOCUMENTATION

[OBJECTIVES 29, 30, 31]

A critical skill for paramedics is documentation of patient care. As with other skills, documentation is best done with practice and instruction. EMS documentation serves many purposes. First and foremost, a prehospital care report (PCR) is a medical record. It is vital to the care and treatment of the patient. In addition, PCRs are used for quality improvement and the retrospective evaluation of the quality of patient care. Other important functions of PCRs are for data collection and research. PCRs also are critical to billing and reimbursement in systems that charge and collect fees for their services. Finally, PCRs are legal documents. They often are central pieces of evidence in court cases, reimbursement audits, provider disciplinary cases, and other legal actions.

Your documentation should be well organized. In general, documentation should follow a chronologic sequence of the incident from dispatch, to arrival on scene, to patient assessment, to treatment and, finally, to disposition or transport of the patient. Special circumstances should be documented as well. These may include, for example, delays in reaching or accessing the patient because of entrapment or other obstacles.

Your documentation should be completed as close to the time of the delivery of patient care as possible. PCRs written while the call is still fresh in your mind typically are the most accurate and reliable. These PCRs offer the most protection to you in the event of a court case or other legal action down the road. Some states regulate the amount of time in which a PCR must be completed after a call. Many states also require reporting of PCRs or, at least, certain data elements from PCRs, to a state or regional EMS oversight agency.

Case Scenario SUMMARY

1. *What is your general impression of this patient?* High priority. In addition to a significant mechanism, this patient appears to have experienced a loss of consciousness, is pale, and may have respiratory compromise.

2. *What additional assessment will be important in the evaluation of this patient?* A rapid trauma assessment should be performed before moving the patient. A more detailed mental status examination, evaluation of respiratory function, more complete assessment of skin and pulses, and vital signs will help in the initial assessment. A head-to-toe physical examination should be completed en route the hospital.

3. *What intervention should you initiate at this time?* Manual spinal immobilization, high-flow oxygen, movement of the patient to a spine board.

4. *What are this patient's potential injuries?* Probably right chest trauma, possible right pneumothorax, potential lumbar spine injury, compensated shock, and a concussion.

5. *What additional treatment should be initiated?* Spinal immobilization, intravenous line initiation, and transport to the trauma center.

6. *If the patient continues to refuse after your best effort to convince him, should you leave him at the scene or transport him against his will? Why?* EMS organizations can transport two types of patients against their will. Patients who lack the *legal capacity* to make decisions because they are not adults, are in custody, or have transferred their medical decisions to another party may be transported against their will. Patients who lack *mental capacity* to make decisions on their own behalf also can be transported against their will. The lack of mental capacity must be identified by tests of orientation, logical thought processes, and ability to understand the consequences of actions. The presence of intoxication also casts doubt on a patient's mental capacity. Competent adults who are alert, oriented to person, place, time, and event who have logical thought processes and understand the consequences of their actions have the right to refuse care. This patient meets those criteria.

7. *What strategies should be used to attempt to convince the patient to accept treatment and transport?* First, start simple. Attempt to determine *why* the patient is refusing. Sometimes the issue is easily resolved, such as when the patient refuses transport because of an assumption that he or she will be taken to a particular hospital or because the patient does not have a way to get home after the emergency department visit is over. Sometimes financial concerns play a role and may be relieved by offering to take the patient to a hospital that offers a significant amount of charity care. If these approaches fail, informed consent is the best tool to help patients make medical decisions in their own best interests. Informed consent has three parts: knowledge about potential injuries, understanding of the benefits of treatment, and acceptance of possible consequences of not being treated. In this case the patient should have been informed, in lay terms, of the potential cerebral, spinal, and thoracic injuries. Benefits of treatment and transport (identification and treatment of potentially severe brain injury, improved oxygenation, identification and treatment of potentially severe thoracic injury, prevention of permanent paraplegia, and management of shock) should be clearly described with

Continued

clear identification of the severe limitations of a paramedic examination compared with that of an emergency physician. Finally, the potential complications of not receiving treatment (cerebral swelling, permanent brain damage or death, permanent damage to the brain or heart from hypoxia, severe lung injury causing lung and/or heart failure, paraplegia requiring permanent incapacity and/or dependence on a wheelchair and caregivers, and death) should be clearly articulated. Do not lie or exaggerate, but include all potential complications.

8. *What role, if any, does the base hospital physician play in this situation?* Emergency physicians play several roles in dealing with patient refusals. At the least, the physician offers a resource for the paramedic to discuss the case with to be sure that all potential strategies have been exercised to adequately inform the patient of the possible consequences of nontransport. In some cases the physician may actually speak to the patient personally, offering a "higher level" of judgment that may convince the patient to accept care. In some EMS systems consultation with the ED physician is required to ensure that steps were taken to protect the safety and health of the patient.

9. *Who has "control" of this patient? Who decides whether this patient is transported?* Do not be confused: the patient has control of the patient. Political or organizational differences should never interfere with the patient's ability to make decisions concerning his or her own health. Do not worry about the "formal" transfer of care between paramedics at different agencies; work *together* to help the patient make the right decision about care.

10. *Do you believe this patient has the "right" to refuse? Why or why not?* Yes. He has both legal and mental capacity. No evidence exists that he is intoxicated or that he lacks the comprehension necessary to make an informed choice.

11. *What documentation should be performed related to a patient refusal?* In essence, the documentation should mirror the informed consent process. Document your evaluation of the patient's mental status in a way that demonstrates his orientation, logical thought process, and capacity to make decisions. Document the injuries found, the description of benefits of treatment, and the patient's understanding of the potential consequences of nontreatment. In some systems the refusal form includes spaces for the paramedic to document this information and a space for the patient to sign that he or she understands the possible injuries, the benefits of treatment, and the potential consequences of nontreatment.

12. *As the fire paramedic, do you have legal responsibility for the refusal decision once you have transferred care to the transporting paramedic?* As noted before, multiagency efforts on the scene of a patient refusal should cooperate in providing informed consent and attempting to help the patient make the best decision. If true disagreement occurs between organizations on scene regarding the patient's legal or mental capacity, the emergency department physician should be consulted as the final authority. The presence of documentation between organizations that attempts to blame the other organization for a patient's nontransport clouds the true issues of the case and may increase legal liability for both organizations if an investigation ensues. The best legal protection EMS organizations can get is the daily practice of cooperative efforts to aid patients in making decisions in their best interests.

Chapter Summary

- Paramedics have legal duties and ethical responsibilities.
- Paramedics are subject to operational policies, clinical protocols, and other state and local requirements.
- EMS law comes from the three branches of government: legislative, judicial, and executive.
- A scope of practice is a predefined set of skills, interventions, or other activities that paramedics are authorized to perform.
- Standard of care is the conduct expected of a reasonably prudent paramedic.
- Medical direction or physician oversight of paramedic practice includes the development of clinical practice standards, such as training curricula and protocols.
- Concurrent medical direction occurs when a paramedic consults a physician by phone, radio, or other electronic means on the scene or during transport.
- Retrospective medical direction occurs after the fact. It includes quality improvement programs and case reviews.
- Licensure through state or local levels is thought of as recognition of minimal competency and completion of prescribed training.
- Certification through state or local levels is thought of as evidence of competency in certain skills or tasks.
- Liability is the legal responsibility of a person for the consequences of his or her acts or omissions.

- Negligence is the failure to act as a reasonably prudent or careful person.
- The following are four elements of a paramedic's malpractice case:
  - Legal duty (or duty to act): the obligation of the paramedic to act with due regard for the patient and to uphold an applicable standard of care
  - Breach of duty: the paramedic violated the standard of care applicable to the circumstances
  - Damages: compensable harm or other losses suffered because of negligence
  - Causation: proof that negligence by the paramedic caused or created the harm sustained by the plaintiff
- Many states recognize immunity provisions or Good Samaritan laws to protect paramedics.
- Paramedics may also be subject to intentional torts, which encompass battery, assault, false imprisonment, invasion of privacy, defamation, libel, and slander.
- Consent is the informed permission (expressed or implied) given by a patient or another person legally responsible for decision making for the care and transportation provided by EMS providers.

- Refusal of care occurs when a competent patient, after being properly informed of risks and benefits, refuses medical care and/or transportation.
- HIPAA requires that all individually identifiable health information be safeguarded and used only for purposes specifically permitted by the regulation.
- EMTALA requires a hospital to provide medical screening examinations and stabilizing treatment to anyone who comes to that hospital.
- Advance directives document instructions for care in case a person becomes incapacitated or unable to make decisions.
- DNR patients direct healthcare professionals to withhold cardiac compressions, intubation, artificial ventilation, resuscitative drugs, defibrillation, and other invasive resuscitative measures.
- Paramedics play a vital role in organ donation by maintaining viability until organs can be harvested.
- Providing care is the paramedic's first priority regardless of crime or accident scene responsibilities.
- Accurate documentation from incident to transport is a crucial step for any paramedic.

REFERENCE

National Highway Traffic Safety Administration. (1998). *Paramedic national standard curriculum.* Retrieved April 26, 2008, from http://www.nhtsa.dot.

SUGGESTED RESOURCES

Barnum, B. S. (1997). Licensure, certification and accreditation, *Online Journal Issues in Nursing.* Retrieved from http://www.nursingworld.org.

Cocanour, C. S., Ursic, C, & Fischer, R. P. (1995). Does the potential for organ donation justify scene flights for gunshot wounds to the head? *Journal of Trauma, 39,* 968.

Doyle, T. J., & Vissers, R. J. (1999). An EMS approach to psychiatric emergencies, *Emergency Medical Services, 28*(6), 87, 90-3, 1999.

Federation of State Medical Boards. (2005). *Assessing scope of practice in health care delivery: Critical questions in assuring public access and safety.* Retrieved April 26, 2008, from http://www.fsmb.org.

National Cancer Institute. (2007). *Advance directives.* Retrieved April 26, 2008, from http://www.cancer.gov.

Transweb. (2000). *Top 10 myths about donation & transplantation.* Retrieved April 26, 2008, from http://www.transweb.org.

USINFO. (2000). *U.S. legal system.* Retrieved April 26, 2008, from http://usinfo.state.gov.

Winmill, D., & Clawson, J. (1990). Seize the moment: The EMS role in organ donation. *Journal of Emergency Medical Services, 15,* 48.

Wolfberg, D. (2000). Sign here and we're gone—practical tips for handling patient refusals. *Journal of Emergency Medical Services, 25,* 3.

Wolfberg, D., & Wirth, S. (2005). *The ambulance service guide to HIPAA compliance* (3rd ed.), Mechanicsburg, PA: PWW Publishing.

Chapter Quiz

1. An area of law in which an individual is prosecuted on behalf of society for violating laws designed to safeguard society is called _____ law.

2. True or False: A paramedic's standard of care is the range of duties and skills he or she is legally allowed to perform when necessary.

3. List the four elements that must be present to prove negligence.

   _____

   _____

   _____

   _____

Chapter Quiz—continued

4. HIPAA legislation pertains to_____.
   a. patient abandonment
   b. patient privacy
   c. motor vehicles
   d. organ donation

5. List four examples of intentional torts.

   _____

   _____

   _____

   _____

6. Confinement or restraint of a person against his or her will or without appropriate legal justification best defines_____.
   a. assault
   b. battery
   c. invasion of privacy
   d. false imprisonment

7. List three sources that may be used to establish a paramedic's standard of care.

   _____

   _____

   _____

8. True or False: Most insurance policies generally will not cover punitive damage awards in a malpractice case.

9. What is the difference between battery and assault?

   _____

   _____

   _____

10. True or False: To be considered valid, expressed consent must be given verbally.

Terminology

Abandonment Terminating care when it is still needed and desired by the patient and without ensuring that appropriate care continues to be provided by another qualified healthcare professional.

Administrative law A branch of law that deals with rules, regulations, orders, and decisions created by governmental agencies.

Advance directive A document in which a competent person gives instructions to be followed regarding his or her healthcare in the event the person later becomes incapacitated and unable to make or communicate those decisions to others.

Assault A threat of imminent bodily harm to another person by someone with the obvious ability to carry out the threat.

Battery Touching or contact with another person without that person's consent.

Breach of duty Violation by the defendant of the standard of care applicable to the circumstances.

Case law Interpretations of constitutional, statutory, or administrative law made by the courts; also referred to as *common law* or *judge-made law*.

Causation In a negligence case, the negligence of the defendant must have caused or created the harm sustained by the plaintiff; also referred to as *proximate cause*.

Certification Recognition of minimal competency in certain skills or tasks.

Chemical restraints Agents such as sedatives that can suppress a patient's neurologic and/or motor capabilities and reduce the threat to the paramedic; also known as *pharmacologic restraints*.

Civil law A branch of law that deals with torts (civil wrongs) committed by one individual, organization, or group against another.

Concurrent medical direction Consultation with a physician or other advanced healthcare professional by telephone, radio, or other electronic means, permitting the physician and paramedic to decide together on the best course of action in the delivery of patient care.

Confidentiality Protection of patient information in any form and the disclosure of that information only as needed for patient care or as otherwise permitted by law.

Consent Permission.

Contributory negligence An injured plaintiff's failure to exercise due care that, along with the defendant's negligence, contributed to the injury.

Criminal law A branch of law in which the federal, state, or local government prosecutes individuals on behalf of society for violating laws designed to safeguard society.

Damages Compensable harm or other losses incurred by an injured party (plaintiff) because of the negligence of the defendant.

Defamation The publication of false information about a person that tends to blacken the person's character or injure his or her reputation.

Defendant The person or institution being sued; also called the *respondent*.

DNR Do not resuscitate orders.

Due process The constitutional guarantee that laws and legal proceedings must be fair regarding an individual's legal rights.

Duty to act A legal obligation (created by statute, contract, or voluntarily) to provide services.

Emancipated minor A self-supporting minor. This status often depends on the minor receiving an actual court order of emancipation.

Emergency Medical Treatment and Active Labor Act (EMTALA) A federal law that requires a hospital to provide a medical screening examination to anyone who comes to that hospital and to provide stabilizing treatment to anyone with an emergency medical condition, without considering the patient's ability to pay.

Expressed consent Permission given by a patient or his or her responsible decision maker either verbally or through some physical expression of consent.

False imprisonment Confinement or restraint of a person against his or her will or without appropriate legal justification.

Immunity Protection from legal liability in accordance with applicable laws.

Implied consent The presumption that a patient who is ill or injured and unable to give consent for any reason would agree to the delivery of emergency healthcare necessitated by his or her condition.

Intentional tort A wrong in which the defendant meant to cause the harmful action.

Invasion of privacy Disclosure or publication of personal or private facts about a person to a person or persons not authorized to receive such information.

Involuntary consent The rendering of care to a person under specific legal authority, even if the patient does not consent to the care.

Jurisprudence The theory and philosophy of law.

Liability The legal responsibility of a party for the consequences of his or her acts or omissions.

Libel False statements about a person made in writing that blacken the person's character or injure his or her reputation.

Licensure Recognition of minimal competency and the completion of prescribed education or training in a profession or occupation.

Malfeasance Performing a wrongful act.

Medical direction Physician oversight of paramedic practice; also called *medical control*.

Medical practice act Legislation that governs the practice of medicine; may prescribe how and to what extent a physician may delegate authority to a paramedic to perform medical acts; varies from state to state.

Minor In most states, a person younger than 18 years.

Misfeasance Performing a legal act in a harmful manner.

Negligence The failure to act as a reasonably prudent and careful person would under similar circumstances.

Negligence per se Conduct that may be declared and treated as negligent without having to prove what would be reasonable and prudent under similar circumstances, usually because the conduct violates a law or regulation.

Nonfeasance Failure to perform a required act or duty.

Pharmacologic restraints Agents such as sedatives that can suppress a patient's neurologic and/or motor capabilities so that the threat to the paramedic is reduced; also known as *chemical restraints*.

Physical restraints Straps, splints, and other devices that prevent movement of all or part of the patient's body.

Plaintiff The person who initiates a lawsuit by filing a complaint; also known as a *claimant, petitioner*, or *applicant*.

Professional malpractice A type of tort case addressing whether a professional person failed to act as a reasonably prudent and careful person with similar training would act under similar circumstances.

Prospective medical direction Physician development of standards such as training curricula and protocols that establish, in advance, the parameters for EMS practice and set forth the expectations that EMS providers must satisfy in the delivery of patient care.

Res ipsa loquitur Latin phrase meaning "the thing speaks for itself." In negligence cases, this doctrine can be imposed when the plaintiff cannot prove all four components of negligence, but the injury itself would not have occurred without negligence (such as a sponge left in a patient after surgery).

Respondeat superior Latin phrase meaning "let the master answer." Under this legal doctrine, an employer is liable for the acts of employees within their scope of employment.

Retrospective medical direction Physician oversight that evaluates the effectiveness of care given through quality improvement programs, case reviews, and similar approaches.

Scope of practice A predefined set of skills, interventions, or other activities that the paramedic is legally authorized to perform when necessary; usually set by state law or regulation and local medical direction.

Slander False statements spoken about a person that blacken the person's character or injure his or her reputation.

Terminology—continued

Standard of care Conduct exercising the degree of care, skill, and judgment that would be expected under like or similar circumstances by a similarly trained, reasonable paramedic in the same scenario.

Statute A law passed by a legislature.

Statute of limitations A law that sets the time limits within which parties must take action to enforce their rights.

Statutory law Statutes and ordinances enacted by the U.S. Congress, state legislatures, and city councils.

Tort A wrong committed on the person or property of another.

Unintentional tort A wrong that the defendant did not mean to commit; a case in which a bad outcome occurred because of the failure to exercise reasonable care.

Ethics

Objectives *After completing this chapter, you will be able to:*

1. Define the terms *ethics, morals, unethical,* and *medical ethics.*
2. Distinguish ethical from moral decisions.
3. Identify the premise that should underlie the paramedic's ethical decisions in prehospital care.
4. Discuss the kinds of ethical dilemmas that paramedics typically encounter in the field.
5. Analyze the relation between the law and ethics in EMS.
6. Discuss the rights of patients.
7. Compare the criteria that may be used in allocating scarce EMS resources.
8. Identify the issues surrounding the use of advance directives in making a prehospital resuscitation decision.
9. Discuss the basic virtues that are most essential in EMS professionals.

Chapter Outline

What Are Ethics?
The Nature of EMS Professionals
Common Dilemmas for Paramedics
Codes of Ethics
Responsibilities of EMS Professionals

Patients' Rights
Professional Accountability
Basic Virtues
The Best Test
Chapter Summary

Case Scenario

A hospice nurse has contacted your ambulance company to arrange transport of a hospice patient to the emergency department for evaluation of possible pneumonia. Because the patient had some difficulty breathing, the dispatcher believed that a "life threat" might be present and requested an emergent response to the patient's home for fire, police, and ambulance. On arrival, you and your partner find a disorganized scene. The patient, a 70-year-old man with irreversible kidney failure, is difficult to arouse and breathing irregularly at a rate of approximately 8 to 10 breaths/min. His skin is pale and yellowish-blue. He is thin and very frail looking. Auscultation reveals bilateral wheezing. He is in a hospital bed in the living room of the home, surrounded by medications and medical devices. His wife is frantically trying to find his do not resuscitate (DNR) paperwork. The first-response EMS personnel are poised to begin ventilation and start an intravenous line.

Questions

1. *What is your general impression of this patient?*
2. *What treatment will you initiate if the patient's wife does find the DNR documents? What if she does not find the DNR documents?*
3. *What do you believe is in this patient's best interests? What role do you have in ensuring that those interests are met?*

People routinely trust paramedics with their lives, their bodies, their belongings, and the most intimate truths about their lives. That kind of trust is an award, not an entitlement. It absolutely mandates a paramedic's adherence to a set of rules and values that any patient or family member could look at and say, "yes, that seems fair to me."

This chapter is offered as such a tool. It comes from this author as well as numerous other caregivers practiced in and dedicated to the art of helping others. Collectively, its principles have helped serve people well.

WHAT ARE ETHICS?

[OBJECTIVES 1, 2, 3]

Ethics are societal principles of conduct that people or groups of people adopt as guidelines for personal behavior. **Morals** are values that help a person define right (what a person ought to do) versus wrong (what a person ought not to do). Morals are derived from teachings from parents, grandparents, mentors, and religious beliefs. **Unethical** refers to conduct that does not conform to approved standards of social or professional behavior.

Ethics is like a set of tools that paramedics use to solve the kinds of practical dilemmas that routinely arise in the field. Consider this example: A paramedic crew is called for a man found unresponsive in an alley. A quick assessment reveals he is breathing and has a pulse. The body odor coming from the patient is overwhelming. It appears he has not changed clothes or bathed in days. Even with gloves on, no one wants to touch him. Two hospitals are nearby. Hospital ABC is a nationally known, state-of-the-art facility that is 2 miles away. Hospital XYZ is 12 miles away. It has frequent staff turnover and the grounds have fallen into a state of disrepair. Both hospitals have emergency departments with appropriate staff and equipment to receive this patient. Based on the patient's untidy appearance, the crew decides to transport the patient to Hospital XYZ.

Was this decision ethical? Was it made in the patient's best interests? Ethics is not concerned with what the crew *does*, except to compare it with what they *ought* to do. The *ought* point of view is a judgment—a moral point of view. In this situation, the crew's actions were unethical because the patient should have been transported to the closest appropriate facility, Hospital ABC.

> **PARAMEDIC** *Pearl*
>
> The word *ethics* comes from the Greek root "ethos," which means *character*. Moral comes from the Latin root "mos," which means *custom*. Ethics relate to personal standards or character. Morals relate to social standards or customs.

Medical ethics is a field of study that evaluates the decisions, conduct, policies, and social concerns of medical activities. Principles of medical ethics include the following:

- *Primum non nocere*. Latin for "first, do no harm," from the Hippocratic Oath (discussed later in this chapter). Some consider this principle the most important of all the principles of medical ethics.
- *Beneficence*. Doing good for others. A healthcare professional has an obligation to act in the patient's best interests.
- *Autonomy*. The patient's right to choose or refuse care. Autonomy may be thought of as "control over one's destiny" and is the basis for the practice of informed consent. Freedom (of choice)—even to make the wrong decision—is the right of any adult patient who is competent.
- *Justice*. In medical ethics, justice refers to the fair distribution of healthcare resources and decisions regarding who gets what treatment.

- *Truthfulness and honesty*. The patient deserves to know the truth about his or her illness or injury and medical treatment.

> **PARAMEDIC** *Pearl*
>
> Medical ethics is based on the notion that a healthcare professional serves people in crisis who are vulnerable and forced to trust strangers with their well-being, intimacy, and immediate life choices. No greater form of trust exists, and it warrants profound respect.

Paramedics routinely witness and cope with the effects of heinous offenses. Some people can butcher a loving spouse, gun down a room full of people eating their lunches, or drown their own children in a bathtub without a moment of remorse. Clearly these acts are unethical, immoral, and illegal. Ethics differs from the law (or a body of law). Although the law applies to all people and penalties usually are prescribed for those violating the law, ethics is stricter and more serious than the law. Ethics is intended to acknowledge that the responsibilities of a professional are greater than those of the average citizen.

THE NATURE OF EMS PROFESSIONALS

When patients are sick, they trust that those treating them are competent and possess some degree of goodness that warrants confidence. Such evidence is typically seen several times every shift, when a paramedic asks permission to start an intravenous (IV) line. Patients almost always consent despite their worry about the pain they will surely suffer. Gloves or no gloves, their consent presupposes that the paramedic washed his hands the last time he or she went to the bathroom. Regardless of the risks, as soon as you mention that IV, patient after patient extends an arm.

Another example commonly occurs when paramedics find themselves in patients' bedrooms. A person's bedroom is his or her most private place. No one but a lover or a close family member is welcome there at 2 AM, and sometimes no one is welcome at all. No one, that is, but the paramedic. Paramedics find themselves not only welcome, but invited there. They will marvel throughout their careers at the willingness of perfect strangers to bare their bodies for examination and answer questions about the most intimate details of their lives.

A patient who shares those kinds of details presumes that you will never share them with anyone unless required for immediate care, and then never again. The patient also presumes that you are competent, your certifications are up to date, and you can perform risky procedures. They are never suspicious unless your actions give them cause to wonder. That kind of trust is a great honor, and you will find yourself impressed by it again and again. You need to respect this trust, *always*. Your integrity in those circumstances must be beyond reproach.

Being a paramedic necessitates that by your very nature and in your everyday life, you are a person of integrity. A person of integrity is honest, sincere, and truthful.

Much more is involved in a patient's well-being than his or her *medical* well-being, including financial status, state of fear, physical comfort in all its forms (warmth, body position, freedom from pain, thirst, hunger, fatigue, need to go to the bathroom, concern for family members), and spiritual peace. Many people who access 9-1-1 for help simply have no one else to turn to and no one who cares whether they live or die.

PARAMEDIC*Pearl*

A paramedic has to be more than a fast-moving mechanic with a few emergency skills and some education in medicine. A paramedic must be a professional: quick-witted and possessed of good hands, but also perceptive, caring, and always worthy of the public's trust—both privately and professionally. That is a significant challenge, considering that no human caregiver in history has ever been perfect.

COMMON DILEMMAS FOR PARAMEDICS

[OBJECTIVES 4, 5]

One of the most difficult things about being a paramedic is that patients generally believe they are always right. We know they are not. Yet, our responsibility is to make them feel as though we have met their needs. The following are examples of no-win situations in which our sense of ethics is absolutely essential.

Sometimes what the patient needs us to do conflicts with what we are authorized to do or have the power to do. For instance, some EMS systems do not authorize paramedics to perform a nasal intubation or surgical cricothyroidotomy. You are almost guaranteed to encounter patients whose most urgent need is one of those skills.

Often, what you are supposed to do conflicts with what the patient (or guardian) wants you to do. For example, Veterans Administration (VA) patients typically ask for transport to VA hospitals—despite the fact that many of those facilities do not have licensed emergency departments. Paramedics are supposed to talk the patient into accepting transport to the closest emergency department. That can mean major costs later on, regardless of his or her VA benefits.

Sometimes what the patient wants conflicts with what the patient's family wants. Paramedics struggle daily to resolve arguments between patients who do not want transport to a hospital and family members who insist on transportation.

Patients have a right to live, but they also have a right to die. Paramedics routinely find themselves confronted with apneic, pulseless patients in their 90s who are emaciated, bedridden, and quite ill and do not have a DNR order—and someone on the scene expects a miracle.

Paramedics commonly encounter questions about patients' health insurance from patients or guardians who will clearly make a medical choice on that basis. This is a trap, although an unintended one. Health insurance coverage is extremely complex, and paramedics should avoid giving advice about it. Paramedics traditionally have been taught that money should never enter into patient's medical choices. This is unrealistic. EMS patients of today *do* make their medical choices based on health insurance, if they are lucky enough to have it.

PARAMEDIC*Pearl*

In the United States, paramedics need to respect the fact that millions of ordinary people are one medical emergency away from bankruptcy, and those people worry about that situation.

Case Scenario—continued

The patient's wife is unable to find the DNR documentation, so as the EMTs begin assisting ventilation you contact medical direction. After quickly explaining the situation, the physician tells you "I have never confronted a situation like this" and reluctantly orders you to intubate the patient, provide oxygen and an inhaled bronchodilator, start an IV, check the patient's glucose level, and give naloxone for the patient's possible "oversedation." You remind the physician of the patient's hospice status, but he repeats his orders. Despite the loud protests of the patient's wife, you follow the physician's orders and transport the patient emergently to the emergency department.

Questions

4. *Do you believe the treatment you provided was in the patient's best interests? The patient's family's? The emergency department's? Who was served by this course of action?*
5. *Could you have handled the situation differently and achieved a different result? How?*
6. *Are you required to follow the physician's orders even if you believe they are harmful to the patient? Could you have refused to follow these orders? How would you have done that?*

CODES OF ETHICS

Historical Codes of Ethics

A **code of ethics** is a guide for interactions between members of a specific profession (such as physicians, nurses, or paramedics) and the public. Some disagreement has always been present regarding the value of ethical codes. What keeps them relevant? Faced with a dilemma, is a healthcare professional likely to even think of guidance written centuries, even thousands of years ago? Maybe not. But wisdom is by definition relevant, and it is an absolute necessity for anyone involved with society's emergencies.

Reliance on codes to govern the behaviors and practices of healthcare professionals had its beginnings at least as far back in history as Hammurabi in Mesopotamia (1700 BC), Hippocrates in Athens (400 BC), and Aulus Celsus in Rome (AD 2). Although Hippocrates (ca. 380-460 BC) generally receives credit for posing the first body of medical ethics (the Hippocratic Oath), many sources dispute his authorship and his adherence to all its principles. The oath consists of two parts. The first lists a medical student's responsibilities to the teacher. The second describes a physician's responsibility to a patient. In the days of Hippocrates, the egotistical approach to medicine was used. It was based on the following: "I will use MY abilities and judgment . . . " There was no mention of the patient's judgment by Hippocrates. Informed consent is a modern, Western notion that dictates patients are their own best advocates and a competent patient has the right to make his or her own decisions. This is important to understand, even when patients make decisions that you, as a paramedic, may not necessarily agree with. However relevant it was to the medical practice of its day, much of the Hippocratic Oath still makes good human and medical sense and deserves respect. Modern graduating physicians still recite various versions of this promise today. The classic version is shown in Box 5-1.

Modern Codes of Ethics

A renewed interest in medical ethics has arisen during recent years. Technologic advances have raised questions about the moral implications of resuscitation, the boundary between life and death, the intricacies of early life, and the real effects of many cures once considered standard. In addition, economic pressures worldwide have blurred the edges of medicine to the extent that many physicians have less time for human contact with their patients.

In addition to the Hippocratic Oath, several newer codes of ethics are used in EMS. One of these is the EMT Code of Ethics, written by Charles Gillespie, MD, and adopted by the National Association of EMTs in 1978 (Box 5-2).

The American Nurses Association has two similar documents, both published as books: *The Nurses Code of Ethics* and *Nursing's Social Policy Statement*. In addition, the International Council of Nurses, a federation of nursing associations from 120 nations, first published its Code of Ethics in 1953 and last revised it in 2005. This document is simple, presented in four sections intended to remind nurses how to regard their practice, profession, patients, and colleagues (International Council of Nurses, 2006).

The American Medical Association (AMA) Code of Ethics (based on nine principles of medical ethics) (2001) is 155 years old. The AMA's Principles of Medical Ethics are listed in Box 5-3.

The American College of Emergency Physicians (2006) Code of Ethics for Emergency Physicians is lengthy and rich in detail. It acknowledges the complexities of dealing with people in crisis and stresses the physician's role as a member of a team, specifically one that includes

---

| BOX 5-1 | Hippocratic Oath |

I swear by Apollo Physician and Asclepius and Hygeia and Panacea and all the gods and goddesses, making them my witnesses, that I will fulfill according to my ability and judgment this oath and this covenant:

To hold him who has taught me this art as equal to my parents and to live my life in partnership with him, and if he is in need of money to give him a share of mine, and to regard his offspring as equal to my brothers in male lineage and to teach them this art—if they desire to learn it—without fee and covenant; to give a share of precepts and oral instruction and all the other learning to my sons and to the sons of him who has instructed me and to pupils who have signed the covenant and have taken an oath according to the medical law, but no one else.

I will apply dietetic measures for the benefit of the sick according to my ability and judgment; I will keep them from harm and injustice.

I will neither give a deadly drug to anybody who asked for it, nor will I make a suggestion to this effect. Similarly I will not give to a woman an abortive remedy. In purity and holiness I will guard my life and my art.

I will not use the knife, not even on sufferers from stone, but will withdraw in favor of such men as are engaged in this work.

Whatever houses I may visit, I will come for the benefit of the sick, remaining free of all intentional injustice, of all mischief and in particular of sexual relations with both female and male persons, be they free or slaves.

What I may see or hear in the course of the treatment or even outside of the treatment in regard to the life of men, which on no account one must spread abroad, I will keep to myself, holding such things shameful to be spoken about.

If I fulfill this oath and do not violate it, may it be granted to me to enjoy life and art, being honored with fame among all men for all time to come; if I transgress it and swear falsely, may the opposite of all this be my lot.

Reprinted from Edelstein, L. (1943). *The Hippocratic oath: Text, translation, and interpretation*, Baltimore: Johns Hopkins Press.

prehospital professionals. Its conclusion seems particularly relevant (Box 5-4).

BOX 5-2	**EMT Code of Ethics**

Be it pledged as an Emergency Medical Technician, I will honor the physical and judicial laws of God and man. I will follow that regimen which, according to my ability and judgment, I consider for the benefit of my patients and abstain from whatever is deleterious and mischievous, nor shall I suggest any such counsel. Into whatever home I enter, I will go into them for the benefit of only the sick and injured, never revealing what I see or hear in the lives of men.

I shall also share my medical knowledge with those who may benefit from what I have learned. I will serve unselfishly and continuously in order to help make a better world for all mankind.

While I continue to keep this oath unviolated, may it be granted to me to enjoy life, and the practice of the art, respected by all men, in all times. Should I trespass or violate this oath, may the reverse be my lot. So help me God.

Reprinted from Gillespie, C. B. (1978). *EMT code of ethics*. Retrieved August 24, 2006, from http://www.naemt.org/aboutNAEMT/EMTCodeOfEthics.htm.

BOX 5-3	**The American Medical Association Principles of Medical Ethics**

1. A physician shall be dedicated to providing competent medical care, with compassion and respect for human dignity and rights.
2. A physician shall uphold the standards of professionalism, be honest in all professional interactions, and strive to report physicians deficient in character or competence, or engaging in fraud or deception, to appropriate entities.
3. A physician shall respect the law and also recognize a responsibility to seek changes in those requirements which are contrary to the best interests of the patient.
4. A physician shall respect the rights of patients, colleagues, and other health professionals, and shall safeguard patient confidences and privacy within the constraints of the law.
5. A physician shall continue to study, apply, and advance scientific knowledge, maintain a commitment to medical education, make relevant information available to patients, colleagues, and the public, obtain consultation, and use the talents of other health professionals when indicated.
6. A physician shall, in the provision of appropriate patient care, except in emergencies, be free to choose whom to serve, with whom to associate, and the environment in which to provide medical care.
7. A physician shall recognize a responsibility to participate in activities contributing to the improvement of the community and the betterment of public health.
8. A physician shall, while caring for a patient, regard responsibility to the patient as paramount.
9. A physician shall support access to medical care for all people.

Reprinted from American Medical Association. (2001). *Principles on medical ethics*. Retrieved August 24, 2006, from http://www.ama-assn.org.

RESPONSIBILITIES OF EMS PROFESSIONALS

A universal rule of medicine, no matter where you go in the world, is ***primum non nocere:*** Latin for "first, do no harm." This is more than a phrase; it is based on many centuries of wisdom and has engendered widespread support in the disciplines of medicine and law. A paramedic who bases a decision on that rule has made a sound decision. Of course, paramedics are responsible for doing much more than not harming people. Their primary responsibility obviously is to help people.

Primum non nocere is the primary reason why a paramedic must sometimes question a physician order or refuse it if necessary. This type of situation should always be handled respectfully by both members of the healthcare team. A paramedic is responsible for questioning any order that does not make sense or does not seem to be in the patient's best interests, even after the physician has explained it. The first thing a paramedic should suspect when that happens is the possibility that the physician does not understand the situation. By far the most common reason for that is poor communication

---

BOX 5-4	**Conclusion to the American College of Emergency Physicians Code of Ethics**

Serving patients effectively requires both scientific and technical competence, knowledge of what can be done, and moral competence, knowledge of what should be done. The technical emphasis of emergency medicine is slowly being eclipsed by the ethical. Increasingly, the profession is being asked to help patients die comfortably rather than secure life at all costs. In the next millennium, the difficult questions of the specialty may not be scientific so much as moral.

In spite of future uncertainties and challenges, ethics will remain central to the clinical practice of emergency medicine. Both technical and moral competence can and should be nurtured through advanced preparation and training. The time and information constraints inherent in emergency practice have made reflection on important ethical principles and values difficult at the bedside. This Code is offered both for thoughtful consideration away from the bedside and as a resource when issues arise in clinical practice. The principles of emergency medical ethics identified herein may serve as a guide for the masters and students of this developing art. Through the process of moral reflection and deliberation, emergency physicians may be empowered to base future time-sensitive decisions on a sound moral framework.

Reprinted from American College of Emergency Physicians. (2006). *Code of ethics for emergency physicians*. Retrieved August 24, 2006, from http://www.acep.org.

regarding the situation, which can result from sender error, receiver error, or equipment problems. At any rate, this is an important safety procedure.

PARAMEDIC Pearl

As a paramedic, you are the patient's advocate. Question a physician's order if he or she orders an action that:

- You believe is contraindicated for the patient
- You believe is medically acceptable but not in the patient's best interests
- You believe is medically acceptable but morally wrong

Handle these situations professionally and respectfully.

There is quite a difference between doing things *for* people and doing things *to* them. Patients are not mannequins posing for the benefit of our skills practice. The "S" in EMS stands for service; paramedics are supposed to do things *for* people. Sadly, you do not have to look hard to find colleagues starting IVs and intubating people so they can "get their sticks" or "get their tubes" without considering who ends up paying the costs for that equipment (and accepting the risks of those services).

Patients and their families (not paramedics) decide what constitutes an emergency and what does not. When a person dials 9-1-1 in the middle of the night and the circumstances do not seem impressive, he or she is not "abusing the system."

PATIENTS' RIGHTS

[OBJECTIVE 6]

Over the last 30 years, many organizations devoted to serving the public have developed instruments such as patient bills of rights. In 1997, President Bill Clinton appointed an Advisory Commission on Consumer Protection and Quality in the Health Care Industry. As part of its work, the Commission issued a document that contained eight principal rights and responsibilities aimed at protecting consumers and improving the quality of care. This document, the Patients' Bill of Rights, has been adopted by many health plans, including all the plans sponsored by the federal government (Box 5-5).

PROFESSIONAL ACCOUNTABILITY

[OBJECTIVES 7, 8]

Paramedics are accountable to a number of entities for their decisions, effect, appearance, and behaviors. Sometimes the interests of those entities conflict with one another. When that happens, feelings of frustration are normal because pleasing everyone at the same time is impossible. Some examples include the following:

Organizations: Paramedics typically answer to supervisors, fire officers, police officers, medical directors,

BOX 5-5   Patients' Bill of Rights

I. **Information Disclosure.** You have the right to receive accurate and easily understood information about your health plan, health care professionals, and health care facilities. If you speak another language, have a physical or mental disability, or just don't understand something, assistance will be provided so you can make informed health care decisions.

II. **Choice of Providers and Plans.** You have the right to a choice of health care providers that is sufficient to provide you with access to appropriate high-quality health care.

III. **Access to Emergency Services.** If you have severe pain, an injury, or sudden illness that convinces you that your health is in serious jeopardy, you have the right to receive screening and stabilization emergency services whenever and wherever needed, without prior authorization or financial penalty.

IV. **Participation in Treatment Decisions.** You have the right to know all your treatment options and to participate in decisions about your care. Parents, guardians, family members, or other individuals that you designate can represent you if you cannot make your own decisions.

V. **Respect and Nondiscrimination.** You have a right to considerate, respectful, and nondiscriminatory care from your doctors, health plan representatives, and other health care providers.

VI. **Confidentiality of Health Information.** You have the right to talk in confidence with health care providers and to have your health care information protected. You also have the right to review and copy your own medical record and request that your physician amend your record if it is not accurate, relevant, or complete.

VII. **Complaints and Appeals.** You have the right to a fair, fast, and objective review of any compliant you have against your health plan, doctors, hospitals, or other health care personnel. This includes complaints about waiting times, operating hours, the conduct of healthcare personnel, and the adequacy of healthcare facilities.

Reprinted from the Advisory Commission on Consumer Protection and Quality in the Health Care Industry. (1997). *Patients' rights and responsibilities.* Retrieved January 29, 2008, from http://www.hcqualitycommission.gov/cborr.

government administrators, hospital staff, and patients' families. Sometimes they do not all want the same thing at the same time, and sometimes what they do want is clearly not in the best interests of a patient. For example, a 24-year-old man has been shot in the chest. He apparently was the victim of a drive-by shooting. The patient has pale, sweaty skin, difficulty breathing, and a rapid heart rate. You realize that time is of the essence; you need to be en route to the hospital *now*. A police officer on the scene approaches. He wants a statement from the

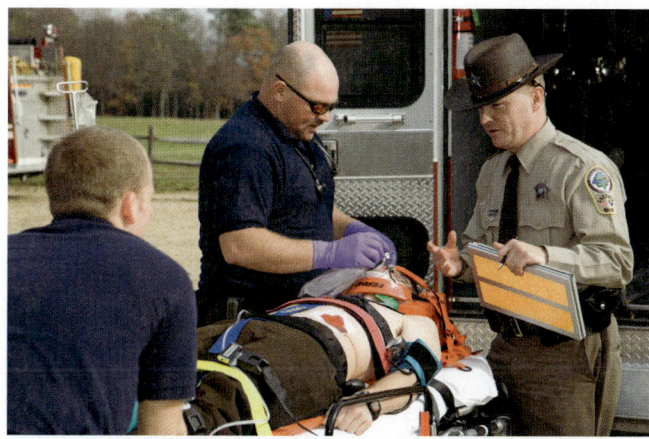

Figure 5-1 Paramedics typically answer to supervisors, fire officers, police officers, medical directors, government administrators, hospital staff, and patients' families, all of whom may have conflicting interests.

patient about what has happened (Figure 5-1). What should you do?

Peers: No paramedic agrees with another paramedic all the time. Occasionally, being a good patient advocate means disagreeing with a colleague, and sometimes that disagreement is key to the well-being of the patient. For example, you and your partner arrive at the home of a 73-year-old man who fell. You find the patient lying on the floor. His right hip is laterally rotated. The patient says he went to sit on the bed and slipped to the floor. He reports severe pain that he rates a 9 on a scale of 0 to 10. His blood pressure is 150/95 mm Hg, pulse is 76 beats/min, and respirations are 18 breaths/min. As your partner prepares to immobilize the patient's hip for transport, you tell your partner that you will start an IV and contact medical direction to give the patient something for pain. Your partner says, "Why do you want to do that? The hospital is only 10 minutes away. He'll be fine." What should you do?

Students: Sometimes a student's needs are outweighed by a patient's needs, such as when the patient really needs an IV and the student cannot seem to hit a garden hose. In those cases, the patient's needs always take priority. In this situation, the paramedic should start the IV instead of the student.

Legal: Some ethical decisions may be illegal. Some legal decisions may be unethical. Some modern areas of debate include abortion, cloning, and physician-assisted suicide. A paramedic is responsible for thoroughly knowing the law as it evolves in his or her area, especially those pertaining to patient refusals and advance directives. Consider a 50-year-old patient with cancer whom you find in his bed. He is not breathing and has no pulse. You see no obvious signs of death. The cardiac monitor shows what appears to be a viable rhythm. His female roommate says he had a seizure tonight but has been in good health otherwise. As you begin resuscitation efforts, a woman arrives who identifies herself as the patient's ex-wife. She franti-

cally protests your resuscitation efforts. She says the patient has terminal cancer and does not want to be resuscitated. She seems unfamiliar with the concept of a DNR document. A heated argument ensues between the two women. The patient does not show any obvious signs that he is suffering from the advanced stages of cancer. You do not have time to argue. What do you do?

Moral: What seems right or wrong to one person may not seem the same to another. Because of their position of public trust, paramedics are generally held accountable to a higher standard of ethical behavior (especially in public) than most people are. For example, while having lunch at a local restaurant, a man walks up to you and your partner and asks if he can have a moment of your time. He quickly explains that he is new to the area and his wife needs surgery. He mentions the name of a surgeon and asks if either of you know anything about him. Immediately recognizing the name, your partner says, "Whoa—find another doctor! I wouldn't let him operate on a member of my family." Even if you agree with your partner's opinion of the surgeon, is his response appropriate?

Paramedics also are personally accountable to themselves and their families as professionals. Following are actions a professional does routinely, simply because he or she is a professional:

1. *Staying certified.* A paramedic is responsible for numerous certificates, depending on governmental, agency, and national registry requirements. Most commonly these include National Registry of Emergency Medical Technicians paramedic certification; a state paramedic license or certificate; an emergency vehicle operator's license (if required); and certification in cardiopulmonary resuscitation, advanced cardiac life support, and pediatric advanced life support (or equivalent). These are a paramedic's tools. Maintaining a personal system for keeping them current is important.
2. *Staying educated* (Figure 5-2). Imagine yourself standing at a patient's bedside, explaining that the reason you made a medication error was that you did not know much about the drug you gave. Once again, paramedics practice *medicine.* This action is incompetence and has no excuse—especially if someone gets hurt as a result.
3. *Reading.* An EMS professional maintains his or her own personal awareness of changes and trends in the profession, even apart from medicine.
4. *Looking (and acting) the part.* Professionals are supposed to *look* professional. What does that mean? It means good grooming, polished leather, and clean, pressed uniforms. Believe it or not, every paramedic call is a public performance. The public may not know how to calculate a dopamine drip, but they do know a slob when they see one compared with a professional (Figure 5-3).

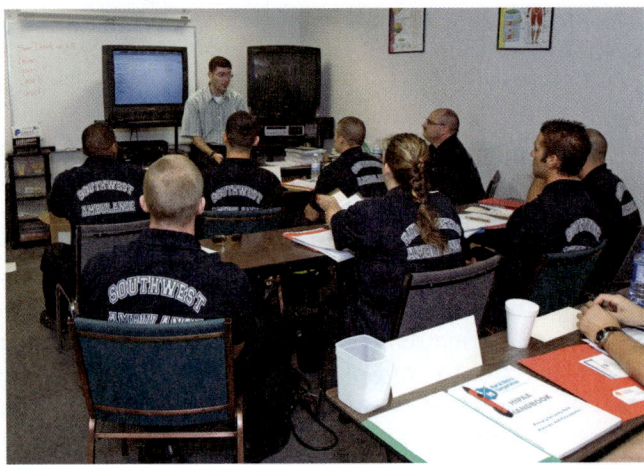

Figure 5-2 Paramedics have a responsibility to stay educated.

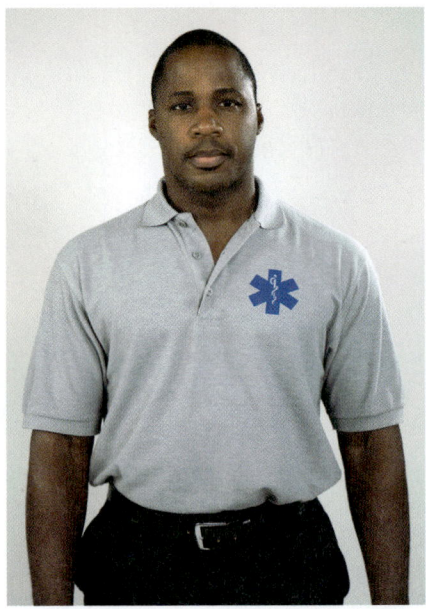

Figure 5-3 Presenting a neat appearance and making a good first impression help inspire confidence in patients and bystanders.

Case Scenario CONCLUSION

In the emergency department, the patient became alert after several doses of naloxone. His respiratory rate and depth increased as he awakened, and he was extubated within minutes of arriving at the hospital. His pain (related to his kidney failure) was excruciating. You and your partner were ordered back to the hospital to transport him back to the in-patient hospice for pain control. He died 3 days later in great pain. The family was furious and reported the incident to the hospital and EMS authority for review.

Looking Back

7. When the EMS agency and your medical director review this case, do you believe they will find fault with your actions? Why or why not?
8. Would this situation have been different had the wife pled with you to "save her husband"? How?
9. What alternatives exist in EMS systems for situations when patient needs are in conflict with system protocols?

BASIC VIRTUES

[OBJECTIVE 9]

Basic virtues are a paramedic's tools—or the tools of anyone whose role depends on the public's trust. The concept of ethics is based on a few basic virtues, some of which have been recognized and valued in most civilizations throughout history. Following are some examples of virtues that are especially important for caregivers.

Courage. Many elements of a paramedic's job require courage, whether it is the courage to stand for what you know is right or the courage to face physical danger. Paramedics face pressure to support decisions by their colleagues, and courage is required to speak a dissenting opinion. Driving an emergency vehicle is fraught with danger from other drivers whose actions are unpredictable. No call is more dangerous than an incident involving a violent patient who needs to be restrained. All these situations are part of the job.

Honor (Integrity). Every action in medicine is subject to the scrutiny of superiors and peers. This reality is not intended to be insulting or oppressive. It simply reflects accountability for the trust you are given. As a result, telling the truth when questioned should be a natural response.

Humility. More than anything else, a paramedic must be humble. Not much glory is found in having a woman throw up on your uniform or extricating a man from a couch after he has lain in his own feces for a week. However, great power is found in humility.

Kindness. Kindness, caring, and consideration are gifts that cannot simply be learned from a teacher (even a good teacher). These gifts are important because many people a paramedic has contact with are having the worst day of their lives; in fact, many are terrified. People in crisis tend to be quite aware of their caregivers. A paramedic who does not care, does not want to be there, and is not concerned about the patient's fear may as well have stayed home for the day. People in crisis are difficult to fool.

Respect. A good caregiver must have respect for people; in fact, it helps to genuinely like them. Why? Because people respond to crisis in many ways—by lying, drugging themselves, losing their tempers, assigning blame to others, praying, or trying to escape (including by self-destructive means). In the process, sometimes they simply are not very nice to caregivers. Nice or not, you still have to be nice to them. That can be difficult if your baseline regard for them in the first place is disrespect or even dislike.

THE BEST TEST

Experience has shown that when paramedics know what it feels like to be treated with dignity and respect, they do a better job of showing dignity and respect to others. Is what you are doing right now ethical? Try "the best test": Could you stand in front of your patient, look him or her in the eye and say, "I did my very best for you"? Better yet, can you do that in front of the person who loves that patient more than anyone else in the world?

Practical tips for ethical behavior are shown in Box 5-6.

BOX 5-6 | **Practical Tips**

1. Ask yourself: Am I doing this for my patient, or am I doing it for me?
2. Remind yourself: Caring counts, kindness cures, and service elevates (Rosen, 1998).
3. Ask yourself: Am I doing this *for* my patient, or *to* them?
4. Picture yourself facing that person you see in your mirror every day.

Case Scenario SUMMARY

1. *What is your general impression of this patient?* This patient is critical based on his level of responsiveness, color, and respiratory rate and pattern. However, his condition also is consistent with his hospice status and provides information that will be useful when deciding how to respond in the absence of DNR documentation.

2. *What treatment will you initiate if the patient's wife does find the DNR documents? What if she does not find the DNR documents?* The legal issues vary somewhat by state and jurisdiction. However, for the most part, resuscitative care is not required for patients with adequate DNR documentation. However, comfort care is allowed, so careful handling, pain medication (not necessary in this case), and oxygen are useful therapies to make patients more comfortable during transport. When DNR documentation is not available, local protocols vary. However, several facts are fairly universal:
   - Hospice patients have been admitted to hospice, and their treatment is guided by the hospice orders. In this way, hospice patients are more similar to interfacility transport patients (who have transport orders) than traditional 911 calls (which are unexpected without any preexisting medical "orders").

   - As in cases of interfacility transports, EMS care should be provided within the context of the hospice orders, which nearly always include DNR orders.
   - Keeping this in mind, the patient must be confirmed as a hospice patient. This can usually be done based on hospice paperwork within the home and can be confirmed by calling the hospice nurse on call and/or simply looking at the environment: hospital bed, patient who appears chronically ill, family statements, and so forth.

3. *What do you believe is in this patient's best interests? What role do you have in ensuring those interests are met?* Not all paramedics agree on the answer to this question, but most believe that resuscitation (intubation, drug therapy, etc.) is not in this patient's best interests. Provision of safe and comfortable transport to the hospital for evaluation—the reason the ambulance was called in the first place—is most likely what is in this patient's best interests.

4. *Do you believe the treatment you provided was in the patient's best interests? The patient's family's? The emergency department's? Who was served by this course of action?* Unfortunately, this situation did not meet anyone's needs. The patient was subjected to

Continued

Case Scenario SUMMARY—continued

unnecessary pain, the family to unnecessary stress and expense (in a time that is already expensive and stressful enough), and the emergency department to receipt of a patient it could not help and a family that was angry.

5. *Could you have handled the situation differently and achieved a different result? How?* Again, paramedics believe differently about this situation, as do medical directors. Although nearly everyone believes that, as this chapter has discussed, the paramedic, physician, and EMS system have an ethical responsibility to ensure that patients are not harmed, many are reluctant to discuss how that responsibility might be carried out. One opportunity to avoid this situation occurs during dispatch. Calling for an emergent response for a hospice patient is rarely appropriate, especially when the hospice nurse (who is knowledgeable about the patient's needs) is the individual placing the call. Once on the scene, the paramedic could have contacted the hospice nurse first then called the emergency physician to confer, armed with further information about the patient's status, medication requirements, and so forth. This additional information may help a physician feel more confident in authorizing paramedics to withhold resuscitation in the absence of DNR paperwork.

6. *Are you required to follow the physician's order even if you believe it is harmful to the patient? Could you have refused to follow this order? How would you have done that?* This idea offers an alternative to the paramedic in this case, although it is a last resort. All healthcare providers are ethically bound to not provide treatment that they believe will harm the patient. In a more black-and-white case, all paramedics would agree that withholding medication from a patient with a history of severe allergy to the medication is appropriate, even if a physician ordered it. For some paramedics and physicians, the care ordered in this case was just as inappropriate. However, if you choose to refuse a physician's order, remember that—no matter how the patient responds—*you* are responsible for your choice. You may be suspended or even terminated (even if you did the "right" thing), and the patient may deteriorate because of

your refusal to provide the medication. Either way, you made the choice and are responsible for the consequences.

7. *When the EMS agency and your medical director review this case, do you believe they will find fault with your actions? Why or why not?* In most cases no fault will be found because you followed the protocols. But does that mean you did the right thing for the patient? Sometimes legal and ethical "rules" conflict. What will you do then? Answering that question for yourself is one of the goals of this chapter and this case scenario. Incidentally, the inquiry in this case did not find fault with the paramedic (who tried hard to avoid resuscitation) but did find fault with the emergency department physician who insisted on treatment that was highly unlikely to benefit the patient.

8. *Would this situation have been different had the wife pled with you to "save her husband"? How?* Yes. In the absence of DNR paperwork, you are left to make decisions based on available information. In the actual case, the patient's condition, the presence of hospice paperwork and cards throughout the house, and the wife's requests were all consistent. If the patient had appeared healthy and robust, or no hospice paperwork was present, or the wife had begged you to resuscitate her husband, the choice would have been much more difficult and the ethical demand to do what was in the patient's best interests would have become more consistent with resuscitation.

9. *What alternatives exist in EMS systems for situations when patient needs are in conflict with system protocols?* Fortunately these cases are somewhat unusual. But when they do occur they are managed better if EMS systems acknowledge that sometimes the protocols are not in the patient's best interests and establish strategies for paramedics and physicians to use to make mutually acceptable decisions. These strategies must be in place system wide. When paramedics are not supported by emergency department physicians in their attempts to meet patient needs (as occurred in this case), conflicts result that may compromise patients.

Chapter Summary

- Ethics are societal principles of conduct that people or groups of people adopt as guidelines for personal behavior.
- Morals are values that help a person define right (what a person ought to do) versus wrong (what a person ought not to do). Morals are derived from teachings

from parents, grandparents, mentors, and religious beliefs.
- *Unethical* refers to conduct that does not conform to approved standards of social or professional behavior.
- Protection of patient privacy is paramount.

- Honesty and respect for humanity are essential traits for the paramedic.
- Medical codes of ethics throughout history and in modern times focus on first doing no harm and the responsibilities of healthcare professionals to the patient.
- Patients' rights are based on their intrinsic autonomy and dignity.

- Professional accountability includes staying current with certificates and maintaining healthy relationships with oneself and colleagues while always placing the patient's best interests foremost.
- Basic virtues exemplify the basis of ethical behavior and are evident in how paramedics treat each other as well as their patients.

REFERENCES

American College of Emergency Physicians. (2006). *Code of ethics for emergency physicians*. Retrieved August 24, 2006, from http://www.acep.org.

American Medical Association. (2001). *Principles on medical ethics*. Retrieved August 24, 2006, from http://www.ama-assn.org.

Brown, M., Craig, B., Dick, J., Dick, T., Federoff, L., Garcia, B., et al. (1987). *Hartson standards of care*, San Diego, CA: Hartson Medical Services.

Gillespie, C. B. (1978). *EMT code of ethics*. Retrieved August 24, 2006, from http://www.naemt.org.

Hippocratic oath—classical version. Retrieved August 24, 2006, from http://www.pbs.org.

International Council of Nurses. (2006). *The ICN code of ethics for nurses*. Retrieved August 24, 2006, from http://www.icn.ch.

Rosen, P. (1998). *Emergency medicine: Concepts and clinical practice* (4th ed.), St. Louis: Elsevier.

SUGGESTED RESOURCES

Dick, T., Berry, S., Forster, J., & Smith, M. (2005). *People care: Career-friendly practices for professional caregivers*, Los Angeles: Summer Communications.

Kingma, D., & Markova, D. (2002). *Random acts of kindness*, New York: Conari Press.

Chapter Quiz

1. Describe "the best test" in your own words.

_____
_____
_____

2. Explain the meaning of *primum non nocere*.

_____

3. A paramedic should strive to do things _____ patients instead of _____ them.

4. What is a code of ethics?

_____
_____
_____

5. Name at least one good excuse for incompetence by a paramedic.

_____

6. Define *ethics*.

_____
_____

7. Which of the following are listed in this chapter as basic virtues that every paramedic should possess? (You may choose more than one.)
   a. Honor
   b. Intelligence
   c. Accountability
   d. Ethics
   e. Humility

8. The first half of the Hippocratic Oath is concerned with a student's responsibilities toward a teacher of medicine. What does the second half of the oath focus on?

_____
_____

Terminology

Code of ethics A guide for interactions between members of a specific profession (such as physicians) and the public.

Ethics Societal principles of conduct that people or groups of people adopt as guidelines for personal behavior.

Medical ethics A field of study that evaluates the decisions, conduct, policies, and social concerns of medical activities.

Morals Values that help a person define right (what a person ought to do) versus wrong (what a person ought not to do).

Primum non nocere Latin for "first, do no harm."

Unethical Conduct that does not conform to approved standards of social or professional behavior.

Medical Terminology Review

Objectives *After completing this chapter, you will be able to:*

1. Explain why using correct medical terminology in medical settings is important.
2. Identify and describe the three word parts that make up medical terms.
3. State why understanding how each word part functions is important.
4. Pronounce various medical terms correctly by applying the appropriate pronunciation guidelines.
5. Correctly change various medical terms from their singular to plural form.
6. Define and give an example of a homonym, an antonym, and a synonym.
7. Describe the impact on patient care when paramedics have a solid grasp of the correct medical terminology.

Chapter Outline

Origins of Medical Words
Components of Words
Using a Medical Dictionary
Plurals
Antonyms

Synonyms
Abbreviations
Practice
Chapter Summary

Case Scenario

As part of your internship, you are riding on a paramedic unit. The unit has been called to the home of a 52-year-old man. He states, "I just don't feel right." On further questioning, he complains of weight loss as well as weakness, nausea, and vomiting for the past 3 days. The patient is responding to questions quickly and easily in complete sentences. Additionally, the patient describes that he has had an increase in his urination, he is constantly thirsty, and he "eats all the time." During the physical examination, you note that the patient has dry mucous membranes and fast, deep respirations and becomes dizzy when standing.

Questions

1. *What are the appropriate medical terms for (1) an increase in urination, (2) excessive thirst, and (3) excessive hunger?*
2. *What is the appropriate medical term for fast, deep respirations?*
3. *From class, you have learned that medical professionals use medical terminology; however, you note that your preceptor uses lay terms with the patient. Why does the preceptor do this?*

[OBJECTIVE 1]

The language used in medicine and healthcare is known as *medical terminology*. Medical terms are used to describe and record every aspect of patient care. This includes a patient's medical history, assessment results, treatment, and outcomes. By understanding the origin of medical terms (words), the components (parts) of those terms, and the guidelines for using them, you will be able to identify and use medical terms correctly. This chapter provides a review of medical terminology.

If a paramedic uses the incorrect medical terminology on the job, consider the following situations that could result:

- The patient could be given an ineffective or even harmful treatment at the hospital as a result of a term being incorrectly used in a radio report or documented on the patient care report.
- The patient could lose trust in the paramedic's ability to care for him or her appropriately.
- A lawsuit could be filed.

ORIGINS OF MEDICAL WORDS

The majority of medical terms come from Greek and Latin words. In general, medical terms that refer to disease are usually derived from Greek words. Words that refer to anatomic structures are usually derived from Latin words. The original words and their meanings are often interesting. For example, the word *muscle* comes from a Latin word for mouse. The movement of a muscle under the skin was thought to resemble the scampering of a mouse. The coccyx, the lower end of the spine, is named for the Greek word for cuckoo because it resembles the cuckoo's bill.

Greek	Disease	Latin	Anatomic
nephro-	nephritis	ren-	kidney/renal
glossa-	glossitis	lingua-	tongue/linguistic

Language used in medicine comes from a combination of Greek and Latin words as well as from eponyms and terms that have resulted from modern medical advances, such as fiberoptic and pacemaker. An **eponym** is a word that has been named for a specific person, place, or thing. You use eponyms every day and may not even be aware of them. For example, the sandwich is named for the Earl of Sandwich, who asked his servant to bring him a serving of meat between two pieces of bread. In medicine, certain diagnostic and surgical procedures, diseases, instruments, and parts of the anatomy are eponyms (Box 6-1).

Furthermore, medical terminology provides one word for a concept that might otherwise take many words to describe. For example, you can say "arthritis" more quickly than you can say "inflammation of the joint." Understanding where medical terms come from, or their origins, can help you begin to decipher their meanings.

BOX 6-1   Medical Eponyms

Specific People*
- McBurney point
- Foley catheter
- Babinski's reflex
- Crohn's disease
- Cesarean section
- Hodgkin's disease

Specific Things
- Athlete's foot
- Pinkeye
- Tennis elbow

*As can be seen, medical eponyms sometimes appear in the possessive form and sometimes not (e.g., Hodgkin disease, Hodgkin's disease).

Case Scenario—continued

Oxygen is applied to the patient as well as pulse oximetry and capnography. His oxygen saturation is 98%, and end-tidal carbon dioxide is 20 mm Hg. His pulse is 110 beats/min, respirations are 32 breaths/min, and blood pressure is 98/64 mm Hg. He has clear lung sounds. Further evaluation of the patient reveals a blood glucose level of 328 mg/dL. This prompts the preceptor to inform the patient that he has high blood sugar. You suggest applying the cardiac monitor, which reveals flattened P waves and peaked T waves. The patient is told his blood gasses are altered and chemical substances in his body are abnormal. An intravenous line is initiated and a fluid bolus of 250 mL is administered while getting the patient ready for transport.

Questions

4. *What is the appropriate medical term for high blood sugar?*
5. *What medical terms would be appropriate to describe this patient's pulse and blood pressure?*
6. *Are there more accurate ways of describing the findings of the physical examination than the terms used with the patient?*

COMPONENTS OF WORDS

[OBJECTIVES 2, 3]

When you encounter a new word, try to break it up into its components, or smaller parts. Some medical terms are quite long; they can be less intimidating if you break them into their smaller parts. If you can figure out the meaning of each part of a word, then you can combine the meanings to determine the full meaning of the word. Many medical words consist of two or three parts. The beginning of the word is known as the prefix. The middle, or foundation, of the word is the word root. Finally, the end of the word is the suffix (Box 6-2).

Word Roots

The **word root** establishes the basic meaning of the word. Prefixes are added to the beginning of a word root, and suffixes are added to the end of a word root. Some word roots are complete words by themselves, but not all are. Further-

BOX 6-2 Word Building

Pericardium
- *peri-* is a prefix meaning around.
- *cardi-* is a word root meaning heart.
- *Pericardium* is a membrane around the heart. (The pericardium is a sac that encloses the heart, holding in fluid.)

Pericarditis
- *peri-* is a prefix meaning around.
- *cardi-* is a word root meaning heart.
- *-itis* is a suffix meaning inflammation.
- *Pericarditis* means inflammation around the heart. (In pericarditis, the pericardium becomes inflamed as a result of a microorganism or a variety of other causes.)

Myocardium
- *my/o* is a combining form meaning muscle.
- *cardi-* is a word root meaning heart.
- *Myocardium* means heart muscle. (The myocardium is the middle and thickest tissue of the heart, which is composed of cardiac muscle.)

Endotracheal
- *endo-* is a prefix meaning inside of.
- *trache/o* is a combining form for trachea, or the windpipe.
- *trache/al* means pertaining to the trachea.
- *Endotracheal* means pertaining to the inside of the trachea. (In endotracheal intubation, a tube is inserted through the mouth or nose into the trachea to open an airway.)

Pyromania
- *pyr/o-* is a combining form meaning fire.
- *-mania* is a suffix that means excessive preoccupation.
- *Pyromania* is excessive preoccupation with fire. (A mania is a type of psychosis characterized by inappropriate overactivity.)

Pyrophobia
- *pyr/o-* is a combining form meaning fire.
- *-phobia* is a suffix meaning abnormal fear.
- *Pyrophobia* is abnormal fear of fire.

TABLE 6-1 Common Word Roots

Word Root	Meaning	Word Root	Meaning
arthr-	joint	later-	side
brachi-	arm	mel-	limb
bucc-	cheek	my-	muscle
cardi-	heart	nas-	nose
carp-	wrist	nephr-	kidney
cephal-	head	occipit-	back of head
chondr-	cartilage	ophthalm-	eye or eyes
cost-	rib	oss-	bone
cyst-	bladder	ot-	ear
cyt-	cell	phleb-	vein
encephal-	brain	pulm-	lungs
enter-	intestine	rhin-	nose
faci-	face	somat-	body
fibr-	fibers	splen-	spleen
gastr-	stomach	thorac-	chest
gloss-	tongue	ventr-	front
gnath-	jaw	viscer-	viscera
hist-	tissue		

means inflammation. Therefore the combined word *osteoarthritis* means inflammation of the bone joints.

Prefixes

A **prefix** introduces another thought or explains the word root (Table 6-2). It is added before, or at the beginning of, the word root. The prefix does not change the meaning of the root word; however, it does change the meaning of the medical term. In other words, prefixes describe the what, how, why, and when of the root word. For example, the prefix *sub-* in subcutaneous means below. The word root *cutaneous* means skin; therefore *subcutaneous* is below the skin. Another word, atypical, which means not typical, can easily be understood when you know that it is formed by adding the prefix *a-*, which means not, to *typical*, which is the word root.

Examples of Prefixes

The word root *-pnea* means breath. If you add the prefix *a-*, which means not, you have the new word *apnea*, which means without breath. The word root *-logy* means study of. If you add the prefix *bio-*, you have the new word *biology*, which means the study of life.

Suffixes

A **suffix** is added at the end of a word root. It changes or adds to the word's meaning or provides further definition (Table 6-3). For example, the suffix *-ase* indicates an

more, the same word root may have different meanings in different fields of study. You may have to consider the context of a word before assigning its meaning.

Some words contain more than one word root. These words are called **compound words.** In compound words each word root retains, or keeps, its basic meaning (Table 6-1). Simple examples of compound words containing two word roots are frostbite and bedpan. A more complicated example is osteoarthritis. The combining form *osteo* comes from the word root *ost-*, meaning bone. The word root *arthr-* means joint or joints. The suffix *-itis*

TABLE 6-2	Common Prefixes	
Prefix	**Meaning**	**Example**
a-, an-	without, from	apnea (without breath), asepsis (without infection)
ab-	away from	abnormal (away from normal)
ad-	toward, to, near	adhesion (something stuck to)
aden-	pertaining to gland	adenitis (inflammation of gland)
ana-	up, toward, apart	anastomosis (joining of two parts)
ante-	before, in front of, forward	antenatal (occurring or formed before birth)
anti-	against, opposing	antiseptic (against or preventing sepsis)
bi-	two, double, twice	bilateral (both sides)
circum-	around, about	circumoral (around the mouth)
contra-	opposed, against	contraindication (indication opposing usually indicated treatment)
derma-	skin	dermatitis (inflammation of the skin)
dia-	through, completely	diagnosis (knowing completely)
dys-	difficult, bad, painful	dyspnea (difficulty breathing)
ecto-	outer, outside	ectopic (out of place)
edem-	swelling	edema (swelling)
endo-	within, inner	endometrium (within the uterus)
ep-, epi-	upon, on, over	epidermis (on the skin)
erythro-	red	erythrocyte (red blood cell)
hemi-	half	hemiplegia (paralysis of one side of the body)
hyper-	excessive, above	hyperplasia (excessive formation)
hypo-	under, deficient	hypotension (low blood pressure)
infra-	below, beneath	infrascapular (below the scapular bone)
inter-	between	intercostal (between ribs)
intra-	within	intralobar (within the lobe)
macro-	large	macroblast (abnormally large cell)
micro-	small	microdrip (small drop)
para-	beside, beyond, after	parathyroids (alongside the thyroid)
per-	through, excessive	perforation (a breaking through)
peri-	around	periosteum (covering of bone)
poly-	many, much, excessive	polyuria (excessive urine)
post-	after, behind	postpartum (after childbirth)
pre-	before, in front of	prediastolic (before diastole)
retro-	backward, behind	retroflexion (bending backward)
semi-	half	semilunar (half moon)
sub-	under, beneath	subdiaphragmatic (under the diaphragm)
supra-	above, superior, excess	supraventricular (above the ventricles)

enzyme. Lipase (*lip-*, which means fat, plus *-ase*) is an enzyme that digests fats. Gastritis, which means inflammation of the stomach, is a combination of the word root *gastr-*, which means stomach, and the suffix -*itis*, which means inflammation. Suffixes are able to change the medical term to a noun or adjective as needed.

Examples of Suffixes

The word root *neur-* means nerve. If you add the suffix *-algia*, which means pain, you have the new word *neuralgia*, which means pain along a nerve. The word root *psych* means the mind. If you add the suffix *-osis*, which means condition, you have the new word *psychosis*, which means condition of the mind.

TABLE 6-3　Common Suffixes

Suffix	Meaning	Examples
-algia	pain	neuralgia (pain along a nerve)
-cyte	cell	leukocyte (white blood cell)
-dipsia	thirst	polydipsia (excessive thirst)
-ectomy	cutting out	tonsillectomy (cutting out of tonsils)
-emia	blood	anemia (lack of blood)
-esthesia	sensation	anesthesia (without sensation)
-genic	causing	carcinogenic (cancer causing)
-gram	record	angiogram (record or graph of vessels of heart)
-itis	inflammation	tonsillitis (inflammation of the tonsils)
-logy	science, study of	biology (study of life)
-ostomy	creation of an opening	gastrostomy (artificial opening of)
-oma	tumor	neuroma (nerve tumor)
-osis	condition of	psychosis (condition of the mind)
-paresis	weakness	hemiparesis (one-sided weakness)
-phagia	eating	polyphagia (excessive eating)
-plegia	paralysis	hemiplegia (one-sided paralysis)
-pnea	breathing	apnea (no breathing)
-phasia	speech	aphasia (inability to speak)
-phobia	fear	hydrophobia (fear of water)
-rhythmia	rhythm	arrhythmia (variation from normal rhythm)
-rrhea	flow or discharge	pyorrhea (discharge of pus)
-taxia	order, arrangement of	ataxia (without muscle coordination)
-uria	to do with urine	polyuria (excessive secretion of urine)

Combining Forms and Vowels

Some word roots cannot combine with other word roots and/or suffixes without help (Table 6-4). For example, *gastr-*, which means stomach, cannot gracefully combine with *megaly*, which means enlargement. The resulting term, gastrmegaly, is not a word. A hyphen at the end of a word root indicates that it is not a completed word. A **combining form** is a word root with an added vowel, known as a **combining vowel.** Thus adding a vowel at the end of the word root, in this case an *o* at the end of *gastr*, solves the problem. The result, *gastro-*, is referred to as a combining form because it is used when combining the root with other roots or suffixes. *Gastr + o + megaly* makes *gastromegaly*, or enlargement of the stomach. In this chapter, word roots with combining vowels are indicated with a slash, as in *gastr/o.*

When adding combining vowels to root words, use the following guidelines:

- Use a combining vowel before a suffix that begins with a consonant (e.g., cyt/o/pathology).

TABLE 6-4　Common Combining Forms

Combining Form	Meaning	Combining Form	Meaning
brachi/o-	arm	pil/o-	hair
cardi/o-	heart	steth/o-	chest
carp/o-	wrist	thorac/o-	chest, thorax
cephal/o-	head	thyr/o-	thyroid gland
cervic/o-	neck	trache/o-	trachea
encephal/o-	brain	ureter/o-	ureter
faci/o-	face	vas/o-	vessel
gloss/o-	tongue	vesic/o-	bladder, blister
nas/o-	nose	viscer/o-	viscera
ot/o-	ear		

- Use a combining vowel to join other root words (e.g., gastr/o/enteritis).
- Do not use a combining vowel before a suffix beginning with a vowel (e.g., gastritis, not gastroitis).

Examples of Combining Forms and Vowels

cardi + *o* + *logy* = cardiology (study of the heart)
neur + *o* + *logy* = neurology (study of the nervous system)

Case Scenario CONCLUSION

En route to the hospital, you continue to monitor and assess the patient. His symptoms have not changed. After the bolus, his lungs remain clear and his blood pressure is 108/72 mm Hg. Two additional boluses of 250 mL are administered without further change in the patient's condition. At the hospital a handoff report is given, including the history of the event, physical findings, treatment administered, and response to treatment.

Questions

7. When you compare your call report to your preceptor's, you notice that your preceptor used several medical terms, yet the preceptor never used those terms during the call. You also recall the terms being used during the handoff report. Why would the preceptor choose to use the terms in these instances, particularly when the preceptor did not use them during the call?
8. What medical terms could have been used in the handoff and written report based on the interaction with this patient?

USING A MEDICAL DICTIONARY

During your paramedic program and throughout your career as a paramedic, you will find a medical dictionary to be quite useful. When choosing a medical dictionary, look for one that includes abbreviations, symbols, and pronunciations.

Pronunciation and Spelling

[OBJECTIVE 4]
A helpful way to familiarize yourself with a medical term is to say it aloud several times. This will help you learn to pronounce it correctly. Soon it will become part of your vocabulary.

Vowels

In most cases, if a **vowel** (*a, e, i, o, u,* and sometimes *y*) in a word is followed by another vowel, then the first vowel receives a long pronunciation. A macron (¯) is placed over the vowel. For example, tray is pronounced (′trā).

Vowel	Word	Phonetic Symbol
a	tray	ā
e	bean	ē
i	pie	ī
o	goat	ō
u	cue	ū
y	bye	ȳ

In general, when a vowel in a word is followed by a consonant, the vowel receives a short pronunciation. A breve (˘) is placed over the vowel. For example, umbrella is pronounced (ŭm-′bre-la).

Vowel	Word	Phonetic Symbol
a	addict	ă
e	endless	ĕ
i	injury	ĭ
o	son	ŏ
u	umbrella	ŭ

Consonants

Pronunciation guidelines also exist for consonants. Some consonants are referred to as sounding soft or hard.

Consonant	Word	Pronunciation
Soft *c* if before *e* or *i*	face	s
Soft *g* if before *e* or *i*	gel	j
Hard *c* if before *a, o,* or *u*	cake	k
Hard *g* if before *a, o,* or *u*	gate	g

Unusual Pronunciation

When two consonants are together in a word, or an *x* is the first letter, the word may have an unusual pronunciation, as in the following:

Consonants	Word	Pronunciation		
ch	chromosome	k		kro
ph	pharynx	f		fay
pn	pneumatic	n		noo
ps	psychology	s		sye
pt	ptosis	t		toh
eu	euthyroid	ū		yoo
x	xeroderma	z		zeer
gn	gnathalgia	n		nuh

Helpful Hint

Notice how the words *suffix*, *prefix*, *affix*, and *fixation* all have *fix* as their word root.

You also should know how to make singular medical terms plural as well as how to distinguish homonyms, antonyms, and synonyms to ensure you are using the correct word.

PLURALS

[OBJECTIVES 5, 6]

A **plural** is a noun that refers to more than one of something. Sometimes when making a noun plural, standard English rules apply. However, most of the medical terms that are nouns stem from Greek or Latin words and therefore require different plural endings. As in any rule, exceptions exist.

Forming Plural Words from English Nouns

A plural is formed by adding an *s* to the singular form, as follows:

- muscle to muscles
- hand to hands
- digit to digits

For nouns ending in an *s*, *ch*, or *sh*, add *es* to the singular form, as follows:

- sinus to sinuses
- church to churches
- sash to sashes

For nouns ending in a *y* preceded by a consonant, change the *y* to *i* and add *es*, as follows:

- capillary to capillaries
- ovary to ovaries

For nouns ending in *o*, add *s* or *es*, as follows:

- tomato to tomatoes
- auto to autos

For nouns ending in *f* or *fe*, drop the *f* or *fe* and add *ves*, as follows:

- half to halves
- calf to calves

Forming Plural Words from Latin and Greek Nouns

For nouns ending in *a*, add an *e*, as follows:

- stria to striae
- petechia to petechiae

For nouns ending in *ax* or *ix*, change the *x* to *c* and add *es*, as follows:

- thorax to thoraces
- appendix to appendices

For nouns ending in *en*, drop the *en* and add *ina*, as follows:

- lumen to lumina
- foramen to foramina

For nouns ending in *ex*, change to *ices*, as follows:

- cortex to cortices

For nouns ending in *is*, change to *es* or *ides*, as follows:

- psychosis to psychoses
- epididymis to epididymides

For nouns ending in *ma*, change to *mata*, as follows:

- sarcoma to sarcomata (could add an *s* to form sarcomas)
- carcinoma to carcinomata

For nouns ending in *nx*, *anx*, *inx*, or *ynx*, change to *nges*, as follows:

- phalanx to phalanges
- larynx to larynges

For nouns ending in *on*, change to *a*, as follows:

- phenomenon to phenomena
- spermatozoon to spermatozoa

For nouns ending in *um*, change to *a*, as follows:

- diverticulum to diverticula
- ovum to ova

For nouns ending in *us*, change to *i*, as follows:

- bronchus to bronchi
- alveolus to alveoli

For nouns ending in a *y* preceded by a consonant, change the *y* to *i* and add *es*, as follows:

- myopathy to myopathies
- artery to arteries

In medical professions, spelling is especially critical because misspelled words can cause confusion and even lead to a misdiagnosis. If you are unsure of a word's spelling, consult a medical dictionary. Be aware that some medical terms sound alike but are spelled differently and have different meanings. These are called **homonyms.** For example, ileum (il'e-um) is a part of the small intestine and ilium is a part of the pelvic, or hip, bone.

If you misspell a medical term, you may completely alter the meaning of what you are trying to express. For example, hyperglycemia (hi'per-gli-se'me-ah) is too much blood sugar, and hypoglycemia (hi'po-gli-se'me-ah) is too little blood sugar. In addition, words spelled correctly but pronounced incorrectly may easily be misunderstood. For example, urethra (ur-re'thrah) is the urinary bladder to the external surface, and ureter (u-re'ter) is one of two tubes that lead from the kidney to the urinary bladder.

> Definitions and spoken pronunciations of commonly used medical terms are available online at *http://evolve.elsevier.com/Aehlert/paramedic*.

ANTONYMS

[OBJECTIVE 6]

Antonyms are root words, prefixes, or suffixes that have the opposite meaning of another word. Examples of words and their antonyms are as follows:

good	eu	bad	mal
right	dextro	left	sinistro
toward	ad	away from	ab

SYNONYMS

[OBJECTIVE 6]

Synonyms are root words, prefixes, or suffixes that have the same or almost the same meaning as another word, prefix, or suffix. Following are examples of synonyms used in the medical setting:

- *pulmon/o*: lung (as in pulmonologist)
- *pneumo*: lung (as in pneumonia)

Both prefixes mean lung, but they are not interchangeable. For example, pneumologist is not an accepted term; pulmonologist is the correct term.

ABBREVIATIONS

Some **abbreviations** are standard and used universally, such as OH for Ohio and Dr. for doctor. In addition, some abbreviations have found their way into spoken language, such as *ASAP*.

Abbreviations used in the medical field are fairly universal. However, check with your local EMS provider or hospital for its approved list of abbreviations. When in doubt about whether to use an abbreviation, write out the term in full. Table 6-5 lists some of the most common medical abbreviations used in the prehospital environment.

TABLE 6-5 Common Medical Abbreviations and Symbols

Abbreviation	Meaning	Abbreviation	Meaning
ā	before	AV	atrioventricular
ACLS	advanced cardiac life support	bid	twice a day
abd	abdomen	BM, bm	bowel movement
ABG	arterial blood gases	BP	blood pressure
ac	before meals	BSA	body surface area
ACS	acute coronary syndrome	c̄	with
ADL	activities of daily living	C	centigrade, Celsius
ad lib	as much as needed, as desired	Ca	calcium, cancer, carcinoma
AIDS	acquired immunodeficiency syndrome	CAD	coronary artery disease
ALS	advanced life support	cath	catheter, catheterization
am	morning	CBC	complete blood count
AMI	acute myocardial infarction	cc	cubic centimeter(s)
ARC	AIDS-related complex	CC	chief complaint
ARDS	acute respiratory distress syndrome	CCU	cardiac care unit, coronary care unit, critical care unit
ASA	aspirin	CHF	congestive heart failure
ASHD	arteriosclerotic heart disease	cm	centimeter(s)

TABLE 6-5 **Common Medical Abbreviations and Symbols**—continued

Abbreviations		Abbreviations	
Abbreviation	**Meaning**	**Abbreviation**	**Meaning**
CNS	central nervous system	ICP	intracranial pressure
CO	carbon monoxide	ICU	intensive care unit
COPD	chronic obstructive pulmonary disease	IDDM	insulin-dependent diabetes mellitus
c/o	complains of	Ig	immunoglobulin
CO_2	carbon dioxide	IM	intramuscular
CPAP	continuous positive airway pressure	IMS	incident management system
CSF	cerebrospinal fluid	IPPB	intermittent positive-pressure breathing
CT	computed tomography	IV	intravenous
CVD	cerebrovascular disease	IVP	intravenous push, intravenous pyelogram
CVP	central venous pressure	kg	kilogram(s)
D_5W	5% dextrose in water	KVO	keep vein open
D/C	discontinue	L	liter(s)
DJD	degenerative joint disease	lb	pound(s)
DTs	delirium tremens	LBBB	left bundle branch block
Dx, dx	diagnosis	LLQ	left lower quadrant
EC	emergency center	LR	lactated Ringer's solution
ECG or EKG	electrocardiogram	LUQ	left upper quadrant
ED	emergency department	LOC	level of consciousness
EEG	electroencephalogram	m	meter(s)
ER	emergency room	MAP	mean arterial pressure
F	Fahrenheit	mcg	microgram(s)
fx	fracture	MCI	multicasualty incident
g, gm, Gm	gram(s)	MICU	mobile intensive care unit
GB	gallbladder	mg	milligram(s)
GCS	Glasgow Coma Scale	MI	myocardial infarction
GI	gastrointestinal	mL	milliliter(s)
gr	grain	mm	millimeter(s)
GSW	gunshot wound	mm Hg	millimeters of mercury
gtt	drops	MRI	magnetic resonance imaging
GU	genitourinary	NG	nasogastric
Gyn, GYN	gynecologic	NICU	neonatal intensive care unit
h	hour	NKDA	no known drug allergies
Hb, hgb	hemoglobin	NPO	nothing by mouth
HBV	hepatitis B virus	noc	night
HIV	human immunodeficiency virus	NS	normal saline
HPI	history of present illness	NSTEMI	non–ST-segment elevation myocardial infarction
hs	hours of sleep	O_2	oxygen
hx	history	OB	obstetrics

Continued

TABLE 6-5 **Common Medical Abbreviations and Symbols**—continued

Abbreviation	Meaning	Abbreviation	Meaning
OR	operating room	S&S	signs and symptoms
os	mouth	SA	sinoatrial
OTC	over-the-counter	SIDS	sudden infant death syndrome
oz	ounce(s)	SL	sublingual
P	pulse, phosphorus	SOB	shortness of breath
p̄	after	sol, soln	solution
pc	after meals	stat	immediately
PCR	patient care record	STEMI	ST-segment elevation myocardial infarction
PE	physical examination, pulmonary embolus	STD	sexually transmitted disease
PICU	pediatric intensive care unit	Sub-Q	subcutaneous
PID	pelvic inflammatory disease	tab	tablet
pm	evening	T	temperature
PMH	past medical history	TIA	transient ischemic attack
PMS	premenstrual syndrome	tid	three times a day
PND	paroxysmal nocturnal dyspnea	TKO	to keep open
PO	orally	TPR	temperature, pulse, and respirations
post	posterior	tsp	teaspoon
prep	preparation	UA	unstable angina
prn	as needed, as desired, whenever necessary	URI	upper respiratory infection
pt	patient	USP	U.S. Pharmacopeia
q̄	every	UTI	urinary tract infection
qd	every day	VC	vital capacity
qh	every hour	VS	vital signs
q2h	every 2 hours	WNL	within normal limits
qid	four times a day	wt	weight
qm	every morning	x-ray	radiograph
qn	every night	**Symbols**	
R	respiration, rectal	**Symbol**	**Meaning**
RBBB	right bundle branch block	=	equal to
RDS	respiratory distress syndrome	+	positive
RL	Ringer's lactate solution	−	negative
RLQ	right lower quadrant	↑	increased
R/O	rule out	↓	decreased
ROM	range of motion	°	degree
RUQ	right upper quadrant	#	pound
Rx	drug, prescription, therapy	♀	female
RR	respiratory rate	♂	male
s̄	without		

Case Scenario SUMMARY

1. *What are the appropriate medical terms for (1) an increase in urination, (2) excessive thirst, and (3) excessive hunger?* The appropriate medical term to describe an increase in urination is *polyuria* (poly [excessive] + uria [related to urine]). The correct medical term for excessive thirst is *polydipsia* (poly [excessive] + dipsia [thirst]). The correct medical term for excessive hunger is polyphagia (poly [excessive] + phagia [hunger]).

2. *What is the appropriate medical term for fast, deep respirations?* The appropriate medical term for fast, deep respirations is *hyperpnea* (hyper [excessive] + pnea [breathing]).

3. *From class, you have learned that medical professionals use medical terminology; however, you note that your preceptor uses lay terms with the patient. Why does the preceptor do this?* Patients are rarely familiar with medical terminology. Therefore if you use such terms while conducting a patient interview, you will not likely get an adequate history because the patient will not understand your questions. When you interview a patient, use lay terms. For example, because this patient is reporting weakness as well as dizziness when he stands, determine if he has fainted or passed out. In most patients, asking about "a syncopal episode" would be less effective than asking about "fainting." However, in some geographic areas this may not even work; if you ask the patient if he or she "fell out" (or sometimes "fell up"), you may receive the correct information. As a paramedic, you must be familiar with terms and phrases that are common in the geographic area in which you work.

4. *What is the appropriate medical term for high blood sugar?* The appropriate medical term for high blood sugar is *hyperglycemia* (hyper [excessive] + glyclo [glucose] + emia [in the blood]).

5. *What medical terms would be appropriate to describe this patient's pulse and blood pressure?* This patient is experiencing tachycardia (tachy [rapid] + cardio [heart]) and hypotension (hypo [deficient, below, under] + tensions [pressure]).

6. *Are there more accurate ways of describing the findings of the physical examination than the terms used with the patient?* The use of medical terms would provide a more accurate description of findings in this patient and provide valuable baseline information for other healthcare providers. However, in the event that the paramedic does not know the appropriate medical term to use, he or she should use lay terms to provide an accurate description of the patient. This would help avoid an incorrect medical term being used, which might cause incorrect information to be given to the next person providing care.

7. *When you compare your call report to your preceptor's, you notice that your preceptor used several medical terms, yet the preceptor never used those terms during the call. You also recall the terms being used during the handoff report. Why would the preceptor choose to use the terms in these instances, particularly when the preceptor did not use them during the call?* Every group has its own language and terminology unique to that group. In fact, this is one of the defining factors of a group. The language of medicine is known as medical terminology. As previously mentioned, this terminology is not appropriate to use with most patients. However, when you use it among others in the medical profession, it provides valuable information to those who will be caring for the patient next. Moreover, it provides quick and efficient communication regarding conditions, findings, and treatments. Additionally, it provides a method of recording obscure patient statements, such as, "I just don't feel right."

8. *What medical terms could have been used in the handoff and written report based on the interaction with this patient?* The following terms could have been used accurately to describe findings in this patient:

   - *Malaise*: A general feeling of discomfort, illness, or lack of well-being sometimes accompanied by a feeling of exhaustion or of not having enough energy.
   - *Polyuria*: Excretion of an abnormally increased volume of urine.
   - *Polydipsia*: Excessive thirst or an abnormal increase in thirst.
   - *Polyphagia*: Excessive eating.
   - *Kussmaul's respirations:* Abnormally fast and deep respirations.
   - *Orthostatic hypotension*: A reduction in blood pressure when a person rises from a supine or sitting position; often accompanied by a sensation of dizziness.
   - *Hypocapnia or hypocarbia*: Lower-than-normal levels of carbon dioxide.
   - *Hyperglycemia*: Higher-than-normal glucose levels in the blood.
   - *Hyperkalemia*: Higher-than-normal serum levels of potassium.

PRACTICE

[OBJECTIVE 7]

Medical terms can sometimes be long and complex. Consequently, improving your understanding of how they are put together can be helpful. Medical terms are made up of combinations of word roots, prefixes, and suffixes. A helpful tactic is to get into the habit of breaking down complex words into their separate parts.

As you use various word roots, prefixes, and suffixes, you will better understand, interpret, and define new medical terms. In addition, make a practice of looking up new terms in a glossary or dictionary when studying. Spelling and pronunciation are essential elements of effective communication with other healthcare professionals; errors endanger the patient and the paramedic's reputation. So much is involved in medical terminology that it is regarded as a separate course of study in itself.

Take the time and effort to practice building medical terms. Moreover, practice their correct pronunciations. Your proficient use of medical terms demonstrates professionalism to your patients, their families, and other healthcare providers, thereby establishing your credibility.

Chapter Summary

- Paramedics use medical terminology daily, so you must know how to determine the meaning of medical terms.
- The word parts used to build medical words are root words, prefixes, and suffixes.
- Understanding the function of the word parts can help you determine the meaning of unfamiliar medical terms.
- Practice makes perfect. Use flashcards, practice writing and saying the word parts and their meanings, and look up unfamiliar word parts in a medical dictionary if necessary.
- Practice pronouncing difficult medical terms.
- You may have to change a medical term from its singular to plural form to record it. Knowing the guidelines for changing English, Greek, and Latin words from singular to plural will help.
- A homonym is a word that has the same pronunciation as another word but a different spelling and meaning.
- An antonym is a word that has the opposite meaning of another word.
- A synonym is a root word, suffix, or prefix that has the same or almost the same meaning as another root word, suffix, or prefix.
- The correct use of medical terminology creates a good impression and builds credibility with your patients and their families.

Chapter Quiz

1. How can you build a medical vocabulary?
   _____
   _____

2. Why is memorizing every medical term unnecessary?
   _____
   _____

3. What legal and ethical situations could arise from using incorrect medical terminology when recording information on patient care reports?
   _____
   _____
   _____
   _____

4. What is the best way to break down a medical term to determine its meaning? Why?
   _____
   _____

5. Paramedics Bayless and Sartori responded to the home of a 66-year-old woman who was reporting dizziness. The following is the narrative portion of the patient care report they submitted to the emergency department nurse on arrival. Identify all the mistakes this report contains.

   "Mrs. Ramos complained of feeling dizzy with some fertigo for 3 days. On questioning, Mrs. Ramos stated that she was febrille 2 days ago with some gastroentestinal symptomes, such as darhea and nausea. She also complained of laryngetes. Her blood pressure is controlled by medication. She has no complaints of chest pain or anjina, nor does she have dispnea, although she does have some orthapnea. She does have some syanosis of the hands and feet but does not complain of pain in these areas. Her sinuses are painful. Her current diagnosisses are sinisitus, athuroscleroisis, possible streptocokki infection, gastrointeritis, and faringitis."

   _____
   _____
   _____
   _____

6. Define the following terms:

ab- _____

ante- _____

anti- _____

bi- _____

erythro- _____

hemi- _____

hyper- _____

my- _____

para- _____

Terminology

Abbreviation A shorter way of writing something.

Antonym A root word, prefix, or suffix that has the opposite meaning of another word.

Combining form A word root followed by a vowel.

Combining vowel A vowel added to a word root before a suffix.

Compound word A word that contains more than one root.

Eponym A word that derives its name from the specific person, place, or thing for whom or what it is named.

Homonyms Terms that sound alike but are spelled differently and have different meanings.

Plural A noun that refers to more than one person, place, or thing.

Prefix A sequence of letters that comes before the word root and often describes a variation of the norm.

Suffix A sequence of letters that comes at the end of the word root and often describes a condition of or act performed on the word root.

Synonym A root word, prefix, or suffix that has the same or almost the same meaning as another word, prefix, or suffix.

Vowel The letters *a, e, i, o, u,* and sometimes *y.*

Word root The foundation of a word; establishes the basic meaning of a word.

Body Systems: Anatomy and Physiology

Objectives   *After completing this chapter, you will be able to:*

1. Define *anatomy, physiology,* and *pathophysiology* and discuss the importance of human anatomy and physiology to the paramedic profession.
2. Define *homeostasis.*
3. Describe the anatomic position.
4. Describe the sagittal, midsagittal, transverse, and frontal planes.
5. List the structures that comprise the axial and appendicular regions of the body.
6. Name the body cavities, membranes, and some organs within each cavity.
7. Define the function of cellular structures.
8. Describe the cytoplasm.
9. Describe the function of the cell organelles.
10. State the function of the nucleus.
11. Describe how cells reproduce.
12. Discuss input and output of aerobic and anaerobic cellular metabolism.
13. Discuss mechanisms that move substances across cell membranes, including diffusion, facilitated diffusion, osmosis, and active transport.
14. Describe the function of epithelial tissue and how it can be classified on the basis of shape or arrangement.
15. Describe the functions of connective tissue and relate them to the function of the body or an organ system.
16. Explain the basic differences in skeletal, smooth, and cardiac muscle.
17. Describe nervous tissue.
18. Define the 11 major organ systems of the human body. Be prepared to label a diagram listing their major anatomic features, function, and interrelations to the other body systems.
19. State the functions of the integumentary system.
20. Name the two layers of the skin.
21. Describe the function of hair and nails.
22. Describe the functions of the sebaceous and sweat glands.
23. Describe the function of the skeleton.
24. List the parts of the axial and appendicular skeleton.
25. Describe the bones of the upper and lower extremities.
26. Explain how joints are classified. Give an example of each and describe the possible movements.
27. Describe the purpose of the muscular system.
28. List and describe the four basic properties of muscles.
29. State the three primary functions of muscles.
30. Describe the process of muscle movement.
31. Name the three main functions of the nervous system.
32. Name the divisions of the nervous system and state their general functions.
33. List and describe the three layers of the meninges.
34. State the locations and functions of the cerebrospinal fluid.
35. List and describe the three divisions of the brainstem.
36. Describe the diencephalons of the brain.
37. Describe the cerebrum, cerebellum, and spinal cord.
38. Describe the peripheral nervous system.
39. List the groups of cranial nerves and describe them.
40. List and describe the two branches of the autonomic nervous system.
41. Identify the primary endocrine glands and list the major hormones they secrete.
42. List the two parts of the circulatory system.
43. List the parts of the cardiovascular system.
44. Describe the parts of the blood.
45. Describe the location of the heart.
46. State the Frank-Starling law and explain why increased preload will increase myocardial contractility and cardiac output.
47. Discuss the relations among blood pressure, peripheral vascular resistance, cardiac output, stroke volume, and heart rate.
48. Name the great vessels and their functions.
49. Name and describe the chambers and valves of the heart.
50. Trace the pathway of blood flow through the heart and pulmonary circulation.
51. Describe the coronary circulation.
52. Describe the coronary conduction system and cardiac action potential.
53. Describe the systemic circulation.
54. Describe the structure and function of arteries, veins, and capillaries.
55. Describe the functions of the lymphatic system.
56. List the parts of the respiratory system.
57. Describe the pathway of the respiratory system, including nasal cavities, pharynx, and larynx.
58. Describe the structure and function of the larynx.
59. Describe the lower airway structures.
60. State the roles of the visceral and parietal pleura in respiration.
61. Describe the general function of the digestive system and name its major divisions.
62. Describe the structure and function of the parts of the gastrointestinal tract.
63. Describe the essential functions of the urinary system.
64. Describe the location and general function of each organ in the urinary system.

65. Name the parts of a nephron.
66. List the essential and accessory organs of the male and female reproductive systems and give the general function of each.
67. Describe the sense of smell.
68. Describe the sense of taste.
69. Name the parts of the eye and explain their functions in sight.
70. Name the parts of the ear and explain their functions in hearing.
71. Define *isotonic, hypotonic*, and *hypertonic*.

72. Describe the mechanisms that affect distribution of body water between the intracellular and extracellular spaces.
73. Define *ion, electrolyte, anion*, and *cation*.
74. Identify the principal intracellular and extracellular anions and cations.
75. Describe the physiologic mechanisms used to maintain acid-base balance.
76. Given values for pH and $PaCO_2$, determine the acid-base imbalance present.

CHAPTER OUTLINE

Review of Anatomy and Physiology
Characteristics of Life
Organizational Structure
Cell Structure
Tissues
Organ Systems
Integumentary System
Skeletal System
Muscular System
Nervous System

Endocrine System
Circulatory System
Respiratory System
Digestive System
Urinary System
Reproductive System
Special Senses
Body Environment
Chapter Summary

Case Scenario

You and your ambulance partner respond with the fire department for a "truck versus motorcycle" crash on a two-lane highway. On arrival, you learn that a three-quarter-ton pickup truck was stationary in the left-turn lane waiting for traffic to clear. A motorcycle with a single rider was moving toward him at highway speeds in the opposite lane of traffic when it drifted across the yellow line and struck the truck in the center of the front bumper/grill area. The collision caused the truck to be pushed back 10 feet in the turn lane. The motorcycle rider was ejected from the bike and collided with the truck windshield, after which the rider rolled to the ground. The motorcycle rider is face down on the pavement next to the front driver's door of the pickup truck, unconscious and unresponsive. You apply manual cervical spine stabilization and, with assistance, logroll the patient onto his back. You immediately note that the patient is pale and sweaty, and his breathing fast and deep. His upper teeth have been knocked out and his eyes are swollen shut.

Questions

1. *What anatomic areas of the body may be injured as a result of this collision?*
2. *Which anatomic areas of the body may present with life-threatening injuries in this scenario?*
3. *What is the appropriate term for "pale and sweaty"? What is happening in the body to cause it, and what does it mean?*
4. *Given the broken upper teeth and facial swelling, what body structures may have been injured?*

REVIEW OF ANATOMY AND PHYSIOLOGY

[OBJECTIVES 1, 2, 3]

As a paramedic, you must understand human anatomy and physiology. **Anatomy** is the study of the body's structure and organization. An understanding of anatomy will help you in many ways. First, it will give you the ability to organize a physical examination. Second, it will help you describe areas of the patient's body as those areas relate to the patient's injury or symptoms. Third, it will help you locate areas of the body on which to perform procedures.

Physiology is the study of how the body functions. An understanding of physiology will help you identify normal and abnormal physiology in relation to disease processes. Moreover, it will aid you in understanding the various treatments and procedures for patients in specific situations. **Pathophysiology,** which is addressed in Chapter 8, is the study of the functional changes that occur with a particular syndrome or disease.

Homeostasis refers to the general stability in the internal environment of the body regardless of the external environment. This balance is naturally maintained by the body's adaptive responses that help promote healthy survival. Various sensing, feedback, and control mechanisms help keep the body in this steady state. Some of the bodily functions controlled by homeostatic mechanisms are heartbeat, blood pressure, body temperature, respiration, and glandular secretion.

Terminology

[OBJECTIVE 3]

In medicine, directional terms are used to refer to the human body. The **anatomic position** describes the position of a person being examined who is standing erect with his or her feet and palms facing the examiner. A patient lying **supine** is on his or her back (face up). A patient in the **prone** position is lying face down (on his or her stomach). A patient in the **lateral recumbent** position is on his or her left or right side. Always describe the patient in reference to the anatomic position (Figure 7-1). Directional terms such as *up* (superior) or *down* (inferior), *front* (anterior or ventral) or *back* (posterior or dorsal), and *left, right,* or *medial* also are expressed in anatomic terminology. The terms used always refer to the patient, not the examiner (Table 7-1).

Anatomic Planes

[OBJECTIVE 4]

Anatomic planes are used to describe the relation of internal body structures to the surface of the body. These planes are imaginary straight line divisions of the body (Figure 7-2). The **sagittal plane,** for example, runs vertically through the middle of the body, creating right and left sections (or halves). The **transverse (horizontal) plane** divides the body into **superior** (top) and **inferior** (bottom) sections. The **frontal plane** divides the body into ventral **(anterior)** and dorsal **(posterior)** sections. The midsagittal plane is the exact middle of the sagittal plane that divides right and left.

Body Regions

[OBJECTIVE 5]

The body is composed of regions. These body regions organize the anatomic structures. The **axial skeleton** is composed of the head, neck, thorax, and abdomen. The

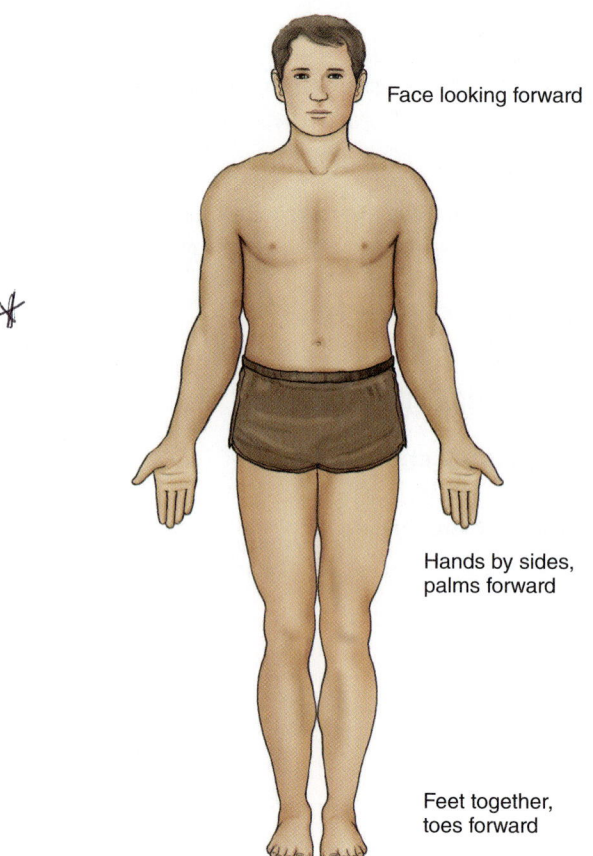

Face looking forward

Hands by sides, palms forward

Feet together, toes forward

Figure 7-1 Anatomic position. Note that the palms face forward.

appendicular skeleton is composed of the extremities (limbs), including the arms, pelvic bones, and legs.

Body Cavities

[OBJECTIVE 6]

Although the body may appear as one large cavity, it is composed of cavities that keep organs contained in specific areas. The organs contained in a cavity are collectively referred to as the viscera. Each of the body's cavities is lined by a **serous membrane.** These membranes are composed of two layers: the parietal membrane and the visceral membrane. The parietal membrane adheres to the cavity wall, and the visceral membrane adheres to the organ. Between these two layers a small amount of lubricating fluid is produced to reduce friction during the movement of the organ.

PARAMEDIC*Pearl*

The term *visceral* is always used in reference to organs. This gives rise to the term *visceral pain,* which is pain associated with an organ. This type of pain is common but is diffuse and difficult for patients to localize.

TABLE 7-1 Important Directional Terms

Term	Definition
Anterior	The front, or ventral, surface
Caudal	A position toward the distal end of the body; usually inferior
Cephalic	A position toward the head; usually superior
Distal	A position farther from the attachment of a limb to the turnk
Dorsal	Referring to the back of the body; posterior
Inferior	Toward the feet; below a point of reference in the anatomic position
Lateral	A position away from the midline of the body
Left	A position toward the left side of the body
Medial	A position toward the midline of the body
Posterior	The back, or dorsal, surface
Proximal	A position nearer to the attachment of a limb to the trunk
Superior	Situated above or higher than a point of reference in the anatomic position; top
Right	A position toward the right side of the body
Ventral	Referring to the front of the body; anterior

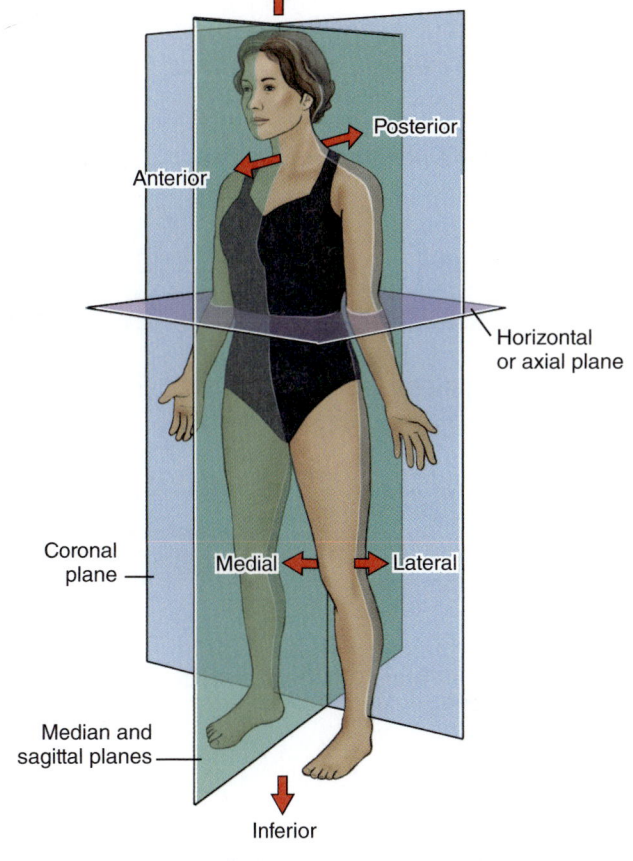

Figure 7-2 Anatomic planes are imaginary straight line divisions of the body.

The body is divided into two main cavities: the ventral cavity and the dorsal cavity. These cavities are further subdivided into smaller subcavities.

The ventral cavity contains the majority of the organs and is divided into the thoracic cavity and the abdominopelvic cavity.

The thoracic cavity is contained in the upper part of the ventral cavity and is further subdivided into the right and left **pleural cavities,** which contain the right and left lungs (or pleura). Separating the two pleural cavities is a space called the **mediastinum.** The mediastinum includes the trachea, esophagus, thymus gland, heart, and great vessels (Figure 7-3). Within the mediastinum the heart is contained in the **pericardium,** which is composed of two layers of fibrous tissue. The visceral pericardium, or epicardium, is the innermost layer and covers the heart itself. The outer layer, the parietal pericardium, surrounds the heart. It is often referred to as the *pericardial sac.* The potential space between these two layers, or membranes, is referred to as the **pericardial cavity.** The inferior border of the thoracic cavity is delineated by the **diaphragm** (Figure 7-4).

The diaphragm is also the superior border of the second subdivision of the ventral cavity, the abdominopelvic cavity. This cavity is a combination of the abdominal and

pelvic cavities because no physical barrier is between them. To help locate organs in the abdominopelvic cavity, visualize this cavity as being divided into four quadrants: two upper quadrants (right and left) and two lower quadrants (right and left). Organs contained in the four quadrants are shown in Figure 7-5. Many of the organs of the abdominopelvic cavity are covered by a double-layered serous membrane called the **peritoneum.** The parietal peritoneum lines the abdominal cavity, and the visceral peritoneum covers the organs. The space between these two layers is called the peritoneal space, or the **peritoneal cavity.** Organs surrounded by the peritoneum are considered **intraperitoneal.** Although these organs are sometimes referred to as *in the peritoneal cavity,* this is slightly inaccurate because no organs are within the peritoneal cavity. Organs are either encased by the peritoneum (intraperitoneal) or behind the peritoneum **(retroperitoneal).** The intraperitoneal organs are held in place by several layers of connective tissue called the *mesentery.* The mesentery is an extension of the peritoneum, which anchors the organs to the posterior wall of the cavity and contains the blood vessels, lymphatic vessels, and nerves that supply the intestines. This is an important concept for the paramedic to understand because mesenteric infarction causes diffuse visceral

✗ Know visceral & parietal

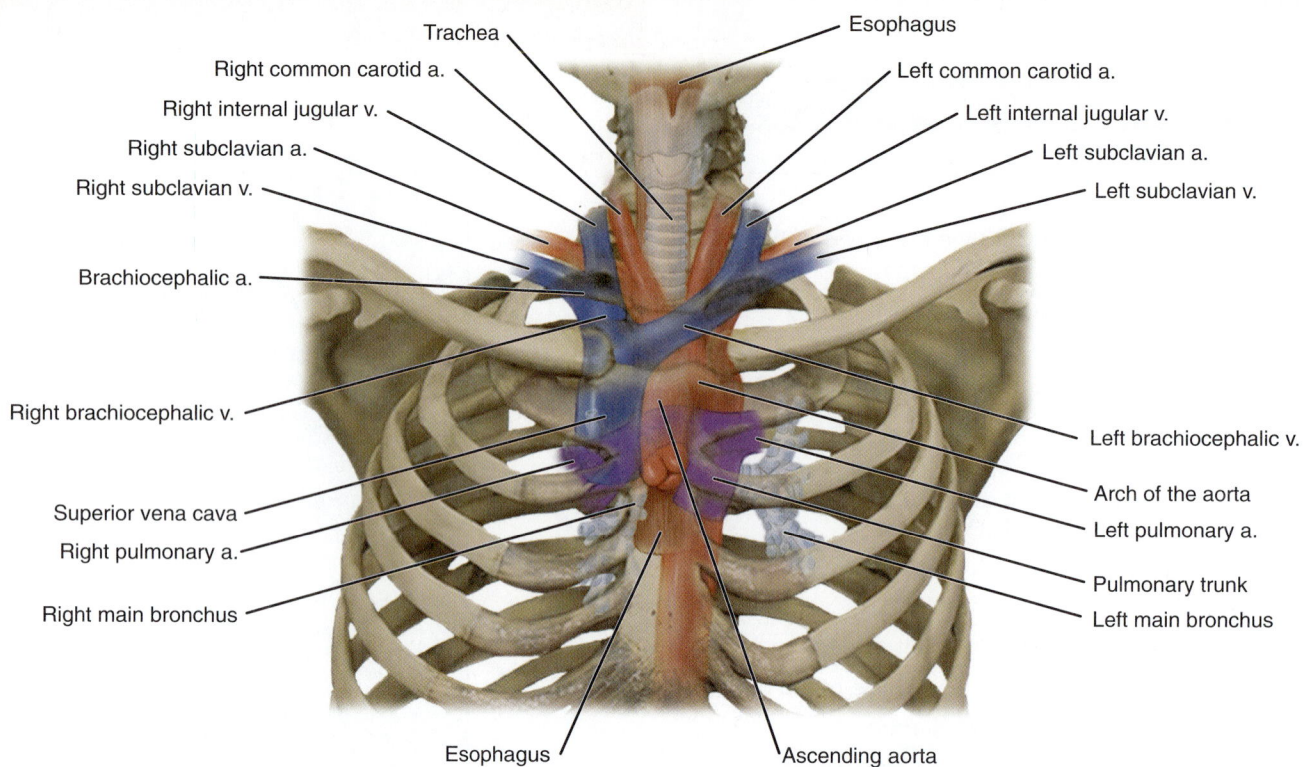

Trachea
Right common carotid a.
Right internal jugular v.
Right subclavian a.
Right subclavian v.

Brachiocephalic a.

Right brachiocephalic v.

Superior vena cava
Right pulmonary a.

Right main bronchus

Esophagus
Left common carotid a.
Left internal jugular v.
Left subclavian a.
Left subclavian v.

Left brachiocephalic v.
Arch of the aorta
Left pulmonary a.

Pulmonary trunk
Left main bronchus

Esophagus

Ascending aorta

Figure 7-3 The mediastinum includes the trachea, esophagus, thymus gland, heart, and great vessels.

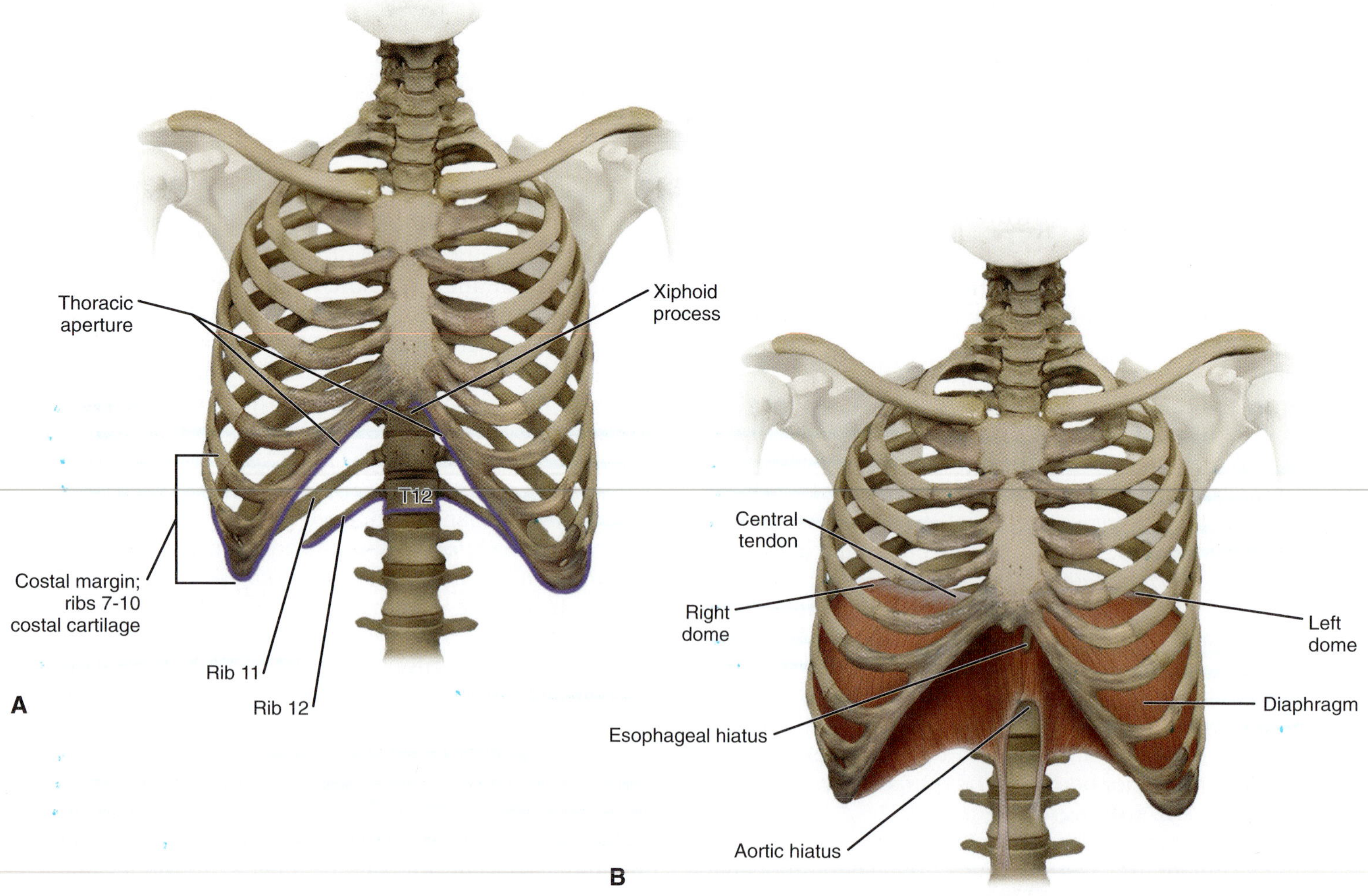

Thoracic aperture

Costal margin; ribs 7-10 costal cartilage

Rib 11

Rib 12

Xiphoid process

T12

A

Central tendon

Right dome

Esophageal hiatus

Aortic hiatus

Left dome

Diaphragm

B

Figure 7-4 The thoracic cavity is separated from the abdominal cavity by the diaphragm.
A, Inferior thoracic aperture. **B,** Diaphragm.

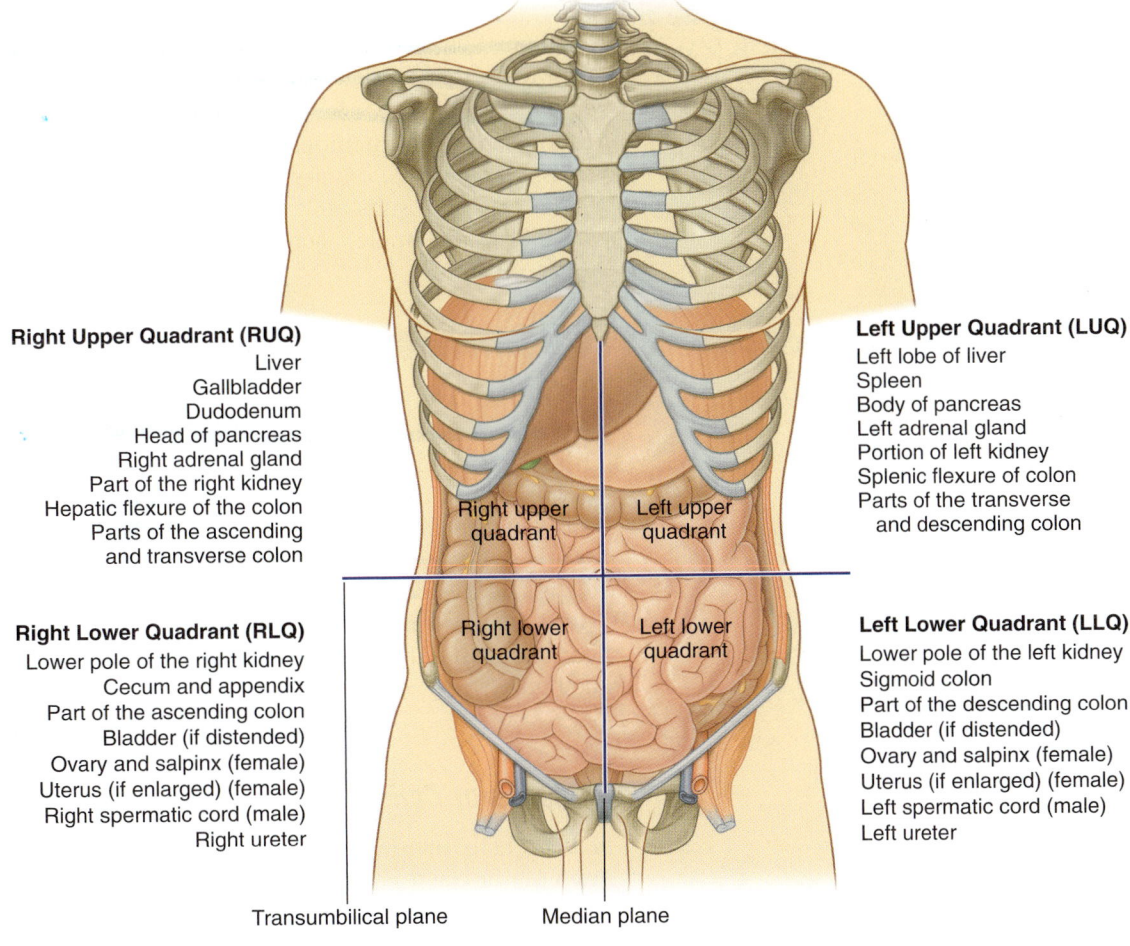

Right Upper Quadrant (RUQ)
Liver
Gallbladder
Dudodenum
Head of pancreas
Right adrenal gland
Part of the right kidney
Hepatic flexure of the colon
Parts of the ascending
and transverse colon

Left Upper Quadrant (LUQ)
Left lobe of liver
Spleen
Body of pancreas
Left adrenal gland
Portion of left kidney
Splenic flexure of colon
Parts of the transverse
and descending colon

Right Lower Quadrant (RLQ)
Lower pole of the right kidney
Cecum and appendix
Part of the ascending colon
Bladder (if distended)
Ovary and salpinx (female)
Uterus (if enlarged) (female)
Right spermatic cord (male)
Right ureter

Left Lower Quadrant (LLQ)
Lower pole of the left kidney
Sigmoid colon
Part of the descending colon
Bladder (if distended)
Ovary and salpinx (female)
Uterus (if enlarged) (female)
Left spermatic cord (male)
Left ureter

Right upper quadrant
Left upper quadrant
Right lower quadrant
Left lower quadrant

Transumbilical plane   Median plane

Figure 7-5 Organs contained in the four abdominal quadrants.

abdominal pain. Organs located behind the peritoneum that are not suspended by the mesentery are referred to as *retroperitoneal.* These organs are held in place, or trapped, between the peritoneum and posterior wall. Intraperitoneal and retroperitoneal organs are listed in Box 7-1.

The dorsal cavity contains the structures of the central nervous system. Subcavities of the dorsal cavity include the cranial cavity, which is the space inside the skull that contains the brain, and the spinal cavity, which is the space inside the spinal column that contains the spinal cord. The structures contained within these cavities are surrounded by three membranes: the dura mater, the arachnoid membrane, and the pia mater (described later).

CHARACTERISTICS OF LIFE

To understand why the body is designed the way it is and functions as it does, a review of the characteristics shared by all living things, as follows, is beneficial:

- *Movement:* the ability of the organism to move from location to location, change its position, or move internal structures
- *Growth:* the ability to increase in size
- *Respiration:* the ability to use food sources in combination with oxygen to release the energy contained within those sources
- *Digestion:* the ability to convert food sources into simpler compounds that can be used in the process of respiration
- *Absorption:* the ability to absorb materials through various membranes, such as the absorption of material through the digestive tract
- *Excretion:* the ability to excrete waste materials that result from metabolism
- *Responsiveness:* the ability to respond to internal and external stimuli
- *Circulation:* the ability to move substances in the body by way of body fluids
- *Reproduction:* the ability to create new cells, such as in cellular reproduction, or the ability to create new organisms, such as offspring

| BOX 7-1 | Intraperitoneal and Retroperitoneal Organs |

Intraperitoneal Organs

- Stomach
- Liver
- Gallbladder
- Spleen
- Uterus
- Ovaries
- Jejunum
- Ileum
- Transverse colon
- Sigmoid colon

Retroperitoneal Organs

- Kidneys
- Adrenal glands
- Pancreas
- Urinary bladder
- Ureters
- Duodenum
- Ascending colon
- Descending colon
- Rectum
- Inferior vena cava
- Abdominal aorta

ORGANIZATIONAL STRUCTURE

To achieve the functions listed previously, the body is organized to ensure the organism as a whole works together toward those goals. This is one of the most important concepts to understand in anatomy and physiology; in fact, the term *organism* itself indicates that organization is crucial. Basic units of organization include the following:

- The cell is the smallest unit of structure and function in the human organism. Each of the 75 to 100 trillion cells in the body has a specific purpose or function. Often the shape of the cell indicates its purpose. For example, the shape of a nerve cell alone indicates its ability to conduct electrical impulses.
- Tissues are created when several cells with common functions join together. For example, many muscle cells join to create muscle tissue.
- Organs are created when several types of tissue join to perform a function. For example, the heart contains muscle tissue as well as epithelial and nervous tissue.
- Organ systems are created when several organs combine to perform a common function.
- The organism is the combination of all lower levels of organization working together to ensure survival.

Although not a structural level of organization, the chemical level of organization must also be appreciated. Without an appropriate amount and concentration of atoms, molecules, electrolytes, and other chemicals, the body would be unable to function and survive. The level of organization includes inorganic substances such as salts, electrolytes, oxygen, carbon dioxide, and water as well as organic substances such as lipids, proteins, carbohydrates, and nucleic acids.

CELL STRUCTURE

[OBJECTIVE 7]

Cells are the basic functional unit of the body (Figure 7-6). They are highly organized structures surrounded by a cytoplasmic membrane **(plasma membrane).** Numerous structures are within the cell. These structures together are referred to as **organelles** and are suspended within a substance called the **cytoplasm.** Most of the cells of the body also contain a **nucleus.** In the nucleus, the genetic material is stored, allowing reproduction and new cell growth.

Classes of Cells

Living cells of multicellular organisms are divided into two major classes according to the way the genetic material is organized inside them: eukaryotes (which means "true nucleus") and prokaryotes (which means "before nucleus"). All human body cells are eukaryotes.

Eukaryotes have an extensive intracellular anatomy. They have a separate membrane-bound nucleus that holds the genetic material (i.e., chromosomes, DNA). The prokaryote is a much simpler cell. In these cells the genetic material and enzymes required for energy production, cell growth, and cell division are contained in the jellylike cytoplasm.

General Cellular Functions

The cells of the human body are extremely varied in their shape and function. Over time cells mature, or differentiate. Through this process of **differentiation,** cells become specialized to perform a specific function. For example, muscle cells are specialized cells that enable the body to move. Cells perform the following seven general functions:

1. Movement (muscle cells)
2. Conductivity (nerve cells)
3. Metabolic absorption (kidney and intestinal cells)
4. Secretion (mucous gland cells)
5. Excretion (all cells)
6. Respiration (all cells)
7. Reproduction (most cells)

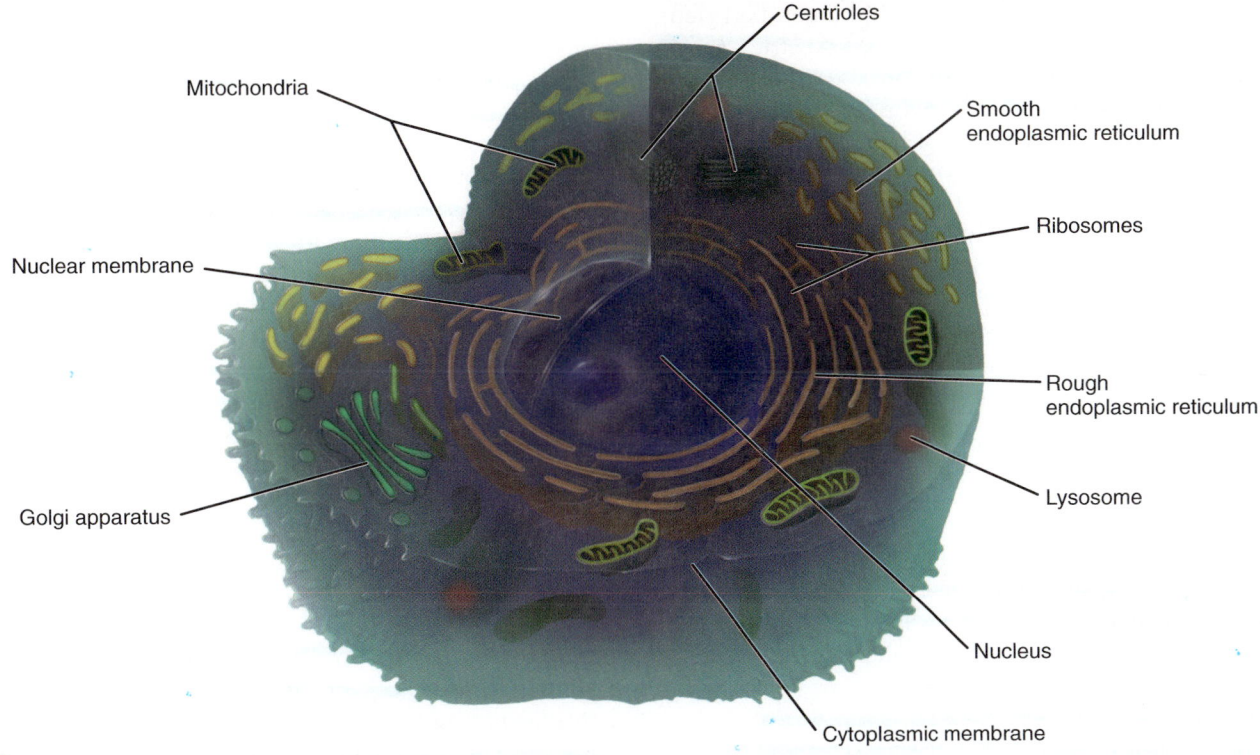

Figure 7-6 Cell structure. Cells are the basic unit of the body.

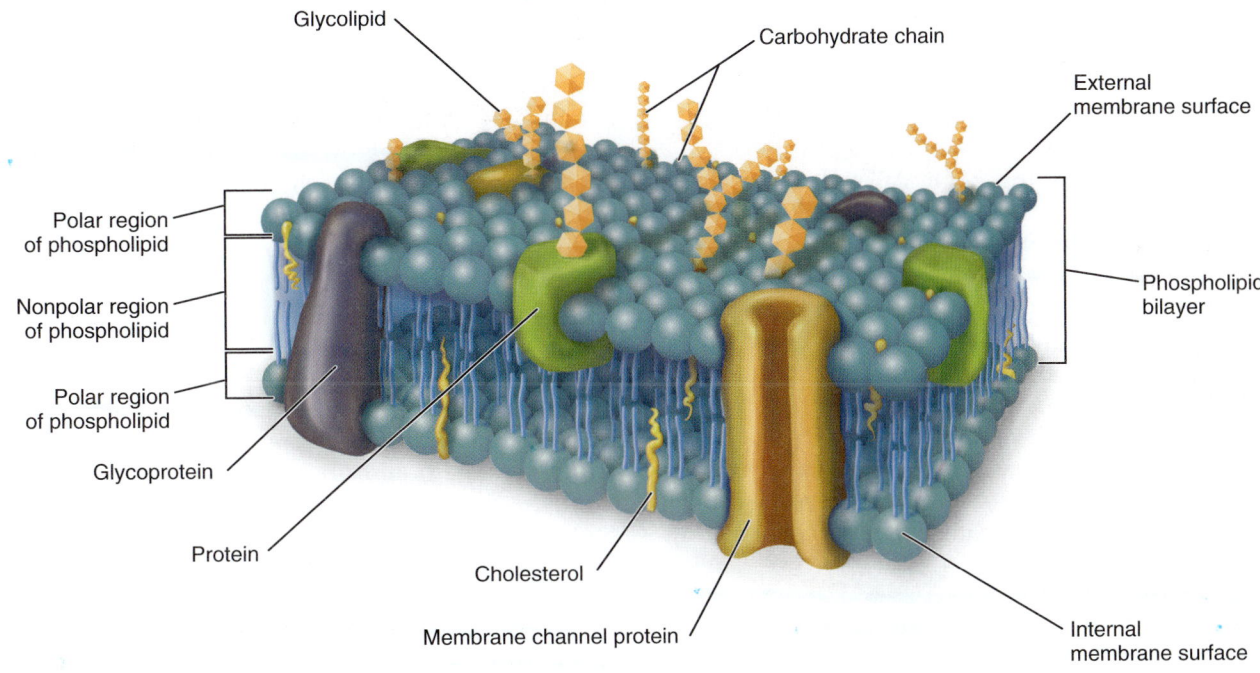

Figure 7-7 Cytoplasm is the fluidlike material within which the organelles are suspended.

Cytoplasmic Membrane

The **cytoplasmic membrane** encloses the cytoplasm and its organelles. Within this enclosed space, most cellular activity takes place. The cytoplasmic membrane is composed of two layers, referred to as a *bilayer*. The bilayer is composed of phosphate and fat molecules called

phospholipids (Figure 7-7). This bilayer forms a fluidlike framework for the membrane. The membrane also forms the outer border of the cell and separates the interior of the cell from the interstitial fluid surrounding the cell. Any substances within this membrane are called **intracellular**, and substances outside this membrane are referred to as **extracellular**. In addition to providing physical isolation between the intracellular compartment and extracellular compartment, one of the major functions of the cytoplasmic membrane is to regulate the transfer of substances in and out of the cell. This is accomplished by the structure of the membrane. Visualize the membrane as a series of balloons with their strings tied together and the balloons facing outward. This is the design of the membrane, with the balloons representing the phosphate molecules and the strings representing the lipid molecules. The phosphate molecules are hydrophilic and attract water, whereas the lipid molecules are hydrophobic and repel water. This results in a selectively permeable membrane in which gases, alcohol, and other substances that are lipid soluble freely pass through the membrane, whereas water and water-soluble substances are unable to pass through the membrane itself. The transport of substances in and out of the cell is discussed in more detail later in the chapter.

The cytoplasmic membrane also has several proteins, known as *membrane proteins,* embedded and floating within it. These proteins serve the following functions:

- Channel proteins act as a pore through the membrane that allows the passive passage of substances into the intracellular compartment. One such example is the manner in which water enters and leaves the cell. As previously mentioned, water is unable to cross the membrane itself; however, because of the amount of channel proteins that allow the passage of water, it can essentially freely enter and exit the cell. The fact that the water is not crossing through the membrane itself is important. Another category of channel proteins are gated ion channels. These channels open and close at specific times and generally only allow specific substances to pass through. Calcium, for example, passes through calcium channels, and sodium passes through the sodium channels. Both are examples of voltage-gated ion channels. Through a variety of medications (such as calcium channel blockers or sodium channel blockers) the paramedic is able to alter transport through membrane channel proteins, causing a dramatic effect on cellular function.
- Enzyme receptors act as sites where enzymes can bind. This binding occurs inside the cell and the enzyme acts as a catalyst for a reaction to take place in the cell itself.
- Proteins that act as receptor sites have their binding site on the outside of the cytoplasmic membrane. The majority of these receptor sites are specific to certain molecules; when the correct molecule binds to the receptor site a change in cellular function occurs. These changes are crucial to the proper function of the cell; however, the paramedic also uses these sites. For example, the administration of a narcotic or narcotic antagonist

results in the medication binding to narcotic receptor sites.

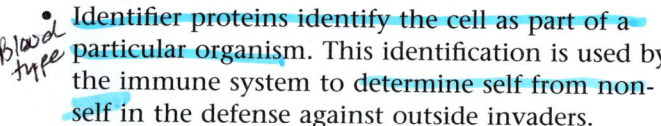

- Identifier proteins identify the cell as part of a particular organism. This identification is used by the immune system to determine self from non-self in the defense against outside invaders.
- Carrier proteins bind to substances and transport them across the cytoplasmic membrane. This is generally an active process. For example, the sodium-potassium pump moves sodium out of the cell and potassium into the cell.
- The shape of a cell is a function of some membrane proteins attaching to the cytoskeleton of the cell. Other membrane proteins adhere to membrane proteins of adjacent cells, allowing tissues to form.

Cytoplasm

[OBJECTIVE 8]

The cytoplasm is the fluidlike material within which the organelles of the cell are suspended. It lies between the cytoplasmic membrane and the nucleus. The fluid contained within the nucleus is called the *nucleoplasm.* The organelles within the cytoplasm work as little factories within the cell. These little factories perform a series of specific functions (Table 7-2). In addition to containing the organelles, many chemicals and compounds are dissolved in the cytoplasm. These include glucose and proteins, among others, which are essential for cell metabolism. As a result many of the chemical reactions necessary for life take place within the cytoplasm. One of the most important of these reactions is glycolysis, the first step in cellular respiration. Cellular respiration is discussed in detail later in the chapter.

Organelles

[OBJECTIVE 9]

Ribosomes are organelles in which new protein is synthesized. They are made of complex strands of macromolecules of protein and ribonucleic acid. Ribosome chains form the framework for the genetic blueprint and the synthesis of proteins. Ribosomes may be found free floating within the cytoplasm or attached to the endoplasmic reticulum.

The **endoplasmic reticulum (ER)** is a chain of canals and sacs that wind through the cytoplasm, connecting the nuclear membrane to the cytoplasmic membrane. This system of canals and sacs works as a circulatory system within the cell that moves substances and proteins through the cell. The ER also plays a part in the detoxification process. ER is either smooth or rough based on the presence or absence of ribosomes on its surface. Smooth ER lacks ribosomes and is found in cells that handle or produce fatty substances and certain hormones, such as the sex hormones. Rough ER has ribosomes on its surface and is found in cells that produce protein to

TABLE 7-2   Cell Structures and Function

Cell Structure	Function
Membrane	Contains cellular contents; regulates what enters and leaves the cell
Cytoplasm	Surrounds and supports organelles; medium through which nutrients and waste move
Nucleus	Contains genetic information; control center of the cell

Endoplasmic reticulum
  Rough
  Smooth
	Transports material through the cytoplasm
	Contains the ribosomes where protein is synthesized
	Site of steroid synthesis

Mitochondria	Convert energy in nutrients to ATP (power plants of the cell)
Golgi apparatus	Packages protein in membrane; puts the "finishing touches" on protein
Ribosomes	Sites of protein synthesis
Lysosomes	"Housekeeping" within the cell; digests cell waste through powerful enzymes
Cytoskeleton	Provides intracellular shape and support
Centrioles	Help separate the chromosomes during mitosis

Modified from Herlihy, B. (2007). *The human body in health and illness (3rd ed.)*. St. Louis: Mosby.
ATP, Adenosine triphosphate.

be excreted for use outside the cell. After creating proteins the ribosomes transfer the protein into the rough ER for transport to the Golgi apparatus, where it will be further processed.

The **Golgi apparatus** is a series of flattened sacs that resemble a stack of pancakes. They are often found attached to the ER; their function is to concentrate and package material for secretion out of the cell. When the material is ready to be secreted, a small vesicle breaks off the Golgi apparatus and travels to the cytoplasmic membrane, where its contents are released outside the cell. An example of a Golgi apparatus product is mucus.

Vesicles are the shipping containers of the cell. They are simple in structure, consisting of a single membrane filled with liquid. They transport a wide variety of substances inside the cell, referred to as endocytotic vesicles, and to the exterior of the cell, referred to as exocytotic vesicles.

Lysosomes are membrane-walled organelles created by breaking off from the Golgi apparatus and contain enzymes. The enzymes contained within these structures help digest nucleic acids, fats, proteins, polysaccharides, and lipids. Certain white blood cells (leukocytes) have large amounts of lysosomes that contain enzymes designed to digest bacteria. Lysosomes also digest nonfunctional organelles.

Perioxomes contain chemicals that combine hydrogen and oxygen to form hydrogen peroxide, which detoxifies substances that would be harmful to the cell. As the main organ of detoxification, the liver contains a large amount of perioxomes.

Mitochondria are the power plants of the cell and the body. They are the site of aerobic respiration, which results in the synthesis of **adenosine triphosphate (ATP),** which serves as a source of energy throughout the body. The mitochondria are composed of two membranes. The outer membrane gives the organelle its shape, and the inner membrane creates several folds called *cristae*. These two membranes are important in cellular respiration (discussed later in this chapter) because they are the location of the two steps of aerobic respiration. Tissues of the body with high energy needs, such as muscle and nerve tissue, typically have large numbers of mitochondria.

Centrioles are paired, rodlike structures that lie at right angles to each other. These structures exist in a specialized area of the cytoplasm known as the **centrosome.** The centrioles play an important role in the process of cell division.

Cilia are organelles described as hairlike projections from the cytoplasmic membrane of some epithelial cells. Cilia function to create a wave of motion, or a current, that moves fluid over the surface of the cell. The cells that line the respiratory tract have a large number of cilia to move particles that have been inhaled and trapped in the mucus into the oropharynx to be swallowed or expelled.

Flagella are singular organelles that project from the cell and are used for propulsion. The male sperm cell is the only cell in the human body that has a flagellum.

Microvilli are projections from the cytoplasmic membrane that increase surface area for absorption. The lining of the small intestine has a large amount of microvilli to increase the rate of absorption of digested food.

Nucleus

[OBJECTIVE 10]

The nucleus is usually a large structure located near the center of a typical cell. The nucleus is surrounded by a membrane called the **nuclear membrane.** This membrane (similar to the cell's cytoplasmic membrane) encases the nucleoplasm. Within the **nucleoplasm** are specialized structures that carry the genetic material that the cell uses for reproduction. This material serves as a blueprint for function. **Deoxyribonucleic acid (DNA)** resides on threads of chromatin (Figure 7-8). Chromatin are tangles of chromosomes that contain thousands of hereditary

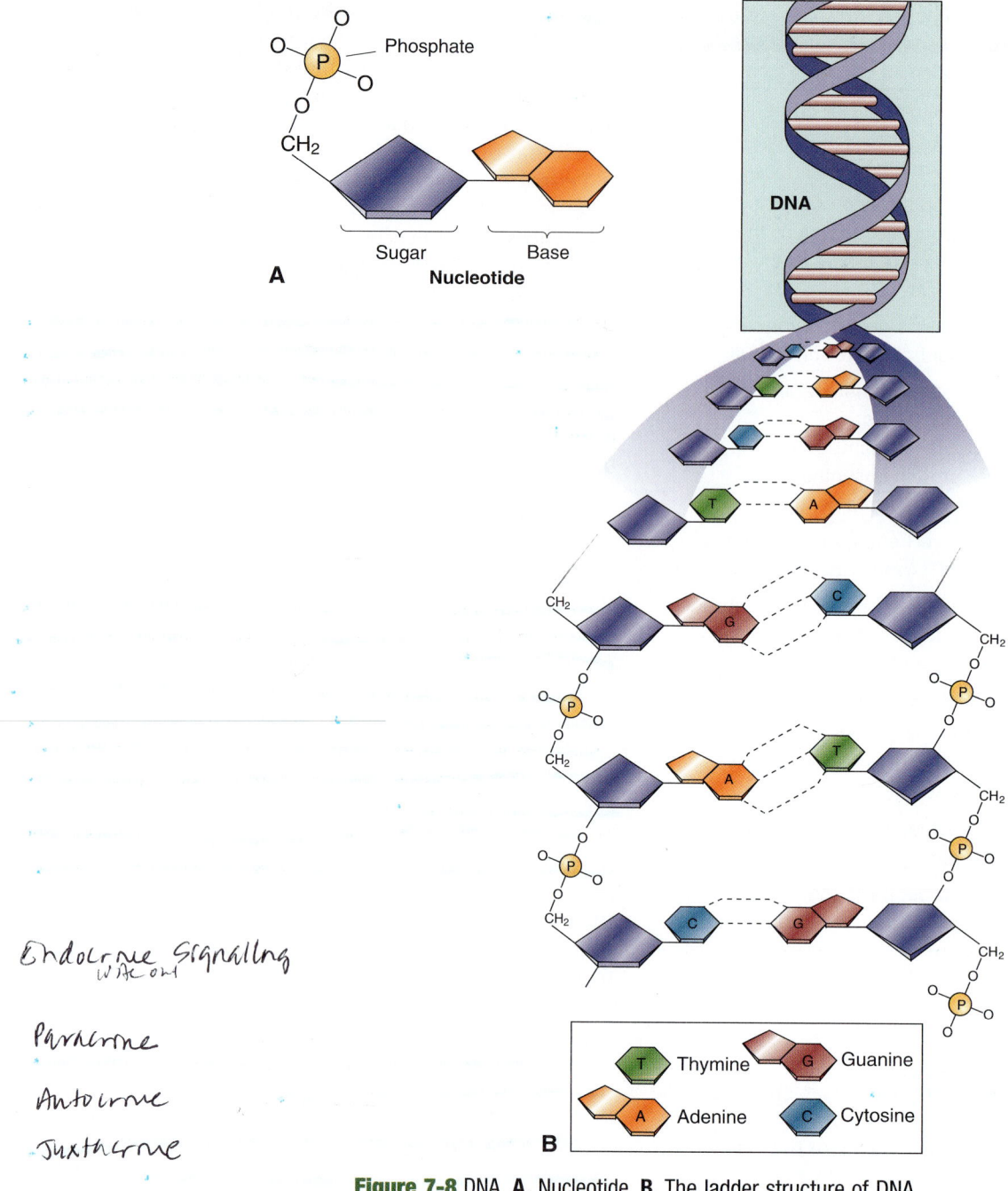

Figure 7-8 DNA. **A,** Nucleotide. **B,** The ladder structure of DNA.

Endocrine Signalling
w/sk out

Paracrine

Autocrine

Juxtacrine

Synaptic

units called genes. The nucleus also contains a suborganelle called the nucleolus, which is nonmembranous. The nucleolus is densely packed with **ribonucleic acid (RNA)** and surrounded by chromatin. RNA is responsible for ribosome production. Ribosomes are then passed through pores in the nuclear envelope (the outer boundary between the nucleus and the rest of the cell) to the ER for protein synthesis. RNA and DNA are considered the blueprint of the cell. Because of this the function, products, appearance, reproduction, and all other aspects of the cell are controlled by the nucleus. Cells without a nucleus, such as red blood cells, have a limited lifespan.

Cell Reproduction

[OBJECTIVE 11]

Most of the cells of the human body, with the exception of reproductive (sex) cells and red blood cells, reproduce by **mitosis.** In this process of division and multiplication, one cell divides to become two new cells that are identical to the original cell (the two cells are referred to as **daughter cells**). This process is continuous. Many cells of the body reproduce in this fashion throughout life (e.g., skin and bone marrow cells). Other cells divide until near birth (e.g., nerve and skeletal cells).

Cellular Communication

To work collectively as a cohesive unit, cells must be able to communicate with other cells and within individual cells. Cells have the ability to generate and respond to a variety of signals, called cellular signaling, to maintain homeostasis, fight infection, reproduce, and perform other normal functions. Alterations in signals also can lead to dysfunction. Some tumors and cancers are believed to be the result of disruptions in this signaling process. Examples of signaling include the following:

- Endocrine signaling occurs when cells respond to hormones released by the endocrine system. This type of signaling mechanism affects the entire body.
- Paracrine signaling occurs when one cell sends a chemical message to surrounding cells.
- Autocrine signaling occurs when a cell sends a message to itself.
- Juxtacrine signaling occurs when a cell sends a message to the cells immediately adjacent to it.
- Synaptic signaling occurs in response to a neurotransmitter across a synaptic gap.

[handwritten: acetylcholine or norepinephrine crosses synaptic cleft]

Cellular Metabolism

[OBJECTIVE 12]

As evidenced by the structural hierarchy of the human body, the ability of the tissues, organs, and organ systems to function depends on the function of individual cells; as a result, cells are constantly breaking substances down and building substances necessary for the survival of the organism. Metabolism is the sum of all physical chemical changes that occur in the body. Metabolic processes include both anabolism and catabolism. In addition, cellular respiration must occur to provide needed energy for body functions.

Anabolism

Anabolism is the building of larger substances from smaller substances, such as the building of proteins from amino acids. One example of anabolism is dehydration synthesis. In this process two molecules are joined together by the removal of hydroxyl (—OH) groups and hydrogen (H) atoms. The removed products combine to form water (H_2O), and the new molecule is joined by a common oxygen atom that remains after the process has taken place.

Catabolism

Catabolism is the breakdown of larger molecules into smaller ones that the body can use for its own needs. An example of catabolism is hydrolysis. This is essentially the opposite of dehydration synthesis. In this case, water is broken into an H atom and an OH group. The H atom then combines with part of the larger molecule, and the OH group combines with the other part, thereby creating two smaller molecules (Figure 7-9).

Cellular Respiration

Almost all metabolic functions require energy. The major source of energy for the cells is the 6-carbon sugar, glucose ($C_6H_{12}O_6$). Utilization of glucose by the cell is called *oxidation*, and the end result is carbon dioxide (CO_2), water (H_2O), and the high-energy molecule ATP. ATP is the true source of cellular energy because of the high energy bonds contained between its phosphate molecules. When needed for cellular function, these bonds are broken to release their stored energy. However, despite the large amount of energy contained in these bonds, glucose contains an even higher amount of energy. If glucose molecules were to be broken down in one step, much of this energy would be lost to heat, with minimal production of ATP. As a result, cellular respiration occurs in three stages to maximize the number of ATP molecules created for each molecule of glucose.

Glycolysis

[handwritten: Anaerobic metabolism - people in cardiac arrest/severe asthma]

As the first step in cellular respiration, glycolysis occurs in the cytoplasm and does not require oxygen. It is therefore an anaerobic process. After the glucose molecule moves into the cell two phosphate molecules, gained from breaking two ATP molecules, immediately attach to it in separate steps. This prevents both the glucose from leaving the cells and the concentration of glucose inside the cells from becoming higher than the concentration outside the cells. It also prepares the glucose molecule for further breakdown. Next, a series of complex steps occurs to break down the glucose molecule into its final product, two molecules of pyruvic acid. During this phase of cellular respiration two molecules of pyruvic acid and four molecules of ATP are formed. However, recall the expenditure of two ATP molecules in the early steps of this process; therefore the net result of glycolysis is two molecules of pyruvic acid and two ATP molecules. This is obviously an inefficient use of glucose, but fortunately the process does not end here.

Krebs Cycle

The second step in cellular respiration is the Krebs cycle, also known as the *citric acid cycle* or the *tricarboxylic acid cycle*. The key to this stage in the breakdown of glucose is the presence or absence of oxygen because it only occurs in the presence of oxygen. As a result, this is termed *aerobic respiration*. After occurring in the matrix of the mitochondria, the pyruvic acid formed during glycolysis undergoes a complex series of steps that produces several products, including three carbon dioxide molecules and one ATP molecule. Because two molecules of pyruvic acid are produced during glycolysis, the Krebs cycle occurs twice for each molecule of glucose oxidized. Therefore the end result of the Krebs cycle is six carbon dioxide molecules (this becomes important in later discussions of capnography) and two ATP molecules for every glucose molecule. To summarize ATP production thus far in cellular respiration, a net total of four

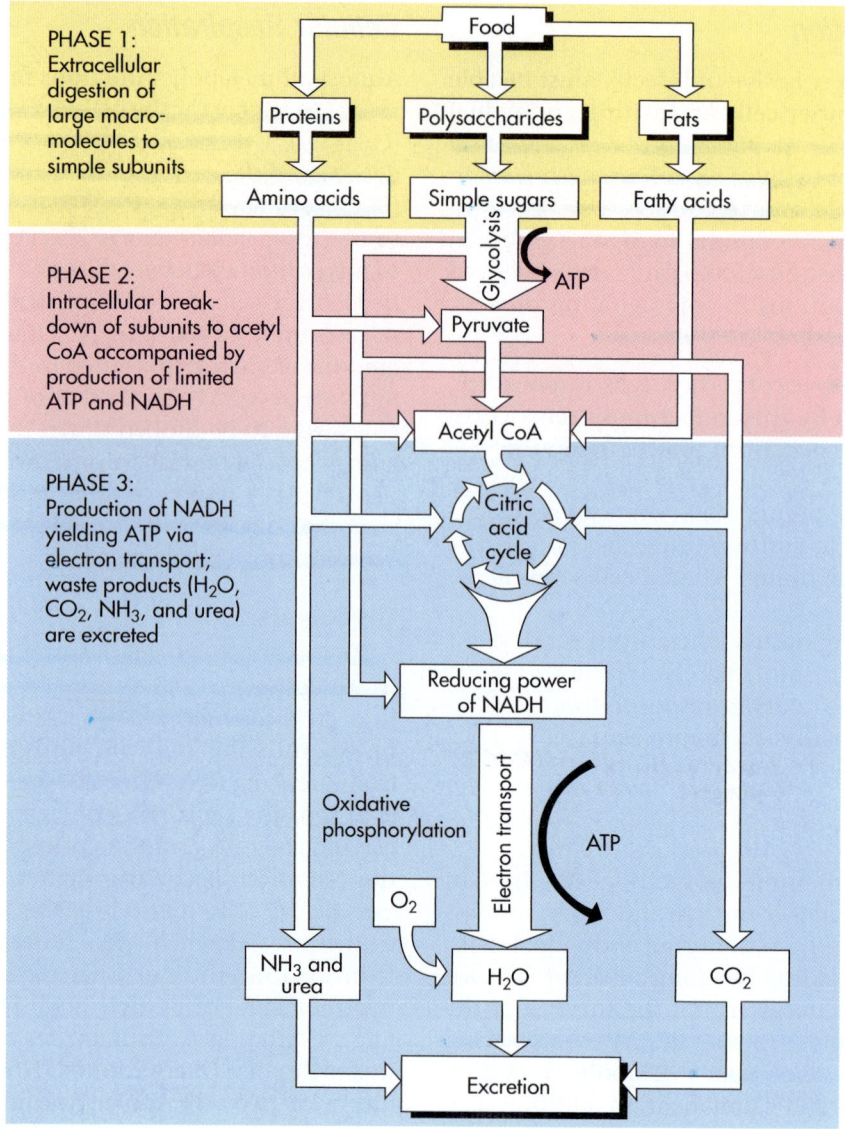

Figure 7-9 Three phases of catabolism, which leads from food to waste products. These reactions produce adenosine triphosphate (ATP), which is used to drive other processes in the cell. *CoA,* Coenzyme A; *NADH,* nicotinamide adenine dinucleotide.

molecules of ATP have been produced, two from glycolysis and two from the Krebs cycle, and only a minimal amount of energy has been gained from the original glucose molecule.

Electron Transport System

The final step in the oxidation of glucose is the electron transport chain, which occurs on the inner cristae of the mitochondria. During this step ATP production truly takes place. In addition to the production of ATP and carbon dioxide from glycolysis and the Krebs cycle, several other products are created during these two steps. After moving to the inner cristae, these products transfer their electrons during a series of reactions that ultimately produces 34 ATP molecules. Because this process depends on the Krebs cycle, the electron transport system is considered a part of aerobic respiration.

Total Results of Cellular Respiration

At the completion of all steps of cellular respiration, 38 ATP molecules are produced: two molecules from glycolysis and 36 molecules from aerobic respiration (two from the Krebs cycle and 34 from the electron transport system). Although this represents an efficient use of the energy contained in one molecule of glucose, it is not 100% efficient because some energy is lost in the form of heat.

Aerobic versus Anaerobic Respiration

As described previously, the presence of oxygen is crucial to the efficient oxidation of glucose by the cells. When it is present, the majority of the respiration that takes place is aerobic respiration (Figure 7-10). However, in certain situations oxygen may not be available to the

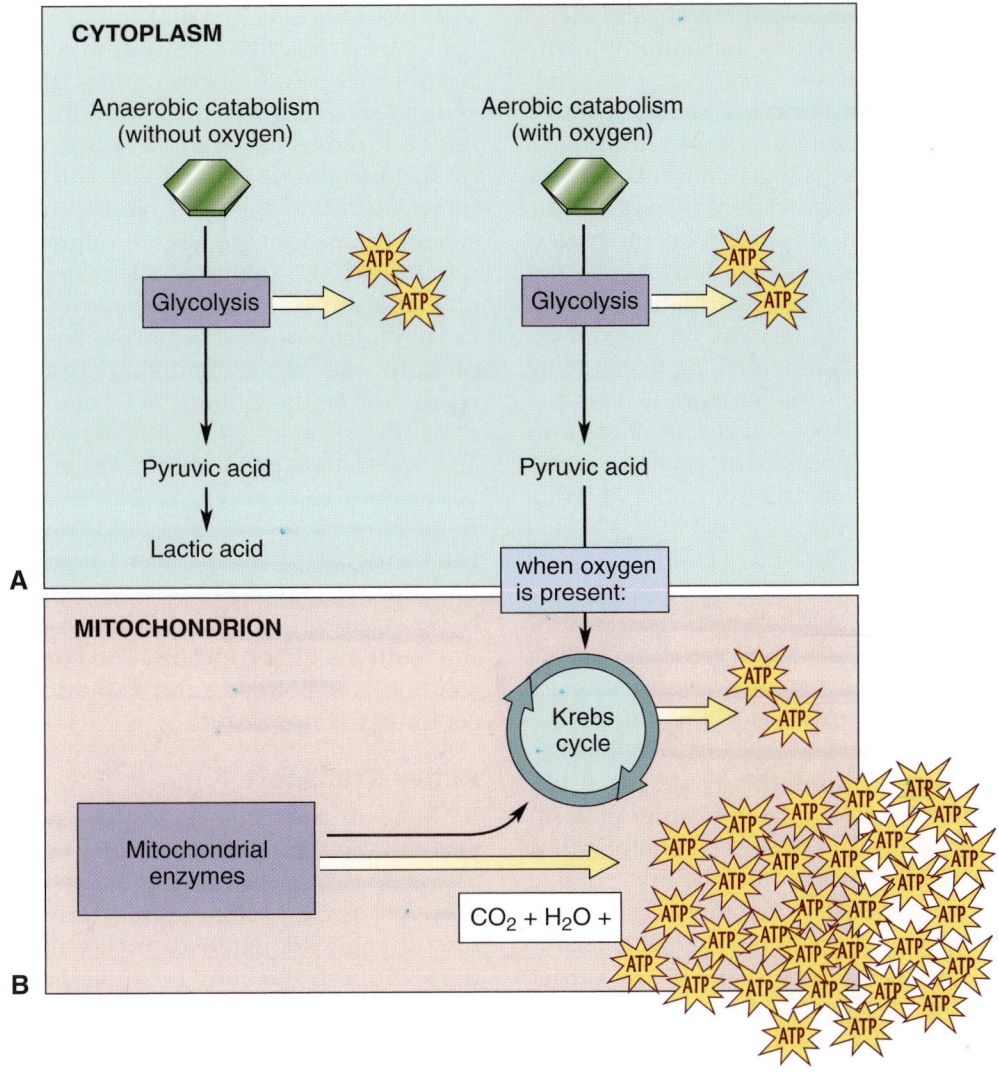

Figure 7-10 Breakdown of glucose. **A,** Anaerobic: to lactic acid. **B,** Aerobic: to carbon dioxide, water, and adenosine triphosphate (ATP).

cells for this portion of respiration to take place. In this situation, called *anaerobic respiration,* glycolysis occurs as it normally would. However, because of the absence of oxygen, pyruvic acid cannot be oxidized in the Krebs cycle. As a result, the pyruvic acid quickly converts to lactic acid and can result in a condition known as lactic acidosis. This occurs in situations such as shock, in which sufficient oxygen is not available to the cells. Fortunately, when oxygen is restored to the cells, lactic acid is converted back to pyruvic acid and aerobic respiration can resume. It is often said that anaerobic respiration starts during a lack of oxygen; however, a more accurate statement is that aerobic respiration stops during a lack of oxygen because anaerobic respiration (glycolysis) is the first step in cellular respiration, regardless of the presence of oxygen. However, by itself anaerobic respiration is a highly inefficient use of glucose, resulting in a net gain of only two ATP molecules compared with a gain of 38 ATP molecules when both anaerobic and aerobic respiration take place.

Transport of Substances Across the Cell Membrane

[OBJECTIVE 13]

As previously described, the cytoplasmic membrane is semipermeable, allowing lipid-soluble substances to move in and out of the cell freely while not allowing water-soluble substances to cross the membrane. However, to sustain life both types of substances must be allowed to enter and exit the cell. This exchange takes place between the intracellular and interstitial fluid. Several methods of transport take place to allow this; however, they all depend on the integrity of the cytoplasmic membrane. Disruption of the membrane causes alteration in the movement of fluid and can lead to cellular swelling or dehydration.

Diffusion

Diffusion is the process of particles moving from an area of higher concentration to an area of lower concentration along a concentration gradient until an equilibrium is achieved. This process does not require energy and therefore is considered a passive transport mechanism. In the human body substances that can freely cross the cell membrane, such as oxygen and carbon dioxide, move by the process of diffusion. For example, blood returning to the lungs from the body has a high concentration of carbon dioxide and a low concentration of oxygen. The lungs, however, have a high concentration of oxygen and a low concentration of carbon dioxide. As the blood passes through the pulmonary vasculature, carbon dioxide leaves the blood and enters the lungs until an equal amount of carbon dioxide is present in both. By the same process oxygen leaves the lungs and enters the blood until an equal amount of oxygen is present in both. By this principle, the amount of expired carbon dioxide is nearly equal to the amount of carbon dioxide contained in the arterial blood.

Facilitated Diffusion

Facilitated diffusion is a passive transport mechanism similar to diffusion in that it involves particles moving from an area of higher concentration to an area of lower concentration. However, in this type of diffusion the molecule entering the cell cannot enter without the assistance of a carrier protein. During this process the substance needed in the cell binds with the carrier protein, and one of two processes takes place. The combination of the molecule and carrier protein may be lipid soluble and pass through the cytoplasmic membrane, or the two may enter the cell through a membrane protein. This is possible either because of the new shape of the carrier molecule combination, or the combination of the two can attach to a binding point in the membrane protein. The membrane protein then changes shape to allow passage of the carrier molecule combination into the cell. Once in the cell the carrier protein breaks off from the molecule and returns to the surface of the membrane to transport other molecules into the cell. Glucose enters the cell by this process. Glucose is not lipid soluble and therefore cannot cross the cytoplasmic membrane; it is also too large a molecule to cross through the membrane proteins. By attaching to a carrier protein, glucose is allowed to enter the cell. Insulin is a hormone that increases the movement of glucose into the cell by a factor of 10 to 20.

Osmosis

Osmosis is another passive transport mechanism. However, unlike diffusion, in osmosis the particles themselves do not move. To understand osmosis, the concepts of solutions, solvents, and solutes must be appreciated. Solutions contain both a liquid (solvent) and particles suspended in the liquid (solutes). In the body the primary solvent is water, which is considered the universal solvent. Within this solvent are several solutes, many of which cannot cross the cytoplasmic membrane because of the property of selective permeability. However, because of the membrane proteins previously discussed, water (the solvent) does have the ability to pass in and out of the cell. This results in a situation in which the solvent will move across the membrane from an area of lower concentration to higher concentration; however, the solute does not move. For example, if the solution on one side of the membrane has 25 sodium ions and 100 water molecules (25% solution), and a solution on the other side of the membrane has 50 sodium ions and 100 water molecules (50% solution), the water will move from the area of lower solute concentration to higher solute concentration in an effort to reach an equal concentration on both sides of the membrane. In this example the end result will be 25 sodium molecules and 66 water molecules on one side (37%), and 50 sodium molecules and 134 water molecules on the other (37%). A solution's concentration, or ability to draw or give water, is referred to as its *tonicity,* and the difference in concentrations from one side of a selectively permeable membrane to the other is called the *osmotic gradient*. Solutions that have an equal concentration are called *isotonic*. A solution with a higher concentration compared with another solution is hypertonic, and a solution with a lower concentration is hypotonic.

Active Transport

In some situations, ions and molecules must be transported against their concentration gradient, or from an area of low concentration to an area of high concentration. As a result of this "uphill" movement, the expenditure of energy is required. For example, the majority of the sodium in the body is contained in the extracellular fluid, whereas the majority of the potassium in the body is contained in the intracellular fluid. Sodium enters the cell through simple diffusion when the sodium channels open, and potassium leaves the cell by the same process when the potassium channels open. To move sodium out of the cell or potassium into the cell, these channels cannot simply be opened again because a higher concentration of sodium on the outside and potassium on the inside is always present. An active transport process, the sodium-potassium pump, must be used to move these ions against their concentration gradient. As with facilitated diffusion, this process uses a system in which the particle being moved binds with a carrier protein. However, unlike facilitated diffusion, this binding requires the use of energy. Once bound, the particle is transported through the membrane and then released. In this example each cycle of the sodium-potassium pump results in three sodium ions being moved out of the cell and two potassium ions being moved into the cell.

TISSUES

A **tissue** is defined as a group of cells that are similar in structure and function. Tissue results from a process called **differentiation.** This process occurs early in the development of a cell. It is the process by which the cell becomes specialized for a specific purpose. For example, a cell can become specialized as a cardiac cell or a bone cell. The cells in this early stage of development are called **stem cells.** When stem cells undergo mitosis, one daughter cell remains an undifferentiated stem cell while the other differentiates and takes on the characteristics of a particular tissue. The remarkable ability for stem cells to differentiate into many different kinds of cells makes them potentially valuable in treating certain illnesses. Four types of tissue are found in the human body and are classified by their shape, structure, and function. The four types are epithelial tissue, connective tissue, muscle tissue, and nervous tissue.

Epithelial Tissue

[OBJECTIVE 14]

Epithelial tissue covers most of the surfaces of the body (both external and internal surfaces) and the interior of hollow organs. This type of tissue is composed of cells that have little or no intracellular material and has four major functions: protection, such as the skin; absorption, such as the lining of the small intestine; secretion, such as exocrine and endocrine glands; and excretion, such as sweat glands. Epithelial tissue always has one open surface and is attached to underlying tissue by a basement membrane. It can be divided into groups on the basis of its microscopic shape and arrangement. It is classified by shape as squamous (flat and scalelike), cuboidal (cubed), and columnar (taller than wide). Epithelial tissue can also be classified according to arrangement. The arrangement can be simple (single layer), stratified (multiple layers), or transitional (different layers of variously shaped cells).

Connective Tissue

[OBJECTIVE 15]

Connective tissue is the most abundant type of tissue in the body. This type of tissue also is the most widely distributed. Connective tissue is composed of cells separated from each other by a nonliving material called **matrix.** This matrix serves as the cement that gives the connective tissue its basic characteristics (connection of tissue). This tissue can be separated into seven subgroups:

1. **Areolar connective tissue** is loose tissue found in most organs of the body. This tissue consists of weblike collagen, reticulum, and elastin fibers.
2. **Adipose, or fat, connective tissue** stores lipids. Lipids serve as an efficient way for the body to store nutrients (fat takes less space per calorie than do other nutrients). This tissue acts as an insulator and protector of the organs of the body.
3. **Fibrous connective tissue** is composed of bundles of strong, white, collagenous fibers (protein) in parallel rows. Tendons and ligaments

are composed of this type of tissue; they are relatively strong and inelastic.

4. **Cartilage** is composed of cells called *chondrocytes.* These cells are distributed in a somewhat rigid matrix. The exact makeup of cartilage varies depending on its location and function in the body. Hyaline cartilage is part of the human skeleton and is found around the joints of the body. This type of cartilage is smooth and firm. Alternatively, fibrocartilage is found between the vertebrae of the spine. It provides cushion and flexibility to the spine.
5. **Bone** is a specialized form of hard connective tissue. It consists of living cells and a matrix composed of minerals. Bones are classified according to their shape (Figure 7-11). Bones are also classified as either cancellous (spongy) or compact (solid).
6. **Blood** is a connective tissue. It is classified as such because the material between the cells (red blood cells and white blood cells)—the matrix—is liquid (mainly water). This matrix allows transportation of nutrients, oxygen, and waste products.
7. **Hemopoietic tissue** is found in the marrow cavities of bones. This tissue also is found in organs such as the spleen, tonsils, and lymph nodes. This tissue is responsible for the formation of blood cells and the cells of the lymphatic system that are important in the defense of the body.

Muscle Tissue

[OBJECTIVE 16]

Muscle tissue is contractile tissue. It is the basis of the body's movement. Muscle tissue is specialized to contract forcefully (shorten). Muscle tissue is classified by its anatomic location (skeletal, smooth, and cardiac) and function (Figure 7-12; Table 7-3).

- *Skeletal muscle.* This is also called *voluntary muscle* because its use is usually under conscious control. It is connected to the skeletal framework of the body by tendons and allows movement. It is sometimes referred to as *striated muscle* because of the striated appearance of the tissue under a microscope. This appearance is the result of alternating dark, thick bands of myosin and light, thin bands of actin. Skeletal muscle also contains several nuclei per cell, which are visible under a microscope.
- *Smooth muscle.* This is also called *involuntary muscle* because it is located in the walls of hollow internal structures and therefore is not under conscious control. Its main functions include constricting the lumen of blood vessels in response to the needs of the body, aiding in the breakdown and digestion of food, moving fluid through the body, and assisting

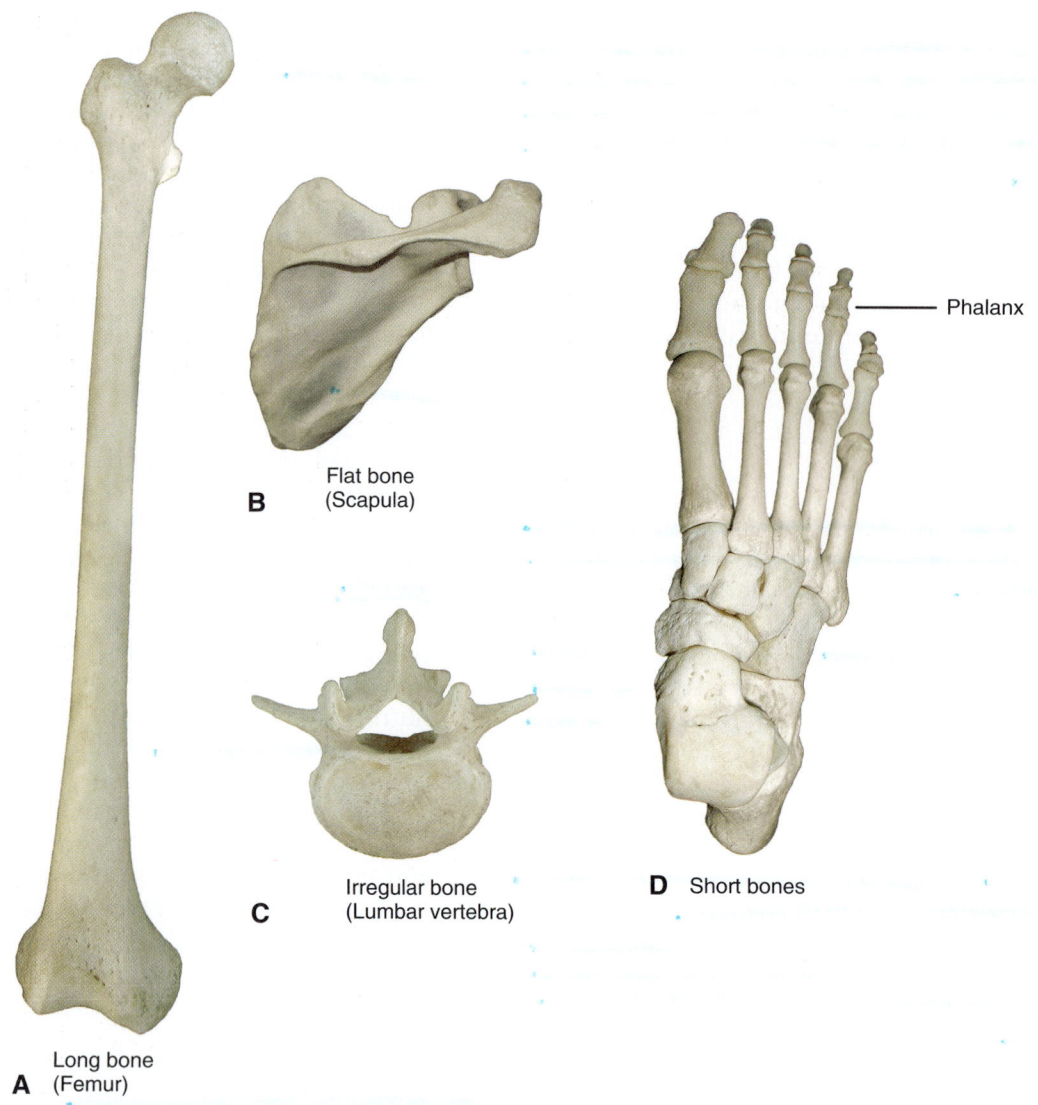

Phalanx

Flat bone
(Scapula)
B

Irregular bone
(Lumbar vertebra)
C

D Short bones

Long bone
A (Femur)

Figure 7-11 Bones are classified according to their shape. **A,** Long bone (humerus). **B,** Flat bone (scapula). **C,** Irregular bone (vertebra). **D,** Short bone (phalanx).

TABLE 7-3	Types of Muscles				
Type	**Control**	**Striations**	**Location**		**Purpose**
Skeletal muscle	Voluntary	Yes	Attached to bone		Produce movement
Visceral muscle	Involuntary	No	In the walls of hollow internal structures and blood vessels		Various: some organ functions, pupil contraction, changes in blood vessel diameter, gland duct operation, hair movement
Cardiac muscle	Involuntary	Yes	Heart		Pump blood

in the elimination of waste products. It is named *smooth muscle* because of its lack of striations under a microscope. This type of muscle has only one nucleus per cell.

- *Cardiac muscle.* The myocardium, the majority of the heart, is cardiac muscle. It is similar to skeletal muscle in that it is striated, yet it differs in its structure. Cardiac cells are generally uninucleate (having one nucleus) and occasionally binucleate (having two nuclei). In addition, the connection between cells is different. These cells form tight connections called intercalated discs. It also differs in that it is not under conscious control but is completely involuntary.

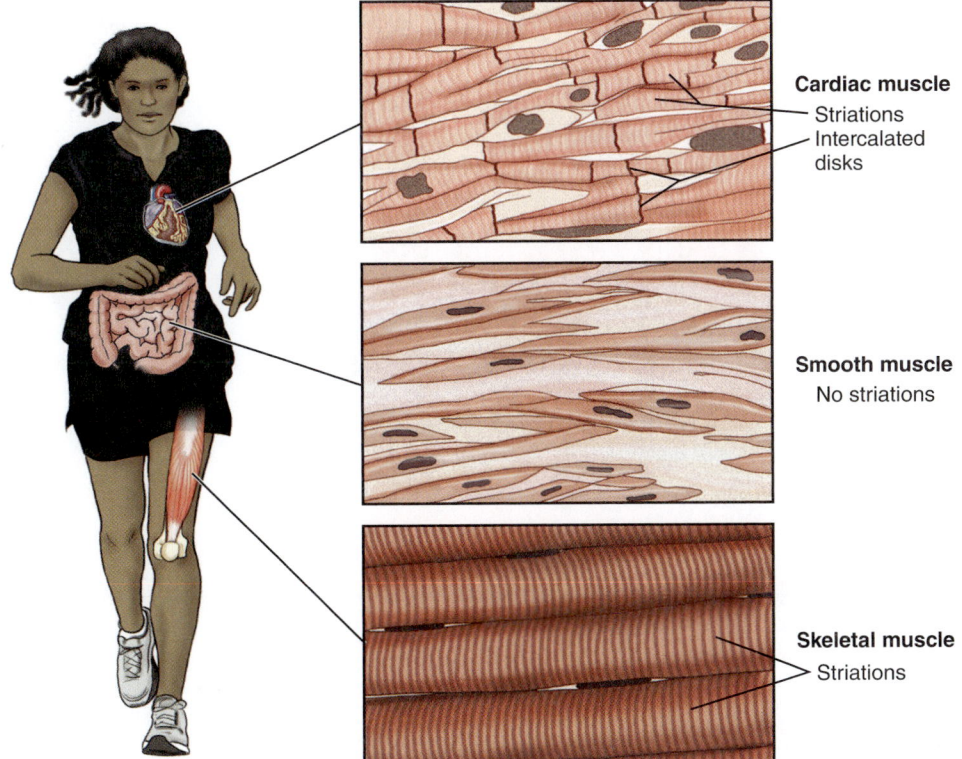

Cardiac muscle
- Striations
- Intercalated disks

Smooth muscle
No striations

Skeletal muscle
- Striations

Figure 7-12 Types of muscle.

These muscle tissues have four basic properties:

1. **Excitability:** the ability to respond to a stimulus
2. **Contractility:** the ability to actively shorten in length
3. **Conductivity:** the ability to conduct an impulse
4. **Elasticity:** the ability to lengthen

Nervous Tissue

[OBJECTIVE 17]

The **nervous tissue** of the body has the ability to conduct electrical impulses that allow communication between body structures and control body functions. Nervous tissue consists of two basic cell types: neurons and neuroglia.

Neurons (nerve cells) are the conducting cells of nervous tissue. Neurons are composed of three parts: the cell body, which contains the nucleus of the cell; one or more dendrites, which carry impulses to the cell body; and one axon, which carries impulses away from the cell body to the dendrites of an adjacent nerve cell. Dendrites and axons of adjacent nerve cells are not in physical contact with each other. Rather, a synaptic gap, or a synapse, is between them. The electrical impulse is transmitted from nerve cell to nerve cell by a neurotransmitter. The paramedic may administer a variety of medications to enhance, slow, or even stop these transmissions.

Axons may be myelinated or unmyelinated. Myelinated axons are surrounded by Schwann cells, which form a white fatty substance called myelin. This appearance leads to the term *white matter*. The myelin sheath acts as insulation along the axon, and gaps between the myelinated regions are called nodes of Ranvier. These nodes speed impulse transmission through the axon because the impulses cannot travel through the insulating myelin, but rather jump from node to node as they travel along the axon. Axons without myelin sheaths are termed gray matter. Because these axons lack the myelin sheath, impulses travel slower than they do in white matter.

Neuroglia are the supporting cells of nervous tissue; however, they do not transmit electrical impulses. The functions of neuroglia include nourishment, protection, and insulation.

ORGAN SYSTEMS

[OBJECTIVE 18]

An **organ** is composed of at least two kinds of tissue. The two kinds of tissue together are organized to perform a more complex task than a single tissue can. A **system** is composed of at least two kinds of organs. Again, these organs together are organized to perform a more complex task than a single organ can. The human body contains the following major organ systems (Figure 7-13):

1. Integumentary
2. Skeletal

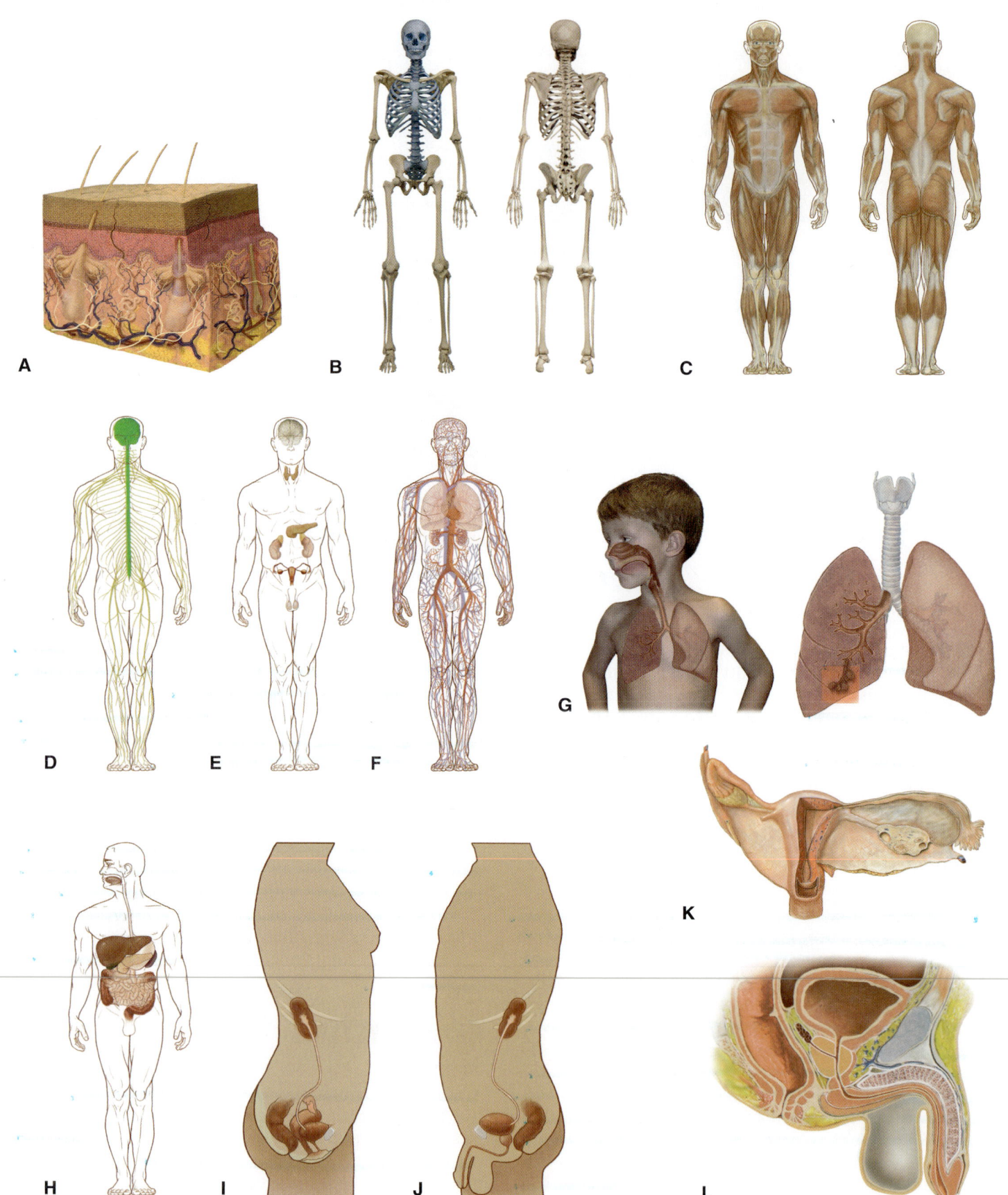

Figure 7-13 Major organ systems in the human body. **A,** Integumentary system, cross section. **B,** Skeletal system, anterior and posterior. **C,** Muscular system, anterior and posterior. **D,** Nervous system. **E,** Endocrine system. **F,** Circulatory system. **G,** Respiratory system. **H,** Digestive system. **I,** Female urinary system. **J,** Male urinary system. **K,** Female reproductive system. **L,** Male reproductive system.

3. Muscular
4. Nervous
5. Endocrine
6. Circulatory (cardiovascular)
7. Lymphatic and immune
8. Respiratory
9. Digestive
10. Urinary
11. Reproductive

INTEGUMENTARY SYSTEM

[OBJECTIVE 19]

The **integumentary system** is the largest and heaviest system of the body. It consists of the skin and accessory structures, such as hair, nails, and glands. The functions of this system include protection, sensation, excretion, fluid regulation, and temperature regulation.

Skin

[OBJECTIVE 20]

The skin is the largest organ of the integumentary system, covering approximately 3000 square inches of surface area. It is composed of two layers, the **epidermis** and the **dermis** (Figure 7-14). The epidermis is the outermost layer of the skin and can be subdivided into five layers. It is composed of tightly packed stratified squamous epithelial cells. The unique junction of the cells of the epidermis gives it flexibility and its continuous nature. This also allows the skin to be an effective barrier against outside organisms. The cells of the outermost layer of the epidermis, the stratum corneum, are dead cells that have had their cytoplasm replaced with keratin, which is a tough, waterproof substance that provides further protection to the underlying tissues from light, heat, microorganisms, and some chemicals. Because cells of the stratum corneum are dead, they are constantly shed and replaced by new cells that move up through the layers of the epidermis. The innermost epidermal layer, the stratum germinativum or stratum basale, is the only location in the epidermis in which the cells are able to undergo mitosis. As the cells are produced they are pushed upward by new cells being produced. These cells work their way through the layers of the epidermis until they are eventually keratinized, become part of the stratum corneum, and are shed. The ability to reproduce allows the epidermis to repair itself if injured, providing further protection against injury and infection. This layer also contains the pigment-producing cells melanocytes, which give skin its color.

The dermis is below the epidermis. These two layers are joined together by the dermal-epidermal junction. One cause of blisters is injury to this junction. The dermal layer consists of two layers and is much thicker than the epidermis. It mainly consists of connective tissue containing

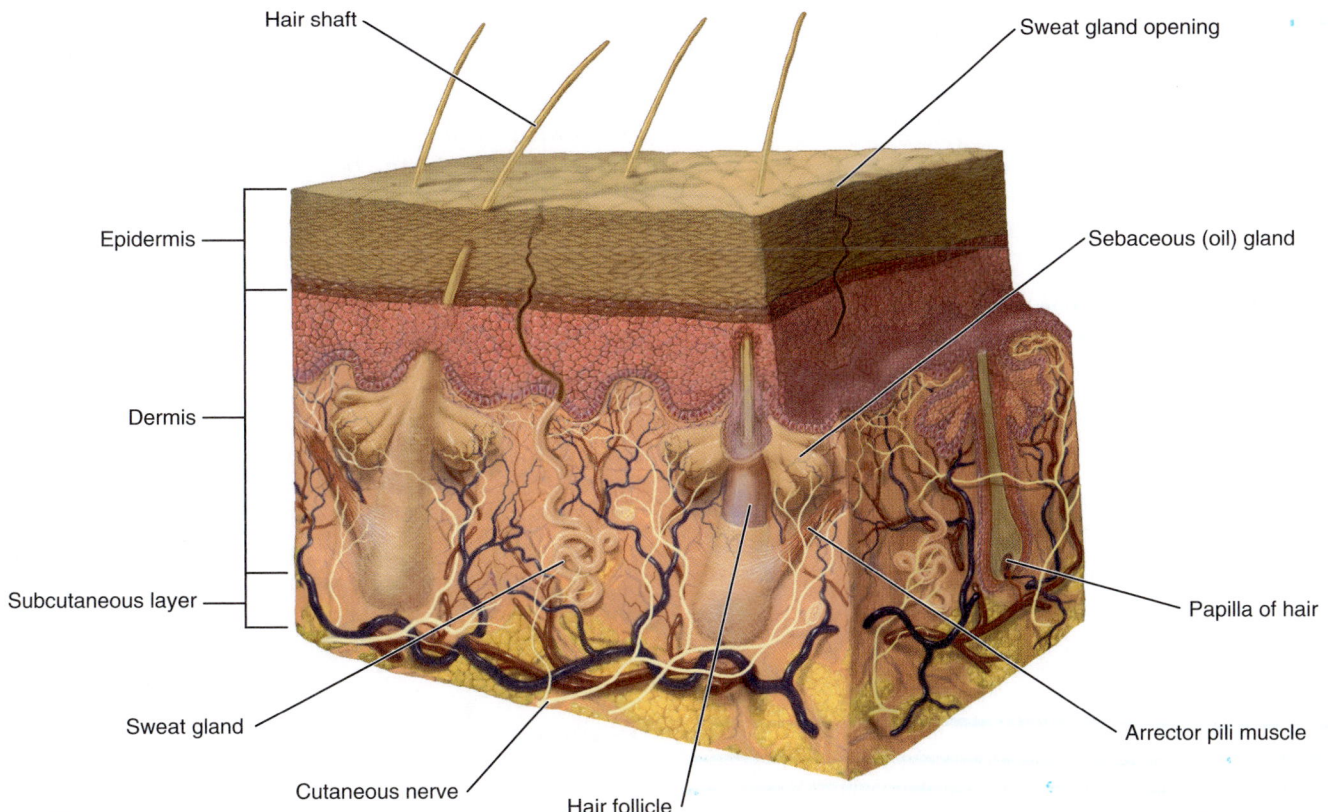

Figure 7-14 Skin is part of the integumentary system.

both collagen and elastin fibers, which connect the cells together. The collagen fibers are tough fibers that give the skin its resiliency, and the elastin fibers give the skin its ability to stretch and (usually) return to normal. Unlike the epidermis, the dermal cells are not closely packed together. The dermis also contains specialized nervous tissue. This tissue provides sensory information, such as pain, pressure, touch, and temperature, to the central nervous system. The dermis also contains hair follicles, sweat and sebaceous glands, and a large network of blood vessels. The size and presence (or absence) of oxygen in these blood vessels cause color variations such as redness or cyanosis. Of note, the epidermis does not have its own blood supply and receives its blood from the dermis.

Between the dermis and the underlying muscle and bone is a thick layer of connective tissue known as **subcutaneous tissue,** or the superficial fascia. This subcutaneous tissue is composed of adipose tissue and areolar tissue. The subcutaneous tissue insulates, protects, and stores energy in the form of fat. Subcutaneous injections are given in this layer.

Hair

[OBJECTIVE 21]

Hair growth begins in a small, tubelike structure called a **follicle.** In each follicle is a small cluster of cells known as the **hair papilla.** The growth of hair begins in this cluster of cells, which is hidden in the follicle, and the cells move upward to become keratinized and form the shaft of the hair. Each follicle is surrounded by **arrector pili.** This is a smooth muscle responsible for "goose bumps," or the pulling upward of the hair and downward of the skin. The main function of hair is protection from physical injury, the sun, or the entry of dust and other particles into the eyes and nose.

Nails

[OBJECTIVE 21]

Nails are produced by cells in the epidermis in an area at the end of the base of the nail called the *nail root.* These cells quickly become keratinized, forming their characteristic hard nature. The bed of skin that lies under the nail (nail bed) contains a high amount of blood vessels and nerves. This is what gives the nail a pink color. Evaluating the nails of a patient for color, shape, attachment, and indentations can provide valuable information during the physical examination.

Glands

[OBJECTIVE 22]

Two types of glands are under the skin: sweat and sebaceous glands. **Sebaceous glands** are found in the dermis. They secrete oil **(sebum)** in the shaft of the hair follicle and the skin. This oil prevents excessive drying of the skin and hair, prevents water loss, and keeps the skin

pliable. The sebum that is secreted also protects the skin from some forms of bacteria. The **sweat glands** (sudoriferous, or odor forming) of the body are of two types: merocrine and apocrine. **Merocrine glands,** also called the *eccrine glands,* are the most numerous and open directly to the surface of the body. When the body's temperature rises, these glands produce a fluid (mainly water). This fluid allows the body to dispel large amounts of heat through the evaporation process. **Apocrine glands** open into hair follicles, including in and around the genitalia, axillae, and anus. These glands secrete an organic substance (which is odorless until acted upon by surface bacteria) into the hair follicles.

SKELETAL SYSTEM

[OBJECTIVE 23]

The skeletal system provides a framework for the body (Figure 7-15). It consists of 206 bones. These bones are as strong as, if not stronger than, concrete but much lighter. The functions of the skeletal system include:

1. **Support.** The skeletal system supports the weight of the body.
2. **Leverage.** Many muscles of the body attach to various locations on the skeletal system. This provides movement through leverage of the attachment sites.
3. **Protection.** The internal structures of the body are protected by the skeletal system.
4. **Storage.** The matrix that gives the bone its strength is composed of calcium phosphate material. This combination of minerals is stored in a usable form of bone. In addition, bone serves as a storage location for yellow marrow, which stores lipids.
5. **Maintenance of calcium levels.** Because 98% of the calcium in the body is stored in the bones and teeth, they are the major regulators of blood levels of calcium. As calcium levels rise the bones absorb the excess calcium; as calcium levels fall, the bones release calcium.
6. **Blood cell production.** The bones have cavities within them that contain red marrow. This red marrow is responsible for making red blood cells, white blood cells, and platelets. The location of the red marrow, or site of blood cell production, varies with age. However, after the age of 4 years, blood cell production is limited to the flat bones (ribs, sternum, pelvis, skull), irregular bones (the spinal column), and the proximal ends of the humerus and femur. Blood cell production is referred to as *hemopoiesis* or *hematopoiesis.*

Structure

Bones are classified on the basis of their shape. The human body has four types of bones: long bones, short bones, flat bones, and irregular bones (see Figure 7-11).

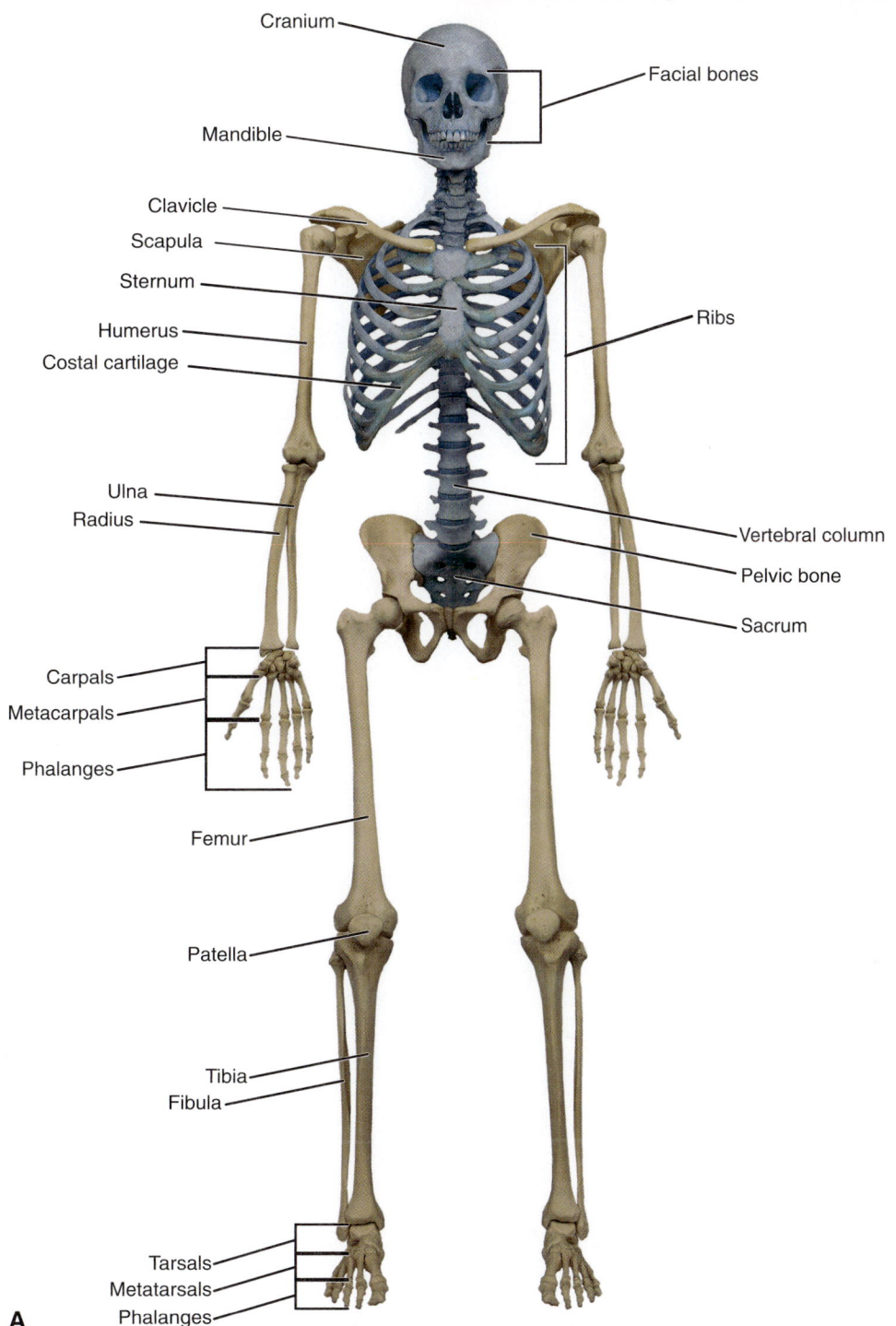

Cranium

Facial bones

Mandible

Clavicle

Scapula

Sternum

Humerus

Costal cartilage

Ribs

Ulna

Radius

Vertebral column

Pelvic bone

Sacrum

Carpals

Metacarpals

Phalanges

Femur

Patella

Tibia

Fibula

Tarsals

Metatarsals

Phalanges

A

Figure 7-15 The skeletal system provides a framework for the body with 206 bones. **A,** Anterior view.

Each type of bone shares common characteristics despite its difference in shape. The long bones are used as an example for this description. Bones are composed of two layers (Figure 7-16). The outer layer of all bones consists of dense, or compact, bone. This layer contains very few spaces and provides structure and support. The diaphysis is the shaft of a long bone and is composed of compact bone. Although long bones look solid, the diaphysis is a hollow tube that serves to lighten the bone while maintaining strength. The hollow area within the diaphysis is called the medullary canal. It is lined with a membrane called the *endosteum,* which contains specialized cells that allow bone growth and repair. The medullary canal contains blood vessels and yellow bone marrow, which is an inactive fatty bone marrow. At each end of the diaphysis is the epiphysis. This area is made of spongy

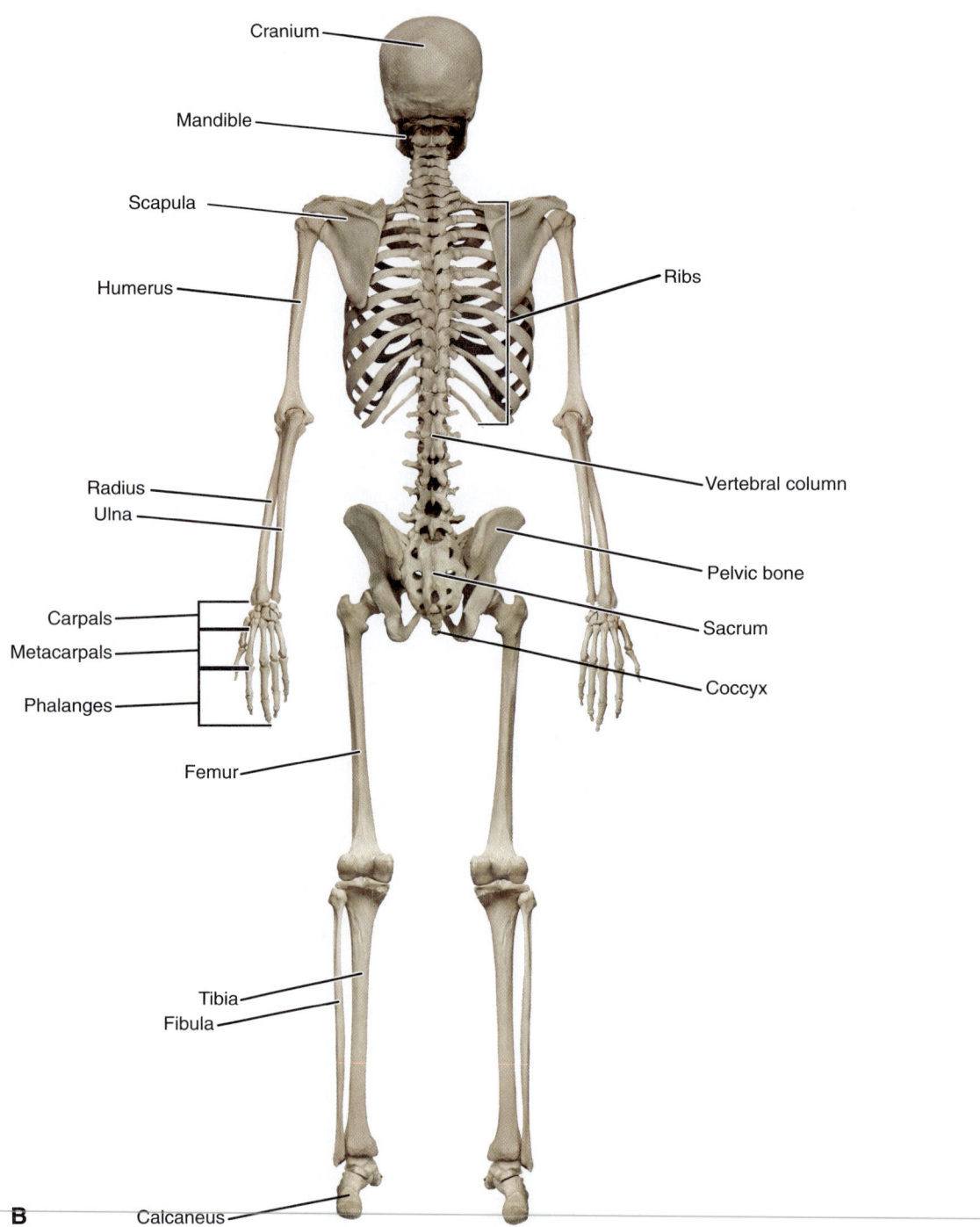

Cranium

Mandible

Scapula

Humerus

Ribs

Radius

Ulna

Vertebral column

Pelvic bone

Carpals

Metacarpals

Sacrum

Phalanges

Coccyx

Femur

Tibia

Fibula

B   Calcaneus

Figure 7-15, cont'd B, Posterior view.

bone, which is composed of several thin plates of bone with spaces between them that contain the red marrow and also serve to lighten the bone. Between and joining the diaphysis and epiphysis is a region called the *metaphysis.* During childhood, when bones are lengthening, this area also contains the epiphyseal plate. This plate consists of cartilage that is replaced by bone as is lengthens. Covering the end of the epiphysis is a thin layer of cartilage called the articular cartilage. The term *articulate,* or articulation, is used where bones come together. This cartilage absorbs shock and reduces friction between bones. The periosteum is a fibrous membrane that covers the entire bone with the exception of areas covered by the articular cartilage. The periosteum is composed of two layers and contains blood vessels, lymphatic vessels, nerves, bone cells, and elastic fibers. Blood supply and nervous intervention to the bone are provided by the periosteum by an extensive network of Haversian canals and Volkmann's canals. These canals also remove waste products from the bone. Blood vessels, lymphatic vessels, and nerves originating in the periosteum enter the compact bone through the horizontal Volkmann's canals. After entering the

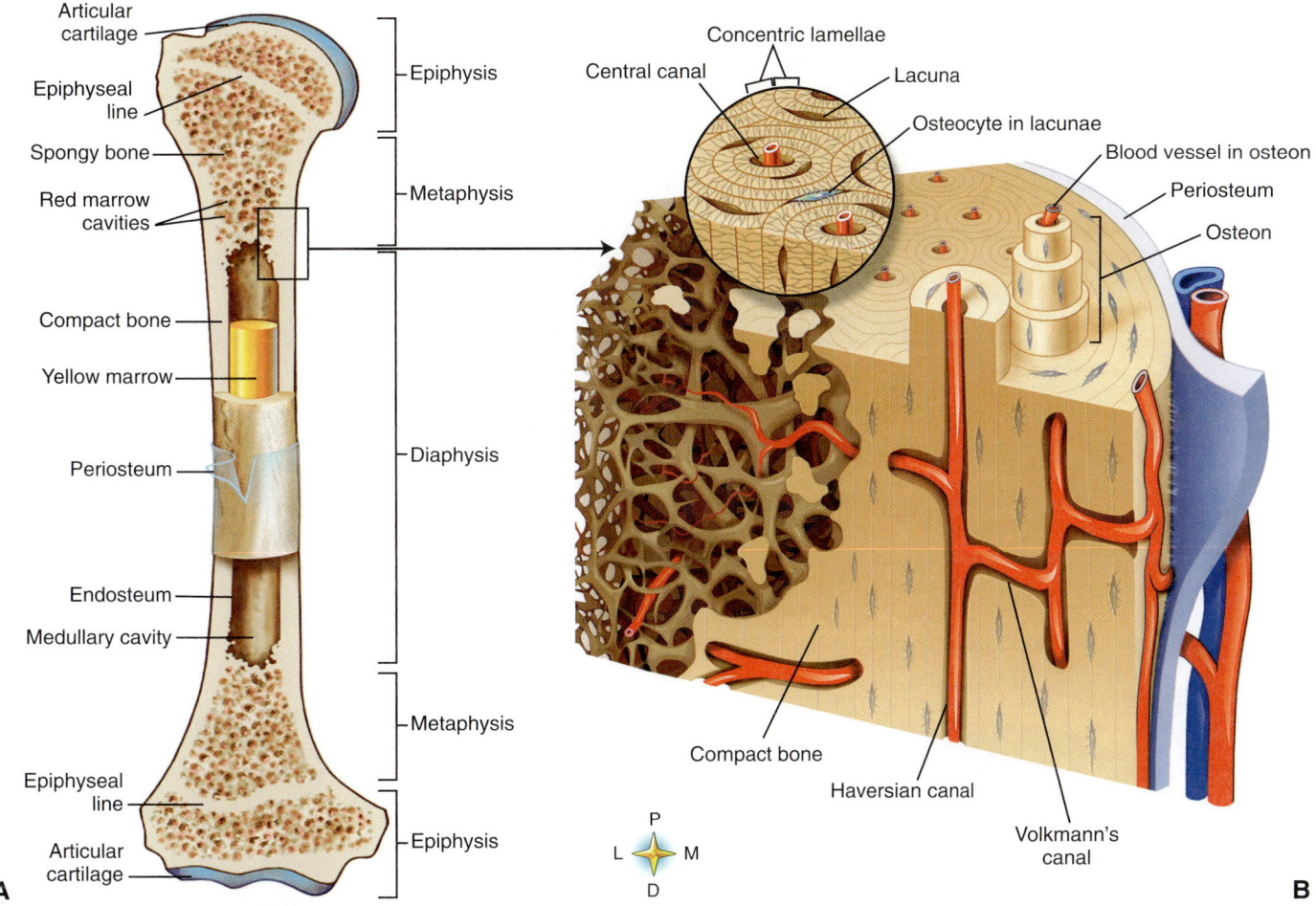

Figure 7-16 Microscopic structure of bone. The longitudinal section of a long bone **(A)** shows the location of the microscopic section illustrated in **B.** Note that the compact bone forming the hard shell of the bone is constructed of cylindrical units called *osteons.* Spongy bone is constructed of bony projections called *trabeculae.*

bone they join with the Haversian canals, which run along the length of the bone, and provide blood and nerve supply to the entire bone.

Axial Skeleton

[OBJECTIVE 24]

The **axial skeleton** is composed of the skull, hyoid bone, vertebral column, and thoracic cage.

The skull is composed of 22 bones divided between the cranial vault and the facial bones. Some sources include the six auditory ossicles (the bones of the ear that function in hearing) in the skull for a total of 28 bones.

The cranial vault consists of eight bones fused together, creating suture lines that surround and protect the brain. They are the parietal (two), temporal (two), frontal, occipital, sphenoid, and ethmoid bones (Figure 7-17). The parietal and temporal bones are considered paired bones because one is on each side of the skull.

The facial bones consist of 14 separate bones that form the structure of the face. These bones protect the entrances to the gastrointestinal system and the respiratory system. The 14 facial bones are the maxilla, mandible (the only freely moving bone in the skull), zygomatic, palatine, nasal, lacrimal, vomer, and nasal concha bones. Both the frontal and ethmoid bones contribute to the cranial fault and the face.

The hyoid bone is a floating bone attached to the skull by muscles and ligaments. It serves as a point of attachment for several important muscles of the neck and tongue.

The vertebral column is approximately 28 inches long in men and 24 inches long in women. It consists of 33 bones divided into five regions: seven cervical vertebrae, 12 thoracic vertebrae, five lumbar vertebrae, five sacral vertebrae (fused during embryonic development), and four coccygeal vertebrae (fused during development or shortly after birth into two or three vertebrae) (Figure 7-18). Two of these vertebrae have unique names and functions. The first cervical vertebra is called the *atlas* and

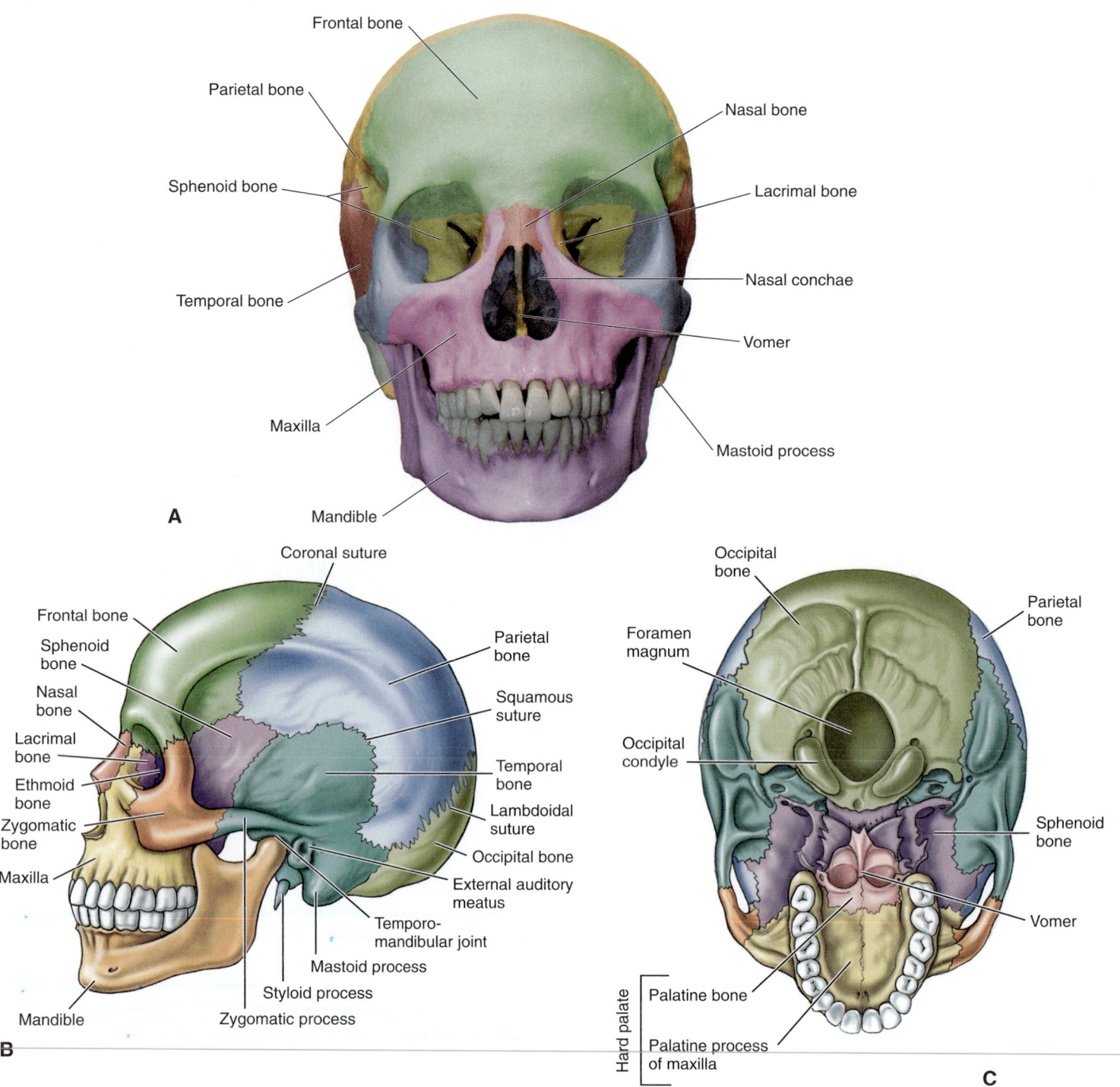

Figure 7-17 Cranial vault. Six bones fuse together, creating suture lines that surround and protect the brain. **A,** Frontal view. **B,** Side view. **C,** Base of the skull.

functions to support the weight of the head. The second cervical vertebra, called the *axis,* has an upward projection called the *odontoid process.* The atlas sits on this process, which acts as a pivot point and allows rotation of the head.

The vertebral column protects the spinal cord and supports the body's weight. To achieve this, each successive vertebral body becomes larger as the cord progresses downward (caudally). To add strength, assist in balance, and prevent injury, the spinal column has four curves: two that curve posteriorly (the cervical and lumbar curvatures) and two that curve anteriorly (the thoracic and sacral curvatures). Variations of these curvatures can exist. Lordosis is an exaggeration of the lumbar curvature, creating a swayback appearance; kyphosis is an exaggeration of the thoracic curvature, causing a humpback appearance; and scoliosis is an abnormal lateral curvature of the spine. The paramedic must be familiar with these

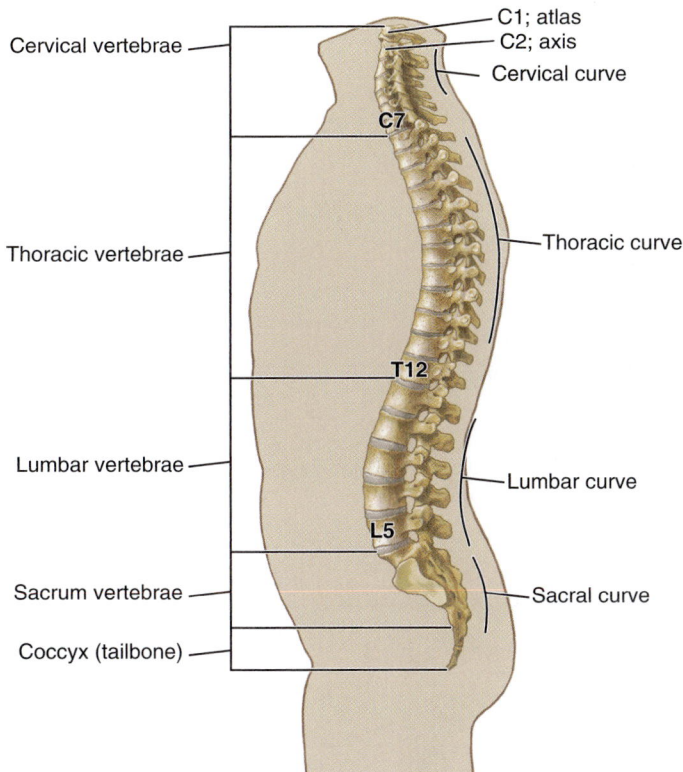

Figure 7-18 Five regions of bones compose the vertebral column.

Labels on figure:
Cervical vertebrae — C1; atlas, C2; axis, Cervical curve, C7
Thoracic vertebrae — Thoracic curve, T12
Lumbar vertebrae — Lumbar curve, L5
Sacrum vertebrae — Sacral curve
Coccyx (tailbone)

conditions because they can affect respiration, immobilization, and other aspects of the patient's condition or care.

Between each vertebra is an intervertebral disk. The intervertebral disks are composed of cartilaginous tissue. This tissue cushions (absorbs shock) and adds space between the vertebrae. The space created by these intervertebral disks allows the spinal nerves to exit the spinal cord. These spinal nerves allow control over the periphery of the body. The vertebral arch and the dorsal, or back, of the vertebral body form a **foramen** (passage) through which the spinal cord passes. This foramen becomes larger as the cord progresses downward. Whereas 95% of the foramen is occupied by the cord in the cervical spine, only 65% of the foramen is occupied by the spinal cord in the lumbar spine. A transverse process extends off either side of the vertebral arch and serves as a point of attachment for muscles. A single spinous process projects from the dorsum (back) of the vertebrae and also is a point of muscular attachment.

The thoracic cage protects the vital organs contained within the thorax. It also prevents the collapse of the thorax during respiration. The thoracic cage consists of the thoracic vertebrae, the ribs, the costal cartilages, and the sternum (Figure 7-19). In anatomic terms the top of the rib cage is called the *thoracic inlet* and is narrower than the bottom of the rib cage, the thoracic outlet. The anatomic terms should not be confused with the clinical condition of thoracic outlet syndrome, in which

neurovascular structures exiting the superior aspects of the thorax, and supplying the upper extremities, are compressed.

The human body has 12 pairs of ribs that articulate with the 12 thoracic vertebrae. The ribs increase in length from rib 1 through 7 and decrease in length through rib 12. Ribs are divided into two categories, true ribs or false ribs, according to their attachment with the sternum. The true ribs (superior seven pairs) articulate directly with the sternum by cartilaginous connections. The false ribs (inferior five pairs) articulate with the thoracic vertebrae, but instead of attaching directly to the sternum they attach through a common cartilage. The eleventh and twelfth ribs are called floating ribs. They attach to the thoracic spine but have no attachment to the anterior surface of the thoracic cage. The spaces between the ribs are called the intercostal spaces and are numbered for the rib above it. In other words, the third intercostal space is below the third rib. These landmarks become important when reporting the location of injuries or when performing procedures. The inferior border of each rib has a costal groove that contains a neurovascular bundle.

The sternum is divided into three parts: the manubrium, body, and xiphoid process. At the most superior point of the manubrium is the suprasternal (jugular) notch. This notch is at the base of the anterior surface of the neck and serves as muscular attachment for the sternocleidomastoid muscles. The point at which the manubrium joins the body of the sternum can easily be felt as a ridge (or a raised part of the sternum). This immovable joint, called the angle of Louis, also serves as an attachment of the second rib's costal cartilage. The xiphoid can be found at the most inferior aspect of the sternum.

Appendicular Skeleton

[OBJECTIVE 24]

The **appendicular skeleton** consists of all the bones not within the axial skeleton: the upper and lower extremities, the pectoral and pelvic girdles, and their attachments (see Figure 7-15, *A*).

Upper Extremities

[OBJECTIVE 25]

The scapula and clavicle form the pectoral girdle, which serves as an attachment for the upper extremities to the axial skeleton. Articulating with the sternum at the sternoclavicular joint, the clavicles are S-shaped bones that function to brace the scapula, holding the shoulders in place. Although the clavicle is one of the most commonly fractured bones in the body, the scapula is extremely difficult to fracture. The scapulae are triangular bones attached to the posterior thorax by muscles. The scapula is divided into two posterior components by a sharp diagonal ridge, or spine, of which the end forms the acromion process and provides muscle attachment of the upper limbs and thorax. The clavicles articulate with

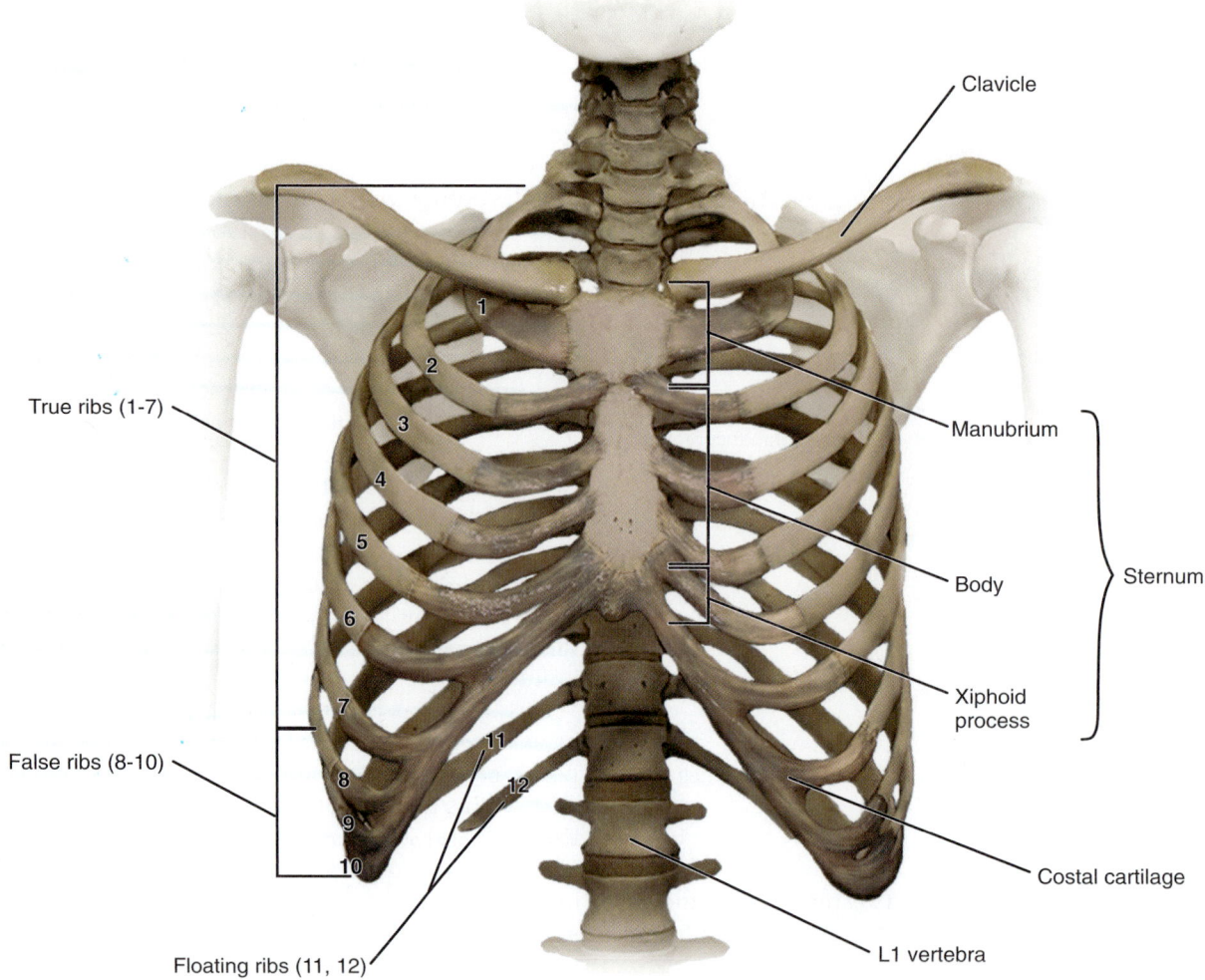

Figure 7-19 The thoracic cage consists of the thoracic vertebrae, ribs, and the sternum.

the scapula at the acromioclavicular joint. Anterior to the acromion process is a projection called the *coracoid process,* which also provides an area for muscle attachment. The area between these two processes is known as the *glenoid cavity,* where the head of the humerus lies.

The upper arm is composed of a single bone, the **humerus** (Figure 7-20). It is the second largest bone in the human body. The proximal portion of the humerus has a head that articulates with the scapula. On this proximal portion of the humerus are two small extensions off either side of the bone (tubercles). These tubercles serve as muscular attachments for the shoulder joint. The distal end of the humerus articulates with the bones of the forearm at the elbow.

The elbow is composed of the distal end of the humerus and the proximal ends of the radius and ulna. The proximal end of the ulna has a large bony process (olecranon process). This bony process forms the tip of the elbow. Lateral to this process, the proximal end of the radius fits and articulates with the humerus. The distal end of the radius articulates with the carpal bones of the wrist. The

distal end of the ulna articulates directly to the radius. This allows a person to twist (supinate and pronate) the wrist (Figure 7-21). The wrist is composed of eight carpal bones. These bones are arranged in two rows of four bones each. Five metacarpals form the bony portion of the hand. There are 14 phalanges in the four fingers and thumb on each hand. The digits are numbered (as a matter of convention). When referring to them, start with the thumb of each hand as 1 and so forth to the smallest finger, which is the fifth digit of each hand.

Lower Extremities

[OBJECTIVE 25]

The pelvic girdle is composed of the pelvis, the sacrum, and the coccyx (Figure 7-22). The pelvis is separated into two coxae (hip bones) that are joined at the pubic symphysis anteriorly and join with the sacrum posteriorly. Each coxa has a fossa, or depression, called the *acetabulum* that articulates with the head of the femur. Through each coxa travels an extensive nerve and vascular supply. This supply, in turn, allows supply to the lower

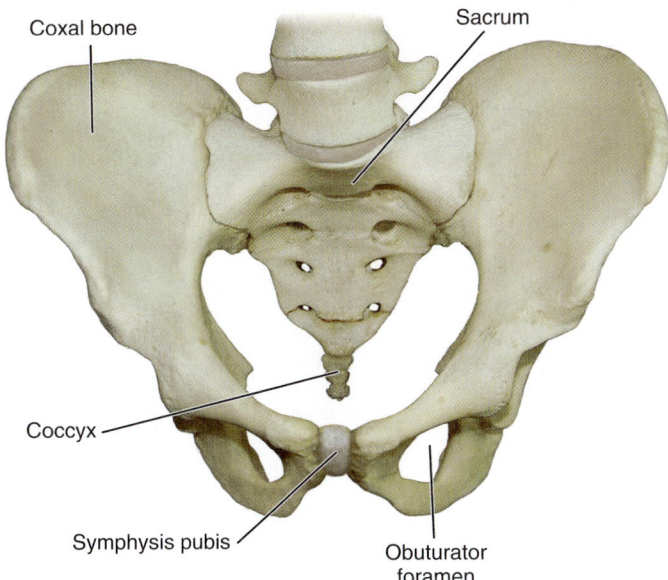

Figure 7-22 The pelvic girdle is composed of the pelvis and the sacrum.

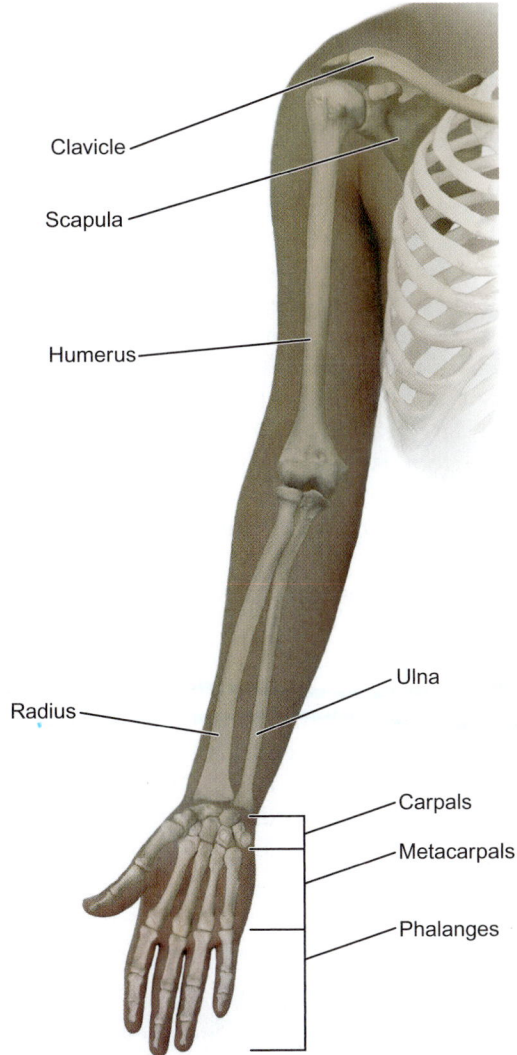

Figure 7-20 Bones of the arm.

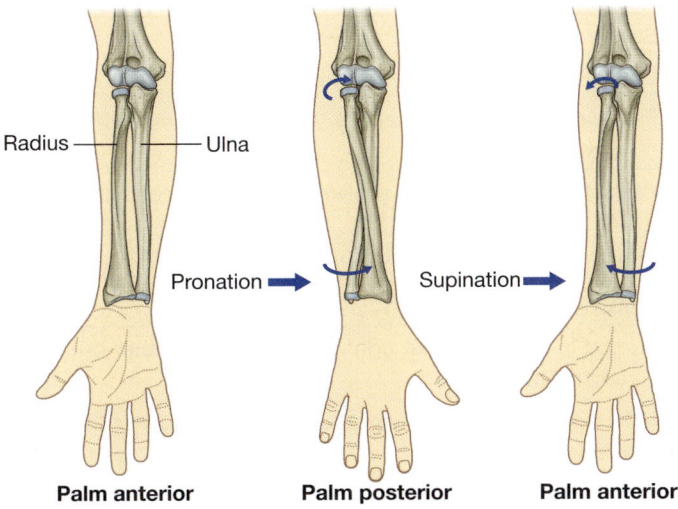

Figure 7-21 Supination and pronation. The distal end of the ulna articulates directly to the radius, allowing the arm to twist.

extremities. The acetabulum is the result of the fact that at birth the hip bones are composed of three parts that eventually fuse into one bone. However, the pelvis commonly is discussed as though it were three individual bones.

- The ilium is the largest portion of the pelvis. Its superior border is called the *iliac crest* and can often be visualized or palpated. Other prominences on the ilium serve as muscular attachment points.
- The ischium is the posterior portion of the pelvis. Several attachment points for muscles are there, including the ischial tuberosity. In addition to being a muscular attachment point, this prominence also supports the weight of the body when sitting. This is also the prominence against which many traction splints are placed to keep them in place.
- The pubis is the anterior portion of the pelvis where the two halves of the pelvis join together. This joint is called the *pubic symphysis* or the *symphysis pubis*. The angle at which these bones come together forms the pubic arch.

The femur (thigh) is the longest bone in the human body (Figure 7-23). It is separated into the head that articulates with the coxae, the neck that redirects the femur at almost a right angle, and a shaft that represents the longest portion of the bone. The neck of the femur has two separate points of muscular attachment, the greater and lesser trochanter. Distally the femur articulates with the tibia and the patella. The patella is a sesamoid bone. It allows the knee joint to travel in its range of motion.

The two bones of the lower leg are the tibia and fibula. The tibia is the larger of the two bones and forms what

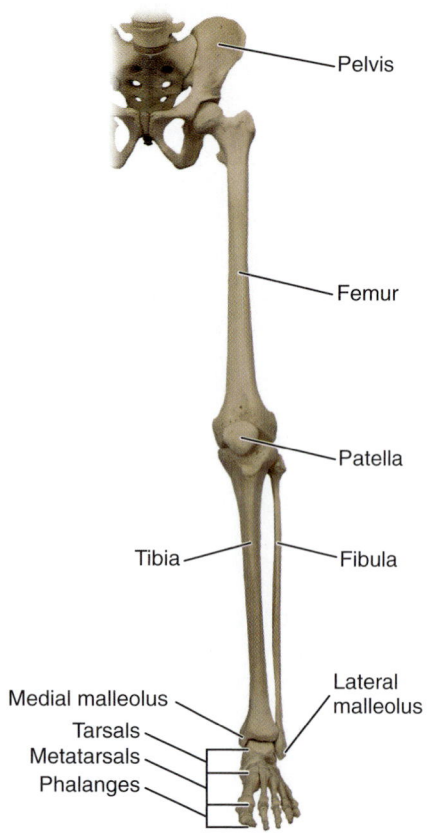

Figure 7-23 Bones of the leg.

Labels: Pelvis, Femur, Patella, Tibia, Fibula, Lateral malleolus, Medial malleolus, Tarsals, Metatarsals, Phalanges

is commonly known as the *shin*. Proximally it articulates with the distal femur and is the weight bearing bone of the leg. The tibial tuberosity is a projection on the anterior surface of the tibia and serves as an attachment point for the patellar ligament. This also is an important landmark for the paramedic to identify before inserting an intraosseous needle into the tibia. Distally the tibia forms the medial malleolus. The fibula is much smaller than the tibia, does not bear any weight, and does not articulate with the femur. It does directly articulate with the tibia. Distally the fibula forms the lateral malleolus on the outside of the ankle.

The foot is composed of seven tarsal bones (Figure 7-24). The largest of these bones is the calcaneus (heel bone). The foot is also composed of metatarsals (foot bones) and phalanges (toe bones). The bones of the foot are arranged in a similar manner to those of the hand.

Articulations

[OBJECTIVE 26]

The joints of the body are areas where two or more bones meet and are made of flexible connective tissue. This type of connection allows movement of the body's extremities that rigid bone would not allow. Joints are divided into several classifications according to structure or function (the type of movement it allows) (Table 7-4). This text uses the classification system based on structure. However,

TABLE 7-4	Classification of Joints	
Type of Joint	**Example**	**Description**
Fibroid (Synarthrosis)		No movement is permitted
Suture	Cranial sutures	United by thin layer of fibrous tissue
Synchondrosis	Joint between the epiphysis and diaphysis of long bones	Temporary joint in which the cartilage is replaced by bone later in life
Cartilaginous (Amphiarthrosis)		Slightly moveable joint
Symphysis	Symphysis pubis	Bones are connected by a fibrocartilage disk
Syndesmosis	Radius-ulna articulation	Bones are connected by ligaments
Synovial (Diarthrosis)		Freely moveable; enclosed by joint capsule, synovial membrane
Ball and socket	Shoulder	Widest range of motion, movement in all planes
Hinge	Elbow	Motion limited to flexion and extension in a single plane
Pivot	Atlantoaxis	Motion limited to rotation
Condyloid	Wrist between radius and carpals	Motion in two planes at right angles to each other but no radial rotation
Saddle	Thumb at carpal-metacarpal joint	Motion in two planes at right angles to each other but no axial rotation
Gliding	Intervertebral: between the articular surfaces of successive vertebrae	Motion limited to gliding

Modified from Seidel, H. M., Ball, J. W., & Dains, J. E. (1999). *Mosby's guide to physical examination* (4th ed.). St. Louis: Mosby.

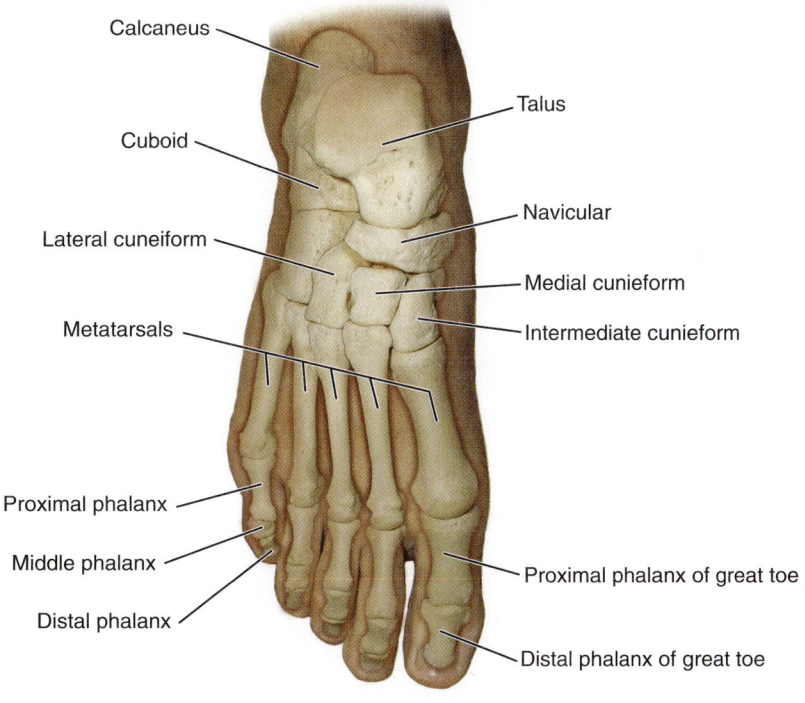

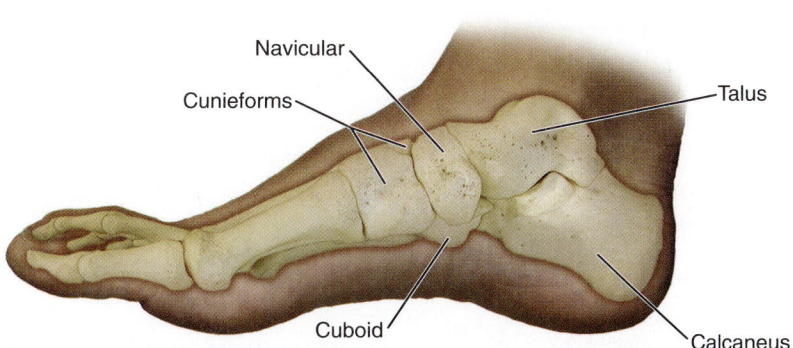

Figure 7-24 The foot consists of seven tarsal bones.

the functional system should at least be mentioned. Functionally, joints fall into three categories. Synarthroses are immovable and include joints such as the suture, gomphosis, and synchondrosis. Amphiarthroses are slightly movable and include joints such as the syndesmosis and symphysis. Diarthroses are movable and include the synovial joints.

Fibrous Joints

Fibrous joints consist of two bones united by fibrous tissue that have little or no movement (Figure 7-25). The joints are further divided on the basis of structure into sutures, syndesmoses, or gomphoses. **Sutures** (seams between flat bones) are located in the skull bones. These may be completely immobile in adults. In the newly born, the sutures have gaps called **fontanels.** These gaps allow the skull to expand or contract during birth. They also allow growth of the head during development. A

syndesmosis is a type of joint in which the bones are united by fibrous connective tissue, forming an intraosseous membrane or ligament. It is a temporary joint in which the cartilage is replaced by bone later in life. The ligaments may provide some movement of the joint. An example is the radioulnar syndesmosis that binds the radius and ulna together (Figure 7-26). **Gomphoses** consist of a peg that fits into a socket. The peg is held in place by fine bundles of collagenous connective tissue. The joints between the teeth and the sockets along the processes of the mandible and maxilla are examples of gomphoses (see Figure 7-26).

Cartilaginous Joints

Cartilaginous joints unite two bones with hyaline cartilage (synchondroses) or fibrocartilage (symphyses). This is a slightly movable joint in which the bones are connected by a fibrocartilage disk or ligaments.

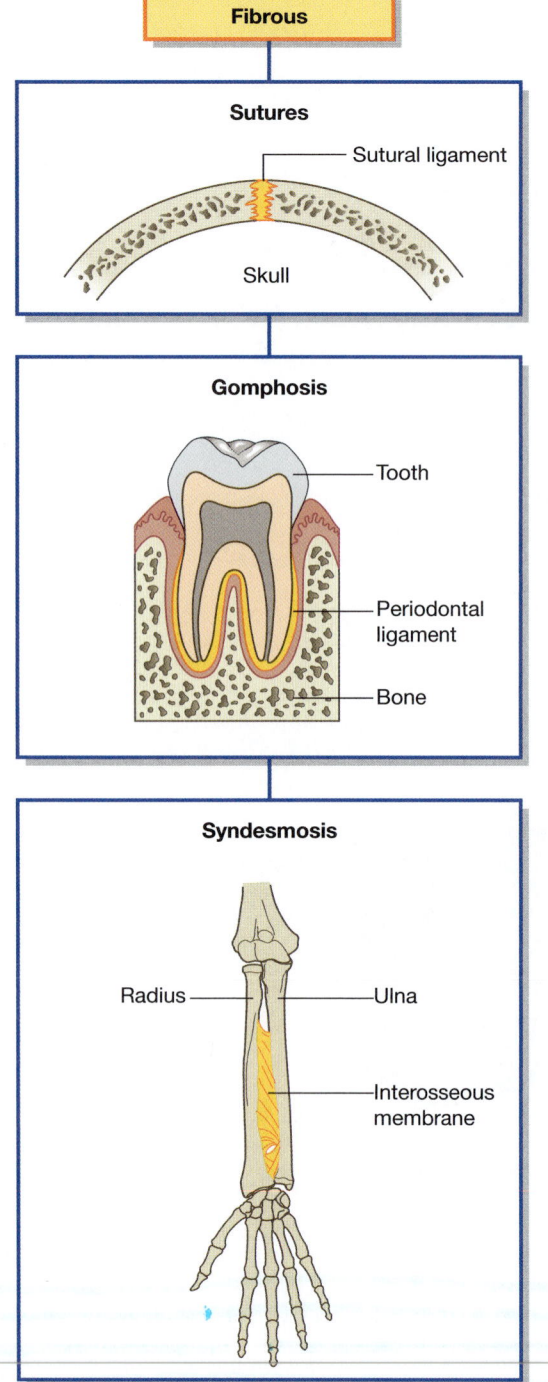

Fibrous

Sutures

Sutural ligament

Skull

Gomphosis

Tooth

Periodontal ligament

Bone

Syndesmosis

Radius

Ulna

Interosseous membrane

Figure 7-25 Fibrous joints are two bones united by fibrous tissue that have little or no movement.

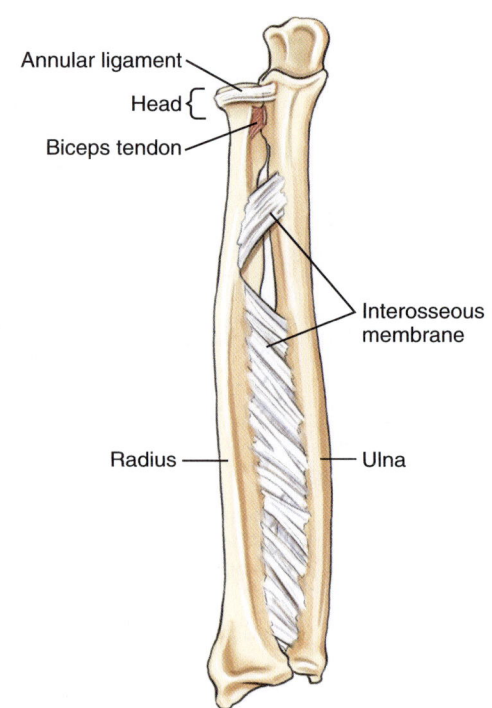

Annular ligament

Head

Biceps tendon

Interosseous membrane

Radius

Ulna

Figure 7-26 Radioulnar syndesmosis binds the radius and ulna together.

capsule lined with a synovial membrane. The synovial membrane secretes synovial fluid, which lubricates the joint and, because cartilage is avascular, removes waste products, microorganisms, and debris. The articular cartilage reduces the friction of movement of the bone ends and absorbs vibrations and shocks. Bones that have synovial joints are connected by ligaments connected to the periosteum of each bone and comprise the outermost layer of the joint capsule. Because the ligaments are flexible they allow movement. However, they are strong enough to resist dislocation. Many ligaments may be present inside or outside the joint capsule. These are considered accessory ligaments and add further structure and support to the joint. To further reduce friction between moving parts, some joints contain bursae. These fluid-filled sacs decrease the friction between bones and also are found between the skin and bones, tendons and bones, tendons and muscles and bones, and any other area where two objects can potentially rub together. Examples of synovial joints include the ball and socket, hinge, pivot, condyloid, saddle, and gliding joints (Figures 7-28 to 7-31).

An example is the symphysis pubis in the pelvis (Figure 7-27).

Synovial Joints

Synovial joints are freely movable joints with articular cartilage between them and are enclosed by a joint

Text continued on p. 142

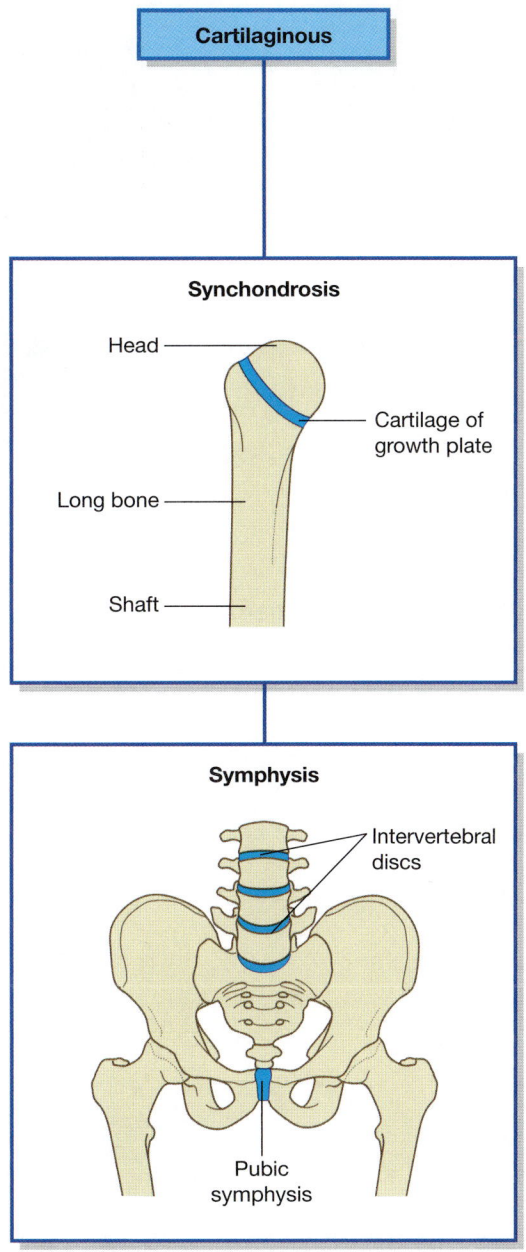

Figure 7-27 Cartilaginous joints unite two bones by means of hyaline cartilage (synchondroses) or fibrocartilage (symphyses). It is a slightly movable joint in which the bones are connected by a fibrocartilage disk or ligaments.

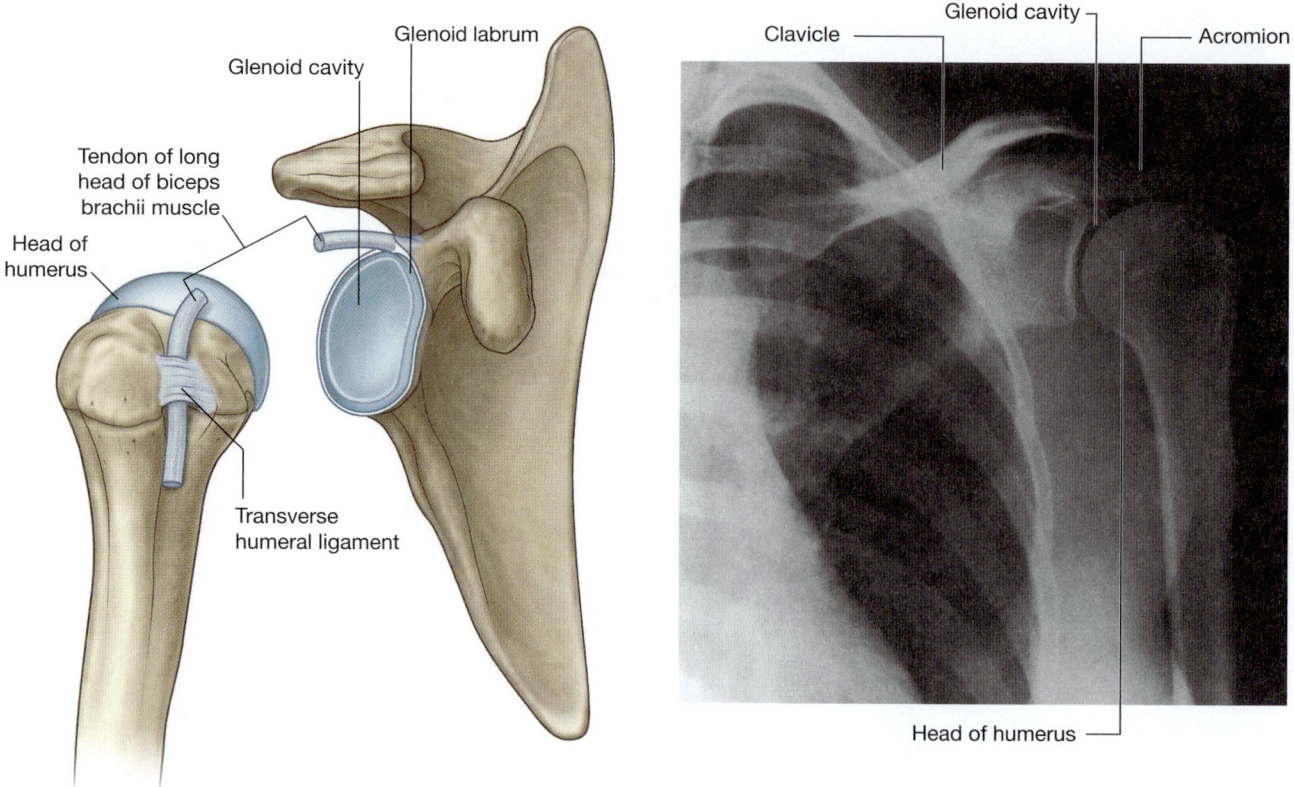

Figure 7-28 The shoulder is an example of a ball-and-socket joint. It has the widest range of motion and can move in all planes.

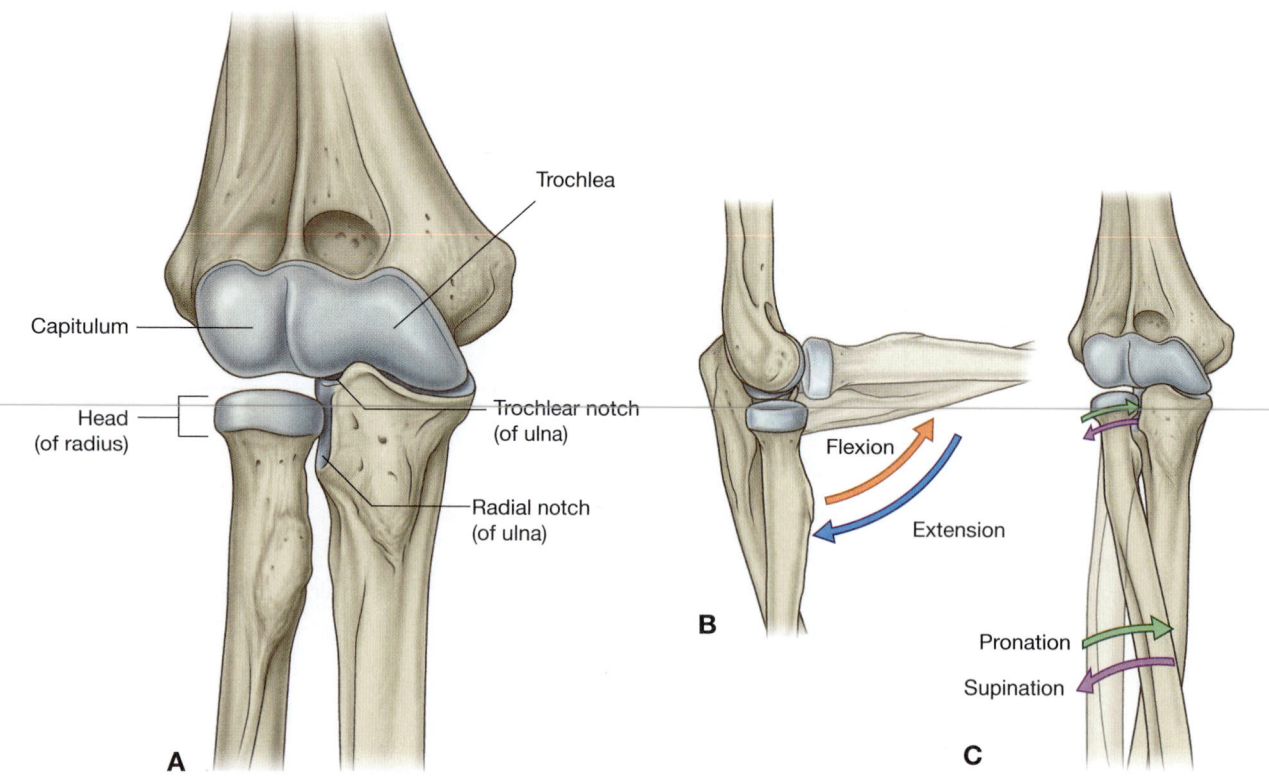

Figure 7-29 The elbow is an example of a hinge joint. Motion is limited to flexion and extension in a plane. **A,** Bones and joint surfaces. **B,** Flexion and extension. **C,** Pronation and supination.

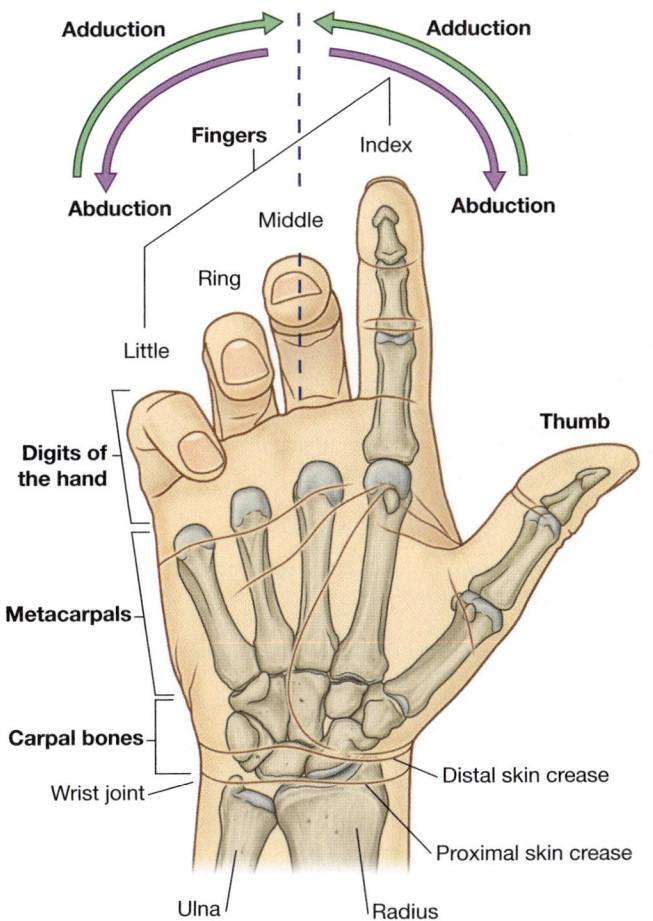

Adduction   Adduction

Fingers   Index

Abduction   Middle   Abduction

Ring

Little

Digits of
the hand

Thumb

Metacarpals

Carpal bones

Wrist joint   Distal skin crease

Proximal skin crease

Ulna   Radius

Figure 7-30 The wrist between the radius and carpals is an example of a condyloid joint. Motion occurs in two planes at right angles to each other, but no radial rotation exists. The thumb at the carpal-metacarpal joint is an example of a saddle joint. Motion is possible in two planes at right angles to each other, but there is no axial rotation.

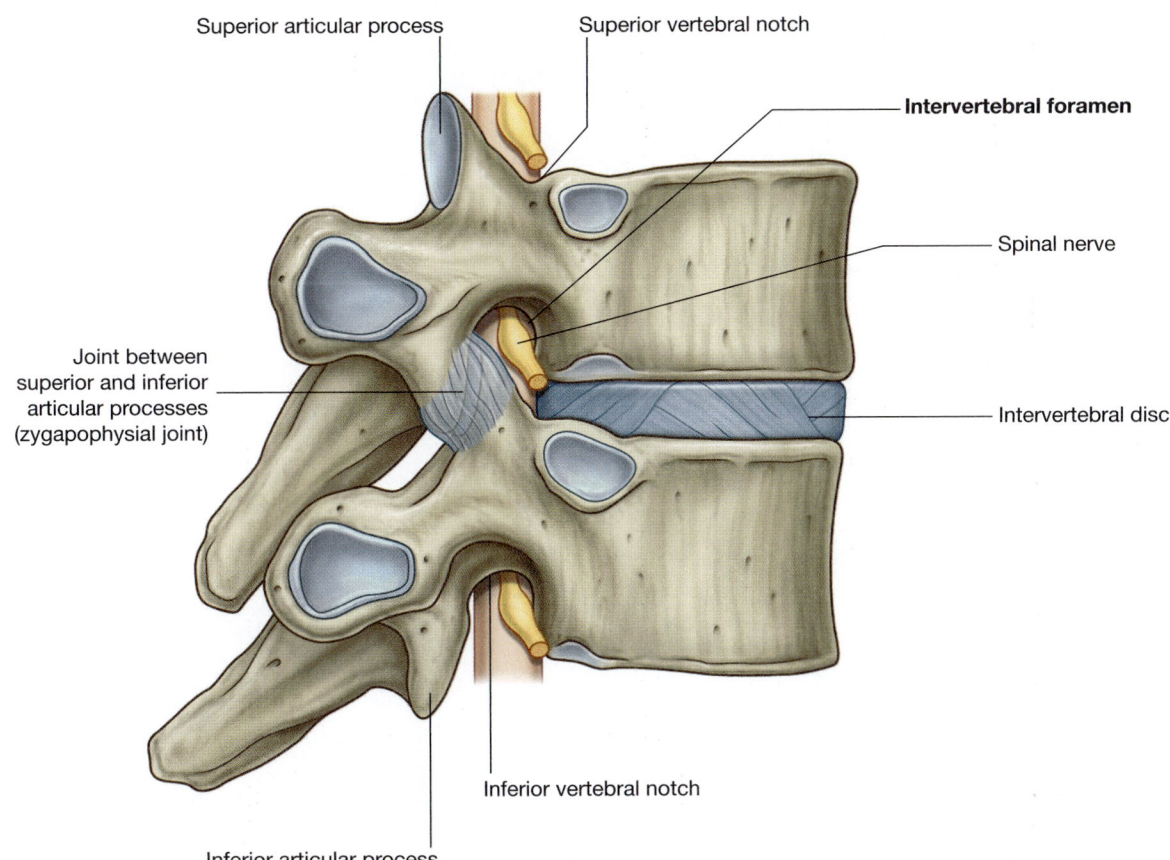

Superior articular process   Superior vertebral notch

Intervertebral foramen

Spinal nerve

Joint between
superior and inferior
articular processes
(zygapophysial joint)

Intervertebral disc

Inferior vertebral notch

Inferior articular process

Figure 7-31 Between the articular surfaces of successive vertebrae (intervertebral) is an example of a gliding joint. Motion is limited to gliding.

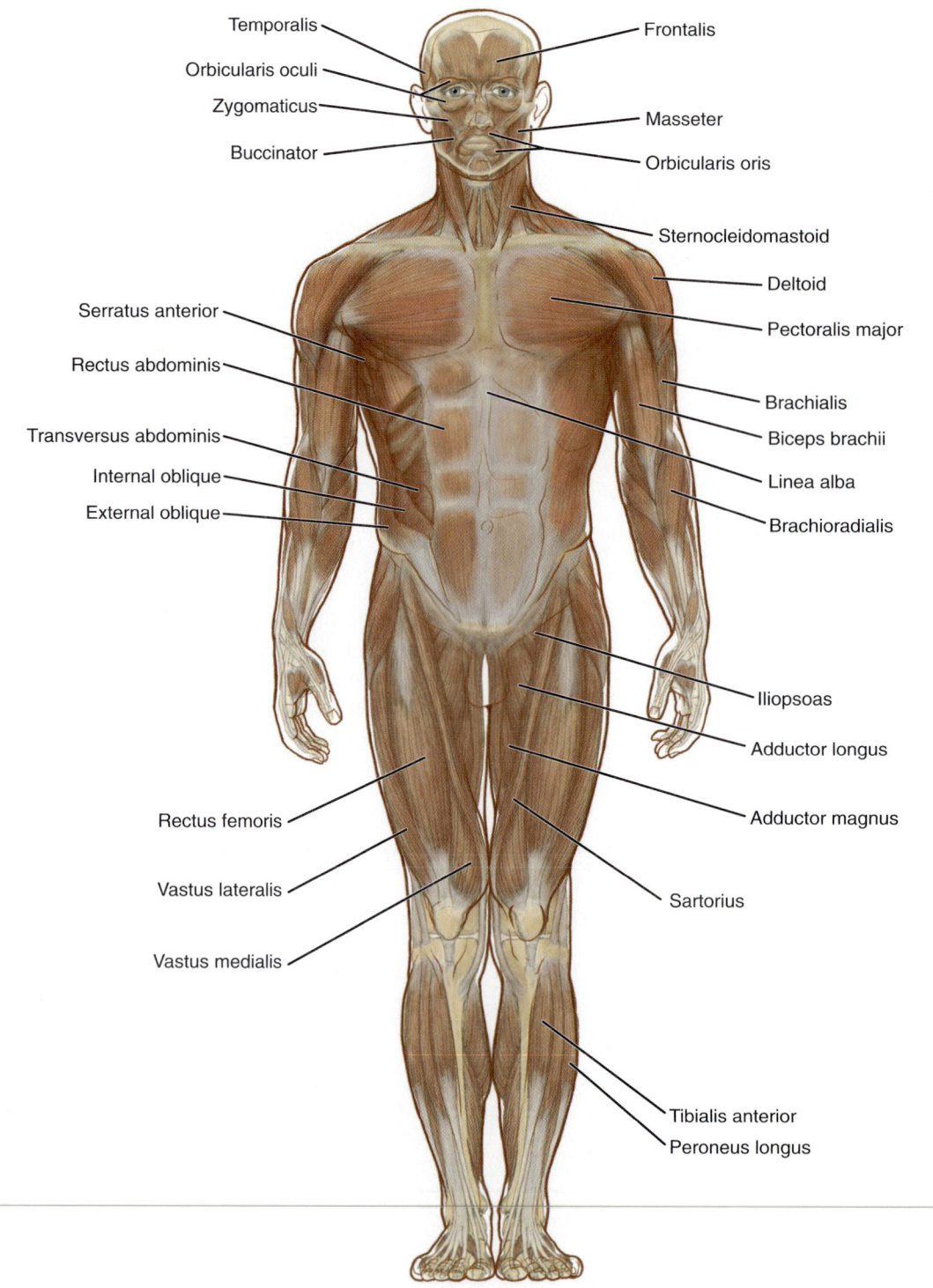

Temporalis
Orbicularis oculi
Zygomaticus
Buccinator
Frontalis
Masseter
Orbicularis oris
Sternocleidomastoid
Deltoid
Pectoralis major
Serratus anterior
Rectus abdominis
Transversus abdominis
Internal oblique
External oblique
Brachialis
Biceps brachii
Linea alba
Brachioradialis
Iliopsoas
Adductor longus
Adductor magnus
Rectus femoris
Vastus lateralis
Vastus medialis
Sartorius
Tibialis anterior
Peroneus longus

A

Figure 7-32 The muscular system. **A,** Anterior view.

MUSCULAR SYSTEM

[OBJECTIVES 27, 28, 29]

As previously discussed, the body contains three types of muscles: skeletal, smooth, and cardiac. They all share the properties of excitability, contractility, extensibility, and elasticity. The muscular system provides movement for the body (Figure 7-32), and although locomotion is the most obvious function of the muscular system, it is also responsible for performing everyday autonomic functions such as circulation of the blood and the rhythmic movement of the digestive tract. Of all the functions of

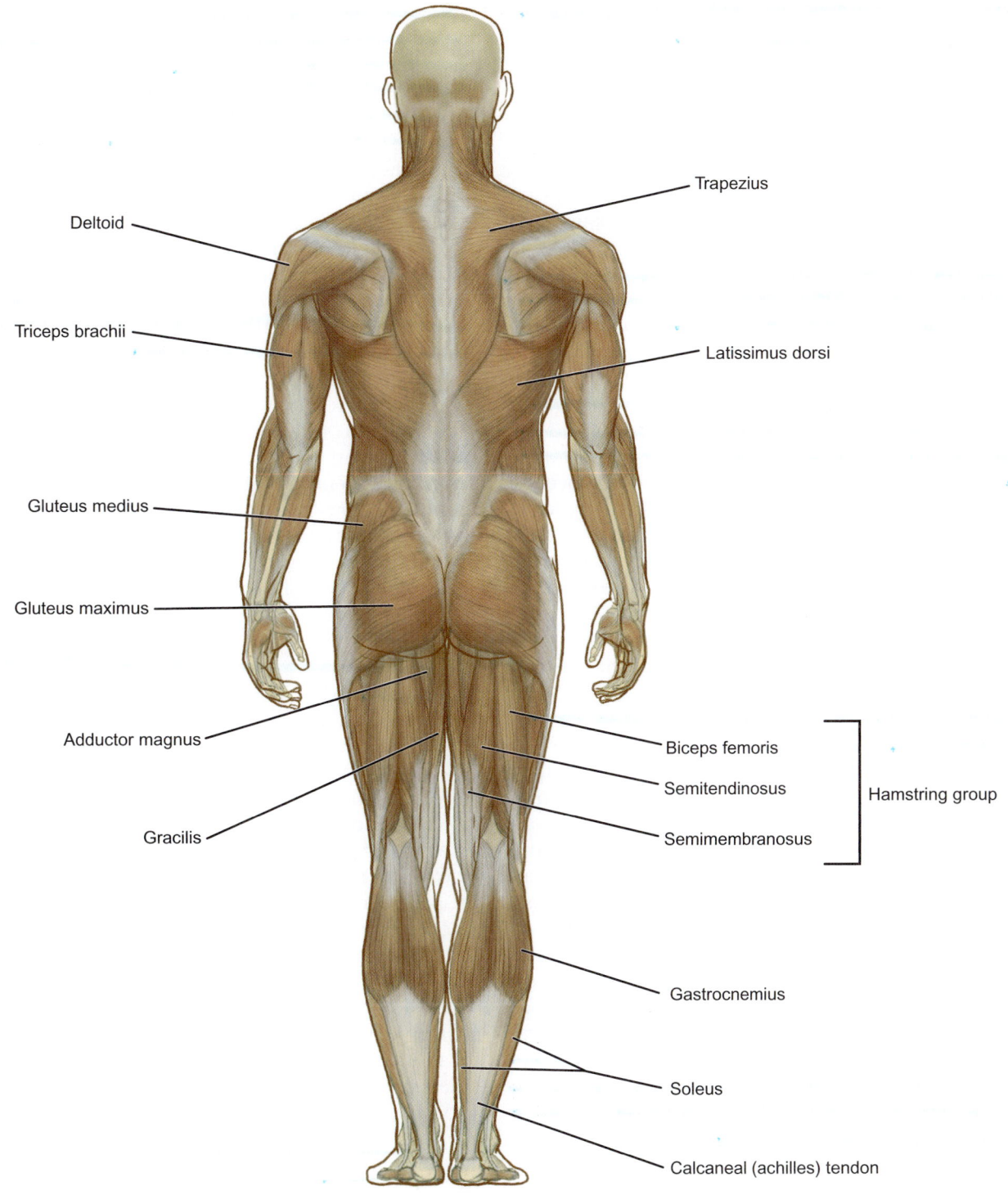

Deltoid

Triceps brachii

Gluteus medius

Gluteus maximus

Adductor magnus

Gracilis

Trapezius

Latissimus dorsi

Biceps femoris

Semitendinosus

Semimembranosus

Hamstring group

Gastrocnemius

Soleus

Calcaneal (achilles) tendon

B

Figure 7-32, cont'd B, Posterior view.

the muscular system, the three primary functions are movement, maintenance of posture, and production of heat.

Muscle Stimulation

To understand how muscles move, you must first understand how they are stimulated. A motor unit is a group of muscle fibers innervated by one motor neuron.

When stimulated, the motor unit contracts as a whole. This contraction is a steady contraction throughout the muscle because motor neuron axons are present throughout the muscle belly. The impulse that stimulates muscle contraction enters the muscle fibers at the neuromuscular junction. At this junction the muscle fibers of the motor unit create the motor end plate, which has receptors for the neurotransmitter acetylcholine.

Before being stimulated, the muscle cells are at their resting membrane potential, or polarized. This is a result of the distribution of electrically charged particles called *ions*. Outside the cell membrane are more positively charged sodium ions (Na^+) than are inside the cell, whereas inside the cell are more positively charged potassium ions (K^+) than are outside the cell. Although both of these ions are positively charged, the ratio is such that a relative negative charge is inside the cell compared with that outside the cell.

When the nervous impulse reaches the synaptic gap between the motor neuron and the motor unit, the neurotransmitter acetylcholine is released. Acetylcholine causes the Na^+ channels in the muscle cell membrane to open, flooding the cell with Na^+ and creating a positive charge inside the cell. This process is depolarization, which causes the muscle cell to generate its own impulse, or action potential, which is then conducted along the motor unit. As a paramedic you may administer a class of medications called *paralytics*, which block or stop the transfer of acetylcholine, resulting in paralysis of the patient. Myasthenia gravis is an autoimmune disorder in which the immune system attacks the acetylcholine receptors on the motor plate, resulting in muscular weakness or failure. A myasthenic crisis is a life-threatening presentation of this disorder in which weakness of the respiratory muscles can lead to respiratory failure or arrest.

Repolarization is the process of the cell returning to its polarized state. This begins with the opening of the K^+ channels, allowing K^+ (and its positive charge) to flow out of the cell and making the inside of the cell slightly more negative than it was at the end of depolarization. This process does not completely restore the resting membrane potential, however. To restore this potential, the Na^+ and K^+ must be returned to their original positions outside and inside the cells, respectively. Because the concentrations of extracellular Na^+ and intracellular K^+ are always higher, simply opening their channels again will cause further influx of Na^+ into the cell and K^+ out of the cell. To move these ions against their concentration gradient the sodium-potassium pump is used. Once the sodium-potassium pump has restored the resting membrane potential, muscle contraction stops and the cell is ready to be stimulated again.

Muscular Movement

[OBJECTIVE 30]

Muscle fibers contain two types of proteins: thick filaments of myosin and thin, light filaments of actin. As previously mentioned, the overlap of these filaments, or striations, can be seen in skeletal muscle, which leads to the name striated muscle. They cannot be seen in involuntary muscle, which leads to the name smooth muscle. When the muscle is in its resting state the actin filaments are surrounded by two substances, troponin and tropomyosin. These substances keep the actin and myosin filaments from interacting with each other. However,

when the muscle is depolarized special organelles in the muscle cells, called the *sarcoplasmic reticulum*, release large amounts of calcium (Ca^{++}). In the presence of Ca^{++} the actin and myosin filaments create cross bridges and pull themselves toward each other, thereby shortening their length and causing contraction. This process continues as long as Ca^{++} is present. Ca^{++} is restored to the sarcoplasmic reticulum by the calcium pump when the resting membrane potential of the muscle is reached and the muscle relaxes and, through the property of elasticity, returns to its original shape.

Contraction is either isometric or isotonic. During isometric contraction the length of the muscle remains unchanged during the contraction. However, during this type of contraction the tension along the muscle dramatically increases. This results in an increase in the tone and firmness of the muscle. Examples include pushing or pulling on an immovable object. During isotonic contraction the length of the muscle changes but the tension along the muscle remains constant. Examples of this include the movement of the extremities and digits. The contractile cells of the muscle need large amounts of energy to accomplish this. As a result, unusually high amounts of mitochondria are located along the length of the fiber.

Movement of the skeleton is the result of isotonic contraction. Muscles are attached to bone by tendons. The origin of a muscle is the stationary attachment of the muscle to a bone, whereas the insertion of a muscle is the moveable attachment to bone. For example, the origins of the biceps (the biceps and some other muscles have two origins) are within the shoulder girdle, whereas the insertion is at the radius. When the bicep is flexed the lower arm moves, not the shoulder. Muscles always work in pairs because only the contraction of a muscle causes movement; relaxation does not. Continuing with the biceps as an example, after it contracts and the arm is bent it will eventually need to be straightened again. Relaxation does not cause this—rather, contraction of the triceps straightens the arm. Although identifying each group of muscles responsible for various movements is beyond the scope of this text, identifying types of muscles responsible for various movements is valuable, as follows:

- Flexors are muscles responsible for decreasing a joint angle.
- Extensors are muscles responsible for increasing a joint angle.
- Abductors are muscles that move limbs away from the body.
- Adductors are muscles that move limbs toward the body.
- Rotators are muscles that rotate a limb.

Maintenance of Posture

Muscle tone is the amount of tension that is constantly in a muscle. It is the result of a constant state of partial contractions in the body. As some motor units contract,

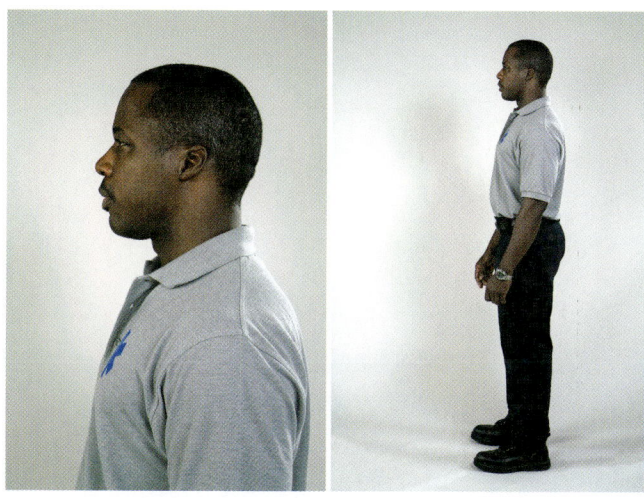

Figure 7-33 Posture. Muscular tension allows the head to stay upright and the back to remain straight.

others relax. Muscle tone in the skeletal muscles helps maintain balance and body position. In the maintenance of posture, muscle tone allows the head to stay upright and the back to remain straight (Figure 7-33). In the smooth muscle, tone maintains the size of the blood vessels and aids in digestion.

Heat Production

Muscles need a great deal of energy to contract. This energy is delivered in the form of ATP. The energy required by muscular contraction is developed during the breakdown of ATP (breaking of bonds). One of the byproducts of this breakdown is heat, which is used to maintain a normal body temperature. If the body's temperature drops below a set point, the nervous system stimulates the muscles to start shivering (a form of rapid contractions). This, in turn, generates heat used to elevate the body's temperature.

NERVOUS SYSTEM

[OBJECTIVES 31, 32]

The nervous system, along with the endocrine system, provides a coordinated response to changes in a person's environment. This system provides a rapid, but often fleeting, response to changes (maintenance of homeostasis). The nervous system is complex in its organization and versatile in its design. Following are the main functions of the nervous system:

1. Monitoring internal and external environments
2. Integrating sensory information
3. Coordinating voluntary and involuntary responses

The nervous system has two anatomic divisions: the central nervous system and the peripheral nervous system

(Figure 7-34). The **central nervous system (CNS)** consists of the brain and the spinal cord. The CNS is responsible for the integration and coordination of sensory information and motor responses. The CNS also is responsible for higher functions: thought, memory, and intelligence. The peripheral nervous system (PNS) is responsible for communication between the CNS and the rest of the body.

Central Nervous System

The CNS is composed of the brain and the spinal cord. The brain has four primary areas: the brainstem, diencephalon, cerebrum, and cerebellum (Figure 7-35). The **meninges** form a covering over the brain and spinal cord.

Meninges

[OBJECTIVES 33, 34]

Three distinct layers compose the meninges: the dura mater, arachnoid mater, and pia mater (Figure 7-36). The **dura mater** is the toughest of the three layers (dura mater means "tough mother"). This tough layer has two layers: a parietal layer and a visceral layer. The parietal layer is tightly adhered to the cranial vault, and the visceral layer lies over the CNS. In some areas of the CNS, the parietal and visceral layers of the dura are fused. The dura mater has two projections. The falx cerebri is a vertical projection that separates the two hemispheres of the brain. The tentorium cerebelli is a horizontal projection of the dura mater that separates the cerebellum from the occipital lobes. The temporal lobes are positioned on an opening in the tentorium cerebelli, which is called the *tentorium incisura*, or tentorial notch. This opening allows passage of the midbrain and occulomotor nerves. These structures play an important role in increased intracranial pressure and herniation of the brain. Above the dura is a potential space referred to as the **epidural space.** Within this epidural space run arterial vessels, in particular the middle meningeal artery. These arterial vessels can become injured during traumatic events. Below the dura is a space referred to as the **subdural space.** This space contains large venous vessels and drains. The **arachnoid mater** is the second meningeal layer. Between the arachnoid and the dura, the subdural space, is a small amount of serous fluid. The last meningeal layer is the **pia mater** ("fine mother"). The pia mater tightly adheres to the CNS (it normally cannot be dissected from the living tissue).

Between the arachnoid and pia mater circulates **cerebrospinal fluid (CSF).** CSF bathes, protects, and nourishes the CNS. CSF is continually made in the areas of the brain referred to as ventricles. Within these ventricles are a group of specialized cells called the **choroid plexus.** The choroids plexus filters blood through cerebral capillaries to create the CSF. The majority of the CSF is made in the large lateral ventricles and then circulates through the smaller third and fourth ventricles. CSF then continu-

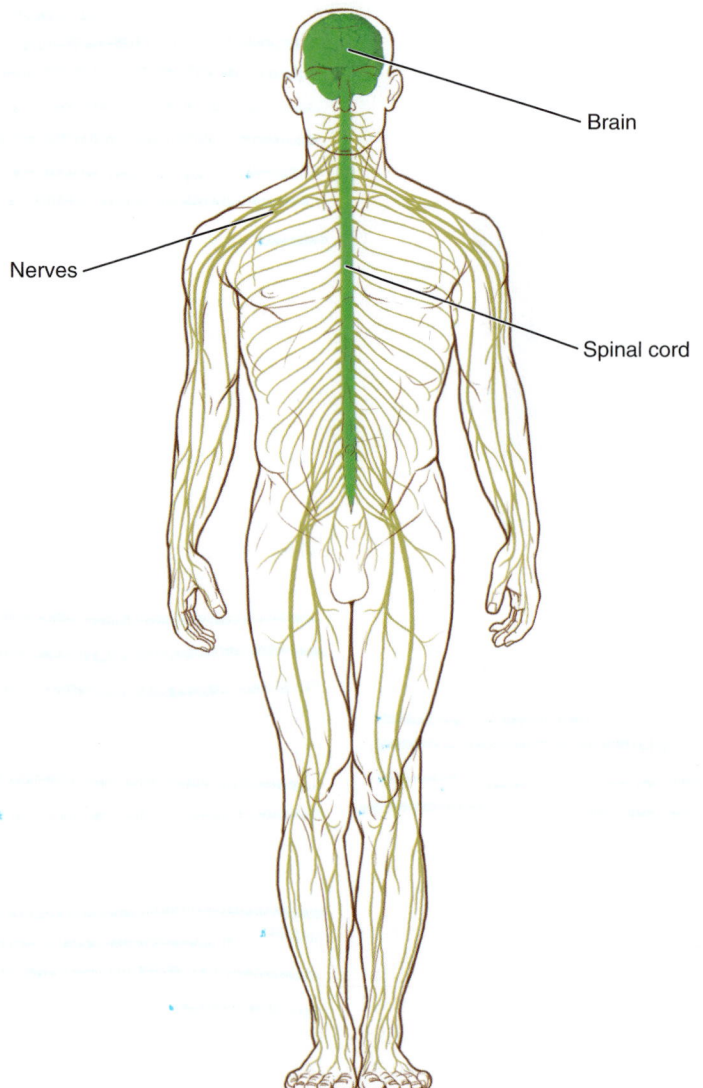

Brain

Nerves

Spinal cord

Figure 7-34 Central nervous system *(CNS)* and peripheral nervous system *(PNS)*. The CNS consists of the brain and the spinal cord. The PNS consists of all neural tissue outside the CNS.

ally circulates through the entire CNS; excess is eliminated through the dural sinuses. Because the brain and spinal cord essentially float in the CSF, one of its main functions is to absorb outside forces that might otherwise be transmitted to the CNS, causing damage. The CSF also plays a role in the delivery of nutrients and elimination of waste products and also helps maintain a stable environment. Pressures in the ventricles remain fairly constant because of the absorption and elimination of CSF. However, in some situations drainage through the dural sinuses can be impeded, causing an increase in the amount of CSF in the CNS and enlargement of the ventricles. This condition, known as *hydrocephalus*, can lead to increased intracranial pressure and the risk of herniation of the brain. Treatment for this condition includes the placement of a ventriculoperitoneal shunt. This shunt is a plastic catheter that is inserted into the ventricles to drain CSF into the peritoneum.

Brainstem

[OBJECTIVE 35]

The divisions of the **brainstem** are the medulla, pons, and midbrain (Figure 7-37). The brainstem connects the brain to the spinal cord. It is responsible for many of the autonomic functions the body requires to survive (called **vegetative functions**). The **medulla** is the most inferior part of the brainstem and lies just above the foramen magnum. The foramen magnum is a large hole in the occipital bone of the skull that allows passage of the spinal cord into the spinal foramen. It is responsible for some vegetative functions and contains the cardiac center, the vasomotor center, and the respiratory center. It also has conduction pathways (tracts) of ascending (afferent, sensory) and descending (efferent, motor) nerve fibers.

The **pons** serves as a relay of both afferent and efferent nerve fibers, which transmit impulses to and from the

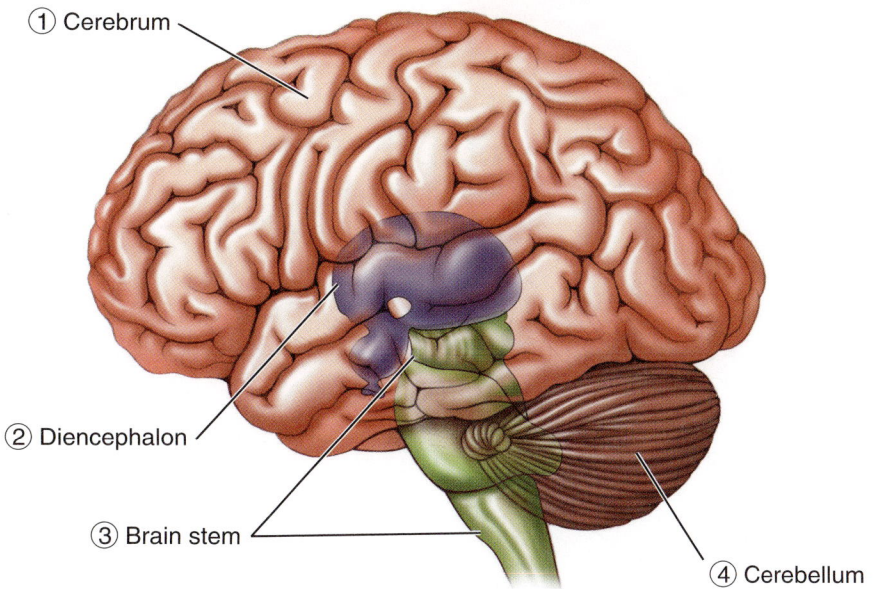

① Cerebrum

② Diencephalon

③ Brain stem

④ Cerebellum

Figure 7-35 The four primary areas of the brain are the brainstem, diencephalon, cerebrum, and cerebellum.

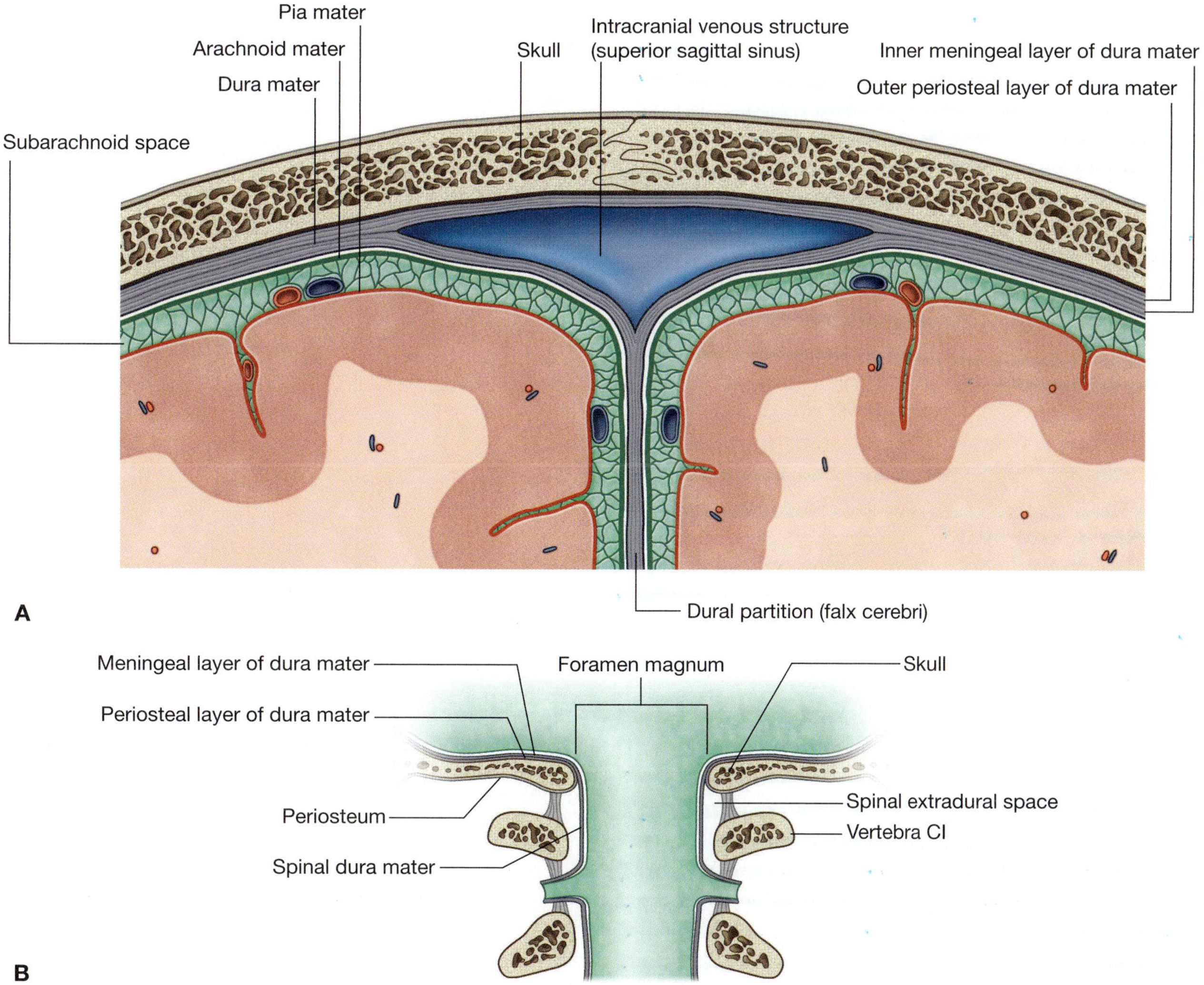

Pia mater

Arachnoid mater

Dura mater

Skull

Intracranial venous structure (superior sagittal sinus)

Inner meningeal layer of dura mater

Outer periosteal layer of dura mater

Subarachnoid space

Dural partition (falx cerebri)

A

Meningeal layer of dura mater

Foramen magnum

Skull

Periosteal layer of dura mater

Periosteum

Spinal dura mater

Spinal extradural space

Vertebra CI

B

Figure 7-36 The dura mater, arachnoid mater, and pia mater are the three layers of the meninges. **A,** Superior coronal view. **B,** Continuity with the spinal meninges.

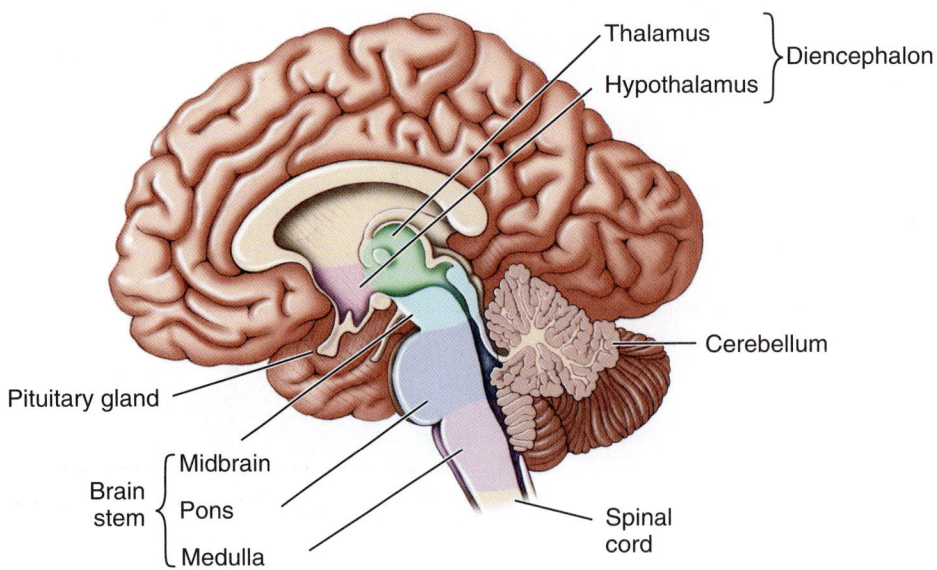

Figure 7-37 Diencephalon, brainstem, and cerebellum. The medulla, pons, and midbrain are the divisions of the brainstem.

medulla and the cerebrum. Additional fibers transmit impulses from the cerebrum to the cerebellum. The pons contains the apneustic and pneumotaxic centers that, along with the medulla, control breathing and play a role in the arousal and sleep cycles of the body.

The **midbrain** (mesencephalon) is involved in hearing and visual reflexes that allow the tracking of the eyes. The midbrain is also involved in the coordination of motor activity and muscular tone and serves as a relay for impulses from the cerebral cortex to the pons and spinal cord. The midbrain contains a group of specialized neurons (nuclei) called the **reticular activating system (RAS).** More of a network than a structure, the RAS is a mixture of gray and white matter and extends from the spinal cord into the diencephalon. The major function of the RAS is to distribute impulses to the appropriate location in the cerebral cortex, resulting in arousal. Because of this, the RAS is involved in sleep-wake cycles and allows a person to maintain consciousness. Damage to the RAS can result in a coma.

Diencephalon

[OBJECTIVE 36]

The **diencephalon** is located above the brainstem and between the cerebral hemispheres. The diencephalon is composed of the thalamus and the hypothalamus (Table 7-5). The thalamus receives and relays sensory information to the cerebral cortex. The hypothalamus plays a key role in the emotions and sexuality of the body through the limbic system. The hypothalamus also contains the temperature regulatory centers of the body, controls the pituitary gland, and is the site of integration of the nervous system and the endocrine system.

TABLE 7-5	Hypothalamic Functions
Function/regulation	**Description**
Autonomic	Regulates involuntary body functions, including the activity of the cardiac muscle, smooth muscles, and glands
Endocrine	Regulates pituitary gland secretions and affects metabolism and sexual development and functions
Emotional	Influences psychosomatic illness and stress-related conditions, fear and rage, body functions
Eating and drinking	Promotes and inhibits eating through the hunger and satiety centers, promotes drinking through thirst
Muscular	Stimulates shivering in some muscles and controls muscles responsible for swallowing
Sleep	Regulates responses to the sleep-wake cycle in coordination with other areas of the brain
Temperature	Regulates temperature through sweat to promote heat loss and shivering to promote heat generation

Cerebrum

[OBJECTIVE 37]

The **cerebrum** is the largest part of the brain. It is divided into right and left hemispheres, which are connected by a structure called the *corpus callosum*. Recall that the cerebral hemispheres are separated by a vertical projection of the dura mater called the *falx cerebri*. Each hemisphere is divided into four lobes, and each lobe has primary functions (Figure 7-38).

The **frontal lobes** are the anterior portion of the brain and play a key role in the voluntary motor function of the body as well as language production, judgment, memory, sexual behavior, socialization, spontaneity, and emotions, including aggression, motivation, impulse control, and mood. Inhibition of the frontal lobe, such as from traumatic injury or alcohol abuse, can cause alterations in these areas of function.

The **parietal lobes** are located superior and posterior in the cerebrum. They are responsible for sensation and perception and for the integration of most of the sensory information from the body, particularly with the visual system. The parietal lobes are also responsible for the ability to perform mathematical calculations and recognize and manipulate numbers as well as the processing of language and understanding speech. Damage to the parietal lobes can result in right-left confusion, difficulty with math, language disorders, the misperception of objects, the loss of voluntary control of gaze, and the inability to reach for objects accurately.

The **temporal lobes** are located inferior to the frontal and parietal lobes and superior to the cerebellum. They receive and evaluate olfactory (smell) and auditory input. The temporal lobes play a key role in memory and an integral role in abstract thought and judgment. The

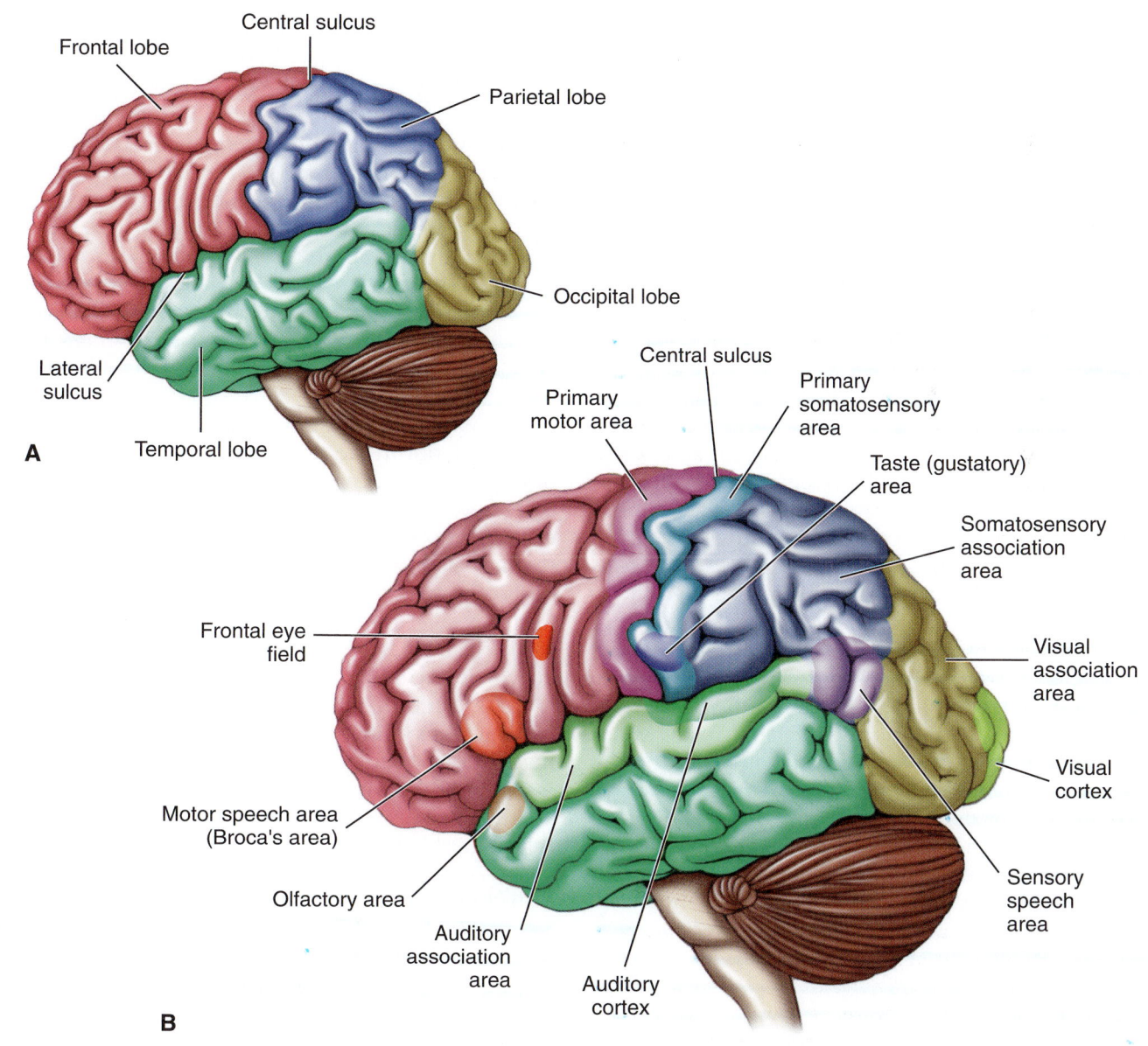

Figure 7-38 A, The lobes of the cerebrum: frontal lobe, parietal love, temporal lobe, and occipital lobe. **B,** The functional areas of the cerebrum.

left temporal lobe is associated with the memory of verbal material, whereas the right is associated with non-verbal memory such as music and art. Temporal lobe seizures tend to be complex partial seizures, meaning they do not result in a loss of consciousness, but the patient does lose awareness of his or her surroundings. Temporal lobe seizures also may result in complex repetitive behavior. Damage to the temporal lobes can result in disturbance of auditory sensation and perception, disturbance of selective attention of auditory and visual input, disorders of visual perception, impaired organization and categorization of verbal material, disturbance of language comprehension, and impaired long-term memory.

The **occipital lobe** forms the posterior section of the cerebrum and contains the center for vision. Areas of this lobe are responsible for color vision, spatial perception, and the recognition of movement. Images from the eyes travel to the occipital lobe by the optic nerves and the optic radii for interpretation. Damage to the occipital lobe can result in visual disturbances such as hallucinations, scotomas (or scotomatas), inability to perceive color, spatial and size misperceptions, and hemianopsias (or hemianopias). Be sure to note that these findings may be associated with damage outside the occipital lobe as well. Central retinal artery occlusion or damage to the retina, optic nerve, optic radii, or optic chiasm are other conditions that can cause these visual disturbances.

Cerebral Cortex

The surface of the cerebrum is composed of a layer of gray matter known as the *cerebral cortex,* which follows the contours of the cerebrum. The cerebral cortex, along with the RAS, is responsible for consciousness. Damage to either of these two structures can result in an altered level of consciousness, including coma. In addition to maintaining consciousness the cerebral cortex is responsible for the distribution of nervous impulses to the appropriate portion of the cerebrum. Three distinct areas of function of the cerebral cortex have been identified: the motor area, sensory area, and association area.

The motor area of the cerebral cortex is located in the frontal lobes (except for the anterior portion) and can be divided into two portions. Just in front of the division of the frontal lobe and parietal lobe is a small strip known as the *primary motor center,* or the *motor strip.* This area provides the impulses for precise muscular control of the voluntary muscles. Impulses from the motor strip are conducted down the spinal cord to the muscles of the body. Specific portions of the motor strip are responsible for certain areas of the body. These locations have been charted in a map known as the *homunculus.* Just anterior to the motor strip is the premotor area. The premotor area is responsible for muscular coordination after the decision to perform a certain movement has been made. As an example of how these two areas work together, imagine the decision to turn to the next page of this text. After the decision has been made, the premotor area

determines what muscles must be used and transmits that information to the motor strip. The motor strip then transmits impulses by way of the spinal cord to the specific muscles of your arm and hand, allowing you to turn the page.

The frontal lobe contains other motor areas as well. One of importance to the paramedic is Broca's area. Located in the inferior left frontal lobe just anterior to the motor cortex, Broca's area is responsible for the muscular actions associated with speech. Patients who have damage to this area, such as from a stroke, may have an expressive aphasia. Patients with this condition are able to understand what they hear and have cognitive knowledge of what they want to say, but they are unable to physically form the appropriate words.

The primary sensory area is a strip that lies just posterior to the motor strip. However, sensory areas are distributed across the cerebral cortex. These areas receive sensory stimulus from the body and interpret what they mean or what actions are needed. For example, the primary sensory area receives sensations from the skin. Other sensory areas contained in the visual cortex of the occipital lobe interpret visual stimulus. Wernicke's area is located at the junction of the temporal and parietal lobes. This is the sensory area for speech recognition and allows comprehension and understanding of speech. Broca's area and Wernicke's area are physically connected and work together to allow verbal communication. Damage to Wernicke's area can result in a receptive aphasia. Patients with this condition can form words but cannot understand what they hear. As a result, the quality of their speech is unaffected, but what they say is not appropriate to the situation.

The association areas of the cerebral cortex are located in the anterior frontal lobe as well as the lateral portions of the temporal, occipital, and parietal lobes. These areas are responsible for the analysis and interpretation of sensory information the brain receives and allow effective interaction with the environment. The association areas of the frontal lobes deal with judgment, concentration, abstract thought, and problem solving. Areas within the parietal lobes are used in the understanding of speech and choosing words to express emotions. The temporal lobe association areas interpret complex sensory information such as reading, visual memory, and the understanding of speech. The visual association area is located in the occipital lobe near the visual cortex. This provides the ability to analyze visual patterns and combine visual information with other sensory information.

Limbic System

The **limbic system** is composed of portions of the cerebrum and diencephalon. This system is involved in mood, emotions, and the sensations of fear and pleasure. Often referred to as raw emotions, the limbic system constantly generates emotional impulses filtered by the anterior portions of the frontal lobe (referred to as the conscience, or judgment). Inhibition of the frontal lobe can stop this filtering process and allow these emotions to be displayed. This may present in many ways, including aggression (verbal or physical), emotional outbursts, language choices, or behavior the individual would not normally display.

Cerebellum

[OBJECTIVE 37]

The **cerebellum** is located inferior to the occipital lobes and is involved in both fine (small muscle groups) and gross (major muscle groups) coordination. The cerebellum is responsible for interpreting actual movement and correcting any movements that interfere with coordination and body position. To accomplish this, the cerebellum receives information from the sensory and motor cortexes regarding the movement to be made. The cerebellum determines the direction, force, and duration of the movement and sends this information back to the motor cortex. The loss of function of the cerebellum often results in a lack of coordination and the inability to make fine motor movements, a condition called *cerebellar ataxia*.

Spinal Cord

[OBJECTIVE 37]

The **spinal cord** is the part of the CNS that connects the brain to the periphery of the body. It is approximately 17 to 18 inches long and is inside the foramen of the spinal vertebrae. Recall that the average spinal column is 24 to 28 inches long. This is because the spinal cord stops at approximately the level of the first or second lumbar vertebra. The terminal point of the spinal cord is called the *conus medullaris*. The nerve roots that extend beyond this point, yet are still within the spinal column, are termed the *cauda equina*, or "horse's tail." The spinal cord is composed of a central core of gray matter organized in the shape of an H. The neurons of the gray matter are surrounded by white matter containing the spinal nerve tracts. These tracts are referred to as *ascending* (afferent) *tracts*; they conduct impulses up the spinal cord to the brain, and *descending* (efferent) *tracts*, which conduct impulses from the brain to the body. These tracts are described in detail in Chapter 23. The white matter consists of a dorsal root (posterior, back) that moves afferent information and a ventral root (anterior, front) that conveys efferent motor information.

The spinal cord contains the main reflex centers of the body. These reflexes include autonomic regulation as well as stretch (arc) reflexes that allow rapid adjustments to sensory information. A stretch reflex produces a muscle contraction after it is stretched as a result of stimulation of that muscle. Tendon reflexes work in this manner. The reflexive arcs are protective mechanisms that do not require the involvement of the brain. An example of this is the patellar reflex. When the tendon is stretched, such as a collapsing knee when walking, the reflex is to straighten the knee to avoid a fall. If this process required the involvement of the brain, the fall would likely occur

before the conscious thought of straightening the knee could occur. In this example, as the tendon is stretched, impulses travel by afferent axons to the dorsal root ganglia. This impulse is then transmitted through an interneuron and directly to the anterior horn. From that point the impulse travels by efferent axons to the skeletal muscles. Reflexes are often crude movements because they do not involve the refinement of the motor cortex or the cerebellum.

Once an impulse from the brain has reached the spinal cord, it is transmitted to the spinal nerves to be transferred to the skeletal muscles. (The spinal nerves are part of the peripheral nervous system and start in the spinal cord and terminate in the skeletal muscles.) The neurons of the spinal cord are considered upper motor neurons, and the neurons of the spinal nerves are considered lower motor neurons. This concept is important for the paramedic to understand the differences in upper and lower motor neuron diseases and the differences in their physical findings. For example, when the upper motor neurons are affected, the reflexes (which depend on the lower motor neurons) become more brisk as the fine coordination of the upper motor neurons is lost. However, when the lower motor neurons are affected, the reflexes diminish. Muscle weakness without associated pain is a classic finding of any type of motor neuron disease, either upper or lower.

Peripheral Nervous System

[OBJECTIVE 38]

All communication between the CNS and the rest of the body occurs through the **PNS** (see Figure 7-34). The PNS consists of all neural tissue outside the CNS, including the cranial nerves and the spinal nerves. It is divided into two divisions: the **afferent** and **efferent** divisions. The afferent division carries information, mainly sensory, to the CNS for integration. The efferent division carries motor information away from the CNS to muscles and organs of the body. Within the efferent division are two more subdivisions: the **somatic** (voluntary) **nervous system** and the **autonomic** (automatic) **nervous system.** The somatic nervous system maintains voluntary control of body movements through the action of skeletal muscles (e.g., locomotion). In addition, it enables the reception of external stimuli, which helps keep the body in touch with its surroundings (e.g., touch, hearing, sight). The autonomic nervous system provides autonomic (unconscious) control of smooth muscles, organs, and glands within the body.

Spinal Nerves

The PNS is composed of 31 pairs of spinal nerves named for the vertebra at which they exit the spinal column. All the spinal nerves, except for the first cervical nerve (C1), exit from beneath their associated vertebrae. C1 exits between the skull and the first cervical vertebrae. Because of this, there are eight cervical nerves even though the body has only seven cervical vertebrae. The remaining number of nerves for each section of the spinal column matches the number of vertebrae in that section. The cauda equina is generally composed of the nerve roots for three pairs of lumbar nerves, five pairs of sacral nerves, and one pair of coccygeal nerves. These fibers continue down the spinal column and also exit below their respective vertebrae. Each spinal nerve (except C1) has a detailed area of cutaneous sensation. This association of the spinal nerves and the cutaneous areas covered can be seen in a dermatome map (Figure 7-39). The dermatome associations help isolate the area of a spinal cord injury. For

instance, a complete injury to the spinal cord at the fifth thoracic vertebra results in the lack of sensation below the nipple line. A spinal nerve is formed when two roots (on each side) exit the spinal column. The dorsal root contains afferent nerves that conduct impulses to the spinal cord, whereas the anterior root contains efferent nerves that conduct motor impulses to the body. These two roots join by an interneuron to form a spinal nerve that communicates with the spinal cord.

The spinal nerves combine in three areas of the body to form plexuses. These are areas of convergence and divergence where spinal nerves come together and are organized to transmit their impulses to areas of the body through a common nerve. This principle allows several spinal nerves to control one area of the body. The main plexuses in the body are the cervical plexus, the brachial plexus, and the lumbosacral plexus. Damage to these areas can result in widespread neurologic deficit because a large number of nerves will be affected.

Cranial Nerves

[OBJECTIVE 39]

The 12 cranial nerves are pairs of nerves that originate in the brainstem. The exception to this is the first pair, which originates in the cerebrum. Cranial nerves are referred to by their name or abbreviated as CN I, II, and so forth. They are divided into sensory, somatomotor, proprioception, and parasympathetic nerves (Tables 7-6 and 7-7). The sensory cranial nerves include CN I and CN II. CN V and VII also contain some sensory distribution. The somatomotor cranial nerves are CN III, IV, V, VI, VII, IX, XI, and XII. The only cranial nerve responsible for balance (proprioception) is CN VIII. CN X carries parasympathetic fibers to the body and has an important motor function in the neck and soft palate. One important characteristic of cranial nerves is that they affect the same side of the body from where they originate.

Autonomic Nervous System

[OBJECTIVE 40]

The autonomic nervous system has two branches, the **parasympathetic** and the **sympathetic nervous system,** that control the involuntary functions of the body. These two branches of the autonomic nervous system are in a constant battle with each other because they both innervate the majority of the organs in the body. In these organs, one system activates the organ and the other has an inhibitory effect. Exceptions to this include the blood vessels and sweat glands, which are exclusively under the control of the sympathetic nervous system. The parasympathetic system normally is in control of the daily functions of the body. However, in times of stress the sympathetic system takes over. This system allows the body to increase heart rate and metabolism, for example (Table 7-8). The nervous pathways of the autonomic nervous system contain two neurons. Neural fibers called *preganglionic neurons* leave the CNS and travel to a synapse within the autonomic ganglion.

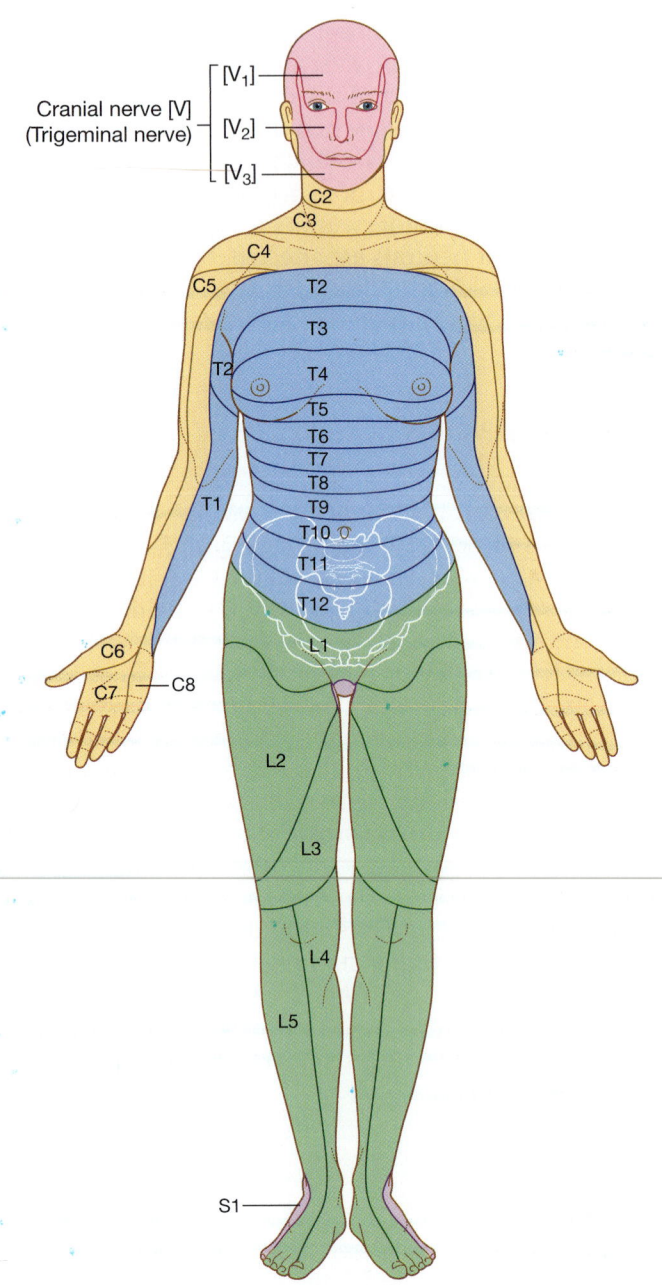

Cranial nerve [V]
(Trigeminal nerve)
[V₁]
[V₂]
[V₃]

Figure 7-39 Dermatome map showing the association of the spinal nerves and the cutaneous areas of the body.

TABLE 7-6	Cranial Nerves		
Mnemonic	**Nerve**	**Type**	**Function**
On	I, Olfactory	Sensory	Sense of smell
Old	II, Optic	Sensory	Sense of sight
Olympus	III, Oculomotor	Motor	Movement of eyeball, raising of eyelid, change in pupil size
Towering	IV, Trochlear	Motor	Movement of eyeball
Tops	V, Trigeminal	Mixed	Chewing of food; sensations in face, scalp, cornea (eye), and teeth
A	VI, Abducens	Motor	Movement of eyeball
Finn	VII, Facial	Mixed	Facial expressions; secretion of saliva and tears; taste; blinking
Viewed	VIII, Vestibulocochlear	Sensory	Sense of hearing and balance
Germans	IX, Glossopharyngeal	Mixed	Swallowing, secretion of saliva and tears, taste; part of the gag reflex
Vaulting	X, Vagus	Mixed	Visceral muscle movement and sensations, especially movement and secretion of the digestive system; sensory for reflex regulation of blood pressure
And	XI, Accessory	Mixed (mostly motor)	Head and shoulder movement
Hopping	XII, Hypoglossal	Mixed (mostly motor)	Speech and swallowing

Modified from Herlihy, B. (2007). *The human body in health and illness* (3rd ed.). St. Louis: Mosby.

The postganglionic fibers leave the autonomic ganglion and form a synapse at the organ it innervates. The length of these fibers, location of the autonomic ganglion, and neurotransmitters used depend on the specific nervous system.

Parasympathetic Nervous System. The parasympathetic nervous system is the system of primary control in nonstressful situations or when the body is recovering from a stressful situation. This system controls functions associated with digestion, rest, and slowing of the heart rate. The preganglionic fibers of the parasympathetic nervous system originate in the cranial nerves and spinal nerves exiting the sacrum, leading to the name *craniosacral system*. Preganglionic fibers are long fibers that join with autonomic ganglia near the organ that will be innervated. Short postganglionic fibers leave the autonomic ganglion and innervate the organ. The neurotransmitter acetylcholine is used at both the preganglionic synapse and the postganglionic synapse. Parasympathetic postganglionic fibers that release acetylcholine are called *cholinergic fibers*. As a paramedic, you will administer a variety of cholinergic and anticholinergic medications that affect impulse transmission of cholinergic fibers. Cholinergic receptors include nicotinic receptors and muscarinic receptors.

Sympathetic Nervous System. The sympathetic nervous system is responsible for the body's response to stress. These responses include increased heart rate, constriction of the majority of the blood vessels, dilation of the blood vessels to the skeletal muscles, pupil dilation, secretion of adrenalin, and slowing of digestion. This response often is referred to as the *fight-or-flight response*. The preganglionic fibers of the parasympathetic nervous system originate in the spinal nerves exiting thoracic and lumbar portions of the spine. The alternate name for this is the *thoracolumbar system*. Preganglionic fibers are short fibers that innervate a structure known as the *paravertebral chain*, which is a chain of autonomic ganglia near and parallel to the spinal column. The long postganglionic fibers leave the paravertebral chain and innervate their respective organs. As with the parasympathetic nervous system, the neurotransmitter acetylcholine is used at the preganglionic synapse. *Adrenergic fibers* release norepinephrine. Sympathetic postganglionic fibers release norepinephrine, except those that innervate sweat glands and some blood vessels in the skin and skeletal muscles. As with the parasympathetic nervous system, a variety of medications affect the sympathetic nervous system. Adrenergic receptors include alpha$_1$, alpha$_2$, beta$_1$, beta$_2$, and beta$_3$ receptors. Stimulation of these receptors has the following effects:

- **Alpha$_1$** receptors primarily cause vasoconstriction and cause mild bronchoconstriction.
- **Alpha$_2$** receptors generally cause smooth muscle contraction, inhibition of insulin release, induction of glucagon release, and neurotransmitter inhibition.
- **Beta$_1$** receptors are found in the heart and cause an increase in heart rate (positive

TABLE 7-7 **Cranial Nerve Lesions**

Cranial Nerve	Clinical Findings	Example of Lesion
Olfactory nerve (I)	Loss of smell (anosmia)	Injury to the cribriform plate; congenital absence
Optic nerve (II)	Blindness or visual field abnormalities, loss of papillary constriction	Direct trauma to the orbit; disruption of the optic pathway
Oculomotor nerve (III)	Dilated pupil, ptosis, eye moves down inferiorly and laterally (down and out), double vision	Pressure from an aneurysm arising from the posterior communication, posterior cerebral, or superior cerebellar artery; pressure from a herniating cerebral uncus (false localizing sign); cavernous sinus mass or thrombosis
Trochlear nerve (IV)	Inability to look inferiorly when the eye is adducted (down and in), double vision	Along the course of the nerve around the brainstem; orbital fracture
Trigeminal nerve (V)	Loss of sensation and pain in the region supplied by the three division of the nerve over the face; loss of motor function of the muscles of mastication on the side of the lesion	Typically in the region of the trigeminal ganglion, though local masses around the foramina through which the divisions pass can produce symptoms
Abducens nerve (VI)	Inability to move eye laterally, double vision	Brain lesion or cavernous sinus lesion extending onto the orbit
Facial nerve (VII)	Paralysis of facial muscles below the eye; paralysis of facial muscles	Damage to the branches within the parotid gland
	Abnormal taste sensation from the anterior two thirds of the tongue; dry conjunctivae	Injury to temporal bone; viral inflammation of nerve
	Paralysis of contralateral facial muscles below the eye	Brainstem injury
Vestibulocochlear nerve (VIII)	Progressive unilateral hearing loss and tinnitus (ringing in the ear)	Tumor at the cerebellopontine angle
Glossopharyngeal nerve (IX)	Loss of taste to the posterior third of the tongue and sensation of the soft palate	Brainstem lesion; penetrating neck injury
Vagus nerve (X)	Soft palate deviation with deviation of the uvula to the normal side; vocal cord paralysis	Brainstem lesion; penetrating neck injury
Accessory nerve (XI)	Paralysis of sternocleidomastoid and trapezius muscles	Penetrating injury to the posterior triangle of the neck
Hypoglossal nerve (XII)	Atrophy of ipsilateral muscles of the tongue and deviation toward the affected side; speech disturbance	Penetrating injury to the neck and skull base pathology

Modified from Drake, R., Vogl, W., & Mitchell, A. (2004). *Gray's anatomy for students.* New York: Churchill Livingstone.

chronotropy), strength of cardiac contraction (positive inotropy), and cardiac conduction (positive dromotropy).

- **Beta₂** receptors are found in several locations in the body. The site of primary importance to the paramedic is the lungs, where the receptors cause bronchodilation. These receptors also cause mild vasodilatation; glycogenolysis; and relaxation of the intestines, bladder, and uterus.
- **Beta₃** receptors have only recently been discovered and much remains unknown about

them. They appear to play a role in lipolysis in the adipose tissue. The clinical significance of beta₃ receptors is unknown at this time.

Some of the effects of these receptors are in opposition to each other. In a setting in which all the receptors are stimulated, the vasoconstrictive effects of the alpha₁ receptors outweigh the vasodilatation caused by the beta₂ receptors. Conversely, the bronchodilation caused by the beta₂ receptors outweighs the bronchoconstriction caused by the alpha₁ receptors.

TABLE 7-8 Autonomic Nervous System

Organ	Sympathetic Response	Parasympathetic Response
Heart	Increases rate and strength of contraction	Decreases rate; no direct effect on strength
Bronchial tubes	Dilates (increases airflow)	Constricts (reduces airflow)
Iris of eye	Dilates (pupil enlarges)	Constricts (pupil becomes smaller)
Blood vessels	Constricts	No innervation
Sweat glands	Stimulates	No innervation
Intestine	Inhibits motility	Stimulates motility and secretion
Uterus	Relaxes muscle	No effect
Adrenal medulla	Stimulates secretion of epinephrine and norepinephrine	No effect
Salivary glands	Stimulates thick secretion	Stimulates watery secretion
Urinary System		
Bladder wall	No effect	Contracts muscle
Internal sphincter	No effect	Opens sphincter

Reprinted from Herlihy, B. (2007). *The human body in health and illness (3rd ed.).* St. Louis: Mosby.

Transmission of Nervous Impulses

The transmission of nervous impulses is essentially the same process as previously described for the stimulus of muscular movement. When the cell is at its resting metabolic potential, greater concentrations of extracellular Na$^+$ and intracellular K$^+$ are available. Also in the cell is the negatively charged ion chloride (Cl$^-$). This ion results in a relative negative charge inside the cell compared with the outside. As with the muscle cell, depolarization of the nerve cell results from the opening of the Na$^+$ channels and the influx of Na$^+$ into the cell. This influx creates a positive charge inside the cell, causing an action potential inside the cell. This process creates a wave of depolarization along the nerve fiber as each cell depolarizes when stimulated by the prior neuron. Repolarization occurs as K$^+$ leaves the cell in an attempt to restore the negative charge inside the cell. Repolarization is complete when the sodium-potassium pump restores Na$^+$ and K$^+$ to their original positions. As the wave of depolarization continues, it eventually reaches the end of the nerve fiber at the synaptic gap. This may be the junction of an axon and the dendrite of another neuron or the neuromuscular junction where the nerve impulse stimulates muscular contraction. Transmission of nervous impulses across a synaptic gap depends on neurotransmitters, which were previously discussed. Neurotransmitters of the somatic nervous system include acetylcholine; neurotransmitters of the autonomic nervous system include acetylcholine and norepinephrine; and neurotransmitters of the CNS include dopamine, serotonin, and gamma-aminobutyric acid, among others. Once released from the presynaptic terminal the neurotransmitter binds with receptor sites on the postsynaptic membrane, triggering an impulse that is propagated in the manner described above. The neurotransmitters are quickly deactivated by substances such as acetylcholinesterase (which breaks down acetylcholine) and monoamine oxidase (which breaks down monoamines such as norepinephrine). After being broken down, these substances are reabsorbed by vesicles in the presynaptic terminal, where the neurotransmitters are recreated.

ENDOCRINE SYSTEM

[OBJECTIVE 41]

The endocrine system is the other controlling system of the human body. It communicates with every cell of the body through **hormones.** Hormones are chemicals that reach cells through the circulatory system. The nervous system is like a telephone system. It communicates through a complex system of hard wires. This works well for crisis management and when quick fixes or corrections are required. However, when long-term management is required, the endocrine system starts to work. The nervous system's "hard wiring" reaches only a percentage of the body. In contrast, the endocrine system and its hormones reach every cell of the body, enabling a cellular control not possible with the nervous system. This hormonal control is relatively slow compared with the control exerted by the nervous system. The two controlling systems of the body operate in parallel lines toward a common goal: homeostasis.

Hormones

Hormones are manufactured in **endocrine glands** (Figure 7-40) within the body and are released directly, without ducts, into the circulatory system. Then they travel to specific target cells, which have receptors that,

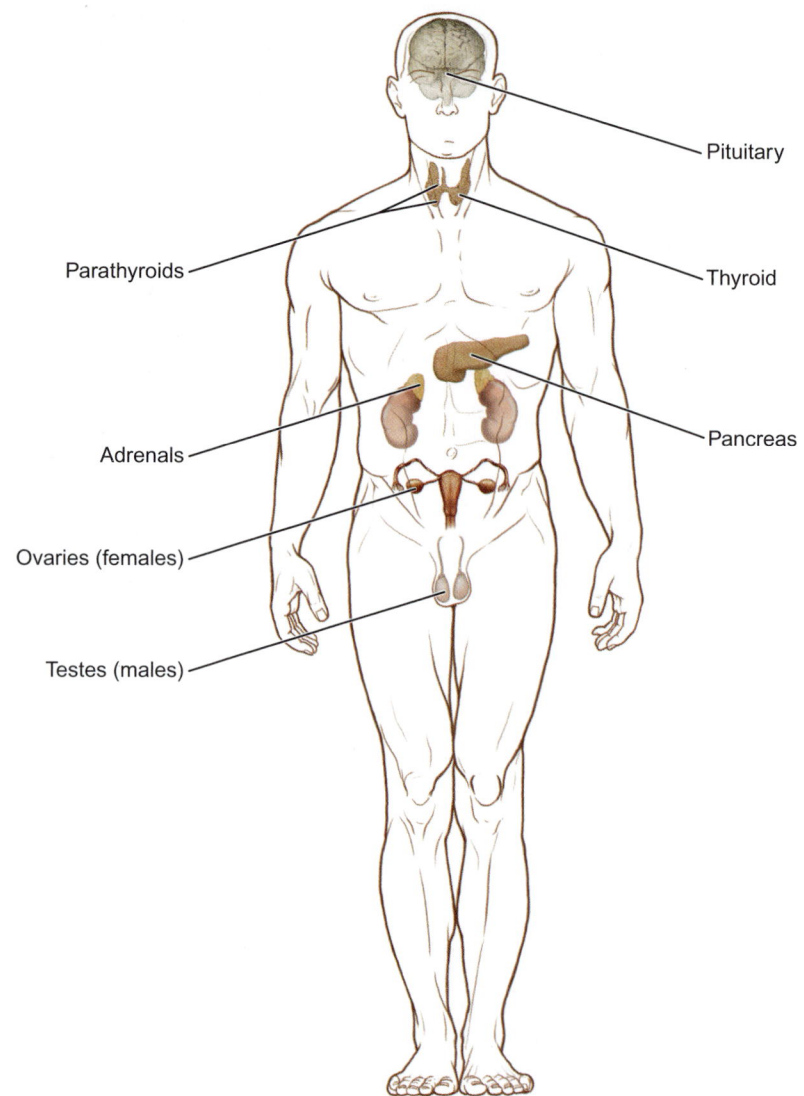

Figure 7-40 The endocrine system communicates with every cell of the body through hormones made in the endocrine glands.

when exposed to the specific hormone for which they are designed, carry out a complex set of instructions and actions. These target cells can exist anywhere in the body. Effects to an individual cell are more gradual and have a longer effect (duration) than the effects of the nervous system.

Hormones work by stimulating or altering the actions of cells. This may include increasing or decreasing cellular production, increasing or decreasing the absorption of materials by the cells, or performing any number of other alterations in cellular metabolism. They typically exert these effects through negative feedback mechanisms. In this type of system an effort is made to negate a certain action or effect in the body. In the case of the endocrine system, as hormones reach a certain level in the body other hormones are produced to stop their production; as the production of the original hormone falls, the inhibitory hormone is no longer produced, allowing the original to be produced again. For

example, gland A produces hormone X. As hormone X reaches the needed level, gland B produces hormone Y. Hormone Y inhibits gland A, reducing the production of hormone X. As levels of hormone X fall, gland B stops producing hormone Y. This allows the levels of hormone X to rise again, and the process repeats itself. Further description of feedback mechanisms can be found in Box 7-2.

The endocrine system is composed of several glands spread throughout the body that are not physically connected. Each gland is responsible for creating specific hormones that create specific responses in specific target cells. Two types of hormones are produced by the endocrine system: steroid hormones and protein hormones.

Steroid hormones are lipid soluble and can cross the cell membrane. Once inside the cell, they combine with a protein receptor to form a steroid-protein complex. This complex enters the nucleus, causing the cell to create proteins used as enzymes. An example of a steroidal med-

BOX 7-2 | Feedback Systems

Feedback systems are used by the body to maintain homeostasis. The majority of the feedback systems in the body are negative feedback systems. In this system, an effort is made by the body to negate the original stimulus. A normal example of this is the way in which hormones function, as described in the section detailing the endocrine system. The body also uses negative feedback systems to negate the effects of a harmful stimulus. For example, in the setting of compensated shock, compensatory efforts such as increased heart rate, increased respiratory rate, and vasoconstriction occur to counteract the effects of shock.

Positive feedback mechanisms are those in which an effect leads to or causes another effect. Normal positive feedback mechanisms in the body include cascade systems, such as the clotting cascade, and childbirth. Positive feedback mechanisms also can occur in harmful situations. In decompensated shock the lack of perfusion to the tissues leads to failure of the cardiac and vasomotor centers, which leads to decreased heart rate and decreased vasoconstriction. This leads to further decreases in perfusion, which further depress the body's ability to combat the shock, thereby creating a vicious cycle.

ication administered by paramedics is methylprednisolone sodium succinate (Solu-Medrol). This medication enters the cell and the enzyme created inhibits the inflammatory system.

Protein hormones are not lipid soluble and therefore are unable to cross the cell membrane. These hormones attach to receptor sites on the cell membrane. This, in turn, creates a reaction in the cell. This reaction activates a second messenger in the cell, such as cyclic adenosine monophosphate, which starts a chain of events resulting in cellular change. These may include changes in the permeability of the cellular membrane, changes in the shape of the cell, or an increase or decrease in cellular production. Insulin and epinephrine are examples of protein hormones that also may be administered as medications. Insulin binds with the cell membrane and causes an increase in the absorption of glucose, whereas epinephrine binds with alpha and beta receptors, causing vasoconstriction, bronchodilation, increased heart rate, and other effects specific to these receptors.

Hypothalamus

Recall that the hypothalamus is the site of integration between the nervous system and the endocrine system, often referred to as the *neuroendocrine system*. The primary function of the hypothalamus is in the control of the anterior pituitary gland. Hormones created by the hypothalamus can be classified as hypothalamic releasing hormones or hypothalamic inhibitory hormones. These either stimulate the anterior pituitary to create hormones or inhibit the creation of hormones by the anterior pituitary (negative feedback mechanisms). Hormones of the hypothalamus include growth hormone–releasing hormone, growth hormone–inhibiting hormone, thyrotropin-releasing hormone, corticotropin-releasing hormone, gonadotropin-releasing hormone, prolactin-releasing hormone, and prolactin-inhibiting hormone.

Endocrine Glands

The pituitary gland is located at the base of the brain, just below the optic chiasm. Two lobes compose the pituitary gland, the anterior lobe and the posterior lobe, which is connected to the hypothalamus by the pituitary stalk. The anterior lobe is made of glandular epithelial cells and is controlled by hormones released from the hypothalamus. Because the anterior lobe is not physically connected to the hypothalamus, these hormones are released into circulation and absorbed in the anterior lobe by the hypophyseal portal veins. When stimulated by the hypothalamus, the anterior lobe produces growth hormone, prolactin, thyroid-stimulating hormone, adrenocorticotropic hormone, follicle-stimulating hormone, and luteinizing hormone. These hormones are inhibited when the hypothalamus releases the appropriate inhibitory hormone. The posterior lobe releases antidiuretic hormone and oxytocin. These hormones are created in the hypothalamus and move to the posterior lobe through the pituitary stalk. There they are stored in vesicles until nervous stimulation from the hypothalamus stimulates their release.

The thyroid gland is located at the level of the thyroid cartilage and consists of two lobes, one on the right and one on the left. These lobes are connected by a band of tissue called the *isthmus*. This large gland is highly vascular and covered by a layer of connective tissue. The cells of the thyroid create secretory spheres called *follicles*. These follicles are lined with epithelial tissue that secretes the thyroid hormones and contain a fluid called *colloid*. The primary function of the thyroid is controlling metabolism. It does this through the creation of the hormones triiodothyronine (T_3) and thyroxine (T_4). The release of these hormones is controlled by the anterior pituitary gland by thyroid-stimulating hormone and ultimately by the hypothalamus by thyroid-releasing hormone. Of the hormones released by the thyroid, T_3 is the more powerful; however, much more T_4 is released. The majority of the T_4 released becomes T_3. The thyroid also produces calcitonin, which decreases calcium release from the bones and increases the excretion of calcium by the kidneys. Calcium levels in the blood are decreased in this manner.

The four parathyroid glands are found on the posterior aspects of each lobe of the thyroid gland. Parathyroid hormone is released by the parathyroid glands and causes an increase in the calcium levels in the blood by stimulating the bones to release calcium and inhibiting excretion of calcium by the kidneys.

The adrenal glands are located on top of each kidney and are composed of two layers, the outer cortex and the inner medulla. The adrenal cortex produces hormones classified as corticosteroids. These hormones are critical to life function and include the following:

- Aldosterone, a mineralocorticoid, which inhibits the excretion of sodium and enhances the excretion of potassium by the kidneys.
- Cortisol, a glucocorticoid that helps regulate glucose concentrations, stimulating other sources of energy. Cortisol also acts as an antiinflammatory agent.
- Testosterone, estrogen, and progesterone are produced in the adrenal cortex. These hormones are responsible for secondary sexual development in both sexes as well as sperm development, egg maturation, and changes associated with pregnancy.

The hormones of the adrenal medulla are epinephrine and norepinephrine, with the majority of secretions being epinephrine. These hormones are responsible for the fight-or-flight response of the sympathetic nervous system as previously described and affect alpha and beta receptors.

The pancreas is located midline in the retroperitoneal space. It is a unique organ that performs both endocrine and exocrine functions. The endocrine functions arise from specialized groups of cells called the *islets of Langerhans*. The alpha cells of the islets secrete glucagon and the beta cells secrete insulin. These two hormones work in opposition to each other to maintain glucose levels in the blood between 60 and 120 mg/dL. In the setting of increased blood glucose, parasympathetic stimulation causes the release of insulin, which promotes the movement of glucose into the cells, the storage of glucose as glycogen, and the stimulation of adipose tissue to create fat, all of which reduce the blood glucose level. Parasympathetic stimulation causes the release of insulin, and sympathetic stimulation causes the release of glucagon. In the setting of decreased blood glucose, sympathetic stimulation causes the release of glucagon, which stimulates the conversion of glycogen to glucose, thereby increasing blood glucose levels. These two hormones compose a negative feedback system; when the level of one rises, the level of the other lowers. The delta cells of the islets of Langerhans produce somatostatin, which inhibits insulin and glucagon production, decreases the motility of the digestive system, and decreases absorption and secretion in the digestive system.

The thymus gland is located in the mediastinum. This organ is large in children and shrinks in size with aging. Thymosin is produced by the thymus gland, which functions in the creation of T cells. These specialized lymphocytes function in the cell-mediated response of the immune system, which is discussed in more detail in Chapter 8.

Case Scenario—continued

As you continue your evaluation you find rapid, irregular respirations and unequal, nonreactive pupils. The patient's arms are flexed across his chest and his hands are tightly fisted. He has a large abrasion in the middle of his left chest just below the clavicle. On examining his abdomen, you find rigidity on both sides of the abdomen just below the umbilicus. When you press on the patient's pelvis, you feel instability and grinding. He has deformity and a large laceration on the lower right leg immediately above the inner ankle bone.

Questions

5. What is the best way to describe the location of the injury on the left chest?
6. What is the best way to describe the location of the rigidity in the abdomen? What organs are located here?
7. What might the instability in the pelvis indicate?
8. What is the best way to describe the location of the deformity and injury on the right leg?

CIRCULATORY SYSTEM

[OBJECTIVE 42]

The circulatory system has two parts: the cardiovascular system and the lymphatic system. The cardiovascular system is composed of many parts that operate together to move nutrients to the cells of the body and waste products away from those cells. This movement of nutrients and waste products is necessary for the cells within the body to function (recall all those little organelles [factories] within each cell). The vasculature, or vessel system, of the body extends to every cell. The vessels are responsible for bringing nutrients (oxygen, carbohydrates, proteins, and fats) to cells and transporting waste products away for elimination (e.g., carbon dioxide, nitrogen waste products). The fluid that moves within the cardiovascular system is called *blood*. Blood also plays a key role in the regulation of temperature and fluid

TABLE 7-9 Blood Cell Functions

Blood Cell	Purpose
B lymphocyte	Antibody creation
Basophil	Inflammatory response
Eosinophil	Parasite defenses
Erythrocyte	Oxygen transport
Monocyte	Immune defenses
Neutrophil	Immune defenses
Platelet	Blood clotting
T lymphocyte	Immune response (cellular)

balance in the body and helps protect the body from pathogens.

Cardiovascular System

[OBJECTIVE 43]

Following are the components of the cardiovascular system:

- **Blood** transports nutrients and waste products throughout the body.
- The **heart** works as a pump that provides the force needed to move the blood around the body.
- **Blood vessels** provide the internal piping of the body. They allow the blood to be circulated to every cell.

Blood Components

[OBJECTIVE 44]

Blood is a form of connective tissue. It consists of cells, collectively referred to as *formed elements,* and a matrix called **plasma** (Table 7-9). Although determining the exact amount of blood in the human body is difficult, estimates range between 5 and 6 L, accounting for approximately 8% of the total body weight.

Plasma. **Plasma** is a pale yellow material composed of approximately 92% water and 8% dissolved molecules. It constitutes 54% of the total blood volume. The plasma contains several plasma proteins such as albumin, globulins, prothrombin, and fibrinogen as well as dissolved electrolytes.

Albumin accounts for 60% of the plasma proteins and is responsible for the oncotic pressure in the vasculature, or the attraction of water. Microfiltration, which is described in more detail below, is the process by which oxygen, nutrients, and water leave the vasculature at the arterial side of the capillary because of hydrostatic pressure (the pressure exerted by a fluid because of its weight). However, albumin is too large to escape the vasculature and continues to the venous side of the capillary. The oncotic pressure it exerts essentially pulls water back into

the vasculature along with carbon dioxide and other cellular waste products. Albumin may be administered as an intravascular volume expander. Hydrostatic and oncotic pressure are discussed in more detail in Chapter 8.

Globulins are divided into several categories and account for 36% of the plasma proteins. The most important globulins for the paramedic to be aware of are the gamma globulins. These are produced in the lymphatic tissue and include proteins that act as antibodies in the immune system. Gamma globulins may be administered to patients to assist in the defense against infectious organisms.

Prothrombin and fibrinogen account for 4% of the plasma proteins and play an integral role in the clotting cascade (Figure 7-41). This process is described in more detail in the following section disscussing platelets.

Formed Elements. Three **formed elements,** accounting for 46% of the total blood volume, are found in the bloodstream: **erythrocytes** (red blood cells), **leukocytes** (white blood cells), and **thrombocytes,** or **platelets.** Blood cell production, or hemopoiesis, starts in the yolk sac, liver, and spleen during fetal development. After birth this production takes place exclusively in the red marrow of the bones; after the age of 4 years it is limited to the marrow cavities of the flat bones (ribs, sternum, pelvis, skull), irregular bones (the spinal column), and the proximal ends of the humerus and femur. The cells produced during hemopoiesis are termed *pluripotential hemopoietic stem cells.* These cells have the ability to differentiate into any type of blood cell the body needs at a particular time (Figure 7-42). For example, at high altitude a greater number of erythrocytes are produced, and during times of illness a greater number of leukocytes are produced.

In the presence of the hormone erythropoietin (released from the kidneys and a lesser amount from the liver), the pluripotent hemopoietic stem cells differentiate into erythrocytes. Erythrocytes account for approximately 45% of the total blood volume, and their measurement is termed the *hematocrit.* The average circulating amount of erythrocytes is between 4.2 and 6.2 million cells/mm^3. This number depends on the individual and his or her oxygen demand and is slightly higher in males than in females. An excess of erythrocytes is called *polycythemia,* and a deficiency is called *anemia.* The erythrocytes are anucleated round cells with hollowed-out centers that carry oxygen to the cells (biconcave cells). The oxygen binds to hemoglobin, an iron-containing compound, for transport, which gives these cells their red color. In addition to being anucleated, the red blood cells also do not contain mitochondria. The average lifespan of red blood cells is 120 days because they do not contain a nucleus and incur damage while they travel through the small structures of the cardiovascular system.

The leukocytes contain nuclei yet contain no coloration—hence the name *white blood cells.* They function in the inflammatory and immune systems to help the body defend against infection. These two systems are

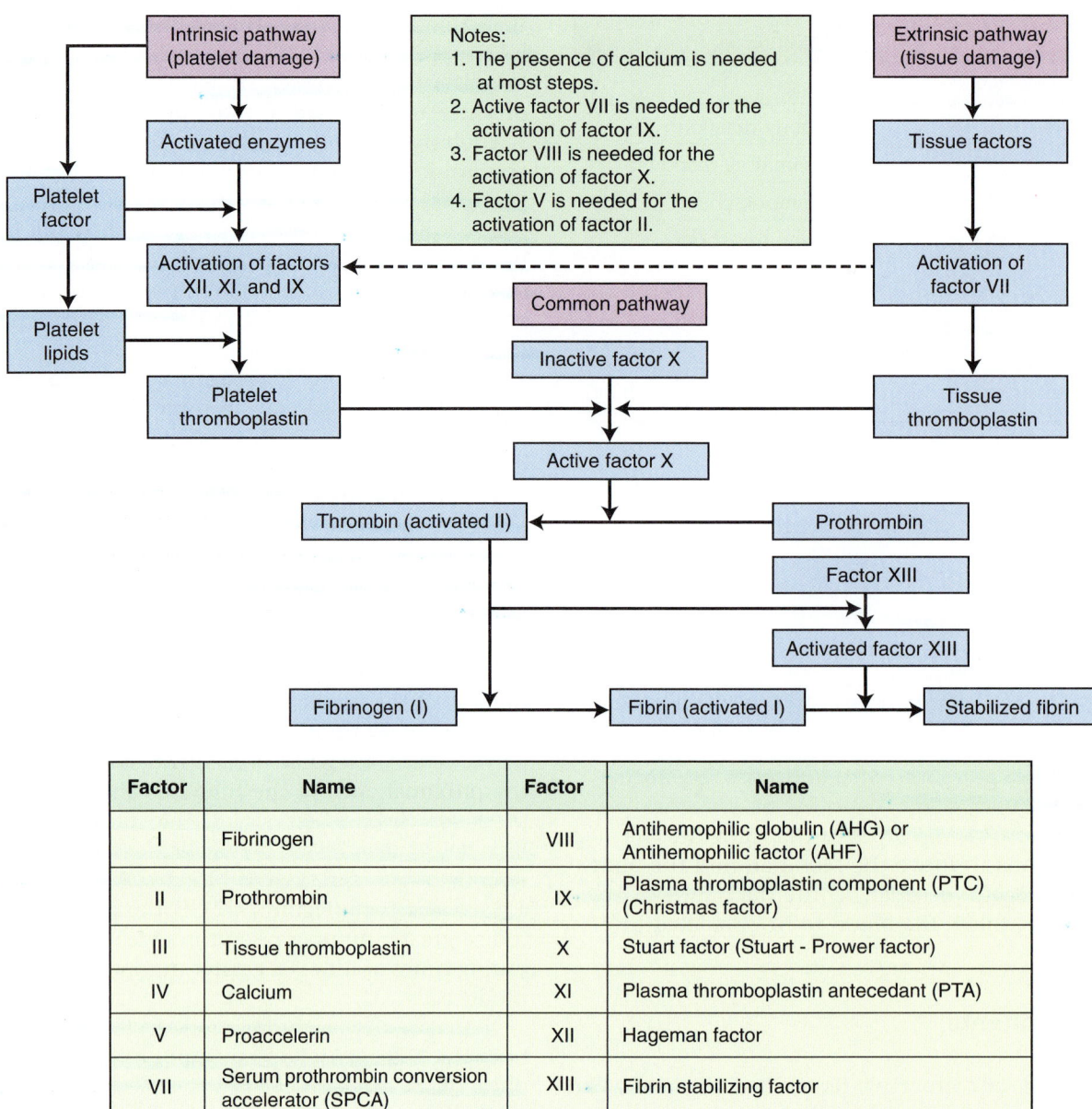

Figure 7-41 Clotting cascade.

Factor	Name	Factor	Name
I	Fibrinogen	VIII	Antihemophilic globulin (AHG) or Antihemophilic factor (AHF)
II	Prothrombin	IX	Plasma thromboplastin component (PTC) (Christmas factor)
III	Tissue thromboplastin	X	Stuart factor (Stuart - Prower factor)
IV	Calcium	XI	Plasma thromboplastin antecedant (PTA)
V	Proaccelerin	XII	Hageman factor
VII	Serum prothrombin conversion accelerator (SPCA)	XIII	Fibrin stabilizing factor

explained in detail in Chapter 8. Leukocytes along with the platelets, account for 1% of the total blood volume and are present in various amounts in circulating blood. The total white blood cell count averages between 5000 and 10,000 cells/mm³ in a healthy person and is elevated during an inflammatory and/or immune response. *Leukopenia* refers to abnormally low white blood cell counts; *leukocytosis* refers to abnormally high white blood cell counts.

Neutrophils account for 54% to 62% of the circulating leukocytes. They are the first cells to respond to an infection and leave the vasculature by a process called *diapedesis*. The primary function of neutrophils is phagocytosis, or the ingestion of foreign particles. These cells contain a large amount of lysosomes, which then destroy the ingested matter. Another function of the neutrophils is

the release of macrophage-stimulating factor, which causes monocytes to develop into macrophages.

Monocytes account for 3% to 9% of the circulating leukocytes. When stimulated by macrophage-stimulating factor, monocytes develop into macrophages. Macrophages are large phagocytic leukocytes capable of ingesting much larger particles than the neutrophils. As with the neutrophils, they leave the vasculature by diapedesis and contain a large amount of lysosomes for destroying ingested particles. Another function of macrophages is to act as antigen-presenting cells. After digesting an invading organism, the macrophages then present parts of the invading organism on their cell membranes (antigen presenting cells) and simultaneously release a cytokine (chemical messenger) called *interleukin-1* that attracts the helper T cell. The interaction of the antigen-presenting

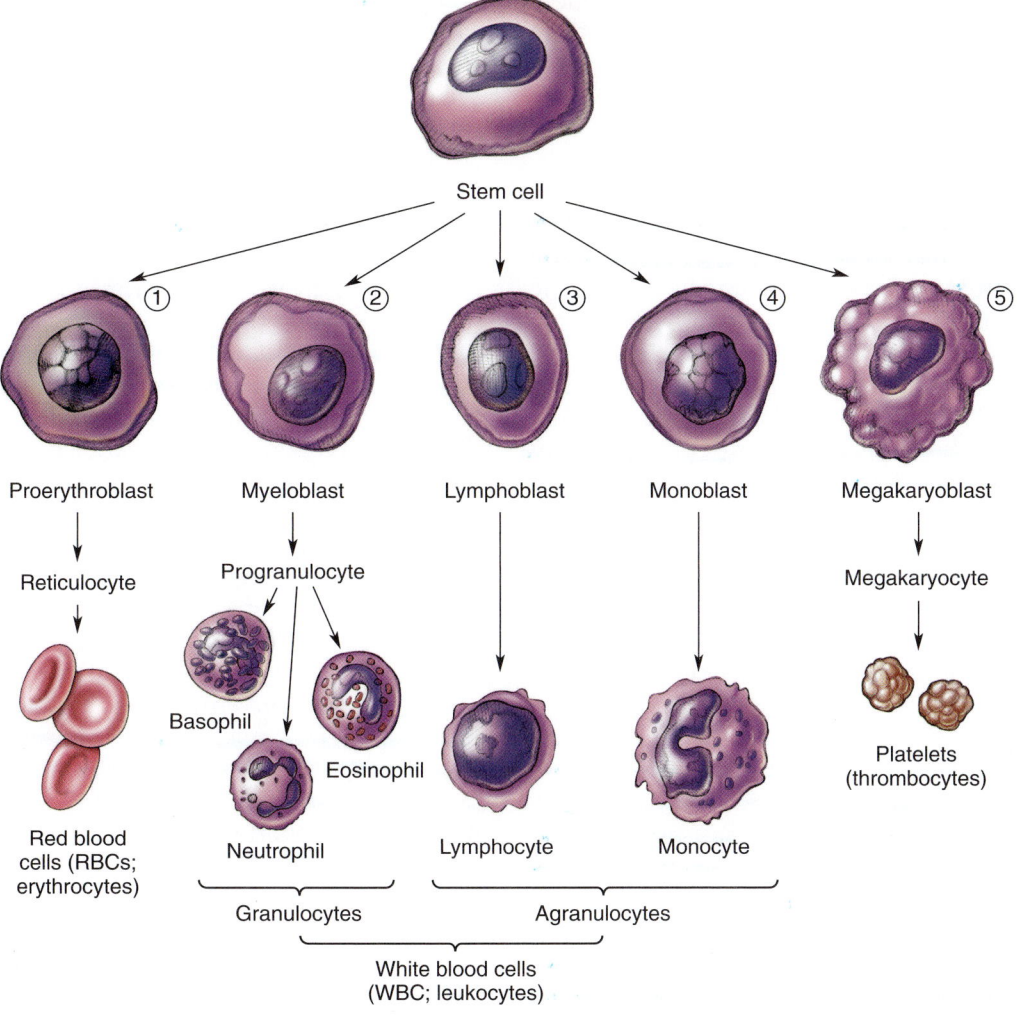

Figure 7-42 Lines of cell differentiation.

cell and the helper T cell stimulates the immune response, which is described in Chapter 8.

Eosinophils account for 1% to 3% of the circulating leukocytes and are mildly phagocytic. The primary function of these cells is a chemical attack on parasites. These cells also control inflammation and allergic reactions by producing antihistamines.

Basophils account for less than 1% of the circulating leukocytes and are involved in allergic reactions. When activated they release histamine, serotonin, and heparin.

Lymphocytes account for 25% to 33% of circulating leukocytes. Lymphocytes are divided into T cells and B cells and are responsible for the immune response. T cells directly attack invading organisms, whereas B cells produce plasma cells, which then produce antibodies (see Chapter 8).

Platelets, or thrombocytes, are responsible for a positive feedback mechanism known as the *clotting cascade* or *coagulation cascade*. The normal platelet count has a wide range of 130,000 to 360,000 per mm³. When the platelets encounter a break in the vasculature, they begin to clump together in an attempt to stop the escape of blood. The

clotting cascade results from the interaction of 12 clotting factors and calcium. The extrinsic pathway is the result of damage to the tissues, which then release clotting factors. These factors react with other clotting factors and calcium with the final product being tissue thromboplastin. The intrinsic pathway is the result of damaged platelets releasing clotting factors. These factors also react with other clotting factors and calcium, with the final product being platelet thromboplastin. These two pathways occur simultaneously. Both tissue thromboplastin and platelet thromboplastin join together at the common pathway, where they convert inactive factor X to active factor X. Active factor X converts prothrombin to thrombin, which converts *fibrinogen* to insoluble fibrin. The long, interwoven fibrin fibers, or fibrin mesh, create what is known as a clot. The paramedic must understand the steps of the common pathway to understand many of the causes of hemophilia and the actions of anticoagulants (medications that inhibit the clotting mechanism). The dissolving of a clot is known as *fibrinolysis*. This occurs naturally in the body after the damaged tissue is repaired and plasma proteins dissolve the fibrin fibers of the clot. The paramedic may administer fibrinolytic medications, such as tissue plasminogen activator, to dissolve clots that occur in the coronary arteries during a myocardial infarction.

Heart
[OBJECTIVE 45]

The heart is a pump that consists of four chambers: two receiving chambers called **atria** and two pumping chambers called **ventricles.** Located in the mediastinum, the heart is approximately 3.5 inches wide, 5 inches long, and 2.5 inches thick—approximately the size of the body's fist. The heart lies behind and slightly to the left of the sternum and just superior to the diaphragm (Figure 7-43). The tip of the heart is called the **apex,** and the top of the heart is called its **base.** The base lies at approximately the area of the second intercostal space, and the apex (bottom) lies at approximately the fifth intercostal space along the midclavicular line. The apex of the heart creates the point of maximal impulse, which may be palpable through the chest wall. An abnormally located point of maximal impulse may indicate a change in the size of the heart or displacement of the heart.

The heart is enclosed by a two-layered serous membrane. The outermost layer is a fibrous, nondistensible sac called the *fibrous pericardium,* which is attached by ligaments to the sternum, diaphragm, and spinal column. The fibrous pericardium surrounds a two-layered serous membrane called the *pericardium.* The inner layer of the pericardium is divided into two additional layers. The innermost of these two is a thin membrane called the *visceral pericardium,* which is attached to the outer layer of the heart (the epicardium) itself at the apex. The outer layer is called the *parietal pericardium,* which forms the inner layer of the fibrous pericardium. The space between the visceral and parietal pericardium is called the *pericardial cavity* and contains a small amount of serous fluid called pericardial fluid. This fluid reduces friction between the layers caused by the motion of the heart. An abnormal accumulation of fluid in this space can create pressure on the heart, reducing cardiac output.

Three distinct layers compose the walls of the heart. The innermost layer, the endocardium, is made of epithelial and connective tissue. This surface is quite smooth so as not to disrupt blood flow or platelets as they pass through the heart. This lining is continuous with the innermost lining of the blood vessels of the body. The middle layer of the heart, the myocardium, is the thickest layer of the heart and consists of cardiac muscle. This layer is responsible for cardiac contraction and efficient ejection of blood from the heart. The myocardium has a large capillary supply to meet the oxygen demands of the heart; in fact, most areas of the myocardium have a 1:1 ratio of capillaries to muscle cells. The thickness of the myocardium varies depending on the workload of the chamber. The atria have a thin myocardial layer, and the ventricles have a much thicker layer. The left ventricle has the thickest myocardial layer because it must pump blood to the entire body. The outermost layer of the heart is the epicardium. This layer functions as a protective layer and consists of epithelial tissue, connective tissue, and fat. The epicardium is the first entry point of the coronary arteries and receives oxygenated blood before the arteries continue into the myocardium. This layer also contains capillaries, components of the lymphatic system, and nerves.

Cardiac Muscle
[OBJECTIVE 46]

As previously described, cardiac muscle is unique to the heart. However, like other muscles, contraction occurs when calcium interferes with troponin and tropomyosin,

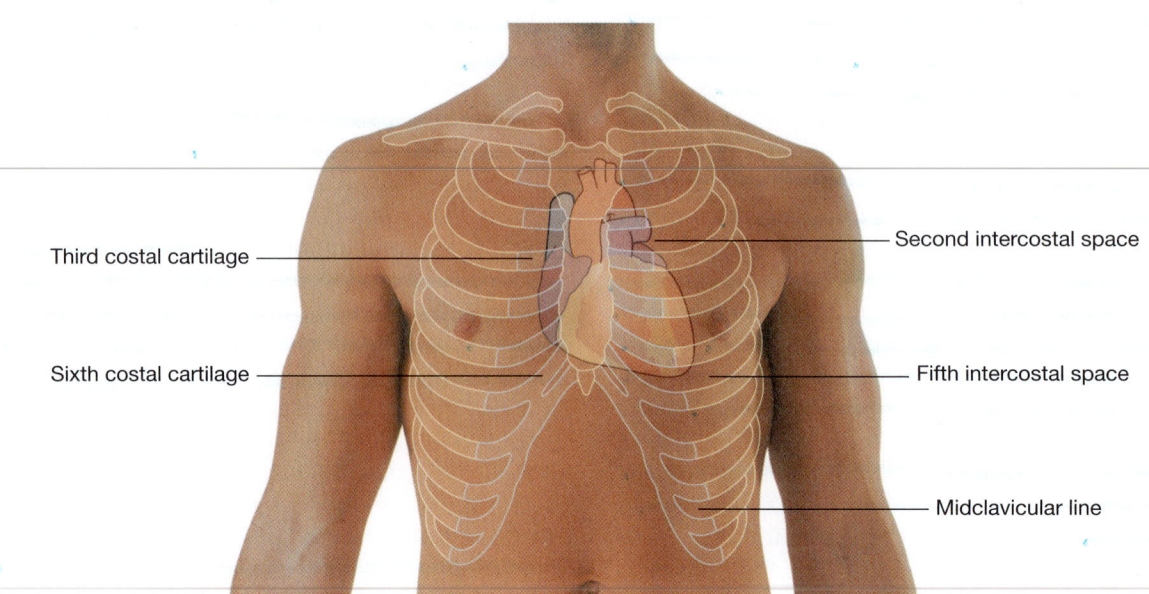

Third costal cartilage

Sixth costal cartilage

Second intercostal space

Fifth intercostal space

Midclavicular line

Figure 7-43 The heart lies in the mediastinum, slightly left of the sternum.

allowing the actin and myosin fibers to create cross links that pull against each other to shorten, or contract. (Refer to the section on muscles in this chapter for further information regarding this process and the role of electrolytes.)

Cardiac muscle shares many properties with other muscle, but it does have unique properties. Troponin is common to all muscles, but the presence of cardiac troponin within the bloodstream is indicative of a myocardial infarction. Although this test was previously possible only in the hospital, it can now be done by paramedics in the prehospital setting. Cardiac muscle fibers are long branching cells that fit together tightly at junctions called *intercalated disks*. The arrangement of these tight-fitting junctions gives an appearance of a syncytium, that is, resembling a network of cells with no separation between the individual cells. The intercalated disks fit together in such a way that they form gap junctions. Gap junctions allow cells to communicate with each other; they function as electrical connections and permit the exchange of nutrients, metabolites, ions, and small molecules. As a result, an electrical impulse can be quickly conducted throughout the wall of a heart chamber. This characteristic allows the walls of both atria (likewise, the walls of both ventricles) to contract almost at the same time. The heart consists of two syncytiums: atrial and ventricular. The *atrial syncytium* consists of the walls of the right and left atria. The *ventricular syncytium* consists of the walls of the right and left ventricles.

One final unique property of cardiac muscle is referred to as the *Frank-Starling mechanism,* or Starling's law of the heart. This law states that, within physiologic limits, the greater the stretch of the cardiac muscle, the greater the resulting contraction. Because of this relationship, an increase in preload (the amount of blood returning to the right atrium) will cause an increase in the forcefulness of the next ventricular contraction because the muscle fibers were stretched further, resulting in a stronger contraction.

Cardiac Output

[OBJECTIVE 47]

Cardiac output (CO) is defined as the amount of blood the heart ejects each minute. This is a function of both the stroke volume (SV) and the heart rate (HR), which is mathematically expressed as $CO = SV \times HR$.

The SV is the amount of blood ejected with each contraction and is a function of the end-diastolic volume (EDV) and end-systolic volume (ESV). This can be mathematically expressed as $SV = EDV - ESV$. At the end of **diastole** the amount of blood contained in the ventricles (EDV) ranges from 110 to 120 mL, whereas at the end of **systole** the amount of blood in the ventricles (ESV) ranges from 40 to 50 mL. This results in a SV of 60 to 80 mL while at rest. The ESV compared with the EDV, or percentage of blood ejected with each contraction, is the ejection fraction (EF). The mathematical expression of this is $EF = SV/EDV$. The normal EF is greater than 50%; an EF of less than 40% is impaired. When an increase in blood flow is needed, such as exercise or stressful situations, an increase in preload can increase the EDV to 150 to 180 mL. Because of Starling's law, this increase in stretch will increase the force of contraction, and ESV can decrease to 10 to 20 mL. This ability allows the heart to have an SV range of 60 to 170 mL when needed.

The heart rate is calculated as the number of contractions of the heart per minute. This generally is expressed as *beats per minute* or *bpm*. The normal heart rate is 60 to 100 beats/min. Cardiac output can be calculated with the above formulas and concepts. For example, assuming cardiac output is 70 mL and the HR is 80 beats/min, cardiac output would be 70 mL × 80 beats/min, or 5600 mL/min (5.6 L/min). Normal cardiac output ranges between 4 and 8 L/min; however, this can range widely depending on the patient's needs. Maximum cardiac output of the average person is 13 L/min. With external stimulus, or in the case of well-conditioned athletes, this can increase to a maximum of 30 L/min. The following factors affect cardiac output:

- An increase in SV without a change in HR will increase cardiac output.
- A decrease in SV without a change in HR will decrease cardiac output.
- An increase in HR without a change in SV will increase cardiac output.
- A decrease in HR without a change in SV will decrease cardiac output.
- An increase in both SV and HR will increase cardiac output.
- A decrease in both SV and HR will decrease cardiac output.

When both SV and HR are altered, the resulting change in cardiac output may not be so obvious. For example, if the SV increases but the HR decreases, cardiac output may decrease, increase, or not change. Along the same lines, a decrease in SV and an increase in HR may result in a decrease, increase, or no change in CO. The degree of change in cardiac output, if any, depends on how much SV and HR change.

The final concept that must be appreciated is the effect of HR on SV. As HR increases, the length of both systole and diastole shorten, which results in decreased ventricular filling time and therefore a decrease in SV. In the average person the maximum effective heart rate is 150 to 180 beats/min. Rates above this result in such a small SV that cardiac output drops despite the increased HR. By the same token, an extremely slow HR will cause cardiac output to decrease despite an increase in SV. With all the above principles in play, the paramedic must always evaluate the effectiveness of the cardiac output of each individual patient.

Blood Pressure. One method of evaluating the effectiveness of cardiac output is the measure of blood pressure (BP). This finding reflects the mechanical function of the heart and measures the pressures exerted on the vascular walls during both systole and diastole. BP is a function of CO and peripheral vascular resistance (PVR) and is mathematically expressed by the formula $BP = CO \times PVR$. The following factors affect blood pressure:

- A decrease in cardiac output without a change in PVR will decrease BP.
- An increase in cardiac output without a change in PVR will increase BP.
- A decrease in PVR without a change in cardiac output will decrease BP.
- An increase in PVR without a change in cardiac output will increase BP.
- A decrease in both cardiac output and PVR will decrease BP.
- An increase in both cardiac output and PVR will increase BP.

As with cardiac output, when both factors are changing in different directions, the results may not be as predictable. For example, the cardiac output will increase (primarily by an increase in HR) in the setting of a decreased PVR in an attempt to maintain BP. This may result in no change, an increase, or a decrease in BP. Conversely, PVR will increase in an attempt to maintain BP if the cardiac output decreases. This may or may not be effective. Again, the paramedic must evaluate each patient individually to determine the effectiveness of the cardiovascular system. *Afterload* is the term used to describe the pressures the heart must pump blood against to perfuse the organs. Afterload is a function of BP.

Great Vessels
[OBJECTIVE 48]

The large vessels that carry blood to the heart include the **superior** and **inferior venae cavae** (vessels that return venous blood from the upper and lower parts of the body to the right atrium), and the **pulmonary veins** (vessels that return oxygenated blood from the lungs to the left atrium). The large vessels that carry blood away from the heart include the **aorta** (which delivers blood from the left ventricle to the body) and the **pulmonary trunk**, or **pulmonary arteries** (which deliver unoxygenated blood from the right ventricle to the lungs) (Figure 7-44). Although not a large vessel, the coronary sinus returns blood from the coronary circulation to the right atrium.

Heart Chambers and Valves
[OBJECTIVE 49]

The heart is divided into right and left halves by a tough piece of tissue called the **septum.** The septum dividing the atria is called the **interatrial septum.** The septum dividing the ventricles is the **interventricular septum.**

The valves separating the atria and ventricles are called the *atrioventricular* (AV) *valves* (Figure 7-45). The right AV valve is called the **tricuspid valve,** and the left AV valve is called the **bicuspid valve,** or the **mitral valve.** These valves direct the flow of blood between the chambers. They also prevent backward flow during ventricular

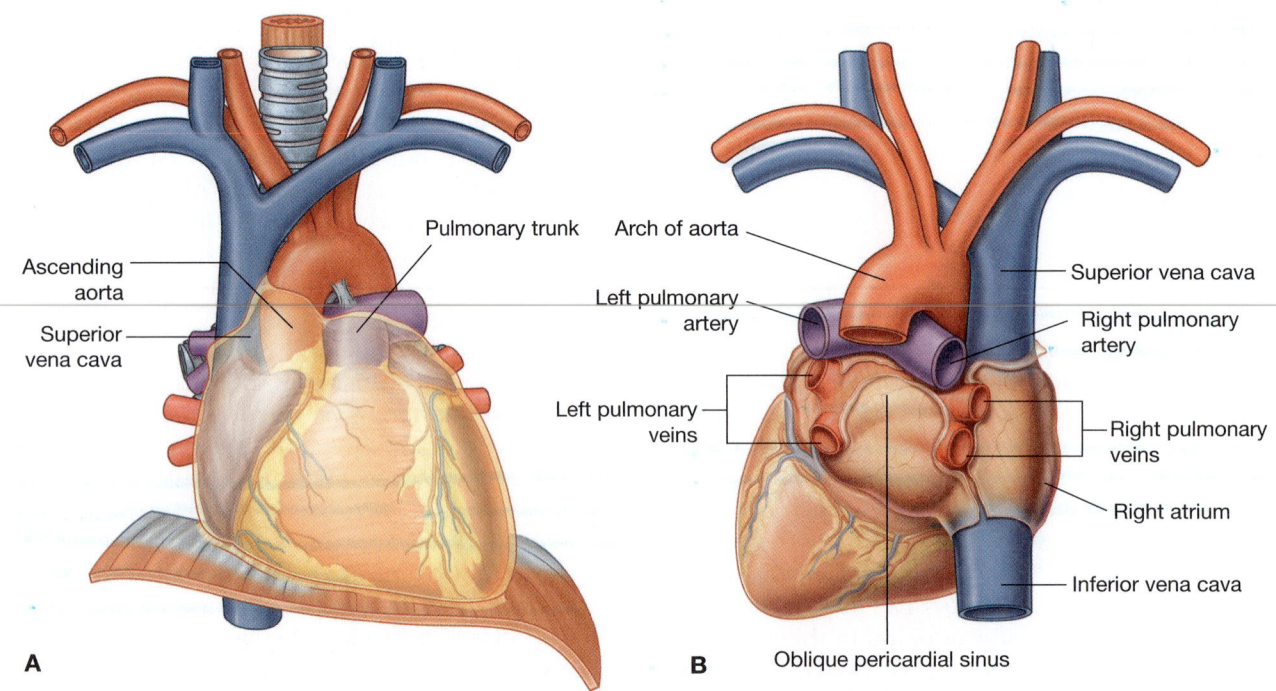

Ascending aorta

Superior vena cava

Pulmonary trunk

A

Arch of aorta

Left pulmonary artery

Left pulmonary veins

Superior vena cava

Right pulmonary artery

Right pulmonary veins

Right atrium

Inferior vena cava

Oblique pericardial sinus

B

Figure 7-44 The great vessels carry blood to and from the heart. **A,** Anterior view. **B,** Posterior view.

contraction (called **regurgitation**). The valves have fibrous bands of tissue called **chordae tendineae** attached to each part, or cusp, of the valve. Attached to the chordae tendineae and the endocardium of the ventricles are **papillary muscles.** During ventricular systole the AV valves are closed because of the increase in pressure in the chamber. The papillary muscles also contract during ventricular systole, providing counterpressure to the cusps of the AV valves. This pressure prevents the AV valves from "blowing out" or being forced open into the atria. During ventricular diastole, the ventricles and the papillary muscle relax and the AV valves open by the force of blood flowing downward from the atria to the ventricles. Closure of these valves creates the S1 heart tone. The valves separating the ventricles and their associated great vessel are called the **semilunar valves.** These valves each have three cusps. The right semilunar valve is called the **pulmonic valve.** It separates the right ventricle and the pulmonary trunk. The semilunar valve on the left is the **aortic valve.** This valve separates the left ventricle from the aorta. These valves have no tendon or muscular support. Moreover, they function only by the relative pressure differences between the ventricles and great vessels they separate. When the ventricle contracts, the pressure in the ventricle exceeds the pressure in the trunk; therefore the valve opens, allowing blood to enter the great vessel. When the pressure in the great vessel exceeds the ventricle's pressure, the valve closes. Closure of these valves creates the S2 heart tone.

Blood Flow through the Heart and Pulmonary Circulation
[OBJECTIVE 50]

Blood enters the right atrium by way of the superior and inferior venae cavae and the **coronary sinus** (the venous drain for the coronary circulation) (Figure 7-46). This blood, approximately 70% to 80%, enters the right ven-

tricle through the tricuspid valve passively. The remaining 20% to 30% is forced into the right ventricle during atrial contraction (this is called the **atrial kick**). Upon ventricular contraction the blood moves from the right ventricle into the pulmonary circuit for oxygenation through the pulmonic valve, and into the pulmonary trunk. This is called **pulmonary circulation.** The blood becomes oxygenated and then is delivered through the pulmonary veins to the left atrium. Again, approximately 70% to 80% of the blood moves passively into the left ventricle through the mitral valve. The remaining 20% to 30% of the blood is forced into the ventricle through the atrial kick. The blood is then ejected from the left ventricle, through the aortic valve, and into the aorta for systemic distribution. The heart can be thought of as a two-sided pump, with the low-pressure right side being responsible for pulmonic circulation and the high-pressure left side being responsible for systemic circulation. However, the paramedic must realize that the atria function together and the ventricles function together because of the presence of the atrial syncytium and ventricular syncytium previously described. As both atria undergo systole the ventricles are in diastole; conversely, as both ventricles undergo systole the atria are in diastole.

Coronary Circulation
[OBJECTIVE 51]

At the base of the aortic valve is the inlet to the coronary arteries. These arteries are the first vessels that receive blood after left ventricular contraction; they fill during ventricular diastole and are compressed during systole. No valve is between the coronary vessels and the aorta, and although these are the first vessels filled, coronary circulation depends on pressures within the aorta and in the thoracic cavity. The coronary circulation is divided

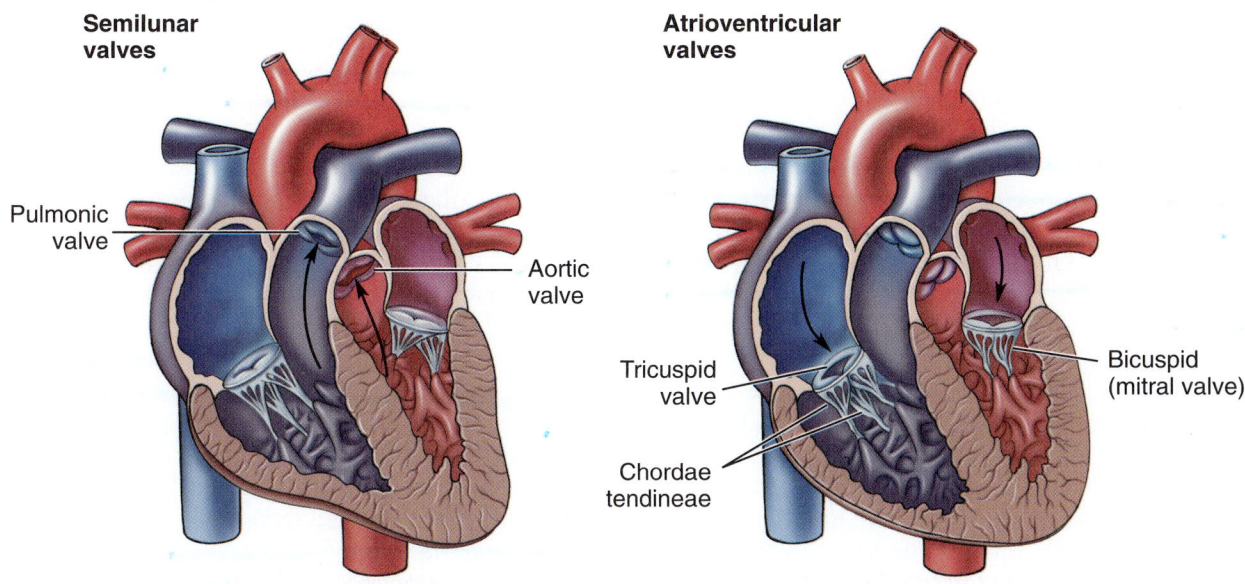

Figure 7-45 Blood is circulated through the chambers and valves of the heart.

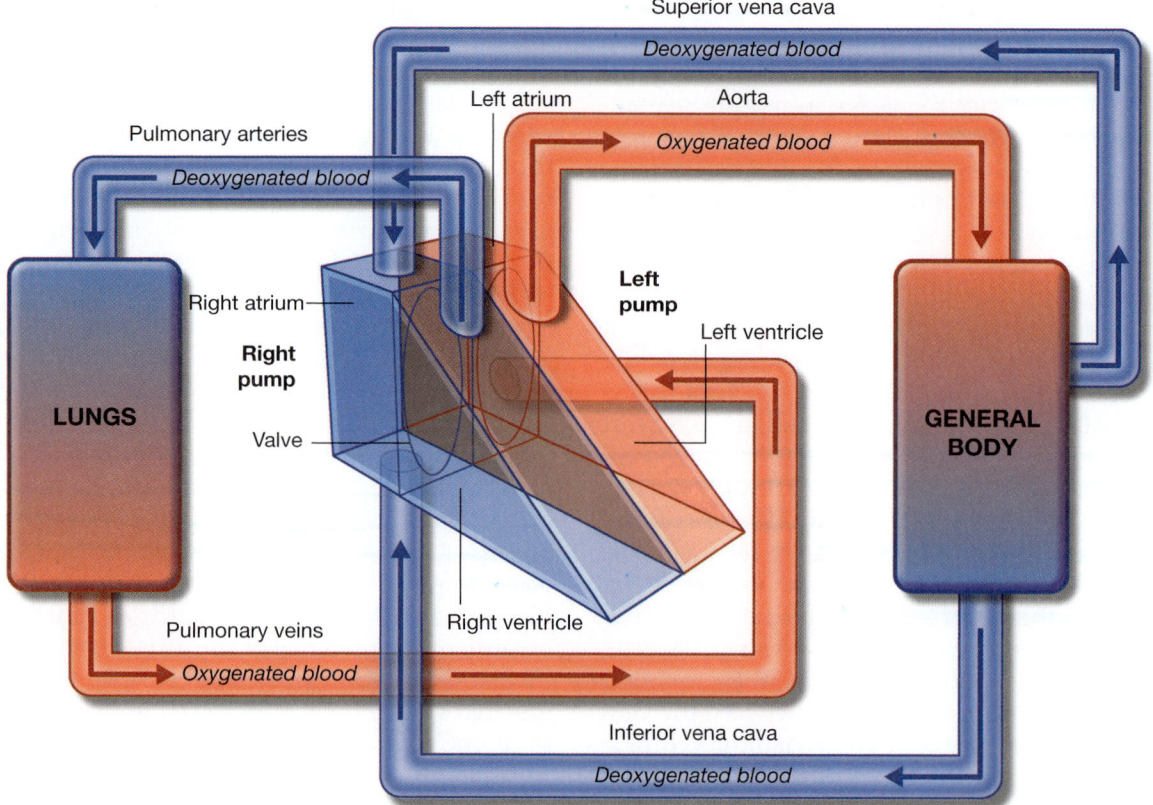

Figure 7-46 Blood flows through the heart and pulmonary circulation.

into the **right coronary artery** and **left coronary artery** (Figure 7-47). The left coronary artery further divides into the anterior descending artery and the circumflex artery. These coronary arteries then continue to bifurcate (divide) into smaller and smaller branches, feeding every area of the heart with blood supply. As previously mentioned, venous blood from the coronary circulation is drained directly into the right atrium through the main coronary sinus.

Cardiac Action Potential
[OBJECTIVE 52]

As previously discussed, for an electrical stimulus to be conducted cells must create an action potential. The heart contains two types of cells—pacemaker cells, which are capable of producing their own impulse or action potential (a property called *automaticity* that is unique to cardiac pacemaker cells), and myocardial cells, which respond to impulses from the pacemaker cells by contracting.

Myocardial working cells are considered to be polarized when they are at their resting membrane potential. Recall that this potential is the result of the imbalance of charges on the outside and inside of the cell from the distribution of Na^+ and K^+, respectively. While at rest the inside of the myocardial working cell has a charge of −90 mV compared with the outside of the cell. This is partly because of the large concentration of Na^+ outside the cell and the concentration of K^+ inside the cell. In addition, the slow leakage of K^+ out of the cell, and the inability of negatively charged ions such as phosphate to leave the cell, contributes to this imbalance of charges. In this state the cell is ready to be stimulated. The process of depolarization and repolarization of the myocardial cells occur in five stages, as shown in Figure 7-48.

Phase 0: Depolarization. The rapid entry of Na^+ into the cell is largely responsible for phase 0 of the cardiac action potential. Phase 0 represents depolarization and is called the rapid depolarization phase. Phase 0 also is called the *upstroke, spike,* or *overshoot.* Phase 0 begins when the cell receives an impulse. Na^+ moves rapidly into the cell through the Na^+ channels. K^+ leaves the cell and Ca^{++} slowly moves into the cell through Ca^{++} channels. The cell depolarizes and cardiac contraction begins. Phase 0 is represented on the electrocardiogram by the QRS complex. The cells of the atria, ventricles, and the Purkinje fibers of the conduction system have many sodium channels. The sinoatrial and AV nodes of the heart have relatively few sodium channels. If the flow of Na^+ through the Na^+ channels is slowed or blocked, the heart rate slows, the cells become less excitable, and the speed of conduction decreases. Phase 0 of the cardiac action potential is immediately followed by repolarization. Repolarization is divided into three phases.

Phase 1: Early Repolarization. During phase 1 of the cardiac action potential, the Na^+ channels partially close, slowing the flow of Na^+ into the cell. At the same

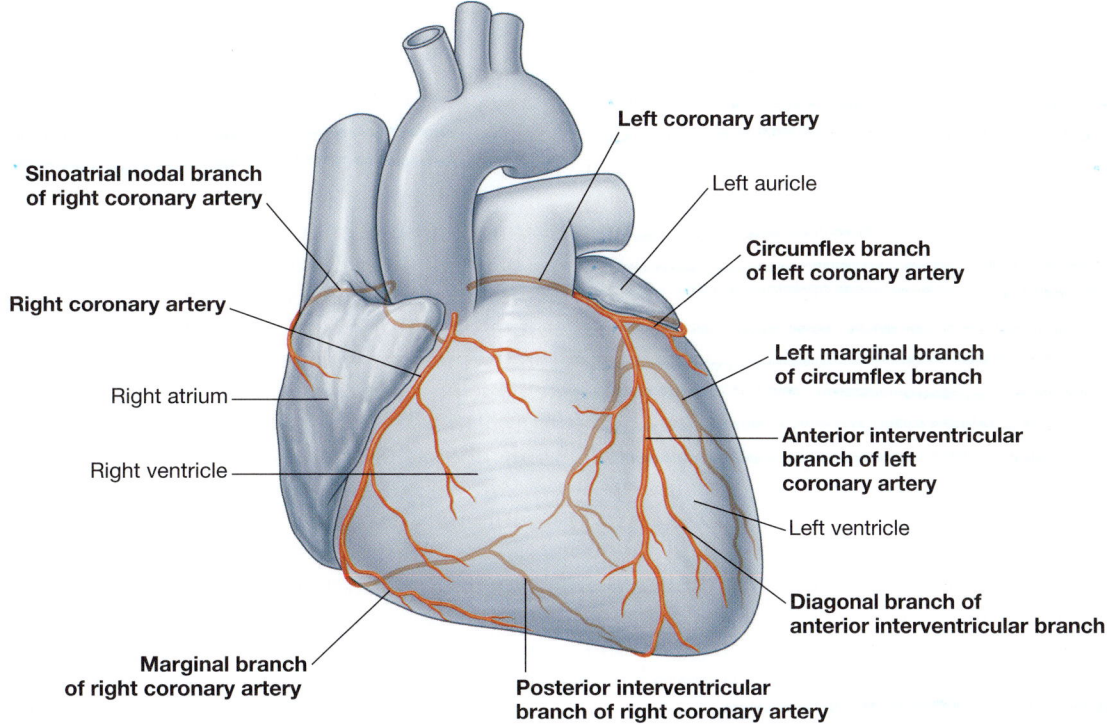

Figure 7-47 Blood oxygenates the heart through the coronary circulation.

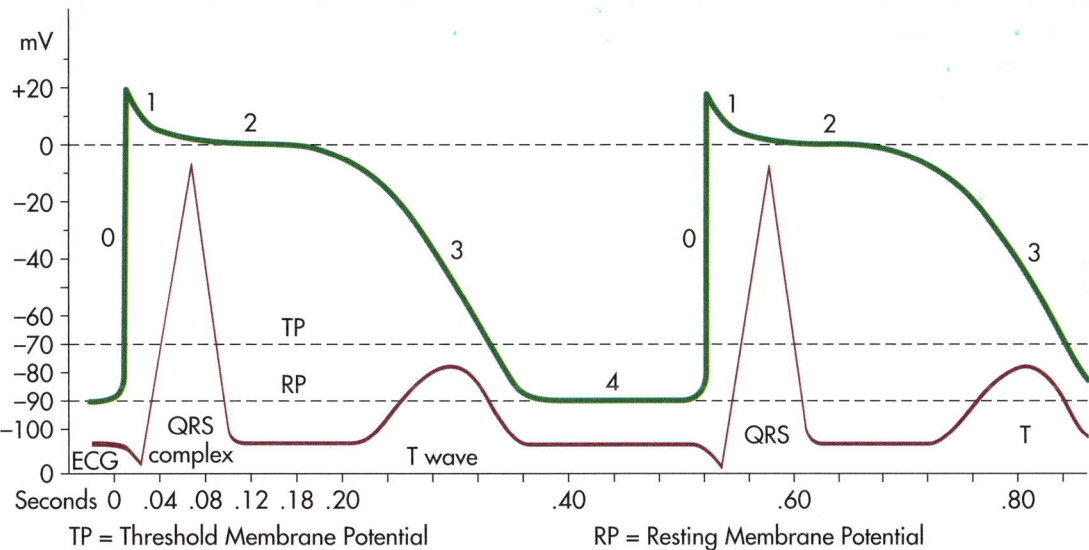

Figure 7-48 Myocardial action potential.

time, Cl⁻ enters the cell and K⁺ leaves it through K⁺ channels. The result is a decrease in the number of positive electrical charges within the cell. This produces a small negative deflection in the action potential.

Phase 2: Plateau Phase. Phase 2 is the plateau phase of the action potential. During this phase, Ca^{++} slowly enters the cell through Ca^{++} channels. The cells of the atria, ventricles, and the Purkinje fibers of the conduction system have many Ca^{++} channels. K⁺ continues to leave the cell slowly through K⁺ channels. The plateau phase allows cardiac muscle to sustain an increased period

of contraction. The cells of the atria, ventricles, and Purkinje fibers spend less time in phase 2 if the flow of Ca^{++} through Ca^{++} channels is slowed or blocked. Phase 2 is responsible for the ST segment on the electrocardiogram. The ST segment reflects the early part of repolarization of the right and left ventricles.

Phase 3: Final Rapid Repolarization. Phase 3 begins with the downslope of the action potential. The cell rapidly completes repolarization as K⁺ quickly flows out of the cell. Na⁺ and Ca^{++} channels close, stopping the entry of Na⁺ and Ca^{++}. The rapid movement of K⁺ out of the cell causes the inside to become progressively more electrically negative. The cell gradually becomes more sensitive to external stimuli until its original sensitivity is restored. Phase 3 of the action potential corresponds with the T wave (ventricular repolarization) on the electrocardiogram. Repolarization is complete by the end of phase 3. If potassium channels are blocked, the result is a longer action potential. The time from the beginning of phase 0 to a point in phase 3 where the cell is at −70 mV is termed the *absolute refractory period*. During this time the cell cannot respond to another impulse because it has not yet recovered from the original depolarization. Once the cell reaches −70 mV in phase 3, it can depolarize again in response to a stronger-than-normal impulse. This is called the *relative refractory period*. At the end of phase 3 the inside of the cell has reached −90 mV relative to the outside of the cell. However, the cell is not considered to be at its resting membrane potential because of the placement of Na^+ and K^+. Although the cell is capable of depolarizing, repetitive depolarizations are not possible without the restoration of the Na^+ and K^+ balance. This process takes place during phase 4.

Phase 4: Resting Membrane Potential. Phase 4 is the resting membrane potential (return to resting state). During phase 4 an excess of Na^+ is inside the cell and an excess of K^+ is outside the cell. The sodium-potassium pump is activated to move Na^+ out of the cell and K^+ back into the cell. The heart is polarized during this phase (ready for discharge). The cell remains in this state until the cell membrane is reactivated by another stimulus.

Pacemaker cells undergo a similar set of phases in their repolarization and depolarization process (Figure 7-49). The primary difference between pacemaker cells and myocardial cells occurs in phase 4.

Phase 4 is the most important phase for the pacemaker cell because it is responsible for automaticity. Because of this, phase 4 is always generating an action potential to stimulate a working cell. Beginning with a charge of −60 mV inside the cell, phase 4 is a slope that is moving more positive because of Ca^{++} and a small amount of Na^+ moving into the cells. As Ca^{++} moves in, it slows the movement of K^+ leaving, making the inside of the cell more positive. This process, called *spontaneous diastolic depolarization*, causes a gradual lessening of the resting membrane potential (it becomes less negative). In this manner Ca^{++} is responsible for the slope of phase 4 and ultimately heart rate. When the resting membrane potential reaches its threshold potential at −40 mV, the action potential spontaneously generates and phase 0 starts again. Because phase 0 begins at a less-negative resting membrane potential (−40 mV as opposed to −70 mV in the myocardial cell), the rate of rise of phase 0 is slower than that seen in the myocardial cells. The slow rate of rise of phase 0 in the cells of the sinoatrial node and AV junction depends on the accelerated entry of Ca^{++} and possibly Na^+ through the slow channels.

The slope of phase 4 has direct effects on the heart rate. As the slope becomes steeper, the threshold potential is reached faster and the heart rate is faster. Conversely, as the slope flattens out, the threshold potential is reached slower and the heart rate is slower. Sympa-

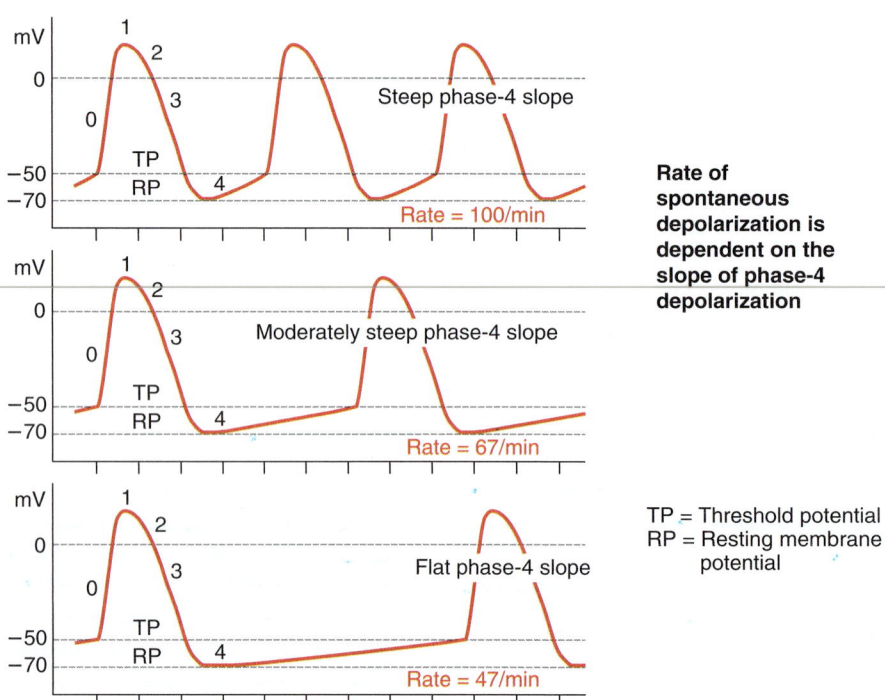

Figure 7-49 Pacemaker action potential.

thetic stimulation makes the slope steeper, whereas parasympathetic stimulation flattens the slope. The paramedic may administer a class of medications called *calcium channel blockers* to slow certain fast heart rates.

Cardiac Conduction System. The pacemaker impulses described above generally start in the primary pacemaker site of the heart, the **sinoatrial node.** This specialized bundle of tissue is located in the upper right atrium (Figure 7-50). The impulse then rapidly travels to the **atrioventricular node (AV node)** by way of the internodal pathways and to the left atrium by way of Bachman's bundle. As the impulse travels through the conduction system, a wave of depolarization is created in the entire heart. This is attributable to the principle of conductivity, in which each myocardial cell can transmit the impulse to adjoining cells. For this reason cells of the conduction system are not required to innervate every myocardial cell. The AV node is a group of cells composed of thin fibers located in the floor of the right atrium immediately behind the tricuspid valve and near the opening of the coronary sinus. The function of the AV node is to delay the impulse, allowing atrial systole to occur before ventricular systole starts. After passing through the AV node, the electrical impulse enters the **bundle of His,** located in the upper portion of the interventricular septum. Unlike the thin fibers of the AV node the bundle of His is composed of thick fibers, causing the impulse to travel rapidly toward the ventricles. The AV node and bundle of His are collectively referred to as the AV junction. After passing through the bundle of His the impulse is conducted down the right and left bundle branches and then through the **Purkinje fibers** found in the ventricles. After reaching the apex of the heart the Purkinje fibers travel back up the lateral walls of each ventricle. This conduction is the "nervous system" of the heart, rapidly moving electrical impulses from the sinoatrial node (located in the upper right atrium) and down to the apex of the left ventricle. This electrical conduction system allows the organized mechanical action known as the **heartbeat** to occur. Because of the arrangement of the Purkinje fibers and the spiral nature of the myocardium, the heart contracts in a "wringing" motion from the apex toward the base.

Although the sinoatrial node is the primary pacemaker of the heart, other sites within the conduction system are capable of automaticity. These additional pacemaker sites provide redundancy in the event the sinoatrial node fails to discharge. The reason the sinoatrial node is the primary pacemaker site is simply because it has the fastest rate of depolarization. Each cell capable of automaticity moves toward its threshold potential, and the first one to reach this is the first to depolarize the rest of the heart. When this occurs, the remainder of the pacemaker cells are also depolarized and must start the process again. One excep-

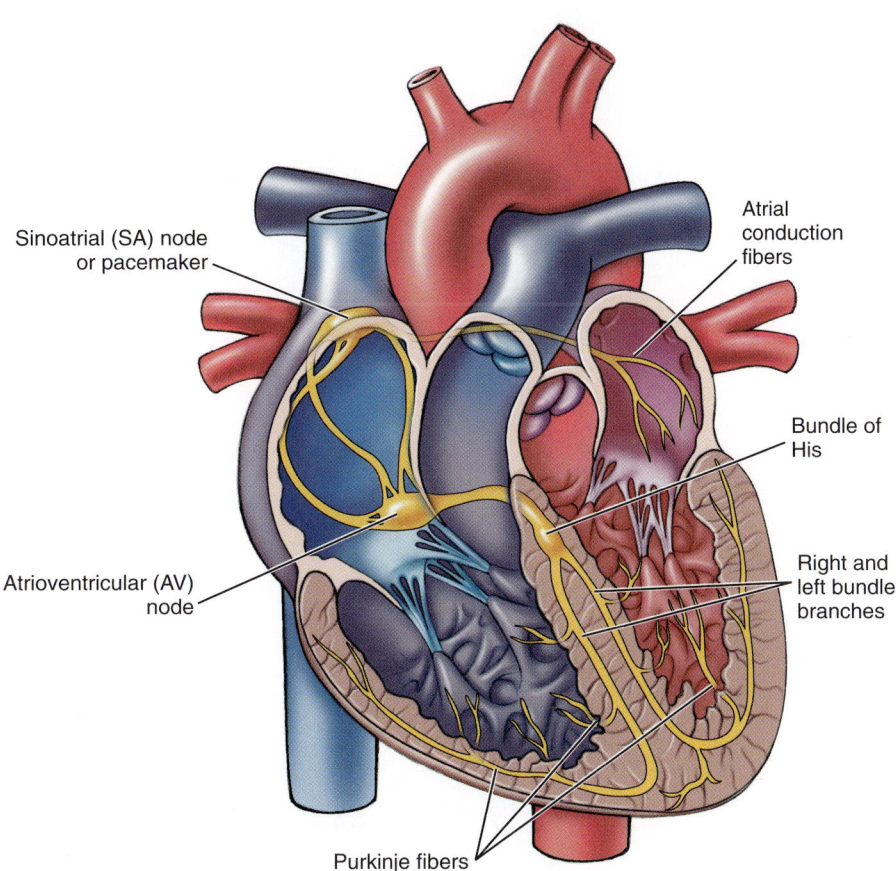

Sinoatrial (SA) node or pacemaker

Atrial conduction fibers

Bundle of His

Atrioventricular (AV) node

Right and left bundle branches

Purkinje fibers

Figure 7-50 Conduction system of the heart.

tion to this is when the pacemaker cells of the Purkinje fibers initiate an impulse; these generally do not depolarize the atrial tissue.

The intrinsic rates of the various pacemaker sites are as follows:

- Sinoatrial node: 60 to 100 impulses/min
- AV junction (specifically the bundle of His): 40 to 60 impulses/min
- Purkinje fibers: 20 to 40 impulses/min

Additional pacemaker cells in the atrium are capable of producing an impulse; however, these cells generally are not considered part of the redundancy system. However, they can be an ectopic source of cardiac depolarization.

Systemic Circulation

[OBJECTIVES 53, 54]

The oxygenated blood is pumped by the left ventricle to the general (systemic) circulation through the aorta. The aorta and other large arteries then continually branch into smaller arteries and **arterioles.** The arterioles eventually end in the capillary beds. The arterial blood is then circulated to all the tissues of the body (Figure 7-51). The capillaries are vessels that deliver blood to each cell in the body. The blood that has been circulated to the tissues of the body is then returned through the small **venules.** These small venules gradually become larger veins and drain all the blood into the right atrium by way of the inferior and superior venae cavae.

Arteries and Veins. Blood vessels are composed of different layers of an elastic tissue and smooth muscle called **tunics.** The innermost layer is the **tunica intima.** It is composed of a single layer of epithelial cells and provides almost no resistance to blood flow. The middle layer is called the **tunica media.** This middle layer is mainly composed of smooth muscle that alters the diameter of the lumen of the vessel. The smooth muscle of the tunica media is under sympathetic control. Thus it enables the body to adjust the blood flow quickly to meet immediate needs. The outermost layer of the vessels is called the **tunica adventitia.** This layer is mainly composed of elastic connective tissue. It allows the vessel to expand to great pressure or volume.

The large arteries of the body, the aorta and the pulmonary trunk, are called **conducting arteries.** These vessels have more elastic tissue and less smooth muscle. These large vessels are required to stretch under great

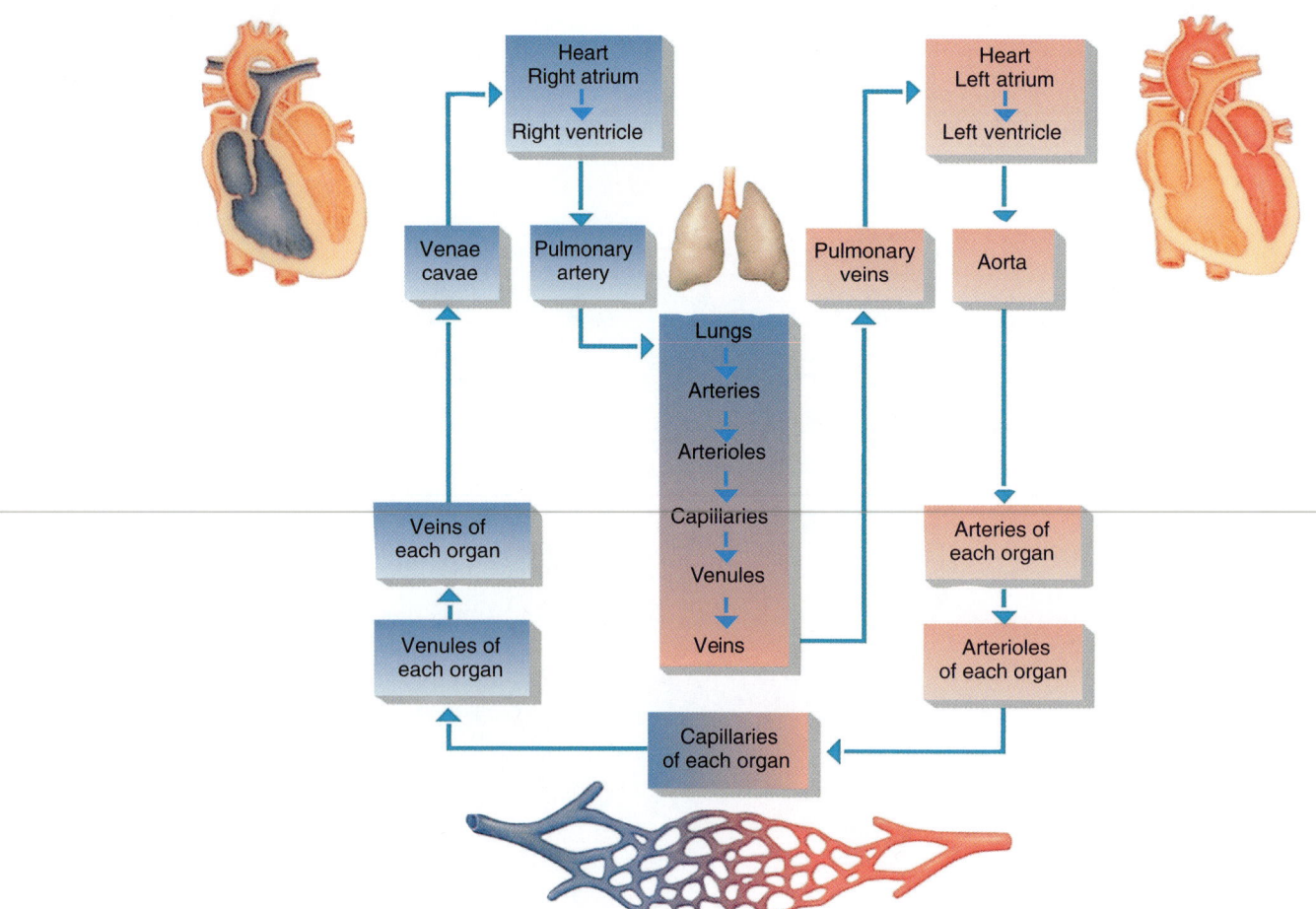

Figure 7-51 Blood flows through the cardiovascular system.

pressures and quickly return to their original shape. Medium and small arteries are called **distributing arteries.** These arteries have well-defined adventitia layers, but they also have larger amounts of smooth muscle. This gives the body the ability to alter blood flow. The smallest of the arteries are called *arterioles*. These vessels supply blood to the capillary beds.

Venules are the smallest of the venous vessels. They have very little smooth muscle in their middle layer. Venules are called **capacitance vessels** because they are capable of holding large amounts of volume. Although the majority of the blood is contained in the venous system, in times of stress, such as shock, these vessels constrict in an attempt to maintain blood pressure. The venules gradually increase in thickness and become medium-sized vessels. These medium-sized veins have valves within them that prevent a backward flow of blood. They gradually increase in size until they become the central veins. The central veins direct the blood into the right atrium. These central veins have no valves and rarely collapse.

Capillary Network (Beds). Small arterial vessels called arterioles supply oxygenated blood to the capillaries (Figure 7-52). This blood then is returned through small venous vessels called venules. Flow in the capillary bed is regulated through smooth muscles called **sphincters.** These sphincters are located at the entrances to the capillaries and are called **precapillary sphincters.** These sphincters are responsive to local tissue needs (e.g., pH changes and oxygen demands). The precapillary muscle relaxes when the tissues require oxygen or have a change in pH. Blood then is allowed to flow into the capillary beds, providing nutrients to the tissue.

Capillary Filtration. The exchange of nutrients and waste products between the intravascular space and the intracellular space is crucial to survival. The majority of substances, such as oxygen and carbon dioxide, pass between these spaces by way of diffusion, facilitated diffusion, and osmosis. However many substances depend on the process of capillary filtration for this exchange to take place. This process depends on three factors: capillary membrane permeability, arterial hydrostatic pressure, and venous oncotic pressure. Blood entering the arterial side of the capillary is forced out of the capillary bed, along with the nutrients it carries, by hydrostatic pressure and into the interstitial space. This pressure is the result of the systemic blood pressure. Exchange between the intracellular and extracellular compartments takes place in the interstitial space. As the plasma portion of the blood leaves the capillaries, the plasma proteins remain in the capillary beds because they are too large to escape. This creates an oncotic, or osmotic, pressure that draws the fluid back into the venous side of the capillary. Approximately 24 L of fluid is forced out of the arterial capillaries per day, and approximately 20 L are reabsorbed by the venous capillaries. The remaining fluid is absorbed by the lymphatic system and rejoins central circulation by the thoracic duct or the right lymphatic duct. Capillary filtration also allows communication between all fluid compartments of the body, which is essential in the fight against foreign particles and organisms.

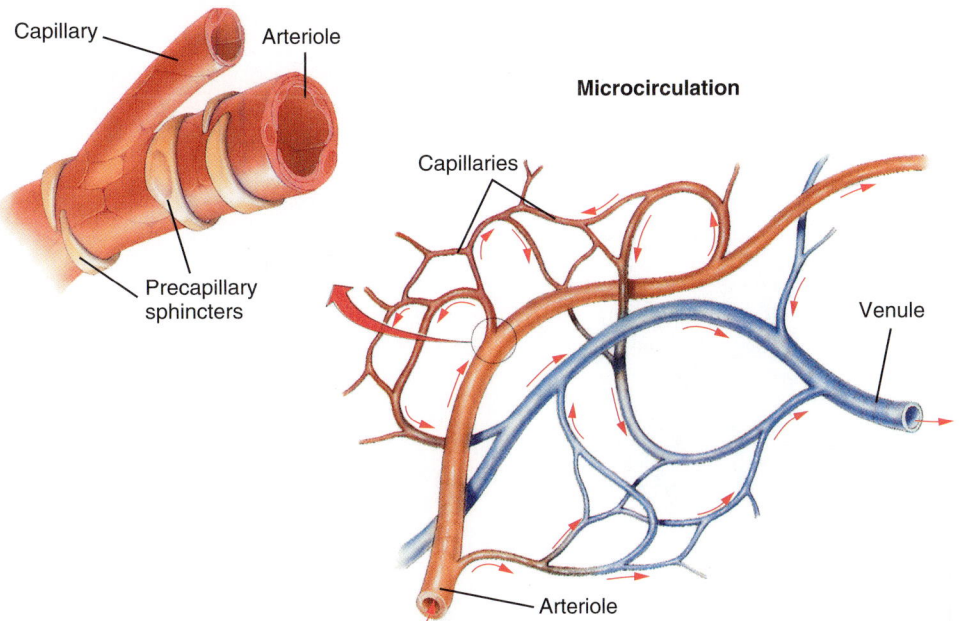

Figure 7-52 Capillary network. Blood circulates through small vessels called arterioles and venules.

Lymphatic System

[OBJECTIVE 55]

The **lymphatic system** is considered part of the circulatory system of the body (Figure 7-53). This system is composed of a series of unidirectional vessels called **lymphatic vessels** and several lymphoid organs. The fluid within these vessels is called *lymphatic fluid,* or **lymph.** The lymphatic system drains fluid from the tissues of the body and returns it to the general circulation. The lymphatic capillaries are interspersed throughout the interstitial fluid (the fluid that surrounds the cells and is in

neither the intravascular nor the intracellular spaces) and lie in close proximity to the cells. These closed-ended vessels are composed of a single layer of epithelial tissue that allows the absorption of fluids and particles from the interstitial space. The capillaries are closed-ended because flow through the lymphatic system is unidirectional—toward central circulation. As the lymphatic capillaries merge and grow, they form the lymphatic vessels. These vessels are constructed much like veins and also contain valves that maintain the unidirectional flow. As lymph flows back to central circulation it passes through a series of lymphoid organs, or lymph nodes. The lymph is evalu-

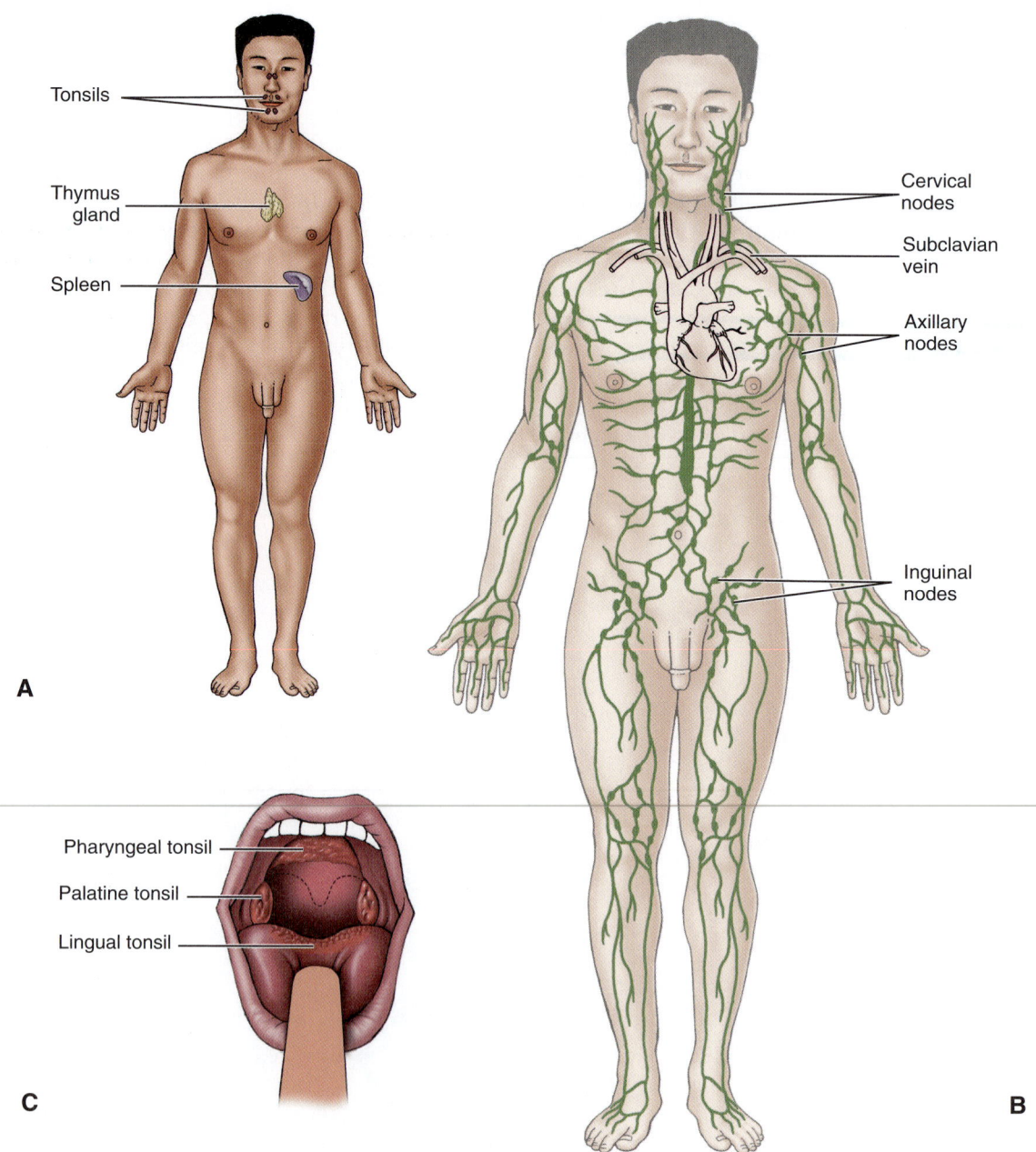

Figure 7-53 Location of lymphoid tissue. **A,** Lymphoid organs. **B,** Distribution of lymph nodes. **C,** Tonsils.

ated by components of the immune system while in these nodes (see Chapter 8). As the lymphatic vessels move toward central circulation they combine to form the lymphatic trunk and, eventually, the lymphatic collecting ducts. The thoracic duct is the larger of the two ducts and collects lymph from the lower body, the left side of the head and neck, and the left arm. This duct returns lymph to central circulation by a connection with the left subclavian vein. The right lymphatic duct collects lymph from the right arm and the right side of the head and neck. This duct returns lymph to central circulation by a connection with the right subclavian vein. The lymphatic system has the following three primary functions:

1. Removal of excess fluid from tissues of the body and the recovery of fluid needed to maintain the proper balance of water required. The lymphatic capillaries are found in the tissues of the body, with the exception of the CNS, bone marrow, and the tissues without blood vessels (e.g., tendons, cartilage). These lymphatic capillaries serve as a series of valves. They allow fluid to be drained into them but prevent the backward flow of fluid into the tissue. The lymph is drained from the tissues and returned to the cardiovascular circulation (Figure 7-54).

2. The production and circulation of lymphocytes. These lymphocytes are produced within lymphoid organs, which provide a significant portion of the body's immune function.

3. Distribution of various products unable to enter the bloodstream directly, such as nutrients and some hormones.

Various body dynamics, such as respiratory pressure changes, muscular contractions, and movement of organs surrounding lymphatic vessels, combine to pump lymph through the lymphatic system. This network also transports fats, proteins, and other substances to the circulatory system and restores 60% of the fluid that filters out of the capillaries into interstitial spaces during normal metabolism.

RESPIRATORY SYSTEM

[OBJECTIVE 56]

The cells of the body must have energy to function. This energy is produced through a series of complicated steps that require oxygen. The primary function of the respiratory system is to bring oxygen into the body and eliminate the waste product carbon dioxide (CO_2). This system also provides nonspecific defenses against disease, helps control pH, and permits vocalization. The

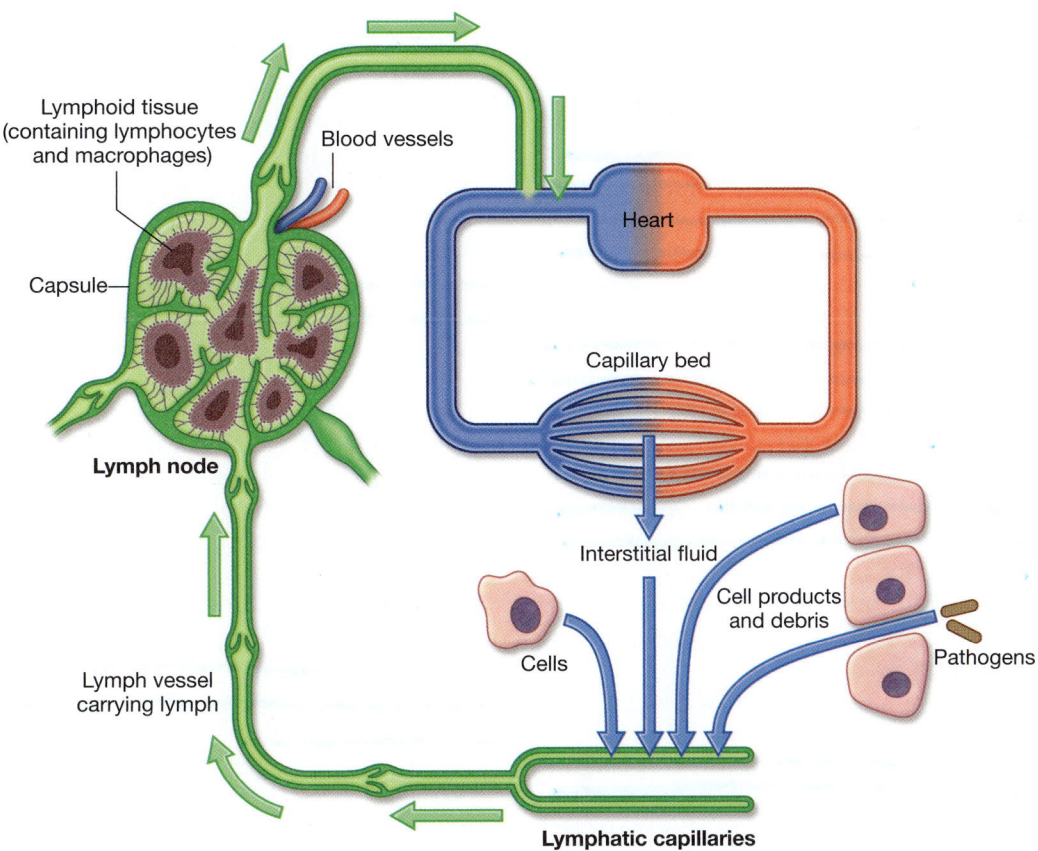

Figure 7-54 Lymphatic vessels mainly collect fluid lost from vascular capillary beds during nutrient exchange processes and deliver it back to the venous side of the vascular system.

respiratory system is composed of the following parts (Figure 7-55):

1. **The respiratory tract,** which consists of passages to move air to and from the exchange surfaces
2. **The respiratory membrane,** where gas exchange takes place (oxygen is picked up in the bloodstream and CO_2 is eliminated through the lungs)
3. **The lungs,** which allow the mechanical movement of air to and from the respiratory membrane

The airway is separated into upper and lower structures. The upper and lower structures can be distinguished on the basis of their location above or below the glottis.

Upper Airway Structures

[OBJECTIVE 57]

The entrance to the respiratory tract begins at the nasal and oral cavities (Figure 7-56). The area between the nasal cavity and the larynx and posterior to the oral cavity is referred to as the *pharynx*. The pharynx allows passage of air to the lower airway and food to the esophagus. It is referred to as having three sections, although no physical structures separate these sections.

Nasopharynx

Air passes into the nasal cavity through the nares. The nasal cavity is separated into right and left halves by the nasal septum. This septum is rich in blood supply, as are the nasal turbinates, or nasal conchae. The nasal turbinates are three horizontal projections of tissue from the lateral walls of each nostril that cause turbulence in airflow, making inhaled particles stick to the mucus-coated walls of the nostrils. This combination of vascular supply and turbulence warms, filters, and humidifies the air as it is inhaled. These structures are of particular importance to the paramedic because they can be damaged easily and bleed profusely with nasal airway management procedures. Within the nasopharynx is the **olfactory tissue.** This tissue contains receptors that give a person the ability to smell (olfaction). **Sinuses** are cavities within the bones of the skull that connect to the nasal cavity (Figure 7-57). These sinuses are hollow areas that lessen the weight of the head; they also give a person's voice resonance. The back of the nasal cavity opens into the **oropharynx.**

Oropharynx

At the uvula the nasopharynx ends and the oropharynx begins. The anterior oropharynx opens into the oral cavity. This cavity is composed of the lips, cheeks, teeth, tongue, and hard and soft palates. The back of the oral cavity opens into the oropharynx. The oropharynx extends down to the epiglottis.

Laryngopharynx

The laryngopharynx extends from the epiglottis to the glottis. The epiglottis is a flaplike structure that closes over the glottis to prevent the passage of foreign matter into the trachea. The glottis is an opening between the vocal cords that has the ability to close when swallowing.

Larynx

[OBJECTIVE 58]

The **larynx** lies between the pharynx and the lungs. The larynx has three purposes: to facilitate the passage of air; as a sphincter, to prevent foreign material (solids and liquids) from entering the lungs; and to produce speech.

The larynx protects and supports the vocal cords and is composed of an outer case of nine cartilages (Figure 7-58). These cartilages are connected by muscles and ligaments. The largest of these cartilages is the thyroid cartilage, or Adam's apple.

The most inferior cartilage is the **cricoid cartilage.** This cartilage is the only complete ring in the larynx.

Within the larynx are the false vocal cords and the vocal cords. The false vocal cords are folds of tissue that help close the glottis during swallowing; however, they have no function in the production of speech. The true vocal cords are folds of tissue that also contain elastic fibers. Vibration of these cords creates the sounds of speech.

Lower Airway Structures

Below the glottis is the lower airway. The structures of the lower airway include the trachea, bronchial tree, alveoli, and lungs.

Trachea

[OBJECTIVE 59]

The **trachea** is the air passage that connects the larynx to the lungs. The trachea is composed of connective tissue and smooth muscle supported by 15 to 20 pieces of cartilage that form C shapes. These rings protect the trachea and prevent it from collapsing. The adult trachea is approximately 2.5 cm in diameter and 9 to 15 cm in length. The trachea is anterior to the esophagus. It extends from the larynx to the bifurcation **(carina)** of the trachea into the right and left mainstem bronchi. The trachea is lined with columnar epithelial tissue and goblet cells. The goblet cells produce large amounts of mucus, which traps foreign particles that are able to make it into the lower airway. The epithelial cells are ciliated and sweep the mucus and trapped particles up to the pharynx to be swallowed or expelled.

Bronchial Tree

The bronchial tree begins at the carina, separating into the right and left mainstem bronchi. Each bronchi directs air into its respective lung. An external landmark for the carina is the junction of the body and manubrium of the

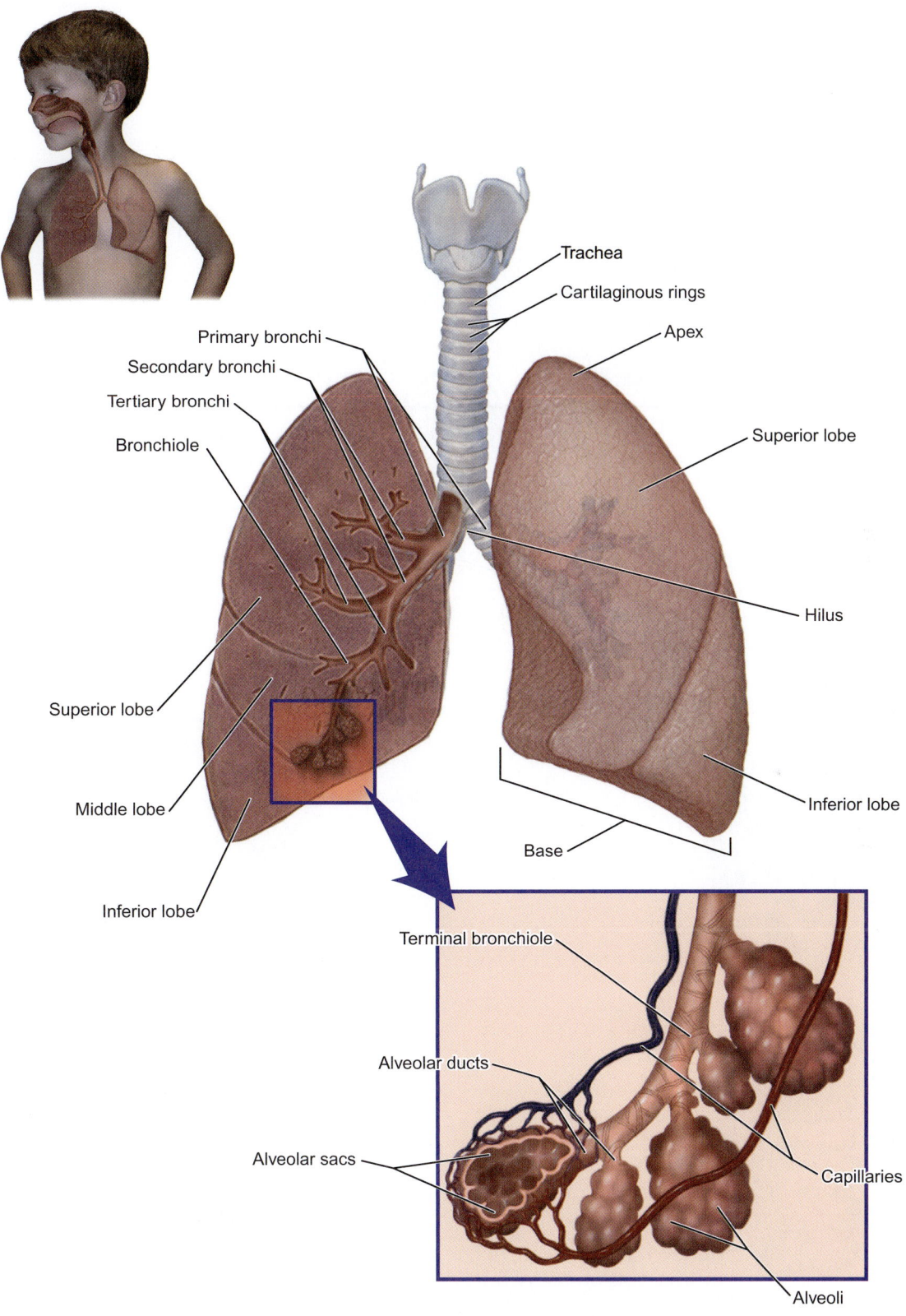

Figure 7-55 The respiratory system.

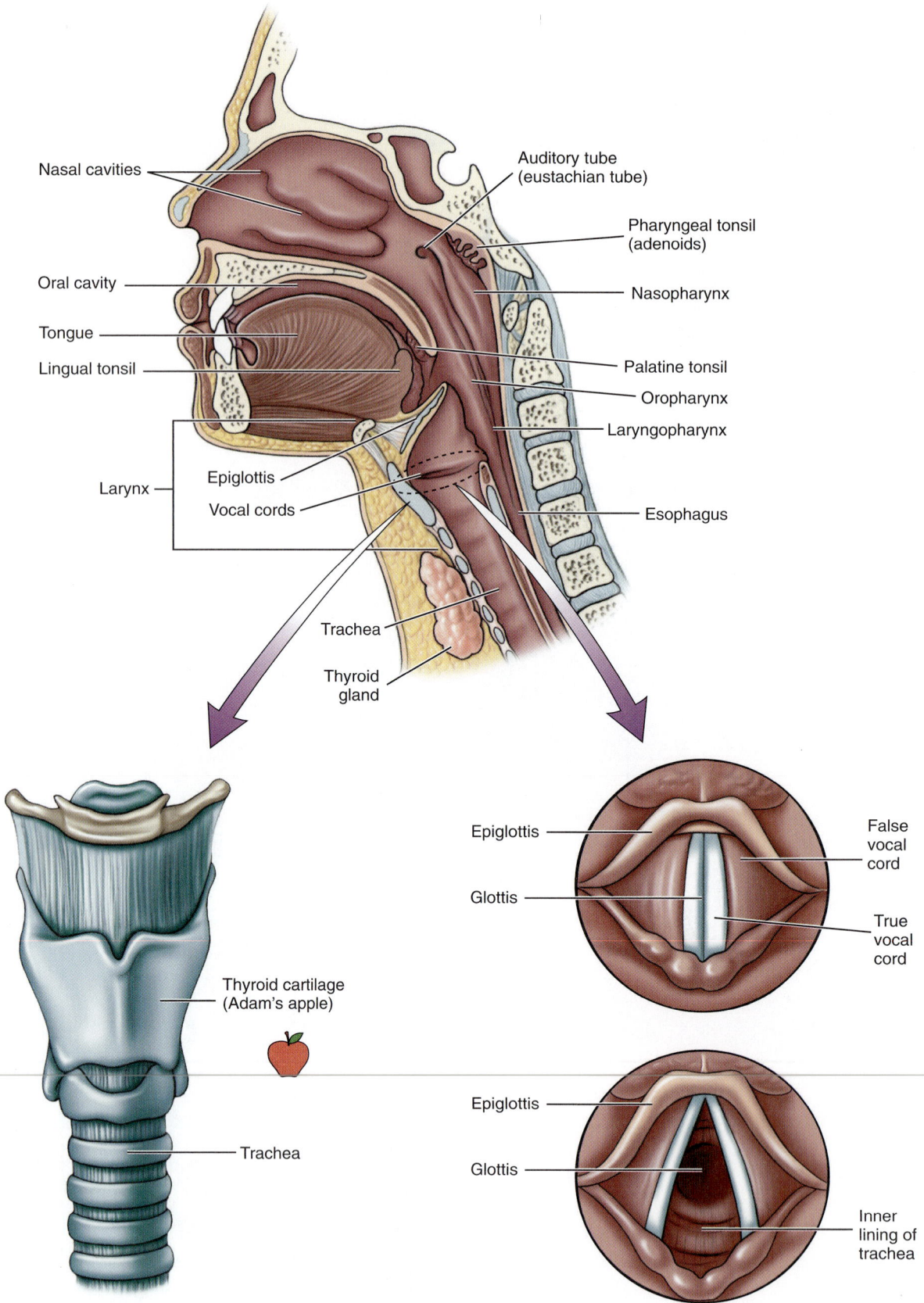

Figure 7-56 Anatomy of the upper airway.

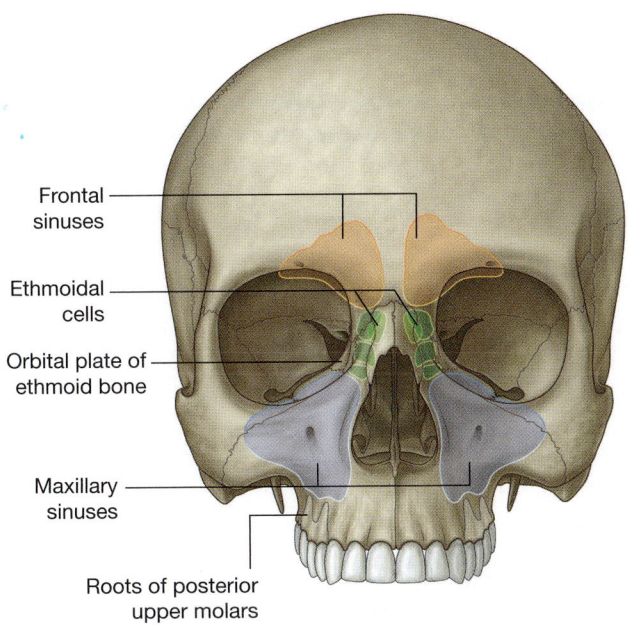

Figure 7-57 Sinuses are cavities within the bones of the skull that connect to the nasal cavity.

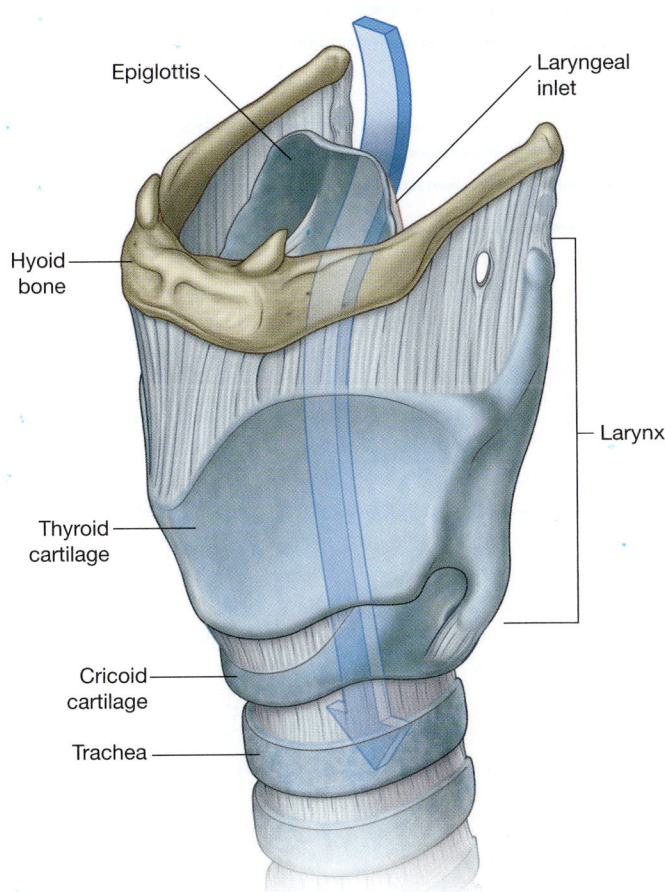

Figure 7-58 The larynx is composed of an outer cage of cartilages that protect and support the vocal cords.

sternum, referred to as the angle of Louis. The right mainstem bronchus is shorter and wider than the left and leaves the carina at a less-acute angle than the left. This is important to the paramedic because an endotracheal tube passed beyond the carina is more likely to pass into the right mainstem bronchus than the left mainstem bronchus. Like the trachea, the bronchi are lined with ciliated epithelial cells and goblet cells to prevent the inhalation of foreign particles.

The bronchi begin to branch into progressively smaller subdivisions. They end in respiratory bronchioles that lead to alveolar sacs. As the bronchi begin to branch, they begin to lose their supporting cartilage and gain increasing amounts of smooth muscle. This smooth muscle is under autonomic control, enabling the body to alter air flow. The smallest of these air passages are called **bronchioles.** The bronchioles are supported only by smooth muscle. The bronchioles become respiratory bronchioles that end in alveolar ducts. The alveolar ducts direct air into **alveoli,** where the majority of gas exchange takes place.

Alveoli

The alveoli are the functional units of the respiratory system (see Figure 7-55). Alveoli compose the majority of lung tissue. Approximately 150 million alveoli are found in each lung. The alveoli allow the exchange of respiratory gases (oxygen and CO_2). The alveolar walls consist of a single layer of epithelial tissue and elastic fibers. These elastic fibers allow the alveolus to expand and recoil during breathing. Each alveolus is surrounded by a network of capillaries. Only a fine respiratory membrane separates the alveolus from the vascular bed. The distance between the air-containing alveolus and the vascular bed is important in the gas exchange that must take place. In pulmonary diseases such as emphysema, lung cancer, and pulmonary edema, this distance is two to three times its normal 0.5 to 1 μm. This distance prevents adequate gas exchange from taking place. The alveoli are coated with a thin layer of pulmonary **surfactant.** This surfactant is made by specialized cells within each alveolus and keeps the alveoli from collapsing.

Lungs

[OBJECTIVE 60]
The lungs are two large, paired structures located within the pleural cavities. The lungs expand and contract as a result of the changes in the intra-thoracic pressure during the respiratory cycle. During inspiration, the diaphragm, scalene muscles, and parasternal muscles contract. This action increases the volume in the thoracic cage, causing the intrathoracic pressure to decrease compared with the air pressure outside the body. This allows outside air to rush in (through whatever opening is available, typically the mouth and nose). During exhalation, the diaphragm and the accessory muscles of respiration relax, enabling the intra-thoracic pressure to increase above the air pressure outside the body. This causes the air to exit the mouth and nose.

The lungs are attached to the heart by the pulmonary trunk (arterial) and the pulmonary veins. The point of entry for bronchial vessels, bronchi, and nerves in each lung is called the **hilum.** An average adult lung weighs less than 2.2 kg. The base of each lung rests on the diaphragm, and its apex extends approximately 2.5 cm above each clavicle. The apex of the left lung is slightly more superior than that of the right. The right lung is divided into three lobes: the upper, middle, and lower. The left lung has only two lobes, one upper and one lower. The left lung has a notch where the heart lies (cardiac notch). Each lobe is composed of separated lobules; these lobules can be surgically removed, leaving the rest of the lung intact.

Each lung is contained within its individual pleural cavity. This serous cavity is lined by a membrane called the **pleura.** The **parietal pleura** is tightly attached to the interior of the chest cage, and the **visceral pleura** tightly adheres to the lung surface. This design is important in the physiology of respiration. The parietal and visceral pleurae are separated by a thin layer of pleural fluid (less than 5 mL). The surface tension caused by the fluid between the two layers causes the layers to stick together. As a result, when the parietal pleura moves with the chest wall, it takes the visceral pleura with it, expanding the lungs. The pleural fluid also allows the movement of each lung with little friction. This fluid occasionally can become infected, causing an irritation of the surface of the lung with respiratory movement (called pleuritis or pleurisy). This potential space between the two layers of the pleura can fill with fluid, air (pneumothorax), or blood (hemothorax).

Collectively, the lungs are capable of holding a total of 5800 mL of air. This is referred to as the *total lung capacity,* which can be subdivided into four distinct categories referred to as *pulmonary volumes,* or lung volumes, as follows:

- Tidal volume (V_T) is the amount of air inhaled or exhaled during a normal breath. The normal tidal volume is 500 mL.
- Inspiratory reserve volume (IRV) is the additional amount of air that can be inhaled after the normal V_T has been reached. The average person can inhale an additional 3000 mL of air when needed in times of physiologic stress.
- Expiratory reserve volume (ERV) is the additional amount of air that can be exhaled after the normal tidal volume is expelled. The average person can exhale an additional 1100 mL of air when needed in times of physiologic stress.
- Residual volume (RV) is the amount of air that remains in the lungs after maximal exhalation. This serves to prevent atelectasis by keeping the alveoli slightly inflated. In the average person the residual volume is 1200 mL.

These individual volumes can be combined to further express pulmonary function. When one or more volumes are combined, the term *pulmonary capacity* is used. Combined volumes include the following:

- Inspiratory capacity (IC) is equal to the tidal volume plus the inspiratory reserve volume (IC = V_T + IRV). This represents the maximal amount of air that can be inhaled when starting the inhalation with the ERV and RV intact. The IC in an average person is 3500 mL.
- Functional residual capacity (FRC) is the expiratory reserve volume plus the residual volume (FRC = ERV + RV). This represents the amount of air in the lungs at the end of a normal exhalation. The FRC in an average person is 2300 mL.
- Vital capacity (VC) is the inspiratory reserve volume, plus the tidal volume, plus the expiratory reserve volume, or the inspiratory capacity plus the expiratory reserve volume. Mathematically this can be expressed as VC = IRV + V_T + ERV or as IC + ERV. This represents the total amount of air that can be moved in and out of the lungs after maximal exhalation followed by maximal inhalation, followed again by maximal exhalation. In the average person this is 4600 mL.
- Total lung capacity (TLC) is the vital capacity plus the residual volume. Mathematically this is expressed as TLC = VC + RV. This represents the total amount of air the lungs can hold with maximal inhalation. In the average person this is 5800 mL.

One of the critical determinants in the effectiveness of ventilation is the amount of air moved in and out of the respiratory system in 1 minute. This is referred to as *minute volume* (MV), which is the respiratory rate (RR) multiplied by the tidal volume. Mathematically this is expressed as MV = RR × V_T. Using a respiratory rate of 12 ventilations per minute and a tidal volume of 500 mL, the average MV is 6000 mL (12 × 500 mL). However, the entirety of this 6000 mL does not reach the alveoli and is not available for exchange with the red blood cells. The amount of air contained in the trachea and conducting airway cannot be exchanged because of the nature of these structures. This space is referred to as the *anatomic dead space* (V_D) and accounts for approximately 150 mL of air. To determine the amount of air that reached the alveoli with each breath, V_D must be subtracted from V_T. The amount of air that actually reaches the alveoli is referred to as the minute alveolar volume (MV_A). Mathematically, this is expressed as MV_A = RR × (V_T − V_D). Continuing with the previous example, 12 × (500 mL − 150 mL) or 12 × 350 mL, the MV_A would be 4200 mL.

The final consideration in the amount of air actually reaching the alveoli is physiologic dead space. This is a function of the amount of damaged alveoli that cannot participate in gas exchange. Unlike anatomic dead space, which is fairly constant among patients, the physiologic dead space varies widely based on medical history and exposure to toxins that damage the alveoli, among other factors. Physiologic dead space is the anatomic dead space plus the amount of space occupied by damaged alveoli and can be as much as 1 to 2 L of volume. Although physiologic dead space cannot be measured in the prehospital setting, the paramedic must keep this principle in mind and apply it to an individual's history and presentation when determining the effectiveness of ventilation.

Physiologic dead space is an example of a ventilation-perfusion mismatch. This situation occurs when an area of the lung is either ventilated but not perfused or perfused but not ventilated. Respectively, these are situations in which oxygen is in the alveoli but no blood flow can pick up the oxygen, or blood flow to the alveoli is present but no oxygen is to be absorbed. Regardless of the cause of the ventilation-perfusion mismatch (lack of oxygen or lack of blood flow), the condition that occurs is called a *right-to-left shunt*. In essence the unoxygenated blood from the right atrium is returning to the left atrium in an unoxygenated state.

Gas Exchange

Inspired air is a mixture of 78% nitrogen, 21% oxygen, 0.04% carbon dioxide, and a nominal amount of other gases exerting a pressure of 760 mm Hg at sea level. Each gas represents a portion of the air mixture and therefore exerts a partial pressure. The sum of the partial pressures is equal to the total pressure of the mixture. In inspired air nitrogen exerts a partial pressure of 593 mm Hg, oxygen exerts a partial pressure of 160 mm Hg, and carbon dioxide exerts a partial pressure of 0.3 mm Hg. Because gases are lipid soluble, they freely cross the cell membrane and move by diffusion. Partial pressures of the air mixture are responsible for diffusion across cell membranes.

Of the gases dissolved in the venous blood returning to the lungs, carbon dioxide exerts a high partial pressure and oxygen exerts a low partial pressure. This is in contrast to the high partial pressure of oxygen and low partial pressure of carbon dioxide in the lungs. As a result carbon dioxide diffuses out of the venous blood into the lungs and oxygen diffuses out of the lungs and into the arterial blood, where it combines with the hemoglo-

bin molecule of the red blood cell for transport. On reaching the tissues the arterial blood has a high partial pressure of oxygen and a low partial pressure of carbon dioxide. This is in contrast to the interstitial and intercellular fluid, which has a low partial pressure of oxygen and a high partial pressure of carbon dioxide. On reaching the capillaries, oxygen diffuses out of the arterial blood and into the interstitial fluid (and eventually into the intracellular fluid), whereas carbon dioxide diffuses out of the interstitial fluid and into the venous blood.

In addition to the partial pressures of gases, other factors enhance gas exchange, including the acid-base balance, or pH, of the blood. When carbon dioxide (an acid) diffuses out of the blood and into the lungs, the pH of the blood increases (becomes more alkaline). This change results in enhanced attachment of oxygen to the hemoglobin (an increase in oxygen uptake). When the blood reaches the cells, where carbon dioxide is in high concentration, the pH is reduced (becomes more acidic). This change causes oxygen to be released from the hemoglobin (more efficient offloading). This is an important concept for the paramedic to understand because acidosis, such as in states of shock, decreases oxygen delivery to the tissues even in the setting of high partial pressures of oxygen. This is because the ability of oxygen to bind with hemoglobin is reduced in acidic blood.

Transport of Carbon Dioxide

Unlike oxygen, which is transported by the hemoglobin, carbon dioxide is transported by one of three methods by the venous blood. Carbon dioxide may be dissolved in the blood (7%), attached to the hemoglobin (23%), or be present in the form of bicarbonate ions (73%), which are created when carbon dioxide combines with water. ($CO_2 + H_2O = H_2CO_3$). Of note, the carbon dioxide that is attached to the hemoglobin attaches to amino groups, whereas oxygen attaches to iron atoms. Because of this the two molecules may both be carried simultaneously without competing for binding sites on the hemoglobin.

Case Scenario **CONCLUSION**

You and your partner provide high-flow oxygen and assisted ventilation as the patient is immobilized for transport. En route to the hospital, you successfully intubate the patient and establish venous access. You note that the patient's posture has changed. His arms are extended, his toes are pointed, and his back is arched. By the time you arrive at the trauma center (approximately 25 minutes) his heart rate has slowed to 42 beats/min. Despite your efforts and those of the emergency department, the motorcycle rider dies approximately 15 minutes after arrival.

Looking Back

9. *Visualizing the airway during intubation is difficult because of bleeding from the patient's facial injuries. What anatomic structures could be used during a difficult intubation such as this one?*

10. *What is the most likely cause of the slowing pulse in this patient?*

DIGESTIVE SYSTEM

[OBJECTIVE 67]

The **digestive tract** is a series of muscular tubes. These tubes are designed to move food and liquid from its entrance into the body (typically the mouth) to its elimination from the body through the anus (Figure 7-59). The digestive system also is composed of several accessory organs that produce and secrete enzymes, which are chemicals that increase the speed of reactions, and juices essential in the digestive process. The digestive system is responsible for the following six related processes:

1. **Ingestion** is the process of bringing food into the digestive tract.

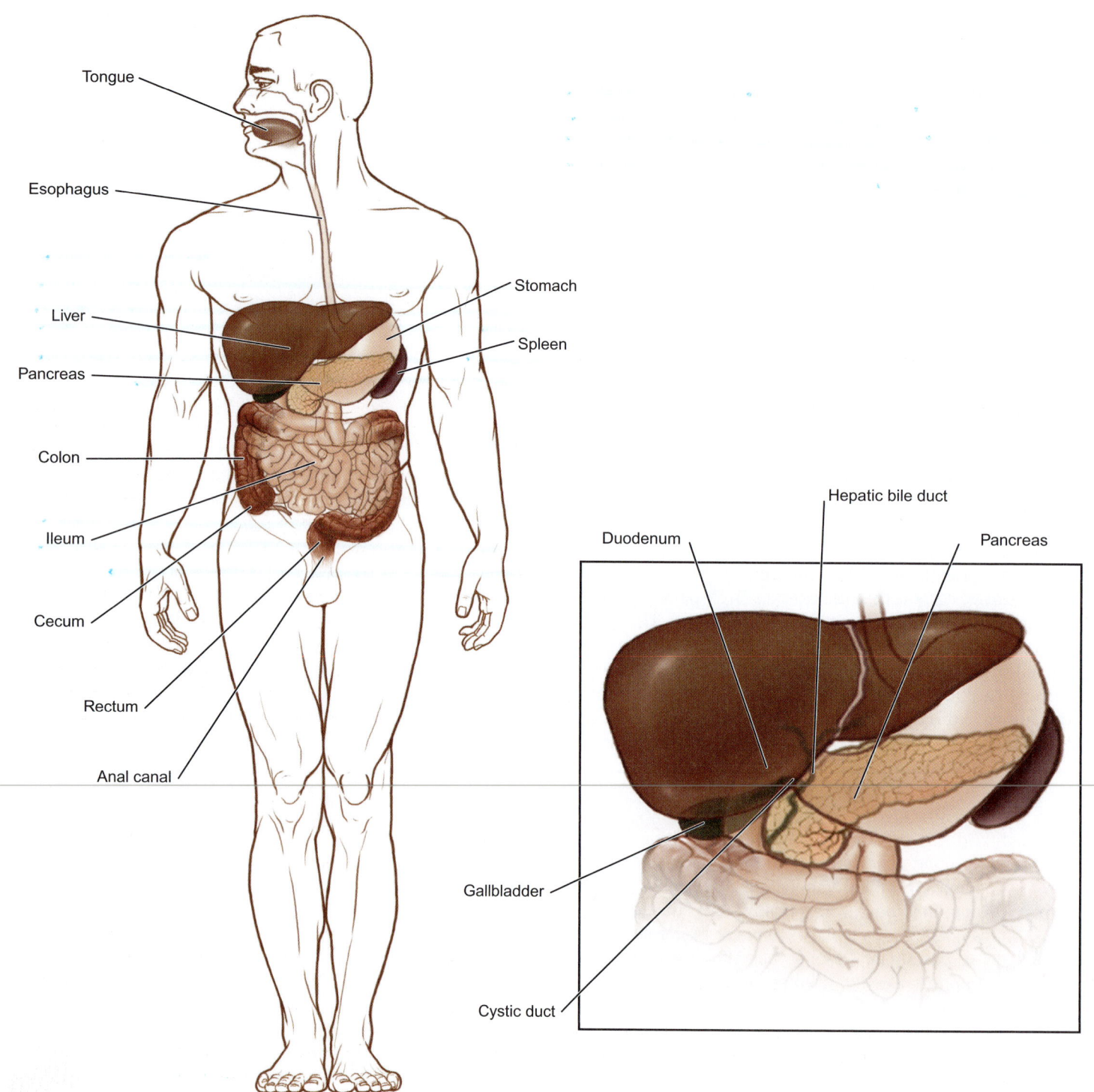

Figure 7-59 The digestive system.

2. **Mechanical processing** is the physical manipulation and breakdown of food.
3. **Digestion** is the chemical breakdown of food material into smaller fragments that can be absorbed into the circulatory system.
4. **Secretion** is the release of water, acids, enzymes, and buffers that aid in the breakdown and digestion of food in the digestive tract. This secretion comes from both the digestive tract and the accessory organs.
5. **Absorption** is the movement of small organic molecules, electrolytes, vitamins, and water across the digestive tract and into the circulatory system.
6. **Excretion** is the removal of waste products from the body. Within the digestive tract, these waste products are compacted and removed from the body by the process of defecation.

Gastrointestinal Tract

[OBJECTIVE 62]

The first part of the gastrointestinal (GI) tract is the **oral cavity.** Within the oral cavity are the salivary glands, teeth, and tongue. The **salivary glands** produce saliva and are composed of two types of cells. The serous cells produce amylase, a salivary enzyme that begins the digestive process of starchy food material. The mucous cells produce mucus that binds and lubricates material placed in the mouth, such as food. The **teeth** masticate (chew) food products in preparation for entry into the stomach. The **tongue** is a muscular organ that provides the sensation of taste. The tongue also directs the food toward the esophagus. The oral cavity opens posteriorly into the pharynx. The pharynx opens inferiorly into the esophagus. The **esophagus** is a tube surrounded by smooth muscle that propels material into the stomach by a series of wavelike contractions called *peristalsis.* Peristalsis is not limited to the esophagus; it is responsible for movement throughout the GI tract. At the inferior end of the esophagus is the **stomach.** The entrance into the stomach is surrounded by the **cardiac sphincter.** The cardiac sphincter is a circular muscle that controls the movement of material into the stomach.

The stomach is a large storage vessel surrounded by multiple layers of smooth muscle (Figure 7-60). The stomach also has cells within it that produce acid. This **acid,** along with the muscular motion of the stomach, breaks down the food material within it into a substance called **chyme.** Chyme is the semifluid mass of partly digested food. Chyme is expelled by the stomach into the **duodenum,** the first part of the small intestine. In the duodenum are important accessory structures that digest various types of nutrients. The next segment of the small intestine is the **jejunum,** a major site of nutrient absorption. The last segment of the small intestine is the **ileum.** The ileum is an area of similar, but decreased, absorption where the chyme is prepared for entry into the large intestine.

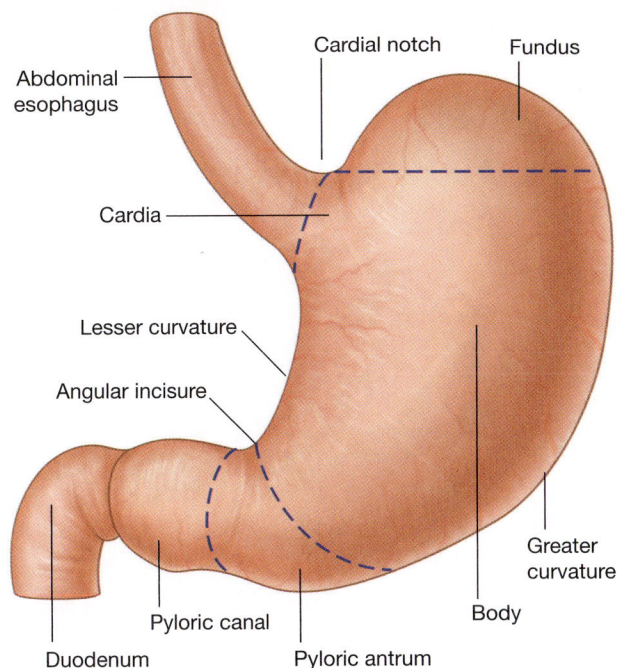

Figure 7-60 The stomach is a large storage vessel surrounded by multiple layers of smooth muscle.

The **large intestine** is where a large amount of water and electrolytes is absorbed (Figure 7-61). It also is where undigested food is concentrated into feces. The first segment of the large intestine (bowel) is the **cecum** and its accessory structure, the **appendix.** The cecum is followed by the **ascending, transverse, descending,** and **sigmoid** parts of the **colon.** Fluid reabsorption occurs in the colon. The sigmoid colon leads into the **rectum,** where feces are further compacted into waste. The rectum joins the **anal canal,** which ends at the **anus.** The anus has two sphincters (internal and external). The **internal anal sphincter** (under autonomic control) has stretch receptors that give the sensation of the need to defecate. The **external anal sphincter,** which is under voluntary control, allows a controlled bowel movement.

Accessory Structures

The accessory organs of the GI system include the liver, gallbladder, and pancreas.

Liver

The **liver** is the largest internal organ of the body. It is located just under the diaphragm, mainly in the right upper quadrant of the abdomen. The liver is a major detoxifier in the body. To accomplish this detoxification, many biochemical processes must occur. The liver is a highly vascular organ through which 100% of the body's blood circulates. This vascular supply has two sources: the **hepatic artery** and the **portal vein.** The hepatic artery is how the liver receives its blood and nutrient

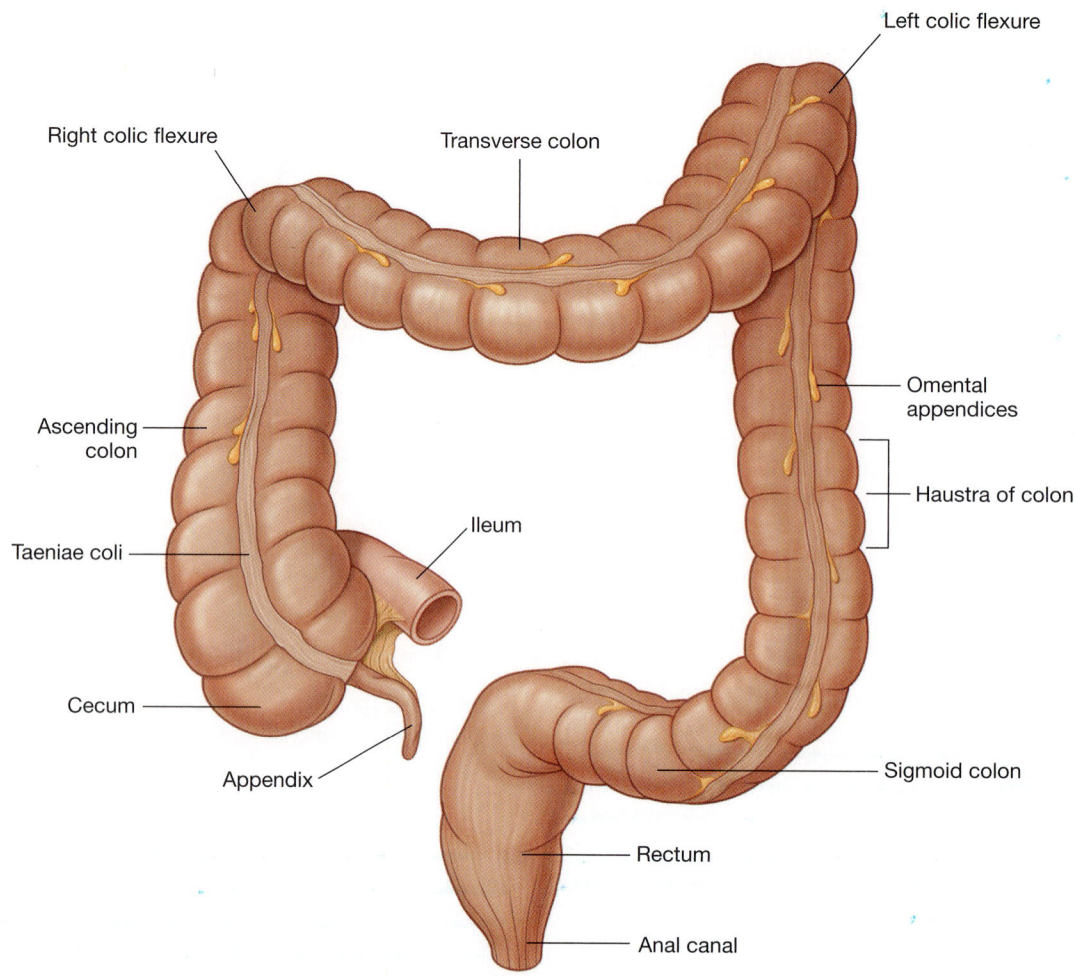

Figure 7-61 The large intestine is where a large amount of water and electrolytes is absorbed and undigested food is concentrated into feces.

supply from the circulatory system. The portal vein is composed of a group of vessels that originate from the digestive system. These vessels ensure that all nutrients absorbed from the intestinal tract first get detoxified in the liver before their release into the general venous circulation (first pass). The liver is responsible for the manufacturing of **bile salts.** These bile salts are composed of electrolytes and iron recovered from red blood cells (RBCs) when they die. Bile emulsifies fats, allowing their digestion and absorption. The liver also is responsible for the manufacturing of blood proteins (albumin, fibrinogen, and globulins) and clotting factors, which allow the body to seal off damaged vessels to prevent blood loss.

Gallbladder

Bile is secreted from the liver into the gallbladder. The gallbladder is located underneath the liver. It is connected to the common bile duct via the cystic duct. The liver connects to the common bile duct via the **hepatic duct.** Bile helps to emulsify fat.

Pancreas

The pancreas is an exocrine gland as well as an endocrine gland. The exocrine cells of the pancreas produce pancreatic juice. This juice is a critical digestive enzyme secreted into the duodenum. It consists of sodium bicarbonate (to neutralize the hydrochloric acid from the stomach), amylase, and digestive enzymes. The amylase continues the digestion of starchy material begun in the mouth.

URINARY SYSTEM

[OBJECTIVES 63, 64, 65]

The **urinary system** eliminates dissolved organic waste products by urine production and elimination (Figure 7-62). Other essential functions of the system include the following:

1. Regulation of blood volume and blood pressure
2. Regulation of the concentrations of electrolytes

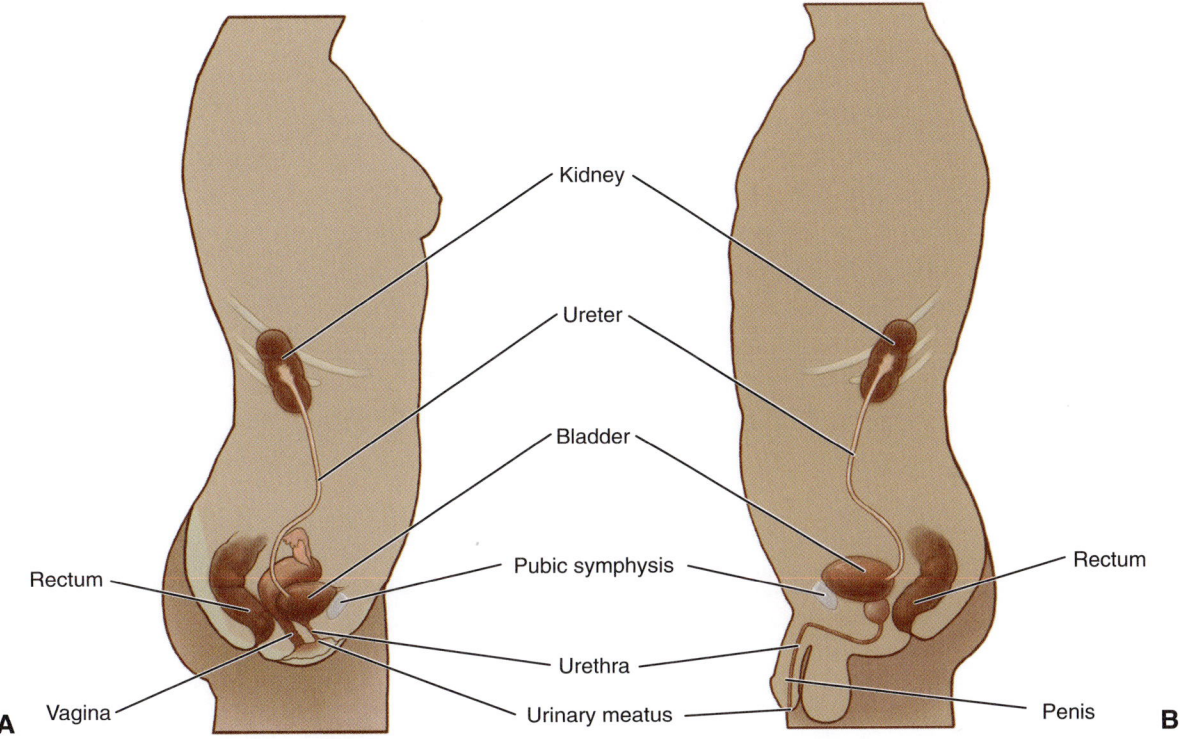

Figure 7-62 The urinary system. **A,** Female. **B,** Male.

3. Homeostasis of blood pH by controlling the loss of hydrogen ions and bicarbonate ions in the urine
4. Conservation of valuable nutrients and the elimination of organic waste products

Kidneys

Two kidneys are found in the retroperitoneal space under the inferior portion of the rib cage (Figure 7-63). A fibrous capsule surrounds each kidney. Moreover, an adipose layer protects the kidney from injury. The kidney consists of a cortex (outer portion) and a medulla. The medulla consists of a number of divisions called **renal pyramids.**

The basic functional unit of the kidney is the **nephron.** The nephron is composed of several parts, with a large terminal end called the **renal corpuscle.** The renal corpuscle is composed of a capsule called **Bowman's capsule** and a network of capillaries called the **glomerulus.** Bowman's capsule is where the initial filtrate is formed that will become urine. Blood pressure forces fluid out of the capillary bed and into the capsule where the filtrate is made. The remaining portions of the nephron are the proximal tubule, the loop of Henle, and the distal tubule. The distal tubule empties into a collecting duct. This duct carries urine from the nephron to the urinary tubes (calyces).

Ureters, Urinary Bladder, and Urethra

The **ureters** drain urine from the calyces to the **urinary bladder** (Figure 7-64). The urinary bladder is a hollow organ that stores urine. It is surrounded by smooth muscle. Stretching of the urinary bladder provides the stimulation for **micturition** (urination). The bladder empties into the **urethra,** which is an opening at the end of the bladder. The junction of the urethra and the bladder has two rings of smooth muscle: the **internal urinary sphincter** and the **external urinary sphincter.** The internal sphincter is under autonomic control. The external sphincter is under voluntary control. The urethra in a female is much shorter than the urethra in a male. This predisposes females to urinary tract and bladder infections.

REPRODUCTIVE SYSTEM

[OBJECTIVE 66]

The purpose of the male reproductive system is to make **spermatozoa.** The organs of the male reproductive system also are designed to transfer the spermatozoa to the female. The purpose of the female reproductive system is to make **oocytes.** The organs of the female reproductive system are designed to receive the spermatozoa for fertilization, conception, and birth.

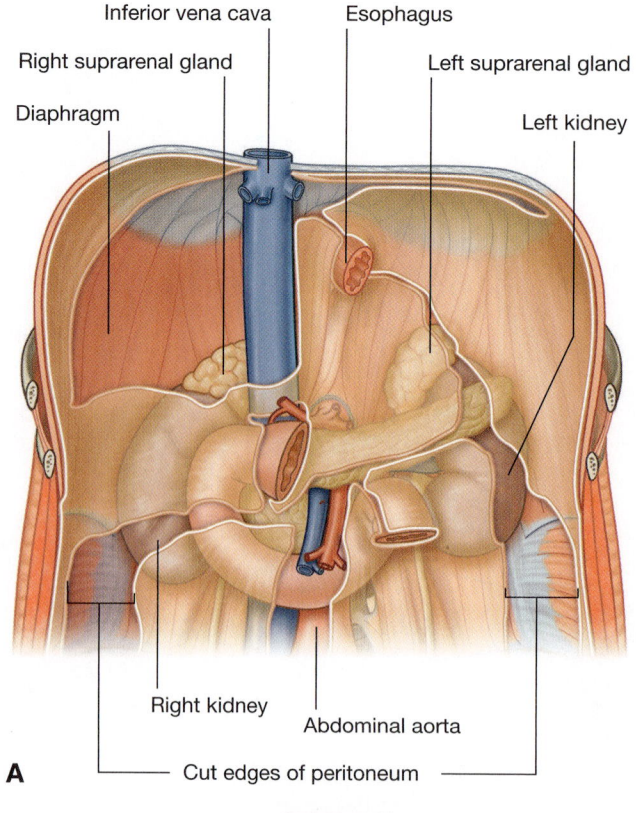

Inferior vena cava

Right suprarenal gland

Diaphragm

Esophagus

Left suprarenal gland

Left kidney

Right kidney

Abdominal aorta

A Cut edges of peritoneum

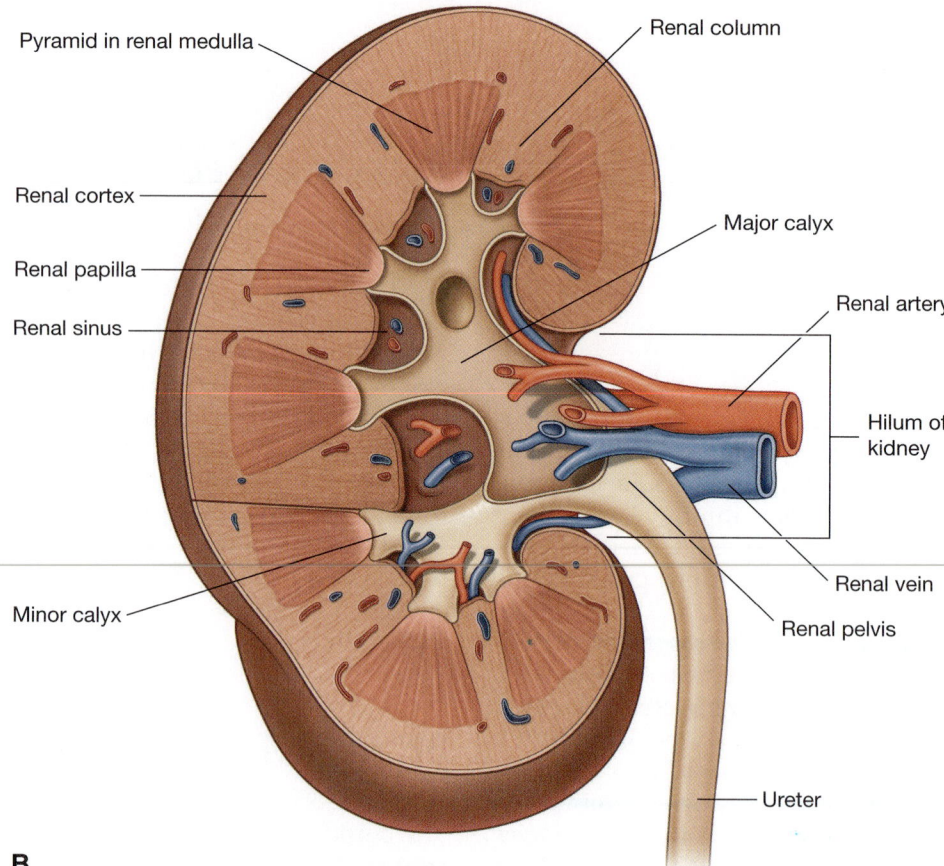

Pyramid in renal medulla

Renal cortex

Renal papilla

Renal sinus

Minor calyx

Renal column

Major calyx

Renal artery

Hilum of kidney

Renal vein

Renal pelvis

Ureter

B

Figure 7-63 The kidneys are found in the retroperitoneal space under the inferior portion of the rib cage. **A,** Retroperitoneal position. **B,** Kidney.

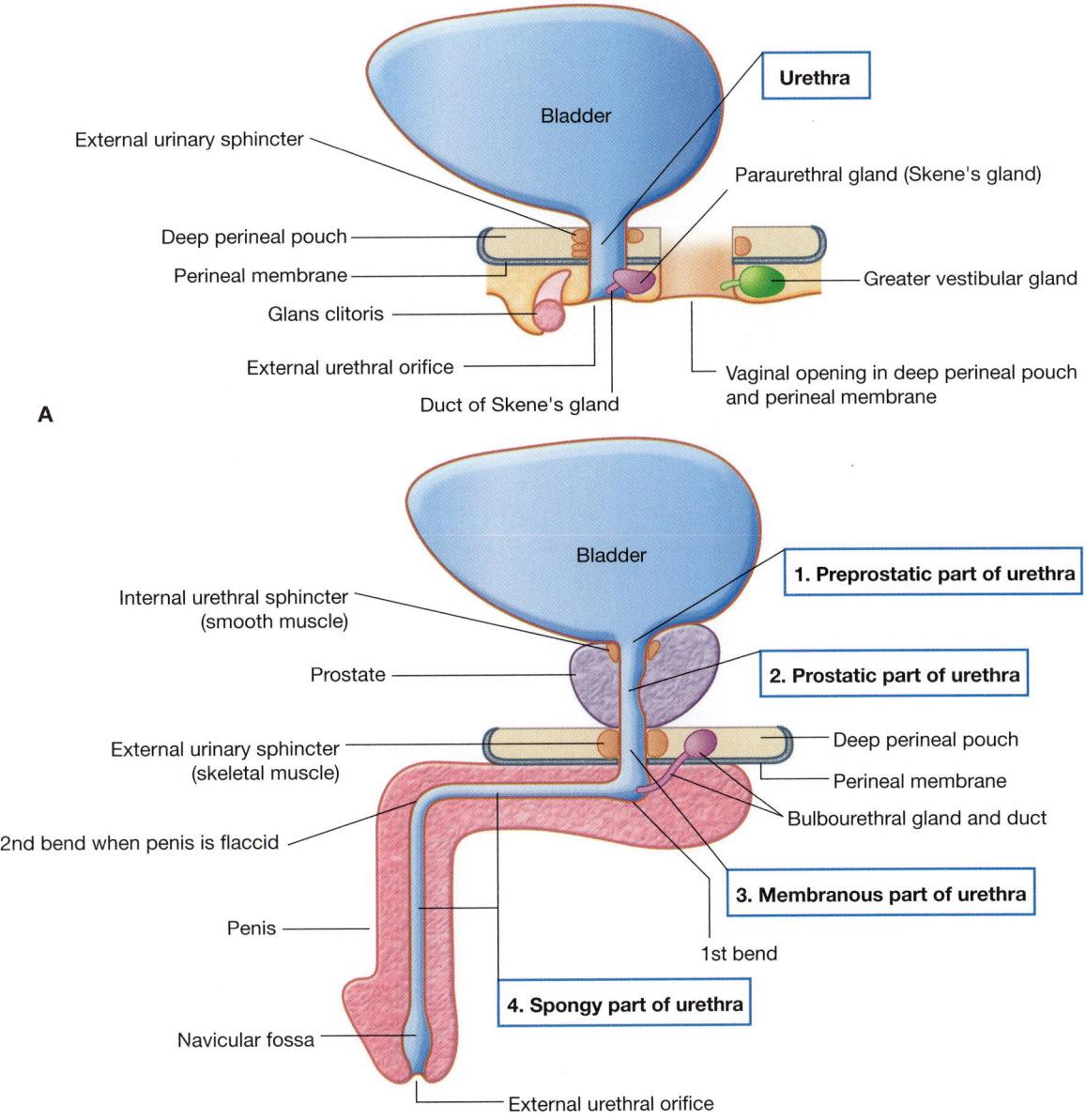

Figure 7-64 The ureters, urinary bladder, and urethra empty urine from the body. **A,** Urethra in women. **B,** Urethra in men.

Male Reproductive System

The male reproductive system consists of the testes, epididymis, ductus deferens, urethra, seminal vesicles, prostate gland, bulbourethral glands, scrotum, and penis (Figure 7-65).

The **testes** are organs suspended within the scrotum. Interstitial cells within the testes secrete the male hormone **testosterone.** At puberty, testosterone levels increase and spermatozoa production begins. The spermatozoa mature in the **epididymis.** The epididymis is a convoluted series of tubes located in the posterior portion of the scrotum.

The **ductus deferens (vas deferens)** extends from the end of the epididymis and travels through the **seminal vesicles.** The seminal vesicles produce **seminal fluid.** This ductus surrounded by nerves, blood vessels, and smooth muscle. The ductus deferens, testicular artery and vein, lymphatic vessels, and nerves compose the **spermatic cord.** The smooth muscle surrounding the vas deferens helps propel sperm through the duct.

The **urethra** is a passageway for both urine and male reproductive fluids. The **prostate** is found dorsal to the symphysis pubis and at the base of the urinary bladder. The prostate is composed of glandular tissue that produces prostatic fluid and a muscular portion that contracts during ejaculation to prevent urine flow.

The **bulbourethral glands** are a pair of small glands that manufacture a mucuslike secretion. This secretion

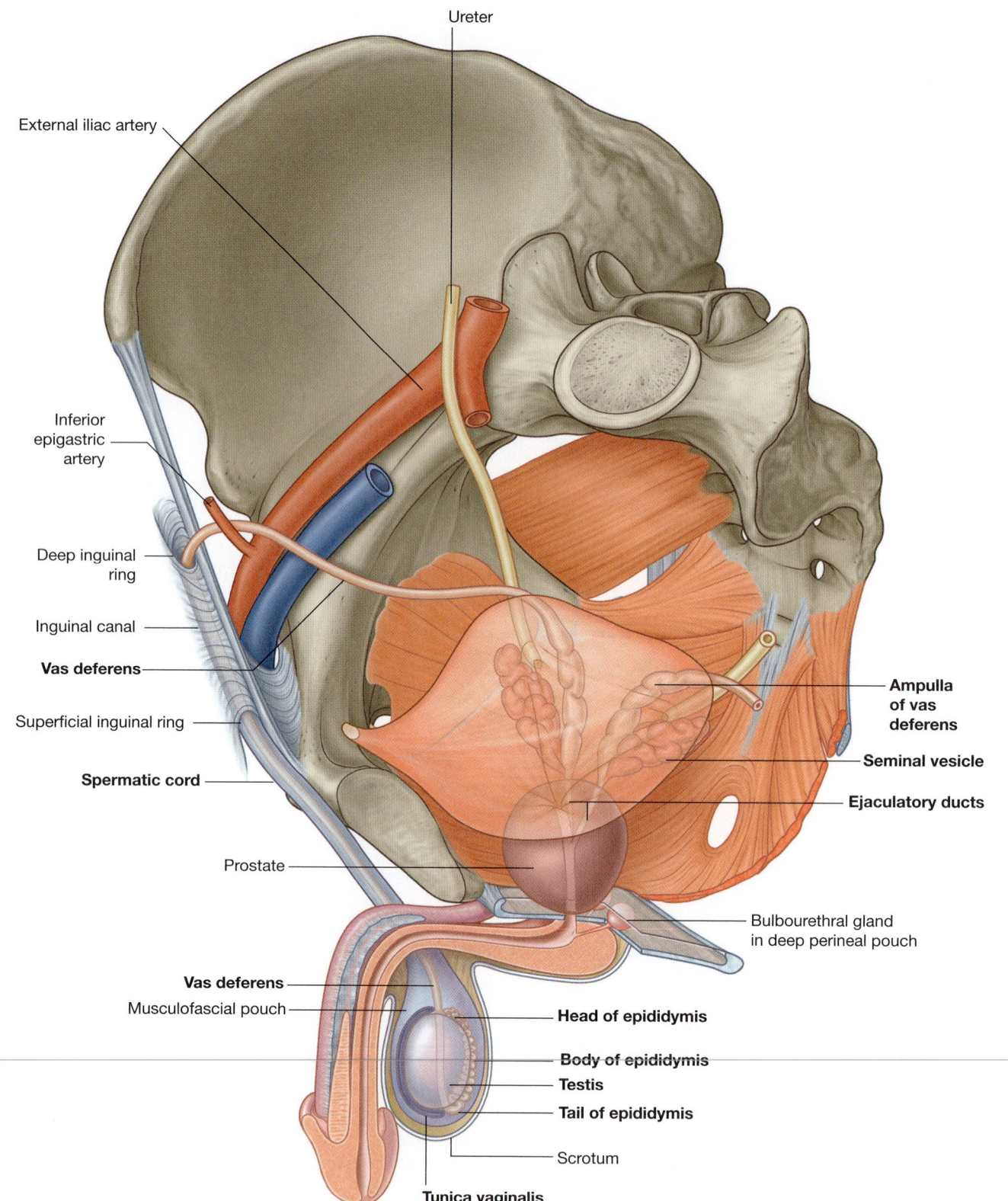

Ureter

External iliac artery

Inferior epigastric artery

Deep inguinal ring

Inguinal canal

Vas deferens

Superficial inguinal ring

Spermatic cord

Prostate

Vas deferens

Musculofascial pouch

Ampulla of vas deferens

Seminal vesicle

Ejaculatory ducts

Bulbourethral gland in deep perineal pouch

Head of epididymis

Body of epididymis

Testis

Tail of epididymis

Scrotum

Tunica vaginalis

Figure 7-65 Male reproductive system.

unites with the prostatic fluid and the spermatozoa to form **sperm.**

The **scrotum** is a loose layer of connective tissue that supports the testes. The dartos muscle—a thin layer of smooth muscle fibers within the scrotum—is important in the regulation of the temperature in the testes, which is necessary for spermatozoa formation **(spermatogenesis).**

The **penis** consists of three columns of erectile tissue. When this tissue is engorged with blood the penis becomes enlarged and firm, causing an erection. The penis transfers sperm during copulation.

Female Reproductive System

The female reproductive organs consist of the ovaries, uterine tubes (fallopian tubes), uterus, vagina, external genital organs, and the mammary glands. The internal reproductive organs lie in the pelvic cavity (Figure 7-66).

The **ovaries** are the site of egg production **(oogenesis).** They are suspended in the pelvic cavity by ligaments. Each ovary has an outer cortex and an inner portion called the **ovarian medulla.** Within the cortex are small vesicles called **follicles.** Each follicle contains an **oocyte** (the female gamete).

The **uterine tubes (fallopian tubes)** extend from each side of the superior end of the body of the uterus to the lateral pelvic wall. The distal portion of the uterine tube is suspended over the ovary (opening into the peritoneal cavity). When an oocyte is released from the ovary, it is picked up by the uterine tube and transported to the uterus by cilia and peristaltic contractions.

The **uterus** is a muscular organ roughly the size of a pear (Figure 7-67). It is designed to grow with the developing fetus. The superior aspect of the uterus is called the **fundus,** and the inferior portion is called the **cervix.** Major ligaments support the uterus within the pelvic cavity.

The **vagina** is the female organ of copulation. It receives the erect penis during intercourse. The vagina extends from the cervix to the outside of the body. The vagina provides a passage for childbirth and menstrual flow.

The external genitalia are called the **vulva.** The entrance to the vagina is concealed by the labia minora and labia majora. A small erectile structure called the **clitoris** is at the entrance to the vagina (Figure 7-68).

The **mammary glands** are the organs of milk production. They are located within the breast tissue (mammae). The breasts have nipples connected by a lactiferous duct to lobules that produce milk (Figure 7-69).

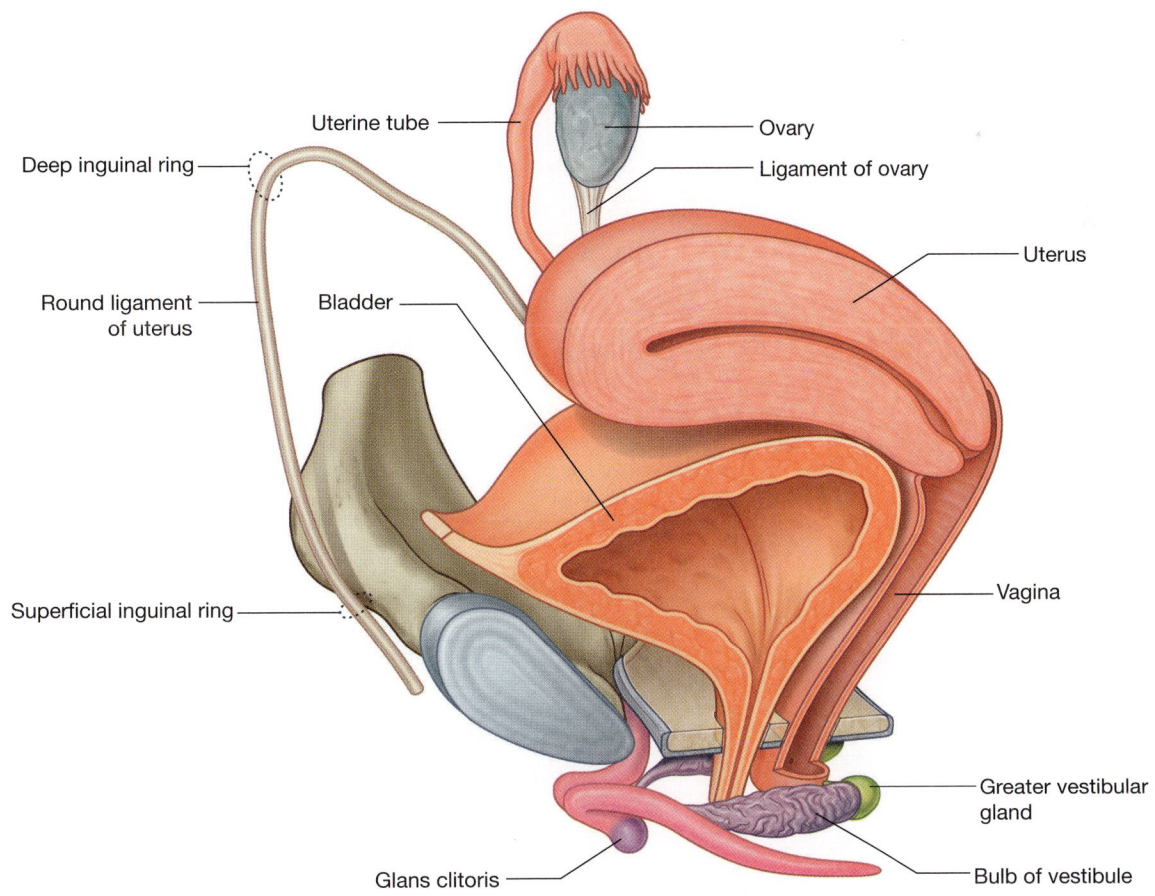

Figure 7-66 Female reproductive system.

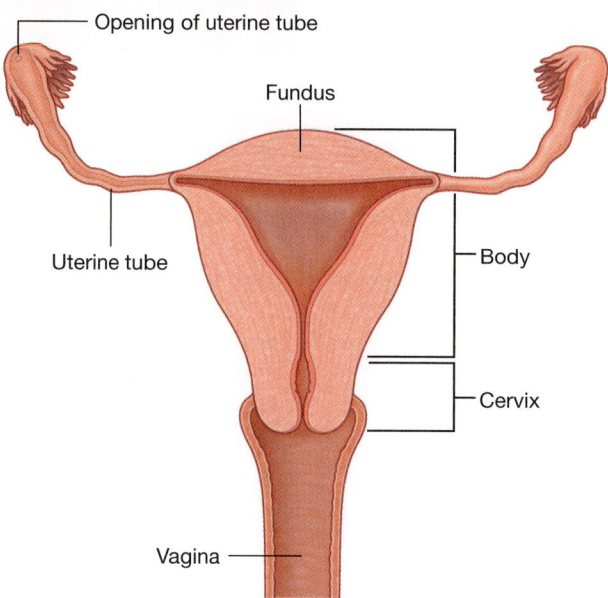

Opening of uterine tube

Fundus

Uterine tube

Body

Cervix

Vagina

Figure 7-67 The uterus is a muscular organ approximately the size of a pear.

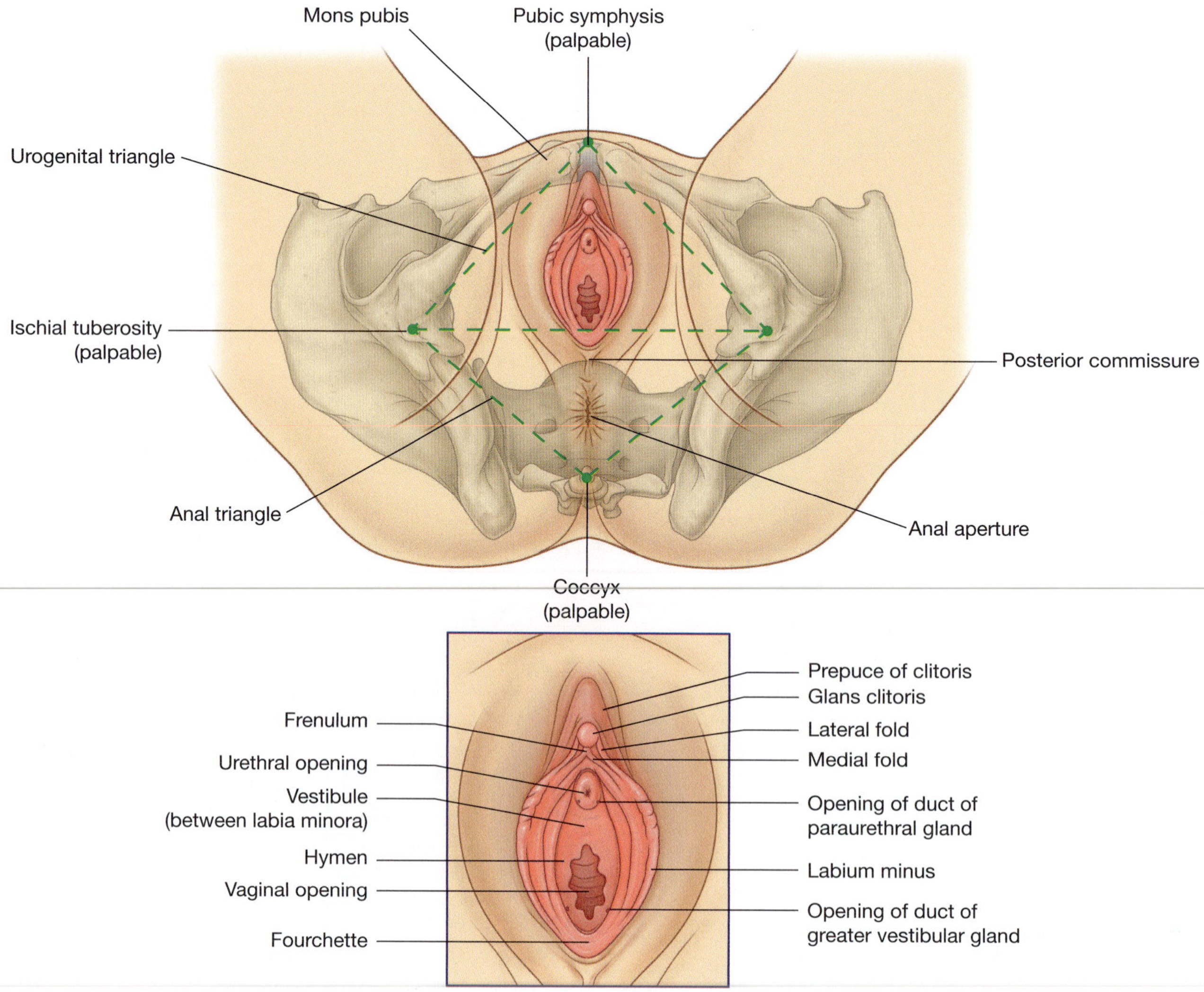

Mons pubis

Pubic symphysis
(palpable)

Urogenital triangle

Ischial tuberosity
(palpable)

Posterior commissure

Anal triangle

Anal aperture

Coccyx
(palpable)

Prepuce of clitoris

Glans clitoris

Frenulum

Lateral fold

Urethral opening

Medial fold

Vestibule
(between labia minora)

Opening of duct of
paraurethral gland

Hymen

Labium minus

Vaginal opening

Opening of duct of
greater vestibular gland

Fourchette

Figure 7-68 External female genitalia.

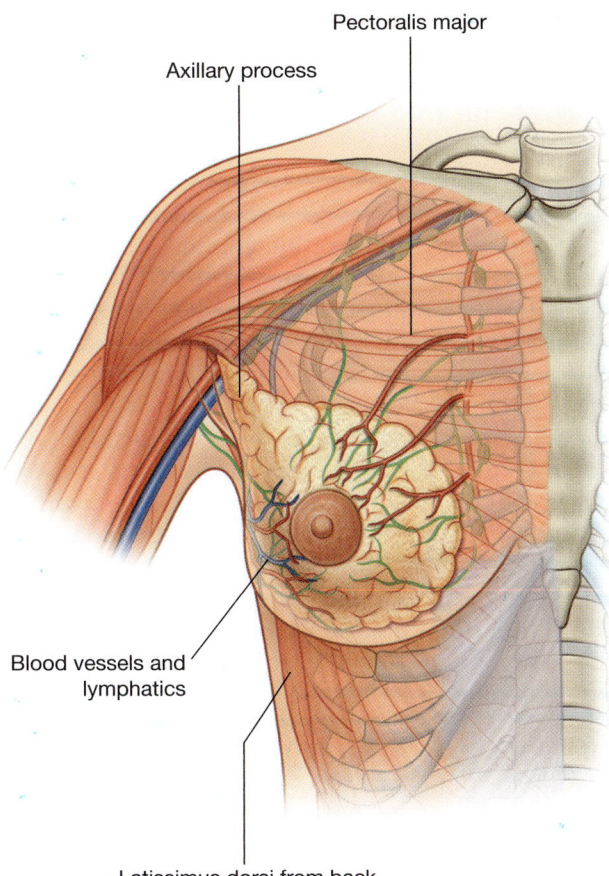

Figure 7-69 Mammary glands are located inside the breast tissue with the blood vessels and lymphatics.

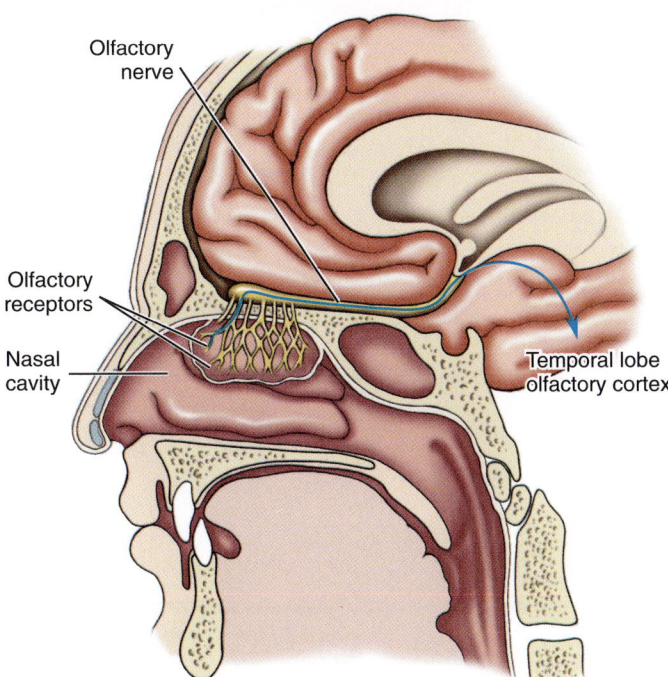

Figure 7-70 Sensations of smell are transmitted from the nasal cavity to the olfactory bulb in the brain.

SPECIAL SENSES

The special senses provide information to the brain about the outside environment.

Olfaction

[OBJECTIVE 67]

The sense of smell **(olfaction)** is controlled by the first cranial nerve (CN I) with nerve fibers that lie in the upper part of the nasal cavity (Figure 7-70). The dendrites of the olfactory neurons extend from the olfactory bulb (in the brain) to the upper part of the nasal cavity. Molecules in the air stimulate these nerve fibers in the nasal cavity. The resulting impulses travel through the olfactory nerves to the olfactory centers in the brain. These centers in the brain interpret these impulses as odors. The nerves are sensitive but fatigue quickly.

Gustation

[OBJECTIVE 68]

The sense of taste **(gustation)** is ruled by parts of the seventh and ninth cranial nerves (CN VII and IX). These nerve fibers are located in taste buds on the surface of the tongue, palate, lips, and throat (although most are located on the tongue) (Figure 7-71). The taste impulses are relayed to the gustation centers in the brain.

Sight

[OBJECTIVE 69]

The sense of sight is conducted by the second cranial nerve (CN II). It is facilitated by the eyes, accessory structures, the optic nerve, and the tracts that conduct the impulses to the brain.

The Eye

The eye is composed of three layers (Figure 7-72). These layers include the fibrous tunic, which consists of the sclera and cornea; the vascular tunic, which consists of the choroids, ciliary body, and the iris; and the nervous tunic, which contains the retina.

1. **The fibrous tunic.** The **sclera** is a firm, opaque, white outer layer of the eye. The sclera helps maintain the shape of the eye. It also serves as an attachment for the muscles that move the eye and is in line with the meningeal layers that extend along the optic nerve. The **cornea** is an avascular, transparent structure that permits light through to the interior of the eye.

2. **The vascular tunic** contains most of the vasculature of the eye. Anteriorly the vascular tunic consists of the ciliary muscles and the iris. The **ciliary body** consists of muscles that change the shape of the lens and a network of capillaries that produce aqueous humor. The **iris** is the colored

part of the eye. It consists of a ring of smooth muscle that surrounds the **pupil,** which is the central opening in the iris. Light enters through the pupil, and the iris controls the size (diameter) of the pupil.

3. The **retina** consists of an outer pigmented area and an inner sensory layer that responds to light. The sensory part of the retina contains cells called **photoreceptor cells.** These photoreceptor cells (rods and cones) relay impulses to the optic nerve. Cones are used for day and color vision, and rods are used for night vision.

The eye is composed of an anterior compartment and a posterior compartment. These compartments are separated by the **lens.** The lens is a transparent, biconvex elastic disc suspended by ligaments. The anterior chamber is filled with **aqueous humor** that maintains **intraocular pressure.** This fluid circulates through the canal of Schlemm. This canal drains from the anterior chamber into the anterior ciliary veins. Because of this circulation the aqueous humor is replaceable. The posterior chamber is filled with a jellylike material called **vitreous humor.** In addition to maintaining the eye's shape, the fluid helps hold the retina in place. Vitreous humor is not replaceable.

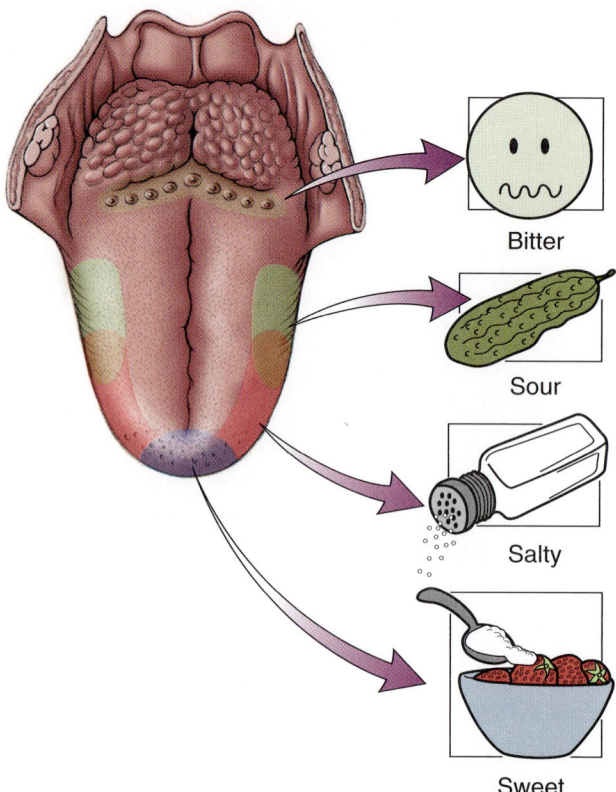

Figure 7-71 The surface of the tongue is sensitive to taste in various regions.

Bitter

Sour

Salty

Sweet

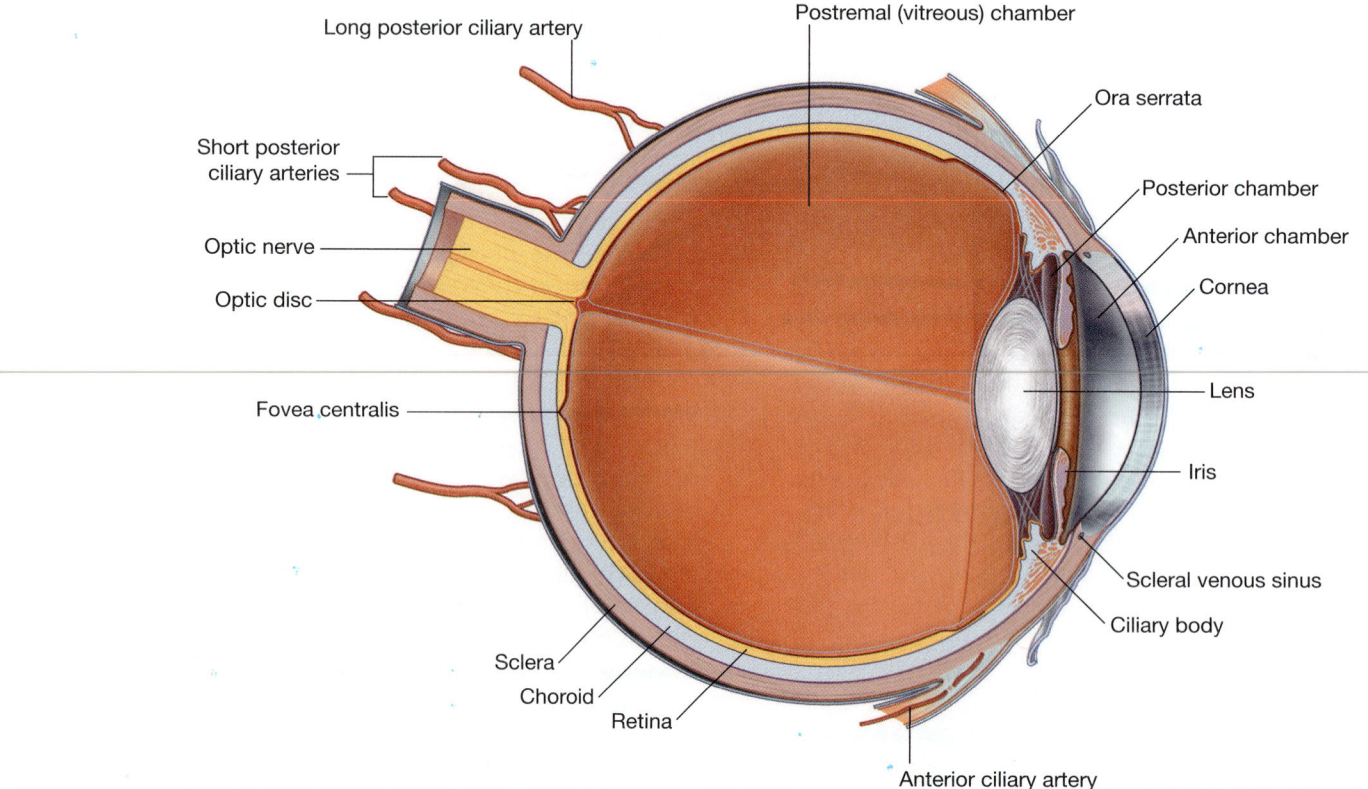

Long posterior ciliary artery

Postremal (vitreous) chamber

Ora serrata

Short posterior ciliary arteries

Posterior chamber

Optic nerve

Anterior chamber

Optic disc

Cornea

Fovea centralis

Lens

Iris

Scleral venous sinus

Ciliary body

Sclera

Choroid

Retina

Anterior ciliary artery

Figure 7-72 The globe-shaped eyeball occupies the anterior part of the orbit.

Accessory Structures

The accessory structures of the eye protect, lubricate, move, and aid in the function of the eye. These structures include the eyebrows, eyelids, conjunctiva, and lacrimal gland.

Eyebrows protect the eyes by providing shade and preventing foreign material (e.g., sweat, dust) from entering the eye from above.

The **eyelids** protect the eyes from foreign objects. Blinking lubricates the eyes by spreading tears over the eye's surface.

The **conjunctiva** is a thin, transparent mucous membrane. It covers the inner surface of the eyelids and the outer surface of the sclera.

The **lacrimal gland** is one of a pair of glands situated superior and lateral to the eye bulb (Figure 7-73). It makes **lacrimal fluid.** This fluid is a watery, slightly alkaline secretion that consists of tears and saline that moisten the conjunctiva. The fluid leaves the gland and covers the surface of the eye by the action of blinking. Lacrimal fluid also contains enzymes that help protect the eye from protein material (e.g., bacteria). Excess fluid is collected at the medial corner of the eye and drains into the nasal cavity through the **nasolacrimal duct.** The nasolacrimal duct is a superficial structure on the outer lateral aspects of the nose. Superficial lacerations to this area can disrupt these ducts, which can lead to life-long problems with the drainage of tears. Patients with injuries to this

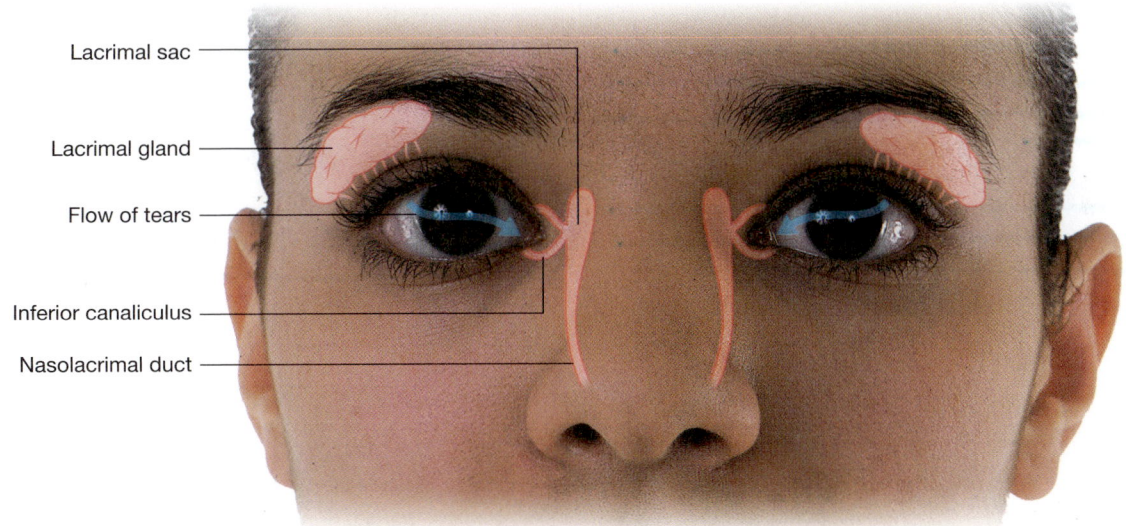

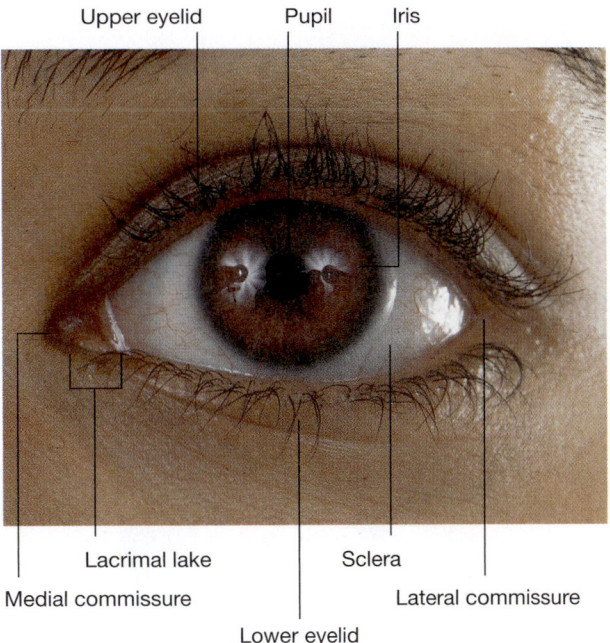

Figure 7-73 Accessory structures of the eye. The accessory structures of the eye include the eyebrows, eyelids, conjunctivae, and lacrimal glands.

area who are not transported should be encouraged to follow-up with a physician to evaluate possible damage to this structure.

Hearing and Balance

[OBJECTIVE 70]

The organs of hearing are divided into three portions: **external, middle,** and **inner ear** (Figure 7-74). The external and middle ear are involved in hearing only. The inner ear functions in both hearing and balance, which occur by way of the eighth cranial nerve (CN VIII).

The external ear includes the **auricle** (pinna) and the **external auditory canal.** The external canal is lined by hair and **ceruminous glands.** These glands produce **cerumen** (earwax). This external canal ends at the **tympanic membrane** (eardrum).

The middle ear is an air-filled chamber within the temporal bone. The middle ear contains the **auditory ossicles.** These are three small bones (malleus, incus, and stapes) that articulate with each other to transmit sound waves to the cochlea.

The inner ear holds the sensory organs for hearing and balance. The inner ear is composed of a series of bony tunnels called the **labyrinth.** This labyrinth is filled with a fluid called **endolymph.**

The external ear's auricle is designed to collect sound waves directed toward the tympanic membrane. Sound waves cause this membrane to vibrate. This vibration is transmitted to the middle ear, causing the ossicles to vibrate. This vibration is transmitted to the inner ear. The bony labyrinth of the inner ear is separated into three areas, the **vestibule,** the **cochlea,** and the **semicircular canals** (Figure 7-75). The vestibule (space or cavity that serves as the entrance to the inner ear) and the semicircular canals (three bony fluid-filled loops) are involved in balance. The cochlea (bony structure resembling a tiny snail shell) contains the organ of hearing, the **organ of Corti.**

BODY ENVIRONMENT

For the cells, tissues, organs, and organ systems to perform their functions efficiently certain parameters must be maintained. These include the amount, distribution, and movement of body fluids; electrolyte balance; and the amount of hydrogen ions, or acid-base balance. Alterations in these items are pathophysiologic.

Distribution of Body Fluids

[OBJECTIVES 71, 72]

The most prevalent fluid in the human body is water. Water accounts for approximately 60% of the total body weight and is an essential part of all the chemical reactions that regularly occur in the body. Patients with

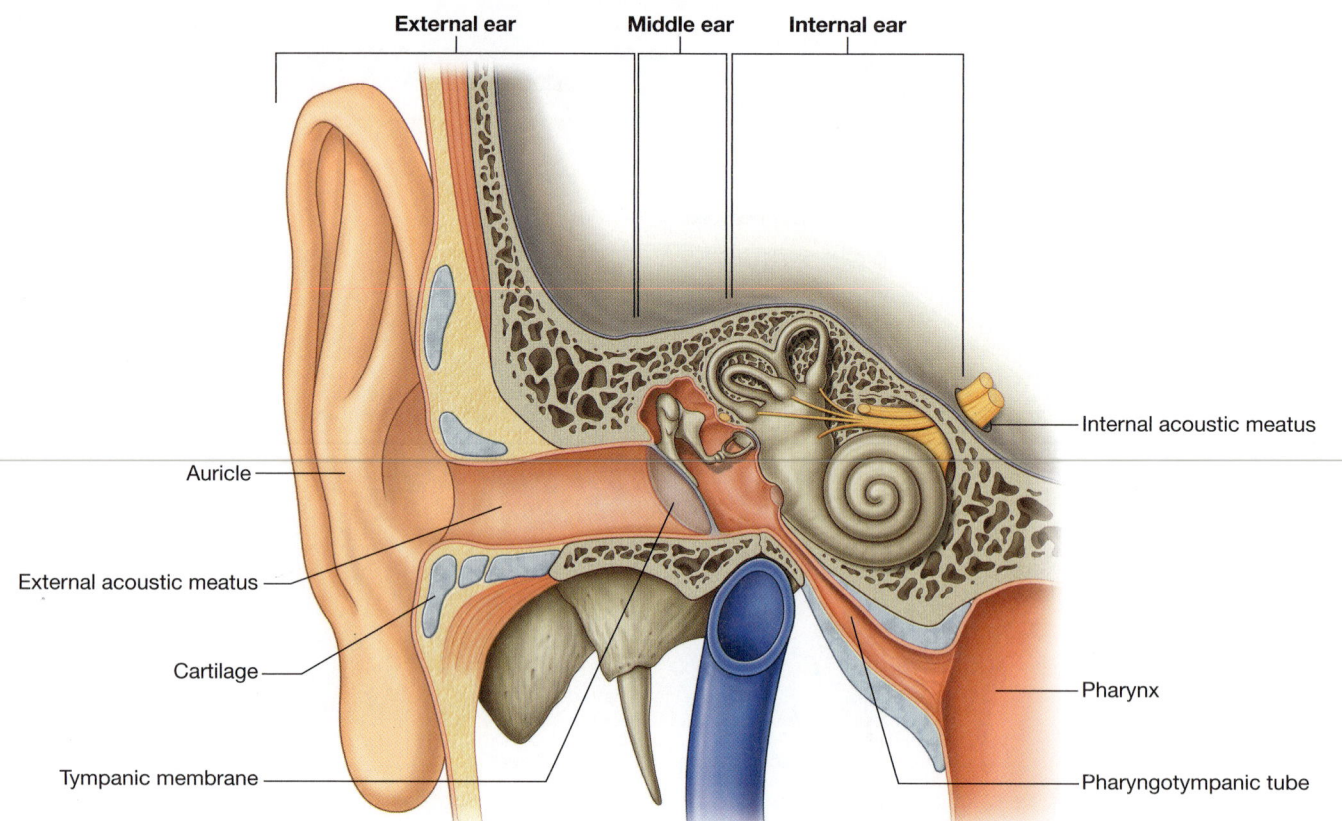

External ear   Middle ear   Internal ear

Internal acoustic meatus

Auricle

External acoustic meatus

Cartilage

Tympanic membrane

Pharynx

Pharyngotympanic tube

Figure 7-74 The organs of hearing are divided into three portions: external, middle, and inner ear.

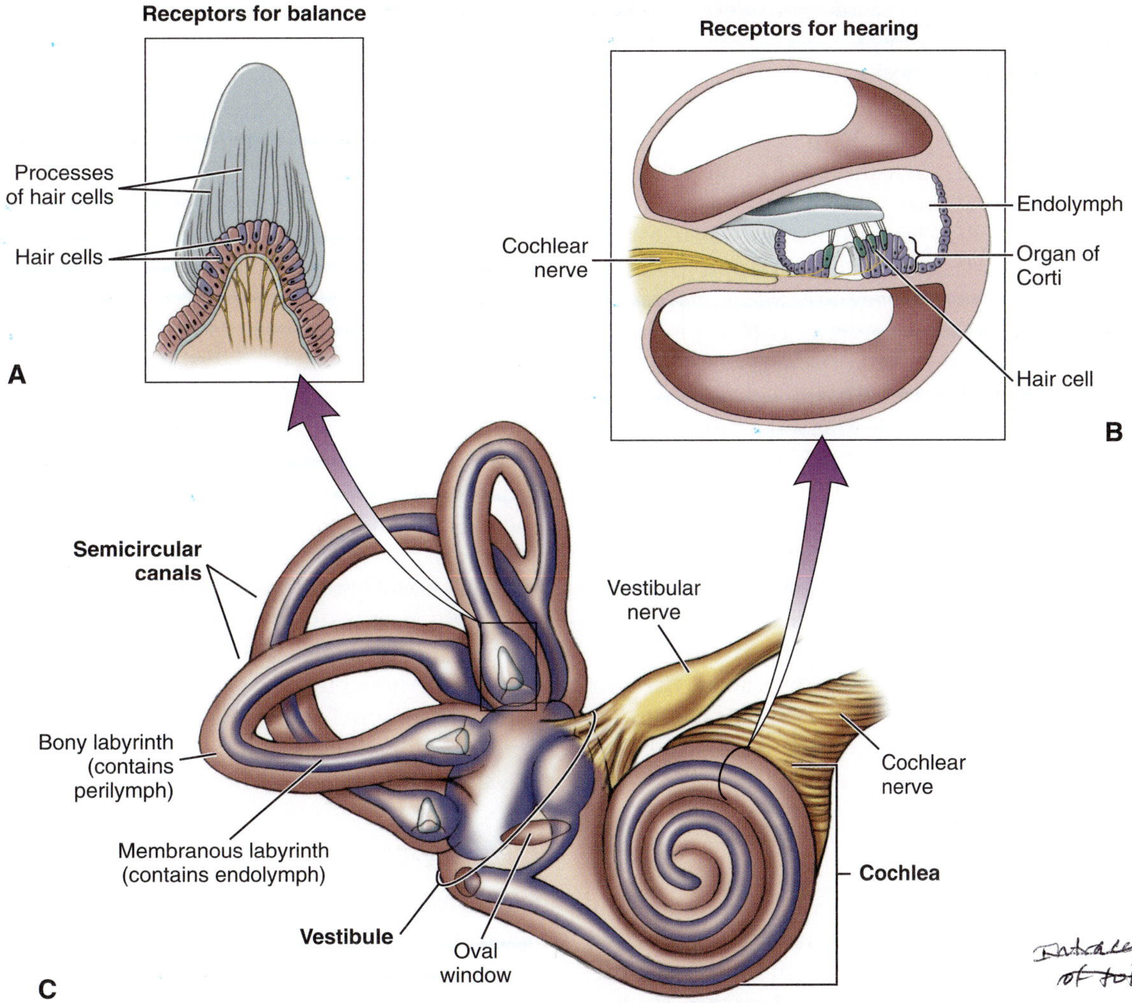

Receptors for balance

Processes of hair cells

Hair cells

A

Receptors for hearing

Cochlear nerve

Endolymph

Organ of Corti

Hair cell

B

Semicircular canals

Vestibular nerve

Bony labyrinth (contains perilymph)

Membranous labyrinth (contains endolymph)

Cochlear nerve

Cochlea

Vestibule

Oval window

C

Intracellular 70% of total body water

Figure 7-75 Inner ear. **A,** Hair cells. **B,** Receptors for hearing. **C,** Structures of the inner ear.

less fluid reserve are more likely to be affected when fluid balance is disrupted. The total amount of fluid in the body at any given time is referred to as **total body water (TBW).** The TBW as a percentage of total body weight decreases with age. This fluid is distributed throughout several compartments in the human body.

The two main classifications of these compartments are **intracellular fluid (ICF)** and **extracellular fluid (ECF).** ICF consists of the fluid found within the cells. This compartment contains approximately 40% of total body weight. The balance is distributed extracellularly between the **intravascular, interstitial,** and **transcellular** compartments (Figure 7-76). The intravascular component is the fluid that is outside cells but inside the circulatory system. The majority of intravascular fluid is plasma, or the fluid component of blood. It accounts for approximately 5% of total body weight. The interstitial component is composed of fluid that is outside cells and the circulatory system, not including the transcellular fluid. It accounts for approximately 15% of total body weight. The transcellular fluid can be classified as extracellular, but it is distinct in that it is formed from the

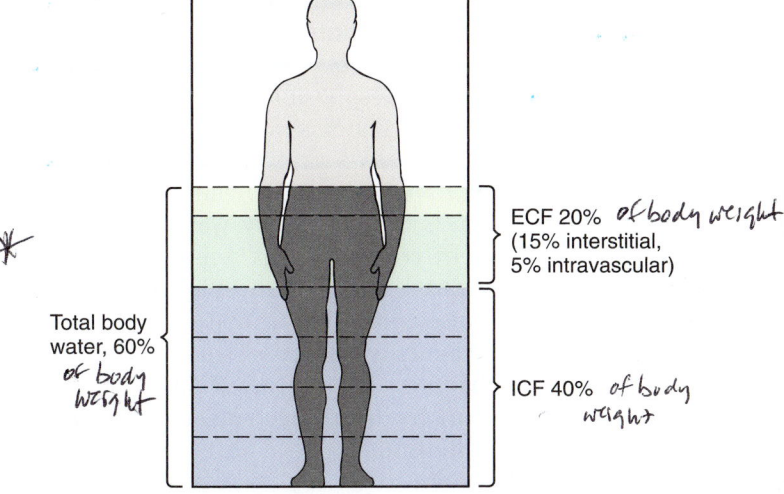

ECF 20% *of body weight*
(15% interstitial, 5% intravascular)

Total body water, 60% *of body weight*

ICF 40% *of body weight*

Figure 7-76 Total body water. *ECF,* Extracellular fluid; *ICF,* intracellular fluid.

interstitial (between cells) - 20-22% of total body water

cell

7% Intravascular

70% Intracellular

100% body water

Renin secreted by kidney → angiotensin I → angiotensin II
Ace Inhibitor (pril)
In stress situation, body can move up to 1L per hour
from interstitial to intravascular space

194 **Chapter 7** Body Systems: Anatomy and Physiology ↓BP

transport activities of cells. Cerebrospinal fluid, bladder urine, the aqueous humor, and the synovial fluid of the joints are considered transcellular (McCance & Huether, 2002). The electrolyte composition of these fluids also is unique and quite different from the rest of the body.

At birth, the total body percentage of fluid is higher than that of an adult at approximately 75% to 80%, with proportionately more ECF in adults. This percentage decreases during the first year of life to approximately 67%. Infants lose body water for physiologic reasons as they adjust to their new environment. This age group is at an increased risk for negative consequences of excessive fluid losses (**dehydration**) because of their greater metabolic rate and higher body surface area. By the time the child reaches adolescence, the TBW drops to 60% to 65%, or normal adult values. This trend continues throughout a person's life. As the body ages and the amount of muscle mass and adipose tissue (fat) changes, the TBW decreases because muscle mass is composed of more water than adipose tissue, which repels water. As individuals age, the amount of muscle mass decreases and the amount of adipose tissue increases. This can lower the TBW to as low as 45% to 55%. This age group also is at risk for deadly consequences from fluid and electrolyte imbalances.

Normal Hydration

The human body tries to maintain a constant level of fluid. To accomplish this ongoing task, the amount of water entering the body must equal the amount of water leaving the body. The process of taking in fluids with the normal daily output is referred to as **hydration.** Hydration is maintained by several mechanisms.

Intake. The average male adult takes in approximately 2400 to 3200 mL of water every day. This water comes from a variety of sources. The most obvious source is from drinking, which usually accounts for approximately 1400 to 1800 mL. The second source of water is through food consumption, which is responsible for approximately another 700 to 1000 mL. Water is pulled from solid food during digestion. The third source of water is through oxidative cellular metabolism, which comprises another 300 to 400 mL. The amount of body water distributed between the different compartments remains relatively constant regardless of the daily variances in the intake or losses of fluid because of the movement of body water between the compartments (discussed below). The body uses several mechanisms to increase TBW. The most important of these are the thirst mechanism, antidiuretic hormone, and aldosterone.

- The **thirst mechanism** is activated by cells in the hypothalamus. These cells, called osmoreceptors, activate when they detect an imbalance in body water, creating the sensation of thirst. As the body is replenished by drinking fluid, the osmoreceptors sense a return to baseline and turn off this mechanism.

secreted by post. pituitary

- **Antidiuretic hormone (ADH)** is released in response to detected loss of body water. This hormone works by preventing further losses of water through the urinary tract. It does this by promoting the reabsorption of water into the blood from the kidney tubules. Reabsorb more Na so reabsorb more water → ↓urine output
- **Aldosterone** is a hormone responsible for the reabsorption of sodium and water from the kidney tubules. When a fluid deficit is detected in the body, aldosterone is released and fluid is then retained at higher levels, raising the TBW.

secreted by kidney

Output. As previously described, the amount of output should roughly equal that of input, approximately 2400 to 3200 mL. Output comes from several sources, including urine, stool, skin, and lungs. Urine is responsible for the largest amount of output, accounting for 1400 to 1800 mL. Urine is made in the kidneys and is used to remove waste. Stool is solid waste produced in the GI tract. It is responsible for approximately 100 mL of fluid output per day. The balance of normal output occurs through insensible losses—water vapor expelled during exhalation, which produces 600 to 800 mL of loss, and perspiration from the skin, which produces 300 to 500 mL of water loss per 24-hour period (see Table 7-1).

Electrolytes

[OBJECTIVES 73, 74]

Electrolytes are substances that dissociate into charged particles when dissolved in water. The ability of the body to perform normal functions, such as nervous impulse transmission, depends on appropriate amounts of these substances being present. A cation is a positively charged electrolyte. The primary cations in the body are sodium (Na^+), potassium (K^+), calcium (Ca^{++}), and magnesium (Mg^{++}). Anions are negatively charged electrolytes. The primary anions in the body are chloride (Cl^-), bicarbonate (HCO_3^-), and phosphate (HPO_4^{3-}). This section provides a brief overview of these substances and their functions. A more detailed discussion of electrolyte imbalances is presented in Chapter 8.

Sodium is the primary extracellular cation, and its normal concentration levels range from 135 to 145 mEq/L. The primary functions of sodium include the regulation of water levels, particularly in the extracellular fluid, and the transmission of nervous impulses. Sodium levels are regulated by the kidneys. When sodium retention is needed, aldosterone is released from the kidneys and antidiuretic hormone from the posterior pituitary gland. Both substances cause the kidneys to retain sodium. If sodium needs to be excreted, the release of these hormones is suppressed.

Potassium is the primary intracellular cation, and its normal concentration levels range from 3.5 to 5.0 mEq/L. The primary roles of potassium are in cardiovascular and neuromuscular function. Potassium also plays a role in the maintenance of normal pH levels by being exchanged for hydrogen ions as needed. Serum potassium levels rise in acidosis and fall in alkalosis. Potassium levels also are maintained by the kidneys, and 80% of the daily excretion of potassium is through the urine.

Calcium is involved in a number of metabolic functions, including muscle contraction, the transmission of nerve impulses, and the growth of bones. Normal calcium levels are 4.5 to 5.5 mEq/L. Calcium is regulated by the release of calcitonin and parathyroid hormones. The kidneys are the primary method of excretion of calcium, filtering up to 10 g/day.

Magnesium is the second most abundant intracellular cation after potassium. The major roles of magnesium include DNA and protein synthesis, the transmission of nervous impulses, and the binding of hormones to receptor sites. Normal magnesium levels are 1.8 to 2.4 mEq/L. Control of magnesium is not well understood; however, the kidneys are the primary regulator of levels.

Chloride plays a primary role in balancing the positive charges of the cations. It also functions in the maintenance of fluid balance and renal function.

Bicarbonate is the principal chemical buffer of the body through the bicarbonate buffer system. It neutralizes hydrogen ions by combining with them to form carbonic acid. Bicarbonate also transports the majority of the carbon dioxide in the venous blood. Normal bicarbonate levels are 22 to 26 mEq/L.

Phosphate plays an important role in the formation of energy bonds and DNA. It also is involved in maintaining normal pH levels through the phosphate buffer system. Phosphate is excreted in the urine and stool.

Acid-Base Balance

[OBJECTIVES 75, 76]

For the body to maintain normal function it must maintain a normal acid-base balance. Acidity is caused by hydrogen ions and is expressed as power of hydrogen, or pH. The pH scale ranges from 0 to 14, with 7.0 being neutral. A pH less than 7 is acidic and a pH greater than 7 is alkalotic, or basic. Because pH is defined as the negative logarithm of the hydrogen concentration, the hydrogen ion concentration changes by a factor of 10 for every unit of change on the pH scale. The normal pH of the blood is 7.35 to 7.45, or slightly basic in nature. For the purposes of medicine a blood pH of less than 7.35 is associated with acidosis and a pH greater than 7.45 is associated with alkalosis. However, some components of the body normally are acidic, such as stomach acid, and some components normally are alkalotic, such as bile. To maintain normal pH levels the body balances both respiratory and metabolic factors to adjust the levels of carbon dioxide (an acid) and bicarbonate ions (a base). Normal carbon dioxide levels are 35 to 45 mm Hg. In situations in which the body retains carbon dioxide, the pH will fall and respiratory acidosis occurs. In situations in which the body eliminates too much carbon dioxide, the pH will rise and respiratory alkalosis occurs. Normal bicarbonate levels are 24 to 26 mEq/L. These ions bind with or dissociate from hydrogen ions in the setting of metabolic acid-base disturbances. In metabolic acidosis the bicarbonate level falls as the ions are bound with hydrogen. In metabolic alkalosis the bicarbonate level rises as carbonic acid is broken into hydrogen ions and bicarbonate ions in an attempt to increase the acid in the body.

Acid-base disorders and compensation are described in detail in Chapter 8. However, in brief, the body compensates for these disorders through three main mechanisms. The fastest response is the bicarbonate buffer system. As described previously, during acidosis bicarbonate ions bind with hydrogen ions to form carbonic acid. This is a weak acid that is easily dissociated into water and carbon dioxide. During alkalosis carbonic acid dissociates into hydrogen and bicarbonate ions. The next response is by the respiratory system, which attempts to eliminate carbon dioxide in metabolic acidosis and retain carbon dioxide in metabolic alkalosis. The final, and slowest, response is by the renal system. Bicarbonate ions are conserved or eliminated as needed to compensate for acidosis or alkalosis. Additional compensatory mechanisms include the phosphate buffer system and the movement of potassium in and out of the cell in exchange for hydrogen ions.

Case Scenario SUMMARY

1. *What anatomic areas of the body may be injured as a result of this collision?* Face, skull, brain, thoracic cavity, limbs, spine.

2. *Which anatomic areas of the body may have life-threatening injuries in this scenario?* Airway, brain injury, bilateral or single femur fractures, and mediastinum injury or insult.

3. *What is the appropriate term for "pale and sweaty"? What is happening in the body to cause it, and what does it mean?* Pallor and diaphoresis best describe "pale and sweaty." These signs are caused by vasoconstriction, a compensatory mechanism for shock and other physiologic insults. Physiologically, vasoconstriction is caused by the release of epinephrine. Practically

Continued

Case Scenario **SUMMARY**—continued

speaking, pallor and diaphoresis are indicators of shock.

4. *Given the broken upper teeth and facial swelling, what body structures may have been injured?* The maxilla (upper jaw) and zygomas (cheekbones).

5. *What is the best way to describe the location of the injury on the left chest?* Injury to the superior chest at the left midclavicular line.

6. *What is the best way to describe the location of the rigidity in the abdomen? What organs are located here?* Bilateral rigidity of the lower quadrants. The large and small intestine, bladder, and (in women) ovaries and uterus are located in the lower quadrants.

7. *What might the instability in the pelvis indicate?* This finding typically indicates a pelvic fracture and the potential for significant internal bleeding.

8. *What is the best way to describe the location of the deformity and injury on the right leg?* Deformity and laceration just proximal to the right medial malleolus.

9. *What is the correct name for the extended arms, pointed toes, and arched back posture the patient assumed? What is its clinical significance?* Decerebrate posturing or abnormal extension. It is a progressive sign of increasing intracranial pressure, occurring after abnormal flexion and before the patient becomes flaccid.

10. *What is the most likely cause of the slowing pulse in this patient?* Increased intracranial pressure, which ultimately was the cause of this patient's death.

Chapter Summary

- The paramedic must understand human anatomy. This understanding will help the paramedic organize a patient assessment by body regions. Mastering the anatomy of the human body also will help the paramedic communicate illness and injury information for the continuity of care for the patients he or she encounters.

- Having an understanding of physiology will help the paramedic predict injury and illness patterns.

- The anatomic position refers to a patient who is standing erect with his or her palms facing the examiner.

- Directional terms are used to discuss the body. Such terms include *superior, inferior, anterior,* and *posterior.* These terms are used to give direction to findings during assessments.

- The appendicular skeleton is composed of the extremities, including the arms, pelvic bones, and legs. The *axial skeleton* refers to the head, neck, thorax, and abdomen.

- The abdomen is divided into four quadrants: upper right, lower right, upper left, and lower left.

- The major cavities of the human body are the ventral and dorsal cavities. These are further divided into subcavities, including the thoracic cavity, the abdominopelvic cavity, the cranial cavity, and the spinal cavity.

- The thoracic cavity contains the trachea, esophagus, thymus, heart, great vessels, lungs, and the cavities and membranes surrounded by them. The abdominopelvic cavity is surrounded by membranes and contains organs and blood vessels.

- The cytoplasm lies between the cytoplasmic membrane and the nucleus. Specialized structures in the cell (organelles) are located in the cytoplasm. These organelles perform jobs that are key to the survival of the cell. The nucleus controls all other organelles in the cytoplasm.

- Most human cells reproduce by a process known as *mitosis*. In this process, cells divide to multiply.

- Four types of tissue comprise the many organs of the body: epithelial, connective, muscle, and nervous. Epithelial tissue covers surfaces and forms structures. Connective tissue is composed of cells separated from each other by intercellular material known as the extracellular matrix. Muscle tissue is contractile tissue and is responsible for movement. The nervous tissue has the ability to conduct electrical signals known as *action potentials*.

- A system is a group of organs arranged to perform a more complex function than any one organ can perform alone. The 10 major organ systems in the body are the integumentary, skeletal, muscular, nervous, endocrine, circulatory (cardiovascular and lymphatic/immune), respiratory, digestive, urinary, and reproductive.

- The integumentary system consists of the skin and accessory structures such as hair, nails, and a variety of glands. It protects the body against injury and dehydration, defends the body against infection, and regulates the body's temperature.

- The skeletal system consists of bone and associated connective tissue, including cartilage, tendons, and ligaments. The skeletal system provides a rigid framework for support and protection. It also provides a system of levers on which muscles act to produce body movements.

- The three primary functions of the muscular system are movement, the maintenance of posture, and the production of heat.
- The nervous and the endocrine systems are the major regulatory and coordinating systems of the body. The nervous system rapidly sends information by means of nerve impulses conducted from one area of the body to another. The endocrine system sends information more slowly by means of chemicals secreted by ductless glands into the bloodstream.
- The heart and cardiovascular system are responsible for circulating blood throughout the body. Blood carries carbon dioxide and waste products away from tissues as well as hormones produced in endocrine glands to their target tissues. Blood regulates temperature, balances fluid, and protects the body from bacteria and foreign substances.
- The lymphatic system is composed of lymph, lymphocytes, lymph nodes, the tonsils, the spleen, and the thymus gland. The lymphatic system has three basic functions: to help maintain fluid balance in tissues, absorb fats and other substances from the digestive tract, and assist the immune defense system of the body.
- The organs of the respiratory system and the cardiovascular system move oxygen to cells. They move carbon dioxide from cells to where it is released into the air. The respiratory system begins at the nasal cavity, with the nasopharynx, oropharynx, laryngopharynx, and larynx. The glottis is located at the lower airway, which leads to the lungs and consists of the trachea, the bronchial tree, the alveoli, and the lungs.
- The digestive system provides the body with water, electrolytes, and other nutrients needed to ensure the best use of the body's cells. Associated accessory organs (mainly glands) secrete fluid into the digestive tract.
- The urinary system works with other body systems to maintain homeostasis. It does this by removing waste products from the blood and helping maintain a constant body fluid volume and composition. The structures of the urinary system include two kidneys, two ureters, the urinary bladder, and the urethra.
- The purpose of the male reproductive system is to make and transfer spermatozoa to the female. The purpose of the female reproductive system is to make oocytes and receive the spermatozoa for fertilization, conception, gestation, and birth.
- The male reproductive system consists of the testes, epididymis, ductus deferens, urethra, seminal vesicles, prostate gland, bulbourethral glands, scrotum, and penis. The female reproductive organs consist of the ovaries, uterine/fallopian tubes, uterus, vagina, external genital organs, and mammary glands.
- The senses provide the brain with information about the outside world. Four senses are recognized as special senses: smell, taste, sight, and hearing and balance.

SUGGESTED RESOURCES

Herlihy, B. (2007). *The human body in health and illness* (3rd ed.). St. Louis: Mosby.

Thibodeau, G. B., & Patton, K. T. (2007). *Anatomy and physiology* (6th ed.). St. Louis: Mosby.

Chapter Quiz

1. The layer of skin that contains nerve endings is the _____.

2. Water accounts for what percent of total body weight?

3. The difference in concentration between solutions on opposite sides of a semipermeable membrane is called _____.

4. The organ system that virtually controls all body functions is the _____ system.

5. As the thoracic cavity begins to expand, the intrathoracic pressure will _____.

6. Physiologically, the term respiration refers to _____.

7. When swallowing, the structure that occludes the tracheal opening to prevent aspiration of food and liquids is the _____.

8. The relative shortness of the _____ in the female and its proximity to the vaginal canal enable bacteria to enter the bladder easily.

9. The _____ is a series of tubes located in the posterior portion of the scrotum.

10. The trachea divides into the right and left mainstem bronchi at the _____.

11. What is the purpose of the cervical spine?

12. The largest portion of the brain, which provides for consciousness and higher mental functions, is the _____.

13. Minute volume is best described as _____.

Chapter Quiz—continued

14. The skeletal muscles that provide for voluntary movement are controlled by the _____.

15. The release of the neurotransmitter acetylcholine results in ____.

16. An increase in carbon dioxide production will trigger an increase in _____.

17. The structure that filters blood into a nephron is the _____.

18. The anterior-most organ in the pelvis of men and women is the _____.

19. The exchange of gases between a living organism and its environment is called _____.

Terminology

Absorption Movement of small organic molecules, electrolytes, vitamins, and water across the digestive tract and into the circulatory system. Also, the movement of a drug from the site of input into the circulation.

Acid Fluid produced in the stomach; breaks down the food material within the stomach into chime.

Adenosine triphosphate (ATP) Formed from metabolism of nutrients in the cell; serves as energy sources throughout the body.

Adipose, or fat, connective tissue Tissue that stores lipids; acts as an insulator and protector of the organs of the body.

Afferent division Nerve fibers that send impulses from the periphery to the CNS.

Alveoli Functional units of the respiratory system; area in the lungs where the majority of gas exchange takes place; singular form is alveolus.

Amylase Enzyme in pancreatic juice.

Anal canal Area between the rectum and the anus.

Anatomic plane The relation of internal body structures to the surface of the body; imaginary straight line divisions of the body.

Anatomic position The position of a person standing erect with his or her feet and palms facing the examiner.

Anatomy Study of the body's structure and organization.

Anterior The front, or ventral, surface.

Anus The end of the anal canal.

Aorta Delivers blood from the left ventricle of the heart to the body.

Aortic valve Semilunar valve on the left of the heart; separates the left ventricle from the aorta.

Apex Tip of the heart.

Apocrine glands Sweat glands that open into hair follicles, including in and around the genitalia, axillae, and anus; secrete an organic substance (which is odorless until acted upon by surface bacteria) into the hair follicles.

Appendicular skeleton Consists of all the bones not within the axial skeleton: upper and lower extremities, the girdles, and their attachments.

Appendix Accessory structure of the cecum.

Aqueous humor Fluid that fills the anterior chamber of the eye; maintains intraocular pressure.

Arachnoid mater Second layer of the meninges.

Areolar connective tissue A loose tissue found in most organs of the body; consists of weblike collagen, reticulum, and elastin fibers.

Arrector pili Smooth muscle that surrounds each follicle; responsible for "goose bumps," which pull the hair upward.

Arterioles Small arterial vessels that supply oxygenated blood to the capillaries.

Ascending colon Part of the large intestine.

Atria Two receiving chambers of the heart; singular form is atrium.

Atrial kick Remaining 20% to 30% of blood forced into the right ventricle during atrial contraction.

Atrioventricular node (AV node) A group of cells that conduct an electrical impulse through the heart; located in the floor of the right atrium immediately behind the tricuspid valve and near the opening of the coronary sinus.

Auditory ossicles Three small bones (malleus, incus, and stapes) that articulate with each other to transmit sounds waves to the cochlea.

Auricle Also called the *pinna*; outer ear.

Autonomic nervous system Provides unconscious control of smooth muscle organ and glands.

Axial skeleton Made up of the skull, hyoid bone, vertebral column, and thoracic cage.

Base Top of the heart.

Bicuspid valve Left atrioventricular valve in the heart; also called the mitral valve.

Bile salts Manufactured in the liver; composed of electrolytes and iron recovered from red blood cells when they die.

Blood Liquid connective tissue; allows transport of nutrients, oxygen, and waste products.

Bone Hard connective tissue; consists of living cells and a matrix made of minerals.

Bowman's capsule Located in the renal corpuscle.

Brainstem Part of the brain that connects it to the spinal cord; responsible for many of the autonomic functions the body requires to survive (also called vegetative functions).

Bronchioles Smallest of the air passages.

Bulbourethral glands Pair of small glands that manufacture a mucous-type secretion that unites with the prostate fluid and spermatozoa to form sperm.

Bundle of His Fibers located in the upper portion of the interventricular septum; connects the AV node with the right and left bundle branches.

Capacitance vessels Venules; have the capability of holding large amounts of volume.

Capillaries Tiny vessels that connect arterioles to venules; deliver blood to each cell in the body.

Cardiac sphincter Circular muscle that controls the movement of material into the stomach.

Carina Area in the bronchial tree that separates into the right and left mainstem bronchi.

Cartilage Connective tissue composed of chondrocytes; exact makeup depends on the location and function in the body.

Cartilaginous joints Unite two bones by means of hyaline cartilage or fibrocartilage.

Caudal A position toward the distal end of the body; usually inferior.

Cecum First segment of the large intestine; appendix is its accessory structure.

Central nervous system (CNS) The brain and spinal cord.

Centrioles Paired, rodlike structures that exist in a specialized area of the cytoplasm known as the centrosome.

Centrosome Specialized area of the cytoplasm; plays an important role in the process of cell division.

Cephalic A position toward the head; usually superior.

Cerebellum Area of the brain involved in fine and gross coordination; responsible for interpretation of actual movement and correction of any movements that interfere with coordination and the body's position.

Cerebrospinal fluid Fluid that bathes, protects, and nourishes the central nervous system.

Cerebrum Largest part of the brain; divided into right and left hemispheres.

Cerumen Earwax.

Ceruminous glands Glands lining the external auditory canal; produce cerumen or earwax.

Cervix Inferior portion of the uterus.

Chordae tendineae Fibrous bands of tissue in the valves that attach to each part or cusp of the valve.

Choroid plexus Group of specialized cells in the ventricles of the brain; filters blood through cerebral capillaries to create the cerebrospinal fluid.

Chyme Semifluid mass of partly digested food expelled by the stomach into the duodenum.

Ciliary body Consists of muscles that change the shape of the lens in the eye; includes a network of capillaries that produce aqueous humor.

Clitoris Small, erectile structure at the entrance to the vagina.

Cochlea Bony structure in the inner ear resembling a tiny snail shell.

Conception The act or process of fertilization; beginning of pregnancy.

Conducting arteries Large arteries of the body (e.g., aorta and the pulmonary trunk); have more elastic tissue and less smooth muscle; stretch under great pressures and then quickly return back to their original shapes.

Conjunctiva Thin, transparent mucous membrane that covers the inner surface of the eyelids and the outer surface of the sclera.

Connective tissue Most abundant type of tissue in the body; composed of cells that are separated by a matrix.

Contractility Ability to shorten in length actively.

Cornea Avascular, transparent structure that permits light through to the interior of the eye.

Coronary sinus Venous drain for the coronary circulation into the right atrium.

Cricoid cartilage Most inferior cartilage of the larynx; only complete ring in the larynx.

Cytoplasm Fluid-like material in which the organelles are suspended; lies between the plasma membrane and the nucleus.

Cytoplasmic membrane Encloses the cytoplasm and its organelles; forms the outer border of the cell.

Daughter cells Two cells that result from mitosis.

Deoxyribonucleic acid (DNA) Specialized structure within the cell that carries genetic material for reproduction.

Dermis Located below the epidermis and consists mainly of connective tissue containing both collagen and elastin fibers; contains specialized nervous tissue that provides sensory information, pain, pressure, touch, and temperature, to the CNS; also contains hair follicles, sweat and sebaceous glands, and a large network of blood vessels.

Descending colon Part of the large intestine.

Diaphragm Muscle that separates the thoracic cavity from the abdominal cavity.

Diaphysis Shaft of the bone where marrow is found that forms red and white blood cells.

Diastole When the ventricles of the heart relax and fill with blood.

Diencephalon Portion of the brain between the brainstem and cerebrum; contains the thalamus and hypothalamus and the temperature regulatory centers for the body.

Differentiation Process of cell maturation.

Digestion Chemical breakdown of food material into smaller fragments that can be absorbed into the circulatory system.

Digestive tract Series of muscular tubes designed to move food and liquid.

Distal A position farther from the attachment of a limb to the trunk.

Distributing arteries Blood vessels that have well-defined adventitia layers and larger amounts of smooth muscle; capable of altering blood flow.

Dorsal Referring to the back of the body; posterior.

Ductus deferens Also known as *vas deferens;* tubes that extend from the end of the epididymis and through the seminal vesicles.

Duodenum First part of the small intestine; has important accessory structures that help digest various types of nutrients.

Dura mater Toughest layer of the meninges; top layer.

Efferent division Nerve fibers that send impulses from the central nervous system to the periphery.

Elasticity Ability of muscle to rebound toward its original length after contraction.

Endocrine gland Where hormones are manufactured.

Endolymph Fluid that fills the labyrinth.

Endoplasmic reticulum (ER) Chain of canals or sacs that wind through the cytoplasm.

Epidermis The outermost layer of the skin; made of tightly packed epithelial cells.

Epididymis Convoluted series of tubes located in the posterior portion of the scrotum; final maturation of sperm occurs here.

Epidural space Potential area above the dura mater; contains arterial vessels.

Epiphysis Either end of the bone where bone growth occurs during the developmental years.

Epithelial tissue Covers most of the internal and external surfaces of the body.

Erythrocytes Red blood cells.

Esophagus Tube surrounded by smooth muscle that propels material into the stomach.

Excitability Ability to respond to a stimulus.

Excretion Removal of waste products from the body.

Extensibility Ability to continue to contract over a range of lengths.

External anal sphincter Muscle under voluntary control that allows a controlled bowel movement.

External auditory canal Tube from the external ear to the middle ear; lined with hair and ceruminous glands.

External ear Includes the auricle and external auditory canal.

External urinary sphincter Ring of smooth muscle in the urethra under voluntary control.

Extracellular Outside the cell or cytoplasmic membrane.

Eyebrows Protect the eyes by providing shade and preventing foreign material (e.g., sweat, dust) from entering the eyes from above.

Eyelids Protect the eyes from foreign objects.

Fibrous connective tissue Composed of bundles of strong, white collagenous fibers (protein) in parallel rows; tendons and ligaments are composed of this type of tissue; relatively strong and inelastic.

Fibrous joints Two bones united by fibrous tissue that have little or no movement.

Fibrous tunic Layer of the eye that contains the sclera and the cornea.

Follicle Small, tubelike structure in which hair grows; contains a small cluster of cells known as the hair papilla.

Follicles Vesicles within the cortex of the ovary.

Fontanelles Membranous spaces at the juncture of an infant's cranial bones that later ossify.

Foramen Open passage.

Formed elements Located in the bloodstream; erythrocytes, leukocytes, and thrombocytes, or platelets.

Frontal lobe Section of cerebrum important in voluntary motor function and the emotions of aggression, motivation, and mood.

Frontal plane Imaginary straight line that divides the body into anterior (ventral) and posterior (dorsal) sections.

Fundus Superior aspect of the uterus.

Glomerulus Network of capillaries in the renal corpuscle.

Golgi apparatus Substance that concentrates and packages material for secretion out of the cell.

Gomphoses Joint in which a peg fits into a socket.

Great vessels Large vessels that carry blood to and from the heart; superior and inferior venae cavae, pulmonary veins, aorta, and pulmonary trunk.

Gustation Sense of taste.

Hair papilla Small cluster of cells within a follicle; growth of hair starts in this cluster of cells, which is hidden in the follicle.

Heartbeat Organized mechanical action of the heart.

Hemopoietic tissue Connective tissue found in the marrow cavities of bones (mainly long bones).

Hepatic artery The artery that supplies the liver with blood and nutrients from the circulatory system.

Hepatic duct Connects the gallbladder to the liver; secretes bile into the gallbladder.

Hilum Point of entry for bronchial vessels, bronchi, and nerves in each lung.

Homeostasis A state of equilibrium in the body with respect to functions and composition of fluids and tissues.

Hormones Chemicals within the body that reach every cell through the circulatory system.

Ileum Last segment of the small intestine; area of decreased absorption where chyme is prepared for entry into the large intestine.

Inferior Toward the feet; below a point of reference in the anatomic position.

Inferior vena cava Vessels that return venous blood from the lower part of the body to the right atrium.

Ingestion Process of bringing food into the digestive tract.

Inner ear Holds the sensory organs for hearing and balance.

Integumentary system The largest organ system in the body, consisting of the skin and accessory structures (e.g., hair, nails, glands).

Interatrial septum Septum dividing the atria in the heart.

Internal anal sphincter Muscle under autonomic control; has stretch receptors that provide the sensation of the need to defecate.

Internal urinary sphincter Ring of smooth muscle in the urethra that is under autonomic control.

Interventricular septum Septum dividing the ventricles in the heart.

Intracellular Inside of the cell or cytoplasmic membrane.

Intraperitoneal Abdominopelvic organs surrounded by the peritoneum.

Iris Colored part of the eye; ring of smooth muscle that surrounds the pupil; controls the size (diameter) of the pupil.

Jejunum Second part of the small intestine; major site of nutrient absorption.

Labyrinth Series of bony tunnels inside the inner ear.

Lacrimal fluid Watery, slightly alkaline secretion that consists of tears and saline that moisten the conjunctiva.

Lacrimal gland One of a pair of glands situated superior and lateral to the eye bulb; secretes lacrimal fluid.

Large intestine Organ where a large amount of water and electrolytes is absorbed; also where undigested food is concentrated into feces.

Larynx Lies between the pharynx and the lungs; outer case of nine cartilages that protect and support the vocal cords.

Lateral A position away from the midline of the body.

Lateral recumbent Lying on either the right or left side.

Left A position toward the left side of the body.

Left coronary artery Vessel that supplies oxygenated blood to the left side of the heart muscle.

Lens Transparent, biconvex elastic disc suspended by ligaments.

Leukocytes White blood cells.

Limbic system The part of the brain involved in mood, emotions, and the sensation of pain and pleasure.

Liver Largest internal organ in the body; serves as a major detoxifier in the body.

Lungs Organs that allow for the mechanical movement of air to and from the respiratory membrane.

Lymph Fluid within the lymphatic system.

Lymphatic system The network of vessels, ducts, nodes, valves, and organs involved in protecting and maintaining the internal fluid environment of the body; part of the circulatory system.

Lymphatic vessels Unidirectional tubes that carry fluid or lymph within the lymphatic system.

Lysosomes Membrane-walled structures that contain enzymes.

Mammary glands Female organs of milk production; located within the breast tissue.

Matrix Nonliving material that separates cells in the connective tissue.

Mechanical processing Physical manipulation and breakdown of food.

Medial A position toward the midline of the body.

Mediastinum Area that includes the trachea, esophagus, thymus gland, heart, and great vessels.

Medulla Most inferior part of the brainstem; responsible for some vegetative functions.

Meninges Covering of the brain and spinal cord; layers include the dura mater, arachnoid, and pia mater.

Merocrine glands Sweat glands that open directly to the surface of the body; produce a fluid (mainly water) when the temperature rises that allows the body to dispel large amounts of heat through the evaporation process.

Mesentery Layers of connective tissue found in the peritoneal cavity.

Micturition Urination.

Midbrain Section of the brainstem involved in hearing and visual reflexes as well as coordination of motor activity and muscular tone; contains reticular activating system.

Middle ear Air-filled chamber within the temporal bone; contains the auditory ossicles.

Mitochondria Power plant of the cell and body; site of aerobic oxidation.

Mitosis Process of division and multiplication in which one cell divides into two cells.

Mitral valve Left atrioventricular valve in the heart; also called the bicuspid valve.

Muscle tissue Contractile tissue that is the basis of movement.

Nasolacrimal duct Opening at the medial corner of the eye that drains excess fluid into the nasal cavity.

Terminology—continued

Nephron Functional unit of the kidney.

Nervous tissue Tissue that can conduct electrical impulses.

Neuroglia Supporting cells of nervous tissue; functions include nourishment, protection, and insulation.

Neurons Conducting cells of nervous tissue; composed of cell body, dendrites, and axon.

Nuclear membrane Membrane in the cell that surrounds the nucleus.

Nucleoplasm Protoplasm of the nucleus as contrasted with that of the cell.

Nucleus Area within a cell where the genetic material is stored.

Occipital lobe Section of cerebrum that is the center for vision.

Olfactory tissue Located within the nasopharynx; contains receptors that enable the ability of smell (olfaction).

Oocyte The female gamete; product of the female reproductive system.

Oogenesis Egg production.

Oral cavity First part of the gastrointestinal tract; includes salivary glands, teeth, and tongue.

Organ A structure composed of two or more kinds of tissues organized to perform a more complex function than any one tissue alone can.

Organ of Corti Organ of hearing located in the cochlea.

Organelles Numerous structures within the cell.

Oropharynx Starts at the uvula; back of the oral cavity that extends down to the epiglottis.

Ovarian medulla Inner portion of the ovary.

Ovaries Site of egg production in females.

Papillary muscles Muscles attached to the chordae tendineae of the heart valves and the ventricular muscle of the heart.

Parasympathetic nervous system The subdivision of the autonomic nervous system usually involved in activating vegetative functions, such as digestion, defecation, and urination.

Parietal lobe Section of the cerebrum responsible for the integration of most sensory information from the body.

Parietal pleura Lining of the pleural cavity attached tightly to the interior of the chest cage.

Pathophysiology Functional changes that accompany a particular syndrome or disease.

Penis Male sex organ; has three columns of erectile tissue; transfers sperm during copulation.

Pericardial cavity The potential space between the two layers of the pericardium.

Pericardium Two-layer serous membrane lining the pericardial cavity.

Peripheral nervous system All of the nerves outside of the central nervous system.

Peritoneal cavity The space between the parietal and visceral peritoneum; also called the *peritoneal space*.

Peritoneum Double-layered serous membrane that lines the abdominal cavity and covers the organs located in the abdominopelvic cavity.

Photoreceptor cells Rods and cones contained in the sensory part of the retina; relay impulses to the optic nerve.

Physiology Study of how the body functions.

Pia mater Last meningeal layer; adheres to the central nervous system.

Plasma Pale, yellow material in the blood; made of approximately 92% water and 8% dissolved molecules.

Plasma membrane The outer covering of a cell that contains the cellular cytoplasm; also known as the *cell membrane*.

Platelets One of three formed elements in the blood; also called *thrombocytes*.

Pleura Serous membrane that lines the pleural cavity.

Pleural cavities Areas that contain the lungs.

Pons Area of the brainstem that contains the sleep and respiratory centers for the body, which along with the medulla control breathing.

Portal vein A vein is composed of a group of vessels that originate from the digestive system.

Posterior The back, or dorsal, surface.

Precapillary sphincters Smooth muscle located at the entrances to the capillaries; responsive to local tissue needs.

Prone Position in which the patient is lying on his or her stomach (face down).

Prostate Glandular tissue that produces prostatic fluid and muscular portion that contracts during ejaculation to prevent urine flow; dorsal to the symphysis pubis and the base of the urinary bladder.

Proximal A position nearer to the attachment of a limb to the trunk.

Pulmonary circulation Blood from the right ventricle is pumped directly to the lungs for oxygenation through the pulmonary trunk; blood becomes oxygenated and then is delivered through the pulmonary arteries for the left atrium.

Pulmonary trunk Vessels that deliver blood from the right ventricle of the heart to the lungs for oxygenation.

Pulmonary veins Vessels that return blood to the left atrium of the heart.

Pulmonic valve Right semilunar valve; separates the right ventricle and the pulmonary trunk.

Pupil Central opening in the iris.

Purkinje fibers Fibers found in both ventricles that conduct an electrical impulse through the heart.

Rectum End of the sigmoid colon; feces are further compacted into waste here.

Regurgitation Backward flow of blood through a valve during ventricular contraction of the heart.

Renal corpuscle Large terminal end of the nephron.

Renal pyramids Number of divisions in the kidney.

Respiratory membrane Where gas exchange takes place; oxygen is picked up in the bloodstream and carbon dioxide is eliminated through the lungs.

Respiratory tract Passages to move air to and from the exchange surfaces.

Reticular activating system Group of specialized neurons in the brainstem; involved in sleep and wake cycles; maintains consciousness.

Retina Outer pigmented area and inner sensory layer that responds to light.

Retroperitoneal Abdominopelvic organs found behind the peritoneum.

Ribonucleic acid (RNA) Specialized structures within the cell that carry genetic material for reproduction.

Ribosome Substance in organelle where new protein is synthesized; forms the framework for the genetic blueprint.

Right A position toward the right side of the body.

Right coronary artery Blood vessel that provides oxygenated blood to the right side of the heart muscle.

Sagittal plane Imaginary straight line that runs vertically through the middle of the body, creating right and left halves.

Saliva Mucus that lubricates material like food that is placed in it; enzymes begin the digestive process of starchy material.

Salivary glands Located in the oral cavity; produce saliva.

Sclera Firm, opaque, white outer layer of the eye; helps maintain the shape of the eye.

Scrotum Loose layer of connective tissue that support the testes.

Sebaceous glands Found in the dermis; secrete oil (sebum) in the shaft of the hair follicle and the skin.

Sebum Oil secreted by the sebaceous glands in the shaft of the hair follicle and the skin; prevents excessive drying of the skin and hair; also serves to protect from some forms of bacteria.

Secretion Release of water, acids, enzymes, and buffers that aid in the breakdown and digestion of food in the digestive tract.

Semicircular canals Three bony fluid-filled loops in the internal ear; involved in balance of the body.

Semilunar valves Valves separating the ventricles of the heart from the associated great vessels (e.g., pulmonary trunk and aorta).

Seminal fluid Liquid produced in the seminal vesicles.

Seminal vesicles Ducts that produce seminal fluids.

Septum Tough piece of tissue that divides the left and right halves of the heart.

Serous membrane Membrane that lines the thoracic, abdominal, and pelvic cavities; composed of the parietal membrane, which adheres to the cavity wall, and the visceral membrane, which adheres to the organ.

Sigmoid colon Part of the large intestine.

Sinoatrial node Pacemaker site of the heart; where impulse formation begins in the heart.

Sinuses Cavities within the bones of the skull that connect to the nasal cavity.

Sodium bicarbonate Neutralizes hydrochloric acid from the stomach.

Somatic nervous system Division of the peripheral nervous system whose motor nerves control movement of voluntary muscles.

Sperm Mucuslike secretion made of prostatic fluid and spermatozoa.

Spermatic cord Nerves, blood vessels, and smooth muscle that surround the vas (ductus) deferens.

Spermatogenesis Spermatozoa formation.

Spermatozoa Product of the male reproductive system.

Sphincters Smooth muscles that regulate flow through the capillary beds.

Spinal cord Part of the central nervous system that connects the brain to the periphery of the body; contains the main reflex centers of the body.

Stomach Organ located at the inferior end of the esophagus; large storage vessel surrounded by multiple layers of smooth muscle; cells within it produce acid.

Subcutaneous tissue Thick layer of connective tissue found between the layers of the skin; composed of adipose tissue and areolar tissue; insulates, protects, and stores energy (in the form of fat).

Subdural space Area below the dura mater; contains large venous vessels, drains, and a small amount of serous fluid.

Superior Situated above or higher than a point of reference in the anatomic position; top.

Superior vena cava Vessel that returns venous blood from the upper part of the body to the right atrium of the heart.

Supine Position in which the patient is lying on his or her back (face up).

Surfactant Specialized cells within each alveolus that keep it from collapsing when little or no air is inside.

Sutures Seams between flat bones.

Sweat glands Odor-forming glands in the body; two types are merocrine and apocrine.

Sympathetic nervous system Division of the autonomic nervous system that prepares the body for stress or the classic fight-or-flight response.

Symphysis Cartilaginous joint; unites two bones by means of fibrocartilage.

Terminology—continued

Synchondroses Cartilaginous joint; unites the bones by means of hyaline cartilage.

Syndesmosis Joint in which the bones are united by fibrous, connective tissue forming an intraosseous membrane or ligament.

Synovial joint Freely movable; enclosed by a capsule and synovial membrane.

System At least two kinds of organs organized to perform a more complex task than can a single organ.

Systole Contraction of the ventricles of the heart that causes the ejection of blood.

Teeth Provide mastication of food products in preparation for entry into the stomach.

Temporal lobe Section of the cerebrum that receives and evaluates smell and auditory input; plays a key role in memories.

Testes Male reproductive organs suspended within the scrotum.

Testosterone Male hormone secreted within the testes.

Thrombocytes One of three formed elements in the blood; also known as *platelets*.

Tongue Muscular organ that provides for the sensation of taste; also directs food material toward the esophagus.

Trachea Air passage that connects the larynx to the lungs.

Transverse colon Part of the large intestine.

Transverse plane Imaginary straight line that divides the body into top (superior) and bottom (inferior) sections; also known as the horizontal plane.

Tricuspid valve Right atrioventricular valve of the heart.

Tunica adventitia Outermost layer of the blood vessel; made of mainly elastic connective tissue; allows the vessel to expand to great pressure or volume.

Tunica intima Innermost layer of the blood vessel; composed of a single layer of epithelial cells; provides almost no resistance to blood flow.

Tunica media Middle layer of the blood vessel; mainly composed of smooth muscle; functions to alter the diameter of the lumen of the vessel; under autonomic control, which enables the body to adjust blood flow quickly to meet immediate needs.

Tunics Layers of an elastic tissue and smooth muscle in the blood vessels.

Tympanic membrane Eardrum.

Ureter Tube that drains urine from the kidney to the bladder.

Urethra Passageway for both urine and male reproductive fluids; opening at the end of the bladder.

Urinary bladder Hollow organ that stores urine; surrounded by smooth muscle.

Urinary system Eliminates dissolved organic waste products by urine production and elimination.

Uterine tubes Also known as *fallopian tubes*; extend from each side of the superior end of the body of the uterus to the lateral pelvic wall; pick up egg released by ovary and transport it to the uterus.

Uterus Muscular organ about the size of a pear; grows with the developing fetus.

Vagina Female organ of copulation; extends from the cervix to the outside of the body.

Vas deferens Also known as *ductus deferens*; tubes that extend from the end of the epididymis and through the seminal vesicles.

Vascular tunic Layer of the eye that contains most of the vasculature of the eye.

Vegetative functions Autonomic functions the body requires to survive.

Ventral Referring to the front of the body; anterior.

Ventricles Two pumping chambers in the heart.

Venules Small venous vessels that return blood to the capillaries.

Vesicles The "shipping containers" of the cell. They are simple in structure, consisting of a single membrane filled with liquid, and transport a wide variety of substances both inside and outside the cell.

Vestibule Space or a cavity that serves as the entrance to the inner ear.

Visceral pleura Lining of the pleural cavity that adheres tightly to the lung surface.

Vulva External female genitalia.

Pathophysiology

Objectives *After completing this chapter, you will be able to:*

1. Discuss cellular adaptation.
2. Describe cellular injury and cellular death.
3. Describe the factors that lead to disease in the human body.
4. Describe the systemic manifestations that result from cellular injury.
5. Describe the cellular environment.
6. Discuss familial diseases and their associated risk factors.
7. Describe environmental risk factors.
8. Describe aging as a risk factor for disease.
9. Discuss the process of analyzing disease risk.
10. Discuss the combined effects of risk factors and the interactions among risk factors.
11. Discuss hypoperfusion.
12. Define cardiogenic, hypovolemic, neurogenic, anaphylactic, and septic shock.
13. Describe multiple organ dysfunction syndrome.
14. Define the characteristics of the immune response.
15. Discuss activation of the immune system.
16. Discuss fetal and neonatal immune function.
17. Discuss aging and the immune function in the elderly.
18. Describe the inflammation response.
19. Discuss the role of mast cells as part of the inflammation response.
20. Describe the plasma protein system.
21. Discuss the cellular components of inflammation.
22. Describe the systemic manifestations of the inflammation response.
23. Describe the resolution and repair from inflammation.
24. Discuss the effect of aging on the mechanisms of self-defense.
25. Discuss hypersensitivity.
26. Describe deficiencies in immunity and inflammation.
27. Discuss the interrelations among stress, coping, and illness.
28. Describe neuroendocrine regulation.

Chapter Outline

Alterations in Cells and Tissues
Cellular Injury
Cellular Death and Necrosis
Cellular Environment
Role of Electrolytes
Electrolyte Imbalances
Acid-Base Balance
Genetics and Familial Diseases
Analyzing Disease Risks
Hypoperfusion
Types of Shock
Multiple Organ Dysfunction Syndrome

Immune System and Resistance to Disease
Characteristics of the Immune Response
Activation of the Immune System
Humoral Immune Response
Immunoglobulins
Inflammation
Variances in Immunity and Inflammation
Stress and Disease
Stress Response
Stress, Coping, and Illness Interrelations
Chapter Summary

Case Scenario

You and your partner respond to a home in a rural area for a "man with the flu." On arrival, you find a 58-year-old man sitting upright in a chair. He reports having flu symptoms with diarrhea and vomiting for 1 week. He has diabetes and has reduced his daily insulin dose for the past 3 days because he has been unable to keep food down. The patient is awake, alert, and oriented to person, place, time, and events. His color appears good and he speaks without difficulty.

Questions

1. What is your general impression of this patient?
2. What conditions could lead to these symptoms?
3. How would these patient findings affect the patient's glucose levels?
4. What physiologic complications would you expect from nausea, vomiting, and diarrhea for 1 week?

The anatomy and physiology, or structure and function, of the body are described in Chapter 7. An alteration in these normal functions by disease or abnormal conditions is known as *pathophysiology*. Pathology is the study of diseases caused by pathophysiologic changes. Diseases associated with structural changes within the body are organic diseases, whereas those that cause disturbances in function without structural changes are called functional diseases. An understanding of pathophysiology and pathology is essential for the paramedic to make accurate treatment decisions and evaluate the effects of treatment.

ALTERATIONS IN CELLS AND TISSUES

The ability of cells and tissues to adapt and change is essential for the survival of the organism. These changes can result from a change in the internal environment of the body or from an external stressor. The adaptation of a cell can occur to protect the cell from injury or as a result of a normal physiologic process (Figure 8-1).

Cellular Adaptation

[OBJECTIVE 1]

Changes in structure and function regularly occur throughout the human body. Most of these changes occur without a person's knowledge. Some of the changes, however, can be quite obvious. Once a cell has undergone successful adaptation, meaning that the cell has changed and achieved a sense of homeostasis with its environment, the cell's function may be enhanced. However, cells that undergo adaptation may instead have reduced functionality. Whether the adaptation has occurred as a result of a pathologic process or an increased functional demand is sometimes difficult to tell. The most common forms of adaptation include **atrophy, hypertrophy, hyperplasia, dysplasia,** and **metaplasia.**

Atrophy

Atrophy is defined as the shrinkage of cells. Shrinkage can occur for a variety of reasons. The cause of the atrophy may be temporary, as is the case with most cellular adaptations. The most common pathologic causes of atrophy include conditions such as denervation of muscle tissue, diminished blood supply, and nutritional deficiencies

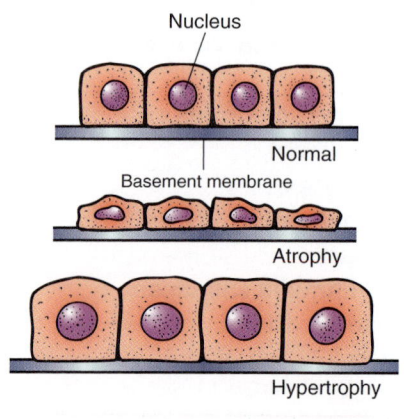

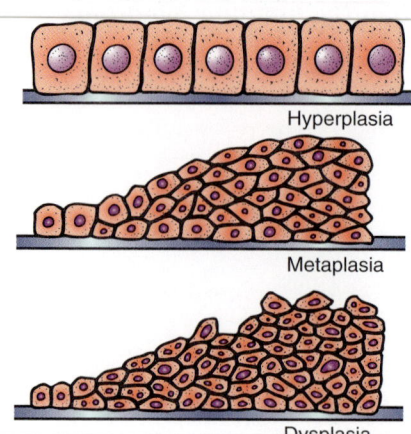

Figure 8-1 Adaptive changes in cells.

(Yeldani et al., 1996). Cellular atrophy also has physiologic causes. These usually include a decreased workload or a change in the needs of the body, such as the reduction in the size of the uterus after childbirth or the reduction in the size of an extremity while immobilized in a cast.

If a cell undergoes atrophy for one of these physiologic reasons, it is an effort to realign the energy requirements of that cell to the function it is performing. For example, an assembly line with hundreds of workers is not necessary if the goal is to produce one bicycle a day. The amount of resources used to accomplish the end product would not be efficient. Likewise, the cells in the body try to run as efficiently as possible. The extra resources, such as oxygen and glucose, are diverted to where the need is more pressing.

Hypertrophy ✳

The term *hypertrophy* refers to the increase in the size of a cell, tissue, or organ. This traditionally occurs in response to an increase in the workload or the demand placed on the cell. In cells that cannot divide, such as skeletal muscle and cardiac muscle, growth is the only option to meet the increased demands. This increased size usually is a temporary condition. The cells revert to their original size if the workload returns to normal or the causative factor is removed. For example, a bodybuilder lifts weights to gain muscle mass. This gain occurs because the cells that compose the muscle undergo hypertrophy in response to the increased demand. Once cells begin this process, they require a greater amount of resources such as oxygen and glucose. Once the bodybuilder stops regularly lifting weights, the muscle mass begins to decrease.

Hyperplasia ✳

This form of adaptation is the result of cellular division that occurs to increase the number of a specific type of cell. As with atrophy, physiologic and pathologic reasons exist for why this can occur. These reasons generally are part of the normal growth and maturity of the human body. The pathologic reasons for this multiplication of cells are much more sinister. For instance, the growth of many neoplasms (tumors) is a result of hyperplasia. This may occur in various places throughout the body. The tumors can be benign (noncancerous) or malignant (cancerous). Common presentations include endometrial hyperplasia (thickening of the lining of the uterus) in women and benign prostatic hyperplasia (an enlarged prostate) in men.

Dysplasia ✳

Dysplasia is a form of adaptation that is closely related to hyperplasia. It sometimes is referred to as atypical or abnormal hyperplasia. In this type of adaptation the cells take on an abnormal size, shape, and organization as a result of ongoing irritation or inflammation. This can be reversed sometimes if the irritation is removed in the early phases. This type of cellular adaptation is great

cause for concern. Many of these occurrences are considered precancerous conditions and can progress to a malignant formation.

Metaplasia ✳

Metaplasia is defined as the transformation of one type of mature differentiated cell into another type of mature differentiated cell. Again, normal physiologic causes for this type of adaptation exist. For instance, cartilage can change into bone. Pathologic reasons also exist, such as the change that occurs in the bronchial lining of long-term smokers. This tissue is lined with ciliated cells used to trap and remove foreign substances. Smoking causes the loss of cilia, and the cells transform into cells that can better withstand the toxins found in cigarette smoke. This may sound beneficial, but these changes cause a decrease in moisture and a reduction in the ability to clean the bronchial lining. This, in turn, can lead to infection and increased mucus production.

CELLULAR INJURY

[OBJECTIVE 2]

Cells face constant assault. For the most part they are well prepared for the task, but occasionally they can be overwhelmed. Cellular injury occurs when the cell is negatively altered or damaged to the point that normal function suffers or is permanently impaired. Following are the most common forms of cellular injury:

- Hypoxic
- Chemical
- Infectious
- Immunologic and inflammatory
- Genetic
- Nutritional imbalance
- Physical agent

Hypoxic Injury ✳

Hypoxic injury is the most common and probably most studied form of cellular injury. This form of cellular injury can be categorized as reversible or irreversible. Moreover, this form of injury can be caused by a variety of events. Whether caused by a reduction of oxygen in the air, a loss of hemoglobin or hemoglobin function, a decrease in the number of red blood cells, or a reduction in the effectiveness of the respiratory or cardiac systems, the result is the same. The most common cause of hypoxia is a reduction in oxygenated blood. Reversible hypoxic injury also is referred to as ischemic injury. This type of injury is only reversible when the duration of the hypoxic event is short. Ischemic insult usually results from the following pattern:

- *Impaired aerobic respiration*. This occurs in the mitochondria, the "power plant" of the cell and the site of adenosine triphosphate (ATP) production.

- *Anaerobic glycolysis*. With the lack of oxygen, glucose is not metabolized aerobically. This leads to a marked decrease in ATP production and an increase in harmful byproducts. This also is known as anaerobic metabolism.
- *Decreased ATP*. This occurs because of the lack of available oxygen.
- *Increased lactic acid*. Also known as lactate, this is a byproduct of metabolism that builds up inside the cell. This buildup occurs at a faster rate during anaerobic metabolism.

respiratory, cardiac ineffectiveness

Energy (i.e., ATP) is required to maintain cell wall integrity and the active transport of electrolytes across the cell membrane. Therefore a change in ATP production causes major issues. The reduction in cell wall integrity makes keeping sodium out of the cell difficult. The buildup of intercellular sodium leads to **cellular swelling.** The buildup of lactate inside the cell as a result of anaerobic metabolism increases the amount of cellular swelling. If the cycle of hypoxia continues, the mitochondria may become swollen and the cell will progress to irreversible damage. If the hypoxia is corrected, the cell may return to its normal functioning without any long-term effects.

Irreversible damage occurs when the hypoxic event lasts for a longer period. The exact point at which this occurs, sometimes called the *point of no return,* is unknown. The buildup of lactate eventually breaks down the membrane of the lysosomes. Once this occurs, powerful digestive enzymes are released inside the cell. This damages the other organelles, including the nucleus, the mitochondria, and the cellular cytoskeleton. When this happens, even if the cell is reoxygenated, the cell is too damaged to recover. As oxygen is reintroduced to the cell, an additional sodium influx occurs, causing the cell destruction to continue.

Chemical Injury   *common, environmental*

Chemical injury occurs when a toxic substance is introduced into the body. All types of chemicals can cause injury, alteration, death of cells and, ultimately, death of the organism. These can include common toxins, such as alcohol, drugs, and carbon monoxide, as well as environmental toxins, such as certain insecticides and herbicides. When this injury occurs, the toxins create a biochemical reaction with either the plasma membrane of the cell or one of its organelles. After damaging the cell wall, sodium, water, and calcium rush into the cell and damage continues along the same path as hypoxic injury.

Infectious Injury

Virulence is a term used to refer to the relative pathogenicity of an infectious agent, that is, the relative ability of the agent to damage the host. The virulence of a bacterium, virus, or other agent is determined by its ability to invade and destroy cells, produce toxins, or produce hypersensitivity reactions.

Bacteria

Bacteria are one of the oldest life forms on the planet. These single-celled prokaryotic organisms are responsible for many functions in both the human body and the environment as a whole. The majority of bacteria do not cause adverse effects or disease states in the human body. In the human body, bacterial cells outnumber human cells approximately 10 to 1 (Sears, 2005). This type of nonthreatening bacteria is referred to as **normal flora.** This chapter focuses on the way in which bacteria work to infect the human body and the mechanisms by which they cause people harm.

As with other prokaryotes, bacteria lack the organized intracellular structures common to eukaryotes. Without an organized nucleus, the genetic material floats freely inside the cell's cytosol. This does not, however, inhibit reproduction. Bacteria are capable of independent reproduction; however, they cannot survive without the assistance of a host cell. They rely on the host cell for a stable environment and a constant supply of nutrients (McCance & Huether, 2002). Bacteria are classified according to their appearance and properties identified under microscopic examination. In medicine, identification of the type of bacteria causing the patient's illness is important. This gives the healthcare provider the information needed to select the best treatment. Bacteria are generally classified as **gram positive** or **gram negative** depending on the type of cell wall. This classification is determined by applying different dyes called *Gram stains* that stain the bacteria either red or blue. If the bacteria stain blue, they are gram positive. If they stain red, they are gram negative. This process was first introduced in 1884 by Christian Gram, a Danish physician. Over a century later, it still is the most widespread method for classifying bacteria. Additional classifications of bacteria are based on their shape and grouping. A coccus is a bacterium that is essentially round (plural, *cocci*). Rod-shaped bacteria are bacilli, and a bacterium with a spiral or corkscrew appearance is a spirillum, or spirochete. Further information regarding bacteria can be gained from its arrangement. Bacterial arrangements can be single, paired (diplo), grouped in fours (tetrad), clustered (staphylo), or chained (strepto). All these factors can provide a fairly accurate description of a bacterium. For example, gram-positive staphylococci are round bacteria arranged in clusters that respond to the Gram stain test. Gram-negative streptococci are round bacteria arranged in chains that do not respond to a Gram stain test.

The ability of bacteria to survive and grow in a host organism is directly related to the effectiveness of the host organism's defense mechanisms and the specific properties of the bacteria involved. Not all bacteria have the same properties. Bacteria can be aerobic or anaerobic; some of them can, or prefer to, live without the presence of oxygen, whereas others need oxygen to survive. Bacterial cells create an outer layer called a glycocalyx for protection. The glycocalyx of some of the heartier bacteria is a coating called a **capsule.** In the human host, the capsule protects and prevents the bacteria from being destroyed or digested. The glycocalyx of other bacteria forms as a slime layer. This loose, slippery layer protects the bacteria from the loss of water and nutrients. Bacteria can produce substances harmful to cells and tissues. These substances are called **exotoxins, endotoxins,** and exoenzymes.

Exotoxins are proteins released during bacterial growth. They include enzymes with specific, and possibly systemic, effects. Endotoxins are contained in the cell wall of gram-negative bacteria. These substances are generally released during the destruction of the bacteria by either the host organism's defense mechanisms or by treatment with medications. Endotoxin release also can occur during the growth phase of bacteria. If this occurs, treatment with medication will be ineffective on the endotoxin. Bacteria that release endotoxins are called **pyrogenic** bacteria because of the inflammatory response and fever that follow the release (McCance & Huether, 2002). Exoenzymes are secreted by many microorganisms, including bacteria, during their normal life cycle. These enzymes generally cause the destruction of tissues and include mucinase, keratinase, collagenase, hyaluronidase, coagulase, and the kinases. Streptokinase was one of the earlier thrombolytic medications developed.

The medications used to combat bacterial infection are known as *antibiotics*. These medications were once thought to be the answer to all infectious diseases. However, this was quickly discovered not to be the case. Many other pathogens, including viruses, do not respond to antibiotic treatment. Antibiotics work on some bacteria by destroying the cell wall, inhibiting protein synthesis, or interfering with bacterial reproduction. This allows the body's defenses to digest and eliminate the bacteria. Unfortunately, because of the overuse and misuse of antibiotics, some bacteria have been able to evolve into antibiotic-resistant strains. If the way antibiotics are prescribed and/or used is not revised, the number of drug-resistant bacterial strains is projected to increase dramatically.

Once a large amount of bacteria and toxins reach the bloodstream, a condition called **septicemia** occurs. Also known as sepsis or bacteremia, this is a serious medical condition. It is characterized by vasodilation that leads to hypotension, tissue hypoxia, and eventually cardiogenic shock. Septicemia is usually caused by gram-negative bacteria, but this is not always the case. Blood tests called cultures are used to diagnose septicemia and its cause. By growing the bacteria in a laboratory, the type of bacteria and the best treatment option can be determined.

Viruses   *can't function on their own*

Viruses are the most common cause of infection in the human body. These pathogens are much smaller than bacteria and more adept at causing infections. In fact, viruses can infect bacterial cells. Viruses work differently from other pathogens. They survive and replicate by taking over the metabolic machinery of the host cell. Viruses can avoid being detected and can bypass the body's defense systems because they hide inside normal cells and do not produce endotoxins or exotoxins.

Viruses can be aggressive or nonaggressive. Aggressive viruses replicate quickly. They move from cell to cell to survive. In some instances this can be a good thing. As the virus moves from cell to cell, the immune system develops defenses that eventually stop the virus (discussed later in this chapter). Thus the infection is self-limiting. Other aggressive viruses can cause severe and irreversible damage in short periods, and some may remain hidden or dormant for months or years until they receive a trigger to replicate. These pathogens have a symbiotic relationship with the host cell and do not cause immediate cellular death. In some cases the host's immunity may be strong enough to limit the scope of infectious outbreak or prevent it altogether. Viral infections can result in the death of the host, the death of the virus as a result of the host defense mechanism, or a chronic carrier state. In this last scenario the virus does not kill the host, but the host defense mechanisms are unable to eradicate the virus.

Viruses are not structured like bacteria. They are smaller and lack the structures of either prokaryotic or eukaryotic cells. Without the organelles used for metabolism, these pathogens completely depend on the host cells for replication and survival. Small particles of viruses are called **virions.** Viruses contain strands of nucleic acid (either DNA or RNA) that are surrounded by a protein coat called a **capsid.** The capsid may or may not have an outer envelope surrounding it. Viruses without an outer envelope are called *naked nucleocapsids;* those that do are called *enveloped nucleocapsids.* These envelopes have a series of projections, or spikes, on their outer surface that play a role in attachment to the host cell. The viral nucleic acid must enter the host cell to begin the replication process. Viral replication is composed of five steps: absorption, penetration, replication, maturation, and release. The method of absorption into the host cell is a function of the type of capsid the virus has. Viruses with a naked nucleocapsid bind to the host cell and the nucleic acid is absorbed into the host cell without the virus itself entering the cell. Viruses with an enveloped nucleocapsid bind to the host cell by inserting its spikes into the membrane of the host cell. The entire virus is then absorbed into the host cell, where it is uncoated, releasing the viral nucleic acid into the cell. Once this task has been accomplished, the virus makes multiple copies of itself. Then it prepares the copies for release so they can infect other cells. In contrast, some viruses integrate their genetic material with that of the host cell and become a permanent resident. When this occurs, the virus replicates through the subsequent division of the host cell (McCance & Huether, 2002).

Release of the matured viruses from the host cell is a function of the original nucleocapsid. Viruses that originated in a naked nucleocapsid form a new nucleocapsid inside the host cell and then cause lysis, or bursting, of the host cell to be released. This results in the death of the host cell. Viruses that originated in an enveloped nucleocapsid exit the host cell by a process called budding. As part of the maturation process of these viruses, protein spikes are inserted on the cell membrane of the host cell. As the virus exits the host cell, it takes part of the cell membrane and these spikes along with it, which become the spiked envelope of the new virus. This is one theory behind autoimmune disorders. The protein spikes left by the virus alter the cell membrane of the host cell. This makes it appear as a foreign cell to the immune system, which then initiates an attack to eradicate the supposed foreign invader.

Few medications can combat viruses. To eliminate a virus, the host cell also must be eliminated. This can be quite problematic. Identifying cells that have been infected and targeting pharmacologic agents to attack only those cells are nearly impossible. In addition, the ability of viruses to change, or **mutate,** continues to baffle even the best efforts.

Fungi

In addition to bacterial and viral infections, fungi can cause pathologic conditions in human beings. Fungi are relatively large organisms. They either can grow as single-celled yeasts or multicelled molds. These pathogens have thick cell walls that are distinctly different from those of bacteria and are able to resist the typical treatments designed to disrupt cell wall integrity. Fungi are generally parasitic in nature. They grow on or near the surface of the skin or mucous membranes. Diseases caused by fungi are called **mycoses.**

Protozoa

Protozoa are single-celled organisms that possess a complex cell structure, including a nucelus and organelles. They move by means of flagella, cilia, or by shifting protoplasm. Examples of diseases caused by protozoa include giardiasis and malaria.

Parasites

A **parasite** is a plant or animal that grows, feeds, and is sheltered on or in another plant or animal. It usually causes harm to the host. Endoparasites live inside their hosts. Examples of endoparasites include the following:

- Helminths, such as ascarids (roundworms), cestoda (tapeworms), and *Enterobius vermicularis* (pinworm)
- Fungi, such as ringworm
- Protists (Protozoa), such as *Giardia lamblia* and *Trichomonas vaginalis*

Ectoparasites live on, but not in, their hosts. Examples of ectoparasites include fleas, ticks, lice, and some mites.

Prions

A **prion** is an infectious agent composed of only protein. Known prion diseases affect the structure of the brain or other nervous tissue in animals and human beings. Prion diseases are also known as *transmissible spongiform encephalopathies.* These diseases include bovine spongiform encephalopathy ("mad cow" disease) in cattle, Creutzfeldt-Jakob disease in human beings, scrapie in sheep, and chronic wasting disease in deer and elk. Much about transmissible spongiform encephalopathy diseases is unknown. Because prions are composed of only protein, they are quite difficult to eradicate. The only way to do this is to denature the protein through heat, chemical, or other methods that also would kill the infected cells.

Immunologic and Inflammatory Injury

The human immune system is fascinating and complex. It is designed as protection of the body. Because of this, it is potent and sometimes dangerous. When cells come in direct contact with one of the cellular or chemical components of the immune system, they can be irreversibly damaged. Permanent damage is associated with loss of cell wall integrity. Whether this happens because of phagocytes (neutrophils, lymphocytes, and macrophages), histamine, antibodies, or lymphokines, once cell wall integrity is compromised the appropriate exchange of electrolytes is altered and water enters the cells. As this process continues, the cells begin to swell and cellular death is imminent.

Injurious Genetic Factors
[OBJECTIVE 3]
Genetic injury to cells can result from a defect passed from a parent to child. It also can occur from environmental factors (induced mutations) or spontaneous mutations of genes. These types of defects can cause a change in a cell's nucleus and cell wall structure, shape, receptors, or transport mechanism. Any changes in the structure of the cell can cause changes in the way it works. Furthermore, such changes can lead to a disease state in the host. Examples include sickle cell anemia and muscular dystrophy.

Injurious Nutritional Imbalances

All cells need the proper amount of electrolytes to function. These and other nutrients are acquired through the diet and transported to cells for use. When this does not occur, a wide range of disease states can manifest. In the United States, most of these diseases have been reduced or eliminated. For example, beriberi, scurvy, and rickets are usually only found in other parts of the world. In contrast, an excessive amount of certain nutrients also can cause cellular damage. This imbalance ultimately may lead to cell death. An example of this second type of imbalance prevalent in the United States is excessive carbohydrate intake, which can lead to obesity (McCance & Huether, 2002).

Injurious Physical Agents

Many physical agents are capable of causing significant damage to the cells and tissues of the body. The following list is a sampling of such agents and should not be considered complete; even some of the therapies and treatments used to diagnose and heal can cause damage.

- *Temperature extremes.* Prolonged exposure to extreme heat or cold can damage the skin and underlying tissue (e.g., burns and frostbite). More prolonged exposure can result in hypothermia and hyperthermia.
- *Changes in atmospheric pressure.* This type of injury can result from even brief periods of exposure to dramatic changes in pressure (e.g., diving injuries and altitude sickness).
- *Radiation.* Exposures to ionizing radiation such as x-rays can cause damage over a prolonged period. Other types, such as nuclear radiation, can be more damaging in a shorter time span depending on the level of exposure.
- *Illumination.* This type of injury is a result of exposure to light. The types of injuries normally associated with light are eye strain and certain skin cancers.
- *Mechanical stresses.* These can range from traumatic injury to repetitive use injuries to hearing loss, depending on the agent.

Manifestations of Cellular Injury

As cells are injured, several processes occur. These processes can result in structural and functional changes within the cell. As individual cells change, systemic manifestations follow. The two most common changes to cells as a result of injury are cellular swelling and changes in **lipid accumulation** (Yeldani et al., 1996).

Normal cellular function can be impaired as a result of injury. Processes such as **anabolism** and **catabolism** can be altered to the extent that they harm the cell. When this occurs, certain substances can infiltrate and build up inside cells. This can occur in healthy cells in some situations, but it is more common once a cell has been injured. These substances, such as fluids and electrolytes, lipids, glycogen, calcium, uric acid, protein, melanin, and bilirubin can come from many sources and may even be normally found in cells. A strict balance of these substances is essential for proper cell function. If this imbalance lasts long enough, the cell can be permanently damaged. The accumulation of these substances comes from one of the following three sources:

1. An **endogenous** substance produced in excess or at an accelerated rate
2. An **endogenous** substance not broken down at the correct rate
3. Harmful **exogenous** substances accumulated by inhalation, ingestion, or infection

As the cell tries to compensate for the abnormal levels of the substance that has accumulated, metabolites (products of catabolism) are expelled from the cell into the extracellular environment. When this occurs the body identifies the area as injured. The body then sends phagocytes called macrophages to ingest damaged cells and foreign extracellular substances. As this process continues and more macrophages arrive, the tissue begins to swell. The more phagocytosis occurs, the more evident the damage becomes.

Cellular Swelling

The cellular swelling that goes along with injury is a result of a more permeable cellular membrane. This increased permeability allows potassium to leak out of the cell and sodium to move into the cell. This exchange alters the osmotic gradient. This means that water will move into the cell. Most cellular swelling is considered nonlethal and is reversible.

Lipid Accumulation

In certain parts of the body lipids accumulate in cells as a result of the failure or inadequate performance of the enzyme that metabolizes fats. This can happen in several places. However, the most common site of lipid buildup, also known as *fatty change,* is the liver (Yeldani et al., 1996). This makes sense because the liver is the chief site of fat metabolism in the body. As this accumulation continues, lipids begin to push the normal intracellular contents, such as the nucleus, aside and disrupt normal cellular function. One of the most common causes of a fatty liver is alcohol abuse. These changes can be reversible if the alcohol intake ceases, preventing the progression to cirrhosis of the liver.

Systemic Manifestations
[OBJECTIVE 4]

As previously described, if the cellular injury is not halted or mediated, systemic manifestations can occur. Common systemic signs and symptoms of cellular injury include fever, fatigue, malaise, appetite disturbances, increase in heart rate, pain, and altered laboratory results (e.g., increased white blood cell [WBC] count and enzymatic changes). The increased WBC count is a result of the inflammatory response, and enzyme changes may be specific to the site of the injury.

CELLULAR DEATH AND NECROSIS

Cellular death (necrobiosis) can occur as a result of spreading irreversible injury. It also can occur as a preprogrammed response for tissue regeneration or as a response to atrophy.

The preprogrammed death of cells is called *apoptosis,* which happens in response to cellular damage or injury that results in a nonfunctioning cell. Apoptosis is the body's way of ridding itself of these cells. It is generally considered normal. Lysosomes release their digestive enzymes inside the damaged cells, and they begin to digest the cellular debris. This process is called *autolysis*. It can occur from normal or pathologic stimuli. Necrosis is the sum of cellular changes after local cell death (McCance & Huether, 2002). Necrosis differs from apoptosis in that it is always a result of a pathologic condition. Following are the four primary types of necrosis:

- *Coagulative necrosis* generally occurs in the kidneys, heart, and adrenal glands. It gets its name because of the intracellular change of the protein albumin from a gelatinous form to a firm, opaque state. This usually is caused by hypoxia.
- *Liquefactive necrosis* is most common in neural tissue. Because of their design, **neurons** are rich in hydrolytic enzymes and lipids; these cells are easily liquefied and walled off from healthy tissue.
- *Caseous necrosis* is a combination of the coagulative and liquefactive forms. The most common cause of this type is tuberculosis. The cells are not completely digested and have an appearance similar to cottage cheese. Again, these cells are walled off from healthy tissue.
- *Fat necrosis* occurs in the breast and abdominal structures. Fatty acids combine with certain electrolytes to form soaps. This process is called **saponification.** Pancreatic infarction can lead to this type of necrosis.

Gangrenous necrosis, commonly called *gangrene,* is a widespread area of tissue death. Gangrenous necrosis is categorized into three types. *Dry gangrene* is generally a result of coagulative necrosis. The tissue shrivels, dries, and changes color to brown or black. *Wet gangrene* is a result of the liquefactive necrosis of internal organs. *Gas gangrene* is caused by the bacteria *Clostridium perfringens*. It results in the formation of gas bubbles inside cells, including those of the blood. When the body tries to defend itself, it can destroy the membranes of red blood cells. This creates a deficit in the oxygen-carrying capacity of the blood and can put the patient in a hypoxic state that, if uncorrected, can lead to shock and death.

CELLULAR ENVIRONMENT

[OBJECTIVE 5]

The cells of the human body depend on their environment for survival. This environment consists of varying levels of fluid and electrolytes. The balance of these two factors is necessary for survival as well as adequate function and communication. Many serious conditions result from an inadequate balance in the internal environment. If the imbalance is severe, the organism itself may be in danger of fatal consequences.

Water Movement between Intracellular Fluid and Extracellular Fluid

Water can move without much difficulty from the intracellular fluid (ICF) and extracellular fluid (ECF) compartments and vice versa, depending on the needs of the body. Each of the body's compartments is separated by a membrane. The amount of water in each compartment generally is tightly regulated in an effort to maintain the osmolality of total body water (TBW) in equilibrium.

Osmolality is defined as the number of osmotically active particles in a kilogram of water. The body uses several mechanisms to accomplish a balanced osmolality in each of the body's compartments. The following sections explain osmosis, diffusion, and mediated transport.

Osmosis

Osmosis is the movement of water (solvent) across a semipermeable membrane from an area of lower solute concentration to an area of higher solute concentration to minimize the difference in concentration. In the human body, the solute consists of electrolytes, such as sodium and potassium, and molecules, such as glucose. Water can generally move without much difficulty between the different compartments of the body because the membranes that separate the compartments are permeable to water. This membrane is called *semipermeable* because it also is selectively permeable to certain solutes (Figure 8-2).

Selective permeability is accomplished through pores in the membrane that are selective on the basis of the size, shape, or electrical charge of the molecule. The body tries to maintain an equal solute concentration and therefore osmolality on each side of the membrane. When this balance exists, it is **isotonic.** When an imbal-

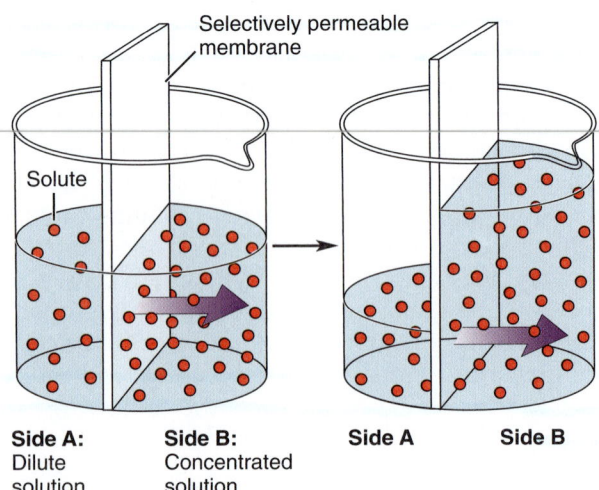

Figure 8-2 Osmosis. The glass is sectioned into side A and B by a membrane that is permeable only to water. The water moved from side A to side B, thereby creating unequal volumes.

ance exists in the ionic concentration from one side of the membrane to the other, the side with the higher concentration is **hypertonic.** The side with the lower concentration is **hypotonic.** The difference in the concentration from one side to the other is called the **osmotic gradient** (McCance & Huether, 2002).

Diffusion

The second way that the body can maintain the balance between compartments is **diffusion.** Diffusion is defined as the spreading of molecules from an area of higher concentration to an area of lower concentration. This property applies to solids and gasses. The human body has examples of both. By moving some of the solute from one side of the membrane to the other, the body reduces or eliminates the concentration gradient and creates balance. This is the body's natural tendency and is referred to as moving with the concentration gradient. Complete elimination of concentration gradients is impossible because ions and molecules are always in motion in a random pattern. This means that concentration gradients come and go. However, the natural tendency is to create equilibrium as much as possible, and the net change is close to zero. This is how the body is able to move some nutrients and waste products into and out of the cell. With gasses, the molecules are spread farther apart and

the diffusion rate depends on the weight of the gas. The body is able to exchange oxygen and carbon dioxide in the lungs because of diffusion (Figure 8-3).

Mediated Transport

It is sometimes necessary to move molecules across a membrane that either cannot use diffusion or must move against the concentration gradient. In these situations, the movement occurs by **active transport** or **facilitated diffusion.** Active transport is used to move substances against the concentration gradient or toward the side with a higher concentration. This type of transport, just as it sounds, requires the use of energy by the cell but is faster than diffusion. This is similar to operating a car in that the car can roll down a hill in neutral without being on, but it would have to be running and in gear to go up the hill.

Facilitated diffusion is the movement of substances across a membrane by binding to a helper protein integrated into the cell wall and allowing only substances to cross the membrane. Once bound to the protein, the resulting molecule changes shape and is allowed to pass through the membrane. After passing through the membrane, the original molecule is released. This is the mechanism the body uses to transport glucose, a large molecule, into cells. It is similar to regular diffusion in

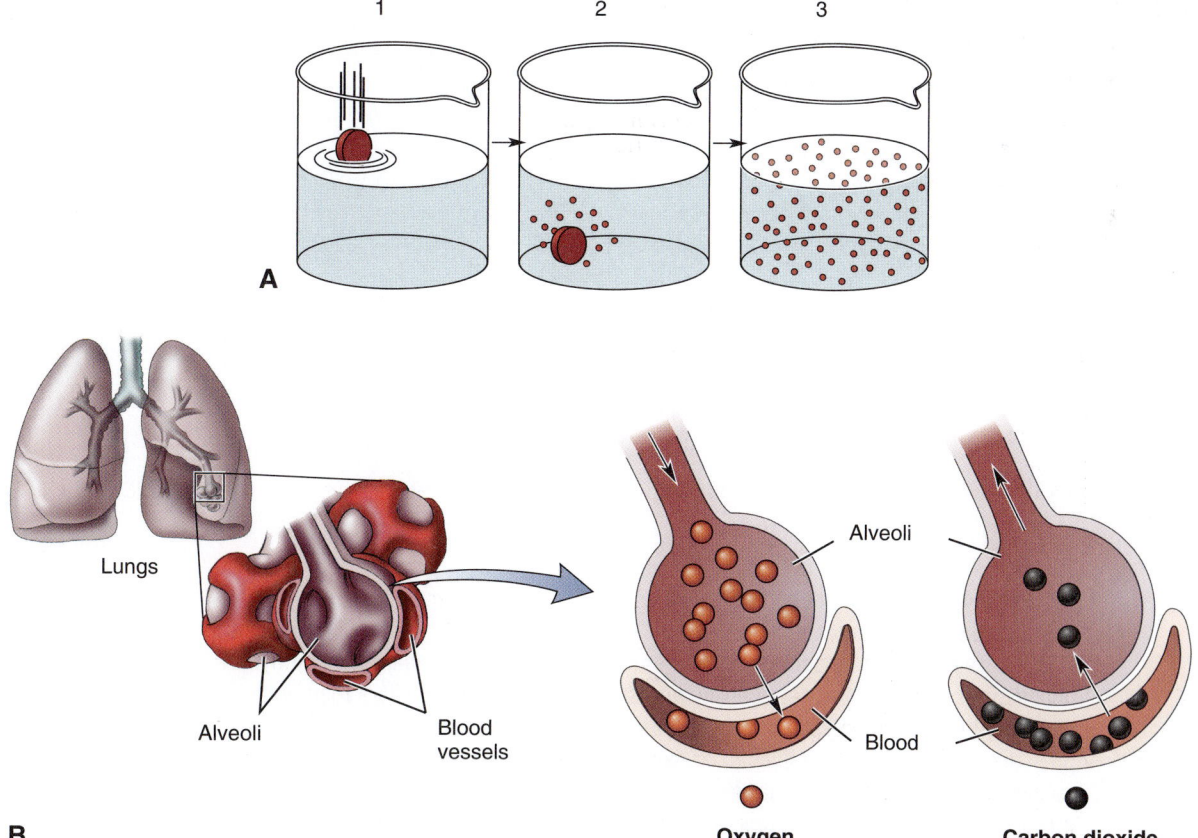

Figure 8-3 Diffusion. **A,** A red tablet is placed in glass 1. Given enough time, the red dye diffuses until it is evenly distributed throughout glass 3. **B,** Diffusion of oxygen and carbon dioxide in the lung.

that it works with the concentration gradient (i.e., from a higher concentration to a lower concentration) and does not generally require energy. As with active transport, facilitated diffusion occurs more quickly than regular diffusion.

Water Movement between Plasma and Interstitial Fluid

The movement of water between the plasma in the intravascular compartment and the interstitial space is a result of pressure. This occurs at the capillary level by a process known as filtration (Figure 8-4). Filtration is the movement of fluid from intravascular fluid under high pressure to interstitial fluid, which generally is under lower pressure. This happens when the hydrostatic and oncotic pressures are favorable. **Hydrostatic pressure** is the pressure exerted by a fluid because of its weight. **Osmotic pressure** is the pressure exerted by the concentration of a particular solute. In the capillary beds two opposing osmotic gradients are present. The pressure from the colloidal proteins in the blood plasma is opposed by the pressure from the tissue proteins in the interstitial space. The net effect of these two pressure gradients is the oncotic pressure. This is important because the capillary beds are the interface in the human body where oxygen, nutrients, and waste products are exchanged. The capillary beds are the vasculature that joins the arterioles to the venules. The precapillary side is arterial and the postcapillary side is venous. The hydrostatic and oncotic pressures differ from one side of the capillary to the other. With higher hydrostatic pressure and lower oncotic pressure on the

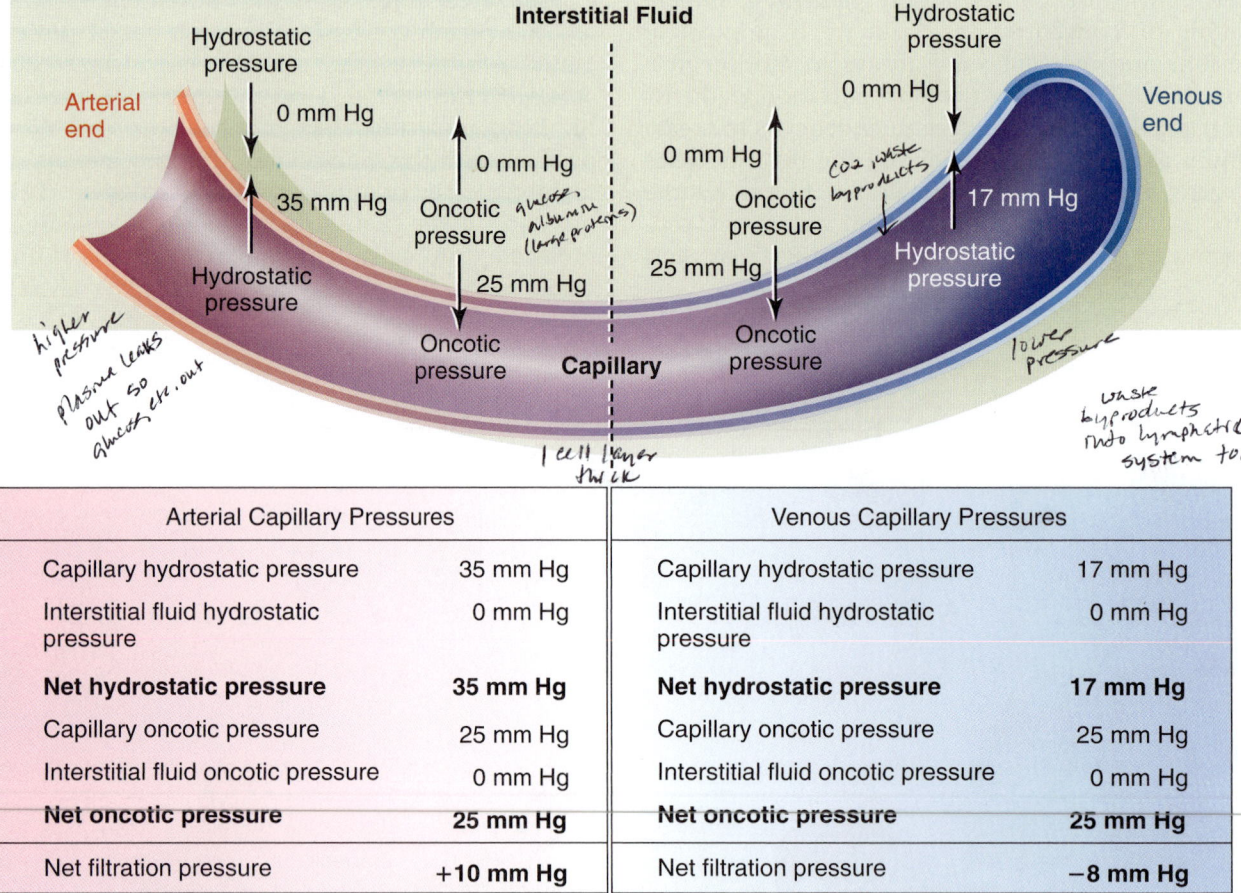

Arterial Capillary Pressures		Venous Capillary Pressures	
Capillary hydrostatic pressure	35 mm Hg	Capillary hydrostatic pressure	17 mm Hg
Interstitial fluid hydrostatic pressure	0 mm Hg	Interstitial fluid hydrostatic pressure	0 mm Hg
Net hydrostatic pressure	**35 mm Hg**	**Net hydrostatic pressure**	**17 mm Hg**
Capillary oncotic pressure	25 mm Hg	Capillary oncotic pressure	25 mm Hg
Interstitial fluid oncotic pressure	0 mm Hg	Interstitial fluid oncotic pressure	0 mm Hg
Net oncotic pressure	**25 mm Hg**	**Net oncotic pressure**	**25 mm Hg**
Net filtration pressure	**+10 mm Hg**	Net filtration pressure	**−8 mm Hg**

Figure 8-4 Capillary filtration forces. Water, electrolytes, and small molecules freely exchange between the vascular compartment and the interstitial space at the site of capillaries and small venules. The rate and amount of exchange are driven by the physical forces of hydrostatic and oncotic pressures and the permeability and surface area of the capillary membrane. The two opposing hydrostatic pressures are capillary hydrostatic pressure and interstitial hydrostatic pressure. The two opposing oncotic pressures are capillary oncotic pressure and interstitial oncotic pressure. The forces that favor filtration from the capillary are capillary hydrostatic pressure and interstitial oncotic pressure, and forces that oppose filtration are capillary oncotic pressure and interstitial hydrostatic pressure. The sum of their effects is known as net filtration pressure. In the example of normal exchange above, a small amount of fluid moves to the lymph vessels, which accounts for the net filtration difference between the arterial and venous ends of the capillary.

arteriole side of the capillary, fluid is forced into the interstitial space. On the venule end of the capillary, the opposite is true and fluid reenters the capillary. Note that sphincters are located at the precapillary entrance and the postcapillary exit of the capillary bed. These sphincters help maintain this relation and therefore the necessary pressure gradients. This process is called net filtration and is described by Starling's hypothesis:

Net filtration = Forces favoring filtration –
Forces opposing filtration

The net filtration at the capillary level is close to zero. As the fluid moves out of the intravascular space, the relative concentration of solute increases. By the time it reaches the end of the capillary bed, the gradient is such that fluid moves back into the capillary before exiting back into the venous system.

Capillary and Membrane Permeability

The movement of fluid described in the preceding section is effective but depends on membrane integrity. Many conditions can lead to a change in the integrity of the capillary membrane, including sepsis, bacterial infection, and shock. Regardless of the cause, the result is an increase in the interstitial osmotic pressure by plasma proteins, which causes a fluid shift from the intravascular space into the interstitial compartment.

Alterations in Water Movement

Edema

Edema is the collection of water in the interstitial space. It can occur as a result of several factors, all of which alter the forces that keep the net filtration in the capillary bed at zero. Edema is not necessarily a problem of fluid overload but rather a problem of fluid distribution. The four most common causes of edema are increased hydrostatic pressure, decreased plasma oncotic pressure, increased capillary membrane permeability, and lymphatic obstruction (McCance & Huether, 2002).

- *Increased hydrostatic pressure.* This can be caused by any mechanism that occludes or diminishes venous flow. Recall that the capillaries empty into the venous system. If fluid exit from the capillary becomes more difficult, the pressure inside will increase. If this problem persists, the pressure will build until capillary leakage occurs, resulting in edema. Any situation that causes an increase in the retention of salt and water will increase hydrostatic pressure. This is common in conditions such as congestive heart failure and renal insufficiency. In these situations the problem is compounded by a true fluid overload.
- *Decreased plasma osmotic pressure.* As previously explained, the osmotic pressure of the fluid in the intravascular space is caused by the solute found there. When the proteins found in the plasma are reduced, the associated pressure decreases. As the fluid passes through the capillary bed, the concentrations of solute may not be enough to pull all the water out of the interstitial space. This is common in diseases that involve the liver or kidneys.
- *Increased capillary membrane permeability.* This type of change is usually associated with the inflammation and immune response, which is examined later in this chapter. Inflammation can be caused by traumatic events such as burns and crushing injuries. It can also result from medical conditions such as an allergic reaction. Either way, the volume of solutes in the interstitial space becomes greater than that of the vascular space and fluid increases in the former, resulting in edema. Plasma proteins also escape the intravascular space and move to the interstitial space. This increases edema by a twofold effect. Venous oncotic pressure is reduced and oncotic pressure in the interstitial space is increased. This is the opposite of the oncotic pressure differential in normal microfiltration.
- *Lymphatic obstruction.* The lymphatic system is a mechanism by which some of the fluid and proteins that cross over into the interstitial spaces are removed. When these pathways are blocked, the fluid is returned to the interstitial space and the resulting edema is called **lymphedema.** This type of blockage is almost always caused by an infection, but it also can be caused by the removal of lymph nodes during surgery.

Clinical Manifestations. Edema can appear in a localized region or be generalized throughout the body. The type of presentation depends on the cause. In localized trauma, such as a sprained ankle, edema is isolated to the area of the injury. Localized edema can also occur in the chambers surrounding the brain, lungs, heart, and intestines. Generalized edema can present as a result of a disease process or systemic infection. It presents as dependent edema, meaning that gravity plays a role in the location of the edema. A person in the sitting or standing position may have edema in the lower extremities, and a person found in the supine position may have presacral edema.

Dependent edema can be measured and sometimes is called *pitting edema.* Pitting edema can be measured by pushing on the edematous area over a bone with the fingers. When the fluid is displaced and the fingers are removed, a pit is formed. Some clinicians clock the amount of time required for the pit to disappear as a measure of the degree of edema present in the tissues. Unfortunately, this method is not scientific and its accuracy is questionable.

Even localized edema can be life threatening if it is located in certain parts of the body, such as the brain, lungs, and tissues of the airway. However, generalized edema can cause many problems. As previously identified, this generally is a problem of fluid distribution. The condition can become severe enough that the patient becomes dehydrated. As the amount of fluid increases in the interstitial space (referred to as *third spacing* because this fluid is not available for metabolism), it can begin to hinder the effective exchange of oxygen and nutrients with the waste products in the tissues. If the condition continues without treatment, the pressure in the tissues can become so great that fluid can be forced through the skin to the outside of the body. This is commonly referred to as *weeping*.

The definitive treatment of edema involves treating the underlying medical condition that caused the edema, including altering the patient's nutritional status by a reduction in salt intake and improved overall balance of the patient's diet, the use of medications called diuretics to promote the elimination of fluids through the urine, and positional therapy. Limiting the amount of time the patient is in a particular position limits the amount of dependent edema. However, in the prehospital setting the treatment options are limited.

Case Scenario—continued

The patient denies chest pain or shortness of breath. He denies any blood in his vomitus or diarrhea. During your examination you note that he is very warm to the touch. His vital signs are pulse, 150 beats/min; blood pressure, 97/62 mm Hg; respirations, 16 breaths/min; temperature, 104.4° F. Pulse oximetry is 92% on room air, blood glucose is 484 mg/dL, and the cardiac monitor shows sinus tachycardia with no ectopy or signs of myocardial ischemia or injury. With the exception of poor skin turgor, the remainder of the examination is normal.

Questions

5. What is this patient's primary problem? How will you treat it?
6. What is the clinical significance of the patient's fever? Does it relate to the other symptoms? How?
7. Is this patient's blood glucose level what you expected given his history? Why or why not?
8. Given the history and vital signs, would you expect this patient's urine output to be higher or lower than normal? Why?

ROLE OF ELECTROLYTES

Water balance is greatly affected by the concentration and distribution of electrolytes. Electrolytes are acquired through the diet and eliminated in the urine. You must grasp this important concept to understand the effects of disease processes such as malnutrition and renal insufficiency.

Sodium is the chief extracellular **cation** (positively charged ion), accounting for approximately 90% of all cations in this space (Rose & Post, 2000). It serves many functions in the body. It maintains water balance by working with other ions to regulate osmotic forces, maintains neuromuscular irritability by working with potassium and calcium, and helps maintain acid-base balance.

Chloride is the major **anion** (negatively charged ion) in ECF. It provides a neutrality or counterbalance to sodium and other cations in the body. Because it is so closely related to the sodium level, the chloride level changes proportionally with the sodium level. If the sodium level increases, the chloride level generally follows. The reverse also is true. In addition, the level of chloride is somewhat inversely proportional to the level of sodium bicarbonate (HCO_3^-) located in the extracellular space.

Sodium and Chloride Balance

The level of sodium in the human body normally is regulated within a narrow range. The normal level for sodium concentration is between 135 and 145 mEq/L. This level is maintained by the kidneys and accomplished by the following mechanisms:

- *Aldosterone* is released in response to a decreased sodium level or an increased potassium level. It controls these levels in the kidneys by increasing the reabsorption of sodium through the distal tubules of the nephron while ensuring that potassium is excreted.

- *Renin* is an enzyme released from the juxtaglomerular cells in the kidneys in response to a decrease in renal blood flow. In the blood renin converts angiotensinogen (a precursor molecule) to angiotensin I (an inactive polypeptide). Angiotensin I is then converted to angiotensin II in the lungs by angiotensin-converting enzyme. Angiotensin II then acts as a hormone and causes the release of aldosterone and vascular constriction. It also causes the release of antidiuretic hormone (ADH). This substance stimulates the kidneys to reabsorb sodium

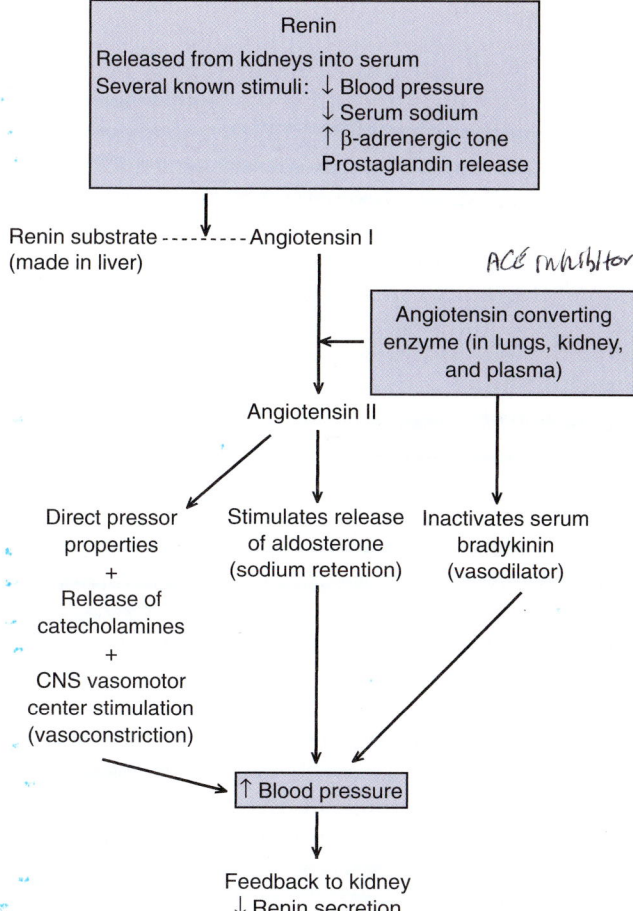

Figure 8-5 Renin-angiotensin-aldosterone system. *CNS,* Central nervous system.

(handwritten annotations in figure: "ACE inhibitor")

and water. These processes raise the sodium and water levels in the body and return the renal blood flow to acceptable levels. Once this happens, the secretion of renin ceases. This chain of events is called the *renin-angiotensin system* (Figure 8-5).

- *Natriuretic peptides* are hormones produced in the heart to control volume and sodium levels. Atrial natriuretic peptide is made in the atria. It is released when the volume of the heart increases. This, in turn, decreases blood pressure and increases the excretion of sodium and water.

Alterations in Sodium, Chloride, and Water Balance

Changes in sodium balance are closely related to water balance in the body because of the inevitable change in the osmotic gradient with the increase or decrease in sodium. On the other hand, if a dramatic change in the TBW occurs, a relative change in the sodium concentration also will occur, and the osmotic gradient shifts again.

Dehydration

Dehydration is a state in which the body loses a large amount of fluid from the tissues. These losses can be classified as isotonic, hypernatremic, or hyponatremic. *Isotonic dehydration* is a state in which the body loses water and sodium in equal proportions. This normally is caused by long-term illness with diarrhea or vomiting or by systemic infections. Worldwide, dehydration caused by diarrheal illness is the leading cause of infant and child death. Hypernatremic dehydration is a state in which the body loses water at a disproportionately higher rate than sodium. As the relative sodium concentration increases in the blood, fluid will shift from the extracellular space into the intravascular space. Hyponatremic dehydration is a state in which the body loses salt at a higher rate than water. When this occurs, the serum sodium level drops and the body's water shifts into the extracellular space, furthering some of the signs and symptoms of the process. The treatment for dehydrated patients is fluid replacement. However, it should be in amounts aligned with correcting the underlying cause.

(handwritten margin note: "Not for KST")

Overhydration

Overhydration is a state in which the body accumulates water faster than it can eliminate it. It is rarely caused by increased water intake. The chief cause of this condition is the failure of the kidneys to eliminate excess fluid as a result of a cardiac condition, impaired renal function, or excessive administration of intravenous (IV) fluids. Hyponatremia can be associated with overhydration as the sodium concentration becomes diluted. The treatment of overhydration is aimed at reducing water intake and promoting elimination. Once the cause is determined, medications such as diuretics may be given to treat the patient. The cause or result of dehydration and overhydration may be an electrolyte imbalance. If this is the case, the treatment is directed at correcting the problem.

ELECTROLYTE IMBALANCES

All electrolytes are affected by changes in the water balance because all the body's electrolytes work together to ensure proper function. Changes in the balance of electrolytes such as sodium, potassium, calcium, and magnesium can have harmful effects on normal physiologic functioning. The signs and symptoms of electrolyte imbalances are traditionally seen in the central nervous system, the peripheral nervous system, and the heart (Rose & Post, 2000).

Sodium

Sodium is the primary extracellular cation. Its normal concentration level ranges from 135 to 145 mEq/L. The primary functions of sodium include the regulation of water levels, particularly in the ECF, and the transmission of nervous impulses. Sodium levels are regulated by the kidneys. When sodium must be retained, aldosterone is released from the kidneys and antidiuretic hormone is released from the posterior pituitary gland. Both substances cause the kidneys to retain sodium. If sodium must be excreted, the release of these hormones is suppressed.

Hypernatremia

Hypernatremia is a serum sodium level above 145 mEq/L caused by either the gain of sodium in excess of water or the loss of water in excess of sodium. The latter is often referred to as *hypernatremic dehydration,* which is the more common cause of hypernatremia. Hypernatremia almost never found in an alert patient who has an intact thirst mechanism and access to water. The signs and symptoms of hypernatremia are primarily seen in the nervous system and may include irritability, tremors, lethargy, stupor, delirium, seizures, and coma. If the cause is excessive loss of water, the patient also may have signs of dehydration, including polydipsia, tachycardia, dry and sticky mucous membranes, poor skin turgor, flat neck veins, and oliguria or anuria.

Treatment for these patients in the prehospital setting is primarily supportive. Address any life-threatening conditions and treat with standard therapy. Isotonic saline is hypotonic compared with the condition of the body and should be administered on the basis of the patient's needs (e.g., vital signs, condition, mental status). As always, when administering fluids the lungs should be closely monitored.

Hyponatremia

Hyponatremia is a serum sodium level below 135 mEq/L and is a condition with many causes. The most common is the retention of water resulting in low sodium concentrations. Hyponatremia also may be caused by the loss of sodium alone or the loss of sodium in excess of water, referred to as hyponatremic dehydration. As with hypernatremia, the signs and symptoms of hyponatremia are seen in the nervous system. These may include difficulty concentrating, lethargy, apathy, confusion, headache, and seizures. Other signs and symptoms may include muscle cramps, tachycardia, nausea, and vomiting. Because hyponatremia causes cerebral edema, signs and symptoms of increased intracranial pressure may be present.

As with hypernatremia, treatment of hyponatremia is primarily supportive. Address and treat any life-threatening conditions and treat with standard therapy. Hyponatremic seizures respond poorly to benzodiazepines; the sodium concentration ultimately must be corrected. However, correction of sodium levels can be dangerous in the prehospital setting or emergency department. Administration of high concentrations of sodium in the emergency setting is rare. Sodium balance is generally restored over a period that extends beyond the time the patient has been transferred from the emergency department to the floor or intensive care unit.

Potassium

Potassium is the chief intracellular cation. It has many functions in the body, including the maintenance of fluid and pH balance inside cells, normal neurologic function, cardiac function, muscle contraction, and storage of glycogen in the liver and skeletal muscle. It accomplishes some of these functions by ensuring that a resting membrane potential exists so that cells can depolarize. Nearly 98% of the body's potassium is intracellular, which equates to an intravascular level of 3.5 to 5.0 mEq/L.

Hyperkalemia

Hyperkalemia is a state in which the body has an abnormally elevated potassium level. The most common cause of this condition is the failure of the body to eliminate potassium at the proper rate. This can be caused by acute or chronic renal failure (most commonly), urinary obstruction, burns, crush injuries, severe infection, and acidosis. In addition to this list, certain medications can cause the condition (e.g., acute digitalis toxicity, beta-blockers, succinylcholine). Note that not all hyperkalemic states occur as a result of an increase in total body potassium. Some causes simply stimulate the redistribution of potassium from inside cells to the vasculature. The signs and symptoms of hyperkalemia present in the neuromuscular system and the cardiac conduction system. The most common sign of hyperkalemia is vague muscle weakness (early) leading to flaccid paralysis (late). Other signs include tetany, paresthesias, generalized fatigue, oliguria, nausea, and diarrhea. Cardiac signs and symptoms can include dysrhythmias, bradycardia, the development of tall, peaked T waves, widening of the QRS complex, and flattening of the P waves.

Patients are usually treated for hyperkalemia in the hospital and critical care settings; however, this condition can be life threatening and may need to be treated immediately. Emergency management of this condition consists of the administration of medications such as calcium, albuterol, sodium bicarbonate, insulin, and dextrose (McCance & Huether, 2002). Calcium can increase the threshold potential, thereby restoring the electrical gradient inside and outside cells. Sodium bicarbonate, albuterol, or insulin administered with dextrose forces potassium back into cells. Kayexalate is a resin that can be given orally or through a gastric tube to reduce the potassium level through the intestines. In extreme cases hemodialysis may be needed. Recall earlier discussions regarding the exchange of potassium and hydrogen ions between the intracellular space and the intravascular space. Because of this principle, hyperkalemic patients also may be acidotic.

Hypokalemia

Hypokalemia is a state in which the level of potassium in the serum falls below 3.5 mEq/L. Although the body receives electrolytes through the diet, hypokalemia from a dietary deficiency is rare. Some of the more common causes are insulin administration, prolonged episodes of vomiting, renal disease, the use of non–potassium-sparing diuretics, and alkalosis. The most common cause in the United States is the use of diuretics. Most patients who have been prescribed one of these medications also are placed on a potassium supplement. The signs and symptoms of hypokalemia include muscle weakness, hyporeflexia, and cardiac dysrhythmias.

The treatment of hypokalemia is directed at replacing potassium and typically occurs in the hospital. The IV replacement of electrolytes can be challenging. It must be done slowly to have a positive effect. Rapid replacement results in the patient eliminating a large quantity of the potassium (or other electrolytes) on the first pass of the kidneys, or it may result in problematic effects for the patient.

Calcium

The body uses calcium for many purposes. It plays a role in the stability of the cell membrane and its permeability, hormone secretion, contraction of muscles, and the transmission of nerve impulses. Calcium also is needed in several chemical reactions of the clotting cascade. Most of the calcium in the human body (99%) is located and stored in the bones. As the body's demand for calcium increases, it is released from the bone into the bloodstream. When it is released, half is bound to albumin (approximately 2.5 mEq/L) and is not used for most of the functions normally associated with calcium. The other half (approximately 2.4 mEq/L) is free ionized calcium and is available for use. The normal level of total calcium is 4.5 to 5.5 mEq/L or 8.4 to 10.2 mg/dL (Rose & Post, 2000). Calcium often has an inverse relation with phosphate. This means an elevation in the calcium level will trigger a drop in the level of phosphate in the body, and vice versa.

Hypercalcemia

Hypercalcemia is a state in which the body has an abnormally high level of calcium. Hyperparathyroidism is the most common cause because parathyroid hormone (PTH) is essential for calcium release into the circulation. Elevated calcium levels also can be caused by tumors (some of which cause elevated PTH), cancers affecting the bone, excessive administration of vitamin D, or the use of diuretics. The body uses vitamin D to stimulate the release of PTH, and some patients receive vitamin D in the treatment of osteoporosis. The signs and symptoms associated with hypercalcemia are sometimes vague. They may include fatigue, weakness, lethargy, nausea, renal stones, and behavioral changes. Treatment is generally directed at correcting the underlying cause.

Hypocalcemia

Hypocalcemia is a state in which the body has an abnormally low calcium level. It can be caused by a lack of PTH in the body. PTH is essential for calcium release from the bone. PTH also activates vitamin D in the kidneys to promote calcium reabsorption. This means that renal failure also can cause decreased calcium levels. The amount of circulating albumin also is important in maintaining calcium levels. If the albumin level falls, calcium also decreases. The body always tries to keep the level of bound calcium and ionized calcium in proportion. Other causes of hypocalcemia include hypomagnesemia and sepsis. If the patient is receiving large amounts of banked blood, the calcium level may drop as a result of increased citrate levels. Citrate is used to prevent coagulation in banked blood by binding calcium. Signs and symptoms of hypocalcemia include nausea and vomiting, diarrhea, numbness and tingling sensations around the mouth or in the fingers and toes, and muscle cramps (particularly in the back and lower extremities) that may progress to carpopedal spasm/tetany, abdominal pain, weakness, headaches, behvioral changes, and seizures.

Treatment is directed at replacing calcium and preventing further losses. Oral replacement is optimal, but IV infusion can be used in an emergency situation. Long-term care includes the restriction of phosphate because of the inverse relation between the two and the maintenance of vitamin D levels.

Magnesium

Magnesium is needed and used in approximately 300 different chemical reactions in the human body, including helping the body absorb and use other electrolytes. Like calcium, it provides a supportive role in muscle and neurologic function. It also is important in the function of the heart. In fact, the relaxation of cardiac muscle depends on a consistent magnesium level. In addition, it helps the body regulate blood glucose level and plays a role in protein synthesis. Somewhere between 40% and 60% of magnesium is stored in muscle and bone, with 30% found inside cells. Only a small percentage (approximately 1%) is found in the blood, for a normal serum concentration of 1.8 to 2.4 mEq/L.

Hypermagnesemia

Hypermagnesemia is a state in which the body has an abnormally elevated concentration of magnesium in the blood. It is a rare condition and is usually associated with a reduction in renal function or a significant increase in dietary intake. In addition, certain medications can increase the serum magnesium levels. The signs and symptoms of hypermagnesemia include nausea and vomiting, muscle weakness, decreased level of consciousness, bradycardia, and hypotension. Treatment may include IV administration of calcium, which buffers the magnesium. For extreme cases the only definitive treatment option is hemodialysis.

Hypomagnesemia   *alcoholics, preeclampsia*

Hypomagnesemia is a state in which the body has an abnormally low serum concentration of magnesium. It may be caused by excessive gastrointestinal (GI)

TABLE 8-1 | Signs and Symptoms of Electrolyte Imbalance

Electrolyte	Disturbance	Central Nervous System	Peripheral Nervous System	Heart
Potassium	Hyperkalemia	Hyperreflexia and tremors	Oliguria, nausea, diarrhea	Cardiac disturbances (including cardiac arrest)
	Hypokalemia	Hyporeflexia	Weakness	Cardiac dysrhythmias
Calcium	Hypercalcemia	Fatigue, nausea, behavioral changes	Weakness, renal stones, lethargy	Cardiac dysrhythmias (including heart blocks)
	Hypocalcemia	Nausea and vomiting, headaches, behavioral changes, seizures	Muscle cramps, abdominal pain, diarrhea, weakness, paresthesia, carpopedal spasm, tetany	Decreased cardiac contractility, prolonged QT interval
Magnesium	Hypermagnesemia	Vomiting, decreased level of consciousness	Muscle weakness	Bradycardia, conduction delays, hypotension
	Hypomagnesemia	Depression, confusion, seizures	Hyporeflexia, muscle weakness	

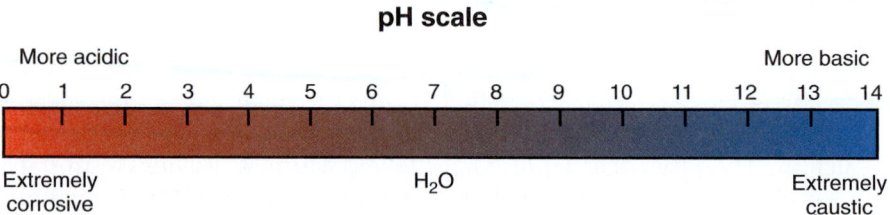

pH scale

Figure 8-6 The pH scale.

losses; excessive renal losses, including those induced by diuretics; alcoholism; malnutrition; and certain chronic disease states such as diabetes. The signs and symptoms of a low magnesium level mimic those of **hypocalcemia.** They may include depression, confusion, hyporeflexia, muscle weakness, and seizures (Table 8-1). The treatment for hypomagnesemia is the IV infusion of magnesium.

ACID-BASE BALANCE

Acid-base balance refers to the delicate balance between the body's acidity and alkalinity. To comprehend the following, you must first understand basic definitions of acids and bases. According to the Bronsted-Lowry classification of acids and bases, an acid is a hydrogen ion or proton donor, and a base is a hydrogen ion or proton acceptor. The form in which this balance is expressed is pH. Measured on a scale of 0 to 14, a pH of 0 represents the most acidic, 14 represents the most alkaline, and 7 represents neutrality. Water has a pH of 7.0. The human body normally is slightly alkaline, with a pH between 7.35 and 7.45. The body's ability to maintain a precise balance is imperative. Even a slight change may cause significant problems throughout various organ

systems because hydrogen ions are important in maintaining the membrane integrity and the efficacy of enzymatic reactions (Figure 8-6).

Hydrogen Ion and pH

The relation between hydrogen ion concentration and pH is inversely proportionate; as the hydrogen ion concentration in the body goes up, the pH goes down, and vice versa. Because hydrogen is an acid, as the concentration rises in the body, the body becomes more acidic. In contrast, if the hydrogen concentration drops, the body becomes more basic, or alkaline. The abbreviation pH (power of hydrogen) is an expression for the negative logarithm of the hydrogen ion concentration in a solution. This means that a change of one unit in the pH (e.g., 7.0 to 8.0) translates into a tenfold change in the hydrogen ion concentration (Rose & Post, 2000).

Changes in the body's acidity can occur from an increase in the intake of acidic compounds, increased production, or a decrease in the elimination of the same. It also can be caused by a decrease in the level of base compounds in the body. Decreases in base compounds can occur because of a decrease in intake or production or an increase in elimination. The body tries to maintain a 1:20 ratio between acids (carbonic acid) and bases (bicarbonate). It does this through several mechanisms collectively called **buffer systems.**

Buffer Systems

The body constantly monitors its pH balance and quickly responds to correct any disturbance. This is accomplished by three primary mechanisms. The carbonic acid–bicarbonate buffer system, protein buffering, and renal buffering are closely related compensatory mechanisms. These systems act together to control the pH. All these systems depend on adequate organ function. Therefore they can be hampered or even rendered ineffective with a significant insult on the body.

Carbonic Acid–Bicarbonate Buffering   *80-85% of time (in plasma)* ✱

Carbonic acid–bicarbonate buffering is the most rapid acting of all the compensatory mechanisms. It works almost immediately after identifying the disturbance. As hydrogen and other acids are produced as a normal byproduct of metabolism, the body will move to neutralize or eliminate them to maintain balance. It does this by combining acids with bases to create a weaker acid. For example, hydrogen (H^+) will combine with bicarbonate (HCO_3^-) to form carbonic acid (H_2CO_3). In addition, carbon dioxide (CO_2) will combine with water (H_2O) to again form carbonic acid. This is done with the help of the enzyme carbonic anhydrase, represented in the following equation:

$$H^+ + HCO_3^- \leftrightarrow H_2CO_3 \leftrightarrow H_2O + CO_2$$

Bicarb   *Carbonic acid*   *lungs*

The equation works in both directions depending on the needs of the body. Elevation of hydrogen ions causes the equation balance to move to the right. CO_2 elevation moves the equation balance to the left. Carbonic acid is an unstable acid, and the conversion to one side or the other of the equation will happen rapidly. This means that an increase of hydrogen ions will increase the carbon dioxide level, and vice versa. The carbonic acid–bicarbonate system then works with protein buffering and renal buffering to eliminate the problem.

Protein Buffering   *15% of time (in cells)*

Some proteins in the intracellular and extracellular space are negatively charged and can serve as a buffer for hydrogen (Figure 8-7). Most are inside the cell, so this system ✱ mainly operates there. Because hemoglobin easily binds to hydrogen and carbon dioxide, it is the most common method of acid elimination in this system. As the blood is circulated throughout the body into the tissues, gases are exchanged at the capillary level. Oxygen is dropped off to the cells of the tissues, and carbon dioxide and hydrogen are bound with the hemoglobin for the return trip to the lungs. Once this blood makes it to the alveolar capillaries, gas exchange again occurs, releasing the carbon dioxide and hydrogen into the lung tissue. Hydrogen is bound with bicarbonate to create carbonic acid, which quickly dissociates into CO_2 and H_2O. The lungs

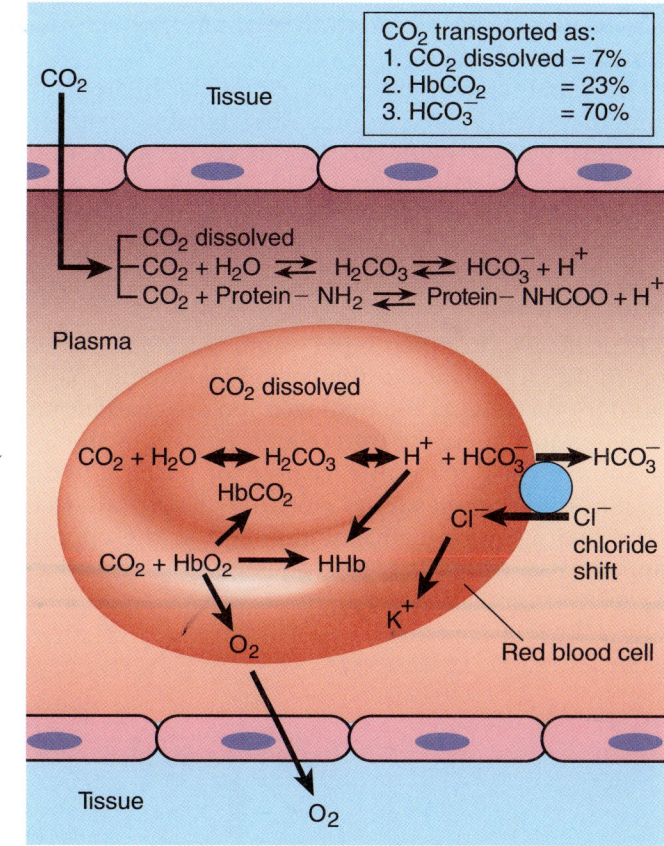

Figure 8-7 Buffering of hydrogen with hemoglobin and carbon dioxide (CO_2) transport. CO_2 is produced in tissue cells and diffuses to plasma, where it is transported as dissolved CO_2, or it combines with water to form carbonic acid (H_2CO_3), or it combines with protein from which hydrogen has been released. Most of the CO_2 diffuses into the red blood cell and combines with water to form H_2CO_3. The H_2CO_3 dissociates to form hydrogen (H^+), bicarbonate (HCO_3^-) shifts into the plasma, and chloride (Cl^-) shifts into the red blood cell to maintain electroneutrality. Hydrogen combines with hemoglobin that has released its oxygen to form ionized hemoglobin, which buffers the hydrogen and makes venous blood slightly more acidic than arterial blood.

(O_2 Hb) → $CO_2 + H_2O$

then eliminate the excess carbon dioxide through exhalation.

This mechanism depends on the respiratory system working effectively. Changes in respiratory rate and depth can have beneficial or adverse consequences. Because of this, the respiratory system is chiefly driven by the level of the blood pH and not oxygen. *Keep CO_2 in 35-45 range while bagging. Don't over ventilate, will blow off CO_2*

Renal Buffering   *Takes days to work   5% of time*

The third primary compensatory mechanism for maintaining acid-base balance is the renal system. This is the slowest method for returning the pH to a normal range. Days are sometimes required to accomplish the task. The kidneys regulate the pH by monitoring the elimination of hydrogen and the reabsorption of bicarbonate in the tubules of nephrons. If the body is too acidic, it will increase the amount of hydrogen eliminated in the urine and recover bicarbonate. If not enough hydrogen (alkalosis) is present, the kidneys will retain to hydrogen and eliminate bicarbonate.

The renal system also can eliminate hydrogen if ammonia (NH_3) is present. The kidneys combine ammonia with a hydrogen ion to create ammonium (NH_4^+) (Rose & Post, 2000). This substance is easily excreted in the urine, thereby decreasing the acidity of the body.

Other Buffers

As explained in Chapter 6, potassium has a unique relation to the pH balance in the body. Potassium is mainly found inside cells. As the hydrogen ion concentration in the blood increases, the intracellular potassium shifts to the intravascular space in exchange for pushing hydrogen ions into the cell so that protein buffering can occur. If the hydrogen ion concentration is low, the opposite happens. Patients with acid-base disturbances must have their potassium levels closely monitored to avoid potentially lethal consequences.

Acid-Base Imbalances

Acid-base disturbances can be caused by respiratory or metabolic issues or a combination of the two. As previously described, anything that increases the hydrogen level or decreases the bicarbonate level causes acidosis. In the body, this is a pH of less than 7.35. Anything that increases the bicarbonate level or decreases the hydrogen level causes alkalosis. This is a pH of 7.45 or greater. A patient may present with a mixed disturbance, which means acidosis and alkalosis have different origins. This is normally one condition trying to compensate for the other.

Metabolic Acidosis

Acidosis is caused by an increase in the level of acids or a loss of bases. Acidosis can result from several metabolic causes, such as lactic acidosis, diabetic ketoacidosis, or renal failure. A loss of base can occur from diarrhea and vomiting. In this type of disturbance the pH decreases but the carbon dioxide level at first remains normal. With

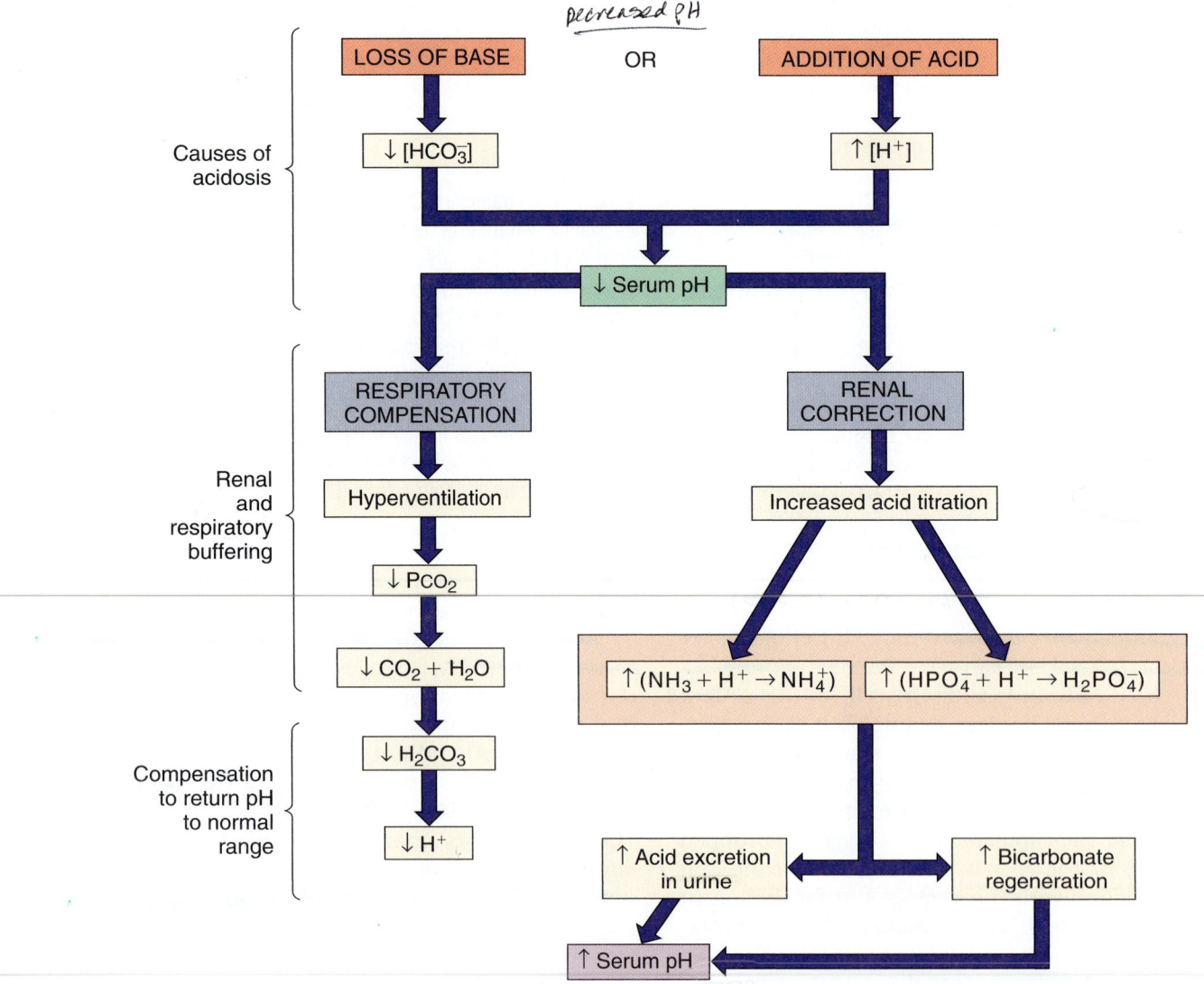

Figure 8-8 Metabolic acidosis with compensation and correction.

a relative increase in carbonic acid (either a true increase or a decrease in bicarbonate), the equation representing this shift is expressed as follows:

$$\uparrow H^+ + HCO_3^- \rightarrow \uparrow H_2CO_3 \rightarrow H_2O + \uparrow CO_2$$

Patients with this type of acid-base disturbance can present with nonspecific symptoms involving multiple organ systems, including the neurologic, cardiac, pulmonary, and GI systems. The signs and symptoms are usually indicative of or directly related to the underlying cause of the acidosis (e.g., poor perfusion causing lactic acidosis or renal failure). The treatment is generally directed at the underlying pathologic condition. Intravenous infusion of sodium bicarbonate is usually reserved for only the most severe cases (Figure 8-8).

Metabolic Alkalosis

Metabolic alkalosis is less common than metabolic acidosis. It occurs when a loss of metabolic acids or an increase in bicarbonate occurs. The most common causes of this disturbance are excessive vomiting and long-term diuretic use. As a general rule, the body loses more acids through vomiting and more bases through diarrhea. In this condition, the pH is increased but the CO_2 level remains within acceptable limits. The equation representing this shift is expressed as follows:

$$\downarrow H^+ + HCO_3^- \rightarrow \downarrow H_2CO_3 \rightarrow H_2O + \downarrow CO_2$$

Patients with metabolic alkalosis can have nonspecific signs and symptoms. However, the severity depends on the degree of the disturbance. This condition is usually associated with an electrolyte imbalance, so the patient may show signs of **hypokalemia** and/or hypocalcemia. The treatment for alkalosis depends on the underlying cause of the condition and volume status of the patient. If the volume status of the patient is low, the treatment is directed at correcting volume with a sodium chloride solution. If excessive vomiting is a concern, the use of antiemetics may be indicated. If the patient has a volume overload (as in congestive heart failure), he or she may be treated with a potassium-sparing diuretic and/or a carbonic anhydrase inhibitor (Figure 8-9).

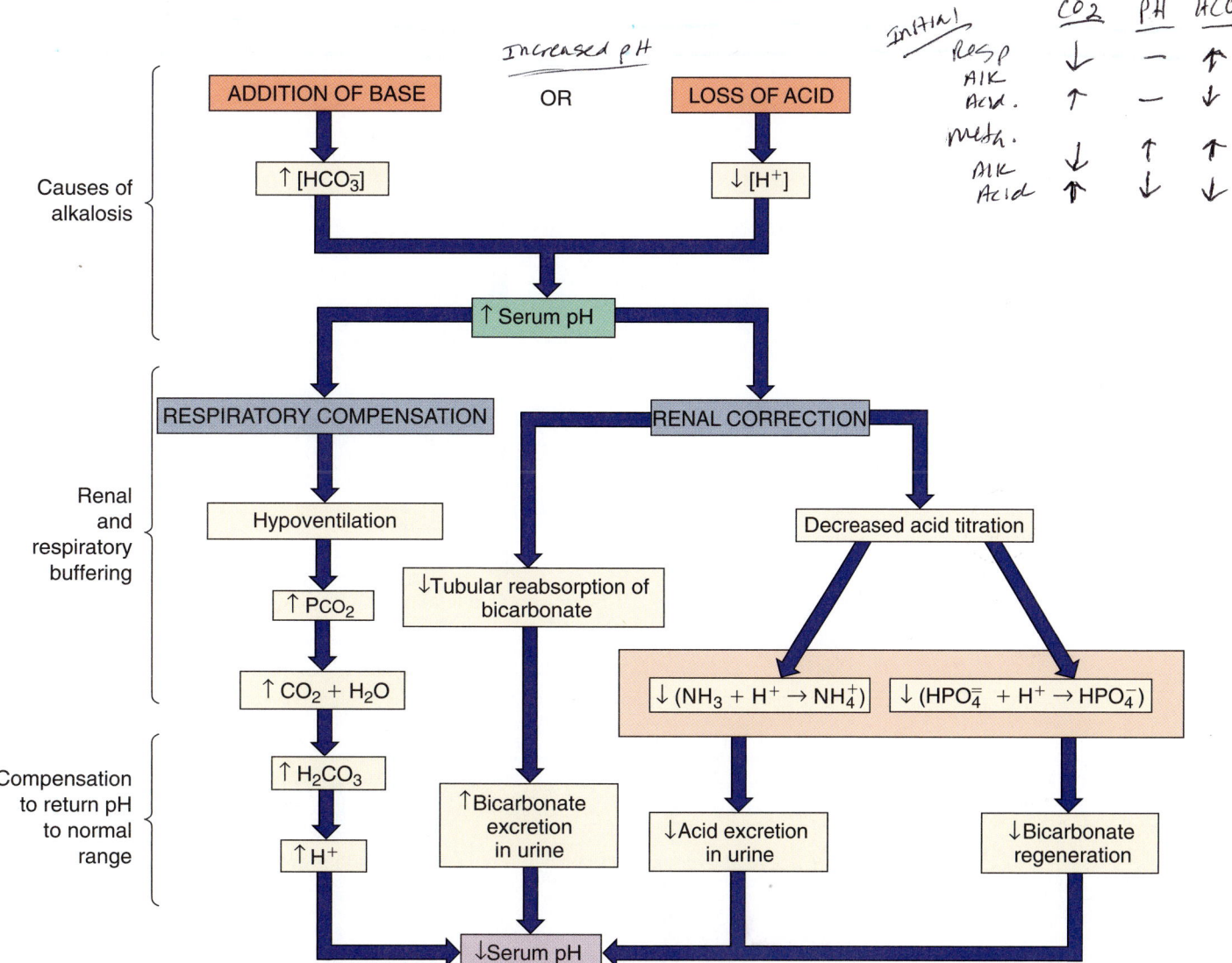

Figure 8-9 Metabolic alkalosis with compensation and correction.

[handwritten notes: Asthma, COPD, Addicts — Give O₂ & assist w/ breathing — Normal pH or ↓, ↑CO₂]

Respiratory Acidosis

Respiratory acidosis is a condition closely linked with the body's ability to eliminate CO_2 through alveolar ventilation. Any condition that causes a decrease in the respiratory rate or volume will lead to acidosis, including respiratory insufficiency or failure, respiratory arrest, and cardiac arrest. Increased levels of CO_2 result in elevated carbonic acid production. Without the ability to eliminate the CO_2 in the lungs, the body must rely on the renal buffering system for compensation. As previously mentioned, this could take days to work, and the prevailing acidotic state could have lethal consequences before the body corrects the problem. In respiratory acidosis, the CO_2 level is increased and pH is decreased. This type of disturbance is represented by the following:

$$\downarrow Respiration = \uparrow CO_2 + H_2O \rightarrow \uparrow H_2CO_3 \rightarrow \uparrow H^+ + HCO_3^-$$

A patient in respiratory acidosis shows signs and symptoms of the underlying cause but is almost always hypoxic. Treatment is directed at the underlying cause and at correcting ventilatory status. By ensuring adequate ventilation and oxygenation, you can promote the elimination of carbon dioxide and reduce the carbonic acid level in the body (Figure 8-10). Unlike metabolic acidosis, the administration of sodium bicarbonate to a patient in respiratory acidosis is contraindicated and will increase the respiratory acidosis.

Respiratory Alkalosis

As with respiratory acidosis, this condition is closely linked to the respiratory system and the elimination of CO_2. In respiratory alkalosis, the issue is the excessive elimination of CO_2. This can be caused by any number of situations that cause an increase in the respiratory rate, such as hyperventilation syndrome, anxiety, hysteria, and altitude acclimation as well as metabolic causes such as fever. In this type of disturbance, the CO_2 level is decreased and the pH is elevated, as represented by the following:

$$\uparrow Respiration = \downarrow CO_2 + H_2O \rightarrow \downarrow H_2CO_3 \rightarrow \downarrow H^+ + HCO_3^-$$

The patient with respiratory alkalosis may show signs and symptoms ranging from minimal changes that do not require intervention to serious issues in the critically ill patient. The most common signs and symptoms include paresthesia, circumoral numbness, chest tightness, dyspnea, dizziness, confusion, and tetany. Treat-

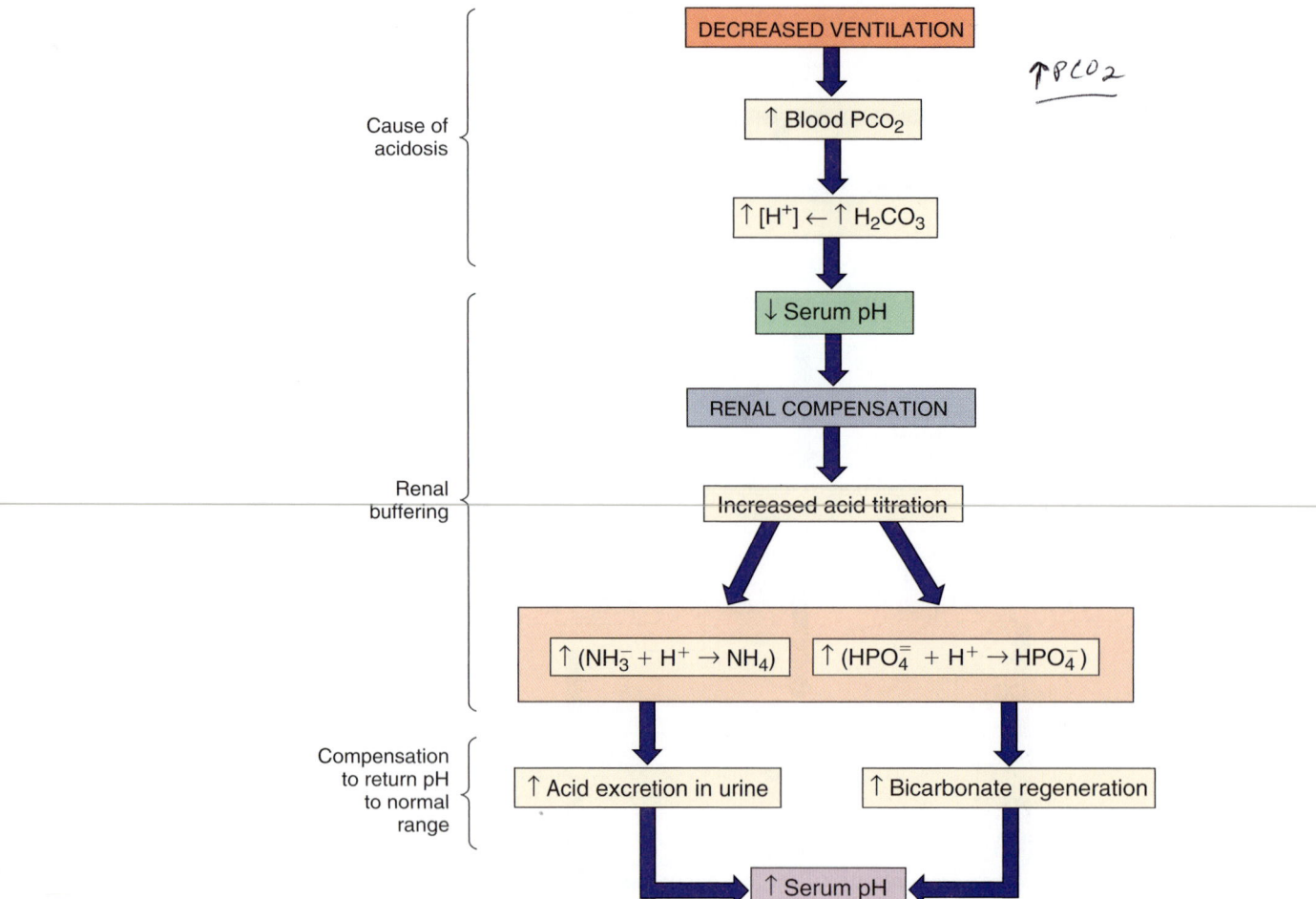

Figure 8-10 Respiratory acidosis with compensation.

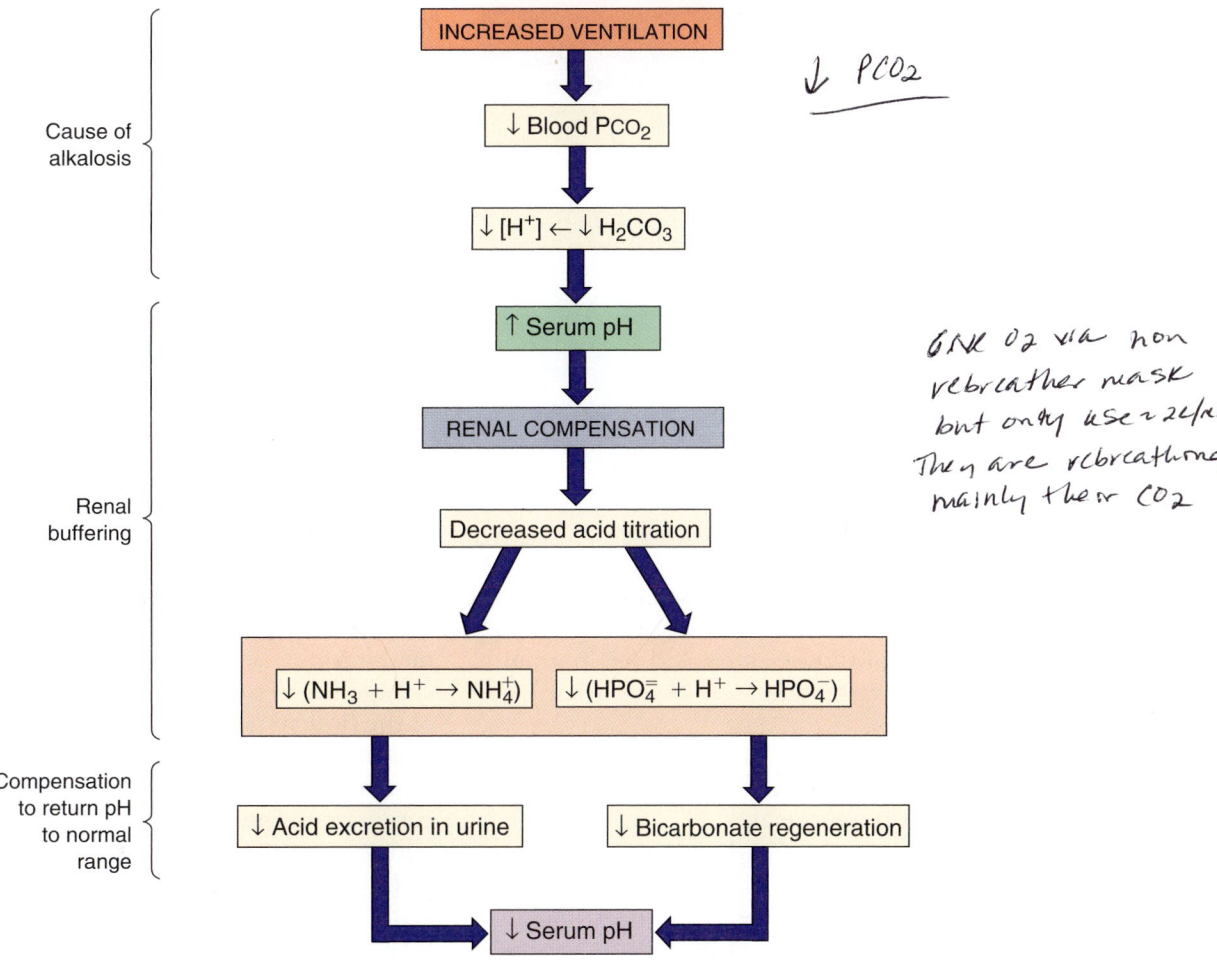

$\downarrow PCO_2$

Give O2 via non rebreather mask but only use 2 2L/min. They are rebreathing mainly their CO2

Figure 8-11 Respiratory alkalosis with compensation.

ment is directed at correcting the underlying cause. This can range from coaching the patient's breathing to administering sedative medications to placing the patient on a ventilator in extreme cases (Figure 8-11).

Mixed Acid-Base Disturbances

As previously mentioned, patients may have a mixed acid-base disturbance. Examples of these types of problems include the following:

- Respiratory and metabolic acidosis
- Respiratory acidosis and metabolic alkalosis
- Respiratory alkalosis and metabolic acidosis
- Respiratory and metabolic alkalosis

To identify any acid-base disturbance accurately, the clinician must use arterial blood gas levels as a guide. In the past these values were not obtainable in the field but sometimes were available for interfacility transports. With advances in technology such as the i-STAT (Abbott Laboratories, Abbott Park, Ill.), these values are now obtainable in the field. These values are used to determine the need for changes in treatment, such as ventilator settings. Even in the absence of actual values the

BOX 8-1	Normal Ranges of Arterial Blood Gases

PaO_2 = 80 to 100 mm Hg
$PaCO_2$ = 35 to 45 mm Hg
pH = 7.35 to 7.45
HCO_3^- = 22 to 26 mmol/L

paramedic should be able to combine the patient's history and presentation with likely acid-base disturbances and provide appropriate treatment (Boxes 8-1 and 8-2).

Compensation in Acid-Base Disorders

In its attempt to maintain a normal pH balance, the body will attempt to compensate for any disturbance in the acid-base balance through the mechanisms previously described.

The initial alteration in these levels is considered an acute situation, meaning compensation has not yet restored the normal pH. This is recognized by an abnormal pH and an abnormality in one other component (CO_2 or bicarbonate), as follows:

BOX 8-2	General Rules of Interpretation of pH Disturbance

pH < 7.35 = Acidosis
High $PaCO_2$ = respiratory
Low $PaCO_2$ = metabolic

pH > 7.45 = Alkalosis
Low $PaCO_2$ = respiratory
High $PaCO_2$ = metabolic

- Acute respiratory acidosis = decreased pH, increased CO_2, normal bicarbonate
- Acute respiratory alkalosis = increased pH, decreased CO_2, normal bicarbonate
- Acute metabolic acidosis = decreased pH, normal CO_2, decreased bicarbonate
- Acute metabolic alkalosis = increased pH, normal CO_2, increased bicarbonate

In these conditions identifying the original problem or the initial cause of the change in the pH is simple because only one component is abnormal.

As the body attempts to correct the pH, compensation occurs. Partial compensation is the situation in which these mechanisms are functioning, but the pH has not yet been restored. This is identified by abnormal values for all three components of the acid-base balance. In attempting to restore a normal pH, compensation occurs in the opposite direction of the original alteration. In other words, metabolic acidosis is compensated by respiratory alkalosis, respiratory acidosis is compensated for by metabolic alkalosis, and so on, as follows:

- Partially compensated respiratory acidosis = decreased pH, increased CO_2, increased bicarbonate
- Partially compensated respiratory alkalosis = increased pH, decreased CO_2, decreased bicarbonate
- Partially compensated metabolic acidosis = decreased pH, decreased CO_2, decreased bicarbonate
- Partially compensated metabolic alkalosis = increased pH, increased CO_2, increased bicarbonate

Because both components are abnormal in partially compensated states, determination of the original problem and the compensatory change is not as obvious as in acute changes. However, it can be discovered easily by determining the direction of the pH (acidotic or alkalotic) and looking for the component that has changed in the same direction on the acid-base scale. For example, suppose the pH is 7.2 (acidotic), the CO_2 level is 80 (acidotic), and the bicarbonate is 28 (alkalotic). In this situation both the pH and the CO_2 level are acidotic, representing respiratory acidosis being compensated for by metabolic alkalosis.

Complete, or total, compensation occurs when the body restores the pH to normal. However, the CO_2 and bicarbonate levels will remain abnormal. These generally are chronic conditions, as follows:

- Completely compensated respiratory acidosis = normal pH, increased CO_2, increased bicarbonate
- Completely compensated respiratory alkalosis = normal pH, decreased CO_2, decreased bicarbonate
- Completely compensated metabolic acidosis = normal pH, decreased CO_2, decreased bicarbonate
- Completely compensated metabolic alkalosis = normal pH, increased CO_2, increased bicarbonate

Complete compensation represents the most challenging situation when attempting to determine the original problem and the compensatory change because the pH cannot be used as in partial compensation. The key to determining the original problem and the compensatory change lies in the patient's history and an understanding of the human body. For example, suppose the patient has a normal pH, an increased CO_2 level, and increased bicarbonate level. This could represent either a completely compensated metabolic alkalosis or a completely compensated respiratory acidosis. If the patient has a history of prolonged vomiting (resulting in the loss of stomach acid), then metabolic alkalosis is the original problem. However, if the patient has a history of chronic obstructive pulmonary disease (a disorder in which CO_2 is retained), then respiratory acidosis is the original problem. Even in the absence of actual acid-base values the paramedic should be able to predict the acid-base status of the patient on the basis of history to provide the most appropriate care. Causes of acid-base imbalances are listed in Box 8-3.

GENETICS AND FAMILIAL DISEASES

[OBJECTIVES 5, 8]

Since early in human history, individuals have attempted to discover the causes of diseases and find effective treatments. In the 1600s, Anton van Leeuwenhoek began the development of **germ theory.** This theory was refined over the course of time by well-known scientists such as Louis Pasteur in the 1860s and Alexander Fleming in the 1920s. The theory states that some disease processes are caused by microorganisms. At first this theory was highly controversial. However, by the early 1900s it was accepted as fact. Then it was touted as the single most important contribution to medical science in history. It has provided the answers and understanding for many of the infectious diseases faced by human beings today.

The next major hurdle is understanding the genetics involved with disease acquisition and progression. With

BOX 8-3 Causes of Acid-Base Disturbances

Respiratory Acidosis

- Asthma
- Chronic obstructive pulmonary disease
- Trauma
  - Pneumothorax
  - Hemothorax
  - Flail chest
  - Pulmonary contusion
- Respiratory arrest
- Respiratory depression
- Anaphylaxis
- Pulmonary edema
- Infection
- Pneumonia
- Airway obstruction
- Neuromuscular disease affecting ventilation

Respiratory Alkalosis

Hyperventilation secondary to any cause, such as:
- Hypoxia
- Anemia
- Central nervous system disorders
- Medications
- Infection
- Psychogenic causes
- Pulmonary disorders
  - Pneumonia
- Pulmonary embolus

Metabolic Acidosis

- Carbon monoxide exposure
- Cyanide exposure
- Alcoholic ketoacidosis
- Toluene exposure
- Methanol exposure
- Uremia
- Diabetic ketoacidosis
- Poisoning
- Paraldehyde ingestion
- Infection
- Isoniazid ingestion
- Iron intoxication
- Lactic acidosis
- Ethylene glycol
- Salicylate overdose
- Hyperkalemia
- Diarrhea

Metabolic Alkalosis

- Ingestion of bicarbonate (e.g., antacids)
- Loss of stomach acids
- Diuretic use
- Aldosteronism
- Mineralocorticoid use
- Adenocarcinoma
- Bartter syndrome
- Cushing syndrome
- Cystic fibrosis
- Hypokalemia

---

the advancement of the Human Genome Project, many more answers are available today than even as recently as 10 years ago. A significant number of disease processes have been identified as having a genetic or environmental origin. As the ability to identify genetic or familial causes of disease continues to progress, the medical and scientific communities must focus on developing treatments that can correct or influence DNA and other genetic components of the body. Other factors such as age and gender have also been shown to be factors.

Genetic Factors

Genetics and heredity are determined by the order in which chromosomes are sorted in the sperm and egg. This occurs randomly, and the traits a person receives from his or her parents are a matter of chance (McCance & Huether, 2002). At conception, an embryo receives 23 chromosomes from the mother and 23 from the father. Disease or the propensity for a disease process can arise when an abnormality exists in a specific part of a

chromosome (gene). With more than 100,000 genes in a person's genetic profile, the chances and variations of possible abnormalities are enormous.

Diseases ranging from Down syndrome to hemophilia and sickle cell anemia have been identified as arising from specific genes or extra copies of genes. Others, such as Alzheimer's disease and depression, may have a genetic component; strong and convincing evidence exists for this but has not yet been proven. Not all genetic abnormalities are thought to be congenital (present from birth). Some indications exist that some genetic changes occur as a result of environmental factors along with a genetic predisposition.

Environmental Factors

[handwritten note: Asthma on SE side of Chicago— people die there at higher rate than anywhere else in world]

[OBJECTIVE 7]

Few disease states are thought to be purely environmental in nature. A large number of diseases are not inherited; however, the predisposing factors are considered genetic. This explains why people exposed to the same environmental stimulus can have quite different consequences.

For example, a health-conscious person can develop heart disease; whereas a person who smokes, eats a high-fat diet, and is obese may seem immune to the effects. Another example of this is type 2, or adult-onset, diabetes. This disease is strongly tied to genetics and family history but sometimes does not manifest until middle age. Onset has been strongly linked to a high-fat diet and a lack of exercise, which both lead to obesity. Obesity is a known risk factor for the development of type 2 diabetes.

Many environmental factors are important in the development of different disease processes. These include microorganisms and immunologic exposures, personal habits and lifestyle, chemical substances, physical environment, and psychosocial environment. Once a genetic predisposition or an environmental trigger is identified, the treatment for these diseases includes, as much as possible, the reduction of risk factors.

Age and Gender

[OBJECTIVE 8]

In addition to genetic and environmental factors, age- and gender-specific factors play a role in the development of disease. Certain disease processes are specific to the hormonal and anatomic differences between men and women, such as breast cancer in women and testicular cancer in men. Another example is the higher occurrence of heart disease in men compared with women before menopause. With changes in the hormonal balance in women after menopause, the occurrence of heart disease approaches that of men. In addition, the changes in human metabolism with age can play a role in the effect of disease processes. Hypertension and the vascular and metabolic conditions associated with it often are found in older patients.

ANALYZING DISEASE RISKS

[OBJECTIVE 9]

When studying how disease processes work in the human body, you need to understand the scope of the problem on society. This quantifies the issue and can give clues to the causes and potential treatments for a specific disease or group of disorders. The people responsible for collecting this type of data are called *epidemiologists*. They try to define the disease rate and conduct risk factor analyses to determine the likely causative factors.

Disease Rates

When epidemiologists looks at the effects of a disease on a population group, they traditionally use at least three common statistics: the **incidence rate,** the **prevalence** and the **mortality rate.** The incidence of a disease is equal to a fraction of the population that contracts a given disease during a certain period. In other words, this is the rate at which new cases are diagnosed in a population group. The prevalence of a disease is the fraction of the population that currently has a certain disease. This is different from incidence rate, which only looks at the rate of contraction of a disease versus how many are currently sick with the disease. The mortality rate is the number of patients who have died from a disease in a given period. Note that the incidence rate and the mortality rate are based on a specified time period. The prevalence, as described here, is based on a particular instant in time and is called the *point prevalence.* The period prevalence is based on an extended time comparable to the incidence and mortality rates. For the consistency of reporting and analyzing, the time period most commonly used is 1 year.

Risk Factor Analysis

Risk factors can be classified into two categories: causal and noncausal. A causal risk factor is a risk factor that can determine outcome. Eliminating or reducing the exposure by a person to this type of risk factor can slow the progression of disease or completely prevent it. A noncausal risk factor is a risk factor that can be helpful in predicting the development of a disease, but its removal does not affect whether the person will acquire the illness.

Combined Effects and Interaction of Risk Factors

[OBJECTIVE 10]

Risk factors are clearly defined occurrences or characteristics associated with the increased rate of a disease. Some risk factors by themselves have a minimal impact on a person's chances of acquiring a disease, but combined with other risk factors they can significantly increase the likelihood. Two of the most common risk factor interactions are familial tendencies and age.

Familial Tendency

[OBJECTIVE 6]

Most people know that some diseases tend to run in families. A large contributor to this phenomenon is genetics. Environmental factors also play a large role. For example, children who live in a house with parents who smoke are exposed to the toxins of secondhand smoke and thus share their parent's environmental risk factor for cancer. Another example are families who live in unsuitable living environments or share high-fat diets. The choices or life circumstances of parents tend to dictate certain risk factors for their children. Familial tendency is not a certainty. Simply because a person has a familial risk factor does not mean that he or she is doomed to have the disease. Most diseases with a genetic aspect also involve environmental risk factors and choices that can help avoid the development of the disease process.

Aging and Age-Related Disorders

[OBJECTIVE 8]

Age is a risk factor in many of the disease processes seen in society (e.g., heart disease). Most people who have heart disease are affected later in life. Although a genetic predisposition may be present, in a large percentage of cases long-term exposure to environmental risk factors is the determining element. Other disease processes, such as Alzheimer's and other degenerative diseases, mainly affect older patients. Although the exact causes of some of these diseases remain elusive, metabolic and other changes associated with aging are theorized to play a role (McCance & Huether, 2002). In certain other situations the period required for the disease to appear and produce signs and symptoms is closely related to the age of the patient.

Common Familial Diseases and Associated Risk Factors

As mentioned previously, some of the more common diseases have been linked to genetics and shared risk factors. Again, the exact causes of some of these diseases are still unknown.

Immunologic Disorders

Several immunologic disorders have shown a tendency to present in familial groups. This leads researchers to assume a genetic component or predisposition to these disorders, although environmental risk factors are clear. Disorders such as rheumatic fever, allergies, and asthma are some of the more commonly seen conditions.

Rheumatic fever is the result of the body's attempt to respond to a bacterial infection. It is an inflammatory disease and not an infection. It occurs in patients after being exposed to streptococci. Antibodies produced as one of the body's natural defense mechanisms attack the bacteria but also cause inflammation because the antibodies attack the body's own tissues. It has been associated with environmental factors such as diet and living conditions. This disorder was once quite prevalent in the pediatric population of the United States. However, with the advances in antibiotic therapy, the disorder now is fairly uncommon.

Allergies are an exaggerated response by the immune system to a stimulus. They can be caused by food, medications, or other environmental stimuli. Although no definitive evidence shows that a specific allergy is inherited, evidence suggests a genetic component to allergies. A child has a 30% greater risk of developing an allergy if one of his or her parents has allergies. If both parents have allergies, the risk dramatically increases. If the allergen is known, a simple change in lifestyle to reduce exposure can solve the problem.

Two types of *asthma* exist: allergic (involving intrinsic factors) and nonallergic (involving extrinsic factors). The signs and symptoms of the two are quite similar. In fact, the only real difference in the presentation seems to be the causative agent. Allergic asthma accounts for the majority of patients. This type of asthma is triggered by an allergen that is inhaled, such as pet dander, pollen, or mold. Nonallergic asthma can be triggered by anxiety, stress, exercise, cold air, dry air, or smoke. Although the propensity for developing asthma is inherited, other factors such as an allergen or other environmental factors must be present for the signs and symptoms to develop.

Cancer

The most common cancerous condition found in women is breast cancer. As with other cancers, breast cancer has been shown to have a strong familial relationship (clusters are found in families). Women with a first-degree relative (i.e., mother or sister) with breast cancer have a risk of developing cancer double that of other women with similar environmental risk factors. In addition, if that first-degree relative developed the cancer earlier in life or if the cancer affected both breasts, the risk is even greater. Research has yielded many advances regarding the genetic origin and early detection of breast cancer. It may be due to these advances that breast cancer is no longer the leading cause of cancer death in women.

In the United States colorectal cancer is second only to lung cancer in the number of cases diagnosed each year. As with breast cancer, a familial relationship appears to exist. People with at least one first-degree relative with the disease have a twofold to threefold risk of acquiring the cancer. This pattern of clustering within families was identified in the 1800s. The identification of the genetic abnormalities associated with the development of colorectal cancer has explained many of the questions regarding the specific cluster patterns. Some cases are linked to specific gene defects, whereas others appear to have a complex interaction of risk factors.

The leading cause of lung cancer is smoking. Other environmental causes, such as asbestos, have been implicated in many cases. Several studies have indicated that genetics may play a role in a person's susceptibility to developing lung cancer. Several genes on chromosome 6 have been identified as potential factors. All the studies show that smokers with this type of genetic predisposition have a greater risk than the general population, which may explain the familial connection with the disease process.

Endocrine Disorders

Diabetes mellitus is the most common of the endocrine disorders found to have a familial tendency. Although the cause is not completely understood, it has been linked to certain genetic abnormalities. In the United States diabetes is the leading cause of blindness, heart disease, and renal failure. The two major types of diabetes are type 1 and type 2.

Type 1 diabetes (previously called *juvenile diabetes* or *insulin-dependent diabetes*) is usually diagnosed early in life. However, it can occur as late as age 40 years. It accounts for 10% to 20% of all diabetes cases and affects men slightly more often than women. In this type of diabetes the insulin-producing beta cells in the pancreas are believed to be destroyed by the lymphocytes of the body. This, in turn, drastically reduces or eliminates insulin-producing capabilities. Another theory holds that the destructive culprit is a virus. Either way, these patients depend on daily insulin injections for normal metabolism and function. The risks associated with a family history are substantially elevated over the general population. A person with a sibling who has type 1 diabetes has an approximately 6% risk of developing the disease as opposed to only a 0.3% to 0.5% risk in those without a family history.

Type 2 diabetes (previously called *adult-onset* or *non–insulin-dependent diabetes*) accounts for the remaining 80% to 90% of cases. This type of diabetes has many distinguishing features. Almost all these patients have some endogenous insulin production. This means that usually the condition can be controlled with dietary changes and/or oral medications. Another difference between the two types is that type 2 diabetics tend to develop an insulin resistance or a difficulty using the insulin produced in the body. Other than the identified familial tendency, environmental risk factors that can significantly increase a person's chances of developing the disease include body habitus and lifestyle. Obesity has been found to have a strong link to the disease and increased insulin resistance, poor diet, and a lack of exercise tend to lead to obesity. A person with a first-degree relative with the disease has a 10% to 15% greater chance of acquiring the disease than does the general population.

Hematologic Disorders

Many blood-related disorders, such as hemophilia and hemochromatosis, have been clearly identified as having a genetic origin. Although the causes of some of these diseases have been found, long-term treatment is the best the medical community can do in most cases.

Hemophilia is a hereditary disease that inhibits the blood's ability to clot, causing excessive bleeding in some patients. Several different types of hemophilia exist, but they all involve a deficiency of certain clotting factors necessary in the clotting cascade. Types A and B hemophilia are caused by a defect on the X chromosome inherited through the mother. Women are mainly carriers of the disease, and it almost exclusively affects their male children. Female children can become carriers of the disease and pass it to their children. The signs and symptoms of this disease are seen early in life (sometimes from birth) and can range from mild to severe. Most patients with hemophilia are treated with concentrated clotting factors.

Hemochromatosis also is a genetic disorder. It causes the body to absorb and store iron in excess. Most healthy people absorb approximately 10% of the iron the body receives through the diet. This is adequate to meet the body's needs. The body uses iron in the formation of the hemoglobin molecules used to transport oxygen. When iron is stored in excess, it settles in organs. This primarily occurs in the heart, liver, and pancreas. If left untreated, excess iron deposition leads to organ failure. A child who inherits the defective gene from both parents has a high probability of developing the disease. If only one of the parents has the defective gene, the child will become a carrier but is not likely to develop the disease. People with the disease have it from birth, but the signs and symptoms will not likely develop until adulthood. Men are five times more likely to develop hemochromatosis than are women. The treatment of choice for hemochromatosis is the removal of blood from the body at defined time intervals depending on the progression of the disease.

Hemolytic anemia is a condition in which red blood cells are prematurely destroyed and removed from the bloodstream, leading to a reduction in the number of red blood cells. The two main types of hemolytic anemia are inherited and acquired. People with this condition do not normally appear to be anemic until stressors, such as an infection, affect the body. Drug-induced hemolytic anemia is an acquired form of anemia. It can be induced by medications such as penicillin and some antiinflammatory and antihypertensive medications. The treatment is directed at discontinuing the causative agent. Steroid therapy may be indicated for some patients. In extreme situations blood transfusions may be required.

Cardiovascular Disorders

Many of the cardiovascular diseases seen in the United States have been proven to have a hereditary link. Conditions such as a prolonged QT interval and mitral valve prolapse have been shown to run in families. A prolonged QT interval has been linked to an issue with the ion pumps in the heart. This can lead to problems with the repolarization of the myocardial tissue. This, in turn, can cause a decrease in cardiac output and potentially lethal arrhythmias such as torsades de pointes, a type of ventricular tachycardia that can quickly lead to ventricular fibrillation and cardiac arrest.

Mitral valve prolapse is a condition in which the valve between the left atrium and left ventricle does not close as it should. It billows upward, allowing a backflow of blood into the left atrium. Some forms of prolapse have a genetic link and are related to disease processes such as Marfan syndrome. The majority of patients with mitral valve prolapse do not show any signs or symptoms. Treatment is reserved for only the most severe cases.

The development of coronary heart disease in a person heavily depends of the number of risk factors that person has. These risk factors are classified as genetic (those that cannot be controlled) and environmental (those that can be controlled). A family history of coronary heart disease is one of the most important genetic risk factors. It greatly increases a person's risk of developing the disease. In addition, the earlier in life a parent was diagnosed with coronary heart disease, the greater the risk to the child. A family history of diseases and conditions such as hypertension and stroke are important risk factors that cannot be overlooked. Although these factors can potentially be controlled, they are important to identify and point toward a genetic predisposition.

Hypertension is a well-known risk factor for many conditions and disease processes. It is defined as having a consistent blood pressure of 140/90 mm Hg or greater. Although no definitive proof exists regarding the cause of essential hypertension, it is thought to have a heredity link. On the other hand, secondary hypertension is a condition caused by another disorder, such as Cushing syndrome or an adrenal gland tumor. Regardless of the cause, it is one of the leading comorbid conditions in disease processes such as renal failure and stroke. The treatment for hypertension may be as simple as dietary modifications and exercise. It may also involve any of a number of medications that can lower blood pressure.

Renal Disorders

The kidneys are responsible for maintaining a stable internal environment for cell and tissue metabolism. They accomplish this through mechanisms such as balancing water and solute, excreting metabolic wastes, conserving nutrients, and maintaining acid-base balance. Many of the disorders that interfere with the renal system's ability to perform these functions have been linked to genetics. For example, men are one and one half times more likely than women to develop a chronic renal disease, and African Americans are four times more likely than whites to develop a chronic renal disease. In addition to the genetic factors, diabetics and patients with hypertension are at a much greater risk than the rest of the population of developing renal failure. Gout is a condition that causes a buildup of uric acid in the body and has been linked to the inability of the kidneys to filter out the excess. This condition tends to run in families and is a risk factor for developing kidney stones. People with a family history of kidney stones have a much higher risk of developing them. Any renal disorder can lead to changes in electrolyte and fluid balance, increasing the risk of developing other life-threatening conditions.

Gastrointestinal Disorders

A wide variety of GI disorders exists. Some are thought to have a genetic link, whereas the causes of others are not clearly understood and are thought to be associated with environmental risk factors. Some evidence exists that certain disorders may be a combination of the two. *Lactose intolerance* results from a deficiency of the enzyme lactase. This is the enzyme responsible for the breakdown of lactose into simpler forms that can be easily absorbed by the body. In many cases this deficiency is present from birth. In others, it results from damage to the small intestine, which is the location of lactase production. No mechanism is currently available to increase lactase production in the body. Although lactose intolerance can seem like a serious problem for the patient, the effects of the disorder usually can be easily treated and controlled through dietary modification and are never life threatening.

Crohn's disease is an ongoing disorder that causes inflammation in the GI tract. Although it can affect any part of the GI tract from the mouth to the anus, it mainly is found in the small intestine. The swelling associated with this disorder usually extends deep into the tissue and causes the patient extreme discomfort and usually frequent diarrhea. All the layers of the bowel may be involved, but healthy tissue can be found between layers of diseased tissue. The exact cause of the disease is unknown, but a genetic link is probable because it tends to run in families. Approximately 20% of patients with the disease have a close relative with some form of inflammatory bowel disorder. The main theory of causation involves the immune system. It mistakes food or bacteria for invaders, which it then attacks. In this process, WBCs gather in the lining of the intestine, causing inflammation. Many other theories exist regarding what causes the disorder, but no theory has yet been proven correct.

Peptic ulcers are sores that form in the lining of the stomach or upper part of the small intestine called the *duodenum*. If they form in the stomach, they are called *gastric ulcers*. In the duodenum they are called *duodenal ulcers*. The majority of patients have more than one ulcer, and the ulcers can be present in both locations. The ulcers form when a breakdown in the lining occurs from one of several causes. The most common are the *Helicobacter pylori* bacteria and certain medications classified as nonsteroidal antiinflammatory drugs, such as aspirin and ibuprofen. *H. pylori* accounts for approximately 66% of the cases, with nonsteroidal antiinflammatory drugs making up most of the rest of the cases. Other conditions rarely can cause ulcers to develop. Almost all these cases are easily treated with medications and the ulcers can be cured.

Cholecystitis is an inflammation of the gallbladder or blockage of the duct leading to the common bile duct. This blockage causes a backup or concentration of bile that results in an irritation or pressure buildup in the gallbladder. In severe cases it can lead to a bacterial infection and even perforation of the gallbladder. The causes include severe illness or alcohol abuse, but the most common is gallstones (accounting for approximately 90% of all cases). These have been shown to have a possible genetic connection. Gallstones are more common in women than men, and Native Americans have a higher incidence than other populations.

Obesity is a serious problem in the United States that is said to affect more than 25% of the adult population and more than 14% of the adolescent population. According to the Centers for Disease Control and Prevention, the number of adolescents who are obese has tripled since 1980. It is the second leading cause of preventable death after smoking. Obesity is usually defined by body mass index. This is not an absolute measure of body fat, but it considers the patient's height and weight. For most people this is a fairly accurate measure. The causes of obesity are varied. Some studies show a clear hereditary connection, giving a person a predisposition to store fat. As with most genetic predispositions, this does not mean obesity is predetermined. Environmental factors play a strong role regarding whether a person will develop the condition. In addition, some cases clearly have no genetic connection and are purely related to environmental factors.

Neuromuscular Disorders

Many neuromuscular disorders are thought to have or are known to have a genetic link in addition to having environmental risk factors. *Huntington chorea* is a devastating degenerative brain disorder for which no treatment or cure is currently available. The signs and symptoms traditionally do not appear until a person is between the ages of 30 and 45 years, but onset in children has been seen. Children who develop a form of the disease do not normally live into adulthood. Early symptoms of the disease consist of cognitive decline, personality changes, and motor problems. In the advanced stages, patients are not able to care for themselves and die from complications of the disease.

Muscular dystrophy is a grouping of similarly disabling neuromuscular diseases that have a well-established genetic link. Muscular dystrophy is an X-linked disorder that is seen almost exclusively in males. Depending on which disease a person inherits, the onset of signs and symptoms can range from early childhood to middle age. All these diseases result in the progressive weakening of muscles. Each has a slightly different pattern of progression. Some of them are fatal in short order, whereas others may take many years to decades to become fatal. Death from Duchenne muscular dystrophy is typically the result of respiratory failure or related disease, such as pneumonia in the second decade of life. A tremendous amount of research is being done to identify effective treatments but currently no cure is available.

Multiple sclerosis is a chronic neurologic disorder that affects the central nervous system. Its exact cause is unknown, but it is suspected to be hereditary because it seems to cluster in families. This disease results in the body attacking the myelin sheath that surrounds the axons of some neurons. When this damage occurs, the transmission of neural messages is affected and signs and symptoms appear. These can be mild, such as occasional numbness, to more severe, such as double vision, cognitive decline, and weakness that can lead to a decrease in mobility. Multiple sclerosis is more common in women than men and is normally diagnosed between the ages of 30 and 50 years. Treatment options are available for those affected, but no cure has been found.

Alzheimer's disease is a progressive, degenerative neurologic disorder. It is estimated to account for 50% to 70% of all causes of dementia. This disease is especially devastating. It begins with mild memory loss and progresses to the total elimination of a lifetime of memories and even self-awareness. Contrary to popular belief, this disease is eventually fatal if the person does not have any other conditions and succumb to them first. Several theories exist regarding how it is caused, including a genetic defect, because the disease seems to be more prevalent in families. Medications can be used to slow the progression of the disease to a point, but none currently can stop it.

Psychiatric Disorders

Schizophrenia is a chronic, and sometimes severe, brain disease. It can render its victim completely disabled. A high prevalence is found worldwide, and more than 2 million Americans have the disease at any given time. This disease affects men and women in approximately the same numbers. However, men generally show signs and symptoms much earlier (in the late teens to early 20s compared with the late 20s to early 30s in women). These patients have auditory hallucinations, paranoia, and delusions. They may have strange speech patterns and tend to be withdrawn and isolate themselves from society out of fear. People with the disease may have only one acute episode and live fairly normal lives, or the condition can be chronic and crippling. The cause of schizophrenia is unknown, but ongoing research points toward a genetic abnormality. The disease has no cure; however, medications can greatly reduce the signs and symptoms.

Bipolar disorder is a condition characterized by broad mood swings between depression and mania. Mania is euphoria or exaggerated excitement. Although the incidence of bipolar disorder is equally split between men and women, women tend to have a higher incidence of rapid cycling. Men tend to have a higher incidence of early-onset bipolar disorder, which generally leads to a more severe condition. The signs and symptoms can be mild, with only a few episodes over the course of a person's life. For another person, however, the symptoms can be severe to the point that he or she cannot function in society. The cycles or acute episodes of the condition are unpredictable. Medications can be used to reduce the impact of these episodes, but no cure exists. A genetic component to the disease seems to exist, but many environmental and possibly immune system risk factors are thought to play a role.

HYPOPERFUSION

Shock is hypoperfusion at cellular level (lack of O₂, nutrients)

[OBJECTIVE 11]

To understand hypoperfusion fully, adequate perfusion must first be understood. The term perfusion is technically defined as the pouring of liquid over or through. In medicine, this translates into the act of pumping fluid (blood) through a vessel into a tissue or an organ. Adequate perfusion means that this movement of blood into the tissue or organ is of a sufficient amount, with adequate nutrients and oxygen, to support the physiologic functions of the area (see Chapter 34).

Hypoperfusion, and its extreme case, shock, is the result of inadequate oxygen available to tissue. Poor perfusion can result from lower than adequate values for any variable described by the Fick principle. The Fick principle was developed in 1870 by Adolf Eugen Fick to describe the volume of oxygen available to meet the demands of an organism. Available oxygen for perfusing tissue is proportional to the (1) amount of hemoglobin, (2) cardiac output, and (3) ability of the pulmonary system to load the hemoglobin with oxygen and ability of the tissue to offload the oxygen. A slightly lower value for one variable can be compensated for by the other variables, but if the net effect of the three variables is an inadequate oxygen volume, hypoperfusion results (Parker, 2007).

Hypoperfusion can occur in isolated tissues or organs; however, it is more commonly a systemic problem that can arise from a number of medical or traumatic conditions. Examples of problems associated with prolonged hypoperfusion include damage to the hepatocytes, leading to liver failure, and tubular necrosis in the kidneys, leading to renal failure. Prolonged hypoperfusion also damages tissues, which can trigger the widespread formation of clots and deplete the body's clotting factors. In addition, as clots break down they release split fibrin products into the bloodstream. Both processes interfere with the clotting mechanism and can lead to a condition called disseminated intravascular coagulation. If hypoperfusion is not corrected, it ultimately leads to death.

Pathogenesis

Every cell in the body needs oxygenated blood for survival. Oxygen is used to drive the metabolic engines in the cells that extract energy from nutrients. In addition to delivering needed oxygen and nutrients, a constant flow of blood is needed to remove the waste products of metabolism, such as carbon dioxide, and maintain homeostasis. Anything that interferes with this flow can lead to hypoperfusion. The most important determinant of this blood flow is cardiac output.

The ability of the patient to compensate for and recover from hypoperfusion depends on the underlying medical condition. For example, the elderly often have diffuse peripheral vascular disease that results in marginal blood flow to body tissues. A brief episode of hypoperfusion can decrease the delivery of oxygen and nutrients to areas already affected by peripheral vascular disease below the level needed to cause cell death and tissue necrosis. A paramedic must continually evaluate each patient and monitor for the onset and effects of hypoperfusion. The paramedic also must be aware of the concept of relative hypotension. In the patient with a history of hypertension, such as an elderly patient, the body may become dependent on the higher blood pressure for adequate perfusion of the tissues and organs. If the patient's blood pressure becomes what is considered "normal" (e.g., 120/80 mm Hg), he or she may not be able to perfuse the tissues adequately, resulting in a state of hypoperfusion. Signs and symptoms of hypoperfusion may not be present or only be subtle in pregnant patients because of the 40% increase in blood volume from the pregnancy. Therefore a greater amount of blood loss occurs before signs and symptoms present. As the pregnant patient compensates for hypoperfusion, blood is shunted from the placenta because it is seen as a nonvital organ. Because of this, the patient may appear asymptomatic, yet the placenta may remain hypoperfused. Pediatric patients have strong cardiovascular systems, which have a faster and more efficient ability to compensate for hypoperfusion. Therefore, unlike adults who may present with a steady deterioration, pediatric patients compensate with minimal signs and symptoms; however, when they are no longer able to compensate, they rapidly deteriorate.

circulate entire volume of blood each minute (4.9L)

Decreased Cardiac Output

CO = amt of blood heart puts out

ave = 70 ml/beat at rest

The ways in which the body accommodates for a decrease in cardiac output are varied and involve multiple systems. Changing the amount of preload or afterload can have a dramatic effect on cardiac output. One of the ways the body monitors cardiac output is through baroreceptors. The receptors are located in the carotid sinus and the arch of the aorta. They are quite sensitive to changes in pressure and respond to even minor changes in either direction of normal. When they detect an increase in arterial pressure, they respond to decrease blood pressure and reduce cardiac output. Decreases in arterial pressure stimulate the opposite effect. These receptors function within a range of pressures. Dramatic changes in the body require the assistance of other mechanisms, such as the central nervous system, catecholamine release, and the renal system, which is responsible for renin production, hormonal mechanisms, and the shifting of fluids (McCance & Huether, 2002).

Changes in the perfusion status in the lower portion of the brain can cause a compensatory response. Two types of vasomotor neurons are found in this part of the brain. One is responsible for ensuring that the brain and the heart receive blood at the expense of all other organs. The other is responsible for ensuring that other organs, including the heart, receive blood at the expense of blood flow to the brain. These two types of neurons work together to maintain internal homeostasis for the longest time frame possible when faced with hypoperfusion.

Epinephrine and norepinephrine are chief chemical mediators of the sympathetic nervous system. When released by the adrenal medulla, they increase sympathetic stimulation. The effect of these catecholamines is not as powerful as that of the central nervous system, but

Low ejection fraction is bad (should be 70-80%)

they do last longer. The sympathetic stimulation causes an increase in the heart rate, contractility, and peripheral vasoconstriction in an attempt to improve perfusion and raise blood pressure. This is represented in the following equation:

$$Blood\ pressure = CO \times PVR$$

where *CO* is cardiac output and *PVR* is peripheral vascular resistance. As previously described, renin is released by the kidneys in response to hypoperfusion. This mechanism starts a chain of chemical events that result in production of angiotensin II. This production of angiotensin II causes vasoconstriction to increase preload, an elevation in blood pressure, and the release of aldosterone. Aldosterone stimulates the kidneys to retain salt and therefore water as a way to conserve volume and increase preload. This mechanism tends to work within 20 to 30 minutes.

In addition to aldosterone release, additional hormonal compensation comes in the form of ADH. It is released in response to a decrease in the blood flow or an increase in solute concentration in the kidneys. When this happens, the hypothalamus is stimulated to send a signal to the pituitary gland with instructions to release ADH. This hormone works quickly to constrict blood vessels and promotes the reabsorption of water by limiting urine production in the kidneys. Again, this increases preload and cardiac output in an attempt to raise systemic blood pressure.

In addition to these mechanisms, fluid shifts from the interstitial spaces into the vascular space during periods of hypoperfusion. This is enabled by the change in the ion concentration gradient with the loss of intravascular volume. This change occurs along with a drop in the hydrostatic pressure at the capillary level. These fluid shifts can be large; estimates range from 0.25 to 0.35 mL/kg/min. This can equate to 1 L/hr or more in the average adult. Fluid, or rather blood, also can shift from other places in the body. The spleen is a highly vascular organ. It contains a microcirculation called the splenic sinuses. It can store several hundred milliliters of blood at any time. In states of hypoperfusion, this blood can be expelled into the general circulation when needed.

The body clearly has many compensatory mechanisms that work together to protect it in states of hypoperfusion. When the body is not successful at limiting the effects of hypoperfusion, it will progress to a shock state. This is a widespread state of lack of perfusion to the tissues of the body.

Cellular Metabolism Impairment

As described in Chapter 7, the cells of the body require energy to function properly. This energy is derived from the utilization of oxygen and glucose in cellular respiration. In a state of hypoperfusion and hypoxia, the body relies more and more on glycolysis, which produces 18 times less ATP that does aerobic metabolism. This, in turn, creates large amounts of lactic acid, which leads to metabolic acidosis. As the body tries to compensate for the acidosis, vasodilation and electrolyte shifts make homeostasis more difficult to maintain. As potassium shifts extracellularly, the electrochemical gradient, and therefore resting membrane potential, are dramatically altered. This leads to a state in which cellular swelling occurs. This also leads to the activation of lysosomes that indiscriminately attack and destroy cells in the area. As a result, irreversible cellular damage leading to cell death is inevitable.

TYPES OF SHOCK

[OBJECTIVE 12]

Shock is traditionally classified according to the agent causing the shock: cardiogenic shock (caused by the heart), hypovolemic shock (caused by loss of volume), neurogenic shock (caused by damage to the nervous system), anaphylactic shock (caused by an allergen), and septic shock (caused by an infection). In recent years the terms for describing the types of shock have occasionally taken different forms related more toward mechanisms. For example, some clinicians may refer to these as cardiogenic shock (failure of the heart), hypovolemic shock (loss of volume), obstructive shock (mechanical obstruction preventing preload), dissociative shock (inability of hemoglobin to bind with or release oxygen), and distributive shock (massive vasodilatation reducing distribution of the blood). Brief descriptions of the different types of shock follow.

Cardiogenic Shock   *Pump is bad*

Cardiogenic shock is the result of the heart's inability to supply the cells of the body with the blood they need to maintain normal metabolism. This type of shock most commonly is caused by damage to the muscle of the left ventricle from an acute myocardial infarction or other insult and the resulting drop in cardiac output. Damaged or dead cardiac muscle does not contract with the same force as healthy tissue. Thus this reduces blood flow to the body, including the heart itself. This condition becomes a type of positive feedback loop as the body tries to compensate and worsens the situation. Even though the body interprets and responds as if the problem is one of volume, the true issue is not volume but the ability to transport the blood to the tissues. As blood flow drops, the heart tries to compensate by increasing the rate and force of the contractions. This increases the oxygen demands of the heart and further worsens the damage sustained by cardiac tissue. When this occurs, the cardiac output drops further. The treatment for cardiogenic shock consists of airway management, oxygen therapy, and possibly several medications designed to inhibit the aggravating mechanisms and promote the effective pumping of the heart. In some cases the use of cardiac assist devices, such as the intraaortic balloon pump or ventricular assist devices, may be indicated.

Hypovolemic Shock
[handwritten: not enough blood]

Hypovolemic shock is the result of approximately 25% to 30% of intravascular fluid volume loss. Again, this type of shock is classified the same way in either classification system. Intravascular volume loss can occur as a result of many causes. The most common cause is from blood loss either internally or externally as a result of trauma. Other causes include plasma loss from extensive burns and medical causes such as extreme dehydration and fluid shifts in the body from the intravascular space into the interstitial spaces. The body tries to compensate by the previously described mechanisms, but it may have little success. A loss of only 15% of intravascular volume can produce the initial symptoms of shock, specifically rapid pulse, pale skin, dizziness, nausea, and thirst. In addition to appropriate airway management and oxygen therapy, the goal of treatment is directed at fluid or blood replacement and correction of the source of fluid loss.

Neurogenic Shock

Neurogenic shock causes a relative hypovolemia in the body because of the loss of nervous control of the vasculature. This is usually a result of a traumatic injury to the brain or spinal cord. The loss of nervous control of the vasculature causes the vessels to dilate, increasing the capacity of the system and creating a state in which proportionally less volume is present without volume loss. Blood pools in the extremities of the body and reduces the amount returning to the heart. This causes some of the signs and symptoms of hypovolemic shock, but the body may not have the capacity to compensate because of the structures affected by the trauma. This means that decompensation may occur at an accelerated rate because of the inability of the compensatory mechanisms to constrict vessels, release catecholamines, or increase the heart rate and stroke volume because neurologic impulses are inhibited by the injury. Prehospital treatment for neurogenic shock consists of administering high-flow oxygen, managing the airway when indicated, and considering a volume infusion of isotonic fluids such as normal saline (0.9% sodium chloride) or Ringer's lactate. In addition, the use of vasoconstricting medications such as dopamine may be indicated to address the effects of the neurologic injury.

Anaphylactic Shock
[handwritten: Acute allergic reaction]

Anaphylactic shock is the result of an extreme allergic reaction called *anaphylaxis*. When the body is exposed to an allergen, the immune system responds to defend the body against the effects of the invader. In the majority of cases this response goes unnoticed by the affected person. The body is constantly sampling the internal environment and responding to change. In other cases the response can produce the signs and symptoms of an allergic reaction. In the most extreme cases this reaction progresses to anaphylaxis and shock. This type of reaction can be caused by many different agents, from foods such as nuts, peanut oil, and shellfish, to environmental causes such as envenomation by stinging insects, such as bees and wasps.

Anaphylactic reactions are systemic and affect more than one organ system. The effect of these reactions on the cardiovascular system is vasodilatation. Anaphylactic shock occurs when hypotension develops as a result of this vasodilatation. In addition to the standard signs and symptoms of shock, urticaria (hives) and constriction of the airway can occur. These reactions can be severe, with an acute onset and rapid progression. Although rare, anaphylactic shock can occur without associated signs and symptoms other than cardiovascular collapse. If left untreated, the patient can die within minutes. Treatment for anaphylactic shock includes providing high-flow oxygen; aggressively managing the airway because of the rapid nature of the condition; and administering medications such as epinephrine, antihistamines such as diphenhydramine, and corticosteroids (e.g., Solu-Medrol) if indicated. Fluid infusion, and in extreme cases vasoconstrictive drugs, can be used.

Septic Shock
[handwritten: Fluid moves from intravascular to interstitial (also distributive shock)]

The precursor to septic shock is an infection in the blood called *sepsis*. The infection travels throughout the body and spreads into the tissues. As the infection continues to develop, toxins are released by the substance causing the infection. Additional toxins are released from dying gram-negative bacteria. Eventually this leads to the body's inability to fend off the infection, and systemic signs and symptoms appear. Septic shock is the most common cause of multiple organ dysfunction syndrome. The signs and symptoms may not become obvious until the infection is widespread. This means that once the illness is identified, the progression of the illness can happen quickly. Patient presentation may differ depending on the organ systems involved. Prehospital treatment consists of administering oxygen and managing the airway. IV fluids and vasoconstricting medications may be needed to support blood pressure. Definitive treatment for this condition is IV antibiotics specific to the causative agent.

[handwritten: obstructive shock - cardiac tamponade, tension pneumothorax]

MULTIPLE ORGAN DYSFUNCTION SYNDROME

[OBJECTIVE 13]

Multiple organ dysfunction syndrome (MODS) is the progressive impairment of two or more organ systems. This is usually the result of an uncontrolled inflammatory

[handwritten: dissociative shock - No RBCs to carry O2 (bleed out but replace IV fluids) (anemia)]

response from severe illness or injury, such as sepsis, trauma, or severe burn injuries. As previously mentioned, the most common cause of this syndrome is sepsis or septic shock. The severe complications of MODS make it the leading cause of death in patients admitted to intensive care units in the United States. MODS is estimated to be associated with a 60% to 90% mortality rate (McCance & Huether, 2002). This pattern of deterioration was first identified in 1975 and initially was termed multisystem organ failure. It was later renamed MODS in the early 1990s. This was a result of a better understanding of the syndrome and how it affects physiologic processes.

Pathogenesis

The pathophysiology of MODS is poorly understood. It is believed to be a result of the adaptive processes at the cellular level in response to injury or insult. In other words, when the body is damaged, part of the response is inflammation. According to one theory, severe injury or illness produces an inflammatory response that is unable to localize the problem, and systemic inflammation ensues. The most prevalent theory of MODS is that a cascade of events occurs, leading to systemic inflammation and the deterioration of organ function. Regardless of the true cause of the condition and the advances made in diagnosing MODS, the mortality rate over the last 20 years has not improved. MODS can be a primary condition (the organ injury is directly related to a specific insult causing ischemia and hypoperfusion) or secondary condition (as a result of the inflammatory response).

In primary MODS, the injury or infection leads to both a stress and inflammatory response. This response is not thought to be severe and may go unnoticed in the clinical setting. In the body macrophages, neutrophils, and mast cells are thought to be primed, or made ready to respond to the next insult, by cytokines. The next insult usually comes in the form of additional ischemia or infection. This sets off a chain of events that leads to secondary MODS.

In secondary MODS, the body releases inflammatory mediators. These mediators cause a disproportionate reaction to this secondary insult. These mediators and/or the endotoxins released from bacteria cause vascular endothelial damage. Mediators such as cytokine tumor necrosis factor stimulate a proinflammatory state when interacting with the damaged vascular endothelium by causing adhesion of neutrophils. These neutrophils then work their way into the tissue, causing an increase in inflammation. This damage causes the permeability that permits fluid to leak from the vascular system into the interstitial spaces. Increased permeability along with the effects of nitrous oxide release (a potent vasodilator) from endothelial cells can lead to profound hypotension and hypoperfusion.

In response to this state, the neuroendocrine system is activated. This system tries to compensate by releasing catecholamines and other hormones into the circulation. However, the body is unable to compensate at this point. In fact, these factors only contribute to a worsening of the condition by creating tachycardia, hypermetabolism, and increased oxygen demands of the body. Some of the hormones released in the stress response, such as endorphins, only increase the state of hypoperfusion by reducing vascular resistance even further.

The inflammatory mediators released cause the activation of certain plasma protein cascades known as the complement, coagulation, and kallikrein/kinin systems. The activation of the complement system causes a release of chemicals that increases the level of neutrophil aggregation and promotes the release of histamine from mast cells. Both contribute to further vasodilation and hypoperfusion. The kallikrein/kinin system, once activated, releases bradykinin (also a potent vasodilator) that furthers hypotension. Coagulation factors become activated as a result of the endothelial damage. Because the damage is extensive, these form microemboli that cause blockages in the microcirculation of organs, furthering ischemia (McCance & Huether, 2002).

One of the hallmarks of MODS is ineffective vascular function. Vasodilation, increased permeability, microvascular thrombi, and selective vasoconstriction all lead to the end result of the condition—multiple organ failure and death. Selective vascular vasoconstriction is the result of the interaction between two chemicals with opposing vascular effects that become inappropriately distributed in varying amounts throughout the body. This leads to an inadequate distribution of systemic blood flow and organ perfusion.

Other changes that go along with the systemic progression of MODS include a hypermetabolic state, an imbalance in oxygen demand and supply, and tissue hypoxia that leads to cellular changes resulting in organ dysfunction. All the changes previously described contribute to a hypermetabolic state that leads to a more rapid depletion of oxygen supply and a reduction in ATP production, which is the body's fuel supply. Without an adequate supply of ATP, the cells, tissues, and organs of the body are unable to perform the necessary tasks to maintain life.

Clinical Progression

Although no specific treatment is available for MODS, early identification of the signs and symptoms of the condition can give the clinician a chance to implement prevention strategies that may improve outcome (Table 8-2). Since the identification of this pattern of progression, hospital therapy has been directed at prevention. Because which patients will develop the condition cannot be predicted, this is the best approach with all patients at risk.

TABLE 8-2 Progression of MODS

Time	Symptoms And Signs
24 hours after resuscitation	Fever Tachycardia Dyspnea Altered mental status Hypermetabolic state
72 hours after resuscitation	Pulmonary failure (ARDS may develop)
7 to 10 days after resuscitation	Hepatic failure begins Intestinal failure begins Renal failure begins
14 to 21 days after resuscitation	Renal failure progresses Liver failure progresses
After 21 days	Hematologic failure Myocardial failure Death

MODS, Multiple organ dysfunction syndrome; *ARDS*, acute respiratory distress syndrome.

IMMUNE SYSTEM AND RESISTANCE TO DISEASE

The human body is capable and well suited to defend itself against attacks from pathogens in the environment. These include disease-producing microbes such as bacteria, viruses, fungi, protozoa, parasites, and prions. The human body is exposed to these pathogens on a daily basis, and yet its defense systems are able to combat most of these invaders without a person even knowing the battle has ever occurred. The ability of the human body to prevent the reproduction of a pathogen is known as disease **resistance.** The opposite of resistance is **susceptibility.** This term indicates a vulnerability or weakness. This is generally the situation when a person gets sick. The body has several lines of defense against attack. Two intrinsic systems work independently and together to provide the best overall approach to defense.

The first of these systems is called the *natural* or *nonspecific system.* This system responds and attacks almost immediately. The first lines of defense in this system are the anatomic barriers of the body. Intact skin and mucosal membranes try to prevent the entry of microbes. The second line of defense is a chemical attack by certain cells in the body called into action when the anatomic barriers are penetrated. The most important process in the second line of defense is *inflammation.* The third line of defense against invading pathogens is the second intrinsic system, called the *acquired* or *adaptive system.* This system is slower to respond and targets specific antigens.

When all the body's defense mechanisms are intact and working as they should, a pathogen has great difficulty gaining entry to the body and establishing a presence. With the ability to physically block entry, mobilize a broad-spectrum chemical attack, and engineer a specific chemical attack, the human body is one of the most amazing and adaptive organisms.

Three Lines of Defense

The first lines of defense against pathogens are anatomic barriers. At the surface of the skin the epidermis is composed of both living and nonliving cells. These cells work together to prevent a pathogen from entering the body. The dead skin cells are immune to the effects of the pathogen, and some of the living cells lack the appropriate receptor for the pathogen to gain a foothold. As the body periodically sheds the dead epidermal cells, the microbes also are removed from the surface of the skin. This layer is a tightly packed and highly keratinized sheet of epithelial tissue. When intact, it provides a highly effective line of defense against most microbes (Figure 8-12).

In addition to the physical barrier of the skin, the body also produces secretions that work with the anatomic barriers to prevent microbes from entering. Mucosal surfaces have a mucous layer responsible for trapping pathogens and preventing entry into the body. It accomplishes this goal because of its viscous consistency. Once pathogens are trapped in the mucous layer, the body expels the mucus, thereby removing the invader. The skin also contains sebaceous glands, which secrete an oily substance called sebum. Sebum coats the skin and can inhibit the growth of certain pathogens. Perspiration also flushes microbes from the surface of the skin. All these systems are effective but not foolproof. The skin is easily penetrated by traumatic insult. Moreover, the mucosal layer can become overwhelmed by large enough quantities of the pathogen. Most viruses enter the body through the mucosal route.

Internal barriers exist to prevent infection as well. These mainly consist of layers of epithelial cells that separate the blood from the tissues. They work to keep the pathogen from gaining access to vital areas such as the brain and placenta. These cells have a low permeability to pathogens. Therefore they are protective in nature, and a large number of pathogens generally are required to gain access.

The second line of defense involves different types of chemical and cellular reactions. These reactions occur as a result of an attack from a pathogen. The human body produces *antimicrobial proteins* that live in the blood and interstitial fluid that work together to inhibit growth of certain microbes. In addition, **natural killer cells** and **phagocytes** work together through separate processes to destroy and digest certain microbes.

The most important process in this phase of defense is the inflammatory response. It occurs as a result of tissue injury, heat, chemical insult, or infection by pathogens such as bacteria, viruses, and fungi. It also is an innate or natural response, with the primary goals of preventing the spread of damaging agents to adjacent tissues, dispos-

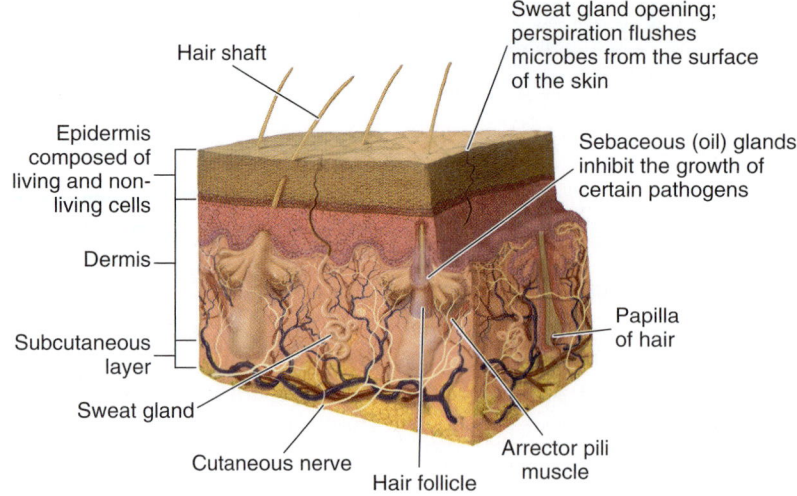

Figure 8-12 Layers of the skin.

ing of debris and pathogens, and preparing the affected area for tissue repair.

#3 ✱ The third line of defense is the immune response. As described, this type of response acts much more slowly and is specific in nature. It can confer long-term immunity to specific organisms. This type of immunity can be a result of the body's natural exposure to an organism or can be induced by vaccinations. Vaccines are made by using organisms, or portions of organisms, that are altered to a less-virulent form but that still initiate the immune response. When the body is exposed to a specific antigen, this antigen sets off a chain of events that work with the inflammatory process to defend the body. This type of response is limited to one type of serum protein (immunoglobulin), which is known as an antibody, and one type of blood cell, which is known as a lymphocyte.

CHARACTERISTICS OF THE IMMUNE RESPONSE

[OBJECTIVE 14]

The immune response can be classified in several ways depending on the type of antigen and the type of response it causes; it can be natural or acquired, active or passive, primary or secondary, and humoral or cell mediated. The following section explores each of these types of responses.

Natural versus Acquired Immunity

✱ As the name implies, this type of defense is natural or *innate*. This means that it is with the body from birth because it is part of the genetic profile. This system has many components, and all of them offer almost immediate protection from invading pathogens. Innate defenses do not have what is referred to as immunologic memory. This means that they do not remember the antigen, resulting in a more rapid response the next time the

organism is exposed. Most of these types of defenses are specific to the species. For example, human beings are naturally immune to diseases that may affect other animal species, such as canine distemper. This type of immunity exists in other species as well. Thus some diseases that affect human beings are harmless to certain animals.

✱ Acquired immunity develops after birth. It is developed after a person is exposed to a certain antigen that causes an immune response. The two types of acquired immunity are active acquired and passive acquired. Active acquired immunity is developed after the host is either naturally exposed to a certain antigen or has been vaccinated against a certain antigen. Passive acquired immunity is not developed as a result of the host's immune system; it can occur with the mother passing the immunity to an unborn child or with medical treatment. For example, a person can receive preformed antibodies from a donor to treat certain conditions, such as snakebite or rabies.

Primary versus Secondary Immune Response

Primary and secondary immune responses are examples of actively acquired immunity that occurs in two separate phases. Primary immunity is developed when the host is ✱ exposed to an antigen. After exposure, the B-type lymphocytes produce a certain type of blood protein called an *immunoglobulin,* or *antibody.* Five types of antibodies are identified in this chapter. This is how the body fights a foreign invader.

These antibodies grow in number after exposure and are eventually broken down when the threat has ceased. However, the level will be elevated from the preexposure state. This process also forms immunologic memory, which is responsible for the secondary immune response. ✱ This means that the next time the host is exposed to this specific antigen, the body will respond much more quickly and with a specific attack. This memory for the antigen and the elevated levels can last for years.

[handwritten notes at top of page: B cells from bone marrow — Antibodies formed after 1st exposure - memory for next exposure in blood. T cells from thymus - Thymus stops growing at sexual maturity - cell mediated immunity - Phagocytic - work on their own]

Formation of Lymphocytes

When a pluripotential hemopoietic stem cell follows the lymphocyte line, an immature lymphocyte is formed that does not have the ability to create an immune response. To participate in the immune response the lymphocyte must be preprocessed. This takes place in the bone marrow and the thymus gland. Cells that are preprocessed in the bone marrow become B cells (B lymphocytes), and those preprocessed in the thymus gland become T cells (T lymphocytes).

While in the thymus gland and bone marrow, the cells develop into mature lymphocytes capable of reacting to specific antigens. They achieve this ability by randomly exchanging gene segments with other immature lymphocytes, which causes them to develop the ability to react to only one type of antigen. Because of this random exchange of gene segments, millions of single-antigen responses can be created from only several hundred to a few thousand genes. This process is called *clonal diversity*.

Because this process is random, a B cell or T cell may develop to respond against the body's own tissues, or self-antigens. Before being released from the thymus or bone marrow, the cells are exposed to all the autoantigens in the body to ensure no response. If the lymphocyte does respond, it is immediately destroyed so it cannot cause an autoimmune response.

Once the lymphocyte has been processed, it is then released into circulation where the majority migrate to the lymph nodes. If the lymphocytes encounter the antigen they have been programmed for during clonal diversity, they are activated. They immediately begin to increase in number by dividing and proliferating. The process by which a specific lymphocyte is chosen in response to a specific antigen is called clonal selection. These two processes allow the initiation of the immune system and are stimulated by portions of the inflammatory response.

Humoral versus Cell-Mediated Immunity

Humoral immunity is a result of the differentiation of lymphocytes into B cells. These cells have minimal ability to recognize antigens when they enter the body and cannot perform a direct attack on an antigen. Instead, the majority of B cells are activated by a specific type of T cell called a helper T cell. Once this occurs the B cells begin to divide, antibodies ultimately are formed, and the defense of the body begins. The antibodies perform the actual "attack" of the humoral immune system. This also is the point at which memory formation begins and immunity occurs.

Cell-mediated immunity is the result of the differentiation of lymphocytes into T cells. They have some ability to recognize the antigen when it enters the body, but they are primarily activated by components of the inflammatory system that interact with helper T cells.

The helper T cells in turn activate both the humoral immune response and the remainder of the cell-mediated response. Unlike B cells, cytotoxic T cells, or killer T cells, they are able to mount a direct attack against the antigen (Figure 8-13).

ACTIVATION OF THE IMMUNE SYSTEM

[OBJECTIVE 15]

The immune system in the body is in a constant state of readiness. Once a stimulus or trigger activates the system, it responds with the appropriate mechanisms to defend the body. Most of the time this occurs automatically without the knowledge of the host.

Antigens and Immunogens

[handwritten notes: Every Antigen is not an Immunogen. Every Immunogen is an Ag]

An antigen is a protein marker on a cell that identifies the cell as self or nonself and identifies the type of cell. All cells have these protein markers. Recall that several of the proteins on the cell membrane are identifier proteins, or antigens. Self-antigens are present in the body as part of the major histocompatibility complex, or the histocompatibility locus, and allow self- and nonself-recognition. Foreign antigens are on any cell not intrinsic to the body. If a foreign antigen triggers an immune response, the antigen binding site of the antibodies binds with the antigen, forming an antigen-antibody complex. However, the body's immune system does not become active and stimulate a response to every foreign antigen. An *immunogen* is an antigen that reacts with the immune system and causes an immune response. In other words, not all antigens are immunogens. Several factors determine whether an antigen will be immunogenic: foreignness, size, complexity, and quantity.

The foreignness of the antigen is important because the body does not want to attack a substance it is using for other functions and that is normally found in the body. These self-antigens are not usually identified as a foreign invader and are therefore tolerated. This tolerance is established by several mechanisms, with the two chief ones being the elimination of the B cells and T cells that react to self-antigens and the prevention of recognition of these useful substances (McCance & Huether, 2002). In this way the body differentiates self-antigens from a foreign substance.

The size of the molecule is used in many situations to determine the immunogenic properties of a substance. Molecules such as proteins, polysaccharides, and nucleic acids are more likely to be identified as invaders. Smaller or low-molecular-weight molecules such as monosaccharides, amino acids, and fatty acids are much less likely to be seen as immunogenic. These substances, however, can combine with larger molecules to become haptens, which are then identified as foreign and immunogenic.

The complexity, quantity, and route of entry of an antigen also determine the response, or lack of response, from the immune system. A more complex molecule (the

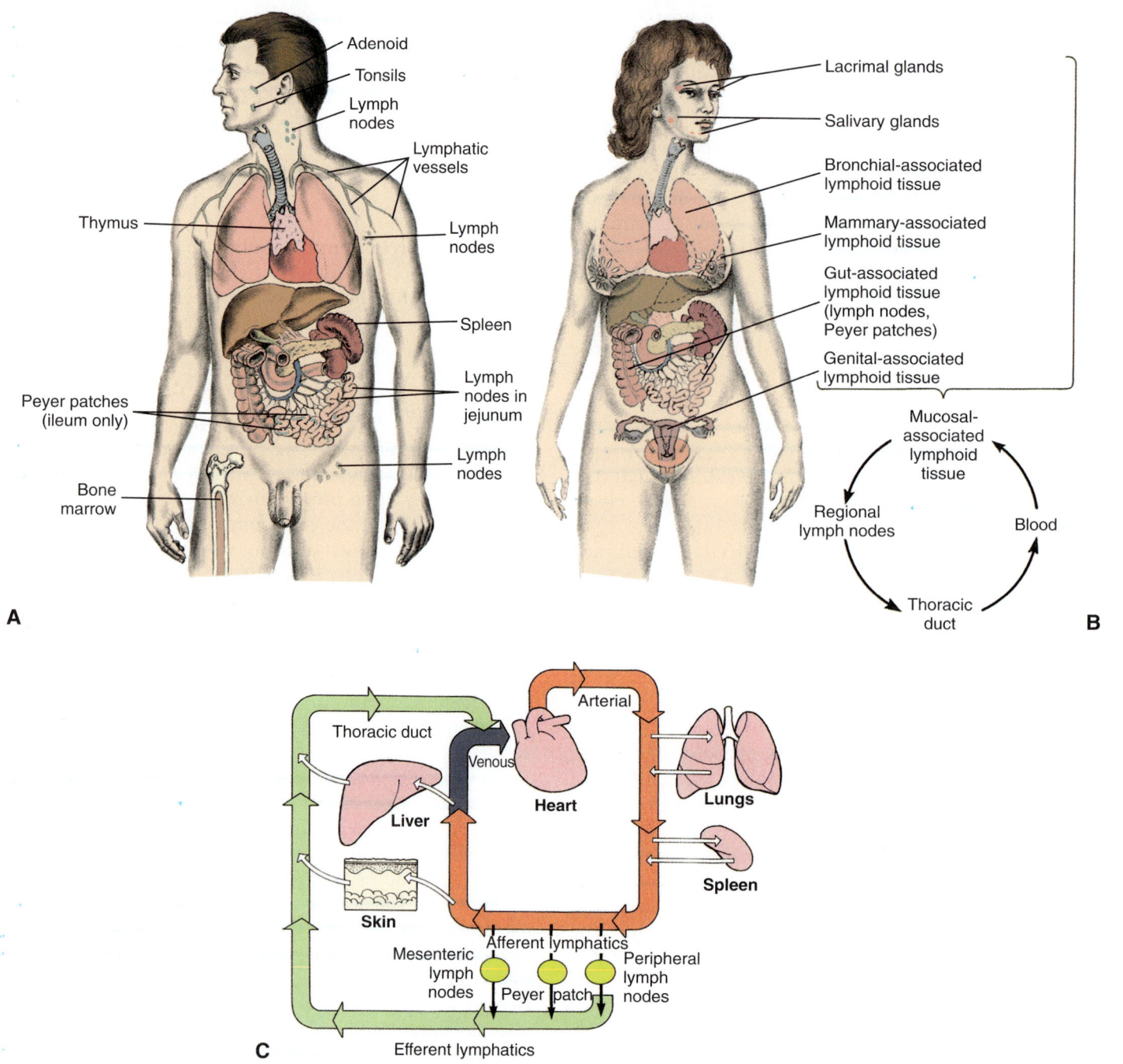

Figure 8-13 Lymphatic tissues: sites of B-cell and T-cell differentiation. **A,** Immature lymphocytes migrate through central (primary) lymphoid tissues: the bone marrow (probable central lymphoid tissue for B lymphocytes) and the thymus (central lymphoid tissue for T lymphocytes). Mature lymphocytes later reside in the T and B lymphocyte–rich areas of the peripheral (secondary) lymphoid tissues. **B,** Lymphocytes from the mucosal-associated lymphoid tissues circulate throughout the body in a pattern separate from other lymphocytes. For example, lymphocytes from the gut-associated lymphoid tissue circulate through the regional lymph nodes, the thoracic duct, and the blood and return to other mucosal-associated lymphoid tissues rather than to lymphoid tissue of the systemic immune system. **C,** Pathways of lymphocyte travel.

more antigenic binding sites it has) is more likely to be seen as immunogenic. The host's genetic profile also plays a large role in the immune response. Histocompatibility locus antigens (HLAs) are how the body determines whether a substance is self or foreign. The major genetic source of these antigens is in a section of chromosome 6 known as the major histocompatibility complex. These antigens are located on all the cells in the body except red blood cells (McCance & Huether, 2002).

Blood Group Antigens

Just as antigens are found on cells other than erythrocytes, some antigens are found only on red blood cells. Dozens of these antigens are grouped in many different blood systems. They form the bases for the ABO and Rh classification systems.

ABO System

The ABO classification of blood is based on the antigen groups that cause the largest humoral response. Four different blood types result from two primary antigens called A and B. The blood types are A, which carries the A antigen on the erythrocytes; B, which carries the B antigen; AB, which carries both the A and the B antigen; and O, which carries neither the A nor the B antigen. The body recognizes the antigens of the host's blood as normally occurring. Thus it will not initiate an immune response. Conversely, the host with type A blood also carries type B antibodies. This means that if the host receives type B or AB blood, the immune response will be almost immediate. This holds true for a host carrying

type B blood and type A antibodies if he or she receives A or AB blood.

AB blood has the antigens for A and B, but no antibodies are present. This means that AB blood hosts can receive any type of blood in small amounts without causing an immune response. Large amounts of unmatched blood can begin to cause a reaction in which the red blood cells begin to clump, resulting in a transfusion reaction. Because of this, hosts with this blood type have the title of universal recipient. Hosts with type O blood do not carry either the A or the B antigen, but they do have both the A and B antibodies. This host is unable to receive any other blood type than O, and because of the lack of antigens this donor is termed the *universal donor*. (Figure 8-14).

Rh System

Rh antigens are one of the groups of antigens identified in rhesus monkeys. These antigens are also present in human beings. The Rh antigen D, also called the *Rh factor*, determines an immune response. Hosts with Rh-positive blood have the antigen; Rh-negative means that the antigen is not present. Approximately 85% of the population in North America is Rh-positive. If a host that is Rh-negative receives Rh-positive blood, a primary immune response is induced. The second time the host is exposed, a massive immune response may occur.

In today's world, with the technology available in the emergency departments in the United States, this type of hemolytic reaction is rare. Most patients needing blood receive type O-negative blood until a definitive blood match can be made. In addition to transfusion, this type

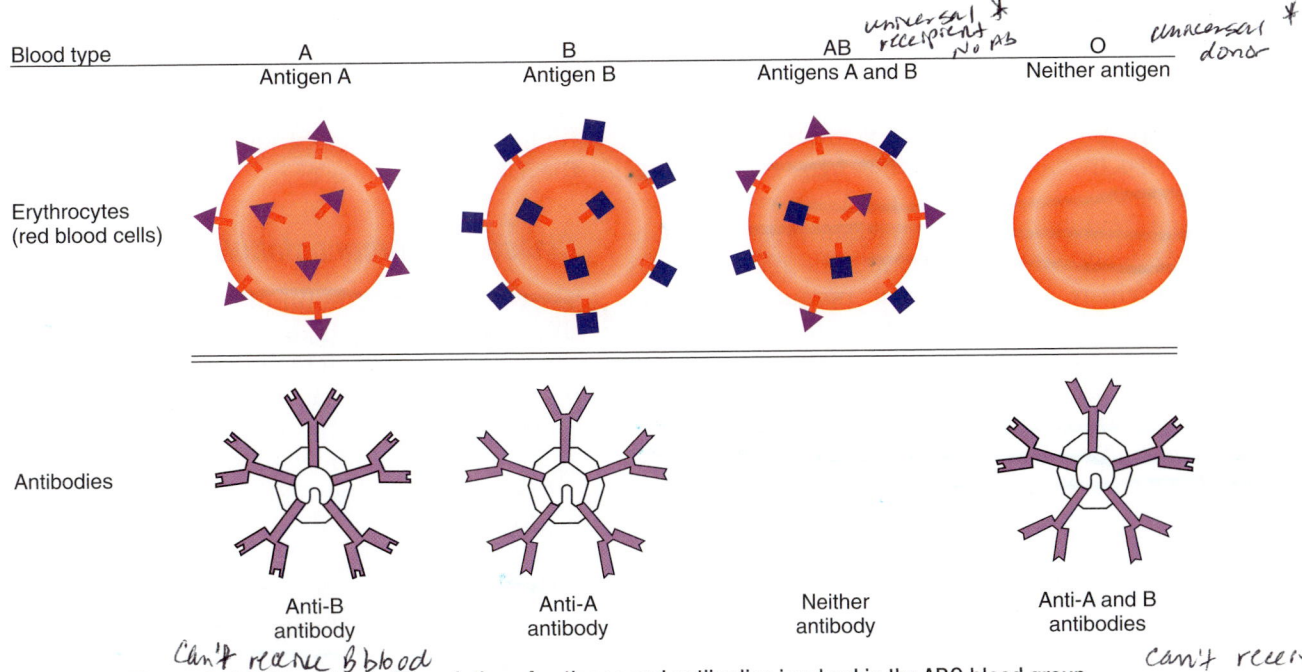

Figure 8-14 Blood types. The relation of antigens and antibodies involved in the ABO blood group system.

of mismatch can occur between mother and fetus. A mother who is Rh-negative and who has a fetus that is Rh-positive can induce a primary immune response that may set the stage for a serious reaction if she has a second Rh-positive fetus. In this situation, the mother develops antibodies that can cross the placental barrier and attack the red blood cells of the fetus. Fortunately, this type of reaction is not common.

Case Scenario CONCLUSION

You and your partner provide oxygen by nonrebreather mask, establish an IV line, and begin infusing normal saline at 30 mL/hr. As you stand the patient up to pivot him onto the stretcher, he becomes lightheaded and requires assistance to remain standing. A quick check of his vital signs while he is standing reveals a pulse of 162 beats/min and blood pressure of 80/58 mm Hg. En route to the hospital, you infuse approximately 500 mL of normal saline. In the emergency department a variety of laboratory tests are performed before his admission. They reveal the following information: elevated sodium, potassium below normal, blood glucose 596 mg/dL, and elevated WBCs. He is admitted to the hospital with a diagnosis of sepsis and septic shock.

Looking Back

9. Do you think you should have administered more than 500 mL of normal saline to this patient? Why or why not?
10. How are the changes in his laboratory values related to his condition and medical history?

HUMORAL IMMUNE RESPONSE

The humoral immune response is the function of B lymphocytes. In noninfected states the B cells are located in the lymph nodes and are dormant. Immunogens that enter the body initially cause a response of the immune system that includes the macrophages. When these immunogens circulate through the lymph nodes, they are engulfed by the macrophages by a process called *phagocytosis*. The macrophages then present parts of the immunogen on their cells membranes (antigen-presenting cells) to both the B cells and T cells. This causes slight activation of the B cells and significant activation of helper T cells. The primary activation of the B cells is in response to B-cell growth factor released by the helper T cells. In fact, without the helper T cells the immune system essentially does not function.

Once activated the B cells immediately differentiate into memory cells and plasmablasts. The memory cells do not participate in the current immune response; rather, they provide memory of the particular immunogen. This leads to the rapid secondary immune response if the body is reexposed to the same immunogen in the future. The plasmablasts mature into plasma cells that produce antibodies. These antibodies are the functional unit of the humoral immune system.

IMMUNOGLOBULINS

The terms *antibody* and *immunoglobulin* are used somewhat interchangeably, which may not be the most correct use of these terms. Whether all immunoglobulins are antibodies has not been determined. Although both antibodies and immunoglobulins are serum glycoproteins, only antibodies have specificity for a particular antigen.

Structure of Immunoglobulins

Antibody molecules consist of four polypeptide chains. The different amino acids that come together to form these chains, and the subsequent shapes of the antigen-binding portion of the molecule, determine specificity. The substitution of one critical amino acid can change the antigen with which the molecule is designed to interact. Although slight differences exist between immunoglobulins, they all seem to have a Y-type structure, with the antigen-binding sight located at the tips of the Y.

Classes of Immunoglobulins

The ways in which immunoglobulins are grouped or classified are based on their structure and function. Each of the classes of immunoglobulins shares a common heavy polypeptide chain that determines shape and therefore function. Although most of the functions of immunoglobulins are well understood, this is not the case for all the classes. Following are the five major classes of immunoglobulins (Ig):

- *IgG.* This class is the most common immunoglobulin in the human body. It accounts for 80% to 85% of all the circulating immunoglobulins. It is responsible for the memory formation aspect of the immune response and is the molecule most often found in

largest group in body

fetal blood as a result of selective transport across the placenta.

- *IgA.* Two subclasses of IgA are found in the body. IgA1 is normally found in blood. IgA2 is normally found in body secretions. IgA2 is structurally altered from IgA1 to protect it from the enzymes in the secretions of the body. *Saliva & mucus*
- *IgM.* This class is the largest of the immunoglobulins. It is responsible for the primary immune response and is produced early in the life of the host.
- *IgD.* The function of IgD is not yet clearly understood. It is found in low concentrations in the blood and appears on the surfaces of B lymphocytes during development.
- *IgE.* This class of immunoglobulins is responsible for the allergic response. It also is found in the lowest concentration in the blood. It has been identified in the defense of parasitic infections.

Function of Antibodies

An antibody can exert one of two effects on an antigen that it encounters. It circulates in blood or remains in body secretions until it binds to an antigen. It has either a direct effect on the antigen or an indirect effect. Both methods result in the neutralization or destruction of the antigen. This binding of antibody and antigen form a complex called the immune complex. The direct effects of an antibody on an antigen include agglutination, precipitation, and neutralization. *opsonization*

Agglutination is the process by which a soluble antibody interacts with an insoluble antigen. This causes the antigen to clump together with other antigens, making identification and destruction of phagocytes easier. Precipitation is the process by which the antibody-antigen complex is moved from the blood and removed by the fluids of the body. Neutralization is the process by which the antibody deactivates the binding sites of the antigen, making binding with the cells of the body of the host impossible for the antigen. Which of these actions occurs is based on the class of the antibody and the antigen encountered.

Indirect effects of antibodies on antigens include the enhancement of phagocytosis and the activation of plasma proteins that will attack and destroy the antigen. This occurs as a coordinated effort that involves the inflammatory response and the proteins of the complement cascade. Whether antibodies take the direct approach or the indirect approach, the basic goal is the same: defend the body. This occurs by the neutralization of bacteria, neutralization of viruses, opsonization of bacteria, and activation of the inflammatory response (McCance & Huether, 2002).

The neutralization of bacteria is accomplished by forming an antibody-antigen complex. In this case, the antigen is the toxin released by the bacteria. When this complex is formed, the antigenic sites of toxin are occupied and rendered harmless to the host. In addition,

precipitation may occur, allowing more effective phagocytosis. Some vaccinations work in this manner. For example, tetanus and diphtheria bacteria are chemically altered to make them less toxic but retain the immunogenic qualities so that the body will act and promote immunity.

Antibodies do have the capability to defend against certain viruses. This is accomplished by reducing the ability of the virus to attach to and enter a cell. The body subsequently induces agglutination or phagocytosis to eliminate the invader. If a virus is successful at entering the cell, in most cases it can be shielded and protected from antibodies by the cell wall. This is because the virus does not circulate through the bloodstream but rather spreads by direct cell-to-cell interaction. This means that antibodies are of lesser importance once certain viral infections have occurred. Recurrent infections also are less apt to be prevented in some cases. Some viruses (polio and influenza) do spread through cell-to-cell interaction in the blood. In these cases, antibodies may have an impact on the scope of the infection.

Antibodies also have the ability to perform a process by which bacteria become susceptible to phagocytosis—opsonization. Bacteria often have an outer capsule to protect them from phagocytes. Once an antibody is produced against certain bacteria, it will begin to make the bacteria susceptible to attack from phagocytes and try to neutralize the infection. It also will activate certain components of the complement system that assist in opsonization.

The immune response occurs when an antibody encounters an antigen in the body. The antibody attaches to the antigen by its Y-shaped antigen-binding site. The opposite side of the antibody is the location for adjuncts of the inflammatory system, such as the complement cascade.

Antibodies as Antigens

As valuable as antibodies are to the host in which they are found, they usually are seen as an antigen and are immunogenic in the body of another host. This also is true in situations of cross-species contamination. If a human antibody were introduced to a dog, it would be identified as an antigen and subsequently attacked by the canine immune system. Antibodies can be classified into one of three groups when referring to antigenic properties:

- *Isotypic antigens* are species specific. They are common between hosts of the same species but foreign to other species. This is a common way of determining the species of origin in a blood sample.
- *Allotypic antigens* are slightly different within a species. The difference is found in one or more of the polypeptide chains. These differences are called *alleles.* Significant numbers of alleles exist among the different possible chain arrangements, meaning that

a host of the same species can recognize the antibody of the other host as an antigen.

- *Idiotypic antigenic determinants* are differences in antibodies of the same class in a single host. For example, an IgG subclass 3 antibody that develops specificity for the mumps virus is different from an IgG subclass 3 antibody that develops specificity for the tetanus toxoid. This is because of the change of a few key amino acids in the structure.

Monoclonal Antibodies

When the body responds to an antigen, it produces antibodies considered to be polyclonal; they are produced from multiple clones of B lymphocytes. This is because a typical antigen has multiple antigenic determinant sites that may stimulate a wide range of B lymphocytes to respond. Monoclonal antibodies have been developed in laboratories that are specific to one antigenic determinant. They are more pure and quite specific, which is useful in the early diagnosis and identification of a viral invader. The body produces a spectrum response that can cloud the identity of the invader, but exposure to a monoclonal antibody in the laboratory can clarify the situation. This type of technology also is being used in the experimental treatment of some cancers.

Secretory Immune System

In addition to the humoral response described, a separate but closely related system called the *secretory immune system* also protects the body. This system involves tears, sweat, saliva, breast milk (provides passive immunity to the neonate), the GI tract, and the respiratory tract. Its job is to stop invaders before they enter the body or protect the body after invaders have been inhaled or ingested. These antibodies are produced in a slightly different way than are the B lymphocytes. They are similarly passed through lymphatic tissue and nodes but in a different region of the body. This path ensures that the secretions of the body are used to identify and protect the body before the entry of the antigen.

Instead of being passed through the spleen, these lymphocytes are passed through the lacrimal and salivary glands, lymphoid tissue in the breast, bronchi, intestines, and genitourinary tract. These lymphocytes provide local protection to the area in which they are produced. Although several types of antibodies are present in the secretory immune system, the primary immunoglobulin produced is IgA. In this way the body tries to prevent attachment and invasion of the antigen through the mucous membranes. As previously mentioned, the mother gives passive immunity to the fetus before it is born. In addition, the child gains passive immunity after birth by the passage of the IgA, IgM, and IgG antibodies through breast milk. The secretory immune system, although technically different from the standard humeral response, is quite important in the defense of the body. It serves as one of the first lines of defense when faced with a foreign antigen.

Cell-Mediated Immune Response

The lymphocytes that take the pathway through the thymus gland are destined to become T lymphocytes. These cells are the backbone of the cell-mediated immune response. As they pass through the thymus gland, they are inundated with thymic hormones. These hormones are responsible for the maturation of the cells into one of five kinds of mature T lymphocytes. The five types include (1) memory cells that induce the secondary immune response; (2) lymphokine-producing cells, known as transfer delayed hypersensitivity cells, which activate macrophages; (3) cytotoxic cells that attack antigens directly; (4) helper T cells; and (5) suppressor T cells, which affect the cell-mediated immune response and the humoral immune response. Transfer delayed hypersensitivity cells are believed to be a subset of helper cells responsible for activating both T cells and the B cells of the humoral immune response.

Once the T lymphocytes exit the thymus gland, they are mature and able to interact with a foreign antigen. When this occurs, T cells are stimulated to proliferate. This means that a large number of T cells with different functions are capable of attacking an antigen in different ways. Following are four main ways in which these cells respond to an antigen:

- *Cytotoxicity.* This is the direct attack of infected cells by a T cell. The cytotoxic cell, through direct binding, releases toxic substances to attack cells that have been infected with a virus, tumor cells, or the cells of foreign grafts (transplants).
- *Delayed hypersensitivity.* Transfer delayed hypersensitivity cells are a part of the inflammatory response and produce mediators called lymphokines that influence other cells.
- *Memory.* These cells are responsible for the secondary immune response. They are able to prepare the body for a response if it is exposed to an antigen for a second or subsequent time.
- *Control.* The helper T cells and suppressor T cells exert control over both humoral and cell-mediated response by activation (helper T cells) and suppression (suppressor T cells).

Cellular Interactions in Immune Response

The cells of the immune system and the processes in which they participate do not operate alone. They must interact to defend the body. This is accomplished with three basic interactions: antigen-presenting cells (macrophages) with T helper cells, T helper cells with B cells, and T helper cells with cytotoxic cells (Box 8-4).

Cytokines

Cytokines are secreted proteins that generally act over a short distance for a short period and at low concentrations. These proteins are released in response to an immune stimulus. Cytokines alter the function of cells by binding to a receptor site and releasing a second messenger inside the cell. This messenger causes an increase or a decrease in the expression of membrane proteins. This process occurs with nearby cells and also can alter the cell that initiated the secretion of the protein. This type of function is called *autocrine action*.

The name *cytokine* is a general name that includes several different kinds of proteins. If a cytokine is released from a lymphocyte, it is called a *lymphokine*. If it is released from a monocyte, it is called a *monokine*. Only two of a growing number of proteins are classified as cytokines. Many ongoing studies at the DNA level are determining that many more proteins with similar functions have yet to be found.

Antigen Processing, Presentation, and Recognition

As previously described, three basic interactions must occur in the immune response. For those to begin, the body must activate these interactions through processing the antigen and presenting it to the immune system; the immune system must then recognize the presentation and respond appropriately. The key to this process is the action of macrophages. These cells are responsible for ingesting and destroying invading organisms. In doing so, they also process the antigens, taking fragments into the endoplasmic reticulum of the cell and forming a complex that is then transported to the surface of the macrophage.

The combination of the antigen complex and the self-antigen presenting on the surface of the macrophage alerts the T helper cells to its presence. Once the T helper cells recognize the macrophage has both antigens on its surface, they are activated. The T helper cells are activated on the basis of the type of receptors on the surface. Two kinds of receptors respond—T-cell receptors, which are antigen specific, and CD receptors, which respond regardless of the antigen type.

HLAs are either class I or class II. Class determines the type of cells that respond to the presented antigen. T helper cells respond only to class II HLA antigens. Class I HLA antigens activate cytotoxic T cells and suppressor T cells. Antigen receptor interaction is crucial to the process, but macrophages also release interleukin-1, which has many functions that assist in the immune response, including elevating body temperature and increasing the production of interferon (Figure 8-15).

T-Cell and B-Cell Differentiation and Control

The differentiation of both T cells and B cells only occurs once an antigen is identified in the body. Once this occurs, the act of processing and the presentation of the antigen complexes on the surface of the macrophage begins. As previously explained, depending on the type of antigen and the subsequent complex presented, the body responds in one of several ways.

If the antigen interacts with the T-cell receptors, it will differentiate into one of the following based on the type of receptor and antigen that has the interaction: helper cells, cytotoxic cells, transfer delayed hypersensitivity cells, or suppressor cells. B cells, on the other hand, produce antibodies in the form of IgM, IgG, IgA, IgE, or IgD, depending on whether the precipitating interaction is direct recognition or through a helper T cell.

The process of controlling T-cell and B-cell differentiation and proliferation generally falls to the suppressor cells. The need to control this process is itself a defense mechanism. By controlling the immune system, the body is preventing an attack from itself through inhibition. Two theories exist regarding how this control takes place. The first is to alter antigen recognition, thus inhibiting a response. The second is through altering the response to an identified antigen (McCance & Huether, 2002).

Fetal and Neonatal Immune Function

[OBJECTIVE 16]

The immune system of the newborn is underdeveloped at birth. When the fetus is in the mother's womb in the last trimester of pregnancy, it is developing the primary

---

BOX 8-4	Overview of the Immune Response

The immune system is highly complex, and the immune response can often be difficult to visualize. Following are the primary activities that occur in the immune response.

When a foreign invader enters the body, the inflammatory response occurs. As part of the inflammatory response, the neutrophils begin phagocytosis of the invader. During this process they also release macrophage-stimulating factor, which causes monocytes to become macrophages, which also participate in phagocytosis. When the macrophages engulf the invader they become antigen-presenting cells and present portions of what they have engulfed on their cell membranes to B cells and helper T cells. The stimulus for the helper T cell to join with the antigen-presenting cell is the result of the secretion of IL-1 by the antigen-presenting cell. If the helper T cell does not recognize what is being presented as an immunogen, no immune response occurs. If a helper T cell does recognize what is being presented as an immunogen, it will secrete IL-2 and B-cell growth factor. IL-2 initiates the cell-mediated response, whereas B-cell growth factor initiates the humoral immune response.

IL, Interleukin.

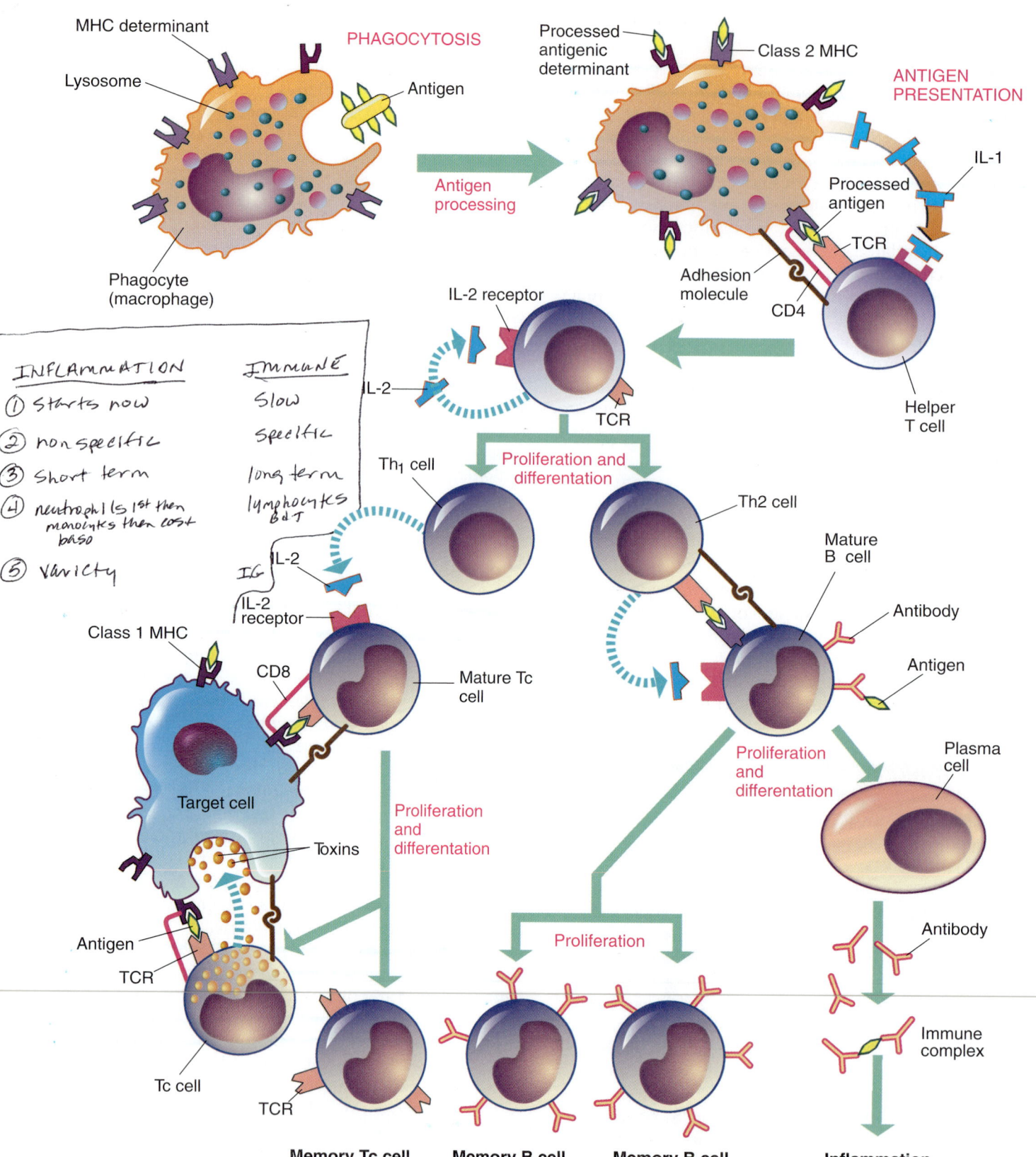

Figure 8-15 Model of cellular interaction and the immune response showing antigen processing, activation, and differentiation of T- and B-cell immune response. *Solid arrows* indicate differentiation steps. *Hashed arrows* indicate indirect effects through cytokines. *MHC,* Major histocompatibility complex; *TCR,* T-cell receptor; *IL,* interleukin.

function of the immune system, almost exclusively creating IgM antibodies. This is the extent of its abilities, and it must rely on the mother's immune system to provide protection. This occurs when maternal antibodies from the mother's blood are transferred to the fetus by the umbilical cord through the placenta. A layer of specialized cells called *trophoblasts* are responsible for the active transport of immunoglobulins across the membrane. These molecules are too large to diffuse by themselves.

This protection stays with the fetus until birth. Once the infant can no longer receive antibodies from the mother's blood, the levels begin to drop over the course of several months. At this time infants may have an increase in the number of infections they contract. The child's immune system continues to mature from this point forward, and the levels of antibodies produced approach normal levels.

Aging and the Immune System

[OBJECTIVE 17]
As with most other body systems, the function of the immune system deteriorates with age. The changes in the immune system are noticeable mainly in the T cells. The thymus gland reaches its maximal size around the time of sexual maturity. From this point forward, it deteriorates until middle age. By the age of 45 to 50 years the thymus gland has lost 85% of its maximal size. This means that although the number of circulating T cells may not decrease, their ability to function may be affected.

INFLAMMATION

[OBJECTIVE 18]
The inflammatory process is designed to serve two main functions. First, it defends the host organism against infection. Second, it facilitates tissue repair and healing. This is accomplished through components found in the circulatory system. These components are together known as *exudate* once they move into the affected tissue to perform their functions. This pattern of movement occurs as a result of several steps.

The first step in the inflammatory process is the dilation of blood vessels at the site of injury to increase blood flow. Second, vascular permeability increases to permit plasma movement into the tissues. WBCs then adhere to the vessel walls and migrate into the affected tissues. This process occurs in phases. The early and late phases of inflammation are different, but they work together to accomplish the same goals: (1) attack and destroy injurious agents, (2) confine these agents by walling them off to prevent effects on the host, (3) stimulate the immune system, and (4) promote healing (Figure 8-16).

The inflammatory response is methodical in its function. It responds the same way regardless of the stimuli. It does not have the ability to create memory for specific antigens and responds in similar fashion regardless of the number of exposures. This may seem quite different from the immune response and, in fact, it is. The fact still remains that these systems are linked, and the inflammatory response is integral to the initiation of the immune system.

Acute Inflammatory Response

The acute phase of the inflammatory response occurs almost immediately after the injury. The injurious agent, as previously described, can come in the form of trauma, hypoxia, genetic defects, chemical agents, microorganisms, temperature, or radiation. The immediate response is vasoconstriction followed by vasodilation to increase blood flow to the microcirculation. The increase in pressure allows exudate to escape into the tissues, causing edema and swelling. In addition, biochemical stimulation of the endothelial cells to retract creates additional space between the cells. The retraction of the endothelial lining of vessel walls allows the leukocytes to penetrate the tissues. These cells are responsible for the phagocytosis of bacteria or cellular debris. This, in conjunction with mast cells and platelets, begins the healing process.

Mast Cells

[OBJECTIVE 21]
Mast cells are one of the most important parts of the inflammatory response. They are structurally similar to basophils in that they are fundamentally large sacs of granules. They differ in that they are not found in the bloodstream, but rather in the connective tissues outside the vessels. Mast cells activate the inflammatory response in two ways. The first is degranulation, in which the cell drops its granules into the extracellular matrix. The second is the synthesis of chemical mediators that furthers the inflammatory response.

Degranulation of Vasoactive Amines and Chemotactic Factors

Degranulation is the process by which mast cells empty themselves of the granules located on the inside of the cell. This process is stimulated by one of the following events:

- Physical injury, such as radiation or heat
- Chemical agents, such as toxins, insect or snake venom, certain enzymes, and proteins released from neutrophils
- Immunologic processes, such as the production of IgE as a result of an allergic reaction

The granules released as a result of this process include preformed biochemical mediators. These include histamine, neutrophil chemotactic factor, and eosinophil chemotactic factor. These substances work within seconds to exert their effect. Platelets also release a powerful biochemical mediator, serotonin.

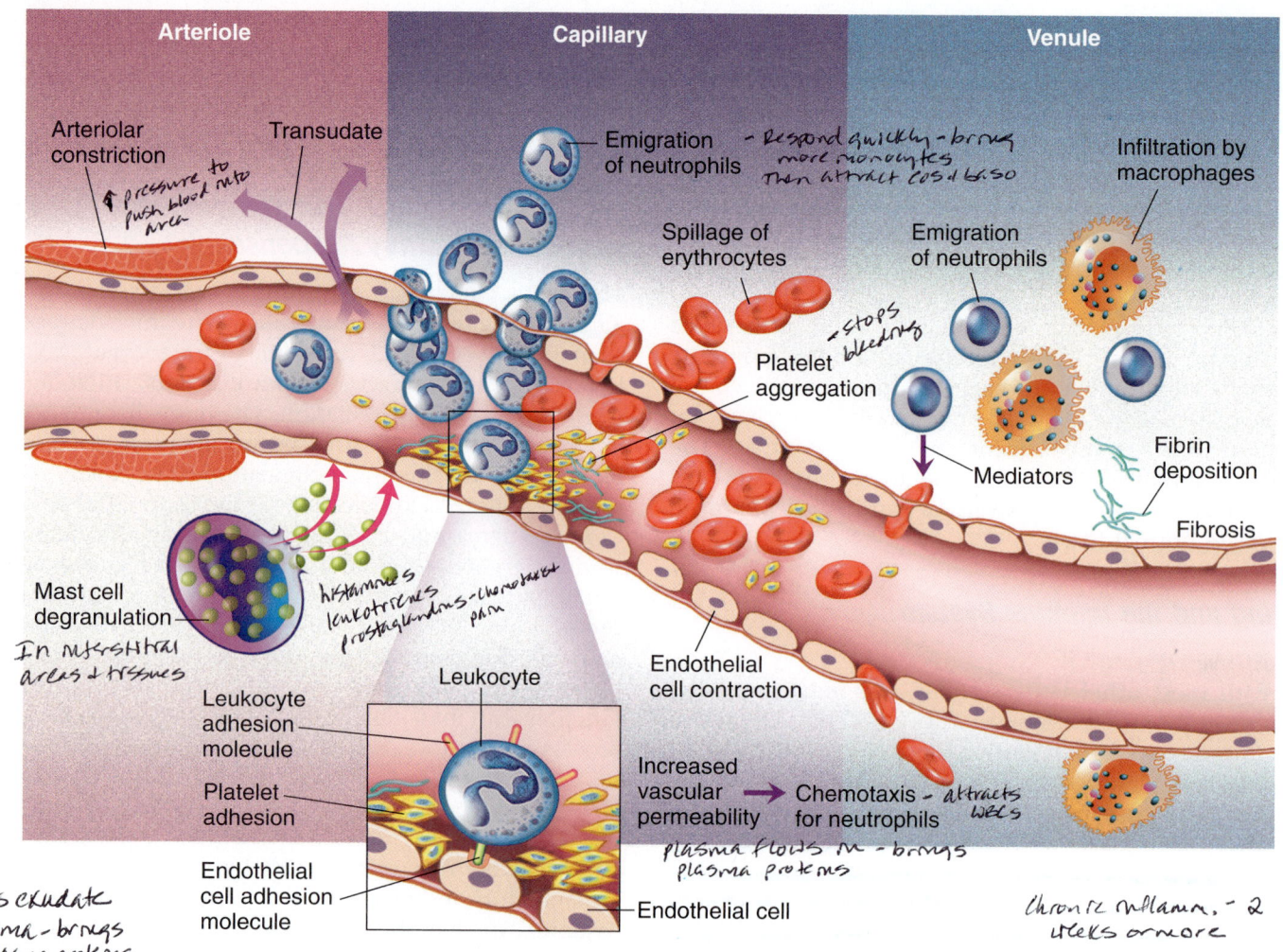

Handwritten annotations on figure:
- ↑ pressure to push blood into area
- Respond quickly - brings more monocytes then attract eos & baso
- stops bleeding
- histamines leukotrienes prostaglandins - chemotaxis pain
- In interstitial areas & tissues
- attracts WBCs
- plasma flows in - brings plasma proteins
- Serous exudate plasma - brings plasma proteins
- Chronic inflamm. - 2 weeks or more

Figure 8-16 Sequence of events in the process of inflammation.

The vasoactive amines include histamine and serotonin. These substances work together to alter the diameter of the vasculature. Within seconds they cause a temporary constriction of the smooth muscle of the large vessel walls. This action, along with the dilation of the postcapillary sphincter, causes an increase in blood flow to the microcirculation. They also cause an increase in the permeability of the vasculature. This is a result of the retraction of the endothelial cells. Chemotactic factors are responsible for attracting leukocytes to the site of inflammation. The definition of chemotaxis is the attraction of WBCs. These factors attract the type of cell for which they are named. Neutrophils account for the majority of the leukocytes that arrive in the early phases of acute inflammation because they are responsible for most of the work during this part of the process. Eosinophils are responsible for several functions during the acute inflammatory response. They are mildly phagocytic in nature and the body's chief defense against parasites. Even though these are important functions, the most important function of eosinophils is to regulate the intensity and duration of the acute phase. They release enzymes that deactivate or control the effects of histamine and leukotrienes, limiting the response.

Synthesis of Leukotrienes and Prostaglandins

Leukotrienes are synthesized by mast cells. They have an effect similar to the vasoactive amines. However, leukotrienes are more important in the later stages of inflammation because of their slow, long-lasting effects. They also are known as slow-reacting substances of anaphylaxis. They promote vasoconstriction, increased permeability, and chemotaxis.

Prostaglandins are synthesized and released from mast cells. As with other substances in this process, they serve more than one purpose. They promote vasoconstriction, increased permeability, and chemotaxis. They also are responsible for pain at the site of inflammation. Like eosinophils, prostaglandins play an inhibitory role as well. They suppress the release of histamine and lysosomal enzymes (Figure 8-17).

Plasma Protein Systems

[OBJECTIVE 21]

The plasma protein system has several important components. Three primary systems play a role in the inflammatory process: the complement system, the coagulation system, and the kinin system. Each system works on the cascade theory; each step in the process depends on the

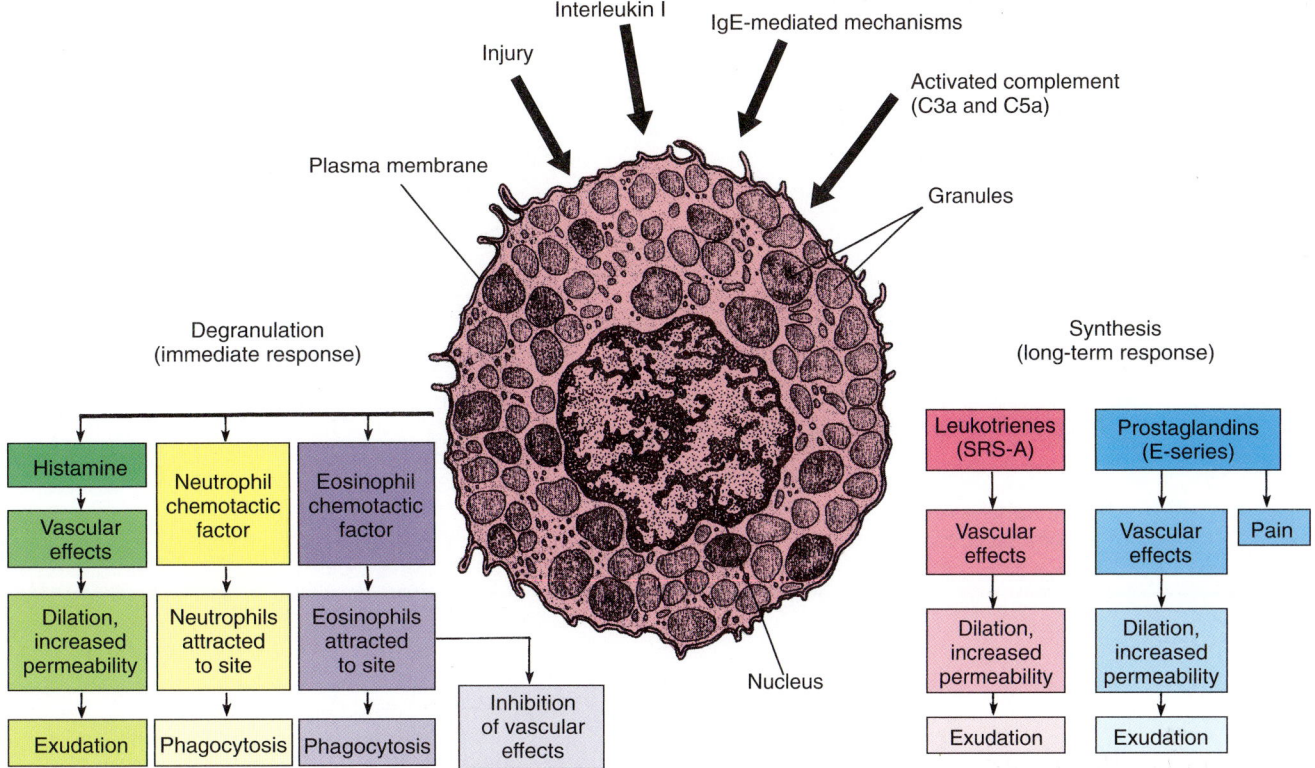

Figure 8-17 The effects of degranulation *(left)* and synthesis *(right)* by mast cells. The electron micrograph of a tissue mast cell shows darkly stained granules in the cytoplasm (× 9200). *SRS-A*, Slow-reacting substances of anaphylaxis.

step before it. Step two cannot happen without step one, and so on.

Most of the chemical reactions in these systems and the effects they cause are normally short lived because they are quickly deactivated by other plasma proteins found in the body.

Complement System. The complement system consists of at least 20 proteins that account for approximately 5% of all the plasma proteins found in the circulation. This system is a nonspecific mechanism that mediates inflammation. Thus it plays a role in almost every inflammatory response. It is considered by some to be the most important plasma protein system. It can be activated by antigen-antibody complexes, byproducts released from invading bacteria, or components of other plasma protein systems.

Once activated, a cascade of events begins, resulting in the creation of complexes that have a role in almost every phase of the inflammatory response. The last few proteins in the complement cascade can attack and destroy invading bacteria. This makes this system one of the body's most potent defenders against bacterial infection. The complement system can be activated by two pathways: the classic pathway and the alternative pathway (Figure 8-18).

Classic Pathway. The activation of the classic pathway is preceded and induced by the formation of an antigen-antibody complex. This complex interacts with the C-1 complement factor to begin the cascade. The

process can be induced by even a small stimulus. The activation of C-1 through C-5 produces substances that enhance inflammation by opsonization of bacteria, chemotaxis, and promotion of degranulation of mast cells. C-6 through C-9 are responsible for increasing the permeability of the cell wall, thereby allowing water and ions to rush into the cell, causing the death and destruction of the bacterial cell.

Alternative Pathway. This pathway of activation occurs without the stimulus of an antigen-antibody complex. In this scenario the invading microorganism produces substances that can interact with the complement factors B and D. This interaction can cause the activation of the C-3 complement factor. If this occurs, the remainder of the cascade follows in normal fashion. This process occurs more quickly because the system does not need to wait for the formation of the antigen-antibody complex.

Coagulation System. The coagulation system has several functions. These functions are accomplished by the formation of fibrin, which is the end product of the cascade in this system that forms a fibrinous mesh responsible for the following:

- Preventing the spread of infection and the inflammation to adjacent tissues
- Keeping microorganisms at the site of greatest phagocytotic activity

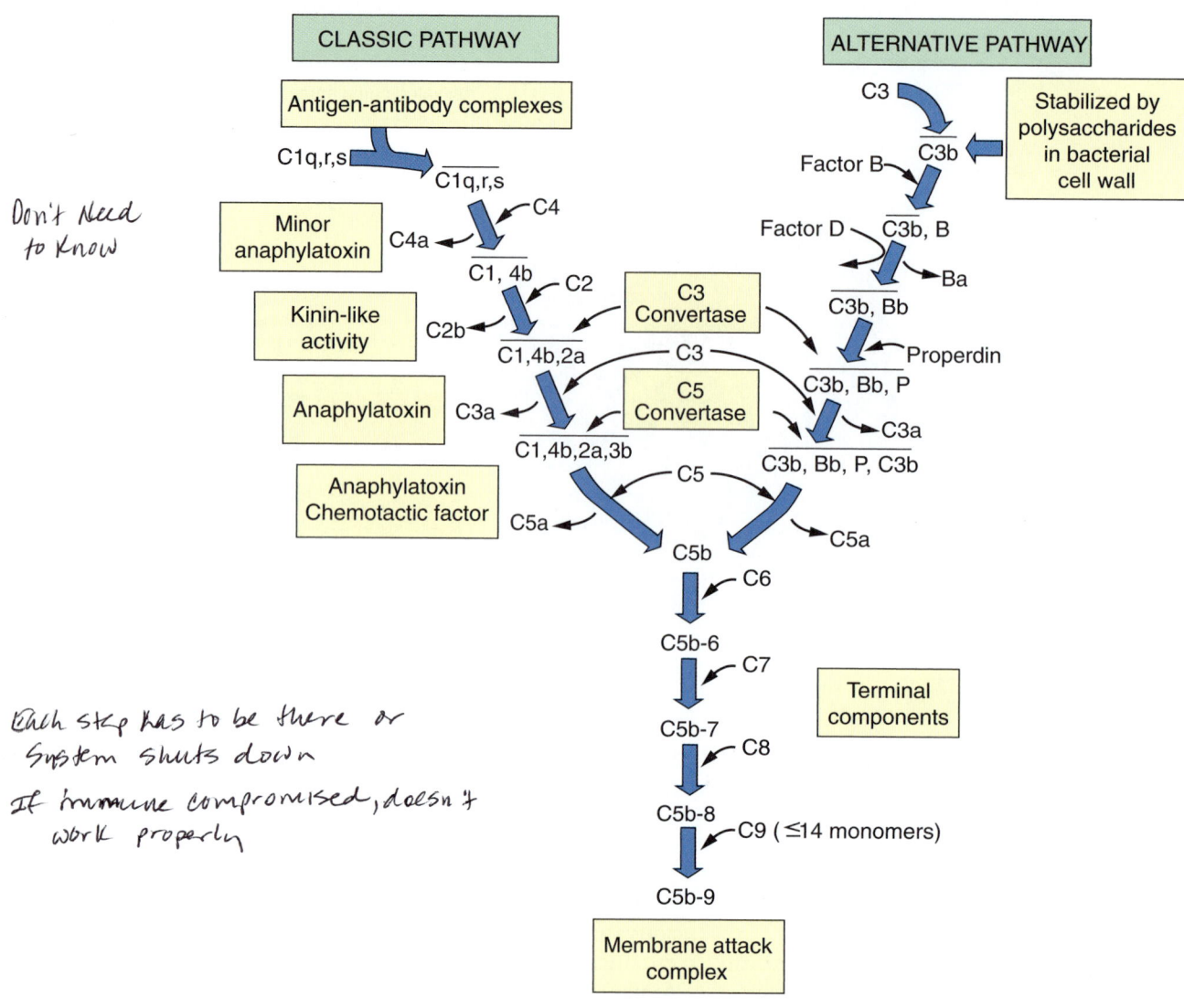

Don't Need to Know (handwritten note)

Each step has to be there or System shuts down (handwritten note)

If immune compromised, doesn't work properly (handwritten note)

Figure 8-18 Pathways of activation of the complement cascade. Complement components are cleaved into fragments, or subcomponents (denoted by *lowercase letters*), during activation. Many of the subcomponents are biochemical mediators of inflammation. The larger activated fragment is usually converted into an active enzyme (indicated by the *bar* above the fragment) and forms a complex with the preceding components in the cascade. By one nomenclature, the small fragments are the "a" fragments, and the large fragments are the "b" fragments (e.g., C3b is the larger fragment from C3 and Bb is the activated form of factor B), although historically the small C2 fragment has been designated the "b" fragment, as indicated here. The classic pathway is usually activated by antigen-antibody complexes through component C1, whereas the alternative pathway is activated by many agents, such as bacterial polysaccharides, through component C3b. Both pathways produce C3 convertases and C5 convertases, which are enzymatically active complexes that activate C3 and C5, respectively.

- Forming a clot that stops bleeding and creates a framework for tissue repair and healing

Just as in the complement system, the clotting system can be activated by two separate pathways. These pathways, just as in the complement system, converge at a common point and proceed on a common course to the end of the cascade. These pathways are called the *intrinsic and extrinsic pathways.* The extrinsic pathway is activated when damage has occurred to the vascular wall or surrounding tissues. The intrinsic pathway is activated by the exposure to collagen or other activators in the blood as a result of vessel damage. Both pathways end with the production of fibrin and the promotion of the inflammatory response, increased permeability, and chemotaxis.

Kinin System. The last of the three plasma protein systems is the kinin system. Bradykinin is the primary kinin; it causes vasodilation, extravascular smooth muscle contraction, and increased permeability. Evidence exists that it also promotes chemotaxis. The smooth muscle contraction associated with bradykinin is a slower response than that of histamine. It is generally believed to play a role in the prolonged phase of inflammation.

The kinin system is activated by factors in the coagulation cascade. The cascade that follows activation is a conversion of factors that eventually results in the production of kinin. Kinin has other sources, including saliva, sweat, tears, urine, and feces. These are together called tissue kallikreins, which are the precursors to kininogen, which converts to kinin. Regardless of the source, the end product is the same—predominantly bradykinin (McCance & Huether, 2002).

Control and Interaction of the Plasma Protein System. The plasma protein system produces powerful substances. Moreover, it is quite important to the protection of the host. As such, controlling this system is critical for the following reasons:

1. The inflammatory process is important for protection and is therefore full of fail-safe mechanisms to ensure proper activation. In other words, more than one way exists to initiate inflammation.
2. The mediators created during inflammation are so powerful that they are potentially harmful to the host; if they are not contained to the injured site the host may be harmed.

Therefore more than one mechanism is necessary to regulate or deactivate the system.

Control of the plasma protein system occurs at many levels throughout the inflammation process. Naturally occurring enzymes can inactivate components of the complement system, and eosinophilic enzymes modulate or have an antagonistic effect on histamine and leukotrienes. Other natural inhibitors, or antagonists, exist for histamine, kinins, complement components, and other components of the inflammatory response.

The actions of histamine are controlled by the receptors on the host's target cells. At least two types of histamine receptors are found in the human body: H_1 and H_2 receptors. The H_1 receptors are responsible for promoting inflammation. These are primarily located on cells of smooth muscle, especially those of the bronchi. When activated, they cause bronchial constriction. H_2 receptors are responsible for suppression of leukocyte function and mast cell degranulation. H_2 receptors are located in large quantities in the stomach mucosa and are responsible for the production of gastric acids when stimulated. Although these receptors are found in some areas more than others, both receptors are found on the same cell in several places. In this instance, the receptors can accomplish either agonistic or antagonistic effects based on the receptor that is stimulated.

Most of the processes involved in the inflammatory response tend to interact with one another. In other words, the activation or inactivation of one plasma protein system tends to have a similar effect on the others.

A classic example of this interaction is seen in patients with a genetic C-1 esterase inhibitor deficiency. These patients can have recurrent episodes of edema in the GI tract, respiratory tract, and skin. In the worst-case scenario, death can occur as a result of laryngeal edema. With the absence of the C-1 esterase inhibitor, the activation of plasmin and the three plasma protein cascades can occur as a result of some stressor. Without the normal controls in place, the effects of inflammation go unchecked and the results can be fatal. This clearly illustrates the interdependent nature of these systems.

Cellular Components of Inflammation

[OBJECTIVE 21]
The inflammatory process begins with vascular changes, resulting in increased blood flow to the affected site and increased permeability of the capillaries.

Function of Phagocytes
Neutrophils and macrophages are the primary phagocytes of the inflammatory response. They both are normally found in the circulation. They remain there until activated by the inflammatory process to move toward the affected site and become part of the exudate. When they arrive, these cells become sticky and adhere to the vessel wall by a process known as **margination.** While this process occurs, the endothelial cells of the vessel wall begin to contract, allowing gaps to develop. This act allows the exudate, including WBCs, to escape into the tissues. This process is called **diapedesis.** Once through the vessel wall, they are attracted by chemotactic factors specific to each of them and trapped in the fibrin meshwork, where they begin the process of phagocytosis (Figure 8-19).

Although these cells are similar in function, they are different in many ways. Neutrophils arrive at the site of inflammation faster than macrophages, but they do not remain active for as long a period. In addition, they are attracted by unique chemotactic factors, and their lysosomes each carry different enzymes. The process by which they destroy the invading organism follows the same pattern.

Phagocytosis is the process by which invading microorganisms are engulfed and destroyed. Following are the four basic steps in this process:

1. Recognition of the invader and the process of the phagocyte adhering to the microorganism.
2. Engulfment of the microorganism; this is the process of ingesting the invader into the phagocyte.
3. Fusion of the phagocyte's lysosomes with the invader in an effort to kill it.
4. Destruction of the target microorganism by the lysosomal enzymes of the phagocyte.

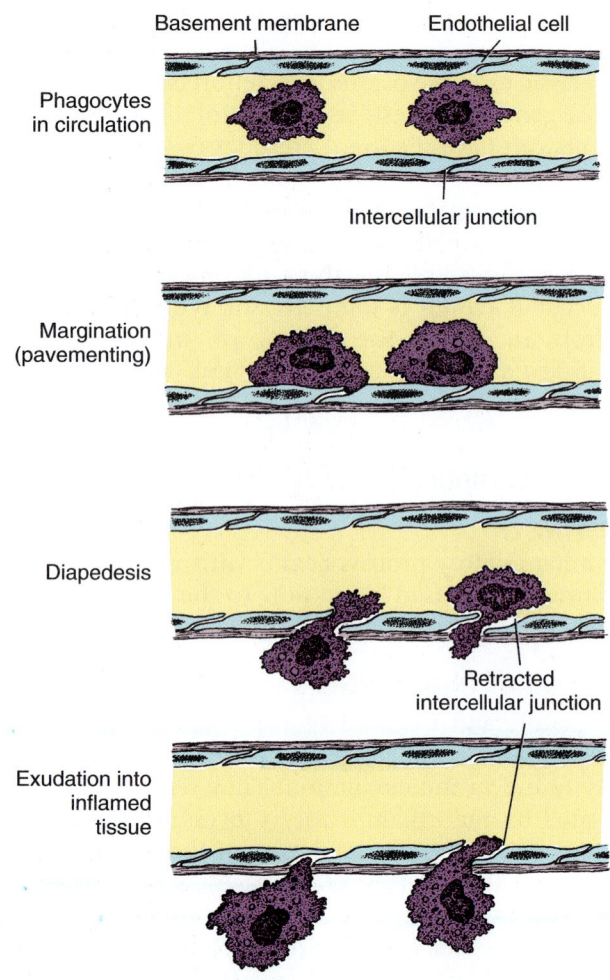

Basement membrane   Endothelial cell

Phagocytes in circulation

Intercellular junction

Margination (pavementing)

Diapedesis

Retracted intercellular junction

Exudation into inflamed tissue

Figure 8-19 Diapedesis of a phagocyte. Phagocytes are capable of ameboid movement, which allows them to squeeze through intercellular junctions and migrate to inflammatory lesions.

During the process of phagocytosis, the target organism and lysosomal enzymes are contained within the confines of the membrane-bound vesicle. This ensures that the phagocyte is protected from any harmful effects of the invader.

Polymorphonuclear Neutrophils

In the early phase of the inflammatory process, the predominant phagocyte at the site of inflammation is the neutrophil, or polymorphonuclear neutrophils. They arrive within the first 6 to 12 hours because of the strong draw of the chemotactic factors. These cells are usually short lived because of the properties of the cells themselves. They have a varied role depending on the type of lesion that has occurred. In lesions such as burns, they are responsible for removing debris and preparing the site for the next phase in the process. In the face of bacterial infection, they begin the process of phagocytosis.

Monocytes and Macrophages

Monocytes are the precursors of macrophages. These cells usually arrive at the site of inflammation several days after the neutrophils. Neutrophils are the most abundant white blood cells in circulating blood, and when exposed to a foreign invader they release macrophage-stimulating factor, which causes monocytes to develop into macrophages. They are more closely associated with the chronic inflammatory response than the acute phase. These cells are attracted by chemotactic factors released by the neutrophils in the early stages of the process. In addition, these cells move slower than neutrophils.

Macrophages differ from neutrophils in many ways. These differences make them a stronger candidate for long-term protection against invading microorganisms. Macrophages are capable of surviving the acidic environment of the inflammatory site for a much longer period. Furthermore, unlike neutrophils, they are able to perform cell division.

The roles of macrophages in the inflammatory process are varied and span the course of the process. They include responding to lymphokines, presenting antigens to lymphocytes, stimulating the production and differentiation of granulocytes and monocytes in the bone marrow, and even participating in the healing process by releasing chemicals that promote the regrowth of tissues.

Eosinophils

Eosinophils are granulocytes packed with lysosomes. These cells are the body's primary response to parasitic infection. Unlike the cells previously described in this section, these cells do not work by phagocytosis. They bind tightly to the invading parasite rather than engulf it. Once bound, they release their granules, which contain a caustic protein that destroys the surface of the parasite, thereby killing it. In this way eosinophils are capable of defending against invaders that are multicelled and much larger than themselves, such as worms. In addition to the defense against parasitic invaders, these cells release biochemical mediators that control the vascular effects of serotonin and histamine. Thus they limit the inflammatory response and prevent the negative effects of the process on the host.

Cellular Products

In the defense of the body, cells produce soluble chemicals that communicate between cells and contribute to the nonspecific defense. These chemicals are generally referred to as *cytokines*. Cytokines can further be subdivided into lymphokines, which are produced by lymphocytes, and monokines, which are produced by monocytes and macrophages. Cytokines come in many forms and are produced by many different types of cells. These cells can interact in a synergistic manner. This means that the effect of two or more agents acting together is greater than the sum of the effects of the agents acting independently. In addition to a synergistic effect, they can inhibit one another as well. The cytokines primarily involved in the inflammatory and immune response are interleukin, lymphokines, and interferon.

Interleukins

Interleukins are chemical mediators produced by both lymphocytes and macrophages in response to either an antigen or products of the inflammatory response. More than one type of interleukin exists. Moreover, they can be activated by other means than antigen stimulation. Interleukin-1 (IL-1) is a lymphocyte-stimulating factor. This means that in addition to assisting the T helper cells in responding to antigens and the stimulation of IL-2, it induces a process called neutrophilia. This is the proliferation or an increase in the number of circulating neutrophils.

Lymphokines

These cells are produced by the T lymphocytes in the body's response to antigen presentation. Like interleukins, they come in several different forms. In general, they stimulate the transformation of monocytes into macrophages. A specific lymphokine called *migration inhibitory factor* is responsible for ensuring that the macrophages remain in the area of inflammation and do not spread to surrounding tissues. Another, called the *macrophage activating factor,* is responsible for enhancing the phagocytosis provided by macrophages. Some lymphokines perform functions such as stimulating the production and proliferation of more lymphokines; others, in contrast, inhibit their function.

Interferon ✗ *Have flu like symptoms all the time*
Body is in inflamm. process from it

These cytokines are critical in the body's defense against viral infections. Their chemicals do not kill viruses and they do not have an effect on cells that have already been infected. Interferon is a small, low-molecular-weight protein released by the host's cells that have been infected. Interferon then spreads to other host cells in the area that have not been infected and binds to them. Although this does not prevent infection of the other cells, it causes them to produce a blocking protein that blocks the virus ✗ from taking over the host cell once inside. Therefore the newly infected cell does not reproduce the virus.

Systemic Responses of Acute Inflammation
[OBJECTIVE 22]

Three main systemic responses to the acute inflammatory process are possible: fever, leukocytosis (an increase in the number of circulating lymphocytes), and an increase in the number of circulating plasma proteins. Fever may be caused by stimulation of the hypothalamus by endogenous pyrogens, which are similar to IL-1 and are released by neutrophils and macrophages after the initiation of phagocytosis. Fever can also be induced by endotoxins released from bacteria or an antigen-antibody complex. This can be a beneficial or harmful response depending on the situation. An increase in body heat can prove harmful to some invading microorganisms, but it also makes the host more susceptible to certain bacterial infections.

During the course of an infection, the number of circulating leukocytes in the body increases. Neutrophils account for a majority of this increase. The ratio of immature neutrophils to mature neutrophils changes and is commonly referred to as a shift to the left. When the body increases the number of immature neutrophils, called bands, to the number of mature neutrophils, called segs, the body is preparing to proliferate itself with neutrophils. This is caused by a number of factors, including components of the complement system and chemicals released by phagocytes, which will, in addition to neutrophils, increase the number of eosinophils and basophils.

The last of the systemic responses is the increase in the number of circulating plasma proteins. In the acute phase, plasma proteins called acute phase reactants are produced in the liver. These proteins are released and contribute to the control of the inflammatory process.

Chronic Inflammatory Response

The simplest way to distinguish between acute and chronic inflammation is by the length of the response. Chronic inflammation is defined as an inflammatory response lasting longer than 2 weeks, regardless of the cause. It can be a result of an unsuccessful acute inflammatory response or as a distinct process independent of an acute response. In other words, a wound with a foreign object such as a splinter can progress to chronic inflammation.

In addition, certain bacteria, such as those that produce tuberculosis, have cell walls that can withstand the onslaught of phagocytes. Because of the high lipid and wax content of the cell wall, it is resistant to the normal degradation of phagocytosis. Because these types of bacteria persist in the system, the inflammatory response is constantly stimulated. Certain bacteria produce toxins that can cause tissue damage even after they are dead.

Chronic inflammation is characterized by a high concentration of lymphocytes and macrophages. If the macrophages are unable to defend the host from the invading microorganism, they attempt to isolate it to minimize the damage inflicted. This process forms a pocket called a *granuloma* at the site of infection. It generally occurs with infection of certain bacteria, fungi, and parasites as a result of macrophage differentiation. These cells have varied roles. Some take up cellular debris and others fuse into giant cells capable of phagocytosis. The process continues while the outside of the granuloma is coated with collagen that will become calcified to prevent escape of the microorganism. Once this occurs, giant cells eventually liquefy, releasing all their contents inside the granuloma. The microorganism is eventually destroyed and the contents of the granuloma are absorbed and eliminated. The granuloma itself may persist for the life of the host.

Local Inflammatory Response

Regardless of the cause of inflammation, the fact that it is a nonspecific defense mechanism means that it will follow a similar pattern of manifestation. All the changes seen in the local inflammatory response are a result of vascular changes and exudation. The pain and swelling associated with this process are a result of the process of exudation, whereas the redness and heat are a result of the increased blood flow from vascular changes. The reason for these changes is to allow the cellular components of inflammation to get to the site of injury.

Exudate has three primary functions:

1. To dilute the toxins produced by bacteria and toxic products released by dying cells
2. To carry plasma proteins and leukocytes (both phagocytes and lymphocytes) to the site of injury
3. To carry away bacterial toxins, dead cells, debris, and other products of inflammation

The type and content of the exudate found at the site of inflammation greatly depends on the phase of the inflammatory process. In the early stages the exudate is watery, with few plasma proteins or leukocytes. This is called *serous exudate.* As the process continues and more of the cellular components arrive, the composition of the exudate changes to a thick and clotted state referred to as fibrinous exudate. If the inflammation is the result of persistent bacterial infection, the exudate may consist of pus. This pus is called *purulent* or *suppurative exudate.* If bleeding is present it is considered *hemorrhagic exudate.*

How the inflammation proceeds or forms lesions varies depending on the part of the body involved. For example, in cardiac tissue dead tissue is replaced with scar tissue. In the brain, however, the dead tissues liquefy and are contained in an abscess or a cyst. In the liver, dead cells stimulate the regeneration of liver cells. Inflammation is only possible in areas in which blood flow is possible. Areas that have no blood flow, such as gangrenous lesions, are incapable of inflammation and healing.

Phases of Resolution and Repair

[OBJECTIVE 23]

After the body has received an insult, the healing process begins almost immediately with the onset of acute inflammation. The process can continue for many months or even a few years. The body has multiple ways in which it can repair itself, and each of these meets with varying degrees of success, depending on many factors. The preferred outcome is a complete return to normal structure and function. This is called *resolution.* Resolution is accomplished through regeneration, which is the proliferation of the remaining cells in the damaged tissue.

However, because of many factors, resolution is not always possible. Some of these factors include excessive tissue damage or damage in an area incapable of resolution because of granuloma formation. In these cases a process known as repair takes place. In this process damaged tissue is replaced with scar tissue by filling in the lesion with collagen. This process does not result in a return of the normal function of the tissue. However, it does provide structure and strength to the area.

Regardless of which path the body takes to heal the damaged tissue, the initial actions are the same. Debridement is the cleaning up of the area in preparation for healing. This process involves enzymes that dissolve fibrin clots or scabs. Once this is complete, the body continues to clean the area by ridding it of exudate and any toxins. The vascular effects, including dilation and permeability, are reversed and the body then follows one of the two pathways previously described.

Some wounds that involve minimal tissue damage heal easily and leave minimal long-term evidence of their existence. In these wounds the edges are close together and tissue loss is minimal. These types of wounds are said to be healed by primary intention. Wounds that do not meet these criteria because of the extensive nature of the damage can take much longer to heal. Wounds that require significant tissue replacement and scar formation are said to heal by secondary intention. Regardless of whether wounds heal by primary or secondary intention, other factors play a role in the length of time necessary for the process to be completed.

Both resolution and repair occur in two overlapping phases. Reconstruction is the first phase. It begins 3 to 4 days after the initial injury and can last up to 2 weeks. It is characterized by the proliferation of connective tissue cells. The second phase is known as *maturation;* it begins weeks after the injury and can last up to 2 years. This phase is characterized by continued cellular differentiation, scar formation, and contraction of the wound.

Reconstructive Phase

In the initial phases of reconstruction, the wound is sealed off through the formation of a blood clot. This clot contains fibrin and trapped blood cells, both erythrocytes and leukocytes. This process is the first part of the coagulation cascade, and it begins to create a cross-linked mesh of fibrin. The mesh then traps platelets that have been activated by the initial insult to create a plug. This plug provides a protective barrier against bacterial and other infections. It also gives the wound a framework from which to begin the healing process. As previously described, this fibrin clot is then slowly dissolved as the body begins the process of debridement. It is then replaced by either normal tissue or scar tissue.

Reconstruction continues with a process known as granulation. In this phase, the healthy tissues surrounding the site of injury show signs of growth of a special tissue called granulation tissue. This tissue grows inward toward the center of damage. The job of this tissue is to revascularize the area. Capillary buds begin to form and continue to grow into the area of injury that has been debrided. These capillary buds then differentiate into arterioles and venules. They form fragile loops that anastomose into complete capillary beds. Lymphatic vessels grow in a similar fashion. Macrophages and the biochemical mediators they bring perform the following three primary functions in this phase of healing:

- Stimulation of fibroblasts to enter the area and secrete the collagen precursor known as *precollagen*
- Stimulation of vascular endothelial cells to cause capillary buds to form and grow
- Stimulation of the epithelial cells to grow over and seal the wound's surface (i.e., the next phase, epithelialization)

The process of epithelial cells growing over the wound follows a similar pattern to that of granulation tissue. Similarly, it proceeds from the outer edges of the injury toward the middle. These cells, which are stimulated by an unknown factor believed to be released by macrophages, continue to proliferate slowly, separating the scab from the wound. This proliferation continues until the cells meet the edges of the tissue coming from other directions and the wound is sealed. Once the sealing process is complete, the proliferation of cells stops. However, the differentiation of these cells continues until the various layers of the skin are formed.

The final phase of reconstruction is called *contraction*. It is accomplished by specialized cells called myofibroblasts. These cells have the ability to exert a contractile force on the edges of the wound, pulling them closer together. This process usually begins within 6 to 12 days of the initial injury, and the edges contract at a rate of approximately 0.5 mm/day. This process is especially important in wounds that heal by secondary intent.

Maturation Phase

As previously described, the reconstructive phase is rarely complete by the time the maturation phase begins. As a result, they usually overlap, even for years. In this phase healing scar tissue is remodeled and the vascular tissue disappears, leaving an avascular scar that strengthens over time. This tissue never regains the strength of the original healthy tissue, but it can achieve approximately 75% of its original strength within a few weeks. The best possible outcome still only achieves approximately 80% of the original strength.

Only a few tissues can regenerate by reproducing the original tissue found at the site of injury. These tissues include epithelial, hepatic, and bone marrow tissues. Most areas of the body produce tissue that is similar but not an exact duplication. The function of the tissue can vary from the original as well on the basis of many variables (Figure 8-20).

Dysfunctional Wound Healing

The healing of wounds can be altered and, as a result, dysfunctional healing can occur at any phase of the process. This is usually the result of a predisposing condition such as diabetes mellitus or an acquired condition such as hypoxia. Even the presence of many drugs in the body can be the cause of such dysfunction. The dysfunction can range from insufficient repair to excessive repair or infection. Keep in mind that continued attempts to repair a wound delay the healing process by reactivating the inflammatory process.

Dysfunction during the Inflammatory Response

One of the major concerns during the inflammatory response is continued bleeding. This can lead to many problems with wound healing. First, continued bleeding at the site of injury can produce clots that take up valuable space. In addition, these clots make granulation more difficult. Second, the clotting can create a barrier to oxygen exchange and delay the process. Furthermore, accumulating blood can provide a haven for bacteria; subsequent infection can lead to further delays in the healing process.

The accumulation of excess fibrin at the site of injury also can alter wound healing. If this fibrin is not eventually reabsorbed into the body, it can organize into adhesions, which are fibrous bands that can bind tissues and organs together inappropriately. Most adhesions are clinically insignificant unless they are located in the pleural, pericardial, or abdominal cavities. In those spaces they can cause significant dysfunction of primary organs.

Another factor that can cause dysfunction during the inflammatory response is hypovolemia. Again, this can lead to hypoperfusion, which leads to delayed healing. Poor nutrition, the development of an infection, and antiinflammatory medications can all promote dysfunction as well.

Dysfunction during the Reconstructive Phase

Of the many problems that can occur during the reconstructive phase, the most common are associated with impaired collagen synthesis, impaired epithelialization, wound disruption, and impaired contraction. The synthesis of collagen is essential for healing and can be altered by nutritional deficiencies. On the other end of the spectrum, collagen production can be excessive, leaving raised scars and leading to improper healing.

The most common causes of impaired epithelialization include the use of antiinflammatory medications, hypoxia, and ionizing radiation. *Wound disruption* is a term used to describe the pulling apart of the wound. This can occur as a result of various stresses placed on the body during healing. Impaired contraction occurs when excessive myofibroblast activity is more than normal. This can occur as a result of burns and other conditions that cause a deformity called a contracture. Several approaches can be taken to prevent dysfunctional wound

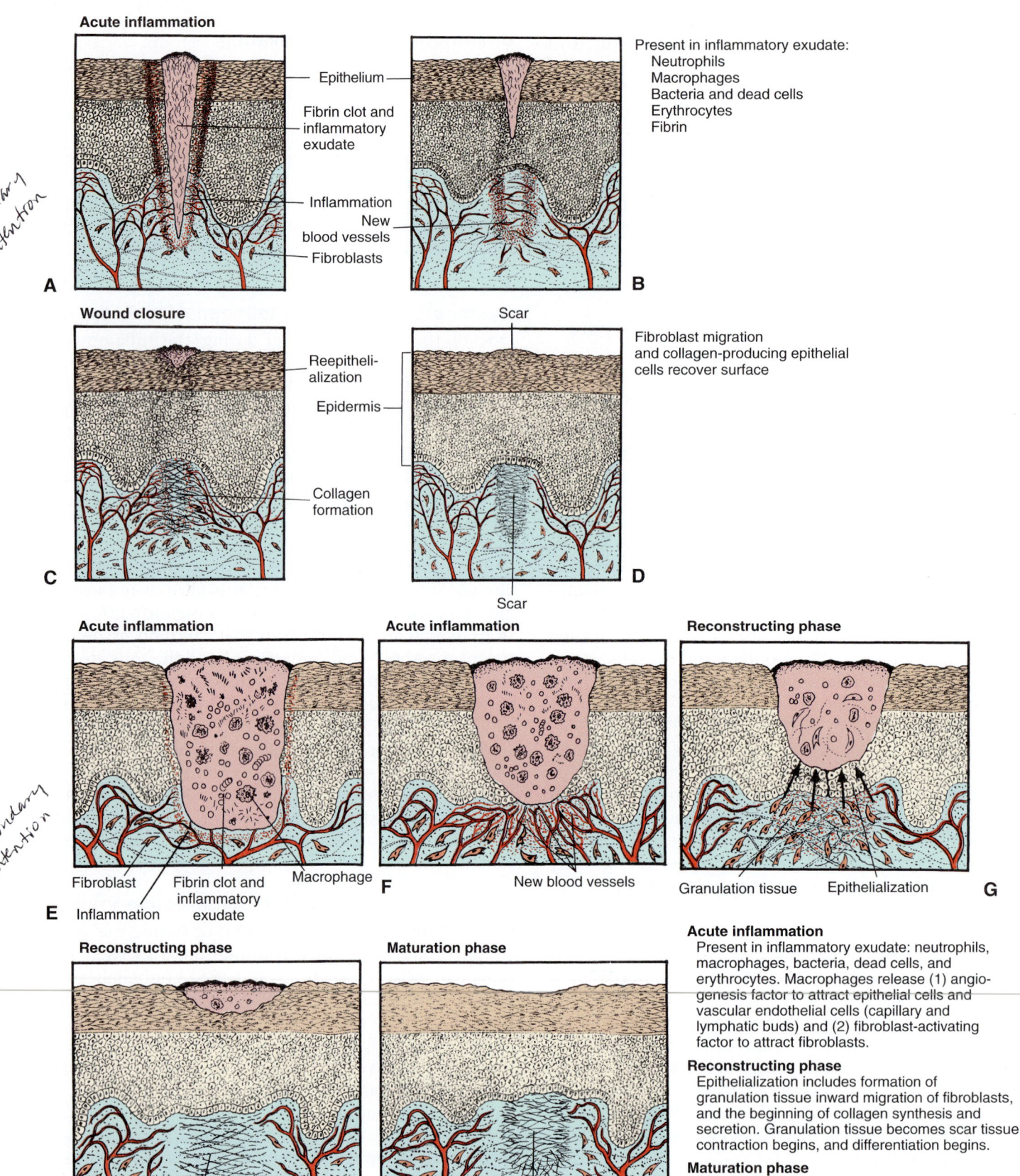

Primary Intention

Acute inflammation

— Epithelium

— Fibrin clot and inflammatory exudate

— Inflammation
New blood vessels
— Fibroblasts

A

B

Present in inflammatory exudate:
Neutrophils
Macrophages
Bacteria and dead cells
Erythrocytes
Fibrin

Wound closure

Scar

— Reepitheli-alization

Epidermis —

— Collagen formation

C

D

Scar

Fibroblast migration and collagen-producing epithelial cells recover surface

Secondary Intention

Acute inflammation

Fibroblast   Fibrin clot and inflammatory exudate   Macrophage

Inflammation

E

Acute inflammation

New blood vessels   **F**

Reconstructing phase

Granulation tissue   Epithelialization   **G**

Reconstructing phase

Collagen fibers

H

Maturation phase

Scar tissue

I

Acute inflammation
Present in inflammatory exudate: neutrophils, macrophages, bacteria, dead cells, and erythrocytes. Macrophages release (1) angiogenesis factor to attract epithelial cells and vascular endothelial cells (capillary and lymphatic buds) and (2) fibroblast-activating factor to attract fibroblasts.

Reconstructing phase
Epithelialization includes formation of granulation tissue inward migration of fibroblasts, and the beginning of collagen synthesis and secretion. Granulation tissue becomes scar tissue, contraction begins, and differentiation begins.

Maturation phase
This phase includes completion of contraction, differentiation and remodeling of scar tissue, and disappearance of capillaries from scar tissue.

Figure 8-20 Wound repair by primary or secondary intention. **A** to **D,** Healing by primary intention. **E** to **I,** Healing by secondary intention.

healing, including range-of-motion exercises, positioning, medications, and surgery.

Aging and Self-Defense Mechanisms

[OBJECTIVE 24]

Regarding the body's ability to defend and heal itself, two specific populations traditionally have difficulty. These populations are neonates and the aged. In the neonate group, this difficulty seems to be mainly a function of immature immune systems and a relative deficiency of some of the most critical factors necessary for defense. In addition, neonates appear to have a transient depression in the inflammatory response that has been linked to an altered response to chemotactic factors that can predispose the child to certain bacterial infections.

In the elderly population many factors can inhibit defense and healing. No evidence has shown that aging causes a natural degradation of the ability to heal. However, failure to heal certainly has been linked to long-term disease processes and conditions found within this population. For example, consider the patient who has long-term effects of diabetes and cardiovascular disease. The elderly population undergoes physiologic changes that predispose them to impaired healing. Changes in the skin, the reduction of the amount of subcutaneous fat, loss of surface vasculature, and decreased ability to fight off infections can all contribute to dysfunctional healing.

VARIANCES IN IMMUNITY AND INFLAMMATION

The following section addresses what occurs in the body when the immune system works too well, becomes misdirected, or does not work as expected.

Hypersensitivity, Allergy, Autoimmunity, and Alloimmunity

[OBJECTIVE 25]

A **hypersensitivity reaction** is an immune response that is excessive and beyond the bounds of normalcy. This type of reaction typically does not occur at the time of first exposure. For this reaction to occur, the host must first be exposed to the pathogen and sensitized, or have an immunologic response. The second time the host is exposed, the hypersensitivity reaction occurs. It develops as a result of an exaggerated inflammatory response and can become life threatening. One common example of this type of reaction is the allergy to bee or wasp stings. Once a person is stung, a systemic chain of events begins that leads to vascular changes and constriction of the airway that, when left untreated, can lead to death. Hypersensitivity is categorized into the following three

subdivisions on the basis of the type of antigen against which the reaction is directed:

- *Allergy:* hypersensitivity to an environmental antigen such as venoms and pollens.
- *Autoimmunity:* the failure of the body to recognize its own tissues as self, resulting in an attack by the immune system. The body can, even in healthy hosts, produce antibodies to self-antigens. This may be considered normal at low levels. *[lupus rheum. arth.]*
- *Alloimmunity:* a condition in which the host acquires immunity against itself from the tissue of a member of the same species. It can occur in response to organ transplants, blood transfusions, or the fetus during pregnancy.

The exact mechanisms that initiate a hypersensitivity reaction are not well understood. However, the concept that it may be a result of genetic and/or environmental factors individually or together is generally accepted. Most disease states that occur as a result of hypersensitivity can be linked to one or more of the following variables:

- The initial insult that disturbs or alters the body's tolerance to self-antigens
- The individual's genetic makeup, which can determine susceptibility to specific antigens
- An immunologic process that can amplify or exaggerate the insult

Targets of Hypersensitivity

Hypersensitivity is an exaggerated response to an allergen. The targets of hypersensitivity responses are based on the type of allergen encountered. These allergens come from the environment, the host, or another person's antigens.

Allergy

[from outside]

Allergens are environmental in nature and can cause a hypersensitivity reaction. They include pollens, molds, and fungi; foods such as peanuts, milk, and shellfish; animal sources such as dander; and cigarette smoke and dust. Some allergens are so large that the phagocytes cannot destroy them, or they are surrounded by a protective nonallergenic coat. Thus the allergen is not released until the coating is broken down by enzymes.

In certain situations an allergen can bind with the components of host tissue. This action forms a new antigen known as a neoantigen. The new antigen is seen as a foreign substance by the body, and the tissue is attacked and destroyed. In people who are predisposed to hypersensitivity reactions from penicillin, a metabolite binds to tissue and creates a neoantigen. The body then attacks the tissue, in this case red blood cells, which are then destroyed, potentially leading to anemia.

Mechanisms of Hypersensitivity

The mechanisms of hypersensitivity can be categorized by the substances that initiate the inflammation and the damage to healthy tissue that follows. Four distinct categories exist: type I, or IgE-mediated allergic reactions; type II, or tissue-specific reactions; type III, or immune complex–mediated reactions; and type IV, or cell-mediated reactions. Even though this system of classification may seem straightforward, hypersensitivity reactions often are mixed.

Hypersensitivity reactions also are classified as either immediate or delayed on the basis of the time necessary for the reaction to cause a secondary immune response. Immediate hypersensitivity reactions manifest in a matter of minutes, whereas delayed hypersensitivity reactions may take hours.

Immunoglobulin E–Mediated Allergic Reactions

Immunoglobulin E–mediated allergic reactions are associated with the production of antigen-specific IgE after exposure to the antigen. This is the most common reaction in response to an environmental antigen. The IgE antibodies are produced by B lymphocytes, which then bind to receptors on the plasma membrane of mast cells. If the exposure is repeated and the dose of allergen is significant enough in quantity, the IgE antibodies cause a degranulation of the mast cells, releasing histamine into the body.

Histamine is the most important mediator of the IgE-mediated hypersensitivity reaction. Two specific receptor sites react to histamine. H_1 receptor sites respond to histamine by constricting the smooth muscle around bronchioles, increasing capillary permeability, and causing vasodilation, which begins the inflammatory process. On the other hand, H_2 receptor sites mediate this type of response by increasing gastric secretions and inhibiting the release of histamine by mast cells. In this way the body tries to maintain control of the histamine response. This also explains why certain medications used in the treatment of a hypersensitivity response are so effective.

The ways in which an IgE-mediated hypersensitivity reaction manifests in the body are largely a result of the histamine release and its effects. The distribution of the reactive receptors and target tissues is wide and includes the GI tract, skin, and respiratory system. In the GI tract the reaction traditionally is stimulated by an allergen that has entered through the mouth. Foods are one example. GI signs and symptoms include vomiting, diarrhea, and abdominal pain. The skin can show signs of a hypersensitivity reaction with the development of urticaria (hives). These are caused by isolated areas of edema. They appear as white, fluid-filled blisters surrounded by an area of redness. Urticaria is commonly associated with skin itching. The respiratory system begins to manifest bron-

chiole constriction. In addition, an increase in mucus production and subsequent edema can cause a wide range of reactions, such as mild respiratory distress to extreme respiratory compromise, depending on the severity of the reaction. Many other systems may show evidence of the reaction, including the cardiovascular system. The signs and symptoms may include an increase in heart rate and, as previously described, vasodilation (Figure 8-21).

Some populations are more prone to allergies than others. These people are known as *atopic individuals*. This predisposition to allergic reactions results from the production of a larger amount of IgE in response to an allergen. The origin for this appears to be genetic. It also appears to be a heritable trait. In families with one parent who has an allergy, approximately 40% of the children will develop an allergy. This number doubles to 80% in families in which both parents are involved.

Because allergic reactions can progress to anaphylaxis, a life-threatening condition, individuals who have these allergies must be aware of the specific allergen to which

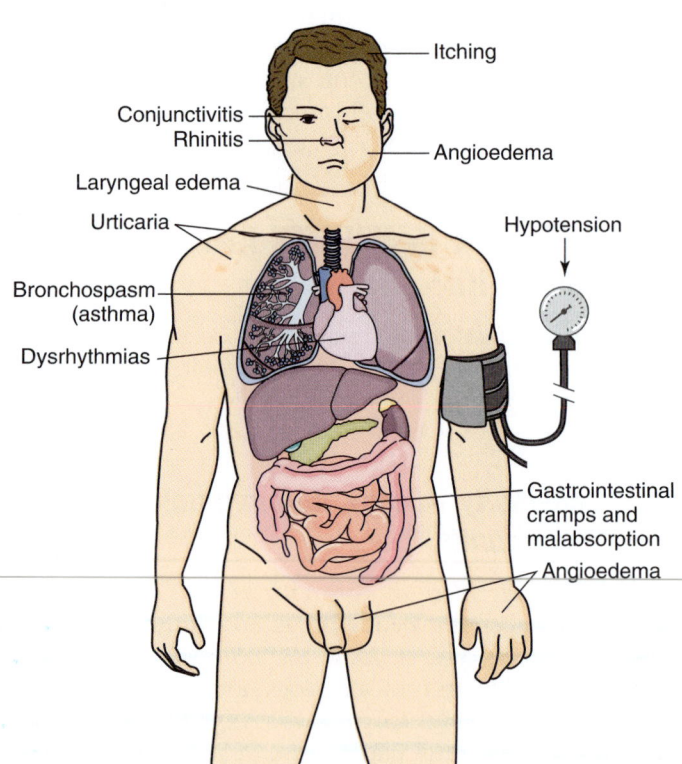

Figure 8-21 Type I hypersensitivity reactions. Manifestations of allergic reactions as a result of type I hypersensitivity include itching, angioedema (swelling caused by exudation), edema of the larynx, urticaria (hives), bronchospasm (constriction of the airways in the lungs), hypotension (low blood pressure), dysrhythmias (irregular heartbeat) from anaphylactic shock, and gastrointestinal (GI) cramping caused by inflammation of the GI mucosa.

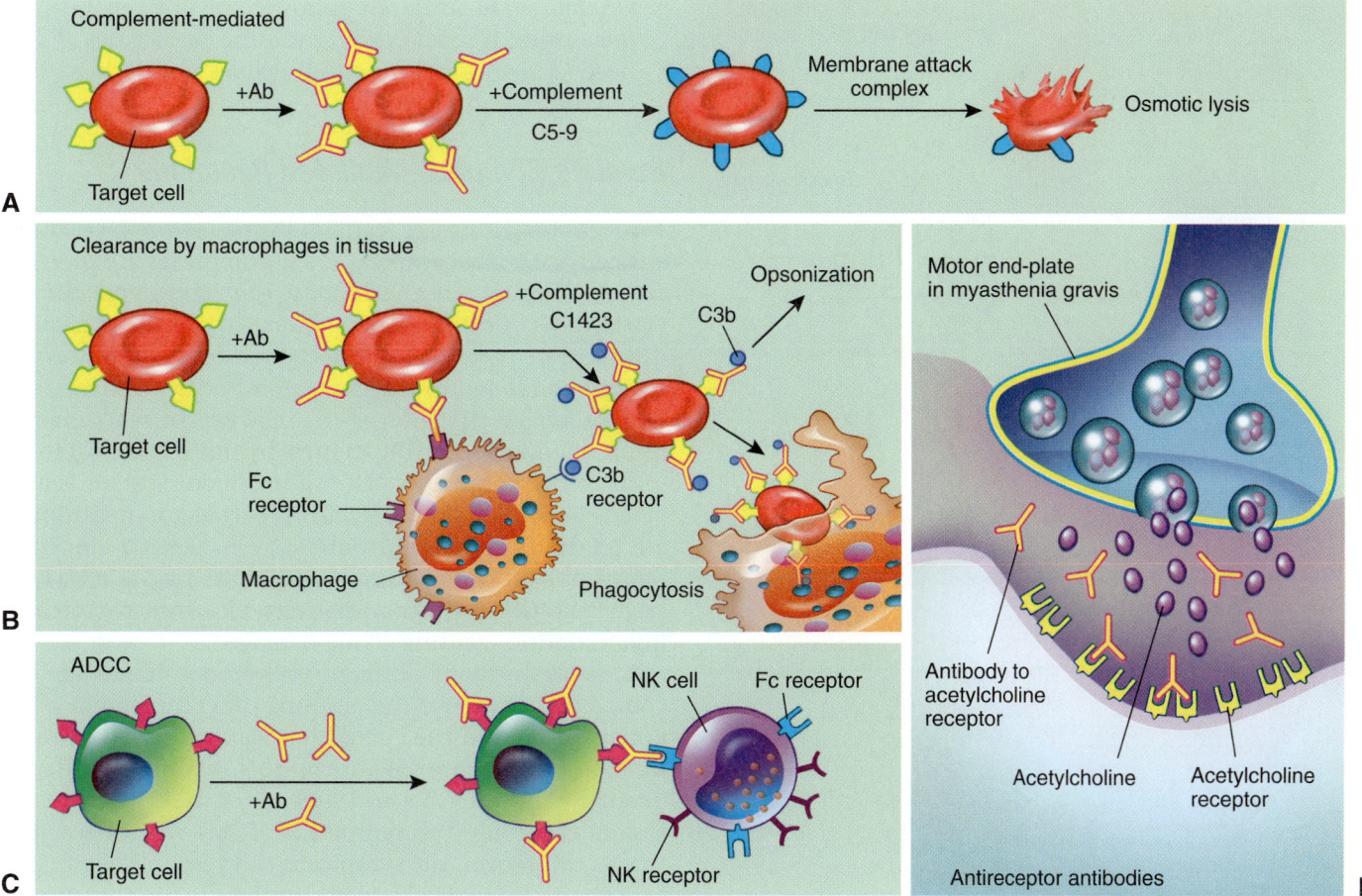

Figure 8-22 Mechanism of type II, or tissue-specific, reactions. **A,** Antigens in the target cell bind with antibodies and are destroyed or prevented from functioning by complement-mediated lysis. **B,** Clearance by macrophages in tissue. **C,** Antibody-dependent cell-mediated cytotoxicity *(ADCC).* IgG-coated target cells are lysed by cells that have Fc receptors for IgG (e.g., natural killer cells, macrophages). **D,** Antireceptor antibodies modulate or block the normal function of receptors. This example shows myasthenia gravis, in which acetylcholine receptor antibodies block acetylcholine from attachment to its receptors on the motor end plates of skeletal muscle, impairing neuromuscular transmission and causing muscle weakness.

they are sensitized and attempt to avoid the substance. Several options exist for testing sensitivity to a specific allergen. In addition, once the allergen has been identified, treatment options aimed specifically at desensitizing the patient may be available. Desensitization has met with some success. It is accomplished by exposing the patient to increasing doses of the allergen over a long period.

Tissue-Specific Reactions

Most cells in the body have tissue-specific antigens in addition to the HLA antigens that define it as a self-antigen. For example, platelets express an antigen specific to platelets and no other cells. In this type of hypersensitivity reaction, only the cells presenting a specific antigen are affected (Figure 8-22). The distribution of these cells determines the extent of the reaction. This type of reaction can alter or damage target cells by the following four mechanisms:

- *The complement system.* An antibody binds to the antigen on the cell's plasma membrane, subsequently activating the complement system, which causes the plasma membrane to dissolve.
- *Phagocytosis.* The target cell becomes a preferential target by macrophages because of interaction with the tissue-specific antigen.
- *Cytotoxins.* The antibody binds to the antigen, which then binds to cytotoxic cells and destroys the target cells.

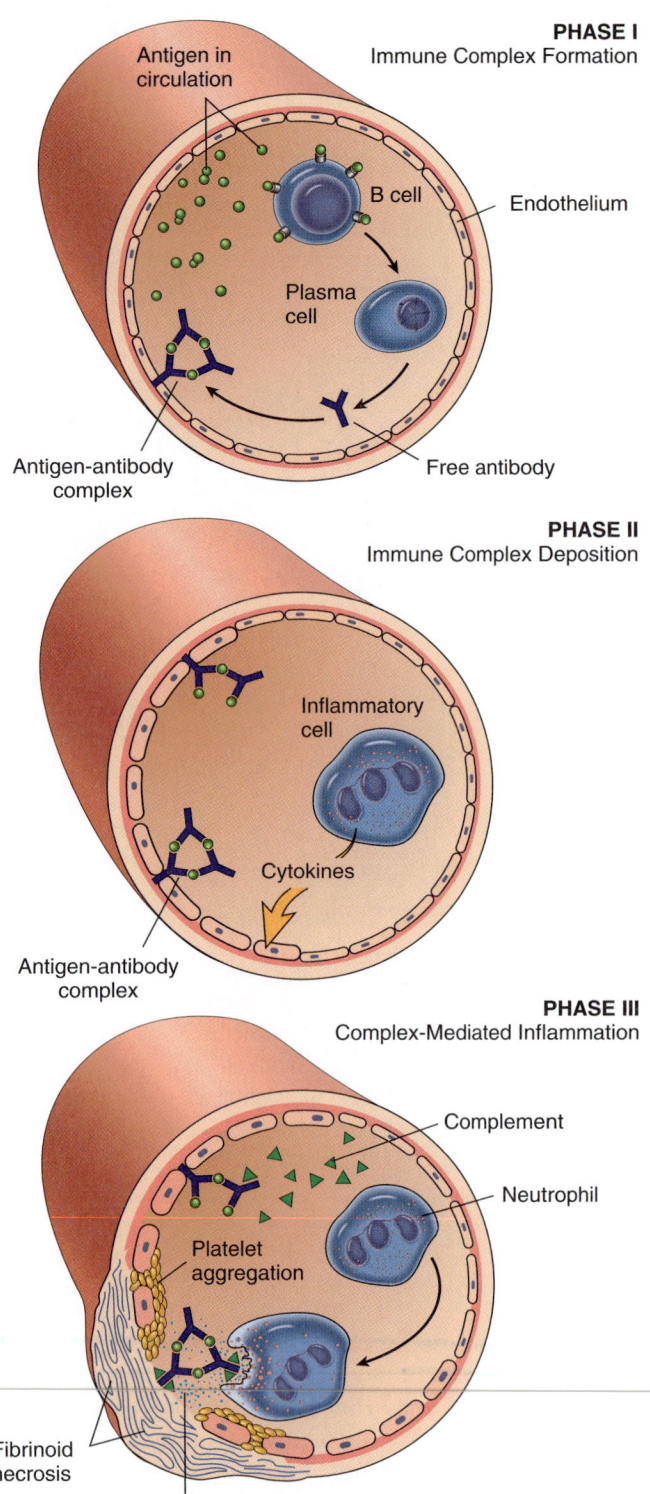

PHASE I
Immune Complex Formation

Antigen in circulation

B cell

Endothelium

Plasma cell

Antigen-antibody complex

Free antibody

PHASE II
Immune Complex Deposition

Inflammatory cell

Cytokines

Antigen-antibody complex

PHASE III
Complex-Mediated Inflammation

Complement

Neutrophil

Platelet aggregation

Fibrinoid necrosis

Neutrophil lysosomal enzymes

Figure 8-23 Mechanism of type III, or immune complex–mediated, reactions. Three sequential phases include phase I with immune complex formation, phase II immune complex deposition, and phase III activation of the complement cascade and generation of complement fragments, including C5a. C5a is a chemotactic for neutrophils, which migrate into the inflamed area and attach to IgG and C3b in the immune complexes. The neutrophils degranulate a variety of degrading enzymes that destroy healthy tissues.

- *Disabling.* The antibody binds to the antigen, preventing it from binding to other molecules needed for normal function. It does not destroy the cell, but incapacitates it.

Immune Complex–Mediated Reactions

Type III reactions are caused by the formation of an antigen-antibody complex. These complexes are then circulated throughout the bloodstream and deposited on vessel walls or other tissue. Because of this unpredictable distribution pattern, the effects of these complexes are seldom correlated to the entry point of the antigen. The tissue damage that occurs in this type of reaction is a result of an unsuccessful attempt by the neutrophil to rid itself of the complexes. The complement system is activated, and chemotactic factors specific for neutrophils are released. These neutrophils try to destroy the complexes but do not succeed. This results in the release of large quantities of lysosomal enzymes into the area of inflammation, causing tissue damage.

Because antibody-antigen complexes can activate the complement system, the amounts of complement components found in the circulation vary at any given time. In addition, the ratio of antigen to antibody, quality and quantity, and the class and subclass of the antigen in the system can cause the symptoms of this type of reaction to vary. Moreover, the symptoms can vary in severity and can change drastically over the course of the disease process (Figure 8-23).

Immune complex disease processes can be localized or systemic. An example of a systemic disease is serum sickness. In this process, blood vessels, joints, and kidneys are generally affected. Serum sickness was first seen with the administration of foreign serum into a host, such as when the horse tetanus toxin was used. Today foreign serum is rarely used in the clinical setting. However, the disease process is still seen on repeated administration of other antigens present in some medications. The clinical manifestations of serum sickness may include swollen lymph nodes, fever, rash, and pain at the site of inflammation. One form of serum sickness is called *Raynaud's phenomenon.* This condition is caused by the precipitation of temperature-dependant immune complexes in the capillary beds of the peripheral circulation. It manifests as localized pallor and numbness followed by cyanosis (McCance & Huether, 2002).

An example of a localized immune complex–mediated reaction is an Arthus reaction, which is caused by repeated exposure to an environmental antigen. This antigen can enter the body through ingestion, injection, or inhalation. The symptoms typically begin within the first hour of exposure. Signs and symptoms usually peak within 6 to 12 hours and include inflammation, increased vascular permeability, and accumulation of neutrophils, edema, hemorrhage, clotting, and tissue damage. These are commonly seen in the skin after inoculations, in the GI tract after the ingestion of wheat products, or in the respira-

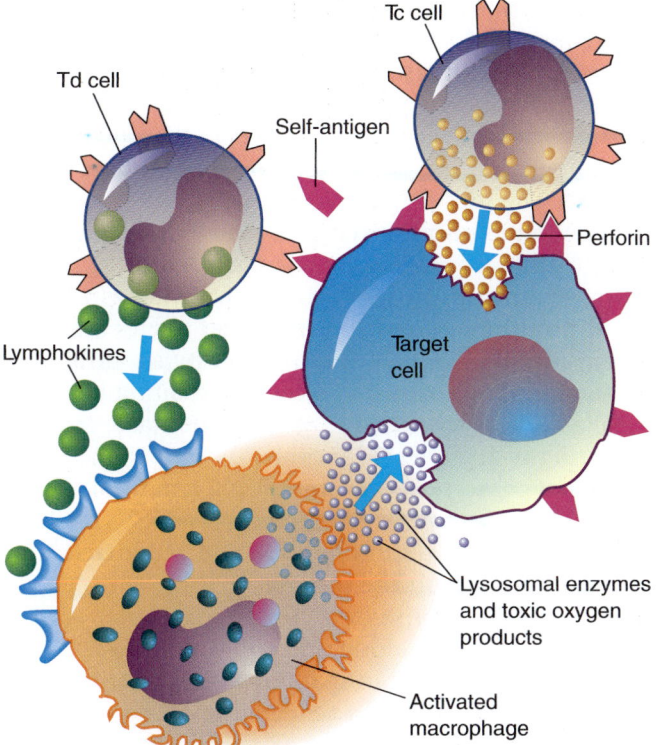

Figure 8-24 Mechanism of type IV, or cell-mediated, reactions. Self-antigens from target cells stimulate T cells to differentiate into cytotoxic T cells, which have direct cytotoxic activity, and T cells involved in delayed hypersensitivity. Delayed hypersensitivity cells, a form of T helper cells, produce lymphokines, some of which attract and activate macrophages. The macrophages and enzymes released by them are responsible for most of the tissue destruction.

tory system after inhalation of moldy hay or pigeon feces.

Cell-Mediated Tissue Reactions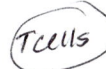

Cell-mediated tissue reactions differ from the previously described reactions in that they do not occur as a result of antibody actions. This type of reaction is mediated directly by T lymphocytes that have been specifically sensitized. The damage that follows the beginning of this reaction occurs in one of two ways. The first pathway is that of cytotoxic T lymphocytes. They can attack and destroy cellular targets directly. The second pathway is that of transfer delayed hypersensitivity cells, which produce lymphokines that attract phagocytic cells such as macrophages (Figure 8-24).

Classic examples of this type of reaction include the rejection of grafts and allergies such as poison ivy. This type of reaction also is used as a diagnostic tool in clinical medicine. In fact, this reaction creates a positive tuberculosis skin test. Cell-mediated reactions also have been linked to autoimmune disease processes

such as rheumatoid arthritis and insulin-dependent diabetes.

Autoimmunity

The newborn develops a tolerance to antigens marked as self-antigens. The loss or breakdown of this tolerance to self-antigens, in which the body begins to see these self-antigens as foreign, is known as *autoimmunity*. In this situation the body begins to attack and destroy essential cells and tissues. Autoimmune diseases are typically seen in females. The mechanisms that cause this condition are mainly unknown in most disease states. In a few of these, however, the mechanism has been identified as one of the following:

- *A previously sequestered antigen exposed to the body.* During the development of the fetus, antigens are exposed to the fetal immune system to be tolerated after birth. Some antigens are never exposed to the immune system, because they exist in parts of the body that are separated from the immune system, because they are not drained by the lymphatic system. Examples of this include the cornea of the eye and the testicles. These are called *immunologically privileged sites.* If they are never exposed, they cannot become a tolerated antigen. In situations such as trauma, these antigens can be introduced into the system and cause an extreme reaction.
- *Development of a neoantigen.* As previously described, this is a situation in which a new antigen is formed when an antigen binds to host tissue. This neoantigen is seen as a foreign substance and subsequently is attacked by the immune system, damaging healthy tissue.
- *Complications of infectious diseases.* Certain infectious diseases can cause a hypersensitivity reaction, usually by one of two mechanisms. First, the microorganisms can create an immune complex that will precipitate in the tissues of the host. This is seen in the kidneys, where these complexes can deposit and cause an inflammatory response leading to tissue damage and complications such as glomerulonephritis. The second mechanism by which this can occur is when the foreign antigen alters the self-antigens in the body such that it confuses the immune system and normal tissues become seen as foreign, again leading to damage. As previously discussed, an example of this is the insertion of viral spikes into a cell's membrane during the viral replication process.
- *Forbidden clone.* During the development of the fetus, the maturing lymphocytes are exposed to self-antigens. In this theory, if a lymphocyte becomes reactive to a self-antigen, its clones are prevented from maturing. The autoimmune response occurs as a result of survival of one of the clones that triggers the event. This theory is under investigation and

currently has not been linked to a specific disease process.

- *Suppressor cell dysfunction.* T suppressor cells are theorized to be responsible for suppressing autoimmune responses. If the T suppressor cells are not functioning properly, they can form clones that initiate an autoimmune response.

Some of the immune diseases are caused by predictable mechanisms, such as medications. Others are caused by recent viral infections, such as rubella, leading to autoimmune encephalitis. Many other autoimmune disease processes are impossible to link to a cause. These are theorized to have been caused by a past infection that can no longer be traced in the system of the host.

Autoimmune diseases that have a genetic cause are easier to find than those caused by a pathologic agent, because most of these processes tend to run in families. The disease process may vary among affected members of the family, but they all are likely to have hypersensitivity responses.

Alloimmunity

Alloimmunity hypersensitivity reactions are caused by one individual's immune response to the antigens of another individual. The two most often seen are mothers who have a reaction to the Rh antigens of the fetus and the immune system's response to grafted or transplanted tissues, including blood transfusion reactions.

Autoimmune and Isoimmune Diseases

Autoimmune and isoimmune disorders can affect many different parts of the body. The nervous, muscular, endocrine, and GI systems are common sites. The following disease processes are some of the more commonly identified disorders:

- *Graves' disease* is characterized by nervousness, rapid heart rate, increased appetite, increased blood pressure, and weight loss. Occasionally other signs such as bulging eyes and lumpy, reddish thickening of the skin over the shins, known as *pretibial myxedema,* can occur. The cause of this condition has been theorized to be an antibody that triggers a release of excessive amounts of thyroid hormone. This hyperthyroidism also has been linked to the formation of an enlarged thyroid gland, called *goiter.* It is found in women more often than in men, as is the case with most autoimmune diseases. Moreover, it can potentially be transmitted to a fetus.
- *Rheumatoid arthritis* is a chronic condition that causes an inflammation in the joints of the body. This condition eventually causes joint destruction and loss of function, but patients may have periods without symptoms. The exact cause is unknown, but it is considered an autoimmune disorder and is theorized to be caused by an antibody reaction in the collagen of the joints.
- *Myasthenia gravis* is a condition that affects the neuromuscular junction of skeletal and cardiac muscle. The presynaptic neuron releases acetylcholine into the synapse, which finds a receptor site on the motor end plate, causing impulse transmission into the target tissues. In this condition the receptors on the target tissues are desensitized to the neurotransmitter by an antibody to the self-antigen on the receptor, resulting in weakness. It is theorized that this is heritable to offspring of the affected mother.
- *Immune thrombocytopenic purpura* is a condition that results in a decrease of circulating platelets. This is theorized to be a result of antibodies that attack the self-antigens on the platelets, resulting in a phagocytic response from mononuclear macrophages. This, along with a decrease in platelet production, can manifest signs and symptoms that include a tendency to bleed, easy bruising called purpura, and extravasation of blood from the capillaries into the skin, which appears as petechiae.
- *Isoimmune neutropenia* is a condition in which the body develops antibodies to the host's neutrophils. This results in a predisposition to infection by bacteria found in the mouth and GI tract. These antibodies can pass from mother to fetus, thereby destroying the neutrophils of the fetus. Most cases of this condition do not require treatment. Moreover, most appear with little in the way of physical signs and symptoms. Severe cases and those with severe infections can usually be treated with medication.
- *Systemic lupus erythematosus* is one of the most complex, common, and potentially destructive of the autoimmune diseases. Because it affects multiple organ systems and can present with a wide variety of signs and symptoms, diagnosis is quite difficult. It is characterized by a large production of antibodies to nucleic acids, erythrocytes, proteins involved in coagulation, phospholipids, lymphocytes, platelets, and many other tissues. It is more commonly seen in women. The signs and symptoms usually manifest by ages 20 to 40 years. The symptoms are usually episodic in nature and include arthritis, vasculitis and rash, renal problems, hematologic conditions such as anemia, and cardiovascular disease. It has been shown to cause congenital heart problems in the offspring of affected mothers.
- *Rh and ABO alloimmunization,* as previously described, is a condition in which the mother and fetus have differing antigens on their blood cells. It stimulates the production of antibodies that can be damaging to both mother and fetus.

Immunity and Inflammation Deficiencies

[OBJECTIVE 26]

Disorders that occur from a deficiency in immunity or inflammation are caused by impaired function in one of the components of the immune system or the inflammatory process. This deficiency can involve B cells, T cells, phagocytic cells, or complement components. These conditions are considered primary (congenital) or secondary (acquired).

Congenital Immune Deficiencies

Primary immune deficiencies are caused by a change or cessation of the development of lymphocytes in the fetus. They can occur at any stage in the development or maturation of the stem cells that differentiate into B cells or T cells. The point at which this happens to a certain degree establishes which type of disorder exists. For example, if the change occurs in the stem cells, it could affect one or both of the lymphocyte lines. If both lines are affected, it interferes with both humoral and cell-mediated immunity. Patients with this type of disorder are said to have severe combined immune deficiencies.

Congenital deficiencies include DiGeorge syndrome, Bruton agammaglobulinemia, bare lymphocyte syndrome, and chronic mucocutaneous candidiasis. Depending on which condition the patient has, the effect on the body is a change in the number of either B or T lymphocytes, which can lead to fatal infections in children and the inability to respond to a specific antigen (McCance & Huether, 2002).

Acquired Deficiencies

Secondary immune deficiencies develop after birth and are not linked to a genetic cause. Many different conditions can lead to a secondary deficiency, including pregnancy, infections, malnutrition, diabetes, and medications. The most prominent deficiency of interest in the last 25 years is acquired immunodeficiency syndrome (AIDS). Most acquired deficiencies can be placed into one of the following categories:

- *Nutritional deficiencies.* The nutritional state of the host is important in the immune system's ability to function. Patients who have critical nutritional deficits, as in starvation, have a decreased number of T cells. Moreover, the T cells they do have do not function normally. Patients deficient in zinc have altered function in both T and B cells.
- *Iatrogenic deficiencies.* These types of deficiencies are a result of medical treatment. Certain medications, such as chemotherapeutic agents, can suppress blood cell formation in the bone marrow. Others can cause the destruction of granulocytes by initiating an immunologic response. The medications that can

induce this response include analgesics, antithyroids, anticonvulsants, antihistamines, antimicrobials, and tranquilizers. Patients who receive radiation therapy along with chemotherapeutic medications are at a higher risk. In recent decades the immunosuppressive medications given to transplant recipients or those receiving cancer treatments have been identified as suppressing the function of both B cells and T cells. This lowers the defense capability of the body. In addition, patients who have received anesthesia for surgery have a reduction in the efficacy of both T and B cells. Specific surgeries, such as a splenectomy, can result in a decreased ability to defend against encapsulated bacteria because of a suppression of the humoral response.

- *Deficiencies caused by trauma.* The classic example of this type of deficiency is the severely burned patient. This patient has several challenges. First, the body's first line of defense, the skin, is destroyed. This allows foreign invaders access to the body. In addition, thermal burns have been linked to a decrease in neutrophil function, decreased complement function, a decrease in cell-mediated immunity, and a decreased primary humoral response. All this occurs in the face of an increase in immunosuppressive function because of the sera developed by burn patients.
- *Deficiencies caused by stress.* The conclusion that stress or emotional disturbance can increase the incidence of illness and depress immune function has been, until recently, empirical at best. Research into this theory is ongoing. In fact, several researchers have come to the conclusion that intense stress, such as the death of a loved one, divorce, or long periods of ongoing stress can cause an increased level of corticosteroids in the circulation. These increased levels can contribute to suppressed immune function. More research is needed to define the conditions in which this and other factors can contribute to immunosuppression.
- *AIDS.* This is the most well known of the acquired immune dysfunctions. With improved treatment options since the mid-1990s, AIDS is not necessarily the same death sentence that it was before that time. The number of deaths from this syndrome has been dramatically reduced in the United States, but in other parts of the world, such as sub-Saharan Africa, the disease is rapidly spreading. Furthermore, the successful treatments used in the United States are not widely available.

AIDS is caused by a retrovirus known as *human immunodeficiency virus* (HIV). This virus carries genetic material in RNA rather than DNA. Retroviruses infect a target cell by binding to receptors on the cell wall and injecting its RNA to the interior of the cell. Through a viral enzyme, this genetic material becomes part of the genetic code of the host cell. If the cell is activated, it can proliferate, spreading the infection in the host and destroying cells. This can cause a profound suppression of the immune system, predisposing the host to infections from many sources. Many studies are ongoing into the spread and treatment of this syndrome. One of the greatest fears among those involved is that because the current treatments do not kill the virus but merely suppress its spread, the virus will develop into a strain resistant to current therapies. This has been seen to some degree. Certain patients undergoing therapy suddenly stop responding to treatment, requiring a change in their cocktail of multiple medications.

Replacement Therapies for Immune Deficiencies

The following therapies have been devised to address immune deficiencies:

- *Gamma-globulin therapy*. This therapy has been successful in treating patients with B-cell deficiencies, such as hypogammaglobulinemia and agammaglobulinemia.
- *Transplantation and transfusion*. As previously described, patients with severe combined immune deficiencies have a lack of stem cells to create B and T cells. Certain patients who have the disorder because of a lack of thymus function or enzyme deficiencies can be treated with transplanted tissue or blood transfusions to replace the missing factors. This has proven effective in certain patients.
- *Gene therapy*. The replacement of defective genes with cloned versions in the laboratory has been proven to be effective. These clones are placed in a viral vector that is then inserted into the body. The retrovirus used is harmless to the host, and the clones proliferate and have shown, in limited cases, to restore immune function. This type of therapy is in its infancy. Thus much more research is needed to develop the process.

STRESS AND DISEASE

[OBJECTIVE 27]

The concept of stress is not new for most of the world today. Most people have experienced a stressful situation or period in their lives. During this time, they probably were well aware of the physiologic and psychological effects of stress on the mind and the body. Although these are separate responses, they are undeniably linked.

Concepts of Stress

The link of mind and body has not always been understood or even, quite frankly, believed to exist. Not until the 1940s did a physician named Hans Selye discover the cause and effect of stress and disease. In fact, it was an incidental finding in his quest to discover a new sex hormone.

General Adaptation Syndrome

Selye's experiments involved injecting crude ovarian extracts into rats. As with any valid experiment, the results must be repeatable to be considered valid. The results of his study consistently produced a triad of structural changes in the bodies of his subjects: (1) enlargement of the cortex of the adrenal gland, (2) atrophy of the thyroid gland and other lymphoid structures, and (3) the development of bleeding ulcers of the stomach and duodenal lining.

After he began exposing the rats to other noxious stimuli, such as cold, surgical injury, and so forth, he achieved the same results. He discovered that his findings were attributable to the stressors placed on the subjects and not specifically to the agent he was using. He termed this triad the general adaptation syndrome (GAS) and later refined his theory to include the following three successive stages:

- *The alarm stage* is the initial stage of the GAS process. It manifests as a sympathetic response (increased heart rate, blood pressure, and respirations).
- *The resistance or adaptation stage* initially contributes the sympathetic response, but the body eventually returns to homeostasis as the stress hormones return to normal and the body adapts to the changes. In most situations this will be the last stage of the process unless the situation is not resolved or the stressor is not removed.
- *The exhaustion stage* occurs when the stressor continues. At this point the person can no longer cope or resolve the situation and stops trying. At this point the immune system is compromised and illness can occur.

Selye further explained that "physiologic stress is a chemical or physical disturbance in the cells or tissue fluid produced by a change, either in the external environment or within the body itself, that requires a response to counteract the disturbance" (McCance & Huether, 2002). He identified three components of physiologic stress: (1) the exogenous or endogenous stressor that initiates the disturbance, (2) the chemical or physical disturbance produced by the stressor, and (3) the body's counteracting response to the disturbance.

Psychologic Mediators and Specificity

The work by Selye in the 1940s undoubtedly was pioneering. Others who followed him used his conclusions as the basis to continue the study of stressors and the psychologic and physiologic responses. This research, which continues today, has further elucidated the mind/body link and determined that stress, as a strictly physiologic response, is a rather narrow view. In the 1950s researchers discovered that the adrenal cortex in human beings could be activated in response to a psychological stressor. Furthermore, in the 1960s researchers discovered that an individual's plasma cortisol levels increased with exposure to films about war and decreased with exposure to Disney nature films.

Other researchers challenged Selye's views that stress causes a general or nonspecific response. They later proved that the physiologic response to stress was strongly linked to the psychological state of the subject. This was seen in studies that showed large increases in sensitivity of the pituitary gland and adrenal cortex to emotional, psychological, and social influences. Furthermore, in situations in which psychological triggers were minimized, physical stressors did not appear to induce a response from either the pituitary or adrenal cortex in a nonspecific way. In other experiments the body was exposed to physical stresses (e.g., heat), and it showed a reduction in adrenocortical hormone levels because of the care taken to avoid discomfort in the subjects.

Homeostasis as a Dynamic Steady State

Homeostasis is the body's ability to maintain a fairly constant internal environment. The body is in a constant state of change; however, it maintains what is known as a *dynamic steady state.* This means that even though reactions constantly occur—and the levels of various chemicals, electrolytes, gases, and so forth change from one moment to the next—the net effect is relatively consistent levels. This constant state of flux is named *turnover.* Stress on the body can alter this dynamic steady state, and if the alteration is chronic it is considered a sign of disease.

STRESS RESPONSE

[OBJECTIVE 28]

Psychoneuroimmunologic regulation is the theory that all immune-related diseases are a result of the interaction of multiple systems in the body. These interactions or interrelations include the nervous system (both psychologically and physiologically), the endocrine and immune systems, and behavioral factors.

The stress response is physiologically initiated in the body by the release of corticotropin-releasing factor (CRF) from the hypothalamus, which then activates the sympathetic nervous system, the pituitary gland, and the adrenal gland. All the physiologic responses previously described must first be triggered by a psychological response to a stressor transmitted to the central nervous system. This activation of neuroendocrine responses then affects the immune system.

Neuroendocrine Regulation

Neuroendocrine regulation of the stress response involves many factors. First, as described, it involves the release of CRF from the hypothalamus, which then stimulates the release of catecholamines, cortisol, and other hormones that can affect the immune system.

Catecholamines

After stimulation from the stress response, the sympathetic nervous system sends signals to the adrenal medulla to release catecholamines (epinephrine, norepinephrine, and dopamine) into the circulation. The majority of the hormones, approximately 80%, released by the adrenal medulla are epinephrine, and the balance, or approximately 20%, is norepinephrine. When these catecholamines reach their targets, they mimic the effects of sympathetic stimulation.

Norepinephrine raises blood pressure by constricting peripheral vasculature, inhibits GI activity, and dilates the pupils of the eye. Epinephrine has similar effects to those of norepinephrine. However, it also has a stronger effect on cardiac function and is primarily responsible for metabolic rate. Catecholamines are able to create change through the stimulation of specific receptor sites on the various organs of the body. These receptors are of two classes: alpha-adrenergic and beta-adrenergic receptors.

The alpha-adrenergic receptors are further subdivided into alpha$_1$ and alpha$_2$ receptors. Alpha$_1$ receptor sites, once stimulated, cause smooth muscle to constrict, resulting in the constriction of blood vessels, mild bronchoconstriction, and increased glycogenolysis. Stimulation of the alpha$_2$ receptor sites results in the relaxation of smooth muscle because it has an inhibitory effect. They turn off the release of norepinephrine once a certain concentration is achieved. The beta-adrenergic receptors also are subdivided into beta$_1$ and beta$_2$ receptors. Beta$_1$ receptor sites are responsible for an increase in heart rate, cardiac contractile force, and automaticity once stimulated. Beta$_2$ receptors cause bronchodilation and, to a certain degree, vasodilation. The physiologic effects of catecholamines are listed in Table 8-3.

Cortisol

During periods of stress, the activation of the neuroendocrine mechanisms and the release of CRF also stimulate the release of adrenocorticotropic hormone (ACTH) from the anterior pituitary gland. ACTH is responsible for stimulating the adrenal cortex to release glucocorticoid hormones, primarily cortisol. Once released, it enters the circulation and either binds to transcortin, the main plasma-binding protein, forming a protein complex, or remains free and active, playing a role in gathering substance for cellular metabolism.

TABLE 8-3 Physiologic Effects of Catecholamines

Organ	Effect
Brain	Increased blood flow Increased glucose metabolism
Cardiovascular system	Increased rate and force of contractions Peripheral vasoconstriction
Pulmonary system	Increased oxygen supply Bronchodilation Increased ventilation
Skin	Decreased blood flow
Muscle	Increased glycogenolysis Increased contraction Increased dilation of skeletal muscle vessels
Liver	Increased glucose production Increased gluconeogenesis Increased glycogenolysis Decreased glycogen synthesis
Adipose tissue	Increased lipolysis Increased fatty acids and glycerol
Skeleton	Decreased glucose uptake and utilization (insulin release decreased)
Gastrointestinal and genitourinary tracts	Decreased protein synthesis
Lymphoid tissue	Increased protein breakdown (lymphoid tissue shrinks)

Cortisol has many functions, primarily stimulation of gluconeogenesis, the creation of glycogen from sources such as amino acids or free fatty acids in the liver. It also enhances the elevation of blood glucose levels promoted by other hormones and inhibits the uptake and oxidation of glucose by some of the cells in the body. This further contributes to higher blood glucose levels.

Protein metabolism is increased with the release of cortisol because it increases the rate of synthesis of proteins and RNA in the liver while increasing catabolism of proteins in muscle, lymphoid tissue, adipose tissue, skin, and bones. The overall net of protein metabolism and catabolism produces a net increase in the level of circulating amino acids. Cortisol promotes the uptake of these amino acids in the liver, where they are converted to even more glucose.

High levels of cortisol in the body have proven to suppress the immune system by suppressing the synthesis of proteins and primarily immunoglobulins or antibodies.

Cortisol also can have an effect on the number of eosinophils, lymphocytes, and macrophages. In addition, it can promote atrophy in the lymphoid tissue of the thalamus, spleen, and lymph nodes. It causes a change in the lymphocyte numbers and can promote apoptosis of these cells. It also can, in high concentrations, cause a suppression of the T helper cells, leading to a suppression of the T cell–mediated immune response.

Despite the many harmful effects of cortisol on the immune system, the fact that the stress response causes an increase in the levels found in the body indicates potential positive or beneficial effects as well. Research into this is ongoing but is not yet understood. Several theories relate to the increased glucose levels and the body's need for glucose during a stress reaction; the immunosuppression is to prevent a prolonged immune response that could damage the body. Table 8-4 lists the physiologic effects of cortisol.

Other Hormones

As previously described, many hormones are released during the stress response. Many have both positive and negative effects on the body. Some substances appear to have a stronger effect one way than the other. In addition to catecholamines and cortisol, other hormones such as endorphins, growth hormone, prolactin, and testosterone are involved in the stress response.

Beta-endorphins are released from the pituitary gland along with ACTH as a result of stimulation by CRF. These endorphins relieve pain and promote emotional well-being. The classic example of this is called a *runner's high,* which is experienced by long-distance runners. Subjects describe this as immediate relief from the pain felt from the repeated painful stimuli of running once a certain threshold is achieved. These endorphins work off of opiate receptors. Evidence exists that beta-endorphins may play a role in the regulation of ACTH, thereby limiting the stress response.

Growth hormone (GH) plays a role in protein, lipid, and carbohydrate metabolism. It also plays a role in tissue repair and healing. Evidence shows that GH levels fluctuate during certain experiences. Certain surgery patients and those subjects who anticipate certain events have presented with elevated levels. In contrast, those with long-term stress have shown to have reduced GH levels.

Prolactin is also released from the anterior pituitary gland. It has the primary role of breast development and lactation. Prolactin levels are seen to rise after certain surgical procedures and during events such as skydiving. Unlike other hormones, prolactin levels do not seem to rise during traditional exercise; they require more intense stimulation. Several classes of lymphocytes have receptors from prolactin. This has lead investigators to believe that prolactin has a direct effect on the immune system.

TABLE 8-4	Physiologic Effects of Cortisol
Function	**Effects**
Protein metabolism	Increased protein synthesis in the liver and depressed synthesis in muscle, lymphoid tissue, adipose tissue, skin, and bone; increases levels of amino acids in plasma
Carbohydrate metabolism	Diminished peripheral uptake and use of glucose; promotes gluconeogenesis and elevates blood glucose levels
Inflammatory effects	Decreased circulating eosinophils, lymphocytes, and macrophages; decreases the concentration of lymphocytes at the site of injury or inflammation and delays healing
Lipid metabolism	Lipolysis in extremities and lipogenesis in the face and trunk
Immune reserves	Decreases tissue mass of all lymphoid tissues; inhibits production of IL-1 and IL-2 and blocks cell-mediated immunity
Digestive function	Promotes secretions and ulcer formation
Urinary function	Enhances urine secretion
Connective tissue function	Decreases proliferation of fibroblasts in connective tissue, resulting in delayed healing
Muscle function	Maintains normal contractility and maximal work output for skeletal and cardiac muscle
Bone function	Decreases bone formation
Cardiovascular function	Maintains normal blood pressure, assists arteriole constriction, optimizes myocardial function
Central nervous system function	Modulates perceptual and emotional function; essential for normal daytime arousal and activity

IL, Interleukin.

Testosterone is a hormone traditionally thought of as a strictly male sex hormone. However, in addition to being produced in the male testicles, it also is produced in the adrenal cortex of both men and women. The role of testosterone in the stress response is still under investigation because the evidence presents a mixed and confusing picture. In many situations stress will lead to a decrease in testosterone levels, whereas other stressful stimuli, such as certain sports activities, show an increase in these levels.

Role of the Immune System

Evidence shows that many immunologic diseases and conditions are linked to stress and the stress response. Unfortunately, no concrete evidence exists that specifically points to cause and effect of many of the most commonly seen processes. The immune, nervous, and endocrine systems are theorized to communicate through complex pathways. These pathways are considered complex because they do not appear to be linear but are more of a circular progression or pathway in which regression is possible. Table 8-5 lists some of the more common conditions that have a possible link to stress.

STRESS, COPING, AND ILLNESS INTERRELATIONS

The link has been established between an individual's ability to cope with the stimuli associated with stressful situations and the likelihood that he or she subsequently becomes ill. Those with inadequate coping mechanisms are much more likely to become ill. The type of stress on the individual also can contribute to the outcome.

Physiologic stresses have a direct effect on the body, such as traumatic injury or heat and cold injury. Psychological stresses are caused by unpleasant emotions, such as the loss of a loved one or divorce. The way in which each of these contributes to the overall well-being and health of the person depends on his or her ability to cope with the stressor and other mitigating factors, such as the use of alcohol and drugs and any preexisting illness.

Potential Effects of Stress Based on Effectiveness of Coping

The potential effects of stress and a person's ability to cope with stressors have a strong relation to the health of the individual. In a healthy person with effective

TABLE 8-5	Examples of Stress-Related Diseases and Conditions
Target Organ or System	**Disease or Condition**
Cardiovascular system	Coronary artery disease
	Hypertension
	Stroke
	Disturbances of heart rhythm
Muscles	Tension headaches
	Muscle contraction backache
Connective tissue	Rheumatoid arthritis (autoimmune disease)
	Related inflammatory disease of connective tissue
Pulmonary system	Asthma (hypersensitivity reaction)
	Hay fever (hypersensitivity reaction)
Immune system	Immunosuppression or deficiency
	Autoimmune disease
Gastrointestinal system	Ulcer
	Irritable bowel syndrome
	Diarrhea
	Nausea and vomiting
	Ulcerative colitis
Genitourinary system	Diuresis
	Impotence
	Frigidity
Skin	Eczema
	Neurodermatitis
	Acne
Endocrine system	Diabetes mellitus
	Amenorrhea
Central nervous system	Fatigue and lethargy
	Type A behavior
	Overeating
	Depression
	Insomnia

coping mechanisms, this stress may lead only to a transient effect on the immune system, with a quick return to a normal state and no illness. In healthy people with ineffective coping mechanisms, stress response can be significant, leading to increased incidence of distress and illness.

Patients who are symptomatic of disease processes with effective coping mechanisms may show little or no effect on their preexisting conditions. Yet those with ineffective coping mechanisms manifest a worsening of the symptoms. In patients undergoing medical treatment, a variety of outcomes have been seen as well. In patients who perceive their treatment as helpful

or beneficial, a positive effect on the stress symptoms, as well as their underlying illness, has been seen. In contrast, those who did not see their treatment as beneficial had a negative impact on their disease process.

Many healthcare providers and facilities have seen the effects of coping and the recovery of the patients receiving treatment. Because of this, many institutions have put a special emphasis on counseling both the patient and his or her family in the postoperative and intensive care settings. This focus on treating the entire patient, not just the disease process, has been found to improve patient outcomes and shorten hospital stays.

Case Scenario SUMMARY

1. *What is your general impression of this patient?* Given mental status, skin color, and respiratory status, he does not appear to be a high priority patient at this time.

2. *What conditions could lead to these symptoms?* This patient may have a simple case of influenza. Other potential causes of diarrhea and vomiting include food poisoning, viral gastroenteritis, complications of alcohol or drug use, or gastric ulcers. Vomiting and diarrhea also could lead to dehydration, electrolyte abnormalities (caused by dehydration and diabetes), complications of diabetes, or acidosis.

3. *How would these patient findings affect the patient's glucose levels?* Depending on severity, illnesses such as this tend to cause the release of stored sugars (gluconeogenesis and glycogenolysis), resulting in a temporary increase in blood sugar despite his lack of dietary intake. Dehydration also concentrates the blood, further increasing the blood glucose level.

4. *What physiologic complications would you expect from nausea, vomiting, and diarrhea for 1 week?* Dehydration and electrolyte abnormalities.

5. *What is this patient's primary problem? How will you treat it?* Further examination has demonstrated that this patient is sicker than he initially appeared. His vital signs (tachycardia and hypotension) and skin turgor demonstrate decompensated shock. This shock or hypoperfusion is potentially caused by dehydration and hyperglycemia. Assuming no evidence of congestive heart failure exists, this patient requires significant infusion of isotonic fluids to treat hypovolemia and hypoperfusion.

6. *What is the clinical significance of the patient's fever? Does it relate to the other symptoms? How?* Until proven otherwise, assume the fever is caused by infection related to sepsis. He may have septic shock in addition to his hypovolemic shock. At the present time the initial cause of his vomiting and diarrhea is unknown; the presence of the fever may suggest an infectious origin. This dramatically increases the potential for further shock and additional complications in many patients.

7. *Is this patient's blood glucose level what you expected given his history? Why or why not?* Many paramedics may have expected this patient to be hypoglycemic because of his history of reduced food intake and insulin administration. However, as previously noted, illnesses such as this one cause *all* patients to release stored sugars (fight-or-flight response). For nondiabetic individuals, this response is accompanied by the release of insulin. For diabetic individuals, the blood sugar will climb unless they actually *increase* their insulin dose.

8. *Given the history and vital signs, would you expect this patient's urine output to be higher or lower than normal? Why?* One of the ironic features of dehydration and shock related to hyperglycemia is an *increase* in urine output. Most dehydrated patients have a significant decrease in urine output as the body works to retain fluids. However, the body draws fluid from the interstitial and intracellular spaces in the bloodstream to attempt to dilute the glucose in the blood. This causes an increase in intravascular volume and an increase in urine output. Diabetics with hyperglycemia become dehydrated because of an elevation of urine output, a finding that can help confirm your field diagnosis of hyperglycemia and/or diabetic ketoacidosis.

9. *Do you believe you should have administered more than 500 mL of IV fluids to this patient? Why or why not?* Yes. Based on this patient's presentation, there is no reason to run this IV at 30 mL/hr and every reason to open it up. The patient has a history consistent with dehydration, is hypotensive, tachycardic, and has poor skin turgor. He also has no history or physical findings suggestive of renal failure or congestive heart failure. He needs some significant IV fluid infusion to restore his lost volume and further dilute his blood glucose.

10. *How are the changes in his laboratory values related to his condition and medical history?* Dehydration has led to increased concentration of the blood, elevating the sodium (and further elevating his blood glucose). Potassium is lost in both diarrhea and urination (remember, he is urinating excessively as a result of hyperglycemia). The elevated WBC count demonstrates his body's response to whatever the source of infection is.

Chapter Summary

- The human body is a fascinating and complex organism.
- The cell is the basic unit of life.
- Tissues are groupings of similar cells that perform a common function.
- Organs are composed of tissues that work together to accomplish specific functions.
- All the organs of the body work to maintain the homeostasis of the organism.

- Changes in the structure and function of cells can be helpful or harmful to the host. These changes occur as a result of a stimulus. The most common forms of adaptation include atrophy, hypertrophy, hyperplasia, dysplasia, and metaplasia.
- The most common forms of cellular injury are hypoxia, chemical injury, infectious injury, immunologic and inflammatory injury, genetic factors, nutritional imbalances, and physical agents.
- Cellular death can occur as a result of spreading irreversible injury, called *necrosis,* or it can be a preprogrammed response for tissue regeneration, called *apoptosis.*
- Viruses are the most common cause of infections in the human organism.
- Water in the body is distributed between intracellular and extracellular compartments. The proper distribution of fluid between these compartments is essential for proper function.
- The movement of water and other substances between the various compartments of the body occurs by osmosis, diffusion, and mediated transport.
- Water balance is greatly affected by the distribution and concentration of electrolytes.
- The proper electrolyte balance is essential for the body systems to function.
- Upsetting the proper balance of electrolytes generates signs and symptoms, primarily in the central nervous system, peripheral nervous system, and the heart.
- The body strives to maintain a constant concentration of hydrogen ions. This concentration is known as pH. The pH should be between 7.35 and 7.45. Anything greater than 7.45 is known as *alkalosis,* and anything less than 7.35 is called *acidosis.*
- Acid-base derangements can be respiratory or metabolic in nature. The body attempts to compensate for any change through the carbonic acid–bicarbonate buffer system, protein buffering, and renal mechanisms.
- Hypoperfusion is a state of inadequate tissue perfusion. To maintain adequate perfusion, the body must be able to deliver oxygen and remove cellular waste products from the tissues. The most important determinant of adequate blood flow is cardiac output.
- MODS is the progressive impairment of two or more organ systems. This is usually the result of an uncontrolled inflammatory response from severe illness or injury, such as sepsis, trauma, or severe burn injuries. The cause of this condition is largely unknown. However, clinicians' ability to identify patients at high risk is improving.
- The human immune system has multiple mechanisms to defend the body against foreign invaders. The first of these are the anatomic barriers, such as the skin. The second line of defense includes certain chemical attacks and the inflammatory response. The third line includes the adaptive mechanism.
- When the immune system produces an exaggerated response to a stimulus, it can be harmful to the body. This type of response is known as a *hypersensitivity reaction.*
- Research is ongoing into the effects of stress on the body and its link to disease. The communication between the immune system, the nervous system, and the endocrine system is believed to play a role in the progression of disease as it relates to the stress response.
- You should understand the way in which cells interact in the various tissues in the body. This knowledge will assist you in understanding the physiologic basis of the condition of your patient as well as the best approach for treatment.

REFERENCES

McCance, K., & Huether, S. (2002). *Pathophysiology: The biological basis for disease in adults and children* (4th ed.). St. Louis: Mosby.

Parker, M. (2007). *The Fick principle.* Retrieved January 9, 2008, from http://athome.harvard.edu.

Rose, D. B., & Post, T. (2000). *Clinical physiology of acid-base and electrolyte disorders* (5th ed.). New York: McGraw Hill.

Sears, C. (2005). A dynamic partnership: Celebrating our gut flora. *Anaerobe, 11*(5), 247-251.

Yeldani, A. U., Kaufman, D. E., & Reddy, J. K. (1996). *Cell injury and cellular adaptations* (10th ed.). St. Louis: Mosby.

SUGGESTED RESOURCE

Gould, B. (2002). *Pathophysiology for the health professions* (2nd ed.). Philadelphia: Saunders.

Chapter Quiz

1. Which type of cellular adaptation is a great cause of concern because it involves a change in the size or shape of the cell and is closely linked to the development of cancer?
   a. Atrophy
   b. Dysplasia
   c. Hyperplasia
   d. Metaplasia

2. The most common form of cellular injury is_____.
   a. hypoxia
   b. infectious injury
   c. nutritional imbalances
   d. physical agents

3. Which of the following is the most common cause of infection in human beings?
   a. Bacteria
   b. Fungi
   c. Parasites
   d. Viruses

4. The preprogrammed death of cells for the purpose of regeneration of tissues is known as_____.
   a. apoptosis
   b. coagulation
   c. liquefaction
   d. necrosis

5. Which of the following ions is the chief intracellular cation responsible for pH and water balance inside cells?
   a. Chloride
   b. Magnesium
   c. Potassium
   d. Sodium

6. The substance needed for the body to release stored calcium into the bloodstream is_____.
   a. citrate
   b. lymphocytes
   c. PTH
   d. vitamin C

7. The normal blood pH of the human body is_____.
   a. 6.25 to 7.45
   b. 7.00 to 7.50
   c. 7.35 to 7.45
   d. 7.85 to 8.00

8. The normal ratio between bases and acids required to maintain balance in the body is_____.
   a. 10:1
   b. 10:2
   c. 15:3
   d. 20:1

9. You are transferring a patient who has a pH of 7.30, a $PaCO_2$ of 55 mm Hg, and an HCO_3^- of 24. The most likely acid-base disturbance with these laboratory values is_____.
   a. metabolic acidosis
   b. metabolic alkalosis
   c. respiratory acidosis
   d. respiratory alkalosis

10. Water balance in the body primarily is regulated by which of the following substances?
    a. Antidiuretic hormone
    b. Chloride
    c. Epinephrine
    d. PTH

11. The chief extracellular cation is_____.
    a. magnesium
    b. phosphorus
    c. potassium
    d. sodium

12. A molecule or compound that reacts with the preformed components of the immune system is known as a(n)_____.
    a. antibody
    b. antigen
    c. leukocyte
    d. macrophage

13. The inadequate delivery of blood, oxygen, and nutrients to the cells of the body is known as_____.
    a. hyperreflexia
    b. hypoperfusion
    c. hypotension
    d. necrosis

14. Which cells are responsible for the release of vasoactive amines such as histamine?
    a. Mast cells
    b. Osteocytes
    c. Phagocytes
    d. Stem cells

15. The process of phagocytes adhering to capillary and venule walls in the early phases of inflammation is known as_____.
    a. diapedesis
    b. margination
    c. neutropenia
    d. opsonization

16. Inflammation caused by a trauma to tissue that lasts for 6 weeks is known as_____.
    a. acute inflammation
    b. chronic inflammation
    c. granuloma
    d. septicemia

17. The phase of the general adaptation syndrome in which the central nervous system is activated is known as_____.
   a. homeostasis
   b. the alarm stage
   c. the stage of resistance
   d. the stage of exhaustion

18. The primary substance released as a result of stimulation of the adrenal cortex by ACTH during stress is_____.
   a. cortisol
   b. GH
   c. prolactin
   d. testosterone

Terminology

Acid-base balance Delicate balance between the body's acidity and alkalinity.

Active transport A process used to move substances against the concentration gradient or toward the side that has a higher concentration; requires the use of energy by the cell but is faster than diffusion.

Aldosterone A hormone responsible for the reabsorption of sodium and water from the kidney tubules.

Anion A negatively charged ion.

Antidiuretic hormone (ADH) A hormone released in response to detected loss of body water; prevents further loss of water through the urinary tract by promoting the reabsorption of water into the blood.

Anucleated Cells of the body that do not have a central nucleus, such as those in cardiac muscle.

Atrophy Decrease in cell size that negatively affects function.

Buffer systems Compensatory mechanisms that act together to control pH.

Capsid Layer of protein enveloping the genome of a virion; composed of structural units called the capsomeres.

Capsule A membranous shell surrounding certain microorganisms, such as the pneumococcus bacterium.

Catabolism Process of breaking down complex substances into more simple ones.

Cation A positively charged ion.

Cellular swelling Swelling of cellular tissues, usually from injury.

Chromatin Material within a cell nucleus from which the chromosomes are formed.

Chromosomes Any of the threadlike structures in the nucleus of a cell that function in the transmission of genetic information; each consists of a double strand of DNA attached to proteins called histones.

Cytosol Liquid medium of the cytoplasm.

Dehydration A state in which the body has an excessive water loss from the tissues.

Deoxyribonucleic acid (DNA) Genetic material passed on to the cell from the parent cell.

Diapedesis Migration of phagocytes through the endothelial wall of the vasculature into surrounding tissues.

Differentiation Process by which the cell becomes specialized for a specific purpose, such as a cardiac cell versus a bone cell.

Diffusion Spreading out of molecules from an area of higher concentration to an area of lower concentration.

Dysplasia Abnormal cell growth; cells take on an abnormal size, shape, and organization as a result of ongoing irritation or inflammation.

Edema A collection of water in the interstitial space.

Endogenous Produced within the organism.

Endotoxin A substance contained in the cell wall of gram-negative bacteria, generally released during the destruction of the bacteria by either the host organism's defense mechanisms or by treatment with medications.

Eukaryotes One of the two major classes of cells found in higher life forms (more complex in structure).

Exogenous Produced outside the organism.

Exotoxin Proteins released during the growth phase of the bacteria that may cause systemic effects.

Extracellular fluid (ECF) The fluid found outside the cells.

Facilitated diffusion Movement of substances across a membrane by binding to a helper protein integrated into the cell wall and highly selective about the chemicals allowed to cross the membrane.

Gangrenous necrosis Tissue death over a large area.

Gene The biologic unit of inheritance, consisting of a particular nucleotide sequence within a DNA molecule that occupies a precise locus on a chromosome and codes for a specific polypeptide chain.

Germ theory Controversial theory developed in the 1600s in which microorganisms were first identified as the possible cause of some disease processes.

Glycolysis Process by which glucose and other sugars are broken down to yield lactic acid (anaerobic glycolysis) or pyruvic acid (aerobic glycolysis). The breakdown releases energy in the form of ATP.

Gram-negative bacteria Bacteria that do not retain the crystal violet stain used in Gram's stain and that take the color of the red counterstain.

Gram-positive bacteria Bacteria that retain the crystal violet stain used in Gram stain.

Homeostasis Balance; a stable environment in the human body.

Hormones Broad-reaching chemical mediators released in one part of the body but with an effect in another part of the body.

Hydration Process of taking in fluids with the normal daily output.

Hydrophilic Attracts water molecules.

Hydrophobic Repels water molecules.

Hydrostatic pressure Pressure exerted by a fluid from its weight.

Hypercalcemia A state in which the body has an abnormally high level of calcium.

Hyperkalemia A state in which the body has an abnormally elevated potassium level.

Hypermagnesemia A state in which the body has an abnormally elevated concentration of magnesium in the blood.

Hyperplasia Abnormal cell division that increases the number of a specific type of cell.

Hypersensitivity reaction An immune response that is excessive beyond the bounds of normalcy to a point that it leads to damage (as with endotoxins) or is potentially damaging to the individual.

Hypertonic In a membrane, the side with the higher concentration in an imbalance in the ionic concentration from one side to the other.

Hypertrophy Enlargement or increase in the size of a cell(s) or tissue.

Hypocalcemia A state in which the body has an abnormally low calcium level.

Hypokalemia A state in which the level of potassium in the serum falls below 3.5 mEq/L.

Hypomagnesemia A state in which the body has an abnormally low serum concentration of magnesium.

Hypotonic In a membrane, the side with the lower concentration when an imbalance exists in the ionic concentration from one side to the other.

Incidence rate The rate of contraction of a disease versus how many are currently sick with the disease.

Intercalated discs The cell-to-cell connection with gap junctions between cardiac muscle cells.

Interstitial compartment Area consisting of fluid outside cells and outside the circulatory system.

Intracellular fluid (ICF) Fluid found within cells.

Intravascular compartment Area consisting of fluid outside cells but inside the circulatory system; the majority of intravascular fluid is plasma, which is the fluid component of blood.

Isotonic A balance in the ionic concentration from one side of the membrane to the other.

Lipid accumulation Accumulation of lipids in cells, usually as a result of the failure or inadequate performance of the enzyme that metabolizes fats.

Lymphedema Edema that follows when lymphatic pathways are blocked and fluid accumulates in the interstitial space.

Margination Process of phagocytes adhering to capillary and venule walls in the early phases of inflammation.

Metabolism Sum of all physical and chemical changes that occur within an organism.

Metaplasia The transformation of one type of mature differentiated cell into another type of mature differentiated cell.

Mitosis The process of cell division.

Mortality rate The number of patients who have died from a disease in a given period.

Mutate To change in an unusual way.

Mycoses Diseases caused by fungi.

Natural killer cells Specialized lymphocytes capable of killing infected or malignant cells.

Neuroglia Support cells that do not transmit nerve impulses but are critical to proper function.

Neuron A highly specialized cell responsible for converting stimuli into nerve impulses that move throughout the body.

Normal flora Nonthreatening bacteria found naturally in the human body that, in some cases, are necessary for normal function.

Nuclear envelope The outer boundary between the nucleus and the rest of the cell to the endoplasmic reticulum for protein synthesis.

Oncotic pressure The net effect of opposing osmotic pressures in the capillary beds.

Organ A grouping of similarly functioning tissues that work together to accomplish certain functions (e.g., the heart).

Organelles Structures within cells that perform specialized functions.

Organism An entity composed of cells and capable of carrying on life functions.

Organ systems The coordination of several organs working together.

Osmolarity The number, or concentration, of solutes per liter of water.

Osmotic gradient The difference in the concentration from one side of a membrane to the other in the presence of an imbalance in the ionic concentration.

Osmotic pressure The pressure exerted by the concentration of the solutes in a given space.

Phagocytes Cells that are part of the body's immune system that play a predominant role in the destruction of invading microorganisms.

Phospholipid bilayer A double layer composed of three types of lipid molecules that comprise the plasma membrane.

Terminology—continued

Plasma membrane Outer surface of the cell.

Prevalence rate The fraction of the population that currently has a certain disease.

Prokaryotes One of the kingdoms of cells; simpler in structure and found in lower life forms such as bacteria.

Pyrogenic Substances, such as endotoxins from certain bacteria, that stimulate the body to produce a fever.

Resistance The ability of the body to defend itself against disease-causing microorganisms.

Ribonucleic acid (RNA) Genetic material responsible for ribosome production.

Saponification A form of necrosis in which fatty acids combine with certain electrolytes to form soaps.

Septicemia A serious medical condition characterized by vasodilation that leads to hypotension, tissue hypoxia, and eventually shock; usually caused by gram-negative bacteria; diagnosed by blood tests called cultures.

Stem cells Formative cells whose daughter cells may give rise to other cell types.

Stimuli Anything that excites or incites an organism or part to function, become active, or respond.

Susceptibility Vulnerability or weakness; the opposite of resistance.

Thirst mechanism Sensation activated by cells in the hypothalamus when cells called osmoreceptors detect an imbalance in body water; as the body is replenished by drinking fluid, the osmoreceptors sense a return to baseline and turn off this mechanism.

Tissue A group of cells that are similar in structure and function.

Total body water (TBW) The total amount of fluid in the body at any given time.

Transcellular compartment Compartment classified as extracellular but distinct because it is formed from the transport activities of cells; cerebrospinal fluid, bladder urine, the aqueous humor, and the synovial fluid of the joints are considered transcellular.

Virions Small particles of viruses.

Virulence A term to describe the relative pathogenicity or the relative ability to do damage to the host of an infectious agent.

Life Span Development

Objectives *After completing this chapter, you will be able to:*

1. Describe the body system developmental milestones, characteristics, and vital signs of infants, toddlers and preschoolers, school-age children, adolescents, early adults, middle adults, and late adults.
2. Distinguish the unique psychosocial characteristics of infants, toddlers and preschoolers, school-age children, adolescents, early adults, middle adults, and late adults.
3. Explain the psychosocial development of children and adolescents that results from parenting styles, sibling and peer relationships, and environmental factors.
4. Explain the physiologic characteristics and emotional challenges faced when treating older adults.

Chapter Outline

Infants
Body and Organ Systems
Toddlers and Preschoolers
School-Age Children
Adolescence

Early Adulthood
Middle Adulthood
Late Adulthood
Chapter Summary

Case Scenario

You and your paramedic engine company respond to an apartment complex during the middle of a very cold night for a "possible carbon monoxide poisoning." On arrival, you find a family of five gathered outside their apartment, bundled in coats and robes, shivering. The family includes parents in their mid thirties, a son aged 3 years, a daughter who is 15 years old, and the grandfather who is 74 years old. They have been living in a tiny, rundown, drafty one-bedroom apartment. Because their apartment became very cold, the family moved mattresses into the kitchen and started the stove to provide warmth. Although this seemed to work, both parents awoke at 3 AM with severe headaches and remembered a recent public service television announcement about the signs of carbon monoxide poisoning. To get the family out of the cold, you move the family into two ambulances.

Questions

1. *What developmental stages are the children in? How will knowing this affect your approach to these patients?*
2. *What developmental stages are the parents and grandfather in? How will knowing this affect your approach to them?*
3. *When you consider how to divide the family between the two ambulances, should particular members of the family be kept together? Why?*

All people are different. Nobody knows that better than prehospital professionals. Although all children grow and develop at different rates and adults age differently, most share some common characteristics. By understanding normal child and adolescent development and understanding how adults age, you will be better able to recognize health and related problems early on and to take action before they become bigger problems.

To help you prepare for interacting with the wide range of patients EMS professionals are called on to treat, this chapter provides a brief overview of some of the common developmental characteristics and behaviors that mark normal development in children and the expected changes that aging adults undergo.

INFANTS

[OBJECTIVE 1]

The term *infant* is used to describe a baby until the age of 1 year. Infants who are a few hours old are referred to as *newly born;* until they are 1 month old they are called *neonates.*

Growth is rapid during infancy. The infant's size, shape, and organs undergo change. As these physical changes occur, the infant gains new abilities.

PARAMEDIC*Pearl*

Pediatric Age Classifications

- Newly born: neonate in the first minutes to hours after birth
- Neonate: Birth to 1 month
- Infant: 1 to 12 months of age
- Toddler: 1 to 3 years of age
- Preschooler: 4 to 5 years of age
- School age: 6 to 12 years of age
- Adolescent: The period between the end of childhood (beginning of puberty) and adulthood (18 years of age)

Vital Signs

Immediately after birth, an infant has a heart rate of 160 to 180 beats/min, although heart rates as high as 200 beats/min are not unusual. This is because newborns have a blood volume of 300 mL, but require approximately 500 mL/min to meet their metabolic demands. To meet this demand, their heart rate is increased to circulate the blood quickly. Within the first 30 minutes of birth, the heart rate should drop to less than 160 beats/min, and by the time the infant has reached 1 year of age, normal heart rate averages 120 beats/min.

As with heart rate, the newborn's respiratory rate is high, typically between 40 and 60 breaths/min, dropping to 30 to 40 breaths/min a few minutes after birth. A respiratory rate of 20 to 30 breaths/min is considered normal for a 1-year-old child. Respiratory tidal volumes should range from 6 to 8 mL/kg initially to 10 to 15 mL/kg by age 1 year.

Blood pressure, which often is difficult to obtain in this age group, is considered normal at 70 mm Hg after birth and 90 mm Hg at 1 year.

Although a normal core temperature is 98° to 100° F, newborns lack the ability to regulate their body temperature. As a result, a wide fluctuation in "normal" temperature may occur depending on the time of day, activity, and sleep. Newborns also lack the ability to generate heat and are susceptible to hypothermia.

Weight

Term babies typically weigh 3 to 3.5 kg (7 to 8 lb) at birth. A newborn loses 5% to 10% of his or her birth weight during the first week but should gain back enough to exceed birth weight by the end of the second week. As rapid growth begins, weight should significantly increase, with a gain of approximately 30 g/day during the first month, doubling by 4 to 6 months and tripling at 9 to 12 months. At this age approximately 25% of weight is the head.

BODY AND ORGAN SYSTEMS

During the first year, physical development mainly involves the infant coordinating motor skills. The infant repeats motor actions that build physical strength and motor coordination.

Cardiovascular System

The most significant differences in the infant's cardiovascular system are the fetal circulatory structures (fetal shunts) of the ductus arteriosus, ductus venosus, and the foramen ovale. These structures normally close at birth or shortly thereafter.

In the fetus, the **ductus arteriosus** shunts blood from the left pulmonary artery to the aorta, bypassing the fetus's lungs, because oxygen for the fetus is provided through the mother's placenta. The high levels of oxygen exposure after birth cause the ductus arteriosus to begin to close, in most cases within 24 hours. Complete constriction of this vessel can take up to 6 months (Van De Graaff, 1998).

In the fetus, the **ductus venosus** connects the left umbilical vein with the inferior vena cava. The ductus venosus is a shunt that allows oxygenated blood from the placenta to bypass the liver and return to the systemic circulation for distribution to the rest of the body. It closes functionally soon after birth, but anatomically it does not close for 15 to 20 days (Meyer & Lind, 1966).

The **foramen ovale** is a small hole located in the atrial septum used during fetal circulation. In the womb, a fetus does not use its own lungs; it relies on the mother to provide oxygen-rich blood from the placenta through the umbilical cord. Therefore blood can travel from the veins to the right side of the baby's heart and cross to the left side of the heart through the foramen ovale, skipping the trip to the baby's lungs. The foramen ovale normally closes at birth with the first breath the baby takes, when increased pressure on the left side of the heart forces a flap of tissue to cover the opening.

At birth, a significant decrease in pulmonary vascular resistance as the lungs expand allows blood to be redirected from the placenta to the lungs. This decrease in pulmonary vascular resistance leads to an eightfold to tenfold increase in pulmonary blood flow. Systemic vascular resistance increases at birth, at least in part from removal of the low vascular resistance bed of the placenta (Steinhorn, 2000).

Respiratory System

The respiratory system in the infant differs in some ways that are important to the paramedic. All passages are smaller and softer or more flexible, making them more susceptible to obstruction. An infant's tongue is large in relation to the mouth. The large tongue and shorter distance between the tongue and hard palate make rapid upper airway obstruction possible. If an infant or small child is placed in a supine position, the neck tends to flex, causing obstruction of the airway. This happens because the anteroposterior diameter of an infant or small child's head is greater than the anteroposterior diameter of the torso. This problem can be prevented by padding under the torso to bring it into alignment with the head and neck.

The nasal passages are soft, narrow, and distensible and have little supporting cartilage and more mucosa and lymphoid tissue than an adult. Infants younger than 6 months are obligate nose breathers. Any degree of obstruction (e.g., swelling of the nasal mucosa, buildup of mucus) can result in respiratory difficulty and problems with feeding. A small degree of airway swelling can be significant because of the small diameter of the airway, resulting in a disproportionately higher resistance to airflow than in an adult. An infant's vocal cords are more cartilaginous than an adult's and are easily damaged.

An infant's chest wall is thin and the bony and cartilaginous rib cage is soft and pliant. Because of an infant's thin chest wall, transmitted breath sounds make localizing a problem area difficult.

Breathing is predominantly a result of diaphragmatic movement. Impaired movement of the diaphragm, such as that from gastric distention, can significantly affect ventilation. With poorly developed accessory muscles that tire easily and ribs positioned more horizontally (already causing the infant to rely on diaphragmatic breathing), the infant quickly experiences early respiratory fatigue when increased respiratory effort is required. An infant's lungs contain proportionally fewer alveoli, decreasing collateral ventilation opportunities (movement of air from one pulmonary segment into the next, occurring through openings between the alveoli), and the tissue is more likely to be injured from **barotrauma** during ventilation.

With higher oxygen demands than those of older children and adults, small respiratory insults can lead to rapidly increasing respiratory rates and a resulting increase in internal heat generation and fluid loss, leading to dehydration.

Renal System

The infant's kidneys are unable to concentrate urine, resulting in excretion of larger volumes of dilute urine and making dehydration from **polyuria** a serious threat.

Immune System

Infants in the first 3 to 6 months of life have an immature immunologic system and are more susceptible than an older infant or child to severe infections and infections by unusual organisms. The infant's immune system is essentially limited to passive immunity, based on maternal antibodies, through the first 6 months of life.

Nervous System

At birth the brain is nearer its adult size than is any other organ; virtually all the neurons of the nervous system are present but they are immature.

> **PEDIATRIC***Pearl*
>
> **Myth:** Young infants do not feel pain. Children's nervous systems are not fully developed, making them unable to perceive and experience pain the way adults do.
>
> **Fact:** The central nervous system of a 26-week-old fetus possesses the anatomic and neurochemical capabilities of experiencing pain (Anand, 1998).

The infant principally has reflexes as the sole physical ability. A reflex is an automatic body response to an involuntary stimulus (i.e., the person has no control over the response). Some reflexes occur in infancy and disappear a few weeks or months after birth. The presence of reflexes at birth is an indication of normal brain and nerve development. Some reflexes, such as the rooting and sucking reflex, are needed for survival. The rooting reflex causes the infant to turn the head toward anything that brushes the face. This survival reflex helps the infant find food, such as a nipple. When an object is near a healthy infant's lips, the infant immediately begins sucking. This reflex also helps the baby get food. This reflex usually disappears by 3 weeks of age.

The startle response (also called the *Moro reflex*) occurs when a newborn is startled by a noise or sudden movement (Figure 9-1). When startled, the infant reacts by flinging the arms and legs outward and extending the head. The infant may cry, drawing the arms together in

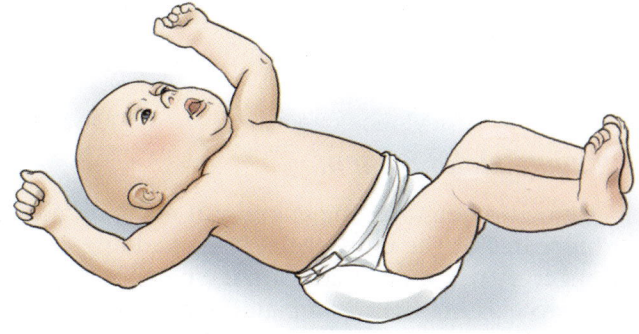

Figure 9-1 Moro reflex.

a hugging motion. This reflex peaks during the first month and usually disappears after 4 months.

The palmar grasp reflex can be observed when the infant's palm is touched and when an object is placed across the palm. The infant's hands grip tightly. This reflex disappears by the first 3 or 4 months after birth.

The Babinski reflex is present in normal babies of term birth. When the sole of the infant's foot is stroked on the outside from the heel to the toe, the infant's toes fan out and curl and the foot twists inward. An abnormal Babinski reflex is present when dorsiflexion of the great toe occurs with or without fanning of the other toes. This response may or may not be present in children younger than 2 years. If present, it is a normal finding; however, the absence of this response is also normal.

The stepping or walking reflex can also be observed in normal term babies. When the infant is held so that the feet are flat on a surface, the infant will lift one foot after another in a stepping motion. This reflex usually disappears 2 months after birth and reappears toward the end of the first year as a learned voluntary behavior.

Motor sequence and growth and physical development are orderly and occur in predictable sequence. The motor sequence (order of new movements) for infants is described in Box 9-1.

During infancy the bones of the cranium are separated by fibrous tissue called **fontanelles.** These fontanelles allow the rapid growth of the brain and permit the skull to undergo changes in shape. The posterior fontanelle closes at approximately 3 months and the anterior fontanelle at 9 to 18 months (Van De Graaff, 1998). Pulsations of the fontanelle reflect the heart rate. A bulging anterior fontanelle may be caused by crying, coughing, vomiting, or increased intracranial pressure from a head injury, meningitis, or hydrocephalus. A depressed anterior fontanelle is seen in dehydrated or malnourished infants.

Sleep needs for infants vary depending on age. Although newborns do sleep much of the time, their sleep is in short segments. As a baby grows the total amount of sleep gradually decreases, but the length of nighttime sleep increases. Newborns initially sleep 16 to 18 hours per day with sleep and wakefulness evenly distributed over a 24-hour period. The longest sleep periods are generally 4 or 5 hours; this is approximately how long they can go between feedings.

Between 2 and 4 months sleeping gradually decreases to 14 to 16 hours per day with a 9- to 10-hour concentration through the night. An infant is normally easily awakened.

Musculoskeletal System

Bones grow in length at the epiphyseal plate, or growth plates, located at the ends of the bones, adding cells to get longer. Bones grow in thickness by depositing new bone onto existing bone material. Bone growth is influenced by growth hormones, thyroid hormones, genetic factors, and general health and nutrition (Van De Graaff, 1998).

BOX 9-1	Motor Sequence for Infants

1. In the first few months after birth, the infant begins head and trunk movement (e.g., lifting the head, tracking objects by rotating the head).
2. At 4 or 5 months, the infant rolls over—first onto the back, then onto the stomach.
3. At 4 to 6 months, the infant develops more strength in the back and neck and sits upright when supported, as in a highchair.
4. The infant gradually develops the muscle strength and control to sit up unassisted.
5. After learning to roll over, the infant crawls with his belly on the floor, using his arms to pull himself forward, and sometimes using his legs to push.
6. After learning to sit unassisted, the infant develops the ability to hitch: while sitting, the infant uses her arms and legs to obtain motion, hitching her buttocks across the floor.
7. As his limbs become stronger, the infant supports his weight on his hands and knees in a motion called creeping.
8. As she gains in strength, the infant stands with assistance
9. Over time, the infant stands on his own with the aid of furniture or walls.
10. As she gains leg strength and coordination, the infant is able to walk, still supported, with more confidence. This is called cruising.
11. The infant can stand up without help.
12. The infant can stand by himself without any support or assistance.
13. The infant can walk by herself without any support or assistance.

Infants' muscles, which are 25% of their weight, continue to grow and strengthen with continued use.

Tooth eruption, or teething, generally begins with front teeth at 5 to 7 months, although some infants are born with erupted teeth and others may not have eruption for 12 months or more.

Psychosocial Development

A long-held concept has been that the first 3 years of life are the most critical for a person's emotional and intellectual development. Indeed, if an infant does not get the proper interaction, the foundation of this emotional and intellectual development is broken for life. Hence **psychosocial development** is critical.

During infancy, some of the most simple bidirectional interactions (reciprocal socialization) such as mother and infant mutual gaze or eye contact have been found to play an important role in early social interaction. These behaviors of mothers and infants create substantial interconnection and synchronization, and synchrony in parent-child relationships has been positively related to children's social competence. Another parental interaction, called *scaffolding*, occurs when a physical situation is artificially modified to support children's efforts, allowing them to be more skillful than they would if they relied only on their own abilities (e.g., helping pick up a rattle). This interaction affects the level of behavior children show in the future. Infancy also is described as the "trust versus mistrust" psychosocial stage of development. Infants who receive proper care, love, and affection from their parents or parent substitutes develop this sense of trust. Without this caring environment, the infant may become suspicious, fearful, and mistrusting of his or her surroundings. These fears can even influence the ability to form relationships as an adult.

Research supports the idea that forming a secure attachment is a critical part of an infant's development and later adjustment. Parents and other caregivers have many opportunities to help the infants in their care develop positive attachments early. Touch—including cuddling, fondling, and holding—greatly increases positive attachment to the parent.

Infants are not able to communicate their needs well and cry to express some of their basic feelings and needs. Caregivers soon learn to tell the difference among all the types of cry an infant uses, primarily the basic or hunger cry used from birth; the anger cry, interpreted by adults as an expression of exasperation or anger; and the pain cry, which is distinct in that it tends to be more prolonged and has periods in which the baby holds his or her breath. Paramedics should be attentive to information that the baby is crying differently that usual because this may be the only indication the infant can give that something is wrong.

As the infant grows, many of the social interactions discussed help develop bonds and relationships between the infant and parents or caregivers. In the first few weeks of life, the infant will not have developed much more than a bond related to feeding, so interactions with strangers tend not to be stressful for the infant. After approximately 1 month, infants begin to recognize and interact with adults who are present, often showing more happiness at the presence of women. By their second month, most infants have a more complex interaction with adults, especially with their mothers, often smiling and making sounds to express their happiness. After 3 months, the infant has formed a need for social interaction with adults that will increase for several years. These interactions increase the bonds, or attachments, between the infant and family members and caregivers.

By approximately 9 months, an infant will cry when separated from the mother or other person with whom he or she has a true attachment. This is called *separation anxiety* and can result in several types of behaviors. One behavior is protest, which results in loud crying, rejection of other adults, and extreme agitation and restlessness. Protest often is followed by despair, with nonstop crying, inactivity, and withdrawal. The third behavior is detachment, when the infant becomes distracted by the surroundings and even ignores the return of the mother. The

separation can sometimes be made easier by ensuring the child has his or her favorite toy or blanket. Separation anxiety is a normal developmental process in which children are fearful because their familiar caregivers are leaving them. See Boxes 9-1 and 9-2 for more specific milestones in infants.

BOX 9-2   Growth and Development: Birth to 1 Year

2 Months
- Tracks objects with eyes
- Recognizes familiar faces

3 Months
- Moves objects to mouth with hands
- Displays primary emotions with distinct facial expressions

4 Months
- Drools without swallowing
- Reaches out to people

5 Months
- Sleeps throughout the night without food
- Discriminates family and strangers

6 Months
- Sits upright in a highchair
- Makes one-syllable sounds (ma, mu, da, di)

7 Months
- Fears strangers
- Quickly changes from crying to laughing

8 Months
- Responds to "no"
- Sits alone
- Plays "peek-a-boo"

9 Months
- Responds to adult anger
- Pulls self to standing position
- Explores objects by mouthing, sucking, chewing, and biting

10 Months
- Pays attention to own name
- Crawls well

11 Months
- Attempts to walk without assistance
- Shows frustration to restrictions

12 Months
- Walks with help
- Knows own name

Emergency Care Implications

- Observe the infant before making contact.
- Keep the infant on the caregiver's lap during the physical examination if possible.
- Handle the patient gently, but firmly, supporting the head and neck. **Do not shake or jiggle the infant.**
- Keep the caregiver in sight if possible to decrease separation anxiety and involve the caregiver in the care of the infant whenever possible.
- Return the infant to the caregiver as soon as possible after procedures; allow the caregiver to comfort the infant.
- Perform least-invasive parts of the examination first.
- Keep the infant warm, warm anything that touches the infant, and keep the environment warm.
- Speak softly and smile; touch, rock, hold, and cuddle if possible.
- Examine from toes to head.
- Provide comfort measures (such as a pacifier).
- Distract with keys, penlight, or musical toy in the infant's field of vision.
- Persistent crying, irritability, or inability to console or arouse patient may indicate physiologic distress.

Case Scenario—continued

All members of the family are alert. Vital signs of the children are as follows:

- 3-year-old: pulse, 120 beats/min; respirations, 35 breaths/min; blood pressure, 90/64 mm Hg.
- 15-year-old: pulse, 98 beats/min; respirations, 16 breaths/min; blood pressure, 110/72 mm Hg.

The family members deny any type of trauma or medical histories, so your examination focuses on mental status and the cardiac and respiratory systems.

Questions

4. *What will your approach be to examining the 3-year-old? How will you evaluate orientation?*
5. *Are the vital signs of the 3-year-old normal? If not, what is abnormal, and what could it be caused by?*
6. *What will your approach be to examining the 15-year-old? How will you evaluate orientation?*
7. *Are the vital signs of the 15-year-old normal? If not, what is abnormal, and what could it be caused by?*
8. *What communication barriers might exist during your interview and evaluation of the grandfather? How can you overcome them?*

TODDLERS AND PRESCHOOLERS

[OBJECTIVE 1]

Toddlers (1 to 3 years old) and preschoolers (3 to 5 years old) can be among the more challenging patients for a paramedic. This age group, which includes the "terrible twos," tends to be apprehensive with strangers and is beginning to develop independence. During the first 2 years the body enlarges faster than at any other time after birth, and these age groups typically add 2 kg each year to their body weight and an average 2 to 3 inches in height. This also is the age during which the child begins to become aware of his or her gender and begins to model actions based on the gender role model.

Vital Signs

The vital signs within this age group vary over a relatively wide range of what is considered normal. Heart rate should range between 80 and 120 beats/min for toddlers and between 80 and 100 beats/min for preschoolers. Toddler and preschooler respiratory rates average 20 to 30 breaths/min. To determine the minimal systolic blood pressure for a child aged 1 to 10 years, the following formula may be used: 70 + (2 × Age in years). Normal systolic blood pressure is approximately 70 to 100 mm Hg for toddlers and 80 to 110 mm Hg for preschoolers. Normal core temperature for both should be 96.8° to 99.6° F.

Cardiovascular System

As children grow, the cardiovascular system continues to grown in strength and function. For example, capillary beds become more developed, allowing better peripheral perfusion and thermoregulation, and hemoglobin levels are more similar to those of an adult.

Respiratory System

The respiratory system of toddlers and preschoolers continues to develop, with passages becoming larger and more rigid and more alveoli developing. The chest becomes less flexible and accessory muscles better developed, so they can rely less on diaphragmatic breathing alone in times of stress. Although their ribs and sternum are pliable and more resistant to rib fractures than those of adults, the force of an injury to the chest is readily transmitted to the delicate tissues of the lung and may result in a pulmonary contusion, hemothorax, or pneumothorax.

Renal System

By age 2 years the kidneys are well developed and are able to concentrate urine, making urinary output, like that of an adult, a better gauge of function. This is the age at which children gain control of bladder and bowel function.

Immune System

By this age, the passive immunity children had as infants no longer protects them. They become more susceptible to minor respiratory and gastrointestinal infections, particularly as they begin to mix with other children in nursery and preschool environments and play groups. Many vaccinations against more serious illnesses are given to this age group.

Nervous System

During these years the brain continues to grow faster than any other part of the body. By age 2 years the brain has reached 90% of the weight of the adult brain and will reach 95% by age 6 years. The grey matter of the brain continues to thicken throughout these years as brain cells continue to add connections. Physical development is typified by an explosion of gross and fine motor skills, influenced by a combination of hereditary and environmental factors. Preschoolers develop a basic understanding of written symbols and arithmetic concepts through informal experiences. Vision and sight should be nearly completely developed by the end of the toddler years.

PEDIATRIC Pearl

Myth: Children tolerate pain better than adults.

Fact: Younger children experience higher levels of pain during procedures than do older children. Children's tolerance for pain increases with age (Broome et al., 1998; Broome et al., 1990).

Musculoskeletal System

Muscle mass and bone density increase, and children begin to develop proportions more like that of adults and start to lose their top-heavy appearance. Their trunk, legs, and arms lengthen, and they lose baby fat. Walking generally occurs by 14 to 15 months of age but may start earlier. All their primary teeth should be erupted by approximately 3 years.

Children younger than 3 years are much less likely to have serious injuries than are older children who fall the same distance. Younger children may better dissipate the energy transferred by a fall because they have more fat and cartilage and less muscle mass than older children.

PEDIATRIC Pearl

A young child's vertebral column may withstand traction and torsion without evidence of deformity while the spinal cord tears (Meller & Shermeta, 1987).

Psychosocial Development

[OBJECTIVES 2, 3]

Toddlers develop a growing awareness of self, and self-control and self-confidence begin to develop at this stage. Toddlers develop a unique personality and set of likes and dislikes by age 2 years. Children can do more on their own and begin to feed and dress themselves as they strive for autonomy. Some have referred to the toddler years as the "age of negativism" as they begin to use their firm "no" as a response to nearly everything. Preschoolers begin to assert their independence and continue to be assertive and take initiative. Playing and hero worshipping are an important form of initiative for children. Children in this stage are eager for responsibility. Preschoolers typically engage in magical thinking, which is a belief that thoughts have power to influence reality. Because preschoolers think magically, they may believe illness or injury is a punishment for something bad they have done or thought.

Parenting styles have a significant impact on the psychosocial development of this age group. Most parenting styles fall into one of the following categories:

Authoritarian parenting: This is a restrictive, punitive style in which the parent exhorts the child to obey, follow the parent's directions, and respect their work and effort. Firm limits and controls are placed on the child, and little verbal exchange is allowed. This style is associated with low self-esteem and socially incompetent behavior in the child.

Authoritative parenting: This style encourages children to be independent but still places limits and controls on their actions. Extensive verbal give and take is allowed, and parents are warm and nurturing toward the child. This style is associated with more successful children who are responsible, more self-reliant, assertive, and socially competent and have more self-esteem.

Permissive-indifferent parenting: Permissive-indifferent parents usually are uninvolved in their children's lives. They have a low level of control and have a low level of responsiveness to their child. They are uninvolved with their children's peer group and fail to monitor their children's activities. This style is associated with children who are dependent and moody and who have low social skills and low self-control.

Permissive-indulgent parenting: These parents are more involved with their children but they place little or no limits or control on their behavior. Little punishment occurs, no guidelines are set, little structure is present, and the parents avoid taking charge. The parent, often referred to as *uninvolved,* spends little time and effort with the child. The child of this parent learns little self-control, has low social skills, and is immature. However, these children often tend to feel that they are especially privileged.

Sibling Rivalry

Sibling rivalry refers to the natural jealousy of children toward a brother or sister. The arrival of a new baby is especially stressful for the firstborn. Not surprisingly, most children prefer to be the only child at this age. In short, they do not want to share their parents' time and affection. The jealousy arises because the older sibling sees the newcomer receiving all the attention, visitors, gifts, and special handling.

When toddlers have older siblings, they watch what happens between the siblings and their parents. The greater the difference in the maternal affection and attention, the more hostility and conflict between the siblings. From age 18 months on, siblings understand how to comfort, hurt, and exacerbate each other's pain; they understand family rules, can differentiate transgressions of different sorts, and can anticipate the response of adults to their own and other people's misdeeds and use that knowledge. If a family deals with sibling rivalry in a productive, nonaggressive, and respectful manner, this can provide the child with critical skills in their development and allow them to learn to compromise, negotiate, and value other people's point of view.

Peer Relationships

Peer relationships are a critical component in the social development of children. At ages 2 to 3 years, children begin to develop basic relationships with other children,

usually beginning with play in the presence of, rather than with, other children. They begin to play more interactively and begin to share, even to take turns. Play progresses to acting out fantasies, using their imaginations to develop simple and then more complex games with rules. Peer group activities help develop problem-solving skills and interpersonal relationship skills, and older preschoolers may begin to create the bonds of lasting friendships.

Divorce

The effects of a divorce on a toddler or preschooler vary widely, largely as a result of the age of the child, his or her social and cognitive development, and the relationship with and dependency on the parents. Although many children do well after a divorce, children of divorced parents have a statistically higher incidence of behavioral problems than do those raised in a two-parent home (Poehlmann & Fiese, 1994). Among the many factors involved for the child, social and economic turmoil, loyalty to a parent, custodial conflicts, and nonparental child care requirements often influence the behavior of the child. Depression, withdrawal, and fear of abandonment are common reactions of the child.

Television Violence

Belief is growing that exposure to violence on television and in video games creates acceptance of that behavior in children. Some research shows that between the ages of 3 and 5 years, television, specifically cartoons, has a profound impact on children. In early childhood self-concept begins to take shape. The child mimics what is seen. By this age they begin to put together plots and find meaning in what they are viewing but do not yet know that the violence is not real. Parents should carefully monitor television viewing and play activities of toddlers and preschoolers.

PEDIATRIC Pearl

Toddlers: Common Fears

- Being left alone
- Interacting with strangers
- Interruptions in usual routine
- Losing control
- Getting hurt (falls, cuts, scrapes)

Preschoolers: Common Fears

- Bodily injury and mutilation
- Loss of control
- The unknown and the dark
- Being left alone
- Being lost or abandoned
- Adults who look or act mean

Emergency Care Implications

Toddler

A typical toddler dislikes strange people and responds to an examination attempt by crying, becoming uncooperative, and fighting. Perform a toddler examination as you would for an infant, with the addition of the following:

- Encourage the child's trust by gaining the cooperation of the caregiver.
- Try not to separate the child and caregiver.
- Address the child by name.
- Smile and speak in a calm, quiet tone.
- Allow the child to participate in care when possible.
- Respect modesty; keep the child covered if possible and promptly replace clothing after examining each body area.
- Allow the child to hold transitional objects.
- Explain that illness or injury is not the child's fault.
- Reassure the child if a procedure will not hurt.
- Do not show needles or scissors unless necessary.
- Avoid procedures on the dominant hand or arm.
- Avoid covering the child's face.
- Involve the caregiver in the treatment whenever possible.
- Persistent irritability and inability to console or arouse the patient may indicate physiologic distress.
- Foreign body airway obstruction continues to be a risk.

> **PEDIATRIC Pearl**
>
> Because children expect their caregivers to protect them, do not ask a caregiver to restrain a child or participate in any way other than to comfort the child.

Preschooler

When examining a preschooler, keep in mind that a child in this stage of development does not separate fantasy and reality. He or she also has an intense fear of injury, pain, and blood loss. Perform the examination as you would for a toddler, with the addition of the following:

- When possible, examine and treat the child in an upright position.
- Explain procedures in brief, simple terms as they are performed.
- Speak quietly in clear and simple language; avoid baby talk and frightening or misleading comments (e.g., shot, deaden, cut, germs).
- Allow the child to hold a transitional object or keep it in sight.

- Tell the child what will happen next and encourage the child to help with his or her care.
- Warn the child of a painful procedure just before carrying it out.
- Offer the child treatment choices if possible.
- Use an adhesive bandage after a procedure or when an injection has been given because the child may fear that "all of my blood will leak out" if a bandage is removed or not applied.
- Respect the child's modesty.
- Keep the child warm.
- Allow the caregiver to remain with the child whenever possible to help relieve the child's fear of separation from his or her caregiver.
- Persistent irritability or inability to arouse the patient may indicate physiologic distress.
- Foreign body airway obstruction risk continues.

SCHOOL-AGE CHILDREN

[OBJECTIVE 1]

School-age children are between the ages of 6 and 12 years. These children continue to grow, adding approximately 3 kg of weight and 2 to 3 inches of height each year. During these years most body functions reach adult levels. See Box 9-3 for developmental milestones for this age group.

Vital Signs

The average heart rate for school-age children is 70 to 110 beats/min, respiratory rate is 20 to 30 breaths/min, and systolic blood pressure is between 80 and 120 mm Hg. Their normal core temperature is 98.6° F.

Nervous System

Brain function continues to increase during this time. In the frontal lobe of the brain (the areas of judgment, personality, organization, planning, strategizing), thickening of gray matter peaks at approximately age 11 years in girls and age 12 years in boys.

> **PEDIATRIC Pearl**
>
> **Myth:** Children will tell you when they feel pain.
> **Fact:** Children may not report pain because of the fear of administration of a painful injection or fear of lengthening their hospital stay. Children with chronic pain may not be fully aware that they are in pain. Children may be developmentally unable to communicate their pain, or parents may not think telling health professionals about the pain is necessary.

BOX 9-3	Developmental Milestones in School-Age Children

- Weight gain is more related to muscle development than fat
- Psychomotor skills and coordination improve
- Body changes related to puberty begin
- Body proportions become more like those of adults
- Child begins to engage in more unsupervised activities
- Child's moral and ethical values and beliefs develop
- Child's sexual interests grow with onset of puberty
- Social skills such as sharing, giving, and receiving are refined

Reproductive System

Puberty, the time when the reproductive system starts to mature, often begins in this age group. Puberty begins when the body releases increasing levels of sex and growth hormones. For both genders, the release of the hormones precedes any external changes to the body. For girls, this process typically begins between the ages of 8 and 13 years; for boys, this occurs between ages 13 and 15 years.

Lymphatic System

The lymphatic system, among other functions, plays a critical role with the immune system in fighting infection and disease. This system continues to grow and undergoes many changes until puberty, when growth slows significantly. In this age group lymphatic tissue remains proportionally larger than that of adults.

PEDIATRIC*Pearl*

You can usually reason with a school-age child.

PEDIATRIC*Pearl*

School-Age Child: Common Fears

- Fear of unknown setting
- Separation from caregiver
- Loss of control
- Pain, loss of function
- Bodily injury and mutilation
- Failure to live up to the expectations of others
- Rejection by peers
- Death
- Being unable to compete in school, sports, or play
- Interruptions in daily routine

Psychosocial Development

[OBJECTIVE 2]

The school-age child is living in an ever-expanding world. At this stage the child learns to master more formal skills of life such as relating with peers according to rules, progressing from free play to play that may be elaborately structured by rules and demand formal teamwork (e.g., baseball), and mastering tasks that require self-discipline, such as school assignments and homework. While still under the general supervision their parents, these children spend less time with their parents and more time with their peers or alone. These also are stressful years for children. As interaction with others increases, so increases their need to be accepted by their peers. They begin to compare themselves to others as they develop more of their self-concept. Self-esteem issues are more common in this age group and often are the result of external factors such as popularity with peers, emotional support from family and friends, and acceptance or rejection from social groups.

Psychosocial development varies greatly in this age group, with some children seeming quite mature while others remain immature. Their behavior varies on the basis of their maturity, life experiences, and predictable stressors such as peer pressure and fear of new situations (e.g., attending a new school).

This is the age when moral development typically occurs. Their behaviors begin to be the result of their beliefs of what is right and wrong and their internal self-control, rather than the external control provided by parents. Many theories of moral development exist; Kohlberg's six stages of moral development are found in Box 9-4. Common among nearly all expert beliefs is the role that a caring, positive, loving environment plays in moral development.

Emergency Care Implications

A school-age child masters the environment through information, can make compromises, and thinks objectively. Conduct the examination as you would for a preschooler, with the addition of the following:

- Enlist the child's cooperation.
- Introduce yourself to the child and approach him or her in a friendly, sympathetic manner.
- Explain procedures before carrying them out.
- Allow the child to see and touch samples of equipment that may be used in his or her care (e.g., blood pressure cuff, stethoscope).
- Tell the child what will happen next and encourage the child to help with his or her care.
- Warn the child of a painful procedure just before carrying it out. *Honesty is particularly important when interacting with school-age children.*

BOX 9-4 Kohlberg's Stages of Moral Development

Premoral or Preconventional Stages (Ages 4-10 Years)

Behavior is motivated by anticipation of pleasure or pain.

- *Stage 1.* Punishment and obedience: avoidance of physical punishment and deference to power. Children obey rules simply to avoid punishment.
- *Stage 2.* Instrumental exchange: "You scratch my back, I'll scratch yours." Child does what is necessary and makes concessions only as necessary to satisfy own needs.

Conventional Morality (Ages 10 to 13 Years)

Acceptance of the rules and standards of one's group.

- *Stage 3.* Interpersonal conformity: good boy/nice girl mentality. Good behavior pleases or helps others within the group. "Everybody is doing it." Earns approval by being conventionally "respectable" and "nice." Failure to punish is "unfair." "If he can get away with it, why can't I?"
- *Stage 4.* Law and order: respect for rules and authority. Responsibility toward the welfare of others. Justice demands that the wrongdoer be punished, that he or she "pay a debt to society," and that law abiders be rewarded.

Postconventional or Principled Morality (Ages 13 Years and Older)

Ethical Principles

- *Stage 5.* Prior rights and social contract: moral action in a specific situation is not defined by a checklist of rules, but from logical application of universal, abstract, moral principles. Individuals have natural or inalienable rights and liberties. Right action tends to be defined in terms of standards that have been critically examined and agreed upon by the whole society, such as the Constitution. The freedom of the individual should be limited by society only when it infringes on someone else's freedom.
- *Stage 6.* Universal ethical principles: an individual who reaches this stage acts out of universal principles based on the equality and worth of all human beings. Having rights means more than individual liberties. It means that every individual is due consideration of his or her own interests in every situation, with those interests being of equal importance to one's own. This is the "golden rule" model. A list of rules inscribed in stone is no longer necessary.

Modified from Crain, W. C. (1985). *Theories of development* (2nd ed.), (pp. 118-136), Upper Saddle River, NJ: Prentice-Hall.

- Offer the child alternatives ("It's OK to yell, but don't move").
- Make a contract with the child ("I promise to tell you everything I am going to do if you will help me by cooperating").
- When speaking with the caregiver, include the child.
- Persistent irritability or inability to arouse the patient may indicate physiologic distress.
- Respect patient modesty.
- Reassure the patient of body integrity.
- Address preoccupation about death when appropriate.

ADOLESCENCE

[OBJECTIVE 1]

Adolescents are 13 to 18 years old. This is the age when the final stages of growth and development occur. Most early adolescents have a rapid, 2- to 3-year growth spurt, beginning with enlargement of the hands and feet, then arms and legs, and ending with the chest and trunk. Bone and muscle mass development is nearly complete, and their bodies now have achieved adult proportions (Figure 9-2). Organs such as the heart, kidneys, liver, and spleen reach their full size, and the skin toughens. For most girls, this growth ends by the time they are 16 years old; for boys, growth typically ends by age 18 years.

Adolescence also is when sexual maturity is reached. In girls, the first external indications of puberty that begin during school age are the development of breast buds, soon followed by enlargement of their breasts. Within 2 years of the development of breast buds, as long as their body fat is at least 18% to 20% of body weight, **menarche,** or first menstruation, occurs.

Two hormones, luteinizing hormone and follicle-stimulating hormone, are secreted from cells in the anterior pituitary. These are called *gonadotropins* because they stimulate the gonads—the testes in males and the ovaries in females. Luteinizing hormone, in turn, stimulates gonadal secretion of the sex steroids testosterone in boys and estrogen and progesterone in girls.

For girls, progesterone affects breast development and estrogen causes secondary sex characteristics such as underarm and pubic hair and addition of subcutaneous fat in the breasts, buttocks, and thighs. Estrogen promotes the buildup of the endometrium in the uterus.

For boys, testosterone causes the development of secondary sexual characteristics such as changes to the scrotum and an increase in the size of the testes. The penis enlarges and assumes an adult shape, and pubic hair grows. At approximately age 14 years, boys experience their first ejaculation. Later in adolescence further changes occur, such as growth of underarm, facial, and chest hair, and deepening of the voice.

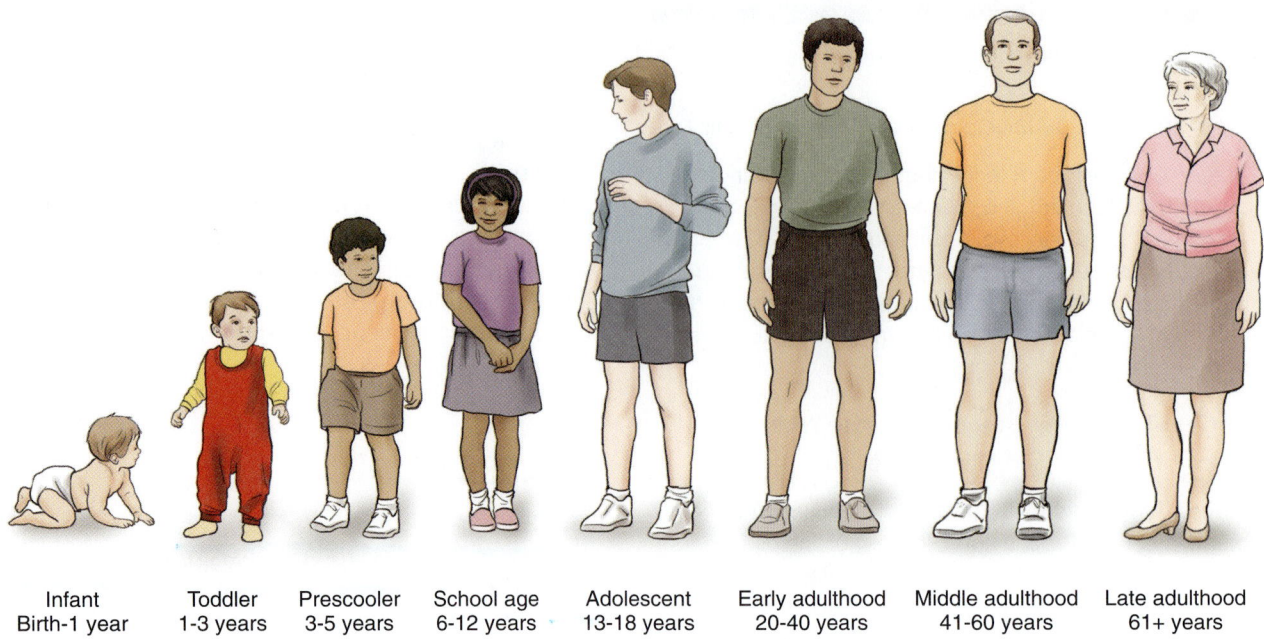

Infant Birth-1 year	Toddler 1-3 years	Prescooler 3-5 years	School age 6-12 years	Adolescent 13-18 years	Early adulthood 20-40 years	Middle adulthood 41-60 years	Late adulthood 61+ years

Figure 9-2 Bodily proportions from fetus to adult.

PEDIATRIC*Pearl*

Adolescent: Common Fears

- Being left out or socially isolated
- Fear they will inherit parent's problems such as alcoholism, mental illness
- Early and violent death
- Loss of control
- Altered body image
- Separation from peer group

Vital Signs

Normal vital signs for adolescents are heart rate, 55 to 105 beats/min; respiratory rate, 12 to 20 breaths/min; systolic blood pressure, 100 to 120 mm Hg; and core temperature, 98.6° F. Blood chemistry is nearly equal to that of adults.

Psychosocial Development

[OBJECTIVE 2]

Chaos and *confusion* are two terms that can be used to describe the psychosocial development of most adolescents. While coping with significant physical changes, adolescents are trying to determine who they are and where they fit into society. The major components of adolescent psychosocial development are establishing identity, autonomy, and intimacy; becoming comfortable with one's sexuality; and working toward future goals.

In addition to the physical changes that mark this time, the adolescent's mind and methods of thinking begin to change as well. This process, known as *cognitive development,* continues well after the physical changes of puberty are complete. For many adolescents, puberty is finished as early as 13 or 14 years of age, and their adult cognitive development is just beginning. Considerable conflict can exist between the adult body and the child's mind, such as not understanding the future consequences of current behavior. An adolescent continues to improve regarding this type of thinking, and at approximately 15 years old this adult cognition is fairly well in place. However, this mental development can continue well into adult life.

Early adolescents (13 to 15 years old) typically display their desire to become independent in an irrational, gut-level manner. A clear indication of developing independence is embarrassment and desire not to be seen with their parents. At this stage they want to be with their same-sex friends more than with their families. This is the age at which parents often become "stupid," a condition that usually resolves in a few years. Adolescents who are a little older are generally finished with most of their pubertal development, and they have begun to use their new "adult" (i.e., abstract) cognitive abilities well. They still want to be with their peers, but now the group includes both sexes. Girls at this stage are deeply involved in their relationships with friends, whereas boys are more likely to want to "hang out" and do things with their friends. Concern about body image is considerable, and subjects such as weight, complexion, body odors, and hair styles can be preoccupying. Eating disorders, depression, and suicide attempts are not uncommon. Parental conflicts are common as adolescents attempt to find their identity through new behaviors, attire, drugs and alcohol experimentation, and sexual experimentation. Toward the end of adolescence, most begin to recognize that their parents may not be infallible, but that parents can be their best friends. Peer groups fade in importance and are replaced by fewer, but closer, friends. The adolescent's interests now focus on an educational or vocational future.

Emergency Care Implications

An adolescent has fragile self-esteem, and body image is important. Respect an adolescent's need for modesty and conduct the examination as you would for school-age children, with the addition of the following:

- Speak in a respectful, friendly manner, as though speaking to an adult.
- Obtain a history from the patient if possible.
- Respect independence; address the adolescent directly.
- Allow the caregiver to be involved in the examination if the patient wishes.
- Explain things clearly and honestly; allow time for questions.
- Involve the patient in treatment whenever possible.
- Respect the patient's modesty.
- Address patient concerns of body integrity or disfigurement.
- Deal with the patient tactfully and fairly.
- Provide discharge instructions to the patient.
- Vital signs approach adult values.
- Consider the possibility of substance abuse and endangerment of self or others.

EARLY ADULTHOOD

Physical Changes

[OBJECTIVE 1]

Early adulthood includes the ages of 20 to 40 years. During this period human beings reach peak conditioning (generally between 19 and 26 years of age), and all body systems operate with optimal performance. Most pregnancies occur in this period. This also is when aging begins, with early signs of diminished hearing and sight and slower reaction times. The leading cause of death for this age group is accidents.

Normal early adults have a heart rate averaging 70 beats/min, respiratory rate between 16 and 20 breaths/min, blood pressure averaging 120/80 mm Hg, and a core temperature of 98.6° F.

Psychosocial Development

[OBJECTIVE 2]

Psychosocial development in the adult stages is much less defined than in the childhood stages, and people differ dramatically. Overall the underlying goal in early adulthood is to achieve some degree of intimacy—to be close

to others as a lover, a friend, a parent, and as a participant in society. Young adults have a much clearer sense of who they are, and this period is not as associated with psychological problems related to well-being despite this age having the highest reported level of job-related stress. Noted psychologist Erik Erikson believed that if a person successfully negotiates this stage of life, he or she will carry for the rest of life the virtue or psychosocial strength he calls love—not only the love found in a good marriage, but the love between friends and the love of one's neighbor, co-worker, and compatriots as well. Leaving the parental home for the first time, learning to live with a marriage or life partner, and raising children are major roles in the psychosocial development during these years.

MIDDLE ADULTHOOD

Physical Changes

[OBJECTIVE 1]

Middle adulthood ranges from 41 to 60 years of age. Aging begins during early adulthood, but these physiologic changes continue and become much more obvious in middle adulthood. Although most systems still have a high level of function, lifestyle and genetics cause varying degrees of mostly gradual degradation. Vision and hearing loss becomes more prominent. Weight gain is typical, the skin may wrinkle, and hair becomes thin and may begin to lose pigment. Bone density decreases, and both cardiac output and kidney function decreases to as little as 50% of that of a 20-year-old. Women typically experience **menopause** between their late 40s and early 50s. Cancer rates increase in this age group, and high cholesterol levels are common.

Normal vital signs for this age group are the same as those for early adulthood, with a heart rate averaging 70 beats/min, respiratory rate between 16 and 20 breaths/min, blood pressure averaging 120/80 mm Hg, and a core temperature of 98.6° F.

Psychosocial Development

[OBJECTIVE 2]

Middle adulthood is a period considerably less stressful than early adulthood or adolescence. Two reasons for this are experience and, for many, the professional and financial status that comes with increasing age. By middle age, people often have less anxiety because they are able, through experience, to anticipate likely outcomes of situations and are more sure of their goals and abilities. For some, however, a concern for the "social clock,"—a concept of societal expectations for the time when people are expected to marry, have children, and accomplish other life tasks—may be a source of stress in the earlier part of middle adulthood.

This is also, however, when most adults begin to focus more on their own mortality, the rapid passing of years, and their physical decline. Middle adults often have to become caregivers for their parents, further emphasizing these points. Their children typically leave home to be on their own during these years, which for some offers a renewed sense of freedom and for others can be a depressing sense of loss (empty nest syndrome). This leads some middle adults to a "midlife crisis," defined as sudden, and occasionally irrational, life changes or purchases.

Case Scenario CONCLUSION

You stay with the grandfather during transport to the hospital. His vital signs and physical examination are within normal limits. As you talk to him, he frequently states, "I've had a good life" and "it would be fine for me to die now."

Looking Back

9. *Given his age, what underlying medical problems would this patient most likely have?*
10. *This patient has no abnormalities and will almost certainly be rapidly discharged from the emergency department. Why would he verbalize a readiness to die in this situation?*

LATE ADULTHOOD

Physical Changes

[OBJECTIVE 4]

Beginning at age 61 years, people are said to have reached late adulthood. Older persons aged 65 years and older represent 13% of the U.S. population—33.9 million persons, or approximately one eighth of all Americans. By 2030, this age bracket is expected to be 70 million, or 19.5% of the population, and the population older than 85 years is expected to increase fivefold (United States Census Bureau, 2006). Although an eventual life span of 120 years is theorized, actual life span is a factor of genetics, environment, health, and other factors.

Physical and systemic deterioration, which has already begun, continues during this age. External changes, such as hair loss and skin changes, include the continued loss of bone and muscle mass that contributes to a loss of height, averaging 1 inch for women and 2 inches for men. Although these changes are obvious, aging has a significant change on all body systems and parts (Box 9-5). Vital signs are expected to be close to those found in middle adults but are more likely to be result of the underlying health of the person in this age group (Figure 9-3). A number of studies of this age group have led to a **"terminal drop"** hypothesis, which states that mental and physical functioning drastically decline only in the few years immediately preceding death.

Cardiovascular System

Aging alters the cardiovascular system. Blood vessels become calcified and the elasticity of the vessel wall decreases. These changes cause thickening and rigidity of the vessels, which results in increased peripheral vascular resistance and reduced blood flow to organs. By 80 years of age, the ability of the arteries to stretch has decreased 50%. Baroreceptors, important in blood pressure regulation, become thick, stiff, and less sensitive

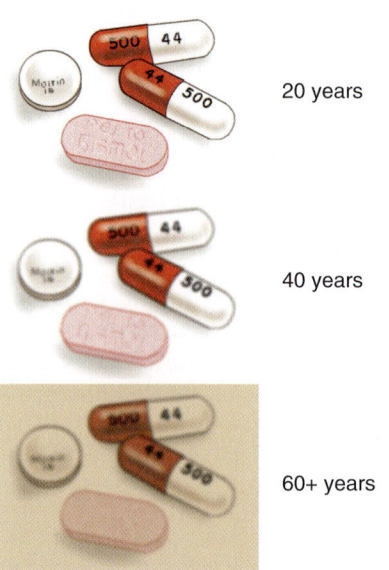

20 years

40 years

60+ years

Figure 9-3 Vision comparison: focus, contrast, glare sensitivity, and color discrimination all decrease with age.

to pressure changes. Decreased baroreceptor sensitivity results in fluctuations in blood pressure. Systolic blood pressure often is increased because of a loss of arterial distensibility. The pulse pressure widens because the diastolic blood pressure remains unchanged or is slightly elevated.

Physiologic changes within the heart itself include stiffening of the heart muscle. The atrioventricular valves become thick and rigid. Within the heart's conduction system, the shell surrounding the sinoatrial node becomes thickened with fibrous tissue and the number of pacemaker cells diminishes. These changes can alter heart rate and rhythm. Tachycardia is not well tolerated in older adults because the left ventricle requires more time for diastolic filling and systolic emptying to be completed. The left ventricle becomes thicker and may become enlarged because it must work harder to pump blood through a rigid aorta. In older adults, cardiac output at

BOX 9-5 Physiologic Changes That Occur with Age

Cardiovascular System
- Decreased muscle strength and efficiency
- Walls of large arteries thicken, vessels become dilated and elongated
- Fewer pacemaker cells

Respiratory System
- Lungs less elastic
- Lung function and capacity decrease
- Coughing becomes less effective because of muscle weakness

Musculoskeletal System
- Decreased muscle mass
  - Legs: hard to rise from sitting or kneeling
  - Hands: hard to manipulate tools, keys, doorknobs
- Decreased calcium in bones
  - Decreased bone mass
  - Increased risk for fractures
- Ligaments and tendons stiffen
  - Decreased flexibility
  - Increased risk for falls

Gastrointestinal System
- Difficulty chewing
- Difficulty swallowing
  - Increased choking on foods and liquids
  - Difficulty holding food in the mouth
  - Increased drooling
- Decreased taste, smell, saliva secretion
- Decreased gastric acidity
- Decreased gastric movements
- Decreased appetite
- Decreased absorption of nutrients
- Increased constipation
- Tooth loss
  - Causes changes in dietary choices

Urinary System
- Bladder sphincter muscle weakens
  - Decreased ability to hold urine, increased trips to the bathroom
- Leaking of urine
- Enlarged prostate (men)
- Increased risk of infection
- Progressive decrease in renal blood flow
  - Up to 50% decrease in renal function

Nervous System
- Nerve cell mass is lost
  - Atrophy of the brain and spinal cord
- Diminished taste, touch, smell, hearing, and vision
- Pain sensation decreases
- Reaction time increases
- Sleep changes occur
  - Increased awakenings and arousals
- Reduced sleep efficiency
  - Effects of sleep disturbance: impaired vigilance, impaired memory, impaired mood, decreased respiratory drive

Skin Changes
- Redistribution of fat
- Skin more dry, flaky, thin, fragile; has more wrinkles
- Skin less elastic
- Nails tougher, brittle and thick

rest usually is unchanged, but physiologic stress, such as exercise, often results in decreased cardiac output. This reduction in cardiac output generally occurs because the heart muscle becomes less efficient with age, its contractile strength decreases, and sensitivity to circulating catecholamines is reduced.

Respiratory System

Changes in the chest wall attributable to aging include calcification of the costal cartilage, which results in increased rigidity and stiffness of the thoracic cage. This requires more work from the respiratory muscles to move air in and out of the lungs. Although the diaphragm does not lose mass with aging, its elasticity diminishes and the inspiratory and expiratory muscles become weaker and contract with less force. As a result, older adults often use accessory muscles of respiration (such as the sternocleido-mastoid, trapezius, and abdominal muscles). The anteroposterior chest diameter increases with age, and curvature of the spine (kyphosis) can result in a shorter thorax, interfering with normal breathing mechanics.

An older adult has decreased upper airway muscle tone, and cough and laryngeal reflexes are diminished. Within the respiratory tree the number of cilia is reduced, and those present are less vigorous in removing material from the lungs. These changes increase the older adult's risk for developing respiratory infections.

The oxygen-carrying capacity of the blood is decreased in older adults. The elasticity of the alveoli diminishes with age, the elastic fibers of the terminal bronchi lose inward elastic recoil, and the lungs become smaller. Although the number of alveoli changes little with age, the number able to participate in gas exchange diminishes. The volume of air moved during the deepest inhalation and exhalation (vital capacity) decreases, and the amount of air that remains in the lungs after exhalation of the maximal possible amount of air (residual volume) increases. Diseases such as emphysema can cause destruction of the alveoli as a result of chronic exposure to tobacco or inhaled agents, significantly affecting respiratory function. The alveolar walls become thin, fewer capillaries are available for gas exchange, and dilation of the proximal bronchioles results in enlargement of the alveoli. Diffusion through the alveoli is diminished because the alveolar surface area available for gas exchange is diminished.

Endocrine System

With age, the pituitary gland decreases in volume by approximately 20%. Although the size of the thyroid gland and thyroid hormone production decrease with age, essentially normal hormone levels are maintained by a reduced metabolic clearance and increased half-life.

Older adults have a delayed and insufficient release of insulin from the beta cells of the pancreas and decreased sensitivity to circulating insulin. The ability to metabolize glucose is reduced. When an older adult is put under stress by a sudden concentration of glucose, the result is higher and more prolonged hyperglycemia.

Circulating levels of testosterone slowly decline with aging in men. More time is needed to become sexually aroused and achieve orgasm. Although sperm production declines, a man at age 80 years is still capable of fathering a child. With age the prostate gland enlarges, becomes stiffer, and may cause urinary frequency or obstruct urine flow. Because of the threat of prostate cancer, annual physical examinations are important.

In women, menopause results when the ovaries cease estrogen and progesterone secretion. Decreased levels of estrogen and progesterone cause the reproductive organs to atrophy. The vaginal walls become thinner and shrink, and some shrinkage of the external genitalia occurs. The vagina decreases in size and the production of vaginal lubricant is reduced and delayed.

Gastrointestinal System

Decreased awareness of cues of hunger and thirst increase an older adult's risk of dehydration, fluid and electrolyte imbalance, and vitamin and mineral deficiencies. Poor sight, difficulty ambulating, and transportation issues may impair an older adult's ability to shop for or prepare food.

Approximately half the population in the United States aged 65 years or older are estimated to wear dentures, although they may not be worn regularly because of poor fit or discomfort. Teeth in older adults often are in poor condition, with stains, flatter surfaces, and varying degrees of tooth decay or gum disease.

Salivary secretion decreases with age and results in decreased taste, increased difficulty clearing food from the oral cavity, and increased difficulty in swallowing foods. Digestion is more difficult because of decreased hydrochloric acid production and gastric secretions in the stomach, fewer digestive enzymes, and decreased

motility of the large intestine. The esophagus becomes slightly dilated with age and esophageal emptying is slower, causing food to remain in the esophagus for a longer period. Relaxation of the lower esophageal sphincter may occur in some older adults. The risk of aspiration is increased in older adults because of a weakened gag reflex and delayed esophageal emptying.

Constipation is a common problem in older adults. Decreased exercise contributes to constipation, and postponing defecation occurs if the older adult does not have access to a toilet. If the older adult must use a bedpan, incomplete bowel evacuation may occur because a bedpan does not permit normal positioning. An age-related loss of tone of the internal sphincter and decreased awareness of the need to evacuate the bowels because of slower transmission of neural impulses to the lower bowel also can affect bowel elimination.

Renal System

The weight of the kidneys decreases with age. Most of the reduction in weight is because of a loss of the renal cortex (which contains the glomeruli, Bowman's capsule, and 85% of the nephrons) rather than a loss of the renal medulla (where the tubules and collecting ducts are located). Atherosclerosis contributes to renal artery narrowing and decreased renal blood flow, which results in a decrease in the filtering ability of the kidneys (glomerular filtration rate). The renal tubules decrease in length and volume with age, reducing the ability to concentrate or dilute urine.

Bladder capacity decreases, involuntary bladder contractions increase, and bladder muscles weaken with age, which can lead to urinary urgency and frequency. In general, older adults get up at least once per night to urinate. In men, prostate enlargement can cause decreased urine flow and/or obstruction. In women, decreased estrogen levels can cause thinning of the urethral mucosa, which can contribute to urinary urgency and frequency. Stress incontinence, a leakage of urine associated with activities that increase intraabdominal pressure (e.g., lifting, bending, coughing, sneezing, laughing), is particularly common in women because of a weakening of the supporting tissues of the pelvis after childbirth.

Nervous System

Age-related changes in the nervous system include a decrease in brain weight and a reduction in the number of functioning neurons. To compensate for this reduction, the number and length of dendrites of the remaining nerve cells increase. Age-related declines in neurotransmitter levels affect the efficiency with which information is transmitted among neurons. For example, extremely low levels of the neurotransmitter dopamine can result in Parkinson's disease.

Short-term memory may decline with age, but long-term memory generally remains intact. Despite these changes, most healthy older adults have reasonable cognitive function and normal behavior.

The sleep-wake cycle of older adults often is disrupted. Studies of older adults show they may have shorter periods of rapid eye movement sleep, which is considered essential for optimal brain functioning. Some older adults have difficulty falling asleep, may awaken more frequently during the night, and have difficulty falling back to sleep. Common reasons for awakening during the night include noise, chest or arthritis pain, coughing, leg cramps, dyspnea, and trips to the bathroom. These disruptions in sleep result in the older adult feeling fatigued. Daytime napping is common and helps supplement the total daily amount of sleep needed by older adults.

Sensory Changes

Perhaps the most noticeable changes associated with aging pertain to a decline in sensory function. The ability to sense pressure, pain, and differences in temperature diminishes with age. Older adults also have more difficulty detecting odors at low concentrations and identifying or recognizing odors. The inability to detect unpleasant odors such as body odor or bad breath can have embarrassing social consequences. A reduction in the sense of smell alters the sense of taste. Taste sensations diminish with age because of atrophy of the tongue, but no conclusive evidence shows that the number or responsiveness of taste buds decreases. Taste also may be affected by poor oral hygiene, decreased saliva production, medications, and medical conditions.

Physiologic changes associated with aging and vision include thinning and yellowing of the conjunctiva, yellowing of the cornea, diminished peripheral vision, diminished upward gaze, and decreased tear production. Depth perception becomes distorted, and the ability to see detail and discriminate different visual patterns (visual acuity) diminishes with age. Consequences can be significant, such as misjudging the height of curbs and steps and difficulty reading medicine labels.

Important structural changes associated with vision include a decrease in the amount of light that passes through the eye and in the eye's ability to adjust and focus (accommodation). Loss of accommodation is caused by an increase in the size of the lens and increased density and rigidity of the lens. Consequences can include an inability to see small details, such as a buttonhole, or pose problems during driving, such as changing focus from the instrument panel to the road. Yellowing of the lens and impaired transmission of light through the retina makes discriminating colors such as blue, violet, and green difficult. Some colors may appear to blend together, such as dark brown, black, and dark blue, and pastel or pale colors. If opaque spots (cataracts) develop on the lens, the amount of light transmitted to the retina is significantly limited. Cataracts can be treated by surgical removal and corrective lenses. Less-efficient reabsorption of the fluid in the eye can cause an increase in the pressure within the eye (intraocular pressure), and loss of vision may result. Increased intraocular pressure is a risk factor for glaucoma.

With age, the pupil of the eye becomes smaller and less elastic because of atrophic changes to the muscles of the iris. These changes decrease the ability of the eye to dilate and constrict when adapting to changes in light intensity. As a result, the pupil of an older adult takes longer to adjust when going from dark to light and back to dark. Increasing illumination to see adequately (e.g., increasing the wattage of light bulbs) can produce glare. Because increased sensitivity to glare begins at approximately age 40 years, the need for additional illumination must be balanced with the need to minimize glare.

Physiologic changes associated with aging of the ear include thinning and a loss of elasticity of the tympanic membrane, reducing sound transmission. Cerumen glands atrophy, causing the cerumen (earwax) in the middle ear to be dry. Hardened cerumen, coupled with narrowing of the auditory canal and stiffer, coarser hairs that line the canal can lead to a cerumen impaction, interfering with movement of the eardrum and sound transmission.

Age-related hearing loss is called **presbycusis.** It is most commonly caused by gradual changes in the inner ear but is sometimes caused by abnormalities of the outer ear and/or middle ear. Hearing loss is usually greater for high-frequency tones, such as the nearby chirping of a bird, the ringing of a telephone, or the ability to hear consonants such as *s, z, t, f,* and *g.* The same individual may be able to hear low-frequency sounds clearly, such as vowels or a truck rumbling down the street. An older adult with presbycusis may find conversations difficult to understand especially when background noise is present.

Psychosocial Development

[OBJECTIVES 2, 4]

The psychosocial development stage, especially from the perspective of youth, seems to be the most difficult. The attitudes of society can have a significant effect on those in late adulthood.

Some cultures and social groups hold older persons in high esteem and value their wisdom, whereas others treat them in a manner that makes them seem a burden and diminishes their feelings of self-worth. As the older adult retires and moves out of the workplace environment, a sense of detachment from society grows, as does a decreased sense of usefulness. A sense of biologic uselessness also can develop because the body no longer does everything it used to. Women have gone through a sometimes dramatic menopause. Men often have sexual dysfunction. The illnesses of old age, such as arthritis, diabetes, and heart problems, and concerns about breast, ovarian, and prostate cancers further point out their failings. Fears about things they were never afraid of before start to arise—the flu, for example, or simply falling down. Along with illnesses come concerns of death. Friends die. Relatives die. Spouses die. Of course you, too, will die. Some studies show that 15% to 27% of individuals older than 65 years have depressive symptoms, and white men older than 65 years account for 81% of all suicides annually (Beekman, 2000).

Faced with all this, everyone may seem to feel despair. However, for those who are retired with good health, strong family connections, social involvement and activities, or other purposeful activities, these years may be the culmination of a lifetime of hard work and sacrifice and among the best years of their lives.

Case Scenario SUMMARY

1. *What developmental stages are the children in? How will knowing this affect your approach to these patients?* The 3-year-old is in the toddler/preschool stage and the 15-year-old can be classified as an adolescent. This information can be helpful in planning the approach. Although a toddler/preschooler is beginning to establish some independence from his parents, frightening experiences (such as this one) will likely cause him to regress a little. He is likely to want to stay close to his mother or father. Once within that safe place, he will be somewhat fearful of you, curious about the examination, and terrified that you are going to hurt him. Move slowly, provide reassurance, avoid showing needles or scissors unless absolutely necessary, and replace clothing after you have finished your examination.

   The adolescent daughter shares some characteristics with the 3-year-old—growing independence from the parents and a tendency to regress when stressed. You should take your cues from her regarding how involved she wants to be with her parents. On a normal day, she would likely be fiercely independent, but during this emergency she may cling to her mother or father. She also will be quite concerned about her own health and will be worried about possible scarring. You should speak to her as an adult, ask her whether she would like her parents to be present during the interview and examination, and keep her informed about what you will be doing. Be sure to honor her need for privacy and keep her covered.

2. *What developmental stages are the parents and grandfather in? How will knowing this affect your approach to them?* The parents are in early adulthood, and the grandfather can be classified as late adulthood. Although these development stages do not affect your evaluation and care quite as much as the younger ones, be mindful of a few things. First, remember that the parents will likely be completely focused on the needs of their children. Keep them involved and informed. Second, the grandfather will likely find all the commotion surrounding this event disorienting and may even regress to becoming dependent on his children. Nevertheless, treat him as an adult by speaking with him directly (rather than through his children) and, like his grandchildren, take cues from his behavior to determine how involved to have the other adults in his evaluation.

3. *When you consider how to divide the family between the two ambulances, should particular members of the* family be kept together? Why? In most cases, the 3-year-old should be kept close to his mother or father (whichever one he is clinging to). Most of the other dynamics will be a little harder to predict.

4. *What will your approach be to examining the 3-year-old? How will you evaluate orientation?* As noted above, keep him with his preferred parent. Address him directly but get some of your information from the parent. Remember that no matter how tough he appears, he is pretty scared. Move slowly, talk before you touch, and respect his need for modesty. Orientation in a toddler/preschooler can be evaluated by asking his name (person), location (if he is at home or a frequently attended preschool), and recent or seasonal activities (for time) such as what he is doing in school, what season it is, what holiday is coming up, and so forth.

5. *Are the vital signs of the 3-year-old normal? If not, what is abnormal, and what could it be caused by?* They are fairly normal, although his pulse rate is above normal. This is to be expected because of the stress of this situation.

6. *What will your approach be to examining the 15-year-old? How will you evaluate orientation?* You should speak to her directly and take her lead about how involved to keep her parents. Although she appears grown up, adolescents are quite focused on their bodies and have an unrealistic fear of death and/or disfigurement. Keep her informed of what you find and provide reassurance. Respect her need for modesty. If a female paramedic is available, she might be more comfortable being examined by a woman. You should be able to evaluate orientation for a 15-year-old using the same questions you would for an adult.

7. *Are the vital signs of the 15-year-old normal? If not, what is abnormal, and what could it be caused by?* Her vital signs are within normal limits.

8. *What communication barriers might exist during your interview and evaluation of the grandfather? How can you overcome them?* Many older adults have difficulty hearing, especially in loud environments. Do what you can to limit extraneous noise. Speak clearly and in low tones, and position yourself in front of the patient so he can see your face. Most people with hearing deficits use some lip reading to augment their hearing. In addition, remember to give him a chance to answer your first question before moving on to another.

9. *Given his age, what underlying medical problems would he most likely have?* Normal aging often results in problems related to the heart and lungs. Neurologic abnormalities also are fairly common.

10. *This patient has no abnormalities and will almost certainly be rapidly discharged from the emergency department. Why would he verbalize a readiness to die in this situation?* Mortality is a fairly common theme in aging adults. Remember that, by age 75 years, he likely has experienced the deaths of many friends and family members. In fact, his reality may be that his friends leave home in an ambulance, go to the hospital, and never return. Do not argue with his concerns but do inform him of what you have found—a normal examination that will likely allow him to leave the hospital quickly.

Chapter Summary

- The newborn is a baby in the first few hours of life, and a neonate is younger than 28 days old.
- The typical newborn weighs 3 to 3.5 kg at birth but should triple in weight by the end of a year. Twenty-five percent of the weight is the infant's head.
- The infant is born with several circulatory structures necessary for a fetus that should change shortly after birth.
- Nervous system functions in an infant are primarily reflex actions.
- Toddlers are children aged 1 to 3 years, and preschoolers are aged 3 to 5 years.
- Toddlers and preschoolers grow rapidly and undergo an increase in muscle and bone mass.
- Walking generally occurs by 14 to 15 months of age but may start earlier.
- Parenting styles can have a significant impact on the development of children and adolescents.
- School-age children are from 6 to 12 years old. Brain function increases rapidly, and these children are likely to begin puberty.
- Adolescents are 13 to 19 years old. They have nearly completed their growth, and their form has changed to that of an adult. Adolescents reach sexual maturity.
- Early adulthood is from 20 to 40 years of age. Body systems are at their peak performance. This is the age when love relationships occur and parenting takes place.
- Age 41 to 60 years is considered middle adulthood. This is when menopause occurs and when systems begin to show signs of aging.
- Late adulthood encompasses those older than 60 years. Body system deterioration becomes more apparent at different times for different people in this age group on the basis of genetics, health, and lifestyle.

REFERENCES

Anand, K. J. (1998). Clinical importance of pain and stress in preterm neonates. *Biology of the Neonate, 73,* 1-9.

Beekman, A. (2000). Depression and medical illness in later life. *Journal of Clinical Psychiatry, 2,* 9-14.

Broome, M. E., Rehwald, M., & Fogg, L. (1998). Relationships between cognitive behavioral techniques, temperament, observed distress, and pain reports in children and adolescents during lumbar puncture. *Journal of Pediatric Nursing, 13,* 48-54.

Broome, M. E., Bates, T. A., Lillis, P. P., & McGahee, T. W. (1990). Children's medical fears, coping behaviors, and pain perceptions during a lumbar puncture. *Oncology Nursing Forum, 17,* 361-367.

Meller, J. L., & Shermeta, D. W. (1987). Falls in urban children: A problem revisited. *American Journal of Diseases of Childhood, 141,* 1271-1275.

Meyer, W. W., & Lind, J. (1966). Postnatal change in the portal circulation. *Archives of Diseases in Childhood, 41,* 606-612.

Poehlmann, J., & Fiese, B. H. (1994). The effects of divorce, maternal employment, and maternal social support on toddlers' home environments. *Journal of Divorce and Remarriage, 22,* 121-131.

Steinhorn, R. (2000). *Control and management of pulmonary vascular tone in the newborn.* Retrieved February 13, 2008, from http://www.childsdoc.org.

United States Census Bureau. (2006). *Annual estimates of the population by sex and five year age groups for the United States: April 1, 2000 to July 1, 2005 (NC-EST2005-1).* Washington, DC: United States Census Bureau.

Van De Graaff, K. (1998). *Human anatomy* (5th ed.). Boston: WBC/McGraw-Hill.

SUGGESTED RESOURCES

National Highway Traffic Safety Administration: *EMT-paramedic: National standard curriculum,* Washington, DC: United States Department of Transportation.

Chapter Quiz

1. The term neonate is used to describe a child who is_____.
   a. a few hours old
   b. less than 28 days old
   c. newborn through 6 months of age
   d. newborn through 1 year of age

2. The head of an infant is proportionally large, constituting _____ of the baby's total weight.
   a. 15%
   b. 20%
   c. 25%
   d. 30%

3. The average weight of a newborn is approximately_____.
   a. 3 kg
   b. 5 kg
   c. 8 kg
   d. 12 kg

4. All fontanelles have generally closed by approximately _____ months of age.
   a. 3 to 6
   b. 9 to18
   c. 12 to 24
   d. 24 to 30

5. Puberty usually begins during_____.
   a. preschool age
   b. school age
   c. early adolescence
   d. late adolescence

6. Which type of parenting is restrictive and punitive in style?
   a. Authoritarian
   b. Authoritative
   c. Permissive-indifferent
   d. Permissive-indulgent

7. Sibling rivalry refers to_____.
   a. the natural jealousy of a child toward a brother or sister
   b. when a child becomes competitive in his or her psychosocial development
   c. when a child competes with one parent for another parent's attention
   d. when a child is jealous of another child in his or her peer group

8. _____ are at the age during which they begin to develop independence and have a desire to not be seen with their parents.
   a. Early adolescents
   b. Early adults
   c. Preschoolers
   d. School-age children

9. Menopause generally occurs in women in their_____.
   a. mid to late 30s
   b. late 30s to mid 40s
   c. late 40s to early 50s
   d. mid 50s to early 60s

10. Terminal drop is_____.
    a. a significant decrease in cardiovascular function seen in older adults
    b. the decrease in bone mass that causes older adults to facture bones easily
    c. the drastic mental and physical decline that occurs in the few years immediately preceding death
    d. a sudden weight loss in adolescents caused by anorexia

Terminology

Barotrauma An injury resulting from rapid or extreme changes in pressure.

Ductus arteriosus Blood vessel that connects the pulmonary trunk to the aorta in a fetus.

Ductus venosus Fetal blood vessel that conects the umbilical vein and the inferior vena cava.

Fontanelles Membranous spaces at the juncture of an infant's cranial bones that later ossify.

Foramen ovale The opening in the interatrial septum in a fetal heart.

Menarche A girl's first menstruation.

Menopause Cessation of menstruation in the human female.

Polyuria Excessive urination.

Presbycusis Age-related hearing loss.

Psychosocial development The social and psychological changes human beings undergo as they grow and age.

Terminal drop A theory that holds that mental and physical functioning decline drastically in the few years immediately preceding death.

Public Health and EMS

Objectives *After completing this chapter, you will be able to:*

1. Define the term *public health*.
2. Identify the potential public health roles of EMS providers.
3. Describe opportunities for EMS to enhance access to care.
4. Define the public health role of EMS in emergency preparedness.
5. Explain opportunities to reduce medical costs through the appropriate use of emergency medical services.

Chapter Outline

Definition of Public Health
Immunizations
Screening
Education

Access to Personal Healthcare
Emergency Preparedness
Cost Containment
Chapter Summary

Case Scenario

You are called to a local homeless shelter for a "patient who is coughing up blood." On arrival, you find a 56-year-old man lying on his side on a cot in the sleeping area of the facility. The evening is brutally cold and the shelter is full, with some people sleeping on blankets on the floor. Your patient is alert and oriented to person, place, and time. He is holding a wad of tissues filled with thick white sputum, streaked with blood. He tells you that he has had this cough for a long time and that a couple of years ago a doctor told him that he had tuberculosis (TB) and gave him "a bunch of pills to take." He tells you that he ran out of the pills months ago and has just recently refilled the prescription but does not take them on a regular basis. His major complaint is that he cannot stop coughing and he does not feel like eating anything. In addition, he cannot get any sleep because of "really bad night sweats and the shakes." His skin is warm and wet, and he appears emaciated.

Questions

1. *What is your general impression of this patient?*
2. *What physical assessment findings are most pertinent at this time?*
3. *What is the significance of his noncompliance with the medication regimen?*
4. *What treatment should be immediately initiated?*

Today's world is one of unpredictability. Despite modern technology, attempting to predict Mother Nature is futile, as proved by the Florida hurricanes of 2004 and Hurricanes Katrina and Rita the following year. Likewise, recent terrorist events in New York, Washington D.C., Spain, and England have also demonstrated the impossibility of predicting the destructive capabilities of the human minds of those determined to disrupt society.

Although these disasters, manmade and natural, cause significant damage to property and loss of human life, they also force communities to come together to respond and rebuild. As a result, walls that exist between elements of public service systems are torn down.

Just as disaster brings new challenges and opportunities, so does the ever-changing nature of prehospital care. The new era of EMS is continually being redefined by evolving scopes of care and increasing capabilities and responsibilities of providers. Moreover, the integration of EMS with public health services offers exceptional room for growth of EMS. Public healthcare is poised to be the next frontier in EMS care, promoting community health and welfare. As such, the inherent value of EMS will be enhanced, which will ensure the permanence of prehospital care within the pantheon of public protection. In an era of limited resources, the integration of EMS into the field of public health practice also may yield financial benefits for prehospital providers.

This chapter explores the nature of public health. It also highlights a number of ways in which EMS professionals can enhance their level of service by taking part in public health initiatives.

DEFINITION OF PUBLIC HEALTH

[OBJECTIVE 1]

Defining exactly what an EMS system is or ought to be is sometimes difficult. Similarly, the definition of health, specifically public health, is even more elusive. In the largest sense, the World Health Organization defines **health** as "a state of complete physical, mental, and social well-being and not merely the absence of disease or infirmity" (World Health Organization, 2006). **Public health,** in turn, can be defined as "the science and practice of protecting and improving the health of a community," with a mission to "fulfill society's interest in assuring conditions in which people can be healthy" (*American Heritage Dictionary*, 2004). In a working sense, public health is the discipline that studies the overall health of populations and intervenes on behalf of those populations rather than on behalf of individuals. Most clinicians evaluate and plan the best treatment for individual patients, independent of the effects on others. However, public health professionals examine the overall needs of the population to determine the best use of health resources to enhance the quality of life for the public as a whole.

In the United States, public health services are provided through various means. At the federal level, public health services are a core function of the Department of Health and Human Services. This agency serves the public health community. Key components of the agency include the Centers for Disease Control and Prevention, the National Institutes of Health, the Health Resources and Services Administration, and the Office of Public Health and Science (including Public Health Service Corps programming and the Office of the Surgeon General). Other federal agencies, including the Department of Homeland Security, the Environmental Protection Agency, and the Department of Agriculture, among others, also have an effect on public health services. At the federal level, the influence on public healthcare occurs directly through legislation, funding patterns, and technical guidance (Halverson et al., 1998).

The structure of public healthcare at the state and local levels varies significantly. All states have recognized state health officials. These key officials may reside within an independent department of health or within another executive agency. Public healthcare at the local level may be a function of the state, region, county, or municipality. State and local statutes determine the exact nature of the relation between these entities. As an EMS provider, you must understand the public health infrastructure in your area. This will help you work together effectively with the traditional public healthcare agencies in your area.

The role of a public health agency traditionally has been defined as one that prevents and controls communicable disease and promotes health. The modern public health professional recognizes that this definition includes a wide range of activities. These activities include immunization and nutrition programs for children; environmental health monitoring, regulation, and remediation; community planning; and exploration of the social determinants of health. The notion that the primary mission of public health agencies is to provide clinical services for those who are unable to access services elsewhere is a myth that must be dispelled. Although many public health departments choose to include clinical services as part of their range of offerings, the core activities of public health extend far beyond personal healthcare and have a much greater impact. In fact, the two advances in the past century that have done the most to improve health in the United States have been the provision of clean water and mass immunization. These are good examples of the power of bedrock public health services.

IMMUNIZATIONS

[OBJECTIVE 2]

One of the most visible ways in which EMS professionals have interacted with public health agencies is through the provision of immunizations. Consider how EMS professionals are ideally suited to reach at-risk populations. This is attributable to the credibility of EMS in the community as well as the inherent mobility of EMS. EMS stations are often located in areas of ready community access. Moreover, they can travel with mobile units to reach more widely dispersed populations. This ability may be especially important in rural areas, where clinical vaccination sites may be distant or rare, or where transportation means are a major concern. Furthermore, the positive perception of EMS providers in small communities puts them in an ideal position to approach families who are unable or unwilling to use private or governmental healthcare services.

Many EMS providers have the requisite clinical training in medication security, aseptic technique, medication administration, postinjection care, and other administrative tasks (e.g., obtaining consent for treatment and informing patients of potential side effects). This training makes them ideal candidates to administer vaccines to adults and children. Before starting an immunization program, EMS must work closely with a local public health agency to address the issues of assessing further training needs, vaccine procurement, and liability. In practice, these challenges most often can be readily overcome. Moreover, participation in an aggressive immunization program is extremely satisfying to both EMS providers and the communities they serve.

Many successful immunization programs involve EMS providers. For example, one of the authors of this text experienced remarkable success working with a Florida fire-based EMS unit (Volusia County) to roll out an influenza immunization project. In fact, during the flu vaccine shortage of 2004, this EMS agency was, for a time, the primary provider of influenza vaccine to the community. Likewise, the Pennsylvania MEDICVAX project demonstrated the efficacy of EMS agencies in providing more than 2000 adult influenza vaccinations. Nearly one third of the clients would most likely not have been vaccinated otherwise (Mosesso et al., 2003). In Nova Scotia, the provincial EMS system developed a primary care paramedic credential. These EMS professionals offer flu shots and provide other preventive care services in the community (Emergency Health Services, 2006).

EMS professionals can play a role in traditional vaccination campaigns. However, they can also integrate the screening of influenza vaccination status into their protocol for emergency response, expanding their traditional screening programs and identifying new candidates for vaccination (Shah et al., 2004). Pneumococcal vaccinations in particular have been highlighted as an area for EMS involvement (Hostler et al., 2003). The promotion of pneumococcal vaccination by EMS could become increasingly attractive as the prospect of a future pandemic influenza looms on the horizon. In scenarios in which flu vaccine supply may be limited, the focus may turn to the prevention of lethal complications, such as pneumonia.

Although the literature does not address issues of reimbursement, immunizations certainly represent a potential revenue stream for ambulance services. EMS agencies may be reimbursed directly from patients on a fee-for-service basis, or the agencies may bill Medicare (and in some cases Medicaid and other third-party payers) for administering the vaccine.

SCREENING

Another key component of public health is screening. This is the process of evaluating a population for the presence or absence of disease. In public health, the term expands to include the assessment for risk factors and determinants affecting health. As an EMS professional, you are ideally suited to participate in this process.

An advantage of EMS is its mobility in the community. As a paramedic, you can observe population dynamics, physical environments, and social conditions on scene in the course of EMS activities. As a result, you and your EMS agency are in a unique position to identify at-risk situations in the course of your day-to-day operations. One study found that paramedics were able to screen for dangerous levels of carbon monoxide within a residence by using a hand-held meter. In fact, occult elevations in carbon monoxide levels were found in 3% of homes (Jaslow et al., 2001).

Paramedics also have the opportunity during their interactions with patients to observe potential issues that affect patient health and well-being. For instance, the circumstances in which prehospital patients are found may suggest problems with their physical or emotional well-being. In the course of a prolonged transport time, and after the patient has been stabilized, you may use the additional time to assess the patient's risk factors for problems such as cardiovascular disease or diabetes and to suggest the need for follow-up care. Prehospital professionals also may branch into less-common areas for screening. For example, brief assessments, sometimes limited to one or two questions, may determine whether a patient is at risk for domestic violence, alcohol abuse, or depression (Weiss et al., 2000; Canagasaby & Vinson, 2005; Williams & Vinson, 2001; Bradley et al., 2003; Dill et al., 2004; Corson et al., 2004).

However, the literature suggests that in many cases EMS professionals do not recognize such opportunities. This may even be the case in instances of abuse when patients are in imminent danger. A study of paramedic reporting of child abuse found that 60% of paramedics had no training in the formal recognition of child abuse; although 60% claimed to have reported a case, only one third did so to the correct authorities. The authors of that study concluded that paramedics lack an understanding of their role in the identification and reporting of child abuse (King et al., 1993). Similar findings were noted in a study of elder abuse. A Michigan study noted that although nearly 70% of EMS professionals said they had come across a suspected case of elder abuse or negligence in the prior year, only 27% reported the case to authorities. More than 90% of those surveyed said they had received no formal instruction in elder abuse during their EMS training (Jones et al., 1995). An opportunity clearly exists to enhance the training of EMS staff in identifying hazards to the well-being of those who cannot care for themselves. Training modules, such as one developed to aid rural EMS providers in identifying victims of domestic violence, are a required part of expanding the EMS professional's capabilities to assist those in need (Hall & Becker, 2002).

As emphasized, the training of paramedics in the use of screening methods can be enhanced. In addition, tools to help paramedics follow up on positive results must accompany the use of screening systems. These tools can include such items as referral lists or inventories of community resources to be given to the patient who is at risk. Although the EMS system is not responsible for developing, funding, or scheduling the follow-up plan, the EMS agency must give patients the tools to access the system when they have been identified to be at risk. Moreover, the EMS agency must notify community resources of potential referrals.

EDUCATION

One of the unique aspects of public health is its stated desire to eliminate the need for its services altogether. To illustrate this point, in an environment in which health is optimal, no need for public health would exist. EMS providers share this worldview. In fact, they work hard to educate the community about preventive issues in acute care.

Injury prevention has long been a key focus of EMS interactions with the public. These activities may be formal or informal in nature. The formal part of community education may consist of appearances at health fairs, speeches to community groups, and classroom interactions with schoolchildren. Other examples of formal education include the distribution of bicycle helmets, the use of motor vehicle crash simulators, and the provision of infant and child car seat installation checks. Prehospital providers have initiated many excellent injury prevention programs. Nonetheless, although the majority of EMS providers recognize injury prevention as a core mission of EMS, in practice only an estimated one third of EMS professionals try to educate patients about ways to avoid injury-prone behaviors. Moreover, less than 20% provide instruction on the use

of protective devices. Furthermore, more than one third received no formal instruction of any kind on injury prevention during their training (Jaslow et al., 2003). The EMS system clearly can play a much larger role in injury prevention education.

The informal aspect of public education is perhaps the most effective. This consists of the EMS professional taking advantage of the teachable moment. This moment is that time when people are most open to receiving a health education message. For EMS patients and their families, that moment occurs just after an acute event, when the sense of distress and danger is still very real. At that moment the role of the EMT or paramedic as a caregiver and protector is the strongest. Approaching the patient in a nonjudgmental way during these moments can sometimes be difficult. However, the teachable moment is a time when you can penetrate an individual's usual facade and reach his or her core values.

Another activity that falls under the banner of education is advocacy. In essence, advocacy is education at the level of the policymaker. EMS agencies have an obligation to address issues relevant to their scope of work. Challenges such as seat belt laws, alcohol use, violence, and gun safety are too close to the heart of EMS to be ignored. EMS support of legislation and rules to combat these ills will have a significant impact on public health. As an advocate, you must serve as a role model of the behaviors you espouse.

Case Scenario—continued

The patient's pupils are equal, round, and react to light and accommodation. Chest movement is symmetric and breath sounds are equal. His pulse is 100 beats/min, blood pressure is 90/78 mm Hg, and respiratory rate is 24 breaths/min. He denies any significant major illness other than the TB diagnosis. He does not take any prescription drugs on a regular basis, although he does admit to consuming large quantities of alcohol daily. The patient clearly is underweight. The results of the remainder of the physical examination are within normal ranges.

Questions

5. *Should this patient be isolated? Why or why not?*
6. *How should the coughing be controlled?*
7. *What is the clinical significance of bloody sputum?*
8. *What additional treatment should be provided?*

ACCESS TO PERSONAL HEALTHCARE

[OBJECTIVE 3]

Public health services are not obligated to provide individual healthcare. However, as trustees of the public, they do have a strong desire to ensure that all people have access to care. Expanded EMS scopes of care can help accomplish this goal. EMS agencies can use their stations as community health resources. As such, they can provide medication compliance checks, blood pressure and blood

sugar measurements, and chronic wound care on site. This helps alleviate the need for more costly visiting nurse, physician, and hospital visits.

EMS agencies also may participate in home health visits, providing wound care, assessing the status of home intravenous or injection therapy, and performing well-being checks on those identified by their physicians as at particularly high risk. These actions expand access to healthcare services within the community and also may decrease individual morbidity and mortality rates, prevent healthcare costs that arise from preventable hospitalization, and lessen the overall burden of disease on society. Prehospital personnel also may serve as a cost-effective supplement to hospital emergency department or nursing care staff. In addition, through these activities EMS professionals help build themselves a clinical career ladder as they gain more skills. These activities make them better mentors and teachers and ease any future transition into other health professions. The development of such a career ladder may enhance retention of the EMS professional. As a result, in some states the board of EMS has worked with the nursing profession and educators to develop an articulation plan that would create bidirectional education mobility for registered nurses and paramedics in the state. For example, the Kansas Board of EMS, partnering with members of the Council for Nursing Articulation in Kansas, created a process through which nursing and paramedic programs could cooperate to facilitate the educational progress of graduates from one program to the other with minimal loss of academic credit and duplication of coursework.

Fiscal concerns understandably exist regarding exploring enhanced EMS roles in the provision of nonacute healthcare services. However, the consideration of how much downtime a service has to perform these activities is important, especially in light of the fixed costs required to maintain an EMS presence whether or not the station or unit is currently active in response. Given that EMS salary scales generally are lower than those of other health professionals and the services of EMS are accordingly less expensive, reimbursement opportunities are possible through creative contracting with hospitals, managed care agencies, or other third-party payers. As the volumes of these expanded scope services build and revenues rise accordingly, EMS may find that devoting staff and resources exclusively to these activities during the workday is financially viable.

EMERGENCY PREPAREDNESS

[OBJECTIVE 4]

Preparing for mass casualty incidents has long been a part of EMS operations. However, the events of September 11, 2001, have sharpened the world's focus on **all-hazards emergency preparedness.** The term *all hazards* refers to a cross-cutting approach in which all forms of emergencies, including manmade and natural disasters, epidemics, and physical and biologic terrorism, are managed from a common template that uses consistent language and structure.

A combination of statutory changes, funding streams, and public and political pressure has driven the EMS, law enforcement, and public health communities to work more closely together than ever before. Nonetheless, the manner in which each discipline views the typical emergency incident differs. In general, EMS systems view preparedness as responding to transient and time-limited situations (a classic mass casualty incident) that tempo-

rarily stress the medical care system but have minimal aftereffects on capabilities or infrastructure. By way of contrast, public health agencies adopt a longer term view of preparedness. They focus on the prolonged incident (such as the multiple waves of pandemic influenza) and prolonged recovery periods (as seen in the 2004 hurricanes). Because of these differences in outlook, as well as a traditional independence from each other and infrastructures that often are incompatible, EMS and public health must work together to enhance understanding and promote working relationships well in advance of when an actual emergency arises (Lerner et al., 2005; O'Connor et al., 2004). Only through such advanced preparation will these two professions be able to work together at an optimal level during an actual emergency situation.

Many jurisdictions in the United States use an emergency management model that designates service realms as an **emergency service function (ESF)**. In general, the ESF related to health and medical care is headed by the appropriate state or local health officer. During a time of activation of the local emergency management system, EMS often functions in a subsidiary role to public health within this ESF. Although these lines of command often are blurred in an acute event, during prolonged states of emergency the relationship changes dramatically. Public health authorities may order EMS to assume unaccustomed or nontraditional roles to serve the greater needs of the community. For example, during the Florida hurricane season of 2004, EMS units were used to transport patients with special healthcare needs from homes to shelters and back before and after the storms, move supplies between shelters and within the community, help acquire outside healthcare resources, supply medical gases to oxygen-dependent patients, and conduct on-scene surveys of storm damage. The expanded roles of EMS personnel, especially as primary care providers, also were evident during the sheltering phase of the 2005 response to Hurricanes Katrina and Rita. As provisions were made to house evacuees at sites throughout the United States, EMS agencies transferred displaced persons from staging to reception points, performed medical screening examinations on evacuees, and served in primary care roles as on-site shelter medical staff.

Emergency conditions also require EMS to make changes in its operational philosophies. Prehospital providers may need to stop responding to emergency calls because of staffing or environmental conditions, and they may have to alter triage and transport protocols during times of high demand or lack of personnel. Such changes in the basic functions of EMS must be coordinated with the remainder of the healthcare system to use limited resources in the best possible fashion.

The role of **epidemiology** in emergency preparedness is often overlooked. Taken broadly, epidemiology is the study of the prevalence and spread of disease in a community. In the context of preparedness, it is the ability to interpret incidence and prevalence data to determine the cause, geographic source, and nature of an imminent threat to public health. The earlier a potential biohazard can be detected, the sooner it can be traced to its source and those likely to be at risk can be identified and treated. One manner in which EMS can assist this public health effort is by using dispatch data as a form of syndromic surveillance. In a syndromic surveillance system, information regarding the number and nature of medical cases is compared with an expected volume of calls for the community at a given time and place. If cases exceed the expected volumes, epidemiologists are alerted to the possibility of an outbreak of disease. Consequently, they can promptly begin the investigation process. The speed with which an outbreak can be identified is crucial to the effective management of bioterror incidents, for which a limited amount of time is available to begin vaccination or antibiotic prophylaxis procedures. Since 1998, New York City EMS has piloted a syndromic surveillance system. It has found the system to be useful in monitoring rises in flulike illness as a simulation for a bioterror incident (Greenko et al., 2003).

In addition to investigating an outbreak, public healthcare agencies use the tools of isolation and quarantine to help prevent the spread of disease. These terms describe different public health processes. **Isolation** refers to the seclusion of individuals with an illness to prevent the transmission to others. In contrast, **quarantine** pertains to the seclusion of entire groups of exposed but asymptomatic individuals for monitoring (*Dorland's Illustrated Medical Dictionary*, 2003). Both processes present unique challenges for EMS staff (Erich, 2004). A pilot project in New York City successfully tested the ability of a prehospital system to prevent the transmission of disease by using isolation procedures during field care and transport (Erich, 2004). Experiences in Canada during the 2003 severe acute respiratory syndrome epidemic demonstrated the ability of EMS to assist in this endeavor as well. During that epidemic, a provincial transfer center was established to manage patient movement between hospital facilities to prevent the further spread of the illness. As a result of the screening, command, and control processes, no cases of severe acute respiratory syndrome resulted from interfacility transport, and up to 13 new cases were discovered by clinical criteria before transport (MacDonald et al., 2004).

Case Scenario CONCLUSION

The paramedic team follows local protocol for airborne protection from infectious diseases, donning the appropriate filtration masks and protective clothing. The patient is placed on oxygen by nonrebreather mask at 15 L/min and given a box of tissues and container to place them in. The paramedics alert the emergency department team regarding the diagnosis of TB. On arrival at the emergency department, the paramedics are directed to take the patient to a special isolation cubicle. The patient's mental status is unchanged. His vital signs remain stable.

Looking Back

9. *What actions should be taken to reduce the risk of a community outbreak of TB?*

COST CONTAINMENT

[OBJECTIVE 5]

To ensure that all persons can access healthcare, public health has an interest in making sure that finite resources serve the maximal number of clients. Cost containment is a critical element in the effective use of resources, and EMS can play an important role in this endeavor. Although many EMS systems pursue cost-containment measures for their own fiscal benefit and to decrease staff workload, the overall impact of these efforts on the healthcare system cannot be overlooked.

One of the most dramatic ways in which EMS systems might address cost containment is through revising the traditional paradigm of "triage, treatment, and transport." Some services are experimenting with the idea of triaging callers. With this concept, those who call EMS dispatch centers would possibly be referred to alternate, less-costly forms of care rather than summon EMS response and hospital transport. The Canadian province of Nova Scotia has taken this idea one step further and introduced the concept of primary care paramedic, as previously described. By providing nontransport preventive and primary care services as part of a paramedic-based integrated care model on two remote islands in the province, hospitalizations of residents of the islands were reduced 23% over a 3-year study period (Emergency Health Services, 2006). The published results of alternate triage mechanisms have been mixed, but the process of developing a standardized methodology to explore this issue has begun (Dale et al., 2004; Neely et al., 2000; Schmidt et al., 2003; Schmidt et al., 2004).

Of note, the patient's ability to pay for services may, in and of itself, affect the quality of EMS care. A study in

Canada concluded that a policy that required patients to be billed for the services EMS provided had an adverse effect on patient acceptance of care and outcomes as well as on the actions and attitudes of the EMS provider. The results indicated that the goal of equitable EMS care for all persons was placed at risk when patients were held liable for their bills (Rothe, 2004). EMS must take care that the requirements for reimbursement and the desire for cost containment do not jeopardize the core public service mission of prehospital care.

Case Scenario SUMMARY

1. *What is your general impression of this patient?* Despite the emaciated appearance of the patient, he is stable with warm, wet skin and good mental status. His most apparent high-risk problem is the possibility of active TB as well as the potential for spreading active TB throughout the shelter. TB is a disease caused by bacteria *(Mycobacterium tuberculosis)*. The disease usually affects the lungs but can attack any part of the body, including the brain and the kidneys. If not treated properly, TB can be fatal. TB is an airborne infection, meaning it is spread through the air when the infected person talks, laughs, coughs, or sneezes. People near the infected person can breathe in the airborne bacteria and become infected. The bacteria also are spread by contact with door handles, toilet seats, or handshaking. TB bacteria can float in the air for several hours. Sometimes people can have latent TB—a condition in which they are infected with the bacteria but do not show any signs and symptoms and cannot spread the disease. However, people with latent TB may develop an active case of TB. People with active TB can be treated and cured if they seek medical help. You realize that you will be in contact with the patient for only a short period, using appropriate airborne infection control methods, whereas the other persons in the shelter have been exposed to the patient for hours. You recognize that you have a public health situation that must be dealt with appropriately.

2. *What physical assessment findings are most pertinent at this time?* Signs and symptoms associated with active TB are persistent coughing, bloody sputum, weight loss, night sweats, and chills.

3. *What is the significance of his noncompliance with the medication regimen?* TB usually can be treated with a course of common, or first-line, TB drugs. Patients who do not comply with the medication regimen can develop a strain of TB resistant to the most common TB medications. This is called multi-drug-resistant TB (MDR-TB). MDR-TB takes longer to treat with second-line drugs. In some cases in which patients continue to be noncompliant with medication regimens, extensively drug-resistant TB (XDR-TB) can develop. Because XDR-TB is resistant to first-line and second-line drugs, chances of cure are low. Patients can transmit the drug-resistant forms of TB to others in the same environment.

4. *What treatment should be immediately initiated?* In addition to the care providers using adequate respiratory protection, an appropriate respiratory protection mask should be placed on the patient. High-flow oxygen and strict adherence to airborne infection protocol must be followed. The patient must be removed from the shelter and isolated. Particulate filter respirators certified by the Centers for Disease Control and Prevention's National Institute for Occupational Safety and Health that can be used for protection against airborne *M. tuberculosis* include nonpowered respirators with N95, N99, N100, R95, R99, R100, P95, P99, and P100 filters (including disposable respirators) and powered air-purifying respirators with high-efficiency filters.

5. *Should this patient be isolated? Why or why not?* Yes. TB is a highly contagious airborne pathogen. Although the chances of infecting others depend on many factors, including environmental and underlying health status of those exposed, TB is a major public health threat.

6. *How should the coughing be controlled?* Humidified oxygen may offer some relief to the patient. Placing the patient in a position of comfort also is important.

7. *What is the clinical significance of the bloody sputum?* Bloody sputum combined with weight loss, night sweats, and persistent cough is indicative of active TB.

8. *What additional treatment should be provided?* High-flow oxygen should be continued and his respiratory status monitored. He should be transported to a healthcare facility to be assessed for the presence of active TB. The local health department must provide testing for anyone who was exposed to this patient.

9. *What actions should be taken to reduce the risk of a community outbreak of TB?* In addition to appropriate healthcare for the patient (quickly recognizing the possibility of active TB and taking appropriate protective and containment actions), the local health department should be notified of the possibility of exposure to TB in the homeless shelter's population and volunteers. In most communities the local health department would assume responsibility for contacting potentially exposed individuals for follow-up.

Chapter Summary

- Health is a state of complete physical, mental, and social well-being and not merely the absence of disease or infirmity.
- Public health can be defined as the science and practice of protecting and improving the health of a community.
- In the United States, public health services are provided through various means. At the federal level, public health services are a core function of the Department of Health and Human Services. This agency serves the public health community.
- The role of a public health agency is to prevent and control communicable disease and promote health.
- One of the most visible ways in which EMS professionals have interacted with public health agencies is through the provision of immunizations. EMS personnel also are well positioned to screen the population for the presence or absence of disease, recognize evidence of abuse or addiction, and educate the public on matters of public health and safety.
- EMS professionals are ideally suited to reach at-risk populations because of the credibility of EMS in the community as well as their inherent mobility. EMS stations often are located in areas of ready community access.
- Public health services are not obligated to provide individual healthcare; however, a strong desire exists to ensure that all people have access to care. Expanded EMS scopes of care can help accomplish this goal.
- EMS personnel have the opportunity to enhance access to care by using EMS stations as community health resources. Examples include providing medication compliance checks, blood pressure and blood sugar measurements, and chronic wound care on site.
- EMS agencies also may participate in home health visits, providing wound care, assessing the status of home intravenous or injection therapy, and performing well-being checks on those identified by their physicians as at particularly high risk.
- Prehospital personnel also may serve as a cost-effective supplement to hospital emergency department or nursing care staff.
- The EMS, law enforcement, and public health communities must work more closely together than ever before to be prepared for all-hazard emergencies.
- EMS systems generally view preparedness as responding to transient and time-limited situations that temporarily stress the medical care system but have minimal aftereffects on capabilities or infrastructure. In contrast, public health agencies adopt a longer term view of preparedness, focusing on the prolonged incident (such as the multiple waves of pandemic influenza) and prolonged recovery periods (as seen in the 2005 hurricanes). Because of these differences, EMS and public health must work together to enhance understanding and promote working relationships well in advance of when an actual emergency arises.
- Many jurisdictions in the United States use an emergency management model that designates service realms as an ESF.
- Epidemiology is the study of the prevalence and spread of disease in a community. In the context of preparedness, it is the ability to interpret incidence and prevalence data to determine the cause, geographic source, and nature of an imminent threat to public health. The earlier a potential biohazard can be detected, the sooner it can be traced to its source and those likely to be at risk can be identified and treated.
- Public health care agencies use the tools of isolation and quarantine to help prevent the spread of disease. Isolation refers to the seclusion of individuals with an illness to prevent transmission to others. Quarantine pertains to the seclusion of entire groups of exposed but asymptomatic individuals for monitoring.
- EMS systems may be able to address cost containment by revising the traditional paradigm of "triage, treatment, and transport." Some services are experimenting with the idea of triaging callers. With this concept, those who call EMS dispatch centers may be referred to alternate, less-costly forms of care rather than summon EMS response and hospital transport. In Nova Scotia, primary care paramedics treat patients on site when possible, reducing the need for transport and hospitalization.
- EMS personnel must take care that the requirements for reimbursement and the desire for cost containment do not jeopardize the core public service mission of prehospital care.

REFERENCES

The American heritage dictionary of the English language (4th ed.). (2004). Boston: Houghton Mifflin Company.

Bradley, K. A., Bush, K. R., Epler, A. J., Dobie, D. J., Davis, T. M., Sporleder, J. L., et al. (2003). Two brief alcohol-screening tests from the Alcohol Use Disorders Identification Test (AUDIT): Validation in a female Veterans Affairs patient population. Archives of Internal Medicine, 163(7), 821-829.

Canagasaby, A., & Vinson, D. C. (2005). Screening for hazardous or harmful drinking using one or two quantity-frequency questions. Alcohol, 40(3), 208-213.

Corson, K., Gerrity, M. S., & Dobscha, S. K. (2004). Screening for depression and suicidality in a VA primary care setting: 2 items are better than 1 item. American Journal of Managed Care, 10(11 pt 2), 839-845.

Dale, J., Williams, S., Foster, T., Higgins, J., Snooks, H., Crouch, R., et al. (2004). Safety of telephone consultation for "non-serious" emergency ambulance service patients. *Quality and Safety in Health Care, 13*(5), 363-373.

Dill, P. L., Wells-Parker, E., & Soderstrom, C. A. (2004). The emergency care setting for screening and intervention for alcohol use problems among injured and high-risk drivers: A review. *Traffic Injury Prevention, 5*(3), 278-291.

Dorland's illustrated medical dictionary (30th ed.) (pp. 957-1557). (2003). Philadelphia: W. B. Saunders.

Emergency Health Services. (2006). *Community paramedicine: A part of an integrated health care system*. Retrieved January 30, 2008, from http://www.gov.ns.ca.

Erich, J. (2004). Quarantine angst. What it might mean for EMS, public health. *Emergency Medical Services, 33*(5), 66.

Greenko, J., Mostashari, F., Fine, A., & Layton, M. (2003). Clinical evaluation of the emergency medical services (EMS) ambulance dispatch-based syndromic surveillance system, New York City. *Journal of Urban Health, 80*(2 suppl 1), 50-56.

Hall, M., & Becker, V. (2002). The front lines of domestic violence. Training model for rural EMS personnel. *Journal of Psychosocial Nursing and Mental Health Services, 40*(9), 40-48.

Halverson, P. K., Kaluzny, A. D., & McLaughlin, C. P. (1998). *Managed care & public health* (pp. 11-41), Gaithersburg, MD: Aspen.

Hostler, D., Milspaw, J., & Paris, P. M. (2003). Pneumococcal vaccination: An opportunity for emergency medical services. *Prehospital Emergency Care, 7*(1), 125-135.

Jaslow, D., Ufberg, J., & Marsh, R. (2003). Primary injury prevention in an urban EMS system. *Journal of Emergency Medicine, 25*(2), 167-170.

Jaslow, D., Ufberg, J., Ukaskik, J., & Sananman, P. (2001). Routine carbon monoxide screening by emergency medical technicians. *Academy of Emergency Medicine, 8*(3), 288-291.

Jones, J. S., Walker, G., & Krohmer, J. R. (1995). To report or not to report: Emergency services response to elder abuse. *Prehospital Disaster Medicine, 10*(2), 96-100.

King, B. R., Baker, M. D., & Ludwig, S. (1993). Reporting of child abuse by prehospital personnel. *Prehospital Disaster Medicine, 8*(1), 67-68.

Lerner, E. B., Billittier, A. J. IV, O'Connor, R. E., Allswede, M. P., Blackwell, T. H., Wang, H. E., et al. (2005). Linkages of acute care and EMS to state and local public health programs: Application to public health programs. *Journal of Public Health Management Practices, 11*(4), 291-297.

MacDonald, R. D., Farr, B., Neill, M., Loch, J., Sawadsky, B., Mazza, C., et al. (2004). An emergency medical services transfer authorization center in response to the Toronto severe acute respiratory syndrome outbreak. *Prehospital Emergency Care, 8*(2), 223-231.

Mosesso, V. N. Jr., Packer, C., McMahon, J., Auble, T. E., & Paris, P. M. (2003). Influenza immunizations provided by EMS agencies: The MEDICVAX Project. *Prehospital Emergency Care, 7*(1), 74-78.

Neely, K. W., Eldurkar, J., & Drake, M. E. (2000). Can current EMS dispatch protocols identify layperson reported sentinel conditions? *Prehospital Emergency Care, 4*(3), 238-244.

O'Connor, R. E., Lerner, E. B., Allswede, M., Billittier, A. J. IV, Blackwell, T., Hunt, R. C., et al. (2004). Linkages of acute care and emergency medical services to state and local public health programs: The role of interactive information systems for responding to events resulting in mass injury. *Prehospital Emergency Care, 8*(3), 237-253.

Rothe, J. P. (2004). Patient payment for emergency medical services treatment and its impact on injury control: An Alberta case. *Injury Control and Safety Promotion, 11*(4), 291-295.

Schmidt, T. A., Cone, D. C., & Mann, N. C. (2004). Criteria currently used to evaluate dispatch triage systems: Where do they leave us? *Prehospital Emergency Care, 8*(2), 126-129.

Schmidt, T., Neely, K. W., Adams, A. L., Newgard, C. D., Wittwer, L., Muhr, M., et al. (2003). Is it possible to safely triage callers to EMS dispatch centers to alternative resources? *Prehospital Emergency Care, 7*(3), 368-374.

Shah, M. N., Brooke Lerner, E., Chiumento, S., & Davis, E. A. (2004). An evaluation of paramedics' ability to screen older adults during emergency responses. *Prehospital Emergency Care, 8*(3), 298-303.

Weiss, S., Garza, A., Casaletto, J., Stratton, M., Ernst, A., Blanton, D., et al. (2000). The out-of-hospital use of domestic violence screen for assessing patient risk. *Prehospital Emergency Care, 4*(1), 24-27.

Williams, R., & Vinson, D. C. (2001). Validation of a single screening question for problem drinking. *Journal of Family Practice, 50*(4), 307-312.

World Health Organization. (2006). *About WHO*. Retrieved January 30, 2008, from http://www.who.int.

SUGGESTED RESOURCES

General

National Association of State EMS Officials: http://www.nasemsd.org

National Rural and Frontier Emergency Medical Services Agenda for the Future: http://www.nrharural.org/groups/sub/EMS.html

Office of Emergency Medical Services, National Highway Traffic Safety Administration: http://www.nhtsa.dot.gov/portal/site/nhtsa/menuitem.2a0771e91315babbbf30811060008a0c

Office of Rural Health Policy, Rural Emergency Medical Services & Trauma Technical Assistance Center: http://www.ruralhealth.hrsa.gov/ruralems

Immunizations

Journal Watch. *Influenza vaccine by EMS: An ounce of prevention is worth a pound of cure:* http://emergency-medicine.jwatch.org/cgi/content/citation/2003/514/7

New Hampshire Department of Safety, Division of Fire Standards and Training and Emergency Medical Services. *Immunization program:* http://www.nh.gov/safety/divisions/fstems/ems/documents/NHEMSImmunizationProgram1.pdf

Healthy Housing

Centers for Disease Control and Prevention Healthy Homes Initiative: http://www.cdc.gov/healthyplaces/healthyhomes.htm

National Center for Healthy Housing: http://www.centerforhealthyhousing.org

Screening for Alcohol Abuse

AlcoholScreening.org, Boston University School of Public Health: http://alcoholscreening.org

Medical College of Wisconsin Healthlink. *Screening for alcoholism and alcohol use disorders,* http://healthlink.mcw.edu/article/1031002170.html

Screening for Child Abuse and Domestic Violence

Child Welfare Information Gateway. *Identification, screening, and assessment of child abuse and neglect,* http://www.childwelfare.gov/systemwide/assessment/family_assess/id_can/index.cfm

Injury Prevention

Florida Department of Health. *Injury prevention and control,* http://www.doh.state.fl.us/Workforce/ems1/InjuryPrevention/injurypreventhome.html#Florida%20Injury%20Prevention%20Programs

Kansas Department of Health and Environment. *Injury disability and prevention programs:* http://www.kdheks.gov/idp

Chapter Quiz

1. According to the World Health Organization, how can health be defined?

   _____
   _____
   _____

2. How does the provision of personal healthcare differ from the practice of public health?

   _____
   _____
   _____

3. Who is responsible for public health at a local level?

   _____
   _____
   _____

4. What two advances have improved the quality of health and life expectancy in the United States the most in the past century?

   _____
   _____
   _____

5. Why should EMS participate in immunization campaigns?

   _____
   _____
   _____

6. EMS providers often have the unique chance to identify problems in the community setting. Are EMS personnel trained in identifying child abuse and neglect?

   _____
   _____
   _____

7. What is all-hazards preparedness?

   _____
   _____
   _____

8. Describe syndromic surveillance.

   _____
   _____
   _____

9. What is the difference between isolation and quarantine?

   _____
   _____
   _____

10. How might EMS help control health system costs?

   _____
   _____
   _____

Terminology

All-hazards emergency preparedness A cross-cutting approach in which all forms of emergencies, including manmade and natural disasters, epidemics, and physical and biologic terrorism, are managed from a common template that uses consistent language and structure.

Emergency service function (ESF) A grouping of government and certain private sector capabilities into an organizational structure to provide the support, resources, program implementation, and services most likely to be needed to save lives, protect property and the environment, restore essential services and critical infrastructure, and help victims and communities return to normal, when feasible, after domestic incidents.

Epidemiology The study of the prevalence and spread of disease in a community.

Health A state of complete physical, mental, and social well-being, not merely the absence of disease or infirmity.

Isolation The seclusion of individuals with an illness to prevent transmission to others.

Public health The discipline that studies the overall health of populations and intervenes on behalf of those populations rather than on behalf of individuals.

Quarantine The seclusion of groups of exposed but asymptomatic individuals for monitoring.

PHARMACOLOGY

Basic Principles of Pharmacology

Objectives *After completing this chapter, you will be able to:*

1. Describe historic trends in pharmacology.
2. Differentiate the chemical, generic, and trade names of a drug.
3. List the main sources of drug products.
4. Describe how drugs are classified.
5. List the authoritative sources for drug information.
6. List legislative acts controlling drug use and abuse in the United States.
7. Differentiate Schedule I, II, III, IV, and V substances and list examples of each.
8. Discuss standardization of drugs.
9. Discuss investigational drugs, including the Food and Drug Administration approval process and classifications for newly approved drugs.
10. Discuss the paramedic's responsibilities and scope of management pertinent to the administration of medications.
11. Review the specific anatomy and physiology pertinent to pharmacology with additional attention to autonomic pharmacology.
12. List and describe general properties of drugs.
13. List and describe liquid and solid drug forms.
14. List and differentiate routes of drug administration, including the enteral and parenteral routes.
15. Describe the mechanisms of drug action.
16. List and differentiate the phases of drug activity, including the pharmaceutical, pharmacokinetic, and pharmacodynamic phases.
17. Describe the processes of pharmacokinetics and pharmacodynamics, including theories of drug action, drug-response relation, factors altering drug responses, predictable drug responses, iatrogenic drug responses, and unpredictable adverse drug responses.
18. Discuss special considerations in drug treatment regarding pregnant, pediatric, and geriatric patients.
19. Differentiate drug interactions.
20. Discuss considerations for storing and securing medications.
21. List the components of a drug profile by classification.

Chapter Outline

Historic Trends in Pharmacology
Drug Names
Sources Of Drugs
Drug Classification
Sources of Drug Information
United States Drug Legislation
Standardization of Drugs
Investigational Drugs
Scope of Management
Autonomic Pharmacology

General Properties of Drugs
Drug Forms
Routes of Medication Administration
Mechanisms of Drug Action
Special Considerations in Drug Therapy
Drug Interactions
Drug Storage
Components of a Drug Profile
Chapter Summary

1906- Pure Food & Drug Act

Case Scenario

Your ambulance co-responds with the basic life support fire department to a college dormitory for an "unconscious person." When you arrive, you find a crowd gathered around a 20-year-old woman in the parking lot. She appears unconscious and has profound central and peripheral cyanosis. Two individuals are performing chest compressions and mouth-to-mouth ventilation. You ask that they stop compressions and ventilations so you can perform a primary survey. You discover that she has a slow, faint carotid pulse with no respiratory effort. Your partner and a fire department EMT place an oral airway and then begin bag-mask ventilation. They inform you that lung compliance is poor and that they "can't get very much air in."

Questions

1. What is your general impression of this patient? What treatment will you initiate before continuing your assessment?
2. What potential causes can you think of for the profound cyanosis, respiratory arrest, poor lung compliance, and difficulty in ventilating?
3. What medications might be appropriate to treat the list of potential causes in the previous question?

A **drug** is any substance (other than a food or device) intended for use in the diagnosis, cure, relief, treatment, or prevention of disease or to affect the structure or function of the human body or other animals. **Pharmacology** is the study of drugs, including their actions and effects on the host. In EMS the most important concern is how medications affect human beings. Pharmacology is one of the most advanced and exciting areas of study in medicine. The application and administration of drugs for therapeutic use is entrusted to you as a paramedic. This chapter provides information about the many factors that affect drugs and their applications. The purpose of this chapter is to examine the complex interactions among drug molecules and how they affect the human body.

HISTORIC TRENDS IN PHARMACOLOGY

Ancient Healthcare

[OBJECTIVE 1]

Healers in ancient civilizations believed that illness and disease were caused by hostile sorcerers or evil spirits living in the body. The healing process often involved the use of potions, religious rituals, and crude surgeries. Substances used in healing often were discovered by trial and error. Greater understanding eventually developed that some of the substances used to treat illness had the power to cure it, without the use of rituals or surgery. The information learned was passed on orally to the next generation. The oldest prescriptions known were found inscribed on a clay tablet, written by a Sumerian physician nearly 5000 years ago in what is now known as Iraq.

The Greco-Roman people used many substances in medicinal practices. Asclepius is considered the Greek god of healing. He and his family represented health. His wife, Epione, soothed pain. His daughter Hygeia was the goddess of health and represented the prevention of disease. Another daughter, Panacea, represented treatment. They combined religion and healing in a temple setting to cure the rich and poor of their illnesses. Hippocrates, commonly called the father of medicine, advanced the ideas that disease results from natural causes and the body has the ability to heal itself.

Claudius Galen (AD 131-201) is recognized as the father of pharmacy. He was a Greek physician in Rome who was also a teacher, philosopher, pharmacist, and scientist. Galen believed that illness was caused by an imbalance of blood, phlegm, black bile, and yellow bile. He also believed that blood was continuously being made and used up. To rid the body of disease, he used bloodletting and medicines he prepared from animal and vegetable extracts.

The Renaissance

After the fall of the Roman Empire, medicine in some areas of the world reverted to folklore and tradition. Muslims settling in Egypt, Spain, North Africa, and other areas of the world combined their knowledge of math and science with that of the Greek, Roman, and Jewish people. They introduced many new drugs and preparations, developing formularies. A **formulary** is a book that contains a list of medicinal substances with their formulas, uses, and methods of preparation. These formularies represented the first sets of drug standards. During the same period, religious orders built monasteries. Monasteries became sites for learning, including pharmacy and medicine.

Although the Spanish Emperor Frederick II declared pharmacy separate from medicine in 1240, it was not recognized as a separate specialty until the sixteenth century when the first pharmacopeia was written. A **pharmacopeia** is a book describing drugs, chemicals, and medicinal preparations in a country or specific geographic area. It usually contains information about all approved drugs within an area or country, including a description of the drug, its formula, and **dosage.** Frederick II drafted laws that limited ownership of apothecary shops (pharmaceutical houses) to licensed pharmacists. He also required that drug preparation be overseen by inspectors.

The use of medicines grew during the Renaissance. Paracelsus, a professor of physics and surgery, challenged the beliefs of Galen. Paracelsus believed that illness was the result of the body being attacked by outside agents. He recommended and introduced the use of specific remedies to fight disease. By the seventeenth century, belladonna (later the base of atropine) was being used to treat nausea and vomiting. In eighteenth century England, purple foxglove was one of 20 herbs used in a folk remedy to treat dropsy (excessive swelling). Digitalis, a cardiac glycoside, is derived from the leaves of this plant and is still used today to treat heart failure.

Knowledge of pharmacy, chemistry, physiology, and medicine grew during the nineteenth century. Scientists learned to isolate active ingredients from plants and previously known drugs. Opium was isolated from the flowers of the poppy. Morphine, derived from opium, was used to treat severe pain and is still used today. The antimalarial compound quinine was isolated from the bark of the cinchona tree. Research focused on the effects of active ingredients on the body's organs and tissues. Understanding of the sites of drug action increased and drug dosages became more precise.

Modern Healthcare

Pharmaceutical laws were enacted at the end of the nineteenth and early twentieth centuries to protect the public. Many drugs were developed in the early 1900s that improved the treatment of chronic illnesses. Phenobarbital was discovered and used to treat epilepsy. The treatment of diabetes improved with the development of insulin. Tetanus antitoxin was used during World War I. The discovery of penicillin in the mid 1940s changed the treatment of some bacterial infections. World War II demonstrated the success of early penicillin administration. With the use of penicillin, the loss of life from poor sanitary conditions and large wounds was significantly reduced.

The last 50 years of the twentieth century and the beginning of the twenty-first century have brought about more changes in the area of pharmacology than any other time in history. Today, many different medications exist to improve, suppress, or change body functions.

PARAMEDIC*Pearl*

As a paramedic, you are authorized to give specific medications for specific conditions under the direction of a physician. When used properly, these medications contribute to the advanced medical care you give in the field.

The Present Period of Change

EMS is constantly evolving. Pharmacology is one area of constant development and research. Throughout your paramedic career, you must keep abreast of new medications and technology. This includes medications you give to your patients, new medications your patients may be taking, and new ways in which medications may be packaged or administered.

Healthcare consumers are taking responsibility for their health and disease prevention. This includes educating themselves about signs and symptoms of disease and medication safety. As a healthcare professional, you often will be asked questions about the medications patients are taking or those you give them in the course of care. This means you must know the uses of all drugs that you carry as well as common patient medications. You also must be able to recognize side effects and adverse reactions.

Researchers continually discover new treatments, cures, and methods to prevent disease. **Orphan drugs** are medicines developed for the diagnosis and/or treatment of rare diseases or conditions (Box 11-1). This term was designated by the U.S. Food and Drug Administration (FDA) when the Orphan Drug Act was signed into law on January 4, 1983. As understanding of illness and disease grows, new treatments and medications will be tested and better understood.

BOX 11-1 | **Diseases or Conditions for Which Orphan Drugs Are Being Developed**

- Sickle cell anemia
- Cystic fibrosis
- Amyotrophic lateral sclerosis (Lou Gehrig's disease)
- Tourette syndrome
- Hemophilia
- Acute respiratory distress syndrome
- Juvenile rheumatoid arthritis
- Muscular dystrophy
- Non-Hodgkin lymphoma
- Stomach, pancreatic, and ovarian cancer
- Huntington chorea
- Multiple myeloma

DRUG NAMES

[OBJECTIVE 2]

Chemical Name

The **chemical name** is a precise description of the drug's chemical composition and molecular structure.

Official Name

A drug's **official name** is the name listed in the *United States Pharmacopoeia,* which is discussed later in this chapter.

Generic Name

A drug's **generic name** is the name proposed by the first manufacturer when the drug is submitted to the FDA for approval. In the United States, the United States Adopted Names (USAN) Council officially assigns a drug its generic name. USAN usually accepts the name proposed by the manufacturer. The generic name (also called the **nonproprietary** name) often is an abbreviated form of the drug's chemical name, structure, or formula. This name is used by all companies that manufacture this chemical compound.

Trade Name

A drug's **trade name** (also called the *brand name* or *proprietary name*) is the name given the chemical compound by the company that makes it. When a new drug is developed, the manufacturer patents the drug and its trade name. This gives the manufacturer the sole right to make, market, and sell the drug until the patent expires. This patent protection allows the manufacturer to recoup some of its costs for research, development, and marketing of the drug. A trade name is usually patent protected for 20 years from the date the patent is submitted. As the expiration date of the patent nears, other drug companies apply to the FDA to make and sell generic versions of the drug. Although other drug companies may make the drug when the patent expires, they cannot use the drug's original trade name.

Drug manufacturers try to use trade names that are easily remembered by healthcare professionals and patients or provide a clue about what the drug is used for. For example, Brethine is a bronchodilator and Lopressor lowers blood pressure. Examples of drug names are shown in Table 11-1.

SOURCES OF DRUGS

[OBJECTIVE 3]

Drugs are derived from many different sources, including plants, animals and human beings, minerals or mineral products, synthetic chemical substances, and recombinant DNA technology (Box 11-2).

BOX 11-2 Sources of Drugs

- Plants
- Animals and human beings
- Minerals or mineral products
- Chemical substances
- Recombinant DNA technology

DNA, Deoxyribonucleic acid.

TABLE 11-1 Examples of Drug Names

Generic Name	Trade Name	Chemical Name
amiodarone hydrochloride	Cordarone	(2-butyl-3-benzofuranyl)[4-[2-(diethylamino)ethoxy]-3,5-diiodophenyl]methanone hydrochloride
diazepam	Valium, Diastat	7-chloro-1,3-dihydro-1-methyl-5-phenyl-2H-1,4-benzodiazepin-2-one
thiamine hydrochloride	Vitamin B_1	3-(4-amino-2-methylpyrimidal-5-methyl)-4-methyl-5(beta-hydroxyethyl) thiazolium chloride hydrochloride

Plants

Alkaloids are a large group of plant-based substances that contain nitrogen and are found in nature. They have been used as poisons, substances of abuse, and as lifesaving treatments. Many drugs with names ending in "ine" are alkaloid derivatives (e.g., atropine, caffeine, quinine, morphine, quinidine, nicotine). ↳Belle Donna

A **glycoside** is a compound that yields a sugar and one or more other products when its parts are separated. Digitalis is an example of a glycoside derived from the foxglove plant.

Gums are plant residues used for medicinal or recreational purposes. The most common is opium gum. The plant has a capsule, and the gum is harvested and transferred to a factory where it is turned into morphine or heroin.

Oils are extracted from flowers, leaves, stems, roots, seeds, and bark. They are used as therapeutic treatments. An example is oil of wintergreen (salicylate).

Animals and Human Beings

Pharmaceutical products derived from animals and human beings include hormones and vaccines. An example of a hormone is insulin. Until 1980 insulin was extracted from the pancreases of pigs and cows. Additional hormones derived from animals include thyroid and estrogen. Examples of human components include vaccines, blood, and plasma components.

Minerals or Mineral Products

Minerals are chemical elements or compounds found in the earth and soil. In the body, minerals are present primarily as ions (charged particles). The human body requires relatively large amounts of some minerals (e.g., sodium, potassium, calcium, magnesium) to function properly. Minerals or mineral products are included in many therapies used in medicine. For example, magnesium is found in Milk of Magnesia, gold salts are used in the treatment of rheumatoid arthritis, and bismuth is an active ingredient in antacids.

Chemical Substances

Chemically developed drugs are made in laboratories by scientifically duplicating specific compounds. Drugs that are chemically developed in a laboratory are called **synthetic drugs.** Synthetic drugs are free of the impurities found in natural substances. Insulin is an example of a synthetic drug. Insulin was originally derived from animals and purified for human use. Because of concerns over transmission of infection and tumor-inducing potential, synthetic derivatives were developed. This afforded mass production and virus-free alternatives for diabetic individuals. Other examples of synthetic drugs include barbiturates and oral contraceptives. Semisynthetic drugs are naturally occurring substances that have been chemically changed. Many antibiotics are semisynthetic drugs.

Recombinant DNA Technology

Recombinant DNA technology, or genetic engineering, is the newest source of drugs. This technology enables individual genes and DNA sequences to be changed, resulting in organisms that have been genetically modified to produce the desired medication. Some of the drugs produced by this technique include insulin, alpha-interferon (a cancer drug), erythropoietin (a drug used to treat anemia), and human growth hormone.

DRUG CLASSIFICATION

[OBJECTIVE 4]

Drug classification systems are used to sort or group drugs that have common characteristics. The Anatomical Therapeutic Chemical Classification System is used for the classification of drugs. It is controlled by the World Health Organization Collaborating Centre for Drug Statistics Methodology and was first published in 1976. Although this system uses multiple levels to categorize drugs, the three main areas of classification are body system, **mechanism of action,** and class of agent.

Body System   *Where*

The first level of classification groups drugs according to the organ or body system on which they act. This grouping is sometimes called the *drug's physiologic classification*. Examples of this level of classification include the following:

- Alimentary tract and metabolism
- Blood and blood-forming organs
- Cardiovascular system
- Skin
- Genitourinary system and sex hormones

Mechanism of Action   *How*

The next level of classification sorts drugs by their mechanism of action. This is often called the *drug's therapeutic classification*. With the cardiovascular system group of drugs as an example, the therapeutic classification of the drugs in this category includes the following:

- Cardiac therapy
- Antihypertensives
- Diuretics
- Peripheral vasodilators
- Vasoprotectives
- Beta-blocking agents
- Calcium channel blockers
- Agents acting on the renin-angiotensin system
- Serum lipid–reducing agents

Class of Agent why

The class of an agent refers to a drug's chemical classification. Using calcium channel blockers from the previous list, the chemical classification of this group of drugs includes the following:

- Selective calcium channel blockers with mainly vascular effects
- Selective calcium channel blockers with direct cardiac effects
- Nonselective calcium channel blockers

For example, verapamil is a drug that works on the cardiovascular system (physiologic classification). Its therapeutic classification is calcium channel blocker. It is chemically classified as a selective calcium channel blocker with direct cardiac effects.

SOURCES OF DRUG INFORMATION

[OBJECTIVE 5]

United States Pharmacopeia/ Dispensing Information

The U.S. Federal Food, Drug, and Cosmetics Act designated the *United States Pharmacopeia-National Formulary* (USP-NF) as the official reference source for drugs marketed in the United States. In 1980 the USP and NF were published under the same cover as USP Dispensing Information (USP DI). In 1994 the USP signed an agreement with the American Medical Association (AMA) to combine the information in AMA's Drug Evaluations database with the USP DI database. This resulted in a single product containing drug and therapeutic information. In 1998, USP sold USP DI and its associated products to The Thomson Company.

Physician's Desk Reference

The *Physician's Desk Reference* is a commercially published compilation of information about more than 4000 drugs, including indications, drug interactions and other precautions, mechanism of action, side and adverse effects, dosing information, and dosage forms. It is indexed by brand and generic name, manufacturer, and product category. The information is updated yearly.

American Hospital Formulary Service

The *American Hospital Formulary Service* is published by the American Society of Hospital Pharmacists. It is a collection of information about virtually every drug available in the United States. This resource provides healthcare professionals with information about uses for drugs included in the labeling approved by the FDA and those that are not ("off-label" uses). Off-label uses for the drug may become evident because of studies done before and after the drug is approved by the FDA.

Hospitals may have a formulary specific for their institution. This may be referenced when working in a hospital environment. The formulary may provide information on drug action, dosing, and drug preferences for specific conditions.

Package Inserts

Before a drug is marketed, the Federal Food, Drug, and Cosmetic Act requires the manufacturer to submit information about the drug's safety and effectiveness to the FDA. A complete description of the product and its labeling must be reviewed and approved by the FDA.

The product description and information about appropriate use of the product are then included with each drug as a package insert. Accessing the manufac-turer's Internet site often provides the package insert equivalent.

> **PARAMEDIC*Pearl***
>
> Some drugs have inserts designed to be given to the patient ("patient package insert"). Most package inserts, however, are not meant for this purpose.

Other Sources

Other sources of information about medications include nurses, physicians, and pharmacists. Poison Control Centers also are useful sources. Published sources of drug information also are helpful. Pocket references are literally pocket-sized books that contain abbreviated versions of drug dosing, indications, and contraindications. An example is *Tarascon Pocket Pharmacopoeia* by Tarascon Publishing.

The Internet has a large number of resources. Many Web sites have been set up by pharmaceutical companies and research facilities and provide accurate information. The source must be verified as having a solid reputation. **Information on the Internet is not monitored, and many sites provide misinformation.**

UNITED STATES DRUG LEGISLATION

Laws govern the purchase, distribution, dispensation, and administration of drugs throughout the United States. These laws are federal, state, and local in nature and sometimes include regulations in the municipal agency or healthcare institution in which the paramedic works. Because of these variations, describing specific laws is beyond the scope of this text. However, as a paramedic, you are responsible for knowing the laws and regulations in your area of employment.

Purpose of Legislation

Before 1906 no legal control over any pharmaceutical substance existed. Many remedies had false claims and were mislabeled. Drug legislation was put in place to protect the public from adulterated or mislabeled drugs.

History of Legislation

[OBJECTIVE 6]

Laws governing pharmaceuticals actually began at the beginning of the twentieth century when the U.S. Congress passed the Pure Food and Drug Act. This act was a landmark document in American history. It standardized the name, strength, quality, and purity of drugs. Its purpose was to forbid the mislabeling of drugs. This law was replaced in 1938 with the Federal Food, Drug and Cosmetic Act and has been updated several times since. The Harrison Narcotics Act of 1914 established the word "narcotic" and regulated the importation, manufacture, sale, and use of opium, codeine, and their derivatives and compounds. Precise record keeping by distributors was first required by the Harrison Narcotics Act, and the registration of manufacturers, pharmacists, and physicians was initiated with the federal government. Specific fines and imprisonment were authorized to be imposed for illegal possession or distribution of controlled drugs. This law was eventually replaced by the Controlled Substances Act of 1970.

In 1928 the Durham-Humphrey Amendments required prescriptions for certain drugs. In 1937, 107 deaths (mostly children) occurred after taking an **elixir** that contained a poisonous solvent. Shortly thereafter, the Federal Food, Drug, and Cosmetic Act of 1938 was passed. This was the first legislation to regulate drug safety. It required that all new drugs be tested for toxicity. This law also established the FDA's responsibility for supervising and regulating drug safety; required labels to list side effects, directions, and ingredients; and authorized the FDA to determine drug safety and efficacy before marketing.

The Durham-Humphrey Amendment of 1951 created a category of prescription drugs and specified how prescription drugs could be ordered and dispensed. It also required warning labels about drowsiness, habit-forming potential, and other side effects to be placed on the drug's packaging. Prescription drugs are also called *legend drugs* because they must carry the following label: "Caution: Federal law prohibits the transfer of this drug to any person other than the patient for whom it was prescribed."

Until passage of the Kefauver-Harris Amendment of 1962, a drug was not legally required to be effective. This law was a response to severe fetal deformities attributable to thalidomide, a sedative marketed in Europe. It required proof of the effectiveness and safety of new prescription and over-the-counter drugs before being approved by the FDA for use.

Schedule of Controlled Substances

[OBJECTIVE 7]

The Comprehensive Drug Abuse Prevention and Control Act of 1970 is the legal basis by which the manufacture, importation, possession, and distribution of certain drugs are regulated by the U.S. government. This law established five schedules (classifications) of substances based on their accepted medical use in the United States, abuse potential, and potential for addiction. This law demanded, and still does demand, control and accountability. The list of schedules and their definitions with examples of drugs in each category are provided in Table 11-2.

> **PARAMEDIC*Pearl***
>
> Diligence in handling and accounting for all medications is of critical importance if a paramedic is to function within safe legal boundaries. Medical direction has the last and final word for the prehospital administration of medications.

Food and Drug Administration

The FDA is the governing body that oversees general safety standards in the production of drugs, foods, and cosmetics. It also regulates medical devices (e.g., pacemakers, contact lenses, hearing aids) and radiation-emitting products (e.g., cell phones, lasers, microwaves). The FDA is a part of the U.S. Department of Health and Human Services. The Center for Biologics Evaluation and Research at the FDA is responsible for the regulation of most biologic products, including vaccines; blood and blood products; and cellular, tissue, and gene therapies.

Drug Enforcement Administration

The Drug Enforcement Administration is a part of the U.S. Department of Justice. It enforces controlled substances laws and monitors the need for changing schedules of abused drugs.

Federal Trade Commission

The Bureau of Consumer Protection within the Federal Trade Commission protects consumers by enforcing the nation's truth-in-advertising laws, with particular emphasis on claims for food, over-the-counter drugs, dietary supplements, alcohol, and tobacco as well as on conduct related to high-tech products and the Internet.

STANDARDIZATION OF DRUGS

[OBJECTIVE 8]

Because drugs may vary in their strength and activity, standardization is necessary. An **assay** is a test of a substance to find out its components (amount and purity). A **bioassay** tests the effects of a substance on an organism and compares the result with some agreed standard. In the United States, the *United States Pharmacopeia* is the official public standards–setting authority for prescription and over-the-counter medicines, dietary supplements, and other healthcare products manufactured and sold.

TABLE 11-2   Schedule of Controlled Substances

Schedule	Accepted Medical Use In United States	Abuse Potential	Potential for Addiction	Examples
I	None; used for research, analysis, or instruction only	High	May lead to severe dependence	Heroin, peyote, marijuana (cannabis), lysergic acid diethylamide (LSD)
II	Yes	High	May lead to severe physical and/or psychologic dependence	Morphine, meperidine, codeine, oxycodone, methadone, pentobarbital, amphetamines, cocaine, opium, methylphenidate (Ritalin)
III	Yes	Less abuse potential than drugs in Schedules I and II	May lead to moderate to low physical or high psychologic dependence	Anabolic steroids, hydrocodone with acetaminophen (Vicodin), codeine with acetaminophen (Tylenol 3), and other narcotic, amphetamine, and barbiturate types
IV	Yes	Lower abuse potential compared with drugs in Schedule III	May lead to limited physical or psychologic dependence	Benzodiazepines (diazepam, lorazepam), phenobarbital, chloral hydrate
V	Yes	Low abuse potential compared with drugs in Schedule IV	May lead to limited physical or psychologic dependence	Medications generally used for relief of diarrhea or to suppress cough; contain small amounts of opioid substances; diphenoxylate and atropine combination (Lomotil), promethazine (Phenergan) with codeine, nitrous oxide

[handwritten note beside Schedule IV: more psychological addiction]

INVESTIGATIONAL DRUGS

Prospective Drugs and Evaluation

[OBJECTIVE 9]

Prospective drugs are put through a lengthy evaluation process. Investigation begins with conceptual evidence that a drug will have physiologic benefit. Studies often have been performed on tissue models (in vivo) or animals (in vitro). Specific information is gathered about toxicity, drug absorption, and metabolism.

Food and Drug Administration Approval Process

[handwritten note: Takes 7-12 years to get drug into market]

Phases of Investigation

The FDA approval process for an **investigational drug** has four phases. These phases require specific information about the drug and its effects on human beings. Three phases are conducted before a New Drug Application (NDA) is submitted by the manufacturer to the FDA. The fourth phase follows NDA approval and is not closely monitored by the FDA. The phases are described in Table 11-3.

New Drug Application

The main purpose of an NDA is to provide information and investigational data proving that the drug has promise for treating human beings. During a new drug's early preclinical development, the sponsor's main goal is to find out if the product is reasonably safe for initial use in human beings and if the compound shows pharmacologic activity that justifies commercial development.

An abbreviated NDA is used for generic drugs. As previously discussed, generic drugs are products that are comparable to the original patented medication. They are similar in dosage, form, strength, route of administration, and quality of performance characteristics. Generic drug applications are termed "abbreviated" because they generally are not required to include preclinical (animal) and clinical (human) data to establish safety and effectiveness. As a substitution, these applications must demon-

TABLE 11-3 Phases of the Approval Process for Investigational Drugs

Phase	Description
Preclinical testing	Testing required before the new drug can be used in human beings Drug absorption, distribution, metabolism, and elimination evaluated Drug toxicity and potentially useful effects evaluated
Phase I	Closely monitored by the FDA Initial introduction of an investigational new drug in human beings May be conducted in patients, but usually conducted in 20 to 80 healthy human volunteers Drug metabolism, mechanism of action, and side effects associated with increasing doses evaluated
Phase II	Closely monitored by the FDA Involves a relatively small number of patients, usually several hundred people Preliminary data about the drug's effectiveness for a specific disease or condition evaluated Common short-term side effects and risks associated with the drug evaluated
Phase III	Expanded controlled and uncontrolled trials Involves several hundred to several thousand patients with a particular condition or disease Information gathered about the drug's effectiveness and safety Data gathered used as the basis for predicting results in the general population If analysis of the clinical trial results successfully show the safety and effectiveness of the drug, the manufacturer files a new drug application with the FDA
Phase IV	Postmarketing surveillance New drug released for general use Not closely regulated by the FDA Toxicities voluntarily reported by prescribing physicians

[handwritten annotation next to Phase III: Bigger group of people w/ specific disease]

FDA, U.S. Food and Drug Administration.

strate that their product performs in the same manner as the original patented drug.

SCOPE OF MANAGEMENT
Responsibilities

Safe and Effective Administration
[OBJECTIVE 10]
As a paramedic, you are expected to administer every medication correctly and safely. Before giving any medication, you must assess the scene and patient. Obtaining a history is an important part of medication administration. Knowing and understanding the medications a patient is taking are also important. When obtaining a patient's medical history and history of the present illness, use critical thinking skills to assess for indications and contraindications of medications. Obtaining the patient's pill bottles and copying the information down directly from them are often helpful steps. Asking how the patient takes his or her medications is vital because patients may not take their drugs as directed. Questions that should be routinely asked when taking a medication history are shown in Box 11-3.

Standard precautions should be used at all times for the protection of the patient, yourself, and the crew. Numerous mechanisms ensure safe medication administration, including checking with a partner, using drug references, and rechecking calculations and dosages.

BOX 11-3 Questions for a Medication History

- Do you have any medication allergies or reactions?
- What prescription medications are you taking?
- What over-the-counter medications are you taking?
- Do you take any vitamins, herbs, or natural supplements?
- What are the dosages or strengths of your medications?
- What conditions do you take these medications for?
- Are there any medicines your doctor has told you not to take?

Drug references should be sought if any question arises regarding **dose,** indication, or contraindication. Protocols should be reviewed regularly; if in doubt, contact medical direction for online assistance. This should be standard practice. Use Box 11-4 as a safety guide to medication administration.

Legal, Moral, and Ethical Obligations
As a paramedic, you are permitted to give specific substances to your patients. This responsibility comes with a legal, moral, and ethical obligation to give each substance according to its intended use, indication, and your written protocols.

Maintaining patient confidentiality is the law. Professionalism is critical during any exchange of information with a patient. You are responsible for maintaining patient confidentiality, including the patient's medication and medical history.

AUTONOMIC PHARMACOLOGY

Nervous System Organization and Function

[OBJECTIVE 11]

The nervous system is the body's electrical network. Many medications and therapeutic treatments have been designed to modify the actions of this complex biologic system. The nervous system is divided into the central nervous system and the peripheral nervous system (Table 11-4).

Brain → L2-L3

Central Nervous System ✳

The brain and the spinal cord combine to make up the **central nervous system (CNS).** All the body's electrical impulses are sent, received, or coordinated here.

BOX 11-4	Medication Administration Safety Guide

- Always use standard precautions.
- Take an accurate and thorough history.
- Check and recheck medication selection.
- Evaluate for indications and contraindications.
- Use protocols, drug references, and medical direction authority.
- Document medication administration.
- Keep knowledge base current.
- Maintain professionalism.

Almost every response in the body interfaces with the CNS at some point. The brain is the central processing center for all input and output. The spinal cord is contained in the spinal canal surrounded by bony vertebrae. Peripheral nerves enter the spinal cord between each vertebra. The spinal cord is composed of various tracts (divisions) responsible for the transmission of various types of stimuli, including motor, temperature, vibration, and sensation.

Peripheral Nervous System ✳

The **peripheral nervous system** is composed of all the nerves outside of the CNS. The peripheral nervous system includes the cranial nerves (nerves that come directly from the brain) and the spinal nerves (nerves that carry impulses to and from the spinal cord). Combined, the central and the peripheral nervous systems encompass all the nerves in the body. The motor nerves of the peripheral nervous system are divided into the somatic and autonomic divisions on the basis of their function.

✳ **Somatic Nervous System.** The **somatic nervous system** refers to cranial and spinal nerves that carry messages to skeletal muscles. These nerves are controlled voluntarily and consciously. Motor pathways of the somatic nervous system use one neuron to conduct information from the CNS to the muscle innervated by the nerve. *motor function*

✳ **Autonomic Nervous System.** The **autonomic nervous system (ANS)** is the part of the peripheral nervous system that is not under voluntary control. Nerves in the ANS carry messages to the heart, secretory glands (sweat, salivary, bronchial, and gastric glands), smooth muscles of the gastrointestinal (GI) tract, blood vessels, bronchi, and genitourinary system. The ANS has great relevance to pharmacology. *smooth muscle*

The two main branches of the ANS are the **sympathetic** and **parasympathetic divisions.** These divisions are divided on the basis of how they affect specific organs and their functions. Most organs are innervated by both divisions of the ANS, and they generally have opposite effects from one another.

TABLE 11-4	Summary of the Nervous System		
Main Divisions	**Components**	**Subdivisions**	**Function**
CNS	Brain, spinal cord	None	Sends, receives, and coordinates impulses
Peripheral nervous system	Cranial nerves, spinal nerves	Somatic nervous system	Controls movement of voluntary muscles
		ANS: Sympathetic (adrenergic) division, parasympathetic (cholinergic) division	Regulates many involuntary functions

afferent - from sensory neurons to brain
efferent - from brain to motor neurons

CNS, Central nervous system; *ANS,* autonomic nervous system.

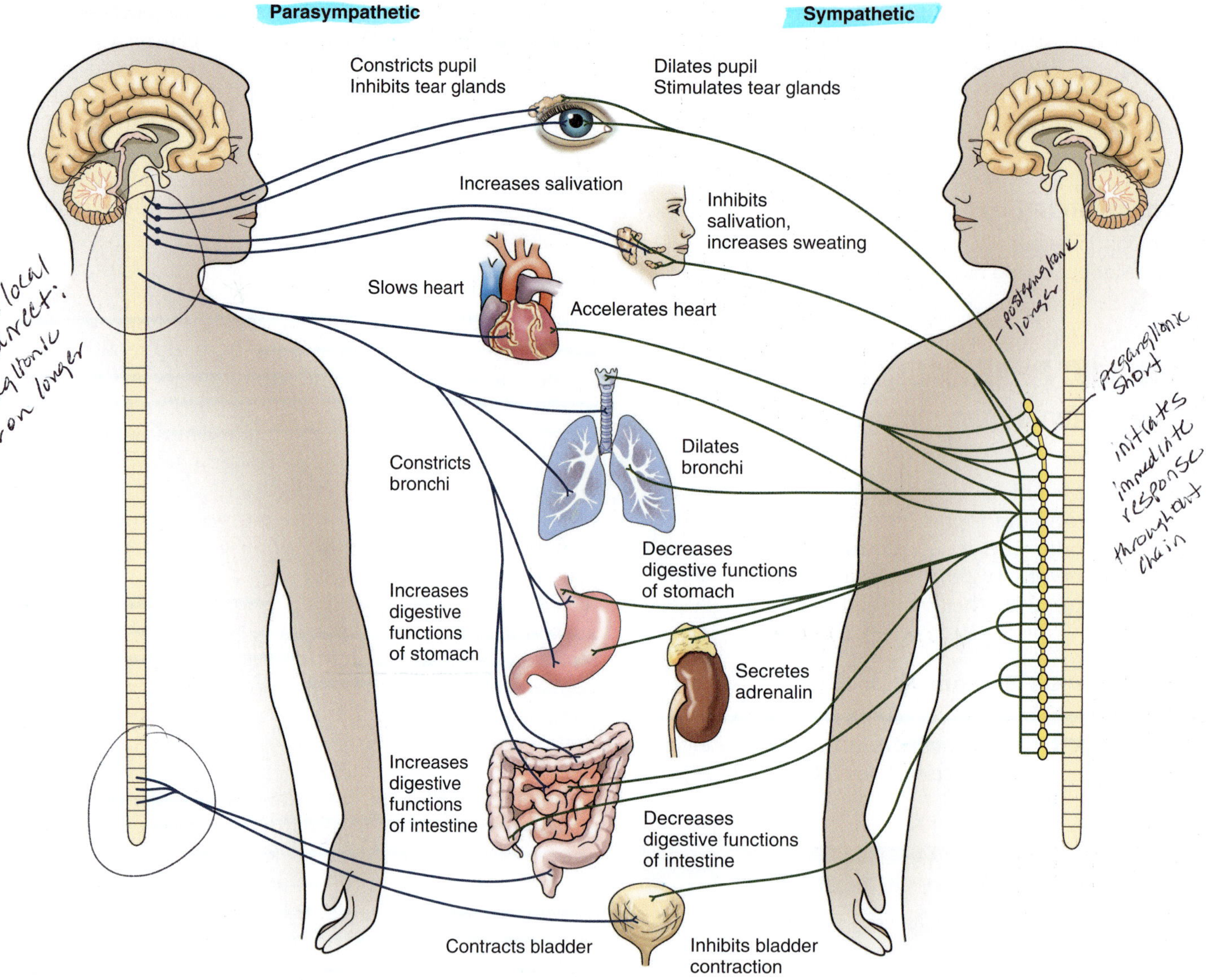

Parasympathetic

Sympathetic

Constricts pupil
Inhibits tear glands

Dilates pupil
Stimulates tear glands

Increases salivation

Inhibits
salivation,
increases sweating

Slows heart

Accelerates heart

more local & direct: preganglionic neuron longer

Constricts bronchi

Dilates bronchi

Decreases digestive functions of stomach

Increases digestive functions of stomach

Secretes adrenalin

Increases digestive functions of intestine

Decreases digestive functions of intestine

postganglionic longer

preganglionic short

initiates immediate response throughout chain

Contracts bladder

Inhibits bladder contraction

Figure 11-1 Effects of stimulation of the autonomic nervous system.

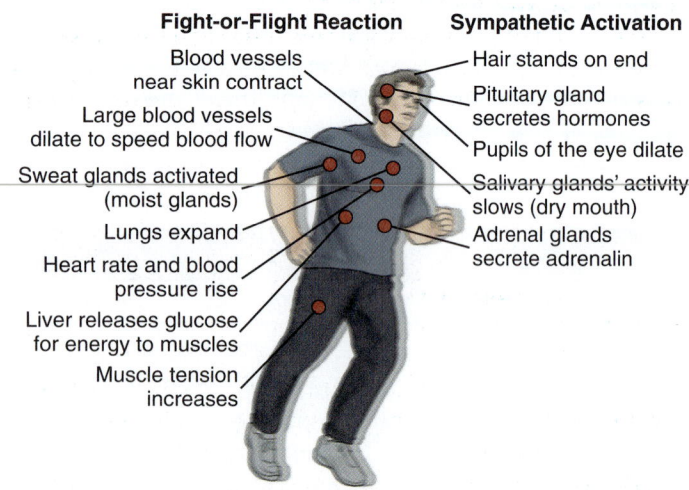

Fight-or-Flight Reaction

Blood vessels near skin contract
Large blood vessels dilate to speed blood flow
Sweat glands activated (moist glands)
Lungs expand
Heart rate and blood pressure rise
Liver releases glucose for energy to muscles
Muscle tension increases

Sympathetic Activation

Hair stands on end
Pituitary gland secretes hormones
Pupils of the eye dilate
Salivary glands' activity slows (dry mouth)
Adrenal glands secrete adrenalin

Figure 11-2 The sympathetic division of the autonomic nervous system mobilizes the body, allowing it to function under stress.

Motor pathways of the ANS use two neurons to send information from the CNS to the effector. An **effector** is the muscle, gland, or organ on which the ANS exerts an effect.

Sympathetic Division. Anatomically, the sympathetic division of the ANS originates from the spinal nerves that leave through the ventral roots in the first thoracic through the second lumbar vertebrae. These nerve cells act peripherally on blood vessels and on the organs of the thorax, abdomen, and pelvis (Figure 11-1).

The sympathetic division (also known as the **adrenergic** division) mobilizes the body, allowing it to function under stress. This "fight-or-flight" response is designed to prepare the body for stress, such as fighting with an enemy or running away (Figure 11-2). During the fight-or-flight response, heart rate increases, blood is shunted from the skin to the muscles, and the bronchi and pupils dilate. Box 11-5 lists the effects of sympathetic stimulation.

BOX 11-5 | **Effects of Sympathetic Stimulation**

- Increased heart rate, force of myocardial contraction, speed of conduction through the heart's conduction system, blood pressure, and cardiac output
- Bronchodilation to improve oxygenation
- Shunting of blood from skin and blood vessels to skeletal muscle
- Mobilization of stored energy to ensure an adequate supply of glucose for the brain and fatty acids for muscle activity
- Pupil dilation
- Increased sweating

BOX 11-6 | **Effects of Parasympathetic Stimulation**

- Reduction in heart rate, myocardial contractility, conduction velocity through the heart, and cardiac output
- Reduced respiratory rate
- Constriction of bronchial smooth muscle
- Constriction of pupils
- Increased digestive secretion (pancreatic and salivary)
- Emptying of bladder and bowel

Parasympathetic Division. The parasympathetic division is composed of several cranial nerves (III [oculomotor], VII [facial], IX [glossopharyngeal], and X [vagus]) and some of the spinal nerves (S2 to S4) that exit the sacrum. Parasympathetic nerves leave the brain by way of cranial nerves and the vertebrae at the sacral level. This division is less widely distributed compared with the sympathetic division. The parasympathetic division causes responses opposite those of the sympathetic division. Most of the functions of the parasympathetic division are involved when the body is relaxed and in no imminent danger (Box 11-6). This is often referred to as the "feed and breed" or "resting and digesting" response of the ANS. The body is taking care of functions such as digestion, growth, healing, and the removal of toxins.

Parasympathetic and Sympathetic Characteristics. Most organs of the body receive both sympathetic and parasympathetic innervation. In general, these divisions oppose one another and serve special functions. Box 11-7 highlights examples of imbalances in the sympathetic and parasympathetic divisions of the ANS.

Neurochemical Transmission

Neurochemical transmission is important to understand, because pharmacology affects the ANS. Each nerve impulse generates an action potential and chemical discharge of either a neurotransmitter or **neuropeptide.**

BOX 11-7 | **Imbalance in the Sympathetic and Parasympathetic Divisions of the ANS**

The sympathetic division of the ANS has neurons that exit at the thoracic and lumbar areas of the spinal cord. The parasympathetic division has neurons that exit by way of the cranial nerves (no involvement of the spinal cord) and the sacral portion of the spinal cord. When caring for a patient with a spinal cord injury, his or her body may not be able to produce a sympathetic response. For example, a pedestrian is hit by a motor vehicle. As a result of the impact, he incurs a spinal cord transection at T1 and is a paraplegic. This patient would typically have a sympathetic response to this event. The brain interprets the injury as a "fight" situation and prepares the body for action. In this situation, the patient's brain sends the appropriate nerve signals, but the cord is severed and the signals cannot make it to the target organs, resulting in improper organ function.

Another example involves patients who have received a heart transplant. The patient who receives a heart has a heart implanted without the pericardial sac and vagus nerves. During harvesting of the donor heart, the vagus nerves are removed from the heart's surface. The vagus nerve (cranial nerve X) runs from the brain to the heart and triggers parasympathetic stimulation. When these nerves (one on each side) are cut from the donor heart, the patient receiving the heart will not have the same parasympathetic stimulation on the heart.

ANS, Autonomic nervous system.

All preganglionic neurotransmitters involve acetylcholine

Synaptic Transmission

All autonomic pathways contain two nerves. The **preganglionic neuron** extends from the spinal cord (the CNS) to the ganglion, and the **postganglionic neuron** (peripheral nervous system) travels from the ganglia to the desired organ or tissue. The autonomic **ganglion** is the location where the CNS and peripheral nervous system connect. For a physiologic action at the target organ to occur, the preganglionic neuron must send an impulse to the ganglia and from the ganglia to the postganglionic neuron. These neurons are not physically connected. The **synaptic junction** is the name given to the space where they meet. Impulses (action potentials) are conducted along these nerves. When they reach their synaptic junction, a neurotransmitter is released. A **neurotransmitter** is a chemical molecule that travels to the other side of the synaptic junction. Neurotransmitters are specific to their junction and thus are the target for pharmacologic intervention. When a neurotransmitter reaches the other side of the junction, it interacts with a **receptor** and a chemical reaction occurs, causing either another nerve impulse or a physiologic action at the target (effector) organ.

parasympathetic – postganglionic ACh (1°)
Sympathetic – postganglionic Norepinephrine (1°) Epi ACh

PARAMEDIC*Pearl*

Sympathetic preganglionic neurons are relatively short, and the postganglionic neurons relatively long. One sympathetic preganglionic neuron may synapse with many postganglionic neurons in many organs. As a result, sympathetic effects are often widespread, affecting many organs. Parasympathetic preganglionic neurons are relatively long, and the postganglionic neurons relatively short that lead to a single organ. Thus parasympathetic stimulation often involves a response by only one organ.

Neurotransmitters

Two major categories of neurotransmitters are involved in these transmissions: **cholinergic** and adrenergic. These neurotransmitters correlate with the two divisions of the ANS. In general, the adrenergic (sympathetic) neurotransmitter is norepinephrine and the cholinergic (parasympathetic) neurotransmitter is acetylcholine. These neurotransmitters react with specific receptors in the synaptic junction (Figure 11-3).

In general, adrenergic neurotransmitters generate a sympathetic response and cholinergic neurotransmitters

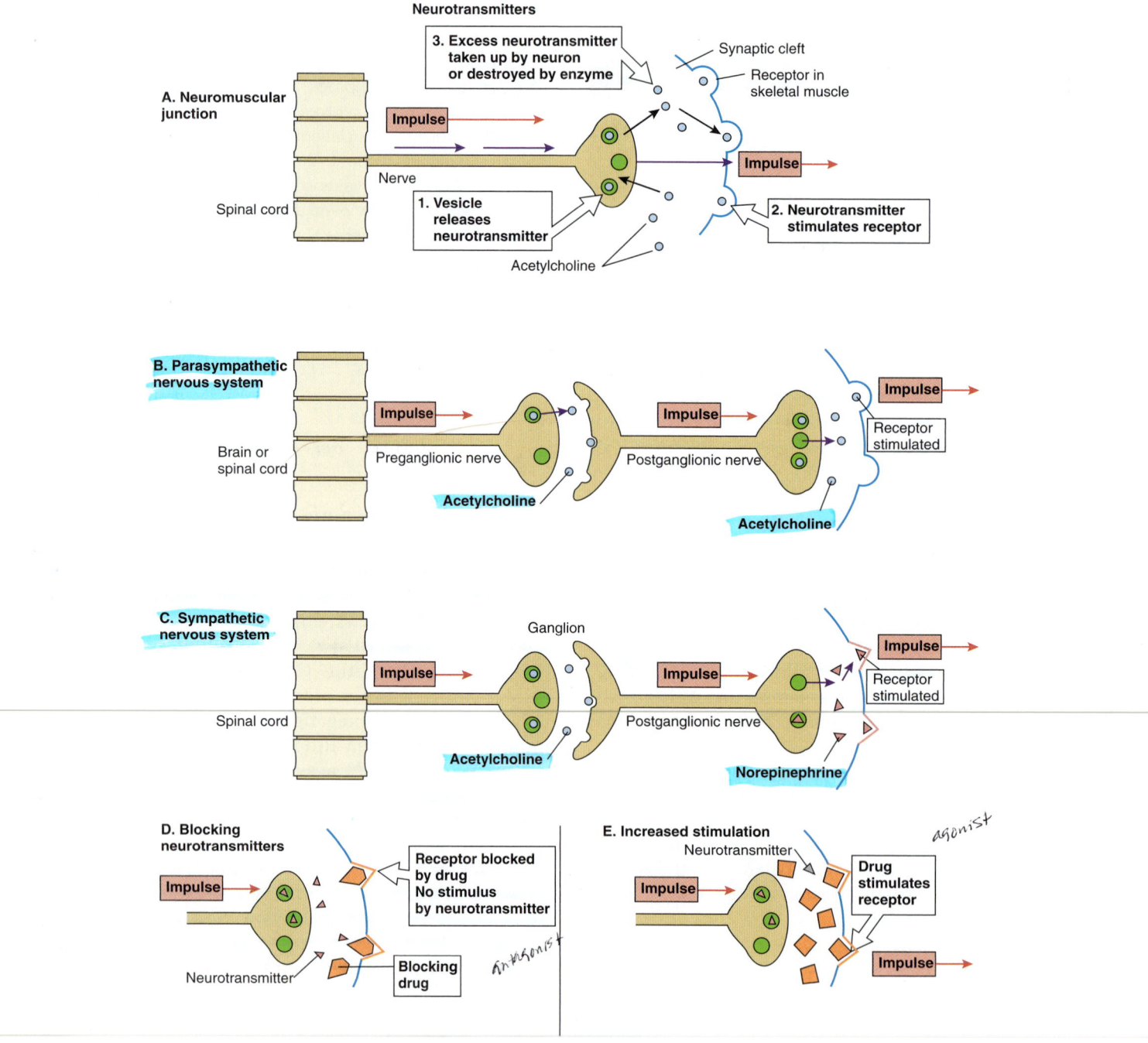

Figure 11-3 Neurotransmitters at the synapse.

muscarinic – organs + smooth muscle

nicotinic – skeletal muscles

generate a parasympathetic response (Figure 11-4). Preganglionic nerves discharge a cholinergic neurotransmitter for both the sympathetic and parasympathetic divisions of the ANS. The postganglionic neurons typically discharge the neurotransmitter of their individual division. For example, the postganglionic nerve discharges acetylcholine in the parasympathetic division of the ANS. In the sympathetic division, the postganglionic nerve discharges norepinephrine. Two exceptions are found in the sympathetic division: the postganglionic neurons that act on sweat glands and those ending on blood vessels in skeletal muscle release a cholinergic neurotransmitter (Table 11-5).

Synaptic Transmission Termination

Termination of the synaptic transmission occurs when the synaptic cleft is cleared of all neurotransmitters. With each discharge of neurotransmitter, it interacts with the recep-

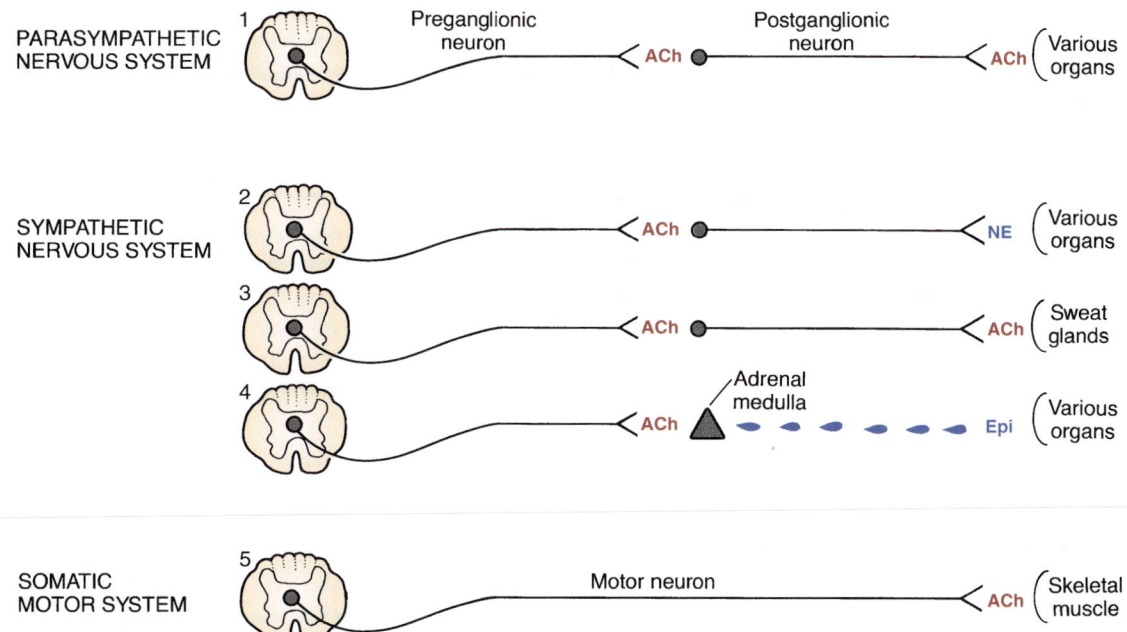

Figure 11-4 Neurotransmitters of the peripheral nervous system. All preganglionic neurons of the parasympathetic and sympathetic nervous systems release acetylcholine as their transmitter. *1,* All postganglionic neurons of the parasympathetic nervous system release acetylcholine as their transmitter. *2,* Most postganglionic neurons of the sympathetic nervous system release norepinephrine as their transmitter. *3,* Postganglionic neurons of the sympathetic nervous system that innervate sweat glands release acetylcholine as their transmitter. *4,* Epinephrine is the principal transmitter released by the adrenal medulla. *5,* All motor neurons to skeletal muscles release acetylcholine as their transmitter. *ACh,* Acetylcholine; *NE,* norepinephrine; *Epi,* epinephrine.

TABLE 11-5	Autonomic Nervous System Neurotransmitters	
Transmitter	**Sympathetic Division**	**Parasympathetic Division**
Preganglionic neurotransmitter	Acetylcholine	Acetylcholine
Postganglionic neurotransmitter	Most postganglionic neurons release norepinephrine Adrenal medulla releases epinephrine Postganglionic neurons that innervate sweat glands release acetylcholine	Acetylcholine

Cholinergic - parasympathic
adrenergic - sympathetic

tor for a finite period. After this interaction, it is either taken up by a reuptake transporter protein or degraded by another enzyme or chemical. The individual pieces of the neurotransmitter are reused to form additional molecules of the neurotransmitter. The neurotransmitter continuously interacts with the receptor and then falls into the synaptic cleft for recycling. The cycle then repeats as long as the brain generates an originating impulse.

Receptors

Neurotransmitters react with receptors and cause a physiologic response. Both the parasympathetic and sympathetic divisions have specific receptors.

Cholinergic Receptors

Two main types of cholinergic receptors are found in the parasympathetic division of the ANS: nicotinic and muscarinic receptors. These receptors received their names by their responsiveness to nicotine (commonly found in cigarettes) and muscarine (found in mushrooms). Nicotinic receptors are found on skeletal muscle, on cells of the adrenal medulla, and on the cell bodies of all postganglionic neurons of the parasympathetic and sympathetic divisions of the ANS (Lehne, 2001). Muscarinic receptors are located in smooth muscle.

When acetylcholine binds to nicotinic receptors, an excitatory response occurs. When acetylcholine binds with muscarinic receptors, the result may be excitation or inhibition, depending on the target tissues in which the receptors are found. Drugs that stimulate these receptors are **parasympathomimetics** (cholinergics). Drugs that block or inhibit their function are **parasympatholytics** (anticholinergics) (Table 11-6).

atropine

Acetylcholine. Acetylcholine interacts with these receptors and causes a physiologic response. Production of acetylcholine occurs in the synaptic junction and is the result of a reaction of choline with acetate. After acetylcholine has bound with its receptor, it must be broken down to make way for a new molecule of acetylcholine. Acetylcholinesterase is the enzyme that breaks down acetylcholine into smaller molecules. The byproducts are recycled and reused to make new molecules of acetylcholine.

Sympathetic Receptors

Sympathetic receptors are called *adrenergic receptors*. When the sympathetic division is stimulated, the adrenal medulla also is stimulated and releases epinephrine into the circulatory system. Epinephrine may cause an action at the nerve terminal or travel through the bloodstream to exert its actions.

Sympathetic receptors are located in different organs and thus have different physiologic actions when stimulated. Medications that stimulate sympathetic receptors are called **sympathomimetics.** Those that block or inhibit their function are **sympatholytics.**

Sympathetic receptors have been categorized into five main types: alpha$_1$, alpha$_2$, beta$_1$, beta$_2$, and dopamine (also called *dopaminergic*). Alpha$_1$ receptors are found in the eyes, blood vessels, bladder, and male reproductive organs. Stimulation of alpha$_1$ receptor sites results in constriction. Alpha$_2$ receptor sites are found in parts of the digestive system and on presynaptic nerve terminals in the peripheral nervous system. Stimulation results in decreased secretions, decreased peristalsis, and suppression of further norepinephrine release.

Beta-receptor sites are divided into beta$_1$, beta$_2$, and beta$_3$. Beta$_1$ receptors are found in the heart and kidneys. Stimulation of beta$_1$ receptor sites in the heart results in increased heart rate, contractility and, ultimately, irritability of cardiac cells. Stimulation of beta$_1$ receptor sites in the kidneys results in the release of renin into the blood. Renin promotes the production of angiotensin, a powerful vasoconstrictor. Beta$_2$ receptor sites are found in the arterioles of the heart, lungs, and skeletal muscle. Stimulation results in dilation. Stimulation of beta$_2$ receptor sites in the smooth muscle of the bronchi results in dilation. Beta$_3$ receptors have also been identified and are believed to be of major importance only in heart failure. Stimulation of beta$_3$ receptor sites results in decreased myocardial contractility (Opie, 2005).

TABLE 11-6	ANS Terminology	
	Sympathetic Division	**Parasympathetic Division**
Stimulation Terms	Sympathomimetic	Parasympathomimetic
	Adrenergic	Cholinergic
	Sympathetic agonist	Parasympathetic agonist
Inhibition (Suppressant) Terms	Sympatholytic	Parasympatholytic
	Adrenergic blocker	Cholinergic blocker
	Sympathetic blocker	Parasympathetic blocker
	Antiadrenergic	Anticholinergic
	Sympathetic antagonist	Parasympathetic antagonist
		Vagolytic

ANS, Autonomic nervous system.

Dopamine receptors are found in the renal, mesenteric, and visceral blood vessels. Stimulation results in dilation. A summary of the most common sympathetic receptors is provided in Table 11-7.

PARAMEDIC*Pearl*

Drugs that stimulate beta$_2$ receptors are often used in respiratory emergencies. For example, albuterol is a drug often used by patients who have reactive airway disease, such as asthma. Albuterol stimulates beta$_2$ receptors, resulting in bronchodilation.

Beta-blockers are drugs that block beta-receptor sites. Some beta-blockers block only beta$_1$ receptors, whereas others are less specific and block beta$_1$ and beta$_2$ receptors. For example, metoprolol (Lopressor) can be used to slow the heart rate of a patient who has reactive airway disease because it is specific for beta$_1$ receptors. Propranolol (Inderal) blocks both beta$_1$ and beta$_2$ receptors. This drug is not typically used to slow the heart rate of a patient who has reactive airway disease because blocking beta$_2$ receptors can constrict the bronchioles, making breathing more difficult.

Sympathetic neurotransmitters (norepinephrine, epinephrine, and dopamine) do not interact with sympathetic receptors in the same way. For example, dopamine receptors respond only to dopamine. They do not respond to norepinephrine or epinephrine. Norepinephrine stimulates alpha$_1$, alpha$_2$, and beta$_1$ receptors but not beta$_2$ or dopamine receptors. A summary of sympathetic neurotransmitters is found in Table 11-8.

Epinephrine and norepinephrine are broken down into inactive compounds by the actions of catecholamine-*O*-methyltransferase and monoamine oxidase. The byproducts are reused to make new molecules of norepinephrine. Monoamine oxidase inhibitors have been used in depression and are discussed in Chapter 11.

Other Neurotransmitters and Receptors

Other neurotransmitters include serotonin, endorphins, and neuropeptides. Serotonin is found throughout the body. A lack of serotonin in the brain is thought to be a cause of depression. In relation to the ANS, receptors for serotonin are found on smooth muscle in the gastrointestinal tract. Stimulation of serotonin receptors stimulates smooth muscle movement in the intestines (peristalsis).

monoamines - epi, norepi, dopamine, serotonin
• monoamine oxidase breaks them down
• MAOI's inhibit breakdown
*   SSRI's more specific for serotonin*

TABLE 11-7	Sympathetic (Adrenergic) Receptors	
Receptor Type	**Location**	**Effects of Stimulation**
Alpha$_1$	Eye	Radial muscle contraction of iris causes increased pupil size
	Arterioles of skin, viscera, mucous membranes	Constriction, increase in peripheral vascular resistance
	Veins	Constriction
	Bladder sphincters	Constriction
	Male reproductive organs	Ejaculation
Alpha$_2$	Digestive system	Decreased secretions, peristalsis
	Presynaptic nerve terminals in peripheral nervous system	Inhibits norepinephrine release
Beta$_1$	Heart	Increase in heart rate Increase in force of contraction Increase in speed of conduction through atrioventricular node Increase in oxygen consumption
	Kidneys	Renin release
Beta$_2$	Arterioles of heart, lungs, skeletal muscle	Dilation, increased organ perfusion
	Bronchi	Dilation
	Uterus	Relaxation
	Liver	Glycogenolysis (breakdown of glycogen to glucose)
Dopamine	Renal, mesenteric, and visceral blood vessels	Dilation

TABLE 11-8	Sympathetic Neurotransmitters and Receptors		
	Neurotransmitter		
	Norepinephrine	**Epinephrine**	**Dopamine**
Receptor			
Alpha$_1$	+	+	
Alpha$_2$	+	+	
Beta$_1$	+	+	
Beta$_2$		+	
Dopamine			+

Modified from Lehne, R. A. (2001). Physiology of the peripheral nervous system. In Pharmacology for nursing care (4th ed.), (p. 109). Philadelphia: Saunders.
+, Stimulates.

BOX 11-8	Neuropeptides

- Gastrin
- Insulin
- Vasopressin
- Oxytocin
- Endorphins
- Glucagon
- Growth hormone–releasing factor

Endorphins are neurotransmitters that function in the transmission of signals within the nervous system. Stress and pain are the two most common factors leading to the release of endorphins. They have similar actions to opiates without the addictive properties.

Neuropeptides are similar to neurotransmitters. They are produced in the neuron and transported through the synaptic junction. They are often hormones and exert their effects locally and systemically. Examples of neuropeptides are provided in Box 11-8.

Effector Cell Response

Receptor Structure

Most drugs exert their effects by binding with protein molecules (receptors) located in the cell membrane. Interactions between neurotransmitters and receptors can occur at the synaptic junction. Hormones circulated through the blood react with receptors on the target organs. Receptor and molecular interaction is determined by their compatibility and fit.

Agonist Gated Ion Channel Receptors

Some receptors regulate ion channels in the cell membrane. An ion-gated channel is a selective pathway in which the membrane allows transfer of specific chemicals across its concentration gradient. A receptor can be coupled with an ion channel. When a specific neurotransmitter interacts with a given receptor, a gate opens and the intended ions enter the cell. For example, some calcium channels in the heart are controlled by this mechanism. Thus when a receptor/neurotransmitter interaction occurs, calcium is allowed to enter the cell. In the case of myocardial cells, calcium influx controls the strength of contraction.

G Protein–Coupled Receptors

Adrenergic and cholinergic receptors belong to a family of receptors called *G protein–coupled receptors* (GPCRs). GPCR systems are composed of chains of proteins that wind back and forth through the cell membrane seven times.

GPCR systems have three main parts: the receptor site itself, G protein, and an effector (such as an enzyme). When the receptor site is stimulated, it in turn stimulates the G protein. Once the G protein is switched on, it initiates a response in the effector.

Second Messengers

A **second messenger** (also called a *biochemical messenger*) is a molecule that relays signals from a receptor on the surface of a cell to target molecules in the cell's nucleus or internal fluid where a physiologic action is to take place. Second messengers can greatly amplify the strength of the signal received. One common second messenger is the calcium ion (Ca^{++}).

Receptor Regulation

Cells have the ability to self-regulate their sensitivity to a substance. When a receptor has long-term exposure to a substance (such as a hormone, neurotransmitter, or drug molecule), the cell may decrease the number of receptors exposed to that substance to reduce its sensitivity. This is called **downregulation.** When a receptor is blocked by a substance long term, the cell will increase the number of receptors exposed to it to improve its sensitivity to the substance. This is called **upregulation.** Drug tolerance and physical dependence (discussed later in this chapter) are influenced by upregulation and downregulation.

Altering Neurotransmission with Drugs

Pharmacology has made great strides in using drugs to interfere with neurotransmission. These drugs are able to produce the biologic effects that may be necessary to help minimize the effects of disease and injury. Some pharmaceuticals are chemically identical to neurotransmitters. Others inhibit the neurotransmitter from stimulating particular receptors. This area of pharmacology is under constant investigation and many new therapies are being developed.

GENERAL PROPERTIES OF DRUGS

[OBJECTIVE 12]

Drugs do not generally give body tissues or organs any new functions. They are designed to take an existing body function and change for a particular advantage. In general, drugs exert multiple actions rather than a single effect. When considering administration of a drug, you must consider all the actions of that medication. For example, morphine is a powerful pain reliever. However, it also dilates blood vessels. When giving morphine for pain relief, you must recognize that the drug also may lower the patient's blood pressure.

Drug action results from a physiochemical interaction between the drug and a functionally important molecule in the body. Some drugs change the activity within the cell membrane. Others combine with small molecules to produce an effect. Most drugs combine with receptor sites on a target cell or within the cell.

DRUG FORMS

[OBJECTIVE 13]

Drugs come in many different forms that have been developed to help with absorption and ease of delivery.

Liquid Drug Forms

Liquid drugs contain medication ground into a powder and mixed with a solvent, often water. A summary of liquid drug forms is given in Box 11-9.

Solid Drug Forms

A solid drug often is swallowed and placed in this form because of its stability and ease of administration. A summary of solid drug forms is given in Box 11-10.

Gas Drug Forms

Gases are substances that are inhaled and absorbed through the respiratory tract. They are commonly used for anesthesia. Medications in a gaseous state at room temperature are not commonly used in EMS. Nitrous oxide ("laughing gas") is used in some EMS systems to relieve moderate to severe pain from specific conditions.

BOX 11-9 Liquid Drug Forms

- **Elixir:** A clear, oral solution that contains the drug, water, and some alcohol
- **Emulsion:** A water and oil mixture containing medication
- **Extract:** A concentrated preparation of a vegetable or animal drug, usually prepared by placing the drug in a water or alcohol solution and evaporating off the excess solvent to a prescribed standard (e.g., liver extract).
- **Solution:** A medication dissolved in a liquid, often water
- **Spirit:** A medication containing volatile aromatic substances
- **Suspension:** Medication suspended in a liquid, such as an oral antibiotic
- **Syrup:** A medication dissolved in water with sugar or a sugar substitute to disguise taste, such as cough syrup
- **Tincture:** A medicine consisting of an extract in an alcohol solution, such as tincture of iodine, tincture of mercurochrome

BOX 11-10 Solid Drug Forms

- **Caplet:** A tablet with an oblong shape and a film-coated covering
- **Capsule:** Small gelatin shell in which a powdered or granule form of medication is placed; easy to swallow, and the shell will not begin to break down until in the GI tract; popular because of reduced adverse taste when swallowing
- **Enteric-coated tablets:** Tablets with a special coating designed to break down in the intestines instead of the stomach
- **Gel cap:** Soft gelatin shell filled with liquid medication
- **Pill:** Dried powder forms of medication in the form of a small pellet; the term *pill* has been replaced with tablet and capsule
- **Powder:** Medication ground into a fine substance
- **Suppository:** Drugs combined to make them a solid at room temperature; when placed in a body opening such as the rectum, vagina, or urethra, they dissolve from the increase in body temperature and are absorbed through the surrounding mucosa
- **Tablet:** Medication pressed into a small form that is easy to swallow; has a specific shape and color and may have engraving for identification

BOX 11-11	**Drug Absorption Time (Fastest to Slowest) Based on Route of Administration**

Enteral

- Sublingual
- Rectal
- Nasogastric
- Oral

Parenteral

- IV, intraosseous, intracardiac
- Tracheal, inhalation, intralingual, intranasal
- IM, **topical**
- Subcutaneous
- Intradermal

IV, Intravenous; *IM,* intramuscular.

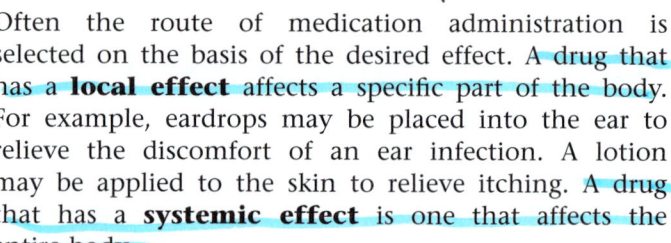

ROUTES OF MEDICATION ADMINISTRATION

[OBJECTIVE 14]

The route of medication administration determines the rate of absorption and onset of action. Many drugs used in emergency care are given by the intravenous route to provide rapid absorption and onset of action. Box 11-11 shows approximate drug absorption times based on the route of administration.

Local versus Systemic Effects

Often the route of medication administration is selected on the basis of the desired effect. A drug that has a **local effect** affects a specific part of the body. For example, eardrops may be placed into the ear to relieve the discomfort of an ear infection. A lotion may be applied to the skin to relieve itching. A drug that has a **systemic effect** is one that affects the entire body.

Route of administration is important in relation to absorption and drug action. Following are the most common routes of administration.

Enteral Routes

An **enteral** drug passes through any portion of the digestive tract. The specific routes of administration that fall into the enteral category are the oral, sublingual, buccal, rectal, and gastric routes.

Case Scenario—continued

The girl's boyfriend informs you that she has told him she has a severe allergy to peanuts. He states that they finished eating in the dorm cafeteria about 1 hour ago (he was unaware of any peanuts). Approximately 20 minutes ago she somewhat abruptly told him that she was sick and that they needed to go to the hospital. They were walking to her car when she collapsed. You orally intubate the patient without difficulty and your partner starts an intravenous line. Ongoing bag-mask ventilation is met with great resistance. Chest wall movement is minimal with positive-pressure ventilation. Her vital signs are pulse, 44 beats/min; blood pressure, 86/40 mm Hg; respirations, 0; and SpO$_2$, 78%. When you consult the base physician, he instructs you to administer epinephrine and diphenhydramine.

Questions

4. *Describe the autonomic innervation of the lungs. What is the effect of epinephrine? How might epinephrine affect the pulse rate, and why?*
5. *Given this patient's condition and assuming no restrictions related to local protocols, what route is most appropriate for the epinephrine? Why?*
6. *What is the brand name of diphenhydramine? What is its drug class? Assuming no restrictions related to local protocols, what route is most appropriate in this case? Why?*

Oral

The **oral** route is used when a drug is given by mouth. This route is one of the most convenient but has one of the slower rates for absorption because of the **first-pass effect.** First-pass effect refers to the breakdown of a drug in the liver and walls of the intestines before it reaches the systemic circulation (Box 11-12).

Sublingual

A drug given by the **sublingual** route is administered directly under the tongue. The drug is then absorbed through the mucous membranes and into the blood vessels. Absorption into the systemic venous circulation is direct because it bypasses the hepatic portal circulation. Advantages of the sublingual route are its accessibility

BOX 11-12 Oral Medication Administration

Advantages

- Readily available route of administration
- Patient acceptance; painless
- Convenient, noninvasive
- Does not generally require special equipment for administration
- No risk of fluid overload, infection, or embolism as with IV medications

Disadvantages

- Limited value in an emergent situation
- Requires a responsive, cooperative patient with an intact gag reflex
- Requires functioning and sufficient gastrointestinal tract for absorption to occur
- Slow or erratic absorption after ingestion
- Possible irritation of gastric mucosa resulting in nausea, vomiting, diarrhea, and/or ulceration
- May cause gagging or aspiration if administered too rapidly

Examples

- Activated charcoal
- Aspirin

Special Considerations

- May require higher doses of a drug for a therapeutic systemic effect
- Do not administer oral medications in solid form (capsules, tablets) to young children because of the danger of aspiration

IV, Intravenous.

BOX 11-13 Oral Transmucosal (Sublingual, Buccal) Medication Administration

Advantages

- Readily available route of administration
- Ease of administration
- Painless
- Rapid onset of action

Disadvantages

- Requires a responsive, cooperative patient with an intact gag reflex
- Unsuitable for young patients who may not understand instructions
- Limited number of medications can be administered by this route
- Variable absorption
- May irritate oral mucosa

Examples

- Nitroglycerin (sublingual)
- Oral glucose
- Some sedatives

Special Considerations

- Mucosal surfaces typically have a rich blood supply, allowing rapid drug transport to the systemic circulation

(easily used by patients who use nitroglycerin tablets or spray) and rapid onset. However, the patient must be adequately hydrated for the drug to be absorbed well.

Buccal

The **buccal** route provides the same mechanism as the sublingual route, except the medication is placed in the mouth between the gum and the mucous membrane of the cheek and absorbed into the bloodstream (Box 11-13).

Rectal

The **rectal** route is typically used for drugs provided in suppository form. This route eliminates some of the first-pass effect. Although the surface area of the rectum is small, it is highly vascular. Drugs given rectally are used for both local and systemic effects. Situations that would benefit from this route include a child who is seizing, when diazepam (Valium) can be given without starting an intravenous line (Box 11-14).

Gastric

The **gastric** route is used when a tube has been placed in the digestive tract, such as a **nasogastric,** orogastric, or gastrostomy tube. This bypasses the voluntary swallowing reflex. This route may be used in patients who cannot take medications orally for long periods or a situation in which the drug needs to be delivered to the gastrointestinal tract but the patient is not cooperative. For example, an orogastric tube may be inserted in a patient who took an overdose. Activated charcoal is then given through the tube and into the gastrointestinal tract to **adsorb** the toxin ingested. A list of the enteral routes of medication administration is shown in Box 11-15.

Parenteral Routes

The **parenteral** route refers to giving a patient a medication that does not pass through the digestive tract. This route of administration avoids the first-pass effect of metabolism so drug absorption is more rapid and complete. Parenteral drug administration includes a variety of specific routes, including intravenous, intraosseous, intracardiac, endotracheal, inhalation, intralingual, intranasal, intramuscular, subcutaneous, transdermal, intrathecal, intradermal, and umbilical routes.

BOX 11-14 Rectal Medication Administration

Advantages
- Route is always available
- More easily accessible route during active seizures than IV route
- Rapid absorption
- Relatively painless

Disadvantages
- Limited number of medications can be administered by this route
- Absorption can be erratic, delayed, or prevented if the drug is not retained in the rectum or if stool is present
- Most patients dislike this route of administration

Examples
- Anticonvulsants
- Antipyretics
- Antiemetics
- Analgesics
- Sedatives

Special Considerations
- Avoid this route in patients with rectal trauma and immunosuppressed patients in whom even minimal trauma could lead to formation of an abscess

IV, Intravenous.

BOX 11-15 Enteral Routes of Medication Administration

- Oral
- Sublingual
- Buccal
- Rectal
- Gastric

BOX 11-16 Intravenous Medication Administration

Advantages
- Immediate onset of action
- Route is easily accessible
- Particularly useful for resuscitation medications and fluids
- Drugs can be given by continuous IV infusion or intermittently in small amounts
- Dosages can be adjusted (titrated) to the patient's response
- Predictable drug absorption; control over the level of the drug in the blood

Disadvantages
- Painful
- Limits patient mobility
- Time consuming
- Requires technical expertise to perform
- Significant potential for causing adverse reactions

Examples
- IV fluids
- Antiarrhythmics
- Antihistamines
- Diuretics
- Sedatives
- Analgesics

Special Considerations
- No barriers to absorption because the drug is administered directly into the circulatory system
- One of the most dangerous routes of medication administration; once a drug is given, stopping or slowing the effects of the drug is difficult because of its rapid action
- Some drugs are incompatible with an existing IV infusion
- The escape or leakage of some drugs from a blood vessel into the surrounding tissue can cause significant tissue damage.
- Do not attempt IV access in a child with respiratory distress unless the procedure is necessary for immediate lifesaving interventions

IV, Intravenous.

Intravenous

When the **intravenous (IV)** route is used, a drug is given directly into the venous circulation. As a result, it offers instantaneous and nearly complete absorption through peripheral or central venous access (Box 11-16).

Intraosseous

The **intraosseous** route is used in emergency situations when peripheral venous access is not established. A needle is passed through the cortex of the bone and the medication is infused into the capillary network within the bone matrix (Box 11-17).

Intracardiac

The **intracardiac** route of drug administration involves injecting a drug directly into a ventricle of the heart during cardiac arrest. This technique is associated with many complications, including laceration of a coronary artery, injection of the drug into the heart muscle instead of a heart chamber, pneumothorax, and cardiac tamponade. The intracardiac route of medication administration is not a paramedic skill.

Endotracheal

The endotracheal route refers to administration of a drug by tracheal tube. Although a large surface area is available for absorption in the respiratory tract, medication absorption by this route is unpredictable. The endotracheal

BOX 11-17 Intraosseous Medication Administration

Advantages
- Rapid onset
- Control over the level of the drug in the blood
- Effective route when venous access is difficult or time consuming
- Useful for resuscitation medications and fluids

Disadvantages
- Painful
- Limits patient mobility
- Requires technical expertise to perform

Examples
- IV fluids
- Antiarrhythmics
- Vasopressors

Special Considerations
- No barriers to absorption
- Onset of action similar to that of IV route

IV, Intravenous.

BOX 11-18 Tracheal Medication Administration

Advantages
- Permits delivery of specific medications into the pulmonary alveoli and systemic circulation by way of lung capillaries

Disadvantages
- Limited number of medications can be administered by this route
- Medication absorption may be negatively affected by the presence of blood, emesis, or secretions in the trachea or tracheal tube
- No fluid resuscitation possible with this route

Examples
- Use the mnemonic "NAVEL": *n*aloxone, *a*tropine, *v*asopressin, *e*pinephrine, *l*idocaine

[handwritten: L] only give 1x every 20 min during cardiac arrest

Special Considerations
- Although this route is not preferred, the endotracheal route can be used for medication administration during resuscitation efforts if an endotracheal tube is in place but IV or intraosseous access is not available.

route is sometimes used to give drugs to a patient in cardiac arrest in whom vascular access has not been obtained (Box 11-18).

Inhalation *[handwritten: Albuterol]*

Inhalation is the route often used for patients in respiratory distress. Drugs may be humidified and nebulized. This process aerosolizes the drug into tiny particles that are taken in directly to the respiratory tract with each breath (Box 11-19).

Intralingual *[handwritten: Narcan]*

The **intralingual** route is the direct injection of a small volume of medication into the underside of the tongue. Naloxone has been used by this route for narcotic overdose when peripheral venous access could not be obtained.

Intranasal *[handwritten: Versed]*

The **intranasal** route offers direct delivery of medications into the nasal passages and sinuses. It is an effective route for treating sinus congestion and cold symptoms with over-the-counter medications without the systemic side effects. Several medications used in emergency care also can be administered by this route (Box 11-20).

Intramuscular

The **intramuscular (IM)** route is an injection of medication directly into a skeletal muscle. The volume of medication is determined by the size of the muscle. Larger muscles may receive a larger volume of medication. This route is useful when IV access is not established. For

BOX 11-19 Pulmonary (Inhaled) Medication Administration

Advantages
- Provides direct action between the drug and receptors in the bronchi
- Painless
- Ease of administration
- Rapid onset of action

Disadvantages
- Limited use with respiratory failure
- Medications used are limited to those with actions on or absorption through the respiratory tract

Examples
- Oxygen
- Bronchodilators
- Nitrous oxide
- Steroids

Special Considerations
- Administration may be difficult if the patient is uncooperative
- Medication delivery is affected by airway size and the degree of obstruction within the airways from mucous plugs, bronchoconstriction, and inflammation

BOX 11-20 Intranasal Medication Administration

Advantages
- Easy to administer
- Rapid, reliable onset of action
- Relatively painless
- Obviates need for painful injections

Disadvantages
- Some medications (such as midazolam) are associated with a burning sensation and tearing of the eyes when given by this route
- Limited number of medications can be administered by this route
- May cause gagging or aspiration if given too rapidly

Examples
- Phenylephrine (Neo Synephrine)
- Fentanyl
- Midazolam
- Lorazepam
- Steroids

Special Considerations
- Intranasal medications are given by spray, drops, or aerosol into the nasal cavity.
- The medication is being given too quickly if the patient sputters, coughs, or swallows during administration.
- Do not give medications by this route if the patient has respiratory distress, copious nasal secretions, or nasal bleeding because of the increased risk of airway obstruction and aspiration.

BOX 11-21 Intramuscular Medication Administration

Advantages
- Readily available route
- Useful route when IV access is not established
- Allows delivery of a variety of medications

Disadvantages
- More painful than Sub-Q injection
- Requires specific knowledge of anatomy and technical expertise to perform
- Volume of medication that can be delivered is limited by the site chosen and patient's size
- Medication is absorbed slightly more rapidly than Sub-Q injection
- Can cause local tissue injury and nerve damage if improper technique is used
- Chronic injections may damage tissue (fibrosis, abscesses)

Examples
- Glucagon
- Sedatives
- Analgesics
- Antihistamines
- Some vitamins

Special Considerations
- Absorption may be rapid or slow depending on the water solubility of the drug and blood flow to the injection site.
- Creates fear and anxiety in some patients (especially children) and may cause a patient to deny pain to avoid further injections of analgesics.
- IM injections alter serum markers (creatine phosphokinase) used to determine presence of myocardial infarction and muscle damage, interfering with interpretation of test results.

IM, Intramuscular; *IV,* intravenous; *Sub-Q,* subcutaneous.

example, a symptomatic patient with a low blood sugar may be given glucagon IM if glucose cannot be given because IV access is delayed (Box 11-21).

Subcutaneous

The **subcutaneous (Sub-Q)** route is an injection of medication in a liquid form placed underneath the skin into the subcutaneous tissue. The Sub-Q route is slightly slower in action than if the drug is placed in the muscle itself (Box 11-22).

Transdermal

The **transdermal** route involves absorption of the medication through the skin barrier. This route offers slow absorption. Be sure to look for transdermal patches or disks when assessing your patient. Nitroglycerin patches are usually found on the upper chest. Nicotine patches may be found on the upper arms or buttocks. Patches used to control nausea, vomiting, or dizziness may be found behind the ear. Estrogen patches may be found on the buttocks or thighs. Medications used for pain relief may be found anywhere on the body, including the arms, thighs, and abdomen.

Intrathecal

The **intrathecal** route of medication administration is the direct deposition of medication into the spinal canal. This route is used during childbirth and for chronic back pain. It lessens the systemic side effects of pain medications. The intrathecal route of medication administration is not a paramedic skill.

Umbilical

The **umbilical** route may be used in newborns. Because the umbilical cord was the primary source of nutrient and waste exchange, it provides an immediate route of access for drug and fluid administration. It often is used only temporarily but is effective in immediate drug absorption for the newborn. Use of this route requires special training and approval from medical direction.

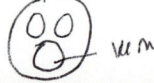

BOX 11-22 | Subcutaneous Medication Administration

Advantages

- Readily available route
- Allows delivery of a variety of medications
- Less painful than intramuscular injection

Disadvantages

- Painful; creates fear and anxiety in most patients
- Requires technical expertise to perform
- Volume of medication that can be delivered is small
- Slower onset and lower peak effects than intravenous route
- Can cause local tissue injury and nerve damage if improper technique used

Examples

- Epinephrine
- Morphine
- Heparin
- Insulin
- Some vaccines
- Allergy desensitization
- Hormone replacement

Special Considerations

- Inappropriate route for medications that are irritating and are not water soluble.
- Absorption may be rapid or slow depending on the water solubility of the drug and blood flow to the injection site.
- The most common sites used are the lateral aspect of the upper arms, the abdomen from the costal margins to the iliac crests, and the anterior thighs.
- Avoid this route of administration if a patient shows signs of shock. Decreased tissue perfusion may radically decrease the rate of drug absorption.

Intradermal

The **intradermal** route of injection is delivery of a medication between the dermal layers of skin. Local anesthetics and allergy testing are examples of uses of this route. A list of parenteral drug administration routes is shown in Box 11-23.

MECHANISMS OF DRUG ACTION

[OBJECTIVE 15]

Once a drug is given, the molecules of the chemical compound must proceed from the point of entry into the body to the tissues with which they react. The extent of the response depends on the dosage and the frequency of doses of the drug in the body. The concentration of the drug at its site of action is influenced by various processes. These processes are divided into three phases of drug activity: pharmaceutical, pharmacokinetic, and pharmacodynamic.

BOX 11-23 | Parenteral Drug Administration Routes

- Intravenous
- Intraosseous
- Intracardiac
- Tracheal
- Inhalation
- Intranasal
- Intralingual
- Intramuscular
- Subcutaneous
- Intrathecal
- Transdermal
- Umbilical
- Intradermal

BOX 11-24 | Four Main Processes of Pharmacokinetics

- Absorption
- Distribution
- Metabolism (biotransformation)
- Elimination and excretion

Pharmaceutical Phase

[OBJECTIVE 16]

Pharmaceutics is the science of preparing and dispensing drugs. During the pharmaceutical phase, a drug is broken down into solution in the body so that it can be absorbed. Because a solid drug must first dissolve into a liquid, oral drugs in liquid form are available more quickly for absorption.

Pharmacokinetics

[OBJECTIVE 17]

[handwritten: How drug moves through body]

Pharmacokinetics is the process by which a drug is ✳ absorbed, distributed, metabolized, and eliminated by the body (Box 11-24).

Modes of Transport

Drugs must be distributed throughout the body to reach the desired receptors on target tissues. To reach these tissues, drugs must cross many tissue barriers, including blood vessel walls, fat tissue, the blood-brain barrier, and even the placental barrier. Depending on the substance, different means of crossing barriers are possible. Some require energy, some carriers, and others simply move because of differences in concentrations.

- **Passive transport** is the ability of a substance to cross a barrier without using energy. Most drug movement occurs by this mechanism. In general, molecules travel down a concentration gradient. The body is working toward equilibrium. When the bloodstream has received a concentration of a drug, it diffuses into the interstitial tissues unless a barrier is present. Diffusion continues until the concentration is equal on both sides of the blood vessel wall. When the concentration is equal this is termed equilibrium or steady state. The term *passive* is used because this occurs without any energy.

- **Diffusion** is the passive transport of solutes (small particles).
- **Osmosis** is the passive movement of water.
- **Facilitated transport** is similar to passive transport. No energy is expended; however, the molecules may only cross the barrier if they find the correct gate. This is generally a protein channel. When they reach the correct gate, they fit like a lock and key and are transported across the barrier. They are still traveling from a high to a low concentration, so no energy is required. This continues until concentrations are equal on both sides.
- **Active transport** is used to move drug molecules and other substances from areas of low concentration to areas of high concentration (against the concentration gradient). Active transport requires an energy source. The classic example of this type of transport occurs with the sodium/potassium pump at the cell membrane.

Stages of Drug Function

A drug goes through four phases of activity after it is given: absorption, distribution, metabolism, and elimination.

Absorption. When a drug is introduced into the digestive system, it must be absorbed into the bloodstream and transported to its intended site of action to produce an effect. Because some drugs can be given by more than one route, factors that affect the speed of **absorption** must be considered. General factors affecting drug absorption include the following (Box 11-25):

- *Nature of the absorbing surface.* A drug that must pass through several cell layers (as in the intestines) is absorbed more slowly than a drug that must pass only through a single layer of cells (such as the skin). The greater the size of the absorbing surface, the greater the absorption and the more rapid its effects. For example, absorption from a small

absorbing surface such as the stomach is slower than from a larger absorbing surface, such as the lungs or small intestine.

- *Blood flow to the site of administration.* The greater the blood supply to an area, the more rapid the absorption. For example, giving albuterol by inhalation, nitroglycerin by sublingual tablet or spray, or epinephrine IV results in rapid absorption and onset of action. Blood flow to an area can be affected by infection, shock, swelling, or a failing heart, among other conditions. The presence of any of these conditions can affect your decision about the best route to administer a drug.
- *Solubility of the drug.* **Solubility** pertains to the ease with which a drug can dissolve. Parenteral drugs dissolved in water or sodium chloride are absorbed more quickly than those dissolved in oily substances. The form of a drug also affects how quickly a drug dissolves.
- *pH.* The acidity of a drug and its surroundings in the body affect absorption. An acidic drug such as aspirin is readily absorbed in an acidic environment, such as the stomach. Alkaline medications are more readily absorbed in the small intestine.
- *Drug concentration.* Drugs given in high concentrations usually are absorbed more rapidly than drugs given in low concentrations. Sometimes a dose higher than the usual dose of a drug (loading dose) is given for one or two doses to achieve the desired effect rapidly.
- *Dosage form.* A drug is absorbed quickly if it is in liquid form. In some situations, a delayed action of a drug is desired. Timed-release or controlled-release drugs are specially made to release their active ingredients slowly or in repeated small amounts over time.
- *Routes of drug administration.* The route by which a drug is given affects how quickly it begins to work and the extent of the response to the drug.
- *Bioavailability.* **Bioavailability** refers to the speed with which and how much of a drug reaches its intended site of action. The presence or absence of food in the stomach, other drugs, and digestive disorders can affect drug absorption and bioavailability. Drugs that are improperly stored may become ineffective. Drugs must be stored properly and their expiration dates routinely checked to ensure patient safety.

Enteric Absorption. A drug may be ingested, and thus absorption occurs through the stomach and intestinal wall into the capillaries. Most drugs are absorbed in the duodenum. Drugs mainly pass this barrier by two routes: across the cell membranes (transcellular pathway) and through the intercellular spaces between the intestinal cells (paracellular pathway). Patients who have had part of their GI tract removed from disease or through bariatric surgery have lost a portion of their surface area and thus have slower absorption. Once a drug moves

---

BOX 11-25 | **General Factors Affecting Drug Absorption**

- Nature of the absorbing surface
- Blood flow to site of administration
- Solubility of the drug
- pH
- Drug concentration
- Dosage form
- Route of drug administration
- Bioavailability

through the intestinal wall, it moves into the capillaries and is carried through the venous system into the systemic circulation.

Parenteral Absorption. A drug that is given by a parenteral route does not enter the GI tract. The drug is absorbed in the bloodstream, delivered to capillaries, and then to the systemic circulation. The drug-specific absorption rate depends on the medicine and which parenteral route was selected. For example, the quickest route of parenteral absorption is direct injection into the systemic circulation. This is why IV access is quickly established and used most often when giving emergency care. When giving a drug by the IM or Sub-Q routes, remember that the greater the blood supply to an area, the more rapid the absorption. For instance, a large muscle group has a greater blood flow because of its higher nutrient requirements. Thus it receives the drug faster and at a higher concentration than a small muscle. Fat tissue does not require as much blood flow, so absorption is slower and thus fat tissue receives a lower amount of the drug.

Distribution. Once a drug is absorbed into the bloodstream, it travels through the blood, lymph, and other body fluids to various body tissues and then to its target site of action. **Distribution** of a drug occurs more quickly to those organs with higher blood flow (such as the brain, heart, liver, and kidneys) than areas with less blood flow (such as the skin, fat, and muscles).

Many drugs attach to protein molecules in the plasma when they enter the systemic circulation. Albumin is the most abundant plasma protein and binds the widest range of drugs. However, because of their large size and inability to leave the bloodstream, plasma proteins serve as a drug reservoir by default. Drugs that bind to plasma proteins are inactive and unable to reach their target organs. When released (unbound) from a plasma protein, the drug can reach its target site and cause its intended effect. As the unbound (free) drug acts on its target site, the level of the drug in the plasma decreases. A fall in the plasma level of the drug triggers the release of some of the bound drug from the plasma protein. By binding to plasma proteins, a drug dose can be stored in the body and released as needed.

Because cell membranes contain a fatty acid layer, drugs that dissolve in fat (fat-soluble drugs) are distributed quickly. They are able to pass through the cell membranes easily and reach their target sites more quickly than drugs that dissolve in water (water-soluble drugs). Water-soluble drugs tend to stay within the blood and the fluid that surrounds the cells (interstitial space).

Many disease states alter distribution. For example, narrowing of the arteries can impair the effects of a drug; fewer drug molecules reach their site of action. Diseases that result in swelling can cause prolonged distribution and delayed clearance of the drug. These disease states include heart failure, liver failure (cirrhosis), and renal disturbances. Additionally, normal physiologic barriers in the body may hamper distribution. Normal barriers include those of the cell wall, the blood-brain barrier, and the placental barrier.

Blood-Brain Barrier. Capillaries in most areas of the body are lined with endothelial cells separated by small gaps. These gaps allow substances to pass between the inside and outside of the vessel. However, in the brain these cells are packed together so tightly that most drugs cannot pass through the interstitial space. Thus a protective barrier of tightly adhered cells is formed, called the **blood-brain barrier.** To pass through this barrier, a drug must be lipid soluble (such as oxygen, carbon dioxide, ethanol, benzodiazepines, and some steroids) or have a transport system to leave the bloodstream and reach a site of action within the brain (such as sugars and some amino acids).

The blood-brain barrier is useful in protecting the brain, spinal cord, and spinal fluid from toxins, bacteria, and viruses. Few molecules can pass through this barrier. Oxygen, water, and small nutrients such as glucose are able to pass with relatively little difficulty and supply the brain with needed nutrients. Conditions such as chronic high blood pressure, multiple sclerosis, trauma, and infection can reduce the effectiveness of the blood-brain barrier.

Placental Barrier. During pregnancy, some drugs can cross the placenta and affect the fetus. The **placental barrier** is composed of many cell layers. It protects the developing fetus from many toxins circulated through the maternal circulation. Small molecules such as nutrients, gases, and wastes are easily transported through the placental barrier. Water- and lipid-soluble drugs also cross the barrier. Some drugs taken by the mother during the first trimester of pregnancy can have a harmful effect on the fetus (although they may be beneficial for the mother). Some substances (such as alcohol and narcotics) may cause harmful effects on both the mother and fetus. The placental barrier is not perfect, but it does slow the transport of many toxins.

Metabolism. **Metabolism** (also called *biotransformation*) is the chemical modification of the original drug by the body. Most drugs must be metabolized before they can be excreted. The liver is the chief organ of metabolism, although other tissues and sites can play an important role for specific drugs. Other sites of drug metabolism include the kidneys, intestinal mucosa, lungs, plasma, and placenta.

When a drug is metabolized, a series of chemical reactions occur that either (1) change an active drug into a less-active or inactive form of the drug, or (2) change a less-active or inactive form of the drug (called a **prodrug**) into a more active drug. Most FDA-approved drugs are transformed into harmless **metabolites** (smaller components) and excreted. Some medications are metabolized to harmful metabolites in certain conditions. When a patient has liver disease, metabolism of medications through the liver is impaired. The amount of the medication given to the patient remains in the bloodstream longer. Repeated doses increase the level of the drug in the blood, predisposing the patient to toxic effects of the drug.

Excretion/Elimination. The kidneys are the site most often used for drug **excretion (elimination).** Other sites for drug excretion include the liver, lungs, sweat, salivary glands, and mammary glands. Most drugs and/or their metabolites not bound to plasma proteins are eliminated in the urine. Patients who have renal disease may have an impaired ability to eliminate drugs by the kidneys.

The liver excretes drugs and/or their metabolites into bile, which is then excreted into the small intestine. Some drugs or metabolites are then excreted in stool. Other drugs are excreted in bile, reabsorbed, returned to the liver (a process called enterohepatic cycling), metabolized, and eventually excreted in urine. This recycling process prolongs the activity of the drug. Drugs or metabolites not recycled are excreted through stool. Patients who have liver disease may have an impaired ability to eliminate drugs by the liver. Patients who have both renal and liver disease may be at risk because of a buildup of the effects of drugs.

The lungs excrete gaseous wastes, such as carbon dioxide, during exhalation. Volatile and gaseous substances such as anesthetics, solvents, and alcohol are also excreted through the lungs. Small amounts of drugs can be eliminated through the sweat glands and saliva. Some drugs taken by nursing mothers can be excreted in breast milk. If a nursing mother must take medication, she should talk with her physician to ensure the drug will not harm her baby.

PARAMEDIC*Pearl*

All drugs undergo the following processes from the time they are given until they produce an effect:

- Entry into the body and then the bloodstream (absorption)
- Movement through the bloodstream to the target organ (distribution)
- Production of an intended effect
- Chemical breakdown (metabolism)
- Removal from the body (elimination)

Pharmacodynamics
How drug works in body

Theories of Drug Action

Drug-Receptor Interaction. Once a drug is distributed to its target tissue, it must interact with other molecules. This interaction causes the physiologic response. Interactions between drug molecules and receptors can be overwhelming and complex. Perhaps the best way to think about this is to imagine a lock and key. The key represents a drug. The lock represents a receptor molecule. Many keys of differing sizes and shapes (different chemical molecules for different drugs) and different locks (different receptors) exist. When a key (drug molecule) of the right size and shape fits into its specific lock (receptor), drug-receptor binding occurs (Figure 11-5). This binding "unlocks" the cell so that the drug can exert a chemical reaction and produce the desired physiologic effect. This lock and key example can also be used to explain the action of hormones and neurotransmitters on specific receptors.

Affinity refers to the intensity or strength of the attraction between a drug and its receptor. If a drug and receptor are not compatible, no physiologic response occurs. Not all drugs can interact with all receptors. **Efficacy** is the ability of a drug to produce a physiologic response after attaching to a receptor. An **agonist** is a drug that causes a physiologic response in the receptor to which it binds. An agonist possesses affinity and efficacy. A **partial agonist** is a chemical molecule that interacts with the receptor but does not cause a significant physiologic response. The key fits the lock but does not provide the full physiologic response. Therefore a partial agonist has affinity and some efficacy. Some research has investigated the theory that in the absence of an agonist, a partial agonist may stimulate the receptor. When a partial agonist and agonist are both present, the partial agonist can actually block the effect of the agonist if the partial agonist has a stronger receptor site affinity.

An **antagonist** is a drug that binds to a receptor and blocks or causes an opposite response in that receptor. Think of this as a key fitting into a lock but

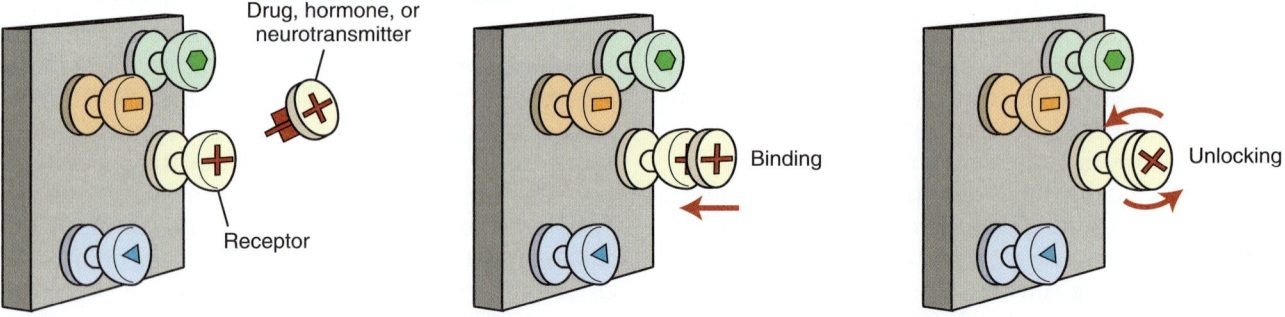

Figure 11-5 Drug-receptor interaction. Think of the key as a drug and the lock as a receptor molecule. When a key of the right size and shape fits in its specific lock, binding occurs. Binding unlocks the cell so that a drug, hormone, or neurotransmitter can exert a chemical reaction and produce the desired physiologic effect.

not being able to turn and open it. Because the first key (antagonist) is occupying space, another key (an agonist) cannot be inserted into the lock (receptor) because it is already occupied. Antagonists often are used in medicine. For example, naloxone is an opioid (narcotic) antagonist used in the treatment of narcotic overdoses. When naloxone is given, it displaces narcotics from their receptor sites. With naloxone now occupying space in the lock (receptor), the narcotic cannot bind to its receptor and exert its effect on body cells. Naloxone does not cause a response in the receptor. The depressant effects of the narcotic are reversed because naloxone displaced the narcotics from their receptor sites.

Drug-Enzyme Interaction. Acetylation is a mechanism in which a drug is processed by enzymes. Research shows that some people are slow acetylators and some are rapid acetylators. Rapid acetylators represent most of the population. Slow acetylators are more likely to experience drug side effects at standard doses.

Nonspecific Drug Interaction. Some drugs do not require receptors or enzymes to produce an effect. For example, an ointment may be applied to the skin to reduce swelling, itching, or pain. Antacids decrease the acidity of the stomach by causing a chemical reaction with the hydrochloric acid present in gastric juice.

Drug-Response Relation

Plasma Level Profile. Rates of absorption, distribution, metabolism, and elimination are unique to each drug. The **therapeutic dose** (also called the *effective dose*) of a drug is the dose required to produce a beneficial effect in 50% of the drug-tested population. A lethal dose and a toxic dose are not the same things. The **median lethal dose,** or LD_{50}, is the dose that kills 50% of the drug-tested population. The toxic dose, or TD_{50}, is the dose at which 50% of test subjects exhibit signs of toxicity. The toxic dose is less than the median lethal dose.

A plasma level profile is a blood test used to monitor and evaluate the effectiveness of a drug. A **plasma level profile** is a description of a drug's activity based on its dosage. When the blood sample is taken, the concentration of the drug in the patient's plasma is measured. Adjustments in dosage may be made on the basis of this measured level.

Half-Life. The therapeutic effect of a drug dose usually is seen when a steady state is reached. **Steady state** refers to an evenly distributed concentration of a drug in the plasma. Steady state is reached when the rate of drug administration is equal to the amount of drug eliminated from the body. The time needed to reach steady state depends on the drug's half-life. The **half-life** of a drug is the time necessary for the concentration of the drug in the blood to be reduced by 50%. Half-life is used to determine when additional amounts of a drug should be given. Concentrations of alcohol and some medications do not reduce by 50%; rather, a specific amount can be eliminated by the body in a certain time frame. The difference in the original concentration is not a factor. For

example, if you took 500 mg of medication X, which has a half-life of 1 hour, after 1 hour 250 mg is left, after 2 hours 125 mg is left, and so forth. On the other hand, if you took 500 mg of medication Y, which the body eliminates at a rate of 25 mg/hr (rate-limited elimination), in 1 hour 475 mg would be left, after 2 hours 450 mg would be left, and so forth.

Therapeutic Threshold. The **therapeutic threshold** (also called the *minimum effective concentration*) is the drug concentration level required to elicit a physiologic therapeutic response in most patients. Any amount less than the therapeutic threshold does not elicit the desired response.

Therapeutic Index. The **therapeutic index (TI)** of a drug pertains to the drug's margin of safety. The TI is derived from the following formula: $TI = LD_{50}/ED_{50}$, where LD_{50} is the lethal dose of a drug for 50% of the population divided by the minimum effective dose for 50% of the population (ED_{50}). The closer the TI is to 1, the more dangerous the medication and more difficult dosing is.

A drug's therapeutic range (TR) is determined by the following formula: $TR = TD_{50} - MEC$, where TD_{50} is the toxic dose of a drug for 50% of the population minus the minimum effective concentration (MEC). A wide therapeutic range means that the drug is relatively safe. A narrow therapeutic range means that the patient's dosage of the drug must be carefully monitored and adjusted.

Factors Altering Drug Responses

Many factors can alter a patient's response to a drug (Box 11-26).

Age. An individual's age affects his or her response to a drug. Because of their immature organs, dosages for infants and children are based on weight or body surface area. An older adult's response to a drug may be affected because of organ degeneration. As a result, the drug concentration level can become toxic with repeated doses at a regular concentration because of impaired excretion.

Gender. The effects of some drugs in women may differ from those of men because of differences in body size and proportions of body fat and water.

BOX 11-26	Factors that Influence Drug Action

- Age
- Gender
- Body weight
- Environment
- General health
- Genetics
- Culture
- Emotional or psychological state
- Time of administration
- Route of administration
- Medication history
- Diet

Body Weight. An adult drug dose is based on an average age (usually 15 to 65 years) and weight (usually approximately 150 pounds). In heavier or leaner adults, the dose must be adjusted to maintain a therapeutic concentration of a drug in the blood. The dose usually is adjusted on the basis of the amount of drug per kilogram of body weight or body surface area.

Environment. Light, moisture, and extreme environmental temperatures can affect the stability of a drug. In high altitudes, the distribution of a drug in the blood is affected because of less available oxygen.

A patient's body temperature can influence how a drug is given or the effects of the drug. For example, IV drugs given to a patient in severe hypothermia are typically given at longer than normal intervals. Drugs such as atropine decrease the body's ability to sweat. Some drugs, such as tricyclic antidepressants, can cause a severe sunburn, hives, or rash if the patient is exposed to sunlight or strong ultraviolet light.

General Health. A person's general health can affect his or her response to a drug. For example, a patient with known cardiovascular disease may be adversely affected when given epinephrine. The same drug may be beneficial in a patient without this condition. Conditions that impair the body's ability to metabolize or excrete drugs (such as liver or kidney disease) can alter a patient's response to a drug and increase the risk of drug toxicity. Acid-base imbalance and electrolyte disorders can also alter a patient's response to a drug.

Genetics. Genetics can influence how well a person's body metabolizes a drug and the time required to metabolize it. **Pharmacogenetics** is the study of inherited differences (variation) in drug metabolism and response. In recent years, an increasing number of genetic variations in drug-metabolizing enzymes and receptors have been identified. Genetic variations influence the rates of drug metabolism, reactions to drugs, and side effects of drugs. For example, some patients metabolize certain drugs more slowly than others do because of an inherited enzyme deficiency. In some cases, these genetic factors have a major impact on an individual's drug sensitivity and adverse reactions. For instance, research shows that some individuals lack aldehyde dehydrogenase. This enzyme is necessary to metabolize ethanol. Patients lacking this enzyme experience the adverse effects of flushing, headache, nausea, and vomiting with the smallest amounts of alcohol ingestion.

Culture. A patient's cultural beliefs may affect his or her willingness to accept or comply with drug therapy. Persons from Native American, Hispanic American, Asian, some African American, and Eastern European cultures may prefer to use folk remedies.

Herbal medicines are used in many cultures to prevent or treat illness. Some herbal medicines can produce potentially serious interactions with prescription drugs. For example, ginseng is a well-known Chinese medicinal herb. It is used to treat many ailments, including indigestion and mental and physical fatigue as well as to improve memory. Ginseng interacts with prescription drugs, including monamine oxidase inhibitors, hypoglycemic drugs, and some anticoagulants. Although knowing the interactions of all herbal remedies with various medications is not feasible, paramedics working in areas with large populations from other cultures should be familiar with herbal remedies common to those cultures and interactions with medications the paramedic may administer as well as interactions with common prescription medications.

Emotional or Psychological State. A person's attitude can influence the effects of a drug. Strong emotions such as fear or extreme worry can affect the actions of a drug because of changes in metabolism. A depressed patient may not respond to a medication or may not take the medication as prescribed. Some patients may be reluctant to take medications because of social acceptability. For example, taking a drug to control high blood pressure is considered by some to be more socially acceptable than taking a drug to treat certain infectious diseases or mental illnesses.

Time of Administration. Food in the digestive tract may increase, decrease, prevent, or delay drug absorption. Some oral medications should be taken on an empty stomach. Others should be taken with food to reduce stomach irritation. Many drugs must be repeated to maintain a therapeutic concentration of the drug in the blood. For example, some antibiotics must be given three times daily to maintain a therapeutic concentration and obtain optimal results.

Route of Administration. The route by which a drug is given affects how quickly the drug's onset of action occurs and may affect the therapeutic response that results. Some drugs reach their therapeutic concentration only if given by a certain route.

Medication History. If a person uses a drug for a long time, the effects of the drug may be reduced because tolerance has developed. On the other hand, long-term use also can result in an increased effect because of a buildup of the drug in the body.

Diet. The affects of some drugs can be altered by certain foods, beverages, mineral or vitamin supplements, and substances such as alcohol or tobacco. Drug-food interactions can usually be avoided by taking the drug 1 hour before or 2 hours after eating. Examples of drug-food interactions are discussed later in this chapter.

Predictable, Iatrogenic, and Unpredictable Drug Responses

When a drug molecule and receptor interact, a specific physiologic response is expected. This response is the basis on which drugs are prescribed and administered. An **adverse reaction** is an unintentional, undesirable, and often unpredictable effect of a drug used at therapeutic doses to prevent, diagnose, or treat disease. Some adverse reactions are predictable, some are iatrogenic, and some are unpredictable. These drug responses and their definitions appear in Table 11-9.

TABLE 11-9 Adverse Drug Responses

Adverse Response	Term/Phrase	Definition/Explanation
Predictable	Desired action	The intended beneficial effect of a drug
	Side effect	An effect of a drug other than the one for which it was given; may or may not be harmful
Iatrogenic	Iatrogenic drug response	An unintentional disease or drug effect produced by a physician's prescribed therapy; *iatros* means *physician; -genic* is a word root meaning *produce*
Unpredictable	Additive effect	The combined effect of two drugs given at the same time that have similar effects
	Adverse effect (reaction)	An unintentional, undesirable, and often unpredictable effect of a drug used at therapeutic doses to prevent, diagnose, or treat disease
	Anaphylactic reaction	An unusual or exaggerated allergic reaction to a foreign substance
	Cross tolerance	Decreasing responsiveness to the effects of a drug in a drug classification (such as narcotics) and the likelihood of development of decreased responsiveness to another drug in that classification
	Cumulative action	Increased intensity of drug action evident after administration of several doses
	Delayed reaction	A delay between exposure and onset of action
	Drug allergy	A reaction to a medication with an adverse outcome; an immunologic reaction to a drug
	Drug antagonism	The interaction between two drugs in which one partially or completely inhibits the effects of the other
	Drug dependence	A physical need or adaptation to the drug with or without the psychological need to take the drug
	Drug interaction	The manner in which one drug and a second drug (or food) act on each other
	Hypersensitivity	Altered reactivity to a medication that occurs after sensitization; response is independent of the dose
	Idiosyncrasy	An unexpected and usually individual (genetic) adverse response to a drug
	Interference	The ability of one drug to limit the physiologic function of another drug
	Potentiation	A prolongation or increase in the effect of a drug by another drug
	Summation	The combined effects of two or more drugs are equal to the sum of each of their effects
	Synergism	The interaction of drugs such that the total effect is greater than the sum of the individual effects
	Tachyphylaxis	The rapidly decreasing response to a drug or physiologically active agent after administration of a few doses; rapid cross tolerance
	Tolerance	Decreasing responsiveness to the effects of a drug; increasingly larger doses are necessary to achieve the effect originally obtained by a smaller dose

Case Scenario CONCLUSION

You administer the epinephrine immediately and give the diphenhydramine en route the hospital. When you arrive in the emergency department (ED), the patient's condition is largely unchanged. The ED physician administers additional doses of epinephrine and diphenhydramine and starts an inline nebulizer of albuterol, with no apparent improvement. She then administers IV atropine and dexamethasone. After an hour of intensive therapy in the ED, the patient's lungs becomes somewhat easier to ventilate, but her blood pressure begins to fall. After administration of dopamine, the patient's blood pressure is stabilized and she is admitted to the intensive care unit, where she has a full recovery.

Looking Back

7. *What drug class is atropine in? How does this class of medications relate to your answer to question 4? What impact would you expect atropine to have on this patient? Why?*
8. *What is dexamethasone? How might its mechanism affect this patient's condition? How fast do you expect it to work?*
9. *The patient became easier to ventilate after receipt of multiple medications. Considering the effects of various medications on the lungs, what could explain this improvement?*
10. *What drug class is dopamine in? How is it typically administered? How does it affect blood pressure?*

SPECIAL CONSIDERATIONS IN DRUG THERAPY

[OBJECTIVE 18]

Pregnant Patients

A number of physiologic changes occur in the body during pregnancy. These changes include increased heart rate and blood volume and changes in body chemistry. These normal changes affect how drugs are metabolized. Some drugs may cross the placental barrier. A **teratogen** is a drug or agent that is harmful to the development of an embryo or fetus. During fetal growth, some medications taken by the mother may cause harm to the fetus or alter normal development. Other medications may be transferred through breast milk after delivery. When a drug is medically necessary for the mother, formula may need to be used to protect the infant.

The FDA has developed a scale that divides medications into five different pregnancy risk categories. The scale ranks the risk of a systemically absorbed drug to cause harm based on available studies in human beings and animals. Each medication is given a specific letter designation for safety and efficacy in pregnancy and lactation (Table 11-10). Although the pregnancy risk category is useful, caution should be used with drugs that fall under those categories for which only animal data are available (categories B and C). In the United States, drugs were not required to have an assigned risk category until after December 1983. Currently all FDA-approved prescription drugs are pregnancy category rated.

Pediatric Patients

Giving medications to the pediatric patient is challenging because of changes that occur from birth through adolescence in body size, physiology, and general health.

These changes affect how the drug is absorbed, distributed, metabolized, and eliminated; where and how much of the drug is deposited in the body, and the therapeutic effects and side effects of the drug.

At birth, the blood-brain barrier is not fully developed. As a result, newborns are vulnerable to the effects of drugs that affect the CNS. An infant's liver does not mature to its full capacity to metabolize drugs until approximately 1 year after birth. Because the liver may not have all the enzymes developed for proper metabolism, infants are especially sensitive to drugs. For the first 6 months of life, the half-life of many drugs is longer than normal because of a decreased filtration and reabsorption rate in the kidneys. The kidneys become functionally mature when a child is approximately 30 months of age.

Drug doses in infants and children are based on weight or body surface area. Because even a small dosing error can cause adverse effects or death, a tool such as the Broselow tape should be used to determine drug doses in infants and children when a patient's exact weight and age are unknown. The Broselow tape is a length-based resuscitation tape that is color coded. To use it correctly, the tape is placed next to the child so that the end of the tape is even with the top of the child's head (Figure 11-6). The child's approximate weight in kilograms is estimated from the point on the tape next to the child's heels. A color is assigned to this length/weight relation that reflects appropriate drug doses and equipment sizes.

Geriatric Patients

Physiologic changes that occur with aging include loss of bone mass, lean muscle mass, and body water. Water-soluble drugs, such as angiotensin-converting enzyme inhibitors, have a smaller area for drug distribution because of the older adult's lower proportion of body

TABLE 11-10	Food and Drug Administration Pregnancy Risk Categories
Category	Description
A	*No evidence of risk exists.* Controlled studies in women failed to demonstrate a risk to the fetus in the first trimester (and there is no evidence of a risk in later trimesters), and the possibility of fetal harm appears remote.
B	*The risk of human fetal harm is possible but remote.* Either animal reproduction studies have not demonstrated a fetal risk or there are no controlled studies in pregnant women, or animal reproduction studies have shown an adverse effect (other than a decrease in fertility) that was not confirmed in controlled studies in women in the first trimester (and there is no evidence of a risk in later trimesters).
C	*Human fetal risk cannot be ruled out.* Either studies in animals have revealed adverse effects on the fetus or there are no controlled studies in women, or studies in women and animals are not available. Drugs should be given only if the potential benefit justifies the potential risk to the fetus.
D	*Positive evidence of human fetal risk exists.* There is positive evidence of human fetal risk, but the benefits from use in pregnant women may be acceptable despite the risk (for example, if the drug is needed in a life-threatening situation or for a serious disease for which safer drugs cannot be used or are ineffective).
X	*Contraindicated during pregnancy.* Studies in animals or human beings have demonstrated fetal abnormalities, or there is evidence of fetal risk based on human experience or both, and the risk of the use of the drug in pregnant women clearly outweighs any possible benefit. The drug is contraindicated in women who are or may become pregnant.
NR	Not rated

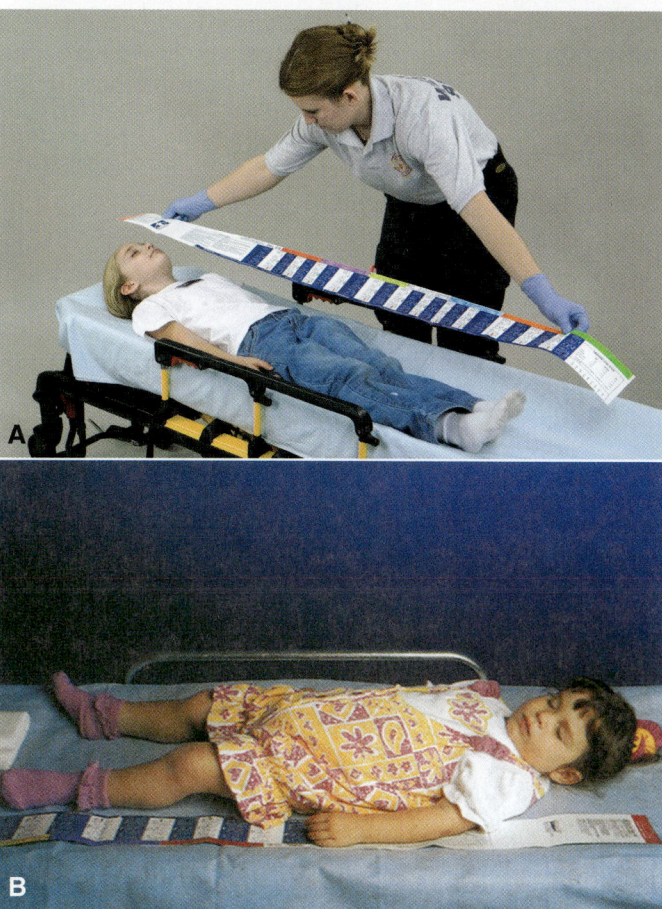

Figure 11-6 The Broselow tape is a length-based tape that is color coded. **A,** To use, unfold the tape. **B,** Place the tape next to the child so that the end of the tape is even with the top of the child's head. The child's approximate weight in kilograms is estimated from the point on the tape next to the child's heels. A color is assigned to this length/weight relation that reflects appropriate drug doses and equipment sizes.

water. This increases the risk for higher drug concentrations in the blood. In contrast, the percentage of fat usually increases. Drugs that dissolve in fat (such as lidocaine and some sedatives) may have a prolonged duration of action in the elderly because of their higher proportion of body fat.

An older adult's response to a drug may be affected because of organ degeneration. To compensate for age-related organ degeneration, doses may need to be reduced or the interval between doses increased. Aging results in decreased blood flow to vital organs, such as the liver. This can be compounded by conditions such as alcoholism, heart failure, or liver disease. With decreased blood flow and function of the liver, increased concentrations of drugs may be in the blood, increasing the risk of toxicity.

Older adults may be taking a number of prescription and over-the-counter medications **(polypharmacy).** An older adult may take multiple medications because he or she has more than one physician, uses more than one pharmacy, has more than one medical condition, or has a complicated illness. The risk of a negative drug interaction increases with the number of medications taken.

Self-medication errors are common in older adults. Errors may occur because the patient took an incorrect dose of a drug, misunderstood instructions, stopped using (or inappropriately continued) medications without consulting the physician, or took a medication for a previous illness or problem. An older adult may stop taking medications because of financial challenges.

PARAMEDIC*Pearl*

When taking a patient's medication history, be sure to ask about *all* the medications the patient is taking. Be alert for possible accidental double dosing of medications. For example, many patients (particularly older adults) may not realize that a prescription bottle labeled "Lasix" contains the same medication as a second bottle labeled "furosemide."

DRUG INTERACTIONS

[OBJECTIVE 19]

Many variables influence drug interaction (Box 11-27). Descriptions of onset of action and therapeutic effects often are described on the basis of healthy human subjects with no variables influencing the drug interaction. Memorizing every medication and the specific interactions that occur would be difficult. However, an understanding of the types of variables that affect drug interactions is important.

Intestinal absorption of any oral medications may be altered by the presence of food. Digestion slows the transit time and thus affects absorption. In contrast, anything that accelerates gastric emptying increases absorption. These factors are independent of the characteristics of the drugs themselves.

Temperature and blood flow are important in determining the rate of absorption. Any state in which body temperature is decreased results in decreased blood flow to the GI tract. Decreased blood flow results in decreased

absorption. Gastric juices may also destroy medications and thus alter their absorption.

Significant competition exists between drugs and other molecules. Drugs can compete with other drugs or with food or nutrients. The competition may occur at the site of absorption, distribution, metabolism, or elimination. In general, the drug that has a higher affinity for any receptor has a higher absorption rate.

Electrolytes may also affect drug interactions. Many drugs rely on the pumps that maintain intracellular and extracellular electrolytes. This is important with some of the antiarrhythmics for cardiac care. Any changes in electrolytes alter the response of these medications.

Metabolism is an area in which significant alterations can occur in the therapeutic effects of medications. Enzymes and their reactions alter medications. This is often done to render them active for therapeutic effects. It may render drugs inactive in preparation for elimination. If considerable competition occurs at the enzymatic sites, one medication may saturate the enzyme. When this occurs, a second medication or toxin may not be able to be metabolized. This may result in toxic levels of a drug or increased circulating levels from the decreased ability to be eliminated.

Drug-Drug Interactions

Most drug-drug interactions involve prescription drugs, but some involve over-the-counter drugs or herbal medicines. Examples of drug-drug interactions are shown in Table 11-11.

Drug-Food Interactions

Intestinal absorption of any oral medication may be altered by the presence of food, including beverages. The significance of a **drug-food interaction** depends on the dose of the drug; when the food is eaten; when the medication is taken; and the patient's age, size, and general health. Examples of food-drug interactions appear in Table 11-12.

BOX 11-27 | **Factors Influencing Drug Action**

- Intestinal absorption
- Drug metabolism or biotransformation
- Action at the receptor site
- Renal excretion
- Alteration of electrolyte balance
- Drug-drug interactions
- Competition for plasma protein binding
- Other drug interactions
  - Drug-induced malabsorption of foods and nutrients
  - Food-induced malabsorption of drugs
  - Alteration of enzymes
  - Alcohol consumption
  - Cigarette smoking
  - Food-initiated alteration of drug excretion
- Drug incompatibilities

DRUG STORAGE

Nitroglycerine sensitive to light, air [handwritten]

[OBJECTIVE 20]

As an EMS professional, you are entrusted with the contents of the drug box. Some medications are volatile and others are medications of abuse. Various protocols exist on how controlled substances are handled and maintained. These protocols must be followed.

Each EMS crew member is responsible for checking the contents of the drug box before the start of each shift. The box should be evaluated for contents, expiration dates, quantity, and locking mechanisms. This action is critical and should never be skipped or overlooked. Occasionally a substance may be out of date or missing. Out-of-date medications must be replaced. Any missing

TABLE 11-11   Examples of Drug-Drug Interactions

Drug	Drug	Interaction
Aspirin	Blood thinners (anticoagulants)	Increases effects, increasing bleeding risk
Antacids	Aspirin	Decreases effect
	Blood thinners	Slows absorption
	Tetracycline (antibiotic)	Interferes with absorption
Antihistamines	Barbiturates, tranquilizers, some prescription pain relievers	Can increase sedative effects
Diazepam (Valium)	Vasodilators	Can increase effects
Diphenhydramine (Benadryl)	Tricyclic antidepressants, monoamine oxidase inhibitors	Increased anticholinergic (drying) effect
	Alcohol, narcotics, sedative/hypnotics	Increased CNS depression
Diphenoxylate and atropine (Lomotil)	Diazepam	Increased sedative effect
Dopamine (Intropin)	Monoamine oxidase inhibitors	Tachycardia, severe hypertension
	Phenytoin (Dilantin)	Hypotension, bradycardia
Epinephrine	Beta-blockers	Block therapeutic effect
	Albuterol	Increased bronchodilator action
Ipratropium bromide (Atrovent)	Anticholinergics	Increased effects
Magnesium sulfate	Antipsychotics, narcotics, barbiturates	CNS depression
Meperidine (Demerol)	Glaucoma medication	Can increase effects
Nitroglycerin	Antihypertensives, beta-blockers, calcium channel blockers	Increased hypotensive effects of nitroglycerin
	Sildenafil (Viagra), tadalafil (Cialis)	Increased hypotensive effects of nitroglycerin
Nonsteroidal anti-inflammatory drugs	Diuretics	Reduced effectiveness of diuretic
Norepinephrine (Levophed)	Tricyclic antidepressants	Severe hypertension, dysrhythmias
Oral hypoglycemics	Beta-blockers	Decreased effect of oral hypoglycemics; increased frequency and severity of low blood sugar episodes

controlled substance must be reported to authorities per protocol.

Storage of medications also is important. Many drugs are subject to degradation and lose their therapeutic effect when exposed to natural factors such as humidity, light, and extremes of temperature. Others simply lose their effects over time. All environmental factors for medications must be checked regularly. Box 11-28 gives instructions from the Occupational Safety and Health Administration for the protection and storage of nitroglycerin.

PARAMEDIC Pearl

Nitroglycerin is one of the more common drugs that patients often have that is outdated or expired.

COMPONENTS OF A DRUG PROFILE

[OBJECTIVE 21]

Drug profiles contain a complete description of a drug. The components of a drug profile are shown in Box 11-29.

TABLE 11-12 **Examples of Drug-Food Interactions**

Food/Substance	Drug	Interaction
Acidic foods (tomatoes, fruits, vegetables, some fruit juices)	Erythromycin, penicillin G	Hasten breakdown of the drug in the intestines
Aged or fermented foods (cheese, bananas, yogurt, sour cream)	Antihypertensives	Enhance release of norepinephrine resulting in vasoconstriction, hypertension
Alcohol	Verapamil	More rapid absorption of alcohol
	Nitroglycerin	Severe hypotension
	Morphine	Increased CNS depression, respiratory depression, hypotension
Grapefruit juice	Caffeine	Insomnia, seizures, tachycardia
	Calcium channel blockers	Flushing, headache, tachycardia, hypotension
	Lovastatin (Mevacor)	Headache, liver and muscle toxicity
	Midazolam (Versed)	Increased sedation
Milk products, calcium supplements	Tetracycline	Reduced absorption, loss of antibacterial drug effects
Swiss cheese, tuna	Isoniazid (INH)	Severe headaches, redness and itching of eyes and face, chills, palpitations, pulse rate changes
Tobacco	Theophylline, phenytoin	Increased drug metabolism
Vitamin C	Atropine, quinidine	Increased excretion of drug, decreased drug activity
	Aspirin	Decreased rate of drug excretion
Vitamin K–containing foods (broccoli, Brussels sprouts, spinach, kale)	Warfarin (Coumadin)	Increased risk of blood clotting
Wheat bran, sunflower seeds	Digoxin (Lanoxin)	Significant decrease in drug absorption

---

BOX 11-28 **Nitroglycerin Storage Requirements**

Nitroglycerin is used frequently in the treatment of angina pectoris as well as chest pain associated with acute myocardial infarction. Nitroglycerin warrants special consideration for storage. The containers should be airtight. Temperature should be controlled and it should be kept in a dark environment. Listed below is an excerpt from the Occupational Safety and Health Administration (OSHA) Web site on nitroglycerin and its reactivity and storage.

Storage

Nitroglycerin should be stored in a cool, dry, well-ventilated area in tightly sealed containers labeled in accordance with OSHA's Hazard Communication Standard [29 CFR 1910.1200]. Containers of nitroglycerin should be protected from physical damage, ignition sources, shocks (or jolts), and ultraviolet radiation and should be stored separately from strong acids (such as hydrochloric, sulfuric, and nitric) or ozone (NIOSH, 1994a; NJDH, 1986, p. 4).

Reactivity

1. Conditions contributing to instability: Heat, flames, shock, or ultraviolet radiation may cause explosive or violent reactions to occur.
2. Incompatibilities: Contact of nitroglycerin with strong acids (such as hydrochloric, sulfuric, and nitric) or ozone may cause violent reactions.
3. Hazardous decomposition products: Toxic gases and vapors (such as oxides of nitrogen) may be released in a fire involving nitroglycerin.
4. Special precautions: None reported.

The National Fire Protection Association has assigned a flammability rating of 2 (moderate fire hazard) to nitroglycerin.

Reprinted from Occupational Safety and Health Administration. *Occupational Safety and Health guideline for nitroglycerin.* Retrieved August 28, 2005, from http://www.osha.gov/SLTC/healthguidelines/nitroglycerin/recognition.html.

BOX 11-29 Components of a Drug Profile

- Generic and trade names of the drug
- Classification
- How supplied
- Mechanism of action
- Pharmacokinetics (onset, peak effects, duration, half-life)
- Indications
- Dosage
- Contraindications

- Precautions
- Side effects/adverse effects
- Route(s) of administration
- Drug interactions
- Pregnancy risk category
- Antidotes (if applicable)
- Special considerations (pediatric patients, geriatric patients, pregnant patients, other special patient groups)

Case Scenario SUMMARY

1. *What is your general impression of this patient? What treatment will you initiate before continuing your assessment?* This patient is extremely high priority. You should perform no additional assessment or treatment until you get her airway established, begin ventilation, and ensure that she has adequate perfusion.

2. *What potential causes can you think of for the profound cyanosis, respiratory arrest, poor lung compliance, and difficulty ventilating?* Although cyanosis can have many causes, the presence of poor lung compliance and an inability to ventilate significantly narrow the options. Upper airway obstruction, lower airway obstruction, severe bronchospasm, and tension pneumothorax can all cause poor lung compliance and an inability to ventilate.

3. *What medications might be appropriate to treat the list of potential causes in the previous question?* Nontraumatic upper airway obstruction (related to anaphylaxis or croup) and severe bronchospasm may respond to drugs that cause vasoconstriction (to reduce swelling), reductions in cellular leakage (to reduce swelling), and bronchodilation. Epinephrine, corticosteroids, and albuterol (or other bronchodilators) work in this way.

4. *Describe the autonomic innervation of the lungs. What is the effect of epinephrine? How might epinephrine affect the pulse rate? Why?* The lungs are innervated by both the sympathetic and parasympathetic nervous systems. Bronchodilation may be caused by stimulation of beta$_2$ receptors in the sympathetic nervous system or by parasympathetic blockade. Conversely, parasympathetic simulation or beta$_2$ sympathetic blockade may result in bronchoconstriction. Beta$_2$ sympathetic stimulation also increases respiratory rate and depth; beta$_1$ sympathetic stimulation increases the pulse rate and cardiac stroke volume (as well as cardiac oxygen consumption).

5. *Given this patient's condition and assuming no restrictions related to local protocols, what route is most* appropriate for the epinephrine? Why? This patient's condition is life threatening, so IV administration is most appropriate because absorption is much more rapid than other routes. Sub-Q or IM administration, may be ineffective for two reasons. First, even in healthy individuals, absorption by these routes is much slower. In addition, this patient's fight-or-flight sympathetic response has caused significant peripheral vasoconstriction, a condition that makes IM or Sub-Q absorption even slower and more unpredictable because of the hypoperfusion of muscle.

6. *What is the brand name of diphenhydramine? What is its drug class? Assuming no restrictions related to local protocols, what route is most appropriate in this case? Why?* Benadryl is the trade name for diphenhydramine. Diphenhydramine is an antihistamine. It blocks cellular histamine response but does not prevent histamine release. Histamine release has many effects, including the release of fluids into the interstitial space. This causes edema in the skin and, importantly, the upper and lower airways. So administration of an antihistamine reduces the release of fluids into the interstitial space and upper airway edema. Because of this patient's grave condition, the diphenhydramine should be administered IV.

7. *What drug class is atropine in? How does this class of medications relate to your answer to question 4? What impact would you expect atropine to have on this patient? Why?* Atropine is a parasympathetic blocker (also known as a parasympatholytic). Effects of parasympathetic blockage include drying of membranes (the reason it is used preoperatively), increases in the pulse rate (the reason it is used in symptomatic bradycardia), and bronchodilation. Although atropine is rarely used in EMS to treat bronchoconstriction, it is present in a commonly used inhaled bronchodilator (Atrovent).

8. *What is dexamethasone? How might its mechanism affect this patient's condition? How fast do you expect*

Continued

Case Scenario SUMMARY—continued

it to work? Decadron is a corticosteroid, a class of drugs that stabilize cell membranes and reduce leakage of fluid from cells into the interstitial space. In anaphylaxis, this action reduces interstitial edema that causes upper and lower airway narrowing. All IV corticosteroids work fairly slowly, taking effect in approximately 6 to 8 hours. Effects from these drugs are not likely seen during the EMS or ED care of these patients.

9. *The patient became easier to ventilate after receipt of multiple medications. Considering the effects of various medications on the lungs, what could explain this improvement?* This patient received large doses of multiple drugs that could have caused bronchodilation: sympathomimetics (alpha/beta sympathetic stimulators, including epinephrine and albuterol), sympatholytics (atropine), antihistamines (diphenhydramine), and corticosteroids (dexamethasone). Given the doses of all the medications, her ultimate bronchodilation likely was a combination of all.

10. *What drug class is dopamine in? How is it typically administered? How does it affect blood pressure?* Dopamine is a medication that has multiple dose-dependent effects on the sympathetic nervous system. In low doses, dopamine primarily stimulates dopaminergic receptors that increase renal and intestinal blood flow. At higher concentrations, dopamine stimulates beta$_1$ receptors, increasing heart rate and the force of cardiac contraction, which may increase blood pressure. At high doses, dopamine stimulates alpha receptors, resulting in peripheral vasoconstriction, increased afterload, and an increase in blood pressure. Alpha stimulation also significantly reduces renal blood flow and may result in damage to the kidneys. Because of these myriad effects, dopamine is administered by continuous IV infusion while carefully monitoring its effect on pulse rate, blood pressure, and overall patient condition.

Chapter Summary

- A drug's trade name is also called its *brand name.* The generic name often is a simplified form of the chemical name. The chemical name represents the chemical structure of the compound.
- Orphan drugs are products used to treat rare diseases or conditions.
- Sources of drugs include plants, animal/human products, minerals, synthetic chemicals, and recombinant DNA technology.
- Three drug classification systems are used in healthcare: body system, class of agent, and mechanism of action.
- Sources of information for drugs include the *Physicians' Desk Reference,* hospital formularies, people (such as physicians, nurses, and pharmacists), pocket references, and package inserts.
- The 1970 Comprehensive Drug Abuse Prevention and Control Act established the schedule of controlled substances.
- The United States Pharmacopoeia is the official public standards–setting authority for all prescription and over-the-counter medicines, dietary supplements, and other healthcare products manufactured and sold in the United States.
- The FDA has an approval process for investigational drugs that totals four phases.
- Safe and effective drug administration is the responsibility of the paramedic. Obtaining a history is crucial for proper administration of medications.

- The nervous system contains the central and the peripheral nervous system. The CNS contains the brain and the spinal cord. The peripheral nervous system contains all the nerves outside the CNS. The somatic nervous system includes nerves under voluntary control. The ANS is automatic and a division of the peripheral nervous system. Two divisions of the ANS have been classified, the sympathetic and parasympathetic.
- The sympathetic division also is called the *adrenergic division* and is responsible for the fight-or-flight response. Neurotransmitters in the sympathetic division include epinephrine and norepinephrine. Receptors in the sympathetic division include alpha$_1$, alpha$_2$, beta$_1$, beta$_2$, and dopaminergic receptors. The parasympathetic division also is called the *cholinergic system* and referred to as the "feed and breed" or "resting and digesting" response of the ANS. The neurotransmitter in the parasympathetic division is acetylcholine. Two receptors are present in the parasympathetic division: muscarinic and nicotinic.
- Synaptic transmission occurs at the synaptic junction. The preganglionic and postganglionic nerves are connected at the ganglion.
- Drugs come in liquid, solid, or gaseous forms.
- The route of drug administration affects the type of effect and onset of action. Enteral drugs enter the systemic circulation by the GI tract. Parenteral drugs enter the systemic circulation by bypassing the digestive tract.

- Medications typically alter a normal body response; they do not generate a new function or response.
- Pharmacokinetics is the process of how drugs are processed in the body. Drugs are absorbed, distributed, metabolized, and finally excreted. Absorption is highly dependent on the route of administration. Distribution depends on a number of physiologic factors, including blood supply, pH, and body temperature. Metabolism may render a drug active, inactive, or ready for excretion. Excretion and elimination are the body's mechanisms for removing the drug or its metabolites from circulation.
- An agonist stimulates a receptor, causing a physiologic response. A partial agonist or antagonist may cause a physiologic response but not to the extent of an agonist. An antagonist binds with a receptor but does not elicit a response.
- The biologic half-life is the time required to eliminate half of a substance from the bloodstream.
- Drugs have been rated for their safety in pregnancy by the FDA. Pediatric patients have different physiologic

functions and thus their response to medications is different from adults. Geriatric patients also have different physiologic characteristics, compounded by multiple medical problems and medications. Their response to medications also is affected.
- A side effect is an effect of a drug other than the one for which it was given. Side effects may or may not be harmful.
- An iatrogenic drug response is an unintentional disease or drug effect produced by a physician's prescribed therapy.
- Many factors may affect drug action, including intestinal absorption, drug metabolism, excretion, electrolytes, drug-drug interactions, and incompatibilities.
- Drug storage is important because certain medications require special storage instructions. Drug storage for controlled substances is critical and is the responsibility of the paramedic.
- A drug profile is a complete description of a drug and its characteristics.

REFERENCES

Opie, L. H. (2001). Mechanisms of cardiac contraction and relaxation. In: D. Zipes, P. Libby, R. Bonow, & E. Braunwald (Eds.), *Braunwald's heart disease: A textbook of cardiovascular medicine* (7th ed.) (p. 470). Philadelphia: Saunders.

Lehne, R. A. (2001). Physiology of the peripheral nervous system. In *Pharmacology for nursing care* (4th ed.) (p. 106). Philadelphia: Saunders.

SUGGESTED RESOURCES

2005 *Physician's desk reference:* http://www.pdrhealth.com.
Atkinson, A. (2001). *Principles of clinical pharmacology,* St. Louis: Elsevier.
Cordell, G. (1992). *Chemistry and pharmacology, vol. 42,* New York: Academic Press.

Food and Drug Administration: http://www.fda.gov.
Mosby's Drug Consult: http://www.mosbysdrugconsult.com.

Chapter Quiz

1. Which of the following names for a drug is used only by the company that manufactures and patents the medication?
   a. Chemical
   b. Generic
   c. Official
   d. Trade

2. List the three drug classification systems.

   _____
   _____
   _____

3. Which of the following schedules of controlled substances contains drugs that have no accepted medical use in the United States and a high potential for abuse?
   a. Schedule I
   b. Schedule II
   c. Schedule IV
   d. Schedule V

4. Which of the following is a true statement regarding the ANS?
   a. It contains the somatic nervous system.
   b. It has three divisions.
   c. It is responsible for involuntary functions.
   d. It is under voluntary control.

5. Which of the following correctly lists enteral routes of medication administration?
   a. Intradermal, intrathecal, umbilical, rectal, and transdermal routes
   b. Intralingual, buccal, intravenous, rectal, and gastric routes
   c. Intramuscular, endotracheal, intraosseous, and subcutaneous routes
   d. Sublingual, buccal, oral, rectal, and gastric routes

Chapter Quiz—continued

6. List the four main processes of pharmacokinetics.

_____

_____

_____

_____

7. Which of the following receptors in the sympathetic system is responsible for controlling heart rate, contraction, and conduction velocity?
  a. Alpha$_1$
  b. Alpha$_2$
  c. Beta$_1$
  d. Beta$_2$

8. Which of the following is a parenteral route?
  a. Intravenous
  b. Oral
  c. Rectal
  d. Sublingual

9. Number the following routes of medication administration from fastest to slowest.
  _____ Endotracheal
  _____ Intradermal
  _____ IM
  _____ IV
  _____ Sub-Q

10. Which of the following stages of drug function is responsible for alteration of the chemical structure of the drug compound?
  a. Absorption
  b. Distribution
  c. Elimination
  d. Metabolism

11. True or False: Distribution of a drug occurs more quickly to the skin and muscles than to the liver and kidneys.

Terminology

Absorption The movement of a drug from the site of input into the circulation.

Acetylation A mechanism in which a drug is processed by enzymes.

Active transport The movement of molecules that occurs with energy input and can occur against concentration gradients.

Additive effect The combined effect of two drugs given at the same time that have similar effects.

Adrenergic Having the characteristics of the sympathetic division of the ANS.

Adsorb To gather or stick to a surface in a condensed layer.

Adverse effect (reaction) An unintentional, undesirable, and often unpredictable effect of a drug used at therapeutic doses to prevent, diagnose, or treat disease.

Affinity The intensity or strength of the attraction between a drug and its receptor.

Agonist A drug that causes a physiologic response in the receptor to which it binds.

Alkaloids A group of plant-based substances containing nitrogen and found in nature.

Anaphylactic reaction An unusual or exaggerated allergic reaction to a foreign substance.

Antagonist A drug that does not cause a physiologic response when it binds with a receptor.

Assay A test of a substance to determine its components.

Autonomic nervous system (ANS) Division of the peripheral nervous system that regulates many involuntary processes.

Bioassay A test that determines the effects of a substance on an organism and compares the result with some agreed standard.

Bioavailability The speed with which and how much of a drug reaches its intended site of action.

Blood-brain barrier A layer of tightly adhered cells that protect the brain and spinal cord from exposure to medications, toxins, and infectious particles.

Buccal An administration route in which medication is placed in the mouth between the gum and the mucous membrane of the cheek and absorbed into the bloodstream.

Caplet A tablet with an oblong shape and a film-coated covering.

Capsule Small gelatin shell in which a powdered or granule form of medication is placed; it is easy to swallow and the shell will not begin to break down until in the GI tract; popular because of a reduced adverse taste when swallowing.

Central nervous system (CNS) Brain and spinal cord.

Chemical name A precise description of a drug's chemical composition and molecular structure.

Cholinergic Having the characteristics of the parasympathetic division of the ANS.

Cross tolerance Decreasing responsiveness to the effects of a drug in a drug classification (such as narcotics) and the likelihood of development of decreased responsiveness to another drug in that classification.

Cumulative action Increased intensity of drug action evident after administration of several doses.

Delayed reaction A delay between exposure and onset of action.

Desired action The intended beneficial effect of a drug.

Diffusion The passive transport of solutes (small particles).

Distribution The movement of drugs from the bloodstream to target organs.

Dosage Administration of a therapeutic agent in prescribed amounts.

Dose The exact amount of medication to be given or taken at one time.

Downregulation The process by which a cell decreases the number of receptors exposed to a given substance to reduce its sensitivity to that substance.

Drug Any substance (other than a food or device) intended for use in the diagnosis, cure, relief, treatment, or prevention of disease or intended to affect the structure or function of the body of human beings or animals.

Drug allergy The reaction to a medication with an adverse outcome.

Drug antagonism The interaction between two drugs with or in which one partially or completely inhibits the effects of the other.

Drug dependence A physical need or adaptation to the drug with or without the psychological need to take the drug.

Drug-food interaction Changes in a drug's effects caused by food or beverages ingested during the same period.

Drug interaction The manner in which one drug and a second drug (or food) act on each other.

Effector The muscle, gland, or organ on which the ANS exerts an effect; target organ.

Efficacy The ability of a drug to produce a physiologic response after attaching to a receptor.

Elimination The process of removing a drug from the body.

Elixir A clear, oral solution that contains the drug, water, and some alcohol.

Emulsion A water and oil mixture containing medication.

Endorphins Neurotransmitters that function in the transmission of signals within the nervous system.

Enteral A drug given for its systemic effects that passes through the digestive tract.

Enteric-coated tablets Tablets that have a special coating so they break down in the intestines instead of the stomach.

Excretion See *Elimination*.

Facilitated transport The transport of substances through a protein channel carrier with no energy input.

First-pass effect The breakdown of a drug in the liver and walls of the intestines before it reaches the systemic circulation.

Formulary A book that contains a list of medicinal substances with their formulas, uses, and methods of preparation.

Ganglion The junction between the preganglionic and postganglionic nerves.

Gases Substances inhaled and absorbed through the respiratory tract.

Gastric The route used when a tube is placed into the digestive tract, such as a nasogastric, orogastric, or gastrostomy tube.

Gel cap Soft gelatin shell filled with liquid medication.

Generic name The name proposed by the first manufacturer when a drug is submitted to the FDA for approval; often an abbreviated form of the drug's chemical name, structure, or formula.

Glycogenolysis Breakdown of glycogen to glucose in the liver.

Glycoside A compound that yields a sugar and one or more other products when its parts are separated.

Gum Plant residue used for medicinal or recreational purposes.

Half-life The time required to eliminate half of a substance from the body.

Hypersensitivity An altered reactivity to a medication that occurs after prior sensitization; response is independent of the dose.

Iatrogenic drug response An unintentional disease or drug effect produced by a physician's prescribed therapy; *iatros* means *physician;* *-genic* is a word root meaning *produce.*

Idiosyncrasy The unexpected and usually individual (genetic) adverse response to a drug.

Inhalation A route in which the medication is aerosolized and delivered directly to the lung tissue.

Interference The ability of one drug to limit the physiologic function of another drug.

Intracardiac The injection of a drug directly into the heart.

Intradermal Route of the injection of medication between the dermal layers of skin.

Intralingual Direct injection into the underside of the tongue with a small volume of medication.

Intramuscular (IM) An injection of medication directly into the muscle.

Intranasal The route that offers direct delivery of medications into the nasal passages and sinuses.

Intraosseous An administration route used in emergency situations when peripheral venous access is not established; a needle is passed through the cortex of the bone and the medication is infused into the capillary network within the bone matrix.

Terminology—continued

Intrathecal The direct deposition of medication into the spinal canal.

Intravenous (IV) Administration route offering instantaneous and nearly complete absorption through peripheral or central venous access.

Investigational drug A drug not yet approved by the FDA.

Local effect The effects of a drug at the site where the drug is applied or in the surrounding tissues.

Mechanism of action The manner in which a drug works to produce its intended effect.

Median lethal dose The dose of a medication that kills 50% of the drug-tested population.

Metabolism The chemical modification of the original drug.

Metabolites The smaller molecules from the breakdown that occurs during metabolism.

Nasogastric The administration route used when a nasogastric tube is in place. This bypasses the voluntary swallowing reflex.

Neuropeptide A protein that may interact with a receptor after circulation through the blood.

Neurotransmitters A chemical released from one nerve that crosses the synaptic cleft to reach a receptor.

Nonproprietary name Generic name.

Official name A drug's name as listed in the *United States Pharmacopeia*.

Oils In medicine, substances extracted from flowers, leaves, stems, roots, seeds, or bark for use in therapeutic treatments.

Oral A route of administration in which the medication is placed in the mouth and swallowed; the drug is absorbed through the GI tract.

Orphan drugs Products developed for the diagnosis and/or treatment of rare diseases or conditions, such as sickle cell anemia and cystic fibrosis.

Osmosis The passive movement of water from a higher to a lower concentration.

Parasympathetic division The division of the ANS responsible for the relaxed state of the body known as "feed and breed."

Parasympatholytics Drugs that block or inhibit the function of the parasympathetic receptors.

Parasympathomimetics Drugs that mimic the parasympathetic division of the ANS.

Parenteral Administration route used for systemic effects and given by a route other than the digestive tract.

Partial agonist A drug that when bound to a receptor may elicit a physiologic response, but it is less than that of an agonist; may also may block the response of a competing agonist.

Passive transport The ability of a substance to traverse a barrier without any energy input; generally occurs from a higher to a lower concentration.

Peripheral nervous system All the nerves outside the CNS.

Pharmaceutics The science of preparing and dispensing drugs.

Pharmacogenetics The study of inherited differences (variation) in drug metabolism and response.

Pharmacokinetics The process by which a drug is absorbed, distributed, metabolized, and eliminated by the body.

Pharmacology The study of the drugs, including their actions and effects on the host.

Pharmacopoeia A book describing drugs, chemicals, and medicinal preparations in a country or specific geographic area, including a description of the drug, its formula, and dosage.

Pill Dried powder forms of medication in the form of a small pellet; the term *pill* has been replaced with *tablet* and *capsule*.

Placental barrier Many layers of cells that form between maternal and fetal circulation that protect the fetus from toxins.

Plasma level profile The measurement of blood level of a medication versus the dosage administered.

Polypharmacy The concurrent use of several medications.

Postganglionic neuron The nerve that travels from the ganglia to the desired organ or tissue.

Potentiation A prolongation or increase in the effect of a drug by another drug.

Powder Medication ground into a fine substance.

Preganglionic neuron The nerve that extends from the spinal cord (CNS) to the ganglion.

Prodrug A substance that is inactive when it is given and is converted to an active form within the body.

Receptor A molecule, such as a protein, found inside or on the surface of a cell that binds to a specific substance (such as hormones, antigens, drugs, or neurotransmitters) and causes a specific physiologic effect in the cell.

Rectal The drug administration route for suppositories; the drug is placed into the rectum (colon) and is absorbed into the venous circulation.

Second messenger A molecule that relays signals from a receptor on the surface of a cell to target molecules in the cell's nucleus or internal fluid where a physiologic action is to take place; also called a *biochemical messenger*.

Side effect An effect of a drug other than the one for which it was given; may or may not be harmful.

Solubility Pertaining to the ease with which a drug can dissolve.

Solution A medication dissolved in a liquid, often water.

Somatic nervous system Division of the peripheral nervous system whose motor nerves control movement of voluntary muscles.

Spirit A medication that contains volatile aromatic substances.

Steady state An evenly distributed concentration of a drug in the plasma.

Subcutaneous Injection of medication in a liquid form underneath the skin into the subcutaneous tissue.

Sublingual Medication placed under the tongue.

Summation The combined effects of two or more drugs are equal to the sum of each of their effects.

Suppository Medications combined to make them a solid at room temperature; when placed in a body opening such as the rectum, vagina, or urethra, they dissolve because of the increase in body temperature and are absorbed through the surrounding mucosa.

Suspension Medication suspended in a liquid, such as an oral antibiotic.

Sympathetic division The division of the ANS that prepares the body for stress or the classic fight-or-flight response.

Sympatholytics Drugs that block or inhibit adrenergic receptors.

Sympathomimetics Drugs that mimic the sympathetic division of the ANS.

Synaptic junction The open space in which neurotransmitters traverse to reach a receptor.

Synergism The interaction of drugs such that the total effect is greater than the sum of the individual effects.

Synthetic drugs Drugs chemically developed in a laboratory; also called *manufactured drugs*.

Syrup A medication dissolved in water with sugar or a sugar substitute to disguise taste.

Systemic effect Drug action throughout the body.

Tablets Medications that have been pressed into a small form that is easy to swallow. They are a specific shape, color, and may have engraving for identification.

Tachyphylaxis The rapidly decreasing response to a drug or physiologically active agent after administration of a few doses; rapid cross tolerance.

Teratogen A drug or agent that is harmful to the development of an embryo or fetus.

Therapeutic dose The dose required to produce a beneficial effect in 50% of the drug-tested population; also called effective dose.

Therapeutic index (TI) The ratio of the amount of drug to produce a therapeutic dose compared with the amount of drug that produces a lethal dose.

Therapeutic threshold The level of a drug that elicits a beneficial physiologic response.

Tincture A medicine consisting of an extract in an alcohol solution; examples include tincture of iodine, tincture of mercurochrome.

Tolerance Decreasing responsiveness to the effects of a drug; increasingly larger doses are necessary to achieve the effect originally obtained by a smaller dose.

Topical On the skin.

Trade name The name given a chemical compound by the company that makes it; also called the *brand name* or *proprietary name*.

Transdermal Through the skin.

Umbilical An administration route that may be used on a newborn infant; because the umbilical cord was the primary source of nutrient and waste exchange, it provides an immediate source of drug exchange.

Upregulation The process by which a cell increases the number of receptors exposed to a given substance to improve its sensitivity to that substance.

Drugs and Chemical Classes

Objectives

1. List and describe drugs that the paramedic may administer according to local protocol.
2. Integrate pathophysiologic principles of pharmacology with patient assessment.
3. Synthesize patient history information and assessment findings to form a field impression.
4. Discuss the analgesic class of medications, including prescription and nonprescription medications.
5. Discuss anesthetics, including types, routes of administration, and indications.
6. Discuss serums, vaccines, and antidotes.
7. Discuss antiinfective agents, including antibiotics, antivirals, antifungals, and antiparasitic agents.
8. Discuss antineoplastic drugs.
9. Discuss vitamins and minerals.
10. Discuss fluids and electrolytes.
11. Discuss and give examples of anxiolytics, antidepressants, mood stabilizers, and antipsychotics.
12. Discuss and give examples of anticonvulsant drugs.
13. Discuss and give examples of muscle relaxants.
14. Discuss central nervous stimulants.
15. Discuss drugs used for Parkinson's and Alzheimer's disease.
16. Discuss drugs affecting the parasympathetic division of the autonomic nervous system.
17. Discuss drugs affecting the sympathetic division of the autonomic nervous system.
18. Discuss drugs affecting the cardiovascular system, including antiarrhythmics, antihypertensives, and vasodilator agents.
19. Discuss anticoagulants, fibrinolytics, and blood components.
20. Discuss antihyperlipidemic drugs.
21. Discuss oxygen, mucokinetic, and bronchodilator drugs.
22. Discuss drugs affecting the renal system.
23. Discuss drugs affecting the gastrointestinal system.
24. Discuss drugs affecting the eyes and ears.
25. Discuss drugs affecting the endocrine system, including hormones.
26. Discuss uricosuric drugs.
27. Discuss drugs that affect the reproductive system.
28. Discuss drugs affecting the immunologic system.
29. Discuss dermatologic preparations.
30. Discuss drugs of abuse, including alcohols and amphetamines.
31. Discuss environmental chemicals, including herbicides, rodenticides, and insecticides.
32. Discuss toxic substances, including alcohols, heavy metals, household chemicals, and hazardous materials.

Chapter Outline

General Information
MEDICATIONS FOR MULTISYSTEM APPLICATION
Analgesics and Antipyretics
Anesthetics
Immunizations, Vaccines, and Immunoglobulins
Antiinfective Drugs
Vitamins and Minerals
Fluids and Electrolytes
DRUGS THAT AFFECT THE NERVOUS SYSTEM
Drugs for Treating Psychiatric Disorders
Anticonvulsants
Muscle Relaxants
Central Nervous System Stimulants
Drugs for Specific Central Nervous System Peripheral Dysfunctions
Drugs Affecting the Autonomic Nervous System
DRUGS AFFECTING THE CARDIOVASCULAR SYSTEM
Antiarrhythmics
Antihypertensives

Anticoagulants, Fibrinolytics, and Blood Components
Antihyperlipidemic Drugs
DRUGS AFFECTING THE RESPIRATORY SYSTEM
Drugs Used for Nasal Congestion
Mucokinetic Drugs and Expectorants
Bronchodilators
Drugs That Affect the Respiratory Center
DRUGS AFFECTING THE URINARY SYSTEM
Renal System Dysfunction
DRUGS AFFECTING THE GASTROINTESTINAL SYSTEM
Antacids
Antiflatulents
Digestants
Antiemetics
Emetics
Cannabinoids
Cytoprotective Agents
H₂ Receptor Antagonists

Case Scenario

You arrive at the scene of a 57-year-old man reporting chest pain. He describes the pain as a burning sensation in the middle of his chest and abdomen. He states that the pain does not radiate and rates it 9 on a 10-point scale. He has a medical history of hypertension and gastroesophageal reflux disease. He states he smokes and has a family history of cardiac disease. You observe that the patient appears to be in mild distress.

Questions

1. What is your impression of this patient?
2. What areas of the medical history are pertinent?
3. What areas of the physical examination will be important?

[OBJECTIVES 1, 2, 3]

Chapter 11 provided the foundation for understanding the important physiologic properties of drugs and their interactions with the human body. This chapter provides information about specific drugs, including specific discussion on medications commonly found in a paramedic's drug box. The mechanisms of action, indications, contraindications, and dosages are discussed. Because you will encounter many other drugs and substances in your practice as a paramedic, these substances are discussed with a focus on pertinent information. This chapter does contain a substantial amount of information and may take some time to comprehend. The more time spent reading and participating in clinical and field internship training, the more familiar the material will become. In addition, this chapter will make an excellent reference for future use.

GENERAL INFORMATION

Understanding Terminology

When discussing the different drugs in this chapter, an understanding of relevant common terms is important. An **indication** is the appropriate use of a drug when treating a disease or condition. A **contraindication** is when using a drug for a condition is not advisable because of potential adverse effects. **Dosage** is the amount of medication that can be safely given for the average person for a specified condition. Many paramedics use *amp* when referring to dose. For example, "Give an amp of D50." This terminology is inaccurate. An amp(ule) is a method of packaging, and a dose is a specific amount of medication that is administered. Drug doses are not cited in this chapter. They may be found in the drug table in Appendix B. Remember that drug doses should *always* be checked against protocols and medical direction.

Overdose

The potential for **overdose** is a possibility for both prescription and nonprescription medications. The effects of taking too much of any medication depend on the properties of the drug and the amount taken. As much information as possible should be obtained at the scene before transporting the patient. The patient may want to commit suicide and may not be willing to provide accurate information. View the scene carefully for signs of bottles, pills, needles, and other items. If the patient is willing to provide a history, obtain information on what was taken, when it was taken, why it was taken, how it was taken, and how much was taken. Bringing pill bottles or any other substances in their original containers is helpful to the receiving facility staff. Consider contacting Poison Control for assistance per local protocol (Box 12-1). You should know the effects of overdose of all medications you administer so that in the event of a medication error you can monitor the patient for these effects.

Treatment

Treatment of a patient who has overdosed is an important part of prehospital care. The patient's airway and vital signs must be monitored. Intravenous (IV) access should be established. The patient should be placed on a monitor with a 12-lead electrocardiogram (ECG) obtained if available. Pulse oximetry should be monitored, as should capnography if available. Patients in overdose

situations may have nausea, vomiting, or seizures. Keep these situations in mind.

Gastric lavage is typically is performed within 1 hour of ingestion. A tube is placed into the stomach and saline is circulated through the tube into the stomach and suctioned back out. Gastric contents are removed through the tubes. The contents are examined for pill fragments. If the patient spontaneously vomits in the ambulance, document pill fragments or bring the emesis.

Activated charcoal is used to bind (adsorb) the toxin physically while it moves through the gastrointestinal tract (Table 12-1). The charcoal mixed with medication is then excreted in the feces. This inhibits absorption along the gastrointestinal tract. It is commonly used, even if the time of ingestion is not known. Some preparations are a sustained release, and the charcoal may still bind some of the medication.

BOX 12-1 | Contacting a Poison Control Center

The American Association of Poison Control Centers is a nationwide organization that can be reached at 800-222-1222. It can be contacted for information or for reporting an exposure. They accept calls 24 hours a day and have access to a large database of toxins, medications, insect stings and bites, reptile bites, and other types of poisonings. Operators can begin by helping the patient manage his or her condition. They can also alert the receiving hospital of the condition of the patient who is going to arrive and how to provide definitive management. Individuals answering these calls are specially trained and have access to a toxicologist. Each patient is carefully followed up by this system.

TABLE 12-1 Activated Charcoal

Generic Name	Charcoal, activated
Trade Name(s)	Actidose, Charcola, SuperChar, InstaChar, Charco-Aide, Liqui-Char
Classification	Adsorbent, antidote
Action	When certain chemicals and toxins are in proximity to the activated charcoal, the chemical will attach to the surface of the charcoal and become trapped.
Indications	Oral poisonings, toxic ingestion
Routes of Administration	Oral, nasogastric tube, orogastric tube
Contraindications	Corrosive materials Caustics (petroleum products) Patients with active gastrointestinal bleeding
Adverse Effects	Nausea, vomiting, abdominal cramping, constipation, or diarrhea Stomach distention (potential risk of aspiration)
Pregnancy	Category C
Special Considerations	Charcoal may be mixed with sorbitol. This mixture is used only on the first dose of charcoal. Sorbitol is a cathartic that speeds the transit time through the intestines. Charcoal only binds large molecules. It is ineffective in binding aspirin, lithium, cyanide, iron, lead, and arsenic.

MEDICATIONS FOR MULTISYSTEM APPLICATION

[OBJECTIVES 3, 4]

ANALGESICS AND ANTIPYRETICS

General

Analgesia is a state in which pain is controlled or not perceived. The treatment of pain is an important part of emergency medicine and prehospital care. Pain should be assessed adequately by taking a thorough and accurate history. Important questions to ask regarding pain are provided in Box 12-2. After assessing pain, decide on an appropriate medication choice. When making this decision, keep in mind the following:

- Interactions with other medications a patient is taking

- Current physiologic status
- Local protocols

Nonprescription Analgesics

Many nonprescription analgesics are available on the market. They are used for a number of different reasons; some are used for pain but have additional features. Some of these features may be desirable and others considered a side effect. Knowing if the patient has taken any of these medications before your arrival is important.

Acetaminophen (Tylenol)

Acetaminophen is an analgesic that may be used alone or combined with many other medications to make effective analgesic preparations (Table 12-2). Acetaminophen also is used to reduce fever (antipyretic). It does not have any antiinflammatory properties, antiplatelet effects, or effect on uric acid levels. When given orally, it takes effect within 30 to 60 minutes. It does have some toxic properties if taken in excess and is one of the more common overdoses (Box 12-3).

Acetylsalicylic Acid (Aspirin)

Aspirin was once used as an analgesic but is now frequently being replaced by **nonsteroidal antiinflammatory drugs (NSAIDs).** It is effective in reducing mild to moderate pain and is currently used frequently for its prevention of clot formation in heart disease and blood clotting disorders. Aspirin inhibits platelet aggregation (antiplatelet effects) and thus blood clot formation. This is a primary treatment for chest pain and one of the few medications that reduces rates of **mortality** and **morbidity** in patients with chest pain (Table 12-3).

BOX 12-2	Important Questions for Assessing Pain

- Where is your pain?
- Do you have pain in any other location?
- Describe the pain (burning, sharp, dull, ache, stabbing, pressure)?
- Does the pain travel or radiate?
- Does anything make it better or worse?
- What were you doing when the pain started?
- On a scale of 0 to 10, what is your pain rated (some may use 0 to 5 scale)?
- Have you taken any medications for your pain?

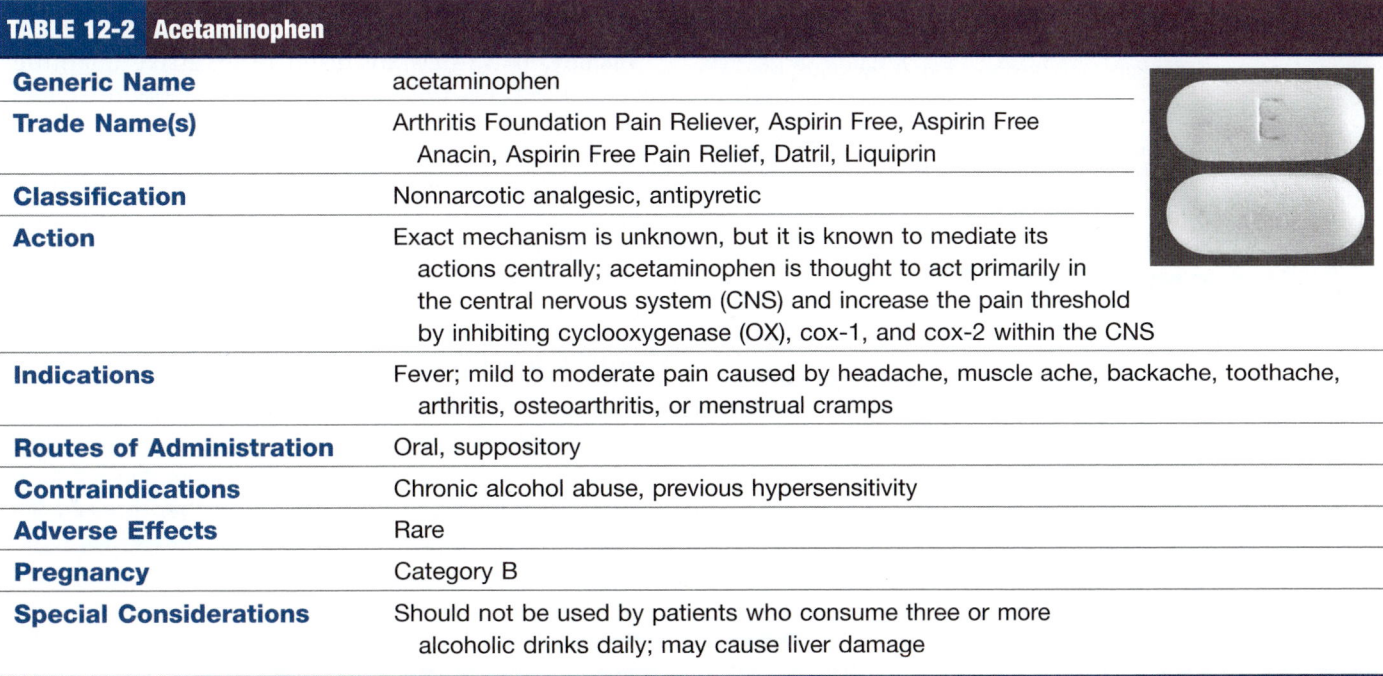

TABLE 12-2	Acetaminophen	
Generic Name	acetaminophen	
Trade Name(s)	Arthritis Foundation Pain Reliever, Aspirin Free, Aspirin Free Anacin, Aspirin Free Pain Relief, Datril, Liquiprin	
Classification	Nonnarcotic analgesic, antipyretic	
Action	Exact mechanism is unknown, but it is known to mediate its actions centrally; acetaminophen is thought to act primarily in the central nervous system (CNS) and increase the pain threshold by inhibiting cyclooxygenase (OX), cox-1, and cox-2 within the CNS	
Indications	Fever; mild to moderate pain caused by headache, muscle ache, backache, toothache, arthritis, osteoarthritis, or menstrual cramps	
Routes of Administration	Oral, suppository	
Contraindications	Chronic alcohol abuse, previous hypersensitivity	
Adverse Effects	Rare	
Pregnancy	Category B	
Special Considerations	Should not be used by patients who consume three or more alcoholic drinks daily; may cause liver damage	

TABLE 12-3	Acetylsalicylic Acid
Generic Name	aspirin, ASA
Trade Name(s)	Aspergum, Bayer, Ecotrin, Empirin
Classification	Nonnarcotic analgesic, antipyretic, antiplatelet, salicylate
Action	Prevents the formation of the chemical thromboxane A$_2$, which causes platelets to clump together, or aggregate, and form plugs that cause obstruction or constriction of small coronary arteries
Indications	Pain, discomfort, fever in adult patients only Chest pain or other signs/symptoms suggestive of an acute coronary syndrome (unless hypersensitive to aspirin) ECG changes suggestive of acute myocardial infarction Unstable angina
Routes of Administration	Oral
Contraindications	Known hypersensitivity to salicylates or other NSAID that has led to hypotension and/or bronchospasm Bleeding ulcer, hemorrhagic states, bleeding disorders (e.g., hemophilia) Children and adolescents (paramedics should not administer aspirin to this age group)
Adverse Effects	Gastrointestinal bleeding, and phylaxis, angioedema, nausea, vomiting
Pregnancy	Category C, except the last 3 months of pregnancy, when it is considered class D
Special Considerations	Large doses of salicylates have a hypoglycemic action and may enhance the effect of the oral hypoglycemics Pediatric chewable aspirin is heat and light sensitive

ECG, Electrocardiogram; NSAID, nonsteroidal antiinflammatory drug.

BOX 12-3	Acetaminophen Toxicity

A risk of liver toxicity exists when acetaminophen is taken in excess either intentionally or accidentally. This drug is easily accessible and does not require a prescription. It is often the drug of choice for suicide attempts. An ingestion of 150 mg/kg or more than 7 g/day may be toxic. The 4-hour level is typically used as a measure of true intoxication. A level of 150 mg/L puts the patient at risk for liver injury. Signs and symptoms of toxicity include nausea and vomiting. After 24 to 36 hours, the patient may have elevated blood liver enzymes, which may lead to coma and death. Treatment is available for acetaminophen overdose and is helpful if administered within 24 hours of ingestion.

Toxicity. Doses of 200 to 500 mg/kg usually produce signs of toxicity. In general, fatal doses are greater than 500 mg/kg. Early symptoms include central nervous system (CNS) stimulation with vomiting, **hyperpnea,** hyperactivity, and possibly seizures. These symptoms quickly progress to depression, coma, respiratory failure, and systemic vascular collapse.

Nonsteroidal Antiinflammatory Drugs

NSAIDs are used to treat acute and chronic inflammatory conditions. They do not contain steroids. They inhibit the synthesis and actions of certain **prostaglandins,** which are responsible for a large part of the inflammatory process and pain (Table 12-4). Each NSAID has chemical differences, even though they are clinically similar. Specific NSAIDs are chosen on the basis of the condition being treated, the dosing interval, and route of administration. The most commonly used over-the-counter NSAIDs are ibuprofen and naproxen sodium (Table 12-5). Ketorolac (Toradol) is commonly used for its systemic analgesic properties.

Toxicity. If NSAIDs are taken in excessive quantities, adverse reactions do occur. Typically, abdominal pain, nausea, vomiting, diarrhea, gastrointestinal hemorrhage, and pancreatitis are the adverse reactions seen with overdose. Even higher doses may trigger CNS involvement, including dizziness, confusion, depression, **nystagmus,** and (rarely) psychosis. Without treatment, the kidneys may be affected by an overdose of any NSAID.

Opioid Agonists

Several types of opioid **agonists** are prescribed; they work similarly and on the same receptors. These drugs are helpful in treating pain and are often classified as analgesics. Many have additional properties helpful for other diseases. The most common drug used in this class is morphine, which is used for pain management, cardiac disease, and pulmonary edema and as a cough suppressant and antidiarrheal. Morphine often is combined with other medications to enhance its effect. Fentanyl is used as an analgesic as well

TABLE 12-4 Ibuprofen

Generic Name	ibuprofen
Trade Name(s)	Advil, Motrin
Classification	Nonnarcotic analgesic, antipyretic, NSAID
Action	Inhibits the synthesis and actions of certain prostaglandins that are responsible for a large part of the inflammatory process and pain
Indications	Arthritis, fever, mild to moderate pain from menstrual cramps, arthritis, joint and muscle pain, headache
Routes of Administration	Oral
Contraindications	Angioedema or previous hypersensitivity to this drug Bronchospasm reactivity to aspirin or other NSAIDs Nasal polyps
Adverse Effects	Nausea, epigastric pain, vomiting, gastrointestinal bleeding, dizziness, headache
Pregnancy	Category B; Category D in third trimester, best to avoid in pregnancy
Special Considerations	Can inhibit platelet aggregation but the effect is less and of shorter duration than that seen with aspirin

NSAID, Nonsteroidal antiinflammatory drug.

TABLE 12-5 Naproxen Sodium

Generic Name	naproxen sodium
Trade Name(s)	Aleve, Naproxyn, Anaprox
Classification	Nonnarcotic analgesic, antipyretic, NSAID
Action	Competitively inhibits both cyclooxygenase (COX) isoenzymes, COX-1 and COX-2 by blocking arachidonate binding, resulting in analgesic, antipyretic, and antiinflammatory pharmacologic effects
Indications	Mild to moderate pain from arthritis, menstrual pain, musculoskeletal pain, acute gout
Routes of Administration	Oral
Contraindications	Previous history of hypersensitivity Asthma or bronchospasm Urticaria (hives) Angioedmea Nasal polyps
Adverse Effects	Nausea, vomiting, gastrointestinal irritation and bleeding
Pregnancy	Should not be used during pregnancy unless clearly needed
Special Considerations	Risk of toxicity may be greater in patients with impaired renal function

NSAID, Nonsteroidal antiinflammatory drug.

as for sedation during rapid sequence intubation. It is a synthetic drug and typically does not affect blood pressure as much as other opioids. Methadone is used for patients with chronic pain. It has a long duration of action. Methadone also is used for people who have had problems with addiction to opioids. Meperidine is an alternate analgesic and may be found in drug boxes around the country. It has a shorter half-life and is not used as frequently as morphine because of its high addiction potential. Table 12-6 lists the different opioid agonists by their chemical class. Tables 12-7, 12-8, and 12-9 describe morphine, meperidine, and fentanyl in detail.

Opioid Analgesic Combination Products

Some prescription products contain combinations of nonprescription analgesics with a lower potency narcotic. These often are oral preparations used for acute pain situations. These medications are abused and often have street value. The narcotic portion may be codeine, pro-

TABLE 12-6	Opioids and Their Classes	
Phenathrenes	**Phenylheptylamine**	**Phenylpiperidines**
Morphine	Methadone	Meperidine — *Demerol*
Hydromorphone		Fentanyl
Oxymorphone		
Codeine		

TABLE 12-7	Morphine Sulfate
Generic Name	morphine sulfate
Trade Name(s)	Duramorph, MS Contin, Roxanol, Astramorph
Classification	Narcotic (opioid) analgesic, Schedule II controlled substance
Action	Binds with opioid receptors; morphine is capable of inducing hypotension by depression of the vasomotor centers of the brain as well as release of the chemical histamine; in the management of angina, morphine reduces stimulation of the sympthic nervous system caused by pain and anxiety; reduction of sympathetic stimulation reduces heart rate, cardiac work, and myocardial oxygen consumption
Indications	Analgesia, especially in patients with an acute coronary syndrome, kidney stones, or burns with moderate to severe pain Cardiogenic pulmonary edema (with or without associated pain)
Routes of Administration	Usually given IV in the field, can be given intramuscularly or subcutaneously Infusion pump should be used for IV infusion
Contraindications	Significant hypotension, head-injured patients, pregnancy, impaired pulmonary function, liver or kidney disease, endocrine disease Use with caution in acute bronchial asthma
Adverse Effects	Hypotension, syncope, tachycardia, bradycardia, euphoria, dry mouth, allergic reaction, hives, itching, nausea, vomiting, respiratory depression
Pregnancy	Category C
Special Considerations	Patients who have demonstrated prior hypersensitivity to morphine should not receive other opioid agonists of the phenanthrene subclass; these patients can be treated with an opioid agonist from the phenylpiperidine subclass (meperidine or fentanyl) or the diphenylheptane subclass (methadone) An opioid antagonist; resuscitative and intubation equipment and oxygen should be readily available Monitor vital signs and pulse oximetry closely Overdose should be treated with naloxone

IV, Intravenous.

poxyphene, or hydrocodone (Box 12-4). They may be combined with acetaminophen, aspirin, barbiturates, and caffeine.

Partial Opioid Agonists

Partial agonists are also called **agonist-antagonists.** These drugs often provide an analgesic effect when given alone. This effect often is less than that of a full agonist. When given in conjunction with a full agonist, it may act like an antagonist and block the receptor, thus rendering the agonist inactive. Examples include butorphanol (Stadol) (Table 12-10), nalbuphine (Nubain) (Table 12-11), and pentazocine (Talwin).

BOX 12-4	Opioid Analgesic Combinations

- Propoxyphene + acetaminophen (Darvocet)
- Hydrocodone + acetaminophen (Vicodin)
- Oxycodone + acetaminophen (Percocet, Tylox)
- Codeine + acetaminophen (Tylenol 3)

Opioid Antagonists

Opioid **antagonists** block the effects of opioid analgesics. They occupy the receptor and do not allow the opioid to elicit its effect. Naloxone (Narcan) is the most commonly used (Table 12-12). This drug is often used in

TABLE 12-8 Meperidine Hydrochloride

Generic Name	meperidine hydrochloride
Trade Name(s)	Demerol
Classification	Narcotic (opioid) analgesic, schedule II controlled substance
Action	Binds to opiate receptors, producing analgesia and euphoria
Indications	Moderate to severe pain, pain with allergies to other opioids
Routes of Administration	Oral, IV
Contraindications	Renal failure, tachycardia Patients taking monoamine oxidase inhibitors, other central nervous system depressants, or alcohol
Adverse Effects	Respiratory depression, nausea, vomiting, delirium, agitation, hallucination, seizures, sinus tachycardia, palpitations, hypertension, hypotension, diaphoresis, shock, syncope, cardiac arrest
Pregnancy	Category C; category D near term
Special Considerations	Use with caution in patients with liver or kidney disease An opioid antagonist; resuscitative and intubation equipment and oxygen should be readily available

IV, Intravenous.

TABLE 12-9 Fentanyl

Generic Name	fentanyl citrate
Trade Name(s)	Sublimaze
Classification	Narcotic analgesic, general anesthetic, schedule II
Action	Binds to opiate receptors, producing analgesia and euphoria
Indications	Pain control, sedation for rapid-sequence intubation, sedation for prolonged intubation
Routes of Administration	IV
Contraindications	Hypersensitivity, myasthenia gravis; use with caution in traumatic brain injury, respiratory depression
Adverse Effects	Hypotension, respiratory depression, nausea, vomiting, apnea, dizziness, sedation, euphoria, sinus bradycardia, sinus tachycardia, palpitations, syncope, diaphoresis
Pregnancy	Category C
Special Considerations	An opioid antagonist; resuscitative and intubation equipment and oxygen should be readily available. Fentanyl is used in the form of a transdermal patch to manage chronic pain.

IV, Intravenous.

patients who are unresponsive and in whom overdose is suspected. The naloxone displaces the opioid from the receptor and reverses the effects of the opioid. This can be life saving in a patient with respiratory depression.

ANESTHETICS

[OBJECTIVE 5]

General

Anesthetics are CNS depressants. In controlled situations, they are reversible. Types of anesthetics include general, regional, and local. These drugs are used to blunt the CNS response to the perception of pain. Patients who undergo surgery receive general anesthesia. Patients who undergo simple procedures, such a cyst removal or laceration repair, may have local or regional **anesthesia.** General anesthesia often is given by inhalation or IV. Regional anesthesia is achieved by injecting an anesthetic near a nerve. When used on toes and fingers this is called a *digital block*; the region of the entire digit receives anesthesia. Local anesthesia often is used directly in a wound and provides anesthesia to a small area so that sutures may be placed without pain. Levels of sedation and analgesia are shown in Table 12-13. Stages of general anesthesia are listed

TABLE 12-10 Butorphanol

Generic Name	butorphanol tartrate
Trade Name(s)	Stadol
Classification	Narcotic agonist-antagonist analgesic, schedule IV controlled substance
Action	Produces analgesia by binding to opioid receptors
Indications	Relief of moderate to severe pain, preoperative anesthetic
Routes of Administration	IV, intramuscular, nasal spray
Contraindications	Respiratory depression, hypersensitivity, active substance abuse
Adverse Effects	Headache, dizziness, hallucinations, palpitations, respiratory depression, nausea, vomiting, bradycardia, hypotension, drowsiness
Pregnancy	Category C
Special Considerations	In patients with liver or kidney impairment, the initial dose of Stadol injection should generally be half the recommended adult dose.

IV, Intravenous.

TABLE 12-11 Nalbuphine

Generic Name	nalbuphine hydrochloride
Trade Name(s)	Nubain
Classification	Synthetic narcotic agonist-antagonist analgesic
Action	Produces analgesia by binding to opioid receptor
Indications	Chest pain, moderate to severe pain, pulmonary edema
Routes of Administration	IV, intramuscular, subcutaneous
Contraindications	Hypersensitivity, hypovolemia, hypotension
Adverse Effects	Sedation, hypotension, bradycardia, facial flushing, respiratory depression, CNS depression, euphoria, blurred vision, nausea, vomiting
Pregnancy	Category B
Special Considerations	Should be used with caution in patients with liver or kidney disease and given in reduced amounts

IV, Intravenous; *CNS,* central nervous system.

TABLE 12-12 Naloxone

Generic Name	naloxone hydrochloride
Trade Name(s)	Narcan
Classification	Opioid narcotic antagonist
Action	Binds to opioid receptors and blocks the effects of narcotics
Indications	Antidote for opioid overdoses Coma of unknown etiology to rule out (or reverse) opioid-induced coma Complete or partial reversal of narcotic depression, including respiratory depression induced by natural and synthetic narcotics and narcotic-antagonist analgesics
Routes of Administration	IV, intralingual, tracheal, intramuscular, subcutaneous
Contraindications	Known hypersensitivity, supraventricular arrhythmias or other cardiac disease, head trauma, brain tumor

TABLE 12-12	Naloxone—cont'd
Adverse Effects	Tachycardia, hypertension, dysrhythmias, nausea, vomiting, diaphoresis, blurred vision, withdrawal symptoms
Pregnancy	Category C
Special Considerations	Not effective when respiratory depression is induced by hypnotics, sedatives, anesthetics, or other nonnarcotic CNS depressants May cause opiate withdrawal Effects may not outlast effects of narcotics Monitor for recurrent respiratory depression Anaphylactic reactions (rare) have been reported

IV, Intravenous; *CNS,* central nervous system.

TABLE 12-13	Levels of Sedation/Analgesia	
Level	**Description**	**Comments**
Minimal	Anxiety reduction; cognitive function and coordination may be impaired Protective reflexes present Able to maintain patent airway independently and continuously Able to respond appropriately to verbal command (e.g., "open your eyes") Ventilatory and cardiovascular functions intact	Equivalent to anxiolysis Examples of minimal sedation/analgesia include peripheral nerve blocks, local or topical anesthesia or a single, oral sedative or analgesic medication given in doses appropriate for the unsupervised treatment of insomnia, anxiety, or pain
Moderate	Minimally depressed level of consciousness Protective reflexes present; able to maintain patent airway independently and continuously Spontaneous ventilation is adequate Able to respond purposefully to verbal command (e.g., "open your eyes"), either alone or accompanied by light tactile stimulation; reflex withdrawal from a painful stimulus is not considered a purposeful response Cardiovascular function is usually maintained	Moderate sedation/analgesia is equivalent to the term "conscious sedation" Risk of potential loss of protective reflexes exists
Deep	Drug-induced state of depressed consciousness Cannot be easily aroused but responds purposefully after repeated or painful stimulation; reflex withdrawal from a painful stimulus is not considered a purposeful response Ability to maintain ventilatory function independently may be impaired Spontaneous ventilation may be inadequate Cardiovascular function is usually maintained	May be accompanied by loss of protective reflexes and ventilatory drive Assistance may be required to maintain a patent airway Positive-pressure ventilation may be required
General anesthesia	Drug-induced state of unconsciousness Unable to maintain patent airway independently Not arousable, even by painful stimulation Ability to maintain ventilatory function independently often is impaired Cardiovascular function may be impaired	Assistance often required to maintain a patent airway Positive-pressure ventilation may be required

in Table 12-14. Types of general anesthetics appear in Table 12-15.

Specific Considerations

Use of anesthetics in the field may be encountered when performing rapid-sequence intubation, **conscious sedation,** and anxiolysis. Etomidate (Amidate) and fentanyl (Sublimaze) are two of these medications. These drugs are used for sedation before performing a rapid-sequence intubation procedure. Fentanyl often is used in trauma and is less likely to cause hypotension compared with other opioids. It also has a short half-life. Etomidate is a short-acting drug that works in the brain to produce anesthesia (Table 12-16).

IMMUNIZATIONS, VACCINES, AND IMMUNOGLOBULINS

[OBJECTIVE 6]

Tetanus

Tetanus is a bacterial disease that can be transmitted through cuts and puncture wounds. The bacteria are found in soil, dust, and manure. The best treatment is prevention. The immunization is a tetanus/diphtheria combination recommended as a booster every 10 years and in the emergency department for anyone with lacerations, abrasions, and puncture wounds if the most recent vaccination was more than 5 years previously. Children who undergo routine immunizations receive the initial series.

TABLE 12-14	Stages of General Anesthesia	
Stage	**Start and End**	**Notes**
1. Analgesia*	Administration of anesthetic until loss of consciousness	Smell and pain are lost before consciousness is lost Hearing is the last sense lost
2. Excitement*	Loss of consciousness to beginning of surgical anesthesia	Reflexes present and may be exaggerated Involuntary muscles are active, breathing irregular Patient may shout, laugh, swear, sing, struggle, or become violent Variability between individuals during this stage because of amount and type of drug used before anesthesia (premedication), anesthetic used, and degree of external sensory stimuli
3. Surgical anesthesia	Lasts until spontaneous breathing stops	Four planes of increasing anesthesia; recognition of different planes determined by reflexes present, pupil size, eyeball movement, and character of respirations
	Plane 1	Corneal reflex present, pupils constricted, eyeball movement increased, regular breathing, blood pressure normal
	Plane 2	Corneal reflex absent, mid-dilation of pupils, eyeball movement decreased or absent, regular breathing, blood pressure normal
	Plane 3	Corneal reflex absent, pupils increasingly dilated, eyeball movement absent, diaphragmatic breathing, blood pressure decreased
	Plane 4	Corneal reflex absent, pupils dilated, eyeball movement absent, absent chest wall breathing, depressed diaphragmatic breathing, blood pressure decreased
4. Medullary depression/ paralysis (toxic stage)	Cessation of breathing to circulatory collapse	This stage of anesthesia is avoided; centers in the medulla that control breathing and other vital functions cease to function; death follows unless the anesthetic is stopped and resuscitation started

*Stages 1 and 2 are known as *induction*.

TABLE 12-15   Types of Anesthetics

Route Of Administration	Form/Type	Example
Inhalation	Gas	cyclopropane nitrous oxide
	Volatile liquids	halothane (Fluothane) desflurane (Suprane) isoflurane (Forane) methoxyflurane (Penthrane) enflurane (Ethrane) sevoflurane (Ultane)
Intravenous	Ultra-short-acting barbiturates	thiopental sodium (Pentothal) methohexital sodium (Brevital)
	Nonbarbiturates	etomidate (Amidate) midazolam (Versed) lorazepam (Ativan) diazepam (Valium) propofol (Diprivan) fentanyl (Sublimaze) sufentanil (Sufenta) alfentanil (Alfenta)
	Dissociative anesthetics	ketamine (Ketalar)
	Neuroleptic anesthetics	droperidol-fentanyl (Innovar)
Local	Topical	benzocaine (Anbesol) dibucaine (Nupercainal) cocaine lidocaine (Xylocaine) tetracaine (Pontocaine)
	Injectable	lidocaine (Xylocaine) procaine (Novocain) bupivacaine (Marcaine)

TABLE 12-16   Etomidate

Generic Name	etomidate
Trade Name(s)	Amidate
Classification	Sedative/hypnotic agent, anesthetic
Action	Exact mechanism is unknown; etomidate appears to have GABA-like effects
Indications	Induction of anesthesia for rapid-sequence intubation, conscious sedation
Routes of Administration	IV
Contraindications	Hypersensitivity; do not use during labor and avoid using in nursing mothers
Adverse Effects	Transient muscle movements, apnea, nausea, vomiting, dysrhythmias, hypotension hiccups, laryngospasm, snoring, tachypnea, hypertension, cardiac arrhythmias
Pregnancy	Category C
Special Considerations	Other medications should be used for prolonged analgesia

IV, Intravenous; *GABA,* gamma-aminobutyric acid.

Signs and symptoms of tetanus include headache, locked jaw, neck stiffness, and muscle rigidity. It a patient has these symptoms, tetanus immunoglobulin should be provided.

Bacterial Immunizations

Immunizations against bacterial infections are commonly given to those who work in close quarters, including prisons, work camps, and the military. Additional vaccines against bacterial infections have been developed to protect children, the elderly, and the immunocompromised.

The *Haemophilus influenzae* type B conjugate was developed and is provided to infants. This has reduced the risk of infection from the bacteria that cause meningitis and other upper respiratory infections. It is also provided to patients who have lost their spleen traumatically and those with sickle cell disease, whose spleens often are not functional.

The *Streptococcal pneumoniae* vaccine has helped reduce the incidence of meningitis in small children. A variant of this vaccine is provided to the immunocompromised and the elderly. Bacterial vaccines also exist for Lyme disease, tetanus, pneumococci, and meningococci.

Viral Immunizations

Viral immunizations protect against hepatitis A and B, influenza, rabies, rubella (German measles), varicella (chickenpox), measles, and mumps. Healthcare providers are encouraged to obtain the hepatitis B series of immunizations, which significantly reduce the chance of disease transmission from body substance exposure. No immunization is currently available for hepatitis C.

Immunoglobulins

Immunoglobulins are preformed antibodies to a specific virus or bacteria. They may be derived from animals or human beings or produced synthetically. They are administered when a patient is exposed to the disease, which works more efficiently than a vaccine. Immunoglobulin is available for hepatitis A, hepatitis B, tetanus, vaccinia, varicella, rabies, respiratory syncytial virus, and Rh immunization.

Antidotes

An antidote is a chemical that counteracts a poison. Antidotes are commonly used in stings and bites. Common antidotes include black widow spider, coral snake, rattlesnake, and some scorpion stings.

ANTIINFECTIVE DRUGS

[OBJECTIVE 7]

Antimicrobials are medications designed to treat infection. Specific medications are designed to treat bacterial, viral, and parasitic infections and are discussed in each following category.

Antibiotics

Antibiotics are medications designed to treat bacterial infections. They may be used locally or systemically. Some antibiotics are bacteriostatic, which means they inhibit bacterial growth and replication. Others are bactericidal, which means they attack and kill existing bacteria. Antibiotics are designed to work against specific types of bacteria, which is why certain antibiotics are used for specific infections and not others.

Penicillins

The penicillin family of antibiotics was the first to be developed. Multiple generations are in use, and they attack different bacteria. Penicillins are effective against gram-positive organisms and some gram-negative organisms. They are often used for infections of the skin, mouth, and respiratory tract. Box 12-5 describes the common prescribing conditions for penicillin. Table 12-17 lists common penicillins.

Cephalosporins

Cephalosporins are related to penicillins but are active against both gram-positive and gram-negative bacteria. They are used to treat infections similar to ones that respond to penicillin as well as those resistant to penicillin. Table 12-18 lists common cephalosporins.

Macrolides

Macrolide antibiotics include erythromycin and erythromycin derivatives (Box 12-6). They are called macrolides because of the large size of their chemical compounds. Macrolides are used to treat respiratory, pharyngeal, skin, and ear infections. They are also effective in treating community-acquired pneumonia.

Tetracyclines

Tetracyclines are antibiotics commonly used to treat respiratory infections and skin infections, including acne (Table 12-19).

Miscellaneous

Many antibiotics do not fit into a specific class. Clindamycin is an antibiotic used for a number of refractory infections. It has good coverage for dental infections and

---

BOX 12-5 | **Medical Conditions Treated with Penicillin**

- Tonsillitis
- Pharyngitis (including streptococcal infections)
- Bronchitis
- Pneumonia
- Dental infections
- Sinusitis
- Otitis media

TABLE 12-17 Common Penicillins

Generic Name	Trade Name	Route of Administration
mezlocillin	Mezlin	IM, IV
azlocillin	Azlin	IV
carbenicillin	Geocillin	Oral, IM, IV
amoxicillin-clavulanate	Augmentin	Oral
bacampicillin	Spectrobid	Oral
amoxicillin	Amoxil, Trimox	Oral
ampicillin	Principen, Polycillin	Oral, IM, IV
methicillin	Staphcillin	IM, IV
penicillin G	Duracillin, Pentids	IM, IV
penicillin V	Pen-VEE-K, V-Cillin	Oral
cloxacillin	Cloxapen, Tegopen	Oral

IM, Intramuscular; *IV,* Intravenous.

TABLE 12-18 Common Cephalosporins

Generic Name	Trade Name	Route of Administration
Cefazolin	Ancef, Kefzol	Oral, IM, IV
Cephalexin	Keflex, Keftab	Oral
Cephapirin	Cefadyl	IM, IV
Cefaclor	Ceclor	Oral
Ceftriaxone	Rocephin	IM, IV

IM, Intramuscular; *IV,* intravenous.

TABLE 12-19 Selected Tetracyclines

Generic Name	Trade Name	Indications for Use
Tetracycline	Achromycin, Sumycin	Rickettsia, *Mycoplasma pneumoniae*
Oxytetracycline	Terramycin	Cholera, Lyme disease, acne, *Chlamydia*
Doxycycline	Vibramycin	Gastrointestinal diseases
Minocycline	Minocin	Acne

BOX 12-6 Examples of Macrolide Antibiotics

- erythromycin (Erythrocin)
- azithromycin (Zithromax)
- dirithromycin (Dynabac)

infections of the pharynx. Vancomycin is an IV antibiotic used for resistant bacteria. Flagyl has good coverage for bacteria that thrive in an anaerobic environment and is used to treat some sexually transmitted diseases, abscesses, and abdominal infections.

Antifungal Agents

Fungal species are found everywhere in nature and in the human body. Some species are naturally found in and on the body, including the mouth, skin, and vaginal area. Treatment of fungal infections is usually necessary when the infection causes distress or occurs in an immuno-compromised individual. Other fungal infections cause distress after antibiotic therapy. The antibiotic destroys natural bacteria that keep the fungus in the appropriate balance, causing symptoms of a fungal overgrowth. Antibiotic therapy is one of the most common causes of yeast vaginitis.

Fungi live best in moist environments and can cause problems in areas of the body prone to perspiration. A good example is athlete's foot (tinea pedis).

Common antifungal preparations are used transdermally or through passage of the mucosal membrane. Thrush may occur in newborns or immunocompromised adults; nystatin is commonly used to coat the mucous membranes of the mouth and pharynx as needed for treatment. Suppositories are used for yeast vaginitis. For tinea capitis, which may be particularly difficult to eliminate, oral medications such as griseofulvin are typically used. Oral or IV antifungals are used for fungal infections that are systemic or affect the lungs in immunocompromised patients. Common antifungal agents are listed in Table 12-20.

Antiviral Agents *Reduce symptoms*

Viruses do not have the capability to replicate and reproduce on their own, but use the human cell as a host. This makes them more difficult to treat. Viral infections range from mild (e.g., warts) to life-threatening (e.g., HIV). Researchers have been working to develop vaccines for viruses that can be particularly dangerous, including influenza, hepatitis B, hepatitis C, and HIV.

Influenza may be serious to fatal in the very young and the elderly. Some advances have been achieved in both the vaccinations and antiviral therapy. One example is amantadine, which, if provided in the first 48 hours of contamination, reduces the length and severity of the influenza illness.

Herpes can cause painful vesicular lesions. Acyclovir has been used to treat these outbreaks. HIV does have a few antiviral drugs that target it specifically. They typically do not work effectively alone, but need to be combined with other medications such as zidovudine (AZT) and lamivudine (Epivir). Protease inhibitors are another form of drug that has been developed to treat HIV. Their mechanism is not clearly understood, but they prohibit the retrovirus from replication. Examples include indinavir (Crixivan), ritonavir (Norvir), and saquinavir (Invirase).

Antimalarial Agents

Malaria is a potentially deadly disease mostly of tropical and subtropical areas caused by a single-celled parasite and transmitted by mosquitoes. The most common areas where malaria is found are Central America, South America, Africa, and Asia. The illness results in recurrent attacks of chills and fever. Drugs used to treat this condition are listed in Box 12-7.

Antituberculotic Agents

Tuberculosis (TB) is a disease caused by the bacterium *Mycobacterium tuberculosis*. It mainly infects the lungs but can spread systemically. It typically is found in the immu-

BOX 12-7	Drugs Used to Treat Malaria

- Chloroquine (Aralen)
- Quinine sulfate
- Hydroxychloroquine (Plaquenil)
- Combination of sulfadoxine and pyrimethamine (Fansidar)
- Mefloquine (Lariam)
- Combination of atovaquone and proguanil (Malarone)
- Doxycycline (Vibramycin)

TABLE 12-20	Selected Antifungal Agents	
Generic Name	**Trade Name**	**Route of Administration**
Systemic Antifungals		
Amphotericin B	Fungizone	IV, topical
Fluconazole	Diflucan	Oral, IV
Nystatin	Mycostatin, Nilstat	Oral
Local Antifungals		
Clotrimazole	Lotrimin, Gyne-Lotrimin	Topical
Econazole	Spectazole	Topical
Miconazole	Monistat	Vaginal
Terbinafine	Lamisil	Topical
Tioconazole	Vagistat	Vaginal
Terconazole	Terazol	Vaginal
Undecylenic acid	Desenex	Topical

IV, Intravenous.

nocompromised and those in underprivileged areas. When a person with untreated TB coughs or sneezes, the air becomes filled with droplets containing the bacteria. Inhaling these infected droplets is the typical way a person contracts TB.

There are different phases of TB. Primary TB is the first part of the infection. Infected individuals may show no signs or symptoms. If symptoms are present, they may include fever and cough. Chest radiographs may be normal or reveal enlarged lymph nodes. Latent TB infection may not cause any symptoms. The patient may have it for years without any symptoms. Routine skin testing for TB may reveal a positive result. Active TB may present with varying symptoms depending on the degree of systemic spread. Patients may report chronic cough, bloody sputum, fever, chills, and weight loss. If it has spread beyond the lungs, it may cause back pain, paralysis, weakness, joint pain, and abdominal pain.

Treatment according to the most current Centers for Disease Control and Prevention (CDC) guidelines include a four-drug regimen of rifampin, isoniazid, ethambutol, and pyrazinamide (CDC, 2003).

Antiamebiasis

An amoeba is a single-celled organism. Many can live in the intestines, but only one type is known to cause disease—*Entamoeba histolytica,* which causes amoebiasis. A patient may contract this disease by drinking contaminated water, often while camping or hiking. These parasites affect the liver and bowel wall. Some patients have no symptoms, whereas others complain of abdominal cramping and watery diarrhea. Medications are directed at eradicating the parasite. The antibiotic metronidazole (Flagyl) is commonly used.

Antihelminths

A helminth is a worm classified as a parasite that lives in human beings. Helminth eggs can contaminate pets, livestock, and water. Human beings can contract helminths by touching contaminated water or an animal and not washing their hands afterwards. They then ingest the eggs, which hatch in the intestine. Common symptoms include fatigue, weight loss, abdominal cramps, nausea, and vomiting. Treatment includes drugs such as albendazole, ivermectin, mebendazole, and pyrantel pamoate. The toxicity of these drugs varies based on the drug but may include gastrointestinal distress, headache, weakness, tachycardia, and hypotension. Types of helminths are shown in Box 12-8.

Leprostatic Agents   5till on malachad, Hawaii

Leprosy is an infectious disease caused by a bacterium characterized by skin lesions, peripheral nerve damage, and progressive debilitation. The disease is uncommon

BOX 12-8	Types of Helminths

- *Enterobius vermicularis* (pinworm), common in United States
- *Trichuris trichiura* (whipworm)
- *Ascaris lumbricoides* (roundworm)
- *Necator* spp. (hookworms)

BOX 12-9	Common Side Effects of Antineoplastic Medications

- Rashes
- Tingling in face, fingers, toes
- Nausea, vomiting, diarrhea, loss of appetite
- Mouth sores
- Easy bruising
- Headache, dizziness
- Hair loss, hearing loss
- Cough, shortness of breath
- Yellowing of the eyes or body (jaundice), dark urine

in the United States but does exist. Treatment includes dapsone. Common adverse effects include gastrointestinal irritation, fever, skin rashes, and hemolysis.

Antineoplastic Agents

[OBJECTIVE 8]

Antineoplastic agents, or chemotherapeutic agents are used to treat cancer. They interrupt the development, growth, or spread of abnormal cells. Cancer chemotherapy is an area of constant growth and change in medicine. For the paramedic, the actual names of antineoplastic drugs are less important than the side effects they may cause. A cancer cell is a normal cell of the body that is growing out of control. It is not a foreign invader; this is what makes treating cancer so difficult. To destroy cancer cells, functioning cells of the body are also destroyed in the process. The specific side effects depend on the actual type of drug and its mechanism of action. Some of the more common side effects are listed in Box 12-9.

VITAMINS AND MINERALS

[OBJECTIVE 9]

Vitamins and mineral substitutes have gained popularity in regard to dieting and weight training and as an anti-cancer therapy. Most essential vitamins and minerals are obtained by eating a well-balanced diet. However, because of certain medications and special medical conditions, some patients require supplementation.

Fat-soluble vitamins are stored in body fat and can cause toxicity if taken in excess. Fat-soluble vitamins include A, D, E, and K. Water-soluble vitamins include vitamin C and the B vitamins (Table 12-21). Certain vitamins are necessary for supplements to be absorbed in the digestive tract. For instance, vitamin C helps iron be absorbed from green vegetables. Vitamin K may interfere with the anticoagulant properties of warfarin (Coumadin). Vitamin K is an antidote for excessive anticoagulation.

Nutritional supplements have been gaining popularity for both weight loss and health changes. Some may have therapeutic benefit. Others may have side effects that may be dangerous to certain individuals with specific medical problems. Always ask patients if they are taking any supplements, and provide this information to the emergency department staff.

FLUIDS AND ELECTROLYTES

[OBJECTIVE 10]

Many crystalloid solutions are used in medicine. The composition of each is slightly different. The two most commonly used crystalloids in prehospital care are normal saline and Ringer's lactate. However, certain medical conditions and medications require the use of other forms of solutions. Table 12-22 provides a brief description of the most commonly used crystalloids.

DRUGS THAT AFFECT THE NERVOUS SYSTEM
DRUGS FOR TREATING PSYCHIATRIC DISORDERS
Anxiolytics

Benzodiazepines

valium
hypnotic sedatives

[OBJECTIVE 11]

Benzodiazepines are used for many medical conditions and have a high therapeutic index. Although taking enough of these medications to reach a lethal dose is difficult, a toxic dose is possible. In this case, overdose effects such as respiratory depression can cause death. However, the cause of death technically is not a lethal dose of the medication; the medication directly results in the cause of death (respiratory depression). This is important to understand so you do not underestimate the potential problems associated with singular benzodiazepine overdose. Even a therapeutic dose of a benzodiazepine can be fatal when mixed with other depressants such as alcohol and narcotics. Benzodiazepines are believed to act on a portion of the brain that affects emotion. These drugs are currently used for four main reasons: to treat anxiety, muscle spasm, and convulsions and to provide sedation. This class of medications has been categorized as Schedule IV because of their abuse

TABLE 12-21	Vitamins
Vitamin	**Function**
A	Growth, bone development, night vision, reproduction, and skin growth
B_1 (thiamine)	Converts blood sugar into energy; involved in metabolic activities of cells of muscles and nerves
B_2 (riboflavin)	Production of energy
B_3 (niacin)	Vasodilation of blood vessels
B_5 (pantothenic acid)	Essential for the metabolism of fats, carbohydrates, and proteins
B_6	Role in nervous system and blood cell production; key treatment in seizures caused by isoniazid overdose
B_{12} (cobalamin)	Production of blood cells, genetic material, and function of nervous system
Folate	Neurotransmitter development and synthesis
C	Antioxidant; important to the production of collagen, basic proteins, bone, cartilage, tendons, and ligaments
D	Maintains healthy bone structure
E	Prevents cell membrane damage
K	Role in blood clotting and prevention of bleeding

TABLE 12-22	Commonly Used Crystalloids					
Solution	**Sodium (Na^+)**	**Chloride (Cl^-)**	**Glucose**	**Lactate**	**Potassium (K^+)**	**Calcium (Ca^{++})**
Normal saline	154	154	0	0	0	0
Ringer's lactate	130	109	0	28	4	3
D_5W	0	0	252	0	0	0
Half normal saline	77	77	0	0	0	0
$D_5{}^{1/2}NS$	77	77	252	0	0	0
D_5NS	154	154	252	0	0	0

potential. Commonly used benzodiazepines are listed in Box 12-10. Tables 12-23 and 12-24 give characteristics of diazepam and lorazepam.

Benzodiazepine Antidote. Flumazenil (Romazicon) is a specific benzodiazepine receptor antagonist that blocks the effects of a benzodiazepine. It is primarily used in large overdoses to reverse respiratory and CNS depression. This drug is not used as often as naloxone. Flumazenil may induce seizures in a patient who has been taking benzodiazepines long term. Once the patient begins to have a seizure, additional use of benzodiazepines for seizure control will not be effective because of the occupation of the receptors by flumazenil. This drug is typically used if a benzodiazepine has been used for a sedation procedure and increased sedation, respiratory depression, or coma occurs. It must be used with extreme caution.

GABA - slow this down w/ antiseizure meds

Barbiturates

Barbiturates were used more often before being replaced by benzodiazepines. Barbiturates are divided into four main classes representing the length of their action (Table 12-25). Phenobarbital occasionally may be used in a patient with a refractory seizure disorder. Pentobarbital is used for refractory seizures when coma induction is necessary for seizure control.

Antidepressants

Overview

Antidepressants are used to treat both depression and bipolar disorder. These are considered mood disorders. Some have beneficial side effects such as assisting with smoking cessation and analgesia and also have antianxiety properties. Patients have depression for a variety of

BOX 12-10	Commonly Used Benzodiazepines

- alprazolam (Xanax)
- chlordiazepoxide (Librium)
- diazepam (Valium)
- midazolam (Versed)
- lorazepam (Ativan)

TABLE 12-23	Diazepam
Generic Name	diazepam
Trade Name	Valium
Classification	Benzodiazepine, anticonvulsant, sedative, anxiolytic, Schedule IV controlled substance
Action	Binds to the benzodiazepine receptor and enhances the effects of GABA; benzodiazepines act at the level of the limbic, thalamic, and hypothalamic regions of the CNS and can produce any level of CNS depression required
Indications	Status epilepticus Transient analgesia/amnesia for medical procedures (e.g., cardioversion, transcutaneous pacing) Management of symptoms of alcohol withdrawal (delirium tremens) Anxiety, skeletal muscle relaxation
Routes of Administration	Oral, IV, rectal
Contraindications	Hypersensitivity to benzodiazepines Substance abuse, alcohol intoxication Children younger than 6 months Coma, shock Acute-angle glaucoma CNS depression from head trauma or increased intracranial pressure Respiratory depression
Adverse Effects	Hypotension, reflex tachycardia, respiratory depression, ataxia, confusion, nausea, drowsiness, fatigue, headache, oversedation
Pregnancy	Category D
Special Considerations	Monitor blood pressure, pulse, and respiratory rate every 5 minutes and before each repeated IV dose. Most likely to produce respiratory depression in patients who have taken other depressant drugs, especially alcohol and barbiturates

IV, Intravenous; *GABA,* gamma-aminobutyric acid; *CNS,* central nervous system.

TABLE 12-24 Lorazepam

Generic Name	lorazepam
Trade Name	Ativan
Classification	Benzodiazepine, anticonvulsant, anxiolytic, Schedule IV controlled substance
Action	Binds to the benzodiazepine receptor and enhances the effects of the brain chemical GABA, an inhibitory transmitter, and may result in a state of sedation, hypnosis, skeletal muscle relaxation, anticonvulsant activity, coma
Indications	Agitation requiring sedation, status epilepticus, alcohol withdrawal, preprocedure sedation induction
Routes of Administration	Oral, intramuscular, IV
Contraindications	Hypersensitivity, substance abuse, coma, shock, severe hypotension, CNS depression, COPD, sleep apnea, acute closed-angle glaucoma
Adverse Effects	Respiratory depression, tachycardia, hypotension, sedation, ataxia, confusion, memory loss, headache, dizziness, euphoria, vertigo
Pregnancy	Category D
Special Considerations	Sedative effect is decreased in heavy smokers

GABA, gamma-aminobytyric acid; *IV,* intravenous; *CNS,* central nervous system

TABLE 12-25 Barbiturates

Barbiturate	Notes
Ultra–Short Acting	
thiopental sodium (Pentothal)	Acts within seconds Used for anesthesia
Short Acting	
secobarbital (Seconal)	Produces an effect within 10-15 minutes
pentobarbital (Nembutal)	Peak 3-4 hours
Intermediate Acting	
amobarbital (Amytal)	Onset of 45-60 minutes
butabarbital (Butisol sodium)	Peak in 6-8 hours
Long Acting	
mephobarbital (Mebaral)	Onset of 60 minutes
phenobarbital (Luminal)	Peak 10-12 hours

BOX 12-11 Examples of SSRI Medications

- citalopram (Celexa)
- escitalopram (Lexapro)
- fluoxetine (Prozac)
- paroxetine (Paxil)
- sertraline (Zoloft)

SSRI, Selective serotonin reuptake inhibitor.

BOX 12-12 Serotonin and Antiserotonin Drugs

Serotonin is a neurotransmitter. Many types of serotonin receptors exist. Serotonin is present throughout the body, but its highest concentration is found in the mucosa of the gastrointestinal tract. Serotonin is present in platelets, but its role in the clotting process (if any) is unclear. Serotonin also is found in the neurons in the brain. Decreased levels of serotonin have been associated with depression. Although the exact mechanism of antiserotonin drugs (also called serotonin antagonists) is unknown, some of these drugs work to inhibit smooth muscle contraction in the gastrointestinal tract and blood vessels.

reasons; some cases are situational or genetic or related to brain chemistry. The classes of drugs in this category are discussed in the following sections.

Selective Serotonin Reuptake Inhibitors

Selective serotonin reuptake inhibitors (SSRIs) have been used for depression, anxiety, obsessive-compulsive disorder, and bulimia (Boxes 12-11 and 12-12). SSRIs block the reuptake of serotonin at the nerve synapse. Symp-

[handwritten: only effects serotonin levels]

toms of overdose include agitation, restlessness, nausea, and vomiting.

Tricyclic Antidepressants   *[handwritten: Not used as much now, not specific enough]*

Tricyclic antidepressants are used to treat depression. They are thought to work by blocking the reuptake of norepinephrine and serotonin at the synapse. This pro-

TABLE 12-26	Examples of Tricyclic Antidepressants
Generic Name	**Trade Name**
amitriptyline	Elavil
amoxapine	Asendin
clomipramine	Anafranil
desipramine	Norpramin
doxepin	Sinequan, Adapin
imipramine	Tofranil
maprotiline	Ludiomil
nortriptyline	Aventyl, Pamelor
protriptyline	Vivactil

longs the life of these compounds and symptoms of depression often resolve. These drugs are life threatening in overdose. The severity depends on the amount of drug absorbed after ingestion. Obtaining an accurate history is crucial, as is bringing the prescription bottles to the emergency department. Time since ingestion, the amount, and age of the patient are critical. Signs of poisoning may produce three major toxic syndromes: anticholinergic, cardiovascular, and seizure. Depending on the dose of the drug, patients may experience some or all of these toxic effects. Clinical findings include ECG changes such as widening of the QRS by more than 0.10 seconds and axis deviation. These patients may require gastric lavage (removal of stomach contents) as well as activated charcoal administration. Tracheal intubation may be required. Initial treatment may include a sodium bicarbonate IV infusion. Contact Poison Control or medical direction. These patients often are placed in the intensive care unit for careful monitoring because these overdoses can be quite serious. Examples of tricyclic antidepressants are given in Table 12-26.

Monoamine Oxidase Inhibitors

Not used as much now due to dietary restrictions

Monoamines are organic compounds that include neurotransmitters in the human brain. These neurotransmitters include dopamine, epinephrine, norepinephrine, and serotonin. Monoamines are moved into or out of cells by proteins called monoamine transporters. Monoamines are believed to contribute to stable moods. Monoamine excess or deficiency is associated with several mood disorders. Monoamine oxidase is an enzyme that metabolizes the neurotransmitters in the brain as well as tyramine, a substance that affects blood pressure. Some evidence has shown that during stressful states monoamine oxidase increases. Monoamine oxidase inhibitors (MAOIs) prevent the breakdown of monoamine neurotransmitters. As a result, neurotransmitter concentrations remain high in the brain, boosting mood (Box 12-13). When monoamine oxidase is blocked, the level of tyramine also begins to rise. If foods and beverages high in tyramine are ingested, a dangerously high increase in blood pressure can result.

BOX 12-13	Examples of Monoamine Oxidase Inhibitors

- isocarboxazid (Marplan)
- phenelzine (Nardil)
- tranylcypromine (Parnate)
- selegiline (Emsam)

Patients who take MAOIs have dietary restrictions limiting their consumption of foods that contain a high level of tyramine, such as certain meats, chocolate, beer, wine, alcohol-free or reduced-alcohol beer and wine, most cheeses, avocados, bananas, eggplant, figs, red plums, raspberries, peanuts, Brazil nuts, and coconuts. In 2006 a transdermal patch form of the drug selegiline (Emsam) was approved by the Food and Drug Administration. The patch is applied to the patient's torso, thigh, or upper arm each day. Because this route of medication delivery bypasses the gastrointestinal system, the dietary restrictions associated with MAOI pills may be reduced when selegiline is taken in low doses.

Other Antidepressants

Some new antidepressants do not fit in a specific class. They are used to treat symptoms of depression and anxiety. Venlafaxine (Effexor) and bupropion (Wellbutrin) are two of these drugs.

Mood Stabilizers

Mania is a component of bipolar disorder. These patients have periods of both depression and mania. Symptoms of **mania** include excessive elation, talkativeness, flight of ideas, motor activity, irritability, accelerated speech, and delusions of grandeur. These patients may engage in dangerous activities such as excessive alcohol intake, drug use, or sexual encounters. These phases may last for days or for months. Episodes commonly occur in early adulthood. Lithium is often used to treat mania and bipolar disorder. It is a cation very closely related to sodium. When lithium is taken, it results in decreased sodium in the cell. This drug has been used with good success. If taken in excess, hemodialysis may be required to remove toxic levels. Charcoal does not bind this cation and therefore makes this drug a challenge in overdose. Valproic acid (Depakote) and carbamazepine (Tegretol), two medications commonly used for seizure control; they are also used for mood stabilization.

Antipsychotics

Haldol — can have extrapyramidal side effects (unusual neuromuscular behavior)

Antipsychotic drugs are used to treat psychosis, which is usually associated with schizophrenia. Schizophrenia is a complex disease with a wide range of symptoms. Changes in neurotransmitter function affect both mood and behavior. Antipsychotic medications are designed to help regulate the neurotransmitters responsible for the symptoms found in schizophrenia. They are often used for Tourette's syndrome and Alzheimer's disease. Their primary action is at dopamine receptors, where they block reuptake so that dopamine remains in the synapse for a longer period. Side effects associated with these drugs are described in Box 12-14. The different classes and names of drugs in those classes are provided in Table 12-27.

ANTICONVULSANTS
Overview

[OBJECTIVE 12]

Anticonvulsants are used to treat seizure disorders. Epilepsy is one of the most common causes of seizures and is caused by recurrent patterns of abnormal neuronal discharges in the brain. When the abnormal discharge occurs, an interruption in the normal level of consciousness and brain function results. Seizures may be associated with increased motor activity, loss or alteration in consciousness, or inappropriate behavior. For specific information on types of seizures, see Chapter 23.

Most medications used for seizures depress the excitability of neurons and terminate abnormal neuronal discharges. Some medications act to prevent seizures, and some are used during a seizure.

Hydantoins

Hydantoins are effective anticonvulsants for most types of seizures, with the exception of absence seizures. Phenytoin (Dilantin) is the most commonly used medication in this class. It is thought to work by limiting the tonic phase of a tonic-clonic (grand mal) seizure. The current theory is that this is accomplished by changes in sodium ion transport. It is used for the prevention and treatment of a variety of seizure disorders. Serum levels currently are measured to ensure the drug level is therapeutic. If excess phenytoin is present in the body, adverse effects such as nystagmus, ataxia, and slurred speech may occur.

BOX 12-14 Side Effects of Antipsychotics

- QT prolongation
- Headache
- Inability to sleep
- Dizziness
- Nausea
- Tardive dyskinesia

TABLE 12-27 Types of Selected Antipsychotic Drugs by Classification		
Generic Name	**Trade Name**	**Selected Indications**
Butyrophenones		
haloperidol	Haldol	Psychotic disorders, hyperexcitability in children
Thioxanthenes		
thiothixene	Navane	Psychotic disorders
Phenothiazines		
chlorpromazine	Thorazine	Psychotic disorders such as schizophrenia
thioridazine	Mellaril	Psychotic disorders, hyperexcitability in children
mesoridazine	Serentil	Schizophrenia, alcohol withdrawal, acute or chronic alcoholism
fluphenazine	Prolixin	Psychotic disorders
Benzisoxazoles		
risperidone	Risperdal	Psychotic disorders
Diphenylbutylpiperidines		
pimozide	Orap	Tourette's syndrome
Thienobenzodiazepines		
olanzapine	Zyprexa	Psychotic disorders
Atypical Antipsychotics		
clozapine	Clozaril	Schizophrenia unresponsive to other antipsychotics

Barbiturates

As previously mentioned, phenobarbital is a barbiturate and a central-acting depressant. It is also a sedative/hypnotic that works as an anticonvulsant in subhypnotic doses. If taken in excess it may cause agitation, confusion, hypoventilation, hypotension, nausea, and vomiting. Pentobarbital is another drug in this class that is used in the hospital for status epilepticus refractory to other treatments.

Succinimides

Succinimides are commonly used to treat seizures. They alter wave spikes. Common drugs in this class include ethosuximide (Zarontin), phensuximide (Milontin), and methsuximide (Celontin).

Benzodiazepines

As previously mentioned, benzodiazepines are often used for initial control of active seizures. Diazepam (Valium), lorazepam (Ativan) and midazolam (Versed) are typically found in the paramedic's drug box.

Others

Valproic acid (Depakote) is often used in seizure disorders as a preventive medication. It is considered a carboxylic acid. Drugs such as carbamazepine (Tegretol), gabapentin (Neurontin), and topiramate (Topamax) are also used to treat seizures. These drugs are not used in prehospital care. In case of overdose, contact Poison Control or medical direction.

MUSCLE RELAXANTS

[OBJECTIVE 13]

Physiology of Muscle Spasticity

Muscle spasticity is a common medical problem. Spasms occur as a result of injury, such as sprain, strain, or fracture. Additional medical conditions also cause spasm, such as overexertion, disc disease of the spine, tetanus, and illness. Many antispasmodics work by decreasing the spasm of the muscle cells. They do not help with healing; they simply ease symptoms.

Central-Acting Skeletal Muscle Relaxants

Many muscle relaxants are centrally acting (Box 12-15). Several types of injuries have a component of muscle spasm, and many new medications are on the market. Emphasis has been on developing nonsedating muscle relaxants. Side effects of these medications include dry mouth, dizziness, drowsiness, lightheadedness, and restlessness. Less-common side effects include nausea, vomiting, headache, heartburn, and weakness.

BOX 12-15	Central-Acting Skeletal Muscle Relaxants

- methocarbamol (Robaxin)
- carisoprodol (Soma)
- cyclobenzaprine (Flexeril)
- chlorzoxazone (Parafon Forte)

Direct-Acting Skeletal Muscle Relaxants

Hydantoin derivatives are direct-acting muscle relaxants. Included in this class are dantrolene and phenytoin. Dantrolene inhibits the release of calcium, so it works directly on the muscle by preventing contraction of the muscle cells. Interestingly, it does not appear to affect cardiac or respiratory muscle function.

CENTRAL NERVOUS SYSTEM STIMULANTS

[OBJECTIVE 14]

CNS stimulants are commonly thought of as street drugs or drugs of abuse. Some of these drugs are prescribed for medical conditions. They typically act by blocking inhibitory neurotransmitters in the brain. Two common types are anorexiants and amphetamines.

Anorexiants

Anorexiants are used to suppress appetite for weight reduction. They work by stimulating a part of the brain that controls appetite. These drugs are not without side effects. Sibutramine (Meridia) is one of the most commonly used on the market. Side effects include headache, back pain, palpitations, chest pain, and allergic reaction.

Amphetamines

Amphetamines stimulate a portion of the brain responsible for alertness. These substances are often abused. The two most common medical conditions for which they are used are narcolepsy and attention deficit disorder. Narcolepsy is a condition characterized by excessive drowsiness. Patients may fall asleep while in school or engaging in other activities. They may even have sudden sleep attacks during the day. Amphetamines help combat this problem. Attention deficit disorder is found most commonly in children. They typically have short attention spans. These medications often help alleviate some of these symptoms. Medications used to treat these conditions include methamphetamine (Desoxyn) and methylphenidate (Ritalin). Patients often have increased energy and even a "high" when taking these drugs. These medications are considered controlled substances.

DRUGS FOR SPECIFIC CENTRAL NERVOUS SYSTEM PERIPHERAL DYSFUNCTIONS

Some diseases cause peripheral dysfunction with movement. These disorders are typically caused by an imbalance with dopamine and acetylcholine neurotransmitters.

Parkinson's Disease

[OBJECTIVE 15]

Parkinson's disease is a brain disorder in which nerve cells become damaged in the area of the brain that controls movement. A decrease in the amount of dopamine produced results in tremor, rigidity, imbalance, and slowness of movement. Because dopamine does not cross the blood-brain barrier, dopamine itself cannot be given to reduce symptoms. Instead, precursors of dopamine, such as levodopa, are given to stimulate production.

Alzheimer's Disease

Alzheimer's disease is a progressive disease of the brain that affects memory and the ability to carry out normal daily activities. The nerves that affect memory undergo destruction, and acetylcholine levels often are decreased. Therapy is directed toward replacing acetylcholine.

Huntington Chorea

Huntington chorea is an inherited disease characterized by progressive dementia and involuntary muscle movement. This disease is thought to be related to an imbalance between dopamine and acetylcholine.

Drugs That Affect Dopamine

Drugs can be used to treat a dopamine deficiency in a number of ways (Table 12-28).

DRUGS AFFECTING THE AUTONOMIC NERVOUS SYSTEM

Drugs Affecting Cholinergic Function

[OBJECTIVE 16]

Cholinergic drugs exert their action by two primary mechanisms. They may stimulate agonist activity at the postsynaptic cholinergic receptor, or they may impede the enzyme acetylcholinesterase, which normally breaks down acetylcholine. This mechanism allows acetylcholine to remain in the synapse longer. Drugs that affect the ganglion, adrenal medulla, and skeletal muscle are responsible for nicotinic effects. Drugs that respond and stimulate at the postganglionic receptor are responsible for muscarinic effects.

These drugs are not typically used therapeutically. Physostigmine (Antilirium) is used to manage extreme cases of atropinelike drug overdoses. Myasthenia gravis is an autoimmune disease in which acetylcholine does not render its normal effects on the postsynaptic membrane. The goal of treatment is to have acetylcholine remain in the synapse longer so that some amount may activate the postsynaptic cleft. Patients with this disease experience excessive muscle fatigue.

TABLE 12-28	Drugs That Affect Dopamine
Drug Classification/Action	**Notes**
Anticholinergics	These drugs block acetylcholine. These drugs help restore the normal acetylcholine-dopamine balance that exists in the brain. Common anticholinergics include benztropine mesylate (Cogentin), trihexyphenidyl (Artane), and orphenadrine citrate (Norflex). Side effects include dry mouth, blurred vision, constipation, nausea, tachycardia, and inability to urinate.
Monoamine oxidase inhibitors	These drugs prevent the metabolism and breakdown of dopamine in the brain.
Dopamine agonists	These drugs mimic the action of dopamine. These drugs include Levodopa and carbidopa (Sinemet). This drug is picked up in the brain and converted to dopamine. Side effects include gastrointestinal disturbances, hypotension, cardiac dysrhythmias, anemia, and musculoskeletal pain.
Dopamine substitute	Bromocriptine mesylate (Parlodel) and pergolide mesylate (Permax) fit into the same receptor as dopamine.
Stimulate dopamine release	Symmetrel (amantadine hydrochloride) is a medication that stimulates the release of dopamine.
Inhibit dopamine breakdown	Selegiline (Eldepryl) is a drug in this class that prevents the breakdown of dopamine. Side effects include nausea, hallucinations, confusion, agitation, and syncope.

Cholinergic Blocking Drugs

Anticholinergic agents are alkaloids from the belladonna plant. They function as a competitive antagonist and occupy the receptor site. The most common example is atropine (Table 12-29). Atropine blocks the cholinergic response and is used to treat symptomatic bradycardia. Synthetic derivatives have been designed to mimic antispasmodic effects on the bowel. Dicyclomine (Bentyl) is used as an antispasmodic and may be used in the emergency department. It is administered by mouth or intramuscular (IM) injection. Glycopyrrolate (Robinul) is used in the emergency department to dry oral secretions.

Ganglionic Stimulants

Ganglionic stimulant drugs stimulate receptors at the autonomic ganglia. They are similar in composition to nicotine and nicotine gum.

Ganglionic Blocking Drugs   *Succinylcholine*

These drugs block the receptors at the ganglia. The most common drug in this class is trimethaphan.

Drugs Affecting Adrenergic Function

[OBJECTIVE 17]

Drugs that affect adrenergic function are designed to produce actions similar to the neurotransmitters norepinephrine and epinephrine.

Adrenergic Drugs

Three natural catecholamines exist: epinephrine, norepinephrine, and dopamine. Norepinephrine is the main neurotransmitter that acts at the synaptic junction (Table 12-30). Epinephrine is released into the bloodstream by the adrenal medulla (Table 12-31). Dopamine is a precursor for both epinephrine and norepinephrine (Table 12-32). Synthetic versions of each of these substances are available and are an integral part of the advanced cardiac life support algorithms.

Adrenergic Blocking Drugs   *Not used*

Adrenergic blocking drugs are classified as alpha- or beta-blockers depending on the receptors they occupy. Some of these drugs are used in medicine and have great thera-

TABLE 12-29	Atropine
Generic Name	Atropine sulfate
Trade Name	Atropine
Classification	Parasympatholytic, antimuscarinic, anticholinergic, parasympathetic antagonist, parasympathetic blocker
Action	Competes reversibly with acetylcholine at the site of the muscarinic receptors; receptors affected, in order from the most to least sensitive, include salivary, bronchial, sweat glands, eye, heart, and gastrointestinal tract
Indications	Symptomatic bradycardia, asystole, pulseless electrical activity, acetylcholinesterase inhibitor poisoning (certain mushrooms, insecticides, nerve gas), refractory bronchospasm
Routes of Administration	IV, tracheal
Contraindications	Tachycardia, hypersensitivity to atropine, obstructive disease of gastrointestinal tract, obstructive uropathy, acute narrow-angle glaucoma, acute MI, myasthenia gravis

Adverse Effects	Anxiety, dizziness, headache, confusion, delirium, hallucinations, coma (low doses cause sedation, high doses cause stimulation)
	Anticholinergic effects:
	  Delirium ("mad as a hatter")
	  Decreased salivation, dry mouth and/or nose, difficulty swallowing/talking ("dry as a bone")
	  Flushed, hot skin ("red as a beet")
	  Blurred vision, photophobia ("blind as a bat")
	  Acute urine retention
	  Nausea, vomiting

Pregnancy	Category C
Special Considerations	Signs and symptoms of cholinergic poisoning = SLUDGEM: **s**alivation, **l**acrimation, **u**rination, **d**efecation, **g**astrointestinal distress, **e**mesis, **m**iosis

IV, Intravenous; *MI,* myocardial infarction.

TABLE 12-30	Norepinephrine
Generic Name	Norepinephrine
Trade Names	Levophed, Levarterenol
Classification	Direct-acting adrenergic agent, inotrope, vasopressor
Action	Norepinephrine is an $alpha_1$, $alpha_2$, and $beta_1$ agonist; alpha-mediated peripheral vasoconstriction is the predominant clinical result of administration, resulting in increasing blood pressure and coronary blood flow; beta-adrenergic action produces inotropic stimulation of the heart and dilates the coronary arteries
Indications	Cardiogenic shock, neurogenic shock, severe hypotension not caused by hypovolemia
Routes of Administration	IV infusion
Contraindications	Hypotension from hypovolemia, patients taking MAOIs
Adverse Effects	Headache, dysrhythmias, angina pectoris, hypertension, dizziness, anxiety, exacerbation of asthma
Pregnancy	Category C
Special Considerations	Should be given by an infusion pump into a central vein or a large peripheral vein to reduce the risk of necrosis of the overlying skin from prolonged vasoconstriction

IV, Intravenous; *MAOI,* monoamine oxidase inhibitor.

TABLE 12-31	Epinephrine
Generic Name	epinephrine
Trade Name	Adrenalin, EpiPen
Classification	Natural catecholamine; sympathomimetic, adrenergic agent, inotrope
Action	Binds strongly with both alpha and beta receptors, producing increased blood pressure, increased heart rate, and bronchodilation
Indications	Cardiac arrest, profound bradycardia, severe bronchospasm, anaphylaxis
Routes of Administration	IV, intramuscular, subcutaneous, tracheal
Contraindications	None in cardiac arrest, hypovolemic shock, coronary insufficiency, closed-angle glaucoma, diabetes, pregnant women in active labor, known hypersensitivity, arrhythmias other than VF, asystole, PEA
Adverse Effects	Cardiovascular: palpitations, tachycardia, hypertension, dysrhythmias, precipitation or exacerbation of myocardial ischemia (even when low doses are administered), angina CNS: tremors, anxiety, headache, dizziness, confusion, nervousness, nausea, vomiting, urinary retention
Pregnancy	Category C
Special Considerations	Epinephrine deteriorates rapidly on exposure to air or light. Solutions that show signs of discoloration should be replaced.

IV, Intravenous; *VF,* ventricular fibrillation; *PEA,* pulseless electrical activity.

peutic value. Alpha-adrenergic blocking drugs may theoretically be used in hypertension. They block the vasoconstricting effect at the alpha receptor and in turn decrease blood pressure.

Beta-blocking drugs are commonly used. They may be selective in their preference for $beta_1$ or $beta_2$ receptors. Cardioselective beta-blockers act on $beta_1$ receptors. Two of the most common cardioselective beta-blockers include metoprolol (Lopressor) and atenolol (Tenormin). They effectively reduce blood pressure and heart rate. They are also used in patients who have an acute coronary syndrome. Nonselective beta-blockers act against both $beta_1$ and $beta_2$ receptors. Examples of nonselective beta-blockers include nadolol (Coreg), propranolol (Inderal), and labetalol (Normodyne).

TABLE 12-32	Dopamine
Generic Name	dopamine hydrochloride
Trade Names	Intropin, Dopastat
Classification	Direct- and indirect-acting sympathomimetic; cardiac stimulant and vasopressor, natural catecholamine; adrenergic agonist; inotrope
Action	Stimulates alpha and beta adrenergic receptors at moderate doses; dopamine stimulates $beta_1$ receptors, resulting in inotrophy and increased cardiac output while maintaining dopaminergic-induced vasodilatory effects; at higher doses, alpha adrenergic agonism predominates, and increases peripheral vascular resistance and vasoconstriction result
Indications	Hemodynamically significant bradydysrhythmias that have not responded to atropine and/or when external pacing is unavailable Hypotension that occurs after return of spontaneous circulation Hemodynamically significant hypotension in the absence of hypovolemia—cardiogenic shock, septic shock, anaphylaxis
Routes of Administration	IV infusion
Contraindications	Hypovolemia, pheochromocytoma, uncorrected tachydysrhythmias or VF, monoamine oxidase inhibitors
Adverse Effects	Tachycardia, palpitations, dysrhythmias especially VF, VT, or other ventricular arrhythmias (from increased myocardial oxygen demand), headache, nausea, vomiting, renal shutdown (at higher doses)
Pregnancy	Category C
Special Considerations	Tissue sloughing may occur with extravasation of the IV

IV, Intravenous; *VF*, ventricular fibrillation; *VT*, ventricular tachycardia.

DRUGS AFFECTING THE CARDIOVASCULAR SYSTEM
ANTIARRHYTHMICS

[OBJECTIVE 18]

General

Antiarrhythmics are used to treat and prevent disorders of cardiac rhythm. They are classified into four groups depending on their mechanism of action (Table 12-33). Because antiarrhythmics are carried in the paramedic drug box, common antiarrhythmics are described in detail in Tables 12-34 through 12-40.

Others

Adenosine ✳

Adenosine often is used to slow supraventricular tachycardias. It is usually a drug of first choice because it has a short half-life and a rapid onset of action (Table 12-41). It slows conduction through the atrioventricular node without affecting myocardial contractility.

Digitalis (Digoxin, Lanoxin)   *more risk of toxicity Narrow T I*

Cardiac glycosides are a closely related group of medications with common specific effects on the heart. *Digitalis* is a term that refers to the entire group of cardiac glyco-

BOX 12-16	Goals of Antihypertensive Therapy

- Reduce workload of the heart *(so heart doesn't thicken as much)*
- Maintain adequate blood pressure for tissue perfusion
- Have no undesirable side effects
- Permit long-term administration

sides. Digitalis is derived from the foxglove plant and has specific effects on the heart. It works by blocking the ion pumps in the cellular membrane, which increases the calcium concentration in the cell. This increases cardiac contraction and affects conduction. Significant side effects are associated with digitalis, particularly if taken in excess (Table 12-42).

ANTIHYPERTENSIVES

Hypertension is a common disease in the United States and is a leading risk factor for acute myocardial infarction. It is also linked to stroke, cerebral hemorrhage, and renal failure. Many recent developments have occurred in antihypertensive therapy. Universal goals for antihypertensive therapy are listed in Box 12-16.

Drugs are classified by their mechanism of action. Some antihypertensives work at the kidney by increasing

Text continued on p. 379.

TABLE 12-33   Classification of Antiarrhythmics

Class	Major Action
IA	Block fast sodium channels in cardiac muscle, resulting in decreased excitability; prolong repolarization
	Examples: quinidine, procainamide, disopyramide
IB	Block fast sodium channels in cardiac muscle, resulting in decreased excitability; shorten repolarization or have little effect
	Examples: lidocaine, tocainide, mexiletine
IC	Profoundly slow conduction
	Examples: flecainide, propafenone
II	Beta-blockers; suppress automaticity and rate of impulse conduction
	Examples: propranolol, esmolol, atenolol
III	Markedly prolong repolarization time, usually by interfering with the outflow of potassium through potassium channels
	Examples: amiodarone, sotalol
IV	Calcium channel blockers; block inward movement of calcium to slow impulse conduction (particularly through the atrioventricular node) and vascular smooth muscle contraction
	Examples: verapamil, diltiazem

Handwritten annotations:
- ✳ (star, top left)
- Vfib (next to IB)
- SVT (next to IV examples)
- ↳ long half life (under verapamil, diltiazem)
- Atenolol & metoprolol are B₁ selective – slows HR which ↓BP
- Now use Adenosine for SVT – drug on it's own – fast half life

TABLE 12-34   Lidocaine

Generic Name	lidocaine hydrochloride
Trade Name	Xylocaine
Classification	Class IB antiarrhythmic
Action	Blocks sodium channels, increasing the recovery period after repolarization; suppresses automaticity in the His-Purkinje system and depolarization in the ventricles
Indications	Ventricular tachycardia, ventricular fibrillation, cardiac arrest, wide-complex tachycardia when amiodarone is not available, preintubation for head trauma or intracranial bleeding
Routes of Administration	IV, tracheal
Contraindications	Hypersensitivity to lidocaine or amide-type local anesthetics Severe degrees of sinoatrial, atrioventricular, or intraventricular block in the absence of an artificial pacemaker Wolff-Parkinson-White syndrome Adams-Stokes syndrome
Adverse Effects	Bradycardia, hypotension; may cause sinoatrial node depression or conduction problems and hypotension in large doses or if given too rapidly; excessive doses in the pediatric patient may produce myocardial and circulatory depression; paresthesias, feelings of dissociation, slurred speech, dizziness, drowsiness, decreased hearing, disorientation, and confusion At higher blood levels, muscle twitching that may ultimately lead to seizures and/or respiratory arrest
Pregnancy	Category B
Special Considerations	Half-life may be prolonged twofold or more in patients with liver dysfunction Lidocaine may be *lethal* in a bradycardia with a ventricular escape rhythm

IV, Intravenous.

TABLE 12-35 Procainamide

Generic Name	procainamide
Trade Names	Pronestyl, Procan SR
Classification	Class Ia antiarrhythmic
Action	Blocks influx of sodium through membrane pores, consequently suppressing atrial and ventricular arrhythmias by slowing conduction in myocardial tissue
Indications	Supraventricular tachycardia, control of rapid ventricular rate in Wolff-Parkinson-White syndrome, wide-complex tachycardia Alternative to amiodarone for stable monomorphic VT with normal QT interval and preserved ventricular function
Routes of Administration	IV
Contraindications	Complete atrioventricular block in the absence of an artificial pacemaker Patients sensitive to procaine or other ester-type local anesthetics Patients with a prolonged QRS duration or QT interval because of the potential for heart block Pre-existing QT prolongation/torsades de Pointes Digitalis toxicity (procainamide may further depress conduction)
Adverse Effects	Hypotension, bradycardia, reflex tachycardia, atrioventricular block, widened QRS, prolonged QT interval, asystole, VF, CNS depression, confusion, seizure
Pregnancy	Category C
Special Considerations	Reduce maintenance infusion rate in liver dysfunction (procainamide is metabolized by the liver) or renal failure (procainamide is eliminated by the kidneys)

VT, Ventricular tachycardia; *IV,* intravenous; *CNS,* central nervous system; *VF,* ventricular fibrillation.

TABLE 12-36 Metoprolol

Generic Name	metoprolol
Trade Name	Lopressor, Toprol XL
Classification	Beta-adrenergic blocker, class II antiarrhythmic
Action	Inhibits the strength of the heart's contractions as well as heart rate; this results in a decrease in cardiac oxygen consumption; also saturates the beta receptors and inhibits dilation of bronchial smooth muscle (beta$_2$ receptor).
Indications	Acute coronary syndromes, supraventricular tachycardia, atrial flutter, atrial fibrillation, heart failure, hypertension, thyrotoxicosis
Routes of Administration	Oral, IV
Contraindications	Heart failure, second- or third-degree heart block, cardiogenic shock, hypotension, bradycardia, bronchospasm, hypersensitivity
Adverse Effects	Bradycardia, atrioventricular conduction delays, hypotension, tiredness, dizziness, diarrhea
Pregnancy	Category C
Special Considerations	The precise mechanism for the beneficial effects of beta-blockers in heart failure is not known

IV, Intravenous.

TABLE 12-37 Propranolol

Generic Name	propranolol
Trade Name	Inderal
Classification	Beta-adrenergic blocker, class II antiarrhythmic
Action	Nonselective beta antagonist that binds with both beta$_1$ and beta$_2$ receptors; propranolol inhibits the strength of the heart's contractions and heart rate; the result is a decrease in cardiac oxygen consumption
Indications	Hypertension, angina pectoris, ventricular tachycardia refractory to other therapy, thyroid storm, migraine headaches
Routes of Administration	Oral, IV
Contraindications	Sinus bradycardia, second- or third-degree atrioventricular block, asthma, cardiogenic shock, pulmonary edema, uncompensated heart failure, known hypersensitivity, sick sinus syndrome
Adverse Effects	Bradycardia, heart block, bronchospasm, dyspnea, dizziness, weakness, nausea and vomiting, visual disturbances
Pregnancy	Category C
Special Considerations	Confusion and skin rashes may occur

IV, Intravenous.

TABLE 12-38 Amiodarone

Generic Name	amiodarone hydrochloride
Trade Name	Cordarone
Classification	Class III antiarrhythmic; although amiodarone is considered a class III antiarrhythmic, it possesses electrophysiologic characteristics of all four classes of antiarrhythmics Amiodarone blocks sodium channels (class I action), inhibits sympathetic stimulation (class II action), and blocks potassium channels (class III action) as well as calcium channels (class IV action)
Action	Acts directly on the myocardium to delay repolarization and increase the duration of the action potential
Indications	Shock-refractory pulseless VT/VF Polymorphic VT, wide-complex tachycardia of uncertain origin VT when cardioversion unsuccessful Adjunct to electrical cardioversion of supraventricular tachycardia/paroxysmal supraventricular tachycardia, atrial tachycardia Rate control of atrial fibrillation or flutter when other therapies ineffective
Routes of Administration	Oral, IV
Contraindications	Known hypersensitivity Severe sinus node dysfunction causing marked sinus bradycardia Second- and third-degree atrioventricular block Syncope from bradycardia (except when used in conjunction with a pacemaker) Pulmonary congestion Cardiogenic shock Hypotension

TABLE 12-38	Amiodarone—cont'd
Adverse Effects	Hypotension (most common side effect), headache, dizziness, bradycardia, atrioventricular conduction abnormalities, flushing, salivation, burning at IV site
Pregnancy	Category D
Special Considerations	In therapeutic doses, amiodarone has only a mild negative effect on myocardial contractility; the reason it appears in multiple algorithms involving patients experiencing dysrhythmias but who have signs of heart failure

VT, Ventricular tachycardia; *VF,* ventricular fibrillation; *IV,* intravenous.

TABLE 12-39	Diltiazem
Generic Name	diltiazem
Trade Name	Cardizem
Classification	Calcium channel blocker (calcium antagonist), class IV antiarrhythmic
Action	Blocks calcium from moving into the heart muscle cell, which prolongs the conduction of electrical impulses through the AV node
Indications	Atrial flutter or atrial fibrillation with a rapid ventricular rate Multifocal atrial tachycardia Supraventricular tachycardia
Routes of Administration	Oral, IV
Contraindications	Wide QRS tachycardia of uncertain origin Poison/drug-induced tachycardias Digitalis toxicity (may worsen heart block) Atrial fibrillation or atrial flutter with an accessory bypass tract (Wolff-Parkinson-White syndrome) Sick sinus syndrome except with a functioning ventricular pacemaker Severe heart failure Second- or third-degree atrioventricular block Hypotension Cardiogenic shock
Adverse Effects	Atrioventricular blocks, bradycardia, hypotension, chest pain, heart failure, peripheral edema, syncope, sweating, nausea, vomiting, dizziness, dry mouth, dyspnea, headache, flushing
Pregnancy	Category C
Special Considerations	Calcium channel blockers decrease peripheral resistance and can worsen hypotension; these medications should not be administered to patients with a systolic blood pressure of <90 mm Hg and should be used with caution in patients with mild to moderate hypotension; monitor blood pressure, heart rate, and ECG closely Avoid calcium channel blockers in patients with wide QRS tachycardia unless it is known with certainty to be supraventricular in origin (may precipitate ventricular fibrillation)

AV, Atrioventricular; *IV,* intravenous.

TABLE 12-40	Verapamil
Generic Name	verapamil
Trade Names	Isoptin, Calan
Classification	Calcium channel blocker (calcium antagonist), class IV Antiarrhythmic
Action	Blocks calcium from moving into the heart muscle cell, which prolongs the conduction of electrical impulses through the AV node; also dilates arteries
Indications	Supraventricular tachycardia Atrial flutter or atrial fibrillation with a rapid ventricular response Unstable angina, chronic angina
Routes of Administration	Oral, IV
Contraindications	Wide QRS tachycardia of uncertain origin Poison/drug-induced tachycardias Digitalis toxicity (may worsen heart block) Atrial fibrillation or atrial flutter with an accessory bypass tract (Wolff-Parkinson-White syndrome) Sick sinus syndrome except with a functioning ventricular pacemaker Severe heart failure Second- or third-degree atrioventricular block Hypotension Cardiogenic shock
Adverse Effects	Dizziness, headache, nausea, vomiting, hypotension, bradycardia, complete atrioventricular block, peripheral edema, CHF, transient asystole
Pregnancy	Category C
Special Considerations	Calcium channel blockers decrease peripheral resistance and can worsen hypotension; these medications should not be administered to patients with a systolic blood pressure of <90 mm Hg and should be used with caution in patients with mild to moderate hypotension; monitor blood pressure, heart rate, and ECG closely Avoid calcium channel blockers in patients with wide QRS tachycardia unless it is known with certainty to be supraventricular in origin (may precipitate ventricular fibrillation)

AV, Atrioventricular; *IV,* intravenous; *CHF,* congestive heart failure; *ECG,* electrocardiogram.

TABLE 12-41	Adenosine
Generic Name	adenosine *6-10 sec half life*
Trade Name	Adenocard
Classification	Endogenous nucleoside, antiarrhythmic
Action	Slows the conduction of electrical impulses at the AV node
Indications	First medication for most forms of narrow QRS supraventricular tachycardia
Routes of Administration	IV
Contraindications	Poison/drug-induced tachycardia Asthma Second- or third-degree atrioventricular block Sick sinus syndrome (except in patients with a functioning pacemaker) Atrial flutter, atrial fibrillation Ventricular tachycardia

AV, Atrioventricular; *IV,* intravenous; *ECG,* electrocardiogram.

TABLE 12-41   Adenosine—cont'd

Adverse Effects	Side effects common but transient and usually resolve within 1-2 minutes
	Facial flushing (common)
	Coughing/dyspnea, bronchospasm (common)
	Nausea
	Headache
	Hypotension
	Chest pressure
	Lightheadedness
	Patients will have a brief period of asystole after administration
	Sense of impending doom
	Paresthesias
	Dysrhythmias at time of rhythm conversion
	Use with caution in patients with emphysema, bronchitis, asthma
Pregnancy	Category C
Special Considerations	Onset of action 10 to 40 seconds
	Discontinue in any patient who develops severe respiratory difficulty
	Must be injected into the IV tubing as fast as possible (over a period of seconds); failure to do so may result in breakdown of the medication while still in the IV tubing
	Follow each dose immediately with a 20-mL normal saline flush. Recommended IV site is the antecubital fossa; use the injection port nearest the hub of the IV catheter; *constant ECG monitoring is essential.*

TABLE 12-42   Digoxin

Generic Name	digoxin
Trade Name	Lanoxin
Classification	Cardiac glycoside
Action	Inhibit sodium-potassium–adenosine triphosphate membrane pump, resulting in an increase in calcium inside the heart muscle cell, which causes an increase in the force of contraction of the heart
Indications	*Limited use in emergency cardiac care*
	Control ventricular response rate in patients with atrial fibrillation or atrial flutter, paroxysmal supraventricular tachycardia, heart failure caused by poor left ventricular contractility
Routes of Administration	Oral, IV
Contraindications	Known hypersensitivity, digitalis toxicity, second- or third-degree atrioventricular block without a pacemaker, VT, VF, sick sinus syndrome, MI
Adverse Effects	Visual disturbances, fatigue, weakness, nausea, loss of appetite, abdominal discomfort, psychological symptoms, dizziness, abnormal dreams, headache, diarrhea, vomiting
Pregnancy	Category C
Special Considerations	Toxic/therapeutic ratio is narrow

IV, Intravenous; *VT,* ventricular tachycardia; *VF,* ventricular fibrillation; *MI,* myocardial infarction.

the excretion of water and electrolytes, which causes a volume reduction. Others work by inhibiting enzymes that help retain intravascular volume. Others cause vasodilatation, thus altering the container, not the amount of fluid. Physicians typically choose these agents on the basis of the physiology of each individual patient. Some of these drugs are used in prehospital emergencies and are discussed in detail the following sections.

Diuretics

General Diuretic → hypernatremic?

Diuretics are based on the premise of volume reduction in the intravascular circulation. They work at the kidney and eliminate water with electrolytes. This reduction immediately pulls fluid from the intravascular space. Water from the extracellular space moves into the intravascular space. Diuretics reduce peripheral swelling by this mechanism. The total effect is a reduction in systemic blood pressure and cardiac workload (preload). A variety of diuretics is prescribed and some combination products have been developed.

Loop Diuretics

Loop diuretics are a common choice for a diuretic. They are located in many paramedic drug boxes. Many patients also take these as prescription medications. They act at the loop of Henle in the renal tubule and prohibit the reabsorption of sodium and water (Figure 12-1). Because loop diuretics can lead to hypokalemia, patients often take a potassium supplement when taking these medications. The most commonly prescribed drug in this class is furosemide (Lasix) (Table 12-43). Other commonly used loop diuretics include bumetanide (Bumex), ethacrynic acid (Edecrin), and torsemide (Demadex).

Thiazide Diuretics

Thiazide diuretics are the most commonly used antihypertensive drugs. This class of medications is used to lower blood pressure and often is encountered as a home medication. Thiazide diuretic drugs work by increasing excretion of sodium, chloride, and water at the distal renal tubule. Some potassium also is excreted. A common example is hydrochlorothiazide (HCTZ).

Potassium-Sparing Diuretics

Potassium-sparing diuretics increase sodium and water loss in the distal renal tubule. At the same time, potassium is reabsorbed instead of being excreted. They are often used as an alternative for patients whose potassium levels have decreased with other diuretics. An example is spironolactone (Aldactone). Patients taking these medications may experience hyperkalemia because they retain potassium.

Osmotic Diuretics

Osmotic diuretics pull fluid into the vascular space by increasing osmotic pressure. Because they are not reabsorbed by the renal tubules, they prevent water reabsorption. Mannitol (Osmitrol) is an example of an osmotic diuretic used to reduce intracranial pressure in cerebral edema.

Adrenergic Blocking Medications

Beta-Blockers

Beta-blockers have been previously discussed in two separate categories, demonstrating how clinically important these medications are in the treatment of a wide variety of medical conditions. These agents are a subclass of adrenergic blocking agents and work by occupying beta-receptors, decreasing cardiac output, and inhibiting renin secretion from the kidneys.

Centrally Acting Adrenergic Inhibitors

These drugs work by blocking the sympathetic stimulation from the CNS. The mechanism is not completely understood; however, they work at multiple receptors. The two most commonly used medications in this class are clonidine hydrochloride (Catapres) and methyldopa (Aldomet). These medications are not commonly seen in prehospital drug boxes but are used in the emergency department and may be part of the home medication regimen for patients.

Peripheral Adrenergic Inhibitors

These agents work similarly to the central acting inhibitors. They exert their effects on peripheral blood vessels, reducing blood pressure. Common medications in this group include guanethidine sulfate (Ismelin), prazosin hydrochloride (Minipress), phentolamine (Regitine), and phenoxybenzamine (Dibenzyline).

Rauwolfia Derivatives. Rauwolfia drugs are derived from tropical trees and shrubs. They are used as antihypertensive agents but not as commonly as other drugs. They work as peripheral adrenergic inhibitors. The most common drug in the class is reserpine (Serpalan). It works by depleting catecholamine storage in the nerve cell. This depletes normal sympathetic activity in the CNS and peripheral nerves. Risks of this medication include toxicity. Increased amounts can cause increased CNS depression, psychiatric depression, cardiovascular toxicity, and gastrointestinal irritation.

Angiotensin-Converting Enzyme Inhibitors

Angiotensin-converting enzyme (ACE) inhibitors affect the renin-angiotensin-aldosterone system. They play an important part of antihypertensive therapy and are car-

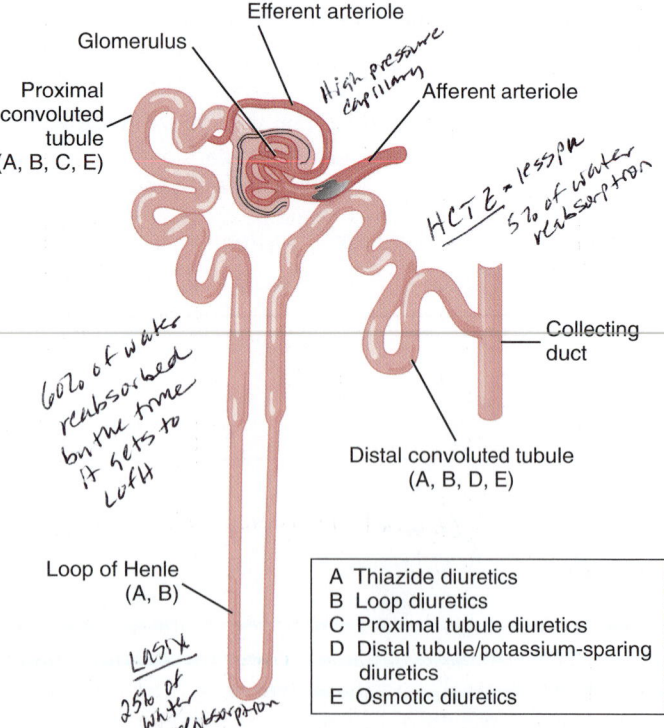

Figure 12-1 The nephron of a kidney and sites of action of diuretics.

TABLE 12-43 Furosemide

Generic Name	furosemide
Trade Name	Lasix
Classification	Loop diuretic
Action	Inhibits the absorption of the sodium and chloride ions and water in the loop of Henle, as well as the convoluted tubule of the nephron; this results in decreased absorption of water and increased production of urine
Indications	Adjunctive therapy in acute pulmonary edema, hypertension, edema associated with cirrhosis and renal disease
Routes of Administration	Oral, IV
Contraindications	Hypersensitivity to furosemide or sulfonamides, hypovolemia, severe electrolyte depletion, hypotension, anuria
Adverse Effects	Hypotension, ECG changes associated with electrolyte disturbances, dry mouth, hearing loss, vertigo, weakness, dizziness, orthostatic hypotension
Pregnancy	Category C
Special Considerations	Can cause excessive fluid loss and dehydration, resulting in hypovolemia and electrolyte imbalance Patients with sulfonamide hypersensitivity or thiazide diuretic hypersensitivity may also be hypersensitive to furosemide Ototoxicity and resulting transient deafness can occur with rapid administration; do not exceed the recommended rate of administration

IV, Intravenous; *ECG,* electrocardiogram.

dioprotective after a myocardial infarction. This system is critical for the maintenance of normal blood pressure and electrolyte balance. When this system is not controlled properly, angiotensin II may be excreted and excessive vasoconstriction may occur. This elevates blood pressure and may put stress on the kidneys. These inhibitors inhibit the cascade, thus blocking the production of angiotensin II. Blood pressure is then lowered. Examples of ACE inhibitors include captopril (Capoten), enalapril (Vasotec), and lisinopril (Prinivil).

Calcium Channel Blocking Agents

Calcium channel blocking agents block calcium entry and prohibit the vasoconstriction of vascular smooth muscle. They were detailed in the section on antiarrhythmics.

Vasodilators

Vasodilators work directly on the peripheral blood vessel wall, causing dilation and inhibiting constriction. This allows for a larger diameter and thus effectively lowers blood pressure without affecting volume. As these drugs exert their effects, a reflex sympathetic response may occur. These medications decrease blood pressure, and the body senses this at the baroreceptors. These receptors stimulate the sympathetic division of the autonomic nervous system, resulting in an increase in heart rate, cardiac output, and renin release. Obviously these medi-

TABLE 12-44 Vasodilators

Arteriolar Dilator Drugs	Arteriolar and Venous Dilator Drugs
diazoxide (Hyperstat IV) hydralazine (Apresoline) minoxidil (Loniten)	sodium nitroprusside (Nipride, Nitropress) nitrates and nitrites amyl nitrate inhalant isosorbide dinitrate (Isordil, Sorbitrate) nitroglycerin sublingual (Nitrostat), nitroglycerin paste IV nitroglycerin (Tridil)

IV, Intravenous.

cations may not be effective when used alone and are often used in combination therapy with medications that may block the reflex sympathetic response. Types of vasodilators are listed in Tables 12-44 and 12-45.

Other Agents

Monoamine oxidase inhibitors were previously described in the antidepressant category. These medications block norepinephrine at the sympathetic junction and thus block vasoconstriction. Because they interact unfavorably with other medications and many food products, they are rarely used strictly as an antihypertensive.

TABLE 12-45	Nitroglycerin
Generic Name	nitroglycerin
Trade Names	Nitrostat, Nitrobid (sublingual); Tridil (IV)
Classification	Vasodilator, organic nitrate, antianginal
Action	Relaxes smooth muscle, thereby dilating peripheral arteries and veins; this causes a pooling of venous blood and decreased venous return to the heart, which decreases preload; nitroglycerine also reduces left ventricular systolic wall tension, which decreases afterload
Indications	Sublingual tablets or spray: Prophylaxis, treatment, and management of patients with angina pectoris Pulmonary congestion from left ventricular failure IV: Ongoing ischemic chest discomfort Management of hypertensive emergencies, particularly if related to volume overload Management of pulmonary congestion from left ventricular failure
Routes of Administration	Sublingual spray, tablet, IV
Contraindications	Viagra (or other PDE inhibitor); use within 24 to 48 hours Suspected inferior wall myocardial infarction with possible right ventricular myocardial infarction Hypotension (systolic blood pressure <90 mm Hg or <30 mm Hg below baseline) Extreme bradycardia (<50 beats/min) Tachycardia (>100 beats/min) Increased intracranial pressure (e.g., head trauma or cerebral hemorrhage) Uncorrected hypovolemia Inadequate cerebral circulation Constrictive pericarditis and pericardial tamponade Known sensitivity Closed-angle glaucoma
Adverse Effects	Primary side effect is hypotension; other side effects include tachycardia, bradycardia, headache, palpitations, syncope
Pregnancy	Category C
Special Considerations	Hypotension may worsen myocardial ischemia. Hypotension usually responds to administration of IV fluids. *Establishing an IV before giving sublingual nitroglycerin is strongly recommended.* When giving nitroglycerin for ischemic chest discomfort, assess the patient's pain, duration, time started, activity being performed, quality. Document the patient's response to the medication. Monitor vital signs and cardiac rhythm closely before, during, and after giving. Significant hypotension may occur in the presence of right ventricular infarction. Nitroglycerin tablets are light, moisture, and heat sensitive. Keep tablets in their original brown glass bottles. Replace metal cap on bottle quickly after opening. Tablets usually lose potency within 3 to 4 months. When giving nitroglycerin spray, do not shake the canister before use. Shaking may produce bubbles within the canister, altering delivery of the medication.

Ganglionic blocking agents are a class of drugs that block both the sympathetic and parasympathetic nervous systems at the ganglia. They decrease peripheral vascular resistance and lower blood pressure. They are not commonly used because of a low safety profile. Examples include trimethaphan (Arfonad), pargyline hydrochloride (Eutonyl), and metyrosine (Denser).

ANTICOAGULANTS, FIBRINOLYTICS, AND BLOOD COMPONENTS

[OBJECTIVE 19]

Anticoagulants and fibrinolytics are frequently used in emergency care to treat strokes and myocardial infarctions.

Anticoagulants

The formation of blood clots is a physiologic process that is protective in many instances. When a blood clot (thrombus) forms intravascularly, it may result in a serious medical condition such as a myocardial infarction or stroke. A blood clot consists of fibrin mesh that holds platelets, blood cells, and plasma. This forms a plug that prevents further bleeding. When a blood clot forms in an artery near the heart, a myocardial infarction may result. If it occurs in a vein, a deep vein thrombosis may occur and may lead to a pulmonary embolus.

Antiplatelet Agents   *81 mg baby aspirin*

These drugs are used to prevent platelets from sticking together. These drugs are commonly used and are often prescribed to prevent clot formation. For instance, a patient with a previous stroke or myocardial infarction may be prescribed one aspirin a day. Other antiplatelet drugs are used before invasive procedures, such as cardiac catheterizations. Types of antiplatelet agents are listed in Box 12-17.

Anticoagulants

Anticoagulants are designed to inhibit a portion of the coagulation cascade in an attempt to prevent blood clot formation. They commonly are used in conditions when a blood clot exists (**deep venous thrombosis [DVT]**) or in an attempt to prevent a clot (e.g., after surgery). These drugs do not break down current clots. They do prevent clots from getting larger or other clots from forming. They are used in DVT, myocardial infarction, atrial fibrillation, and valvular disease. One risk of these drugs is hemorrhage. A careful history and physical is usually taken before giving the drug. This class of medication includes heparin, enoxaparin (Lovenox), and warfarin (Coumadin).
↳ on at home

Fibrinolytic Therapy

Fibrinolytic (thrombolytic) therapy is an area of active research. These medications dissolve clots that have already formed. They are being used to treat myocardial infarction and stroke. The goal of these medications is to reestablish blood flow through the blocked blood vessel. Risks include increased bleeding, including intracranial bleeding. Most institutions have well-defined criteria that must be met before giving these drugs. Common fibrinolytic medications include tissue plasminogen activator (TPA, Activase), reteplase (Retavase), streptokinase (Streptase), urokinase (Abbokinase), and tenecteplase (TNKase).

Antihemophilic Agents

A group of hereditary bleeding disorders affects the clotting cascade. Thirteen proteins are integral in the clotting cascade. Individuals who are affected with these illnesses tend to have problems with clotting and often are missing one of these factors (Table 12-46). When they experience trauma, they may have severe bleeding. These patients often receive medications that provide the missing factor so that the coagulation cascade may proceed and form a clot. Medications in this class include desmopressin (DDAVP), factor VIIa (NovoSeven, NiaStase), factor VII (Advate), and factor IX (BeneFix).

Blood and Blood Components

Two main therapies are used to replace blood components: crystalloids and colloids. Colloids attempt to replace a specific part of the blood contents that may be deficient. Crystalloids attempt to replace volume. Types of colloids are listed in Box 12-18. Crystalloids were previously discussed.

ANTIHYPERLIPIDEMIC DRUGS

[OBJECTIVE 20]

Antihyperlipidemic drugs (also called *hypolipidemics*) are used to reduce elevated cholesterol levels, decreasing the risk of atherosclerosis and coronary artery disease. Many

TABLE 12-46	Types of Genetic Coagulopathies
Hemophilia A	Deficiency factor VIII
Hemophilia B	Deficiency factor IX
von Willebrand disease	Deficiency in von Willebrand factor and factor VIII

BOX 12-17   Types of Antiplatelet Agents

- salicylate (aspirin)
- dipyridamole (Persantine)
- clopidogrel (Plavix)
- ticlopidine (Ticlid)
- abciximab (ReoPro)

BOX 12-18   Types of Colloids

- Whole blood
- Packed red blood cells
- Fresh frozen plasma
- Platelets
- Expanders (Dextran)
- Platelets
- Coagulation factors
- Fibrinogen
- Albumin
- Gamma-globulins

BOX 12-19 | Examples of Antihyperlipidemic Drugs

- atorvastatin (Lipitor)
- fluvastatin (Lescal)
- lovastatin (Mevacor)
- pravastatin (Pravachol)
- simvastatin (Zocor)
- gemfibrozil (Lopid)
- clofibrate (Atromid-S)
- colestipol (Colestid)

BOX 12-20 | Antihistamines

- dimenhydrinate (Dramamine)
- diphenhydramine (Benadryl)
- hydroxyzine (Vistaril)
- promethazine (Phenergan)
- clemastine (Tavist)
- loratadine (Claritin)
- fexofenadine (Allegra)
- cetirizine (Zyrtec)
- desloratadine (Clarinex)

BOX 12-21 | Antitussives

- benzonatate (Tessalon)
- dextromethorphan (Sucrets Cough, Benylin DM, Robitussin DM)
- codeine
- hydrocodone (Hycodan, Histussin)

different types of antihyperlipidemic drugs are available, many of which can be recognized by the word *statin* in their names (Box 12-19). They are not typically used in prehospital care, but many patients name these medications in their home medication list.

DRUGS AFFECTING THE RESPIRATORY SYSTEM
DRUGS USED FOR NASAL CONGESTION

Decongestants

Decongestants help shrink swelling of the nasal mucosa. These medications provide symptomatic relief. Pseudoephedrine is the active ingredient and is found in many over-the-counter brands of cold and allergy medication.

Antihistamines

Histamine is a chemical mediator released during an inflammatory response. It is commonly linked with allergies. Two primary histamine receptors exist; H_1 receptors are found on the blood vessels and bronchioles, and H_2 receptors are found in the gastrointestinal tract. When histamine is released into the bloodstream, it causes increased localized blood flow, increased capillary permeability, and swelling of the tissues. It also affects bronchial tissue by causing contraction. The release of histamine may be localized. This is commonly found in edema, **eczema, rhinitis** (runny nose), urticaria (hives), and asthma. Systemic responses to histamine include **anaphylaxis.**

Antihistamines compete with histamine for the receptor site and may block the effects of histamine by occupying the receptor. If histamine is already attached to a receptor site, the antihistamine will not be effective. Side effects include atropinelike (anticholinergic) effects such as tachycardia, constipation, drowsiness, sedation, and inhibition of secretions. Patients who take antihistamines long term can develop a tolerance. Common antihistamines are listed in Box 12-20. Diphenhydramine, an antihistamine carried in many paramedic drug boxes, is discussed in detail in Table 12-47.

Cough Suppressants

Cough suppressants are used when patients have a cough that disturbs normal daily activities, such as sleep. The cough reflex is a protective mechanism. Its function is to remove irritants and secretions from the airway. Coughing is increased with inflammation that often occurs with bacterial or viral illness. Antitussive agents are available in over-the-counter preparations. Prescription forms often contain narcotics. Common antitussives are listed in Box 12-21.

MUCOKINETIC DRUGS AND EXPECTORANTS

[OBJECTIVE 21]

Mucokinetic Drugs

Mucus is normally produced by the cells of the respiratory tract. The amount of mucus is increased in individuals with allergies and asthma or reactive airway disease. Mucokinetic drugs (also called mucolytics) break down mucus and make it more watery. This helps in the removal of mucus or other secretions from the respiratory tract during coughing or suctioning.

Some mucolytics are given by nebulizer. Others are instilled into the trachea through a tracheal tube or tracheostomy. One of the most commonly used mucokinetic drugs is saline. Saline thins the mucus and helps its expectoration. Dornase alfa (Pulmozyme) is a mucolytic used to relieve the buildup of secretions that occurs in cystic fibrosis.

TABLE 12-47 Diphenhydramine

Generic Name	diphenhydramine hydrochloride
Trade Name	Benadryl
Classification	Antihistamine, anticholinergic, H_1 receptor antagonist
Action	Binds and blocks H_1 histamine receptors
Indications	Phenothiazine-induced dystonic (extrapyramidal) reactions, anaphylaxis, and moderate to severe allergic reactions (after epinephrine); antiemetic
Routes of Administration	Oral, IV, intramuscular
Contraindications	Known hypersensitivity to diphenhydramine Newborn or premature infants; nursing mothers Acute narrow-angle glaucoma Obstructive diseases of the gastrointestinal tract Bronchial asthma Cardiovascular disease or hypertension
Adverse Effects	Cardiovascular: hypotension, reflex tachycardia, palpitations CNS: drowsiness, dizziness, poor coordination, confusion, headache, anxiety, excitement (especially in children), ataxia, vertigo, seizures Respiratory: drying/thickening of bronchial secretions, wheezing, chest tightness, nasal stuffiness, dry nose, throat, mouth Genitourinary: urinary frequency or retention, nausea, vomiting Other: blurred vision, dilated pupils, tinnitus
Pregnancy	Category B
Special Considerations	Do not give subcutaneously because of irritating effects

IV, Intravenous; *CNS,* central nervous system.

BOX 12-22 Examples of Mucolytics/Expectorants

- guaifenesin (Hytussin, Robitussin)
- acetylcysteine (Mucomyst)
- dornase alfa (Pulmozyme)

Expectorants

Expectorants decrease the adhesiveness and surface tension of respiratory secretions, making the secretions easier to cough up. Expectorants such as guaifenesin (Robitussin) are widely available in over-the-counter preparations. Examples of common mucolytics and expectorants are listed in Box 12-22.

BRONCHODILATORS

Bronchodilators remain the primary treatment for obstructive pulmonary disease. This class of diseases includes asthma, chronic bronchitis, and emphysema. Many bronchodilators are given through a small-volume nebulizer or metered-dose inhaler.

Sympathomimetics

Sympathomimetics were previously discussed in regard to other medical conditions and treatments. The drugs that provide the most assistance to respiratory emergencies are beta-selective agonists, with an emphasis on $beta_2$-receptor activation.

Nonselective agonists stimulate both the alpha- and beta-receptors. Some over-the-counter preparations, such as Primatene Mist, contain epinephrine. A prescription form of a nonselective agonist is racemic epinephrine. These medications stimulate all sympathomimetic receptors. They induce bronchodilation by stimulating $beta_2$ receptors in the lungs. They also decrease mucosal edema by stimulating alpha-receptors.

$Beta_2$-selective drugs lessen the incidence of unwanted cardiac effects, putting less stress on the heart. This class of drugs includes albuterol (Proventil, Ventolin), levalbuterol, and terbutaline (Brethine). Albuterol is covered in detail in Table 12-48.

Anticholinergics

When stimulated by acetylcholine, bronchial smooth muscle normally constricts. Anticholinergic bronchodilators block the action of acetylcholine, resulting in smooth

TABLE 12-48	Albuterol
Generic Name	albuterol sulfate
Trade Names	Proventil, Ventolin
Classification	Synthetic sympathomimetic, beta$_2$ agonist, beta-adrenergic stimulator, bronchodilator
Action	Binds and stimulates beta$_2$ receptors, resulting in relaxation of bronchial smooth muscle
Indications	Bronchospasm associated with chronic bronchitis, emphysema, asthma, anaphylaxis
Routes of Administration	Nebulized by mouthpiece or inline by mask, metered-dose inhaler, inline by orotracheal or nasotracheal tube
Contraindications	Hypersensitivity, cardiac dysrhythmias, angioedema
Adverse Effects	Dysrhythmias, palpitations, tachycardia (with excessive use), hypertension, angina CNS: tremors, anxiety, insomnia, headache, dizziness, restlessness, flushing, irritability, nervousness Gastrointestinal: nausea, vomiting, heartburn, irritation of nose and throat Hyperglycemia, hypocalcemia, hypertension
Pregnancy	Category C
Special Considerations	Assess patient's respiratory rate, tidal volume, breath sounds, heart rate, and blood pressure before, during, and after administration Ask the patient about the medications already taken; if the patient has been using an inhaler, find out how often and when the last dose was taken; consult medical direction

- Stops secretions

muscle relaxation and bronchodilation. Ipratropium bromide (Atrovent) is an anticholinergic bronchodilator that is often given in combination with a beta$_2$ agonist, such as albuterol (Table 12-49).

Xanthine Derivatives

Xanthine derivatives act by relaxing smooth muscle. They also stimulate the CNS and cardiac muscle. Examples of xanthine derivatives include caffeine and theophylline. Common names for them include aminophylline (Theo-Dur) and theophylline (Bronkodyl). These medications are not used as often as other types of bronchodilators but may still be encountered in home medications.

Leukotriene Antagonists

Leukotriene inhibitors are drugs that have been developed to help stabilize the cells responsible for inflammation. They are used in patients with severe allergies as well as reactive airway disease. Included in this class is montelukast (Singulair).

Prophylactic Asthmatic Drugs

Steroids often are used to help prevent the inflammatory response. Inhaled steroids localize the effects of these medications without the systemic effects. Some inhalers combine the inhaled steroids with a sympathomimetic for increased patient compliance.

DRUGS THAT AFFECT THE RESPIRATORY CENTER

Oxygen

Although oxygen is found in room air at approximately 21%, it is still classified as a drug when administered at higher concentrations. It is colorless, odorless, and tasteless. It is normally found in the gaseous state. Oxygen increases hemoglobin saturation if ventilation is adequate. It improves tissue oxygenation when circulation is maintained. Oxygen should be given in all cases of cardiac or respiratory arrest, suspected hypoxemia of any cause, and any suspected cardiopulmonary emergency, especially reports of shortness of breath and/or suspected ischemic chest pain.

TABLE 12-49 Ipratropium Bromide

Generic Name	ipratropium bromide
Trade Name	Atrovent
Classification	Bronchodilator, anticholinergic, parasympathetic blocker, parasympatholytic
Action	Antagonizes the acetylcholine receptor on bronchial smooth muscle, producing bronchodilation
Indications	Bronchospasm associated with chronic bronchitis, emphysema, or asthma
Routes of Administration	Nebulized by mouthpiece or inline by mask, metered-dose inhaler
Contraindications	Hypersensitivity to ipratropium bromide or to atropine and its derivatives Closed-angle glaucoma, bladder neck obstruction, prostatic hypertrophy Known sensitivity to peanuts or soybeans
Adverse Effects	Palpitations, dizziness, nervousness, headache, tremor, insomnia, nausea, gastrointestinal distress, dry mouth, cough, skin rash, blurred vision
Pregnancy	Category B
Special Considerations	Assess patient's respiratory rate, tidal volume, breath sounds, heart rate, and blood pressure before, during, and after administration Used either alone or in combination with other bronchodilators, especially beta-adrenergics (such as albuterol) Much of an administered dose is swallowed but not absorbed

Case Scenario—continued

You discover that the patient was supposed to make an appointment for a cardiac stress test. He states he was working in the garage when the pain began. He also began to feel short of breath. The patient describes his discomfort as a "burning" sensation that does not radiate. The pain has lasted 40 minutes and has not improved with rest. Vital signs are blood pressure, 120/74 mm Hg; pulse, 113 beats/min; respirations, 22 breaths/min and labored; lung sounds clear; heart sounds clear; oxygen saturation is 100%. On physical examination you notice that you cannot reproduce the pain with palpation of either the chest wall or the abdomen. His skin is diaphoretic and his extremities are not swollen. The patient's medical history is positive for gastroesophageal reflex disease (GERD) and hypertension. His history is negative for any surgery. He denies diabetes and is unsure of his cholesterol level. He takes famotidine for GERD. He denies drinking alcohol or taking any illegal drugs. He last ate approximately 4 hours ago.

Questions

4. *What do the historical findings indicate?*
5. *What do the physical examination findings indicate?*
6. *What diagnostic and therapeutic interventions should be done?*

Direct Respiratory Stimulants

Analeptics are medications that directly stimulate the medullary center of the brain. They are considered inferior to mechanical ventilation and are rarely used.

Reflex Respiratory Stimulants

Spirits of ammonia are used as a reflex respiratory stimulant. This medication emits a potent vapor that irritates the sensory receptors. Messages are delivered to the brain and respirations are stimulated. This is commonly used on patients who have had a syncopal episode.

Respiratory Depressants

Respiratory depressants are rarely used medically. However, respiratory depression is a common side effect of narcotics and barbiturates.

DRUGS AFFECTING THE URINARY SYSTEM
RENAL SYSTEM DYSFUNCTION

[OBJECTIVE 22]

Many patients have renal function impairments. Many medications are metabolized and excreted through the kidneys. Patients who have renal insufficiency may require smaller or less-frequent dosing. Certain medications are known to induce renal problems. Included in this list are NSAIDs, contrast dye, and aminoglycoside antibiotics.

DRUGS AFFECTING THE GASTROINTESTINAL SYSTEM

[OBJECTIVE 23]

The gastrointestinal tract is important for the absorption of water, nutrients, and medications. Medications used to treat disorders including ulcers, inflammation, nausea, vomiting, constipation, and diarrhea are discussed below.

ANTACIDS

Many medical conditions cause irritation of the gastrointestinal tract. In the stomach, acid is produced as a normal part of digestion. If a patient has gastritis (irritation of the stomach lining), reflux, or ulcer disease, the amount of acid production should be controlled. Antacids buffer the acid content by interacting with the hydrochloric acid secreted in the stomach and helping control systems. Two over-the-counter antacids are Rolaids and Alka-Seltzer.

ANTIFLATULENTS

Increased bowel gas can be painful and uncomfortable. Antiflatulent medications help reduce the formation of gas in the gastrointestinal tract. In infants, gas can cause considerable pain and is thought to be a cause of colic. Simethicone (Mylicon) drops are an example of a medication in this class.

DIGESTANTS

Digestants are drugs given to help the digestive process. For individuals who do not secrete adequate amounts of enzymes, these medications are necessary. An example is pancreatin.

ANTIEMETICS

Vomiting is an involuntary action controlled by the emetic center of the medulla. Nausea and vomiting can have a number of causes. Common antiemetics block

---

histamine, acetylcholine, and dopamine receptors. Examples of antiemetics are listed in Box 12-23.

EMETICS

Emetics are rarely used. In the past, syrup of Ipecac was used to induce vomiting after a toxic ingestion. Different methods are currently used and are discussed under Toxic Substances.

CANNABINOIDS

Cannabinoids are commonly thought of as street drugs. They have been used as an appetite stimulant and as a pain medication. They have been researched in the treatment for increased appetite for cancer patients and for pain control in glaucoma.

CYTOPROTECTIVE AGENTS

Crohn's disease and ulcerative colitis are inflammatory processes of the gastrointestinal tract. Cytoprotective drugs are medications designed to protect the lining of the gastrointestinal tract. These medications also are used to protect against peptic ulcer disease. Examples include sucralfate (Carafate) and misoprostol (Cytotec).

H$_2$ RECEPTOR ANTAGONISTS

The H$_2$ receptor is the main site of action for histamine in the gastrointestinal tract. Medications have been designed to block this histamine release. This blockade reduces the amount of gastric acid secretion and is often used as a treatment for patients with pain. It has also been demonstrated that H$_2$ blockers protect against the development of stress ulcers in hospitalized patients. Examples of H$_2$ receptor antagonists are given in Box 12-24.

LAXATIVES

Laxatives are used to increase the excretion of stool. Constipation is a problem for a significant amount of the population. Constipation may be caused by neurologic

BOX 12-24 H₂ Receptor Antagonists

- cimetidine (Tagamet)
- ranitidine (Zantac)
- famotidine (Pepcid)

BOX 12-25 Types of Antidiarrheals

- Adsorbents
- Pepto-Bismol
- Anticholinergics
- Donnatal
- Opiates
- Codeine
- diphenoxylate (Lomotil)
- loperamide (Imodium)

TABLE 12-50 Types of Laxatives

Type	Example
Saline	Milk of magnesia
Stimulant	Dulcolax, Ex-Lax
Bulk-forming	Metamucil
Lubricant	Mineral oil
Fecal moistening agents	Colace, glycerin suppositories
Prescription	Golytely

BOX 12-26 Types of Medications for Glaucoma

Beta-Blockers
- timolol (Timoptic)
- betaxolol (Betoptic)

Carbonic Anhydrase Inhibitors
- acetazolamide (Diamox)

Prostaglandin Analogs
- latanoprost (Xalatan)

Sympathomimetics
- brimonidine (Alphagan P)

Other
- pilocarpine (Pilocar)

BOX 12-27 Examples of Mydriatic and Cycloplegic Agents

- Atropine ophthalmic
- Cyclopentolate hydrochloride
- Homatropine ophthalmic solution
- Epinephrine

problems, pregnancy, surgery, or the administration of certain medications. Many laxatives and stool softeners are available over the counter. Types of laxatives are listed in Table 12-50.

ANTIDIARRHEALS

Diarrhea may be caused by changes in diet, infection, or other medical conditions. Antidiarrheals are available over the counter but are not recommended without the supervision of a medical professional. Examples of antidiarrheals are listed in Box 12-25.

DRUGS AFFECTING THE EYE AND EAR
DRUGS AFFECTING THE EYE

[OBJECTIVE 24]
Medications applied directly to the eye have many clinical uses. They are used to enhance an eye examination, treat medical conditions, and prevent further eye damage.

Antiglaucoma Agents

Glaucoma is a condition characterized by increased intraocular pressure. The pressure of the fluid in the eye becomes elevated and causes compression or obstruction of the eye's internal blood vessels. This can result in visual loss. Types of medications used to treat glaucoma are given in Box 12-26.

Mydriatic and Cycloplegic Agents

Mydriatic and cycloplegic agents are used to dilate the pupil and suppress the eye's reaction to light. They are used to treat inflammation and pain and allow the eye to rest. They may also be used during routine eye examinations to dilate the pupil for better visualization of the posterior eye. Examples of mydriatic and cycloplegic agents are given in Box 12-27.

Antiinfective and Antiinflammatory Agents

Antiinfective and antiinflammatory agents are used to treat eye conditions such as conjunctivitis and corneal inflammation. These also are used for small scratches to the corneal surface. The most commonly used are antibiotic ointments and liquid drops.

Topical Anesthetic Agents

Local anesthetics reduce pain in the eye without systemic effects. These medications are used when a foreign body has penetrated the corneal surface or when a patient is having trouble opening the eye for examination. They have a short duration of action but a rapid onset. Tetracaine HCl (Pontocaine) and proparacaine HCl (Ophthaine) are commonly used.

Other Ophthalmic Preparations

Artificial tears and lubricants are available over the counter. Patients may use these medications for allergies, dryness, or redness.

DRUGS AFFECTING THE EAR

Many types of medications are designed for the ear canal. Included in this list are antibiotics, antiinflammatory agents, analgesics, and drugs to remove built-up wax.

DRUGS AFFECTING THE ENDOCRINE SYSTEM
OVERVIEW

[OBJECTIVE 25]
The endocrine system is important in maintaining body function. This system is controlled by hormones being released from one organ and traveling to a distant organ, where they exert their effects. Complex cascades are part of the endocrine system.

DRUGS AFFECTING THE PITUITARY GLAND

The hormones of the anterior and posterior pituitary gland exert important effects over the entire body. They affect growth, intravascular volume maintenance, and hormones. Selected drugs that affect the anterior and posterior pituitary gland are shown in Table 12-51.

DRUGS AFFECTING THE PARATHYROID AND THYROID GLANDS

Thyroid function is important in regulating the metabolic rate and is required for normal growth and development. Autoimmune conditions can cause problems with normal thyroid function. Parathyroid hormone is responsible for regulation of calcium. Selected drugs that affect the parathyroid and thyroid glands are listed in Table 12-52.

TABLE 12-51	Selected Drugs That Affect the Anterior and Posterior Pituitary Gland	
Generic Name	**Trade Name**	**Indications for Use**
Anterior Pituitary Gland		
octreotide	Sandostatin	Growth hormone inhibitor
corticotropin	Acthar, ACTH	Diagnostic testing
somatrem	Protropin	Growth hormone deficiency in children
somatropin	Humatrope	Prader-Willi syndrome
sermorelin	Geref	Growth hormone deficiency
Posterior Pituitary Gland		
vasopressin	Pitressin	Diabetes insipidus, acute massive hemorrhage
lypressin	Diapid	Diabetes insipidus
desmopressin	DDAVP	Diabetes insipidus

TABLE 12-52	Selected Drugs That Affect the Parathyroid and Thyroid Glands	
Generic Name	**Trade Name**	**Indications for Use**
Parathyroid Gland		
calcifediol	Calderol	Hypocalcemia
calcitonin-salmon	Calcimar	Hypercalcemia
plicamycin	Mithracin	Hypercalcemia, inhibit bone resorption
Thyroid Gland		
levothyroxine	Synthroid	Synthetic thyroid hormone replacement
liotrix	Euthroid	Synthetic thyroid hormone replacement
potassium iodide	Lugol's iodine	Antithyroid preparation (hyperthyroidism)

Drugs Affecting the Adrenal Cortex

Epinephrine released when stim (handwritten)

The adrenal cortex secretes three major classes of steroid hormones: glucocorticoids (cortisol), mineralocorticoids (primarily aldosterone), and sex hormones. Glucocorticoids increase blood sugar, regulate metabolism of proteins and carbohydrates, and suppress the inflammatory response. Mineralocorticoids regulate electrolyte and water balance. Sex hormones have a small physiologic effect under normal circumstances. Selected steroids and corticosteroids are listed in Table 12-53.

Drugs Affecting the Pancreas

The pancreas functions as an exocrine and endocrine gland. It releases hormones into the bloodstream and enzymes into the digestive tract. It is responsible for the production of insulin, a necessary hormone for the use of glucose. The two major hormones secreted by the pancreas are insulin and glucagon. They are critical to the maintenance of glucose metabolism. Insulin increases the ability of tissue to take up glucose. Glucagon acts on stored liver glycogen, converting it to glucose so that it can be released into the blood and used. It also inhibits the uptake of glucose by muscle and fat tissue.

Glucagon and insulin work together in a balancing act to keep the amount of glucose in the bloodstream relatively steady. Types of insulin preparations are shown in Table 12-54. Dextrose 50% and glucagon are discussed in detail in Tables 12-55 and 12-56.

TABLE 12-53 Selected Steroids and Corticosteroids

Generic Name	Trade Name
Glucocorticoids	
hydrocortisone	Cortef, Cortisol
dexamethasone	Decadron
methylprednisolone sodium succinate	Solu-Medrol
hydrocortisone sodium succinate	Solu-Cortef
methylprednisolone sodium acetate	Depo-Medrol
prednisone	Deltasone, Sterapred
fluticasone	Inhaler: Flovent, Vanceril, Beclovent, Azmacort Aerosol: Flonase, Beconase
Mineralocorticoids	
fludrocortisone	Florinef

TABLE 12-54 Types of Insulin Preparations

Insulin	Onset	Peak Effect	Duration of Action
Rapid Acting			
lispro (Humalog)	15-30 min	30 min to $2\frac{1}{2}$ hours	3-5 hours
aspart (NovoLog)	10-20 min	1-3 hours	3-5 hours
Short Acting			
Regular	30 min to 1 hour	2-5 hours	5-8 hours
Intermediate Acting			
NPH	2 hours	4-12 hours	18-24 hours
Lente	$1-2\frac{1}{2}$ hours	3-10 hours	18-24 hours
Long Acting			
Ultralente	30 min to 3 hours	10-20 hours	20-36 hours
Lantus	$1-1\frac{1}{2}$ hours	Once-per-day preparation with no peak; delivered at a steady level for 20-24 hours	20-24 hours
Combinations			
Humulin 50/50	30 min	3 hours	22-24 hours
Humulin 70/30, Novolin 70/30	30 min	4-8 hours	24 hours

TABLE 12-55	Dextrose 50%
Generic Name	dextrose 50%
Trade Names	Dextrose 50%, $D_{50}W$
Classification	Carbohydrate, hyperglycemic, antihypoglycemic
Action	Increases blood glucose concentrations
Indications	Known hypoglycemia Altered mental status of unknown etiology Seizures of unknown etiology Hyperkalemia
Routes of Administration	IV
Contraindications	Head injury, unless documented hypoglycemia, delirium tremens Known or suspected stroke, unless documented hypoglycemia
Adverse Effects	Hyperglycemia May cause neurologic symptoms in the alcoholic patient Sclerosing effect on peripheral veins Cerebral edema in children when given IV undiluted
Pregnancy	Category C
Special Considerations	Extravasation leads to severe tissue necrosis

IV, Intravenous.

TABLE 12-56	Glucagon
Generic Name	glucagon
Trade Name	Glucagen
Classification	Pancreatic hormone, antihypoglycemic
Action	Converts glycogen to glucose
Indications	Symptomatic hypoglycemia when IV access is delayed Known beta-blocker overdose accompanied by circulatory collapse (check local protocol)
Routes of Administration	IV for beta-blocker overdose, intramuscular or subcutaneous for hypoglycemia
Contraindications	Known hypersensitivity, pheochromocytoma
Adverse Effects	Hyperglycemia, nausea, vomiting, hypotension, sinus tachycardia
Pregnancy	Category B
Special Considerations	Glucagon must be reconstituted before administration

IV, Intravenous.

Case Scenario CONCLUSION

You connect the cardiac monitor to your patient and obtain a 12-lead ECG. It reveals ST-segment elevation in leads V_3 and V_4. Because the patient's oxygen saturation on room air is 100%, you provide supplemental oxygen by a nasal cannula set at 4 L/min. You establish an IV in the antecubital area and begin infusing normal saline at a keep-open rate. The patient is still reporting crushing chest pain.

Looking Back

7. *What are the appropriate pharmacologic interventions?*
8. *What is important to consider during transport?*
9. *What information is essential to document both in the verbal and written reports?*

DRUGS AFFECTING THE MUSCULOSKELETAL SYSTEM

[OBJECTIVE 26]

URICOSURIC DRUGS

Gout is a condition of recurrent episodes of acute arthritis from the deposition of urate in the joints and cartilage. It tends to be genetic and is usually associated with high levels of uric acid in the blood. The treatment of gout is aimed at relieving the symptoms and preventing a recurrence.

Colchicine

Colchicine is an alkaloid substance that acts to suppress the initial immune reaction that precipitates the pain of gout. The drug is absorbed well orally and reaches peak levels within approximately 2 hours. It is metabolized and excreted through the kidneys. This drug does not alter the metabolism or excretion of uric acid crystals. It treats the pain caused by these crystals. Side effects include severe diarrhea, burning throat pain, shock, and **hematuria.**

Nonsteroidal Antiinflammatory Drugs

Indomethacin is an NSAID frequently used for gout. It inhibits the pathway of inflammation and is often used instead of colchicine. Other NSAIDs are also successfully used to treat gout.

Allopurinol   *Gout*

Allopurinol is used to reduce the production of gouty substances. It is an oral medication metabolized by xanthine oxidase, the same substance that metabolizes uric acid. It interacts with xanthine oxidase as a competitive inhibitor. Therefore the uric acid cannot be metabolized and the substances from uric acid that cause gout are decreased. This drug is not generally used by paramedics.

DRUGS AFFECTING THE REPRODUCTIVE SYSTEM
DRUGS AFFECTING THE FEMALE REPRODUCTIVE SYSTEM

[OBJECTIVE 27]

Contraception

The methods of pharmacologic contraception are constantly evolving. Currently the oral birth control pill and patch are a combination of the two main female hormones estrogen and progesterone. These methods are used by many women and have a high success rate at preventing pregnancy when used as directed. Some risks are involved, including DVT development. This is more common in women who are older than 35 years and who smoke cigarettes.

Depo Provera is an injection based on progesterone. It is given intramuscularly every three months and has good results at prohibiting pregnancy. It contains no estrogen and works by inhibiting ovulation.

Ovulatory Stimulants and Drugs Used for Infertility

Considerable research and development in drug therapy for infertility is ongoing. Many new drugs are on the market, including clomiphene citrate (Clomid), which attempts to induce ovulation. These medications are prescribed by infertility experts.

Drugs for Labor and Delivery

Infants born before the development of adequate surfactant in the lungs have significant rates of morbidity and mortality. Several medications are used to stop contractions, including magnesium sulfate, ritodrine (Yutopar), terbutaline, nifedipine (Adalat, Procardia), and indomethacin (Indocin).

Drugs used to increase contractions include oxytocin (Pitocin). This drug is typically used to help the uterus contract after childbirth and prevent postpartum hemorrhage.

Corticosteroid therapy, when given to a woman in preterm labor between 24 and 34 weeks of gestation, is currently the only therapy shown to improve fetal survival (Von Der Pool, 1999).

DRUGS AFFECTING THE MALE REPRODUCTIVE SYSTEM

Testosterone is the major hormone necessary for secondary sexual characteristics. It is also used in a number of medical conditions, including delayed puberty, impotence, and female breast cancer. One common form of testosterone is methyltestosterone (Metandren).

Drugs That Treat Erectile Dysfunction

Erectile dysfunction is a condition in which a man cannot maintain an erection. Many medical causes result in this condition, including peripheral vascular disease. Possible physical causes of erectile dysfunction are listed in Box 12-28. Erectile dysfunction is treated with a class of drugs called *phosphodiesterase* (PDE) *inhibitors*. PDE has many forms or subtypes. As a result, many types of PDE inhibitors are used to treat a variety of conditions. For example, the bronchodilator theophylline and caffeine are nonselective PDE inhibitors. Milrinone is a PDE-3–selective

BOX 12-28	Possible Physical Causes of Erectile Dysfunction

- Alcohol and tobacco use
- Fatigue
- Brain or spinal cord injuries
- Hypogonadism (leads to lower testosterone levels)
- Liver or kidney failure
- Multiple sclerosis
- Parkinson's disease
- Radiation therapy to the testicles
- Stroke
- Surgery

BOX 12-29	Common Immunosuppressants

- Corticosteroids
- Azathioprine
- Cyclophosphamide
- Cyclosporine

inhibitor used for the short-term treatment of cardiac failure. It mimics sympathetic stimulation and increases cardiac output.

PDE-5 is present in the smooth muscle cells lining the blood vessels supplying the corpus cavernosum of the penis and in the smooth muscle of the pulmonary vasculature. Treatment for erectile dysfunction includes the use of PDE-5–selective inhibitors such as sildenafil (Viagra), tadalafil (Cialis), and vardenafil (Levitra). Sildenafil (Revatio) also is used for the treatment of pulmonary arterial hypertension in men and women, a disease in which the blood vessels in the lungs are narrowed. Sildenafil relaxes pulmonary vascular smooth muscle cells. In patients with pulmonary hypertension, this can lead to vasodilation of the pulmonary vascular bed and, to a lesser degree, vasodilation in the systemic circulation.

PDE-5 inhibitors have been shown to potentiate the hypotensive effects of nitrates. Their administration to patients who are using organic nitrates, either regularly and/or intermittently, in any form is contraindicated.

DRUGS AFFECTING THE IMMUNE SYSTEM
OVERVIEW

[OBJECTIVE 28]
Drugs that affect the immune system typically turn off the immune system or regulate its function. "Turning off" the system that protects the body from foreign invaders may seem strange, but it may be necessary if the body is attacking itself or transplanted organs. This is an area of constant development and growth in pharmaceuticals.

IMMUNOSUPPRESSANTS

The immune system defends the body against various forms of foreign invaders. These drugs target the immune system and inhibit the production of immune cells. These drugs are commonly used after organ transplantation. Their goal is to prevent the body from recognizing the new organ as foreign. It is a means of avoiding a rejection reaction, which can be life threatening. Common immunosuppressants are listed in Box 12-29.

IMMUNOMODULATING AGENTS

These medications increase the body's immune system efficiency. Included in this category are vaccines, which help the body build antibodies before an insult, as well as immunoglobulins, which are preformed antibodies to protect against life-threatening infection. These are commonly used in cancer and viral infections.

DERMATOLOGIC DRUGS

[OBJECTIVE 29]
Dermatologic products are medications applied to the skin and work transdermally. This delivery of medication has gained popularity because of its slow absorption and convenience.

Standard dermatologic treatments are aimed at curing problems with the skin, such as eczema and psoriasis. These medications are applied topically to deliver therapeutic effects. Hydrocortisone cream is commonly used for contact dermatitis or insect bites and is a common example of a dermatologic cream or ointment.

Birth control and nitroglycerin are two preparations applied transdermally and used for their systemic effects. The nitroglycerin paste is used both as an inpatient and outpatient medication for vasodilation. The paste lasts approximately 8 hours and then needs to be replaced. It delivers a constant amount of medication and extends the drug's half-life. The birth control patch has been designed for convenience and lasts for 1 week. It delivers hormonal supplementation for contraception and offers convenience over once-a-day dosing of the birth control pill.

DRUGS OF ABUSE AND MISUSE
STIMULANTS/AMPHETAMINES

[OBJECTIVE 30]
Drugs in this class affect areas of the brain that control alertness and attentiveness. A few drugs in this class have medicinal purposes. They are used for narcolepsy, weight

loss, and attention deficit disorder. Although methylphenidate (Ritalin) and sibutramine HCL monohydrate (Meridia) are available by prescription, they may still be abused.

Methamphetamine

Methamphetamine is manufactured in clandestine laboratories. It releases large quantities of the neurotransmitter dopamine. This causes enhanced mood as well as increased alertness, decreased appetite, hyperthermia, and euphoria. It can be taken orally, by IV injection, or be inhalation. It has serious side effects such as convulsions, cardiac **dysrhythmia,** respiratory problems, and even death.

Cocaine

Cocaine is a stimulant found in multiple forms. The drug may be snorted, inhaled, or smoked. The drug is used because it provides a feeling of exhilaration, which is often described as a "rush." Some use it for increased energy. With continued use, addiction may result. Side effects include chest pain, hypertension, paranoia, and hallucinations. Chest pain should be treated seriously because cocaine induces vasospasm (Box 12-30). Intracranial hemorrhage may also result from hypertension.

Drug smuggling is commonly encountered in airports and areas of the country that have international borders. Cocaine body packers wrap cocaine in condoms or other packages and then carefully swallow them. The goal is to get through U.S. Customs and then pass these packs through the feces, where they are retrieved. Packs can rupture and cause a toxic reaction. Signs and symptoms include sympathetic stimulation. Body stuffers are patients who may be interrupted by police or other authorities and rapidly ingest the drugs. These patients are also at risk for toxic side effects.

SEDATIVE/HYPNOTICS

Sedative/hypnotics cause slowing of normal body functions and often induce sleep. The two most common classes are benzodiazepines and barbiturates. These medications are Schedule IV controlled because of their abuse potential. Their side effects were previously discussed in relation to antianxiety and muscle relaxants.

GAMMA HYDROXYBUTYRATE

Gamma hydroxybutyrate (GHB) is a rapidly acting synthetic CNS depressant. It is manufactured in clandestine labs. This drug and Rohypnol are sometimes called "date rape" drugs because they are colorless and odorless and can be mixed into drinks undetected. An average dose takes effect in approximately 15 to 30 minutes and lasts from 3 to 6 hours. The initial state is euphoria or relaxation, which may progress to respiratory depression, nausea, vomiting, coma, and even death. Predicting a person's response is difficult because the actual concentration is unknown and everyone responds differently. These patients may be comatose and the substance ingested may be unknown. Maintaining and monitoring the airway is crucial.

HALLUCINOGENS

Hallucinogens are mind-altering drugs that affect perception of time, reality, and the environment. These drugs can affect the cardiovascular system. The effects are unpredictable; physical findings include dilated pupils, rapid heart rate, incoherent speech, sweating, loss of appetite, sleeplessness, and dry mouth. Table 12-57 lists the different types of hallucinogens and some of their street names.

ETHANOL

Ethanol is a common drug of abuse. It is discussed under Toxic Substances.

BOX 12-30 | **Cocaine Chest Pain**

Chest pain that arises from cocaine use can result from a number of causes. Cocaine causes vasospasm of the coronary arteries and increased myocardial oxygen demand from stimulation of the sympathetic division of the autonomic nervous system. This may result in ischemia of the myocardium. It may also result from the hot gases inhaled from smoking crack cocaine, which can cause pulmonary problems. The treatment for acute coronary syndromes is usually centered on aspirin, oxygen, nitroglycerin, morphine, and beta-blockers. This regimen is slightly altered when a patient has been using cocaine. Beta-blockers are contraindicated in chest pain induced by cocaine use. Cocaine stimulates the sympathetic branch of the autonomic nervous system. When the beta portion of the sympathetic branch is blocked, unopposed alpha stimulation occurs. This may result in increased coronary vasoconstriction. Benzodiazepines are appropriate for heart rate reduction. Be sure to check your local protocols and consult medical direction about patient treatment in these situations.

TABLE 12-57	Hallucinogens	
Hallucinogen	**Street Name**
Phencyclidine (PCP)	Angel dust, crystal dust
Ketamine	Special K, Super K
Lysergic acid diethylamide (LSD) (derived from fungus that grows on rye)	Microdot, white heaven, acid, hit
Jimson weed, wild weed	Angel trumpet

ENVIRONMENTAL SUBSTANCES
HERBICIDES

[OBJECTIVE 31]

Herbicides are used to kill weeds and are toxic to human beings. The main routes of absorption are transdermal, inhalation, and ingestion. Large doses can cause coma and generalized muscle weakness. Kidney and liver dysfunction may also occur. Patients that work around herbicides frequently may develop chronic conditions such as non-Hodgkin's lymphoma. There are two main classes of herbicides: bepridil and chlorophenoxy. Paraquat is the most common of the bepridil class and is discussed in Box 12-31.

RODENTICIDES

Rodenticides are designed to kill mice, rats, and other rodents that may be considered pests. They work by interrupting normal blood clotting functions and cause internal hemorrhage. These chemicals are often mixed with bait. The rodents eat the bait and then over time die from hemorrhage. Warfarin is one common form of rodenticide. This medication is used in human beings to prevent blood clots. Overdose of these types of chemicals should be taken seriously. Small children may ingest this substance accidentally if the chemicals are left on the floor with easy access. If possible, bring the original container to the emergency department with the patient.

INSECTICIDES

Insecticides are used to kill insects. They are often found on farms but are becoming a concern as biologic weapons. There are four main classes of insecticides.

Chlorinated Hydrocarbons

Chlorinated hydrocarbons can be absorbed through the skin as well as by inhalation or oral ingestion. Acute toxicity occurs through disruption of the sodium channel, causing rapid firing in most neurons. Tremor may be the first manifestation, which may progress to convulsions. No direct treatment is available except supportive care.

BOX 12-31	Paraquat

Paraquat has a similar action in both plants and animals. It builds up slowly in the lungs and can cause edema and fibrosis. The first signs and symptoms include gastrointestinal irritation. This is followed by respiratory distress that may be worsened by oxygen. Cyanosis and dyspnea does occur, but oxygen may make the pulmonary injury worse. Discussion with Poison Control or online medical direction is recommended.

Organophosphates

Organophosphates are the most common insecticides and can be readily absorbed through the skin and the respiratory tract, where they exert their effects rapidly. They act by inhibiting acetylcholinesterase, which allows for accumulation of acetylcholine at the nerve junction. The signs and symptoms include excessive stimulation of the parasympathetic nervous system. Increased salivation, lacrimation, abdominal pain and cramping, vomiting, and diarrhea may be seen. When the muscarinic receptors are affected, bronchoconstriction and bronchial secretions increase. When nicotinic receptors are affected, involuntary irregular, violent muscle contractions appear and voluntary muscles grow weak. Death usually results from respiratory failure. Adequate personal protection is important because secondary exposure may be a problem. Decontamination should be done thoroughly. Treatment is established with the use of atropine and 2-pyridine aldoxime methiodide (2-PAM). Atropine helps alleviate the secretions; however, it must be used in very high doses. Adequate atropine may not be available in a standard paramedic drug box. 2-PAM makes atropine more effective and often is located in special bioterrorism drug boxes.

Carbamate

Carbamate compounds inhibit acetylcholinesterase, and the toxic effects are similar to those found with organophosphates. The effects are shorter in duration. Treatment is similar to that for organophosphates, but pralidoxime is not recommended.

Botanicals

The most common botanical insecticide is nicotine. It is rapidly absorbed from mucosal surfaces and interacts with the acetylcholine receptor at the postsynaptic junction.

TOXIC SUBSTANCES
ALCOHOLS

[OBJECTIVE 32]

An alcohol is a substance that contains a molecular group containing oxygen and hydrogen. Alcohols appear in many common substances, including the alcohol consumed in beer and spirits and those used in radiator fluid in vehicles.

Ethanol

Ethanol is found in beer, wine, and spirits. It is a legal substance but is commonly abused. Individuals who drink alcohol may experience euphoria. This, however, may progress to stupor or coma. With extreme excess of ethanol consumption, loss of airway or primitive reflexes such as the gag reflex may occur. This creates a situation in which a patient may aspirate his or her own emesis. The blood alcohol level considered legally drunk is between 0.08 mg/dL and 0.1 mg/dL. The effect of ethanol intoxication depends on the physiology of the individual. Those who drink on a regular basis may have a higher blood alcohol level and not appear intoxicated. The human body eliminates alcohol at approximately 0.025 mg/dL per hour. The treatment for ethanol overdose is supportive care. The patient should be monitored for airway, breathing, and circulation and be placed in the left lateral recumbent position to avoid aspiration in case of vomiting. Finally, other coingestions should be considered.

Isopropyl Alcohol

Isopropyl alcohol, commonly called *rubbing alcohol,* is used as a disinfectant. A bottle typically contains 70% isopropyl alcohol. Poisoning can occur through skin absorption, oral ingestion, or inhalation. Symptoms of toxicity include flushing, headache, dizziness, mental depression, nausea, vomiting, anesthesia, and coma.

Ethylene Glycol

Ethylene glycol is used in antifreeze and in deicing solutions. It is extremely toxic if ingested. It often has a green color and contains fluorescein, which is easily detected with an ultraviolet light source. It may also be detected in urine samples. Because this chemical has a sweet taste, it may be ingested by children and animals. Ethylene glycol may be toxic after ingestion of only a few ounces. The toxic effects may cause renal failure. Other organs are also affected, and pulmonary edema may occur. One of the antidotes to ethylene glycol poisoning is ethanol. These two substances compete for an enzyme, and ethanol has a higher affinity for alcohol dehydrogenase. This enzyme converts ethylene glycol to its toxic metabolite, which is then excreted without any damage to the kidneys. This treatment should be conducted in a controlled environment such as the emergency department. The commercial antidote fomepizole (Antizol) is available. It is an effective alternative and does not cause ethanol intoxication and its associated side effects.

Methanol

Methanol is found in paint remover, glass cleaner, deicing solutions, antifreeze, and shellac. It is toxic when ingested. Small amounts are toxic to children and adults. The symptoms of ingestion include headache, dizziness, drowsiness, and blindness. Patients require supportive care. Dialysis may be needed to correct the metabolic acidosis that occurs with ingestion.

HEAVY METALS

Heavy metals get the name "heavy" because they weigh five times as much as water. Lead, mercury, and arsenic are included in this class. Heavy metals are found in pesticides, batteries, steel, and other alloys. The trace metals are also in this class and include zinc, iron, and copper.

Acute iron toxicity is seen in children and is one of the more common ingestions by children. It can be lethal, which is compounded by the fact that iron is not absorbed by activated charcoal. Severe stages of iron ingestion include gastroenteritis, vomiting, abdominal pain, and diarrhea. Symptoms then progress to shock, dyspnea, metabolic acidosis, and death. Whole bowel irrigation should be initiated in the hospital, and a chelating agent called deferoxamine may be used. This is given systemically, binds the iron, and forces excretion through the urine and feces.

HAZARDOUS MATERIALS

Hazardous materials are found in homes, businesses, schools, and hospitals. A hazardous material in the context of this chapter is classified as any material that may pose a risk to health. (See Chapter 64 for an extensive discussion of hazardous materials.) Some of these chemicals must be considered in terms of their effects on the human body. Recognizing that a hazardous material may be involved in a call is important; it may be obvious, such as an overturned tanker with a placard, or it may be as simple as a patient spilling a chemical on the skin at work. Scene safety for the entire prehospital crew must be ensured. Decontamination is equally important. Information about the chemical should be gathered and brought to the emergency department, including any Material Safety Data Sheets.

Irritants

Irritants are chemicals that cause problems by interacting with the mucous membranes of the respiratory tract, eyes, mouth, and throat. When they combine with moisture, a reaction may create a corrosive substance. The most severe consequences involve the airway and respiratory tract. This should be the paramedic's assessment and treatment focus. Examples of irritants include hydrochloric acid and ozone.

Asphyxiants

Hydrocarbon based cleaners

Asphyxiants are gases that displace oxygen. They dilute the concentration of oxygen in the air. Some interfere with tissue oxygenation. Examples include carbon dioxide, methane, carbon monoxide, hydrogen cyanide, and hydrogen sulfide.

Nerve Agents

These agents are often used in terrorist attacks and during war. They affect the CNS. Their prime target is often the respiratory system.

Carcinogens

Carcinogens are substances that can cause cancer. Their effects may not be seen for many years. These types of substances are found during the combustion of wood and other organic fuels.

HOUSEHOLD AND INDUSTRIAL CHEMICALS

Many chemicals used in households, garages, and industrial settings may be accidentally or intentionally ingested. Some of these chemicals are toxic through absorption by any mucous membrane, the eyes, and even the skin.

Cleaning supplies are commonly found in the home and industrial setting. More than 5000 types of chemicals are estimated to be found in the average home. Patients may ingest these household chemicals as a suicide attempt. When responding to these types of scene calls, follow local protocols and consider consulting both medical direction and Poison Control. The container should be taken to the emergency department. This should be done even if the substance has been removed from its original container so that a pH test can be performed on the substance. The patient should be given nothing by mouth unless directed by medical direction or Poison Control. The patient should receive supportive measures, including oxygen, IV access, and cardiac monitoring.

Certain characteristics affect the types of toxicity of chemicals. These characteristics are described below.

Ignitable Substances

Ignitable substances are chemicals that may burst into flames or explode. They are typically labeled with terms such as *ignitable, combustible,* and *flammable.* These chemicals are exceptionally dangerous around any type of ignition. This may be as simple as a spark, cigarette butt, or lighter. Children often do not realize that they may be around combustible materials while they are playing with matches or a lighter.

Corrosive Substances

Corrosive substances are materials at the extremes of the pH scale. Acids and bases can both cause damage. This generally occurs when they come in contact with the mucous membranes, including the eyes, skin, respiratory tract, and mouth. Examples of extremely acidic components include hydrochloric and sulfuric acid. Examples of extremely basic compounds include caustic soda and ammonia. *Base burns deeper & longer*

Reactive Substances

Reactive substances have an effect when mixed with another substance. It may be as simple as a reaction with water, air, or another substance. For example, an exceptionally toxic combination occurs when bleach is mixed with ammonia.

Toxic Substances

Toxic chemicals harm the body. An immediate or prolonged effect may occur. Toxic chemicals include substances that cause burns, respiratory problems, and even cancer.

Hydrofluoric acid is one of the strongest inorganic acids. It is commonly used in industrial applications for glass etching and in semiconductor plants. This acid, when it makes contact with the skin, may cause a severe burn without much change to the actual skin surface. This is particularly true of concentrations of 50% or greater, which are used in semiconductor plants. As this chemical penetrates deeper into the tissue, it may cause systemic effects, including hyperkalemia, hypocalcemia, and hypomagnesemia. These patients may be in severe pain. Cold packs may be used on skin burns. Be sure to wear proper personal protective equipment before removing the patient's contaminated clothing and placing it in an appropriate container to be disposed of properly. These patients should have oxygen, IV, and cardiac monitoring. The ECG should be monitored closely for signs of QT prolongation caused by electrolyte disturbances. Treatment includes supportive care and application of calcium gluconate gel. This most likely will be accomplished in the emergency department. If this chemical does splash the eyes, treatment includes copious irrigation.

Case Scenario SUMMARY

1. *What is your impression of this patient?* The patient appears in mild distress and describes pain located in his chest and abdominal area. He has some risk factors for coronary disease, including a positive family history of myocardial infarction, hypertension, and smoking.

2. *What areas of the medical history are pertinent?* Medical history can provide significant information. This patient's medical history identifies the risk factors for coronary disease. The most common risk factors include smoking, diabetes, hypertension, a positive family history, and

elevated cholesterol. Patients may also provide helpful information in their past surgical history. If this patient has a history of multiple cardiac stents or a bypass operation, he obviously would have had significant coronary disease. Social history also is important. Smoking is an obvious risk factor for coronary disease. Cocaine abuse is also a significant indicator for morbidity with any kind of chest pain.

3. *What areas of the physical examination will be important?* The examination should encompass a thorough evaluation of the lungs, heart, and abdomen. The chest should be auscultated for abnormal breath sounds. Clicks, rubs, or murmurs should be documented after auscultating heart sounds. The chest wall should be palpated for tenderness or crepitus. The abdomen should be auscultated for bowel sounds. Percussion and palpation should be done to evaluate for abdominal pain, distention, or possible obstruction. The extremities should be palpated for signs of diaphoresis, mottling, or swelling. Swelling in the lower extremities can be a sign of congestive heart failure or possibly DVT.

4. *What do the historic findings indicate?* Evaluating pain with the mnemonic OPQRST is quite helpful. The patient had an onset of pain while doing work and his symptoms did not subside with rest. This indicates the pain may be cardiac in origin and more severe than mere angina. The quality is burning in nature without radiation. The duration is 40 minutes. Cardiac chest pain needs to be a strong consideration in this patient.

5. *What do the physical examination findings indicate?* The vital signs indicate a normal blood pressure, a tachycardic heart rate, dyspnea with increased labor, and good oxygen saturation. The patient is diaphoretic. He has no reproducible pain in the chest wall or abdomen. This patient may be feeling visceral pain. Pain that originates from an organ often does not localize well and is difficult to reproduce. Tachypnea and tachycardia are signs that the patient is in distress.

6. *What diagnostic and therapeutic interventions should be done?* The patient should be placed on a pulse oximeter and cardiac monitor, receive supplemental oxygen, and have venous access established. A 12-lead ECG should be obtained if possible.

7. *What are the appropriate pharmacologic interventions?* This patient is having an anterior wall acute myocardial infarction. Unless contraindicated, the patient should receive an aspirin immediately. He should also receive nitroglycerin. The nitroglycerin may come in the form of a spray or sublingual tablet (some areas may also carry IV nitroglycerin). This should be administered per protocol. Typically the nitroglycerin dose is one tablet or spray given sublingually every 5 minutes for a maximum of three doses. If beta-blockers are available and are not contraindicated (allergy, chronic obstructive pulmonary disease, asthma, hypotension, or bradycardia), these should be considered. Morphine sulfate may also be given for pain control.

8. *What is important to consider during transport?* Continual reassessment is essential. If transport is longer than 15 minutes, a repeat ECG should be performed. The patient should have vital signs repeated approximately 1 to 2 minutes after each dose of nitroglycerin and every 5 to 10 minutes thereafter. The nitroglycerin, morphine sulfate, and beta-blockers can all reduce blood pressure. Beta-blockers can significantly lower heart rate. The patient's pain should also be reassessed during transport.

9. *What information is essential to document in both the verbal and written reports?* The receiving facility should be given the patient's 12-lead ECG findings and the fact that his signs and symptoms are consistent with an acute myocardial infarction. The receiving facility needs this information to have adequate time to prepare for the patient's arrival. Your report should consist of the patient's age, presentation, vital signs, physical examination findings, ECG (and repeat ECG) interpretation, as well medications provided and changes in assessment.

Chapter Summary

- An indication is an appropriate use of a drug. A contraindication is an instance when a drug should not be used.
- Poison Control Centers can be accessed by phone for information on overdose and poisons.
- Gastric lavage is the cleansing of the stomach through a pump and irrigation with water.
- Activated charcoal is used to bind medications so they cannot be absorbed into the systemic circulation.

- Acetaminophen toxicity can affect the liver. Acetaminophen is used as an analgesic and for fever.
- Salicylates can be used as an antiplatelet or analgesic or for fever.
- NSAIDs are used for fever and analgesia.
- Morphine is an opioid. Opioids are narcotics. Some synthetic narcotics, such as fentanyl, do not have a profound effect on blood pressure. Opioid combinations are medications that combine two different types

Chapter Summary—continued

of analgesics. Aspirin or acetaminophen often is combined with a narcotic.

- Partial opioid agonists (agonist-antagonists) provide some effect but block the effect of a full agonist when given together.
- Opioid antagonists block the effects of the agonists.
- Anesthetics are used for deep sedation during procedures, including surgery and rapid-sequence intubation.
- Conscious sedation is a state in which a patient maintains the airway but is not aware of the procedure or pain.
- Benzodiazepines are used for anxiety and to induce sleep.
- Flumazenil (Romazicon) is an antidote for benzodiazepine overdose. It must be used cautiously because of a risk of seizures.
- Anticonvulsants are used to prevent seizure or treat seizure disorders.
- Antidepressants are used to treat both depression and bipolar disorder.
- Most antidepressants are very serious in overdose and can cause cardiac dysrhythmias.
- CNS stimulants include anorexiants and amphetamines.
- Antipsychotics are used to treat schizophrenia.
- Medications have been designed to treat Parkinson's and Alzheimer's disease. They often alter acetylcholine or dopamine levels in the brain.
- Cholinergic drugs are rarely used therapeutically. These drugs include physostigmine, which is used to treat atropine overdose.
- Cholinergic drugs such as atropine are used in advanced cardiac life support.
- Sympathomimetics or catecholamines are used in advanced cardiac life support and in other medical conditions when the sympathetic nervous system needs to be stimulated.
- Antiarrhythmics are used to treat and prevent disorders of cardiac rhythm. Class I antiarrhythmics affect the sodium channel and work on slow conduction. Class II antiarrhythmics are beta-blockers, which block beta-receptors. They slow heart rate and conduction velocity and limit the force of contraction. Class III antiarrhythmics block the potassium channel. Included in this class is amiodarone. Class IV antiarrhythmics block the calcium channel. These are also used for blood pressure control. Adenosine is used to slow supraventricular tachycardias. It is in a class of its own.
- Digitalis is used for dysrhythmias and blocks ion pumps.
- Diuretics often are used to control pulmonary edema and blood pressure.

- Anticoagulants are used to inhibit clot formation. Thrombolytics (fibrinolytics) are used to break up an existing clot.
- Antihemophilic agents are used to treat bleeding after trauma in patients who are deficient in clotting cascade components.
- Bronchodilators are used to help stop bronchospasm and improve respiratory function.
- Mucokinetic drugs are used to loosen mucus so it can be expelled.
- Antihistamines are used to block the release of histamine, which helps reduce tissue edema.
- Antacids treat overproduction of acid and heartburn.
- Antiemetics are used for protracted vomiting and nausea.
- H_2 receptor antagonists are used to block histamine in the gastrointestinal tract.
- Ophthalmic agents are used for the diagnosis and treatment of diseases of the eye.
- Otic preparations are used for analgesia and treatment of diseases of the ear.
- Many hormones are used to treat various endocrine problems.
- Antibiotics are used to treat bacterial infections. Many different types are available.
- Antivirals are used to treat viral infections. Many types are used to treat HIV.
- Antifungals are used to treat fungal infections. Fungal infections can affect the skin as well as the entire systemic circulation.
- Gout is a painful type of arthritis treated with uricosuric drugs, including NSAIDS.
- Vitamins and minerals are necessary for normal body function.
- Crystalloids include normal saline, Ringer's lactate, D_5W, $D_5\frac{1}{2}$ NS, and D_5NS.
- Immunizations are designed to prevent infection.
- Immunoglobulins are used to treat infection; they are preformed antibodies.
- Antidotes are used to treat poisons or toxins.
- Drugs of abuse include stimulants, benzodiazepines, narcotics, hallucinogens, and sedative/hypnotics.
- Ethanol is a common drug of abuse that can cause respiratory depression.
- Herbicides, rodenticides, and insecticides can be highly toxic to human beings.
- Isopropyl alcohol, ethylene glycol, and methanol are in the alcohol family and can be highly toxic if ingested or absorbed.
- Hazardous materials can cause significant toxicity to human beings.

REFERENCES

Centers for Disease Control and Prevention. (2003). Treatment of tuberculosis. *Morbidity and Mortality Weekly Report, 52,* RR-11. Retrieved May 10, 2007, from http://www.cdc.gov.

Von Der Pool, B. A. (1999). *Preterm labor: Diagnosis and treatment.* Retrieved May 10, 2007, from http://www.aafp.org.

SUGGESTED RESOURCES

2005 Physician's desk reference. (2004). Montvale, NJ: Thomson Healthcare.

National Home Infusion Association. *Position statement. United States Pharmacopeia XXVI/National Formulary 21.* Retrieved May 10, 2007, from http://www.nhianet.org.

PDR*Health:* www.pdrhealth.com.

United States Pharmacopeia
12601 Twinbrook Parkway
Rockville, MD 20852-1790
Phone: 800-227-877
Website: http://www.usp.org/aboutUSP

Chapter Quiz

1. Which of the following is an analgesic?
   a. Morphine
   b. Propranolol
   c. Phenytoin
   d. Phenobarbital

2. Which of the following is a definition of a hazardous substance that is at the extremes of the pH scale?
   a. Ignitable
   b. Corrosive
   c. Reactive
   d. Toxic

3. Which of the following is used in glass etching and is one of the strongest inorganic acids?
   a. Sulfuric acid
   b. Lye
   c. Hydrofluoric acid
   d. Bleach

4. Which of the following is a crystalloid solution?
   a. Packed red blood cells
   b. Whole blood
   c. Fresh frozen plasma
   d. Ringer's lactate

5. Which of the following best describes an immunoglobulin?
   a. It is an antigen.
   b. It is an antibody.
   c. It is a special form of antibiotic.
   d. It is an antidote.

6. Which of the following is not an appropriate indication for a sympathomimetic?
   a. Coronary ischemia
   b. Acute asthma attack
   c. Anaphylactic shock
   d. Cardiac arrest

7. Which of the following is an example of a cholinergic blocking drug?
   a. Atropine
   b. Physostigmine
   c. Pyridostigmine
   d. Epinephrine

8. Which of the following is a clinical finding with a tricyclic antidepressant overdose?
   a. Shortening of the QT interval
   b. Prolongation of the QRS complex
   c. Hypertension
   d. Hyperalertness

9. Which of the following is not an indication for acetaminophen?
   a. Fever
   b. Pain
   c. Headache
   d. Cardiac ischemia

10. Which of the following is an accurate definition of an agonist-antagonist?
    a. It is has a partial effect as an agonist and blocks other agonists.
    b. It has only a negative effect in low doses.
    c. It has only a positive effect in low doses.
    d. It is an agonist in certain individuals.

Terminology

Agonist A drug that causes a physiologic response once it reacts with a receptor.

Agonist-antagonist A drug that blocks a receptor. It may provide a partial agonist activity, but it also prevents an agonist from exerting its full effects.

Analgesia A state in which pain is controlled or not perceived.

Anaphylaxis Life-threatening allergic reaction.

Anesthesia A process in which pain is prevented during a procedure.

Angioedema Swelling of the tissues, including the dermal layer; often found in and around the mouth, tongue, and lips.

Antagonist A drug that does not cause a physiologic response when it binds with a receptor.

Conscious sedation A medication or combination of medications that allows a patient to undergo what could be an unpleasant experience by producing an altered level of consciousness but not complete anesthesia. The goal is for the patient to breathe spontaneously and maintain his or her own airway.

Contraindication Use of a drug for a condition when it is not advisable.

Deep venous thrombosis (DVT) A blood clot that forms in the deep venous system of the pelvis or legs. This may progress to a pulmonary embolism.

Dosage The amount of medication that can be safely given for the average person for a specified condition.

Dysrhythmia An abnormal heart rhythm.

Eczema A disorder of the skin characterized by inflammation, itching, blisters, and scales.

Gastric lavage A procedure commonly known as "stomach pumping" in which the stomach is flushed with water; typically used to treat overdose or poisoning.

Hematuria Blood found in the urine.

Hyperpnea Increased respiratory rate or deeper than normal breathing.

Hypersensitivity An exaggerated immune response to a foreign agent.

Indication The appropriate use of a drug when treating a disease or condition.

Mania An excessively intense enthusiasm, interest, or desire; a craze.

Morbidity A disease state.

Mortality A fatal outcome.

Nasal polyps Small, saclike growths consisting of inflamed nasal mucosa.

Nasogastric tube A tube placed by way of the nose into the stomach.

Nonsteroidal antiinflammatory drug (NSAID) Medications primarily used to treat inflammation, mild to moderate pain, and fever.

Nystagmus Involuntary rapid movement of the eyes in the horizontal, vertical, or rotary planes of the eyeball.

Orogastric tube A tube placed by way of the mouth into the stomach.

Overdose The accidental or intentional ingestion of an excess of a substance with the potential for toxicity.

Prostaglandins A class of fatty acids that has many of the properties of hormones.

Rhinitis An inflammation of the mucous membrane that lines the nose.

Tardive dyskinesia A neurologic syndrome caused by the long-term or high-dose use of dopamine antagonists, usually antipsychotic medications; characterized by repetitive, involuntary, and purposeless movements such as grimacing, rapid movements of the face, lip smacking, and eye blinking. Symptoms may last for a significant period after removal of the offending agent.

Withdrawal The termination of drug taking with physiologic symptoms.

Medication Administration

Objectives *After completing this chapter, you will be able to:*

1. List basic mathematic principles.
2. Review mathematic equivalents.
3. Differentiate temperature readings between the Celsius and Fahrenheit scales.
4. Discuss formulas as a basis for performing drug calculations.
5. Discuss applying basic principles of mathematics to the calculation of problems associated with medication dosages.
6. Discuss legal aspects affecting medication administration.
7. Discuss the "six rights" of drug administration.
8. Discuss medical asepsis and the differences between clean and sterile techniques.
9. Describe the use of standard precautions when giving a medication.
10. Describe the use of antiseptics and disinfectants.
11. Describe disposal of contaminated items and sharps.
12. Describe the different oral dosage forms and general principles of giving oral medications.
13. Describe the technique and general principles of rectal medication administration.
14. Describe the technique and general principles of giving medications through a gastric tube.
15. Describe the technique and general principles of giving medications topically.
16. Describe the technique and general principles of giving medications by the inhalation route.
17. Describe the technique for withdrawing medication from an ampule.
18. Describe the technique for withdrawing medication from a vial.
19. Describe the technique and general principles of giving medications by the subcutaneous route.
20. Describe the technique and general principles of giving medications by the intramuscular route.
21. Describe the indications, equipment needed, technique used, precautions, and general principles of peripheral venous access.
22. Describe the indications, equipment needed, technique used, precautions, and general principles of intraosseous needle placement and infusion.
23. Describe the purpose, equipment needed, techniques used, complications, and general principles for obtaining a blood sample.

Chapter Outline

Drug Dosage Calculations
Medical Direction
Principles of Medication Administration
Prevention of Injuries and Exposures
Techniques of Medication Administration

Fibrinolytic Initiation and Monitoring
Blood Infusions
Obtaining a Blood Sample
Chapter Summary

See Written Notes

Case Scenario

You and your partner respond to an office complex for a "man having chest pain." You arrive to find a 52-year-old man sitting upright in a chair complaining of "pressure" in his chest. He is alert and oriented, with pale, diaphoretic skin. He reports that he has a history of angina and that this is the first episode he has had since he was prescribed topical nitroglycerin ointment. He describes his discomfort as "crushing" and rates its severity an 8 on a scale of 0 to 10.

Questions

1. What is your general impression of this patient? What treatment will you initiate before continuing your assessment?
2. What are the advantages of topical drug administration? What are the disadvantages?
3. What protective equipment is appropriate for paramedic use when dealing with nitroglycerin ointment? Why?

Drug calculations are a challenge to most paramedics, but the math can be simple once a few basic formulas are mastered. This chapter eliminates the mystery of drug calculations and replaces it with confidence to learn and achieve ease in calculation.

DRUG DOSAGE CALCULATIONS

Systems of Measurement

Apothecary, Household, and Metric Systems

[OBJECTIVE 1]

Drugs were originally measured according to the apothecary system. The basis of this system was the grain. The weight of a grain of wheat was used as a unit of weight. One ounce equaled 480 grains, 1 pound equaled 12 ounces, which equaled 5760 grains. Linear measures were done in inches, yards, and miles. A liquid (volume) was measured in minims, fluidrams, ounces, pints, and gallons. In the apothecary system, quantities of 20 or less are expressed in lower case Roman numerals. Quantities greater than 20 are expressed in Arabic numbers and fractions. Decimals are not used in the apothecary system.

> **PARAMEDIC Pearl**
>
> Some apothecary measures are still in use today. Aspirin (gr v) and nitroglycerin (1/150 gr) are examples of medications carried in the paramedic drug box whose labels still reflect the apothecary system.

The household system uses the dropper, teaspoon, tablespoon, cup, glass, pint, quart, and gallon for measuring. Household measures are expressed in Arabic numbers and fractions. Decimals are not used.

The metric system is currently used for drug calculations. It is a logical system, organized and based on the basic unit of 10, similar to the U.S. monetary system. One dollar is the basic unit of measurement of the U.S. money system. It is

written as $1.00. One dollar is equal to 10 dimes. One dime is written as $0.10, and is equal to 10 pennies. If you keep this in mind as you calculate drug dosages, the right answer will be much easier to determine.

Just as basic units of measurement in the apothecary system were used for weight, length, and volume, basic units of measurement also are used in the metric system for the same categories. The basic units of measurement in the metric system are the following:

- Weight (solids, or mass): gram (g)
- Length: meter (m)
- Volume (liquid or fluid): liter (L)

Pharmacology Mathematic Equivalents

[OBJECTIVE 2]

Multiple prefixes are used in medicine to distinguish multiples or smaller parts of any of the above units. The four used commonly in drug calculations today are centi, milli, micro, and kilo. The prefix *centi* (c) represents 1/100 of a basic unit. For example:

- 1 centimeter (cm) = 1/100 of a meter
- 1 meter = 100 centimeters, or 1 m = 100 cm
- 1 centimeter = 1/100 of a meter, or 1 cm = 1/100 m

A comparable example in the money system would be that 1 cent = 1/100 of a dollar.

The prefix *milli* (m) represents 1/1000 of a basic unit. For example:

- 1 milligram (mg) = 1/1000 of a gram
- 1 milliliter (mL) = 1/1000 of a liter

Therefore:

- 1 liter = 1000 milliliters, or 1 L = 1000 mL
- 1 milliliter = 1/1000 of a liter, or 1 mL = 1/1000 L
- 1 meter = 1000 millimeters, or 1 m = 1000 mm
- 1 millimeter = 1/1000 of a meter, or 1 mm = 1/1000 m

The prefix *micro* (mc or sometimes the Greek letter μ) represents 1/1,000,000 of a basic unit. For example:

- 1 microgram (mcg) = 1/1,000,000 of a gram

Therefore:

- 1 meter = 1,000,000 micrometers, or 1 m = 1,000,000 mcm
- 1 micrometer = 1/1,000,000 meter, or 1 mcm = 1/1,000,000 m
- 1 gram = 1,000,000 micrograms, or 1 g = 1,000,000 mcg
- 1 microgram = 1/1,000,000 gram, or 1 mcg = 1/1,000,000 g
- 1 millimeter = 1/1000 of a meter, or 1 mm = 1/1000 m

The prefix *kilo* is represents 1000 times a basic unit. Therefore:

- 1 kilogram = 1000 grams, or 1 kg = 1000 g
- 1 gram = 1/1000 kilograms, or 1 g = 1/1000 kg

Table 13-1 shows pharmacology mathematical equivalents for numeric prefixes.

> **PARAMEDIC***Pearl*
>
> Conversions from the apothecary to metric system are inconsistent. For example, 1 gr (one grain) is approximately equal to 64 mg. Some references provide a "range" of approximately equal values from 60 to 65 mg. When you look at the dose of an adult aspirin tablet, you will note that it says, "gr v" and "325 mg." This inconsistency occurs because the apothecary system is not exact.

Metric Conversions

When calculating drug dosages, you must be able to convert milligrams to grams, grams to milligrams, milligrams to micrograms, and micrograms to milligrams.

Again, the U.S. monetary system is a good example. If you want to change a dollar into coins (such as dimes or pennies), you change the larger unit (dollar) into smaller units (dimes or pennies). This means that you would multiply the number of dollars that you have (such as 5 dollars) by the number of dimes or pennies *per dollar.* You will have a greater number of smaller units than larger units. For example, 5 dollars × 10 dimes/dollar = X number of dimes.

$$\frac{5 \text{ dollars}}{1} \times \frac{10 \text{ dimes}}{\text{dollar}} = X \text{ dimes}$$

Remember a basic math principle that says that you can cross out "like terms" if they appear in the **numerator** and **denominator.** In this case, the like term is *dollar.*

$$\frac{5 \; \cancel{\text{dollars}}}{1} \times \frac{10 \text{ dimes}}{\cancel{\text{dollar}}} = X \text{ dimes}$$

Now work the problem: 5 × 10 dimes = 50 dimes. Note that when you convert your pocket full of change into dollar bills, you are changing smaller units (dimes or pennies) into larger units (dollars). You will have fewer larger units (dollars) than smaller units (dimes or pennies).

The same holds true when you convert drug dosages from larger units (such as grams) to smaller units (such as milligrams) or from smaller units to larger units. To convert grams to milligrams, multiply grams by 1000. There are 1000 mg in every gram. This can be written as "1000 mg per g," or more commonly, "1000 mg/g." For example:

TABLE 13-1	Pharmacology Math Equivalents			
Prefix	**Calculation**	**Examples of Equivalents**		**Notes**
centi-	1/100 of a basic unit	1 centimeter = 1/100 meter 1/100 meter = 1 centimeter		*Part* of a basic unit
milli-	1/1000 of a basic unit	1 milligram = 1/1000 gram 1/1000 gram = 1 milligram		*Part* of a basic unit
micro-	1/1,000,000 of a basic unit	1 microgram = 1/1,000,000 gram 1/1,000,000 gram = 1 microgram		*Part* of a basic unit
kilo-	1000 times basic unit	1 kilogram = 1000 grams 1000 grams = 1 kilogram		*Multiple* of a basic unit

Comparable Example

Dollar	Basic unit of U.S. money	1 cent = 1/100 of a dollar 1/100 dollar = 1 cent		*Part* of a basic unit

$$\frac{5\,g}{1}\times\frac{1000\,mg}{1\,g}=X\text{ milligrams}$$

Cross out like terms—in this case, grams:

$$\frac{5\,\cancel{g}}{1}\times\frac{1000\,mg}{1\,\cancel{g}}=X\text{ milligrams}$$

Now work the problem: 5×1000 mg = 5000 mg.

This answer can be quickly determined by moving the decimal point to the right the same number of spaces as there are zeroes in the number. For example, 5 is simply 5. Because there are three zeroes in "1000 mg," move the decimal point in "5" three places to the right: 5 g = 5000 mg.

The same process can be used to convert milligrams (mg) to micrograms (mcg).

"milli-" means "× 1000," or 3 zeroes

"micro-" means "× 1,000,000," or 6 zeroes

To convert milligrams (3 zeroes) to micrograms (6 zeroes), simply move the decimal point three more places to the right, for a total of 6 zeroes: 5000 mg = 5,000,000 mcg. To convert milligrams to grams (smaller to larger), divide the number of grams by 1000 or simply move the decimal point three places to the *left*. This would be the same as changing 100 pennies back to dollars. The 100 actually means "100 cents." Therefore move the decimal point to the left the same number of places as there are zeroes in the equivalent of 1.00 dollar (100 pennies; therefore 2 zeroes, 2 spaces): 100 pennies (cents) = 1.00 dollar.

Temperature Conversions

[OBJECTIVE 3]
Body temperature is measured by two scales: Celsius (centigrade), and Fahrenheit. The scales are compared by their freezing points and their boiling points, as shown in Figure 13-1.

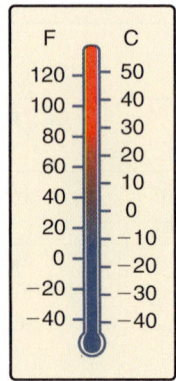

Figure 13-1 Fahrenheit *(left)* and Celsius *(right)* scales used to measure temperature.

A temperature of 5° on the Celsius scale corresponds to 9° on the Fahrenheit scale. The freezing point of water is 0° on the Celsius scale and 32° on the Fahrenheit scale. This information can be used in a simple formula to convert from one scale to the other.

To convert Celsius to Fahrenheit, multiply the Celsius temperature by $\frac{9}{5}$ and then add 32. For example, normal body temperature according to the Celsius scale is 37° C. To determine this value in Fahrenheit:

$$\frac{37°}{1}\times\frac{9}{5}+32=°F$$

$$\frac{(37°\times 9)}{5}+32=°F$$

$$\frac{333}{5}+32=°F$$

$$66.6+32=98.6°F$$

To convert Fahrenheit to Celsius, subtract 32 from the Fahrenheit temperature and multiply by $\frac{5}{9}$. For example:

$$98.6-32=66.6$$

$$\frac{66.6}{1}\times\frac{5}{9}=\frac{333}{9}=37°C$$

PARAMEDIC*Pearl*

Temperature conversion can be done another way. To convert a temperature from Celsius to Fahrenheit, multiply the Celsius temperature by 1.8, then add 32. To convert a temperature from Fahrenheit to Celsius, subtract 32 from the temperature, then divide by 1.8.

Milliliters and Cubic Centimeters

The terms milliliter (mL) and cubic centimeter (cc) are frequently used interchangeably, although this is not technically correct. Milliliter is a measurement of volume (liquids or fluids). A milliliter is 1/1000 of a liter. A centimeter is a measurement of length. A centimeter is 1/100 of a meter. If a little box measured 1 cm × 1 cm × 1 cm in dimension, it would be a "cubic centimeter" box. If the box were filled with 1 milliliter (1 mL) of water at a temperature of 4° Celsius, the water would completely fill the box. Therefore the *volume* is equal to the *space* that was created. Thus 1 cc = 1 mL. This is important to remember because a paramedic may be instructed to give 3 mL of a medication. Alternatively, the same drug may be ordered as 3 cc of medication. These are considered equivalent.

PARAMEDIC*Pearl*

Although 1 mL is equivalent to 1 cc, 1 mL *is not* equal to 1 milligram (mg). *Gram* refers to the weight of powdered drug, not its volume or the space that it occupies.

Weight Conversions

Many drug dosages are based on the patient's weight (not the weight of the drug) in kilograms. One kilogram (kg) is equal to 2.2 pounds. To convert weight in pounds to weight in kilograms, divide the number of pounds by 2.2. Weights are rounded to the nearest tenth of a kilogram. To convert weight in kilograms to weight in pounds, multiply the number of kilograms by 2.2.

Example 1: A patient weighs 154 pounds. How many kilograms does he weigh?

$$\frac{154}{2.2} = 70\,kg$$

Example 2: A patient weighs 50 kg. How many pounds does she weigh?

$$50 \times 2.2 = 110 \text{ pounds}$$

Common metric conversions are shown in Box 13-1.

PARAMEDIC Pearl

To round off a decimal to the nearest tenth, find the tenths place and look at the digit just to the right of it. If the last digit is less than 5, do not change the digit but drop all digits to the right. For example, round 2.43 to the nearest tenth to get 2.4. If the last digit is greater than or equal to 5, add one to the last digit and drop all digits to the right. For example, round 7.45 to the nearest tenth to get 7.5.

Practice Problems

Complete the practice problems below to master the art of converting units of the metric system. The answers are given at the end of this chapter in Box 13-17.

Convert grams (g) to milligrams (mg) and milligrams to grams:

1. 1 g = _1000_ mg
2. 1000 mg = _1_ g
3. 250 mg = _0.25_ g
4. 400 mg = _0.4_ g
5. 500 mg = _0.5_ g
6. 0.75 g = _750_ mg
7. 1.25 g = _1250_ mg
8. 10 g = _10,000_ mg
9. 2 g = _2000_ mg
10. 2500 mg = _2.5_ g

Convert milligrams (mg) to micrograms (mcg) and micrograms to milligrams:

11. 1 mg = _1000_ mcg
12. 500 mcg = _0.5_ mg
13. 250 mcg = _0.25_ mg
14. 400 mg = _400,000_ mcg
15. 200 mg = _200,000_ mcg
16. 800,000 mcg = _800_ mg
17. 800 mg = _800,000_ mcg
18. 200 mcg = _200,000_ mg
19. 1000 mcg = _1_ mg
20. 200,000 mcg = _200_ mg

BOX 13-1 Common Metric Conversions

- 1 g = 1000 mg
- 1 mg = 1000 mcg
- 1 L = 1000 mL or 1000 cc
- 1 kg = 2.2 lb
- 2.5 cm = approximately 1 inch

Conversions applicable to the sizes of bags of intravenous solutions:

21. 1 L = _1000_ mL
22. 1000 mL = _1_ L
23. 500 mL = _0.5_ L
24. 0.5 L = _500_ mL
25. 250 mL = _0.25_ L
26. 0.25 L = _250_ mL
27. 250 mL = _250_ cc

Conversions applicable to drug dosage calculations:

28. 1 mg = _1,000_ mcg
29. 1000 mcg = _1_ mg
30. 500 mcg = _.5_ mg
31. 0.3 cc = _0.3_ mL
32. 0.5 mL = _0.5_ cc
33. 1 g = _1000_ mg
34. 0.5 g = _500_ mg
35. 250 mg = _0.25_ g

Conversions applicable to drug calculation by patient weight:

36. 220 lb = _100_ kg
37. 50 kg = _110_ lb
38. 110 lb = _50_ kg

Conversions applicable to the measurement of wounds:

39. 1 in = _2.5_ cm
40. ~2.5 cm = _1_ in
41. 3 in = _7.5_ cm

Working with Formulas

[OBJECTIVES 4, 5]

Only four basic formulas are necessary to calculate any dosage for patient medications.

Formula 1: Single Dose Calculations

To calculate a single dose of a drug to be given, use what is commonly called the "desire over have" formula, which has three important parts:

- Desired dose (DD): The amount of medication the patient is to receive. This is typically the amount ordered by medical direction or the amount specified by local protocol to be given.
- Dose on hand (DH): The amount (physical weight) of medication present in the medication container (in grams, milligrams, or micrograms).
- Volume on hand (V): The amount of fluid in the medication container in which the medication is dissolved (milliliters).

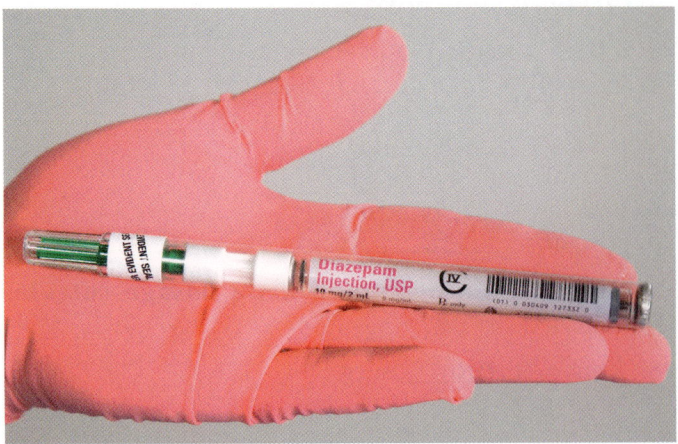

Figure 13-2 Diazepam for injection.

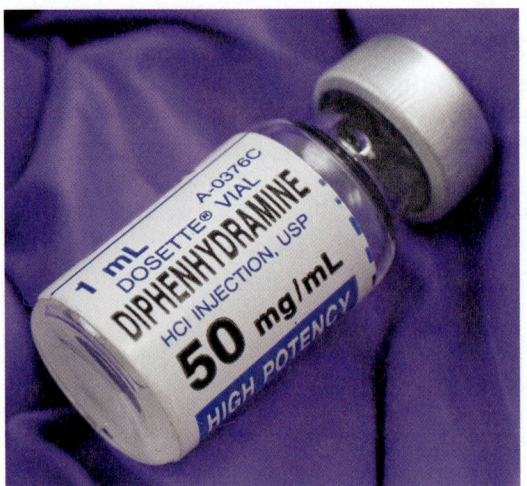

Figure 13-3 Diphenhydramine for injection.

$$\text{Formula: } \frac{DD \times V}{DH}$$

For example, you are instructed to give 2 mg of diazepam intravenously. Diazepam is supplied as 10 mg in 2 mL (Figure 13-2). In this example, the desired dose is 2 mg. The dose on hand is 10 mg. The volume on hand (the amount of fluid in which the drug is dissolved) is 2 mL. To solve the problem, convert different units of measurement to the same unit of measurement if necessary. In this example, the drug weights are in the same unit of measure (mg), so conversion is not necessary. Next, insert the numbers into the formula:

$$\frac{DD \times V}{DH} = \frac{2 \text{ mg} \times 2 \text{ mL}}{10 \text{ mg}}$$

Cross out like terms that appear in the numerator and denominator. Then solve the problem.

$$\frac{2 \text{ mg} \times 2 \text{ mL}}{10 \text{ mg}} = \frac{4 \text{ mL}}{10} = 0.4 \text{ mL}$$

NOTE: Whenever the dosage is less than 1, always place a "0" before the decimal point. In this scenario, 0.4 mL of diazepam should be given to the patient.

Following is another scenario: A 64-year-old woman is enjoying a round of golf on a beautiful spring afternoon when she suddenly steps into a hornets' nest. She is surrounded and bitten multiple times by the insects. Because she is allergic to bee stings, she quickly heads to the clubhouse to seek help. A paramedic unit is summoned. When the paramedics arrive, they find the patient in mild distress. Large hives are present on her face and neck. Because of her age and relatively mild signs and symptoms, the paramedics choose to avoid epinephrine and give diphenhydramine (Benadryl) 25 mg intramuscularly. The prefilled syringe reads: 50 mg/1 mL (Figure 13-3). How many milliliters should they give?

$$\frac{DD \times V}{DH} = \frac{25 \text{ mg} \times 1 \text{ mL}}{50 \text{ mg}} = \frac{25 \text{ mg} \times 1 \text{ mL}}{50 \text{ mg}}$$

$$= \frac{25 \text{ mL}}{50} = 0.5 \text{ mL}$$

A dose of 0.5 mL diphenhydramine should be given to the patient.

Formula 2: Drip (Infusion) Calculations

Intravenous (IV) fluids may be given continuously or over a specific period. "Fluid challenge" is a phrase used to describe a specific amount of fluid to be given over a specific period. The delivery of fluids by the IV route requires a container of IV solution, IV tubing, and an IV catheter. An IV catheter is inserted into the patient's vein. IV catheters are available in different lengths and sizes, which affect the rate and amount of fluid infused. Techniques for inserting IV catheters are covered later in this chapter.

A container of IV solution must be sterile because it will be infused into the patient's venous circulation. IV containers are usually glass bottles or plastic bags. Bags are used in the prehospital setting. An IV bag is marked with calibrations on the side (Figure 13-4). The calibrations allow you to see how much fluid has been infused into the patient and how much has yet to be infused.

Intravenous tubing is also called an *IV administration set*, because it is used to carry the IV solution from the IV container to the patient. Many types of administration sets are available (Figure 13-5). IV tubing is equipped with a roller clamp. The clamp is used to adjust the number of drops that fall into the drip chamber.

When giving IV fluid to a patient, a precise volume of fluid is infused over a specific period. The period of the infusion may be ordered as milliliters per hour, milliliters per minute, or the number of drops (gtt) per minute. **Flow rate** refers to the number of drops per minute an IV administration set will deliver. The size of the inlet in the drip chamber of the IV tubing determines how many drops per milliliter the administration set can deliver. This is called the **drop** (or **drip**) **factor** and is set by the manufacturer of the IV tubing. The smaller the inlet in the drip chamber, the greater the number of drops required to equal 1 mL (Figure 13-5). IV tubing that delivers 60 gtt/mL is called *microdrip* or *minidrip tubing* or a *microdrip administration set*. IV tubing that delivers

fluid expansion (trauma, hypovolemia)

10, 15, or 20 gtt/mL is called *regular* or *macrodrip tubing* or a *macrodrip administration set*.

Consider this scenario: Your paramedic unit is called to attend to an elderly man who has "had the flu" since yesterday. His daughter tells you that he has been throwing up and has had diarrhea for more than 24 hours. The patient is weak, warm to the touch, and has an increased respiratory and pulse rate. His blood pressure is 88/60 mm Hg. His lung sounds are clear bilaterally. Medical direction has instructed you to give a fluid challenge of 200 mL of normal saline over a 20-minute period, reassess the patient after the infusion, then call them back. You select a macrodrip infusion set that delivers 10 gtt/mL. To determine the rate at which to infuse the IV fluid, use the following formula:

$$\frac{\text{Total volume}}{\text{Total time of}} \times \frac{\text{Drops}}{\text{(administration set)}}$$
$$\frac{\text{to be infused}}{\text{infusion in minutes}} \times \frac{\text{(administration set)}}{\text{mL}}$$

Based on the order received from medical direction and the administration you have decided to use, plug numbers into the formula and solve the problem.

$$\frac{200 \text{ mL}}{20 \text{ min}} \times \frac{10 \text{ gtt}}{1 \text{ mL}}$$

Cross out like terms that appear in the numerator and denominator, one for one.

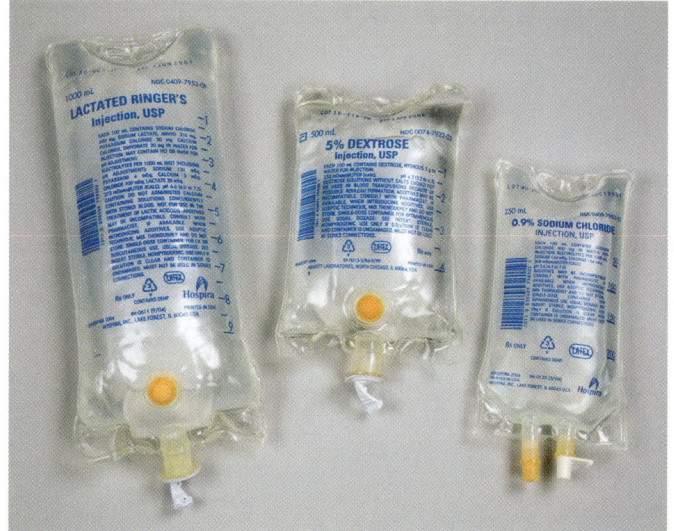

Figure 13-4 IV bags are marked with calibrations on the side of the bag.

DSW – hypotonic
NaCl – isotonic

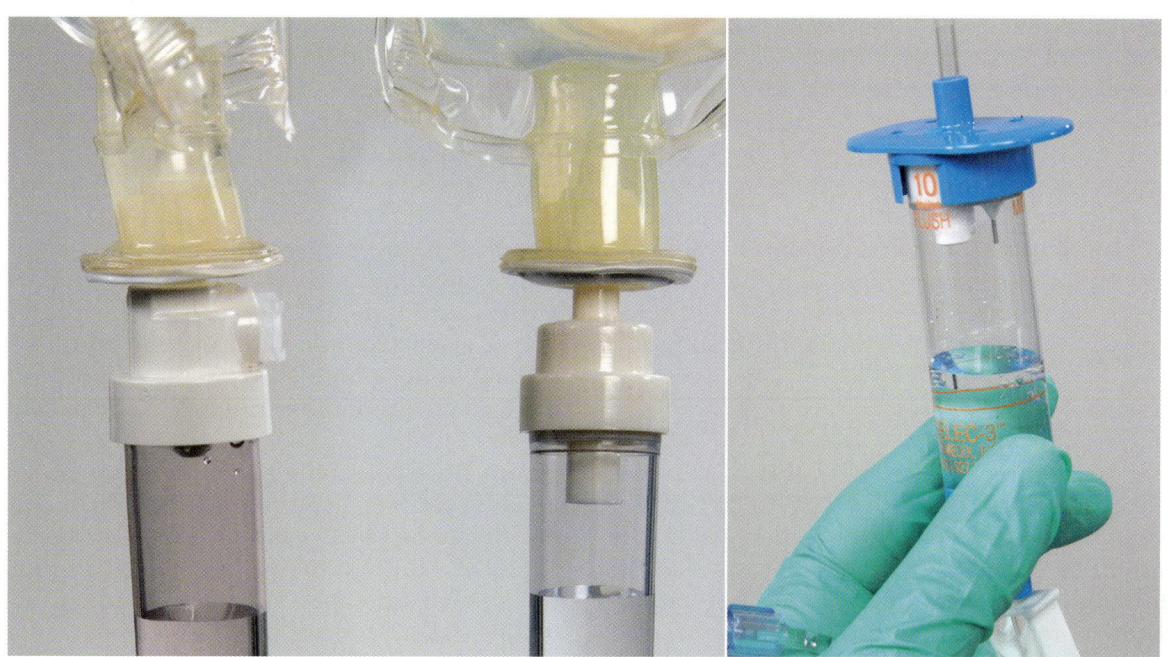

A   B

Figure 13-5 A, The size of the drop delivered by intravenous (IV) tubing is determined by the size of the opening in the drip chamber. **B,** Some IV administration sets can deliver 10, 15, or 60 drops/mL by simply turning the selector top.

$$\frac{200 \ \cancel{mL}}{20 \ \text{min}} \times \frac{10 \ \text{gtt}}{1 \ \cancel{mL}}$$

$$\frac{200 \ \text{gtt}}{2 \ \text{min}} = 100 \ \text{gtt/min}$$

PARAMEDIC*Pearl*

A simple, one-step method can be used to determine drops per minute. If the milliliters per hour rate of the infusion is known, you can figure the flow rate by using a specific division number based on the drop factor of the tubing. For example, if tubing that delivers 10 gtt/mL is used, the ratio between 10 gtt/mL and 60 minutes is 1:6. Divide the milliliters per hour by 6 to determine the flow rate. For 15 gtt/mL tubing, use the number 4. For 20 gtt/mL tubing, use the number 3. For 60 gtt/mL tubing, the drops delivered per minute will be the same as the mL ordered per hour because the ratio of 60 gtt/mL and 60 minutes is 1:1.

Getting the answer in drops per minute (gtt/min) is correct, especially for most tests and classes. However, to make this answer work in reality, you must be able to calculate how many drops per second you need to infuse the solution. To do that, simply remember that there are 60 seconds in 1 minute and then continue the problem:

$$\frac{100 \ \text{drops}/\cancel{min}}{60 \ \text{sec}/\cancel{min}} = \frac{5 \ \text{gtt}}{3 \ \text{sec}} = 5 \ \text{gtt/3 sec}$$

HINT: Avoid reducing to a fraction of a second; that is not practical and cannot be counted.

Formula 3: Drip Not Based on Weight

An **IV bolus** is the delivery of a drug directly into an infusion port on the IV administration set (and subsequently into the patient's venous circulation) with a syringe. After an IV bolus of some medications, a continuous infusion of the drug is needed to maintain the effect of the drug at a consistent level. The dosage of a continuous maintenance infusion is usually given in milligrams per minute or micrograms per minute. The formula used is "desire over have" (formula 1) multiplied by the drops per milliliter of the IV administration set.

$$\frac{DD \times V}{\text{Dose on hand}} \times \frac{\text{gtt}}{\text{mL}} \ (\text{IV administration set})$$

A 65-year-old woman has called you to her home. After shoveling snow, she had severe chest pain. The cardiac monitor revealed dysrhythmias that you successfully treated with IV boluses of lidocaine. Her cardiac rhythm is now normal. Medical direction has instructed you to begin a maintenance infusion of lidocaine at 3 mg/min. You have a peripheral IV in place. You attach a microdrip IV administration to a premixed bag of lidocaine. The information on the bag of lidocaine reads 2 g/500 mL. At how many drops per minute should you run the lidocaine drip to give the proper dose?

$$\frac{3 \ \text{mg/min} \times 500 \ \text{mL}}{2 \ \text{g}} \times \frac{60 \ \text{gtt}}{\text{mL}}$$

Because the dose on hand is in grams and the desired dose is in milligrams, you will need to convert them to like units to solve the problem. Then cross out like terms that appear in the numerator and denominator, one for one.

$$\frac{3 \ \cancel{mg}/\text{min} \times 500 \ \cancel{mL}}{2000 \ \cancel{mg}} \times \frac{60 \ \text{gtt}}{\cancel{mL}} = \frac{90 \ \text{gtt/min}}{2}$$
$$= 45 \ \text{gtt/min}$$

If you looked closely at the premixed bag of lidocaine, you would find that it also indicates that the bag contains 4 mg/mL of lidocaine. With the same formula, this information makes solving the problem much easier:

$$\frac{3 \ \text{mg/min} \times 1 \ \text{mL}}{4 \ \text{mg}} \times \frac{60 \ \text{gtt}}{\text{mL}}$$
$$= \frac{3 \ \cancel{mg}/\text{min} \times 1 \ \cancel{mL}}{4 \ \cancel{mg}} \times \frac{60 \ \text{gtt}}{\cancel{mL}}$$
$$= \frac{180 \ \text{gtt/min}}{4}$$
$$= 45 \ \text{gtt/min}$$

Formula 4: Drip Based on Weight

Some medications, such as dopamine, are administered by continuous IV infusion. However, the drug dose is based on the patient's weight. For example, a typical order for a dopamine infusion is 5 mcg/kg/min. To determine how many drops per minute are needed to infuse the solution at the correct dose, you must first determine the patient's weight. If the patient's weight is known in pounds, you will need to convert it to kilograms by dividing the weight in pounds by 2.2.

You are transporting the elderly woman from the previous scenario to the hospital. En route, her blood pressure begins to drop, even though her cardiac rhythm shows only sinus tachycardia at a rate of 120 beats/min. Medical direction instructs you to begin a dopamine infusion at 5 mcg/kg/min. Prepare the infusion by adding 400 mg of dopamine to a 250-mL bag of normal saline. Use a 60 gtt/mL administration set. The patient states she weighs 110 lbs.

Step 1: Calculate the patient's weight in kilograms by dividing the weight in pounds by 2.2. In this case, you will divide 110 by 2.2, which equals 50 kg.

Step 2: Multiply the patient's weight in kilograms by the desired dose per kilogram (cross out like terms). In this example, the patient's weight is 50 kg and the desired dose is 5 mcg/kg/min. Therefore the desired dose becomes 250 mcg/min.

$$50 \ \cancel{kg} \times 5 \ \text{mcg/}\cancel{kg}\text{/min} = 250 \ \text{mcg/min}$$

Step 3: Prepare the infusion and calculate the dose on hand (concentration on hand):

$$\frac{DD \times V}{DH} \times \frac{gtt}{mL} \text{ (IV administration set)}$$

$$\frac{250 \text{ mcg/min} \times 250 \text{ mL}}{400 \text{ mg}} \times \frac{60 \text{ gtt}}{1 \text{ mL}}$$

Note that the desired dose is in micrograms and the dose on hand is in milligrams. Convert these values to like terms. For this example, convert milligrams to micrograms: 400 mg = 400,000 mcg.

$$\frac{250 \text{ mcg/min} \times 250 \text{ mL}}{400,000 \text{ mcg}} \times \frac{60 \text{ gtt}}{1 \text{ mL}}$$

$$400,000 \text{ mcg/250 mL} = 1600 \text{ mcg/mL}$$
(concentration on hand)

Step 4: Cross out like terms that appear in the numerator and denominator, one for one. Determine the drip rate by a microdrip IV infusion set that delivers 60 gtt/mL.

$$\frac{250 \text{ mcg/min} \times 250 \text{ mL}}{400,000 \text{ mcg}} \times \frac{60 \text{ gtt}}{1 \text{ mL}}$$

$$= \frac{25 \times 25 \times 6 \text{ gtt/min}}{400} = \frac{3750 \text{ gtt/min}}{400}$$

$$= 9.375 \text{ or } 9 \text{ gtt/min}$$

MEDICAL DIRECTION

Legal Considerations

[OBJECTIVE 6]

A paramedic is authorized to give specific medications for specific conditions under the direction of a physician. Federal, state, and local laws govern the purchasing, distribution, dispensing, and administration of drugs in the United States. The organization for which a paramedic works also has policies and procedures pertaining to medication administration. Every paramedic must know what those laws and regulations are in his or her area of employment.

Diligence in handling and accounting for medications is of paramount importance if the paramedic is to be within safe legal boundaries. Medical direction has the final word for the prehospital administration of medications. However, if you know a drug dosage ordered is incorrect, or if a physician orders a drug that you know is contraindicated for the patient situation, do not give the medication. Discuss the situation privately with the prehospital manager and/or physician after the call.

Protocols: Written and Offline

Medical direction is required for paramedics to function. **Protocols** are a written form of medical direction and must be signed by the medical director. Protocols must be filed with the state board of pharmacy on a regular basis. Copies of protocols must be provided to each paramedic, and compliance is required in all instances.

Medical direction may be given by radio or cellular phone when a paramedic is on the scene (online medical direction). However, if communication fails, or in instances in which the paramedic has been given permission to function without radio communication, the written protocol must be followed (offline medical direction). If an event occurs that is not covered by protocol, the paramedic must communicate with medical direction before proceeding.

Protocols often differ among EMS systems. If you are employed by more than one EMS system, you must be especially cautious about knowing each one and only functioning under the appropriate protocol. Be sure to keep current in your knowledge of pharmacology, with emphasis on the medications allowed in your current protocol.

PARAMEDIC*Pearl*

If you are unsure of anything regarding a medication, check it with medical direction first. An injected, inhaled, or tracheally administered drug cannot be retrieved.

PRINCIPLES OF MEDICATION ADMINISTRATION

Safety Considerations and Procedures

Giving medications is an important skill. Indeed, it can save or take a life. Following are some safety considerations regarding medication administration to commit to memory for the duration of your career:

1. Be sure you are familiar with the drug you are giving. This includes knowing the mechanism of action, indications, dosage, contraindications, expected response, and expected side effects of the drug. You must also know the signs and symptoms of an adverse drug reaction and medication interactions.
2. All medications administered by a paramedic require a physician order. Be sure to convey important information about the patient to the online physician. This information should include the patient's age, chief complaint, vital signs, signs and symptoms, allergies, current medications, and pertinent medical history. Although a physician gives the order, you are responsible for assessing the patient and noting any factors that might affect the medication ordered. Medication allergies and pregnancy are two examples of factors that must be considered before giving a drug.
3. Verify the physician's order. When a medication order is received from a physician, repeat the order, including the name and dosage of the drug, back to the physician. Be certain to document the order received.

If the order received does not seem appropriate, tactfully question the order. For example, if the patient is a young child but an adult dose of a medication is ordered, carefully repeat the child's age and the drug dosage as ordered.

If you know a drug dosage ordered is incorrect, or if a physician orders a drug that you know is contraindicated for the patient situation, do not give the medication. Consult a supervisor about the best way to handle this type of situation in your EMS system. In most cases, you will talk privately with the physician at the hospital. In some cases, you may be asked to talk with the prehospital manager at the hospital. The prehospital manager will document your account of what happened and then speak with the physician.

4. Concentrate on the task at hand.
5. Make sure the patient is properly positioned before giving a medication. For example, nitroglycerin may lower a patient's blood pressure. If you are instructed to give nitroglycerin, place the patient in a sitting or supine position before giving the drug.
6. Assemble and use the correct supplies and equipment.
7. Handle all drugs carefully to avoid dropping or breaking.
8. Always use aseptic technique, discussed later in this chapter.
9. Medication errors are common and preventable. Carefully calculate drug dosages.
10. Check for incompatibility with other drugs being given.
11. Monitor for signs of overdose and take corrective measures as necessary.
12. Carefully document the drug given, dose, time, route, and the patient's response to the medication.

PARAMEDIC*Pearl*

If you make a medication error, do not try to hide the fact. You have an ethical and professional responsibility to report the error. Report the error immediately to medical direction or the physician who prescribed the drug. Others may need to be notified based on your EMS agency's policies and procedures. Assess and monitor the patient closely while the patient is in your care. When patient care is complete, reassess how the error could have been avoided and take the necessary steps to ensure the error is not repeated.

The "Six Rights" of Drug Administration

[OBJECTIVE 7]

To ensure you always give a drug with your patient's safety in mind, practice the "six rights" of drug administration (Box 13-2).

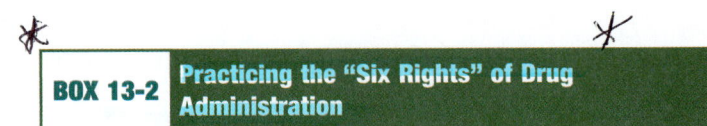

BOX 13-2	Practicing the "Six Rights" of Drug Administration

1. Right drug
2. Right patient
3. Right dose
4. Right route
5. Right time
6. Right documentation

Right Drug

EMS units within an agency typically have drug boxes that are similarly configured. For example, paramedic drug boxes used by City *XYZ* EMS are often of the same type and the drugs located within the container are in the same location—regardless of the location of the EMS vehicles within the city. This allows paramedics within that EMS system to become familiar with the location of the drugs in that drug box.

Many drugs have similar names and/or similar packaging. Always read the label three times before giving a drug. Check the drug label at these times: (1) when removing the drug from the drug box, (2) when preparing the medication, and (3) before giving the medication to the patient. Reading the drug label includes checking the drug's expiration date. When giving a parenteral medication, check the clarity of the solution. Be sure no particulates are present and the solution is not discolored.

PARAMEDIC*Pearl*

Never give an expired drug.

A medication error can occur when drugs are clearly labeled but are packaged similarly to another drug. For example, morphine and epinephrine 1:1000 solution are supplied in **ampules** in many EMS systems. The wrong drug may be given if the label is not checked three times. On more than one occasion, epinephrine 1:1000 solution instead of morphine has been unintentionally given to a patient reporting chest pain. This type of error occurs when a paramedic becomes complacent about his or her responsibilities when giving medications.

Medication errors also occur when a paramedic receives a drug order, prepares the drug to be given, and then hands the preparation to another paramedic who gives the drug. This practice increases the chances of error and the number of persons involved in that error. Consider the following real-life example. Paramedics were called to a high school for an unresponsive 16-year-old boy. The patient was breathing shallowly at approximately 4 breaths/min. His heart rate was 88 beats/min and blood pressure was 104/70 mm Hg. Friends of the patient said he may have been using drugs. An EMT assisted the patient's breathing with a bag-mask device and 100%

oxygen while one paramedic started an IV and another prepared a dose of naloxone, per local protocol. After preparing the dose of naloxone, paramedic No. 1 handed an unlabeled syringe to paramedic No. 2 to administer. As paramedic No. 2 prepared to give the drug IV, he could hear the words of his paramedic instructor echoing in his head, "Never give a drug that you did not prepare yourself without first seeing the container from which it came." He quickly asked paramedic No. 1 to show him the container from which the IV medication was withdrawn. Much to their surprise, paramedic No. 1 held up an empty container of a calcium channel blocker instead of naloxone. In this case, a potentially serious drug error was avoided.

Right Patient

In EMS, you usually know what sort of patient you will treat because you are called to attend to that specific person. Receiving a medication order from medical direction for the wrong patient is possible, however. This may occur when medical direction is provided for multiple agencies or many EMS units request orders at the same time. Question any order that is unclear or that you believe is incorrect. Another way to make the "right patient" applicable in the prehospital setting is to ask yourself if this medication is indicated. For example, "Is this medication indicated for this patient?"

If you are working in a multiple-patient environment such as an emergency department or in a mass casualty situation, be sure to confirm the patient's identity before giving any medication. Remember that patient carts in the hospital are on wheels for easy movement. The person in room 14 may not be the same one who was there 10 minutes ago. Ask the patient his or her name and birth date and check the patient's wristband. Be especially careful if the patient has an altered mental status or is hard of hearing.

Right Dose

In situations involving online medical direction, always repeat the order back to the physician, including the name of the drug, the route, and the dosage. Whether working online or offline, recheck all calculations before giving the drug.

A medication error can occur when the wrong concentration of a drug is given. For example, paramedic drug boxes usually contain epinephrine in different forms. It often is found in a prefilled syringe (epinephrine 1:10,000 solution), a multidose vial (1:1000 solution), and ampules (1:1000 solution). (Medication containers are discussed in more detail later in this chapter.) A 1:10,000 solution is typically used in cardiac arrest. The 1:1000 solution is typically given by intramuscular (IM) injection for some cases of anaphylaxis. Although both solutions contain 1 mg epinephrine, a 1:10,000 solution contains 1 mg epinephrine diluted in 10 mL of solution. A 1:1000 solution contains 1 mg of epinephrine in 1 mL of solution. Therefore a solution of epinephrine 1:1000 is 10 times stronger than a 1:10,000 solution. Giving the wrong concentration of the correct drug can have disastrous results.

Right Time

Many of the medications carried in the paramedic drug box can be administered again if needed within a specific period. For example, some drugs used in the treatment of cardiac arrest can be repeated in approximately 5 minutes. When giving a drug, you must know the correct dosage to give and, if the drug does not produce the desired result, when it may be repeated.

Right time also refers to knowing (and calculating if necessary) the appropriate interval over which a drug should be given and the rate of an IV infusion.

Right Route

The route of medication administration refers to the manner in which a drug is introduced into the body. You must know the **routes of administration** for every drug in the paramedic drug box. You also must know the drugs that can be given by IV bolus and those that are given by IV infusion. For example, 2% lidocaine is given as an IV bolus and is usually followed with an IV infusion. IV bolus medications are usually packaged as prefilled syringes of the medication. Medications given as an intermittent IV infusion are mixed in an IV solution and then "piggybacked" into the patient's main IV administration set. Some medications given as an IV infusion are premixed by the manufacturer and are commonly referred to as "premixed bags" of the drug. Lidocaine is an example of a drug available in a premixed bag for IV infusion. Dopamine is a drug given by IV infusion. It is *never* given as an IV bolus.

Right Documentation

Your medication **documentation** begins when taking a SAMPLE patient history (Box 13-3). The *M* in SAMPLE stands for *m*edications currently being taken by the patient (including **over-the-counter [OTC]** and herbal medications), compliance with those medications, and when they were last taken.

The *A* in the SAMPLE history stands for *a*llergies to medications, food, and environmental substances. Most patients will not have received some of the medications that you might administer. A patient who has several other allergies may be sensitive to a new drug without knowing it. An **atopic** patient has a genetic disposition to an allergic reaction compared with a person who

BOX 13-3	SAMPLE History

Signs and symptoms
Allergies
Medications
(Pertinent) **P**ast medical history
Last oral intake
Events leading to the injury or illness

develops the allergy after one or more exposures. Although this would not stop you from giving a drug, it would be a caution for heightened awareness.

Properly and carefully document the physician's order, patient (correct patient record, especially when dealing with multiple patients such as in an emergency department or in a mass casualty situation), date and time, drug, dose, route, who administered the drug, and the patient's response to the medication. To ensure the continuing care of your patient, this information must be on the patient's record. Following are some additional documentation tips:

- Write out drug names in full; do not use abbreviations.
- Do not use a decimal and a zero after a whole number. For example, use "5 mg" versus "5.0 mg" because the decimal point could be overlooked, resulting in a tenfold misinterpretation of dosing.
- Always use a zero before partial unit doses. For example, use "0.5 mg" instead of ".5 mg" because the decimal point could be overlooked.
- Use the metric system.
- Avoid the use of abbreviations for doses, sites, or routes. In the past medication orders were a challenge to read because many abbreviations and symbols were used. Many of these originated with the apothecary system. However, because the use of abbreviations contributes to medication errors, abbreviations should no longer be used.
- Never document slang terms, such as "1 amp" of medication. Many drugs are supplied in containers of different sizes and strengths. Take extra caution when reading the label for its contents.
- Document your patient assessment of the problem being treated. Include vital signs before and after administration. Include the initial indication and patient status before giving the drug and the patient's response after giving it. An example of proper documentation follows:
  - Before: "06/02/08. 0825 Patient experiencing severe shortness of breath, extremely anxious, and has history of pulmonary edema. BP 124/84, pulse 110 regular, respirations 20 labored."
  - After: "06/02/08. 0830 Morphine sulfate 2 mg slow IV push given per online order from Dr. Scott, ABC Hospital. Patient's breathing less labored. Anxiety level diminished. BP 116/74, pulse 90 regular, respirations 18."

PARAMEDIC*Pearl*

Remember that the prehospital care report is a legal document. Make all documentation legible to anyone trying to read it. If your patient record is ever called into court, it will be displayed to the entire courtroom for evaluation by the judge, jury, and attorneys. What you write—or do not write—can and may be used against you in a court of law.

Medical Asepsis

[OBJECTIVE 8]

Asepsis means to be free of microorganisms. **Medical asepsis** means to be medically clean or using clean technique, not sterile. Medical asepsis is practiced in prehospital care because total asepsis is not always possible. When proper equipment and technique are used, medical asepsis reduces (but does not eliminate) the number of organisms present or reduces the risk of organism transmission.

Source of Infections and Standard Precautions

[OBJECTIVE 9]

Health care involves countless risks of exposure and possible contraction of an illness or infectious disease. To stay healthy, the paramedic must remain cautious in all patient situations. **Standard precautions** refers to the actions required personnel must do every time they are in contact with a patient to prevent exposure to infectious substances from body fluids. Standard precautions are used for all patients, regardless of their diagnosis, and when handling contaminated equipment and materials.

Gloves must be worn when touching a patient's blood, body fluid, secretions, excretions, mucous membranes, nonintact skin, and soiled materials or equipment. Change gloves between tasks and patients.

Frequent and efficient handwashing is important to prevent exposure to infectious disease. Handwashing should be done before and after touching the patient, after touching potentially or actually soiled materials or equipment, and after removing gloves. Handwashing must be done regardless of whether gloves are worn.

Masks and eyewear (goggles or glasses) should always be worn if exposure to body fluids is likely by splashing or spraying. Hair covers and shoe covers are appropriate in many but not all situations. If a patient has a cough, exhibits other signs of respiratory illness, or tells you of a history of tuberculosis, wear an **N-95 particulate mask** to minimize your risk of exposure to infections disease.

Antiseptics versus Disinfectants

[OBJECTIVE 10]

A pathogen is any microorganism capable of producing an infection or a disease. It can be bacteria, which respond to antibiotic treatment, or a virus, which does not. When administering any medication, remember that pathogens can enter the same routes as the medication. Once they enter the bloodstream, complications can occur. They can be as mild as a local skin infection, a more serious condition such as **phlebitis** (inflammation of a vein), or systemic, leading to septic shock and death.

The terms disinfection, antisepsis, and sterilization all have different meanings. **Disinfection** involves the process of cleaning the emergency vehicle, stretcher, and equipment. The substances used are called **disinfec-**

tants. They are toxic to body tissues. **Antisepsis** is the process used to cleanse local skin areas before needle puncture. Alcohol-based or iodine-based products are used for antisepsis.

Sterilization is the process that makes an object free of all forms of life by using extreme heat or certain chemicals. Sterilization is impossible to achieve in a pre-hospital environment. Therefore antisepsis—or in this case, medically clean—is the goal. It begins with proper handwashing and use of gloves. It also includes careful handling of sterile supplies, regular emergency vehicle and stretcher cleaning, and discarding improperly opened or contaminated packages.

Aseptic technique must be a basic part of every paramedic's skills. If a needle becomes contaminated before entering the patient (such as touching the stretcher, patient, yourself, or the outside of the cap), discard it and select a new needle. The cost of a needle or prefilled syringe is considerably less than the cost involved in treating a patient who develops **sepsis.**

Proper Drug Handling

Finally, all medications, whether they are in or out of their protective outer packaging, should be handled with the utmost care. Dropping a box that contains a prefilled glass syringe, for example, could result in the syringe breaking, cracking, or chipping.

The paramedic drug box must be maintained in a clean, neat, and orderly state to allow for quick and easy access to the drugs in an emergency. Drugs must be checked for current date and replaced well before that date arrives. Guidelines from your EMS agency and medical direction will direct the paramedic on these procedures. Drugs such as narcotics require daily accounting. They must be locked and secured with supporting documentation. Some drugs undergo degradation if placed in extreme temperatures (too warm or too cold) or if exposed to direct sunlight. For example, mannitol will crystallize in the cold, and nitroglycerin tablets will lose their potency if exposed to moisture, light, or heat.

Care of the Site

The site of injection for a subcutaneous (Sub-Q) or IM injection or IV cannulation is cleansed by aseptic technique. Cleansing of the area is done with a spiral technique. Begin at the site of injection (the inside of the spiral) and work outward. Rubbing alcohol and/or iodine is used for cleansing depending on local protocol. Check for allergies to iodine before using this agent. By firmly cleansing the skin, dirt, debris, bacteria, and old skin cells are removed and prevented from being injected into the circulation. Allow the skin to dry before proceeding with the puncture. If the skin is unusually contaminated, repeat the cleansing process as needed.

Once the site is prepared, *do not touch the area* with anything, including a gloved finger. Unless you are wearing sterile gloves, you will recontaminate the site.

PREVENTION OF INJURIES AND EXPOSURES

[OBJECTIVE 11]
Paramedics use equipment that falls into the category called *sharps*. For example, all medication and IV needles have the potential for puncturing the skin and directly introducing pathogens into the body or opening the skin for a potential pathway. This can lead to diseases such as hepatitis or AIDS. To avoid injury to yourself or others, use the following simple but critical rules when handling sharps:

- Do not recap needles by hand or otherwise manipulate them before disposal. Use only safe needle devices. Dispose of needles with syringes and other sharp items in puncture-proof containers kept near the point of use.
- Do not overfill sharps containers because someone may be accidentally stuck with a contaminated needle or sharp when trying to use the container. When the container is two thirds full, seal it appropriately.
- Never try to reopen a sharps container or push more in than its capacity. This is a dangerous technique that can lead to a skin puncture. Sharps containers must be disposed of properly per medical direction or agency policy.
- Do not put sharps into the regular trash. Never put a contaminated needle into the patient's mattress or into or on the squad bench. Immediately dispose of them properly.
- Retrieve any sharps that may have been placed on the stretcher and place them in a sharps container. Sharps are often lost in the linen and can result in a needle stick injury when transferring the patient to the receiving facility bed or later to receiving facility staff who had no idea it was there.
- Ensure all sharps are accounted for before removing the patient from the ambulance. During this time movement is increased, as are activities near the floor (hands gathering IV or oxygen tubing, releasing the stretcher, etc.), which increases the risk of injury from an unsecured sharp.

PARAMEDICPearl

Sharps containers are to be used only for contaminated sharps and blood- or body fluid–contaminated objects. Placing items such as wrappings from IV bags or tubing or objects that are not contaminated into these containers is inappropriate. Disposal fees are assessed by weight. Therefore place miscellaneous items into another waste container.

TECHNIQUES OF MEDICATION ADMINISTRATION

Enteral Medication Administration

As discussed in Chapter 11, an **enteral drug** is one that is given and passed through any portion of the digestive tract. An enteral drug is given for its systemic effects. The specific routes of enteral administration are the oral, sublingual, buccal, rectal, and gastric routes.

Giving Oral Medications

[OBJECTIVE 12]

Medications given orally require a responsive, cooperative patient with an intact gag reflex. This route is not used if the patient is vomiting. Aspirin is the most common medication you will give orally in the prehospital setting. Although aspirin can be swallowed, medical direction or your local protocol will usually ask that the patient chew the medication to hasten absorption.

Most oral medications used in the prehospital and emergency department setting are unit-dose medications. A unit-dose medication is packaged as a single dose of medication. Dosage forms of solid and liquid oral medications are shown in Box 13-4. Equipment often used when giving an oral medication is listed in Box 13-5.

BOX 13-4	Dosage Forms of Solid and Liquid Oral Medications

- Capsules
- Elixirs
- Time-released capsules
- Emulsions
- Lozenges
- Suspensions
- Tablets
- Syrups
- Caplets

BOX 13-5	Supplies That May Be Needed for Oral Medication Administration

- Gloves
- Calibrated medicine cup
- Medicine dropper
- Teaspoons
- Oral syringes
- Nipples
- Straws
- Drinking cups
- Water or juice

When giving an oral medication, follow the six rights of drug administration. Ensure you have a physician order to give the drug. Wash your hands and put on gloves. Verify the patient is able to swallow the ordered medication safely. Take the patient's vital signs so you have a baseline with which to compare vital signs taken after the drugs are given.

Ask the patient about allergies as you prepare the medication and again just before giving it. If necessary, calculate the correct dosage of the medication to be given. If the medication is a liquid, carefully pour the medication into a medicine cup. To prevent contamination, do not touch the inside of the medicine cup. Place the cap of the bottle on a countertop with the inside of the lid turned up (Figure 13-6). Recheck the amount of drug to be given.

If the medication is a capsule or tablet in a bottle, be careful not to touch the inside of the bottle cap. Pour the capsule or tablet into the lid of the medication bottle, then into a medicine cup (if available) or the patient's hand (Figure 13-7). Pour water or juice into a drinking cup for the patient to take the medication. Position the patient in a sitting or semisitting position. Before giving the medication, ask the patient again about allergies. Tell the patient the name of the drug you are giving and why. If the patient has no allergies to the drug, give the medication with enough liquid (usually 4 to 8 oz) for swallowing. If you are uncertain whether the patient swallowed the medication, check the inside of the patient's mouth for retention of the medication. Take the patient's vital signs again after giving the drug. Watch the patient closely for signs of an adverse reaction. Documentation should include the dosage, time, route, and patient's response to the medication.

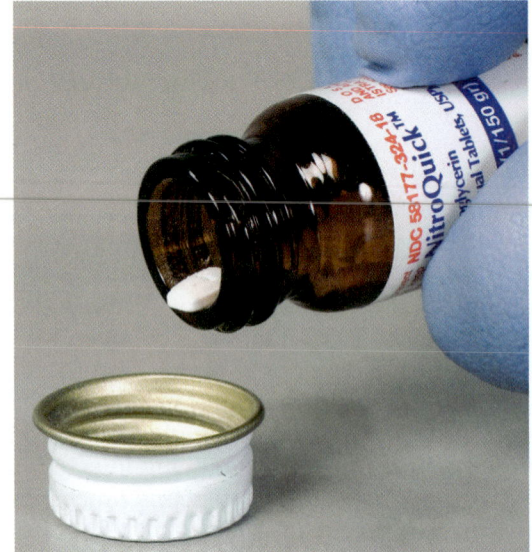

Figure 13-6 When preparing medication from a bottle, place the cap of the bottle on a countertop with the inside of the lid turned up.

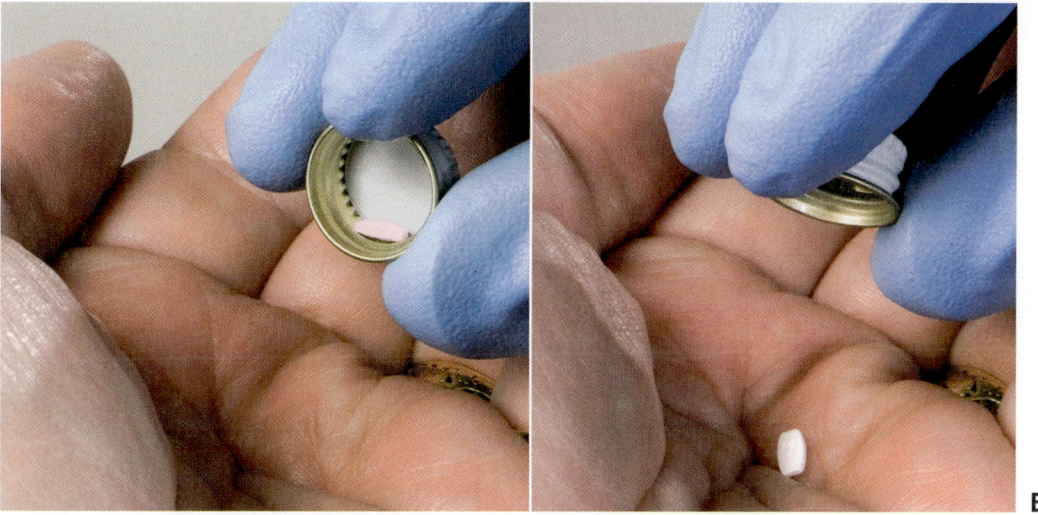

A   **B**

Figure 13-7 Pour a capsule or tablet into the lid of the medication bottle **(A)**. Then pour the capsule or tablet into the patient's hand **(B)**.

Giving Sublingual Medications

A drug given by the **sublingual** route is given directly under the tongue. The drug is quickly absorbed through the mucous membranes of the mouth and blood vessels beneath the tongue. The advantages of the sublingual route are its accessibility and rapid onset. However, the patient must be adequately hydrated for the drug to be absorbed well. The most common medication given by this route in the prehospital setting is nitroglycerin. Nitroglycerin tablets are sensitive to light, moisture, and heat. Quickly replace the cap on the bottle after opening.

When giving a sublingual tablet, place the tablet under the patient's tongue with gloved fingers. Sublingual tablets should not be swallowed. Tell the patient to hold the tablet under the tongue until it is dissolved. The medication should not be spit out or the mouth rinsed for 5 to 10 minutes after administration. Nitroglycerin spray is used in some EMS systems instead of tablets. Skill 13-1 shows the steps used when administering nitroglycerin spray.

Giving Buccal Medications

The **buccal** route differs from the sublingual in that the drug is placed in the pocket between the teeth and the cheek, instead of under the tongue, where it dissolves (Figure 13-8). This route often is used to give **glucose** to a diabetic individual who is need of a rapid increase in blood sugar.

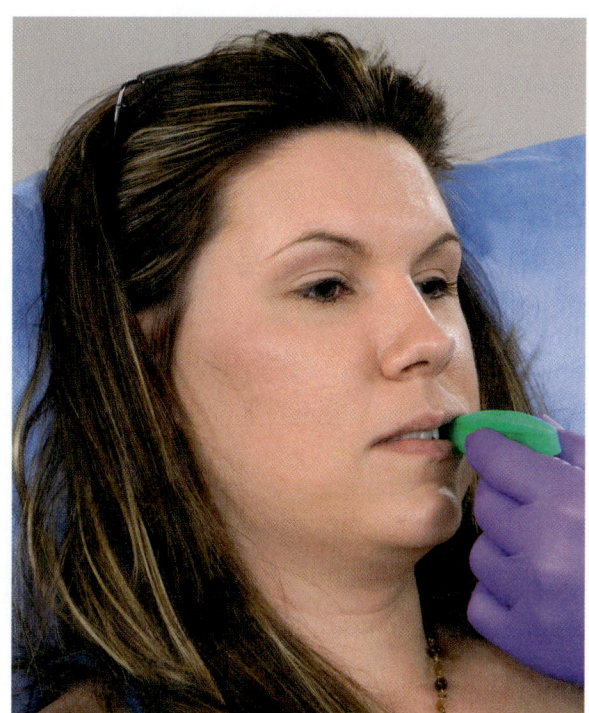

Figure 13-8 Oral glucose is one medication given by the buccal route.

SKILL 13-1 ADMINISTERING NITROGLYCERIN SPRAY

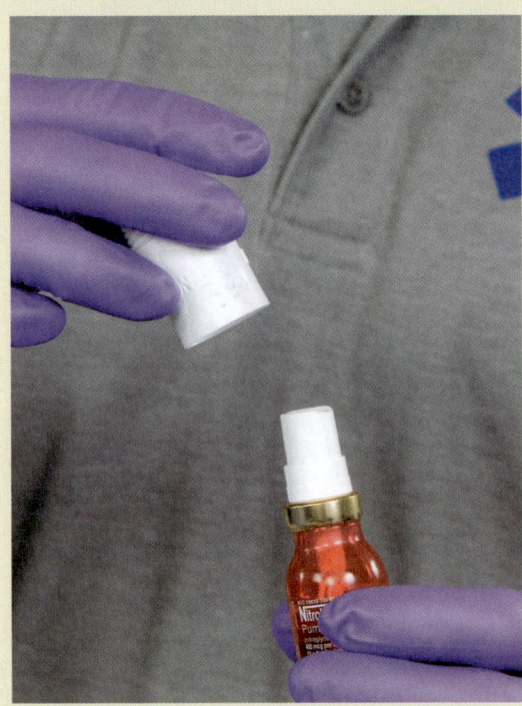

Step 1 When giving nitroglycerin spray, do not shake the canister before use. Shaking may produce bubbles within the canister, altering the amount of medication delivered. Remove the plastic cover from the canister.

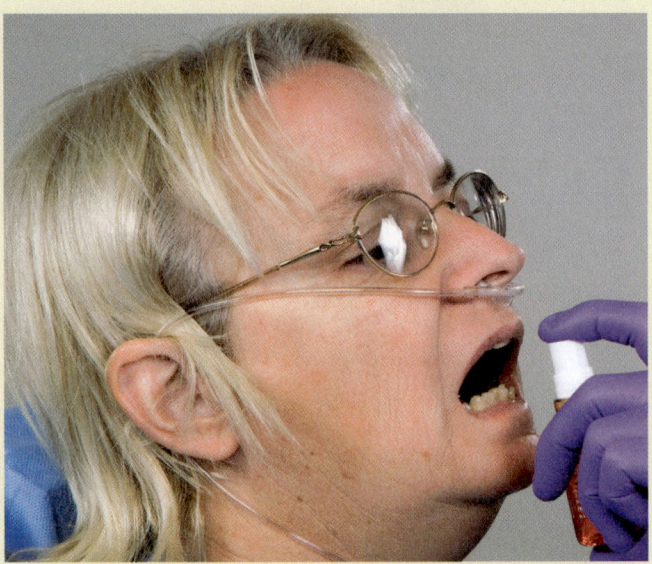

Step 2 Hold the container upright with your index finger on top of the grooved button. Ask the patient to open her mouth. Position the container as close to the patient's mouth as possible without touching it.

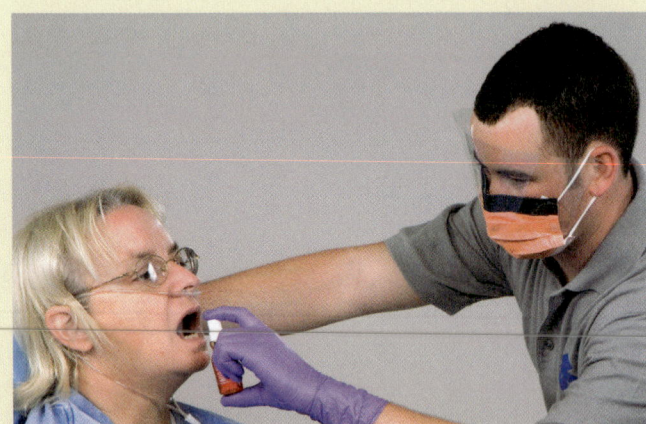

Step 3 Press the button on the canister firmly with your index finger to release the spray under the patient's tongue. Be careful not to inhale the spray.

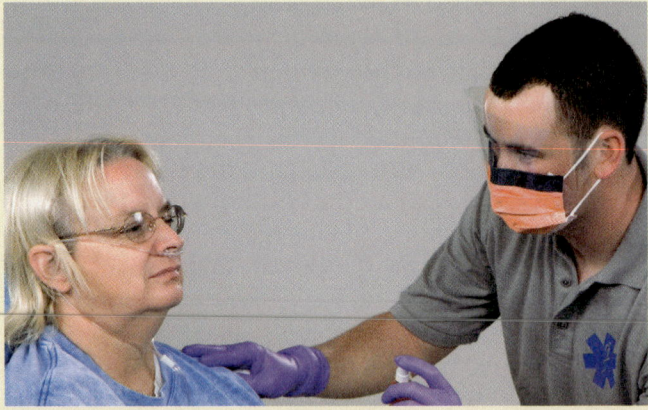

Step 4 Release the button and ask the patient to close her mouth. Tell the patient to avoid swallowing immediately after administering the spray. Replace the plastic cover on the canister.

Case Scenario—continued

After quickly obtaining a SAMPLE history and consulting medical direction, the physician asks that you remove the nitroglycerin ointment and give one dose of sublingual nitroglycerin spray. You and your partner give oxygen by nonrebreather mask, give aspirin, start an IV, and then give the patient a single dose of the nitroglycerin spray. After this treatment, the patient reports being slightly dizzy but states that his pain is now a 5 on a scale of 0 to 10.

Questions

4. Will the sublingual nitroglycerin take effect more quickly or slowly than the cutaneous dose? Why?
5. What information will you want to confirm with medical direction before administering the drug?
6. What protective equipment is appropriate for paramedic use when administering the sublingual nitroglycerin? Why?
7. What is the process for sublingual medication administration?

Giving Medications Rectally

[OBJECTIVE 13]

The rectal route of drug administration is not often used in the prehospital setting. Diastat is a gel formulation of diazepam (Valium) intended for rectal administration in the management of selected patients with acute repetitive seizures (see Chapter 23). Skill 13-2 describes the steps to use when giving Diastat to a child.

Giving Medications by the Gastric Route

[OBJECTIVE 14]

An **orogastric (OG) tube** is a hollow plastic tube placed in the mouth and passed through the esophagus into the stomach. A **nasogastric (NG) tube** is placed through the nose and esophagus into the stomach. An orogastric or nasogastric tube may be used to do the following:

- Decompress the stomach before or after tracheal intubation
- Remove ingested toxins
- Administer nutritional support
- Administer medications

In the prehospital setting, the most likely medication to be given by this route is activated charcoal. Activated charcoal should never be given to a patient who has a depressed gag reflex or altered mental status unless it is administered by an NG or OG tube and the airway is protected by a tracheal tube. Aspiration of charcoal may cause a severe and potentially fatal pneumonitis.

Insertion of an NG tube is usually more difficult in unresponsive patients or patients with altered mental status than in a patient who is alert and cooperative.

NG and OG tubes are available in various sizes. The size of the tube used is related to the patient's age, thickness of the solution given through or removed from the tube, and the length of time the tube will remain in place. Use a length-based resuscitation tape to determine the appropriate size tube for an infant or child. A healthy adult typically requires an NG tube between sizes 10 Fr and 18 Fr. Box 13-6 list the supplies that may be needed for insertion of an OG or NG tube. Skill 13-3 shows the steps of nasogastric tube insertion.

Take care to ensure correct placement of the tube. Trauma to the oropharynx, nasopharynx, or both can result if excessive force is used during insertion of the tube. If a medication or solution is given through a tube that has been incorrectly placed in the trachea, pneumonia may result. A pneumothorax may result if the tube is incorrectly placed in the trachea and forcefully advanced into the lung. Possible complications of NG/OG tube insertion are listed in Box 13-7.

After the correct position of the tube has been confirmed, prepare the correct dose of medication following the six rights of medication administration. Give

BOX 13-6 Supplies That May Be Needed for NG or OG Medication Administration

- Gloves, gown
- Goggles and mask or face shield
- Suction equipment
- Tape
- Towel or sheet
- NG or OG tube
- Cup of water and a straw
- Stethoscope
- 50- to 60-mL irrigation syringe
- Water-soluble lubricant
- Emesis basin

NG, Nasogastric; *OG,* orogastric.

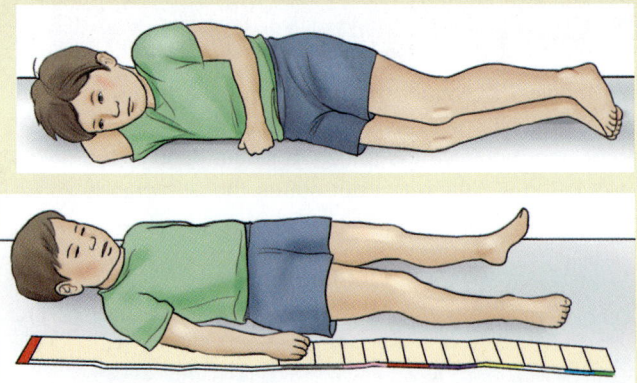

Step 1 Place the child on his or her side, facing you. Measure the child with a length-based resuscitation tape to determine the child's approximate weight.

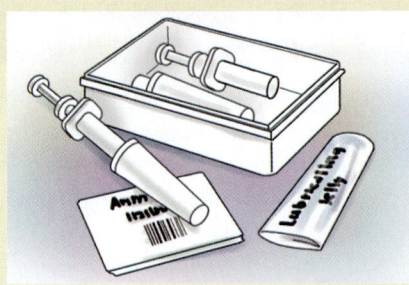

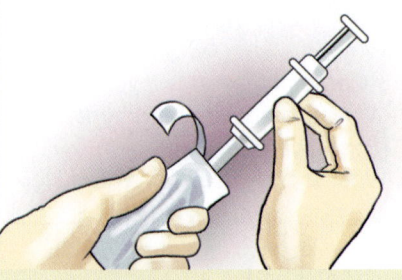

Step 2 Open the medication package and remove the syringe. Remove the protective cover from the syringe tip. Lubricate the syringe tip with water-soluble lubricating jelly.

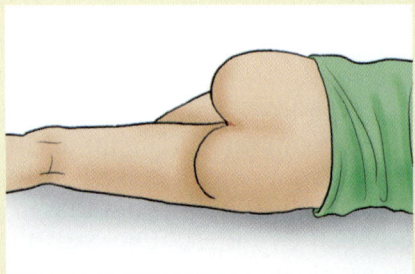

Step 3 Bend the child's upper leg forward so that the knee is close to the chest.

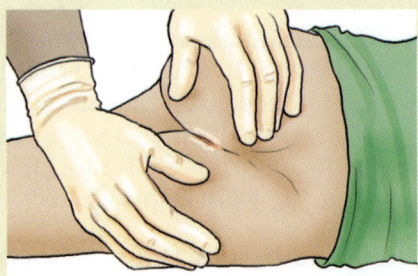

Step 4 Expose the rectum by separating the child's buttocks.

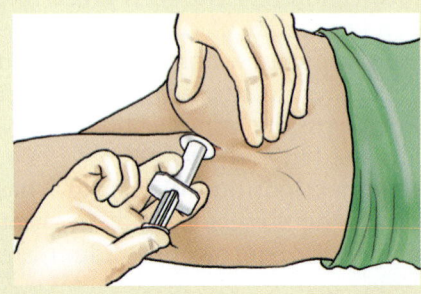

Step 5 Gently insert the lubricated syringe tip all the way into the rectum (the rim of the syringe should be snug against the skin).

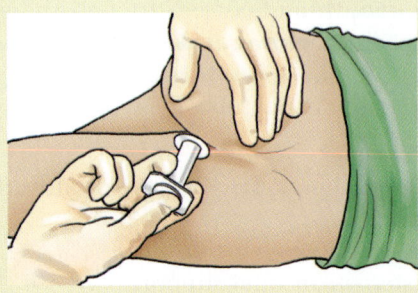

Step 6 Slowly count to three while pushing the plunger in until it stops.

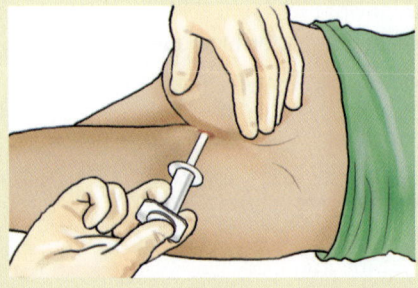

Step 7 Slowly count to three before removing the plunger.

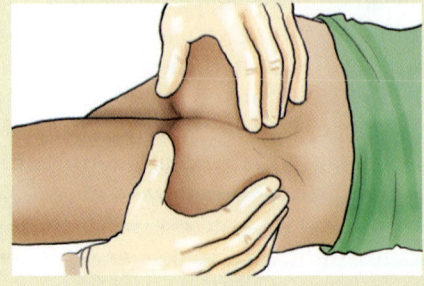

Step 8 Slowly count to three while holding the child's buttocks together to prevent leakage. Keep an eye on the child's respiratory rate and depth. Be prepared to assist breathing as necessary.

SKILL 13-3 NASOGASTRIC TUBE INSERTION

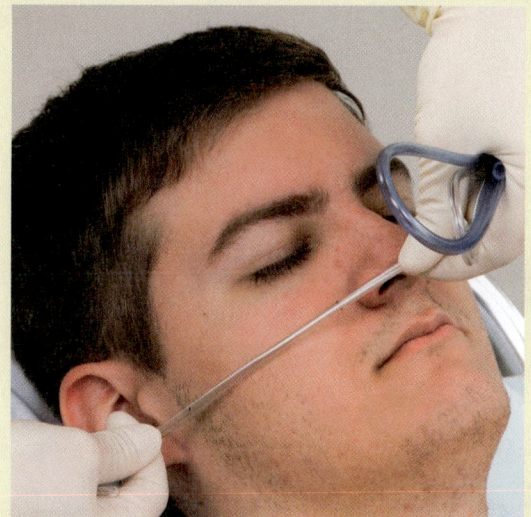

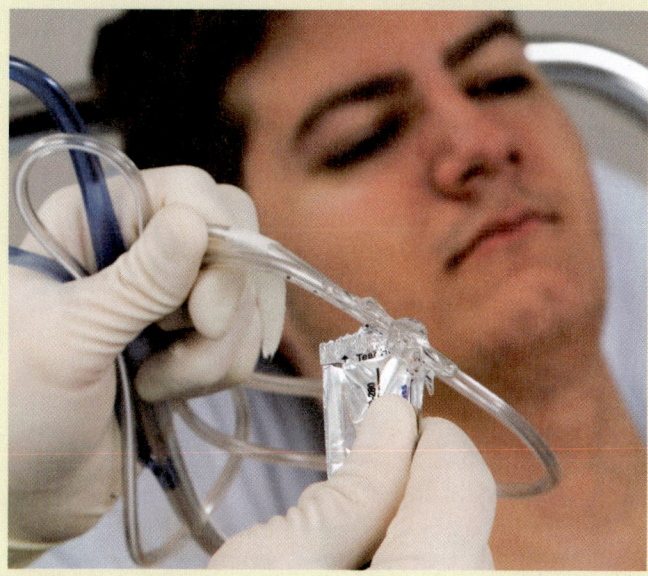

Step 2 Lubricate the first 2 to 3 inches of the tube with water-soluble lubricant.

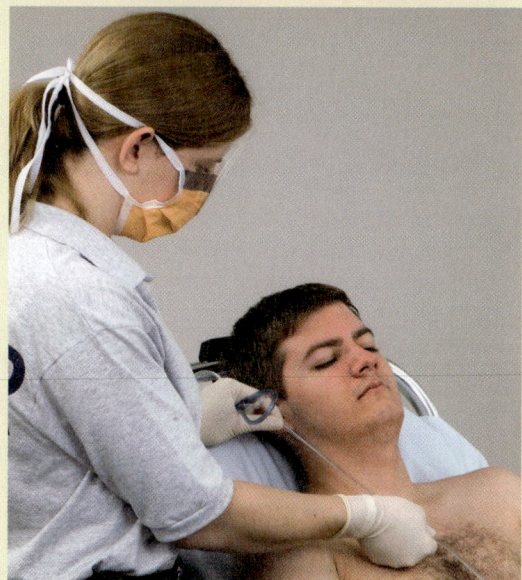

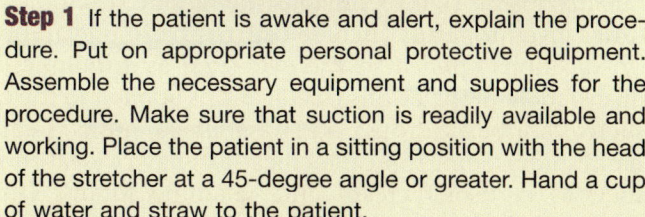

Step 1 If the patient is awake and alert, explain the procedure. Put on appropriate personal protective equipment. Assemble the necessary equipment and supplies for the procedure. Make sure that suction is readily available and working. Place the patient in a sitting position with the head of the stretcher at a 45-degree angle or greater. Hand a cup of water and straw to the patient.

Using the tube to be inserted, determine the distance the tube is to be inserted by measuring from the tip of the nose to the earlobe, then to the patient's xiphoid process. Note the marking on the tube.

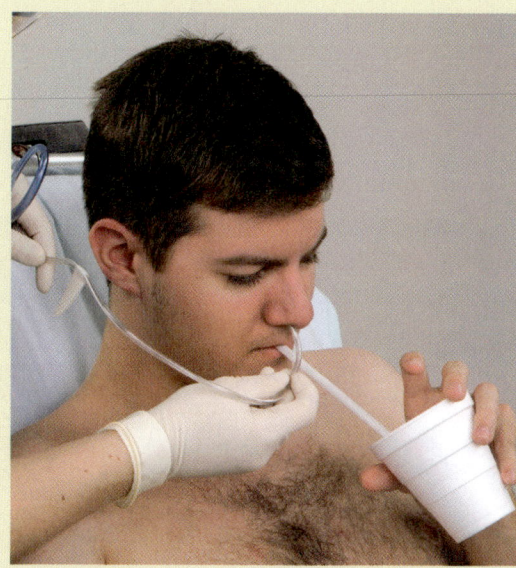

Step 3 Have the patient tilt the head forward, bringing the chin toward the chest. Tell the patient to begin taking sips of water through the straw when you say "swallow."

Continued

SKILL 13-3 NASOGASTRIC TUBE INSERTION—continued

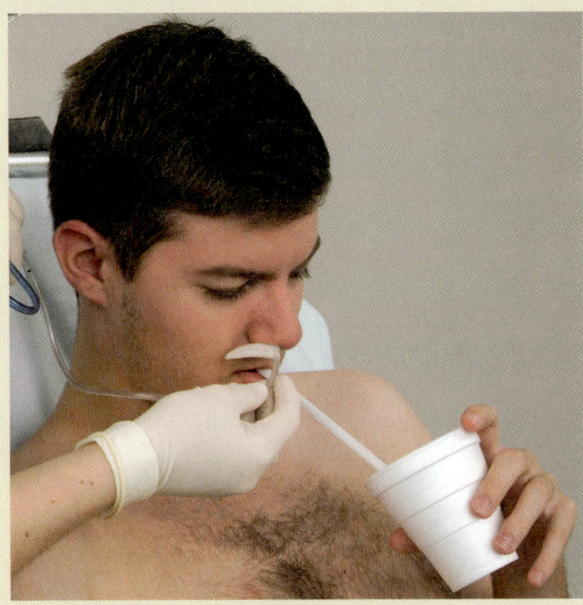

Step 4 Slowly and gently begin inserting the tube into the nostril. Advance the tube along the floor of the nostril as the patient swallows in response to your instructions. Continue gently inserting the tube until the premeasured mark is reached. If resistance is met while advancing the tube, do *not* force the tube. Withdraw the tube slightly and then try gently advancing the tube again. If resistance is met, withdraw the tube and try the other nostril.

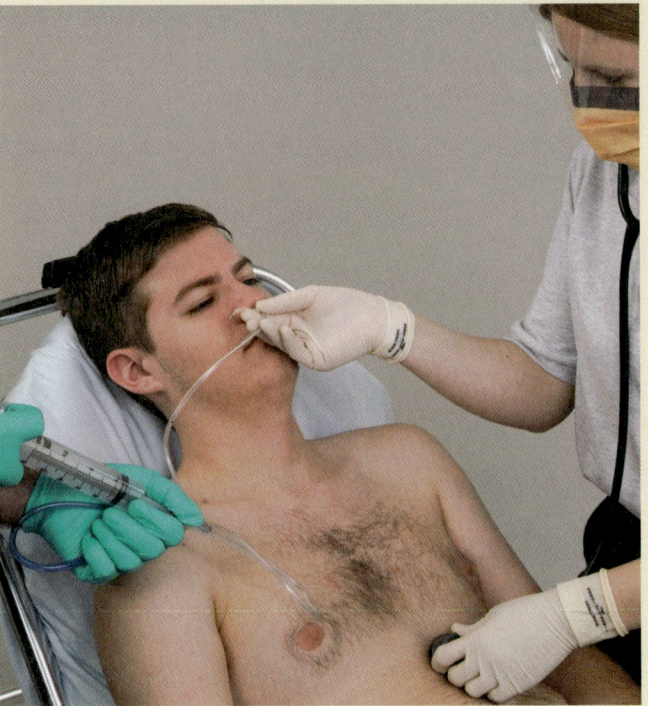

Step 5 Verify placement of the tube by injecting approximately 20 mL of air through the tube while listening over the epigastrium with a stethoscope. A rush of air should be heard if the tube is correctly positioned in the stomach. Tape the tube in place, making sure that the tube does not place pressure on the nostril.

BOX 13-7	Possible Complications of NG or OG Tube Insertion

- Perforation of the esophagus
- Misplacement of the tube into the trachea, resulting in pneumonia or pneumothorax
- Trauma to the oropharynx, nasopharynx, or both

NG, Nasogastric; *OG,* orogastric.

---

the medication through the NG or OG tube and then flush it through the tube with 30 mL water. Watch the patient for any adverse reaction to the medication. Document the reason the tube was inserted, the time the tube was inserted, the size and type of the tube, the name and dosage of the medication given, the time it was given, and the patient's response to the medication.

Parenteral Medication Administration

The parenteral route refers to giving a medication by a route other than the digestive tract. This route of administration is used for systemic effects.

Topical Medications

[OBJECTIVE 15]

A **topical** medication is administered by applying it directly to the skin or mucous membrane. Examples of drugs given topically include **ophthalmic** preparations (medications applied to the eye, such as antibiotic eye drops), **otic** preparations (medications applied to the ear, such as antibiotic drops), and nasal preparations (such as nasal spray). Some topical medications have a local effect, such as cortisone cream and calamine lotion. Other topical medications, such as nitroglycerin ointment, have a systemic effect.

Some EMS systems permit paramedics to prepare and apply nitroglycerin ointment. To administer nitroglycerin ointment, use the following procedure (Figure 13-9):

1. First confirm medical direction's order for nitroglycerin ointment. The order is usually given in inches. Check the patient's vital signs. If the patient's heart rate is less than 50 or more than 100 beats/min or if the systolic blood pressure is less than 100 mm Hg, relay this information to medical

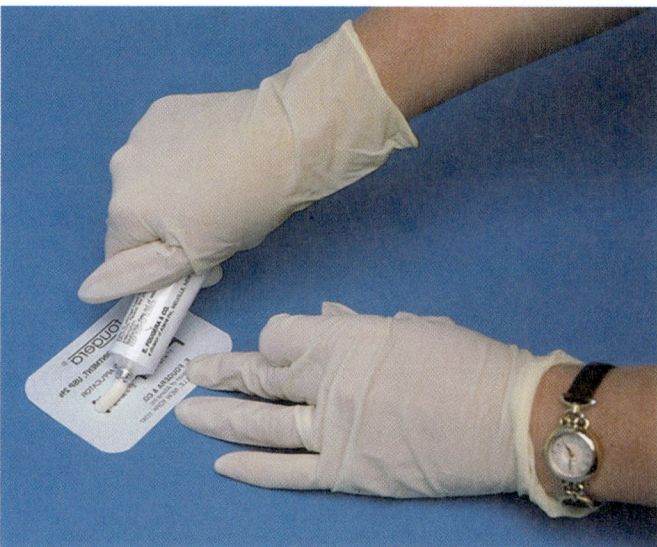

Figure 13-9 Application of nitroglycerin ointment.

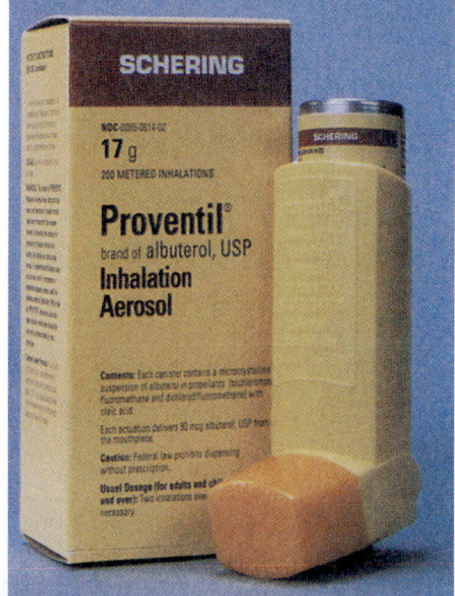

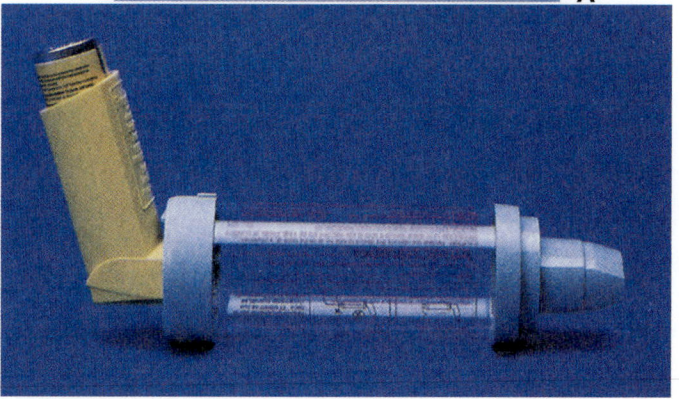

Figure 13-10 Metered-dose inhaler (MDI) **(A)** with spacer attached **(B)**.

direction before giving the medication. Put on appropriate personal protective equipment. Choose an appropriate site for medication administration, usually on the patient's upper chest. Clean and dry the skin of the area selected.

2. Apply the desired amount of nitroglycerin ointment by squeezing the medication directly onto the applicator paper supplied by the manufacturer. Follow the six rights of medication administration.

3. Apply the application paper to the patient's skin with gloved hands. Hold in place for 10 seconds. Apply a piece of tape if needed to hold the paper in place.

4. Observe the patient for desired and adverse effects. Document the procedure and the patient's response to the medication.

PARAMEDIC*Pearl*

It is important to wear gloves when handling nitroglycerin preparations. The medication is easily absorbed through the skin. If you do not wear appropriate equipment, you may experience a severe headache, lightheadedness, and hypotension if exposed to the medication.

Giving Inhaled Medications

[OBJECTIVE 16]

Inhaled medications may be in the form of a gas, spray, powder, or liquid. The medication is rapidly absorbed by the alveoli into the pulmonary capillaries and then into the central circulation. Medications often given by the inhalation route include oxygen, bronchodilators, and steroids.

An **aerosol** is a collection of particles dispersed in a gas. Aerosolized medications, such as albuterol, are given by a metered-dose inhaler or nebulizer.

Metered-Dose Inhalers. A **metered-dose inhaler (MDI)** is a handheld device that directly disperses a measured dose of medication in the form of a fine spray into the airway (Figure 13-10). A dose of medication is delivered by pressing down on the inhaler. For the full amount of the medication to reach the patient's lungs, the patient must breathe in slowly after the inhaler is depressed. Some patients, such as older adults or those with arthritis, may have difficulty depressing the inhaler. Adapters are available to help these patients self-administer the medication. When an MDI is used, much of the medicine is deposited on the tongue or in the back of the throat. To enhance the amount of medication that reaches the bronchioles, a spacer may be used. A **spacer** (sometimes called a *holding chamber*) is a hollow plastic tube that attaches to the MDI on one end and has a mouthpiece on the other (Figure 13-11). Skill 13-4 shows how to administer a medication by MDI.

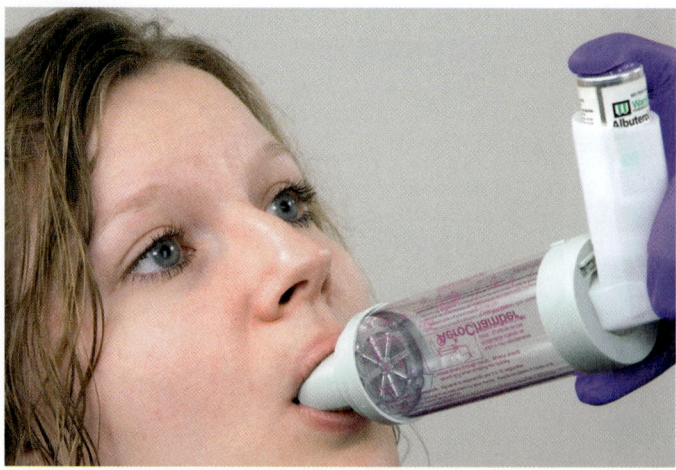

Figure 13-11 A spacer is a hollow plastic tube that attaches to a metered-dose inhaler (MDI) on one end with a mouthpiece on the other.

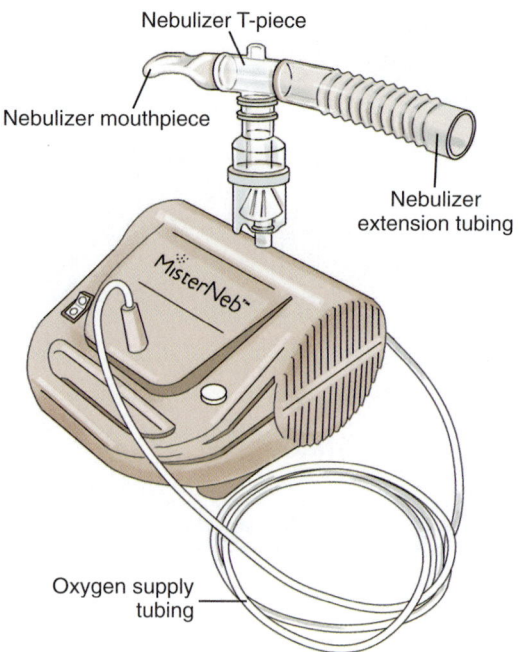

Figure 13-12 Parts of a nebulizer.

Nebulizers. A **nebulizer** (also called a *small-volume nebulizer*) is a machine that turns liquid medication into fine droplets in aerosol or mist form. The droplets are inhaled through a mask or mouthpiece. A disposable nebulizer kit is stocked in many EMS vehicles. A nebulizer kit typically contains the following parts (Figure 13-12):

- Oxygen supply tubing
- Mouthpiece or mask
- T-piece or fitting
- Nebulizer cup (mixing chamber)
- Nebulizer extension tubing (reservoir)

Skill 13-5 shows how to administer a medication by nebulizer.

> ### PARAMEDIC*Pearl*
> The amount of medication delivered by the inhalation route is affected by airway size and the degree of obstruction within the airways from mucus plugs, bronchoconstriction, and inflammation.

Tracheal Medications. The tracheal route refers to giving a medication by means of an endotracheal (ET) tube. This route has a rapid onset of action because of the large surface area available for absorption in the respiratory tract. Once the drug has been instilled in the ET tube, a bag-mask device is used to disperse the drug across the alveoli. The ET route is most often used to give drugs to a patient in cardiac arrest but in whom vascular access has not been obtained. If the patient is an adult, ET medications are generally diluted in 10 mL normal saline. If the patient is an infant or child, the medication should be diluted with approximately 5 mL normal saline. For a newborn, ET medications may be given undiluted and followed with a 0.5 to 1 mL saline flush or diluted to a total volume of 1 mL in normal saline before administration.

If possible, remove the needle from the syringe before instilling medication in an ET tube. This helps prevent accidental detachment of the needle from the syringe and movement of the needle into the bronchial tree. Some ET tubes have a separate medication port that dispenses the medication at the distal end of the tube rather than delivering the medication through the tube. In this case, the needle is needed to penetrate the medication port (unless a Luer port is used by the ET tube manufacturer). Most medications used in cardiac arrest are packaged in prefilled syringes that do not have removable needles. When using a prefilled syringe to give an ET medication, be sure to check that the needle is still attached to the syringe when the procedure is complete. Skill 13-6 shows the necessary steps for ET medication administration.

> ### PARAMEDIC*Pearl*
> ET medication absorption may be negatively affected by the presence of blood, vomitus, or secretions in the trachea or ET tube.

Giving Intranasal Medications

The intranasal route offers direct delivery of medications into the nasal passages and sinuses. Intranasal medications are administered by spray, drops, or aerosol into the nasal cavity. Medications given by this route have a rapid and reliable onset of action.

SKILL 13-4 ADMINISTERING MEDICATION BY MDI

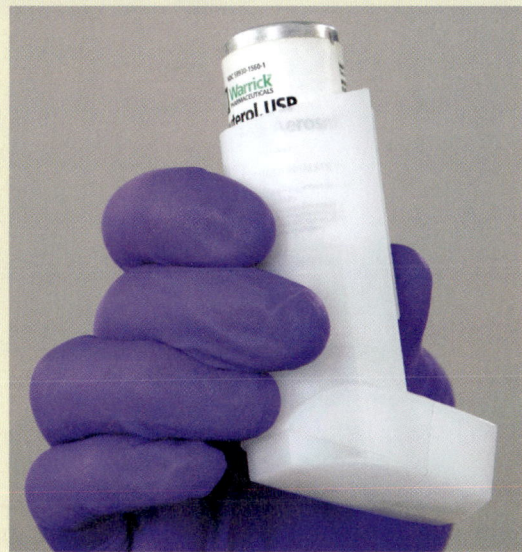

Step 1 Confirm medical direction's order for the medication. Put on appropriate personal protective equipment. Follow the six rights of medication administration. Explain the procedure to the patient. Place the patient in a sitting position. Assemble the inhaler and attach a spacer if available. Shake the inhaler gently several times to make sure the medication particles are aerosolized.

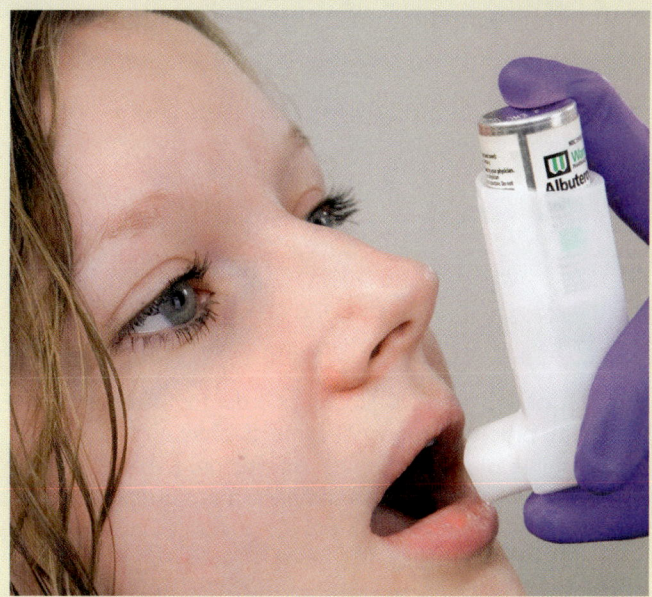

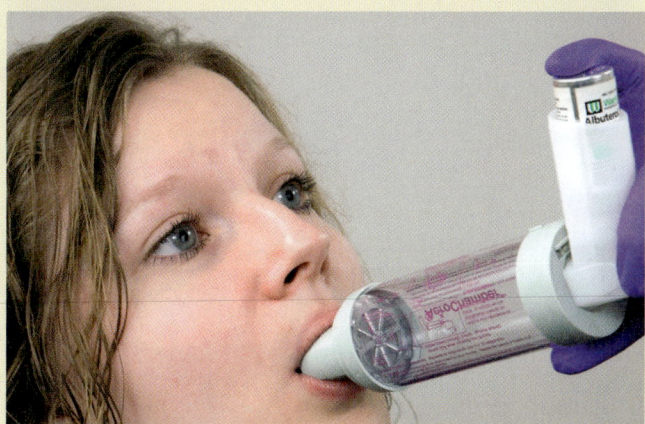

Step 2 Position the inhaler's mouthpiece approximately 2 finger widths from the patient's mouth. If a spacer is used, have the patient place the mouthpiece in the mouth and close the lips around it.

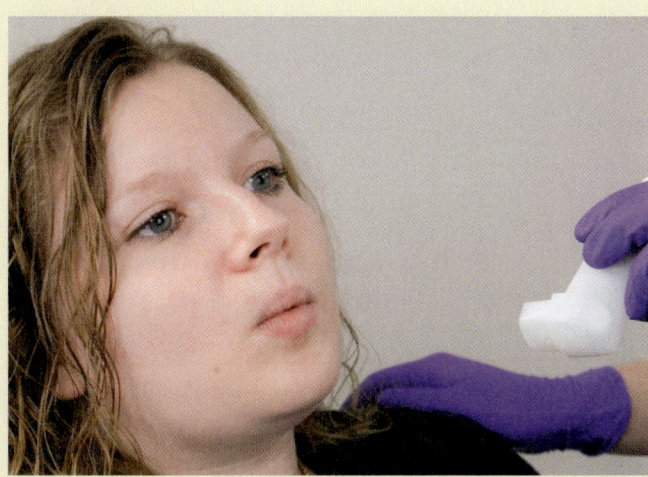

Step 3 Ask the patient to take a deep breath and exhale. Then ask the patient to inhale slowly and deeply while depressing the inhaler. To permit the medication to penetrate the deep structures of the airway, ask the patient to hold the breath for approximately 10 seconds and try not to cough. To help keep the airways open during exhalation, ask the patient to exhale through pursed lips.

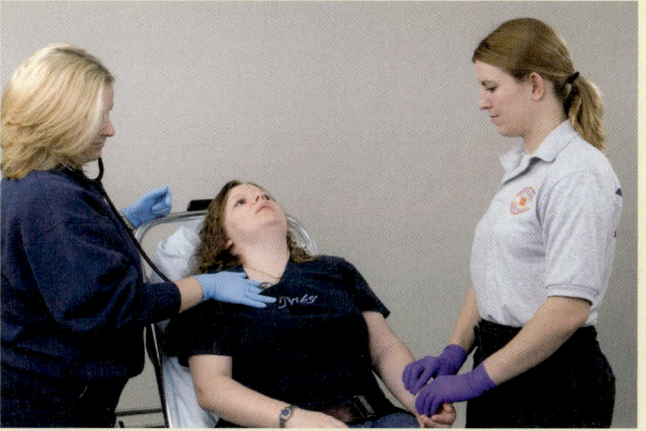

Step 4 Observe the patient for desired and adverse effects. Document the procedure.

SKILL 13-5 ADMINISTERING MEDICATION BY SMALL-VOLUME NEBULIZER

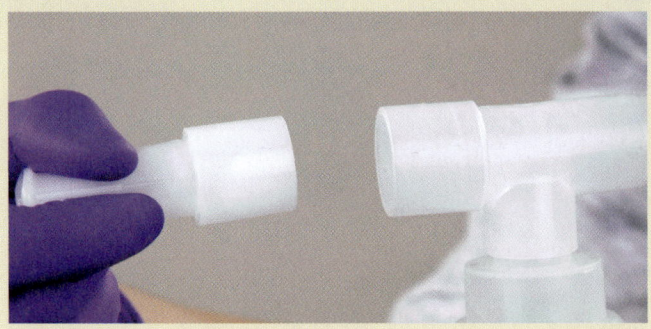

Step 1 Confirm medical direction's order for the medication. Put on appropriate personal protective equipment. Follow the six rights of medication administration. Explain the procedure to the patient. Place the patient in a sitting position. Assemble the small-volume nebulizer. Attach the nebulizer mouthpiece to the large end of the T piece.

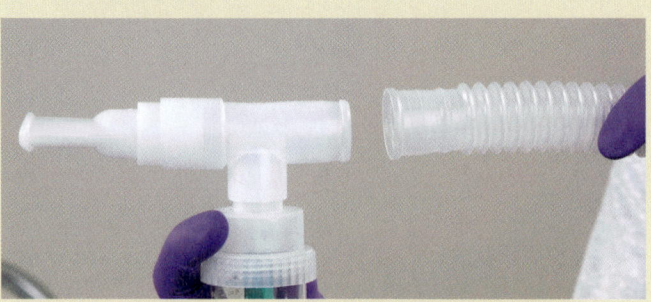

Step 2 Attach the nebulizer extension tubing to the small end of the T piece.

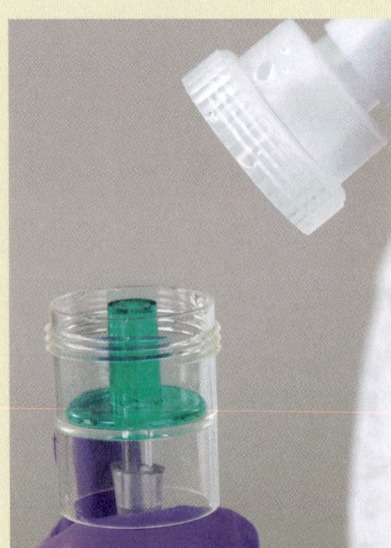

Step 3 Unscrew the top of the nebulizer cup.

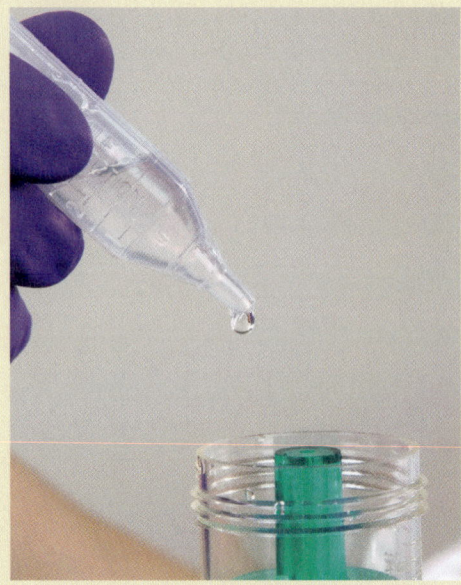

Step 4 Carefully fill the base of the cup with the medication ordered by medical direction. If the drug ordered is a bronchodilator, additional liquid (such as normal saline) may need to be added if ordered.

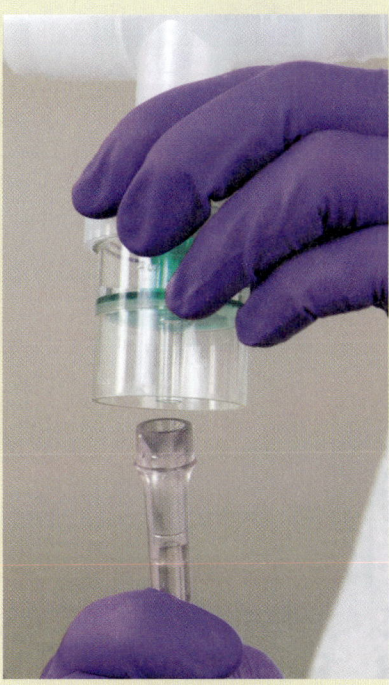

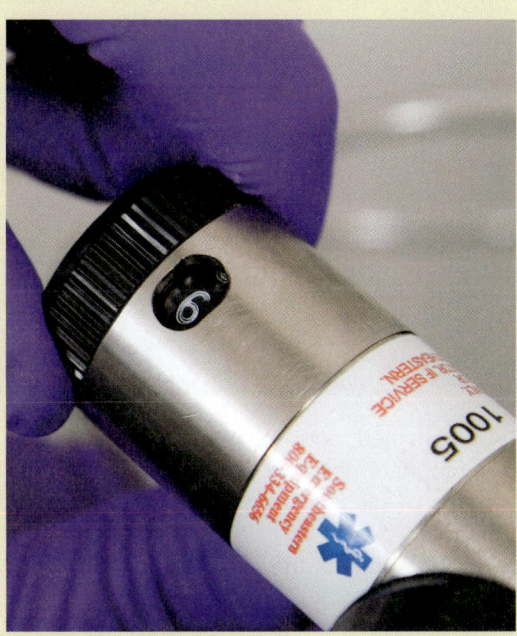

Step 5 Screw on the top of the nebulizer cup and shake to mix the medication and diluent (if used). Attach one end of the oxygen supply tubing to the nebulizer cup. Attach the other end to an oxygen source.

Step 6 Attach the nebulizer cup to the bottom of the T piece. Adjust the oxygen flow rate between 6 and 10 L/min to create a fine mist.

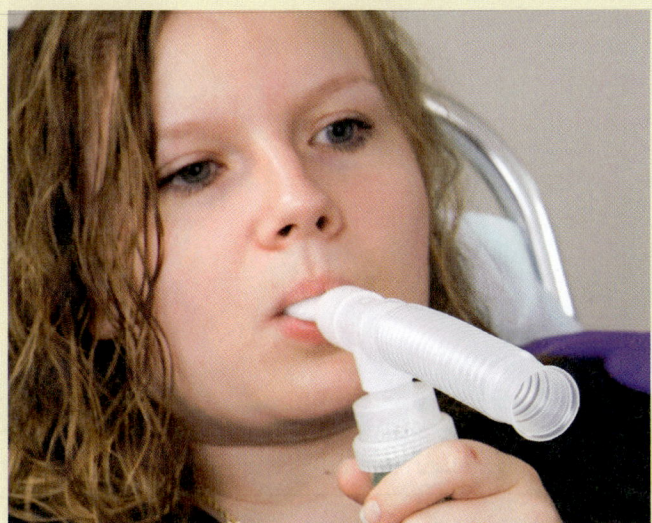

Step 7 Place the patient in a sitting position. If the patient can hold the mask or mouthpiece alone, let her do so. If not, hold it for the patient. Have the patient inhale slowly, pause for 2 or 3 seconds, and then slowly breathe the air out through pursed lips. Continue until all the medication is gone. Observe the patient for desired and adverse effects. Document the procedure.

SKILL 13-6 ET Drug Administration

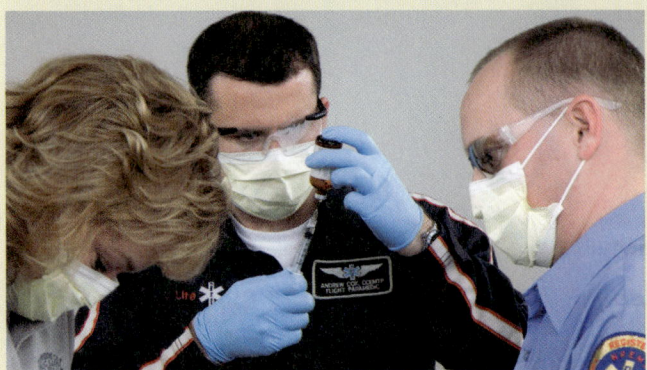

Step 1 Confirm medical direction's order for the medication. Put on appropriate personal protective equipment. Follow the six rights of medication administration. Assemble the appropriate equipment. Ventilate the patient's lungs with several compressions of the bag-mask device.

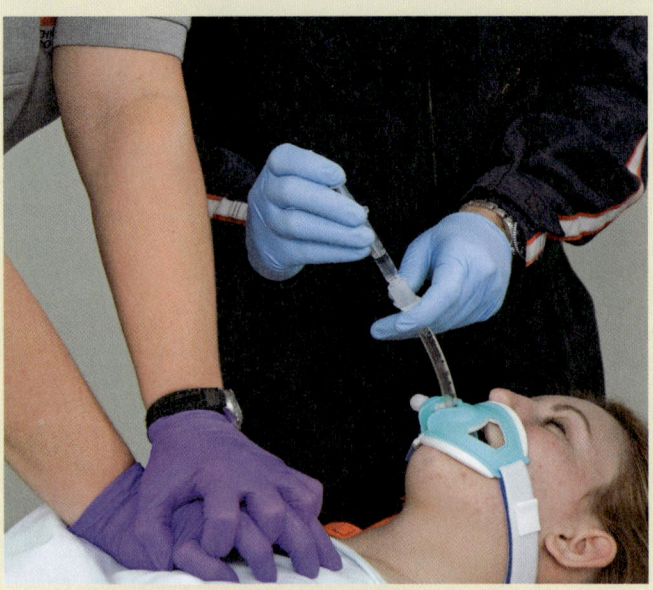

Step 2 Briefly disconnect the oxygen source from the ET tube. Some EMS systems use ET tubes equipped with a drug port. If the ET tube is so equipped, disconnecting the oxygen source from the ET tube to administer medications through the tube is not necessary.

If cardiopulmonary resuscitation (CPR) is being performed, temporarily stop compressions. Instill the medication directly into the ET tube. An alternate method requires passing a suction catheter that extends beyond the tracheal tube. The medication is then instilled into the catheter.

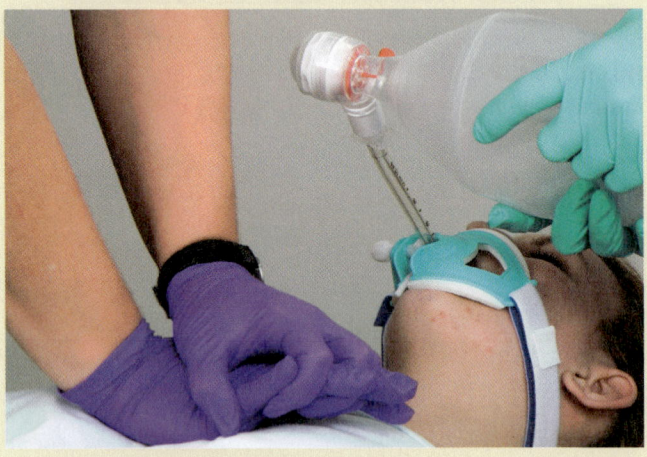

Step 3 After administration, give several positive-pressure ventilations to distribute the medication throughout the tracheobronchial tree and enhance absorption. If CPR was interrupted, resume CPR.

The patient should be placed in a supine position with the head tilted back so that the opening to the nares is almost horizontal (Figure 13-13). The patient should remain in this position for approximately 1 minute after the medication has been instilled to ensure the medication reaches the nasal mucosa. The medication is being given too quickly if the patient sputters, coughs, or swallows during administration. Do not give medications by this route if the patient has respiratory distress, copious nasal secretions, or nasal bleeding because of the increased risk of airway obstruction and aspiration.

A mucosal atomization device (MAD) is used in some EMS systems to give intranasal medications. A syringe is used to prepare the desired dose and volume of medication. The syringe is then connected to the MAD (Figure 13-14). The atomizer is positioned approximately 1.5 cm into the patient's nostril and the medication dispensed. The dose is usually repeated in the patient's other nostril. The device produces a fine-mist spray that targets the nasal mucosa. Naloxone (Narcan) can be given by a MAD for apneic patients who have a pulse and in whom an opiate overdose is suspected. Midazolam (Versed) can be given by an MAD for persistent seizure activity in adults.

Injectable Medications

Equipment

Needles and Syringes. A needle has three parts: the hub, shaft, and bevel (Figure 13-15). The **hub** is the plastic piece that houses the needle and fits onto a syringe.

The **shaft** (also called the *cannula*) is the length of the needle. The needle shaft connects to the hub. The **bevel** is the slanted tip at the end of the needle. An opening is present in the bevel called the **lumen.** Needles are packaged with a plastic shield over them to maintain sterility.

A syringe is a cylinder with a tip on its end that fits into the hub of a needle. The syringe contains a plunger used to withdraw and inject medications. When preparing a needle and syringe for injection, the hub of a needle can be handled to ensure a tight fit on the syringe. However, to maintain sterility, the shaft and bevel of a needle must not be touched.

A needle must be long enough to reach the site chosen for injection. The length of a needle is measured from the point where the needle shaft and hub meet to the tip of the bevel. Needle lengths vary from $\frac{1}{4}$ to 5 inches. Most often, needle lengths of 1, $1\frac{1}{2}$, and 2 inches are used for IM injections in adults. A needle's diameter is also its gauge. The needle gauge selected must be large enough to allow the drug to be injected easily. Needle gauges range from 13 to 30. The larger the gauge, the smaller the needle diameter (Figure 13-16). Factors that affect the needle size used for an injection are shown in Box 13-8. Intradermal and Sub-Q injections require short needles with a small diameter. IM injections usually require a longer needle and larger diameter.

Syringes are available in various capacities and may be packaged with or without a needle. A syringe may be handled by the outside of the barrel and handle of the plunger. To maintain sterility, do not touch the tip of the syringe, shaft of the plunger, or inside of the barrel.

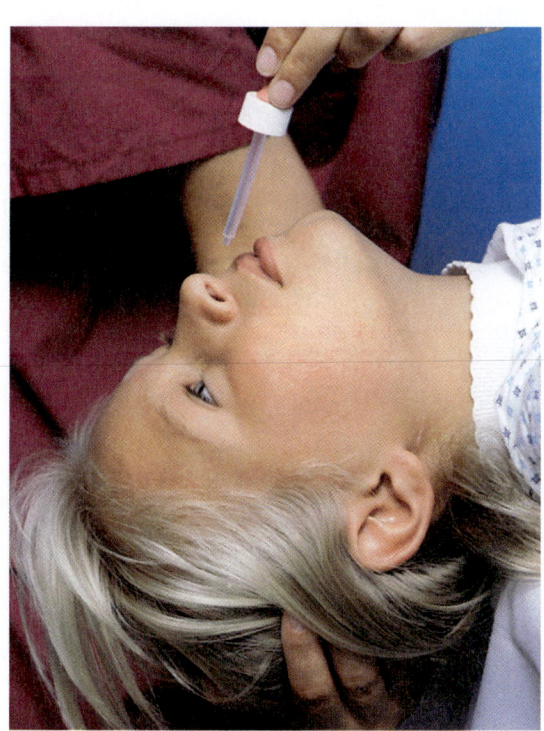

Figure 13-13 Patient positioning for intranasal medication administration.

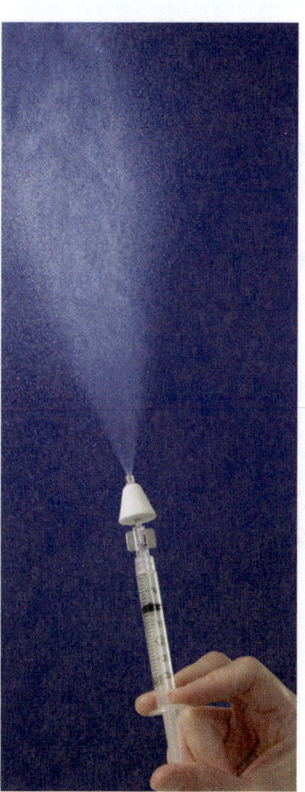

Figure 13-14 Nasal mucosal atomization device (MAD) with syringe (Wolfe Tory Medical, Inc., Salt Lake City, Utah).

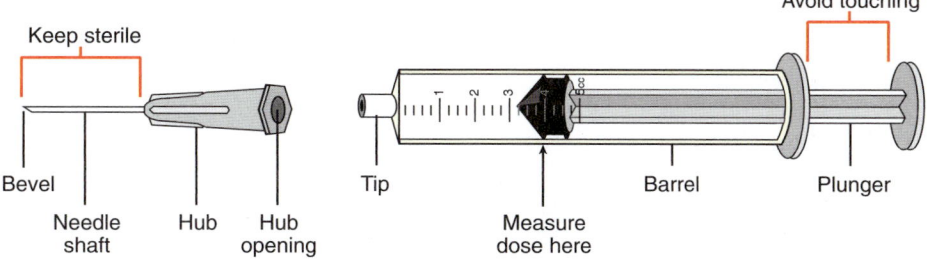

Figure 13-15 Parts of a needle and syringe.

A syringe is marked with calibrations on the barrel for accurately measuring medication dosages. When measuring a dose with a syringe, read the calibration from the top ring of the plunger. A capacity and calibration scale appropriate for the dosage to be given is the prime factor in choosing a syringe. To select a syringe with an appropriate capacity, look to see how many calibrations are in each milliliter. Small-capacity syringes have two scales. One scale typically has calibrations in increments of tenths (or hundredths) of a milliliter. The other scale is calibrated in minims. A tuberculin (TB) syringe is used to measure doses of 1.0 mL or less (Figure 13-17). Because its calibrations are in hundredths, a TB syringe often is used for measuring pediatric dosages. A 3-mL syringe has calibrations in increments of tenths of a milliliter (Figure 13-18). Five-, 6-, 10-, and 12-mL syringes have calibrations in increments of 0.2 mL. Calibrations on a 20-mL syringe are in 1-mL increments.

Needles are not recapped after use to help prevent needle sticks. Contaminated needles must be placed into a sharps container immediately after use. Safety syringes are available that have a protective sheath that covers the needle as it is withdrawn from the skin (Figure 13-19).

PARAMEDIC*Pearl*

Use a TB syringe to measure small dosages accurately.

Parenteral Medication Containers

[OBJECTIVES 17, 18]

Medications used for injection come in liquid or powder form. They may be packaged in small glass containers with narrow necks **(ampules),** glass containers with rubber stoppers at the top **(vials),** or prefilled syringes (Figure 13-20). A vial may contain a single dose (single-dose vial) of a drug or multiple doses (multidose vial). A vial that contains a powder must be reconstituted with a diluent (a specific fluid to dissolve the solid material) before administration. Skill 13-7 shows the steps necessary for withdrawing medication from an ampule. Skill 13-8 shows the steps for withdrawing medication from a vial.

A prefilled syringe is a sterile, disposable syringe and needle combination. The syringe is prefilled with medication. To use a prefilled syringe, the protective cap must be removed from the syringe barrel and the container of medication. The medication container is then screwed into the syringe barrel and the air expelled from the syringe before use.

Intralingual Injections. The intralingual route is the direct injection of a small volume of medication into the underside of the tongue. A 25-gauge, $5/8$-inch needle typically is used for an intralingual injection. The tongue is gently lifted from the floor of the mouth with an oral airway or Magill forceps. The medication is then injected into the ventrolateral surface of the tongue. Naloxone has been used by this route for suspected narcotic overdose when peripheral venous access could not be obtained. In some EMS systems atropine and epinephrine have been

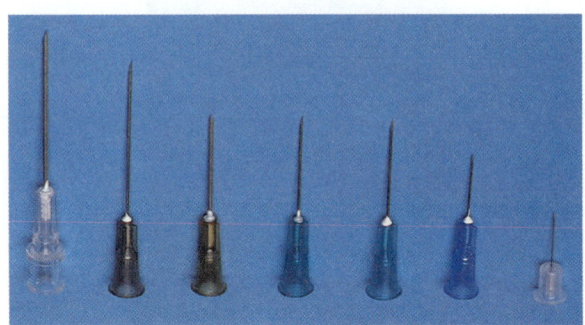

Figure 13-16 Various needle sizes.

BOX 13-8 | **Factors Affecting Needle Size Selection**

- Route of administration
- Patient's size and weight
- Site chosen for injection
- Condition of the tissue at the intended injection site
- Type and thickness of the medication to be injected

Test question

#14 g 1¼"
needle for
max. fluid
infusion

shorter needle =
faster infusion

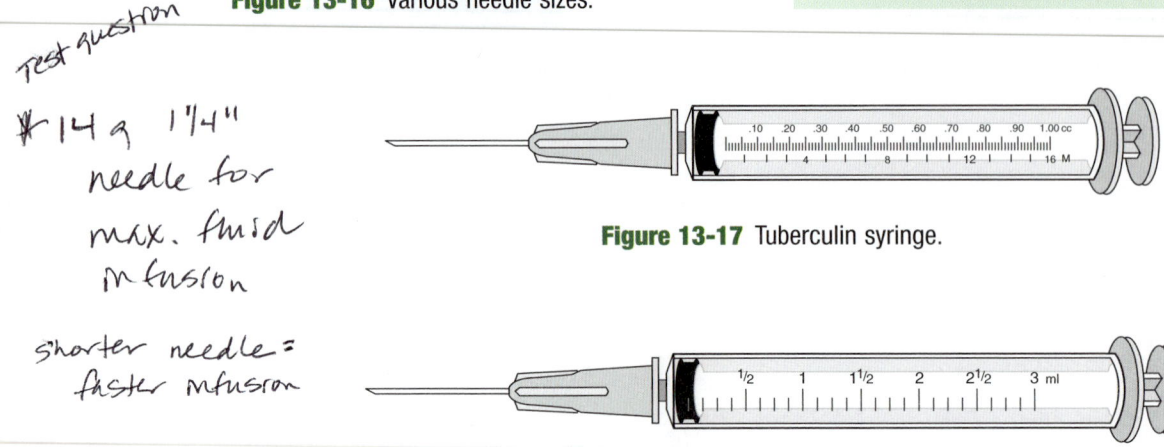

Figure 13-17 Tuberculin syringe.

Figure 13-18 Measurement scale on a 3-mL syringe.

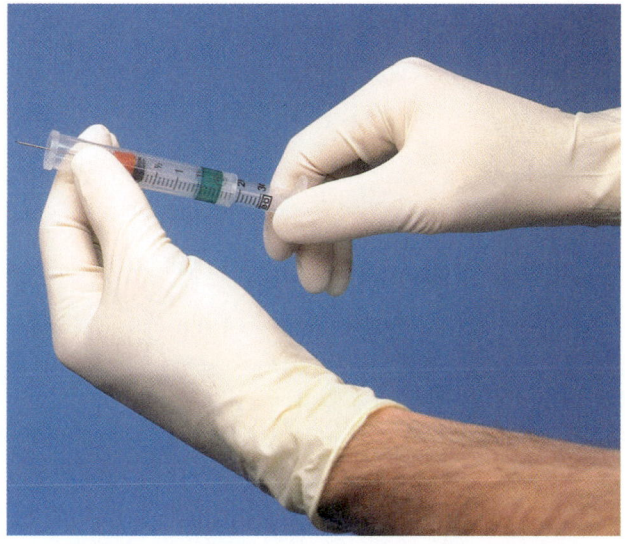

Figure 13-19 Needle with protective sheath.

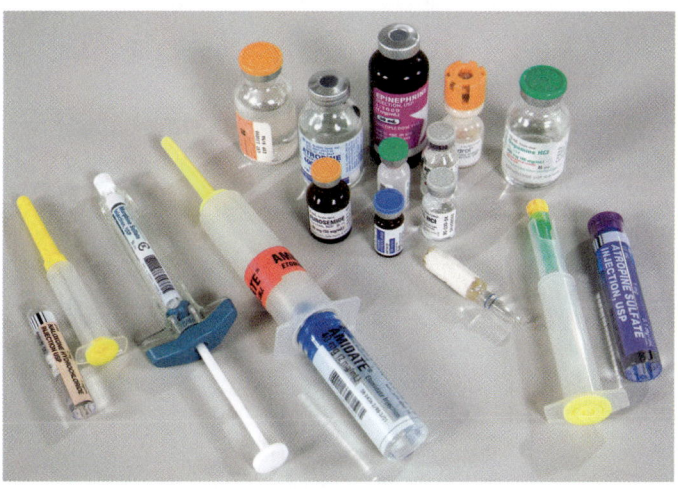

Figure 13-20 Containers of parenteral medication.

SKILL 13-7 WITHDRAWING MEDICATION FROM AN AMPULE

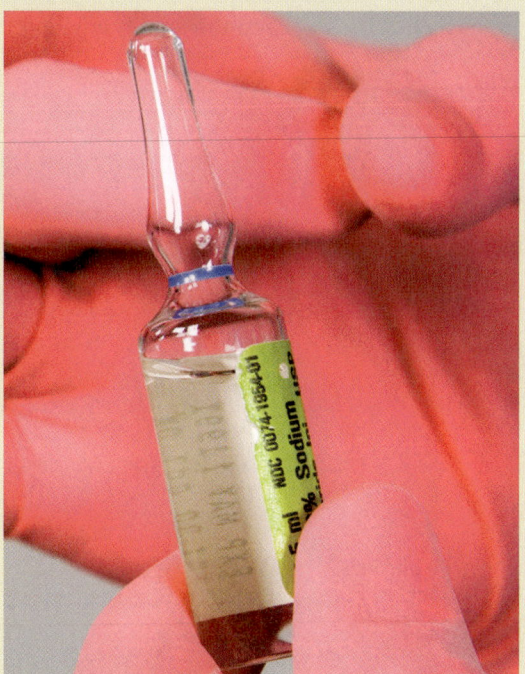
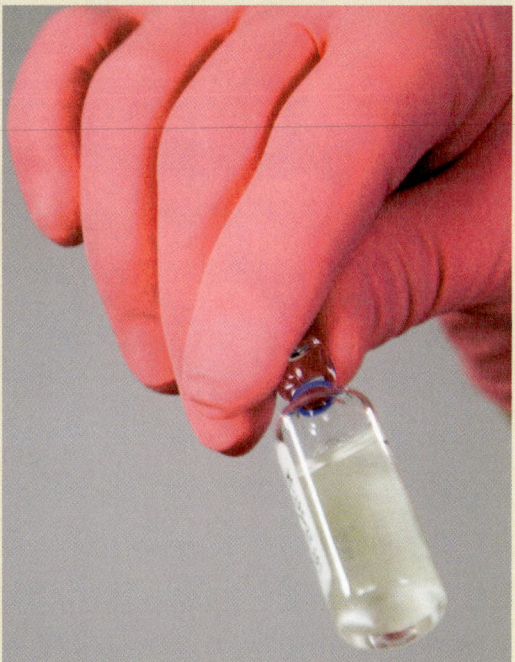

Step 1 Confirm medical direction's order for the medication. Put on appropriate personal protective equipment. Follow the six rights of medication administration. Check the medication for clarity and verify that the drug is not expired. Check the concentration of the medication. To make sure that no medication is wasted when an ampule is opened, clear the contents from the top of it by holding the ampule upright and gently tapping the top of the container with a finger. Alternately, gently swirl the ampule to displace the medication contents from the top of the container.

Continued

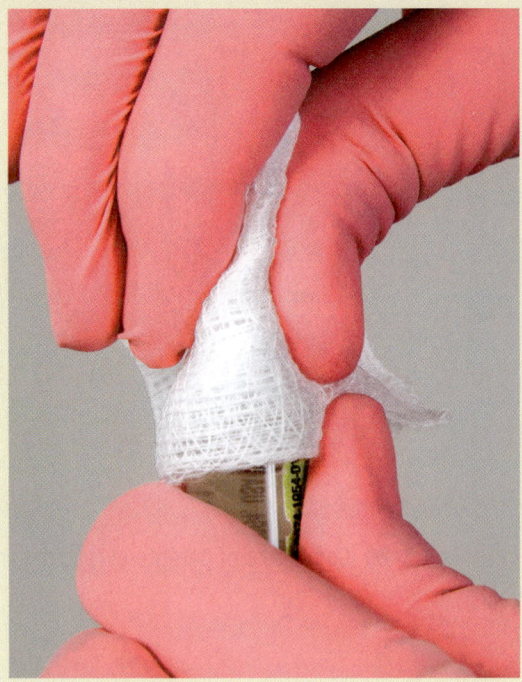

Step 2 Wrap the neck and top of the ampule with an alcohol swab or a 2 × 2 gauze pad.

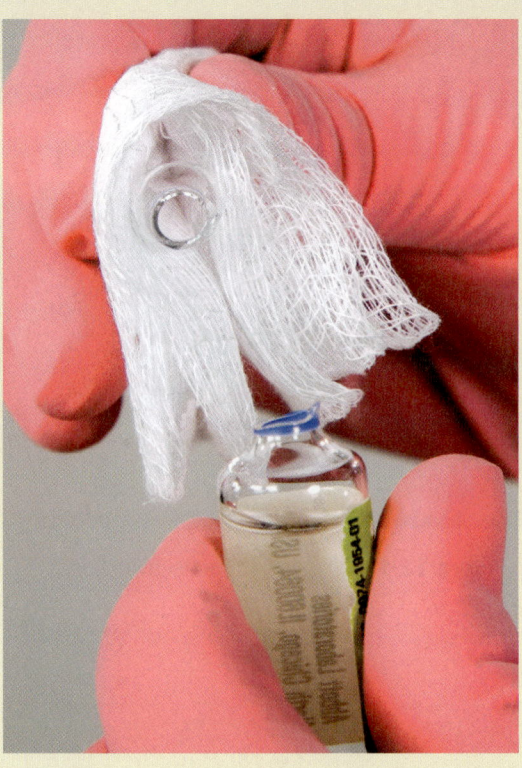

Step 3 To prevent injury, snap the top off the ampule in a direction *away* from you. Replace the sterile needle on the syringe with a filter needle. The filter needle is used to trap glass particles and keep them from entering the syringe.

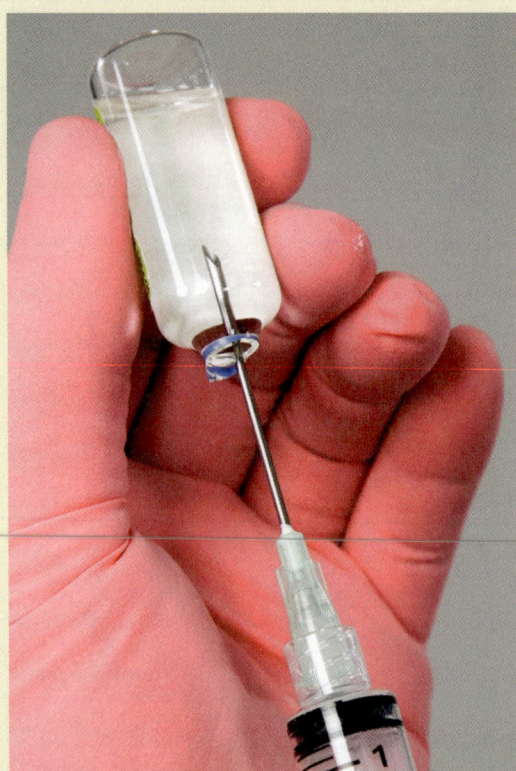

Step 4 With the syringe and filter needle in one hand, place the needle into the solution in the ampule. Be careful not to contaminate the needle by touching the outer surface or rim of the ampule. If the needle is long enough to reach the bottom of the ampule, withdraw the desired dose of medication by pulling back on the plunger. If the needle is not long enough to reach the bottom of the ampule, invert the ampule and withdraw the desired dose. *Do not inject air into an ampule.*

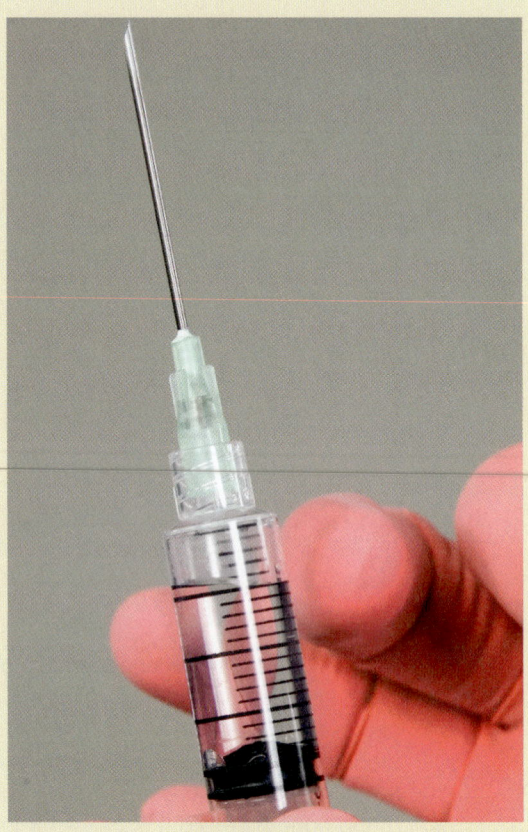

Step 5 Tap the syringe with your finger to remove any air bubbles. Push the plunger to expel the air. Replace the filter needle with the sterile needle that was removed from the syringe. Dispose of sharps in an appropriate container.

SKILL 13-8 WITHDRAWING MEDICATION FROM A VIAL

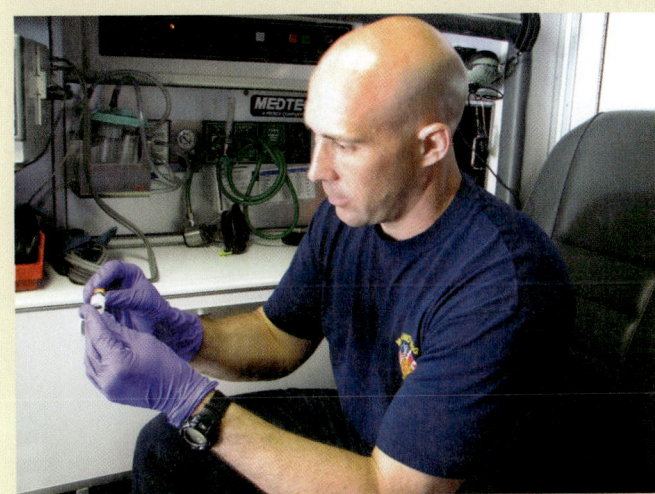

Step 1 Confirm medical direction's order for the medication. Put on appropriate personal protective equipment. Follow the six rights of medication administration. Check the medication for clarity and verify that the drug is not expired. Check the concentration of the medication.

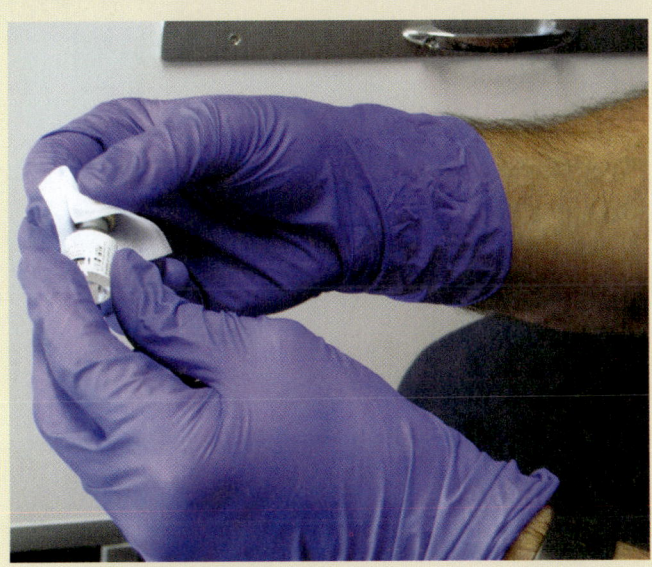

Step 2 If present, remove the protective cover over the vial's rubber stopper. Cleanse the rubber stopper with an alcohol swab. Allow the alcohol to dry.

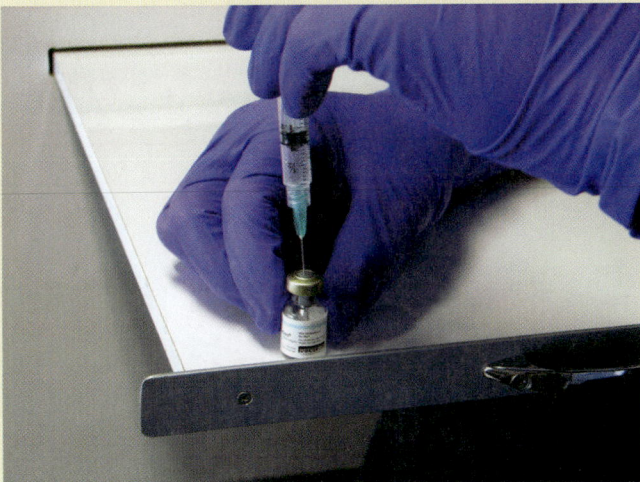

Step 3 With a syringe, pull back the plunger to the desired dose of medication. While securely holding the vial with the thumb and index finger of one hand, insert the needle into the vial. With the needle tip above the level of the solution in the vial, push the plunger on the syringe. This action injects air into the vial equal to the volume of the drug you want to withdraw. This helps prevent the formation of a vacuum in the vial.

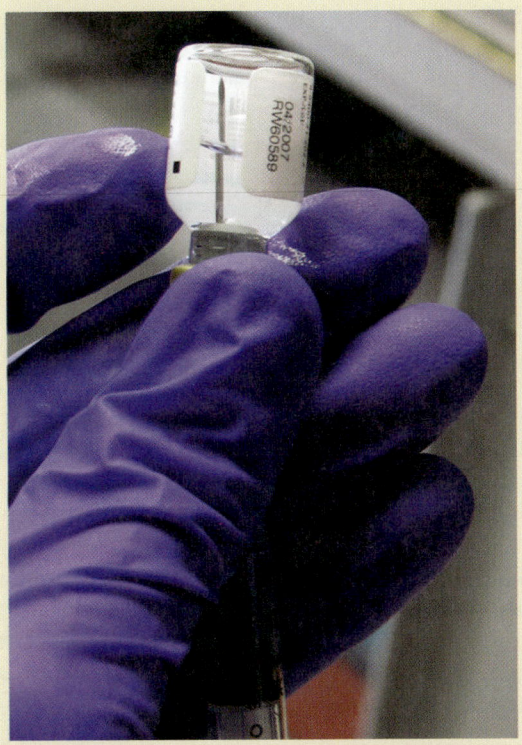

Step 4 Invert the vial and syringe. While holding the vial at eye level, make sure the tip of the needle is below the level of the solution in the vial. If the syringe does not automatically begin to fill with medication, pull the plunger down to the desired dose.

Continued

SKILL 13-8 WITHDRAWING MEDICATION FROM A VIAL—continued

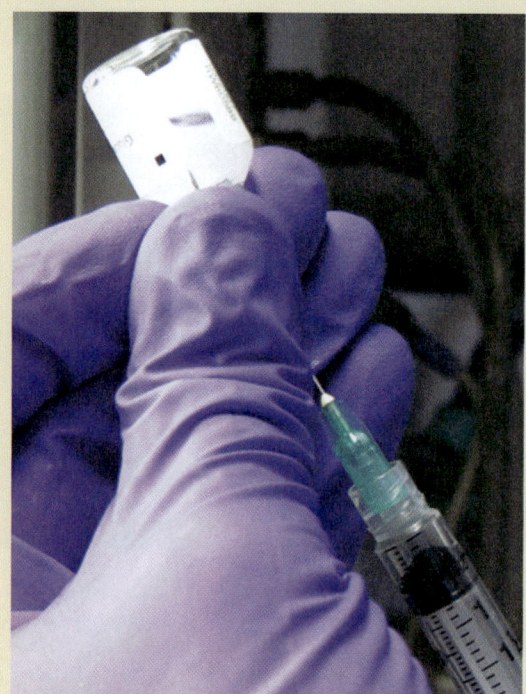

Step 5 Gently tap the syringe with your finger to remove any air bubbles. Push the plunger to expel the air. Adjust the plunger until the exact desired dose is present in the syringe.

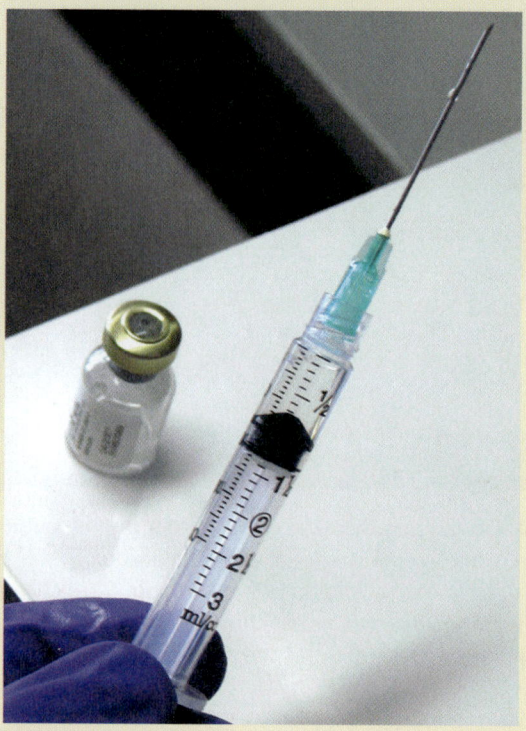

Step 6 Remove the needle from the vial and verify the dose again. Dispose of sharps in an appropriate container.

given intralingually to patients in cardiac arrest when IV or tracheal access is unavailable. After giving an intralingual injection, the patient must be monitored closely for complications such as bleeding or swelling that may compromise the airway. Because the intralingual route is not used by all EMS systems, check with medical direction before administering a drug via this route.

Intradermal Injections. The intradermal route is most often used for tuberculin and allergy testing. Injections are made into the dermal layer of the skin, just below the epidermis (Figure 13-21). Intradermal injections are given with a short ($^3/_8$ to $^5/_8$ inch), small-gauge (26 to 28 gauge) needle and a TB syringe. The dosages used for TB and allergy testing are small but potent. The sites used for injection have a poor blood supply, which permits slow absorption of the solution. Common anatomic sites for allergy testing include the upper chest, upper back just below the shoulder blades, and the inside of the middle to upper forearm. The inside of the middle to upper forearm is commonly used for TB testing.

For an intradermal injection, the needle is inserted at a 10- to 15-degree angle into the dermal layer of the skin. The medication is slowly injected to form a bleb (bump) (Figure 13-22). If a bleb does not form, the medication has been injected into the subcutaneous tissue. Consequently, the test results will be invalid.

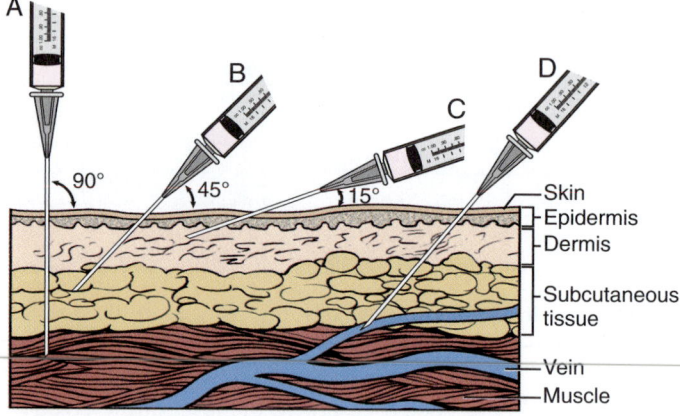

Figure 13-21 Injection routes. *A,* Intramuscular (IM); *B,* subcutaneous (Sub-Q); *C,* intradermal (ID); *D,* intravenous (IV).

Subcutaneous Injections
[OBJECTIVE 19]

When a **subcutaneous (Sub-Q)** injection is given, medication is deposited into the fat or loose connective tissue just under the dermis. Although a $^3/_8$- to $^5/_8$-inch needle typically is used for adults, the needle length depends on the thickness of the patient's subcutaneous tissue. In most cases, the needle is inserted at a 45-degree angle

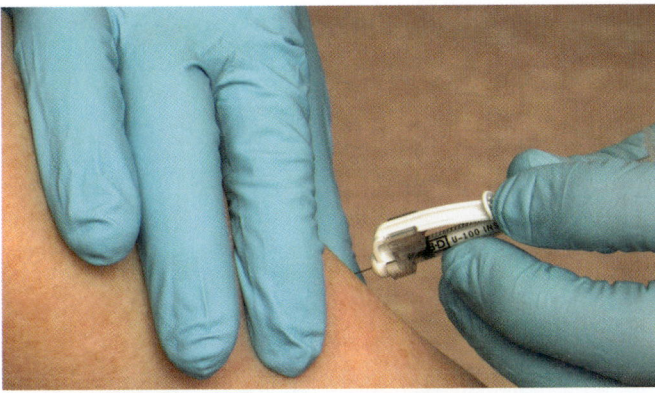

Figure 13-22 Intradermal injection.

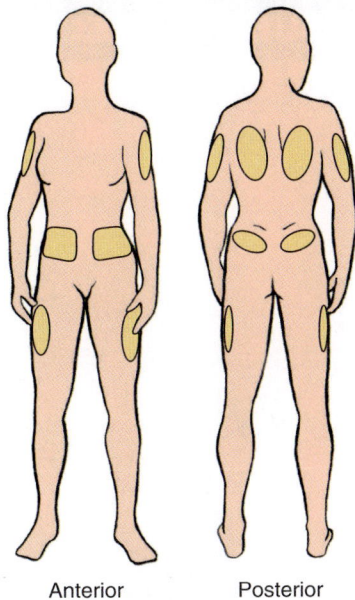

Anterior   Posterior

Figure 13-23 Recommended sites for subcutaneous injections.

BOX 13-9	Supplies for Subcutaneous Injection

- Gloves
- Syringe of appropriate size (3 mL or TB syringe)
- Needle of appropriate size (25 to 28 gauge, ½ to ⅝ inches in length)   *up to 1"*
- Alcohol wipe
- Medication ordered for injection
- Adhesive bandage

TB, Tuberculin.

BOX 13-10	Supplies for IM Injection

- Gloves
- Syringe of appropriate size (3 mL or TB syringe)
- Needle of appropriate size (19 to 23 gauge, 1 to 2 inches in length)   *18*
- Alcohol wipe
- Medication ordered for injection
- Adhesive bandage

IM, Intramuscular; *TB*, tuberculin.

into the subcutaneous tissue. Use a 25-gauge, ½-inch needle for an infant or thin child and a 25-gauge, ⅝-inch needle for a larger child. In a child, the needle is usually inserted at a 90-degree angle, although some healthcare professionals insert the needle at a 45-degree angle if the child has little subcutaneous tissue. Supplies for Sub-Q injection are shown in Box 13-9.

Select an injection site that has relatively few sensory nerve endings and is away from large blood vessels, major nerves, and bony prominences. Recommended sites for Sub-Q injection in adults are shown in Figure 13-23. In children, the most common sites used are the lateral aspect of the upper arms, the abdomen from the costal margins to the iliac crests, and the anterior thighs.

In adults, the maximal volume of medication that can be delivered Sub-Q is 2 mL. In children, the volume is limited to 0.5 to 1.0 mL. The Sub-Q route should not be used to give medications that are irritating to the tissues or are not water soluble. Absorption may be rapid or slow depending on the water solubility of the drug and blood flow to the injection site. Drugs should not be given by this route if the patient shows signs of shock or if the tissue at the selected site is swollen or burned. Skill 13-9 shows the steps to giving a Sub-Q injection.

Intramuscular Injections
[OBJECTIVE 20]

An IM injection penetrates the epidermis, dermis, and subcutaneous tissue into the muscle layer. This route is used when a medication cannot be given orally, a more

rapid onset of action is desired, or the drug is too irritating to be given Sub-Q. Because more blood flows to muscles than to the subcutaneous tissue layer, medications given by the IM route are absorbed more rapidly than those given Sub-Q. Possible complications associated with IM injection include damage to nerves and blood vessels. Nerve damage can result in unnecessary pain and possible paralysis. Damage to blood vessels can result in excessive bleeding.

When selecting a needle for an IM injection, the needle should be of sufficient length to reach the middle of the muscle. The gauge of the needle used depends on the thickness of the medication injected. In general, a 19- to 23-gauge needle is used for an IM injection. A 1- to 2-inch needle is used for most adults. A 1-inch needle may be used for a thin adult. A 2-inch needle may be necessary for a heavy adult. The needle is inserted at a 90-degree angle into the muscle. Supplies needed for an IM injection are shown in Box 13-10.

Multiple sites can be used for an IM injection. The thickness and volume of the medication to be given must

SKILL 13-9 SUBCUTANEOUS INJECTION

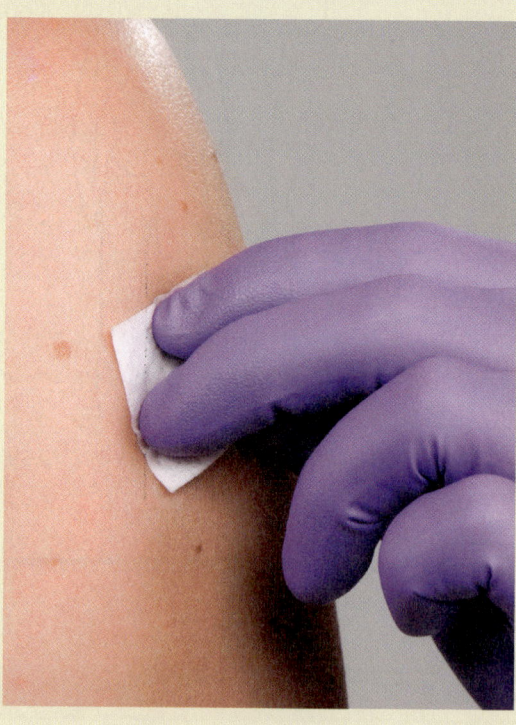

Step 1 Confirm medical direction's order for the medication. Put on appropriate personal protective equipment. Assemble the necessary equipment and explain the procedure to the patient. Follow the six rights of medication administration. Prepare the correct amount of medication. Select an appropriate injection site. Cleanse the site with an alcohol wipe. Use a circular motion, moving from the center of the circle to the outer edge. Allow the alcohol to dry so that alcohol is not injected into the tissue.

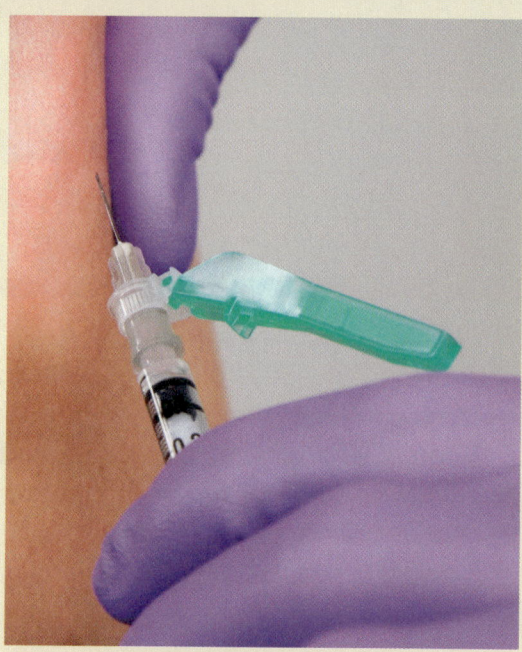

Step 2 Gently pinch the skin and lift the subcutaneous tissue away from the muscle.

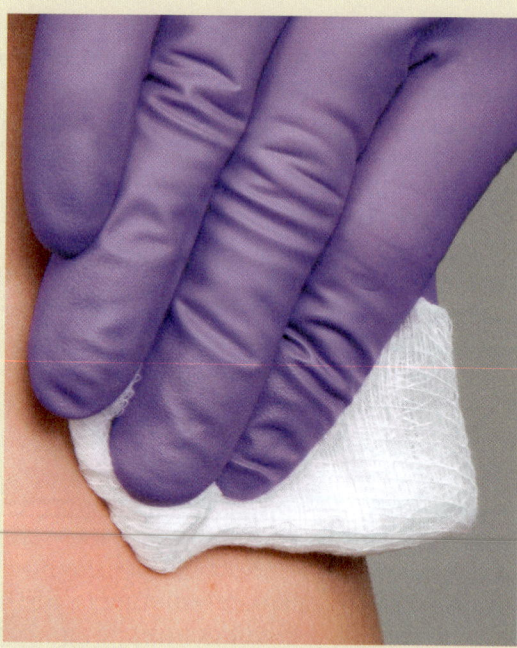

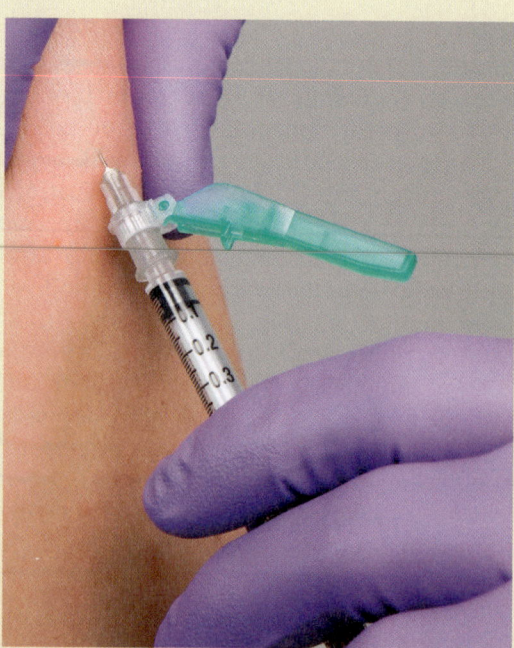

Step 3 Insert the needle into the skin at a 45-degree angle with a quick, darting motion.

Step 4 Release the skin. Pull back slightly on the plunger and check for blood. If blood is present, a blood vessel has been entered; remove the needle. If no blood appears, press the plunger to inject the desired dose of medication. Quickly withdraw the needle. Gently massage the area to disperse the medication into the subcutaneous tissue and hasten absorption unless contraindicated by the medication given. If bleeding is present, apply gentle pressure with a dry gauze pad. Apply an adhesive bandage if necessary. Observe the patient for desired and adverse effects. Dispose of sharps in an appropriate container. Document the procedure.

be considered when selecting an appropriate site. The maximal volume of medication that can be given by the IM route varies by the injection site selected. In an adult, up to 5 mL can be given in some sites. In a child, up to 2 mL can be given depending on the site chosen. See Table 13-2 for information about IM injection sites in children.

Deltoid Site. The deltoid muscle is often used for IM injections in adults because it is easily accessible. Because of its small muscle mass, no more than 2 mL of medication should be injected into the deltoid muscle of an adult. The preferred volume of medication is 0.5 to 1 mL.

The deltoid muscle is triangular shaped. The base of the muscle is attached to the scapula and clavicle. The apex is attached to the humerus. Careful identification of the injection site is important because the radial nerve and brachial artery lie nearby. To identify landmarks, completely expose the upper arm and shoulder. With one hand, find the lower edge of the acromion process (the bony corner of the shoulder) and place your little finger on it (Figure 13-24). Use your other hand to find the lateral aspect of the arm. The injection site is in the base of the upside-down triangle between these two points (approximately 3 finger widths below the acromion process). To lessen the discomfort of a deltoid injection, the patient's forearm should be supported and the elbow bent during the procedure.

Dorsogluteal Site. *Gluteal* refers to the buttocks. The dorsogluteal site is the upper outer quadrant of a buttock.

TABLE 13-2	**IM Injection Sites in Children**			
Site	**Age**	**Needle**	**Considerations**	
Vastus lateralis	Preferred site for infants and children <3 years but may be used in all ages	Use 22- to 25-gauge $\frac{5}{8}$- to 1-inch needle inserted at a 90-degree angle to site	No nearby major nerves or vessels Large, easily accessible muscle Can inject up to 0.5 mL of fluid in infant, 2.0 mL in child	
Ventrogluteal	Consider for children >3 years	Use 22- to 25-gauge $\frac{1}{2}$- to 1-inch needle inserted almost perpendicular to site but angled slightly (10 to 15 degrees) toward iliac crest	No nearby major nerves or vessels Prominent bony landmarks Thin layer of subcutaneous tissue Can inject up to 0.5 mL of fluid in infant, 2.0 mL in child Less painful than vastus lateralis Health care professional often is unfamiliar with site	
Dorsogluteal	Contraindicated in children <3 years and in nonambulatory patients	Use 20- to 25-gauge $\frac{1}{2}$- to 1$\frac{1}{2}$-inch needle inserted perpendicular to surface on which the child in lying when prone	Risk of damage to sciatic nerve Depth of overlying subcutaneous tissue varies between patients Advantage: child does not see needle and syringe Well-developed muscle in older child can tolerate fluid volume of up to 2 mL	
Deltoid	Toddler, preschooler, older child, adolescent	Use 22- to 25-gauge $\frac{1}{2}$- to 1-inch needle inserted at a 90-degree angle to site	Small muscle mass can tolerate only small fluid volume (0.5 to 1 mL) Faster absorption than gluteal sites Easily accessible Less pain than vastus lateralis Possible damage to radial and axillary nerves	

Reprinted from Aehlert, B. (2005). *Mosby's comprehensive pediatric emergency care.* St. Louis: Mosby Elsevier.
IM, Intramuscular.

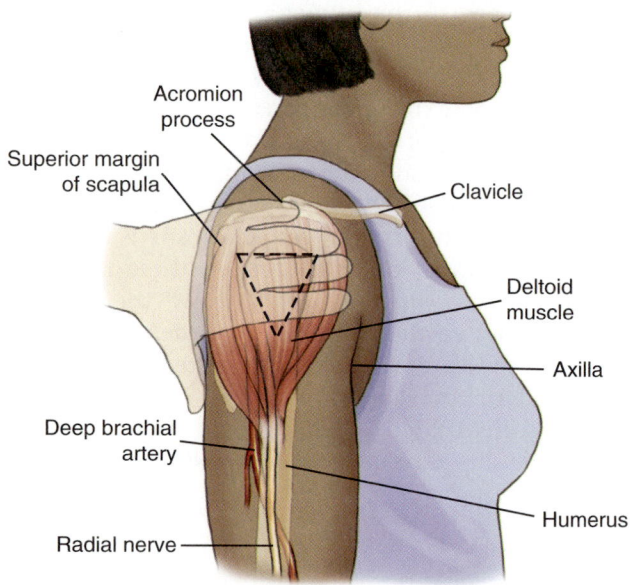

Figure 13-24 Deltoid site for intramuscular injection.

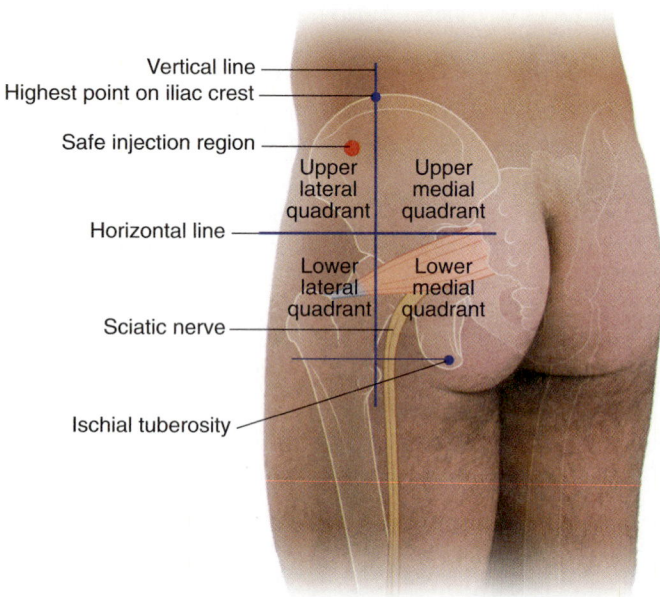

Figure 13-25 Dorsogluteal site for intramuscular injection.

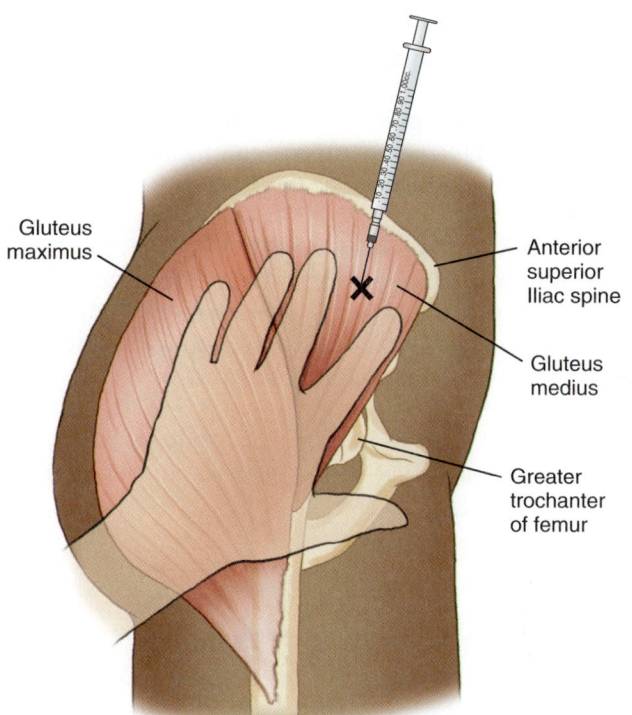

Figure 13-26 Ventrogluteal site for intramuscular injection.

Up to 5 mL of medication can be injected into this site in adults who have well-developed gluteal muscles. The preferred volume of medication is less than 3 mL.

To identify the dorsogluteal injection site, locate the greater trochanter of the femur and the posterior superior iliac spine (Figure 13-25). Draw an imaginary line between the two landmarks. The injection site is above and lateral to the line (the area between the line and the curve of the iliac crest). To lessen the discomfort of a dorsogluteal injection, the patient should be placed in a prone position with the toes pointed inward or on the side with the upper leg flexed at the hip and knee.

Ventrogluteal Site. The ventrogluteal site is preferred over the dorsogluteal site because it has a thick muscle layer and lacks major nerves or blood vessels. To identify the ventrogluteal injection site, place the palm of one hand over the greater trochanter of the femur with the thumb pointing toward the patient's abdomen. Place your index finger on the anterior superior iliac spine. Spread your middle finger toward the iliac crest (Figure 13-26). A V is formed by your index and middle fingers. The ventrogluteal injection site is in the center of the V. To lessen the discomfort of a ventrogluteal injection, the patient should be positioned on the side with the upper leg flexed and forward during the procedure.

Vastus Lateralis and Rectus Femoris Sites. The vastus lateralis and rectus femoris muscles are found in the thigh (Figure 13-27). The vastus lateralis muscle is located on the anterior lateral aspect of the thigh. In adults, it extends from a hand width above the knee to a hand width below the greater trochanter of the femur.

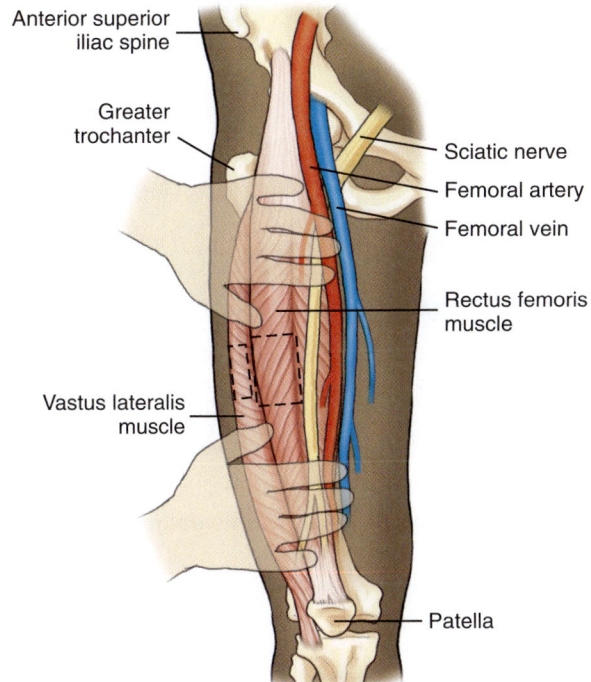

Anterior superior iliac spine
Greater trochanter
Sciatic nerve
Femoral artery
Femoral vein
Rectus femoris muscle
Vastus lateralis muscle
Patella

Figure 13-27 Vastus lateralis and rectus femoris sites for intramuscular injection.

BOX 13-11 Venous Access: Indications

- Maintaining hydration
- Restoring fluid and electrolyte balance
- Providing fluids for resuscitation
- Giving medications
- Giving blood or blood products
- Obtaining blood samples for laboratory analysis

BOX 13-12 Peripheral Venous Access: Advantages

- Effective route for medications during CPR
- Does not require interruption of CPR
- Easier to learn than central venous access
- If an IV attempt is unsuccessful, the site is easily compressible to reduce bleeding
- Results in fewer complications than central venous access

CPR, Cardiopulmonary resuscitation; *IV, intravenous.*

BOX 13-13 Peripheral Venous Access: Disadvantages

- In circulatory collapse, vein may be absent or difficult to access.
- Should be used only for administration of isotonic solutions; hypertonic or irritating solutions may cause pain and phlebitis.
- In cardiac arrest, medications administered from a peripheral vein require 1 to 2 minutes to reach the central circulation.

The middle third of the muscle is the recommended site for injection. Up to 3 mL of medication can be injected into this site in adults. To lessen the discomfort of an injection into the vastus lateralis muscle, position the patient supine with toes pointing toward the midline during the procedure.

The rectus femoris muscle is located on the anterior thigh. Use the middle third of the muscle for injection. Because it is easy to reach, patients who must give themselves an IM injection often use this site. Skill 13-10 shows the steps to give an IM injection.

PARAMEDIC*Pearl*

Because it has few nerves and blood vessels, the vastus lateralis muscle is considered a safe injection site for infants, children, and adults.

Vascular Access
Venous Access
[OBJECTIVE 21]

Various routes may be used for parenteral administration of fluid and/or medications, including the IV route and the intraosseous route. **Intravenous cannulation** is the placement of a catheter into a vein to gain access to the body's venous circulation. **Venipuncture** refers to the piercing of a vein. **Intravenous therapy** refers to administration of a fluid into a vein. IV access may be accomplished by cannulating a peripheral or central vein. A **peripheral vein** is a vein outside the

chest or abdomen. For example, veins of the upper and lower extremities are peripheral veins. The external jugular vein of the neck also is considered a peripheral vein. A **central vein** is a major vein of the chest, neck, abdomen, or pelvis. Examples of central veins include the internal jugular, subclavian, and femoral veins. Indications for venous access are shown in Box 13-11.

Peripheral Venous Access. Peripheral venous access is a commonly performed paramedic skill. It can be performed relatively quickly and, when proper technique and equipment are used, generally results in few complications.

Peripheral venous access is performed much more often than central venous access. Advantages of peripheral venous access are shown in Box 13-12. Disadvantages of peripheral venous access are shown in Box 13-13.

Intravenous Catheters. A peripheral IV line typically consists of a catheter, administration set, and fluid. The most common IV fluids used in the prehospital setting

SKILL 13-10 INTRAMUSCULAR INJECTION

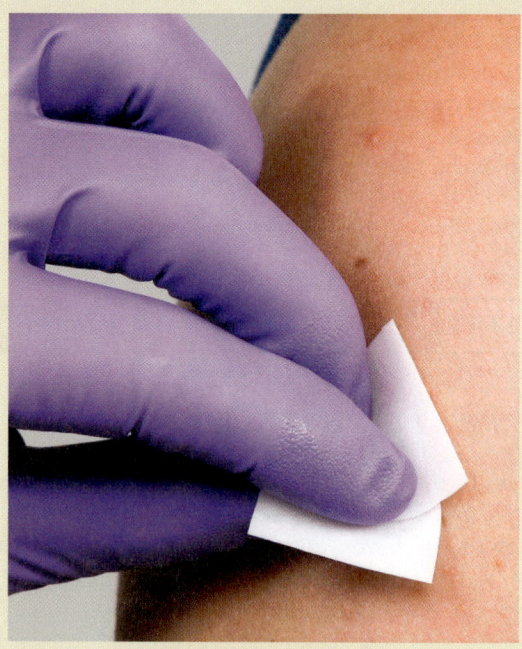

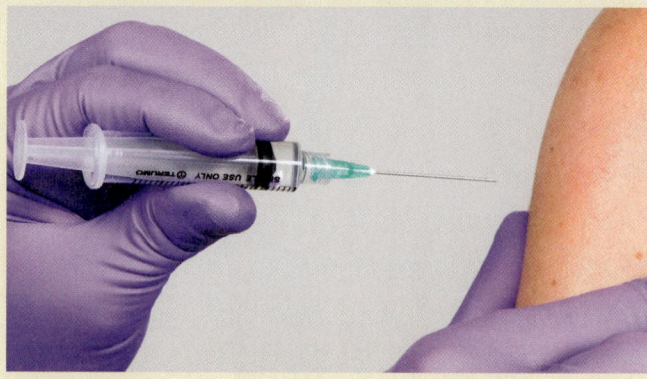

Step 2 Spread the skin at the injection site. This causes less pain and makes insertion of the needle easier.

Step 1 Confirm medical direction's order for the medication. Put on appropriate personal protective equipment. Assemble the necessary equipment and explain the procedure to the patient. Follow the six rights of medication administration. Prepare the correct amount of medication. Select an appropriate injection site. Cleanse the site with an alcohol wipe. Use a circular motion, moving from the center of the circle to the outer edge. Allow the alcohol to dry so that alcohol is not injected into the tissue.

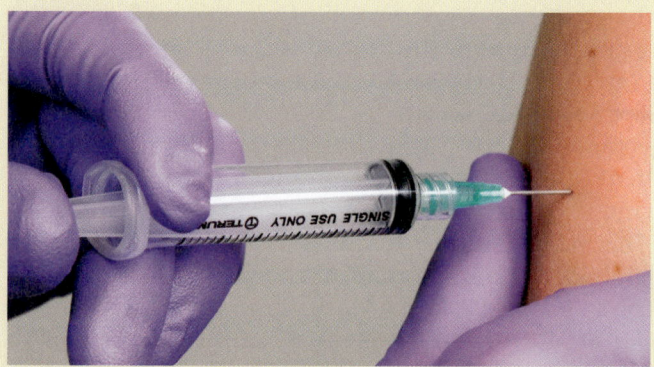

Step 4 Pull back slightly on the plunger and check for blood. If blood is present, a blood vessel has been entered; remove the needle. If no blood appears, press the plunger using a slow, continuous motion to inject the desired dose of medication. Quickly withdraw the needle. Gently massage the area to disperse the medication into the muscle. If bleeding is present, apply gentle pressure with a dry gauze pad. Apply an adhesive bandage if necessary. Observe the patient for desired and adverse effects. Dispose of sharps in an appropriate container. Document the procedure.

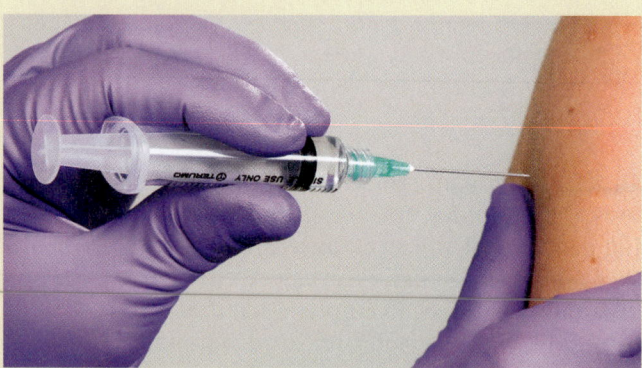

Step 3 While holding the skin taut, insert the needle into the skin at a 90-degree angle with a quick, darting motion.

are normal saline and lactated Ringer's solution. Saline locks are used in some EMS systems (Figure 13-28). A saline lock may be used when a patient requires (or is likely to require) IV medications but does not need a continuous infusion of fluid.

Different types of IV catheters are available. The most commonly used is an over-the-needle catheter (Figure 13-29). The catheter is soft and made of plastic or plastic-like material. The plastic hub of the catheter is color coded. As its name implies, the catheter lies over a hollow metal needle. The length of the catheter is limited by the length of the needle. After the needle enters the vein, the catheter is advanced into the vein and the needle removed. The catheter is left in place to administer fluids. An over-the-needle catheter is available in gauge sizes 10 to 24.

A through-the-needle catheter is mainly used for administration of medications and fluids into the central circulation. A steel needle is used to perform venipuncture. A plastic catheter then slides through the needle and into the vein (Figure 13-30). After the venipuncture is performed, the needle is pulled out of the skin and left attached to the apparatus. A protective device (needle guard) is used to cover the needle to reduce the incidence of catheter shear or trauma to the patient. This type of catheter is rarely used in the field.

A hollow needle IV catheter is also called a *butterfly needle*, *scalp vein needle*, or a *winged infusion set*. It consists of a hollow steel needle with flexible plastic wings and is available in gauge sizes 19 to 27 (Figure 13-31). The wings allow the needle to be taped securely in place. However, a higher risk of fluid or medication seeping out of the vein and into surrounding tissue exists because the needle may puncture the vein after it is inserted.

Like the needles used for Sub-Q and IM injections, IV catheters are available in different gauges and lengths (Table 13-3). Fluid flow rates are proportional to the length of the catheter and its diameter. When rapid volume expansion is needed, use the shortest and smallest gauge catheter possible.

Peripheral Intravenous Sites. Many sites are available for placement of an IV line. Factors to consider when selecting a site include the following:

- Purpose of the infusion
- Amount and type of fluid or medications to be infused
- Accessibility, size, and condition of the vein
- Patient's age, size, general health, hand dominance, and mobility
- Presence of disease, injury, or prior surgery (stroke, burn, mastectomy)
- Presence of a shunt or graft
- Your experience and skill at venipuncture

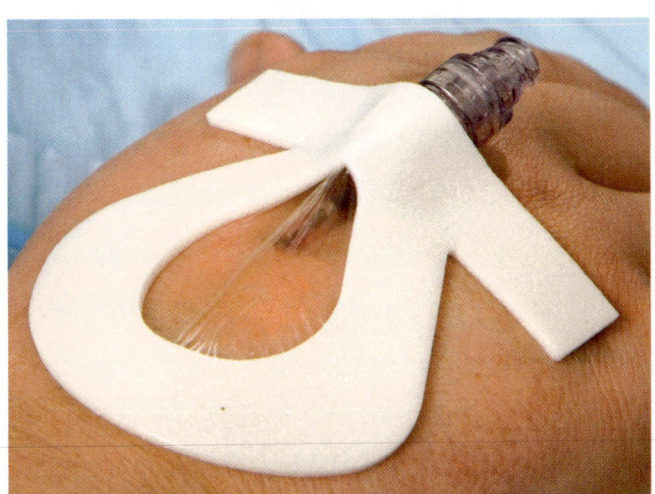

Figure 13-28 Saline lock.

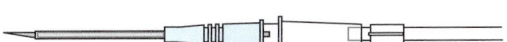

Figure 13-29 An over-the-needle catheter.

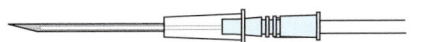

Figure 13-30 Through-the-needle catheter.

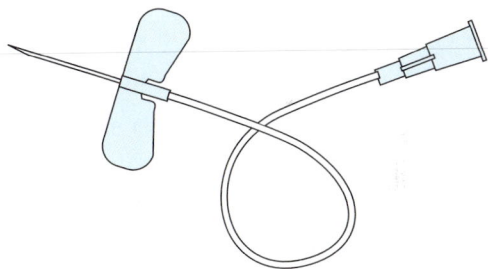

Figure 13-31 Hollow needle, butterfly type.

TABLE 13-3	IV Cannula Selection	
Gauge	Use	Approximate Flow Rate
14 (large bore)	Trauma, surgery, blood administration, administration of thick medications in adolescents and adults	315 mL/min
16 (large bore)	Trauma, surgery, blood administration, administration of thick medications in adolescents and adults	210 mL/min
18	Trauma, surgery; blood administration in older children, adolescents, and adults	110 mL/min
20	Suitable for most IV infusions in older children, adolescents, and adults	65 mL/min
22	Children and elderly patients	38 mL/min
24	Neonates, infants, children, and adults with fragile veins	24 mL/min

Reprinted from Aehlert, B. (2005). *ACLS study guide (3rd ed.).* St. Louis: Mosby.
IV, Intravenous.

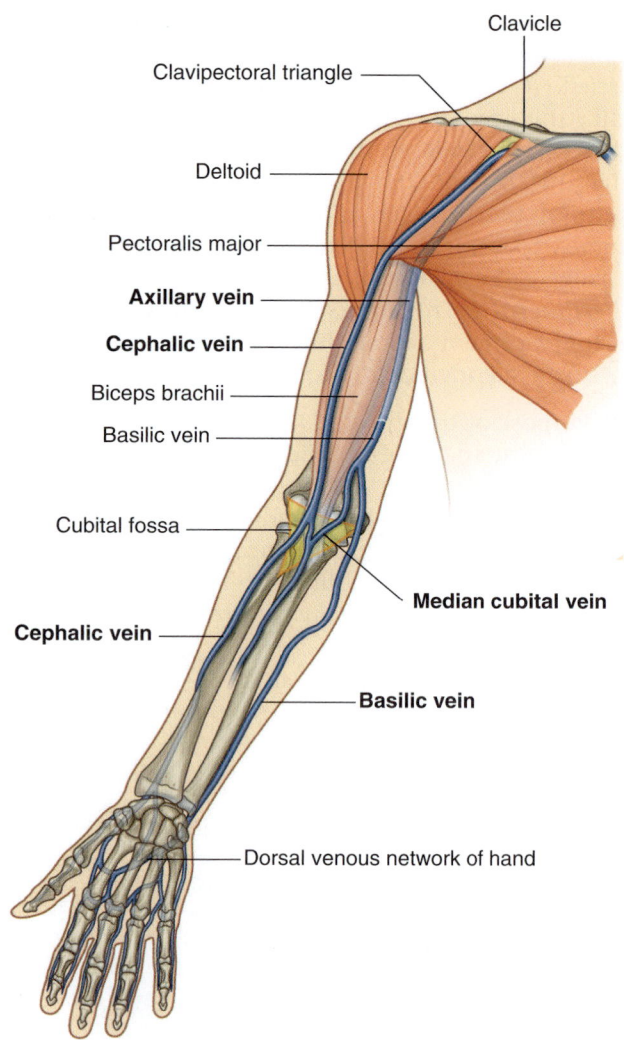

Figure 13-32 Veins of the upper extremity.

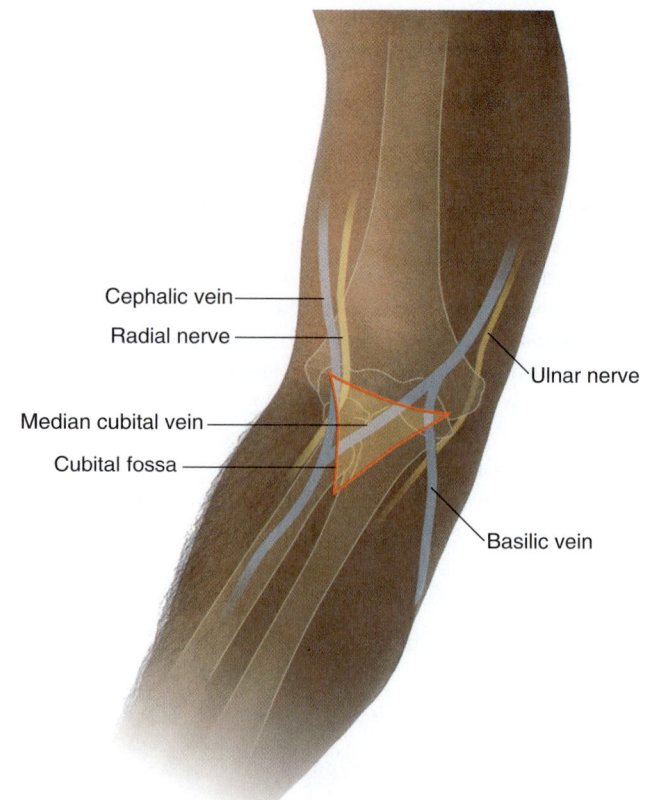

Figure 13-33 The antecubital fossa.

Upper extremity veins are commonly used for peripheral IV access because they usually are the most accessible. The cephalic vein is located on the lateral (thumb) side and the axillary vein on the medial (little finger) side of the forearm (Figure 13-32). The cephalic vein is a large vein that is easy to stabilize and easily accessible. However, movement of the wrist may increase patient discomfort. Irritation to the inner lining of the vessel may result from movement of the cannula. Median veins (cephalic, cubital, and basilic) lie in the antecubital fossa (Figure 13-33). The antecubital vein is usually easily accessible. Cannulation of this vein typically does not interfere with ventilations, chest compressions, or other emergency care. However, accessing the antecubital vein may result in limited movement of the joint and flow restriction if the patient bends the arm. If an attempt to cannulate the antecubital vein is unsuccessful (i.e., it "blows"), distal veins may not be usable. Dorsal hand veins are tributaries of the cephalic and basilic veins (Figure 13-34). If the patient's condition and the condition of the veins allow, assess all veins (instead of simply going for the antecubital vein) and begin distally, working in a proximal direction.

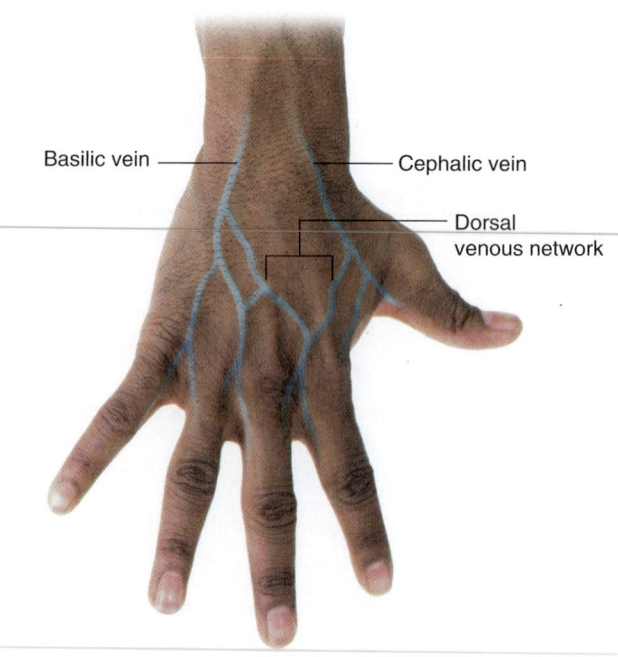

Figure 13-34 Veins of the hand.

Lower extremity veins include the saphenous (Figure 13-35) and dorsal venous arch (Figure 13-36). Because cannulation of the veins of the legs, feet, and ankles may compromise lower extremity circulation, they are not commonly used in the field for IV access. If an IV line must be started in a lower extremity, the saphenous vein is the preferred site.

The external jugular (EJ) vein lies superficially along the lateral portion of the neck (Figure 13-37). It extends from behind the angle of the jaw and passes downward across the sternocleidomastoid muscle and then under the middle of the clavicle to join the subclavian vein. The

EJ vein is usually easy to cannulate because the vein is superficial and easy to see. Pressure and tension applied to the EJ vein just above the clavicle causes the vessel to distend, making cannulation easier. The EJ vein may be difficult to access in emergency situations when healthcare personnel are working to manage the airway. An EJ vein may be easily dislodged and often is positional with head movement.

PARAMEDIC*Pearl*

The EJ vein is considered a peripheral vein.

When selecting a site, avoid placing an IV line in an injured or swollen extremity if an alternate site is available. An IV line should not be placed in an extremity that contains a dialysis shunt or graft or on the side of the body where a radical mastectomy was performed. Avoid starting lower extremity lines if possible, particularly in older adults and patients who have peripheral vascular disease.

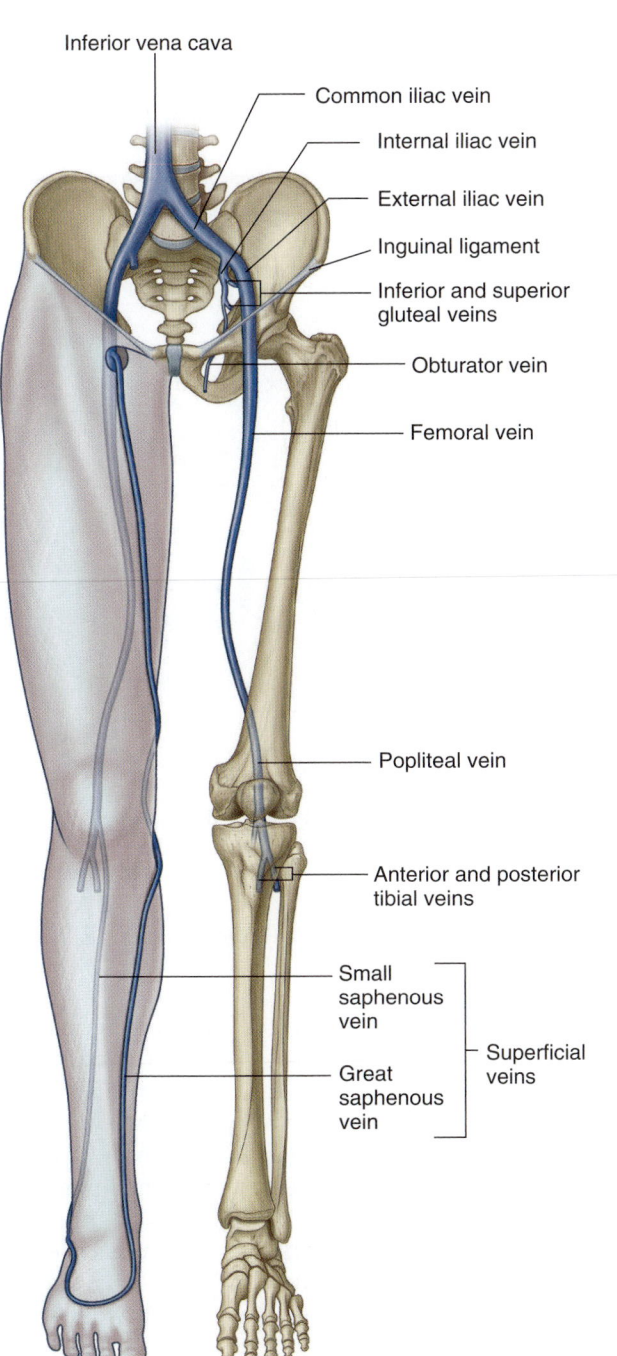

Figure 13-35 Veins of the lower extremity.

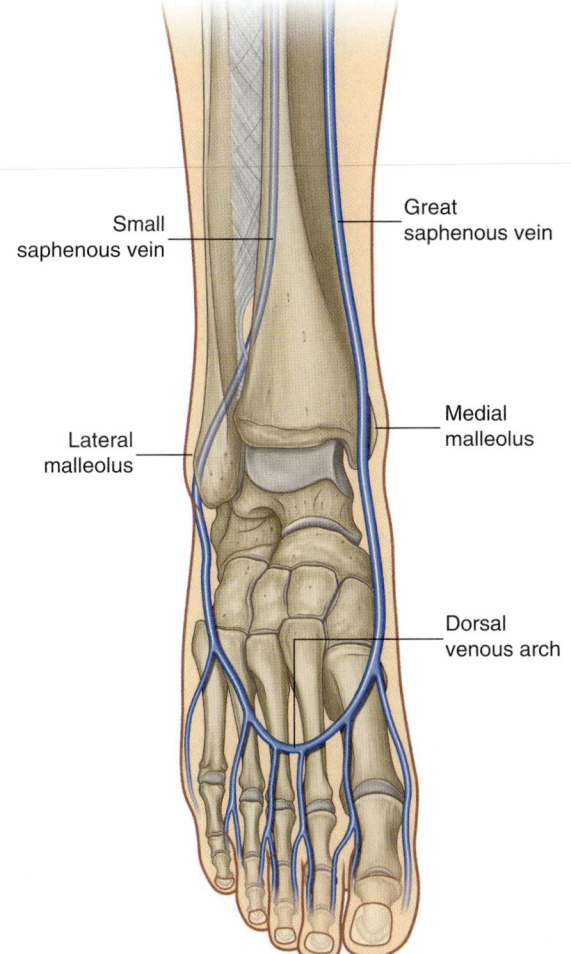

Figure 13-36 Veins of the foot.

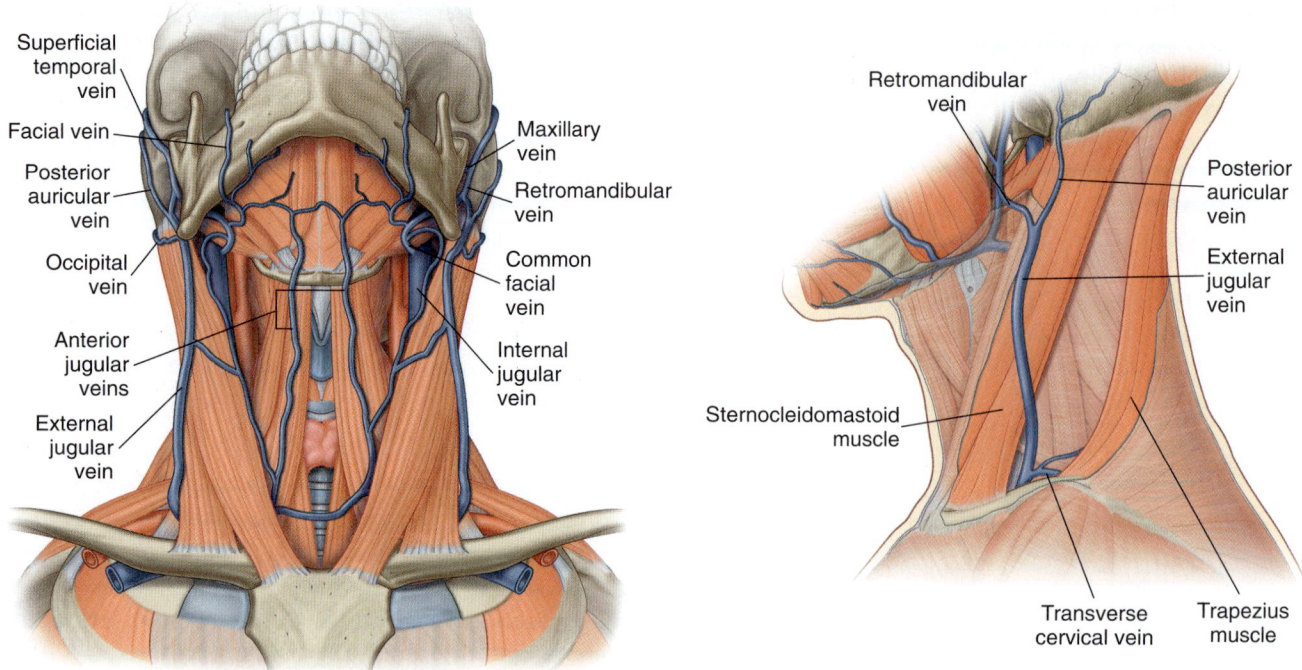

Figure 13-37 Veins of the neck.

BOX 13-14	Supplies Needed for Peripheral Venous Access

- Gloves
- IV catheter
- IV fluid
- IV administration set
- Alcohol or iodine wipes
- Antibiotic ointment (optional)
- Tourniquet (*not* used for EJ cannulation)
- Tape
- Gauze sponges
- Transparent polyurethane dressing (optional)
- Syringes, Vacutainers for blood samples
- Sharps container, biohazard bag

IV, Intravenous; *EJ*, external jugular.

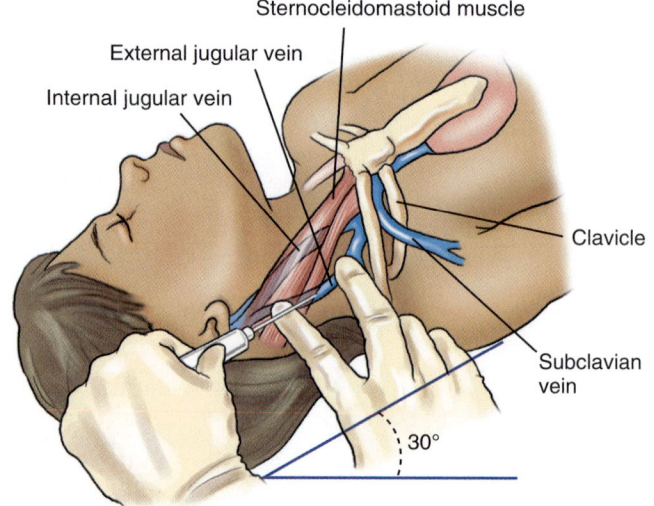

Figure 13-38 Cannulating the external jugular (EJ) vein.

Peripheral Intravenous Insertion. If the patient is awake, explain the procedure and why it is necessary. In addition to taking a SAMPLE history, be sure to ask the patient about allergies to latex, tape, and iodine (if you will be using iodine swabs). Box 13-14 list the supplies typically needed to start an IV line. Skill 13-11 shows the steps to starting an IV line with an over-the-needle catheter in an extremity.

External Jugular Vein Cannulation. To cannulate the EJ vein, the patient ideally should be positioned in a supine, head-down position of 30 degrees. If no head or neck trauma is suspected, turn the patient's head to the left (the right side is preferred for venipuncture), away from the venipuncture site. Cleanse the site. Apply pres-sure to the EJ vein just above the clavicle (Figure 13-38). This temporarily occludes the vessel and causes it to distend, making cannulation easier. Apply slight traction to the vein to stabilize it. Advance the needle at a small angle from the skin plane (approximately 10 degrees) until a "pop" is felt as the needle enters the lumen of the vein. Advance the catheter slightly after feeling the pop to ensure placement within the vessel. Remove the needle and attach a prepared administration set. If the site is patent, adjust the flow of the infusion to the desired rate. Secure the catheter in place.

Central Venous Access. A central venous catheter (also called a *central line*) is inserted into the vena cava

SKILL 13-11 PERIPHERAL VENOUS ACCESS

Follow these steps to start an IV line with an over-the-needle catheter in an extremity.

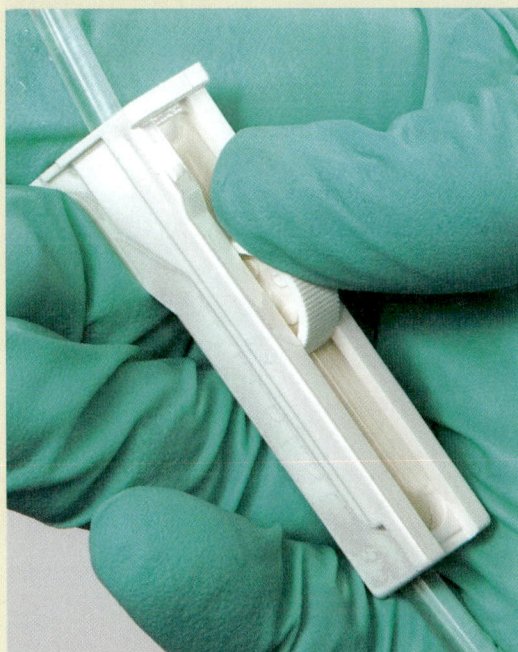

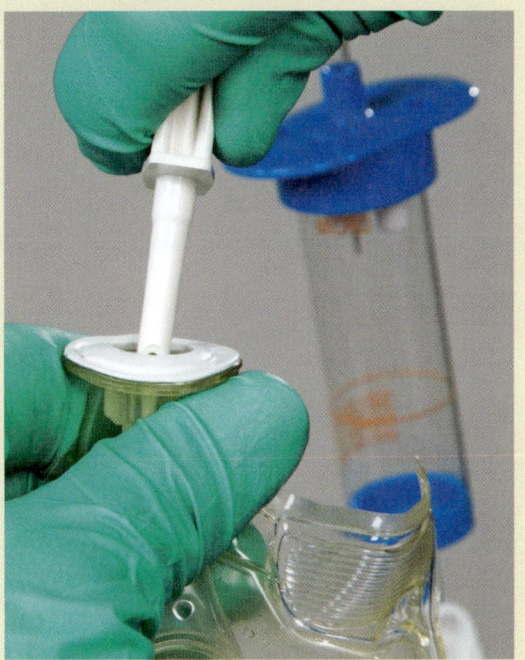

Step 1 Put on appropriate personal protective equipment. Assemble the supplies needed for the procedure.

Make certain that the fluid you will be administering is appropriate for the patient's situation. Check the expiration date on the fluid to ensure that it is not outdated. Check the clarity of the solution and make sure the bag has no leaks.

Select an IV catheter of appropriate length and gauge based on the patient's condition. Select a microdrip or macrodrip administration set appropriate for the patient's condition. Clamp the tubing.

Step 2 Insert the spiked end of the tubing into the bag.

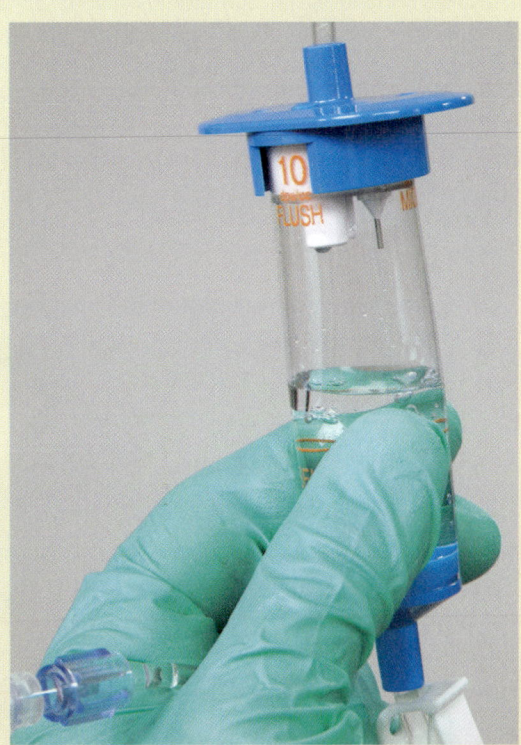

Step 3 Squeeze the drip chamber of the tubing until the chamber fills halfway. Loosen (but do not remove) the protective cap over the needle adapter to allow air to escape. Open the clamp slowly and flush the air from the tubing. Flick the tubing with a finger to remove any air bubbles. Close the clamp and retighten the protective cap.

Continued

SKILL 13-11   PERIPHERAL VENOUS ACCESS—continued

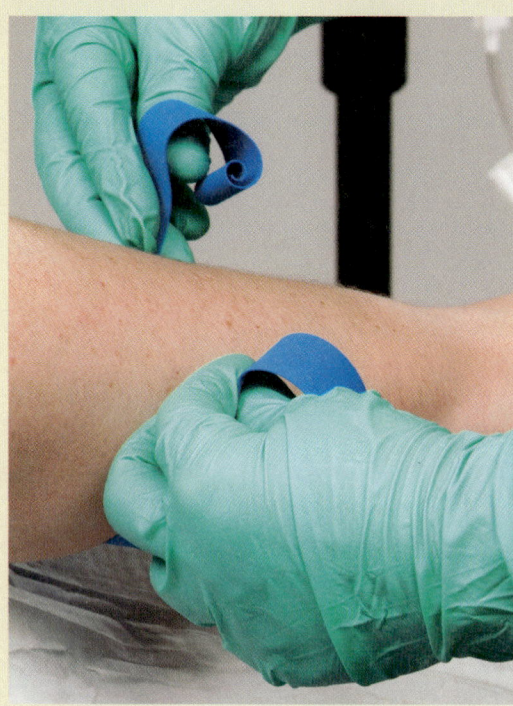

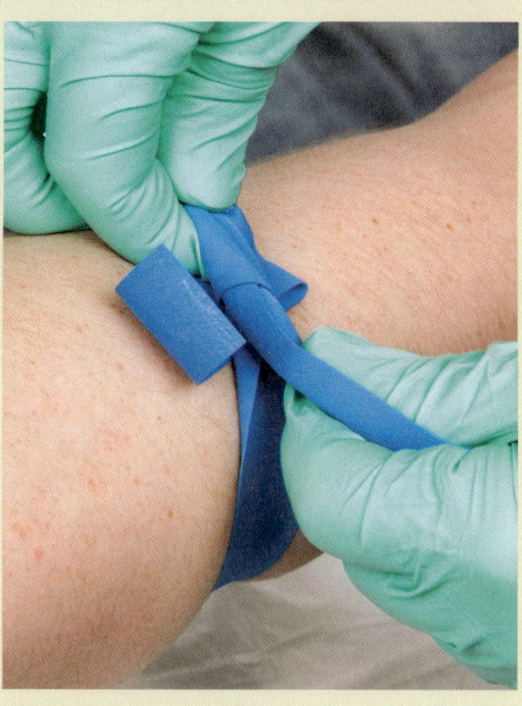

Step 4 Apply a tourniquet approximately 4 inches above the proposed insertion site. The tourniquet (which is actually a venous constricting band) should be applied tight enough to restrict venous blood flow without cutting off the arterial circulation. The tourniquet is too tight if a pulse cannot be felt below the tourniquet site. If the vein is not adequately distended, ask the patient to open and close the fist several times. Cross the ends of the tourniquet and apply tension.

Step 5 Fold the middle portion of one end of the tourniquet under the opposite end to form a loop. Leave the distal portion of the folded end free to allow release of the tourniquet with one hand.

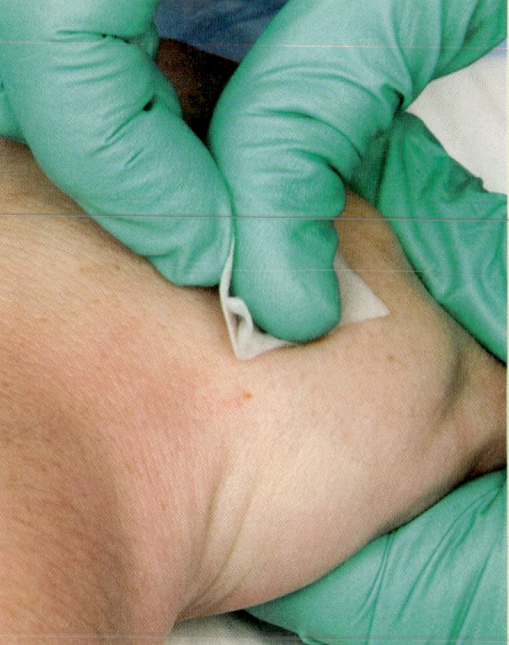

Step 6 Cleanse the intended insertion site according to your EMS agency's policy. This is usually done with a povidone-iodine swab followed by an alcohol swab. Begin in the center and work outward in a circular motion for 2 inches. Allow the area to air dry. Do not fan the area or blow on it because this will deposit microorganisms on the area that was just cleaned.

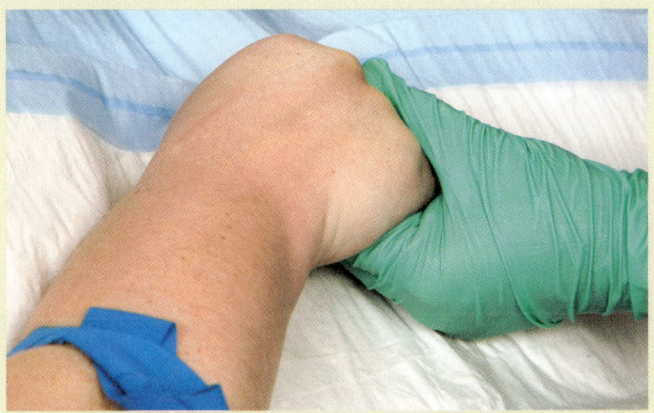

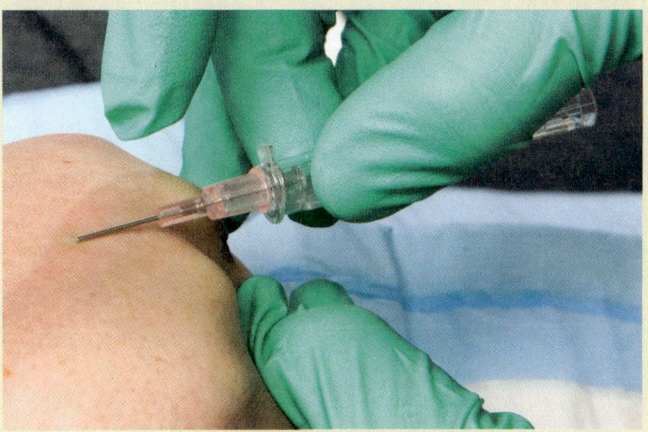

Step 7 With your nondominant hand, anchor the vein by placing your thumb approximately 2 inches directly below the insertion site and hold the skin taut. This is an important step that helps to prevent the vein from rolling. It also helps prevent the skin just below the insertion site from bunching up as the IV catheter is inserted. If the skin is held too tightly, you will be unable to see and/or feel the vein.

Step 8 Puncture the vein using the direct or indirect method of entry. When preparing to puncture the vein, use your dominant hand to hold the IV catheter. To pierce the skin, the IV catheter is held with the bevel up and at a 15- to 30-degree angle to the intended insertion site. Once the skin has been punctured, the IV catheter is quickly lowered so that the catheter's hub is nearly parallel to the skin. Decreased resistance and/or a "pop" may be felt as the needle enters the vein.

Direct method (one-step) Let the patient know he or she will feel a stick. In one continuous motion, enter the skin and vein. This method is useful for large, stable veins.

Indirect method (two-step) Let the patient know he or she will feel a stick. Insert the IV catheter through the skin slightly distal to the site of anticipated vein entry. While keeping the skin taut with your nondominant hand, locate the vein and then gently ease the needle into the vein from the top or the side. This method is useful for smaller veins and is less likely to push the IV catheter completely through the vein.

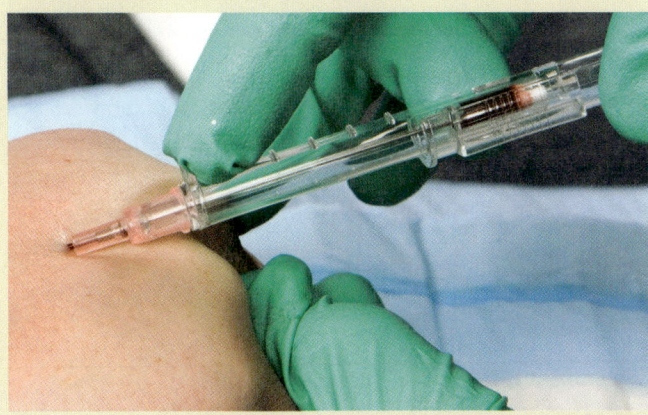

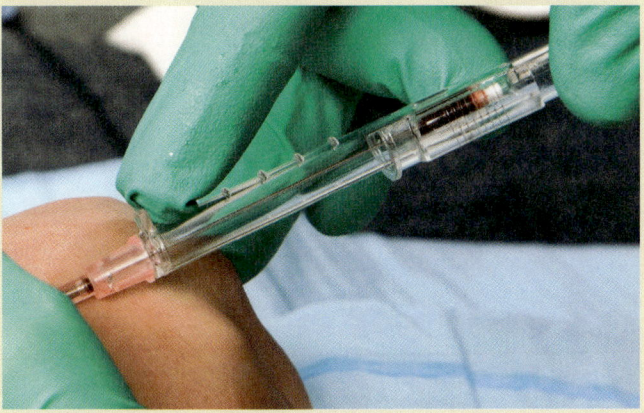

Step 9 If the vein has been successfully entered, a return of blood (flashback) will be visible in the hub of the IV catheter. When the flash of blood is seen, advance the catheter 2 to 3 mm more to make sure it has entered the vein and not just the vein wall. When you are certain the catheter is in the vein, advance the catheter over the needle all the way to the catheter hub.

Step 10 Apply light pressure to the vein proximal to the catheter tip to slow the escape of blood.

Continued

SKILL 13-11 PERIPHERAL VENOUS ACCESS—continued

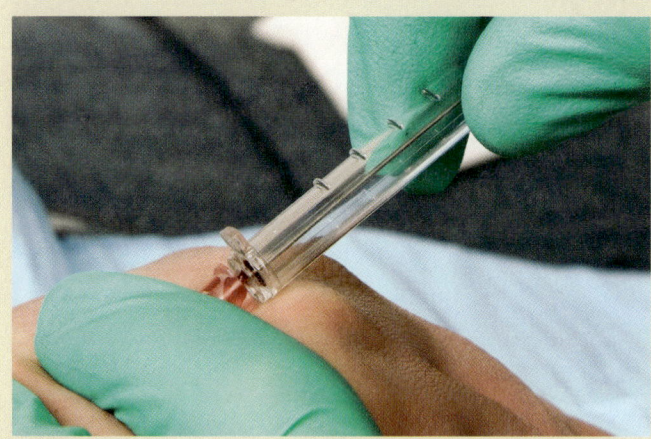

Step 11 Remove the needle portion of the cannula with your dominant hand. Dispose of the needle in an appropriate container.

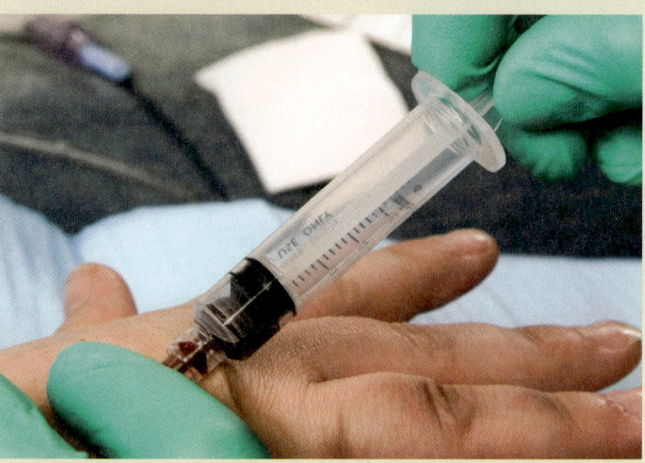

Step 12 Attach a syringe to the IV catheter and withdraw blood if blood samples are needed.

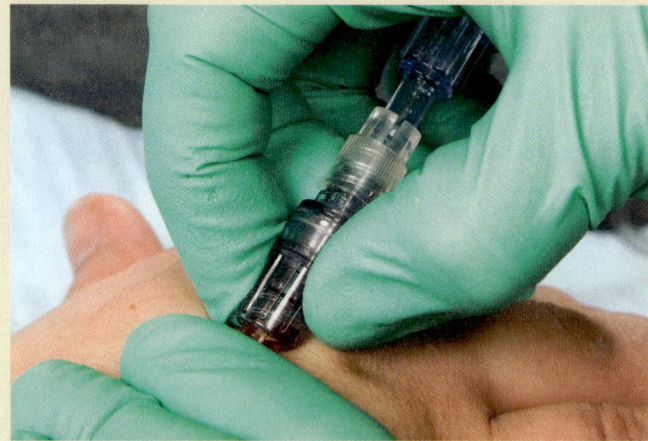

Step 13 Release the tourniquet and connect the administration set to the catheter. Make sure the connection between the catheter and tubing is secure.

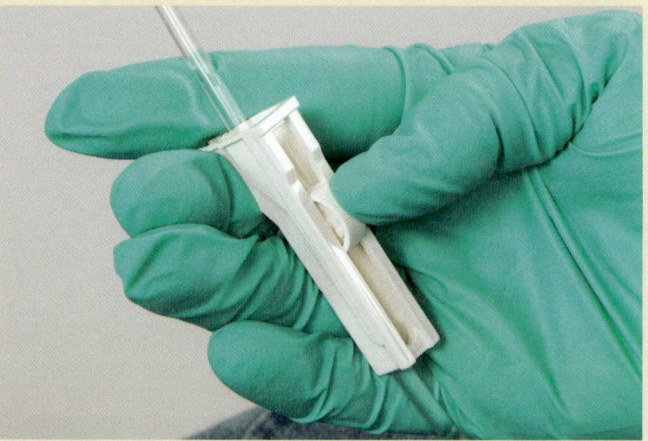

Step 14 Slowly open the clamp on the tubing. Look closely at the site for signs of swelling or leakage of fluid from the site. If the site is patent, adjust the flow of the infusion to the prescribed rate.

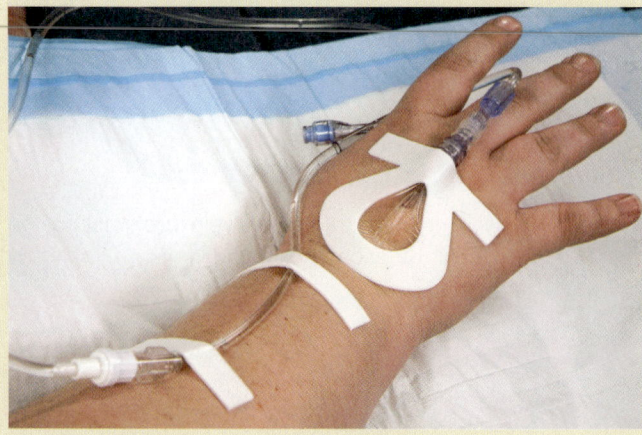

Step 15 Secure the catheter in place.

from the subclavian, EJ, or femoral vein. Indications for central venous access include the following:

- Emergency access to venous circulation when peripheral sites are not readily accessible
- Need for long-term IV therapy
- Administration of large volumes of fluid
- Administration of blood products, hypertonic solutions, caustic medications, or parenteral feeding solutions
- Placement of transvenous pacemaker electrodes
- Central venous pressure monitoring or central venous blood sampling

Central venous access allows rapid volume expansion and delivery of medications closer to their sites of action. It is considered by some to be a more reliable route of venous access than peripheral venous cannulation. However, it has a higher complication rate than peripheral venipuncture. Skill deterioration often occurs because of the infrequency with which this skill is performed in the field. Central venous access requires special training and approval by medical direction. Central venous catheters implanted for long-term use are discussed in Chapter 51.

Complications of Vascular Access.
Local complications of IV therapy are most often seen at or near the insertion site and are more common than systemic complications. Systemic complications occur within the vascular system, usually distant from the insertion site. Some local complications can lead to more serious systemic complications.

Local Complications. Local complications of IV therapy are listed in Box 13-15. A **hematoma** may occur because of advancement of the needle completely through the vein or inadequate application of pressure to prevent leakage of blood from the vein when the needle is removed. Signs and symptoms include bruising over and around the insertion site, pain at the site, swelling and hardness at the insertion site, inability to flush the IV line, or inability to advance the cannula all the way into the vein during insertion.

BOX 13-15 Local Complications of IV Therapy

- Pain and irritation
- Cellulitis
- Phlebitis
- Thrombosis
- Bleeding
- Hematoma formation
- Venous spasm
- Inadvertent arterial puncture
- Nerve, tendon, ligament, and/or limb damage
- Infiltration and extravasation

IV, Intravenous.

Infiltration is the intentional or unintentional process in which a substance enters or infuses into another substance or a surrounding area. Extravasation is the actual (unintentional) escape or leakage of an agent that is irritating and causes blistering (a vesicant) from a vessel into the surrounding tissue. Possible causes include the following:

- Dislodgement of the catheter from the vein
- Puncture of the distal vein wall during venipuncture
- Leakage of solution into the surrounding tissue from the cannula's insertion site
- Poorly secured line
- Poor vein or site selection
- Irritating solution or medication that inflames the intima of the vein and causes it to weaken
- Improper cannula size
- High delivery rate or pressure of the solution or medication

Infiltration is one of the most common complications of IV therapy. If normal saline infiltrates, it is isotonic to tissue fluid and does the least amount of damage. However, if the fluid contains a medication, that drug becomes concentrated in the tissue as opposed to flowing within the bloodstream. If the drug has vasoconstricting properties, it will immediately stop the blood flow to the area, which can lead quickly to tissue death.

Signs and symptoms include coolness of the skin around the site, swelling at the site (with or without pain), sluggish or absent flow rate, an infusion that continues to infuse when pressure is applied proximal to the vein above the cannula tip, or no backflow of blood into the tubing when the clamp is fully opened and the solution is lowered below the site.

If signs and symptoms of infiltration or extravasation are present, immediately discontinue the line. Start an IV line in another site with new equipment. Document and immediately report this when arriving at the emergency department, especially if medication was in the IV bag. A drug that reverses the vasoconstriction can quickly be injected into the area, restoring blood flow.

A **thrombus** (clot) can form if the hematoma remains in place and can result in a **thromboembolism,** meaning that the clot has begun to move within the circulatory system. Thrombosis and thrombophlebitis may be caused by inflammation and injury to the endothelial cells of the vein wall. Signs and symptoms may include a slowed or stopped infusion rate, aching or burning sensation at the infusion site, skin that is warm and red around the site, swelling of the extremity, and/or throbbing pain in the limb.

Venous spasm may be caused by a severe reaction to irritating medications or fluids, administration of cold fluids, or blood. Examples include substances with a high or low pH, diazepam (Valium), phenytoin (Dilantin), and dextrose solutions with concentrations higher than 12.5%. Signs and symptoms include a sluggish or stopped infusion rate when the clamp is completely open, severe pain from the site radiating up the extremity, blanching of the skin over the site, or redness over and around the site.

An **arterial puncture** can occur if you are not careful about the site chosen. If a vessel is pulsating under your fingertips, it is an artery. Two major complications can result. The first is arterial bleeding. The second would occur if you continued to insert the catheter and gave medication directly into the artery. If administered arterially, some medications crystallize and may completely occlude the arterial blood supply distal to the point of injection, resulting in permanent interruption of the blood supply to the affected area.

Cellulitis is a diffuse inflammation and infection of cellular and subcutaneous connective tissue that can lead to abscess formation and ulceration of deeper tissues. Signs and symptoms include pain, tenderness, warmth, swelling, red streaking on skin (if spread to the lymphatic system), roughened appearance of the skin (like that of an orange peel), fever, and chills.

Nerve, tendon, ligament, and/or limb damage may be caused by improper venipuncture technique, improper securing and stabilization of the cannula and line after insertion, extravasated solution, or cellulitis. Signs and symptoms include tingling, numbness, and loss of sensation, loss of movement, cyanosis, pallor, deformity, or paralysis.

Systemic Complications. Systemic complications of IV therapy are listed in Box 13-16. A hypersensitivity reaction can occur as a response to the solution, its preservatives, or medications. The patient may have an allergy to the cannula, antiseptic preparation, or tape. Signs and symptoms can range from mild to severe; affect several body systems; and may develop rapidly, gradually, or be delayed hours after the allergen has been administered.

Speed shock is a systemic reaction to the rapid or excessive infusion of medication or solution into the circulation. Signs and symptoms include flushing of head and neck, apprehension, hypertension, pounding headache, dyspnea, chest pain, chills, loss of responsiveness, and cardiac arrest.

A **pulmonary embolism** may result from a thrombus that forms from trauma to the intima of a vein. Blood flow past the thrombus can cause a portion of the clot to break off and become an embolus. Signs and symptoms may include dyspnea, tachypnea, dysrhythmias, hypotension, diaphoresis, anxiety, and/or a cough.

A **catheter shear/catheter fragment embolism** occurs when the tip of the catheter is literally sheared off while in the patient's vein. To keep this from happening, never try to push the needle back into the catheter once the venipuncture is made and you have attempted to slide the catheter off the needle. Signs and symptoms include sudden, severe pain at the site and/or a reduced or absent blood return when checking placement of the catheter. If the catheter fragment does not travel, the patient may be asymptomatic. If the catheter fragment lodges in a heart chamber or the pulmonary circulation, the patient may experience hypotension, tachycardia, chest pain, cyanosis, and/or a loss of responsiveness.

An **air embolism** occurs when air enters the bloodstream. Air can enter the circulation during catheter insertion, when the tubing is disconnected to replace a solution, or when a container of solution runs dry. The air introduced into venous circulation travels back to the right heart and can impede blood flow through the heart, resulting in shock. A sudden onset of the signs and symptoms of shock is a good indicator of air embolism. These include sudden hypotension; pallor leading to cyanosis; cool and clammy skin; weak, thready, rapid pulse; and diminished level of consciousness.

If you suspect an air embolism, immediate intervention is required. Immediately turn the patient on the left side with the head lower than the rest of the body. Administer high-flow oxygen and notify medical direction. On arrival at the emergency department, a catheter can be inserted into the subclavian vein and passed down through the superior vena cava and into the right heart. The air can then be evacuated.

This complication also can occur with central venous cannulation because the negative pressure of the system can "pull in" environmental air once the venipuncture is made or when the tubing is disconnected from the catheter to replace a bag of solution. Therefore, with a sterile glove, place a finger over the opening until reconnection of the tubing is accomplished.

Intravenous Medications. Intravenous medications may be given as a single dose of medication or by continuous or intermittent infusion.

Intravenous Bolus Medications. An IV bolus is the delivery of a drug directly into an infusion port on an administration set using a syringe. An IV bolus typically is given when a rapid response to a drug is desired. Skill 13-12 shows the steps of administering IV bolus medication.

Intravenous Piggyback. An IV piggyback (IVPB) is also called an *intermittent infusion*. With this method of medication administration, a second solution is "piggybacked" into an already established primary administration set. By piggybacking a second line into

---

BOX 13-16	Systemic Complications of IV Therapy

- Sepsis
- Fluid overload/speed shock
- Hypersensitivity reactions
- Air embolism
- Catheter-fragment embolism
- Pulmonary thromboembolism

IV, Intravenous.

SKILL 13-12 IV BOLUS MEDICATION

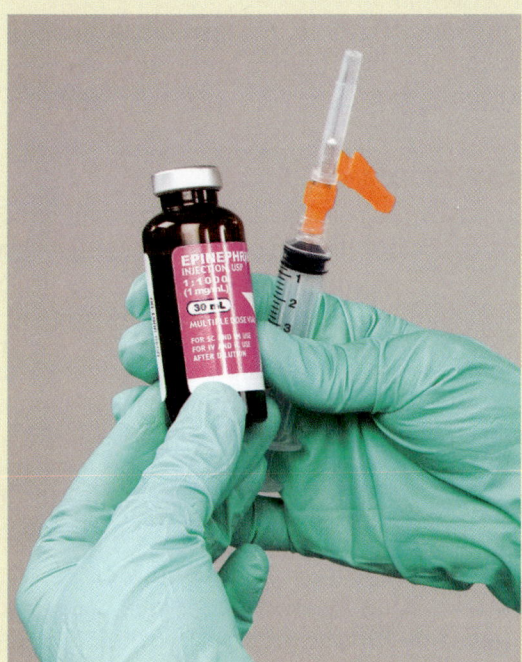

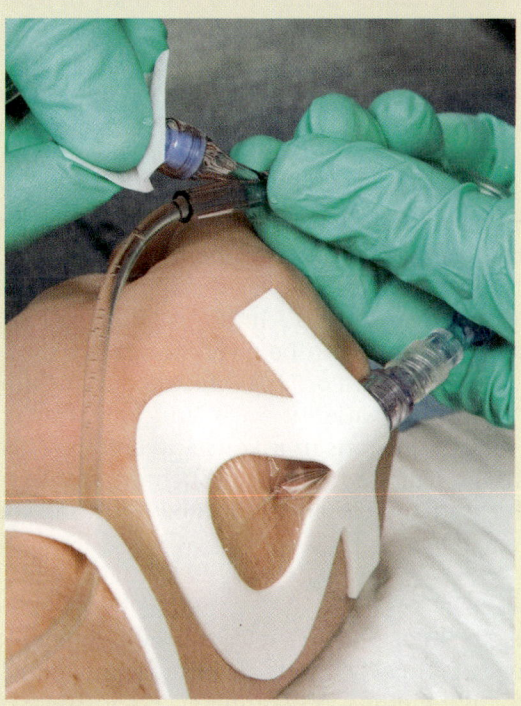

Step 1 Follow the six rights of medication administration. If the patient is responsive, ask about known allergies. Select the correct medication. Check to be sure you have selected the correct concentration of the drug. Check the clarity of the medication and its expiration date.

Calculate and prepare the desired volume of medication to be given. If the entire contents of the syringe are not going to be given, carefully inject only the appropriate amount of drug or squirt out the excess amount according to your EMS agency's protocols.

Step 2 Because some drugs can cause damage to surrounding tissue, check the site for signs of infiltration. If you are certain the catheter is in the vein and no signs of infiltration are present, cleanse the injection port closest to the patient with an alcohol swab. Recheck the medication and dose.

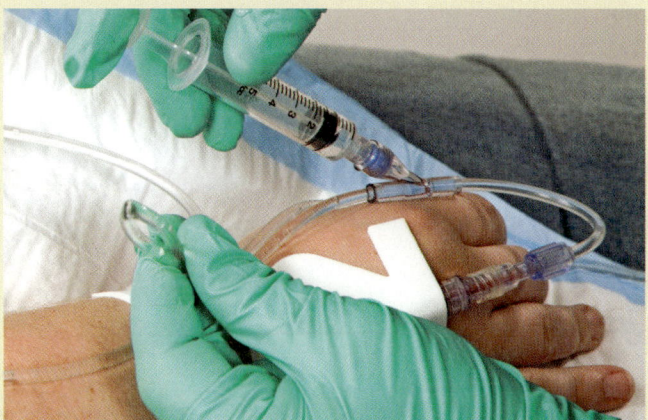

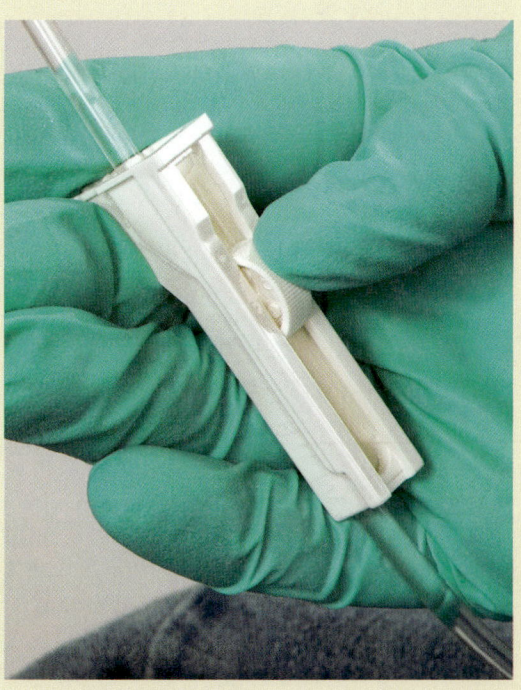

Step 3 Connect the syringe containing the medication to the injection port. Pinch the tubing just above the injection port to temporarily stop the flow. Give the correct dose at the proper push rate. Although the usual push rate is 1 to 3 minutes, some drugs carried in the paramedic drug box are an exception to this rule. If you are uncertain about the rate, check with medical direction or consult a drug reference before giving the drug.

Step 4 Remove the syringe and release the IV tubing. Allow the IV solution to flow at the prescribed rate. Dispose of the syringe in an appropriate container. Observe the patient for desired and adverse effects. Document the procedure.

the first, starting another line to administer the drug in the piggybacked IV line is not necessary.

An IVPB container is hung higher than the primary line. By doing so, gravity forces the second bag to infuse first. If the bags are positioned properly, the piggyback solution should begin infusing and the primary solution should temporarily stop until the secondary bag has infused. IVPB infusion sets (secondary sets) contain a safety feature called a back check valve. This allows the primary line to restart when the secondary infusion is complete without further adjustments. Skill 13-13 shows the steps to prepare an IVPB medication.

Infusion Pumps. An IV infusion pump allows solutions and medications to be given accurately over a set period (Figure 13-39). Portable infusion pumps often are used for home care patients. An IV infusion pump should be used for all infusions in infants and children to avoid inadvertent circulatory overload. Microdrip infusion sets should be used and closely monitored if infusion pumps are not available.

[OBJECTIVE 22]

Intraosseous Infusion. When IV cannulation is unsuccessful or is taking too long, an intraosseous infusion is an alternative method of gaining access to the vascular system. An **intraosseous infusion** is the process of infusing medications, fluids, and blood products into the bone marrow cavity for subsequent delivery to the venous circulation. Any medication or fluid that can be administered IV can be administered intraosseously.

Indications. Indications for an intraosseous infusion include the following:

- Emergency administration of fluids and/or medications, especially in the setting of circulatory collapse, in which rapid vascular access is essential
- Difficult, delayed, or impossible IV access
- Burns or other injuries preventing venous access at other sites

> **PARAMEDIC*Pearl***
>
> Absorption of medications administered by the intraosseous route is more rapid than drugs given by the SubQ or rectal routes.

Sites. Intraosseous infusion traditionally has been accepted as a rapid, reliable method of achieving vascular access under emergency conditions in children. Various sites have been studied to evaluate the effectiveness of intraosseous infusion in adults, including the clavicle, ilium, and tibia, an area proximal to the medial malleolus, and the manubrium.

The most common site used for intraosseous insertion in an infant or child is the anterior tibia (Figure 13-40). Alternate intraosseous infusion sites used in children include the following:

- Distal femur, 2 to 3 cm above the lateral condyle in the midline (Figure 13-41)

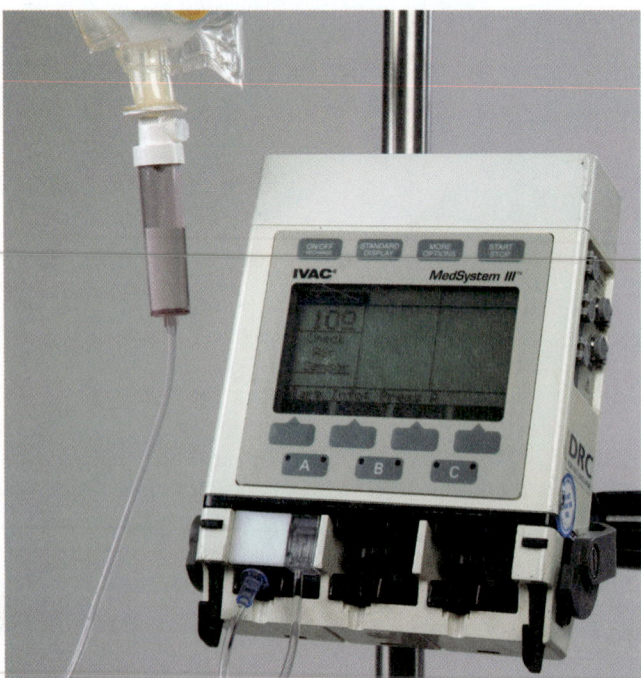

Figure 13-39 Intravenous (IV) infusion pump.

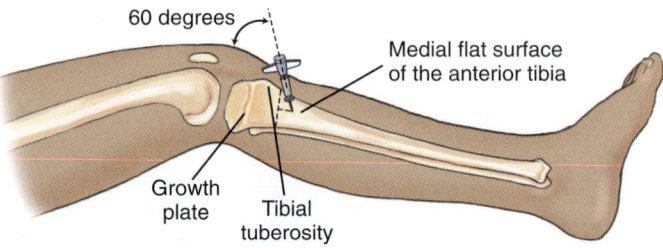

Figure 13-40 Anterior tibial approach for intraosseous infusion.

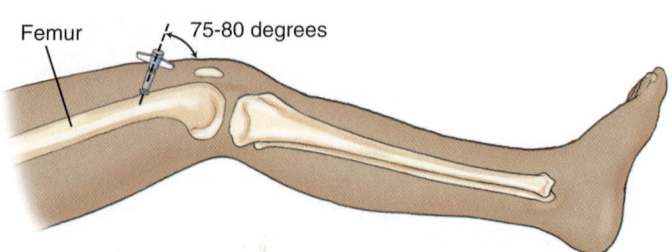

Figure 13-41 Distal femur approach. Insert the intraosseous needle 2 to 3 cm proximal to the external condyle in the midline and direct it superiorly at a 75- to 80-degree angle.

SKILL 13-13 IVPB MEDICATION

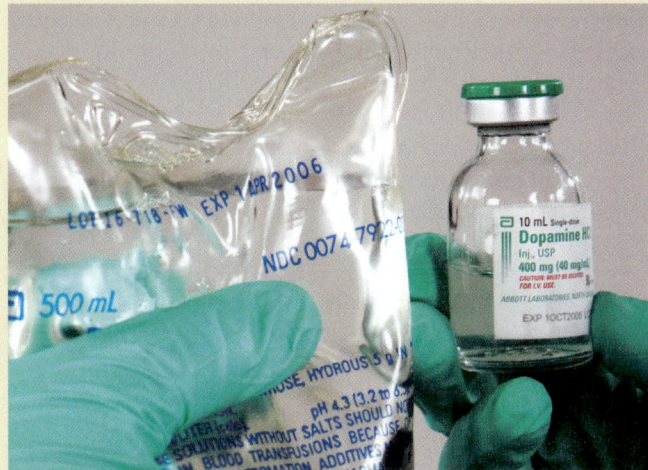

Step 1 Follow the six rights of medication administration. If the patient is responsive, ask about known allergies if not already done. Select the correct medication. Check the clarity of the medication container and IV solution and their expiration dates.

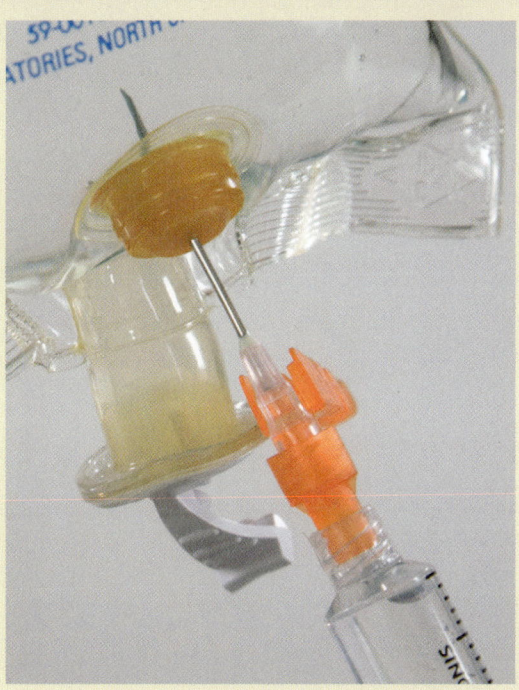

Step 2 Calculate and draw up the desired volume of medication into a syringe. Then calculate the flow rate of the piggyback medication in drops per minute. Cleanse the injection port on the bag with an alcohol swab. Inject the correct volume of medication into the solution. Mix the medication in the solution by gently shaking the bag.

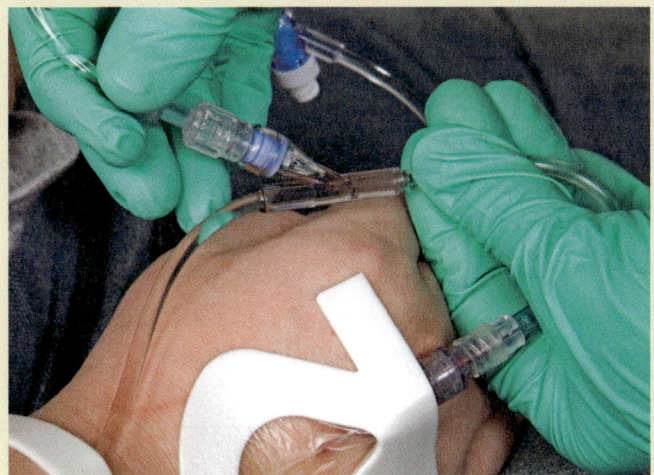

Step 3 Connect a secondary administration set to the medication solution. Fill the drip chamber and flush air from the tubing. Connect the secondary administration set to the tubing of the primary solution.

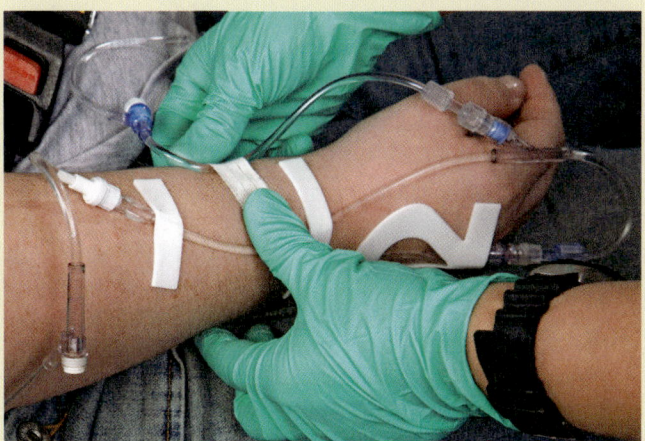

Step 4 Check the site for signs of infiltration. If you are certain the catheter is in the vein and no signs of infiltration are present, prepare to give the piggyback medication. Raise the piggyback solution so that is positioned higher than the primary solution. Securely tape the connection to prevent dislodgement from patient movement.

Continued

SKILL 13-13 **IVPB MEDICATION**—continued

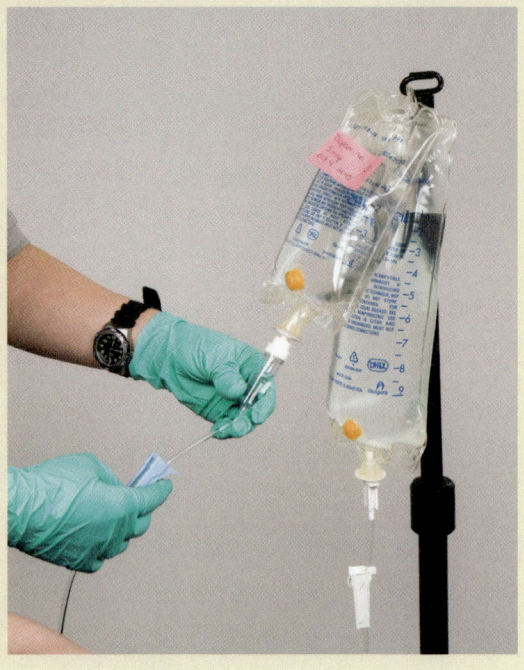

Step 5 Recheck the medication and dose. Open the clamp of the piggyback tubing. Adjust the flow rate to the calculated desired dose. Dispose of any sharps in an appropriate container. Observe the patient for desired and adverse effects. Label the piggyback solution with the date, time, name, amount of medication added to the bag, and the preparer's initials. Document the procedure.

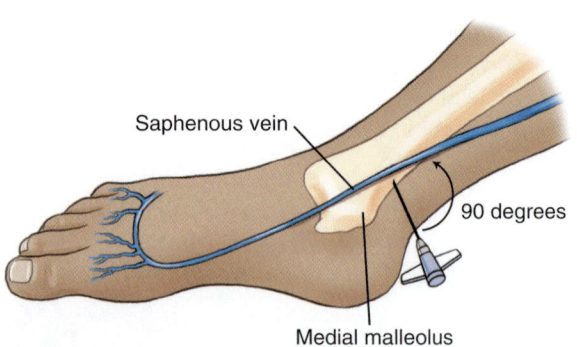

Figure 13-42 Distal tibia approach. Insert the intraosseous needle at a 60-degree angle, just proximal to the medial malleolus and posterior to the saphenous vein.

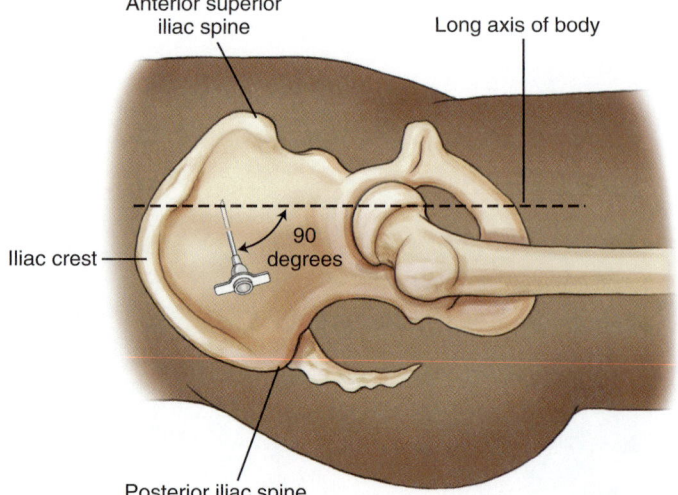

Figure 13-43 Anterior superior iliac spine approach. Insert the intraosseous needle at a 90-degree angle to the long axis of the body.

- Medial surface of the distal tibia 1 to 2 cm above the medial malleolus (may be a more effective site in older children) (Figure 13-42)
- Anterior superior iliac spine (may be a more effective site in older children) (Figure 13-43)

Consult medical direction and your local EMS system protocols before attempting any of these sites. Skill 13-14 demonstrates the proper technique for performing an intraosseous infusion in an infant or child.

The sternum can be used for intraosseous infusion in adults because it is large, thin, and flat; contains a high proportion of vascular red marrow; is easy to penetrate and less likely to be fractured; and is closer to the central circulation. Substances infused into the sternum reach the central circulation by the internal mammary and azygos venous systems within seconds. Alternate sites in adults include the tibia and humeral head.

The First Access for Shock and Trauma (FAST1; Pyng Medical, Richmond, B.C., Canada) device is an example of a sternal intraosseous infusion system. With this device, a handheld introducer is used to insert a flexible infusion tube with a stainless-steel tip to a predetermined

SKILL 13-14   PEDIATRIC INTRAOSSEOUS INFUSION

Step 1 Select the proper IV fluid and prepare equipment. Use personal protective equipment. Place the infant or child in a supine position. Place a towel roll or small sandbag in the popliteal fossa to provide support, optimize positioning, and minimize the risk of fractures.

Step 2 Identify the landmarks for needle insertion. Palpate the tibial tuberosity. The site for intraosseous insertion lies 1 to 3 cm (1 finger width) below this tuberosity on the medial flat surface of the anterior tibia.

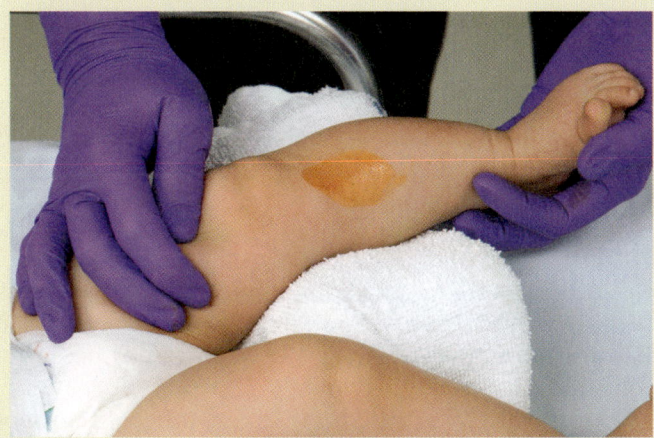

Step 3 Cleanse the intended insertion site. Stabilize the patient's leg. With the needle angled away from the joint, insert the needle using firm pressure. Angling away from the joint reduces the likelihood of damage to the epiphyseal growth plate. Firm pressure pushes the needle through the skin and subcutaneous tissue.

Step 4 Advance the needle by using a twisting motion at an angle of 60 to 90 degrees away from the epiphyseal plate (i.e., toward the toes). A twisting or boring motion is necessary to advance the needle through the periosteum of the bone.

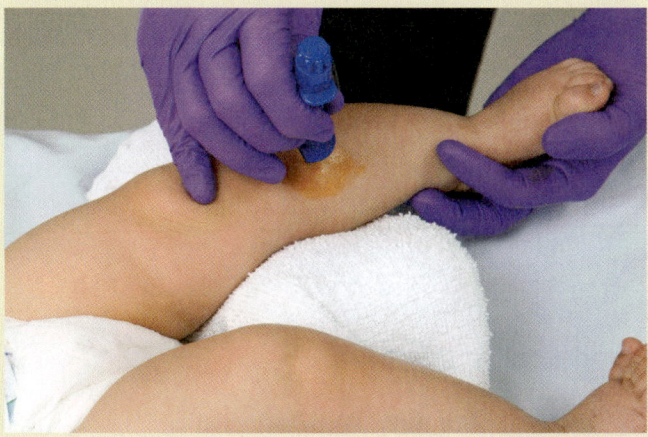

Step 5 Advance the needle until a sudden decrease in resistance or a "pop" is felt as the needle enters the marrow cavity.

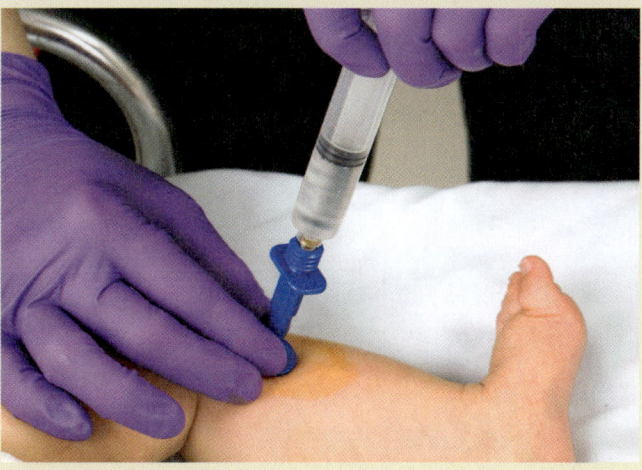

Step 6 Unscrew the cap, remove the stylet from the needle, attach a 10-mL saline-filled syringe to the needle, and attempt to aspirate bone marrow into the syringe. If aspiration is successful, slowly inject 10 to 20 mL of saline to clear the needle of marrow, bone fragments, and/or tissue.

Observe for any swelling at the site. If aspiration is unsuccessful, consider other indicators of correct needle position:

- The needle stands firmly without support.
- A sudden loss of resistance occurred on entering the marrow cavity (this is less obvious in infants than in older children because infants have soft bones).
- Fluid flows freely through the needle without signs of significant swelling of the subcutaneous tissue.

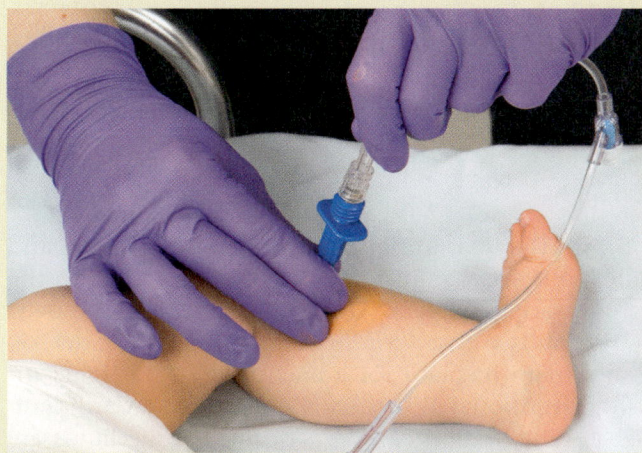

Step 7 If signs of infiltration are present, remove the intraosseous needle and attempt the procedure at another site. If no signs of infiltration are present, attach standard IV tubing. A syringe, pressure infuser, or IV infusion pump may be needed to infuse fluids.

Continued

SKILL 13-14 PEDIATRIC INTRAOSSEOUS INFUSION—continued

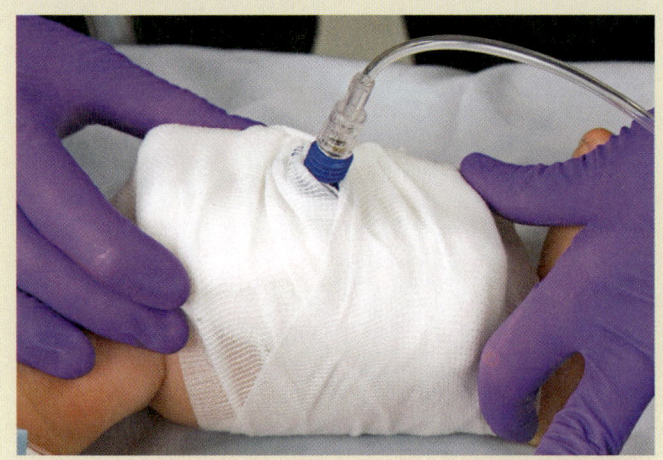

Step 8 Secure the needle and tubing in place with a bulky, sterile dressing and tape. Observe the site every 5 to 10 minutes for the duration of the infusion. Monitor for signs of infiltration and assess distal pulses. Tape a portion of the administration set to the patient's foot so that an accidental pull does not dislodge the needle.

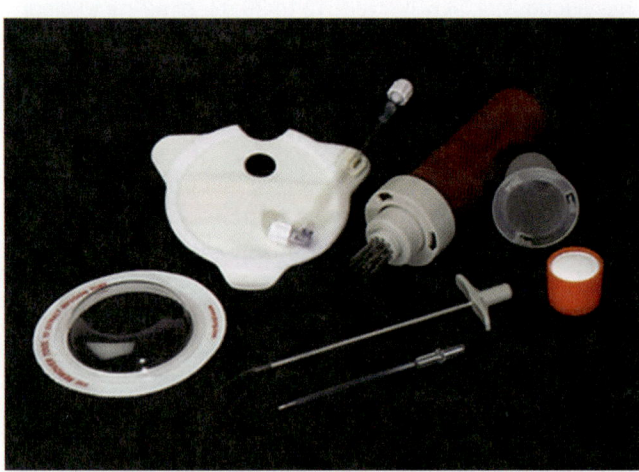

Figure 13-44 The First Access for Shock and Trauma (FAST1; Pyng Medical, Richmond, BC, Canada) intraosseous infusion system.

depth in the manubrium (Figure 13-44). Fluids and medications are administered through the tube into the marrow space. In general, vascular access can be achieved in 60 seconds with a 95% success rate using the device. It can remain in place for a maximum of 24 hours (or until conventional IV access is established). Cardiopulmonary resuscitation can be performed while fluids are being infused. The FAST1 requires a special tool for removal.

The EZ-IO (Vidacare Corporation, San Antonio, Tex.) is another intraosseous device. It consists of a small, battery-powered, intraosseous driver (reusable) and needle set (disposable) (Figure 13-45). For tibial insertion in adults, the EZ-IO is positioned 2 finger widths below the patella and 1 finger width medial (toward the inside) of the tibial tuberosity. An alternate site is the humeral head and distal tibia. The EZ-IO requires no special tool for removal.

Check with your instructor about other intraosseous devices, such as the Bone Injection Gun (WaisMed, Houston, Tex.), that may be used in your area.

Precautions. Use of FAST1 is not recommended in the following situations:

- Patient of small stature
  - Weight less than 50 kg
  - Pathologic small size
- Chest trauma with a suspected fractured sternum
- Significant tissue damage at intraosseous insertion site
- Severe osteoporosis or bone-softening conditions
- Previous sternotomy and/or scar

Use of the EZ-IO device is not recommended in the following situations:

- Fracture of the tibia or femur
- Previous orthopedic procedures
- Preexisting medical condition
- Infection at the insertion site
- Inability to locate landmarks
- Excessive tissue over the insertion site

Contraindications

- Femoral fracture on the same side
- Bone diseases such as osteopetrosis or osteogenesis imperfecta (high fracture potential)
- Fracture at or above the insertion site
- Severe burn overlying the insertion site (unless this is the only available site)

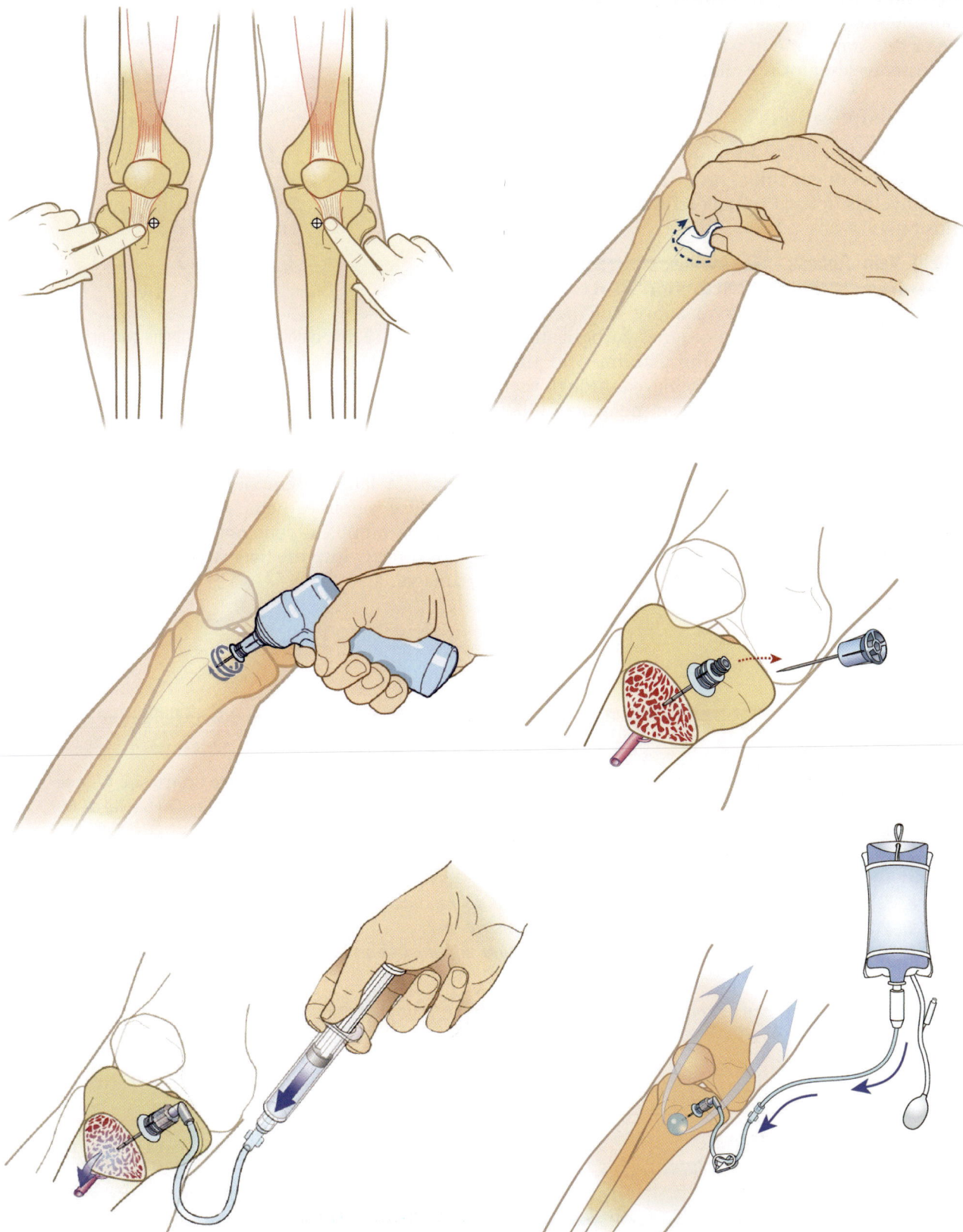

Figure 13-45 The EZ-IO device from Vidacare Corporation (San Antonio, Tex.).

- Infection at insertion site (unless this is the only available site)
- Use of the same bone in which an unsuccessful intraosseous attempt was made

Possible Complications

- Extravasation of fluids into subcutaneous tissue
- Local abscess or cellulitis
- Osteomyelitis (related to long-term intraosseous infusion)

Umbilical Vein Access. A route used to administer drugs to newborns is the **umbilical vein route.** This is a technique that requires training above and beyond initial paramedic training. It also requires authorization from medical direction before being performed in the field. However, when used, access is achieved through the one umbilical vein, which is set between the two umbilical arteries (Figure 13-46). The vein is a thin-walled vessel. The arteries are thicker walled, paired, and often constricted. Insert a typical over-the-needle IV catheter or umbilical catheter through the side of the proximal end of the cord and into the vein. Advance it upward through the translucent wall, attach the selected solution, and begin the infusion at the desired rate. Secure the catheter

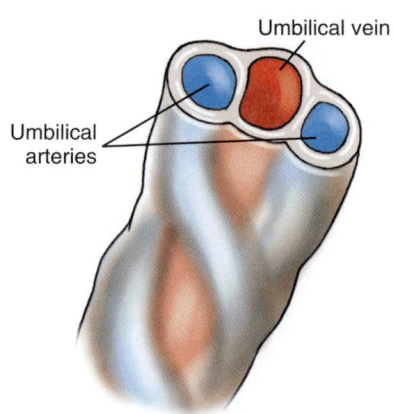

Figure 13-46 The umbilical cord contains two arteries and one vein.

in place with umbilical tape, then tape the tubing to the skin. Infection is one possible complication of this procedure. A fatal air embolus can result if air enters the umbilical venous catheter. Advancing the catheter too far into the umbilical vein may cause infusion of medications directly into the liver with the potential for hepatic damage.

Case Scenario CONCLUSION

En route to the hospital, the patient continues to report chest discomfort. You decide to administer IV morphine as allowed by your standing orders. Within minutes the patient states he feels better. On arrival at the emergency department, he rates his discomfort a 2 on a scale of 0 to 10.

Looking Back

8. *Before administering the morphine, review the six medication rights. What are they?*
9. *What is the process for IV medication administration?*
10. *What are the common side effects of morphine administration, and how could you prevent them?*

FIBRINOLYTIC INITIATION AND MONITORING

Fibrinolytic agents (commonly called *clot busters*) are drugs that dissolve clots. Fibrinolytic therapy is now used commonly and successfully to treat patients with a new onset of acute myocardial infarction and stroke. A timeline is involved because the drug must be given before the clot has disrupted blood flow to such an extent as to cause tissue necrosis. These drugs are being used more often, including for treatment of acute pulmonary embolism, deep vein thrombosis, and peripheral arterial occlusion.

Even though these drugs have serious side effects if given inappropriately or inaccurately, they are used in the prehospital setting in some parts of the United States. A thorough history must be obtained before administration, and extremely careful rate monitoring must continue throughout administration. Some of the fibrinolytic agents include streptokinase (Streptase), tissue plasminogen activator (t-PA, Activase), reteplase (Retavase), alteplase, anistreplase, and tenecteplase. Paramedics should routinely use a focused checklist to assist in the identification of patients eligible for reperfusion therapy. The reperfusion checklist begun in the prehospital setting should be continued and completed on the patient's arrival in the emergency department.

BLOOD INFUSIONS

Implications and Reactions

You may be asked to monitor a patient who is receiving a blood transfusion. Even though every effort is made to **type and crossmatch** the donor's blood with the patient's blood, a transfusion reaction is still possible. You must be keenly aware of the signs and symptoms of this reaction. Transfusion reactions include headache, change in the level of consciousness, flushing of the skin, nausea and vomiting, difficulty breathing, chills, weak and thready pulse with tachycardia, hypotension, and fever.

If these symptoms occur, immediately discontinue the infusion of blood, open the primary IV line, and rapidly infuse the normal saline. Administer high-flow oxygen and continually monitor the patient for changes. If you are in the field, contact medical direction for orders. If you are in a hospital setting, call for the physician or nurse. Save the bag of blood and the tubing because they must be returned to the laboratory for analysis.

OBTAINING A BLOOD SAMPLE

[OBJECTIVE 23]

Purpose

To achieve a true continuum of care, several steps are taken in the prehospital area, beginning with patient assessment. One of the baseline evaluations is obtaining a venous blood sample that can be analyzed (e.g., for blood glucose levels, electrolytes, hemoglobin, hematocrit). It should be obtained before starting any IV lines or giving medications to provide the hospital team with accurate results. It is usually done in conjunction with starting an IV line and may be drawn separately or through the catheter before connecting the solution and removing the tourniquet.

Safety Precautions

Label the tube carefully with the patient's name, date, time, and your initials. Tape the tubes to the back of the bag, or hand them directly to the receiving party in the emergency department. Never lay them down once in the hospital because they may get lost, broken, or confused with another patient.

If for some reason a blood sample must be obtained after an IV line has been started, always choose a site distal to the current site so as to not draw blood that has been mixed with IV solution or medications.

Several different types of blood sample tubes are available and are identified by the color of their stopper. However, different healthcare systems may use different colors of tubes. The paramedic must be familiar with his or her system.

BOX 13-17 Answers to Practice Problems

Convert grams (g) to milligrams (mg) and milligrams to grams:

1. 1 gram = 1000 mg
2. 1000 mg = 1 g
3. 250 mg = 0.25 g
4. 400 mg = 0.4 g
5. 500 mg = 0.5 g
6. 0.75 g = 750 mg
7. 1.25 g = 1250 mg
8. 10 g = 10,000 mg
9. 2 g = 2000 mg
10. 2500 mg = 2.5 g

Convert milligrams (mg) to micrograms (mcg) and micrograms to milligrams:

11. 1 mg = 1000 mcg
12. 500 mcg = 0.5 mg
13. 250 mcg = 0.25 mg
14. 400 mg = 400,000 mcg
15. 200 mg = 200,000 mcg
16. 800,000 mcg = 800 mg
17. 800 mg = 800,000 mcg
18. 200 mcg = 0.2 mg
19. 1000 mcg = 1 mg
20. 200,000 mcg = 200 mg

Applicable to the sizes of bags of IV solutions:

21. 1 L = 1000 mL
22. 1000 mL = 1 L
23. 500 mL = 0.5 L
24. 0.5 L = 500 mL
25. 250 mL = 0.25 L
26. 0.25 L = 250 mL
27. 250 mL = 250 cc

Applicable to drug dosage calculations:

28. 1 mg = 1000 mcg
29. 1000 mcg = 1 mg
30. 500 mcg = 0.5 mg
31. 0.3 cc = 0.3 mL
32. 0.5 mL = 0.5 cc
33. 1 gram = 1000 mg
34. 0.5 gram = 500 mg
35. 250 mg = 0.25 g

Applicable to drug calculation by patient weight:

36. 220 lb = 100 kg
37. 50 kg = 110 lb
38. 110 lb = 50 kg

Applicable to the measurement of wounds:

39. 1 inch = ~2.5 cm
40. ~2.5 cm = 1 inch
41. 3 inches = 7.5 cm

Case Scenario SUMMARY

1. *What is your general impression of this patient? What treatment will you initiate before continuing your assessment?* This patient's chief complaint, pallor, and diaphoresis—coupled with his age and gender—make him a high-priority case. You should immediately provide high-flow oxygen by nonrebreather mask, administer aspirin if no contraindications exist, and expedite assessment and treatment.

2. *What are the advantages of topical drug administration? What are the disadvantages?* Topical medications are easy to administer by either the patient or healthcare professional. Unfortunately, their absorption is somewhat erratic, and they can be quite messy.

3. *What protective equipment is appropriate for paramedic use when dealing with nitroglycerin ointment? Why?* Gloves to prevent absorption of the nitroglycerin ointment through the skin.

4. *Will the sublingual nitroglycerin take effect more quickly or slower than the cutaneous dose? Why?* Sublingual is much faster than cutaneous because of the superior blood flow to the sublingual area.

5. *What will you want to confirm with medical direction before administering the drug?* Confirm the name of the drug, the route, the dose, and that it should be given now.

6. *What protective equipment is appropriate for paramedic use when administering the sublingual nitroglycerin? Why?* Gloves to be certain that the spray is not absorbed into the skin. Some would also advocate wearing protective glasses to ensure that the spray does not get into the eyes.

7. *What is the process for sublingual medication administration?*
   - Step 1. When giving nitroglycerin spray, do not shake the canister before use. Shaking may produce bubbles within the canister, altering the amount of medication delivered. Remove the plastic cover from the canister.
   - Step 2. Hold the container upright with your index finger on top of the grooved button. Ask the patient to open his mouth. Position the container as close to the patient's mouth as possible without touching it.
   - Step 3. Press the button on the canister firmly with your index finger to release the spray under the patient's tongue. Be careful not to inhale the spray.
   - Step 4. Release the button and ask the patient to close his mouth. Tell the patient to avoid swallowing immediately after administering the spray. Replace the plastic cover on the canister.

8. Before administering the morphine, review the six medication rights. What are they?
   - Right drug
   - Right patient
   - Right dose
   - Right time
   - Right route
   - Right documentation

9. What is the process for IV medication administration?
   - Step 1. Follow the six rights of medication administration. If the patient is responsive, ask about known allergies. Select the correct medication. Check to be sure you have selected the correct concentration of the drug. Check the clarity of the medication and its expiration date. Calculate and prepare the desired volume of medication to be given. If the entire contents of the syringe are not going to be given, carefully inject only the appropriate amount of drug or squirt out the excess amount according to your EMS agency's protocols.
   - Step 2. Check the IV site for signs of infiltration. If you are certain the catheter is in the vein and no signs of infiltration are present, cleanse the injection port closest to the patient with an alcohol swab. Recheck the medication and dose.
   - Step 3. Connect the syringe containing the medication to the injection port. Pinch the tubing just above the injection port to temporarily stop the IV flow. Give the correct dose at the proper push rate. Although the usual push rate is 1 to 3 minutes, some drugs carried in the paramedic drug box are an exception to this rule. If you are uncertain about the rate, check with medical direction or consult a drug reference before giving the drug.
   - Step 4. Remove the syringe and release the tubing. Allow the solution to flow at the prescribed rate. Dispose of the syringe in an appropriate container. Observe the patient for desired and adverse effects. Document the procedure.

10. *What are the common side effects of morphine administration, and how could you prevent them?* Morphine commonly causes dizziness and nausea and vomiting. Both side effects may be minimized by administering by slow IV push.

Chapter Summary

Because the administration of drugs by the paramedic can be life saving but equally life threatening (or even lethal), this chapter addresses the critical areas of medication administration.

- Drugs were originally measured according to the apothecary system, which was based on the weight of a grain of wheat.
- The household system uses the dropper, teaspoon, tablespoon, cup, glass, pint, quart, and gallon for measuring. Household measures are expressed in Arabic numbers and fractions. Decimals are not used.
- The metric system is currently used for drug calculations. It is a logical system organized and based on the basic unit of 10.
- The basic units of measurement in the metric system are the following:
  - Weight (solids or mass): gram (g)
  - Length: meter (m)
  - Volume (liquid or fluid): liter (L)
- The four commonly used smaller units in drug calculations today are centi, milli, micro, and kilo. The prefix centi (c) represents 1/100 of a basic unit. The prefix milli (m) represents 1/1000 of a basic unit. The prefix micro (mc or sometimes the Greek letter μ) represents 1/1,000,000 of a basic unit. Kilo means 1000 times a unit.
- When calculating drug dosages, you must be able to convert milligrams to grams, grams to milligrams, milligrams to micrograms, and micrograms to milligrams.
- Body temperature is measured by two scales: Celsius (centigrade) and Fahrenheit.
- Only four basic formulas are necessary to calculate any dosage for patient medications:
  - Formula 1: Single Dose Calculations

  $$\text{Formula: } \frac{DD \times V}{DH}$$

  - Formula 2: Drip (Infusion) Calculations

  $$\frac{\text{Total volume to be infused}}{\text{Total time of infusion in minutes}} \times \frac{\text{Drops (administration set)}}{mL}$$

  - Formula 3: Drip Not Based on Weight

  $$\frac{DD \times V}{DH} \times \frac{gtt}{mL} \text{ (IV administration set)}$$

  - Formula 4: Drip Based on Weight
    - *Step 1:* Calculate the patient's weight in kilograms by dividing the weight in pounds by 2.2.
    - *Step 2:* Multiply the patient's weight in kilograms by the desired dose per kilogram (cross out like terms).
    - *Step 3:* Prepare the infusion and calculate the dose on hand (concentration on hand).
    - *Step 4:* Cross out like terms that appear in the numerator and denominator, one for one. Determine the drip rate by a microdrip IV infusion set, such as one that delivers 60 gtt/mL.

- A paramedic is authorized to give specific medications for specific conditions under the direction of a physician. Federal, state, and local laws govern the purchasing, distribution, dispensing, and administration of drugs in the United States. The organization for which a paramedic works also has policies and procedures pertaining to medication administration. Every paramedic must know what those laws and regulations are in his or her area of employment.
- Protocols are a written form of medical direction and must be signed by the medical director. Medical direction may be given by radio or cellular phone when a paramedic is on the scene (online medical direction). However, if communication fails, or in instances in which the paramedic has been given permission to function without radio communication, the written protocol must be followed (offline medical direction). If an event occurs that is not covered by protocol, the paramedic must communicate with medical direction before proceeding.
- Follow common safety protocols and procedures when giving medications.
  - Be sure you are familiar with the drug you are giving.
  - Be sure to convey important information about the patient to the online physician, including the patient's age, chief complaint, vital signs, signs and symptoms, allergies, current medications, and pertinent medical history.
  - Verify the physician's order. Repeat the order, including the name and dosage of the drug, back to the physician. Be certain to document the order received.
  - Concentrate on the task at hand.
  - Make sure the patient is properly positioned before giving a medication.
  - Assemble and use the correct supplies and equipment.
  - Handle all drugs carefully to avoid dropping or breaking.
  - Always use aseptic technique.
  - Carefully calculate drug dosages.
  - Monitor for signs of overdose.
  - Carefully document the drug given, dose, time, route, and the patient's response to the medication.

Chapter Summary—continued

- The "six rights" of drug administration are the following:
  - Right drug
  - Right patient
  - Right dose
  - Right time
  - Right route
  - Right documentation
- *Standard precautions* refers to the actions required personnel must do every time they are in contact with a patient to prevent exposure to infectious substances from body fluids.
- Disinfection involves the process of cleaning the emergency vehicle, stretcher, and equipment. The substances used are called disinfectants. They are toxic to body tissues.

- Antisepsis is the process used to cleanse local skin areas before needle puncture. Alcohol-based or iodine-based products are used for antisepsis.
- Sterilization is the process that makes an object free of all forms of life by using extreme heat or certain chemicals.
- Observe proper precautions when handling sharps.
- Medications may be given orally, rectally (very rare in the prehospital setting), by gastric tube, topically, by inhalation, by injection, though vascular access, and by intraosseous infusion.
- A blood sample should be obtained before starting any IV lines or giving medications to provide the hospital team with accurate results.

SUGGESTED RESOURCES

Dehn, R. W., & Asprey, D. P. (2002). *Clinical procedures for physician assistants*. Philadelphia: Saunders.

Drake, R. L., Vogl, W., & Mitchell, A. W. M. (2005). *Gray's anatomy for students*. Philadelphia: Elsevier.

Edmunds, M. W., & Mayhew, M. S. (2004). *Pharmacology for the primary care provider* (2nd ed.). St. Louis: Elsevier.

Taber's cyclopedic medical dictionary (17th ed.) (1993). Philadelphia: F.A. Davis.

Chapter Quiz

Practice Problems for Formula 1

1. Give epinephrine (Adrenalin) 0.3 mg of 1:1000 solution Sub-Q. The prefilled syringe reads "1 mg/mL." How many milliliters should you give?

2. Give furosemide (Lasix) 40 mg IV push at a rate no faster than 20 mg/min. The prefilled syringe reads "20 mg/2 mL." How many milliliters should you give?

3. Give atropine sulfate 0.5 mg IV push. The prefilled syringe reads "1 mg/10 mL (0.1 mg/mL)." How many milliliters should you give?

4. Give verapamil (Calan, Isoptin) 5 mg slow IV push. The prefilled syringe reads "5 mg/2 mL (2.5 mg/mL)." How many milliliters should you give?

5. Give adenosine 12 mg rapid IV push. The prefilled syringe reads "6 mg/2 mL." How many milliliters should you give?

Practice Problems for Formula 2

6. Give 60 mL of fluid containing a medication over 10 minutes. The IV infusion set delivers 60 gtt/mL.

7. Give 120 mL of Ringer's lactate as a fluid challenge over 20 minutes. The IV infusion set delivers 20 gtt/mL.

8. Give 150 mL of normal saline over 30 minutes. The IV infusion set delivers 10 gtt/mL.

9. Give 300 mL of Ringer's lactate over 30 minutes. The IV infusion set delivers 10 gtt/mL.

10. Give 1000 mL of normal saline over 5 hours. The IV infusion set delivers 15 gtt/mL.

Practice Problems for Formula 3

11. Give an epinephrine infusion at 4 mcg/min. Add 1 mg of epinephrine to a bag of 250 mL normal saline. Use a microdrip infusion set that delivers 60 gtt/mL.

12. Give a procainamide infusion at 3 mg/min. Prepare the infusion by adding 1 g procainamide to a 250 mL bag of IV solution. What is the drip rate in drops per minute and drops per second?

13. Give an isoproterenol infusion at 4 mcg/min. Prepare the infusion by adding 1 mg isoproterenol to 250 mL of normal saline. What is your drug concentration (i.e., dose on hand)? What is the drip rate if you use an IV infusion set that delivers 60 gtt/mL?

14. Give an epinephrine infusion at 2 mcg/min. Prepare the infusion by adding 1 mg epinephrine to a bag of 500 mL of normal saline. What is the drug concentration (i.e., what is the dose on hand)? What is the drip rate if you use a microdrip infusion set that delivers 60 gtt/mL?

15. Give a lidocaine infusion at 2 mg/min. Prepare the infusion by adding 1 g lidocaine to a 500 mL bag of normal saline. What is the infusion rate if you use an IV set that delivers 60 gtt/mL?

Practice Problems for Formula 4

You have responded to a call at the home of a patient with a long cardiac history. The patient is showing all the signs and symptoms of cardiogenic shock. You have begun all your initial supportive care and have gotten an order to start a dopamine drip to try to increase the patient's blood pressure. The patient's wife tells you that her husband weighed 220 pounds at the doctor's office yesterday.

16. What does the patient weigh in kilograms?

Medical control tells you to add 400 mg of dopamine to a 250-mL bag of normal saline, start the drip at 8 mcg/kg/min, and continue to monitor the level of consciousness and vital signs.

17. Based on his weight in kilograms, what is the desired dose per minute?

18. What is your dose on hand (drug concentration per milliliter in the bag)?

With a microdrip IV administration set, calculate the number of drops per second that will deliver the proper amount of drug to your patient.

19. How many drops per milliliter will your set deliver?

20. How many drops per minute will deliver that dose?

21. How many drops per second must you administer to deliver that dose?

Principles

22. Which of the following would be the fastest route for drug administration?
a. IM
b. IV
c. Sublingual
d. Sub-Q

23. You are treating a patient receiving a blood transfusion who develops headache, change in the level of consciousness, flushing of the skin, nausea and vomiting, difficulty breathing, chills, a weak and thready pulse with tachycardia, hypotension, and fever. Which of the following would be the most consistent with these findings?
a. Air embolism
b. Catheter shear
c. Fluid overload
d. Transfusion reaction

24. In which of the following would the use of tibial intraosseous administration be contraindicated?
a. Adult trauma patient with a pelvic fracture
b. Geriatric cardiac arrest
c. Pediatric hypovolemic shock
d. Pediatric trauma patient with a head injury

25. Which of the following is the preferred site for an IM injection for a child younger than 3 years old?
a. Deltoid
b. Dorsogluteal
c. Vastus lateralis
d. Ventrogluteal

Terminology

Aerosol A collection of particles dispersed in a gas.

Air embolism Introduction of air into venous circulation, which can ultimately enter the right ventricle, closing off circulation to the pulmonary artery and leading to death.

Ampule A sealed sterile container that holds a single dose of liquid or powdered medication.

Antisepsis Prevention of sepsis by preventing or inhibiting the growth of causative microorganisms; in the field, the process used to cleanse local skin areas before needle puncture with products that are alcohol or iodine based.

Arterial puncture Accidental puncture into an artery instead of a vein.

Asepsis Sterile; free from germs, infection, and any form of life.

Atopic A genetic disposition to an allergic reaction that is different from developing an allergy after one or more exposures to a drug or substance.

Bevel The slanted tip at the end of the needle.

Buccal Route of drug administration in which the drug is placed in the pocket between the teeth and the cheek and dissolved.

Catheter shear/catheter fragment embolism Breaking off the tip of the IV catheter inside the vein; the tip then travels through the venous system, where it can lodge in pulmonary circulation as a pulmonary embolism.

Central vein A major vein of the chest, neck, or abdomen.

Denominator The number or mathematic expression below the line in a fraction; the denominator is the sum of parts.

Terminology—continued

Disinfection Process of cleaning the ambulance, the stretcher, and equipment; disinfectant substances are toxic to body tissues.

Documentation Written information to support actions that lead to conclusive information; written evidence.

Drop (or drip) factor The number of drops per milliliter that an IV administration set delivers.

Enteral drug One that is given and passed through any portion of the digestive tract.

Fibrinolytic agent Clot-busting drug; used in very early treatment of acute myocardial infarction, stroke, deep vein thrombosis, pulmonary embolism, and peripheral arterial occlusion.

Flow rate The number of drops per minute an IV administration set will deliver.

Hematoma Collection of blood beneath the skin.

Hub The plastic piece that houses a needle and fits on a syringe.

Infiltration Complication of IV therapy when the catheter tip is outside the vein and the IV solution is dispersed into the surrounding tissues.

Intraosseous infusion The process of infusing medications, fluids, and blood products into the bone marrow cavity for subsequent delivery to the venous circulation.

IV bolus The delivery of a drug directly into an infusion port on the administration set using a syringe.

IV cannulation Placement of a catheter into a vein to gain access to the body's venous circulation.

Intravenous (IV) therapy Administration of a fluid into a vein.

Lumen An opening in the bevel of a needle.

Medical asepsis Medically clean, not sterile; the goal in prehospital care because complete asepsis is not always possible.

Metered-dose inhaler (MDI) A handheld device that disperses a measured dose of medication in the form of a fine spray directly into the airway.

N-95 particulate mask (medical) A facial mask worn over the nose and mouth that removes particulates from the inspired and expired air.

Nasogastric (NG) tube A hollow plastic tube placed through the nose and esophagus into the stomach.

Nebulizer A machine that turns liquid medication into fine droplets in aerosol or mist form.

Numerator The number or mathematic expression written above the line in a fraction; the numerator is a portion of the denominator.

Ophthalmic Route of administration in which medications are applied to the eye, such as antibiotic eye drops.

Orogastric (OG) tube A hollow plastic tube placed in the mouth and passed through the esophagus into the stomach.

Otic Route of administration in which medications are applied to the ear, such as antibiotic drops.

Over-the-counter (OTC) Drugs that can be purchased without a prescription.

Peripheral vein A vein outside the chest or abdomen, such as the veins of the upper and lower extremities.

Phlebitis Inflammation of a vein.

Protocols Written form of medical direction that includes allowable policies, practices, procedures, and drugs; intended to address and include the current standard in the prehospital arena as recognized by the medical community and authorized by the physician medical director.

Pulmonary embolism Movement of a clot into the pulmonary circulation.

Routes of administration Various methods of giving drugs, including oral, enteral, parenteral, and inhalational.

Sepsis Pathologic state, usually accompanied by fever, resulting from the presence of microorganisms or their poisonous products in the bloodstream; commonly called blood poisoning.

Shaft The length of a needle (also called the cannula); the needle shaft connects to the hub.

Spacer A hollow plastic tube that attaches to the MDI on one end and has a mouthpiece on the other; sometimes called a holding chamber.

Standard precautions Precautions used in contact with all patients, regardless of diagnosis, and when handling contaminated equipment or materials; essential with administration of drugs.

Sterilization Process that makes an object free of all forms of life (e.g., bacteria) by using extreme heat or certain chemicals.

Subcutaneous (Sub-Q) Injection of medication in a liquid form underneath the skin into the subcutaneous tissue.

Sublingual Medication placed under the tongue.

Thromboembolism Movement of a clot within the vascular system.

Thrombus Clot formation.

Topical Medication administered by applying it directly to the skin or mucous membrane.

Type and crossmatch Mixing a sample of a recipient's and donor's blood to evaluate for incompatibility.

Umbilical vein route Route of administration that achieves access through the one umbilical vein set between the two umbilical arteries.

Venipuncture Piercing of a vein.

Vials Glass containers with rubber stoppers at the top.

AIRWAY MANAGMENT & VENTILATION

Airway Management

Objectives *After completing this chapter, you will be able to:*

1. Explain the primary objective of airway maintenance.
2. Identify commonly neglected prehospital skills related to airway.
3. Identify the anatomy of the upper and lower airway.
4. Describe the functions of the upper and lower airway.
5. Define *gag reflex*.
6. Define atelectasis.
7. Explain the differences between adult and pediatric airway anatomy.
8. Explain the relation between pulmonary circulation and respiration.
9. List the concentration of gases that comprise atmospheric air.
10. Describe the measurement of oxygen in the blood.
11. Describe the measurement of carbon dioxide in the blood.
12. List factors that cause decreased oxygen concentrations in the blood.
13. List the factors that increase and decrease carbon dioxide production in the body.
14. Describe peak expiratory flow.
15. Define FiO_2.
16. Describe the voluntary and involuntary regulation of respiration.
17. List the factors that affect respiratory rate and depth.
18. Define and differentiate hypoxia and hypoxemia.
19. Define normal respiratory rates and tidal volumes for the adult, child, and infant.
20. Describe causes of respiratory distress.
21. Describe the modified forms of respiration.
22. Identify types of oxygen cylinders and pressure regulators (including a high-pressure regulator and a therapy regulator).
23. List the steps for delivering oxygen from a cylinder and regulator.
24. Explain safety considerations of oxygen storage and delivery.
25. Describe the indications, contraindications, advantages, disadvantages, complications, liter flow range, and concentration of delivered oxygen for supplemental oxygen delivery devices.
26. Describe the use of an oxygen humidifier.
27. Define and explain the implications of partial airway obstruction with good and poor air exchange.
28. Define *complete airway obstruction*.
29. Describe causes of upper airway obstruction.
30. Describe complete airway obstruction maneuvers.
31. Describe manual airway maneuvers.
32. Explain the purpose for suctioning the upper airway.
33. Identify types of suction equipment.
34. Describe the indications for suctioning the upper airway.
35. Identify types of suction catheters, including hard or rigid catheters and soft catheters.
36. Identify techniques of suctioning the upper airway.
37. Identify special considerations of suctioning the upper airway.
38. Describe the indications, contraindications, advantages, disadvantages, complications, equipment, and technique of tracheobronchial suctioning in the intubated patient.
39. Identify special considerations of tracheobronchial suctioning in the intubated patient.
40. Describe the use of an oral and nasal airway.
41. Describe the indications, contraindications, advantages, disadvantages, complications, and techniques for inserting an oropharyngeal and nasopharyngeal airway.
42. Define *gastric distention*.
43. Describe the indications, contraindications, advantages, disadvantages, complications, and techniques for ventilating a patient by the following resuscitation methods:
    - Mouth to mouth
    - Mouth to nose
    - Mouth to mask
    - One-person bag-mask
    - Two-person bag-mask
    - Three-person bag-mask
    - Flow-restricted, oxygen-powered ventilation device
44. Compare the ventilation techniques used for an adult patient with those used for pediatric patients.
45. Explain the advantage of the two-person method when ventilating with the bag-mask.
46. Describe the Sellick (cricoid pressure) maneuver.
47. Describe indications, contraindications, advantages, disadvantages, complications, and technique for ventilating a patient with an automatic transport ventilator.
48. Define, identify, and describe a tracheostomy, stoma, and tracheostomy tube.
49. Define, identify, and describe a laryngectomy.
50. Define how to ventilate a patient with a stoma, including mouth-to-stoma and bag-mask–to-stoma ventilation.
51. Describe the indications, contraindications, advantages, disadvantages, complications, equipment, and technique for inserting a nasogastric tube and orogastric tube.
52. Identify special considerations of gastric decompression.
53. Describe the special considerations in airway management and ventilation for patients with facial injuries.
54. Describe the special considerations in airway management and ventilation for the pediatric patient.
55. Differentiate endotracheal intubation from other methods of advanced airway management.

56. Describe the indications, contraindications, advantages, disadvantages, complications, equipment, and technique for using a dual-lumen airway.
57. Describe the indications, contraindications, advantages, disadvantages, and complications of endotracheal intubation.
58. Explain the risk of infection to EMS providers associated with ventilation.
59. Describe laryngoscopy for the removal of a foreign body airway obstruction.
60. Describe the indications, contraindications, advantages, disadvantages, complications, equipment, and technique for direct laryngoscopy.
61. Describe visual landmarks for direct laryngoscopy.
62. Describe methods of assessment for confirming correct placement of an endotracheal tube.
63. Describe methods for securing an endotracheal tube.
64. Describe methods of endotracheal intubation in the pediatric patient.
65. Describe the indications, contraindications, advantages, disadvantages, complications, equipment, and technique for nasotracheal intubation.

66. Describe indications, contraindications, advantages, disadvantages, complications, equipment, and technique for digital endotracheal intubation.
67. Describe the indications, contraindications, advantages, disadvantages, complications, and equipment for rapid-sequence intubation with neuromuscular blockade.
68. Identify neuromuscular blocking drugs and other agents used in rapid-sequence intubation.
69. Describe the indications, contraindications, advantages, disadvantages, complications, and equipment for sedation during intubation.
70. Identify sedative agents used in airway management.
71. Describe the indications, contraindications, advantages, disadvantages, complications, equipment, and technique for needle cricothyrotomy.
72. Describe the indications, contraindications, advantages, disadvantages, and complications for performing a surgical cricothyrotomy.
73. Describe the equipment and technique for performing a surgical cricothyrotomy.

Chapter Outline

Anatomy and Physiology
Respiratory Assessment
Supplemental Oxygenation
Airway Obstruction
Opening the Airway
Airway Adjuncts
Techniques of Artificial Ventilation

Advanced Airways
Cricothyrotomy
Pulse Oximetry
Exhaled CO$_2$ Monitoring
Continuous Positive Airway Pressure
Chapter Summary

Case Scenario

You and your fire partner respond with an engine company to a "rollover accident, unknown injuries." Upon arrival, you find that a small sedan carrying four college-aged girls has rolled over. Three of the girls are ambulatory; the fourth (the driver) is trapped, with her hips lying under the car. She is unresponsive to deep pain and is lying on her side. Her skin is pale and warm. Her respirations are shallow at 12 breaths/min, and her pulse is irregular and difficult to palpate at 88 beats/min. The engine company has begun blocking and lifting the car and anticipates that the patient will be safely removed within 10 minutes. The engine company assures you that the scene is safe.

Questions

1. What is your general impression of this patient?
2. What additional assessment will be important in the evaluation of this patient? Can you complete any assessments before extrication?
3. What intervention should you initiate at this time?

[OBJECTIVES 1, 2]

From your first cardiopulmonary resuscitation (CPR) course, you learned about the importance of assessing and managing a patient's *a*irway, *b*reathing, and *c*ircula-tion, or the ABCs. Paramedics perform many advanced procedures that are life saving when performed properly and lethal when performed improperly. When managing a patient's airway, your primary objective is to ensure optimal ventilation. You must remember to perform the appropriate basic skills before performing procedures that are more advanced.

In the field, the basics of airway and ventilatory management often are neglected. Examples include failing to maintain a good seal when using a bag-mask device, improper positioning of the patient's head and neck, and failure to reassess the patient. Because failure to address an airway or ventilatory problem can result in brain injury or death in as little as 4 to 6 minutes, you must be vigilant in caring for a patient's airway and ensure effective ventilation.

This chapter begins with a review of the anatomy and physiology of the respiratory system and fundamental basic airway and ventilation skills. A comprehensive discussion of advanced airway management skills follows.

> **PARAMEDIC*Pearl***
>
> Although there are many aspects of paramedic practice, perhaps the most vital of all is airway and ventilatory management.

ANATOMY AND PHYSIOLOGY

[OBJECTIVES 3, 4]

The primary function of the respiratory system is to provide a conduit for oxygen to enter the body and for carbon dioxide, a polluting waste product of metabolism, to leave the body. Respiration is the process by which these gases are exchanged at the functional level of the pulmonary system, the alveoli. If the airway passages are somehow compromised or blocked, life-sustaining oxygen is not made available to the cells of the body and carbon dioxide builds up, unable to exit the body. This chapter assumes knowledge of the material in Chapter 7, however understanding respiratory anatomy and physiology provides the foundation to know when and how to intervene, and more importantly, why. Therefore this chapter provides a brief review of anatomy and physiology. For further explanation or expansion of any of these topics, please refer to Chapter 7.

Upper Airway Anatomy

The upper airway consists of structures located outside the chest cavity, including the nose and nasal cavities, pharynx, and larynx (Figure 14-1). The upper airway functions to filter, warm, and humidify the air, protecting the surfaces of the lower respiratory tract.

Pharynx

[OBJECTIVE 5]

The nasal cavity and the mouth meet at the pharynx (throat). Lining the passages of the pharynx are mucous membranes and cilia. Mucus is a secretion that lubricates and traps fine particulate matter that may enter the airway. Cilia are microscopic hairlike projections. They line multiple segments of the airway and trap and propel particles away from the lower airway, where they are expelled by sneezing or swallowed.

The pharynx extends from the nasal cavities to the larynx and includes three parts: the nasopharynx, oropharynx, and laryngopharynx (or hypopharynx). The pharynx is a passageway common to both the respiratory and digestive systems.

The nasopharynx functions in respiration. Multiple facial bones join to form the nasal cavity on the lateral and superior aspects, and the hard palate serves as the floor of the nasopharynx. The nasal septum divides the nasal cavity into halves.

When air enters the nostrils, nasal hair serves as a first-line filter. Parallel to the nasal floor are the turbinates, bony structures that increase the surface area in the nasopharynx, enhancing the process of filtration, warming, and humidification of the air flowing over them.

The sinuses are small pockets or cavities within the bones of the skull that connect to the nasal cavity. Because the sinuses help trap particles, they are a common source of infection. Because of their closeness to underlying brain structures and the thin nature of the bones forming the sinuses, fractures may lead to leaking cerebrospinal fluid through the nares.

Eustachian tubes, also known as *auditory tubes*, are passages from the inner ear that allow drainage of fluid as well as equalization of pressure that may occur behind the tympanic membrane. Because these tubes are connected to nasal passages, which may contain bacteria, infections can migrate to the middle ear by way of these tubes, especially in toddlers. If you have ever flown in an aircraft or taken an elevator in a high-rise building and noticed pressure within your ears, the auditory tubes provide a release for the buildup of pressure. Yawning or swallowing can help open the tubes, allowing the pressure to release.

Tissues of the nasopharynx are extremely delicate and vascular. Improper or overly aggressive placement of tubes or airways may result in significant bleeding.

> **PARAMEDIC*Pearl***
>
> Because a nostril may serve as an entry point for various tubes, it is important to note that the nasal passageway is directed to the *back* of the head, not toward the top.

Functioning in respiration and digestion, the oropharynx is the portion of the pharynx visible by the mouth. The anterior oropharynx opens into the oral cavity and includes the lips, cheeks, teeth, tongue, and hard and soft palates. The back of the oral cavity opens into the oropharynx, which extends down to the epiglottis.

Within the mouth are several structures that have relevance to the airway, namely the teeth and the tongue.

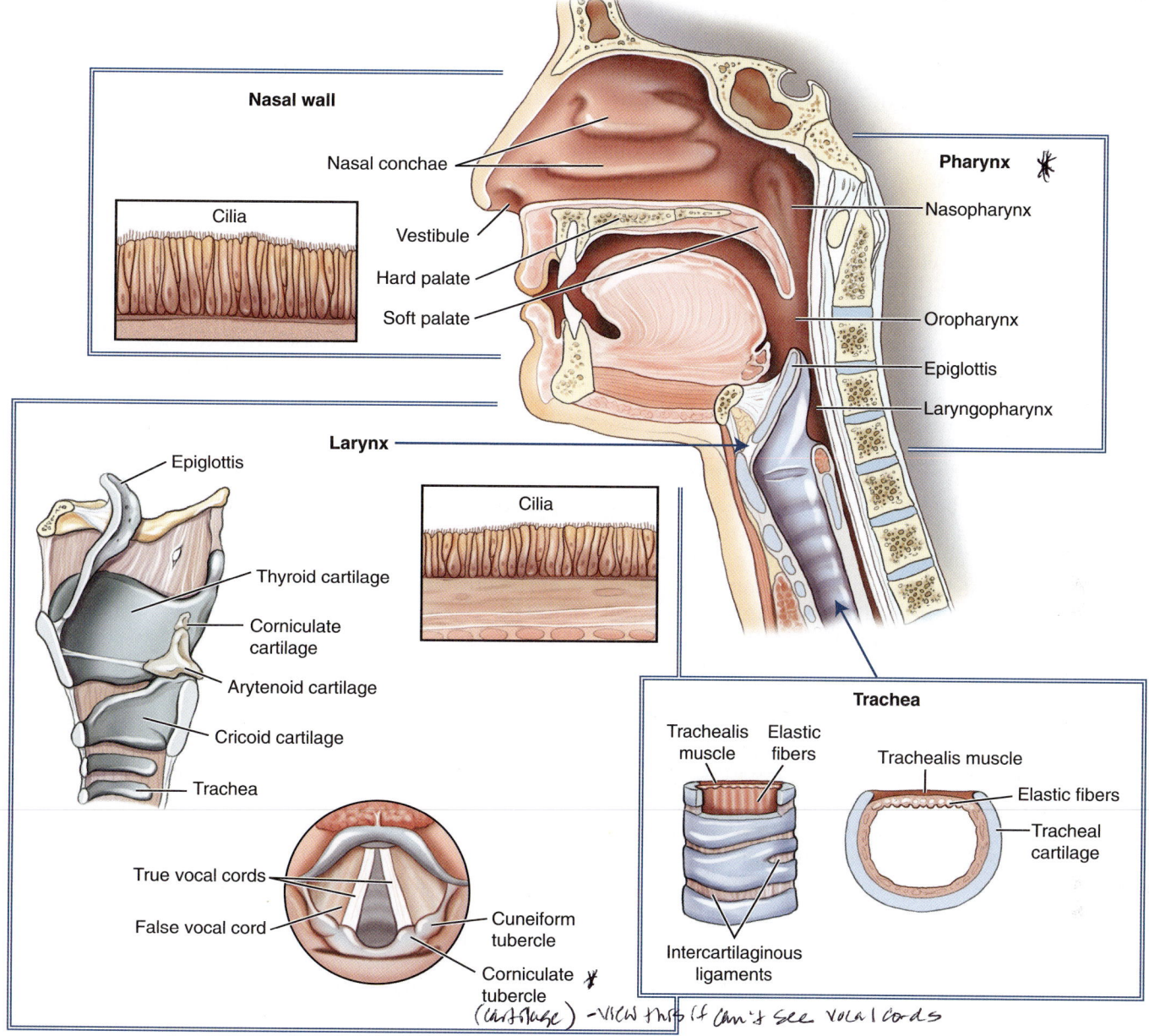

Figure 14-1 Upper airway structures.

Adults who have retained all their teeth normally have 32 teeth. Although significant force usually is necessary to dislodge a tooth, fracture or displacement of a tooth as a result of trauma may result in an airway obstruction. Teeth also provide a supporting structure for the oral cavity and can make artificially ventilating a patient's lungs easier with a bag-mask device.

PARAMEDIC *Pearl*

Avoid inserting your fingers into a patient's mouth whenever possible. You can be injured if a patient bites down or clenches the teeth during certain emergencies, such as a seizure.

The tongue is the leading cause of airway obstruction in an unresponsive patient. The tongue attaches to the mandible (lower jaw) and the hyoid bone. The hyoid bone is buried in the soft tissues behind the chin. It is unique in that it does not articulate with any other bones. Serving as a primary anchor of the tongue, the hyoid bone also allows support of the trachea and larynx by means of several ligaments. On the superior surface (roof) of the mouth are two structures called the *hard and soft palates*. The hard palate serves as a partition between the mouth and the nose. It is formed by the maxilla (upper jaw bone). Extending from the hard palate is an area of tissue that then becomes the soft palate extending downward into the back of the throat. The **uvula** is fleshy tissue resembling a grape that hangs down from the middle of the soft palate. At the uvula, the nasopharynx ends and the oropharynx begins.

The posterior pharynx has a rich supply of sensitive nerves. Stimulation of this area triggers the **gag reflex.** As a protective mechanism, the gag reflex initiates coughing or retching to prevent aspiration. Associated structures in the back of the throat include the tonsils. Tonsils are lymphatic tissue responsible for filtering bacteria and other foreign materials, especially from the mouth and nose. When inflamed and swollen, tonsils become sore and may make swallowing difficult. Two sets of tonsils are located on each side of the throat. The palatine tonsils are larger and more prominent. The adenoids (also called the *pharyngeal tonsils*) are located on the upper rear wall of the oral cavity near the opening of the eustachian tubes. The adenoids, when inflamed, can pose an increased risk of ear infection during childhood because they may block drainage exiting the tube.

The laryngopharynx (sometimes called the *hypopharynx*) functions in respiration and digestion and extends from the epiglottis to the glottis. Two structures located in the laryngopharynx are the epiglottis and vallecula, important landmarks during tracheal intubation. The epiglottis is a leaflike structure composed of cartilage that serves as the gatekeeper into the larynx. During swallowing, the epiglottis prevents food from entering the lower airway. When placing an **endotracheal** tube, the epiglottis is a structure that must be lifted out of the way so you are able to visualize and pass the tube between the vocal cords. More of an anatomical landmark than an actual structure, the **vallecula** (which means "little valley") is the depression (or pocket) between the base of the tongue and the epiglottis.

> **PARAMEDIC*Pearl***
>
> The epiglottis is an important landmark when performing orotracheal intubation with a straight laryngoscope blade. The vallecula is an important landmark when intubating with a curved laryngoscope blade.

Larynx

Serving as a bridge, the larynx (voice box) joins the pharynx to the trachea at the level of the cervical vertebrae. It conducts air between the pharynx and the lungs, prevents food and foreign substances from entering the trachea and houses the vocal cords (involved in speech production). The larynx is composed of an outer case of nine cartilages that protect and support the vocal cords. These cartilages are connected by muscles and ligaments. The largest of these cartilages is the thyroid cartilage. It is shaped like a shield and usually identifiable externally as the Adam's apple. The posterior thyroid cartilage is composed of smooth muscle.

The true vocal cords and the space between them compose the **glottis.** The glottic opening is located directly behind the thyroid cartilage and is the narrowest part of the adult larynx. During tracheal intubation, the paramedic attempts to visualize the glottic opening, flanked on each side by the vocal cords, through which the endotracheal tube must be passed. Patency of the glottis largely depends on muscle tone. Spasm of these muscles can lead to a compromised airway.

The pyramid-shaped arytenoid cartilages also are part of the larynx, serving as a point of attachment for the vocal cords. When intubating, the arytenoid cartilages often serve as an important landmark.

Directly inferior to the thyroid cartilage is the cricoid cartilage. Considered the first cartilage to begin the trachea, it is unique as a complete ring of cartilage, whereas the others are incomplete C-shaped rings on the posterior surface. The C-shaped rings are open to permit the esophagus, which lies behind the trachea, to bulge forward as food moves to the stomach. During **positive-pressure ventilation** with a manually triggered ventilation device or bag-mask device, posterior compression of the cricoid cartilage occludes the esophagus, reducing the risk of aspiration. This technique is called *cricoid pressure*, or the **Sellick maneuver.**

> **PARAMEDIC*Pearl***
>
> The cricoid cartilage is the narrowest diameter of the airway in infants and children younger than 10 years old.

Located between the thyroid and cricoid cartilage is a fibrous membrane called the **cricothyroid membrane.** Anatomically important, the cricothyroid membrane is the location where a needle or surgical (open) cricothyroidotomy is performed, if permitted by your local medical director and state regulations.

Be aware of other associated structures in proximity to the larynx. Avoiding these structures during the performance of certain surgical airway procedures is important. Specifically, the thyroid gland is a bow tie–shaped gland that lies across the trachea just inferior to the cricoid cartilage. Several blood vessels, including the carotid arteries, jugular veins, and several vessels branching off these arteries, run alongside the trachea as well as across it.

Lined with mucous membranes, the larynx is embedded with a rich nerve supply from the vagus nerves. Because the larynx is sensitive to any type of irritation, including suctioning, use of a laryngoscope during intubation and passage of an endotracheal tube may result in forceful coughing or gagging. Stimulation of the vagus nerves can result in bradycardia, hypotension, and decreased respiratory rate. During such procedures, be sure to monitor the patient closely for these effects and discontinue the procedure if they appear.

Lower Airway Anatomy

The lower airway consists of the trachea, bronchial tree (primary bronchi, secondary bronchi, and bronchioles), alveoli, and the lungs (Figure 14-2). The lower airway is where gas exchange occurs. Functionally, oxygen diffuses from the alveoli into the pulmonary capillaries while carbon dioxide diffuses in the opposite direction. Topographic landmarks corresponding to the structures of the lower airway include the fourth cervical vertebrae on the superior margin and, roughly, the tip of the xiphoid process inferiorly.

Trachea

As air moves from the larynx through the glottic opening, it enters the trachea. In an adult the trachea is approximately 10 to 12 cm in length before it divides (bifurcates) into two separate tubes called the *left and right mainstem bronchi.*

Structurally, the trachea is composed of C-shaped cartilaginous rings. The area between the tracheal cartilages is composed of connective tissue and smooth muscle that allow changes in diameter of the trachea.

Internally, the trachea is lined with a mucous membrane containing cilia as well as mucus-producing cells. Recall that cilia sweep foreign materials out of the airway and the mucus can also trap particulate matter that is then expelled during coughing.

PARAMEDIC*Pearl*

Obstruction of the trachea results in death if not corrected within minutes.

Bronchi

The trachea, a single hollow tube, branches into two large tubes called the *right and left mainstem bronchi.* The point where the trachea divides into the right and left mainstem bronchi is called the **carina.** The carina is an important anatomic landmark because the tip of an endotracheal tube often is documented on radiographic study in relation to the carina. The right bronchus serves three lobes and the left serves two lobes of the lung. Anatomically, because the heart occupies space in the left chest cavity, the left mainstem bronchus has an exaggerated angle, whereas the right bronchus is straighter, or less angled. These angles become important for several reasons. First, when intubating, if the tip of the endotracheal tube is inserted too deeply, it will most likely lie within the right mainstem bronchus. When this occurs, your assessment of tube placement when auscultating the chest will reveal good lung sounds on the right and diminished or absent sounds over the left chest. In this situation (referred to as a *right mainstem intubation*), withdraw the endotracheal tube a few centimeters and reassess. Additionally, foreign bodies tend to make their way into the right mainstem bronchus more often than the left.

As the right and left mainstem bronchi enter the lungs at the **hilum** (the point of entry for bronchial vessels, bronchi, and nerves in each lung), they continue to branch into secondary and tertiary bronchi. Think of the bronchi as branches of a tree. As the bronchi continue to divide into the lung tissue and become smaller passageways, they become bronchioles. After multiple subdivisions, the bronchioles attach to the alveoli by alveolar

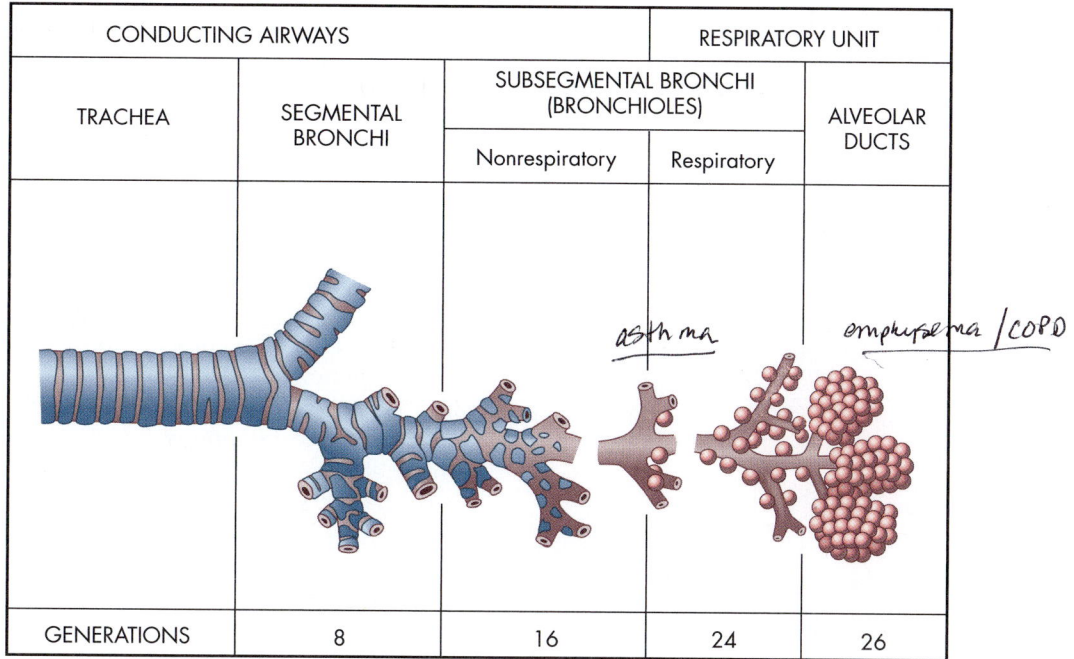

CONDUCTING AIRWAYS				RESPIRATORY UNIT
TRACHEA	SEGMENTAL BRONCHI	SUBSEGMENTAL BRONCHI (BRONCHIOLES)		ALVEOLAR DUCTS
		Nonrespiratory	Respiratory	
GENERATIONS	8	16	24	26

Figure 14-2 Lower airway structures.

ducts, where gas exchange first becomes possible. Stimulation of beta-2 receptor sites in the bronchioles results in relaxation of bronchial smooth muscle.

Alveoli

[OBJECTIVE 6]

Alveolar ducts attach to balloonlike clusters of tiny microscopic air sacs (alveoli) where functional gas exchange takes place through the process of diffusion (Figure 14-3). Each alveolus is composed of multiple alveoli that have very thin walls that become thinner as they expand, making diffusion of oxygen and carbon dioxide possible. Inside the alveoli is a chemical substance called **surfactant.** Surfactant lubricates the alveoli, decreasing surface tension and facilitating ease of expansion. Without surfactant, alveoli collapse and are difficult to inflate, leading to a state of **atelectasis** (alveolar collapse). Alveoli that are collapsed do not participate in gas exchange.

Lungs

Lung parenchyma, the essential or functional unit of an organ, in this case the alveoli, are divided into the inferior, middle, and lower lobes on the right and the upper and lower lobes on the left. Lining the surface of the lung parenchyma, as well as the interior surface of the thoracic cavity, is the pleura. The pleural space is a double-layered membrane with a potential space between

its layers. It contains a small amount of lubricating fluid that prevents friction during the continuous inflation and deflation of the lungs within the thoracic cavity. The visceral pleura is in direct contact with the lung parenchyma. Lining the thoracic cavity is the parietal pleura. Several problems can be associated with the pleura, including an injury, tumor, or pleurisy, an inflammation of the pleura that may be caused by infection. Air (pneumothorax) or blood (hemothorax) may also collect in the pleural space, creating potentially life-threatening conditions.

Differences in the Pediatric Airway

[OBJECTIVE 7]

Though functionally the same as the adult airway but smaller in all aspects, several features of the pediatric airway result in modified airway and ventilatory management strategies. Failure to alter technique can prove disastrous for children.

The heads of infants and young children are large in proportion to the body, with a larger occipital region. Because of the large occiput, the airway will flex when the patient is in a supine position. This condition requires padding be placed under the torso of the pediatric patient to ensure an open airway. Because the cartilaginous rings of the trachea do not fully develop until the patient is eight years old, excessive hyperextension or hyperflexion results in occlusion of the airway.

The pharynx, with a proportionately smaller jaw and larger tongue, means the tongue occupies greater space in the oral cavity. As a result, the tongue often obstructs the pediatric airway. The large tongue provides less space within which to work when performing certain airway procedures. Small infants do not have teeth; when teeth begin to appear, the infant's gum line is especially susceptible to trauma.

The adult epiglottis is broad and flexible. In infants and toddlers, the epiglottis is large, long, and U-shaped. It extends vertically beyond the opening of the cords, making a clear view of the airway difficult. A straight blade typically is used for tracheal intubation in infants and young children because the tip of the straight blade lifts the epiglottis up and out of the line of vision.

In an adult, the larynx is located opposite the fourth to seventh cervical vertebrae (C4-C7). The larynx of the pediatric airway is more anterior and superior in the neck. In a newborn, the larynx is located between C1 and C4. The epiglottis can pass behind the soft palate and lock into the nasopharynx. This creates two separate channels, one for air and one for food (i.e., the infant can breathe and eat at the same time). The connection between the epiglottis and soft palate is constant except during crying and disease. Oral respirations begin at 5 to 6 months. At age 7 years, the larynx level is C3-C5. At this point, the epiglottis no longer connects with the soft palate (i.e., the child does not have two separate channels for food and air).

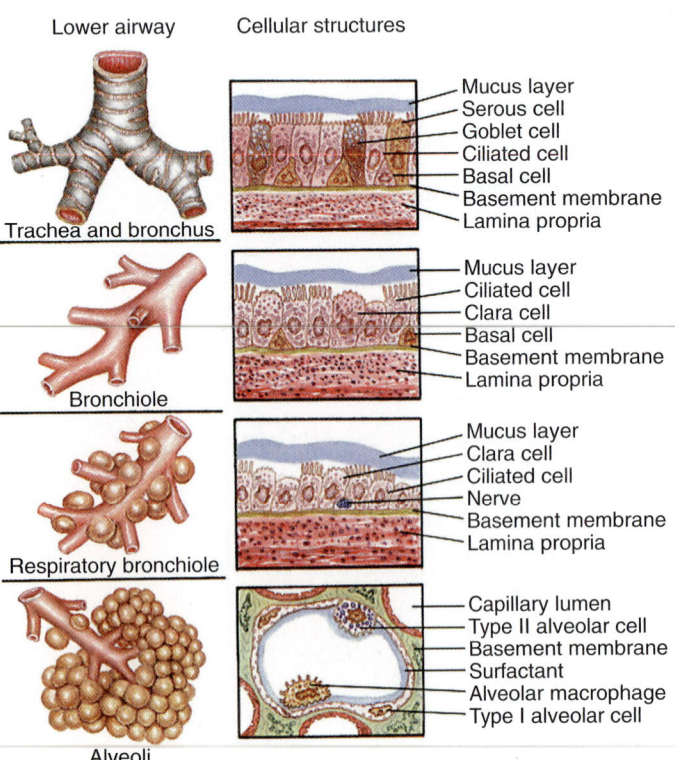

Figure 14-3 Cellular structures of the lower airway.

Lower airway

Trachea and bronchus

Mucus layer
Serous cell
Goblet cell
Ciliated cell
Basal cell
Basement membrane
Lamina propria

Bronchiole

Mucus layer
Ciliated cell
Clara cell
Basal cell
Basement membrane
Lamina propria

Respiratory bronchiole

Mucus layer
Clara cell
Ciliated cell
Nerve
Basement membrane
Lamina propria

Alveoli

Capillary lumen
Type II alveolar cell
Basement membrane
Surfactant
Alveolar macrophage
Type I alveolar cell

Cellular structures

The larynx of the newborn and young child resembles a funnel, with the narrowest portion being at the cricoid ring. This area creates a natural seal (a physiologic cuff) around an endotracheal tube, making cuffed tubes generally unnecessary in children younger than 8 years.

The trachea of an infant and child is smaller and shorter than that of an adult. Movement of an endotracheal tube may occur during changes in head position in a patient of any age. The small, short trachea of an infant and child may result in intubation of the right mainstem bronchus or unintentional removal of the endotracheal tube **(extubation).** Securing an endotracheal tube before movement of any intubated patient is important to prevent tube displacement.

Because the trachea is small, a small change in airway size results in a significant increase in resistance to airflow when swelling or a foreign body is present. A marked increase in airway resistance can result in partial or complete airway obstruction.

In infants and children, the diaphragm is the primary muscle of inspiration. The diaphragm must generate significant negative intrathoracic pressure to expand the child's underdeveloped lungs. The diaphragm is horizontal in infants and results in decreased contraction efficiency. (The diaphragm is oblique in adults.) Efficiency of the diaphragm increases with age. Because this is the main way for pediatric patients to breathe, any compromise is serious. The intercostal muscles are immature and fatigue easily from the work of breathing. The intercostal muscles act more as rib stabilizers and not as efficient rib elevators. Accessory muscles of respiration are quiet during normal breathing but may be activated during periods of respiratory distress. Effective respiration may be jeopardized when diaphragmatic movement is compromised because the chest wall cannot compensate. Restraint for immobilization may impair chest wall movement.

PARAMEDIC*Pearl*

With underdeveloped accessory muscles, children do not have the ability to readily compensate during times of respiratory distress. Hypoxia and fatigue may occur, quickly leading to respiratory failure. For this reason, be vigilant of any pediatric patient with a respiratory complaint.

The chest wall of the infant and young child is pliable because it is composed of more cartilage than bone and the ribs are more horizontal. As a result, the chest wall offers less protection to underlying organs. Significant internal injury can be present without external signs. Because of the flexibility of the ribs, children are more resistant to rib fractures than adults are, although the force of the injury is readily transmitted to the delicate tissues of the lung and may result in a pulmonary contusion, hemothorax, or pneumothorax. Because of their pliability, the ribs may fail to support the lungs, leading to paradoxic movement during active inspiration rather than lung expansion. Children also have fewer and smaller alveoli. Thus the potential area for gas exchange is less.

PARAMEDIC*Pearl*

The thin chest wall of the infant and young child allows for easily transmitted breath sounds. Missing a pneumothorax or misplaced endotracheal tube is easy because of transmitted breath sounds.

Respiratory System Physiology

This discussion of the respiratory system focuses on how these structures work together, with influence from other body systems, to make oxygen available to the body while removing carbon dioxide. Understanding how the respiratory system normally works will help you understand complex pathophysiology. In turn, this supports the "what and why" of interventions when caring for patients.

Ventilation

Ventilation is the mechanical process of moving air into and out of the lungs in two separate phases: inspiration and expiration. The muscles involved in ventilation are shown in Figure 14-4. Many control mechanisms affect ventilation. The primary stimulus to breathe comes from the respiratory center in the medulla oblongata. When considering ventilation, think of it as a mechanical process. Essential to this process is a change in pressures within the thoracic cavity that allow the passive flow of air into and out of the lungs. Of note, nothing in the lung tissues themselves causes us to breathe.

At the end of expiration, but before inspiration, pressures of air in the atmosphere and within the thoracic cavity are essentially equal. No movement of air occurs into or out of the lungs. During inspiration, a nervous impulse is transmitted to the diaphragm by the phrenic nerve. As a result, the diaphragm, considered the major muscle of respiration, contracts and flattens downward toward the abdominal cavity. At the same time, the intercostal muscles contract, causing elevation and expansion of the ribs. Intrapulmonic pressure falls below that in the atmosphere and air is drawn into the lungs like a vacuum. The alveoli inflate, allowing oxygen and carbon dioxide to diffuse across the pulmonary capillary membrane from an area of high concentration to an area of low concentration. Thus oxygen moves from the alveoli into the pulmonary capillaries while carbon dioxide moves into the alveoli for removal from the body. At the end of inspiration the diaphragm and intercostal muscles relax allowing the chest to recoil and a positive pressure is created in the thoracic cavity. As a result air moves out of the lungs.

The **Hering-Breuer reflex** is designed to prevent overinflation of the lungs in a conscious, spontaneously breathing person. Stretch receptors (sensors) are located in the smooth muscles surrounding the large and small airways. When the lungs inflate, these stretch receptors

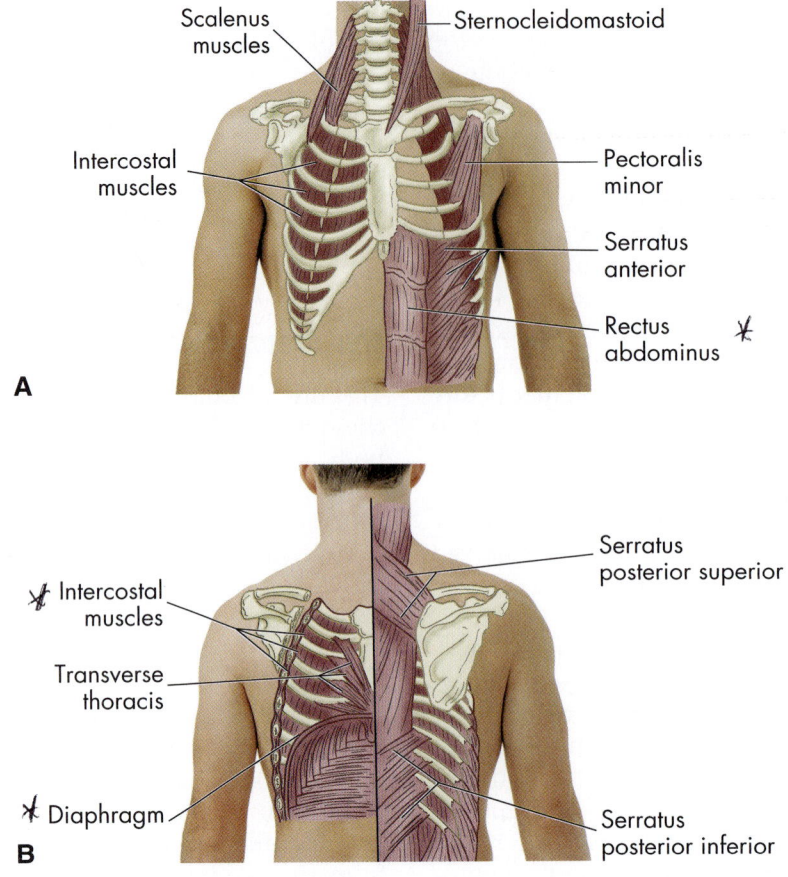

Figure 14-4 Muscles of ventilation. **A,** Anterior view. **B,** Posterior view.

are stimulated and nerve signals are sent to the respiratory center by the vagus nerves to inhibit inspiration. This reflex is active in newborns. In adults, this reflex is active only with increased tidal volumes, such as during exercise, or when the apneustic center in the brain is damaged or non-functional (Huether, 2004).

After inspiration of air into the lungs, expiration occurs. With the diaphragm and intercostal muscles relaxed, intrapulmonic pressure is higher than that in the atmosphere, resulting in air in the lungs being passively expired. Each combination of inspiration and expiration is referred to as a *respiratory cycle*. The normal pulmonary volumes and capacities associated with each respiratory cycle were presented in Chapter 7; however these values vary with the patient's age and sex. The normal tidal volume (V_T) for an adult male is 500 mL, whereas the V_T for a pediatric patient is approximately 8 mL/kg. Because of the smaller volumes of air pediatric patients move, along with their increased metabolic demands, they must maintain a faster respiratory rate than the adult in order to maintain an adequate minute alveolar volume (MV_A). Recall that $MV_A = RR \times (V_T - V_D)$.

Respiration

[OBJECTIVES 8, 9, 10, 11, 12, 13]

Respiration is the exchange of gases between a living organism and its environment. Human respiration provides oxygen to the body while removing carbon dioxide as one of the chief metabolic byproducts of the system.

Respiration is either internal or external. **External respiration** is the exchange of gases between the alveoli of the lungs and the red blood cells traveling through the pulmonary capillaries. Once in the bloodstream, gases exchanged between blood cells and tissues constitute **internal respiration.** Without an intact circulatory system, internal respiration cannot occur.

Exchange of gases occurs as the result of diffusion, that is, the movement of a gas from an area of higher concentration to an area of low concentration. Throughout the capillary beds in the body, cells receive oxygen molecules bound to the **hemoglobin** of red blood cells. As the oxygen is offloaded, cells give up carbon dioxide. The circulatory system operates a continuous transportation system, returning to the alveolus by the pulmonary capillaries and exchanging carbon dioxide for oxygen.

Measuring gases in the bloodstream is a complex process. When multiple gases are present, each gas exerts a pressure. When several gases are contained within the same space, their partial pressures can be measured. **Partial pressure** is the pressure exerted by each individual gas in a mixture. The partial pressure of a gas is not the same as its concentration. Four main gases are found in the earth's atmosphere: nitrogen (N_2), oxygen (O_2), water vapor (H_2O), and carbon dioxide (CO_2). The average total pressure exerted by the gases composing the earth's atmosphere is sufficient to elevate a column of mercury (Hg) 760 mm. 1 mm Hg = 1 Torr. Therefore at sea level the total atmospheric pressure is 760 Torr.

Each of the four gases has a partial pressure within the mixture based on its overall concentration in the atmosphere. For instance, oxygen accounts for roughly 21% of the gas contained in the atmosphere at sea level. Its total partial pressure in relation to the other gases equates to about 160 torr.

When considering the normal lung, normal partial pressure of oxygen in arterial blood is 80 to 100 torr (commonly abbreviated PaO_2). Normal level of carbon dioxide in arterial blood is 35 to 45 torr (commonly abbreviated $PaCO_2$).

Oxygen diffuses from the alveoli into the bloodstream, where approximately 97% is bound to hemoglobin, a protein found on red blood cells that is rich in iron. When hemoglobin has oxygen molecules bound to it, it is referred to as **oxyhemoglobin.** Laboratory analysis of blood samples can provide a measurement of oxygen saturation, which is another way to represent the percentage of hemoglobin bound to oxygen. **Pulse oximetry** is a noninvasive method of measuring the percentage of oxygen-bound hemoglobin. Oxygen saturation values greater than 98% are considered normal.

Carbon dioxide is also found in the bloodstream and can bind with hemoglobin. Approximately 33% of venous hemoglobin is bound with carbon dioxide, and the remaining CO_2 is transported in the blood in the form of bicarbonate ions (HCO_3). In the lungs, as O_2 crosses into the blood, CO_2 diffuses into the alveoli and is expelled from the body.

Several factors can affect the oxygen and carbon dioxide concentrations in the blood. Causes of decreased oxygen concentrations in the blood include the following:

- Decreased hemoglobin concentration in the blood, such as in anemia or hemorrhage
- Lower partial pressures of oxygen in the atmosphere, as is the case in a smoke-filled environment [or high altitude]
- Traumatic conditions, such a pneumothorax or hemothorax, which impair the function of affected alveoli
- Decreased mechanics of respiration as a result of pain, traumatic suffocation, or hypoventilation
- Low inspired oxygen concentrations, as is the case with pulmonary disease such as **chronic obstructive pulmonary disease (COPD)** or respiratory muscle paralysis
- Impaired diffusion across the pulmonary membrane as a result of fluid in the alveoli, as occurs in pulmonary edema or pus associated with pneumonia [Not COPD or asthma] [wet drowning]
- Impaired pulmonary blood flow, as occurs in pulmonary embolism

Each of these conditions can lead to hypoxia and/or hypoxemia. Although often used interchangeably, these terms are not one and the same. *Hypoxemia* refers to a decreased amount of oxygen saturated hemoglobin in the blood stream (measured by the pulse oximeter), while *hypoxia* refers to a decreased amount of oxygen in the tissues. Hypoxemia is the most common cause of hypoxia, but other factors can lead to either one of these conditions. For example, if the patient is anemic he or she may not be hypoxemic, but may very well be hypoxic. This is due to the fact that although all the patient's red blood cells may be saturated with oxygen, there may be too few red blood cells to meet metabolic demands. On the other hand, if the patient has polycythemia vera they may be hypoxemic, but will likely not be hypoxic. This is due to the fact that there are so many red blood cells they will not all be saturated, but there are enough saturated red blood cells to meet the body's demands. The paramedic must evaluate the patient's presentation and past medical history when determining the presence of either or both of these conditions.

The earliest indication of hypoxia is restlessness and anxiety. In cases of severe hypoxemia cyanosis can occur. The bluish discoloration of the skin in cyanosis is the result of circulating deoxygenated blood. Normal concentrations of oxygen bound hemoglobin are 15 mg/dL. Cyanosis occurs when the concentration is 5 mg/dL or less.

Initial management of hypoxia and hypoxemia includes increasing ventilation, providing supplemental oxygen, or a combination of the two. Other options include positive-pressure ventilation and the possibility of medication administration, as may be indicated for a patient with bronchoconstriction caused by asthma or a diuretic for pulmonary edema.

The ability of the body to balance CO_2 levels in the blood is linked to the ability of the respiratory system to "blow off" excess CO_2. Any condition that results in **hypoventilation** increases the carbon dioxide levels in the blood and results in **hypercarbia,** or an excess of CO_2, while blowing off too much carbon dioxide, or **hyperventilation,** leads to **hypocarbia.** Several factors can influence the levels of CO_2.

Causes of hypercarbia include:

- Hypoventilation, which may be associated with drugs such as narcotics
- Decreased elimination of CO_2 secondary to reactive airway disease, or **"air trapping"** in the lungs, as occurs in emphysema
- Increased production of CO_2 that may occur from an increase in metabolism, as with fever or physical exertion

Causes of hypocarbia include:

- Hyperventilation, which lowers CO_2 levels as an increased rate or depth of respiration blows off too much CO_2
- Increased elimination of CO_2, such as in metabolic acidosis
- Decreased cardiac output
- Interference with perfusion or function of the lung(s) such as pulmonary embolus or tension pneumothorax

- Decreased production of CO_2 that may occur from a decrease in metabolism such as hypothermia

Interventions to restore carbon dioxide levels include reversing the underlying cause. Because hyperventilation can have many etiologies, do not have any patient who is hyperventilating breathe into a paper bag. If the patient is hyperventilating secondary to a pulmonary embolus you will worsen any hypoxia that exists. If the patient is hyperventilating in compensation for a metabolic acidosis you will worsen their acidosis. The most effective care for hyperventilating patients is to treat the underlying cause. Psychogenic hyperventilation is a diagnoses of exclusion. If the paramedic determines there is no other cause of the hyperventilation then administering oxygen and coaching patients to slow the rate of breathing and decrease the depth of their breaths is appropriate. However, you should continue to assess the patient to ensure there is not another underlying cause of the hyperventilation.

Lung and Respiratory Volumes

The total lung volume for an average adult man is approximately 6 L. Knowledge of lung volumes is important because they can provide a measure of respiratory function. This information can affect your decision about providing positive-pressure ventilation. When using an automatic transport ventilator, you often must adjust its settings on the basis of a patient's individual needs. **Peak flow meters** are simple devices that assess the maximal amount of air a patient can exhale, expressed in liters per minute. These devices often are used by asthmatics to measure respiratory efficiency. Familiarize yourself with the respiratory capacities and measurements shown in Box 14-1.

Control of Respiration

[OBJECTIVES 14, 15, 16, 17, 18]

Multiple factors influence the rate and depth of ventilation. The respiratory rate is the number of breaths a person takes per minute. Most of the time we give little to no conscious thought to the fact we are breathing. As a process, breathing is an involuntary mechanism that can be consciously altered for a short period. Normally breathing is regulated by a respiratory center in the brain responsible for receiving input through several mechanisms that, in turn, control respiration in an effort to maintain homeostasis of oxygen, carbon dioxide, and hydrogen ion levels.

Primary control of respiration lies in a portion of the brain called the *brainstem* (Figures 14-5 and 14-6). Two components of the brainstem involved in neural control of breathing include the medulla oblongata and the pons. The respiratory center located in the medulla controls involuntary respiration. The impulses for respiration travel from the dorsal and ventral groups of the respiratory center via the respiratory motor neurons to the phrenic nerves (for the diaphragm) and the intercostal

---

BOX 14-1 Lung/Respiratory Volumes

Tidal volume: Represents the volume of gas inhaled or exhaled during a single respiratory cycle. In the average adult male, this is approximately 500 mL (5 to 7 mL/kg).

Dead air space: Not all the air inspired during a breath participates in gas exchange and can be further classified as anatomic or physiologic dead space. In the average adult man this equates to approximately 150 mL. Anatomic dead space includes airway passages such as the trachea and bronchi that are incapable of participating in gas exchange. Physiologic dead space includes alveoli that have the potential to participate in gas exchange but do not because of disease or obstruction, such as in COPD or atelectasis.

Alveolar air volume: In contrast to dead air space, alveolar volume is the amount of air that does reach the alveoli for gas exchange (approximately 350 mL in an adult man). It is the difference between tidal volume and dead-space volume.

Minute Volume: Amount of gas moved in and out of the respiratory tract per minute. Tidal volume multiplied by ventilatory rate equals minute volume. The minute volume is the true measurement of a patient's ventilatory status and is vital in assessing pulmonary function. It ascertains the ventilatory rate and the depth of each inhalation.

Functional reserve capacity: The volume of air remaining in the lungs at the end of a normal expiration.

Residual volume: After a maximal forced exhalation, this is the amount of air remaining in the lungs and airway passages not able to be expelled.

Inspiratory reserve volume: Amount of gas that can be forcefully inspired in addition to a normal breath's tidal volume.

Expiratory reserve volume: Amount of gas that can be forcefully expired at the end of a normal expiration.

FiO_2: The percentage of oxygen in inspired air (increases with supplemental oxygen); commonly documented as a decimal (e.g., $FiO_2 = 0.85$).

Peak expiratory flow: the greatest rate of air flow that can be achieved during forced expiration beginning with the lungs fully inflated.

---

nerves (for the external intercostal muscles). Vagus nerve fibers are richly spread throughout the larynx, trachea, bronchi, and lungs, affecting coughing. During deep suctioning or other airway procedures, the patient's heart rate must be monitored because stimulation of the vagus nerve can result in bradycardia. Another important nerve that innervates the diaphragm, causing its contraction and subsequent inspiration, is the phrenic nerve. As an involuntary pathway, the more impulses transmitted, the more rapid the respiratory rate. If the medulla should fail in its control of respiration, a secondary control center called the *apneustic center* is located in the pons. This center stimulates the inspiratory center prolonging inha-

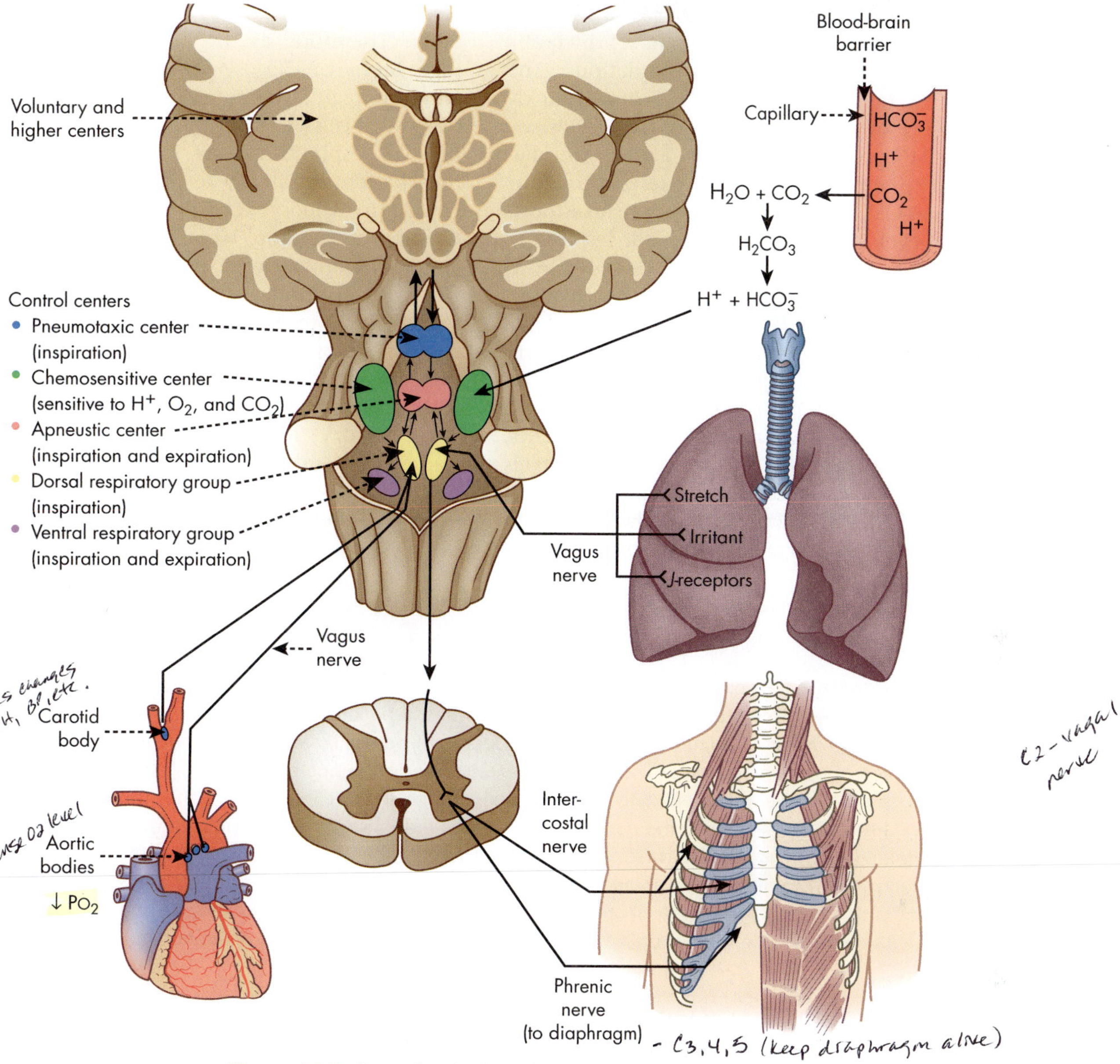

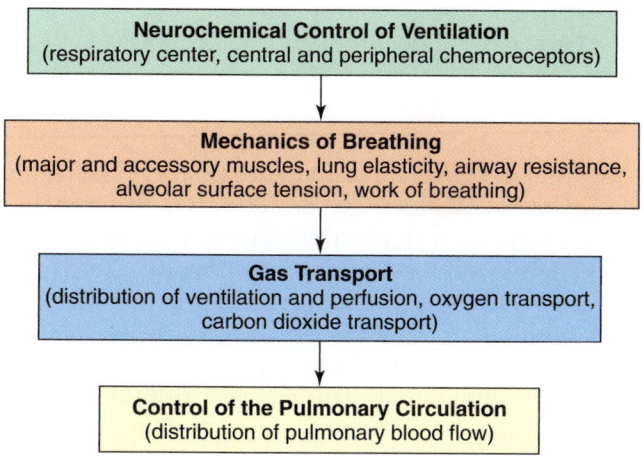

Figure 14-5 Neurochemical respiratory control system.

Control centers
- Pneumotaxic center (inspiration)
- Chemosensitive center (sensitive to H^+, O_2, and CO_2)
- Apneustic center (inspiration and expiration)
- Dorsal respiratory group (inspiration)
- Ventral respiratory group (inspiration and expiration)

Voluntary and higher centers

Blood-brain barrier

Capillary

HCO_3^-

H^+

CO_2

H^+

$H_2O + CO_2$

H_2CO_3

$H^+ + HCO_3^-$

Vagus nerve

Stretch
Irritant
J-receptors

Carotid body

senses changes in pH, pO₂ etc.

Aortic bodies

Sense O2 level

$\downarrow PO_2$

Vagus nerve

Inter-costal nerve

Phrenic nerve (to diaphragm) *– C3,4,5 (keep diaphragm alive)*

C2 – vagal nerve

Neurochemical Control of Ventilation
(respiratory center, central and peripheral chemoreceptors)

Mechanics of Breathing
(major and accessory muscles, lung elasticity, airway resistance, alveolar surface tension, work of breathing)

Gas Transport
(distribution of ventilation and perfusion, oxygen transport, carbon dioxide transport)

Control of the Pulmonary Circulation
(distribution of pulmonary blood flow)

Figure 14-6 Functional components of the respiratory system.

---

lation and inhibiting expiration. Another center, also located in the pons, responsible for control of expiration is the pneumotaxic center. The primary function of the pneumotaxic center is to inhibit inspiration, or act as a "shut off switch" for inhalation. The impulses of the pneumotaxic center normally override the impulses of the apneustic center. When the pneumotaxic center is damaged, a respiratory pattern called *apneustic respirations* may occur. This consists of prolonged inhalation with brief exhalation.

higher in brain stem – affected 1st in swelling

Maintaining proper O_2, CO_2, and pH levels in the body is an essential function of the respiratory system. Receptors designed to monitor each of these substances in the body are called *chemoreceptors*. Chemoreceptors are located in the medulla and in the carotid arteries and the arch of the aorta. Normally an increase in PCO_2 levels sensed by these chemoreceptors results in the respiratory center increasing respiratory rate in an effort to blow off

Sense pH + pCO2 changes

excess CO_2 building up in the body. The pH of the cerebrospinal fluid (CSF) circulating in the brain is principally responsible for respiratory center stimulation. Any changes noted in the PCO_2 of arterial blood are quickly reflected in the pH level of the CSF. When the PCO_2 rises, the pH of the CSF becomes increasingly acidic, stimulating the respiratory center to increase the respiratory rate. Conversely, when CSF pH levels become more alkaline as a result of low levels of PCO_2 in the blood, respiratory rate decreases.

The dominant control of respiration as described above relies on chemoreceptor sensitivity to the level of PCO_2. Secondarily, the respiratory system continuously monitors and can respond when levels of oxygen become low. A patient with a decreased partial pressure of oxygen in the blood is in a state of **hypoxemia.** Some patients, such as those with COPD, tend to retain higher levels of CO_2. As a result, the chemoreceptors become desensitized and no longer respond well to PCO_2 levels in controlling respiration. A backup regulatory mechanism then responds to levels of oxygen in the blood—the hypoxic drive. Therefore, as the body becomes accustomed to high levels of CO_2, it turns to oxygen as the primary stimulus regulating respiration. Breathing is stimulated by low levels of oxygen. As oxygen levels return to normal, respirations slow. Excess oxygen administration in a patient breathing as a result of the hypoxic drive could (in theory) cause respiratory arrest **(apnea).** Caution is therefore recommended when administering supplemental oxygen to a patient who chronically retains CO_2. However, never withhold oxygen from any patient you believe to be hypoxic. If respiratory depression occurs, simply be prepared to support ventilation as necessary.

Multiple other factors influence control of respiratory rates. Factors such as elevated body temperature, central nervous system (CNS) stimulants, pain, emotion, hypoxia, and acidosis cause an increased respiratory rate. Sleep, decreased metabolic states, and CNS depressants, including alcohol, decrease respiratory rate.

Case Scenario—continued

You administer high flow oxygen to the patient and request that your partner prepare the intubation equipment. Your partner also establishes an IV. Examination of the patient's head reveals no gross injuries, and her pupils are midpoint and unresponsive. There appears to be no damage to her mouth or teeth, and her mouth is free of blood or vomitus. There is no visible trauma to her posterior chest or spine, and her chest appears to be symmetrical. One of the other passengers in the car informs you that the driver was not breathing immediately following the accident. She states that she provided mouth-to-mouth breathing for approximately 1-2 minutes, after which the patient began breathing on her own. When the car is lifted off the patient, you move her onto a spine board and immediately perform endotracheal intubation. Transport to the trauma center takes approximately 25 minutes. As you approach the hospital, you note that the patient's lungs have become more difficult to ventilate, although her oxygen saturation stays in the 90s.

Questions

4. *Is this patient's transport a high priority (i.e., lights and siren)? Why or why not?*
5. *What is your preferred method for performing endotracheal intubation in this case? Why?*
6. *What steps will you take to confirm correct positioning of the endotracheal tube?*
7. *What is the significance of the other findings, including the history of respiratory arrest and the unresponsive pupils? Does this affect your treatment plan? How?*
8. *At what rate and depth will you ventilate the patient's lungs en route to the hospital? Why?*
9. *What are some potential causes of the difficulty or resistance in ventilating that you've experienced? What signs or symptoms may assist in differentiating between them? What action should you take at this time?*

RESPIRATORY ASSESSMENT

[OBJECTIVES 19, 20, 21]

As a paramedic, you must be able to identify respiratory problems quickly to provide appropriate and timely intervention. Your patient's outcome may depend on your ability to recognize current or potential problems early in the patient assessment. Be alert for subtle changes and anticipate needs proactively. Assessment of the respiratory system is a constant process of providing support followed by ongoing assessment.

Assessment of age-appropriate respiratory rate, regularity, and work of breathing are essential parameters to evaluate early (and repeatedly) on every patient.

A patient who has breathing difficulty often has a respiratory rate outside the normal limits for his or her age (Table 14-1). An increase in the respiratory rate is an early sign of respiratory distress.

Although some variation in regularity is to be expected, the respiratory cycles should conform to a fairly steady pattern. Any irregularities in respiratory patterns are significant until proven otherwise. Breathing while at rest

TABLE 14-1	Normal Respiratory Rates by Age
Age	**Breaths/min (at Rest)**
Infant (1 to 12 months)	30 to 60
Toddler (1 to 3 years)	24 to 40
Preschooler (4 to 5 years)	22 to 34
School-age (6 to 12 years)	18 to 30
Adolescent (13 to 18 years)	12 to 16
Adult (18 years and older)	12 to 20

Reprinted from Aehlert, B. (2007). *Pediatric life support study guide* (3rd ed.). St. Louis: Mosby.

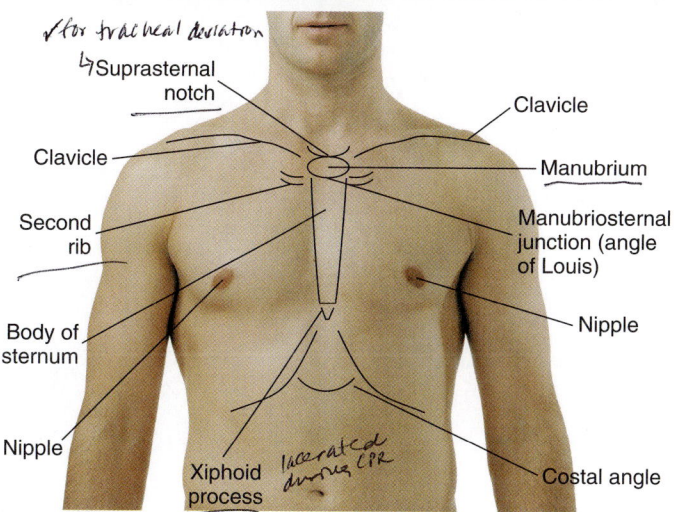

[handwritten annotations on figure: "for tracheal deviation" pointing to Suprasternal notch; "lacerated during CPR" near Xiphoid process]

Labels on figure: Suprasternal notch, Clavicle, Clavicle, Manubrium, Second rib, Manubriosternal junction (angle of Louis), Body of sternum, Nipple, Nipple, Xiphoid process, Costal angle

Figure 14-7 When possible, use topographic landmarks of the chest to describe physical examination findings. These markers include the clavicles, nipples, angle of Louis, suprasternal notch, and costal angle.

should be an effortless process. Observe closely for subtle changes in respiratory rate or effort as a signal of potential problems. Patients with respiratory distress often compensate by instinctively positioning themselves in a manner that will maximize ventilation. Positioning and the use of accessory muscles allow the respiratory system to compensate in some situations. For example, patients with a lower airway obstruction will place themselves in a **tripod position,** while patients with an upper airway obstruction will place themselves in a sniffing position. In a tripod position, the patient sits upright and leans forward, supported by his or her arms, with the neck slightly extended, chin projected, and mouth open which helps maximize airflow through the lower airways. In the sniffing position, the patient will extend the head while flexing the neck to maintain patency of the upper airway. Unless contraindicated, place a patient with respiratory distress in a semi-Fowler's (sitting up with the head at a 45-degree angle) or high Fowler's (sitting upright at a 90-degree angle) position.

Respiratory distress may result from a variety of illnesses and injuries. Either alone or in combination, respiratory distress may be caused by upper and/or lower airway obstruction, inadequate ventilation, impairment of respiratory muscles, or nervous system impairment. **Dyspnea** is an uncomfortable awareness of one's breathing. It may be associated with a change in the patient's breathing rate, effort, or pattern. **Hypoxia,** a lack of oxygen available to the tissues (such as the pulmonary system), is often the result of dyspnea. Conversely, a patient who develops hypoxia may experience dyspnea. When this results in an oxygen deficiency of the blood, hypoxemia, an adequate supply of oxygen is no longer available to the tissues. A total lack of oxygen availability to the tissues is called **anoxia.** Recognizing dyspnea, maintaining an open (patent) airway, and ensuring adequate oxygenation and ventilation are essential to preventing hypoxemia, hypoxia, and anoxic brain injury.

When assessing a patient, you must use all five senses. Additionally, information obtained about the patient's medical history is essential for gaining a complete picture of the patient's airway status. When possible, use topo-

graphic landmarks of the chest to describe your physical examination findings (Figure 14-7). These markers include the clavicles, nipples, angle of Louis, suprasternal notch, and costal angle. The **angle of Louis** is an angulation of the sternum that indicates the point where the second rib joins with the sternum. Because this landmark can be seen and felt, it is used as a starting point from which the ribs and intercostal spaces can be counted. The number of each intercostal space corresponds to that of the rib immediately above it (Seidel, 2003). The **suprasternal notch** is a depression that is easily felt at the base of the anterior aspect of the neck, just above the angle of Louis. The **costal angle** is the angle formed by the margins of the ribs at the sternum. Anatomic landmarks of the chest are used to help localize physical examination findings (Figure 14-8).

When approaching the patient, keep a global perspective; observe the patient's general appearance and level of distress as well as the color of the skin and the patient's posture and surroundings. The presence of cyanosis indicates a serious gas exchange problem requiring immediate corrective action. Look at other physical characteristics that will provides clues regarding the presence of respiratory distress, including gasping, nasal flaring, or pursed-lip breathing.

A number of visual clues help assess a patient's airway and work of breathing. The patient's position, or posture, was previously mentioned. A tripod position is often used by patients in respiratory distress because it reduces airway resistance, maximizes the effectiveness of the diaphragm and accessory muscles, and requires the least amount of effort to maintain the posture. Dyspnea relieved by a change in position (either sitting upright or standing) is called **orthopnea.** Orthopnea indicates possible left ventricular failure or serious pulmonary compli-

[handwritten at bottom: "heart failure / pulmonary edema   "3 pillow orthopnea""]

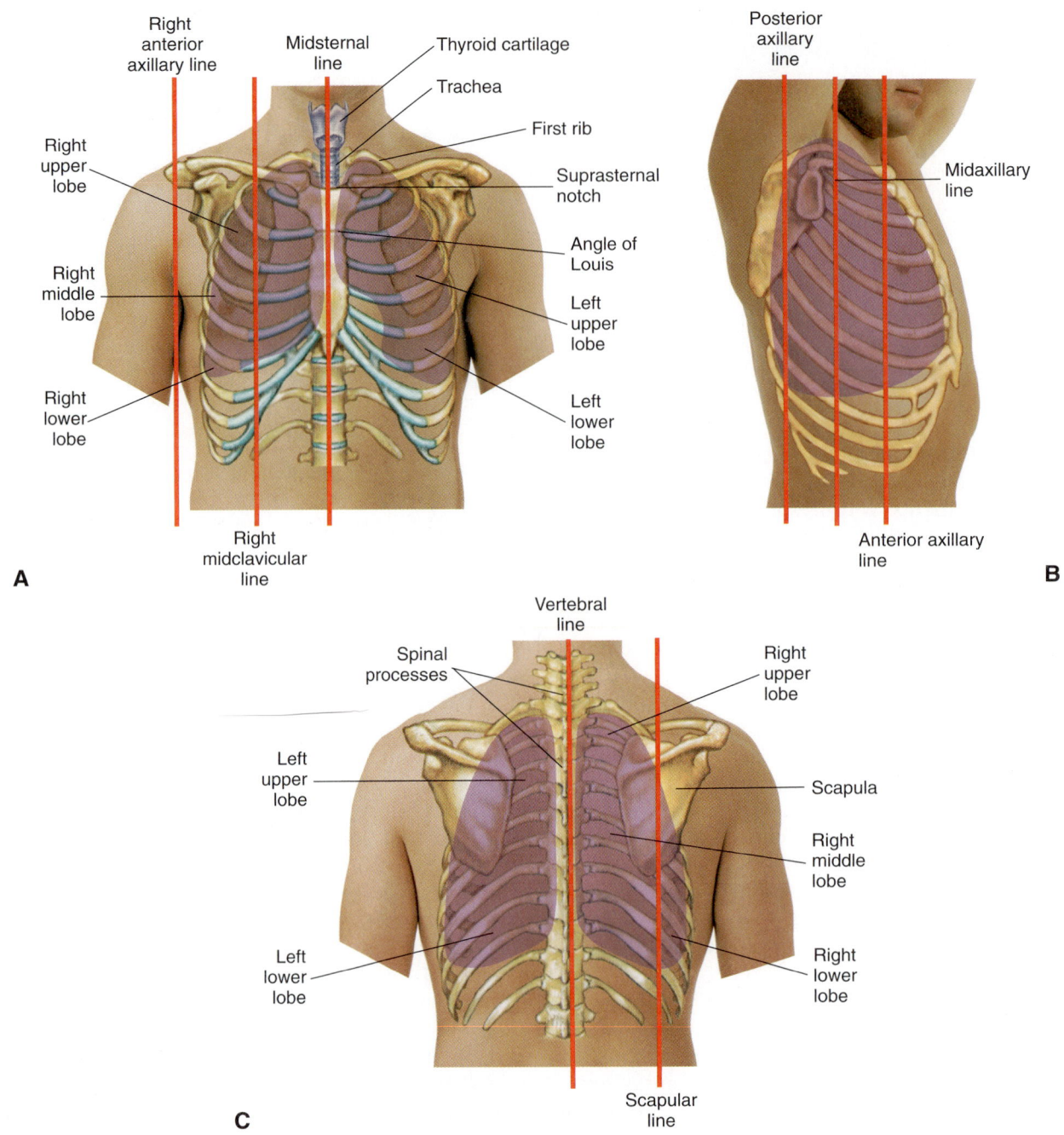

Figure 14-8 Landmarks of the chest. **A,** Anterior chest. **B,** Right lateral chest. **C,** Posterior chest.

cations because of hypoxia and hypoventilation. Patients with orthopnea often sleep propped up on pillows as an aid to improve their respiratory efficiency.

Inspect the chest for full, equal bilateral rise and fall. The entire chest cavity normally moves in unison. **Para-doxic motion** of the chest is movement that can occur when multiple adjacent ribs are broken. During para-doxic motion, a portion of the chest appears to move in the opposite direction of the rest of the chest. For example, a segment of the chest wall moves inward while the rest of the chest is expanding. The affected part of the chest wall is called a **flail segment** (see Chapter 49).

Note the anteroposterior (AP) diameter of the chest (Figure 14-9). The AP diameter of a healthy infant's chest is roughly the same as the lateral diameter. In a healthy adult, the AP diameter of the chest is usually less than the lateral diameter. The presence of a "barrel chest," or an increased AP chest diameter, is common in patients with emphysema (Figure 14-10).

Patients with hypoxia caused by obstructed airways in the bronchial tree use accessory muscles with each breath. The use of the accessory muscles can be seen with retractions of chest and neck muscles. Observe the neck and chest for extra exertion on inhalation and be alert to the

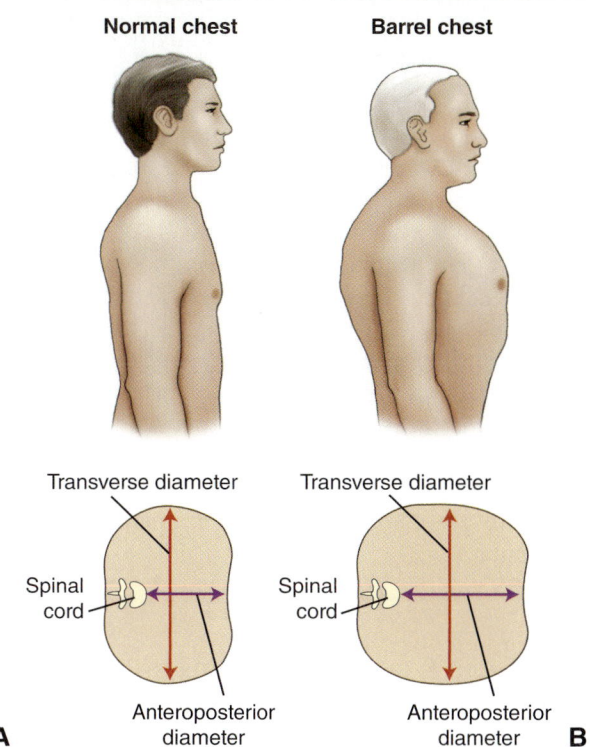

Figure 14-10 Anteroposterior chest diameter. **A,** In a healthy adult, the anteroposterior diameter of the chest is less than the lateral diameter. **B,** Barrel chest. Note the increase in anteroposterior diameter.

"1 to 2 word dyspnea"

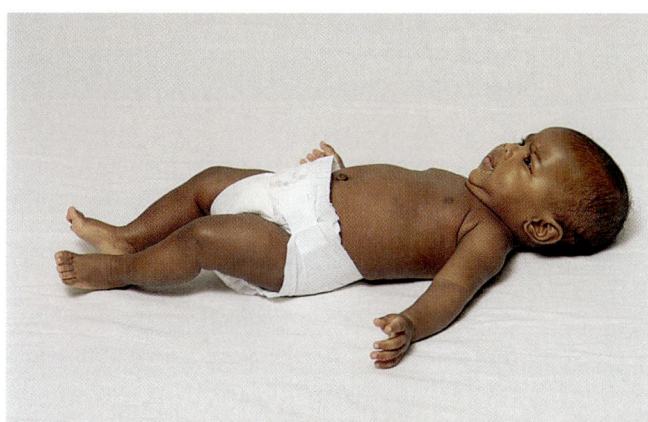

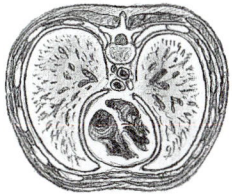

Figure 14-9 The anteroposterior diameter of a healthy infant's chest is about the same as the lateral diameter.

possibility that a patient who does not appear to exert much effort to breathe but appears to be hypoxic (as evidenced by other signs) may be exhausted and in respiratory failure.

Patients who have emphysema often have difficulty expelling air from the lungs. To compensate, they commonly exhale through "pursed lips" with each breath. *slows exhalation* This helps to maintain some back pressure, or self-induced continuous positive airway pressure (CPAP). A small level of CPAP keeps the alveoli inflated longer and allows extra time and surface area for the diffusion of CO_2 out of the body.

Palpation of the chest wall can provide clues, especially about injuries to the chest. The presence of subcutaneous emphysema indicates that air is leaking from the pulmonary system into the soft tissues, often from a pneumothorax. Subcutaneous emphysema produces a "snap, crackle, and pop" sensation that feels like crisped rice cereal under the skin. *Think pneumothorax*

When providing positive-pressure ventilation with a bag-mask device, note the compliance of the patient's lungs. **Compliance** refers to the resistance of the patient's lung tissue to ventilation. The lungs are normally pliable and expand easily. If the lungs feel stiff or inflexible, lung compliance is said to be poor. A tension pneumothorax is an example of a life-threatening condition that presents with poor compliance. Finally, note any **crepitation** (a sign of bone ends grinding together) or tenderness as you palpate the chest.

Careful attention to all sounds that patients make is critical to a complete respiratory assessment. In addition to listening to the patient vocalize and breathe, you must also listen closely inside the patient's body to the sounds the patient is making with each breath. Internal sounds are heard with a stethoscope. Listening with a stethoscope is called *auscultation*. Although auscultation is an important assessment tool, remember to note any audible respiratory sounds as you approach the patient. Any patient with noisy respirations must be assessed for a possible airway obstruction. Physical obstructions generally result in snoring respirations. If the patient is unresponsive, the obstruction is usually caused by the tongue. *snoring* Manual repositioning of the patient's head and insertion of a simple airway adjunct, such as an oral or nasal airway, can quickly relieve this obstruction. A patient who has secretions in the upper airway may exhibit gurgling noises. The presence of gurgling is an indication that immediate suctioning is necessary to maintain an open airway. Stridor, a high-pitched shrill noise that is usually heard on inspiration, is a sign of upper airway compromise and possible impending airway obstruction. *airway burns = insp. + exp. stridor* Many respiratory illnesses have an associated cough, with or without sputum production. A cough that produces sputum is said to be a productive cough. The presence or absence of a cough and the appearance of any sputum can be an important assessment finding.

Auscultating lung sounds is essential for *every* patient with any type of respiratory symptom. The primary goal

BOX 14-2	Sounds That Indicate Potential Respiratory Compromise

Wheezes: A musical, whistling sound heard on inspiration and/or expiration resulting from constriction or obstruction of the pharynx, trachea, or bronchi. Wheezing is commonly associated with asthma.

Crackles (rales): As the name implies, when fluid accumulates in the smaller airway passages, air passing through the fluid creates a moist crackling or popping sound heard on inspiration. Crackles are commonly associated with pulmonary edema.

Rattles *(rhonchi)*: Secondary to inflammation and mucous or fluid in the larger airway passages, rattles, or rhonchi, are descriptive of airway congestion heard on inspiration. Rhonchi are commonly associated with bronchitis or pneumonia.

can palpate rattles

Ronchi - coarse sounds (Pneumonia - congestion)

BOX 14-3	Modified Respirations That Are Variations of Normal Breathing

Coughing: A protective mechanism usually induced by mucosal irritation; the forceful, spastic expiration experienced during coughing aids in the clearance of the bronchi and bronchioles.

Sneezing: Occurs as a result of nasal irritation and allows clearance of the nose.

Gagging: A reflex caused by irritation of the posterior pharynx that can result in vomiting. An emesis basin should be available; prepared to suction as needed.

Sighing: Involuntary and periodic slow, deep breath followed by a prolonged expiratory phase. Occurring about once per minute, the act of sighing is thought to open atelectatic (collapsed) alveoli.

Hiccup (hiccoughing): Intermittent spasm of the diaphragm that results in sudden inspiration with spastic closure of the glottis. Usually annoying, the hiccup serves no known physiologic purpose.

of auscultation is to determine if lung sounds are present and equal bilaterally. Compare sounds from side to side, listening to one lung and then the same place on the other lung. With each stethoscope placement, listen to at least one full inhalation and exhalation. See Chapter 17 for a detailed discussion of normal and abnormal lung sounds.

Sounds that indicate the potential for respiratory compromise are shown in Box 14-2.

PARAMEDIC*Pearl*

When listening to lung sounds, keep in mind that a patient who is in a supine position for a prolonged period will accumulate fluid that may be detected in the posterior and not the anterior lung sound assessments.

The assessment process involves the collection of medical history information from the patient and others. A patient with a chronic respiratory condition will likely be able to paint a fairly clear picture of what has changed with his or her current dyspnea. You must determine what has happened in relation to the patient's difficulty breathing. Has it occurred suddenly, or has it been progressing gradually over time? Is the patient able to pinpoint a trigger that brought on this episode? Also determine whether the problem is constant or recurrent. Ask the patient whether anything seems to make breathing worse or better. Inquiring about other associated symptoms such as a productive cough, chest pain, and fever can help narrow the possibilities of what is wrong with the patient. As you begin to formulate a treatment plan, you must determine what, if anything, the patient may have done to treat his or her condition before your arrival. Patients often follow a predictable pattern, especially with chronic illnesses. Ask if anything like this event has ever happened previously and, if so, what care

was received. Has the patient ever been hospitalized for such a condition? Does he or she take any medications and, if so, as prescribed by the physician? Finally, be certain to ask whether the patient has ever required endotracheal intubation for a prior respiratory problem. Patients who have been artificially ventilated in the past are more likely to require such procedures in the future.

Noting that the purpose of the primary survey is to seek out and find all life threats, recognize that the following assessment parameters in a patient with dyspnea are highly significant and warrant quick attention:

Priority pts.

- Altered mental status
- Cyanosis
- Absent breath sounds
- Stridor
- One- to two-word dyspnea (represents poor minute volume)
- Use of accessory muscles

Failure to intervene and reverse course may have an ominous outcome for your patient.

A change in the rate or rhythm of the respiratory cycle often is an early indication of impending respiratory distress. Some forms of modified respiration are protective in nature or considered a normal variation (Box 14-3). Respiratory pattern changes usually are a sign that a serious condition exists (Box 14-4).

SUPPLEMENTAL OXYGENATION

[OBJECTIVES 22, 23, 24]

Oxygen administered from a supply cylinder through medical tubing is a drug. As such, it requires a thorough understanding for it to be administered safely, just as

BOX 14-4   Common Abnormal Respiratory Patterns

Bradypnea: a respiratory rate that is persistently slower than normal for age; in adults, a rate slower than 12 breaths/min.

Tachypnea: a respiratory rate that is persistently faster than normal for age; in adults, a rate faster than 20 breaths/min.

Hyperpnea (hyperventilation): a respiratory pattern characterized by rapid, deep breathing.

Air trapping: a respiratory pattern associated with an obstruction in the pulmonary tree; the breathing rate increases to overcome resistance in getting air out, the respiratory effort becomes more shallow, the volume of trapped air increases, and the lungs inflate (Seidel, 2003).

Cheyne-Stokes respirations: a pattern of gradually increasing rate and depth of breathing that tapers to slower and shallower breathing with a period of apnea before the cycle repeats itself. Often described as a crescendo-decrescendo pattern or periodic breathing. May occur in children and older adults during sleep, but otherwise occurs in patients with a brainstem abnormality or drug-induced respiratory compromise (Seidel, 2003).

Kussmaul respirations: deep, gasping respirations that may be slow or rapid. Often associated with metabolic acidosis, this breathing pattern is compensatory as it attempts to blow off excess CO_2 built up in the body.

Biot's respirations: irregular respirations varying in rate and depth and interrupted with periods of apnea; associated with increased intracranial pressure, brain damage at the level of the medulla, and respiratory compromise from drug poisoning.

Central neurogenic hyperventilation: similar to Kussmaul respirations; characterized as deep, rapid breathing; associated with increased intracranial pressure.

Agonal respirations: slow, shallow, irregular respirations resulting from anoxic brain injury.

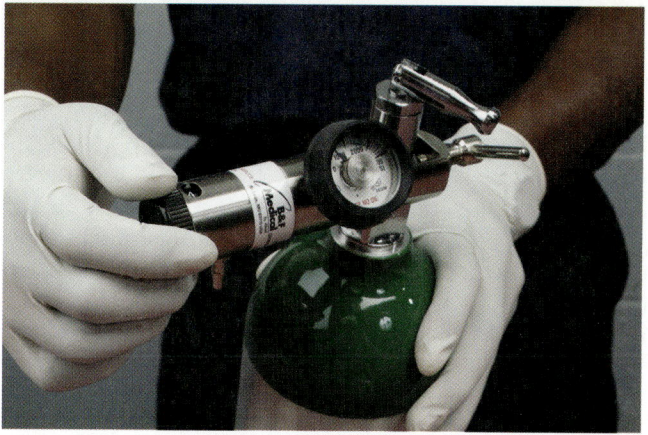

Figure 14-11 Oxygen cylinder with regulator and flow meter attached.

pressure ventilation. For now, this discussion will focus on oxygen delivery devices.

Oxygen Supply

Oxygen is supplied in two available forms, as a compressed gas or liquid. Liquid oxygen offers the advantage of being able to be stored in large quantities in its cooled aqueous state, then converted to a gas during warming. However, upright storage is generally required, and other special requirements are necessary for large volume and cylinder transfer, making liquid oxygen unrealistic for prehospital use.

Compressed gases such as oxygen can also be stored in steel or aluminum cylinders of various sizes. Common oxygen tank sizes include D tanks capable of storing approximately 400 L; jumbo D tanks, storing approximately 640 L; E tanks, storing approximately 680 L, and M tanks, storing approximately 3450 L. D and E cylinders are commonly used for portable purposes in a medic's airway bag, whereas M-sized or larger tanks are for on-board ambulance oxygen supply. Ensuring that your tanks have adequate amounts of oxygen is one of your many equipment responsibilities. To calculate how many minutes of oxygen delivery a tank has remaining, complete the following equation:

$$\frac{\text{Minutes}}{\text{remaining}} = \frac{\text{Tank pressure (psi)} \times 0.28}{\text{flow (L/min)}}$$

With a nonrebreather mask running at 15 L/min, a D-sized tank with 2000 psi will provide approximately 35 minutes of oxygen delivery.

A regulator is an attachment to a cylinder that controls the release of its contents. Two types of regulators include high-pressure regulators, which are used to transfer cylinder gas from tank to tank, and therapy regulators, which are used on cylinders for delivering oxygen to patients (Figure 14-11). A regulator is attached to a cylinder stem decreasing the 50 psi escape pressure to a lower pressure acceptable for oxygen administration.

with any other medication. The administration of oxygen involves side effects, complications, and contraindications, just as with other drugs. Oxygen is essential for the human body to sustain itself. Inadequate amounts of oxygen in the air, inadequate ventilation from shallow or slow breathing, and hypoxia from any cause can rapidly result in a life-threatening medical emergency. Providing supplemental oxygen can improve oxygen diffusion into the blood and diminish the effects of hypoxemia on vital organs.

Many supplemental oxygen delivery methods are available. You must choose the correct option for the patient's circumstances. Remember that when you administer supplemental oxygen to a patient, he or she must have an adequate rate and depth (minute volume) of ventilation. If there is any doubt over the adequacy of ventilation in addition to oxygenation, support the patient with both supplemental oxygen and positive-

Flow meters attached to the regulator allow adjustment and measurement of the amount of oxygen flowing in liters per minute.

Unsafe use of oxygen cylinders can create a dangerous situation. A great force to the stem of a gas-containing oxygen cylinder could cause it to become a projected missile. Although the oxygen itself is a non-combustible gas, oxygen supports combustion. Combustible products in an oxygen rich environment burn very easily. Never use oxygen near an open flame or with a patient who is smoking.

Delivery Devices

[OBJECTIVE 25]

Many devices exist for delivering supplemental oxygen to patients. Devices have various capabilities relating to percentage of oxygen delivery. Your patient's condition will determine the method of delivery as well as the liter per minute flow rate. Some patients will not tolerate a specific device, necessitating an alternate choice. For example, a patient with severe difficulty breathing may not tolerate a nonrebreather mask because of a feeling of suffocation. Sometimes all that is needed is coaching from you when initially beginning oxygen therapy. If coaching is ineffective, a less-optimal delivery device may be required.

Nasal Cannula

A nasal cannula (also called *nasal prongs*) is a piece of plastic tubing with two soft prongs that project from the tubing. The prongs are inserted into the patient's nostrils. The tubing is then secured to the patient's face (Figure 14-12). Oxygen flows from the cannula into the patient's nasopharynx, which acts as an anatomic reservoir. Although the actual inspired oxygen concentration depends on the patient's respiratory rate and depth, a nasal cannula can deliver oxygen concentrations of approximately 25% to 45% at 1 to 6 L/min flow. Flow rates of 6 L/min and more dry the mucous membranes of the nasal cavity and often cause discomfort, including headaches. Advantages and disadvantages of using a nasal cannula are shown in Box 14-5.

Simple Face Mask

A simple face mask is a plastic reservoir designed to fit over the patient's nose and mouth. The mask is secured around the patient's head by an elastic strap. The internal capacity of the mask produces a reservoir effect. Small holes on each side of the mask allow the passage of inspired and expired air. Supplemental oxygen is delivered through a small-diameter tube connected to the base of the mask (Figure 14-13).

At 6 to 10 L/min, the simple face mask can provide an inspired oxygen concentration of approximately 40% to 60%. The recommended flow rate is 8 to 10 L/min. The patient's actual inspired oxygen concentration will vary because the amount of air that mixes with supplemental oxygen depends on the patient's inspiratory flow rate. Advantages and disadvantages of using a simple face mask are shown in Box 14-6.

PARAMEDIC*Pearl*

When using a simple face mask, the oxygen flow rate must be higher than 5 L/min to flush the buildup of the patient's exhaled CO_2 from the mask.

BOX 14-5	Nasal Cannula: Advantages and Disadvantages

Advantages

- Comfortable, well tolerated by most patients
- Does not interfere with patient assessment or impede patient communication with healthcare personnel
- Allows talking and eating
- No rebreathing of expired air
- Can be used with mouth breathers
- Useful in patients predisposed to carbon dioxide retention
- Can be used for patients who require oxygen but cannot tolerate a nonrebreather mask

Disadvantages

- Can only be used in a spontaneously breathing patient
- Easily displaced
- Nasal passages must be open
- Drying of mucosa
- May cause sinus pain

Reprinted from Aehlert, B. (2007). *ACLS study guide* (3rd ed.), St. Louis: Mosby.

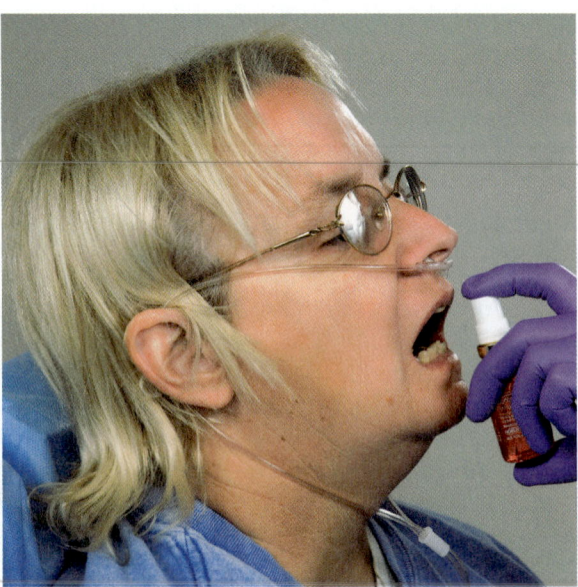

Figure 14-12 Nasal cannula.

6L/min ≈ 40% FiO2   each L adds 2-4 %O2

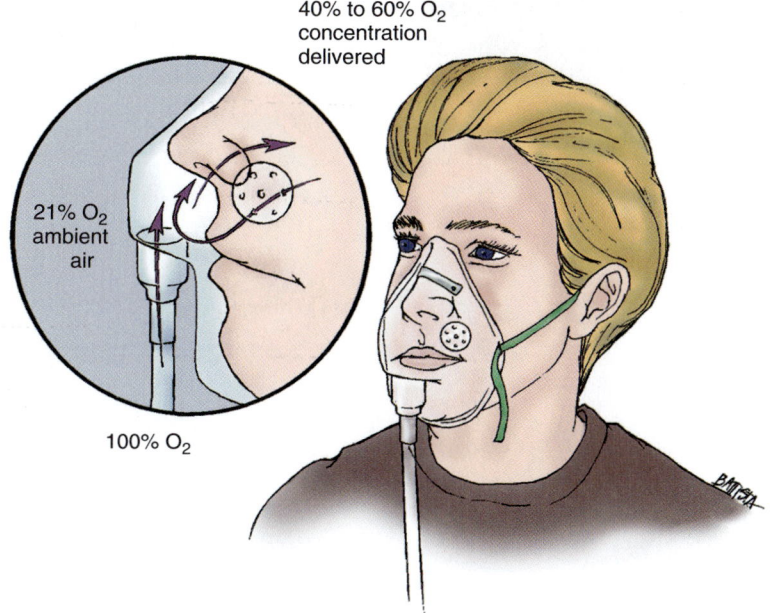

40% to 60% O₂ concentration delivered

21% O₂ ambient air

100% O₂

Figure 14-13 Simple face mask.

Advantages

- Higher oxygen concentration delivered than by nasal cannula

Disadvantages

- Can only be used in a spontaneously breathing patient
- Not tolerated well in severely dyspneic patients
- Can be uncomfortable
- Difficult to hear the patient speaking when the device is in place
- Must be removed at meals
- Requires a tight face seal to prevent leakage of oxygen
- Oxygen flow rates of more than 10 L/min do not enhance delivered oxygen concentration

Reprinted from Aehlert, B. (2007). *ACLS study guide* (3rd ed.), St. Louis: Mosby.

Partial Rebreather Mask

A partial rebreather mask is similar to a simple face mask, but has an attached oxygen-collecting device (reservoir) at the base of the mask that is filled before patient use. One hundred percent oxygen is delivered through oxygen tubing to the reservoir bag. The reservoir collects the oxygen and allows some of the patient's exhaled air (approximately equal to the volume of the patient's anatomic dead space) to enter the reservoir bag and be reused (Figure 14-14).

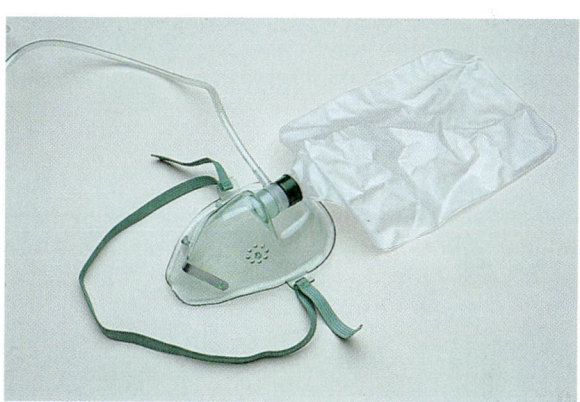

Figure 14-14 Partial rebreather mask.

No flap over vent

The oxygen concentration of the patient's exhaled air, combined with the supply of 100% oxygen, allows the use of oxygen flow rates lower than those necessary for a nonrebreather mask. Depending on the patient's respiratory pattern, oxygen concentrations of 35% to 60% can be delivered when an oxygen flow rate (typically 6 to 10 L/min) is used that prevents the reservoir bag from completely collapsing on inspiration. Advantages and disadvantages of using a partial rebreather mask are shown in Box 14-7.

PARAMEDIC*Pearl*

Do not use a nasal cannula or any type of oxygen mask for a patient who has poor respiratory effort or who is apneic. These patients require positive-pressure ventilation.

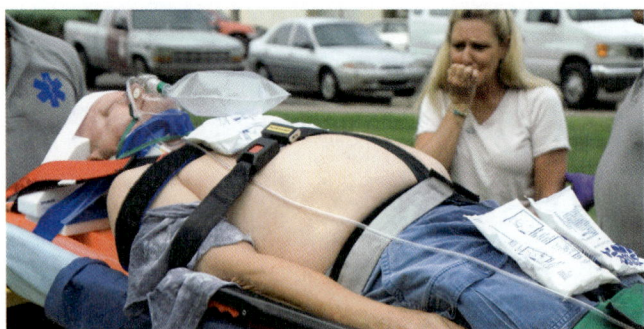

Figure 14-15 Nonrebreather mask.

Nonrebreather Mask

A nonrebreather mask is similar to a partial rebreather mask but does not permit mixing of the patient's exhaled air with 100% oxygen. Rubber flaps cover the side ports on the mask, preventing inhalation of room air. When the patient breathes in, oxygen is drawn into the mask from the reservoir (bag) through a one-way valve that separates the bag from the mask. When the patient breathes out, the exhaled air exits through the side ports on the mask. The one-way valve prevents the patient's exhaled air from returning to the reservoir bag (thus the name nonrebreather). This ensures a supply of 100% oxygen to the patient with minimal dilution from the entrainment of room air (Figure 14-15).

A nonrebreather mask is the delivery device of choice when high concentrations of oxygen are needed in the spontaneously breathing patient. Depending on the patient's respiratory pattern, oxygen concentrations of up to 100% can be delivered when an oxygen flow rate

(typically 10 to 15 L/min) is used that prevents the reservoir bag from completely collapsing on inspiration. Inflate the reservoir bag with oxygen *before* placing the nonrebreather mask on the patient. Advantages and disadvantages of using a nonrebreather mask are shown in Box 14-8.

PARAMEDIC*Pearl*

When using a partial rebreather or nonrebreather mask, ensure that the bag does not collapse when the patient inhales. If the bag collapses, increase the delivered oxygen by 2-L increments until the bag remains inflated. The reservoir bag must remain at least two thirds full so that sufficient supplemental oxygen is available for each breath.

Venturi Mask

A Venturi mask fits over the patient's nose and mouth and contains a short corrugated hose with a jet orifice connected to oxygen supply tubing (Figure 14-16). Oxygen under pressure is forced through a small jet orifice entering the mask. As the oxygen passes through the orifice, it draws room air into the mask. The resulting mixture is delivered to the patient through the face mask.

A Venturi mask typically delivers oxygen concentrations of 24%, 28%, 35%, 40%, or 50% oxygen. The mask is usually supplied with several color-coded adapters that change the rate of oxygen flow past the air entrainment port. The mix of air and oxygen delivered to the patient is adjusted by changing the adapter that attaches to the base of the mask or by having an adjustable, rotating opening that changes the amount of air mixing with

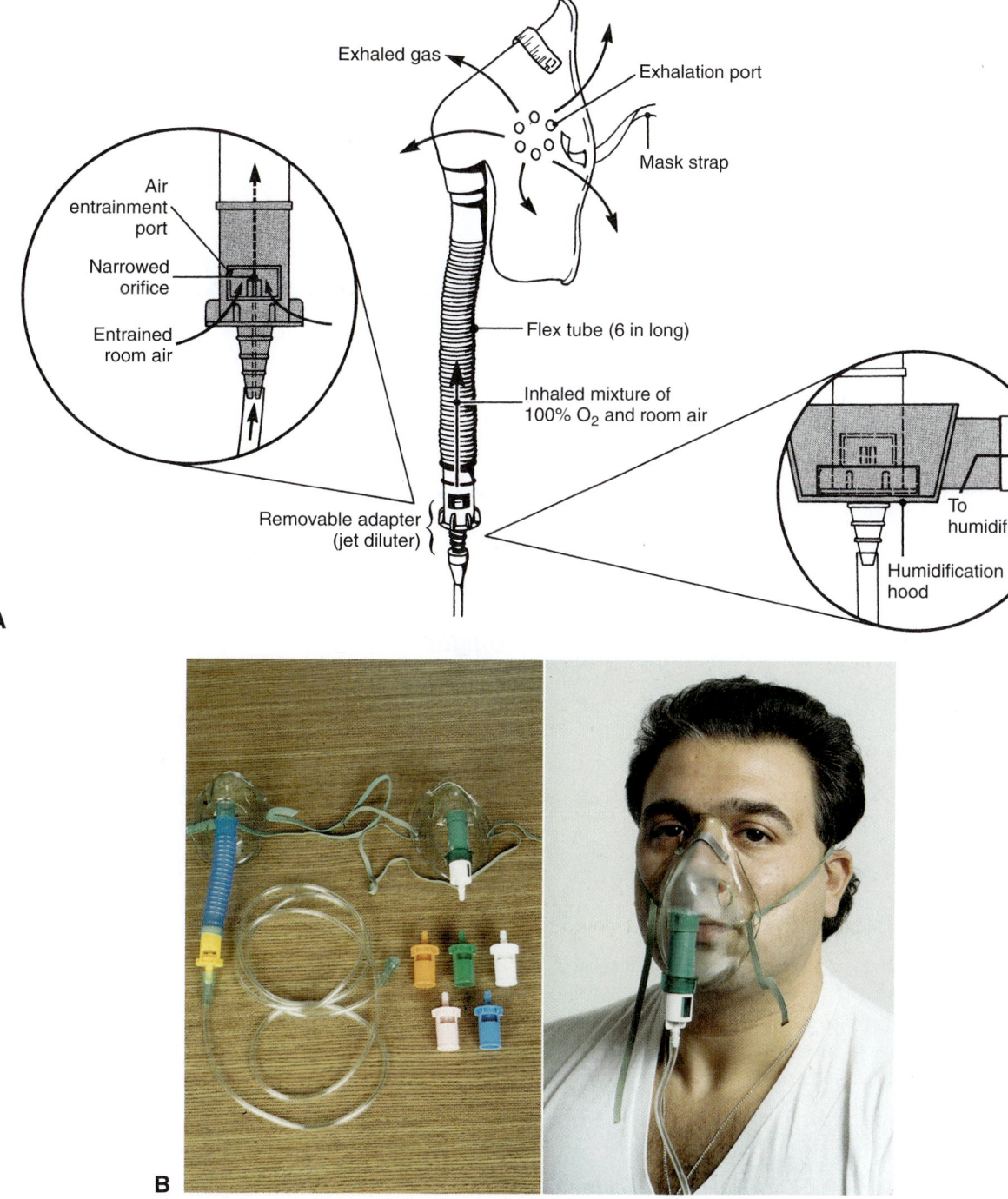

Figure 14-16 A, The Venturi mask fits over the patient's nose and mouth and contains a short corrugated hose with a jet orifice connected to oxygen supply tubing. Oxygen under pressure is forced through the orifice entering the mask. As the oxygen passes through the orifice, it draws ambient air into the mask. The resulting mixture is delivered to the patient through the facemask. **B,** The Venturi mask may be supplied with several color-coded adapters that alter the rate of oxygen flow past the air entrainment port. The mix of air and oxygen delivered to the patient is adjusted by changing either the flow of oxygen or the size of the air entrainment port.

Advantages

- Provides precise inspired oxygen concentration in a selected range
- Recommended for patients who rely on a hypoxic respiratory drive (such as COPD)

Disadvantages

- Can only be used in a spontaneously breathing patient
- Not tolerated well in severely dyspneic patients
- Can be uncomfortable
- Difficult to hear the patient speaking when the device is in place
- Must be removed at meals
- Mask must fit snugly on the patient's face

Reprinted from Aehlert, B. (2007). *ACLS study guide* (3rd ed.), St. Louis: Mosby.
COPD, Chronic obstructive pulmonary disease.

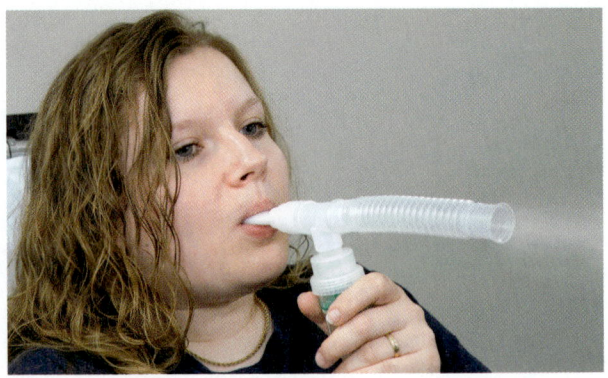

Figure 14-17 Small-volume nebulizer.

oxygen. Advantages and disadvantages of using a Venturi mask are shown in Box 14-9.

PARAMEDIC*Pearl*

Patients breathing on the hypoxic drive benefit from the fine-tuned control of inspired oxygen that the Venturi mask provides.

Small-Volume Nebulizer *6L O2 for nebulizing* ✱

Nebulizers are typically used to aerosolize medications, such as albuterol (Proventil) (Figure 14-17). The aerosol chamber, when attached by oxygen tubing to an oxygen source, creates a fine mist inhaled by the patient and delivers oxygen when attached to a special face mask.

Oxygen Humidifier

[OBJECTIVE 26]

Humidified oxygen is beneficial for patients with croup, epiglottitis, bronchiolitis, or those who are receiving long-term oxygen administration. Humidification helps moisten respiratory mucosa and can aid in loosening thick secretions. Reservoirs are available that attach to the flow meter outlet containing sterile water. During administration, the oxygen is first forced through the water and moistened.

AIRWAY OBSTRUCTION

[OBJECTIVES 27, 28, 29, 30]

Airway obstruction can have many causes. Even a partial blockage of the airway can impair gas exchange to a degree that the patient's life is in jeopardy without quick corrective action. Classifications of airway obstruction include complete obstruction, partial obstruction with poor air exchange, and partial obstruction with good air exchange. Common causes leading to obstruction include the tongue, foreign bodies, laryngeal spasm and edema, trauma, and aspiration.

Tongue

In all unresponsive patients, the tongue is the most common cause of airway obstruction. It is also the easiest to correct. In an unresponsive patient, the muscles that hold the tongue in place become so relaxed that the tongue falls back into the posterior pharynx, blocking the airway. As some air turbulently passes by the obstruction, sonorous respirations are heard. Simple airway maneuvers such as the head tilt/chin lift correctly position the patient's head and jaw, removing the tongue as an obstruction. An oral or nasal airway may be inserted to keep the airway open.

Foreign Bodies

Anything that may be placed in the mouth may, at some point, become a source for an airway obstruction. Food, dentures, broken teeth, toys, and many other items can be implicated. The universal sign of a patient choking includes a person clutching the neck with both hands. Other symptoms associated with a person choking include gagging, stridor, dyspnea, and inability or difficulty speaking.

Patients with a complete airway obstruction should receive emergent basic life support interventions consisting of the Heimlich maneuver, chest thrusts, back blows, and finger sweep as per current guidelines. If basic life support maneuvers fail to relieve the obstruction and the unconscious choking patient cannot be ventilated, a paramedic may perform direct laryngoscopy. With a laryngoscope, the paramedic attempts to visualize the obstruction and, with special forceps called *Magill forceps*, grasps the object and physically removes it from the airway. In a worst-case scenario, the object may actually come to lie beyond the level of the glottis and not be retrievable. In this instance, some medical authorities suggest intubation in an effort to force the foreign body further down the airway (the right mainstem bronchus) so that the patient may be ventilated at least partially on the left. Another option to consider would be the performance of a cricothyrotomy, if trained and authorized to perform by your local medical director.

Laryngeal Spasm and Edema

Several factors can contribute to induce spasm and/or edema of the larynx. Spasm, edema, or a combination can severely constrict the diameter of the airway. In the adult airway, keep in mind that the narrowest portion of the passageway is at the level of the glottis, creating a potentially lethal situation. Edema and spasm may occur because of epiglottitis, anaphylaxis, burns, toxic inhalation, or trauma. Procedurally, intubation can contribute to spasm and edema as well. Overly aggressive intubation can be traumatic and induce spasm. After an endotracheal tube is removed (extubation), swelling and spasm may occur. Administration of an inhaled bronchodilator may help correct the laryngospasm after extubation.

Trauma

Laryngeal tissue is susceptible to both penetrating and blunt trauma. Maintenance of an open pathway involves an intact larynx and supporting muscle tone. Fractured laryngeal tissue decreases muscle tone and results in edema, increasing airway resistance by decreasing airway size.

Aspiration

Vomitus is the most commonly aspirated material. Patients who aspirate face devastating implications, as mortality rate significantly increases. Aspirated material can affect airway structures in a number of ways. In basic terms, aspirated materials may obstruct the airway, thereby preventing adequate oxygenation. Vomitus contains digestive acids and enzymes that destroy delicate bronchiolar tissues. Pathogenic substances may also be introduced that can ultimately lead to a ravaging pulmonary infection. Vigilance on your part to maintain and secure an open airway is important in preventing aspiration.

OPENING THE AIRWAY

Manual Maneuvers

[OBJECTIVE 31]

Basic to any type of airway management procedure is the ability to open a patient's airway manually. Manual maneuvers require no special equipment, are noninvasive, and must not be ignored in lieu of advanced procedures. The first step in every airway procedure, basic or advanced, is to manually open the airway.

The purpose of a manual maneuver is to position the anatomic structures of the patient's airway so that the airway passages are open to the flow of air. Each method helps lift the tongue off the back of the throat, which is the most common cause of a partial airway obstruction in an unresponsive patient. If the patient is breathing, snoring respirations are a sign of airway obstruction from displacement of the tongue. If the patient is not breathing, airway obstruction from the tongue may go undetected until positive-pressure ventilation is attempted. Ventilating an apneic patient with an airway obstruction is difficult. If the airway obstruction is caused by the tongue, repositioning the patient's head and jaw may be all that is needed to open the airway.

An important consideration when determining which maneuver to perform is the possible presence of spinal trauma. Because manual maneuvers manipulate the cervical spine, a modification is required to minimize spinal movement and maintain a neutral spinal position. When opening a patient's airway, the fact you are doing so means that your patient is unable to maintain his or her own airway. You must be prepared with additional equipment such as airway adjuncts and a ventilation device and anticipate the need for suction. Manual airway maneuvers are summarized in Table 14-2.

Head Tilt/Chin Lift

The head tilt/chin lift is the preferred technique for opening the airway of an unresponsive patient without suspected cervical spine injury (Figure 14-18). Following are instructions in performing a head tilt/chin lift:

1. Place the patient in a supine position.
2. Place one hand on the patient's forehead and apply firm pressure with the palm to tilt the patient's head back.
3. Place the tips of the fingers of your other hand under the bony part of the patient's chin and gently lift up and pull the jaw forward. Positioning your fingers under the bony part

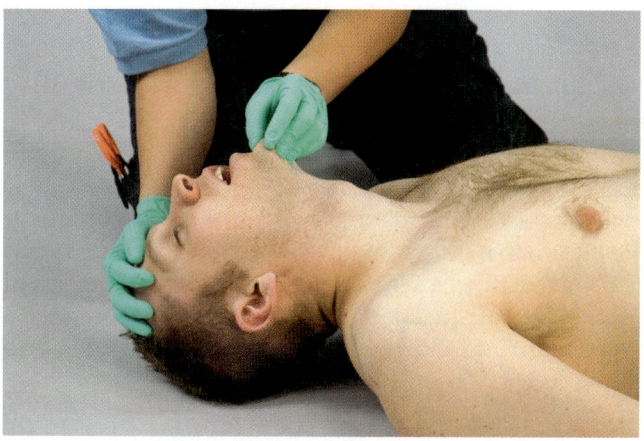

Figure 14-18 Opening the airway with a head tilt/chin lift maneuver.

TABLE 14-2 Manual Airway Maneuvers

	Head Tilt/Chin Lift	Jaw Thrust without Head Tilt
Indications	Unresponsive patient No mechanism for cervical spine injury Unable to protect own airway	Unresponsive patient Possible cervical spine injury Unable to protect own airway
Contraindications	Awake patient Possible cervical spine injury	Awake patient
Advantages	Simple to perform No equipment required Noninvasive	No equipment required Noninvasive
Disadvantages	Does not protect lower airway from aspiration May cause spinal movement	Difficult to maintain Second rescuer needed for bag-mask ventilation Does not protect lower airway from aspiration May cause spinal movement

Reprinted from Aehlert, B. (2007). *ACLS study guide* (3rd ed.), St. Louis: Mosby.

of the patient's chin is important because compression of the soft tissue under the patient's chin can obstruct the airway.

3. Open the patient's mouth by pulling down on the patient's lower lip using the thumb of the same hand used to lift the chin.

Jaw Thrust Maneuver

A jaw thrust maneuver may be performed with or without an accompanying head tilt. For patients who are unresponsive without any risk of spinal injury, perform the following technique:

1. With the patient supine, position yourself above the patient's head or at his side looking at his face.
2. Place your fingers on each side of the lower jaw at the angle of the jaw near the bottom of the patient's ears.
3. Lift the jaw forward toward the patient's face and gently open the mouth.
4. Gently tilt the patient's head while maintaining displacement of the lower jaw.

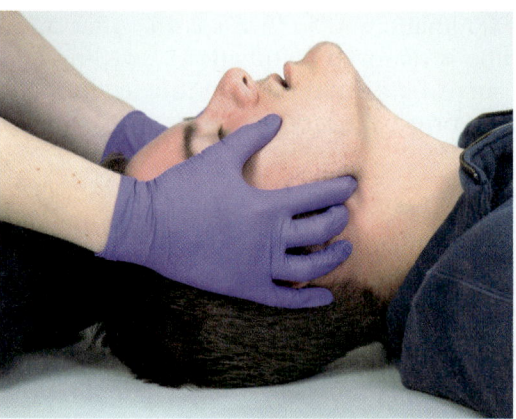

Figure 14-19 Opening the airway with the jaw thrust without head tilt maneuver.

3. While stabilizing the patient's head in a neutral position, grasp the angles of the patient's lower jaw with your fingertips.
4. Displace the lower jaw forward.

Jaw Thrust without Head Tilt Maneuver

The jaw thrust without head tilt maneuver (also called the *modified jaw thrust*) is the technique recommended for opening the airway when cervical spine injury is suspected (Figure 14-19). This maneuver is a difficult technique for one person to manage. In most cases, one rescuer is needed to displace the patient's lower jaw forward. A second rescuer is usually needed to ventilate the patient.

Perform the following for a jaw thrust without head tilt maneuver:

1. Place the patient in a supine position (log roll).
2. Rest your elbows on the same surface on which the patient is lying.

PARAMEDIC*Pearl*

Manual maneuvers *do* cause movement of the cervical spine. Lay rescuers are now taught to open an unresponsive patient's airway with a head tilt/chin lift maneuver for both injured and noninjured victims. The jaw thrust is no longer recommended for lay rescuers.

Healthcare professionals should open the airway with the head tilt/chin lift maneuver if no trauma is suspected. Use a jaw thrust without head tilt if you suspect possible trauma. However, because maintaining an open airway and providing adequate ventilation are a priority in CPR, current resuscitation guidelines recommend using a head tilt/chin lift maneuver if the jaw thrust does not open the airway.

Suctioning

[OBJECTIVES 32 to 39]

Opening the airway may require more than manual maneuvers. In an unresponsive patient, secretions, blood, and vomitus require removal with a suction device before ventilating. Ill patients are often nauseous, and many airway procedures may stimulate vomiting. You must anticipate such situations and have suction within arm's reach to minimize the potential risk of aspiration any time you are managing the airway.

Purpose of Suctioning

Suctioning is performed for the following reasons:

- To remove vomitus, saliva, blood, or other material from the patient's airway
- To improve gas exchange by allowing air to pass to the lower airway
- To prevent atelectasis

Suction Devices

Suction devices are available in many designs, including hand-powered, oxygen-powered, battery-operated, and mounted vacuum-powered in the patient compartment of the ambulance. Refer to Table 14-3 for a comparison of features for each device.

> **PARAMEDIC*Pearl***
>
> For suction units that are battery powered, you must ensure adequate battery life and carry spare batteries. There is nothing worse than reaching for the suction device only to find that it has no power.

Suction Catheters

Suction catheters are essentially one of two types, rigid or soft (Table 14-4). Rigid catheters are also called *hard, tonsil tip,* or *Yankauer catheters.* They are made of hard plastic and angled to aid removal of secretions from the mouth and throat. Because of its size, a rigid suction catheter is not used to suction the nares, except externally. The catheter typically has one large and several small holes at the distal end through which particles may be suctioned.

Soft suction catheters are also called *whistle tip, flexible,* or *French catheters.* They are long, narrow, flexible pieces of plastic primarily used to clear blood or mucus from a tracheal tube or the nasopharynx. A soft suction catheter can be inserted into the nares, oropharynx, or nasopharynx; through an oral or nasal airway; or through an endotracheal tube or tracheostomy tube.

A side opening is present at the proximal end of most catheters that is covered with the thumb to produce suction. (In some cases, suctioning is initiated when a button is pushed on the suction device itself).

Suctioning Technique

The very act of suctioning removes oxygen from the patient. In a patient who requires positive-pressure ventilation, the first priority is to ensure that the patient's airway is clear and open. If the patient needs elective suctioning, preoxygenate the patient before the procedure. In both situations, be sure to oxygenate the patient after suctioning is complete for 30 seconds to 1 minute before repeating the suctioning procedure.

Suction is applied only while withdrawing the catheter. Suction should not be applied for more than 10 to 15 seconds in adults. Limit suctioning in infants and children to no longer than 10 seconds per attempt. In a newborn, do not suction for more than 3 to 5 seconds per attempt. When suctioning to remove material that completely obstructs the airway, more time may be necessary.

Upper Airway. Skill 14-1 shows and explains the steps necessary for suctioning the upper airway.

Lower Airway. A patient who has an endotracheal or tracheostomy tube in place may require suctioning to remove secretions or mucus plugs. These patients are more prone to developing secretions and mucus because

TABLE 14-3	Comparison of Available Suction Devices	
Device Type	**Advantages**	**Disadvantages**
Hand powered	Lightweight, portable, easy to use, inexpensive	Limited volume and manually powered
Portable oxygen powered	Lightweight, small in size	Limited suctioning power and quickly exhausts available oxygen source
Portable battery operated	Lightweight, portable, possesses excellent suction power, easy to use	Must maintain charged batteries (spare batteries important), more complicated mechanics, some fluid contact components are not disposable
Mounted vacuum powered	Extremely strong and adjustable vacuum power, fluid contact components are disposable	Nonportable, no substitute power source and typically not field serviceable

TABLE 14-4	Comparison of Suction Catheters	
	Hard or Rigid Catheters	**Soft or Flexible Catheters**
Size	Standard size	Assorted sizes
Area of use	Oral use with direct visualization	Oropharynx, nasopharynx, ET tube, tracheostomy tube suctioning; may also be used blindly
Diameter	Large diameter Able to remove large volumes of fluid rapidly, as well as some particulate matter	Smaller diameter permits smaller volume to be suctioned; best used for secretions

Modified from National Highway Traffic Safety Administration. (1998). *Emergency medical technician paramedic: National standard curriculum (EMT-P)*, Washington, DC: Department of Transportation.

these tubes irritate the lining of the airway passages. In some instances the mucus can be large and thick, leading to respiratory distress. Only soft catheters are used when suctioning the lower airway, using sterile technique. Skill 14-2 shows and explains the steps necessary for this procedure.

PARAMEDIC*Pearl*

If a patient is intubated and requires suctioning, perform endotrachial suction before suctioning the mouth and throat. The mouth and throat contain more bacteria than the trachea. Suctioning the trachea first leads to less potential for bacterial contamination of the lungs.

Possible Complications

Any patient being suctioned needs to be monitored closely for complications associated with this procedure. Hypoxia and decreased myocardial oxygenation can result in cardiac irritability with resulting dysrhythmias. Stimulation of the vagus nerve can result in slowing of the heart rate and hypotension, especially in children. In the event that coughing or gagging occurs, the patient's heart rate and blood pressure may increase. In some cases a transient rise in intracranial pressure occurs. Be aware of this possibility, particularly in patients you suspect of having a traumatic brain injury. If any of these symptoms occurs during suctioning, pause, oxygenate your patient, and then resume suctioning as necessary. Possible complications of suctioning are shown in Box 14-10.

AIRWAY ADJUNCTS

[OBJECTIVES 40, 41]
Remember that your goal during every patient interaction is to maintain an open airway so that oxygenation can take place, and protect the airway if possible. You must assess your patient to determine what, if any, airway maintenance is required. Airway adjuncts are devices that assist in either maintaining an open passageway, protecting the lower airway from aspiration, or both. Each of

BOX 14-10	Suctioning: Possible Complications

- Hypoxia
- Dysrhythmias
- Increased intracranial pressure
- Local swelling
- Hemorrhage
- Tracheal ulceration
- Tracheal infection
- Bronchospasm
- Bradycardia and hypotension from vagal stimulation
- Tachycardia
- Hypertension

these functions allows air movement to the lower airways thereby facilitating gas exchange.

As evidenced by the many devices available for maintaining an open airway, a positive patient outcome often hinges on your knowledge and skill in selecting appropriate adjuncts for each patient. You must consider the potential risks and benefits of each option available and use the most appropriate adjunct for the specific patient circumstances. The definition of success of any airway procedure is positive patient outcome.

Manual maneuvers facilitate opening an airway, and several devices can assist in keeping it open. Two options specifically designed to prevent the tongue from falling back into the airway and blocking the flow of air are oral and nasal airways.

Oral Airway

An oral airway is also called an *oropharyngeal airway*. Indications for insertion include patients who are unresponsive and have no gag reflex.

An oral airway is a J-shaped plastic device that, when correctly positioned, extends from the patient's lips to the pharynx. The flange of the device rests on the patient's lips or teeth. The distal tip lies between the base of the tongue and the back of the throat, preventing the tongue

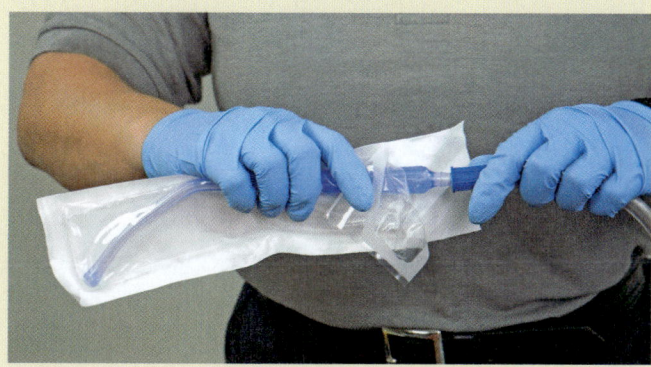

Step 1 Put on appropriate personal protective equipment, including gloves, eye protection, and a face shield. Assemble the necessary equipment, including the suction unit, tubing, and suction catheter. Preoxygenate the patient before suctioning if possible.

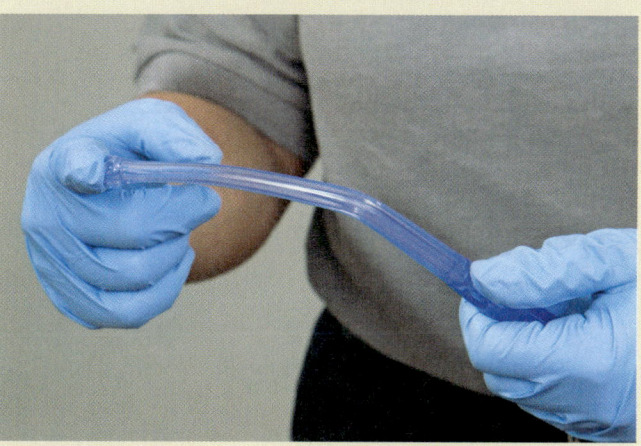

Step 2 Turn on the power to the suction unit. Test for adequate suction by sealing the side port on the catheter with one finger. After confirming adequate suction is present, remove the finger from the port or turn off the suction unit.

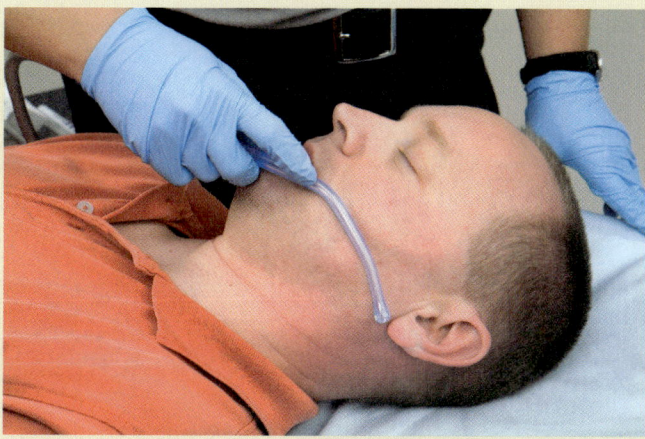

Step 3 To determine the appropriate depth for catheter insertion, measure the catheter from the patient's earlobe to the corner of the mouth.

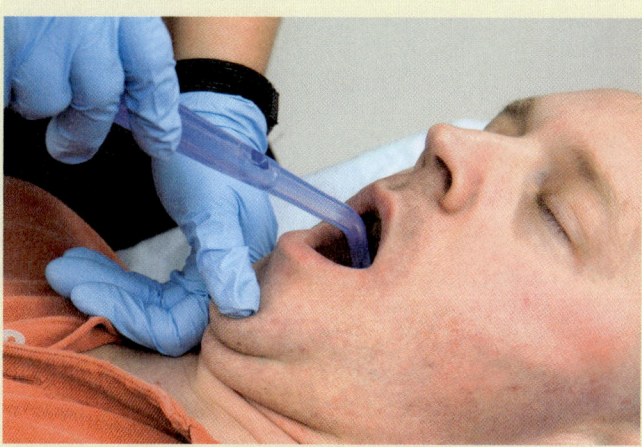

Step 4 Insert the catheter into the patient's mouth to the proper depth *without* applying suction.

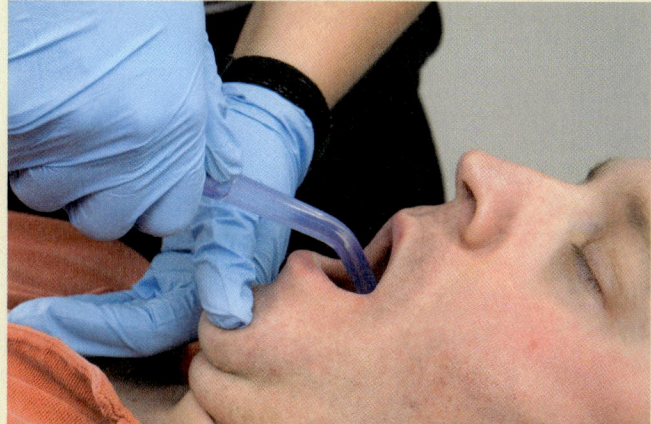

Step 5 To begin suctioning, turn on the power to the suction unit or cover the catheter side port with one finger.

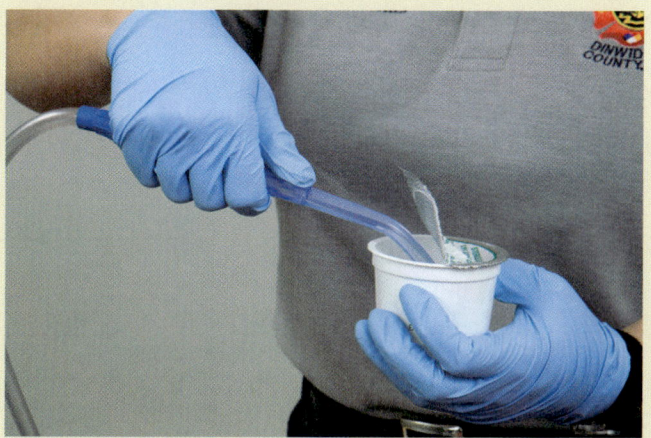

Step 6 Withdraw the catheter while applying suction. In adults, suction should not be applied for more than 10 to 15 seconds. Ventilate the lungs with 100% oxygen for approximately 30 seconds and flush the suction catheter and tubing with saline before repeating the procedure.

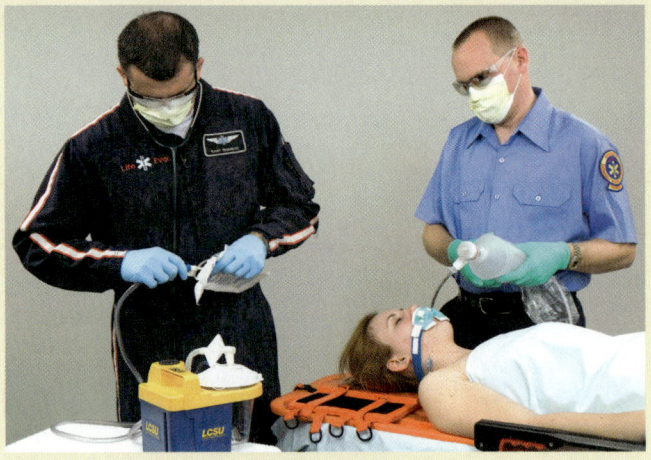

Step 1 Put on appropriate personal protective equipment including gloves, eye protection, and a face shield. Assemble the necessary equipment including the suction unit, tubing, and suction catheter. Preoxygenate the patient before suctioning if possible.

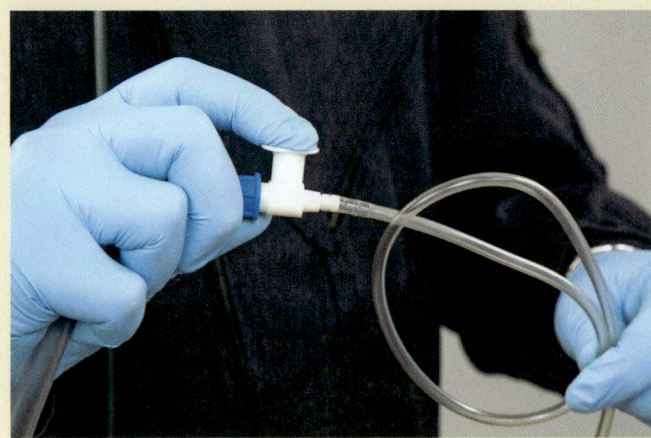

Step 2 Turn on the power to the suction unit. Test for adequate suction by sealing the side port on the catheter with one finger. After confirming adequate suction is present, remove the finger from the port or turn off the suction unit.

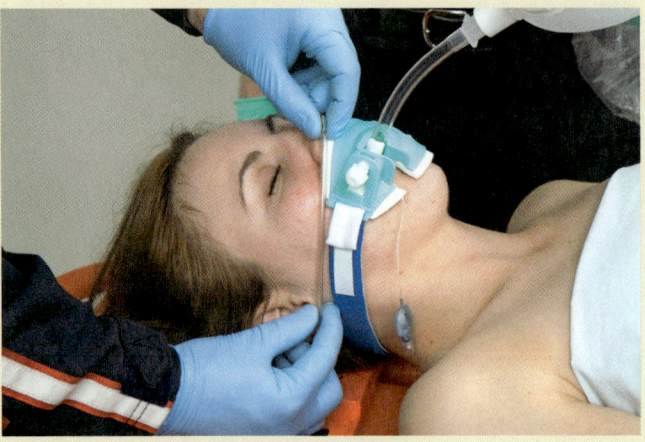

Step 3 To determine the appropriate depth for catheter insertion, measure the distance from the nose to the ear and the nose to the sternal notch.

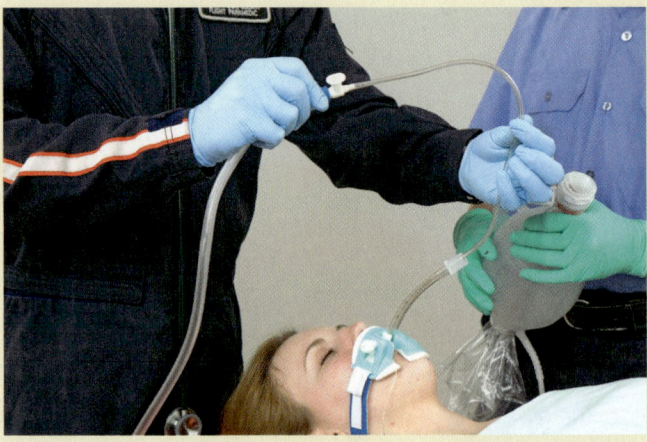

Step 4 Insert the catheter into the ET (or tracheostomy) tube to the proper depth *without* applying suction.

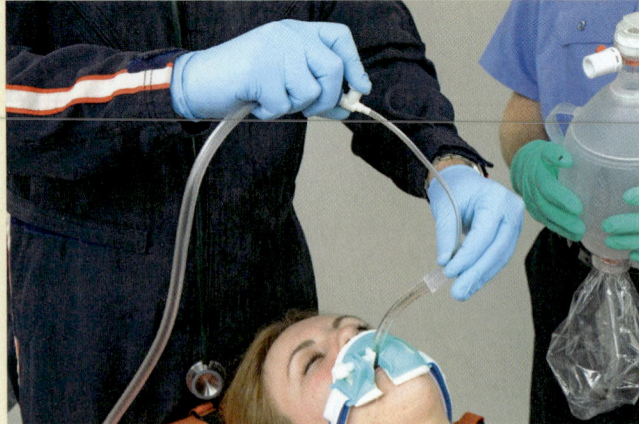

Step 5 To begin suctioning, turn on the power to the suction unit or cover the catheter side port with one finger.

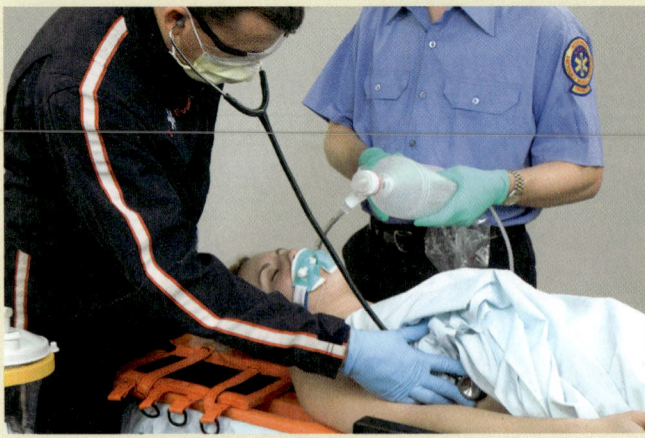

Step 6 Withdraw the catheter while applying suction. In adults, suction should not be applied for more than 10 to 15 seconds. Reevaluate airway patency and auscultate lung sounds. Ventilate the patient with 100% oxygen for approximately 30 seconds and flush the suction catheter and tubing with saline before repeating the procedure.

from blocking the airway. Air passes around and through the device.

Oral airways are available in a variety of sizes ranging from 0 for neonates up to 6 for large adults. The size of the airway is based on the distance, in millimeters, from the flange to the distal tip. Proper airway size is determined by holding the device against the side of the patient's face and selecting an airway that extends from the corner of the mouth to the tip of the earlobe or the angle of the jaw. Proper size is important. If the airway is too long, it may press the epiglottis against the entrance of the larynx, resulting in a complete airway obstruction. If the airway is too short, it will not displace the tongue and may push the tongue further into the airway, as well as advancing out of the mouth. Care during insertion is also necessary to ensure that the tongue is not forced further back in the pharynx, resulting in obstruction. When inserting any device into the airway, never force the device because trauma may result. When inserting an oral airway in pediatric patients, a tongue depressor is recommended to avoid any trauma to the palate.

In addition to its ability to maintain an open airway, the oral airway can help facilitate suctioning of the oral cavity and serve as an effective bite block in patients who might otherwise clench the teeth, thereby limiting your access to the patient's airway by the mouth.

Although the airway is easily inserted and considered noninvasive, it is certainly not without complications. Insertion of an oral airway in a patient with an intact gag reflex may stimulate vomiting and thus increase the risk of aspiration. As an adjunct, the oral airway does not definitively protect from aspiration. Vigilance on your part is necessary to ensure that the oral airway is keeping the tongue off the posterior pharynx. If the patient's gag reflex returns or he or she spontaneously attempts to displace the airway, remove the airway to minimize the risk of aspiration. Skill 14-3 explains the steps for insertion of an oral airway.

Nasal Airway

A nasal airway (also called a *nasopharyngeal airway* or *nasal trumpet*) is a soft, uncuffed rubber or plastic tube designed to keep the tongue away from the back of the throat. Distally, the tube is beveled to help facilitate advancement into the airway. Proximally, the tube takes on a trumpet-shaped appearance that comes to rest on the external surface of the nostril.

Indications for use of a nasal airway include unresponsive patients or those with an altered level of consciousness who continue to have an intact gag reflex. As with any device inserted into the nose, you must be extremely cautious in patients who have sustained any type of facial or head trauma. Such injuries may compromise the bony structures behind the nose and lead to inadvertent placement of the nasal airway in the cranial vault. Patients with known or suspected nasal obstruction or those prone to epistaxis (such as patients on anticoagulant therapy) are not acceptable candidates for a nasal airway.

Nasal airways are available in many sizes varying in length and internal diameter. Proper airway size is determined by holding the device against the side of the patient's face and selecting an airway that extends from the tip of the nose to the angle of the jaw or the tip of the ear. An airway that is too long may stimulate the gag reflex. One that is too short may not be inserted far enough to keep the tongue away from the back of the throat.

Before inserting a nasal airway, use appropriate personal protective equipment and open the airway. Lubricate the distal tip of the device liberally with a water-soluble lubricant to minimize resistance and decrease irritation to the nasal passage. After selecting a nasal airway of the proper size, hold the device at its flange end like a pencil and slowly insert it into the patient's nostril with the bevel pointing toward the nasal septum. Advance the airway along the floor of the nostril, following the natural curvature of the nasal passage, until the flange is flush with the nostril.

The nasal cavity is highly vascular. During insertion, do not force the airway because it may cut or scrape the nasal mucosa and result in significant bleeding, increasing the risk of aspiration. If resistance is encountered, a gentle back-and-forth rotation of the device between your fingers may ease insertion. If resistance continues, withdraw the nasal airway, reapply lubricant, and attempt insertion in the patient's other nostril. Generally the right nostril is the preferred nostril for nasal airway adjuncts. This is because in most patients it is larger and straighter. However, if the procedure is unsuccessful the left nostril may be used. In this case, insert the nasal airway with bevel to the septum, and after the tip of the airway is past the septum rotate it 180 degrees. Indications, contraindications, advantages, and disadvantages of oral and nasal airways are shown in Table 14-5.

Skill 14-4 explains the steps for insertion of a nasal airway.

TECHNIQUES OF ARTIFICIAL VENTILATION

[OBJECTIVES 42, 43]

Adequate oxygenation requires an open airway and adequate air exchange. After the airway has been opened, determine if the patient's breathing is adequate or inadequate. Patients who are apneic or those with inadequate ventilation require artificial ventilation support. Forcing air into the lungs is called **positive-pressure ventilation**, which can be accomplished in the following ways:

- Mouth-to-mouth ventilation
- Mouth-to-nose ventilation
- Mouth-to–barrier device ventilation
- Mouth-to-mask ventilation

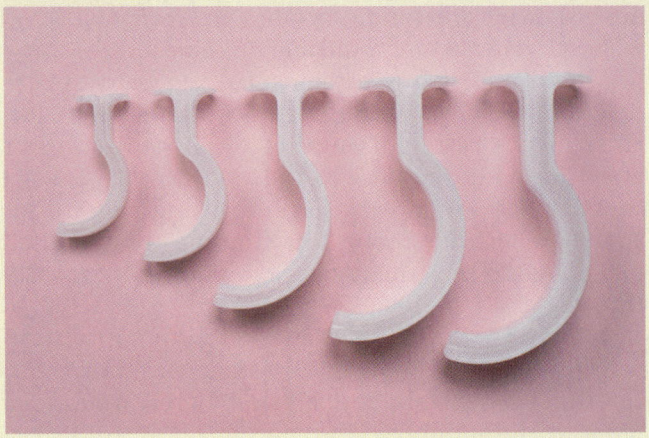

Oral airways are available in a variety of sizes (infant, child, adult). The size of the airway is based on the distance, in millimeters, from the flange to the distal tip.

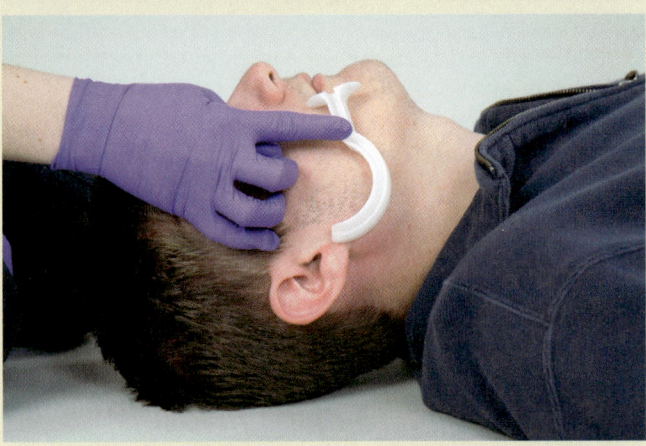

Step 1 Take appropriate standard precautions. Select an oral airway of appropriate size by measuring from the corner of the mouth to the angle of the jaw.

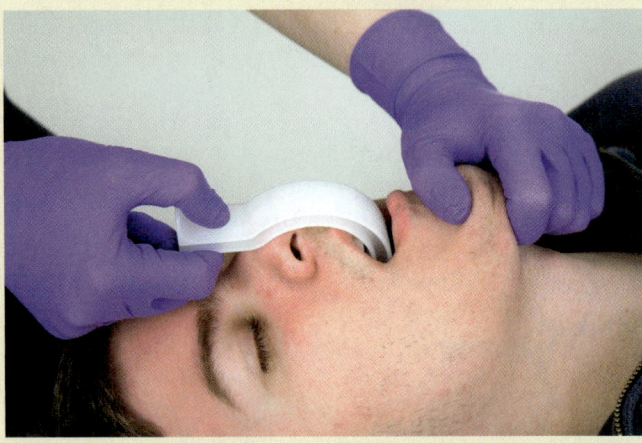

Step 2 Open the patient's mouth. Make sure the patient's mouth and throat are clear of secretions, blood, and vomitus. Suction if needed. Hold the oral airway at its flange end and insert it into the mouth, with the tip pointing toward the roof of the patient's mouth.

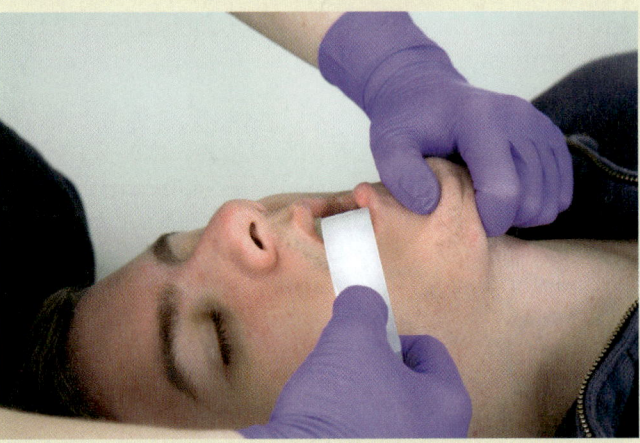

Step 3 Slide the airway along the roof of the mouth. When the distal end nears the back of the throat, rotate the airway 180 degrees so that it is positioned over the tongue.

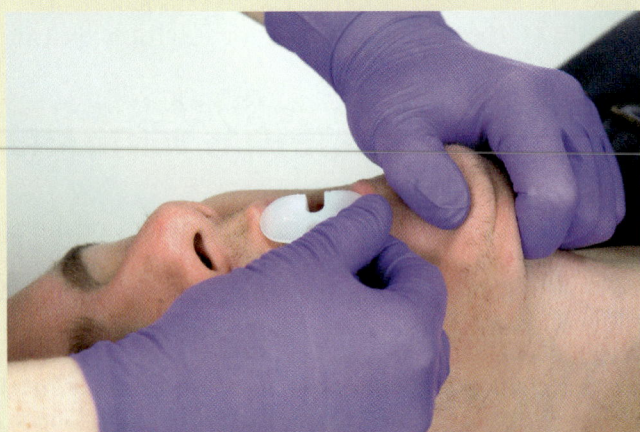

Step 4 When the oral airway is inserted properly, the flange of the device should rest comfortably on the patient's lips or teeth. Proper placement of the device is confirmed by ventilating the patient. If the airway is placed correctly, chest rise should be visible and breath sounds should be present on auscultation of the lungs during ventilation.

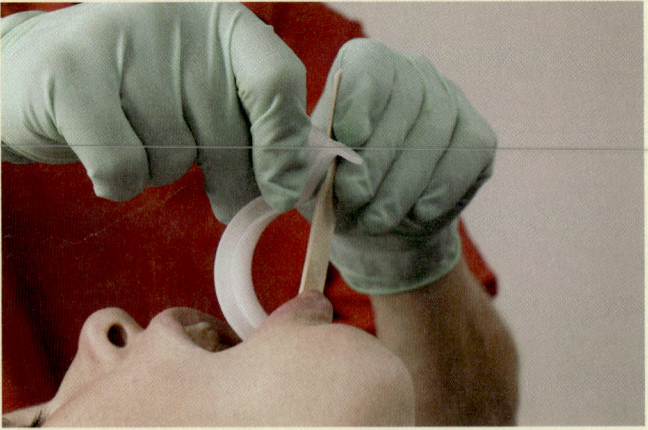

Step 5 Another method of oral airway insertion requires the use of a tongue blade to depress the tongue. If this method is used, the airway is inserted with its tip facing the floor of the patient's mouth (curved side down). Using the tongue blade to depress the tongue, the oral airway is advanced gently into place over the tongue.

SKILL 14-4 NASAL AIRWAY INSERTION

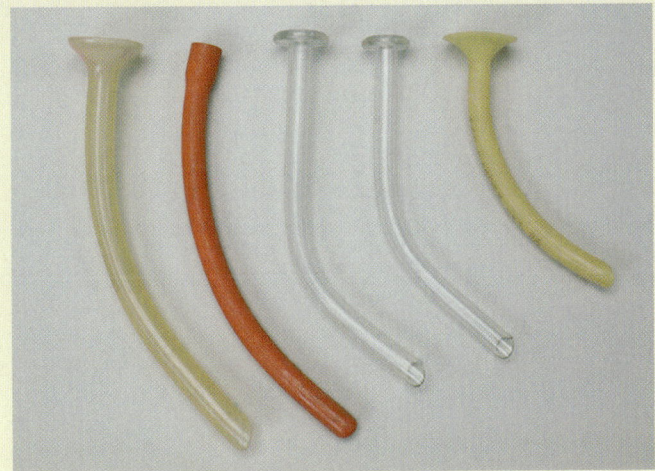

Nasal airways are available in many sizes varying in length and internal diameter.

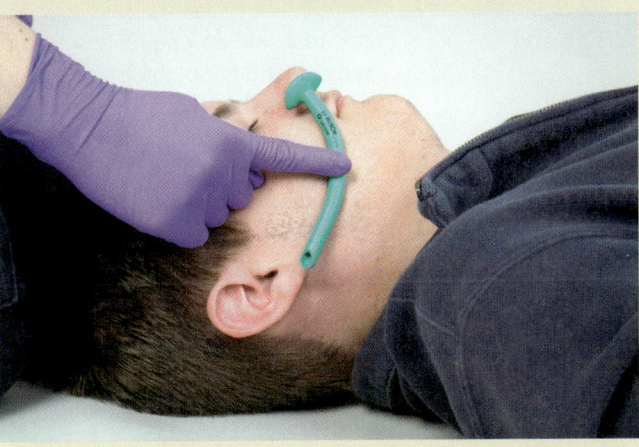

Step 1 Take proper standard precautions. Determine proper airway size by holding the nasal airway against the side of the patient's face. An airway of proper size extends from the tip of the nose to the angle of the jaw or the tip of the ear.

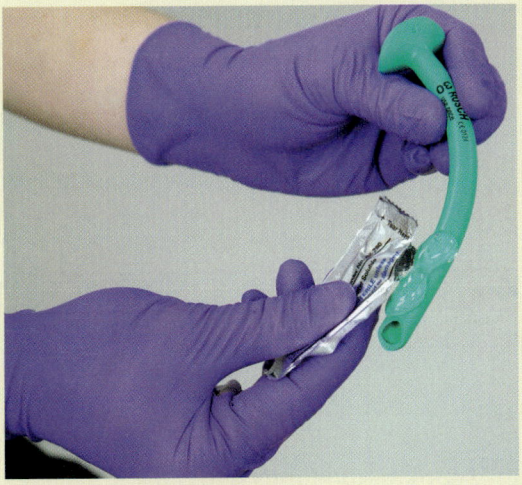

Step 2 Lubricate the distal tip of the device liberally with a water-soluble lubricant to minimize resistance and decrease irritation to the nasal passage.

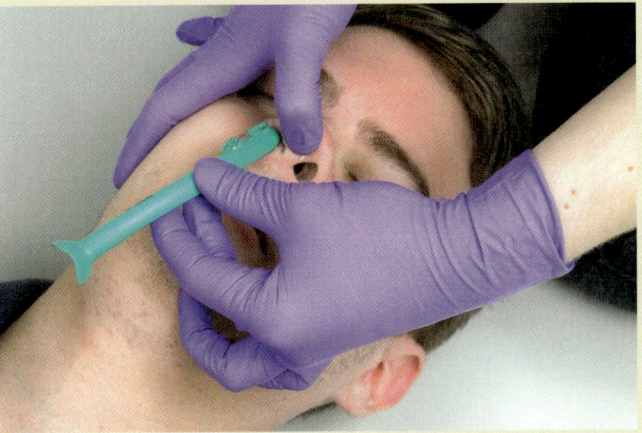

Step 3 Hold the nasal airway at its flange end like a pencil and slowly insert it into the larger of the patient's two nares with the bevel pointing toward the nasal septum.

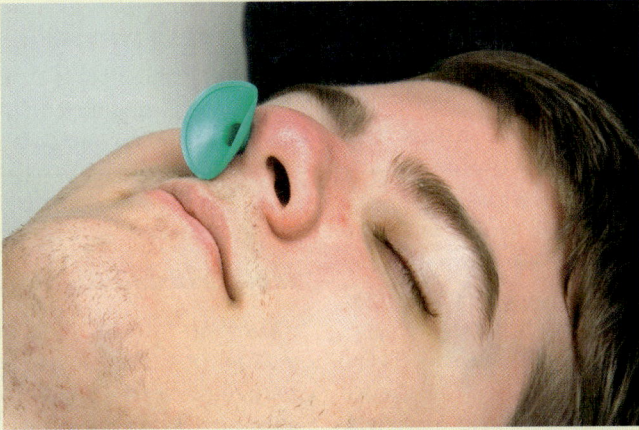

Step 4 Advance the airway along the floor of the nostril, following the natural curvature of the nasal passage until the flange is flush with the nostril.

TABLE 14-5	Oral and Nasal Airways	
	Oral Airway	**Nasal Airway**
Indications	Helps maintain an open airway in an unresponsive patient who is not intubated Helps maintain an open airway in an unresponsive patient with no gag reflex who is being ventilated with a bag-mask or other positive-pressure device May be used as a bite block after insertion of an endotracheal al tube or orogastric tube	Helps maintain an airway when use of an oral airway is contraindicated or impossible Trismus (spasm of the muscles used to grind, crush, and chew food) Biting Clenched jaws or teeth
Contraindications	Responsive patient	Severe craniofacial trauma Patient intolerance
Sizing	Corner of mouth to tip of earlobe or angle of jaw	Tip of nose to angle of the jaw or the tip of the ear
Advantages	Positions the tongue forward and away from the back of the throat Easily placed	Provides a patent airway Tolerated by responsive patients Does not require mouth to be open
Disadvantages	Does not protect the lower airway from aspiration May produce vomiting if used in a responsive or semiresponsive patient with a gag reflex	Does not protect the lower airway from aspiration Improper technique may result in severe bleeding Resulting epistaxis may be difficult to control Suctioning through the device is difficult Although tolerated by most responsive and semiresponsive patients, can stimulate the gag reflex in sensitive patients, precipitating laryngospasm and vomiting
Precautions	Use of the device does not eliminate the need for maintaining proper head position	Use of the device does not eliminate the need for maintaining proper head position

Reprinted from Aehlert, B. (2007). *ACLS study guide* (3rd ed.), St. Louis: Mosby.

- One-person, two-person, or three-person bag-mask ventilation
- Ventilation with an automatic transport ventilator
- Ventilation with a flow-restricted oxygen-powered ventilation device

Regardless of the method used, effective positive-pressure ventilation requires the delivery of an adequate volume of air at an appropriate rate. When considering the need for positive-pressure ventilation, assess the patient's respiratory rate as well as minute volume, which accounts for the rate *and* depth of ventilation.

Providing positive-pressure ventilation is not without complications, and you must be aware of them so you can minimize their occurrence. Of major concern is the potential for **gastric distention,** or forcing air into the stomach instead of the lungs. Gastric distention can result in vomiting, significantly increasing the likelihood of aspiration. An effective seal between the patients mouth and the delivery device with any method used is essential because air follows the path of least resistance. Failure to maintain a good seal means that air will leak

and not ventilate the lungs. Providing effective positive-pressure ventilation requires an open airway, an effective seal, and delivery of an adequate tidal volume while minimizing gastric distention.

PARAMEDIC*Pearl*

Gastric distention is a complication of positive-pressure ventilation that can lead to vomiting and subsequent aspiration. Gastric distention also restricts movement of the diaphragm, impeding ventilation.

Mouth-to-Mouth Ventilation

Mouth-to-mouth ventilation is a basic method for providing positive-pressure ventilation to apneic patients and requires no special equipment to perform. Mouth-to-mouth ventilation is capable of delivering excellent tidal volumes. Because expired air from your lungs contains approximately 16% oxygen, it will also deliver an adequate level of oxygen to the patient.

Patients who are awake or those with a known infectious disease are not acceptable candidates for mouth-to-mouth ventilation. In this day of heightened awareness of communicable diseases, an issue of concern with the use of this ventilation method is direct contact with oral secretions, possibly including blood. For this reason, unless no equipment is immediately available healthcare professionals rarely perform mouth-to-mouth ventilation.

Perform mouth-to-mouth ventilation by opening the patient's airway and pinching the nostrils closed. The paramedic then creates a seal between their mouth and the patient's mouth and exhales into the patient at the desired respiratory rate. Performing mouth-to-mouth ventilation is hard work. Be careful not to cause yourself to hyperventilate and do not hyperinflate the patient's lungs. Adequate ventilation is present if you ventilate with just enough volume to see gentle chest rise.

Mouth-to-Nose Ventilation

The nose can be used as a means by which to deliver artificial ventilation. This may become necessary when a patient's mouth is not able to be opened or is traumatized, making it impossible to create a good seal. Mouth-to-nose ventilation may be performed on any apneic patient. This ventilation method requires no special equipment. Limitations include possible exposure to communicable disease and the psychological hesitation of this ventilatory option. The procedure is similar to mouth-to-mouth ventilation with the exception that the seal is created between the paramedic's mouth and the patient's nose.

Mouth-to–Barrier Device Ventilation

A **barrier device** is a thin film of material, usually plastic or silicone, that is placed on the patient's face and used to prevent direct contact with the patient's mouth during positive-pressure ventilation. One common type of barrier device is a face shield. Face shields are compact, portable, and sometimes equipped with a short tube (1 to 2 inches) that is inserted in the patient's mouth. A one-way valve or filter is present in the center of most face shields that diverts the patient's exhaled air away from you when you lift your mouth off the shield between breaths, reducing the risk of infection. Skill 14-5 shows the steps for mouth-to–barrier device ventilation.

Mouth-to-Mask Ventilation

The device used for mouth-to-mask ventilation is commonly called a **pocket mask,** pocket face mask, ventilation face mask, or resuscitation mask (Box 14-11). A pocket mask is a clear, semirigid mask that is sealed around the mouth and nose of an adult, child, or infant. A pocket mask should have the following characteristics:

- Made of transparent material to allow assessment of the patient's lip color and detection of vomitus, secretions, or other substances
- Capable of a tight seal on the face, covering the mouth and nose
- Equipped with a standard 15-/22-mm fitting that permits connection to a bag-mask (or other ventilation) device

SKILL 14-5 MOUTH-TO–BARRIER DEVICE VENTILATION

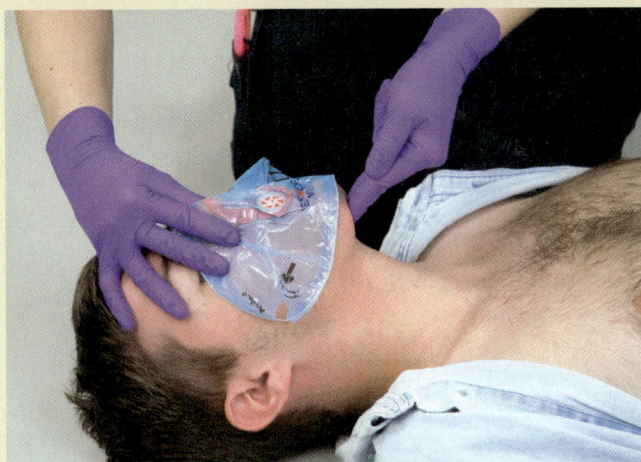

Step 1 Put on appropriate personal protective equipment. Open the patient's airway and place the barrier device over the patient's mouth.

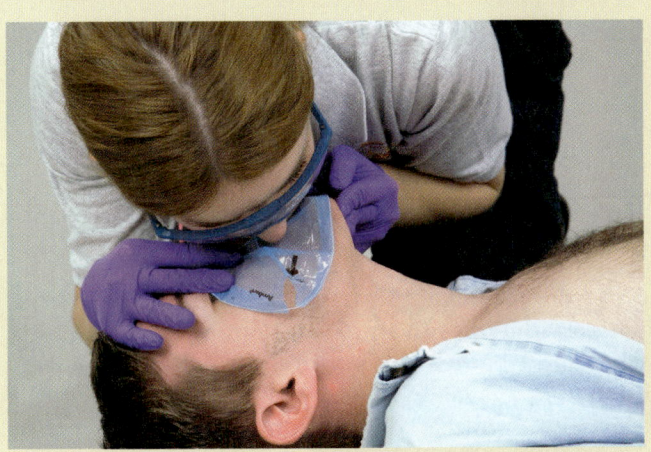

Step 2 Place your mouth over the mouthpiece of the barrier device. Breathe into the device with enough force to cause the patient's chest to rise gently.

BOX 14-11 Mouth-to-Mask Ventilation

Inspired Oxygen Concentration

- Without supplemental oxygen equals approximately 16% to 17% exhaled air
- Mouth-to-mask breathing combined with supplemental oxygen at a minimal flow rate of 10 L/min equals approximately 50%

Advantages

- Aesthetically more acceptable than mouth-to-mouth ventilation
- Easy to teach and learn
- Physical barrier between the rescuer and the patient's nose, mouth, and secretions
- Reduces (but does not prevent) the risk of exposure to infectious disease
- Use of a one-way valve at the ventilation port decreases exposure to patient's exhaled air
- If the patient resumes spontaneous breathing, the mask can be used as a simple face mask to deliver 40% to 60% oxygen by giving supplemental oxygen through the oxygen inlet on the mask (if so equipped)
- Can deliver a greater tidal volume with mouth-to-mask ventilation than with a bag-mask device
- Rescuer can feel the compliance of the patient's lungs

Disadvantages

- Rescuer fatigue
- Gastric distention

Reprinted from Aehlert, B. (2007). *ACLS study guide* (3rd ed.), St. Louis: Mosby.

- Available in one average size for adults, with additional sizes for infants and children
- Equipped with a one-way valve that diverts the patient's exhaled air, reducing the risk of infection
- Fitted with an oxygen inlet to allow the delivery of increased oxygen concentrations to the patient. Some mouth-to-mask devices have an oxygen inlet on the mask, allowing delivery of supplemental oxygen; others do not.

A significant advantage associated with using a mask when providing positive-pressure ventilation is its ability to serve as a barrier between rescuer and victim. With both hands available to seal the mask and open the airway, mouth-to-mask ventilation has been shown to be more effective than bag-mask ventilation for the lone paramedic. Indicated for patients with apnea from any cause, the mask should be readily available. This handy ventilation tool can easily fit into a pocket for quick access. Skill 14-6 shows the steps necessary to perform mouth-to-mask ventilation.

PARAMEDIC*Pearl*

Selection of a mask of proper size is necessary to ensure a good seal between the patient's face and the mask. A mask of correct size should extend from the bridge of the nose to the groove between the lower lip and chin. If the mask is not properly positioned and a tight seal maintained, air will leak from between the mask and the patient's face, resulting in less tidal volume delivery to the patient. Less tidal volume leads to less lung inflation, which leads to less oxygenation. If you do not have a mask of the proper size available, use a larger mask and turn it upside down. Remember: adequate ventilation is present if you ventilate with just enough volume to see gentle chest rise.

Bag-Mask Ventilation

[OBJECTIVE 44]

A bag-valve-mask device may also be referred to as a *bag-mask device*, a *bag-mask resuscitator* (when the mask is used), or a *bag-mask device* (when the mask is not used, i.e., when ventilating a patient's lungs with an endotracheal tube or tracheostomy tube in place). A bag-mask device consists of a self-inflating bag, a nonrebreathing valve with an adapter that can be attached to a mask, tracheal tube or other invasive airway device, and an oxygen inlet valve (Figure 14-20). A bag-mask device should have the following characteristics:

- Consist of a self-refilling bag that is disposable (or easily cleaned and sterilized) and easy to grip and compress
- Have a clear mask to allow evaluation of the patient's lip color and detection of vomitus, secretions, or other substances
- Be capable of a tight seal on the face, covering the mouth and nose
- Have either no pop-off valve (pressure-release valve) or a pop-off valve that can be disabled during resuscitation
- Have standard 15-/22-mm fittings to allow for attachment of the device to a standard mask, tracheal tube, or other ventilation device
- Include a system for delivering high concentrations of oxygen with an oxygen reservoir and supplemental oxygen source
- Have a nonrebreathing valve that does not permit the patient's exhaled gases to escape into the bag
- Perform satisfactorily under all common environmental conditions and temperature extremes

SKILL 14-6 MOUTH-TO-MASK VENTILATION

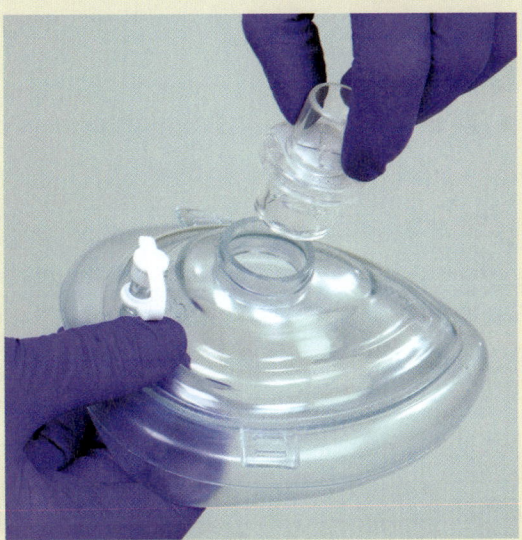

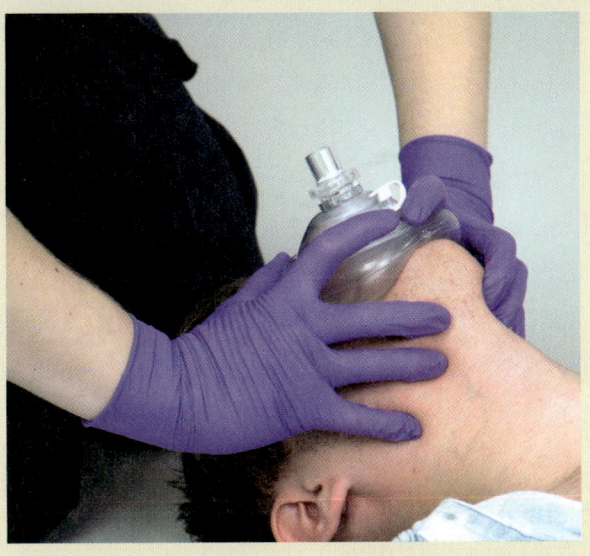

Step 1 Put on appropriate personal protective equipment. Connect a one-way valve to the ventilation port on the mask. If an oxygen inlet is present on the mask and oxygen is available, connect oxygen tubing to the oxygen inlet. Set the flow rate at 10 to 12 L/min.

Step 2 Position yourself at the patient's head. Open the patient's airway. If needed, clear the patient's airway of secretions or vomitus. If the patient is unresponsive, insert an oral airway. Select a mask of appropriate size and place it on the patient's face. Apply the narrow portion (apex) of the mask over the bridge of the patient's nose and stabilize it in place with your thumbs. Lower the mask over the patient's face and mouth. Use your index fingers to stabilize the wide end (base) of the mask over the groove between the lower lip and chin. When in proper position, your thumb and index finger create a C. Use your remaining fingers to maintain proper head position. Your remaining fingers create an E.

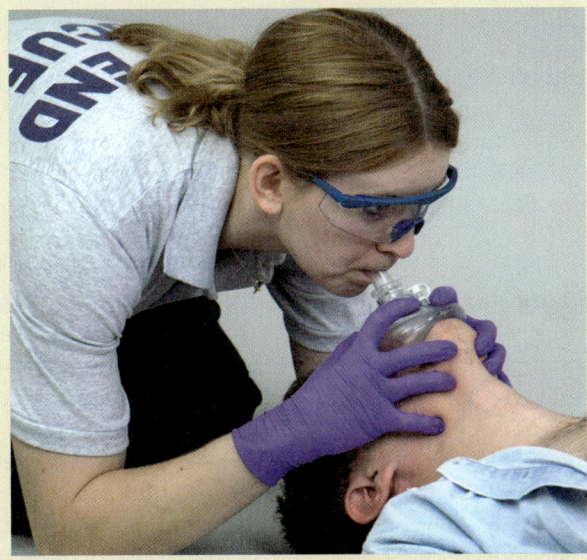

Step 3 Ventilate the lungs through the one-way valve on the top of the mask at an age-appropriate rate.

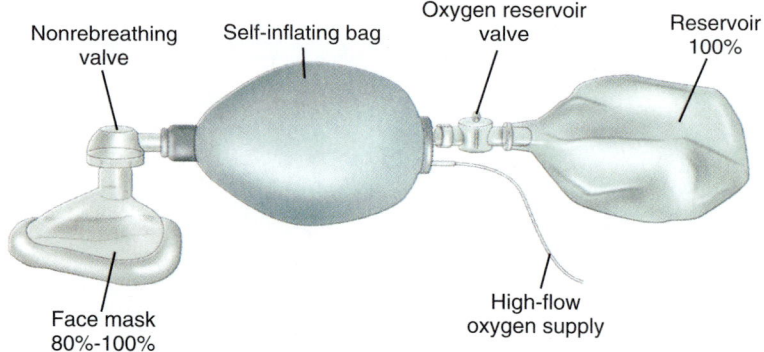

Figure 14-20 Components of a bag-mask device.

- Be available in adult, child, and infant sizes (When selecting equipment, an appropriately sized bag-mask device must be used. Masks are provided in a variety of sizes and bags are available in adult, child, and infant sizes.)

PARAMEDIC*Pearl*

You can deliver a greater tidal volume to the patient with mouth-to-mask ventilation than with a bag-mask device because both your hands can be used to secure the mask in place while simultaneously maintaining proper head position. Your vital capacity can also compensate for leaks between the mask and the patient's face, resulting in greater lung ventilation.

Oxygen Delivery

A bag-mask device used without supplemental oxygen delivers 21% oxygen (room air) to the patient (Figure 14-21). The bag-mask device should be connected to an oxygen source. To do this, attach one end of a piece of oxygen connecting tubing to the oxygen inlet on the bag-mask device and the other end to an oxygen regulator. A bag-mask device used with supplemental oxygen set at a flow rate of 15 L/min delivers approximately 40% to 60% oxygen to the patient (Figure 14-22) when an oxygen reservoir is not used.

Ideally, an oxygen-collecting device (reservoir) should be attached to the bag-mask device to deliver high-concentration oxygen. The reservoir collects a volume of 100% oxygen equal to the capacity of the bag. After squeezing the bag, it re-expands, drawing in 100% oxygen from the reservoir into the bag. A bag-mask device used with supplemental oxygen (set at a flow rate of 15 L/min) and an attached reservoir delivers approximately 90% to 100% oxygen to the patient (Figure 14-23). Advantages and disadvantages of bag-mask ventilation are shown in Box 14-12.

| BOX 14-12 | Bag-Mask Ventilation |

Advantages

- Provides a means for delivery of an oxygen-enriched mixture to the patient
- Conveys a sense of compliance of patient's lungs to the bag-mask operator
- Provides a means for immediate ventilatory support
- Can be used with the spontaneously breathing patient as well as the nonbreathing patient

Disadvantages

- Requires practice to use effectively
- Delivery of inadequate tidal volume
- Rescuer fatigue
- Gastric distention

Reprinted from Aehlert, B. (2007). *ACLS study guide* (3rd ed.), St. Louis: Mosby.

PARAMEDIC*Pearl*

Ventilation of patients in cardiac arrest often requires higher-than-usual airway pressures. Higher-than-usual ventilation pressures may also be needed in situations involving near-drowning, pulmonary edema, and asthma. To effectively ventilate a patient in these situations, the pressures needed for ventilation may exceed the limits of the pop-off valve. Thus a pop-off valve may prevent generation of sufficient tidal volume to overcome the increase in airway resistance. Disabling the pop-off valve, or using a bag-mask device with no pop-off valve, helps ensure delivery of adequate tidal volumes to the patient during resuscitation. To disable a pop-off valve, depress the valve with a finger during ventilation or twist the pop-off valve into the closed position.

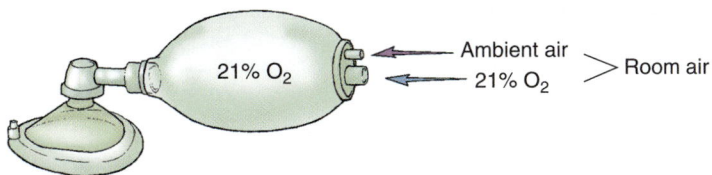

Figure 14-21 A bag-mask device used without supplemental oxygen delivers 21% oxygen (room air).

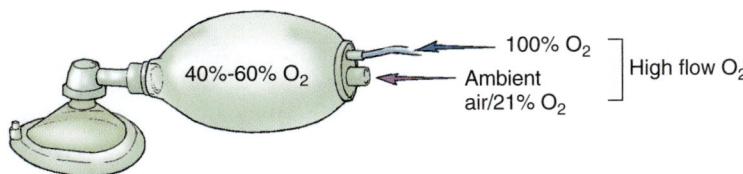

Figure 14-22 A bag-mask device used with supplemental oxygen set at a flow rate of 15 L/min delivers approximately 40% to 60% oxygen to the patient.

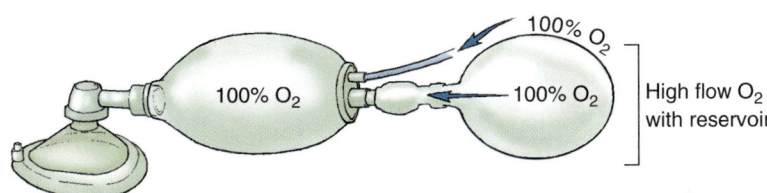

Figure 14-23 A bag-mask device used with supplemental oxygen set at a flow rate of 15 L/min and a reservoir delivers approximately 90% to 100% oxygen to the patient.

Ventilating with a Bag-Mask

[OBJECTIVE 45]

Performing positive-pressure ventilation with a bag-mask device can be quite difficult. Several reasons contribute to this, but none as much as the inability to create a good seal with the mask while simultaneously generating an adequate tidal volume by squeezing the bag. Thus, as a lone rescuer, mastering the technique of bag-mask ventilation may be difficult.

Bag-mask ventilation should be a two- or three-rescuer operation. With two people, one is assigned the responsibility of opening and maintaining the airway while creating a good seal with the mask. That frees a second person to squeeze the bag, ensuring the delivery of an adequate tidal volume. If three people can be assigned to manage the airway, the tasks can be divided even more when ventilating. With three people, one is assigned to open and maintain an airway. If the patient is unresponsive, this rescuer should apply cricoid pressure during positive-pressure ventilation while another person is solely responsible for maintaining a good seal with the mask. Finally, the third person squeezes the bag. Although superior mask seal and volume delivery are possible, it does get somewhat crowded around the airway. As with any form of positive-pressure ventilation, you must remain cognizant of not causing gastric distention or hyperinflation of the lungs. Skill 14-7 shows the steps for one- and two-person bag-mask ventilation.

Cricoid Pressure

[OBJECTIVE 46]

A major issue encountered when providing ventilatory assistance to a patient is gastric distention. As air passes into the lungs, it also overflows into the stomach by way of the esophagus. Collecting in the stomach, air searches for a way to escape and often returns from where it came, bringing other stomach contents with it. Regurgitation then increases the chances of aspirating vomitus into the lower airway, a serious complication that can prove fatal.

Because gas exchange does not occur in the stomach, the air must move in and out of the lungs while keeping chyme and other gastric secretions in the stomach. Therefore, when providing positive-pressure ventilation to an unresponsive patient, apply cricoid pressure (Sellick maneuver) if an assistant is available. This technique takes advantage of the cricoid cartilage, the only rigid cartilaginous ring of the trachea, to occlude the esophagus (Figure 14-24). To perform cricoid pressure, begin by locating the cricoid cartilage. Then apply firm pressure on the cricoid cartilage with the thumb and index or middle finger, just lateral to the midline (Figure 14-25).

SKILL 14-7 BAG-MASK VENTILATION

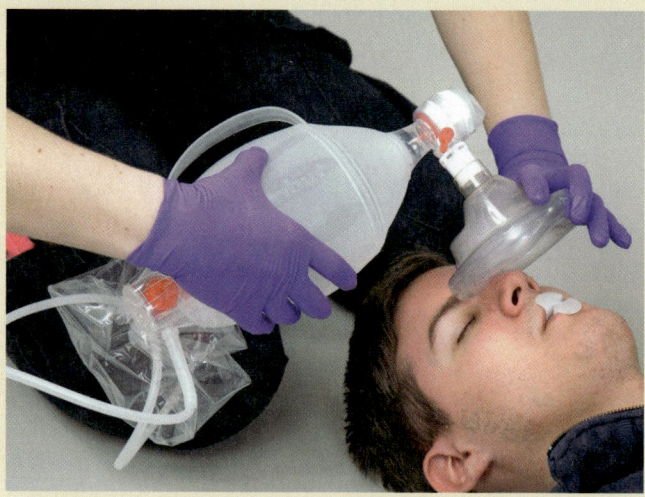

Step 1 Put on personal protective equipment and position yourself at the top of the supine patient's head. Open the patient's airway. If needed, clear the patient's airway of secretions or vomitus. If the patient is unresponsive, insert an oral airway.

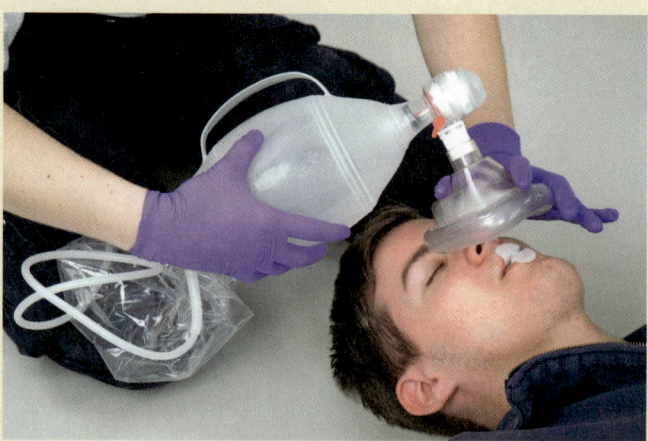

Step 2 Select a mask of appropriate size. Connect the bag to the mask if not already done. Connect the bag to oxygen at 15 L/min and attach a reservoir.

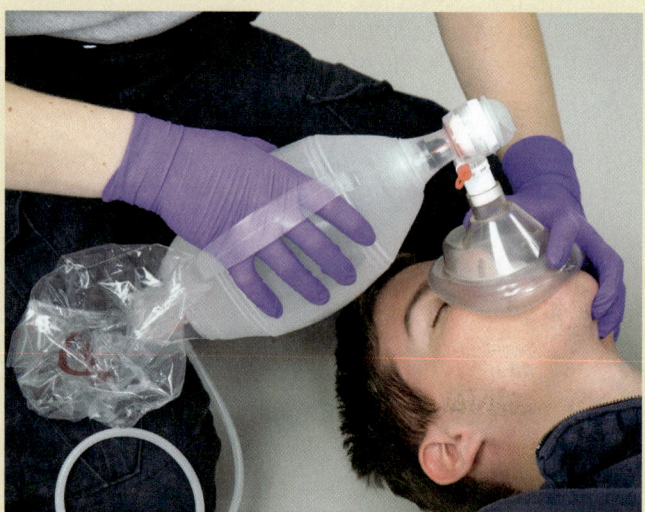

Step 3 Place the mask on the patient's face. Apply the narrow portion (apex) of the mask over the bridge of the patient's nose and the wide end (base) of the mask over the groove between the lower lip and chin. If the mask has a large, round cuff surrounding a ventilation port, center the port over the mouth. Create a good seal using the *E and C* technique with the mask seated over the patient's mouth and nose. *E* serves to control the lower jaw with the small, ring, and middle fingers. The thumb and index finger serve to create a *C* on the mask itself.

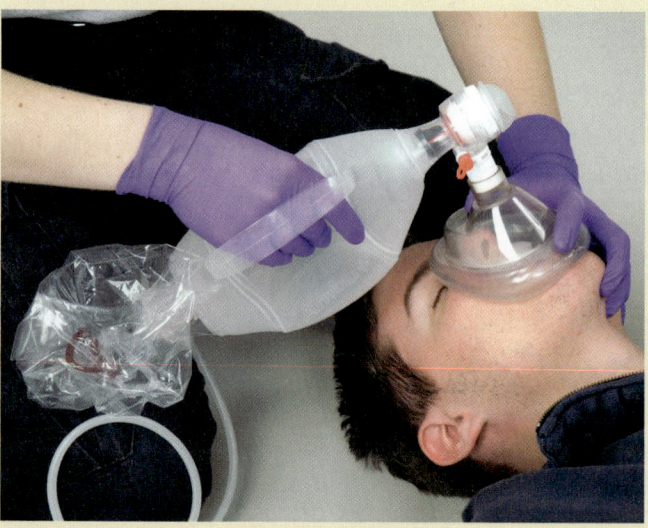

Step 4 If you are alone, squeeze the bag with one hand or with one hand and your arm or chest.

Continued

SKILL 14-7 BAG-MASK VENTILATION—continued

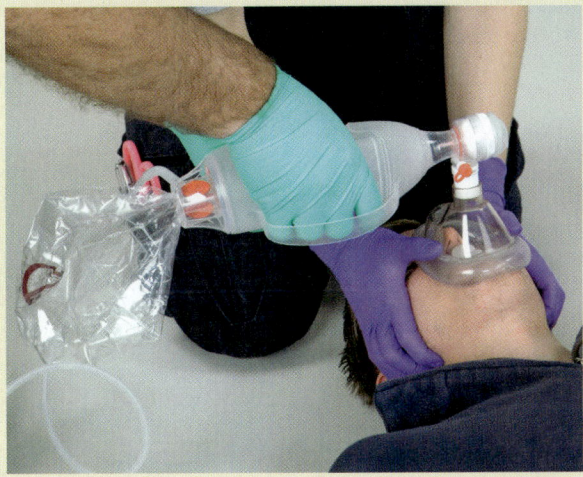

Step 5 If available, ask your partner to squeeze the bag until the patient's chest rises while you press the mask firmly against the patient's face with both hands and simultaneously maintain proper head position.

Observe the rise and fall of the patient's chest with each ventilation. Stop ventilation when you see gentle chest rise. Allow adequate exhalation after each ventilation. Ventilate the patient at an age-appropriate rate.

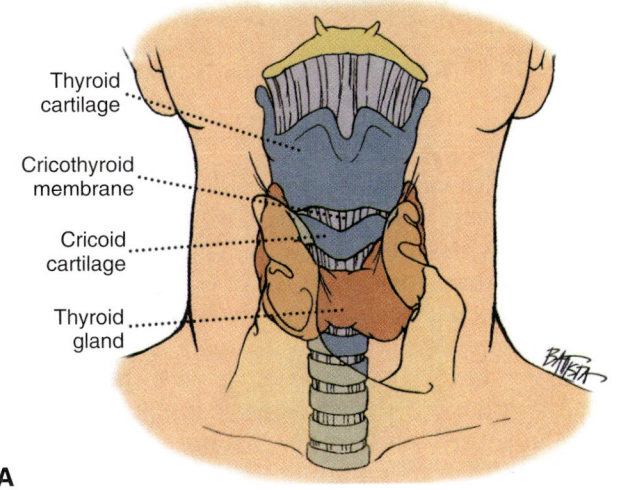

A

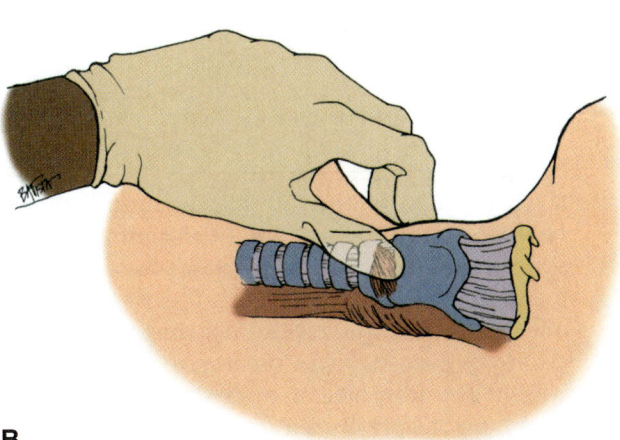

B

Figure 14-24 A, Landmarks of the cricoid cartilage. **B,** When cricoid pressure is applied, the esophagus is compressed between the cricoid cartilage and the cervical vertebrae.

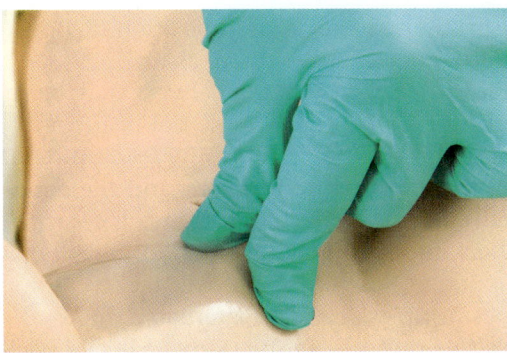

Figure 14-25 To apply cricoid pressure, locate the cricoid cartilage. Apply firm pressure on the cricoid cartilage with the thumb and index finger, just lateral to the midline.

Gentle pressure should be applied with a single fingertip in infants and with the thumb and index finger in older children. By pressing down on the cricoid cartilage, the esophagus is compressed between the cricoid cartilage and the fifth and sixth cervical vertebrae. This helps prevent the overflow of air into the stomach during positive-pressure ventilation, thereby reducing the likelihood of vomiting and aspiration. Cricoid pressure should be maintained as long as artificial ventilation continues. If cricoid pressure is performed during endotracheal intubation, it should be maintained until the endotracheal tube cuff is inflated and proper tube position is verified. However, if vomiting occurs during the procedure, release cricoid pressure to avoid rupture of the stomach or esophagus. Use cricoid pressure with caution if cervical spine injury is suspected.

Complications of this procedure include laryngeal trauma if excessive force is used, obstruction of the airway, especially in small children if too much pressure is applied, and esophageal rupture from unrelieved high gastric pressures.

Troubleshooting Bag-Mask Ventilation

During bag-mask ventilation, remember to avoid overinflation and allow adequate time for exhalation to occur. Also, while ventilating, feel for compliance when ventilating the patient's lungs. If at any time you sense poor compliance, reassess the patient to ensure the airway remains unobstructed and that lung sounds are clear and equal. Another indication that the patient is being well ventilated is improvement of the condition—improved color change, pulse oximeter readings, and responsiveness.

The most frequent problem with bag-mask ventilation is the inability to deliver adequate ventilatory volumes. This is because of the use of poor technique and/or difficulty in providing a leak-proof seal to the face while maintaining an open airway at the same time. If the chest does not rise and fall with bag-mask ventilation, reassess in the following manner:

- Begin by reassessing head position. Reposition the airway and try to ventilate again.
- Inadequate tidal volume delivery may be the result of an improper mask seal or incomplete bag compression. If air is escaping from under the mask, reposition your fingers and the mask. Reevaluate the effectiveness of bag compression.
- Check for an airway obstruction. Lift the jaw. Suction the airway as needed. If the chest still does not rise, select an alternative method of positive-pressure ventilation (such as a pocket mask or an automatic transport ventilator).

Automatic Transport Ventilator

[OBJECTIVES 44, 47]
An automatic transport ventilator (ATV) is a volume-cycled and rate-controlled ventilator. Indications for the use of an ATV include patients requiring ventilatory assistance because of a decreased level of responsiveness or apnea and patients who require extended positive-pressure ventilation. An ATV can be used for breathing and nonbreathing patients as well as intubated and nonintubated patients.

ATVs are compact mechanical ventilators that have become fairly economical and therefore common in prehospital use (Figure 14-26). They are convenient and simple to use, freeing personnel to perform other essential tasks. Typically regulated settings include tidal volume, ventilatory rate, and inspiratory time. Most are set with fixed oxygen flow rates of 100%, though some may be adjustable. A standard adapter allows interfacing with a variety of airway devices.

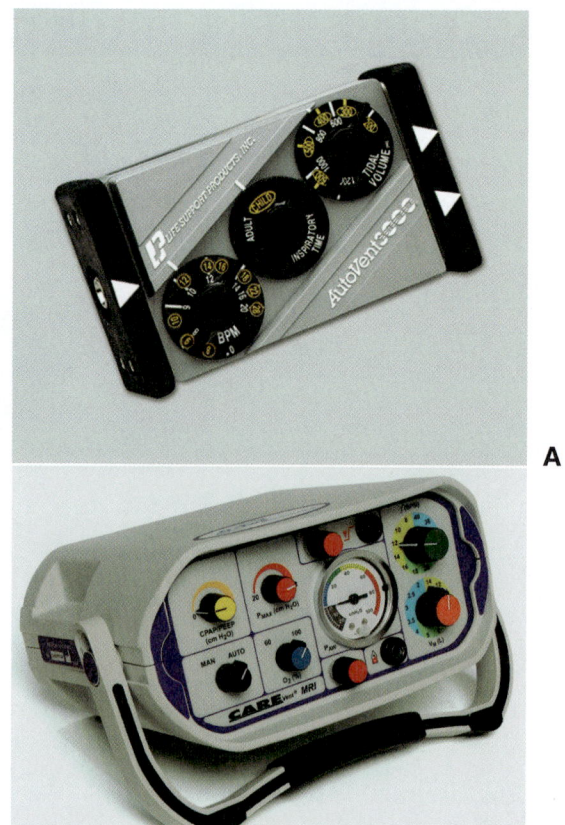

Figure 14-26 Examples of automatic transport ventilators.

Patients with increased airway resistance are not appropriate candidates for this device. Conditions including asthma, adult respiratory distress syndrome, or presence of a pneumothorax are examples of contraindications. In most cases, these simple ventilators do not allow ventilating with pressure controls because a pop-off valve activates to prevent barotrauma. As with the use of any mechanical device, the patient's compliance of chest expansion must be assessed. Advantages and disadvantages of ATVs are shown in Box 14-13.

ATVs should only be used by persons properly trained in the use of the device. Following are instructions for use of an ATV:

1. Test the ATV to ensure it is working properly before using it on a patient
2. If not already set, set the tidal volume and ventilation rate. Adjust the tidal volume to approximately 6 to 7 mL/kg (500 to 600 mL) to make the chest rise with each breath delivered over a 1-second period. Adjust the ventilation rate to deliver 10 to 12 breaths/min. If the patient is unresponsive, an assistant should apply cricoid pressure to reduce the risk of gastric inflation until an advanced airway is in place. If the patient is in cardiac arrest, adjust the ventilation rate to 8 to 10 breaths/min once an advanced airway is in place.

BOX 14-13 Automatic Transport Ventilators (ATVs)

Indications

- Patients requiring ventilatory assistance because of a decreased level of responsiveness or apnea
- Patients requiring extended ventilation

Contraindications

- Airway obstruction
- Increased airway resistance (asthma, adult respiratory distress syndrome, suspected pneumothorax or tension pneumothorax)
- Poor lung compliance (emphysema, significant pulmonary edema)
- Pulmonary overpressurization syndrome (blast injury or water ascent injury)

Advantages

- Lightweight, portable, and durable
- Provides a means for delivery of an oxygen-enriched mixture to the patient
- Can be used for breathing and nonbreathing patients, intubated and nonintubated patients
- Frees the rescuer for other tasks when used in intubated patients
- In patients who are not intubated, the rescuer has both hands free to apply the mask and maintain the airway
- Adjustable settings; once set, provides a specific tidal volume, respiratory rate, and minute ventilation

Disadvantages

- Need for an oxygen source (or sometimes electric power)
- Unable to detect increasing airway resistance
- Hard to secure
- Reliance on oxygen tank pressure
- Some ATVs should not be used in children younger than 5 years old

Reprinted from Aehlert, B. (2007). *ACLS study guide* (3rd ed.), St. Louis: Mosby.

BOX 14-14 Flow-Restricted, Oxygen-Powered Ventilation Devices (FROPVDs)

Indications

- Patients requiring ventilatory assistance because of decreased ventilation or apnea

Contraindications

- Not for use in pediatric patients

Advantages

- Easy to use
- Provides high oxygen concentrations and good volume delivery
- Provides a means for delivery of an oxygen-enriched mixture to the patient
- Can be used for breathing and nonbreathing patients

Disadvantages

- Need for an oxygen source
- Requires high oxygen flow rate, which quickly depletes portable oxygen cylinders
- Inability to monitor lung compliance
- Barotrauma to the lungs (such as a pneumothorax)

Modified from Aehlert, B. (2007). *ACLS study guide* (3rd ed.), St. Louis: Mosby.

8. Monitor the device to ensure delivery of adequate tidal volume and ventilation rate.

Flow-Restricted, Oxygen-Powered Ventilation Devices   *Demand valve*

A flow-restricted, oxygen-powered ventilation device (FROPVD) is capable of delivering 100% oxygen to a patient. An FROPVD consists of high-pressure tubing connecting the oxygen supply and a valve that is activated by a lever, push button, or by negative pressure sensed by the valve when a patient begins to take a breath. When the valve is open, oxygen flows into the patient. The device can be attached to a face mask, tracheal tube, or tracheostomy tube. Oxygen flow from the device is restricted to less than 30 cm H_2O in an effort to minimize gastric distention.

Indications for using an FROPVD include situations in which high-volume, high-concentration oxygen is desirable. It is best used on patients who are awake and able to self-administer. Use in patients who are unresponsive is acceptable, but caution is necessary to avoid barotrauma to the lungs.

When using this device, closely monitor the patient's chest rise during ventilations. Also frequently assess the patient's skin color, lung sounds for equality, and oxygen saturation levels. Indications, contraindications, advantages, and disadvantages of FROPVDs are shown in Box 14-14. Skill 14-8 shows the technique for ventilating the lungs of an unresponsive, nonintubated patient with an FROPVD.

3. Occlude the outlet adapter. An audible pressure limit alarm should sound with the next cycle (breath) to ensure that the pressure limit is intact and the lungs will not be overinflated.

4. Assess lung compliance and chest rise with a bag-mask device. If the patient has COPD, chest rise may not appear full (do not increase the tidal volume control on the ATV past the upper tidal volume limits).

5. Attach the patient valve assembly to the airway device (tracheal tube, mask, or airway adjunct).

6. Assess ventilations, listen for bilateral lung sounds, and look for adequate chest rise.

7. Count the number of ventilator cycles for 1 full minute to ensure proper correlation with the breaths per minute setting on the ATV.

SKILL 14-8 FLOW-RESTRICTED, OXYGEN-POWERED VENTILATION DEVICES

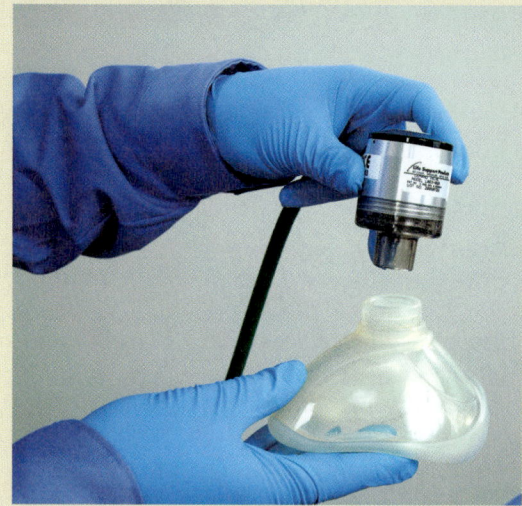

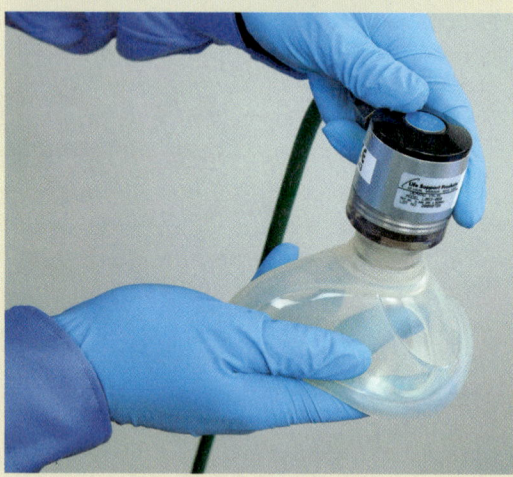

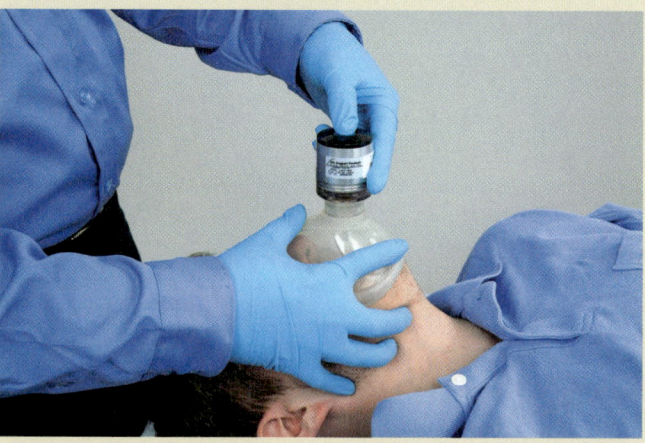

Step 2 Apply the mask to the patient's face and ensure a good seal. Trigger the device until the patient's chest rises. Allow the patient to exhale passively. Repeat once every 5 to 6 seconds.

Step 1 Put on appropriate personal protective equipment. Open the patient's airway. If the patient is unresponsive, insert an oral airway. Attach an FROPVD to the mask.

Special Considerations

Stoma Sites

[OBJECTIVES 48, 49, 50]

A **tracheostomy** is a surgical opening into the trachea between the tracheal rings. The surgical opening created in the anterior neck is called a **tracheal stoma.** It extends from the skin surface into the trachea and connects the trachea with outside air, bypassing the structures of the upper airway. It is the route through which the patient then breathes. The stoma may be temporary or permanent. A tracheostomy may be performed to bypass an upper airway obstruction. It may also be performed in patients who are unable to clear secretions effectively or those who need long-term mechanical ventilation. For example, a patient who has had his larynx

removed (laryngectomy) as a result of cancer would have a tracheostomy.

A tracheostomy tube (or trach tube) may be placed into the stoma (Figure 14-27). Materials used for tracheostomy tubes include silastic (silicone rubber), polyvinylchloride, stainless steel, and silver metals. Most tubes are made of silastic or polyvinylchloride. All tracheostomy tubes have a standard size opening or hub outside the patient's neck to enable attachment of a bag-mask device. Metal tracheostomy tubes require an adapter to make this connection.

A single cannula tracheostomy tube has one lumen used for airflow and suctioning of secretions (Figure 14-28). When changing the tube becomes necessary, a new tube must be quickly inserted because nothing keeps the stoma open once the old tube is removed. All neona-

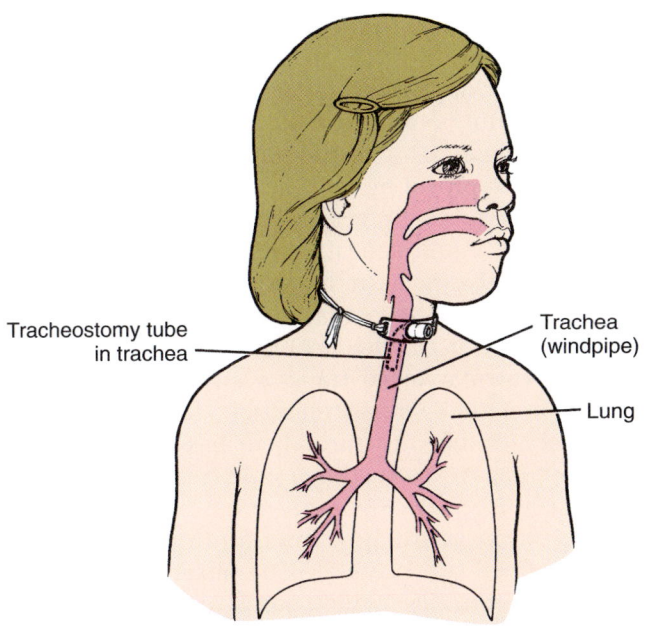

Figure 14-27 A tracheostomy tube in position in the trachea and secured in place.

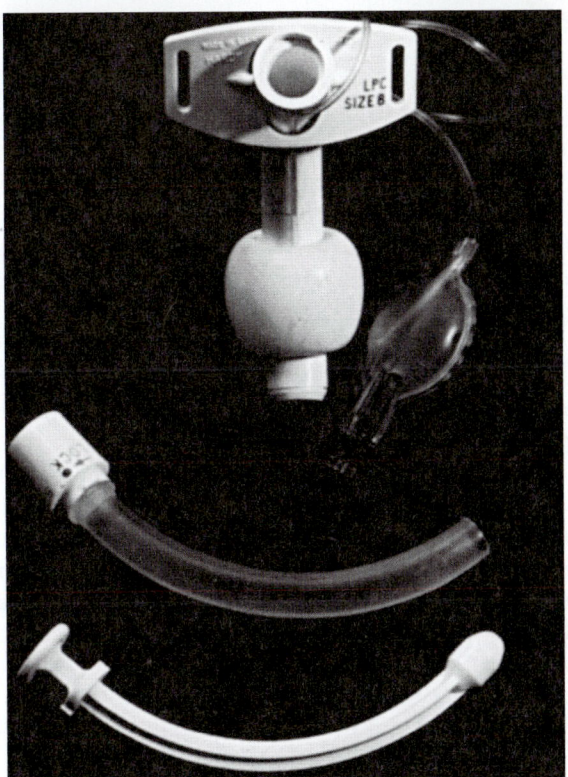

Figure 14-29 Double-cannula tracheostomy tube. Tracheostomy tube *(top)* with inner cannula *(middle)* and obturator *(bottom)*.

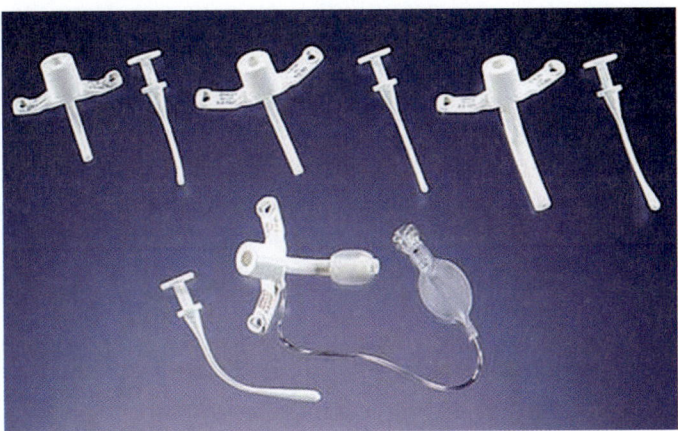

Figure 14-28 Neonatal and pediatric cuffed and uncuffed single-cannula tracheostomy tubes.

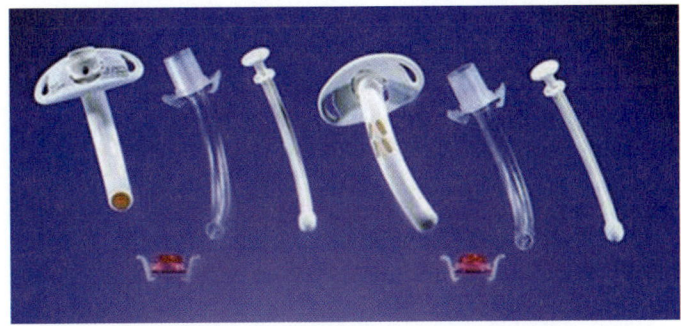

Figure 14-30 Disposable cannula cuffless fenestrated tracheostomy tubes with decannulation caps *(shown in red)*.

tal tracheostomy tubes and most pediatric tracheostomy tubes are single-cannula tubes.

A double-cannula tracheostomy tube consists of an outer cannula (main shaft), inner cannula, and an obturator (stylet) (Figure 14-29). The obturator is used only to guide the outer tube during insertion. When the outer cannula has been inserted, the obturator must be removed to permit ventilation. Once the outer tube is in place, the inner cannula is inserted and locked in place. The inner cannula may be disposable or reusable. A reusable inner cannula must be periodically removed for brief periods for cleaning. When the inner tube is removed for cleaning, the outer tube keeps the patient's airway open.

A fenestrated tracheostomy tube helps the patient learn to breathe through the upper airway, expel secretions, and talk. A fenestrated tube has small holes (fenestrations) in the side of the tube (Figure 14-30). When

a decannulation cap (plug) is attached to the tracheostomy tube, air flow through the stoma is blocked. Air flow is redirected through the holes in the tube, upward past the vocal cords, and out through the nose and mouth. If the patient cannot breathe through the nose or mouth, the decannulation cap must be removed to enable breathing through the stoma.

Patients with a tracheostomy tube have printed instructions on how to maintain it. The most common complications encountered with tracheostomies are dislodgement of the tube, obstruction of the tube, and infection. The upper airway filters and humidifies inspired air. Because a tracheostomy bypasses the upper airway, dried secretions can easily accumulate and occlude the tracheostomy despite regular tracheostomy care. When called to care for a patient who has a tracheostomy and signs

[handwritten: Ban Tube comes out: ① mask over stoma ② finger over stoma, mask to face ③ small ET tube into stoma]

of respiratory distress, assume that the patient has an obstructed tube.

If a patient with a tracheostomy has a dislodged tube, replacing it can be difficult because of swelling and airway narrowing. You can attempt to replace the tube with a tracheostomy tube if available. If a new tracheostomy tube is not available or if replacement attempts are unsuccessful, try to insert a tracheal tube. Insertion of a tracheal tube is a temporizing measure until a tracheostomy tube of the proper size can be replaced (see Chapter 40). Blocked tubes can generally be cleared with suctioning.

If a patient with a tracheostomy tube requires ventilation with a bag-mask device, remember that the trach tube is designed with a universal connector that will attach to any bag-mask device. If a patient no longer has a tracheostomy tube in place with a stoma, positive-pressure ventilation can present some unique challenges. If the larynx has been removed, a connection from the upper and lower airway may or may not exist. Ventilation can be provided by mouth-to-stoma or bag-mask to stoma ventilation. Locate the stoma and create a good seal. Observe for the usual signs that adequate ventilation is occurring. If you note that air is leaking from the nose and mouth, close and seal them while ventilating through the stoma. Special masks are available for supplemental oxygen administration by stoma.

Many patients and family members are knowledgeable of healthcare appliances such as tracheostomies. Other patients may be in assisted living environments or have access to home healthcare agencies, all of which may serve as valuable resources if you encounter a patient with complications associated with a stoma or tracheostomy.

[handwritten: Blood from trach (spurting): pull up on trach to occlude artery / more air into cuff]

Gastric Distention

[OBJECTIVES 51, 52, 53]
In an intubated patient, the trachea is isolated and gases are delivered directly to the pulmonary system. However, when ventilating nonintubated patients, air commonly makes its way into the stomach, causing gastric distention. Air becomes trapped in the stomach, which can lead to regurgitation, increasing the risk of aspiration. As the diameter of the stomach continues to increase, pressure pushes upward on the diaphragm. An increasingly distended abdomen creates less room for full lung expansion, resulting in the potential for compromised gas exchange.

When managing a patient's airway and breathing, your goal is to minimize the potential for gastric distention. Recall that the use of cricoid pressure is meant to minimize this problem and should be used when providing positive-pressure ventilation to an unresponsive, nonintubated patient. Anticipate the possibility for vomiting in any patient who is being artificially ventilated and have suction immediately available.

Once gastric distention has occurred, placing a tube into the stomach for decompression and removal of stomach contents is desirable. Gastric tubes may be

inserted by the nose (nasogastric tube) or the mouth (orogastric tube). In addition to providing a means to alleviate gastric distention, gastric tubes may also be indicated for washing out or pumping the stomach, such as in drug overdoses. This technique is called *gastric lavage* and requires approval by medical direction.

Nasogastric tubes are generally well tolerated, do not interfere with endotracheal intubation, and allow the patient to talk easily. Extreme caution should be used in any patient with suspected facial trauma when using the nasal approach. If gastric decompression is necessary in a patient who has facial trauma, an orogastric tube is generally preferred. Orogastric tubes allow insertion of a larger diameter tube. If your patient has a known or suspected esophageal obstruction, esophageal varices, esophageal cancer, esophageal trauma, or has ingested a caustic substance, defer gastric tube insertion for the controlled environment of the hospital. Complications associated with both approaches include nasal, oral, esophageal, or gastric trauma. During insertion, the tube may be incorrectly positioned, possibly finding its way into the trachea. For this reason, you must confirm the placement of a gastric tube. Tube functionality may be compromised if it becomes twisted or occluded. An added problem that may be encountered with orogastric tubes is a patient who bites or chews on the tube.

Except for the location of insertion, the procedure for placing an orogastric or nasogastric tube is essentially the same. Because of a risk of bleeding from mucosal trauma and vomiting, always wear gloves, protective eyewear, and a face shield. A protective gown, if available, may also be recommended. The procedure for nasogastric tube insertion is discussed in more detail in Chapter 12.

PARAMEDIC *Pearl*

According to the 2005 resuscitation guidelines, if your patient requires placement of an orogastric (or nasogastric) tube and an ET tube, the orogastric (or nasogastric) tube should be inserted *after* placement of the endotracheal tube. If a gastric tube is inserted before the ET tube, the gastric tube can interfere with the gastroesophageal sphincter and may result in vomiting.

Ventilation of Pediatric Patients

[OBJECTIVE 54]
Differences in the anatomy of the pediatric airway mean that some variation is necessary when providing positive-pressure ventilation. For starters, children have a flat nasal bridge that makes achieving a seal with the mask more difficult. Be sure to avoid placing the mask over the child's eyes and use an appropriate size. An effective seal often is best achieved when using the two-person technique and the E-C clamp method.

When performing bag-mask ventilation, be sure to select the appropriate size of bag. Use a bag that holds at least 450 to 500 mL of air (pediatric bag) for term newly born infants, infants, and children. A 250-mL (neonatal) bag should not be used because this size does not provide sufficient volume for term newborns. Use a 1200-mL (adult) bag for larger children and adolescents. A child's lungs can be ventilated with a larger bag as long as proper technique is used; squeeze the bag only until the chest begins to rise, then release the bag. The paramedic must be familiar with appropriate ventilation rates for all ages, and be sure not to hyperventilate the patient.

Remember that the internal airway diameter in infants and small children is proportionately smaller than that of an adult, and the cartilaginous rings of the trachea are not fully developed until the age of eight years old. Therefore positioning is important when maintaining an open airway. Excessive flexion or hyperextension is enough to occlude a child's airway significantly. To compensate for the proportionately large occiput a thin layer of padding placed under the shoulders of a child younger than 3 years may be necessary to obtain a neutral position. If trauma is not suspected, the child can be placed in the sniffing position.

Placing a folded sheet under the occiput of a child more than 3 years old may be necessary to obtain an optimal angle for ventilation (if no trauma is suspected).

In an unresponsive patient, the application of cricoid pressure may help minimize gastric inflation and passive regurgitation. Be careful to not press too firmly and cause a tracheal obstruction, particularly in infants.

Assess your efforts by auscultating lung sounds bilaterally. Pay particular attention to the child's skin color and heart rate. Remember that respiratory compromise is most often the cause of bradycardia and, if present, you must reevaluate the treatment plan.

ADVANCED AIRWAYS

[OBJECTIVE 55]

Advanced airways include the esophageal-tracheal Combitube, the laryngeal mask airway (LMA), and the endotracheal (ET) tube. Insertion of a Combitube or LMA does not require visualization of the vocal cords. In contrast, insertion of an ET tube through a patient's mouth and into the trachea (orotracheal intubation) does require direct visualization of the vocal cords.

Dual Lumen Airway Devices

Dual lumen airway devices consist of two tubes, or lumens, and may be placed in either the trachea or the esphogaus. Because there are two ventilation options of a dual lumen device it is imperative that the paramedic determine placement of the device, esophageal or tracheal. Failure to do so will result in gastric ventilation, hypoxia, and patient death.

Esophageal-Tracheal Combitube

[OBJECTIVE 56]

The esophageal-tracheal Combitube (commonly called the *Combitube* [Tyco-Kedall, Mansfield, Mass.]) allows ventilation of the lungs and reduces the risk of aspiration

of gastric contents. It does not require visualization of the vocal cords (blind insertion) to ventilate the trachea. The Combitube is available in 41 and 37 French (Fr) sizes. The 37 Fr size is used for patients between 4 and 5 feet tall. The 41 Fr size is used for patients taller than 5 feet.

The Combitube is called a *dual-lumen airway* because two separate tubes have been joined together with separate airflow passages. Examination of the tube reveals several key features. Proximally are two tubes with universal adapters; one is longer, blue, and clearly labeled "#1." The second tube is shorter, clear, and labeled "#2." Each tube has a pilot balloon labeled #1 or #2 with the corresponding amount of air that is inserted to fill one of two cuffs. As you progress toward the distal end of the tube, you will see an area that has two solid black rings encircling the device. The black rings become important landmarks indicating proper depth of tube insertion when the teeth/gum line is located between the black lines. Near the center of the tube is a large latex cuff encircling the device called the *pharyngeal cuff*. When inflated, this cuff anchors the Combitube in place and occludes the nasopharynx and oropharynx. This prevents air leaks once the device is properly placed. Toward the distal tip of the tube, a second cuff accomplishes one of two functions. The first function is occlusion of the esophagus (in most cases) to prevent gastric insufflation and minimize the risk of aspiration. Second, if the tube is blindly placed in the trachea, this cuff protects and isolates the lower airway as an ET tube does (Figure 14-31). Between the cuffs on one side of the tube you will note several small holes. These holes facilitate the passage of air into and out of the lungs with an esophageal placement of the Combitube.

Combitube kits also come with a large syringe capable of inflating the pharyngeal cuff, a smaller syringe used to inflate the distal cuff, a flexible suction catheter, and an emesis deflection elbow. The pharyngeal cuff on the small adult tube (37 Fr) is inflated with 80 mL of air, while the pharyngeal cuff on the large adult tube (41 Fr) is inflated with 100 mL of air. The distal cuff is inflated with 15 mL of air on both tubes. Indications, contraindications, advantages, and disadvantages of Combitubes are shown in Box 14-15. Skill 14-9 shows the steps for insertion of a Combitube.

Before insertion of the Combitube test both cuffs to ensure their integrity and lubricate the device. In the trauma patient, leave the patient's neck in a neutral position; in the non-trauma patient the neck can be slightly hyperextended. Grasping the patient's lower jaw and lifting upward, insert the Combitube until the teeth are between the black lines on the device. Inflate the pharyngeal cuff first as the slight upward motion caused by the cuff will seal the device. Inflate the distal cuff second. Initially ventilate the longer blue tube and assess for chest rise, the presence of bilateral breath sounds, and the absence of gastric sounds. If chest rise and bilateral breath sounds are present, the tube is in the esophagus. Ventilate the patient with the blue tube. If there is no

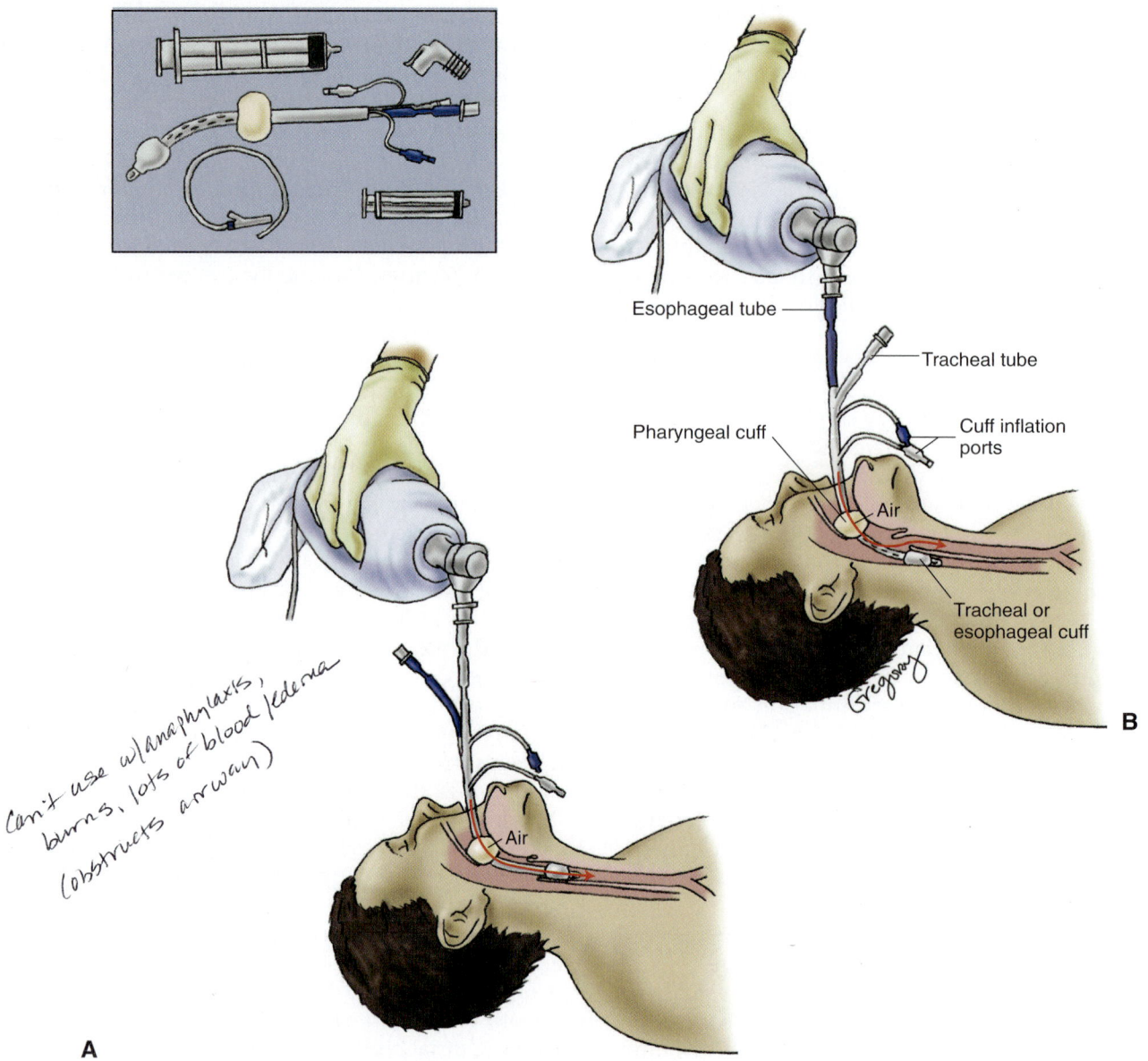

(handwritten note) Can't use w/anaphylaxis, burns, lots of blood/edema (obstructs airway)

Figure 14-31 A, The Combitube inserted into the trachea. **B,** The Combitube inserted into the esophagus.

chest rise, or absent bilateral breath sounds place the bag valve device on the clear tube and ventilate. Reassess for placement. If chest rise and bilateral breath sounds are present, the tube is in the trachea. Ventilate the patient with the clear tube. Measure expired carbon dioxide through the tube that is used for ventilation.

When the Combitube is placed in the esophagus, and gastric distension is present, the stomach can be decompressed by the insertion of a flexible suction catheter into the clear tube. Measure the catheter from the xyphoid process to the top of tube number 3 and mark the length. Lubricate the catheter, insert it through tube number three to the mark, and secure. Alternatively, the emesis deflection elbow has one end that connects to the Combitube and the other end connects to standard suction tubing. The stomach may be allowed to passively decompress, or intermittent suction can be used.

Pharyngeal Tracheal Lumen Airway

The pharyngeal tracheal lumen (PtL) airway is a dual lumen airway device that is similar to the Combitube. The PtL is designed to be either an intubating device, or an esophageal obturator device depending on placement. The PtL consists of a hollow white body with a separate clear tube within it. There are two cuffs, one to occlude the oropharynx, and one to occlude the trachea or esophagus, which are inflated simultaneously. Extending from the top of the device are three tubes, tube number 1 for inflation of the cuffs, tube number 2 for ventilating the patient with esophageal placement (green), and tube number 3 for ventilation with tracheal placement (clear). There is also a stylet in the longer clear tube that acts as an obturator for esophageal placement.

The indications and contraindications of the PtL are listed at the end of this section. To insert the PtL ensure

BOX 14-15 | Combitube

Indications

- Difficult face mask fit (beards, absence of teeth)
- Patient in whom intubation has been unsuccessful and ventilation is difficult
- Patient in whom airway management is necessary but the healthcare provider is untrained in the technique of visualized orotracheal intubation

Contraindications

- Patient with an intact gag reflex
- Patient with known or suspected esophageal disease
- Patient known to have ingested a caustic substance
- Suspected upper airway obstruction from laryngeal foreign body or pathology
- Patient less than 4 feet tall

Advantages

- Minimal training and retraining required
- Visualization of the upper airway or use of special equipment not required for insertion
- Reasonable technique for use in suspected neck injury because the head does not need to be hyperextended
- Because of the oropharyngeal balloon, the need for a face mask is eliminated
- Can provide an open airway with either esophageal or tracheal placement
- If placed in the esophagus, allows suctioning of gastric contents without interruption of ventilation
- Reduces risk of aspiration of gastric contents

Disadvantages

- Proximal port may be occluded with secretions
- Proper identification of tube location may be difficult, leading to ventilation through the wrong lumen
- Soft tissue trauma from rigidity of tube
- Impossible to suction the trachea when the tube is in the esophagus
- Esophageal or tracheal trauma from poor insertion technique or use of wrong size device
- Damage to the cuffs by the patient's teeth during insertion
- Inability to insert because of limited mouth opening

Reprinted from Aehlert, B. (2007). *ACLS study guide* (3rd ed.), St. Louis: Mosby.

both cuffs are fully deflated and the white cap on the inflation port is in place. Unlike other cuffed airway adjuncts, do not test the cuffs as this can weaken their integrity (the integrity of the cuffs are inspected by the manufacturer). Lubricate the device before insertion. In the trauma patient, leave the patient's neck in a neutral position, in the non-trauma patient the neck can be slightly hyperextended. Grasping the patient's lower jaw and lifting

upward, insert the PtL until the flange of the device rests on the patient's teeth and the integrated bite block is between the teeth. Secure the device by placing the attached strap behind the patient's neck and inflate both cuffs simultaneously via tube number 1 with a bag-mask device. Attach the bag-mask device to the number 2 tube (green) and perform ventilation. Assess for chest rise, the presence of bilateral breath sounds, and the absence of gastric sounds. If chest rise and bilateral breath sounds are present, the tube is in the esophagus. Ventilate the patient with tube number 2. If there is no chest rise or bilateral breath sounds, remove the stylet from tube number 3 (clear) and ventilate. Reassess for placement. If chest rise and bilateral breath sounds are present, the tube is in the trachea. Ventilate the patient with tube number 3. Measure expired carbon dioxide through the tube that is used for ventilation.

When the PtL is placed in the esophagus, and gastric distension is present, the stomach can be decompressed by the insertion of a flexible suction catheter into tube number 3. Measure the catheter from the xyphoid process to the top of tube number 3 and mark the length. Lubricate the catheter, insert it through tube number 3 to the mark, and secure. The stomach may be allowed to passively decompress, or intermittent suction can be used.

Indications for the PtL:

- Unconscious patient over the age of 14 years old
- Patient between 5 and 7 feet tall
- Absent gag reflex
- Inability to intubate when airway protection is needed
- Failure of less invasive measures

Contraindications for the PtL:

- Patient is less than 14 years old
- Gag reflex is present
- Known or suspected esophageal disease
- Known or suspected esophageal varices
- Chronic alcohol abuse
- Known or suspected caustic ingestion

Supraglottic Airway Devices

Supraglottic airway devices are those that are not designed to enter the glottis. Unlike the dual lumen airway, there is only one option for placement and ventilation.

Laryngeal Mask Airway

In some EMS systems, the LMA is used as an alternative to endotracheal intubation. The LMA may be used as the primary airway, as a channel for an endotracheal tube, or as an option in the management of a difficult airway in which intubation is unsuccessful.

An LMA consists of a tube that is fused to an elliptical, spoon-shaped mask at a 30-degree angle (Figure 14-32). When inserted, the tube protrudes from the patient's mouth and is connected to a ventilation device by a standard 15-mm inside diameter connector. The mask

SKILL 14-9 COMBITUBE INSERTION

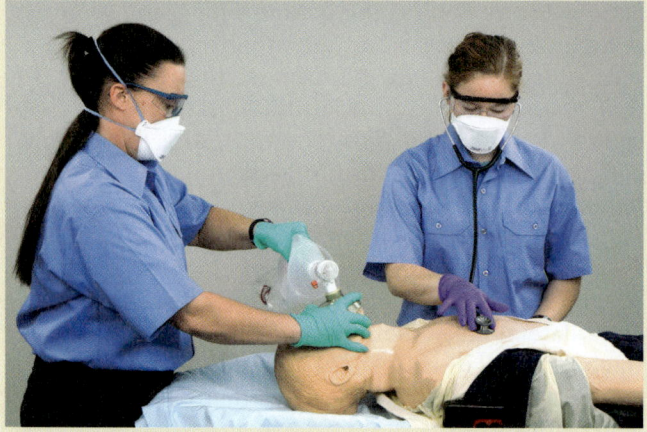

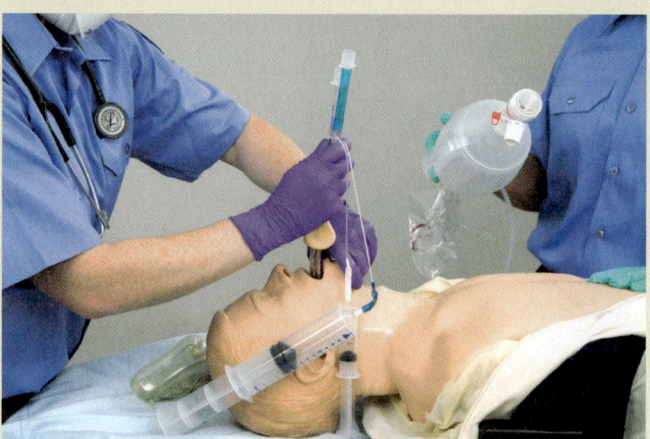

Step 1 Put on appropriate personal protective equipment. Open the patient's mouth and suction if necessary. If an oral airway was inserted, remove it. Auscultate bilateral breath sounds to establish a baseline. Instruct an assistant to pre-oxygenate the patient with 100% oxygen.

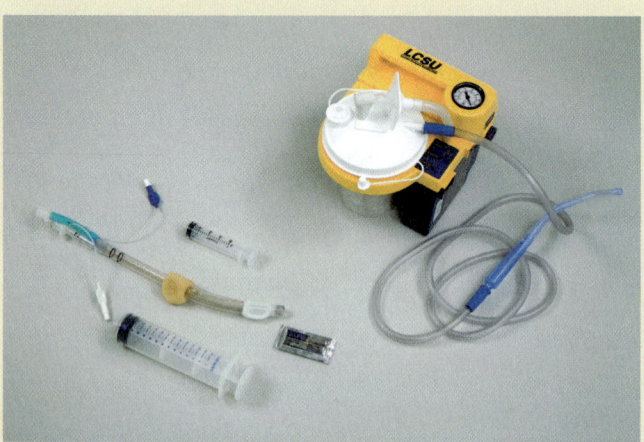

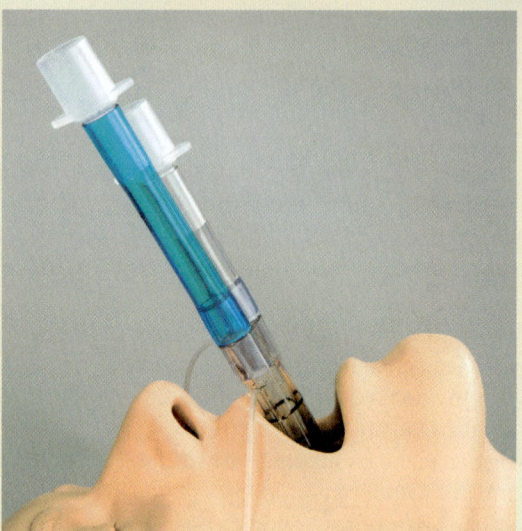

Step 3 Insert the Combitube in the same direction as the natural curvature of the pharynx. Insert the tip into the mouth in the midline and advance it gently along the base of the tongue and into the airway until the line of the patient's teeth (or gums, if the patient lacks teeth) is between the two black lines on the tube. If the tube does not insert easily, do not use force—withdraw and retry.

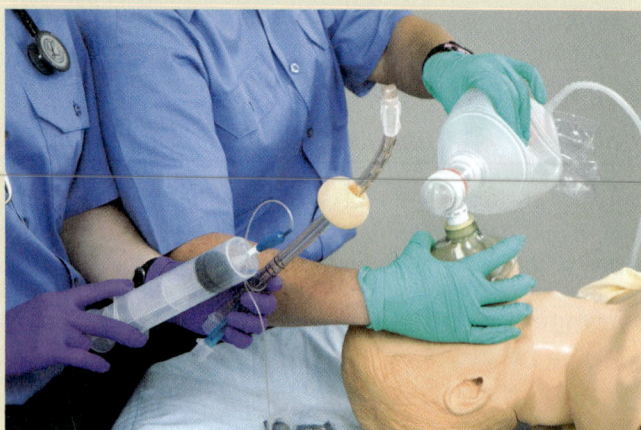

Step 2 Assemble the proper equipment and check the cuffs for leaks. Lubricate the distal tip of the tube with water-soluble jelly.

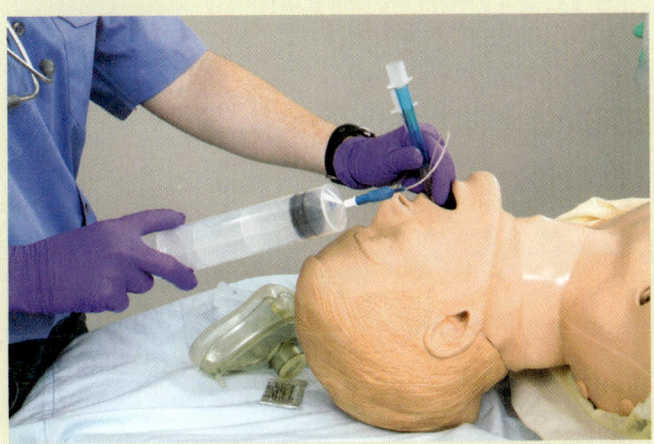

Step 4 Inflate the proximal (pharyngeal) cuff with 100 mL of air through the blue pilot tube marked #1. Once inflated, the pharyngeal balloon holds the device in place and helps prevent the escape of air through the nose or mouth.

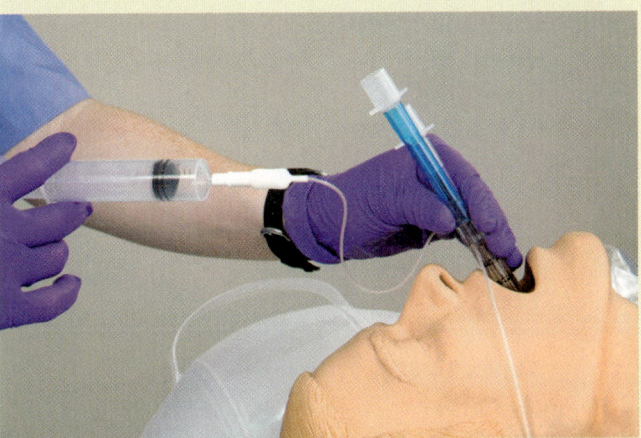

Step 5 Inflate the distal (esophageal) cuff with 15 mL of air through the white pilot tube marked #2. Once inflated, the esophageal balloon seals the esophagus so that air does not enter the stomach, reducing the risk of aspiration of gastric contents.

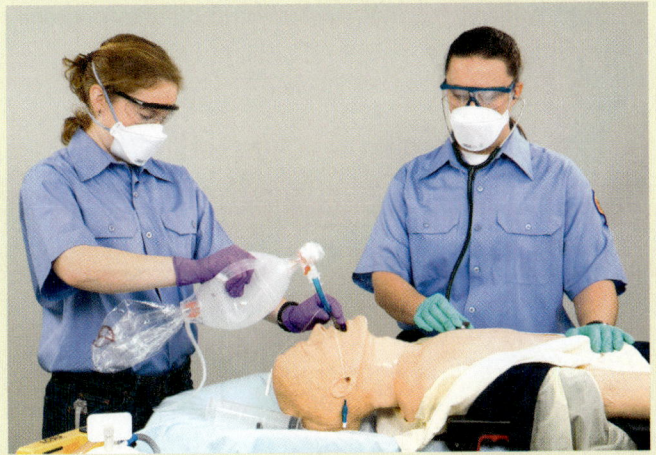

Step 6 Attach a bag-mask device to the longer (blue) connecting tube marked #1 (the esophageal tube) and begin ventilation. Ventilation with the Combitube begins with the esophageal tube because of the high probability of esophageal placement after blind insertion. Confirm placement and ventilation by observing chest rise and auscultating over the epigastrium and bilaterally over each lung. If the chest rises, breath sounds are present bilaterally, and epigastric sounds are absent, the Combitube is in the esophagus. Continue to ventilate through the long (blue) tube. When esophageal tube placement has been verified, the short (clear) tube (marked #2) can be used for gastric suction with the suction catheter provided in the airway kit. Secure the tube in place with a commercial tube holder or tape.

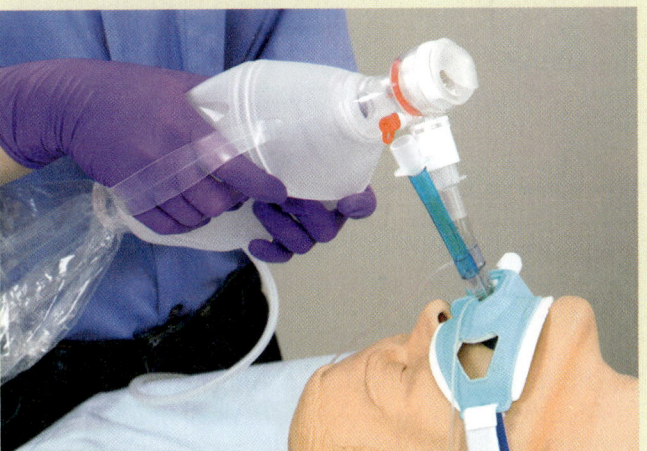

Step 7 If the chest does not rise or sounds are only heard over the epigastrium, attach the bag-mask device to the second (endotracheal) tube and begin ventilation to determine if the Combitube has entered the trachea. If the device is in the trachea, the chest should rise when ventilating through the second (shorter, clear) tube. (The Combitube functions as a standard ET tube when the device is placed in the trachea.) Confirm placement and ventilation by observing chest rise, auscultation over epigastrium, and bilaterally over each lung. If the Combitube is in the trachea and placement has been confirmed, continue ventilation through the second tube. Secure the tube in place with a commercial tube holder or tape.

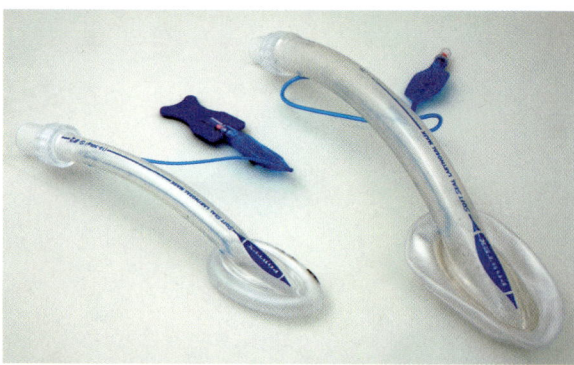

Figure 14-32 Laryngeal mask airways.

resembles a miniature facemask and has an inflatable rim filled with air from a syringe using a pilot valve-balloon system. The tube opens into the middle of the mask by means of three vertical slits that prevent the tip of the epiglottis from falling back and blocking the lumen of the tube.

The LMA is inserted through the mouth and into the pharynx. The device is advanced until resistance is felt. The mask is then inflated, providing a low-pressure seal around the laryngeal inlet. Note that the inflatable LMA cuff does not ensure an airtight seal to protect the airway from aspiration.

The posterior aspect of the tube is marked with a longitudinal black line. When the LMA is correctly placed, the black line on the tube should rest in the midline against the patient's upper lip. Indications, contraindications, advantages, and disadvantages of LMAs are shown in Box 14-16.

Using the Laryngeal Mask Airway. Directions for using the LMA are as follows:

1. Using personal protective equipment, open the patient's mouth and clear the airway of any foreign objects or debris. If an oral airway was inserted, remove it.
2. Auscultate bilateral breath sounds to establish a baseline and instruct an assistant to preoxygenate the patient with 100% oxygen.
3. Assemble the proper equipment and check the cuff and valve for leaks. Deflate the cuff and apply water-soluble lubricant. (Avoid lubricating the anterior surface of the mask because the lubricant may be aspirated.) Position the rim of the mask so that it is facing away from the mask opening. No folds should be near the tip.
4. Place the patient in the "sniffing" position (neck flexed and head extended). During the insertion procedure, maintain this position with your nondominant hand.
5. With the distal opening of the LMA facing anteriorly, insert the tip of the LMA into the patient's mouth (Figure 14-33). Press the tip of the mask upward against the hard palate to flatten it out. With your index or third finger, in one smooth

---

BOX 14-16 | **Laryngeal Mask Airway (LMA)**

Indications

- Difficult face mask fit (beards, absence of teeth)
- Patient in whom intubation has been unsuccessful and ventilation is difficult
- Patient in whom airway management is necessary but the healthcare provider is untrained in the technique of visualized orotracheal intubation

Contraindications

- Healthcare provider untrained in use of LMA
- Contraindicated if a risk of aspiration exists (e.g., patients with full stomachs)

Advantages

- Can be quickly inserted to provide ventilation when bag-mask ventilation is not sufficient and endotracheal intubation cannot be readily accomplished
- Tidal volume delivered may be greater when using the LMA than with face mask ventilation
- Less gastric insufflation than with bag-mask ventilation
- Provides ventilation equivalent to the tracheal tube
- Training simpler than with tracheal intubation
- Unaffected by anatomic factors (e.g., beard, absence of teeth)
- No risk of esophageal or bronchial intubation
- When compared with tracheal intubation, less potential for trauma from direct laryngoscopy and tracheal intubation
- Less coughing, laryngeal spasm, sore throat, and voice changes than with tracheal intubation

Disadvantages

- Does not provide protection against aspiration
- Cannot be used if the mouth cannot be opened more than 0.6 in (1.5 cm)
- May not be effective when respiratory anatomy is abnormal (i.e., abnormal oropharyngeal anatomy or the presence of pathology is likely to result in a poor mask fit)
- May be difficult to provide adequate ventilation if high airway pressures are required

Reprinted from Aehlert, B. (2007). *ACLS study guide* (3rd ed.), St. Louis: Mosby.

movement advance the mask over the hard palate, the soft palate, and as far as possible into the laryngopharynx until resistance is felt. When the LMA has been properly positioned, the cuff tip lies at the base of the laryngopharynx, the sides in the pyriform fossae, and the upper border of the mask at the base of the tongue, pushing it forward.

6. Make sure that the black line on the LMA is in the midline against the patient's upper lip. Failure to make sure that the black line on the LMA is

Supreme LMA has another tube for passing nasogastric tube to decompress stomach

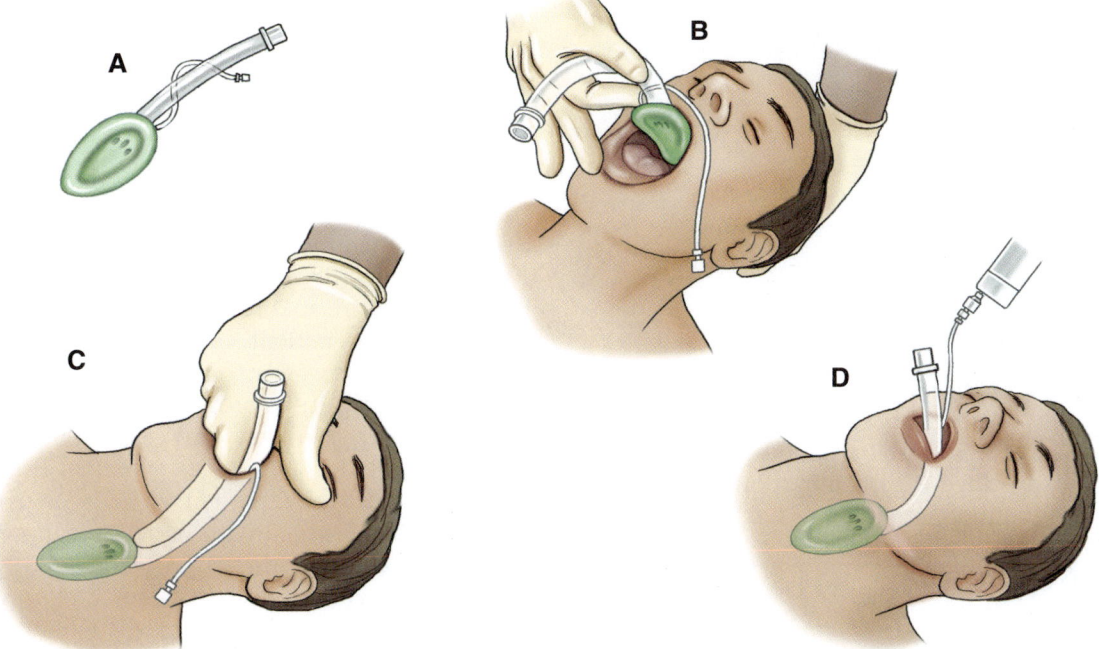

Figure 14-33 A, A laryngeal mask airway (LMA) with the cuff inflated. **B,** LMA placement into the pharynx. **C,** LMA placement using the index finger as a guide. **D,** LMA in place with cuff overlying pharynx.

correctly positioned may result in misplacement of the cuff and a partial airway obstruction. Without holding the tube, inflate the cuff with a volume of air appropriate for the mask size selected. As the cuff is inflated, a slight outward movement of the tube occurs as the cuff centers itself around the laryngeal inlet. This results in slight movement of the thyroid and cricoid cartilages.

7. Confirm placement of the LMA with auscultation, observation of chest rise, and use of an **exhaled CO$_2$ detector.** Secure the LMA and a bite block in place.

King LT-D Airway

The King LT-D airway (King Systems, Noblesville, Ind.) is a single lumen supraglottic airway device. It consists of a curved tube with a proximal and a distal cuff. Along the tube is an orientation/X-ray line that is used when inserting the device and for locating the device on an X-ray. The proximal cuff occludes the oropharynx, while the distal tube occludes the esophagus. Both cuffs are inflated using a single pilot balloon. Unlike dual lumen devices, this device is designed to be placed in the esophagus only. Therefore the paramedic must ensure there is not inadvertent tracheal placement. Ventilations are delivered via a bag-mask device attached to the proximal end of the tube and air escapes through holes in the tube that are located between the two cuffs. An alternate version of the King LT-D airway, the King LTS-D (King Systems), allows

the passage of a flexible suction catheter for gastric decompression. The same principles apply as described for the Combitube and PtL.

The indications and contraindications for both King devices are the same and are listed at the end of this section. Insertion of the device begins with selection of the appropriate size. The King airway devices are available in three sizes. Size 3 is for patients from 4-5 feet tall, and the cuffs are inflated with 45-60 mL of air. Size 4 is for patients from 5 to 6 feet tall, and the cuffs are inflated with 60 to 80 mL of air. Finally, size 5 is for patients greater than 6 feet tall, and the cuffs are inflated with 70 to 90 mL of air. Before insertion of the device, test the cuffs for integrity, remove all the air, and lubricate the tube. Only lubricate the posterior side of the device so the lubricant does not clog the holes from which air escapes. In the trauma patient, leave the patient's neck in a neutral position; in the non-trauma patient the neck can be slightly hyperextended. Grasp the patient's lower jaw and lift it upward. With the device rotated laterally insert the tip into the mouth and advance it behind the tongue. Once past the tongue rotate the device so the orientation line is in the midline of the body. Continue to advance the airway until the bottom of the bag-mask device connector is at the lips or gums. Inflate the cuffs with the appropriate amount of air and connect a bag-mask device to the adapter. Ventilate the lungs while gently withdrawing the device to achieve minimal ventilation pressures. Confirm placement by evaluating for chest rise, confirmation of bilateral breath sounds, and evaluation of expired carbon dioxide. After confirming appropriate placement secure the device and consider the placement of a bite block.

Indications for the King LT-D:

- Unconscious patient over 4 feet tall
- Absent gag reflex
- Inability to intubate when airway protection is needed
- Failure of less invasive measures

Contraindications for the King LT-D:

- Patient is less than 4 feet tall
- Gag reflex is present
- Known or suspected esophageal disease
- Known or suspected caustic ingestion

Endotracheal Intubation

[OBJECTIVE 57]

ET intubation is an advanced airway procedure in which a tube is placed directly into the trachea. Tracheal intubation may be accomplished by using several variations in technique. Presented below is a focus on the traditional procedure of endotracheal intubation, followed by an overview of modified techniques.

Description

Orotracheal intubation requires direct visualization of the vocal cords. A **laryngoscope** is an instrument used to assist in visualization of a number of anatomic markers, such as the teeth, tongue, epiglottis, vocal cords, and the glottic opening. With the laryngoscope, you will be able to view the glottic opening to pass the tip of an ET tube directly through the vocal cords.

Endotracheal intubation requires a high degree of skill and knowledge as well as regular practice to maintain proficiency—and proficiency is an absolute requirement for performing this skill. Regular practice, continuing education programs, and an effective quality management program to monitor skill performance are essential for all paramedics who perform this skill.

Indications

Performing most paramedic procedures is relatively simple once you have perfected your skills. Knowing when to perform (and when not to perform) a skill is not always simple. You will often be faced with "gray" circumstances that require a judgment on your part. Is now the time to take definitive control of the patient's airway by placing an ET tube? Are less-invasive options available? Two important conditions exist for placing an ET tube: patients who have inadequate oxygenation and ventilation and patients who do not possess the ability to maintain the patency of their airway. The latter usually present the greatest challenge of knowing exactly when to intervene. A patient who is unresponsive may be oxygenating well. This may hold

true for the time being, but disaster can strike if the patient begins to vomit and subsequently aspirates.

In general, ET intubation is indicated in patients with apnea, existing or impending respiratory failure, or the inability to protect the airway (Box 14-17). Easiest of all indications is a patient in cardiac or respiratory arrest. An unresponsive patient is often unable to protect his or her airway, thereby necessitating that you take definitive control of the airway by ET intubation.

A patient with an altered mental status is a possible candidate for intubation. One note of caution is to consider the exact patient circumstances when deciding if this procedure is warranted. An unresponsive patient does not have the ability to protect his or her airway. However, a patient with a quickly and easily reversible condition should not be intubated. For example, the airway of an unresponsive diabetic patient who is hypoglycemic should generally be managed with basic life support maneuvers until after dextrose administration. Similarly, a victim of a narcotic overdose with respiratory depression often is

---

BOX 14-17 Endotrachial Intubation

Indications

- Inability of the patient to protect his or her own airway because of the absence of protective reflexes (e.g., coma, respiratory and/or cardiac arrest)
- Inability to ventilate an unresponsive patient with less-invasive methods
- Present or impending airway obstruction/respiratory failure (as in inhalation injury, severe asthma, exacerbation of COPD, severe pulmonary edema, severe flail chest or pulmonary contusion)
- When prolonged ventilatory support is required

Contraindications

- Untrained in endotrachial intubation

Advantages

- Isolates the airway
- Keeps the airway open
- Reduces the risk of aspiration
- Ensures delivery of a high concentration of oxygen
- Permits suctioning of the trachea
- Provides a route for administration of some medications
- Ensures delivery of a selected tidal volume to maintain lung inflation

Disadvantages

- Considerable training and experience required
- Special equipment needed
- Bypasses physiologic function of upper airway (such as warming, filtering, humidifying of inhaled air)
- Requires direct visualization of vocal cords

Reprinted from Aehlert, B. (2007). *ACLS study guide* (3rd ed.), St. Louis: Mosby.
COPD, Chronic obstructive pulmonary disease.

best treated with basic life support airway maneuvers while reversing the underlying cause (administration of naloxone) before considering intubation.

An existing or impending upper airway obstruction is another reason to take control of the airway. Patients with trauma, foreign bodies, burns, or anaphylactic reactions may necessitate early intervention to avoid more drastic procedures later in their care. A burn patient with smoke inhalation and the accompanying swelling of the upper airway that may ensue presents a dilemma: intubate now? Or wait and see how the patient progresses? If you wait too long, the window of opportunity may pass and you are left with a patient with such severe laryngeal swelling that intubation is impossible. You may then have to resort to a cricothyrotomy, an option that is the last resort when controlling an airway. On the other hand you may elect to intubate the patient early and laryngeal swelling does not occur. The decision to manage an airway must be made considering all options, benefits, and risks to the patient.

> **PARAMEDIC*Pearl***
>
> Before performing advanced airway procedures, you must exercise a high degree of judgment and possess the ability to make appropriate decisions after critically analyzing the patient's clinical presentation.

Intubation is used to maintain an open airway and protect it. Intubation also provides the greatest control in improving oxygenation and ventilation. Many conditions that affect the lower airway can result in respiratory distress and severely compromise the patient's ability to exchange gases. Failure to deliver oxygen to the bloodstream results in hypoxemia, with resultant cell, tissue, organ, and ultimately, organism death. Conditions such as COPD, pulmonary edema, pneumonia, asthma, adult respiratory distress syndrome, pulmonary contusion, and thoracic trauma also may necessitate intubation. In some cases, you may have to use medications to facilitate ET intubation. The use of sedatives and neuromuscular blockers is discussed in more detail later in the chapter.

One circumstance that can present a unique challenge is the patient suspected of having epiglottitis. Even minimal manipulation of the epiglottis can result in an immediate, complete airway obstruction requiring a cricothyrotomy. Intubating a patient with epiglottitis is contraindicated unless imminent respiratory failure is likely. Ideally, intubation of these patients would occur in a controlled setting, such as an operating room, with a physician skilled in performing a tracheostomy present. If you have no choice but to intubate, have your most skilled paramedic make one attempt and be sure that you have some alternative means ready by which to manage the airway if an obstruction results. The paramedic should realize that if this occurs, dual lumen and supraglottic airway devices will not be effective, and a cricothyrotomy

is likely the only option of managing the airway. In this situation, you likely will also need a smaller diameter endotracheal tube because of laryngeal swelling. Good practice demands you have at least one half-size smaller and one larger than selected in all patients you are intubating. If any doubt exists when managing a patient with epiglottitis, consult medical direction.

Another consideration when deciding to intubate a patient is to consider his or her wishes. Inquire regarding the status of do not resuscitate orders or other advance directives that may exist.

Equipment

> **PARAMEDIC*Pearl***
>
> ET intubation requires a commitment on your part as a paramedic to maintain skill proficiency. If you fail to maintain your skill with this procedure, you may do more harm than good for the patient.

[OBJECTIVES 58, 59, 60, 61]
Several pieces of equipment are used when performing endotracheal intubation. You must be thoroughly familiar with each item to perform this skill safely and effectively (Box 14-18).

Performance of airway procedures inherently poses risks of exposure to infectious diseases. In particular, advanced airway procedures bring you into close proximity to respiratory secretions. If the patient gags, vomits, or coughs, you are susceptible to exposure if you have not donned proper personal protective equipment. The use of a face shield that prevents splashes to the eyes and oral and nasal mucosa is essential. Wearing medically approved gloves also is necessary.

BOX 14-18	**Endotrachial Intubation: Equipment and Supplies**

- Laryngoscope handle
- Laryngoscope blades
- Extra batteries
- Endotracheal tubes of various sizes
- 10-mL syringe for inflation of the ET tube cuff (if present)
- Stylet
- Bag-mask device with supplemental oxygen and re-servoir
- Suction equipment
- Commercial tube holder or tape
- Water-soluble lubricant
- Bite block or oral airway
- Exhaled CO_2 detector and/or EDD

ET, Endotracheal; *EDD,* esophageal detector device.

Laryngoscope. A laryngoscope is an instrument that consists of a handle and blade used for examining the interior of the larynx. A laryngoscope allows you to manipulate structures in the airway to visualize the glottic opening. A standard laryngoscope is made of plastic or stainless steel. Several companies manufacture variations of laryngoscopes, including fiber optic ones.

The laryngoscope handle contains the batteries for the light source, usually two C-cell alkaline batteries. The end of the handle unscrews to allow battery replacement. Always have a spare set of batteries available. A laryngoscope without a bright light source is of little use when intubating. The laryngoscope handle attaches to a plastic or stainless steel blade that has a bulb located in its distal tip. The point where the handle and the blade attach to make electrical contact is called the *fitting*. The bulb on the laryngoscope blade lights when the blade is attached to the laryngoscope handle and elevated to a right angle (Figure 14-34). Some newer handles also contain the light source, a light bulb that shines brightly through a channel in the blade once it is attached. As an alternative, some light bulbs are located toward the distal end of the blade. In either case, if the bulbs are replaceable you should carry spare bulbs in your airway kit.

A laryngoscope can be used with Magill forceps to remove a foreign body from the upper airway (Figure 14-35). To clear the upper airway with the Magill forceps, use the long forceps with angled tips to literally reach down into the laryngopharynx, grasp the foreign object, and pull it out. This procedure generally should be attempted after basic life support maneuvers to clear an airway obstruction have been unsuccessful.

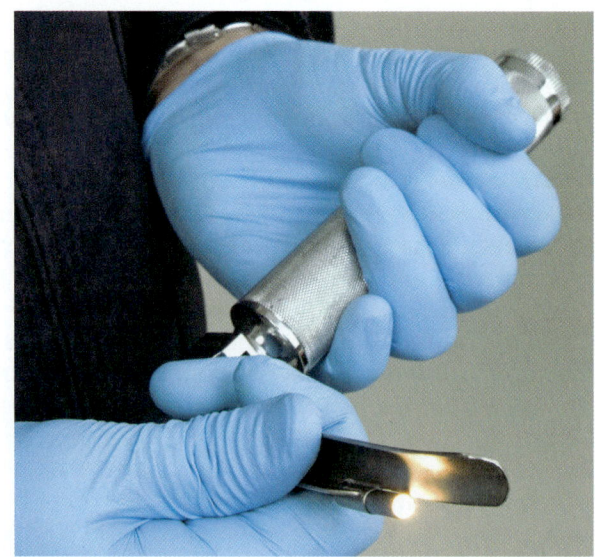

Figure 14-34 The bulb on the laryngoscope blade lights when the blade is attached to the laryngoscope handle and elevated to a right angle.

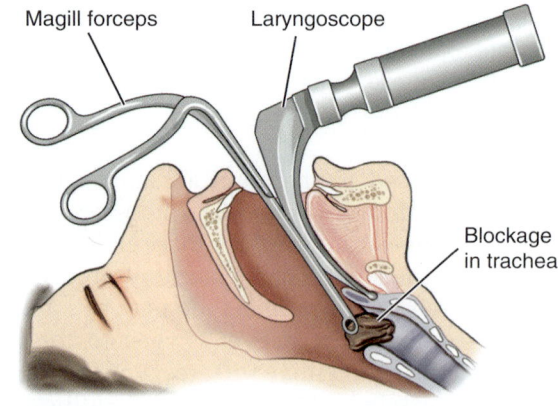

Magill forceps   Laryngoscope

Blockage in trachea

Figure 14-35 Foreign body obstruction removal with direct laryngoscopy and Magill forceps.

> **PARAMEDIC*Pearl***
>
> Because of increasing variability in laryngoscope handles and blades, not all are brands are compatible. As with every device that you use as a paramedic, be sure that you thoroughly know all your equipment and check it out well before you need it.

Laryngoscope blades are available in a variety of sizes ranging from 0 to 4. Size 0 is used for infants. A size 4 blade is used for large adults. Select the appropriate blade size with the laryngoscope blade held next to the patient's face. A blade of proper size should reach between the patient's lips and larynx. If you are unsure of the correct size, select a blade that is too long rather than too short.

Two types of laryngoscope blades are available: straight and curved (Figure 14-36). The straight blade also is referred to as the *Miller, Wisconsin,* or *Flagg blade.* During ET intubation, the tip of the straight blade is positioned under the epiglottis. When the laryngoscope handle is lifted anteriorly, the blade directly lifts the epiglottis out of the way to expose the glottic opening (Figure 14-37). Some paramedics prefer to use a straight blade because they believe it provides greater control of the tongue and

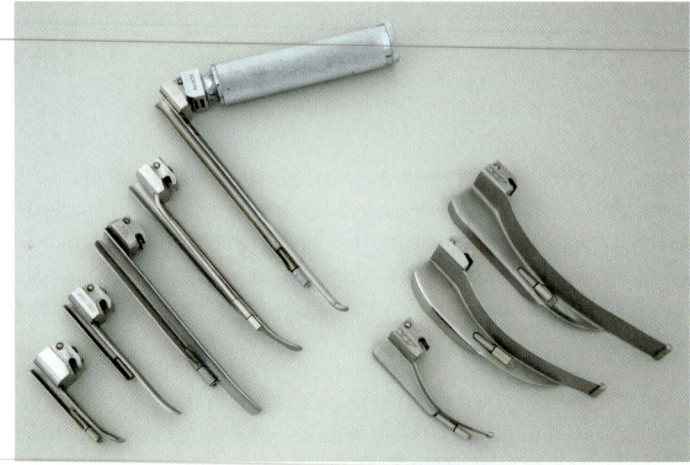

Figure 14-36 Straight and curved laryngoscope blades.

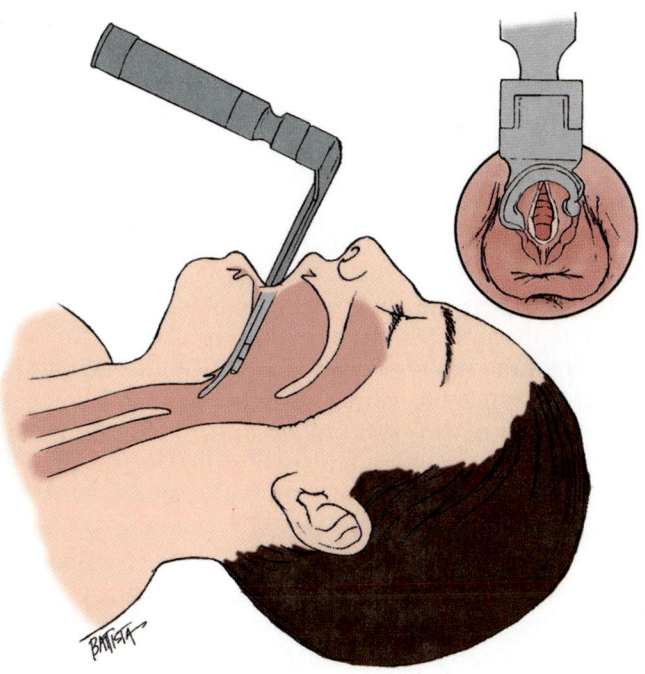

Figure 14-37 The tip of the straight blade is positioned under the epiglottis to expose the glottic opening.

+ trauma

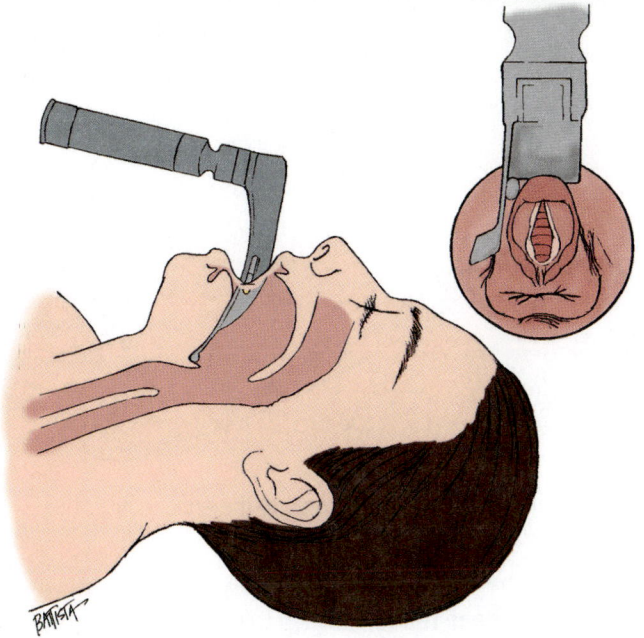

Figure 14-38 The curved blade is inserted into the vallecula, the depression or pocket between the base of the tongue and the epiglottis.

epiglottis. Pediatric patients, for example, have a proportionately larger and floppier epiglottis that is better stabilized with a straight blade. For this same reason, the straight blade may be desirable for some adult patients.

The curved blade also is called the *Macintosh blade*. The tip of the curved blade is inserted into the vallecula. When the laryngoscope handle is lifted anteriorly, the blade elevates the tongue and indirectly lifts the epiglottis, allowing visualization of the glottic opening (Figure 14-38). Many paramedics prefer the curved blade because no direct manipulation of the epiglottis occurs, which is thought to be less traumatic for the patient. Additionally, because the epiglottis is so sensitive, even minimal manipulation can trigger a gag response and reflexive emesis. Because of its shape, the curved blade generally occupies less space, enhancing room to see as well as pass the tube. However, it also has a much larger flange that may pose some extra risk of a broken tooth.

Each of the handles and accompanying blades in your field airway kit and throughout your EMS agency should be interchangeable. Disposable blades are available, and many services are opting to use single-use devices for infection control standards and because of the costs of iatrogenic infections.

During intubation, the laryngoscope is held in the left hand because most laryngoscopes are designed for right-handed individuals. This allows the dominant (right) hand to be used for handling the ET tube. The motion of laryngoscopy is to enter the patient's mouth on the right side and lift the tongue up gently and away in one easy sweep upward and to the patient's left without rotating the scope on a pivot point. Thus you will use the entirety of your left arm without bending your wrist or elbow. Because this motion may be difficult and awkward, a strong tendency exists for using the device as a prying instrument. A prying motion on the scope is dangerous for the patient and largely ineffective because it places the back of the laryngoscope blade in your line of view. Correct performance of the procedure brings several anatomic planes into alignment, resulting in clear visualization and easy passage of the ET tube.

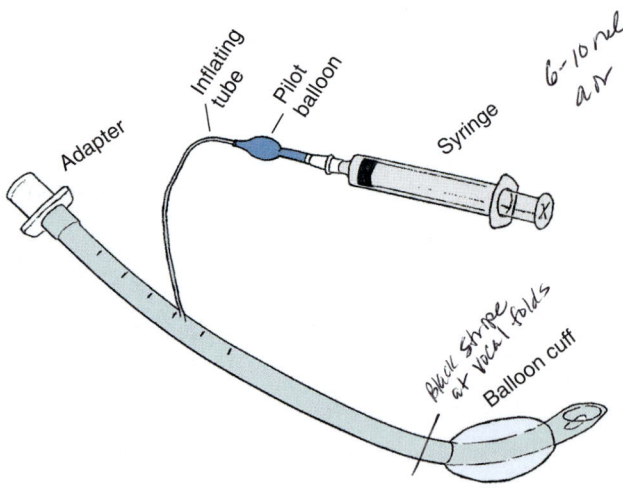

Figure 14-39 Components of the endotrachial tube.

Endotracheal Tubes. An ET tube is a curved tube that is open at both ends (Figure 14-39). A standard 15-mm connector is located at the proximal end for attachment of various devices for delivery of positive-pressure ventilation. The distal end of the tube is beveled to facilitate placement between the vocal cords. In addition to the opening on the distal tip of the tube, an additional hole is located near the tube's end called the *Murphy eye*. If the tip of the tube becomes occluded, this feature allows continued airflow through the tube. Water-soluble lubricant applied to the distal tip of the ET tube promotes ease of passage during intubation and decreases the possibility of trauma. A petroleum-based lubricant should never be used because it may damage the ET tube and cause tracheal inflammation.

Some ET tubes have an inflatable balloon cuff that surrounds the distal tip of the tube. When the distal cuff is inflated, it makes contact with the wall of the trachea as it expands, sealing off the trachea from the remainder of the pharynx and reducing the risk of aspiration. When assembling intubation equipment, ensure that the cuff will hold air because they are prone to leaks and holes. With a syringe, inflate the cuff with approximately 6 to 10 mL of air after tube placement. The cuff is attached to a one-way valve through a side tube with a pilot balloon used to indicate if the cuff is inflated. Be sure to remove the syringe after instilling air into the tube or the pressure exerted from the inflated cuff in the trachea will cause the air to leak out, compromising the ability to prevent aspiration. Cuffed ET tubes are generally unnecessary in children younger than 8 years because narrowing of the cricoid cartilage serves as a natural cuff.

ET tubes are measured in millimeters by their internal diameter and external diameter. They are available in lengths ranging from 12 to 32 cm. Internal tube diameters range from 2.5 to 5.5 mm (uncuffed) and 5.0 to 10.0 mm (cuffed) in half-millimeter increments. Imprinted markings are found along the length of the tube that specifies its internal diameter as well as centi-

meters measured from the distal tip of the tube. A radiolucent line also is present in ET tubes that allow for easy detection of tube placement in radiologic studies. In most respects, except for the absence of a cuff and pilot balloon, the smaller ET tubes are essentially the same as the larger ones. However, at the distal tip of the tube is some type of designation that lets you know how far past the vocal cords to pass the tube into the trachea. Depending on the manufacturer, the distal tip may be blackened. When intubating, pass the tube until the black portion of the tube has disappeared beyond the vocal cords. In some cases, the tube has a series of solid black lines. Closest to the tip is a single black line, and as you move proximally there is a set of two solid black lines. These lines are a point of reference when advancing the tube so that the initial single line is beyond the vocal cords while the double set remains visible.

Selection of an ET tube of the correct size is important. An ET tube that is too small may provide too little airflow and may lead to the delivery of inadequate tidal volumes. A tube that is too large may cause tracheal edema and/or vocal cord damage. Select the largest tube size appropriate for the patient because larger tubes facilitate suctioning of secretions and decrease the work of breathing. Common internal diameters of ET tubes for adults typically range from 7.0 mm to 8.5 mm. Because of the size variation in adults, several sizes of tubes should be on hand. At a minimum, have available an ET tube that is 0.5 mm smaller and 0.5 mm larger than the estimated tube size. When immediate ET tube placement is necessary, most adults can accept an ET tube with an internal diameter of at least 7.5 mm.

When the ET tube has been properly placed, the centimeter markings on the side of the tube should be observed and recorded. This value is typically between the 19- and 23-cm mark at the front teeth.

ET tube manufacturers continually develop new types of tubes for use in intubation. Some tubes have ports that allow for medication instillation into the lungs without interrupting ventilation. Others have built-in controls that allow you to manipulate the distal tip of the tube to facilitate passage into the glottic opening.

PARAMEDIC*Pearl*

Most common ET tube sizes used for adults:
- Adult female: 7.0 to 8.0 mm internal diameter
- Adult male: 8.0 to 8.5 mm internal diameter

Average ET tube depth:
- Adult men = 23 cm at the lips, 22 cm at the teeth
- Adult women = 22 cm at the lips, 21 cm at the teeth

Stylet. A **stylet** is a relatively stiff but flexible metal rod covered by plastic and inserted into an ET tube. It is used for maintaining the shape of the relatively pliant ET tube and "steering" it into position (Figure 14-40). The

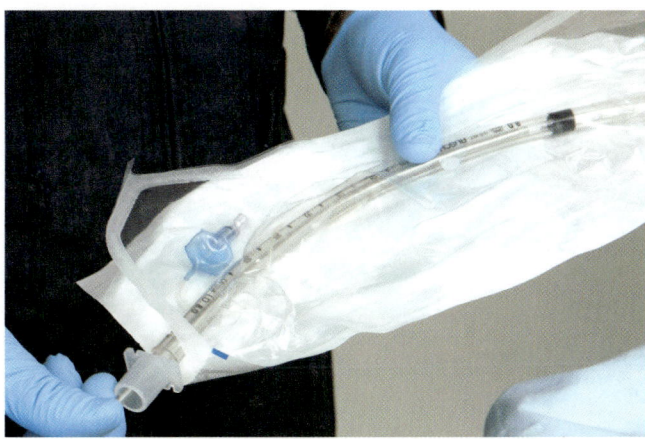

Figure 14-40 Endotracheal tube with stylet.

appropriate size stylet is longer than the selected ET tube and is only approximately 4 mm in diameter so that once lubricated with a water-soluble lubricant, it easily slides in and out of the length of the ET tube.

The functional shape of the stylet can be described as the approximate shape of a hockey stick, or the letter J. Even if you are proficient at performing ET intubations without the aid of a stylet, always have one readily available in the event a patient proves to have a challenging airway to intubate. Many seasoned paramedics always use a stylet, comforted with knowing that they have the greatest control in any situation and in every patient they are intubating.

When a stylet is used, the tip of the stylet must be recessed approximately one-half inch from the end of the ET tube to avoid trauma to the airway structures. To prevent the stylet from slipping down into the ET tube and out of reach, "hook" the manipulation end over the proximal end of the ET tube. Available in a variety of sizes, a stylet may be used while intubating both pediatric and adult patients.

Suction. You never know what you may encounter inside the airway as you make an attempt at intubation. It is best to anticipate needs that may arise. Always have suction readily available. Keep in mind that the patient may regurgitate at any time, and if you are intubating, the airway is already compromised.

Placement Confirmation Devices
[OBJECTIVE 62]
Methods used to verify proper placement of an ET tube include the following:

- Visualizing the passage of the ET tube between the vocal cords
- Auscultating the presence of bilateral breath sounds
- Confirming the absence of sounds over the epigastrium during ventilation

- Visualizing adequate chest rise with each ventilation
- Noting the absence of vocal sounds after placement of the ET tube
- Monitoring for changes in the color (colorimetric device) or number (digital device) on an exhaled CO_2 detector
- Verifying tube placement by an esophageal detector device

Multiple devices are available to assist in confirming placement of an ET tube in the trachea. Capnometry is one such device available to monitor end-tidal CO_2 given off from the lungs during ventilation. Exhaled CO_2 ($ETCO_2$) detection is presented later in this chapter in more detail. Colorimetric $ETCO_2$ devices are relatively inexpensive and provide a visual color indicator representing the range of CO_2 detected. Some detectors are built into bag-mask devices. See specific manufacturer recommendations for the devices you will be using. Because CO_2 may inadvertently enter the stomach, ventilate the patient at least six times before evaluating ET tube placement with an exhaled CO_2 detector to quickly wash out any retained CO_2.

Esophageal detector devices (EDDs) also are available as a means to confirm placement of an ET tube. EDDs are simple, inexpensive, and easy to use. They are used as an aid in determining if an ET tube is in the trachea or esophagus. Two types of EDDs are available—a syringe and a bulb (Figure 14-41). Both are placed on the proximal end of the ET tube immediately after intubation and before the ET tube cuff (if present) is inflated or ventilations are administered. The syringe device is placed on the proximal end of the ET tube with the plunger fully inserted into the barrel of the syringe. The bulb device is compressed before it is connected to an ET tube. The premise behind the devices is that if the tube is indeed in the trachea, the bulb will quickly inflate when releasing a compressed bulb once placed on the tube, or the syringe will meet with little to no resistance when aspirating air while pulling on the plunger. Structurally, the trachea has a cartilaginous framework that is not collapsible. The esophagus is a flabby hollow tube that has a rather small diameter unless swallowing a food bolus. When aspirating on the plunger or observing for the bulb to reinflate, if the ET tube is in the esophagus, the esophagus will be drawn over the tip of the tube. Resistance will be felt when aspirating with the syringe and the bulb will not reinflate. Do not inflate the ET tube cuff before using the EDD. Inflating the cuff moves the distal end of the ET tube away from the walls of the esophagus. If the tube was inadvertently inserted into the esophagus, this movement will cause the detector bulb to reexpand, falsely suggesting that the tube was in the trachea. Conditions in which the trachea tends to collapse can result in misleading findings. Examples of these conditions include morbid obesity, late pregnancy, status asthmaticus, and the presence of profuse tracheal secretions.

[handwritten: 5 intubations to become competent then 12/year]

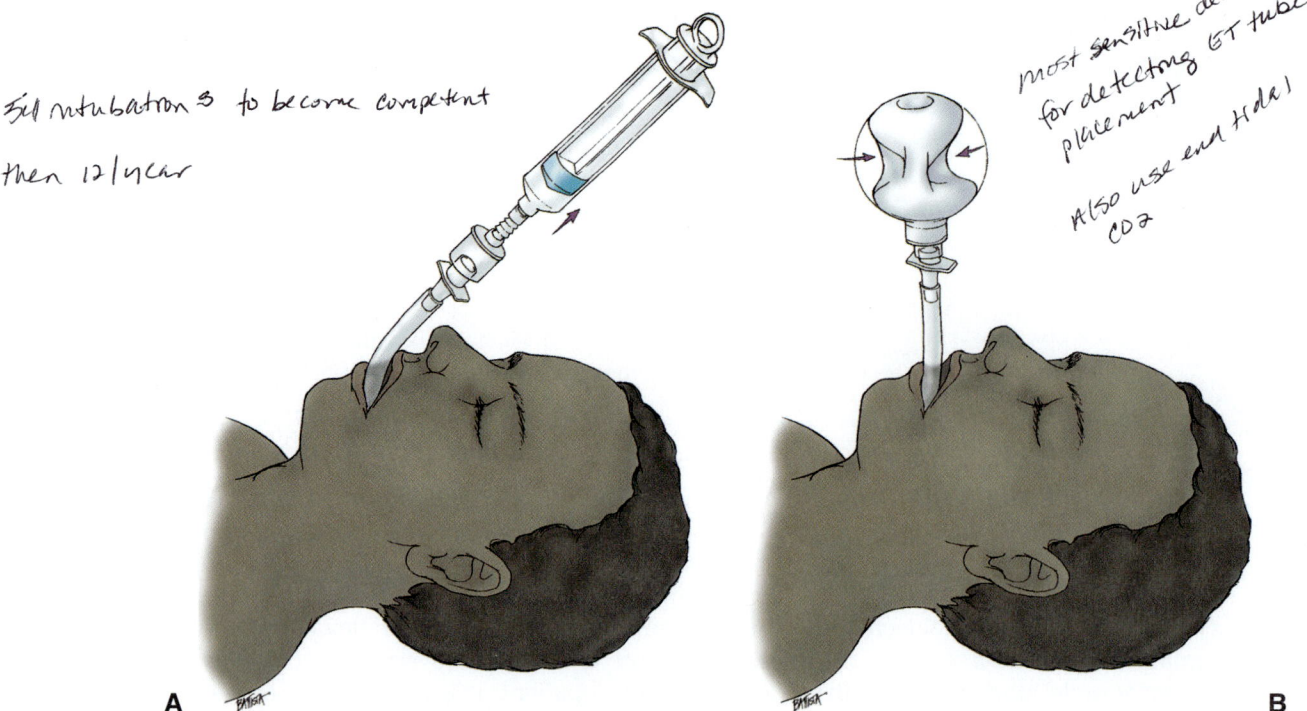

[handwritten: most sensitive device for detecting ET tube placement. Also use end tidal CO2]

Figure 14-41 Esophageal detector device. **A,** Syringe. **B,** Bulb.

PARAMEDIC*Pearl*

Auscultation for breath sounds over the lungs and abdomen and observation of chest rise are not always indicative of correct ET tube placement. After visualizing the ET tube passing through the vocal cords and confirming placement of the tube by auscultation, be sure to verify tube placement by using an exhaled CO_2 detector and/or an EDD.

Securing Devices

[OBJECTIVE 63]

Once proper positioning of the ET tube has been confirmed, secure the tube in place with tape, tube ties, or a commercially available tube holder. Commercial tube holders offer several advantages. They are quick and easy to use and have a built-in bite block, preventing the patient from clenching the teeth and occluding the tube. An added benefit is that they reliably and securely hold the tube in place, minimizing the possibility of dislodgement.

Tubes can be pushed into the airway to a point that the distal tip comes to lie in the right mainstem bronchus, inflating only the right lung. Accidental extubation is a real possibility, especially in the unpredictable environment of EMS. Further, manipulation of the tube can be irritating to patients, causing them to gag and result in increased vagal tone. Increased vagal tone and gagging can result in bradycardia and increased intracranial pressure. Several sources suggest that cervical spine stabilization should be performed to prevent tube movement and possible dislodgement. Rotation or hyperextension of the patient's neck during patient movement

or transfer can cause the tube to inch its way out of the trachea. This movement is why commercial tube holders may add to the possibility of tube displacement. When the ET tube is anchored to the patient's teeth, any movement of the head is transferred directly to the distal end of the tube. Using tube ties or tape allows for a slight amount of absorption of this movement, and while not preventing movement, it can reduce it. Consult your medical director to see whether this is something you should consider.

PARAMEDIC*Pearl*

An advanced airway that is misplaced or becomes dislodged can be fatal. Make rechecking placement of an advanced airway a habit immediately after insertion, after securing the tube, during transport, and whenever the patient is moved. Capnography (discussed later in this chapter) can be used to immediately detect a misplaced or dislodged tube.

Procedure

The steps for orotracheal intubation are as follows and are shown in Skill 14-10:

1. Using personal protective equipment (at a minimum use gloves, protective eyewear, and a mask), open the patient's airway. Ask your partner to preoxygenate the patient while you auscultate bilateral lung sounds to establish a baseline. Ideally,

Text continued on p. 528.

SKILL 14-10 OROTRACHEAL INTUBATION

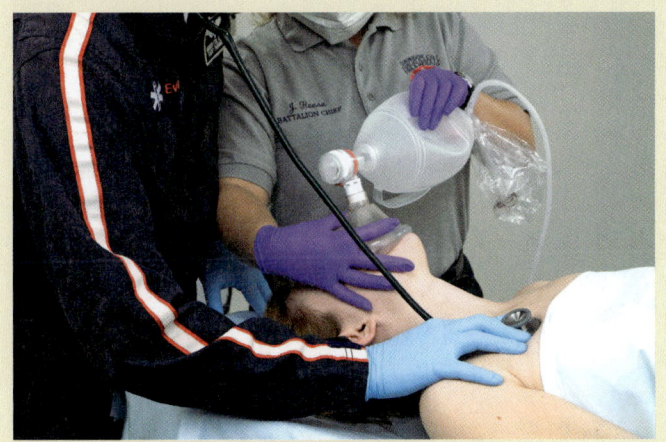 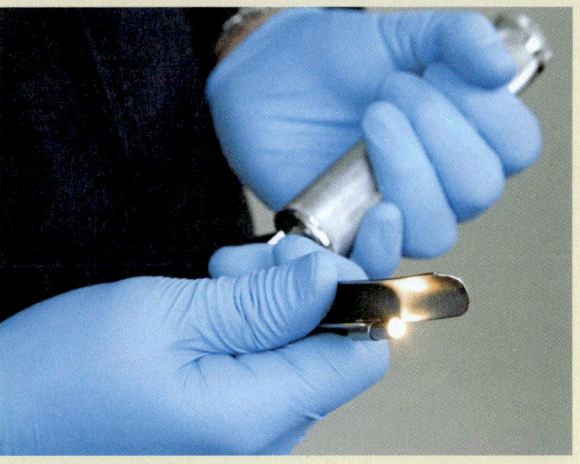

Step 1 Put on appropriate personal protective equipment. Open the patient's mouth and suction if necessary. Auscultate bilateral breath sounds to establish a baseline. Instruct an assistant to preoxygenate the patient with 100% oxygen.

Step 2 While your assistant continues to preoxygenate the patient, assemble and prepare the equipment needed for intubation, including suction equipment. Select the proper size blade and then assemble the laryngoscope. Attach the blade to the handle and check the blade for a white bright light. After verifying that the light is in working order, move the blade to its unlocked position to conserve battery life until the light is needed.

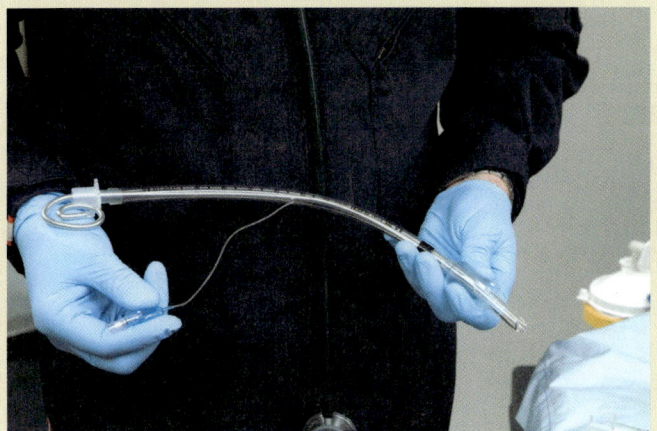 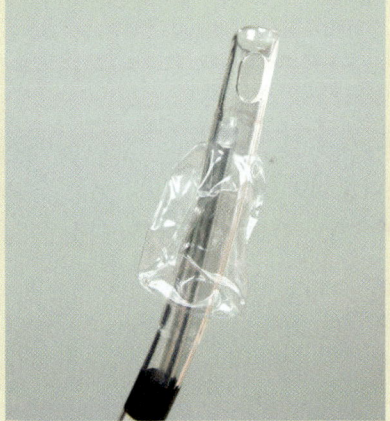

Step 3 Select the proper size ET tube. If a stylet will be used, insert it into the ET tube, making sure that the end of the stylet is recessed at least one-half inch from the tip of the ET tube. Bend the proximal end of the stylet over the ET tube to prevent it from sliding down into the tube.

Test the ET tube cuff for leaks. If there are no leaks, completely deflate the cuff. Leave the syringe filled with air attached to the inflation valve. Lubricate the distal end of the ET tube with water-soluble lubricant.

Continued

Can consider lidocaine if head trauma to decrease intracranial pressure (might ↑ 2° to vagal nerve stim) if stimulate carina, gag-like reflex

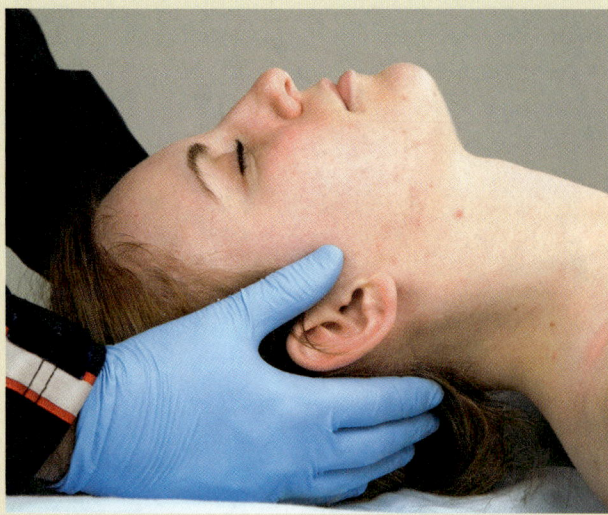

Step 4 Place the patient's head in the sniffing position to align the axes of the mouth, pharynx, and trachea. Open the patient's mouth and inspect the oral cavity. Remove dentures and/or debris, if present. Do not place the patient's head in this position if trauma is suspected. If trauma is suspected, an assistant should manually stabilize the cervical spine in a neutral position.

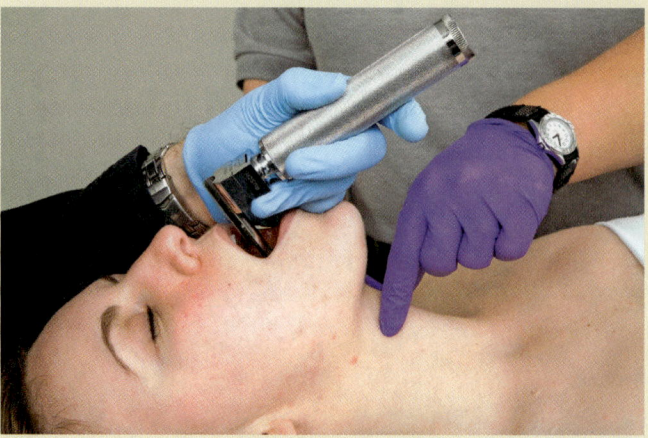

Step 5 Stop ventilations and remove the ventilation face mask and oral airway (if present). Do not exceed 30 seconds from ventilation to ventilation for each intubation attempt. Direct an assistant to apply cricoid pressure and maintain pressure until the airway is secured. If the patient begins to vomit actively, discontinue cricoid pressure until the vomiting stops and the airway has been cleared.

Holding the laryngoscope in the left hand and with the tip of the blade pointing away from you, insert the blade into the right side of the patient's mouth between the teeth, sweeping the tongue to the left. Advance the laryngoscope blade until the distal end reaches the base of the tongue.

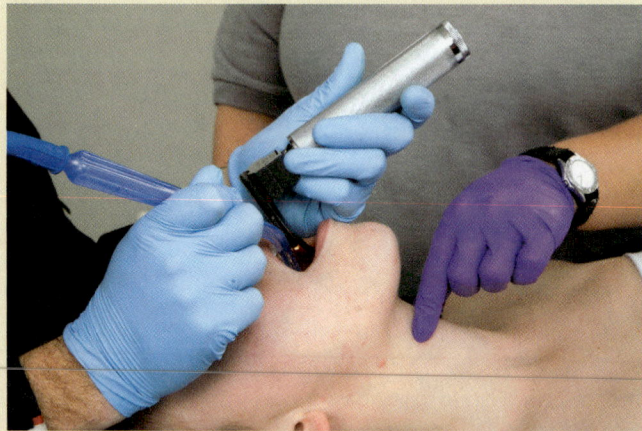

Step 6 Lift the laryngoscope to elevate the mandible without putting pressure on the front teeth and visualize the epiglottis. Do not use the patient's teeth or gums as a fulcrum. Do not allow the blade to touch the patient's teeth. Suction the airway if needed (as shown). After visualizing the epiglottis, identify the vocal cords and place the blade in the proper position. If using a curved blade, advance the tip of the blade into the vallecula. If using a straight blade, advance the tip under the epiglottis.

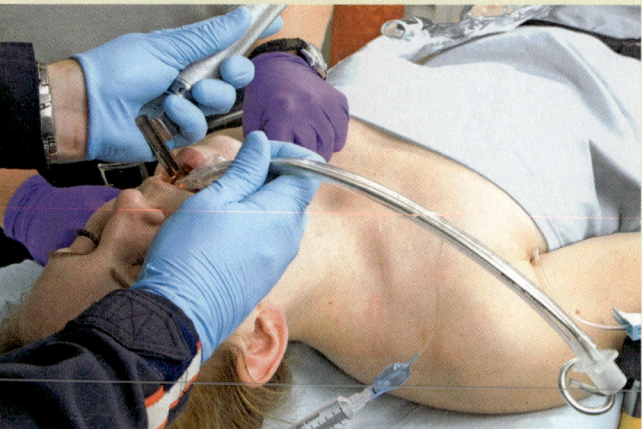

Step 7 Grasp the ET tube with your right hand and introduce it into the right corner of the patient's mouth.

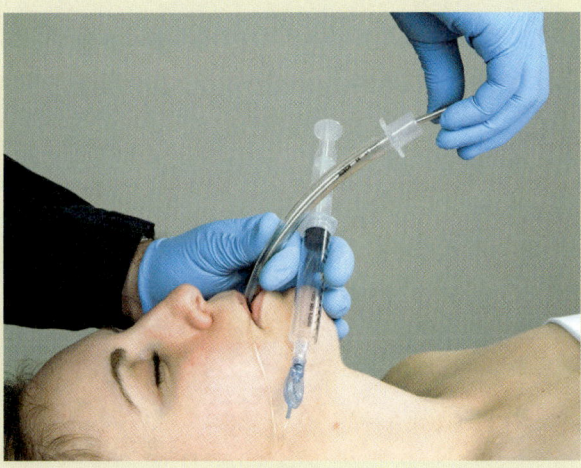

Step 8 Advance the tube through the glottic opening until the distal cuff disappears past the vocal cords. The black marker on the ET tube should be at the level of the vocal cords. Advance the ET tube until the proximal end of the cuff lies $\frac{1}{2}$ to 1 inch beyond the cords. Firmly hold the ET tube, gently withdraw the laryngoscope, and remove the stylet (if used).

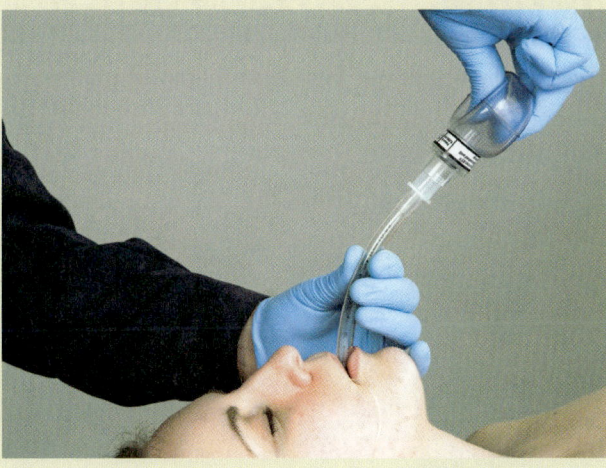

Step 9 If you are using an EDD to confirm placement of the tube, do this now. An EDD must be applied to confirm placement before distal cuff inflation.

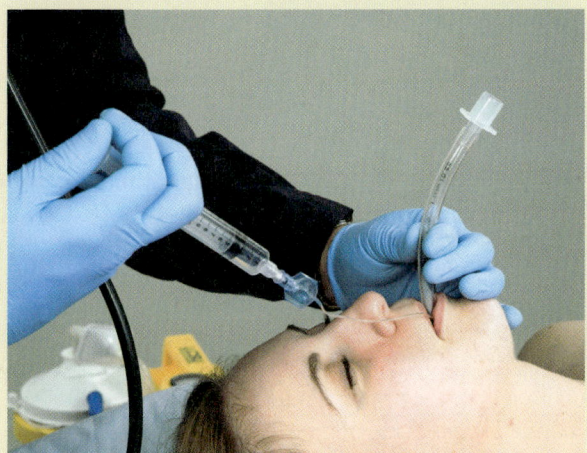

Step 10 If you are using an exhaled CO_2 detector to verify tube placement, the lungs will need to be ventilated at least six times before evaluating ET tube placement to quickly wash out any retained CO_2. While still holding the ET tube, inflate the distal cuff with approximately 6 to 10 mL of air (volume varies depending on cuff size). Disconnect the syringe from the inflation valve.

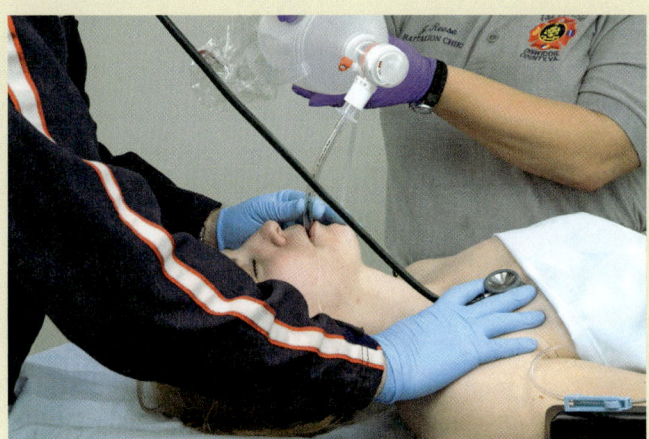

Step 11 Attach a ventilation device to the ET tube and ventilate the patient. Confirm proper placement of the tube by first auscultating over the epigastrium (should be silent) and then in the midaxillary and anterior chest line on the right and left sides of the patient's chest. Observe the patient's chest for full movement with ventilation.

Continued

Confirm
lung sounds (chest rise & fall)
② Esophageal detector
③ End tidal CO₂ (wave form tracing)
① Direct visualization
+/- fogging in tube
↑ HR, improved SPO₂

SKILL 14-10   **OROTRACHEAL INTUBATION**—continued

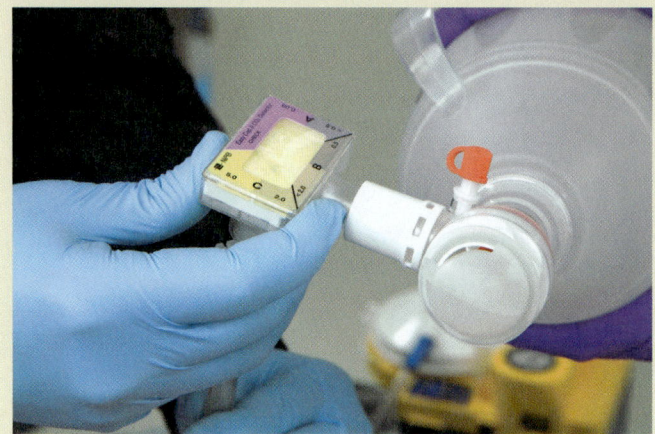

Step 12 Attach an exhaled CO_2 detector to verify tube placement.

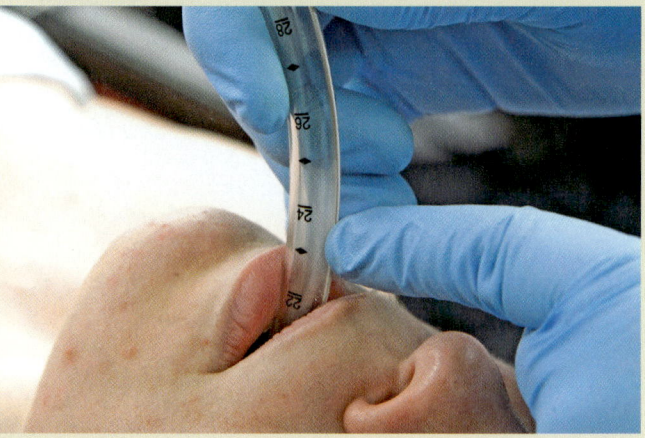

Step 13 Once placement is confirmed, note and record the depth (centimeter marking) of the tube at the patient's teeth.

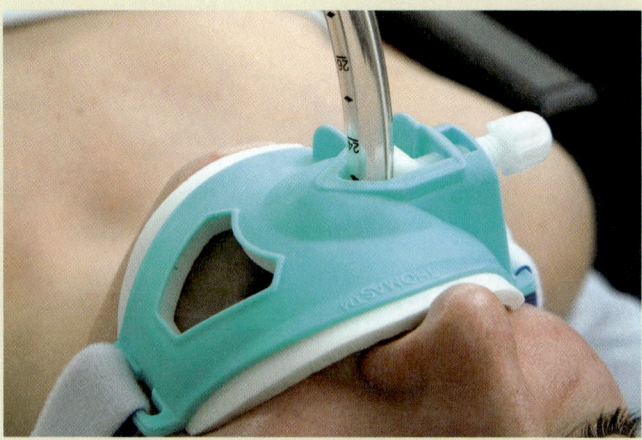

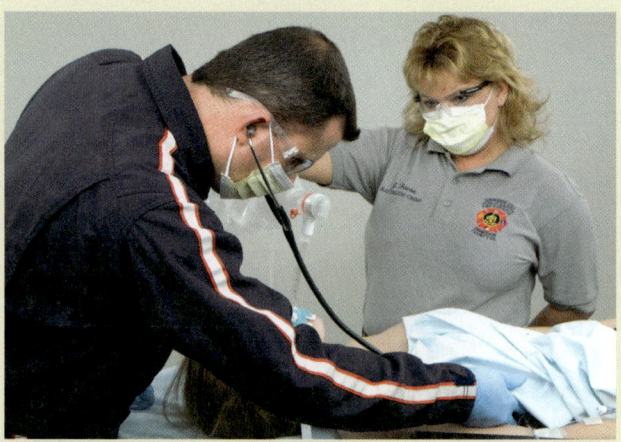

Step 14 After proper tube position is confirmed, secure it with a commercial tube holder or tape and provide ventilatory support with supplemental oxygen. Use of an exhaled CO_2 detector is recommended at this time to monitor tube placement continuously. After securing the tube, recheck (and record) the tube depth at the patient's teeth.

the patient should be preoxygenated for 30 seconds to 1 minute.

2. While your partner continues to preoxygenate the patient, assemble and prepare the equipment needed for intubation, including suction equipment. As the procedure progresses, if you see any vomit, blood, or secretions in the airway, remove them. If available, apply a pulse oximeter and attach the patient to an electrocardiographic monitor.

3. Select the proper size blade and then assemble the laryngoscope. Attach the blade to the handle and check the blade for a bright white light. After verifying that the light is in working order, move the blade to its unlocked position to conserve battery life until the light is needed.

[handwritten: Standard blade: MAC 3 or 4, Miller 5]

4. Select the proper size ET tube and test it for leaks. If there are no leaks, completely deflate the cuff. Leave the syringe filled with air attached to the inflation valve. If a stylet will be used, insert it into the ET tube, making sure that the end of the stylet is recessed at least $1/2$ inch from the tip of the ET tube. Bend the proximal end of the stylet over the ET tube to prevent it from sliding down into the tube. Lubricate the distal end of the ET tube with water-soluble lubricant. Use caution when preparing the endotracheal tube to keep it as medically clean as possible.

5. Place the patient's head in the "sniffing" position to align the axes of the mouth, pharynx, and trachea (Figure 14-42). Open the patient's mouth and inspect the oral cavity. Remove dentures and/

[handwritten: Pt. head at your xyphoid process]

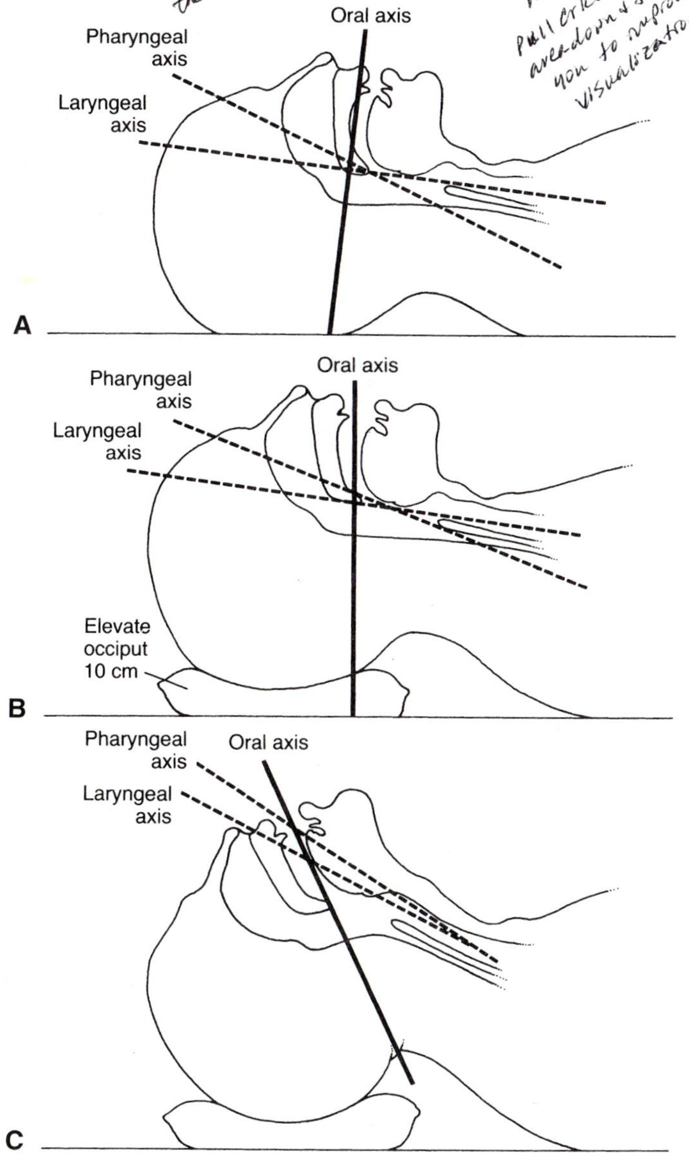

Handwritten notes (top): 3 attempts at intubation then combitube. Bimanual manipulation pull cricothyroid area down & toward you to improve visualization.

Figure 14-42 Head positioning for tracheal intubation. **A,** Neutral position. **B,** Head elevated. **C,** Sniffing position. The sniffing position aligns the axes of the mouth, pharynx, and trachea, creating the shortest distance and straightest line between the teeth and vocal cords.

between the teeth, sweeping the tongue to the left. Controlling the tongue is key to good visualization and room for passing the endotracheal tube. Advance the laryngoscope blade until the distal end reaches the base of the tongue.

9. Lift the laryngoscope to elevate the mandible without putting pressure on the front teeth and visualize the epiglottis. Do NOT use the patient's teeth or gums as a fulcrum. Do not allow the blade to touch the patient's teeth. Suction the airway if needed. *(note: keep wrist locked)*

10. After visualizing the epiglottis, identify the vocal cords and place the blade in the proper position. If using a curved blade, advance the tip of the blade into the vallecula. If using a straight blade, advance the tip under the epiglottis. Viewing the vocal cords may be aided with the use of the BURP (**b**ackward, **u**pward, **r**ightward **p**ressure) technique. With this maneuver, the larynx is displaced in three specific directions: (1) posteriorly against the cervical vertebrae, (2) superiorly as possible, and (3) slightly laterally to the right. Studies have shown that this maneuver improves visualization of the larynx more easily than does simple backpressure on the larynx (cricoid pressure) because the BURP technique moves the larynx back to the position from which it was displaced by a right-handed (held in operator's left hand) laryngoscope.

11. Grasp the ET tube with your right hand and introduce it into the right corner of the patient's mouth. Do not attempt to pass the ET tube through the channel in the laryngoscope blade. Doing so will obstruct your view of the glottic opening. Advance the tube through the glottic opening until the distal cuff disappears past the vocal cords. The black marker on the ET tube should be at the level of the vocal cords. Advance the ET tube until the proximal end of the cuff lies ½ to 1 inch beyond the cords. *(note: Black line on tube)*

12. While firmly holding the ET tube, gently withdraw the laryngoscope and remove the stylet (if used). Use care when removing the stylet so that you do not dislodge the tube from the trachea. If you are using an EDD to confirm placement of the tube, do so at this point. An EDD must be applied to confirm placement before distal cuff inflation.

13. If you are using an exhaled CO_2 detector to verify tube placement, the patient will need to be ventilated at least six times before evaluating ET tube placement to wash out any retained CO2 quickly. While still holding the ET tube, inflate the distal cuff with approximately 6 to 10 mL of air (volume varies depending on cuff size). Disconnect the syringe from the inflation valve.

14. Attach a ventilation device to the ET tube and ventilate the patient. Confirm proper placement of the tube by first auscultating over the epigastrium (should be silent) and then in the midaxillary and anterior chest line on the right and left sides of the

or debris if present. Do *not* place the patient's head in this position if trauma is suspected. If trauma is suspected, an assistant should manually stabilize the cervical spine in a neutral position.

6. Stop ventilations and remove the ventilation face mask and oral airway (if present). Do not exceed 30 seconds from ventilation to ventilation for each intubation attempt.

7. Direct an assistant to apply cricoid pressure and maintain pressure until the airway is secured. If the patient begins to vomit actively, discontinue cricoid pressure until the vomiting stops and the airway has been cleared.

8. Holding the laryngoscope in the left hand and with the tip of the blade pointing away from you, insert the blade into the right side of the patient's mouth

Type I error – thinks tube is in esophagus but actually in trachea – not fatal

Type II error – thinks tube is in trachea but actually in esophagus – fatal

patient's chest. Observe the patient's chest for full movement with ventilation. Unless you suspect underlying pathology that would suggest the presence of unequal lung sounds (such as a pneumothorax or pneumonia), sounds should be equal on both sides of the chest.

15. Attach an exhaled CO_2 detector to verify tube placement. Once placement is confirmed, note and record the depth (centimeter marking) of the tube at the patient's teeth.

16. If baseline breath sounds (i.e., breath sounds before intubation) were equal bilaterally and are absent bilaterally after intubation and gurgling is heard over the epigastrium, the ET tube is most likely in the esophagus. Deflate the ET cuff, remove the tube, and preoxygenate before reattempting intubation.

17. If baseline breath sounds were equal bilaterally, diminished breath sounds on the left side after intubation suggests that the ET tube has entered the right mainstem bronchus. Deflate the ET tube cuff, pull back the tube slightly, reinflate the cuff, and reevaluate breath sounds.

18. Secure the ET tube with a commercial tube holder, tube ties, or tape and provide ventilatory support with supplemental oxygen. After securing the tube, recheck (and record) the tube depth at the patient's teeth. Use of an exhaled CO_2 detector is recommended at this time to continually monitor tube placement. After any movement of an intubated patient, be sure to reassess that the tube has remained in proper position. Any rotation or extension of the patient's head can dislodge the tube from the trachea. Frequently monitor the patient's heart rate and oxygen saturation and reassess the patient and ET tube.

Complications

Intubation has several potential complications. Making yourself aware of the potential complications and being attentive to best practice will help you avoid them.

Used incorrectly, a laryngoscope can break teeth and cause soft tissue trauma. You must exercise care when performing ET intubation to avoid such trauma. The laryngoscope is an instrument used to help align the anatomic structures of the airway so you are able to visualize the glottic opening and pass the ET tube. It is more about finesse than brute force. To avoid using the laryngoscope as a pry bar, consider your arm a locked unit from the shoulder down to the fingertips. Your goal is to lift up and push away without bending your wrist or elbow. Flexion of these joints is what ultimately leads to prying and thus trauma. It may be helpful to think of a rope tied to the bottom of the handle that is pulling the instrument up and toward the patient's feet. Rough handling of the laryngoscope can cause severe bleeding, further compromising an airway in need of definitive management.

Manipulation of any tissue can result in swelling. Laryngeal swelling, if severe, can further obstruct airflow. For example, a patient with an inhalation burn will likely already have laryngeal edema that has led to the need for ET intubation. Be as gentle as possible when intubating to avoid laryngeal trauma and swelling. Unnecessary trauma may further compromise the airway.

Stimulation of laryngeal structures may actually induce spasm of the larynx, especially in a patient with an intact or partially intact gag reflex. Spasm of the vocal cords will make it nearly impossible to pass an ET tube into the trachea. Severe laryngospasm obstructs the airway and further compromises oxygenation. In this situation, if available and approved by your medical director, use of sedation or a neuromuscular blocker may be of benefit.

Direct manipulating the vocal cords with the tip of the laryngoscope blade or traumatically forcing a tube past the vocal cords may lead to nerve or direct cord damage. Permanent voice changes may occur as a result. Be sure that you avoid direct contact with the vocal cords while visualizing and select an appropriately sized ET tube.

Once the tube has been successfully placed in the trachea and properly positioned, the distal cuff is inflated with air to isolate the lower airway and minimize the risk of aspiration. Pressure exerted on the mucosal lining of the airway can interfere with adequate blood flow to the tissues. Without cellular oxygenation, the tissue will die. Do not overinflate the cuff. The volume of air to be used for inflation varies depending on cuff size. In most cases, 6 to 10 mL of air should be sufficient. A good rule of thumb is to inflate the cuff so that the pilot balloon is full but easily compressed between your thumb and index finger.

Once intubated, many options are available for providing artificial ventilation. Whatever device is selected, use caution to not overinflate the patient's lungs. Observe for rise and fall of the chest to know when adequate tidal volumes are being delivered. A bag-mask device is ideal because it allows the person ventilating to feel for lung compliance as the bag is squeezed. Extra care is essential when providing positive-pressure ventilation for a patient with underlying lung pathology, such as emphysema. A weakness may develop in the lung parenchyma called a *bleb*, making the patient particularly susceptible to developing a pneumothorax secondary to positive-pressure ventilation. When the integrity of the visceral pleura has been compromised, air is forced into the pleural space. Positive-pressure ventilation causes air pressure to build, resulting in the life-threatening condition known as *tension pneumothorax*. Tension pneumothorax interrupts venous return to the heart and subsequently compromises cardiac output, further worsening the patient's hypoxemia. Quick recognition and reversal of a tension pneumothorax can prove life saving. Performing needle decompression on the affected side of the chest allows for an escape of air, relieving the pressure.

Unrecognized esophageal intubation and right or left mainstem bronchus intubation are potential complica-

Pt. worsens

D displacement of tube
O obstruction of tube (mucus plug)
P pneumothorax, PE, pulselessness
E Equipment failure

http://evolve.elsevier.com/Aehlert/paramedic   531

tions you must quickly recognize. The purpose of ET intubation is direct access and complete control of the airway to the level of the trachea by the placement of the tube into the tracheal lumen. A misplaced ET tube is worse than having no tube at all, especially in the case of esophageal placement, in which no oxygenation and ventilation can take place. The key principle in regard to tube placement is immediate and continuous assessment of tube placement and the immediate recognition and correction of a misplaced or dislodged tube. Indications that the tube has been placed in the esophagus include the following:

- An absence of chest rise and fall as well as absence of lung sounds during artificial ventilation
- Expansion of the abdomen or presence of gurgling air sounds over the epigastrium on ventilation; over time the abdomen becomes distended
- Worsening respiratory assessment findings, including persistent cyanosis and oxygen desaturation
- A patient who is able to vocalize with the tube in place (the patient should not be able to talk or vocalize sounds with the tube between the vocal cords)
- Presence of vomitus in the ET tube
- Bradycardia

Multiple devices are available for the sole purpose of helping confirm correct tube placement. As previously discussed, you must use at least two means to confirm placement. Auscultation of epigastric and bilateral lung sounds is essential. Also available are EDDs and ETCO$_2$ detection devices. If any question exists regarding whether a tube is in the trachea, remove it immediately, then oxygenate and ventilate the patient with a bag-mask device.

Endobronchial intubation occurs when passing an ET tube too deep into the airway. The most common complication of misplacement occurs when the tube is inserted too far and ends up in the right mainstem bronchus. The tube most commonly enters the right mainstem bronchus because it generally bifurcates at a more oblique angle from the trachea than does the left mainstem bronchus. The primary concern with endobronchial tube placement is that only one side of the pulmonary tree is being ventilated, with resulting hypoxia from inadequate gas exchange on the opposite lung. When confirming placement of an ET tube, hearing lung sounds on only one side may indicate endobronchial placement. When passing the tube, visualize it as you insert it through the vocal cords. The cuff should be 1 to 2 cm beyond the level of the vocal cords. Your goal is that the tip of the ET tube comes to lie a few centimeters above the level of the carina. If you recognize that the tube has come to lie in either the right or left mainstem bronchus, deflate the cuff and slowly withdraw the tube a few centimeters. Reinflate the cuff and reassess the tube for proper placement. Be certain to secure the tube

| BOX 14-19 | ET Intubation: Possible Complications |

- Bleeding
- Laryngospasm
- Vocal cord damage
- Mucosal necrosis
- Barotrauma
- Aspiration
- Cuff leak
- Esophageal intubation
- Right mainstem intubation
- Tube occlusion caused by patient biting the tube or secretions
- Laryngeal or tracheal edema
- Hypoxia from prolonged or unsuccessful intubation
- Dysrhythmias
- Trauma to the lips, teeth, tongue, or soft tissues of the oropharynx
- Increased intracranial pressure

in position adequately so that it does not migrate into or out of the airway.

As an EMS professional, one of your responsibilities includes maintaining functional equipment in preparation for the next call. A laryngoscope is useless without a bright light source, which depends on a power and light source. You should have spare batteries and assorted blades in case you encounter such a failure. Check all your equipment as you prepare to intubate, including the integrity of the ET tube cuff. Possible complications of ET intubation are summarized in Box 14-19.

PARAMEDIC*Pearl*

Failure to recognize a tube that has been misplaced or dislodged from the trachea into the esophagus is an inexcusable fatal error. You only need to use the appropriate clinical skills and adjuncts available to you to confirm, without any doubt, the correct placement of an ET tube.

Special Considerations
Pediatric Intubation
[OBJECTIVE 64]

For prehospital professionals with short transport times, current resuscitation guidelines recommend oxygenation and ventilation of infants and children with a bag-mask device instead of ET intubation because of the high incidence of misplaced and dislodged ET tubes. For situations in which pediatric intubation is warranted, and because the anatomic sizes of pediatric patients varies from neonates to near adult-size adolescents, additional knowledge, understanding, and clinical skill are required to intubate an infant or child and properly manage a pediatric patient who has an ET tube in place (Skill 14-11).

SKILL 14-11 PEDIATRIC (YOUNGER THAN 2 YEARS) VENTILATORY MANAGEMENT

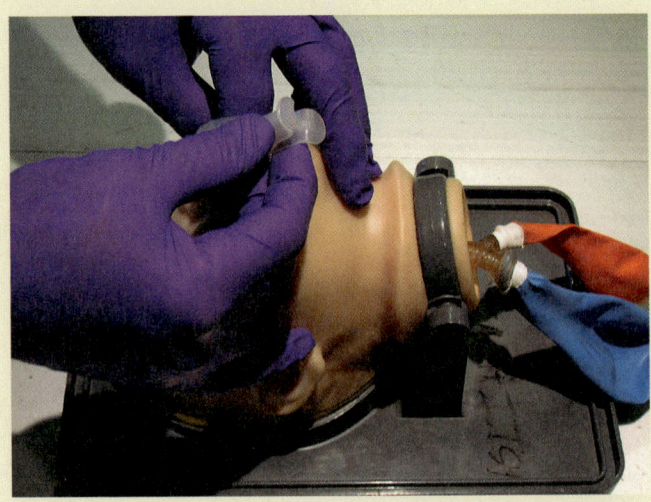

Step 1 Using standard precautions, open the airway and insert an oropharyngeal airway.

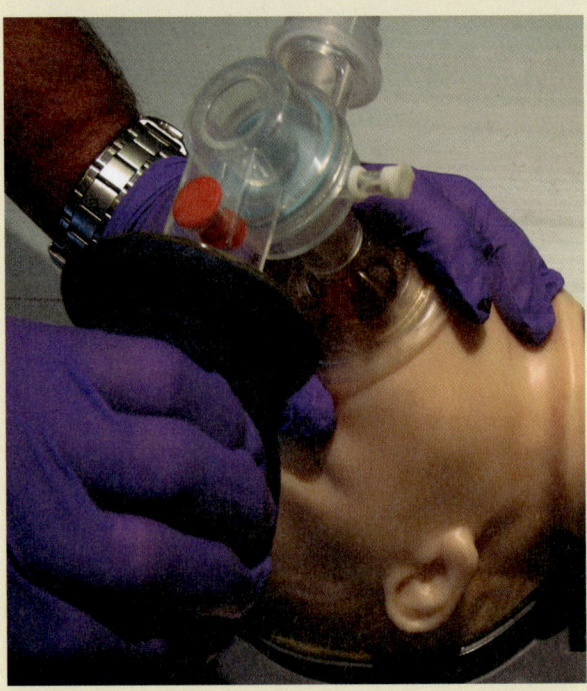

Step 2 Immediately ventilate the lungs 12 to 20 times per minute using a bag-mask device. If oxygen is not readily available, attach an oxygen reservoir connected to high-flow oxygen as soon as it is available.

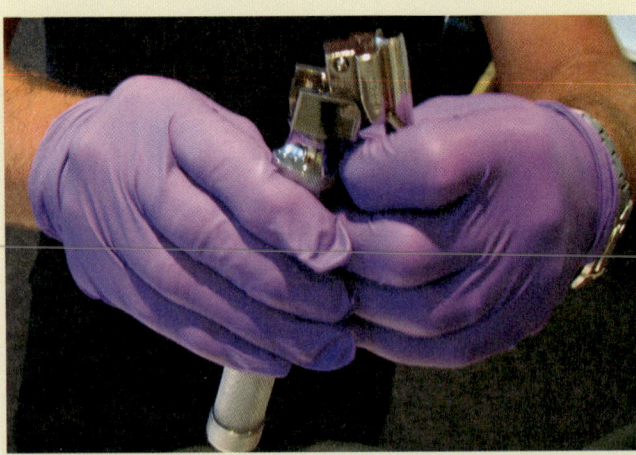

Step 3 Preoxygenate the patient.
Step 4 Prepare proper equipment for intubation.

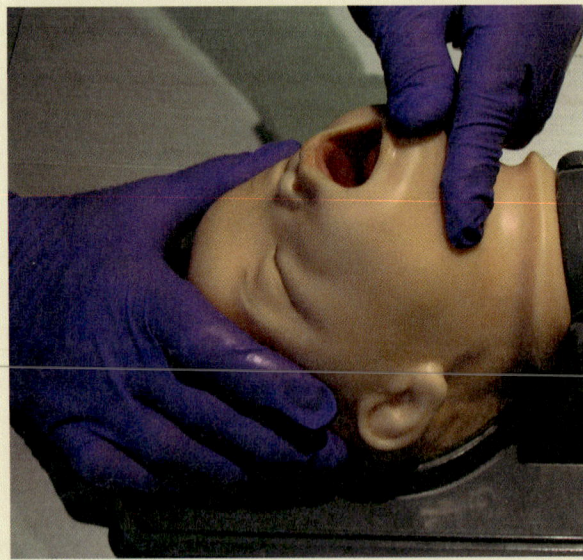

Step 5 Place patient in neutral or sniffing position.

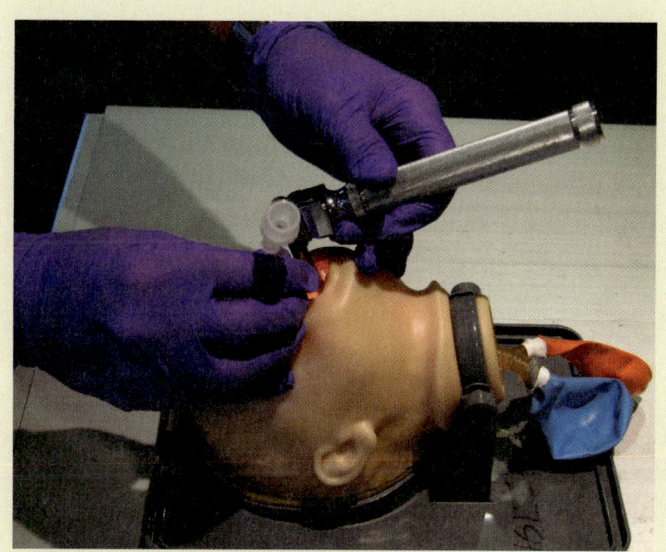

Step 6 Insert the laryngoscope blade while displacing the patient's tongue.

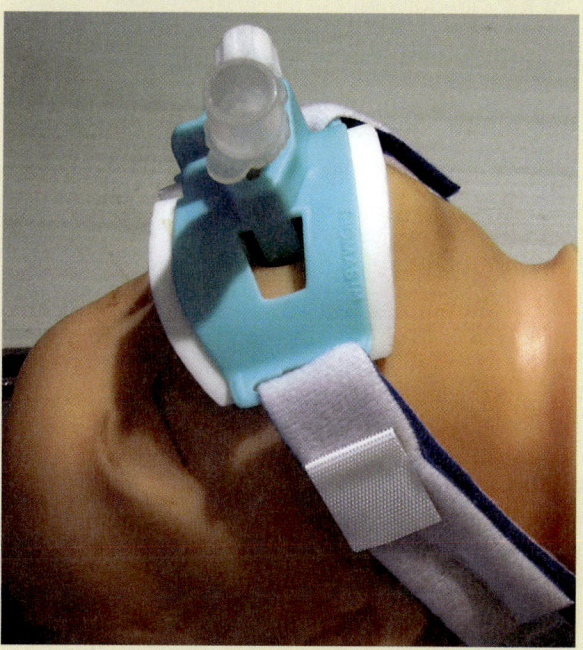

Step 7 Insert the endotracheal tube to the appropriate depth. Ventilate the patient's lungs and confirm proper tube placement by auscultating bilaterally over the lungs and epigastrium. After proper tube position is confirmed, secure the tube and provide ventilatory support with supplemental oxygen.

pinky finger – approx. diameter

The same general technique and equipment are used as for adults but with less force and with proportionately smaller equipment. A discussion of the differences in technique follows.   *100602 x 1 mm*

✱ Preoxygenation before intubation is critical in all patients and particularly important in children because they have less oxygen reserve in their lungs and their metabolic oxygen consumption is proportionately greater than in adults. When intubating a child younger than 8 years, a straight blade is recommended. The straight blade is preferred because it provides greater movement of the large tongue into the floor of the mouth and visualization of the glottic opening. A curved blade may not adequately control and retract a child's longer, more pliable epiglottis to permit a clear view of the glottic opening (Foltin et al. 2002).

As previously mentioned, cuffed tracheal tubes generally are unnecessary in children younger than 8 years because the narrowing of the cricoid cartilage serves as a natural cuff. However, balloon cuffs are available for younger children who require high-pressure ventilation. Some leakage of air is expected with uncuffed ET tubes in children when inspiratory pressures reach 20 to 30 cm H_2O.

Selecting the proper tube size for a pediatric patient is important. When possible, a length-based resuscitation tape should be used to determine the correct ET tube size for children who weigh up to approximately 35 kg. Several formulas may be used to approximate tube size. The following formulas may be used for children 1 to 10 years of age:

✱ $$\frac{16 + \text{Age (years)}}{4} = \begin{array}{l}\textit{Uncuffed} \text{ ET tube size} \\ \text{(internal diameter [mm])}\end{array}$$

$$\frac{\text{Age (years)}}{4} + 4 = \begin{array}{l}\textit{Uncuffed} \text{ ET tube size} \\ \text{(internal diameter [mm])}\end{array}$$

$$\frac{\text{Age (years)}}{4} + 3 = \begin{array}{l}\textit{Cuffed} \text{ ET tube size} \\ \text{(internal diameter [mm])}\end{array}$$

As with adults, several sizes of tubes should be on hand. At a minimum, have available an ET tube that is 0.5 mm smaller and 0.5 mm larger than the estimated tube size.

Remember that the pediatric trachea is shorter than that of an adult. Failure to approximate the proper depth of tracheal tube insertion may result in hypoxia, perforation, or endobronchial intubation. An ET tube is gener-

BOX 14-20 Nasotracheal Intubation

Indications
- Breathing patient who requires intubation
- Suspected spinal injury
- Inability to access the mouth (e.g., clenched teeth, jaw wired closed)
- Severe jaw or oral trauma
- Glasgow Coma Scale score less than 8 because of trauma or medical condition
- Inhalation injury
- Patients with short, fat necks or other anatomic characteristics making oral intubation difficult or impossible

Contraindications
- Apneic patient
- Untrained in nasotracheal intubation
- Patient age younger than 10 years
- Severe nasal or mid-face congenital or traumatic deformity
- Nasal airway obstruction
- Known or suspected basilar skull fracture (raccoon eyes, Battle's sign, or CSF leakage from nose or ears) (relative contraindication)
- Patients who have hemophilia, liver disease, or are on anticoagulant therapy (increased risk of uncontrolled epistaxis) (relative contraindication)
- Acute hypertension (relative contraindication)
- Suspected increased intracranial pressure (relative contraindication)

Advantages
- Use of a laryngoscope is not required
- Neutral inline neck position can be maintained
- Securing the tube once placed is more easily accomplished
- Patients are not able to bite and compromise tube integrity

Disadvantages
- Procedural limitations, including blind technique and the requirement that the patient be breathing
- Generally a more difficult skill than oral intubation; can be much more time consuming and require a great deal of patience
- Trauma leading to bleeding that is often difficult to control, further compromising the airway
- Introduction of nasal bacteria into the lower airway, increasing the risk of infection
- Increased likelihood of improper placement

Complications
- Bleeding (common)
- Nasal fracture
- Vomiting or aspiration
- Possible intracranial tube placement

CSF, Cerebrospinal fluid.

ally placed to a depth determined with a vocal cord mark on the tube. Alternatively, the proper depth of ET tube insertion (in centimeters at the teeth or lips) is approximately three times the tracheal tube size. This formula assumes that the proper size ET tube is selected. The following formula may also be used to determine proper depth of insertion (from the distal end of the tube to the alveolar ridge of the teeth) for children older than 2 years: (Age in years/2) + 12.

Unfortunately there are no formulas for selecting the appropriately sized laryngoscope blade for a child. The following list contains average sizes based on age. However, these are guidelines and the paramedic should determine the appropriate size for each individual patient.

- Newborn <2 kg—0 Miller
- Newborn >2 kg—1 Miller
- 6 months to 2 years—1 to 2 Miller
- 2 to 8 years—2 Miller
- 8 to 12 years—2 Miller or 2 Macintosh
- >12 years—3 Miller or 3 Macintosh

When confirming ET tube placement, look for bilateral chest movement and confirm the absence of sounds over the epigastrium during positive-pressure ventilation. Listen for lung sounds in the second or third intercostal space in the anterior axillary line. Listen for two breaths on the right side of the chest, then listen to the left side and compare. Check for exhaled CO_2 if a perfusing rhythm is present. If the child has a perfusing rhythm and weighs 20 kg or more, an EDD may be used to check for evidence of esophageal placement. Check oxygen saturation with a pulse oximeter.

Nasotracheal Intubation
[OBJECTIVE 65]

[handwritten: Not done anymore. Done before paralytics]

Nasotracheal intubation is an alternative approach for intubating the trachea. The procedure is performed with the same initial preparatory steps as for orotracheal intubation, but the laryngoscope is not used and the use of a stylet is contraindicated. Nasotracheal intubation is considered a blind procedure because the vocal cords are not visualized. The ET tube is inserted into a nostril and gently passed in an effort to introduce the tube into the trachea. This procedure requires a breathing patient. Alternative approaches, such as the use of rapid-sequence intubation, have made nasotracheal intubation less common. Indications, contraindications, advantages, disadvantages, and complications of nasotracheal intubation are listed in Box 14-20.

Nasotracheal intubation is often a time-consuming procedure when carried out in the best of clinical circumstances. The steps for nasotracheal intubation are as follows:

1. Using personal protective equipment (at a minimum, use gloves, protective eyewear, and a mask), prepare the patient for the procedure. The patient may be positioned supine or even

sitting upright. If spinal injury is suspected, use caution and maintain inline stabilization. Ask an assistant to preoxygenate the patient while you auscultate bilateral lung sounds to establish a baseline. Ideally, the patient should be preoxygenated for 30 seconds to 1 minute.

2. While your assistant continues to preoxygenate the patient, assemble and prepare the equipment needed for intubation, including suction equipment. The laryngoscope and stylet are not needed, though you should have them standing by in case your patient's condition changes, necessitating the oral approach (unless contraindicated). If available, apply a pulse oximeter and attach the patient to an electrocardiographic monitor. Prepare the tube by wrapping it into a circular shape for approximately 1 minute. Lubricate the distal tip of the tube with lidocaine jelly (if approved by medical direction). Whistle devices (such as the Beck Airway Flow Monitor) are available for placement on the proximal end of the tube to signal the distal tube's approach to the larynx during insertion. If such a device is available, attach it to the proximal end of the tube at this time.

3. Select the patient's nostril that appears larger for insertion. Because the ET tube will need to pass easily through the nasopharynx, a tube $\frac{1}{2}$ to 1 size smaller than that used for oral insertion often is necessary.

4. If approved by local medical direction, you may be able to apply a topical anesthetic to the patient's nasal and oral mucosa. An over-the-counter nasal spray, such as phenylephrine, is also helpful because it constricts blood vessels in the nasal mucosa, minimizing potential bleeding.

5. Once you are prepared, ask your assistant to remove any airway adjuncts in place. Be sure to have suction ready in case the patient vomits.

6. Insertion of the tube is accomplished by directing it straight back and down along the nasal floor with the bevel toward the septum. Do not angle the tip of the tube upward toward the skull or downward. If you meet slight resistance, use a slight back-and-forth rotation of the tube to advance it. If you meet significant resistance, remove the tube and attempt insertion in the opposite nostril. Do not force passage of the tube.

7. As the tip of the tube advances past the nasopharynx and turns toward the larynx, begin listening closely to the proximal tip for sounds of airflow. The closer the tip of the tube is to the larynx, the more pronounced airflow becomes.

8. If the patient is unresponsive, gently advance the tube during inhalation. If the patient is responsive, ask the patient to take a deep breath, then gently advance the tube during inhalation. As you get close to the glottic opening and during passage of the tube past the vocal cords, you may notice the patient coughing or gagging. You *must* assess proper placement of the tube in the trachea and ensure that it is not in the esophagus.

9. Holding the tube securely in place, use the same procedures for confirming placement as outlined for orotracheal intubation. If using an EDD, do not yet inflate the distal ET tube cuff. The cuff should be inflated before all other confirmation methods. Indications of proper tube placement include the following:
   - The patient begins coughing.
   - A responsive patient is unable to speak.
   - Lung sounds are present bilaterally on auscultation.
   - Chest rises and falls with positive-pressure ventilation.
   - An exhaled CO_2 detector confirms the presence of CO_2.

10. While continuing to hold the tube in place, inflate the cuff with 6 to 10 mL of air if not already done. Be sure to remove the syringe after inflation or the cuff will deflate.

11. If tube placement has been confirmed, secure the tube in place. Remove the Beck Airway Flow Monitor (if used). Begin positive-pressure ventilation. Exhaled CO_2 monitoring is recommended to evaluate tube placement continuously. Frequently monitor and reassess the patient and the ET tube.

Digital Intubation
[OBJECTIVE 66]
Digital intubation is another blind approach for tracheal tube insertion in which you use your index and middle fingers as a manual guide for placement of the ET tube. Safety requires that the patient be deeply comatose or in cardiac arrest. Even a semiresponsive patient may be stimulated to bite down, and severe injury may result. Use of digital intubation is reserved for situations involving confined spaces when access to the patient for direct visualization is simply not possible or during other circumstances that prevent you from being able to carry out direct visualization.

The steps to prepare the patient for a digital intubation are similar to other intubation methods. However, one important difference is that before the intubation attempt is made, a bite block should be placed between the patient's molars to prevent trauma to your fingers if the patient bites down. Remember that the jaw muscles are the strongest in the body. An oral airway held in place by an assistant, a roll of gauze, or folded 4 × 4 gauze pads make adequate bite blocks.

When inserting your index and middle fingers into the oral cavity, gently "walk them down" the patient's tongue until you feel the epiglottis. Once the patient's epiglottis is located, it can be gently lifted with your middle finger so that the glottic opening becomes accessible to the tube. Using your other hand, pass the tube gently down into the oral cavity with a stylet in place within the tube and the tube curved in a more exaggerated shape of a J. Direct the tube between your index and middle finger and then gently guide the tube with your index finger into the trachea.

Transillumination Technique. Another method of intubation that does not involve direct visualization of the vocal cords is called the *transillumination technique*, or the *lighted stylet technique*. Transillumination is based on the principle of using a very bright light that will be visible through the soft tissues of the neck when placed in the trachea. Transillumination intubation is clearly difficult to perform in brightly lit environments because the light will not be perceptible through the tissues of the neck. A lighted stylet is a flexible piece of plastic-coated wire that can be form shaped attached to a handle containing batteries. Some devices have a sliding locking mechanism that holds the tube firmly in place. As with other stylets, it is inserted into the lumen of an ET tube.

Similar to digital intubation, use your index and middle finger to "walk down" the base of the tongue and locate the epiglottis. Lift the epiglottis and insert the lighted stylet with ET tube attached and light turned on. As the lighted stylet is advanced, observe for the light source emitting through the soft tissues of the patient's anterior neck. Visualization of the bright light underlying the patient's Adam's apple indicates correct placement. Detach the tube from the securing mechanism and remove the stylet while holding the tube in place. A dim, difficult to see, or absent light indicates esophageal placement. Limit your intubation attempt to no more than 30 seconds. Once in place, confirm placement and secure in place. If unsuccessful, remove the lighted stylet and ventilate the patient with a bag-mask device attached to 100% oxygen.

Gum Elastic Bougie. The gum elastic bougie, or bougie, is an adjunct to intubation that is particularly useful in difficult intubations, or patients with anterior airways. The bougie is typically a 60 to 70-cm long flexible plastic shaft with a stiff distal end that is angled upward 30 to 35 degrees. Although it is usually used when only the epiglottis or arytenoid cartilages can be seen, it can be used in any difficult intubation. Direct laryngoscopy is performed as described earlier; however, instead of introducing an endotracheal tube into the trachea the bougie is introduced. The angled distal end assists in placement when only the epiglottis is seen. In this instance the bougie is passed under the epiglottis with an upward angle. The paramedic should feel a series of vibrations, or "clicks" as the distal end of the bougie encounters the tracheal cartilages which indicates endotracheal placement. With the bougie held firmly in place an endotracheal tube is passed over the device and into the trachea. Although the vibrations of the bougie against the tracheal cartilages indicate correct placement, the placement of the endotracheal tube must be confirmed using the techniques described earlier.

Rapid-Sequence Intubation
[OBJECTIVES 67, 68, 69, 70]

As a paramedic, your scope of practice includes the capability of inducing sedation and neuroblockade in responsive patients for making ET intubation easier, or in some cases, possible. This is a critical procedure in which errors and complications are likely to result in a negative outcome or death. Hence, you must be current in your knowledge of this procedure and remain skill proficient to perform this procedure safely. For the purpose of this chapter, all forms of "drug-assisted" sedation or paralysis intubation are called *rapid-sequence intubation*.

Rapid-sequence intubation (RSI) is the use of medications to sedate and paralyze a patient to achieve ET intubation rapidly. In addition to sedatives and paralytics, other medications may be used to minimize or prevent the physiologic responses of intubation such as the cough reflex, gag reflex, cardiac dysrhythmias, increased intracranial pressure, pain, hypoxia, hypertension, and increased ocular pressure.

Patients who require RSI are likely to die or deteriorate inevitably and rapidly without oxygenation and ventilatory support by an ET tube but who also are either conscious or seizing, making intubation highly unlikely or impossible to perform without sedation or paralysis. Possible indications for RSI are shown in Box 14-21.

The steps involved in the RSI procedure can be remembered by the memory aid of the "7 P's of RSI" (Box 14-22). A discussion of each of these steps follows. Possible complications of RSI are shown in Box 14-23.

BOX 14-21 Possible Indications for RSI

- Excessive work of breathing, which may lead to fatigue and respiratory failure
- Combative patients requiring airway control
- Uncontrolled seizure activity (to provide airway control)
- Functional or anatomic airway obstruction
- Head trauma and Glasgow Coma Scale score less than 8
- Severe asthma
- Inadequate central nervous system control of ventilation

BOX 14-22 The 7 P's of RSI

Preparation (zero – 10 minutes)
Preoxygenate (zero – 5 minutes)
Premedicate (zero – 3 minutes)
Paralysis with sedation (zero)
Protect the airway (zero + 15 seconds)
Pass the tube and proof of placement (zero + 45 seconds)
Postintubation management (zero + 60 seconds)

*P*reparation (zero – 10 minutes). Obtain a SAMPLE medical history and perform a focused physical examination. Assess the patient for a possible or likely difficult airway because of the patient's facial and neck anatomy. In particular, patients with oversized heads, short necks, and small chins may be difficult to intubate. There are assessment tools to assist the paramedic in determining if an airway will be difficult. First, look for external indications that the intubation will be difficult. Second, evaluate the ability of the patient to open his or her mouth. The paramedic should be able to fit three fingers between the patient's upper and lower central incisors. You should also be able to fit three fingers between the tip of the chin and the hyoid bone, and two fingers between the bottom of the jaw and the thyroid cartilage. Third, evaluate the Mallampati scale. This is shown in Figure 14-43. Patients who are class 1 or class 2 are candidates for RSI. Alternative methods of airway management should be considered for class 3 and class 4 patients. Fourth, assess for possible airway obstructions. Finally evaluate the mobility of the neck as manipulation (in the nontrauma patient) can make visualization of the vocal cords easier. RSI does not make it considerably easier to perform an intubation on a patient that is anatomically extremely difficult to intubate. Thus remember to always have a fallback plan and equipment ready. Assemble all necessary intubation equipment and ensure that it is in working order (Figure 14-44). Equipment and supplies should include oxygen, a bag-mask device, suction equipment, a laryngoscope with various blade sizes, stylet, an ET tube of appropriate size for the patient plus tubes 0.5 mm larger and smaller, tape or a commercial tube holder, oral and nasal airways, nasogastric tube, and Magill forceps. Alternative airways should be readily available to assist in the management of a difficult airway such as laryngeal mask airways, needle cricothyrotomy equipment, and surgical cricothyrotomy equipment. However, rarely is a cricothyrotomy indicated in the setting of a failed RSI attempt. The use of an alternative airway device should be the first attempt if RSI is unsuccessful. At this time, apply the cardiac monitor and pulse oximeter. If cervical spine injury is suspected, assign an assistant to stabilize the neck manually in a neutral position. Be sure to monitor and document the patient's heart rate, ECG rhythm, blood pressure, and pulse oximeter readings throughout the procedure. Establish an intravenous line. Assemble and draw all medications that will be used during the procedure.

*P*reoxygenate (zero – 5 minutes) with 100% oxygen. The goal of this step is both hyperoxygenation and the washout of nitrogen from the lungs. More often than not a nonrebreather mask is effective in doing this. Be cautious with the use of a bag-mask as this will result in gastric distension. Pressurizing the stomach with subsequent paralysis can lead to

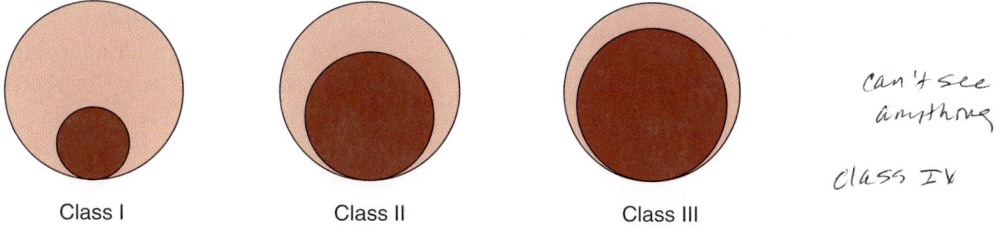

Class I Class II Class III

Can't see anything

Class IV

Figure 14-43 The conceptual basis of the Mallampati Airway Classification is determining the size of the tongue (darker area) relative to the size of the pharyngeal cavity.

BOX 14-23	RSI: Complications

- Prolonged apnea
- Bradycardia
- Fasciculations (muscle twitches)
- Death from anoxia in a patient who cannot be intubated or ventilated
- Hypotension (as a result of sedative administration)
- Hyperkalemia (adverse effect associated with succinylcholine)
- Increased intragastric pressure
- Malignant hyperthermia

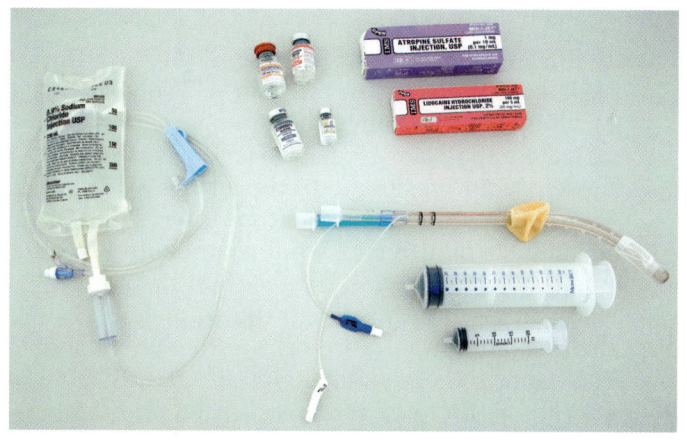

Figure 14-44 Items needed for RSI.

gastric contents spilling into the oral cavity during the intubation attempt.

Premedicate (zero – 3 minutes). The initial medications administered during RSI are used to minimize the physiologic responses sometimes associated with intubation. These medications are referred to *adjunctive medications* or *adjunctive agents*. For example, atropine is given to decrease airway secretions and minimize the bradycardia that may result from vagal stimulation during intubation. For maximal effect at the time of intubation, atropine should be given at least 1 to 2 minutes before the procedure. Alternately, glycopyrrolate (Robinul) may be preferred by your medical director. Like atropine, glycopyrrolate is an anticholinergic used for the same indications as atropine. Lidocaine is given in situations involving a head injury or increased intracranial pressure. It diminishes the cough and gag reflexes and may diminish the rise in intracranial pressure associated with intubation. If indicated, give lidocaine 2 to 5 minutes before the RSI procedure.

Paralysis with sedation (zero). Agents used for sedation (also called *induction*) during RSI vary by EMS system and include barbiturates, benzodiazepines, opiates, nonbarbiturate sedatives, and dissociative agents. Common RSI induction agents include etomidate, thiopental, ketamine, midazolam, diazepam, and lorazepam. The sedative selected should last as long as or longer than the paralytic agent to be administered, or be prepared to administer additional sedation. Administer the sedative *before* the paralytic agent and ensure it has taken effect before administering the paralytic. It is imperative the paramedic understands the time of onset of the sedative agent used. If the patient is not fully sedated when the paralytic is administered the possibility exists of the patient being paralyzed, yet fully conscious and alert, but unable to move or respond. Then administer a paralytic agent. **Once a paralytic has been administered, you assume complete responsibility for maintaining an adequate airway and ventilation.** Examples of medications used during RSI are shown in Table 14-6.

Protect the airway (zero + 15 seconds). To reduce the risk of aspiration, ask an assistant to apply cricoid pressure when the patient becomes unresponsive and before the paralytic has taken effect. Do not release cricoid pressure until the airway is protected. Position the patient for intubation. Open the patient's mouth and, while maintaining direct visualization, insert the ET tube from the right corner of the mouth through the vocal cords.

Pass the tube and prove placement (zero + 45 seconds). Relaxation of the mandible indicates that the patient is ready to be intubated. Insert an ET tube of appropriate size to an appropriate depth. Confirm tube placement. If the ET tube is in the

TABLE 14-6	Medications Used during RSI	
	Onset	**Duration**
Adjunctive Medications		
Atropine	2 to 3 minutes	>30 minutes
Glycopyrrolate	60 seconds	>30 minutes
Lidocaine	2 to 5 minutes	>30 minutes
Sedatives		
Etomidate	30 to 45 seconds	10 to 20 minutes
Fentanyl	Almost immediate	30 to 90 minutes
Ketamine	30 to 60 seconds	5 to 20 minutes
Midazolam	2 to 3 minutes	20 to 30 minutes
Propofol	10 to 30 seconds	3 to 5 minutes
Thiopental	10 to 40 seconds	10 to 20 minutes
Paralytics		
Pancuronium	1 to 2 minutes	45 to 90 minutes
Rocuronium	30 to 60 seconds	30 to 60 minutes
Succinylcholine	30 to 60 seconds	3 to 12 minutes
Vecuronium	1 to 2 minutes	30 to 90 minutes

proper position, release cricoid pressure. If intubation is unsuccessful, maintain cricoid pressure and ventilate the patient with a bag-mask device. After the patient is reoxygenated, either attempt another intubation or use an alternative airway technique.

Postintubation management (zero + 60 seconds). Verify that the ET tube is positioned at the correct depth. Secure the tube in place with tape or a commercial tube holder. Begin positive-pressure ventilation. Reassess the patient's vital signs, including pulse oximetry and ET CO_2 readings. During long transports the administration of additional sedative medications may be necessary. It is crucial that the paramedic be aware of the duration of action of the sedatives administered to ensure the effects of sedation do not wear off before the effects of paralysis. Indications that the sedative agent is no longer effective are subtle and may be limited to an increase in the heart rate and blood pressure. If the paramedic were to wait to re-medicate the patient until the return of motor function, such as intrinsic respirations or biting of the endotracheal tube, there could easily have been a period in which the patient was conscious, alert, and sensing pain.

PARAMEDIC*Pearl*

Paralysis without sedation has been described as comparable to being buried alive. The patient should *never* be awake while paralyzed.

Case Scenario CONCLUSION

As you have experienced more difficulty in ventilating this patient's lungs, you also assess that she does not have jugular venous distention and her blood pressure is consistent at 115/70 mm Hg. Her breath sounds are equal bilaterally, but have become quieter. As you transfer the patient to the ED physician, she has become significantly more difficult to ventilate, and her oxygen saturation has dropped to 87%. Following a chest radiograph to rule out pneumothorax or tension pneumothorax, the ED physician removes the ET tube and finds that there is a partial obstruction of the distal end of the ET tube because of a tooth. Following reintubation the patient is again easy to ventilate and her saturation returns to normal.

Looking back

1. What is the clinical significance of the absence of jugular venous distention or hypotension? What about the bilaterally equal, quiet breath sounds? How does this information impact your further treatment plan?
2. If the patient's drop in saturation had occurred in the ambulance while still en route, what would you have done? Why?
3. What is the procedure for removing and replacing an ET tube in the field?

CRICOTHYROTOMY

Cricothyrotomy is an emergency procedure performed to allow rapid entrance to the airway (by the cricothyroid membrane) for temporary oxygenation and ventilation. It can be effectively accomplished in one of two ways: inserting a needle or commercial device into the cricothyroid membrane (needle cricothyrotomy) or creating an opening into the cricothyroid membrane with a scalpel (surgical cricothyrotomy). Your ability to locate anatomic landmarks on the neck is critical to the success of both procedures. In both cases, you are required to identify the thyroid cartilage and cricothyroid cartilage. Between these structures lies the cricothyroid membrane, the point of insertion for the needle or location for surgical opening with a scalpel. This membrane is approximately 10 mm high, 22 mm wide, and lies approximately 1 cm below the vocal cords. Therefore correct identification of the membrane is crucial to avoid damage to other vital structures. Review and study the topographic landmarks that identify these structures and practice locating them on real people. The thyroid cartilage, or Adam's apple, is usually more prominent in men than women. The solid ring of cartilage directly inferior to it is the cricoid cartilage. Between them is the cricothyroid membrane.

Great skill and knowledge, coupled with continual medical oversight from your medical director, are necessary if you are handed the tools to perform these procedures. Although lifesaving procedures, they can also result in disaster with even the slightest error in judgment. Cricothyrotomy is considered a last resort procedure to be used only when all other alternatives such as head positioning, suctioning, foreign body airway maneuvers, bag-mask ventilation, and endotracheal intubation fail to establish or maintain an open airway. Needle and surgical cricothyrotomy require frequent refresher training to maintain skill proficiency.

Although the specific indications for cricothyrotomy are determined by your medical director, common indications for consideration of performing either technique include the following:

- Conditions in which intubation is difficult or impossible
- Complete upper airway obstruction (Examples may include epiglottitis, acute anaphylaxis, or severe inhalation injury from burns)
- Laryngeal fracture
- Craniofacial abnormalities
- Congenital laryngeal anomalies
- Excessive oropharyngeal hemorrhage
- Massive traumatic or congenital deformities
- Respiratory arrest or near arrest in patients who cannot be tracheally intubated
- Cervical spine fracture with respiratory compromise in patients who cannot be tracheally intubated
- Delayed or inability to ventilate the patient by any other means
- Inability to access the patient's mouth because of clenched teeth or a mass, such as a tumor

Contraindications to performing either technique include:

- Ability to ventilate the patient by less aggressive means
- Inability to identify landmarks
- Primary laryngeal injury
- Infralaryngeal obstruction

Needle Cricothyrotomy

[OBJECTIVE 71]

Needle cricothyrotomy (also called *percutaneous cricothyrotomy, translaryngeal cricothyrotomy,* and *transtracheal cricothyrotomy*) is a method of providing ventilation by insertion of a large-bore, over-the-needle catheter into the trachea through the cricothyroid membrane. This procedure provides temporary (less than 30 to 45 minutes) oxygenation and limited ventilation. Intermittent ventilation with high-flow oxygen is required. To put the limitations of this procedure in perspective, consider this: imagine yourself breathing through a 14-gauge IV catheter. How long would you be able to do so?

Needle cricothyrotomy can be performed on patients of all ages, including pediatric patients. However, this procedure may be extremely difficult to perform in infants and young children because of the mobility of the larynx and trachea and the softness of the laryngeal cartilage in these patients, making palpation of the landmarks for the procedure difficult and collapse of the upper airway with labored breathing more likely (Bower, 1997). An 18-gauge or smaller catheter is used in pediatric patients.

In general, needle cricothyrotomy can be performed quickly. It does not interfere with subsequent attempts at intubation. Needle cricothyrotomy does not isolate and protect the airway from aspiration. Possible complications of this procedure include hypercarbia, bleeding, infection, hematoma, hypoxemia, false placement, catheter dislodgement, subcutaneous and/or mediastinal emphysema, equipment failure, catheter kink, barotrauma, and inadequate ventilation resulting in hypoxia and death.

The equipment needed for needle cricothyrotomy is shown in Box 14-24. A special device called a *jet ventilator* is necessary to be able to deliver oxygen under pressures as high as 50 psi. In the absence of a jet ventilator a bag-mask device can be attached to the catheter using a pediatric endotracheal tube adapter. However, this method of ventilation is unable to generate the pressures needed to ventilate a patient with a needle cricothyrotomy and should only be used when there is no other option. The steps for performing this procedure are shown in Skill 14-12.

There is a variety of commercial percutaneous cricothyrotomy devices available. These devices include those that are placed via direct puncture of the cricothyroid membrane, those that introduce a cannula over a wire through the membrane, and those that use a series of dilators to introduce a cannula through the membrane. While the indications and contraindications for these devices are the same as those listed earlier, the procedure will vary from device to device. The paramedic must be familiar with the techniques used for any commercial device used in their local EMS system.

Surgical Cricothyrotomy

[OBJECTIVES 72, 73]

The technique of surgical cricothyrotomy (also called *open cricothyrotomy*) is similar to needle cricothyrotomy with the exception that an incision is made through the cricothyroid membrane to facilitate passage of a tube into the airway. When performing this procedure, correctly identifying the cricothyroid membrane is crucial to prevent severe injury to other vital structures of the neck. The equipment requirements for the procedure are listed in Box 14-25. Although local protocols may vary, surgical cricothyrotomy is absolutely contraindicated in children younger than 5 years old, and relatively contraindicated in children between 5 and 8 years old because of their anatomic airway differences. Do not perform a surgical airway procedure in the field if the following are true:

- Endotracheal intubation can be accomplished
- You are unable to identify and locate the cricothyroid membrane
- The patient has a crush injury to the larynx or transection of the trachea

BOX 14-24   Needle Cricothyrotomy: Equipment

- Personal protective equipment
- Oxygen source
- Suction equipment
- Antiseptic solution
- High-pressure oxygen source and jet ventilation device (if not using a bag-mask device)
- Adapter from the top of a 3.0-mm endotracheal tube (if using a bag-mask device)
- Bag-mask device (size appropriate for patient) with oxygen tubing
- 14-gauge (or larger) over-the-needle catheter
- 10-mL syringe
- Several 4 × 4 gauze pads
- Tape or commercial tube holder

BOX 14-25   Surgical Cricothyrotomy: Equipment

- Personal protective equipment
- Oxygen source
- Suction equipment
- Antiseptic solution
- Bag-mask device with oxygen tubing
- Scalpel (#10 or #15)
- Hemostat (forceps)
- Several 4 × 4 gauze pads
- Endotracheal tube (6 to 7 mm) or tracheostomy tube (#5 or #6)
- Tape or commercial tube holder

SKILL 14-12 NEEDLE CRICOTHYROTOMY

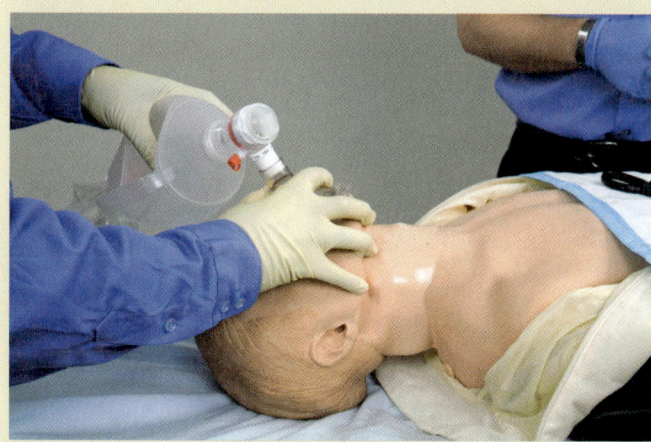

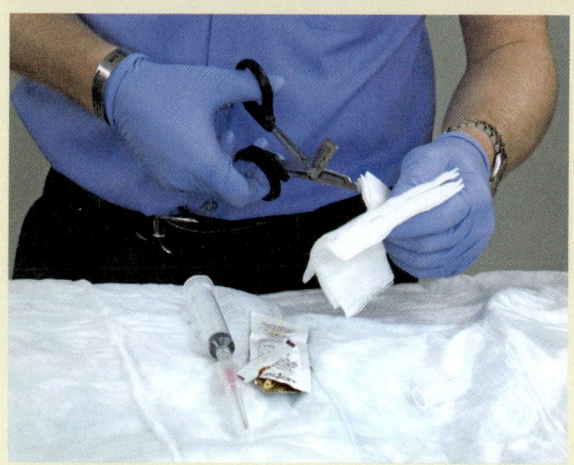

Step 1 Position the patient supine and hyperextend the head and neck (maintain a neutral position if you suspect cervical spine injury). Manage the patient's airway with basic adjuncts and supplemental oxygen. Attach a pulse oximeter and cardiac monitor to the patient. Monitor the patient's vital signs every 5 minutes.

Step 2 Assemble and prepare all equipment.

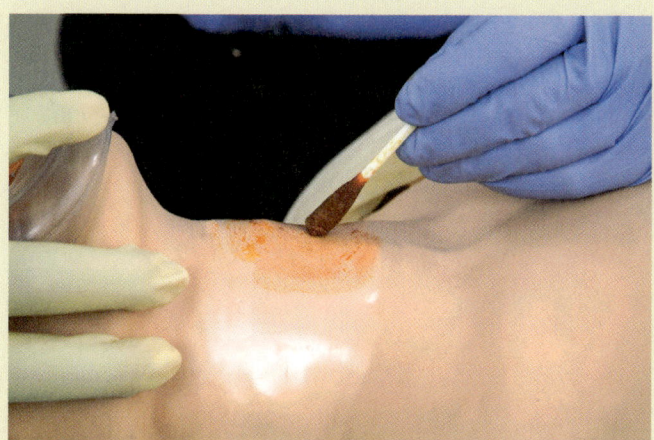

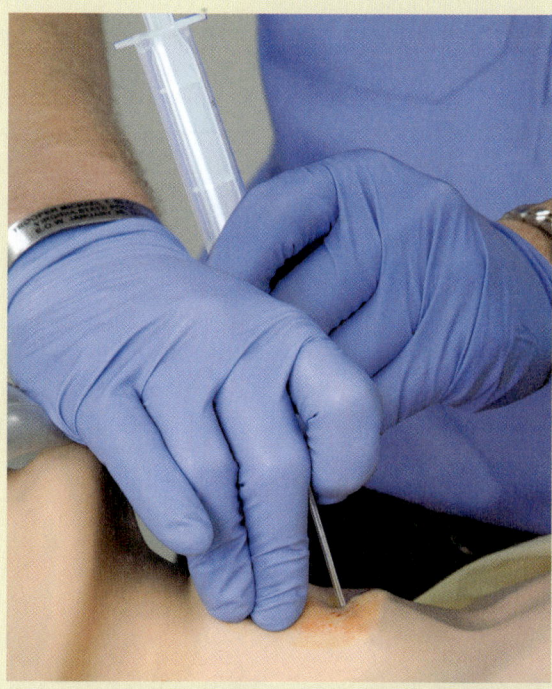

Step 3 Palpate the neck locating the cricothyroid membrane—between the thyroid and cricoid cartilages. Cleanse the site.

Step 4 With the needle attached to a syringe and held in the dominant hand, stabilize the laryngeal cartilages with the thumb and fingers of the other hand. Reconfirm the location of the cricothyroid membrane. Direct the needle and catheter toward the feet at a 45-degree angle.

Continued

SKILL 14-12 NEEDLE CRICOTHYROTOMY—continued

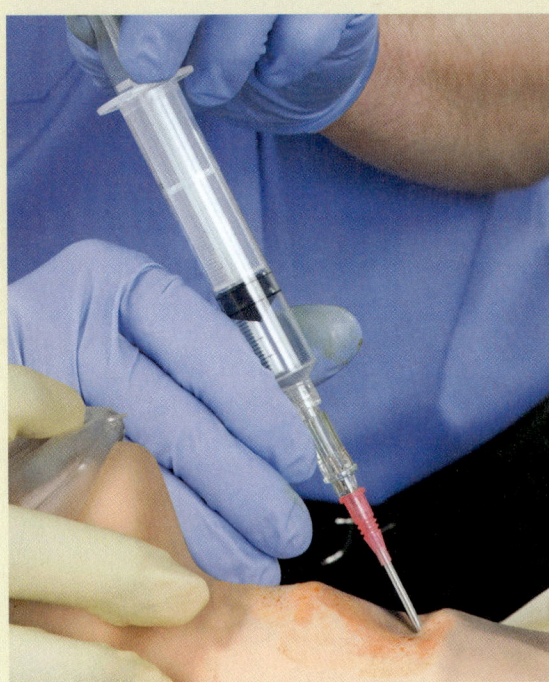

Step 5 Carefully insert the needle and catheter through the cricothyroid membrane, maintaining negative pressure (pulling back) on the syringe as the needle is advanced. Advance slowly while aspirating for air, signifying placement in the tracheal lumen.

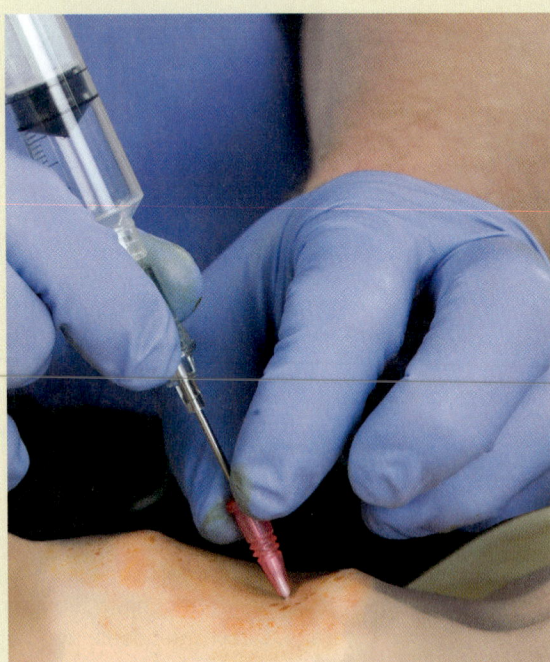

Step 6 Advance the catheter over the needle, being careful to avoid the posterior tracheal wall, until the catheter hub is flush with the skin. Hold the catheter hub in place to prevent displacement and discard the needle in a sharps container.

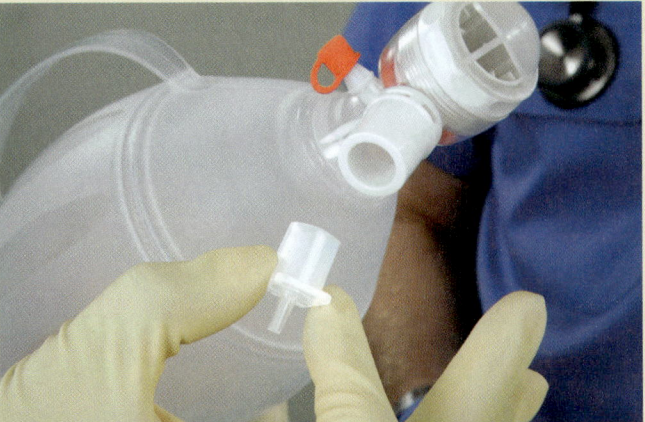

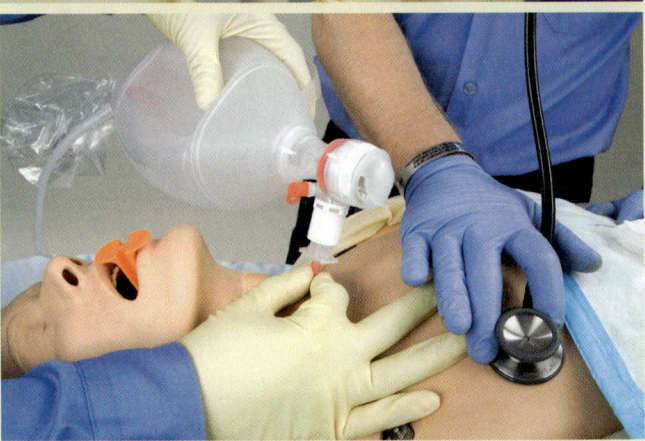

Step 7 If using a bag-mask device, attach a 3-mm ET tube adapter to the bag and then connect to the catheter hub. Alternately, attach the barrel of a 3-mL syringe to the intravenous catheter and an 8-mm ET tube adapter to the syringe barrel, or use a commercially available jet ventilator. Begin ventilation. Inflate for 1 second and allow exhalation for 2 to 4 seconds. Observe for chest rise.

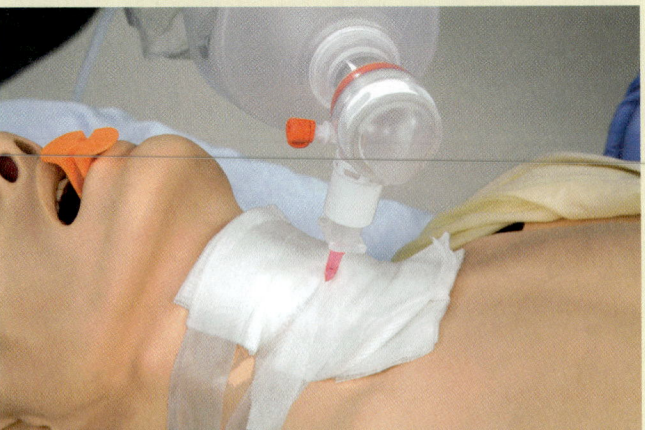

Step 8 Place 4 × 4 gauze pads that have been slit on one side to the middle around the catheter to stabilize it. Then tape in place to secure the catheter hub in the neck. Continue to monitor carefully for chest rise and auscultate for adequate ventilation. Assess $ETCO_2$, pulse oximetry, electrocardiogram, and vital signs at least every 5 minutes.

- An underlying anatomic abnormality exists such as trauma, tumor, or subglottic stenosis
- You lack the skill and knowledge to perform the procedure

Possible complications of a surgical cricothyrotomy include asphyxia, aspiration, creation of a false passage into the tissues, mediastinal emphysema, hemorrhage or hematoma formation, vocal cord paralysis, hoarseness, laceration of the trachea/esophagus, subglottic stenosis, and tube dislodgement. The steps for performing this procedure are shown in Skill 14-13.

PULSE OXIMETRY

Pulse oximetry is a noninvasive measurement of the oxygen saturation of hemoglobin in peripheral tissues. A pulse oximeter (commonly called a *pulse ox*) is a small instrument with a light sensor clip that is easily applied to a fingertip or an earlobe (Figure 14-45). The instrument sensor emits two light frequencies. One is a red beam the approximate color of oxygenated hemoglobin and the other is an infrared beam that is the approximate wavelength of deoxygenated hemoglobin. By measuring the absorption of the two frequencies, the oximeter quickly and accurately calculates the percentage of hemoglobin saturated with oxygen. This calculation is called the **saturation of peripheral oxygen,** or SpO_2. The oximeter displays this value as a percentage and the patient's pulse rate on its screen. The SpO_2 is a generally reliable indicator of the status of the partial pressure of oxygen in the arterial blood (PaO_2). A healthy adult breathing room air at sea level generally has an SpO_2 in the range of 98% to 100%, with a lower range of normal between 93% and 95%. Patients older than 75 years generally have lower SpO_2 values, with 86% to 90% being common. Oxygen saturation measurements of healthy adults at higher altitudes (above 5000 feet) are commonly found in the 88% to 92% range. Patients with SpO_2 values that are significantly lower than normal are likely to be hypoxic.

A number of limitations are associated with pulse oximetry (Box 14-26). Interpret the SpO_2 values cautiously when the measurement is not consistent with the patient's presenting signs, symptoms, and environment. For instance, a patient with severe carbon monoxide poisoning generally has an SpO_2 of 99% to 100% even though the patient is actually severely hypoxic. The false measurement occurs because the carbon monoxide that is bound to the hemoglobin mimics the oxygen absorption reading exactly. Another false reading that occurs much more frequently is when a patient is in an early (compensated) stage of shock in which the patient's peripheral vasculature has constricted and very little blood is perfusing to the fingers, toes, or earlobes. The SpO_2 readings in these patients may be completely unreliable and may indicate that the patient is poorly oxygenated when, in fact, the patient is well oxygenated, but only to the central circulation. Changes in the amount of red blood cells, or hemoglobin, will also affect the readings of the pulse oximeter. As discussed earlier, patients with low hemoglobin or hematocrit, such as anemia or hemorrhage, may have a high percentage of bound hemoglobin, but there is physically not enough oxygen carrying capability to meet the metabolic demand. In this situation the SpO_2 will be high, yet the patient may be hypoxic. In the setting of a high hematocrit, such as in polycythemia, the SpO_2 may be low, yet there is sufficient oxygen delivery to the tissues. Misinterpreting the pulse oximetry reading in these patients may result in unnecessarily aggressive airway management.

> **PARAMEDIC***Pearl*
>
> A pulse oximeter is an adjunct to, not a replacement for, vigilant patient assessment. You must correlate your assessment findings with pulse oximeter readings to determine appropriate treatment interventions for the patient.

BOX 14-26	Causes of False Pulse Oximetry Readings

- Dark or metallic nail polish
- False nails
- Bright ambient light, including sunlight
- Carbon monoxide or cyanide poisoning or other molecules that bind to hemoglobin
- Poor peripheral perfusion from shock, hypotension, or hypothermia
- Medications (such as vasoconstrictors)
- Severe jaundice

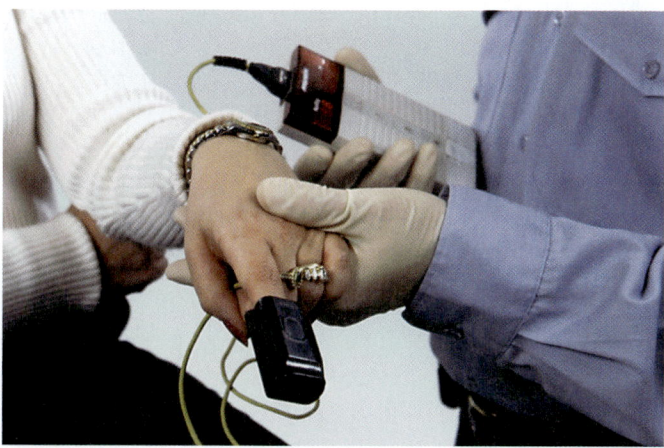

Figure 14-45 A pulse oximeter is a small instrument with a light sensor clip that is easily applied to a fingertip or an earlobe.

SKILL 14-13 SURGICAL CRICOTHYROTOMY

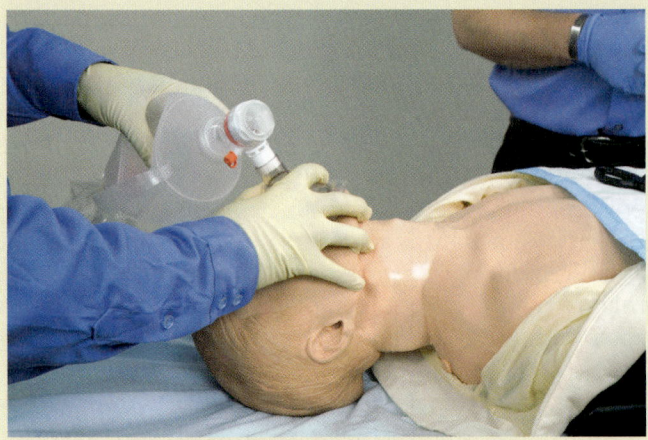

Step 1 Position the patient supine and hyperextend the head and neck (maintain a neutral position if you suspect cervical spine injury). Manage the patient's airway with basic adjuncts and supplemental oxygen. Attach a pulse oximeter and cardiac monitor to the patient. Monitor the patient's vital signs every 5 minutes. Assemble and prepare all equipment.

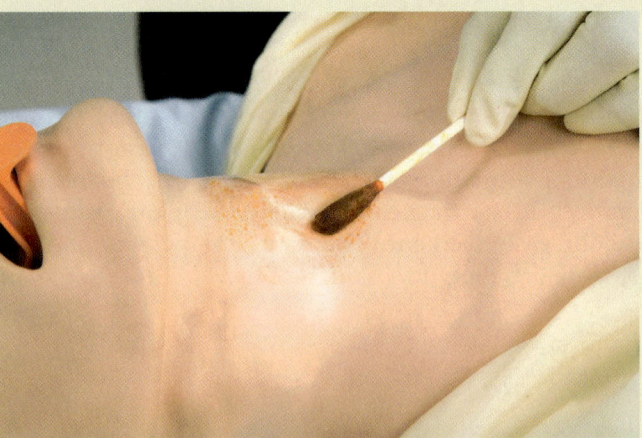

Step 2 Palpate the neck to locate the cricothyroid membrane between the thyroid and cricoid cartilages. Cleanse the site.

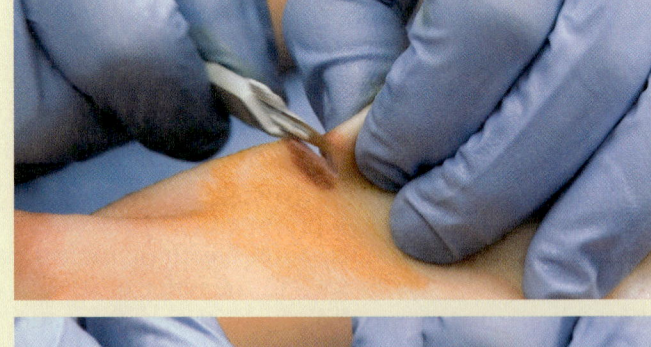

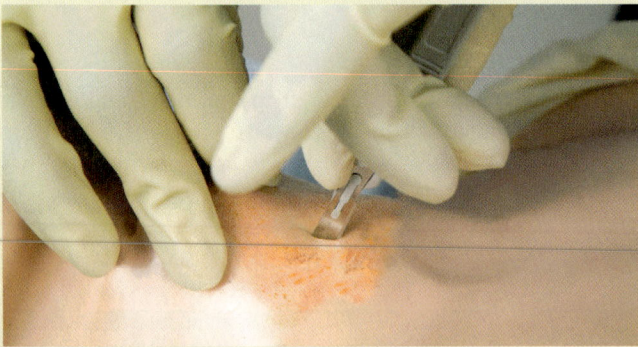

Step 3 Stabilize the laryngeal cartilages with the thumb and fingers of your nondominant hand while reconfirming the location of the cricothyroid membrane. Carefully make a 1- to 2-cm midline and vertical incision with a scalpel through the skin over the membrane (use 4 × 4 gauze pads to control any bleeding).

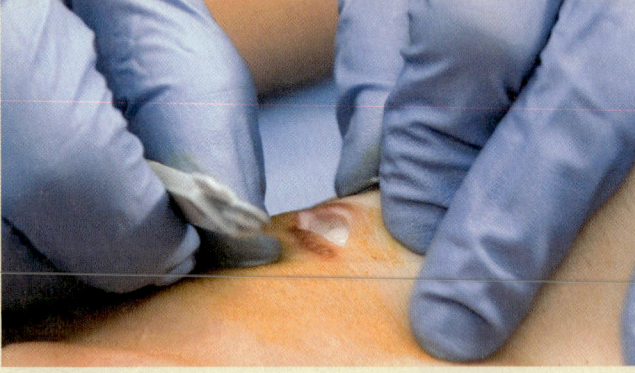

Step 4 Some medical directors prefer that the initial incision be made horizontally (as shown) instead of vertically.

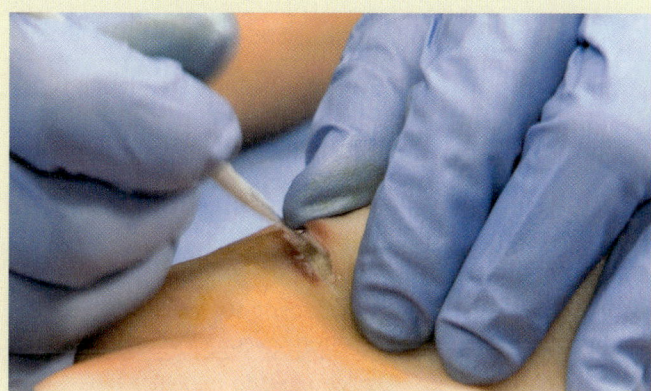

Step 5 Locate the cricothyroid membrane and make a 1-cm incision in the horizontal plane of the membrane. This may be done with the scalpel or punctured with the tip of a hemostat (forceps).

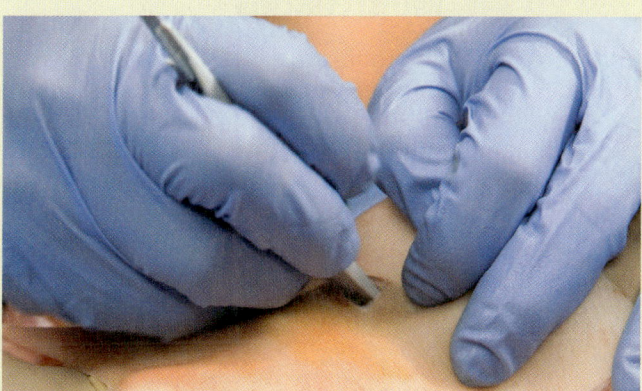

Step 6 Once the cricothyroid membrane has been penetrated, use a curved hemostat or the handle of the scalpel to maintain the surgical opening created and increase the diameter for tube placement. With the hemostat, release and spread apart (like a pair of pliers), increasing the size of the opening, or insert the handle of the scalpel and twist to increase the opening (separating the cartilages).

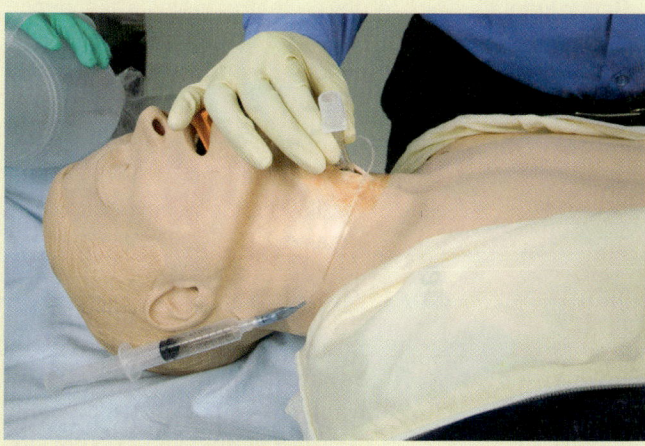

Step 7 Insert an ET tube into the tracheal opening. Direct the tube toward the patient's feet.

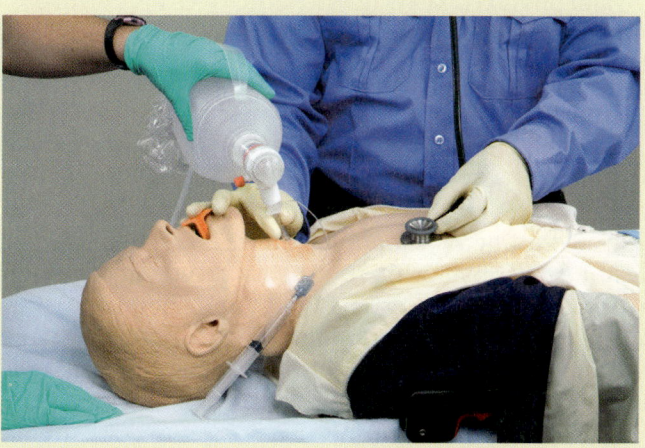

Step 8 Inflate the tube cuff with air using a 10-mL syringe so that the pilot balloon is full. Detach the syringe. While firmly holding the tube, ask an assistant to begin ventilation with a bag-mask device and supplemental oxygen. Confirm correct tube placement—observe chest rise and auscultate lung sounds.

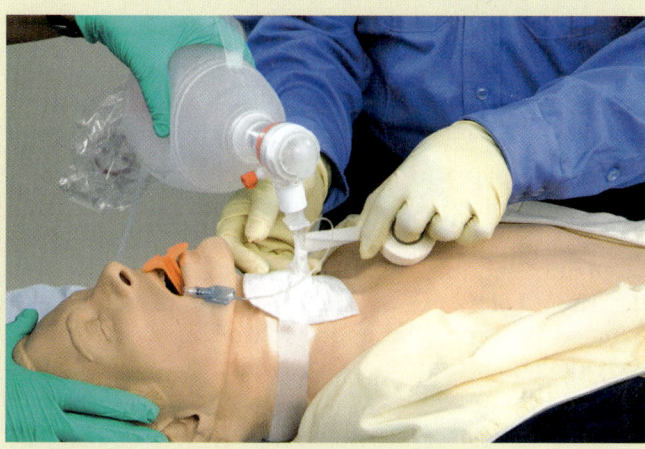

Step 9 Secure the tube. Continue to monitor carefully for adequate ventilation. Assess $ETCO_2$, pulse oximetry, ECG, and vital signs at least every 5 minutes.

Normal blood level = 40
ETCO₂ is little lower

EXHALED CO₂ MONITORING

The ventilatory end product of metabolism is carbon dioxide. The detection of CO_2 in the exhaled breath is a nearly, if not perfectly, 100% reliable indicator that an orotracheal tube (or nasotracheal tube) has been properly placed in the trachea. Because the air in the esophagus normally has very low levels of CO_2, exhaled CO_2 monitoring is a rapid method of preventing unrecognized esophageal intubation.

Exhaled CO_2 monitoring is commonly used in the following situations:

- Verification of ET tube placement
- Evaluation of mechanical ventilation and resuscitation efforts
- Continuous monitoring of ET tube position (including during patient transport)
- Monitoring of exhaled CO_2 levels in patients with suspected increased intracranial pressure
- Assessment of the adequacy of ventilation in patients with bronchospasm, asthma, COPD, anaphylaxis, heart failure, drug overdose, stroke, shock, or circulatory compromise

Remember that proper ET tube placement and exhaled CO_2 are not reliable indicators of oxygenation. Thus exhaled CO_2 detection does not replace pulse oximetry or good clinical assessments of patients, including mental status, lung sounds, pulse rate, and skin color. When using a colorimetric capnometer in the setting of cardiac arrest it is possible for there to be no detection of carbon dioxide. However, this situation is rare when using capnography. Although the amount of exhaled CO_2 may be lower than normal, it should not be absent unless the patient has been in arrest for a prolonged period. The absence of CO_2 detection when using capnography should raise strong suspicions of placement of the ET tube in the esophagus. Capnography, or capnometry, at least, should be used with all ET intubations. Capnography-related terms are given in Table 14-7.

Capnometers and capnographs work differently. A colorimetric capnometer functions through a pH change that occurs with the acidic breath of a patient (Figure 14-46). The patient's breath causes a chemical reaction on pH-sensitive litmus paper housed in the detector. The capnometer is placed between an ET tube or advanced airway device, and a ventilation device (Figure 14-47). The presence of CO_2 (evidenced by a color change on the colorimetric device) suggests placement of the tube in the trachea, however this type of capnometer is qualitative in that it simply shows the presence of CO_2. It has no ability to provide an actual CO_2 reading or indicate the presence of hypercarbia. A lack of CO_2 (no color change) suggests tube placement in the esophagus, particularly in patients with spontaneous circulation. Colorimetric capnometers have been shown to work reliably for only about 15 minutes. These capnometers are susceptible to inaccurate results because of the age of the paper, expo-

TABLE 14-7	Capnography-Related Terms
Term	**Description**
Capnography	Continuous analysis and recording of CO_2 concentrations in respiratory gases
	Output displayed as a waveform
	Graphic display of the CO_2 concentration versus time during a respiratory cycle
	CO_2 concentration may also be plotted versus expiratory volume
Capnometer	Device used to measure the concentration of CO_2 at the end of exhalation
Capnometry	A numeric reading of exhaled CO_2 concentrations without a continuous written record or waveform
	Output is a numerical value
	Numeric display of CO_2 on a monitor
Capnograph	A device that provides a numeric reading of exhaled CO_2 concentrations and a waveform (tracing)
Exhaled CO_2 detector	A capnometer that provides a noninvasive estimate of alveolar ventilation, the concentration of exhaled CO_2 from the lungs, and arterial carbon dioxide content; also called an *end-tidal CO₂ detector*
Colorimetric ETCO₂ detector	A device that provides CO_2 readings by chemical reaction on pH-sensitive litmus paper housed in the detector
	The presence of CO_2 (evidenced by a color change on the colorimetric device) suggests tracheal placement
Qualitative ETCO₂ monitor	A device that uses a light to indicate the presence of ETCO₂

ETCO₂, End-tidal carbon dioxide.

sure of the paper to the environment, patient secretions (such as vomitus), or acidic drugs such as endotracheally administered epinephrine.

Digital capnometers, like the capnography devices described below, use infrared technology to analyze the exhaled gas from the endotracheal tube. These devices provide a quantitative measurement of the exhaled CO_2, in that they provide the exact amount of CO_2 exhaled. This is beneficial as trends in CO_2 levels can be monitored and the effectiveness of treatment can be determined.

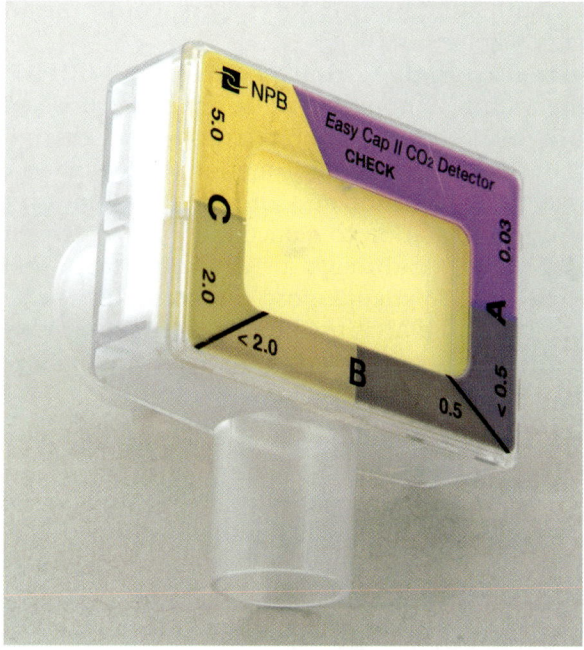

Figure 14-46 Colorimetric end-tidal CO_2 (ETCO$_2$) detector.

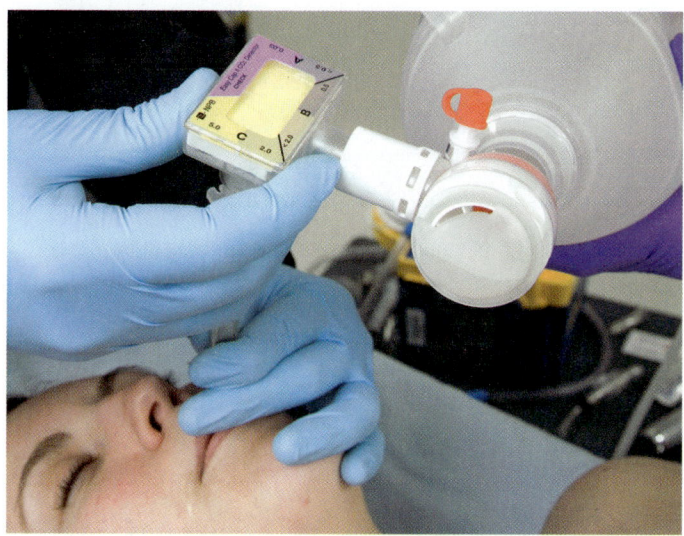

Figure 14-47 Colorimetric end-tidal CO_2 (ETCO$_2$) detector connected to an endotracheal tube.

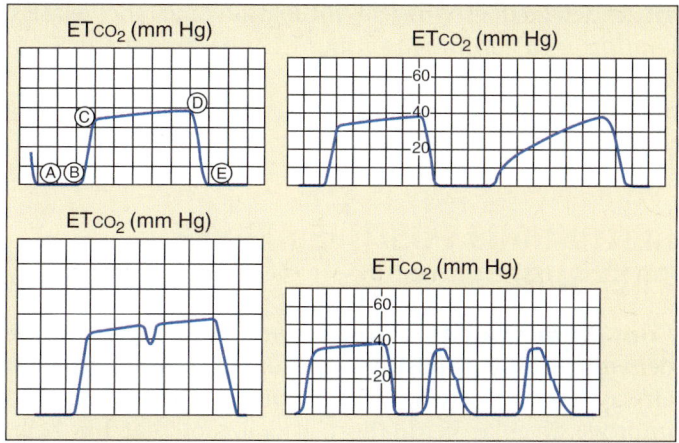

Figure 14-48 Normal capnogram. A capnograph provides a numeric reading of exhaled CO_2 concentrations and a waveform (tracing).

The normal level of exhaled CO_2 is 33 to 43 mm Hg. This is dependent upon adequate ventilation and adequate perfusion. A change in either factor will increase or decrease the amount of exhaled CO_2.

Capnography devices function through infrared technology. In addition to providing quantitative data as the digital capnometer does, they also provide information about air movement in and out of the lungs with a graphical waveform. An example of a normal capnograph waveform is shown in Figure 14-48. Phase I of the wave-

form occurs during the beginning of exhalation when air from the anatomic dead space is being exhaled. Because this air contains undetectable amounts of CO_2 there is no movement of the wave from the baseline. During phase II CO_2 from the larger bronchi is beginning to pass the sensor resulting in the expiratory upslope. This represents a sharp increase in the concentration of CO_2 passing the sensor and results in a rapid departure of the waveform from the baseline. Phase III, or the alveolar plateau, results from CO_2-rich alveolar air passing the sensor. Phase 0 indicates the end of exhalation and the beginning of inhalation in which the levels of CO_2 passing the sensor quickly drop to zero resulting in a quick return of the waveform to the baseline. The space that occurs between waveforms is the result of the pause between respirations. The point at which exhalation ends and inspiration begins is the end tidal CO_2, (ETCO$_2$), which is the number that is reported by most capnometers. Changes in the end tidal CO_2 generally result from changes in perfusion or ventilation rates. Changes in the morphology of the waveform indicate a change in air movement through the lower airways.

With very few exceptions the presence of exhaled CO_2 indicates the placement of the endotracheal tube in the trachea. Endotracheal tubes placed in the esophagus or displaced from the trachea generally result in the absence of CO_2 detection. In the setting of extratracheal placement, with a positive CO_2 reading, the ETCO$_2$ and waveform will be abnormal and erratic. In this setting the placement of the endotracheal tube should be immediately re-evaluated. Conditions that can cause this include placement of the distal end of the tube in the hypopharynx just in front of, but not through, the glottic opening, or the presence of CO_2 in the stomach. In the latter situation CO_2 may be detected for the first six ventilations and will then be absent.

The advantages of capnography include a positive benefit/expense ratio when considering the tragic cost of an undetected esophageal intubation and the relative comfort of a confirmed proper ET tube placement. Capnography devices are compact, light, and disposable and have been shown to work reliably for unlimited periods.

CONTINUOUS POSITIVE AIRWAY PRESSURE

Get on CPAP early—can avoid intubation (CHF, asthma, COPD)

Continuous positive airway pressure (CPAP) is the delivery of slight positive pressure airflow to prevent airway collapse, reduce the work of breathing, and improve alveolar ventilation. It is a tool that has been gaining attention and popularity within the EMS community after positive results of several documented studies. With CPAP, positive pressure is exerted throughout the airway during the entire respiratory cycle (Figure 14-49).

Patients on mechanical ventilation with an ET tube in place have the ability to receive varying degrees of **positive end-expiratory pressure (PEEP).** PEEP indicates the amount of pressure above atmospheric pressure present in the airway at the end of the expiratory cycle. PEEP is measured in centimeters of water pressure. In the field, PEEP should not exceed pressures of 10 cm H_2O. PEEP improves gas exchange by preventing collapse of the alveolar passages, increasing functional residual capacity, and redistributing fluid in the alveoli. In the intubated patient, an increase in PEEP is gained through the use of a PEEP valve. This tubular device is hollow with a weight in the lumen, and is placed between the endotracheal tube and the bag-mask device. As the patient exhales the ball must be lifted for air to escape the lungs, thereby increasing the pressure in the respiratory system. In contrast, CPAP is considered a noninvasive technique using a snugly fitting mask that covers the patient's nose and mouth and is used for spontaneously breathing patients (Figure 14-50).

Bilevel positive airway pressure (BiPAP) is another form of noninvasive positive-pressure ventilation. In BiPAP therapy, two (bi) levels of positive pressure are delivered—one during inspiration (to keep the airway open as the patient inhales) and the other (lower) pressure during expiration to reduce the work of exhalation. BiPAP is delivered through a tight-fitting mask that fits over either the patient's nose or the mouth and nose (Figure 14-51). BiPAP is used in the treatment of patients with chronic respiratory failure. Adjustments are possible

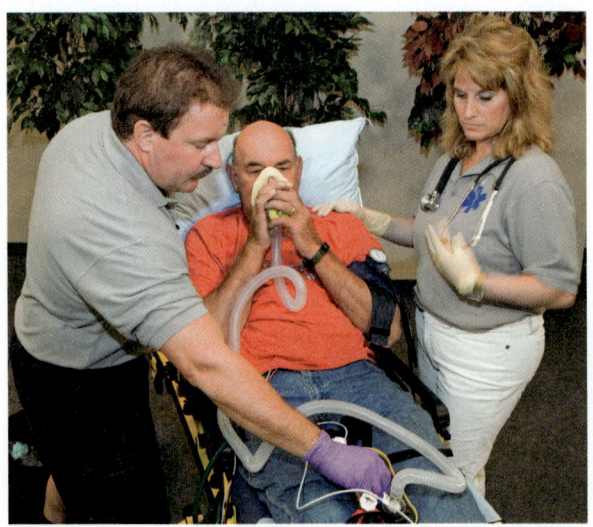

Figure 14-50 Continuous positive airway pressure (CPAP) mask applied.

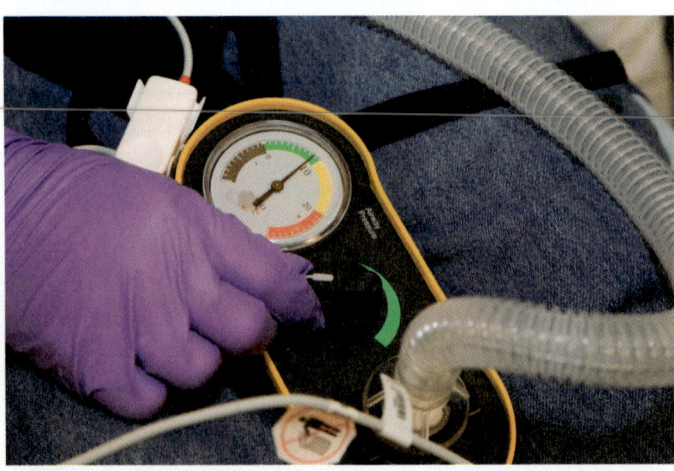

Figure 14-49 Continuous positive airway pressure (CPAP) flow generator.

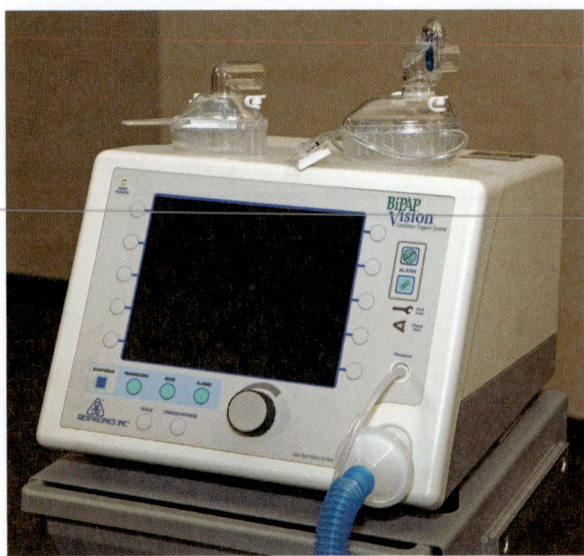

Figure 14-51 Bilevel positive airway pressure (BiPAP) machine.

to use lower pressures during expiration and higher pressure during inspiration.

Indications

Many clinical circumstances are appropriate for the use of CPAP. Pulmonary edema and congestive heart failure are two universally accepted indications for the use of CPAP. When fluid accumulates in the alveoli, surfactant becomes diluted and is no longer able to decrease surface tension within the air sacs. Loss of surfactant requires greater effort to open the alveoli as they become stiff.

As an effective alternative to ET intubation for specific types of patients, CPAP offers several advantages. Avoiding ET intubation when possible decreases the potential complications inherent with intubation. Patients have shorter hospitalizations and may avoid admission to the intensive care unit. Additional advantages of CPAP include the following:

- Improves oxygenation
- Increases alveolar pressure, which helps minimize the shift of fluid from the vascular space into the alveoli
- Reduces work of breathing
- Prevents atelectasis
- Provides positive-pressure ventilation without the need for ET intubation
- Avoids the risks, complications, and expense of ET intubation
- Preserves normal airway defense mechanisms
- Allows greater patient comfort while preserving the ability to talk, eat, and drink
- Increases amount of time for other medical therapies to take effect (such as medications)

Exact parameters for CPAP use are established by your medical director. Common indications include a responsive patient who is in severe respiratory distress from the following suspected conditions:

- Pulmonary edema
- Congestive heart failure
- Acute respiratory distress syndrome
- Drowning
- COPD
- Pneumonia

Contraindications to the use of CPAP include the following:

- Age younger than 14 years
- Upper airway or facial trauma or abnormalities that prevent the mask from sealing
- Open stoma or tracheotomy
- Severe cardiorespiratory instability (such as respiratory or cardiac arrest, penetrating chest trauma, suspected pneumothorax, dysrhythmias)
- Persistent nausea and vomiting
- Active upper gastrointestinal bleeding or history of recent gastric surgery
- Suspected preexisting barotrauma

Although CPAP is generally considered safe and effective, it is not without potential complications. Tolerated well by most patients, some may feel a sense of smothering from the mask. Patients sensitive to claustrophobia may also not tolerate the mask. Venous blood return to the heart may become impaired as high CPAP pressures transfer to increased intrathoracic pressures, with a resultant decrease in cardiac output. As with any device generating positive pressure in the airways, barotrauma is a possibility. Air delivered under pressure also has the ability to enter the gastrointestinal tract, leading to gastrointestinal upset. Monitor the patient closely for this complication. In some instances, your local medical director may encourage the placement of a nasogastric tube to allow gastric decompression. Because airway pressures during the use of CPAP may actually force air into the cranial vault, caution is indicated in patients who may have increased intracranial pressure or those with a suspected basilar skull fracture. The success of CPAP also depends on a cooperative, spontaneously breathing patient and a mask that fits properly, preventing mask leak.

Procedure

Procedurally, many commercial devices and attachments are available when using CPAP. The following steps outline the basic procedure:

1. Set up your equipment and explain the procedure to the patient. Attach a pulse oximeter and cardiac monitor to the patient. Monitor the patient's vital signs every 5 minutes.
2. Connect the CPAP device to a suitable oxygen supply. A CPAP system rapidly depletes an oxygen source. Ensure that your oxygen source is sufficient and that you have a backup source available. Attach the breathing circuit to the CPAP device and ensure the device is functioning properly.
3. Place the patient in a seated position with the head of the bed raised to approximately 45 degrees.
4. Place the breathing circuit mask over the patient's nose and mouth and secure it with the straps provided.
5. Titrate increases in positive airway pressure (measured in centimeters of water) until the patient's pulse oximetry readings and symptoms improve. *Do not exceed pressures of 10 cm H_2O.*
6. Check for air leaks around the mask and monitor the patient's response to treatment.
7. If the patient's respiratory status deteriorates, discontinue CPAP and use an alternative means to manage the patient's airway and ventilation.

Case Scenario SUMMARY

1. *What is your general impression of this patient?* You need no further information to identify this patient as a high priority critical trauma patient.

2. *What additional assessment will be important in the evaluation of this patient? Can you complete any assessments before extrication? Why or why not?* This patient will require a rapid trauma survey. It should be possible to perform the survey from the head to the pelvis, effectively evaluating the critically important neurological, pulmonary, and cardiovascular functions before extrication is completed. The abdominal and pelvic exam, as well as evaluation of the lower extremities, will need to be deferred until the patient has been extricated.

3. *What intervention should you initiate at this time?* Assisted ventilation, oxygenation, and IV access. It may be possible to provide endotracheal intubation (either oral or nasal), although it may be more difficult given the patient's lateral position. If ventilations and oxygenation can be adequately maintained without intubation, it should be delayed until the patient is in a more favorable position.

4. *Is this patient's transport a high priority (i.e., lights and siren)? Why or why not?* This patient is obviously a high priority. She should be extricated, stabilized, and transported to the trauma center as rapidly as possible. Air transport should be considered based on a number of factors that include time of day (traffic) and the location of the incident (such as in a rural area).

5. *What is your preferred method for performing endotracheal intubation in this case? Why?* The answer to this question will vary some among EMS systems. Oral intubation is the method with which most paramedics are comfortable, and it can be safely performed in trauma patients if other rescuers provide manual in-line stabilization to prevent movement of the neck during the procedure. Nasal intubation reduces the movement of the neck, but is associated with a significantly reduced success rate in the prehospital setting. Consult with your local EMS leadership and protocols.

6. *What steps will you take to confirm correct positioning of the endotracheal tube?* All intubations should be followed by several methods of confirmation including chest rise and fall, bilateral breath sounds, the absence of gastric sounds and distension, successful use of the esophageal detector device, normal pulmonary compliance, and fogging in the tube. More importantly, waveform capnography provides accurate, ongoing confirmation of tube position throughout transport.

7. *What is the significance of the other findings, including the history of respiratory arrest and the unresponsive pupils? Does this affect your treatment plan? How?* At this stage of the case, the history of respiratory arrest does not have an obvious cause. It could have been an airway obstruction or related to injury to the brainstem. The unresponsive pupils suggest either prolonged hypoxia or direct brain trauma.

8. *At what rate and depth will you ventilate this patient's lungs en route to the hospital? Why?* Recent research has demonstrated complications related to hyperventilation of trauma patients. This patient's lungs should be ventilated at a rate of 12 to 15 breaths/min, or at a rate and depth that maintains a normal $ETCO_2$ and oxygen saturation.

9. *What are some potential causes of the difficulty or resistance in ventilating that you've experienced? What signs or symptoms may assist in differentiating between them? What action should you take at this time?* Several causes include airway obstruction, bronchospasm, anaphylaxis, or tension pneumothorax. Look for signs of airway obstruction (e.g., blood in the pharynx, broken teeth, vomitus in the ET tube), bronchospasm (wheezing), anaphylaxis (rash, hypotension, wheezing), or tension pneumothorax (unequal or absent breath sounds, jugular venous distension, hypotension) to clarify the cause. If there are no specific findings, suspect airway obstruction.

10. *What is the clinical significance of the absence of jugular venous distention or hypotension? What about the bilaterally equal, quiet breath sounds? How does this information affect your further treatment plan?* These signs dramatically reduce the likelihood that the difficulty ventilating is the result of a tension pneumothorax. Do not needle the chest.

11. *If the patient's drop in saturation had occurred in the ambulance while still en route, what would you have done? Why?* Assuming that you had evaluated and not found the signs identified in question number 9, you would have little choice but to assume that the problem was the airway. You could consider attempting to suction the tube, checking for obstructions when you advance a suction catheter, visualizing with the laryngoscope to confirm that the tube passes through the cords, evaluating for signs of a misplaced tube including subcutaneous air and/or gastric distension. Ultimately, you may need to remove and replace the ET tube.

12. *What is the procedure for removing and replacing an ET tube in the field?* After you have performed the steps discussed in 11 above, it is time to replace the tube.
    - Maintain ventilation throughout
    - If clinically feasible, turn the patient onto their side
    - Prepare a second endotracheal tube for insertion
    - Have suction on hand, assembled, and turned on. You will want the yankauer tip.
    - Deflate the ET tube cuff
    - Gently but rapidly remove the ET tube. Have your partner prepare to provide suction if the patient vomits
    - If vomiting occurs, initiate suction and manual removal of vomitus
    - When vomiting subsides, position the patient and intubate

Chapter Summary

- The upper airway consists of structures located outside the chest cavity, including the nose and nasal cavities, pharynx, and larynx. The upper airway functions to filter, warm, and humidify the air, protecting the surfaces of the lower respiratory tract. The lower airway consists of the trachea, bronchial tree (primary bronchi, secondary bronchi, and bronchioles), alveoli, and the lungs. The lower airway is where gas exchange occurs. Functionally, oxygen diffuses from the alveoli into the pulmonary capillaries while carbon dioxide diffuses in the opposite direction.

- Ventilation is the mechanical process of moving air into and out of the lungs in two separate phases: inspiration and expiration. Respiration is the exchange of gases between a living organism and its environment. The bodies of human beings provide oxygen while removing carbon dioxide, one of the chief metabolic pollutants within our system.

- You must be able to identify respiratory problems quickly so you can provide appropriate and timely intervention. Assessment of age-appropriate respiratory rate, regularity, and work of breathing are essential parameters to evaluate early (and repeatedly) on every patient. When possible, use topographic landmarks of the chest to describe physical examination findings. These markers include the clavicles, nipples, angle of Louis, suprasternal notch, and costal angle.

- Auscultating lung sounds is essential for every patient with any type of respiratory symptom. The primary goal of auscultation is to determine if lung sounds are present and equal bilaterally. Compare sounds from side to side by listening to one lung and then the other in the same place. With each stethoscope placement, listen to at least one full inhalation and exhalation.

- Many supplemental oxygen delivery methods are available. You must choose the correct option for your patient's circumstances. When you administer supplemental oxygen to a patient, an adequate rate and depth (minute volume) of ventilation is necessary. If any doubt exists regarding the adequacy of ventilation in addition to oxygenation, you must support the patient with both supplemental oxygen and positive-pressure ventilation.

- Many devices exist for delivering supplemental oxygen to patients. Devices have various capabilities relating to percentage of oxygen delivery. Your patient's condition determines the method of delivery as well as the liter per minute flow rate.

- Airway obstruction can have many causes. Even a partial blockage of the airway may impair gas exchange to a degree that the patient's life is in jeopardy without quick corrective action. Classifications of airway obstruction include complete obstruction, partial obstruction with poor air exchange, and partial obstruc-

tion with good air exchange. Common causes leading to obstruction include the tongue, foreign bodies, laryngeal spasm and edema, trauma, and aspiration.

- Basic to any type of airway management procedure is the ability to manually open a patient's airway. Manual maneuvers require no special equipment and are noninvasive. The purpose of a manual maneuver is to position the anatomic structures of the patient's airway so that the airway passages are open to the flow of air.

- In an unresponsive patient, secretions, blood, and vomitus require removal with a suction device before ventilating. Ill patients often have nausea and many airway procedures may stimulate vomiting. You must anticipate such situations and have suction within arm's reach to minimize the potential risk of aspiration.

- Several devices can help keep the airway open. Two adjuncts specifically designed to prevent the tongue from falling back into the airway and blocking the flow of air are oral and nasal airways.

- Patients who are apneic or those with inadequate ventilation require artificial ventilation. Forcing air into the lungs is called *positive-pressure ventilation*. Methods by which positive-pressure ventilation may be accomplished include mouth-to-mouth, mouth-to-nose, mouth-to–barrier device, and mouth-to-mask ventilation; one-person, two-person, or three-person bagmask ventilation; ventilation with an ATV; and ventilation using an FROPVD.

- Advanced airways include the Combitube, the LMA, and the ET tube. Insertion of a Combitube or LMA does not require visualization of the vocal cords. In contrast, insertion of an ET tube through a patient's mouth and into the trachea (orotracheal intubation) does require direct visualization of the vocal cords. Nasotracheal intubation is an alternative approach for intubating the trachea. It is considered a blind procedure because the vocal cords are not visualized. RSI is the use of medications to sedate and paralyze a patient to achieve rapid ET intubation. Capnography, or capnometry, at least, should be used with all endotracheal intubations.

- Pulse oximetry is a noninvasive measurement of the oxygen saturation of hemoglobin in peripheral tissues.

- CPAP is the delivery of slight positive pressure to prevent airway collapse, reduce the work of breathing, and improve alveolar ventilation.

- Cricothyrotomy is an emergency procedure performed to allow rapid entrance to the airway for temporary oxygenation and ventilation. It can be accomplished by inserting a needle into the cricothyroid membrane (needle cricothyrotomy) or creating an opening into the cricothyroid membrane with a scalpel (surgical cricothyrotomy).

REFERENCES

Bower, C. M. (1997). The surgical airway. In Dieckmann, R. A., Fiser, D. H., & Selbst, S. M. (Eds.), *Illustrated textbook of pediatric emergency & critical care procedures* (pp. 166-122). St. Louis: Mosby–Year Book.

Foltin, G. L., Tunik, M. G., Cooper, A., Markenson, D., Treiber, M., & Skomorowsky, A. (2002). *Teaching resource for instructors in prehospital pediatrics for paramedics* (p. 29). New York: Center for Pediatric Emergency Medicine.

Huether, S. (2004). *Understanding pathophysiology* (3rd ed.). St. Louis: Elsevier.

Seidel, H. M. *Mosby's guide to physical examination* (5th ed.). St. Louis: Mosby.

SUGGESTED READINGS

Aehlert, B. (2007). *ACLS study guide* (3rd ed.). St. Louis: Mosby.

Aehlert, B. (2005). *PALS pediatric advanced life support study guide* (2nd ed.). St. Louis: Mosby.

Airway section. Retrieved March 13, 2008, from http://www.merginet.com.

American Heart Association. (2005). American Heart Association guidelines for cardiopulmonary resuscitation and emergency cardiovascular care. *Circulation, 112.* Retrieved from http://circ.ahajournals.org/.

Chapter Quiz

1. An abnormal deficiency in the concentration of oxygen in the blood is _____.
   a. hypocarbia
   b. hypoventilation
   c. hypoxemia
   d. hypoxia

2. List at least three indications for cricothyrotomy.
   _____
   _____
   _____

3. Which of the following is the leading cause of airway obstruction in an unresponsive patient?
   a. Edema
   b. Steak
   c. Tongue
   d. Vomitus

4. Which of the following airway structures is unique in that it has a dual function with both the respiratory system and digestive system?
   a. Larynx
   b. Pharynx
   c. Trachea
   d. Vallecula

5. Define *minute volume*.
   _____
   _____
   _____

6. Which of the following lung sounds is associated with fluid accumulating in the smaller airway passages heard on inspiration?
   a. Crackles (rales)
   b. Rattles (rhonchi)
   c. Stridor
   d. Wheezes

7. Which supplemental oxygen delivery system is capable of delivering fairly precise concentrations of oxygen?
   a. Nasal cannula
   b. Nonrebreather mask
   c. Small-volume nebulizer
   d. Venturi mask

8. Describe a common complication encountered when providing ventilatory assistance in a nonintubated patient and a simple maneuver that you can perform to minimize this complication.
   _____
   _____
   _____

9. List at least thee indications for endotracheal intubation.
   _____
   _____
   _____

10. List at least three indications for the use of CPAP.
    _____
    _____
    _____

Terminology

Agonal respirations Slow, shallow, irregular respirations resulting from anoxic brain injury.

Air trapping A respiratory pattern associated with an obstruction in the pulmonary tree; the breathing rate increases to overcome resistance in getting air out, the respiratory effort becomes more shallow, the volume of trapped air increases, and the lungs inflate.

Alveolar air volume In contrast to dead air space, alveolar volume is the amount of air that does reach the alveoli for gas exchange (approximately 350 mL in the adult male). It is the difference between tidal volume and dead-space volume.

Angle of Louis An angulation of the sternum that indicates the point where the second rib joins the sternum; also called the *manubriosternal junction*.

Anoxia A total lack of oxygen availability to the tissues.

Apnea Respiratory arrest.

Atelectasis An abnormal condition characterized by the collapse of alveoli, preventing the respiratory exchange of carbon dioxide and oxygen in a part of the lungs.

Barrier device A thin film of material placed on the patient's face used to prevent direct contact with the patient's mouth during positive-pressure ventilation.

Bilevel positive airway pressure (BiPAP) The delivery of two (bi) levels of positive-pressure ventilation; one during inspiration (to keep the airway open as the patient inhales) and the other (lower) pressure during expiration to reduce the work of exhalation.

Biot respirations Irregular respirations varying in rate and depth and interrupted by periods of apnea; associated with increased intracranial pressure, brain damage at the level of the medulla, and respiratory compromise from drug poisoning.

Bradypnea A respiratory rate that is persistently slower than normal for age; in adults, a rate slower than 12 breaths/min.

Capnograph A device that provides a numerical reading of exhaled CO_2 concentrations and a waveform (tracing).

Capnography Continuous analysis and recording of CO_2 concentrations in respiratory gases.

Capnometer A device used to measure the concentration of CO_2 at the end of exhalation.

Capnometry A numeric reading of exhaled CO_2 concentrations without a continuous written record or waveform.

Carina The point where the trachea divides into the right and left mainstem bronchi.

Central neurogenic hyperventilation Similar to Kussmaul respirations; characterized as deep, rapid breathing; associated with increased intracranial pressure.

Cheyne-Stokes respirations A pattern of gradually increasing rate and depth of breathing that tapers to slower and shallower breathing with a period of apnea before the cycle repeats itself; often described as a crescendo-decrescendo pattern or periodic breathing.

Chronic obstructive pulmonary disease (COPD) A progressive and irreversible condition characterized by diminished inspiratory and expiratory capacity of the lungs.

Compliance The resistance of the patient's lung tissue to ventilation.

Continuous positive airway pressure (CPAP) The delivery of slight positive pressure throughout the respiratory cycle to prevent airway collapse, reduce the work of breathing, and improve alveolar ventilation.

Costal angle The angle formed by the margins of the ribs at the sternum.

Coughing A protective mechanism usually induced by mucosal irritation; the forceful, spastic expiration experienced during coughing aids in the clearance of the bronchi and bronchioles.

Crackles (rales) As the name implies, when fluid accumulates in the smaller airway passages, air passing through the fluid creates a moist crackling or popping sound heard on inspiration.

Crepitation A crackling sound indicative of bone ends grinding together.

Cricothyroid membrane A fibrous membrane located between the cricoid and thyroid cartilages.

Cricothyrotomy An emergency procedure performed to allow rapid entrance to the airway (by the cricothyroid membrane) for temporary oxygenation and ventilation.

Dead air space Not all the air inspired during a breath participates in gas exchange and can be further classified as anatomic or physiologic dead space. In the average adult male this equates to approximately 150 mL. Anatomic dead space includes airway passages such as the trachea and bronchi, which are incapable of participating in gas exchange. Alveoli that have the potential to participate in gas exchange but do not because of disease or obstruction, as in COPD or atelectasis, are referred to as *physiologic dead space*.

Dyspnea An uncomfortable awareness of one's breathing that may be associated with a change in the breathing rate, effort, or pattern.

Endotracheal (ET) Within or through the trachea.

Terminology—continued

Endotracheal intubation An advanced airway procedure in which a tube is placed directly into the trachea.

Exhaled CO_2 detector A capnometer that provides a noninvasive estimate of alveolar ventilation, the concentration of exhaled CO_2 from the lungs, and arterial carbon dioxide content; also called an *end-tidal CO_2 detector*.

Expiratory reserve volume Amount of gas that can be forcefully expired at the end of a normal expiration.

External respiration The exchange of gases between the alveoli of the lungs and the blood cells traveling through the pulmonary capillaries.

Extubation Removal of an ET tube from the trachea.

FiO_2 Fraction of inspired oxygen.

Flail segment A free-floating section of the chest wall that results when two or more adjacent ribs are fractured in two or more places or when the sternum is detached.

Functional reserve capacity At the end of a normal expiration, the volume of air remaining in the lungs.

Gagging A reflex caused by irritation of the posterior pharynx that can result in vomiting.

Gag reflex A normal neural reflex elicited by touching the soft palate or posterior pharynx; the responses are symmetric elevation of the palate, retraction of the tongue, and contraction of the pharyngeal muscles.

Gastric distention Swelling of the abdomen caused by an influx of air or fluid.

Glottis The true vocal cords and the space between them.

Hemoglobin A protein found on red blood cells that is rich in iron.

Hering-Breuer reflex A reflex that limits inspiration and prevents overinflation of the lungs in a conscious, spontaneously breathing person; also called the *inhibito-inspiratory reflex*.

Hiccup (hiccoughing) Intermittent spasm of the diaphragm resulting in sudden inspiration with spastic closure of the glottis; usually annoying and serves no known physiologic purpose.

Hilum The point of entry for bronchial vessels, bronchi, and nerves in each lung.

Hypercarbia An excess of CO_2 in the blood.

Hyperpnea (hyperventilation) A respiratory pattern characterized by rapid, deep breathing.

Hyperventilation Blowing off too much carbon dioxide.

Hypocarbia An inadequate amount of carbon dioxide in the blood.

Hypoventilation Occurs when the volume of air that enters the alveoli and takes part in gas exchange is not adequate for the body's metabolic needs.

Hypoxemia An abnormal deficiency in the concentration of oxygen in arterial blood.

Hypoxia Inadequate oxygenation of the cells.

Inspiratory reserve volume Amount of gas that can be forcefully inspired in addition to a normal breath's tidal volume.

Internal respiration The exchange of gases between blood cells and tissues.

Kussmaul respirations An abnormal respiratory pattern characterized by deep, gasping respirations that may be slow or rapid.

Laryngoscope An instrument used to examine the interior of the larynx; during ET intubation, the device is used to visualize the glottic opening.

Minute volume Amount of gas moved in and out of the respiratory tract per minute. Tidal volume multiplied by ventilatory rate equals minute volume. The minute volume is the true measurement of a patient's ventilatory status and is vital in assessing pulmonary function. It ascertains the ventilatory rate and the depth of each inhalation.

Orthopnea Dyspnea relieved by a change in position (either sitting upright or standing).

Oxyhemoglobin Hemoglobin that has oxygen molecules bound to it.

Paradoxic motion (of a segment of the chest wall) Part of the chest moves in an opposite direction from the rest during respiration.

Partial pressure The pressure exerted by an individual gas in a mixture.

Peak expiratory flow The greatest rate of airflow that can be achieved during forced expiration beginning with the lungs fully inflated.

Peak flow meter A device used to assess the severity of respiratory distress.

Pocket mask A clear, semirigid mask designed for mouth-to-mask ventilation of a nonbreathing adult, child, or infant

Positive end-expiratory pressure (PEEP) The amount of pressure above atmospheric pressure present in the airway at the end of the expiratory cycle.

Positive-pressure ventilation Forcing air into the lungs.

Pulse oximetry A noninvasive method of measuring the percentage of oxygen-bound hemoglobin.

Rapid sequence intubation (RSI) The use of medications to sedate and paralyze a patient to achieve endotracheal intubation rapidly.

Rattles (rhonchi) Attributable to inflammation and mucus or fluid in the larger airway passages, rattles or rhonchi are descriptive of airway congestion heard on inspiration. Rhonchi are commonly associated with bronchitis or pneumonia.

Residual volume After a maximal forced exhalation, the amount of air remaining in the lungs and airway passages not able to be expelled.

Respiration The exchange of gases between a living organism and its environment.

Saturation of peripheral oxygen The percentage of hemoglobin saturated with oxygen (SpO_2)

Sellick maneuver Technique used to compress the cricoid cartilage against the cervical vertebrae, causing occlusion of the esophagus, thereby reducing the risk of aspiration; cricoid pressure.

Sighing Involuntary and periodic slow, deep breath followed by a prolonged expiratory phase. Occurring approximately once per minute, the act of sighing is thought to open atelectatic (collapsed) alveoli.

Sneezing Occurs from nasal irritation and allows clearance of the nose.

Stylet A relatively stiff but flexible metal rod covered by plastic and inserted into an ET tube; used for maintaining the shape of the relatively pliant ET tube and "steering" it into position.

Suprasternal notch A depression easily felt at the base of the anterior aspect of the neck, just above the angle of Louis.

Surfactant Specialized cells within each alveolus that keeps it from collapsing when little or no air is inside.

Tachypnea A respiratory rate persistently faster than normal for age; in adults, a rate faster than 20 breaths/min.

Tidal volume The volume of gas inhaled or exhaled during a single respiratory cycle. In the average adult male this is approximately 500 mL (5 to 7 mL/kg).

Tracheal stoma A surgical opening in the anterior neck that extends from the skin surface into the trachea, opening the trachea to the atmosphere.

Tracheostomy The surgical creation of an opening into the trachea.

Tripod position Sitting upright and leaning forward, supported by the arms, with the neck slightly extended, chin projected, and mouth open to maintain an airway.

Uvula Fleshy tissue resembling a grape that hangs down from the soft palate.

Vallecula The depression or pocket between the base of the tongue and the epiglottis.

Ventilation The mechanical process of moving air into and out of the lungs.

Wheeze A musical, whistling sound heard on inspiration and/or expiration resulting from constriction or obstruction of the pharynx, trachea, or bronchi. Wheezing is commonly associated with asthma.

PATIENT ASSESSMENT

Therapeutic Communication

Objectives *After completing this chapter, you will be able to:*

1. Define *communication*.
2. Discuss the importance of developing effective communication skills.
3. Identify internal and external factors for effective communication.
4. Differentiate sympathetic and empathic responses to elicit the patient's history.
5. Understand the patient interview process, including the identification of verbal and nonverbal cues.
6. Discuss the importance of using open-ended versus direct questions.

7. Describe the use of facilitation, reflection, clarification, confrontation, and interpretation.
8. Identify various interviewing traps and pitfalls that can hinder effective communication.
9. Discuss ways to gather information from sources other than the patient.
10. Identify techniques to develop patient rapport and trust.
11. Discuss and overcome communication barriers between you and your patient.
12. Discuss special situations that require additional effort and diligence to obtain a comprehensive history.

Chapter Outline

Case Scenario

You and your partner respond with the fire department to a low-income housing unit for a "woman with an unknown medical problem." On arrival, you find an 87-year-old woman in a very small but meticulously kept one-bedroom apartment. She is flanked by two middle-aged women who you quickly learn are her daughters. The older woman is your patient. You note that she is aware of your approach, her skin color is good, and she is well groomed. As you begin your interview, she loses her focus as she joins her daughters in scolding the fire personnel and your partner for leaning on breakable items in her tiny apartment.

Questions

1. *What is your general impression of this patient?*
2. *What nonverbal information has been communicated to you at this point?*
3. *How can you improve the patient's ability to focus on you and your interview?*
4. *How can her daughters improve the quality of communication with their mother? How can they impede it?*

[OBJECTIVES 1, 2]

Perhaps one of the most important skills a paramedic must develop is the ability to communicate effectively. **Communication** is the use of words, writing, or other commonly understood symbols to send a message to a receiver, who then provides feedback that indicates the receiver's interpretation of the message. It is more than simply interviewing a patient. Communication involves gathering vital information from a variety of sources to understand the nature of a patient's emergency. It also involves successfully conveying this information to healthcare professionals who assume responsibility for the patient's medical care. Prehospital medicine is unpredictable, unexpected, dramatic, and chaotic and involves an entire spectrum of patients with different medical conditions, educational skills, cultural beliefs, and motivations. As a result, paramedics regularly encounter barriers to effective communication with their patients. This chapter helps you develop improved skills and identify external and internal factors, patients, and special situations that present barriers to effective communication.

COMMUNICATION MODEL

Communication among individuals can be difficult and, although an often-discussed topic, the process is not well understood. Miscommunication is a part of daily life; however, unlike missing an appointment or not completing a task, miscommunication in medicine can result in failure to treat the patient appropriately, a negative outcome, or even death. The communication process is composed of several steps that can be combined into the communication model.

A communicator, or person who has a message to convey, must encode that message to a receiver or the person with whom the communicator wants to communicate. These roles alternate between the patient and paramedic throughout their interaction. The communicator must encode the message in a medium understood by both parties. This could be verbal, written, gestures, or any other medium as long as it is understood by all parties involved. Once the message is encoded, the receiver must decode the message and interpret its meaning. This process takes place hundreds, if not thousands, of times each day. Each time you hear, read, or receive some type of message, someone has communicated with you.

An important component of this process is feedback, which ensures that the intended message was received. Without this step communication does not occur easily. Feedback can be as simple as asking the patient a question to clarify a portion of his or her history to avoid miscommunication. During the feedback process the roles of the communicator and receiver may change, but the process of encoding and decoding must still occur. One example of using feedback is the patient who refuses care or transport. As you have learned, in this situation you must receive an informed refusal. Through the feedback component of communication, you ensure your patient truly understands the benefits of treatment and the risks of refusal.

Feedback helps avoid interference in the communication process that can lead to miscommunication. Interference can come from many sources and can occur during any phase of the communication process. This is the most common cause of miscommunication among people. For example, the message may have been encoded in a manner the receiver did not understand. The use of medical terms when speaking with patients would cause a failure of communication unless the patient is familiar with medical terminology. Alternatively, the interference may be a result of the medium used. A classic example of this is a language barrier.

Interference can be internal or external. External examples include a noisy environment, a patient who is not comfortable answering questions in a public area, and interference from family members or other providers on scene. Internal interference, or the preoccupations of the mind, occurs with both the patient and paramedic. Although it cannot be avoided, efforts should be taken to minimize these situations. Internal interference for the patient may include financial concerns, quality of life issues, fears of permanent disability or death, concerns about the impact of the event on the patient's family, and the patient's trust or mistrust of the quality of care being received. Each of these causes mental distractions that can have dramatic effects on the ability to fully decode the questions being asked. This can in turn lead to answers that unintentionally omit information that would be valuable to the paramedic.

Internal interference for the paramedic can be just as varied. It may depend on the type of shift you have had before the call. Is your mind occupied with a disagreement with your partner or supervisor? Is the last call bothering you? Interference does not have to be caused by factors outside the specific call you are on. As you interview and listen to your patient, you are also thinking of your next questions and making diagnostic, treatment, and transport decisions. Although this is part of the normal patient care process, it also causes a mental "split" among several things. This can lead to miscommunication because subtle information can be missed.

INTERNAL FACTORS FOR EFFECTIVE COMMUNICATION

[OBJECTIVES 3, 4]

To communicate effectively, the paramedic must be open to others without preexisting opinions or bias. The EMS profession is one of helping others, and genuine affection for other people is vital. Your affection for people may be tested during your career; however, personal feelings cannot cloud judgment, compassion, or treatment. The paramedic must understand that each person has individual strengths and weaknesses, and every human being is unique. For example, social skills, educational background, **customs** and **cultural beliefs,** and the ability to display and control emotions differ from person to person. Long before the first patient encounter, paramedics must realize that these individual, internal attributes can have a real (and sometimes negative) effect on the communication process between the paramedic and the patient.

preexisting opinions, bias

For example, paramedics may encounter a patient who abuses alcohol or drugs. Such a patient has the potential to invoke negative emotional responses from the paramedic such as anger, disgust, or apathy. These internal responses are derived from the following sources:

- *Personal beliefs.* "Alcoholics are lazy, weak, and a burden to society."
- *Personal experiences.* Perhaps the paramedic has family or friends with other addiction problems and knows firsthand the problems such diseases can create.
- *Educational and professional beliefs.* "Sure, I'll transport him to the hospital tonight, but we'll be right back here next week for the same thing. This is a waste of my time."

In effect, the paramedic has now labeled this patient as "a drunk" or "a druggie" and put an abrupt end to the communication process because a conclusion has already been reached. This leads to one of many traps of communication: labeling. Once a label has been applied to a patient, the communication process and any further investigation into the current situation have stopped. This mistake may lead to errors, such as failing to identify other causes of the condition—in this scenario, potentially missing the diagnosis of hypoglycemia by labeling the patient as "drunk."

Other situations stir the paramedic's emotions. For example, a paramedic may be faced with the necessity of treating a patient who has just harmed another, such as an intoxicated person in a motor vehicle crash who just killed a child in the other vehicle. As difficult as this situation is, the paramedic must put the personal emotions aside, at least temporarily, to provide appropriate and adequate care to the patient. Outlets are available after the call to discuss these negative emotions. Resources can include simply talking through the emotions with your partner, your supervisor, a mental health professional, or a member of the clergy.

Other internal factors can negatively affect the communication process. Personal relationship or financial troubles, personal illness, or bitterness toward a co-worker or company supervisor can be projected into the patient relationship or encounter. If a patient senses anger or hostility, for whatever reason, a relationship with the paramedic can be hampered. This can lead to miscommunication and an increased risk of errors.

PARAMEDIC*Pearl*

Only a small number of EMS calls provide the chance to save a life, but every patient encounter is a chance to provide compassionate care to an individual in need. Keep in mind that the frail, incontinent, and confused patient transported from a nursing home may be a Nobel Prize winner or a survivor of the Holocaust.

Every day before seeing his or her first patient, the successful paramedic takes a personal inventory of his or her own internal barriers to communication. If the paramedic is facing a negative personal social situation, those emotions must be left at home. He or she must be prepared to face the shift with empathy and respect toward each patient without projecting his or her own negative emotions into the process. If the paramedic encounters a patient with different customs or cultural beliefs, the paramedic must be open to these factors without dismissing them. If the paramedic has a personal illness that affects his or her ability to focus or perform tasks adequately, the paramedic must consider taking time off to recover. The adage "take care of yourself first, then the patient" certainly applies here.

Distinguishing between sympathy and empathy is an important tool in helping develop appropriate rapport with patients. **Empathy** can be defined as understanding the patient's experience of an illness; **sympathy** implies sharing the patient's feelings or emotional state in relation to the illness (Willett, 2005). An empathic statement such as "I could see how this chest pain would make you worried about having a heart attack" reveals to the patient that you can identify with him or her as another human being. Such mutual understanding allows the patient to feel comfortable revealing information to you and often helps improve patient satisfaction with the encounter.

Sympathetic statements, on the other hand, can at times be misconstrued by patients as insincere gestures of comfort. True sympathy is difficult to express unless you have personally experienced what the patient is encountering. However, even if you have experienced the same situation, always realize that every experience is unique to an individual. Although you may have also had a myocardial infarction, for example, your fears, thoughts, reactions, and acceptance may be quite different than your patient's. Patients may feel that your attempt at comforting them is insincere; sometimes asking the patient about his or her emotional response to the illness is a better choice to provide support. Providing empathic responses to patient concerns is an art that can only be learned with time, observation, and practice. Often a simple touch on the shoulder or a reassuring smile is enough to help a patient overcome fears and concerns.

EXTERNAL FACTORS FOR EFFECTIVE COMMUNICATION

[OBJECTIVE 3]

To obtain a good history, you must use the skill of **active listening.** Active listening can be defined as hearing the words that your patient is saying as well as paying attention to the significance of those words to the patient. Recognizing the impact of the patient's words means watching facial expressions and body language, picking up on cultural cues, and attempting to assess the patient's mental status. At the same time you must determine the reliability and accuracy of the history being provided. Becoming a skilled active listener requires focusing your mental energy on the words being heard as well as the way the words are being presented (Feldman & Christensen, 1997).

To improve your ability to be a good active listener, you must eliminate environmental barriers that may be a hindrance to communicating with your patient (Feldman & Christensen, 1997). Try to obtain the patient history in a calm, quiet setting. For example, if you are at a busy accident scene you may want to ask important history questions to meet urgent patient needs. Obtaining a detailed medical history is more appropriate after the patient has been loaded into the ambulance. This offers some privacy from the outside world. Although some questions must be asked in a public venue, make it a practice to repeat those questions in the ambulance. Comments such as "Now that we are alone I can tell you . . ." are not uncommon.

In addition to privacy issues, other environmental factors can impede effective communication. Examples of these situations include the effect of ambient lighting, multiple patients, dangerous conditions, a noisy environment, interference or reactions of family or bystanders, influences from other responders such as law enforcement personnel, and the weather. For example, if a patient is wet and cold, his or her only focus is on getting warm and dry, not on what is being asked. Controlling or removing all external factors is not always possible, but understanding their effects and using techniques to minimize these factors improves the communications process.

Make sure that you maintain good eye contact with your patient and try to stay at the same eye level. If you are towering over a patient, that patient is less likely to feel secure enough to provide information because you are being viewed in an authoritarian role. Bring yourself down to the patient's eye level; he or she will feel more comfortable talking to you. Being below the patient's eye level may be beneficial because it gives the patient a sense of control over his or her situation. This is especially beneficial in children and the elderly. Maintaining eye contact while speaking with the patient shows that you are interested in what the patient has to say. Always respect the patient's **personal space.** In Western cultures this space generally is 1.5 to 4 feet around the patient; intrusion into this space tends to cause discomfort. **Intimate space** is less than 1.5 feet. Obviously, entry into the personal space occurs during the course of patient care. However, the paramedic must be cognizant of the effects this could have on the patient's comfort and subsequent communication. The **social distance** in Western cultures is 4 to 12 feet around the patient and is comfortable for most people. However, attempting to perform a history or provide care from this distance gives the impression the paramedic is not invested in the patient's condition or outcome. The concept of eye contact and personal space varies among individuals and cultures. Addressing all the cultural variations in this text is impossible, so paramedics should be familiar with the cultural variations they are likely to encounter. Always be alert for clues of patient discomfort surrounding the amount of eye contact and appropriate distance when interacting with a patient. Avoid sunglasses when interviewing a patient because they interfere with eye contact and limit nonverbal clues to the patient; they also may give the impression the paramedic is hiding something.

How you present yourself makes a tremendous difference in the confidence your patient will have in you, your compassion, and your ability to provide care. Dressing in a professional manner and making sure that you are well groomed are essential. Maintain good body posture to ensure that patients believe you are interested in what they have to say. If you need to take notes during the interview, try to maintain as much eye contact as possible with the patient. Letting the patient know up front that you may be taking notes during the interview allows the patient to recognize the importance of keeping accurate records of his or her current state of health. Treat the patient with respect, as you would want to be treated, and you will not go wrong.

INTERVIEW PROCESS

[OBJECTIVES 5, 6]

The medical interview begins even before you speak directly with a patient. In most cases the nature of the emergency is conveyed to the paramedic from dispatchers who have taken the call. Important clues about the patient can be obtained, such as the chief medical complaint, the condition of the patient, and the status of the scene. This information allows the paramedic an opportunity to formulate a plan and have a framework with which to begin the communication process.

For example, if the nature of the call is a cardiac arrest, the paramedic already knows that the patient will not be able to communicate and that collection of information regarding the emergency usually will be brief, urgent, and involve other parties, such as family or bystanders. In multiple-patient situations a triage protocol may be needed to assess all patients rapidly and identify those in need of immediate care. On the other hand, if the patient's symptom is weakness, the paramedic may have the option of a more relaxed, open-ended interview involving detailed information gathering.

The next phase of communication is nonverbal—the immediate first impression the paramedic gathers entering the scene. What are the living conditions of the patient? How does the patient look? What is the emotional state of the patient—cooperative, anxious, threatening, tearful? Is the patient in distress—from a medical condition, circumstances of the emergency, pain? Are family members present? Processing these nonverbal cues allows the paramedic to choose the type of interview to conduct and the urgency of collecting further information.

While you assess the nonverbal information obtained from the patient, the patient's family and bystanders are formulating their initial impressions of you and other EMS personnel. If the siren was wailing all the way up the driveway, if radios are blaring, if mud was tracked into their home, or if you are unprofessionally dressed, the patient may have little confidence in your abilities and may not be trusting of your advice. On the other hand, if you are professionally dressed and respectful of being "invited" into the patient's home or personal space, the individual will usually trust you as a professional healthcare provider.

If the patient is conscious, is able to communicate effectively, and is not in a distressed condition either from the medical condition or the circumstances of the emergency, begin the interview by providing a greeting and an open-ended statement. When you first meet the patient, clearly state your name and role to the patient so he or she can begin to establish trust in your abilities. Address patients by their names. If the name is unknown, ask how the patient would prefer to be addressed. Inform the patient what part in the care you will provide. Let them know you are going to obtain a history, perform physical examination skills, and start basic therapy to assist the patient until arrival at the hospital. A good way to begin would be to offer a handshake and say "Hello, sir, my name is Todd, and I am a paramedic here to help you. How can we be of service today (Figure 15-1)?" Such an opening statement denotes a level of respect for the patient and identifies the paramedic as the person in charge. Asking an open-ended question allows the patient

the opportunity to respond freely. Try not to use statements with negative connotations during the introduction. For example, questions such as "What is wrong today?" "What is your complaint today?" or "What is the problem today?" can cast a negative shadow over the entire communication process.

When starting to take the medical history, ask multiple open-ended questions to allow patients to tell their stories in their own words. **Open-ended questions** do not require a yes or no answer. Examples of open-ended questions include the following:

- What can I help you with today?
- What symptoms are you experiencing?

Asking several open-ended questions up front allows the patient to have some control regarding how the encounter will proceed. You are usually able to obtain valuable information from the patient when he or she is allowed to answer questions independently.

Once you have obtained enough basic information and need to obtain more specific details about the patient's symptoms, direct, or closed-ended, questions become important. **Direct questions** can be answered with short responses, such as "yes" or "no." Examples of direct questions include the following:

- Are you experiencing any nausea?
- Did the symptoms get worse this morning?
- Are you allergic to any medications?
- Is the pain located on the right or left side?

Ensure that your questions do not lead the patient toward making a certain response. An example of such a leading question would be, "You are not experiencing any chest pain, are you?" The patient is less likely to answer

Conscious pt.
Greet pt., ask name
Explain paramedic role to pt.
Use open-ended questions
    encourage use of pt.
    own words
Use direct question to clarify

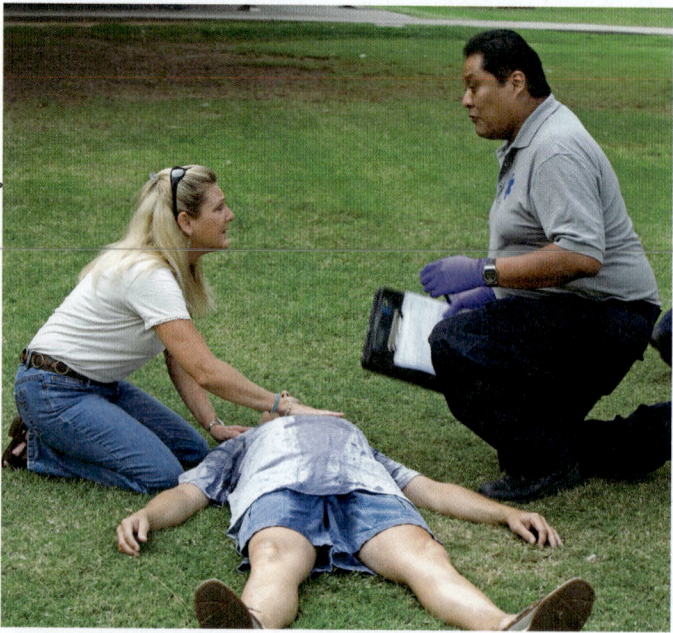

Figure 15-1 Unless circumstances dictate otherwise, most patient interviews should begin with the paramedic providing a greeting and a statement such as "Hello, my name is Todd. I am a paramedic here to help you. How can we be of service today?"

your question honestly because you are implying that chest pain is "wrong" by the way the question was posed.

Open-ended questions encourage patients to talk and provide more general information. They also give patients an opportunity to discuss all information they believe to be relevant to the situation in their own words and at their own pace (Seidel et al., 2006).

Medical interviewers frequently make the mistake of interrupting the patient immediately after asking the first open-ended question. This can lead to tunnel vision because the first symptom that the patient states may not be the most important. Furthermore, other issues may not be obtained if the paramedic focuses on the patient's first words. Finally, when you interrupt the patient, he or she may assume that you have the information you need and may not share something that would be relevant because of this belief. Be sure to ask one question at a time. When simultaneously faced with multiple questions patients often feel overwhelmed or do not know which question to answer. As a result, they may give incomplete answers. Other sources of interruption include family or bystanders taking over the role of answering questions and side conversations with a partner. These situations interfere with the ability of the patient to tell the story of the illness and give the patient the impression that what he or she has to say is not important.

As the paramedic begins to gather information from the patient, he or she needs to narrow the scope of the questions gradually to focus on the problem. This is when the transition to closed-ended questions becomes more useful. For example:

Paramedic: "Hello, sir, my name is Todd, and I'm a paramedic with County Ambulance. How can we help you today?"
Patient: "I called because I'm having chest pain."
Paramedic: "Sir, you say you are having chest pain. Please tell us more about the pain."
Patient: "I don't know, it feels like a weight on my chest, right here in the middle. I get heartburn a lot, but this feels different. And I feel short of breath, too."

Paramedic: "Ok, sir, how long have you been having this pain?"

The open ended-question discovered several useful clues regarding the cause of the patient's pain. The closed-ended question narrowed down the details of the patient's symptoms.

Ultimately, the goal is to obtain a thorough, detailed history, including past medical problems, medications being taken, allergies, and important details of the social or family history relevant to the chief complaint.

Performing other tasks while the interview is being obtained is reasonable and efficient (Figure 15-2). While the interviewer continues the discussion with the patient, other EMS personnel can and should begin assessment and treatment of the patient. Informing the patient of this plan usually helps, such as saying "Mr. Brown, this is my partner, Susan. While you and I continue talking, Susan will need to check your blood pressure and pulse and attach a cardiac monitor."

At the end of the interview, a useful technique is to summarize briefly what was learned from the patient and allow him or her a chance to add any other details not discussed (Maguire & Pitceathly, 2002). For example:

Paramedic: "So Mr. Brown, you called us because you are having chest pain, which I understand started 1 hour ago while you were making dinner. You described this pain as a weight in the middle of your chest, and you have never felt this way before. You mentioned you felt a little short of breath and nauseated. Your pain goes into your left arm. Did I get this information correct? Do you want to add anything else?"

Sometimes the circumstances of the emergency or the patient's condition does not allow a structured, detailed interview. The paramedic should identify people on the scene who can answer questions and provide information. These resources often include a family member. If the scene is unsafe or unstable, remove the patient from the scene before beginning the interview.

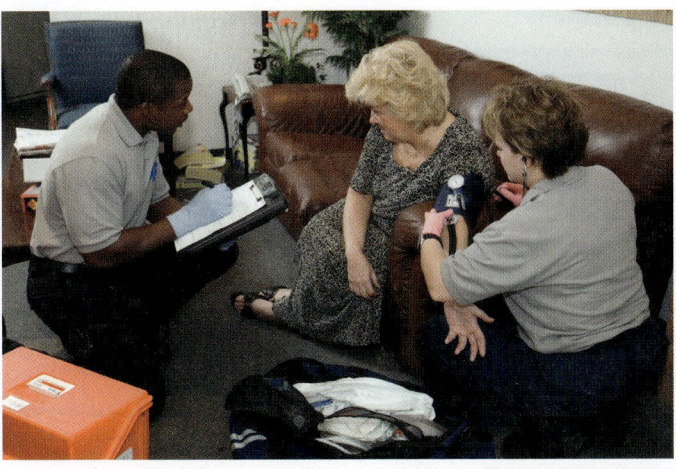

Figure 15-2 Performing other tasks while conducting the interview is reasonable and efficient.

Case Scenario—continued

As you ask the fire personnel to return to your unit to get the stretcher and prepare it for patient transport, one of them informs you that they have encountered this patient before. The fire responder quietly tells you that she always calls for the same problem: "sick." Her nonverbal signals suggest that she doubts how "sick" the patient actually is. As you begin, your patient reports that she's "sick," and has been for many years. She has had two knee replacements that make getting up and down the steps to her apartment difficult. She also requires dialysis twice each week. She is frustrated by the inaccessibility of her dialysis physician, whom she says she can "never" talk to, and states that she would never contact her if she had an emergency "like this." As you attempt to get more information about today's emergency, one of her daughters speaks to her mother in Spanish, then tells you that she is "weak and having trouble breathing—very sick." When you attempt to determine what medications the patient is taking she reports "too many, I don't know their names."

Questions

5. *What barriers to communications exist in this case? What strategies can you use to reduce them?*

6. *One of the daughters seems quite willing to speak on her mother's behalf. Is that the best communication strategy in this case? Why or why not? If you choose to use this method, how can you ensure that you get correct information?*

7. *How can you learn more about the patient's medication history?*

CONTINUING THE INTERVIEW

[OBJECTIVE 7]

Your goal is to obtain the needed medical information in an efficient manner so you can establish priorities of treatment. Directive questions often are used to help continue the patient's story. **Facilitation** can be defined as the use of questions or phrases to allow the patient to continue to tell the story. Essentially, you are facilitating the flow of the interview by using phrases such as the following: "Tell me more about your stomach pain," and "I understand; go on. I'm listening."

Reflection can be defined as repeating words or phrases that the patient stated to allow the patient to continue to talk about that particular concern. For example, a patient may tell you that he or she has had pain in the stomach. Your response to the patient would be "Your stomach?" to encourage the patient to continue to describe the pain in his or her own words. At times you may not understand what a patient is trying to convey. **Clarification,** defined as using a phrase or question in an attempt to clarify any ambiguous statements or words, may be important. An example of clarification is a statement such as "I don't know what you mean by pain in your stomach. Could you please be more specific?"

Understanding how the patient's medical problems affect daily life is vital to have complete understanding of his or her needs. At times, **confrontation,** or using statements to address the patient about his or her feelings, is useful to help figure out how the patient is being affected by medical issues. An example of confrontation is "You appear to be anxious." Going further, **interpretation** infers how the patient may be feeling. A statement such as "I could see how this problem would make you feel frustrated" is an example of interpretation. Picking up on the patient's nonverbal and verbal cues may give you an idea of how the patient is responding to the medical problem. Stating what emotions you observe or identifying how someone would typically respond to a medical problem may give you some insight into how the patient actually feels; such understanding helps develop trust and mutual respect between you and your patient.

As previously described, empathy, or empathic responses, acknowledge patients' feelings and let them know those feelings are acceptable. These responses are important in building a relationship in which the patient believes you can be trusted. When a patient's feelings are recognized and accepted, trust in you is built and the patient provides more in-depth and sometimes personal information without fear of being judged. A patient involved in a motor vehicle accident may be visibly upset while telling you how she saw the tree coming at her and there was nothing she could do. A response of "That must have been very scary for you" lets her know her feelings are acceptable and allows her to continue her description.

CLOSING THE INTERVIEW

Once you have obtained the history from the patient, summarize the information to check for accuracy and see if any information was overlooked. Briefly restate the information the patient has provided; you may choose to do several **summarizations** as you progress through the history or one longer summarization at the end. This often allows you to clarify any ambiguous information and ensure that you did not misunderstand anything the patient may have said. A good question to ask at the end of a summarization is "Is there any information that I did not understand or that I left out?" Summarization may remind the patient to tell you something important to his or her current health status that was not previously mentioned.

Once the history has been obtained, talk with the patient to determine a treatment plan (Feldman & Christensen, 1997). Patients often ask what is wrong with them. If you are reasonably sure you understand the pathophysiology behind the patient's problem, state what procedures or treatments you will provide until the patient arrives at the hospital. Include the patient as much as possible in the decision-making process so he or she will understand what is going to happen and still have some level of control in the situation. Never guess about the patient's condition or provide information that is not accurate. If you are unsure of an answer to a question, inform the patient that you are unsure and will try to make certain someone else addresses his or her concerns. Avoid answers such as "I don't know" because they will cause the patient to question your confidence and wonder if they are receiving quality care. Frequently reassess the patient and ask questions to monitor progress en route to the emergency department; how the patient responds to interventions is a critical piece of the medical history that the medical team needs to know.

NONVERBAL SKILLS

[OBJECTIVE 5]

In addition to verbal techniques used to gather information from a patient, many **nonverbal cues** give useful clues about his or her condition. For example, a patient who exhibits loud, angry, threatening behaviors will be treated much differently than the quiet, sitting, cooperative patient. A patient who sits with arms crossed and answers only one or two words at a time will be more challenging to interview than the patient who looks relaxed and openly and freely enters into conversation.

In a potentially hostile or violent patient, nonverbal cues to be alert for include clenched fists, upright or standing position, pacing, angry facial expression, and tense posture. In a sad or depressed patient, nonverbal cues include tearfulness, withdrawal, quiet tone of voice, and possibly a disheveled appearance. The patient's clothing also can give important information. If the patient is dressed inappropriately for the situation, evaluate why. For example, someone who is wearing a heavy winter coat with shorts on or plaids and stripes together may have an alternative fashion style, but he or she may also have an underlying psychiatric disorder or organic brain syndrome that needs to be considered both for treatment and the manner in which your conversation is conducted.

Just as patients can provide nonverbal cues to their underlying condition, paramedics also bring their own nonverbal skills to the interview. Poor eye contact, crossed arms, rolling eyes, sideways glances at a partner, a standing position, frequent checking of a watch or answering of a cell phone, and shifts in weight from foot to foot can give signals of impatience, indifference, or even boredom. A clean and neat appearance, including a well-kept uniform, conveys a sense of trust and professionalism to the patient.

A good use of nonverbal skills from the paramedic is to sit near the patient at eye level. Maintaining eye contact, keeping arms open, and even assuming a slightly leaned-in position show interest and help keep the patient engaged in the communication process (Maguire & Pitceathly, 2002). When appropriate, physical contact is personal and useful, from shaking hands with the patient to even putting an arm around the patient's shoulders in a gesture of comfort or condolence (Figures 15-3 and 15-4).

CULTURAL *Considerations*

A person's culture can influence the interpretation of verbal and nonverbal communication. For example, several cultures generally prefer to avoid eye contact. Middle Easterners avoid eye contact between men and women out of politeness. Filipinos and Koreans may be insulted if an index finger is used to summon them. Middle Easterners may be insulted if the left hand is used to greet them or hand them something. (In their culture, the left hand is used only for toileting functions.) Many Southeast Asians find viewing the sole of the foot (and by extension the bottom of the shoe) to be insulting because they consider the foot the dirtiest part of the body. Pointing of the foot also is considered offensive by some. In general, sit with your back straight, feet on the ground, with your head and chest turned toward the person with whom you are speaking.

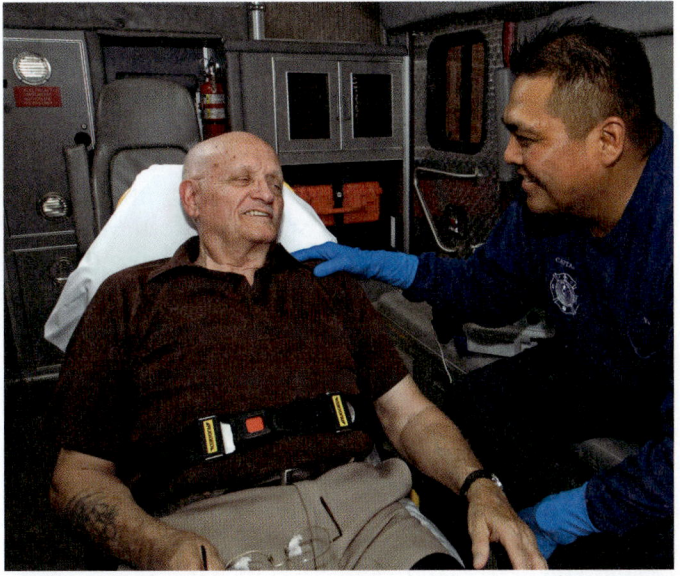

Figure 15-3 Nonverbal cues can express more than what is said with words.

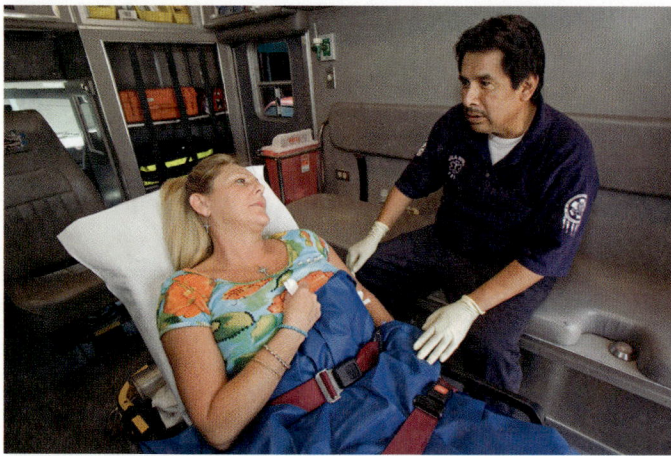

Figure 15-4 Simple gestures can go a long way to building trust with a patient.

TRAPS OF INTERVIEWING

[OBJECTIVE 8]

Several pitfalls may be encountered during the interview process that can lead to inaccurate assessment and treatment errors.

Patronizing Terms of Endearment

Although often done with good intentions, the use of terms such as "dearie," "sweetie," "pal," or "buddy" can be condescending and are signs of disrespect. Addressing an older patient by a first name can have the same effect. A more formal approach, such as Mr. or Ms., can help portray a sense of respect.

Complicated Medical Terms

Avoid using complicated medical terms when discussing care with a patient. Most patients will not know the meanings of these terms. Communication will be more effective if you do not use medical terminology. For example, talk in terms of a "heart attack" rather than a "myocardial infarction," or a "stroke" instead of a "cerebrovascular accident." Knowing the local terminology that your patients are likely to use for specific complaints is important.

Labeling

Labeling is the application of a derogatory term to a patient on the basis of an event, habit, or personality trait and may not be accurate about the underlying condition. As previously noted, labeling someone a "drunk" because of a history of alcohol abuse may lead the paramedic to stop looking for other causes of acute altered mental status, such as hypoglycemia.

Stereotyping

Stereotyping is the attribution of some trait or characteristic to a person on the basis of the interviewer's preconceived notions about a general class of people with similar characteristics. Such a mistake can occur when assuming a distressed or upset patient of a certain ethnicity is behaving in a particular way because "all people of the same ethnicity act that way" in similar situations.

Impatience and Interrupting

If the paramedic has a premature or preconceived **explanation** for the patient's symptoms, the interview may become rushed because he or she has already reached a conclusion. The paramedic may even be tempted to force the questioning to lead to that conclusion.

Allow the patient to provide as much information as possible. The paramedic sometimes takes over the conversation after only a few seconds. For example, once the patient states the symptom is abdominal pain, the paramedic has a series of questions to ask to gain information specific to that complaint. The result is that the patient believes the paramedic has all the information needed and does not feel compelled to offer more information other than cursory responses to questions being directly asked. By allowing the patient time to tell his or her story, the paramedic often gains the same information while affirming to the patient that what he or she has to say is important and valuable.

Another common scenario in which someone other than the patient dominates the conversation is the family member or bystander who answers every question for the patient. Although these individuals can provide important information, the paramedic must ensure the patient is allowed to provide answers whenever possible; after all no one knows better how the patient feels than the patient.

Previous Diagnosis

When confronted with a patient with symptoms of a certain condition that has already been diagnosed, falling into the trap of believing that the current symptom "is more of the same" is easy. For example, assuming that a patient with difficulty breathing and a history of emphysema must be having a worsening of the underlying illness is a simple, but possibly incorrect, conclusion. Other causes of difficulty breathing, such as a heart attack, pneumonia, pneumothorax, or pulmonary embolus can be missed easily.

Failing to Consider Other Sources of Information

[OBJECTIVE 9]

The person who summons help to the scene often is not the patient. Family members, bystanders, law enforcement personnel, or even the patient's physician may have called EMS on behalf of the patient. These other parties can be valuable sources of information regarding the patient. When using alternative sources of information, consider the source, however. Only the patient can truly describe what he or she is feeling or experiencing. Information gained from others will be based on their thoughts, experiences, biases, and needs, not the patient's. This often is done unknowingly by the individual, but the paramedic must understand this tendency of third parties to frame the information they provide. When interviewing others the paramedic also must look for clues of the quality of the relationship between the patient and the individual giving the information. Indications of a good relationship lend credibility to the information being given, whereas clues of a bad relationship may bring the information into question.

Discrimination

Discrimination is the act of treating someone differently because he or she is part of a specific group.

Providing False Assurance

Patients are often able to comprehend the severity of their illness or injury. Falsely assuring a patient that nothing is wrong, or things will be fine, often is detrimental to the provider-patient relationship because the patient may know better and feel patronized. This can lead to questions about the honesty or competency of the paramedic. If patients have doubts in either of these areas, they are unlikely to provide complete information or answers to the questions you ask.

Avoidance

Emergency responses often involve situations in which uncomfortable subjects must be addressed. In this situation it is human nature to avoid the particular topic, and this often is done subconsciously through word choice, body language, or facial expressions. Doing so expresses disinterest in what the patient has to say and discourages the patient from providing what may be the exact information you need to treat the condition correctly. If you find yourself in a situation where you are uncomfortable but the information is relevant to patient care, you must make sure you do not use avoidance techniques. Through experience you will become more comfortable discussing a variety of topics.

Sensitive Topics

Although similar to avoidance, sensitive topics are those with which the patient and/or the paramedic are uncomfortable, such as alcohol use or abuse, physical abuse, or sexual history. Questions regarding sensitive topics should be worked into the conversation as any other question

would. Patients are often accustomed to answering the specific questions from prior interactions with medical personnel. The more comfortable you appear when asking the question, the more comfortable the patient will be answering it.

"Why" Questions

"Why" questions can provide valuable information, but they often are interpreted as a challenge. Many times patients feel as if they must justify what they are feeling or what they have done to try to treat their illness or injury. Asking several why questions in a row results in an interrogation rather than a conversation and may result in the patient becoming defensive. People who are defensive often will not provide in-depth information because they fear having to provide further justification for their statements. These types of questions should be used sparingly and spaced well apart from each other.

Giving Advice

Providing advice to a patient may be beneficial or destructive. In many situations the patient may have initiated an EMS response and is looking for advice. These calls often begin with the patient stating something to the effect of "I am sorry I called, but I was not sure what to do." In these instances the advice is welcome and expected. On the other hand, unsolicited advice can be seen as lecturing or badgering. This can lead to the patient feeling defensive, just as "why" questions do, and have the same negative effect on communication.

DEVELOPING PATIENT RAPPORT

[OBJECTIVE 10]

A paramedic can sabotage the interview process in many ways. The successful paramedic remembers to inventory his or her own emotional and physical condition before the patient encounter, identify nonverbal cues from the patient and provider, minimize the influence of negative external factors that present barriers to communication, treat the patient with respect, and ask open-ended questions (Greene, 1996).

Sometimes the greatest challenge is to gain the patient's trust. This can be done by developing a good rapport with the patient. If the patient seems hesitant to talk or be transported to the hospital even when the medical condition is serious, the first goal of the paramedic is to state simply, and with genuine concern, that the paramedic is there to help and ensure the patient is given the best possible medical care.

Simple gestures can go a long way to building trust with a patient. If the patient is cold, providing a warm blanket is a kind gesture that can promote trust. If the scene is in a public place, taking the patient to a private location also shows respect and promotes good rapport.

Removing the patient from an unsafe or hostile environment serves the same purpose.

Understanding a patient's objections also can help build rapport. Patients may not want medical assistance for a variety of reasons, including the following:

- Fear—of hospitals, losing decision-making ability, or dying.
- Financial concerns—how is he or she possibly going to pay for all this?
- Religious beliefs—"God will take care of me."
- Legal or social concerns—what if an employer finds out that drugs were involved in this accident?
- Seemingly simple concerns—"Who will take care of my pets if I am in the hospital?"

Simply asking the patient, "Why don't you want to go to the hospital when you are clearly having trouble breathing?" and enlisting the help of family, friends, clergy, or neighbors to address these concerns can identify and remove some of these obstacles.

Finally, continue to communicate with the patient during the entire encounter. Telling the patient what is going to happen, and why, improves the level of trust between the patient and the EMS professional. For example, if the treatment plan includes starting an intravenous line, giving medications, and transporting to the hospital, the plan should be carefully explained to the patient before starting the actual procedures.

STRATEGIES TO GET PATIENT INFORMATION

[OBJECTIVE 11]

In some situations the information available from the patient may be incomplete or inaccurate. For example, getting an adequate history of possible loss of consciousness or suspected syncope from the patient alone is impossible. No patient is able to confirm whether he or she lost consciousness or provide vital information related to the period of suspected loss of consciousness (including whether a true loss of consciousness or seizure activity occurred, or the duration of the unresponsiveness). A number of other sources of information are available to the paramedic to gather more details about the patient. Some of these resources include the following:

- *The person who activated the EMS system.* Someone else initiated the call for help if the patient did not. What did that person see? Why did he or she make the call? What was the concern?
- *First responders on the scene.* In many situations, the first providers of prehospital emergency care on the scene may be volunteers, EMTs, law enforcement personnel, lifeguards, or other individuals with varying levels of EMS training. As the advanced life support provider, the paramedic must obtain a report from these other responders on the scene. This is important to gain an understanding of how the patient was doing on contact with the first responder and what treatment was given before the arrival of advanced life support. This may have an effect on subsequent treatment provided by the paramedic. Often a verbal report from the first responder(s) is given to the arriving paramedic. The paramedic is responsible for acknowledging this report and including these details in the medical care record.

- *Family or spouse.* Other family members present usually have good information about the patient's condition, history of the present illness, and medical history. An important detail in critically ill patients may be a living will or "do not resuscitate" directives.

- *Bystanders.* People who witnessed the event may give useful clues about a patient's condition. EMS personnel have a unique opportunity to obtain critical information from these individuals. Bystanders generally do not accompany the patient to the hospital. Bystanders may have left the scene before the emergency department physician needs to contact them for more information. Therefore, especially in situations of suspected loss of consciousness, the paramedic should carefully obtain the critical information from the individuals present when the illness or injury occurred.

- *Medication bottles.* If medication bottles are handy, the prescribed medications can give clues about the patient's medical problems. In addition, the physician who prescribed the medication, which must be printed on every medication label, may be available by telephone for more information.

- *Medical identification bracelets and other personal information.* Many patients with chronic medical conditions, allergies, or implanted medical devices wear a medical identification bracelet or necklace indicating this information to healthcare providers. Sometimes this information can be found in the patient's wallet or other personal belongings. If possible, search through these items, optimally with the assistance of law enforcement personnel. In some states, specific EMS "do not resuscitate" (DNR) bracelets, necklaces, or wallet cards exist. Every paramedic should know his or her state's law regarding the ability to honor DNR orders. They may only be able to honor certain "official" bracelets or other indicators of prehospital DNR status.

Case Scenario CONCLUSION

The fire personnel return with the stretcher and begin moving equipment and furniture in preparation for patient transport. Your partner and one of the fire personnel begin a conversation with one of the daughters while you try to complete your interview and patient assessment. The patient's attention again departs as she abruptly (although shakily) gets to her feet and moves toward her daughter and the fire personnel to better hear what is being said. You abandon further conversation and work with the remainder of the team to secure the patient on the stretcher in preparation for transport to the hospital.

Looking Back

8. *How might you have handled the return of the fire personnel and preparation for transport to better maintain communication with the patient?*

9. *What are your communication priorities for this patient after you arrive in the ambulance and before you depart for the hospital?*

10. *Interpreters are frequently useful in evaluating patients who have limited or no fluency in English. What steps should be taken to ensure the accuracy of translated information?*

METHODS TO ASSESS MENTAL STATUS DURING THE INTERVIEW

Effective communication with a patient requires that the patient understand the questions from the paramedic and respond with appropriate answers. Some situations can cause the paramedic to question the patient's capacity for meaningful communication. This can be caused by the patient's underlying medical condition or other barriers, such as speaking a different language or dealing with a mentally challenged patient.

One technique that is useful in the beginning of the interview process is to ask some simple demographic information questions, such as name, date of birth, and address. Persons with diminished mental capacity or an altered mental status will not be able to comply. If the patient's mental status appears to be altered, you may need to stop the interview process and perform a brief mental status examination. One method is to determine whether the patient is oriented to person, place, time, and event. Does the patient know his or her name, the current location, the day and/or date, and details of the event? If the patient cannot provide correct answers, use other sources for patient information.

Another tool to gauge mental status is simply to ask the patient whether he or she understands the information just presented. Have the patient repeat instructions or summarize the paramedic's information to determine if the information was processed and comprehended. This tool assesses the patient's thought process, attention span, concentration, and comprehension. Assessing the patient's memory of both long-term and short-term events, as well as observing the patient's, affect can also provide valuable information regarding mental status.

SPECIAL INTERVIEW SITUATIONS

[OBJECTIVE 12]

Silence

Patients may be silent during your encounter for a number of reasons, including fear of medical care, embarrassment, avoidance of legal prosecution, or medical or psychiatric conditions that prohibit the patient from communicating at a functional level. You should ensure that the patient understands your questions and a communication barrier does not exist, such as a language barrier, the inability to hear, or the inability to understand the terms you are using. At times silence may be a useful adjunct to allow a patient to continue telling the story in his or her own words; allowing brief periods of silence without having a prolonged interruption in the flow of your interview often results in the patient continuing to talk. Patients may be silent because they are thinking of the best way to tell you what is on their mind or trying to remember details about a question you may have asked. The patient may be deciding whether to trust you with personal details of his or her current medical condition. At times patients become quiet if they are upset over the way they are being treated or sensitive questions you may have asked. In these circumstances, asking the patient if anything you may have said is bothering or upsetting may be appropriate to help establish better rapport. When needed, the paramedic may have to identify other sources of information, ensure privacy for the patient during the interview process, and assure the patient that the paramedic is not there to harm, but to help.

In addition, some patients may appear unmotivated to talk but in fact *cannot* talk because of an underlying medical condition such as a stroke. Despite the inability or lack of desire to communicate verbally, these patients still can understand and comprehend. The paramedic must not stop communicating directly with them. Closed-ended questions, allowing the patient to respond "yes" or "no" either verbally or by moving the head, may allow the paramedic to gather important information.

Overly Talkative Patient

The overly talkative patient can be more difficult than a silent patient. Because the amount of time you have with the patient is limited, you must be able to get as much useful information as possible. Allowing the patient to talk initially may be useful to help determine what issues must be addressed most urgently. Once you have an idea of what must be addressed, ask more directive questions or summarize what you have been told to limit the patient's responses to your questions. Although you do not want to interrupt the patient, you may have to refocus the patient frequently on what you need to accomplish. You may have to lower your expectations somewhat, accepting a less-than-perfect summary of the history given the time allowed. Frequently summarizing and checking conveys to the patient that you are listening to what he or she is saying, ultimately giving you more control over the interview.

Hostile Patients

When faced with a hostile patient, the prime concern for EMS providers is of course personal safety. Law enforcement personnel must be present before confronting a hostile patient. Once personal safety has been ensured, the next step is to try to de-escalate the situation. The potential sources of stress on scene contributing to the patient's hostility should be identified. If a family argument has occurred, have law enforcement personnel remove the patient or bystanders from the scene. An exit, such as an open doorway, should always be closest to the EMS provider (the patient ideally should not feel cornered and have an exit available as well).

Patients may be angry or upset for a number of reasons; they may be angry at their current medical condition if it has been recently diagnosed or unsuccessfully treated. They may have been in an altercation or be intoxicated and in trouble with the law. Perhaps they are having issues with a significant other or are being physically or verbally abused. Unfortunately, these feelings of anger often get displaced toward the healthcare provider. If you encounter a patient who is angry, try to find out why he or she is so upset. Use a kind, calm, professional demeanor in your interactions with the patient, maintaining eye contact at all times. Resist your temptation to get angry in return, and ensure your actions do not escalate this situation. Acknowledge the patient's apparent emotion, such as "I can see you are very upset, and I would like to help." Taking the extra time to find out what has made the patient so upset often allows the patient to trust in your care and eventually calm down.

Limited Intelligence

Patients with limited intelligence are often overlooked when obtaining information about current state of health. Although you may need to rely on caregivers for some information, include the patient in the interaction as much as possible. You may be surprised how much the patient is able to contribute. Also recall that illiteracy is common and often unrecognized in society. If the patient seems to have problems reading instructions or filling out needed paperwork, ask about level of education and provide assistance as needed. Patients often are embarrassed to tell healthcare providers that they are unable to read or write. These are the same patients who may be labeled as noncompliant with patient instructions; alternative ways of providing instructions, perhaps by using pictures, may allow these patients greater independence in meeting their own healthcare needs.

Children

Interviewing children can pose its own unique set of challenges. The paramedic's knowledge of normal developmental stages will be of tremendous help with these patients, because you will be able to use age-appropriate communication techniques. For example, preschoolers are rooted in the present and will not be able to understand future events such as "we will be going to the hospital." On the other hand, school-age children are able to understand the concepts of past, present, and future, but their timelines often are distorted. Be cautious with terms that could be misunderstood. For example, the phrase "taking a pulse" may indicate to the child you are going to take something and not return it. It would be better to say "check a pulse" or "count a pulse."

Remember that when you are dealing with children you are really dealing with two patients, the child and the parent(s), and rapport must be established with each. To help establish a rapport, be sure to use the child's name and the parent's title. The interview begins with both the child and the parent. If the child is younger than 6 years the parent is the primary focus of the interview, but not to the exclusion of the child because he or she can add some information, especially in relation to physical feelings and sensations. In this situation the paramedic must be aware that the history is from the parent's point of view and that the parent needs to feel as though he or she is doing a good job. Avoid phrasing questions in a manner that could put the parent on the defensive, such as repetitive "why" questions.

When speaking with children, approach them slowly and at eye level so as not to be intimidating, and use a calm, quiet voice. If appropriate for the child's age, toys or other security items can be helpful. Although the interview begins with both the parents and the child, depending on the child's age interviewing each party alone may be beneficial. This is especially true for children older than 6 years because they can add their own perspective and concerns to the history and can more accurately describe signs and symptoms. This is particularly important if you believe the child is withholding information because of the presence of a parent.

Adolescents have a variety of reasons for seeking healthcare that may be initiated by themselves or by a parent. Determining who initiated the EMS response can provide important clues to the adolescent's perspective of the need for healthcare. This population responds better to those who treat them as people rather than cases. As a result, they should be interviewed without their parents when possible. Because of their stage of development the reflexive self-concept is a large component of their thought process. For this reason communication techniques such as reflection, confrontation, and silence should be avoided.

Elderly Patients

Elderly patients can have conditions that lead to permanent cognitive dysfunction, such as dementia. Obtaining information from these patients can be difficult. Medical records, family members, and the patient's personal physician often are needed to gather necessary medical information. Physical changes are part of the normal aging process. These natural changes include narrowing of the visual field, hearing loss starting in the higher frequency ranges, and diminished visual acuity. When communicating with elderly patients the paramedic should be at eye level in front of the patient to ensure being within the patient's visual field. Speak slowly and distinctly in a low voice, as needed. However, note that not all older persons hearing impaired, so avoid the temptation of speaking loudly simply because the patient is elderly. If the patient uses assistive aids for communication, such as a hearing aid or glasses, make every effort to locate the device.

In addition to visual and auditory deficits, other challenges to communication must be considered when speaking with the elderly patient. As patients age, their response time to questions will be slower. To receive accurate information the paramedic must be patient and allow the patient enough time to answer questions completely; prematurely interrupting may stop the patient from giving you necessary information. Elderly patients may downplay or deny symptoms they are experiencing for several reasons. They may simply attribute them to the aging process and not think they are relevant. Taking multiple medications may mask symptoms, or the patient may be concerned about the financial impact of medical care or loss of independence. Finally, many elderly patients believe that patients go to hospitals to die. They may know of many friends and family members who were transported to a hospital and never returned home, which can result in denying symptoms to avoid transport. Any indication that the patient is not completely forthcoming with the entire history should prompt further exploration. Facilitation and confrontation are especially useful in these situations.

Cultural Considerations

Cultural differences include cultural beliefs, foreign languages, colloquialisms, and rules of personal interaction and communication and can present some obstacles to communication. Both the paramedic and the patient bring these to a patient-provider relationship, and their effect must be recognized. When introducing yourself to any patient you should state your name as you wish to be addressed and ask your patient for the same information. This is particularly important with patients from other cultures because using the wrong method of addressing them could be offensive.

As previously mentioned, paramedics should make every effort to become familiar with the cultural aspects of patients they are likely to come in contact with in their communities. Some cultures expect healthcare workers to have all the answers to their questions and illnesses. They may heavily involve family members in the interview, possibly to the point that the patient will not answer questions. The role of handshaking and/or physical contact, eye contact, and personal space, as discussed earlier, and the use of nontraditional treatments for injury and illness may be factors you will have to handle. **Ethnocentrism** and **cultural imposition** should never play a role in the relationship with and care of the patient. Paramedics must be respectful of cultural differences while also explaining the importance of communicating directly with the patient and clarifying unusual responses (Seidel et al., 2006). If confusion arises from what the paramedic says, rephrasing the questions may be necessary.

Language Barriers

Language barriers are often associated with patients of different cultures. Speaking a different language from your patient can be one of the most frustrating situations in medicine. Your ability to gain information to treat your patient is hampered until a common medium of communication is found. Several bilingual questionnaires are available that can be used for this purpose in which questions are written in the language of the paramedic and the patient. Part of the questionnaire includes responses written in the same manner. The paramedic can simply point to the question and the patient can then point to the appropriate response. Other possibilities include telephone translation services in which each party speaks to an interpreter over the phone. Whenever possible, however, you should use a trained medical interpreter who is familiar with the terms and general process used in patient-practitioner communications. It is imperative, however, that the paramedic remember that a few broken words from a patient is inadequate information on which to base treatment, and a better method of communication must be found.

Hearing-Impaired Patients

Much like a language barrier, communicating with a deaf or hearing-impaired patient can prove to be a challenge. The one advantage over a language barrier is that in this case usually both the paramedic and the patient have the same language base; the only difference is the method of expression. Depending on the age of onset of a hearing impairment and the degree of residual hearing the patient has, each patient will have a preferred method of communication. The paramedic should determine what this is and use that method with the patient.

Although many ways of communicating with the deaf or hearing-impaired patient exist, the following general concepts apply to all interactions. Do not raise your voice unless the patient asks you to do so. Depending on the severity of the hearing loss the patient will not hear you anyway or will only hear incomprehensible noise. Visual contact is highly important in deaf culture and should be maintained at all times. Be aware of the importance of light to this population. Events associated with hearing, such as the ringing of a telephone or doorbell, are represented by lights from specialized equipment. Therefore these individuals tend to be sensitive to flashing lights. The emergency lighting of an ambulance or other emergency vehicles on scene can be distracting.

Common methods of communication include sign language, gestures, writing, and lip reading. The method used should be the one that is most effective in each particular situation.

Sign Language

Not all deaf and hearing-impaired patients use sign language. However, if the patient does use it this will most likely be his or her preferred method of communication. If you know sign language, no matter how little, you should attempt to use it if the patient prefers. Even if you are not able to complete the entire conversation with sign language, you can supplement it with another method.

Gestures

Gestures can be an effective communication method when sign language is not known by both parties. Although gestures are not an element of sign language, you often will find that the gesture you use is the correct sign for what you are trying to say. Gestures also may be effective because deaf individuals are much more used to communicating with hearing individuals than hearing

individuals are with deaf individuals. More often than not, it will be easier for the patient to understand the paramedic than for the paramedic to understand the patient.

Writing

Writing is often the best option for clear, effective communication. Although this method may be more time intensive, it eliminates any error or miscommunication that may result from poorly understood gestures or sign language.

Lip Reading

Because lip reading is the least effective method of communication, it should be the last choice when speaking with a deaf or hearing-impaired patient. Lip reading is an acquired skill that takes considerable practice to develop. Contrary to popular belief, many deaf individuals do not use lip reading on a regular basis because they may primarily interact with the deaf community; therefore do not assume that because a patient is deaf he or she is a skilled lip reader. If you are faced with a situation in which lip reading is your only option for communication, be sure both parties look directly at each other and neither person looks directly into a bright light. Remove any objects from your mouth and be sure nothing covers your mouth. Speak at a normal rate and tone, distinctly and clearly. Shouting or exaggerating your words distorts your lip movements and makes lip reading even more difficult.

Use of Interpreters

When faced with a language barrier or a deaf or hearing-impaired patient, the best course of action is to use a medical interpreter. These interpreters are specifically trained for medical interpretation and are familiar with medical terms and the patient interview process. They also remain neutral and do not interject their own thoughts or feelings into the conversation between the patient and provider.

Unfortunately, in the prehospital setting a medical interpreter is rarely available and the patient's family members or friends are the only option for use as an interpreter. In this situation you must appreciate the fact that the person you use as an interpreter has a vested interest in the patient's condition and outcome; just as any other time you use a family member for information, that individual is likely to interject his or her own thoughts and opinions. Inform the person acting as the interpreter to interpret exactly what you say and exactly what the patient says. The interpreter should not paraphrase or add opinions to the conversation. Medical interpreters do not need these instructions because this is strongly emphasized in their training.

Regardless of who is used, remember that the interpreter is simply a conduit for communication and not a participant in the conversation. The following guidelines should be adhered to when you use an untrained individual as an interpreter:

- Speak directly to the patient, not the interpreter. Ask "Where is your pain?" rather than "Can you ask him where the pain is?"
- Maintain eye contact with the patient, not the interpreter.
- Do not think out loud. Patients will wonder what is not being interpreted.
- Speak at a pace that allows time for interpretation.
- Clarify with your interpreter if you want the person to interpret simultaneously (interpreting what is said at the time it is said) or consecutively (waiting until the person is done speaking and then interpreting everything at that time).
- Avoid medical terms that may make interpretation more difficult. Although a medical interpreter may be familiar with medical terms, family and friends who act as interpreters may have difficulty translating medical terms.

Substance Abuse

When patients have an altered mental status, determining whether they may be under the influence of any alcohol or related drug substance is important. In these situations the first priority is to ensure personal safety on the scene. Depending on the level of responsiveness of the patient, direct, closed-ended questions often are needed, limiting the questions to "yes or no" responses. Conducting the interview and examination in a calm, quiet, controlled environment in a nonthreatening manner helps maximize the chances of successful communication.

Many times you will not be able to communicate with the patient and you must rely on witnesses or caregivers to obtain appropriate history. Try to find out what substances the patient possibly used; also determine if the patient has a history of overdosing or abusing substances. Determining whether the overdose was intentional is essential so that appropriate psychiatric treatment can be started once the patient's altered mental status has improved.

Sexually Attractive or Seductive Patients

Clinicians and patients may be sexually attracted to one another. These are normal feelings that should not change the way you interact with the patient in a professional manner. If your patient becomes seductive, remind the patient that your relationship is on a professional, not a personal, level. Making this statement perfectly clear should let the patient know that his or her comments or actions were inappropriate and allows you to continue to provide care for the patient.

If these situations occur or you suspect that they may occur, ensure you are never alone with the patient during the interview or physical examination. Have a partner, other EMS provider, or family member present. When at all possible this person should be of the same sex as the patient. Any inappropriate acts by the patient should be documented, such as on an incident form.

Patient with Multiple Symptoms

Patients may have multiple medical symptoms, some of which may be irrelevant to the current reason for the EMS call. You should list the patient concerns but then prioritize which issues most urgently need to be addressed. You should tell the patient that the other concerns are valid, but in the limited time available you must focus on addressing urgent needs first. Negotiate priorities with patients and they usually will respect your decision to address urgent issues first.

Anxious Patients

Patients seeking medical care naturally are anxious about their medical problems. Picking up on verbal or nonverbal cues that may reveal anxiety is important; respond to these cues with an appropriate empathic gesture to build trust and rapport with the patient. Acknowledging that the patient's anxiety is common goes a long way in helping reassure the patient about concerns.

Depression or Crying

Although crying may be a symptom of depression, patients may be crying for other reasons, such as pain or loss of something or someone important to them. Go the extra step in trying to calm and reassure these patients by providing them with tissues or supportive, empathic statements. Ask the patient why he or she is crying. If the patient does feel depressed, ask if he or she has any suicidal or homicidal thoughts. You must determine the level of risk the patient may pose to himself or herself as well as you.

Case Scenario SUMMARY

1. *What is your general impression of this patient?* This patient's condition appears stable given her good color and normal mental status. However, because her advanced age places her at a greater risk of multiple problems, you should get additional information and perform a more thorough patient assessment to confirm this general impression.

2. *What nonverbal information has been communicated to you at this point?* The patient's grooming and the care of her apartment suggest that she is oriented and capable of performing basic self-care and household tasks. Her insistence on maintaining the order of her home is further evidence of this and demonstrates her pride in her ability to take care of herself.

3. *How can you improve the patient's ability to focus on you and your interview?* First, respect the patient's concerns about her apartment by reducing the number of people in the room. You can also help her to focus by explaining what other EMS personnel will be doing and assuring her that they will be respectful of her home and possessions. It may also be effective to "assign" one of the daughters to the fire personnel, thus ensuring the patient that they are being watched and allowing her to return her focus to you.

4. *How can her daughters improve the quality of communication with their mother? How can they impede it?* The presence of a trusted family member during an interview can be helpful. The daughters can help provide context to the patient's comments and can interpret what their mother has said. However, having other individuals speak on behalf of the patient has a distinct disadvantage: accuracy. Knowing whether the daughters are accurately conveying their mother's symptoms, history, or concerns is impossible. Unless speaking to the patient is impossible, use the daughters to supplement your communication with the patient, not replace it.

5. *What barriers to communications exist in this case? What strategies can you use to reduce them?* This situation presents multiple barriers, including language; potential cultural differences; on-scene distractions; patient frustration with her physician and the health care system; potential EMS personnel responder bias against the patient's frequent use of the EMS system; patient's lack of knowledge about her own health, medications, and symptoms; and multiple different communicators on both the EMS team and the patient's family.

6. *One of the daughters seems quite willing to speak on her mother's behalf. Is that the best communication strategy in this case? Why or why not? If you choose to use this method, how can you ensure that you get correct information?* Having family members assist in communicating with an older adult can be helpful, especially when a language barrier exists. However, family members sometimes communicate their own issues, not those of the patient. Try to get the patient to answer directly whenever possible. Watch the patient's face for signs that she does not understand your questions, then either rephrase or let the family member restate the question for her. Keep an eye on the patient's face to see signs that she does not agree with the conversation. Speak to her directly even when the daughters answer.

7. *How can you learn more about the patient's medication history?* In addition to the patient, the daughters may be useful sources of information. In addition, with the permission of the patient, you may send your partner into the bathroom or bedroom to find medications.

8. *How might you have handled the return of the fire personnel and preparation for transport to better maintain communication with the patient?* The disappearance or reappearance of crew members inherently creates questions in many patients' minds: where are they going? Will they be back? What are they doing, and will it affect me and my home? This uncertainty makes focusing on you and your interview difficult for the patient. A prime strategy is to keep the patient informed. When the crew leaves, inform her (and the daughters) that they are going out to the ambulance to get equipment, including an oxygen tank and the stretcher. Let them know that the crew will be back and what will happen when they return. Then, as they return, interrupt the interview yourself to remind the patient that they have returned and what they are going to do next. This reduces the patient's anxiety about the unknown and may enable her to better focus on you and your questions and examination.

9. *What are your communication priorities for this patient after you arrive in the ambulance and before you depart for the hospital?* As the previous question noted, patients have many questions about what you will do and what will happen next. This uncertainty is, at the very least, stressful. In many cases it will prevent further communication. Providing the patient a summary of what has happened so far and what will happen next is a powerful tool for reducing this stress. Remind her that you have almost completed the interview, that you have transferred her and her purse (or other valuables) to the ambulance, and that you will ensure she is comfortable. Let her know that you will be taking a blood pressure, starting an intravenous line, and transporting her to the hospital (be sure to tell her which one). In some cases you may want to give her information about your planned route, if you know it, because she will be looking out the window trying to figure out where she is. All of these strategies answer her questions about what is happening so that she can concentrate on what you still need to discuss.

10. *Interpreters frequently are useful in evaluating patients who have limited or no fluency in English. What steps should be taken to ensure the accuracy of translated information?* In reality, you cannot ensure the accuracy of translated information because you can only understand half of the conversation. You should focus on ensuring that your communication with the interpreter is clear and concise. Frequently check for understand-ing, then monitor the nonverbal communication that occurs during the conversation between the interpreter and the patient. Ask the interpreter about any apparent confusion or anxiety you see in the patient's face. Restate questions if necessary and, when the anxiety is related to a question the patient may have voiced, be sure to answer that issue before returning to the interview.

Chapter Summary

- The ability to communicate effectively is an essential skill.
- Internal and external factors affect your ability to communicate.
- The interview process begins before actual contact with the patient and is a dynamic process in response to each individual situation.
- Open-ended questions are usually the most effective and efficient means to gather information during the patient interview.
- Nonverbal cues, from both the patient and the paramedic, have an impact on the communication process.

- Building patient rapport, which can be done in several ways, is conducive to good patient communication and care.
- Several traps of interviewing can negatively affect patient communication and care.
- Paramedics must realize and take advantage of other sources of information regarding any call.
- Special situations require adjusting your communication skills to maximize your chances of gathering information and promoting good care.

REFERENCES

Feldman, M. D., & Christensen, J. F. (1997). *Behavioral medicine in primary care: A practical guide.* Stamford, CT: Appleton and Lange.
Greene, H. (1996). *Clinical medicine* (2nd ed.). St. Louis: Mosby.
Maguire, P., & Pitceathly, C. (2002). Key communications skills and how to acquire them. *British Medical Journal, 325,* 697-700.

Seidel, H., Ball, J., Dains, J., & Benedict, G. (2006). *Mosby's guide to the physical examination* (6th ed.). St. Louis: Mosby.
Willett, R. (2005). *Syllabus: Foundations for clinical medicine.* Richmond, VA: Virginia Commonwealth University.

Chapter Quiz

1. List three reasons to obtain a medical history.

   _____

   _____

   _____

2. Which of the following is an example of a direct question?
   a. "Did you take your medication this morning?"
   b. "Tell me about the pain in your stomach."
   c. "What other symptoms are you experiencing?"
   d. "What can I help you with today?"

3. The most effective and efficient method to gather information during the medical interview is to _____.
   a. interview the patient's family only
   b. talk only to the patient's personal physician
   c. use closed-ended questions
   d. use open-ended questions

4. The attribution of some trait or characteristic to one person based on the interviewer's preconceived notions about a general class of people of similar characteristics is known as _____.
   a. discrimination
   b. impatience
   c. labeling
   d. stereotyping

5. When approaching a hostile patient, avoid
   a. identifying and removing sources of stress from the scene;
   b. keeping the patient in a secure location, such as a closed bedroom, to ensure his or her safety and prevent escape;
   c. speaking in a calm, quiet voice while positioned at eye level with the patient;
   d. using law enforcement personnel to ensure a safe scene;

Chapter Quiz—continued

6. List three sources the paramedic could turn to for information when a patient cannot communicate directly with the EMS provider.

_____

_____

_____

7. The best approach to dealing with your own emotions in response to a patient or situation is to
  a. ask for another responder to assume care of the patient, even if it means calling another unit to the scene.
  b. continue to provide appropriate care in a nonjudgmental fashion until the encounter is over, then use appropriate outlets to discuss the emotions.
  c. keep the emotions bottled up until you get home, then let it all out.
  d. tell the patient why you are angry or upset.

8. List three methods of communicating with a hearing-impaired patient.

_____

_____

_____

9. List at least three nonverbal cues that may indicate a patient is hostile or agitated.

_____

_____

_____

10. List three ways to determine if a patient has appropriate mental status during the interview.

_____

_____

_____

11. The application of a derogatory term to a patient on the basis of an event, habit, or personality trait that may not be accurate about the underlying condition is known as
  a. discrimination.
  b. impatience.
  c. labeling.
  d. stereotyping.

12. True or False: Except for the physical examination, the paramedic should never engage in physical contact with a patient, such as hugging or shaking hands.

Terminology

Active listening Listening to the words that the patient is saying as well as paying attention to the significance of those words to the patient.

Clarification Asking to speaker to help you understand.

Closed-ended questions A form of interview question that limits a patient's response to simple, brief words or phrases (e.g., "yes or no," "sharp or dull").

Communication The use of words, writing, or other commonly understood symbols by a sender to send a message to a receiver, who then provides feedback that indicates the receiver's interpretation of the message.

Confrontation Focusing on a particular point made during the interview.

Cultural beliefs Values and perspectives common to a racial, religious, or social group of people.

Cultural imposition The tendency to impose your beliefs, values, and patterns of behavior on an individual from another culture.

Customs A practice or set of practices followed by a group of people.

Discrimination Treatment or consideration based on class or category rather than individual merit.

Direct (closed-ended) questions Questions that can be answered with short responses such as "yes" or "no."

Empathy Identification with and understanding of another's situation, feelings, and motives.

Ethnocentrism Viewing your life as the most desirable, acceptable, or best, and acting in a manner conveying superiority to another culture's way of life.

Explanation Sharing objective information related to the message.

Facilitation Encouraging the patient to provide more information.

Interpretation Stating the conclusions you have drawn from the information.

Intimate space The area within 1.5 feet of a person.

Labeling The application of a derogatory term to a patient on the basis of an event, habit, or personality trait that may not be accurate about the underlying condition.

Nonverbal cues Expressions, motions, gestures, and body language that may be used to communicate other than with words.

Open-ended questions A form of interview question that allows patients to respond in narrative form so that they may feel free to answer in their own way and provide details and information that they believe to be important.

Personal space The area around individuals that they perceive as an extension of themselves. In the United States, personal distance is 1.5 to 4 feet.

Reflection Echoing the patient's message using your own words.

Social distance The acceptable distance between strangers used for impersonal business transactions. In Western cultures, social distance is 4 to 12 feet.

Stereotyping The attribution of some trait or characteristic to one person on the basis of the interviewer's preconceived notions about a general class of people of similar characteristics.

Summarization Briefly reviewing the interview and your conclusions.

Sympathy Sharing the patient's feelings or emotional state in relation to an illness.

History Taking

Case Scenario

You and your partner respond to a private residence for an "unknown medical problem." You arrive to find a 78-year-old man in obvious respiratory distress. He is alert, slumped in a chair, and gray and ashen in appearance. His speech is quiet and hard to hear, and he has two- to three-word dyspnea. His family reports that this episode began 2 days ago and got significantly worse approximately 3 hours before they called 9-1-1.

Questions

1. *What is your general impression of this patient?*
2. *What questions are important to ask to understand the nature of this episode better?*
3. *What additional assessment will be important in the evaluation of this patient?*
4. *What intervention should you initiate at this time?*

Healthcare providers often hear that more than 70% of the time an accurate medical diagnosis can be made on the basis of a comprehensive medical history alone. When combined with proper physical examination techniques, the percentage of correct diagnoses can be increased to 90% or better. However, studies have revealed that even physicians often do not obtain all the information necessary to obtain a complete history (Ramsey et al., 1998). Learning the correct technique for eliciting a comprehensive medical history can be beneficial to your patient's care.

Paramedics are often the patient's first point of contact with the healthcare system. During this initial contact, the foundation for further care must be set by establishing effective rapport with the patient. Making the patient feel comfortable enough to provide valuable information may be crucial to the physician's ability to care for that patient on arrival in the emergency department. This chapter discusses the components of a comprehensive medical history, or comprehensive health history. Also discussed is how to obtain information from your patients in a timely manner. In addition, you will learn tech-

niques for establishing effective rapport with patients, increasing the level of satisfaction with encounters both for you and your patients.

PURPOSE OF MEDICAL HISTORY

[OBJECTIVE 1]

Why is obtaining a comprehensive medical history important? After all, the phrase "medical history" literally means a summary of a *past* state of health, recent or remote. A number of reasons exist why a medical history is an essential component of the patient's medical care.

First and foremost, a good historian is able to gather data about the patient's current medical problems as well as the patient's medical history. Data gathering is not always as easy as it sounds. The reliability of the patient must be determined regarding his or her ability to provide an accurate medical history. If for some reason the patient is unable to provide a reliable history, you must find a caregiver or bystander who can speak to the patient's medical issues. For example, a patient who was involved in a high-speed motor vehicle crash may not be able to provide an accurate history because of alterations in mental status from a head injury. Similarly, a patient who is under the influence of alcohol or other drugs may not be in a state of mind to provide a reliable history. In these situations, finding a relative, caregiver, or witness may be the best method of obtaining information that will be important in regard to care.

Another important aspect of history taking is being able to monitor the patient's progress by direct observation as well as conversation. Repeatedly asking certain questions over time may let you realize how a patient is responding to treatments you begin in the field. For example, an asthmatic patient with dyspnea and wheezing must be asked if the symptoms have improved after the paramedic gives nebulizer treatments on the way to the hospital. Maintaining discussion with the patient after the initial history is complete can help alert you to any changes in the patient's status that may lead to deterioration or improvement in current health. You frequently will find yourself asking additional history questions while performing physical examinations on your patients; such dialogue may allow to you figure out important aspects of the history that were previously unaddressed.

Obtaining a medical history is not a simple collection of facts. The art of being a good historian allows the patient to build trust in you and the care you provide. Establishing rapport with the patient is critical to obtaining accurate and appropriate information. The first impression you make on the patient through questions you may ask or gestures of comfort you may provide sets the tone for the remainder of the patient's encounter with the healthcare system. Recognizing the patient's concerns and providing reassurance make the patient trust your ability to provide care. Patients are often scared and isolated in times of emergency. They are more likely to open up to you and give you the information you need if you ask questions in a way that respects the person's autonomy, privacy, and concerns. Thoughtful history questions allow you to establish effective rapport with your patients.

Finally, the medical history should give you an opportunity to educate patients and include their personal input into treatment plans when appropriate. Patients are more likely to be compliant with treatment plans if they are included in the decision-making process. You may be able to prevent future illness or injury by discussing risk factors appropriate for the patient's symptoms. For example, a discussion of bicycle helmet use with a pediatric patient may prevent a head injury.

OBTAINING A COMPREHENSIVE HEALTH HISTORY

[OBJECTIVE 2]

The medical history is generally the initiation of your relationship with your patient. The ability to obtain a comprehensive history depends on your use of the communication skills described in Chapter 15. A medical history has three main goals: establishing rapport, obtaining data, and educating and motivating patients. In emergency medicine the latter is not as common as the first two goals. The medical professional must analyze the symptoms reported by the patient and make a decision regarding the most likely cause. If poor communication skills lead to symptoms being omitted from the history, the **differential diagnosis** likely will be inaccurate. The history, although often combined with the physical examination in emergency medicine, is crucial because it guides the physical examination. The interrelations among the history, physical examination, and differential diagnosis are unique, and their roles often reverse. Although the differential diagnosis helps guide the history and physical examination, the history and physical examination help narrow the differential diagnosis to the most likely cause of the patient's complaints.

Beginning the Interview

After introducing yourself to the patient, you and the patient should together negotiate priorities for the remainder of the encounter. Inform the patient that you will ask multiple questions about the patient's current and past state of health. Ask the patient what he or she hopes to achieve during the course of the medical visit by offering an open-ended question such as, "What can I help you with today?" Including the patient early in the decision-making process ultimately improves patient compliance and satisfaction.

Because patients often respond best to open-ended questions, this type of approach allows them to describe their symptoms as they relate to the specific situation as well as their concerns, experiences, and questions. In short, how the interview is approached can make or break the therapeutic relationship. Patients must know that you are interested in their condition as a whole and not simply their disease status. More often than not the cause of the patient's symptoms can be determined from the history alone, with the physical examination and diagnostic tests simply confirming the suspected cause or differential diagnosis.

The comprehensive medical history is divided into several components, as described below. You should systematically interview the patient, placing emphasis on areas suggested by the chief complaint. Note that most patients view the history (and associated physical examination) with apprehension and anxiety.

COMPONENTS OF A COMPREHENSIVE HISTORY

[OBJECTIVE 3]

Identifying Data

To document the encounter with the patient properly, the following information should be obtained:

- *Date and time:* Always document the time the encounter with the patient occurred. If you realize you omitted information from your original note, go back and write the date and time that you added additional information to the record.
- *Age*
- *Gender*
- *Race:* The race of your patient is not always important to record. For some medical conditions that have a higher prevalence in certain ethnic backgrounds, this information may be important.
- *Occupation:* Occupation may be important if certain risks exist at the worksite that may make the patient more susceptible to certain injuries or illnesses. Discussing occupation with patients often helps establish rapport because it reveals you are interested in them as a person and not only as a patient.
- *Place of birth:* Although not commonly acquired in the prehospital setting, the patient's place of birth may provide clues to possible disease tendencies or exposures.

Source of Referral

Briefly state where the patient is coming from (e.g., home, physician's office, accident scene) as well as any pertinent information from the referral source. The source of referral is important when the person is not the patient. If the family initiated the call, then the patient may not believe the symptoms are important or warrant evaluation and may be less cooperative in the history-taking process. The goals of expected intervention also differ according to who requested the evaluation. The patient's goals may be different than those of family, law enforcement, or the physician.

Source of History

The patient is often the "historian" for the encounter. If the patient is unable to provide information, record how and from whom you were able to obtain information about the patient's state of health. The source of information could be family members, friends, police, or other healthcare workers. The source of this history is important in determining the value and possible biases of the information you receive about the patient. A medical record may be the only source of information you have during an interfacility transfer or a transfer from an extended-care facility to a hospital.

Reliability

Comment on the reliability of the historian. Relate why the patient or other historians may be unable to provide an accurate history (e.g., altered mental status, intoxication). Reliability of information can depend on several factors, including memory, trust, and motivation.

Remember to judge the reliability of your source of information at the end of your evaluation, not at the beginning. By making such a determination at the beginning, you will not accurately listen to the history and may miss vital information.

Chief Complaint

The **chief complaint** can be defined as the reason the patient has sought medical attention. When possible, the chief complaint should be recorded in the exact words of the patient (Bates et al., 2003). A typical encounter with a patient when obtaining a chief complaint follows:

> *EMS Provider:* What can I help you with today?
> *Patient:* I have had a severe headache for the past 2 days.
> *EMS Provider:* Is there anything else?
> *Patient:* I also have had several episodes of vomiting.

When recording the chief complaint for this example, state that the patient has a history of "severe headache" and "several episodes of vomiting." The patient may have many complaints (i.e., symptoms) but has only one chief complaint. Other complaints are considered associated complaints. When presented with several complaints ask, "What is the one thing that is bothering you the most today?" Each complaint can then be addressed in the order of perceived importance to the overall health of the patient. At times, minor complaints may need to be addressed at future encounters or in the hospital rather than the prehospital setting. Realize that some chief complaints may be misleading regarding the reason the patient is seeking medical care. Patients who are feeling depressed or anxious may have somatic complaints such as headache; even though you may realize the patient is depressed, still record "headache" as the chief complaint.

If the patient does not have a chief complaint, attempt to determine his or her goal in seeking treatment. This may include pain relief or a general evaluation.

History of Present Illness

The bulk of the information obtained concerning the patient's current state of health should be recorded under the **history of present illness,** a narrative detail of the symptoms that the patient is experiencing. The history of present illness should contain a full, clear, chronologic account of the patient's symptoms. For each symptom a number of details will help you better understand what the patient is experiencing. This includes the onset of the symptoms, the setting in which they occurred, their manifestation, aggravating and mitigating factors, and prior attempts at treatment. Finally, determine what the patient thinks is the cause of the symptoms. This can provide valuable information and insight. For example, if a patient has chest pain and states, "I think I may be having a heart attack," you should ask why the patient has that specific concern. A response of, "My father died of a heart attack at my age" will help you understand the patient's mindset more completely than simply knowing he or she has chest pain. Following are typical questions that could be used to determine the attributes of symptoms for a patient with a headache:

- *Location:* "Where is your pain located?" "Does the pain move anywhere else?" "Has the location of the pain changed over time?"
- *Quality:* "How would you describe your pain?" If the patient is unable to describe the pain, offer several suggestions such as sharp, dull, aching, or throbbing to assist in response.
- *Severity:* "On a scale of 0 to 10, where 0 is no pain and 10 is the worst pain you could imagine, how would you rate your pain?" "How is your pain affecting your day-to-day life?" Attempt to determine how the patient tolerates pain. For example, because a 10 typically is defined as the worst pain the patient has ever experienced, find out what that pain experience was. A patient who previously has passed several kidney stones may rate the pain of an acute myocardial infarction lower on a scale of 0 to 10 than would a patient who has never had a significantly painful event.
- *Timing:* "When did the pain start?" "Has the pain changed in intensity over time?" "Are there any times in the day that the pain is worse?" "Does the pain wake you from sleep?"
- *Setting:* "What were you doing when the pain started?" "Is there anything else that you can associate with the onset of the symptoms?"
- *Modifying factors:* "What makes the pain better?" "What makes the pain worse?" Ask each question separately and whether anything else changes the pain level.
- *Associated symptoms:* "Are you experiencing any other symptoms along with your pain?" If the

patient seems unsure, list several symptoms that may be associated with the pain, such as blurry vision, nausea, or vomiting, to provide examples of common symptoms other patients have (Willett, 2005).

Alternately, the mnemonic OPQRST is a memory aid that may be used to explore the patient's signs and symptoms, as follows (Box 16-1):

- *O*nset: Identify events or conditions when the chief complaint (e.g., pain, sensation) began or when the injury occurred.
- *P*rovocation/*p*alliation/*p*osition: Does anything make the chief complaint better or worse (moving, changing position, etc.)?
- *Q*uality: What does the pain, discomfort, or sensation feel like? Can the patient describe the pain, discomfort, or sensation?
- *R*egion/*r*adiation: Does the pain or discomfort stay in one spot, or does it move or radiate to another location? Referred pain is pain in an area different from the injury or illness.
- *S*everity: On a 0 to 10 scale (0 being none and 10 being worst), how bad is the chief complaint?
- *T*iming: How long have the patient's symptoms been present?

BOX 16-1 OPQRST Mnemonic

- *O*nset
- *P*rovocation, *p*alliation, *p*osition
- *Q*uality
- *R*egion and *r*adiation
- *S*everity
- *T*iming (duration)

Case Scenario—continued

The patient is alert and oriented to person, place, time, and event. His respiratory rate is 48 breaths/min and breath sounds are diminished, especially in the bases. He has faint inspiratory and expiratory wheezes in the upper lobes. You can see that he has retractions. He is using his accessory muscles to breathe. Although he tells you that he is "getting tired," he still has a strong gag reflex. The family informs you that he has myasthenia gravis, for which he takes prednisone. Other vital signs are pulse, 110 beats/min, and blood pressure, 164/98 mm Hg. He has no other pertinent medical history.

Questions

5. Does this patient require emergency transport? Why or why not?
6. What is the significance of the history of myasthenia gravis? Is it related to this episode?
7. What additional information could the family and/or patient provide?
8. In a case such as this, what role does prior history and patient/family information play in your decision making? Why?
9. What destination is most appropriate for this patient? Should you transport to the hospital with lights and siren? Why or why not?

Medical History

The **past medical history** (or simply *medical history*) can be defined as a summary of all past health-related events. The following areas within a person's medical history must addressed:

- *Childhood illnesses:* Obtain any history of illnesses contracted as a child, such as chickenpox or measles.
- *Adult illnesses:* Ask about any chronic medical problems for which the patient has received treatment in the past. Include date of diagnosis, severity of symptoms, and current and past treatments. You may need to ask direct questions about specific illnesses. For example, a patient who has respiratory distress should be asked, "Have you ever been diagnosed with asthma?"
- *Psychiatric illnesses:* Although often sensitive information for patients to provide, any current or past psychiatric illnesses should be discussed. A good screening question may be "Have you ever sought the help of a counselor or psychiatrist?" Follow-up with questions about specific common psychiatric diagnoses such as depression may be warranted. Ask about any psychiatric hospitalizations as well.
- *Accidents and injuries:* Ask the patient whether he or she has ever experienced any serious accidents or injuries. Obtain the nature of the injury, when it occurred, and any treatment or residual effects the patient may have experienced.
- *Surgeries:* Ask about the type of surgery as well as any complications that may have been experienced.
- *Hospitalizations:* Most medical issues that require hospitalization are serious and easily remembered by patients when asked. A good question to ask to screen for serious medical issues would be, "Have you ever been hospitalized overnight for any medical problem?"

Current Health Status

can't ask all of this if emergency

The **current health status** focuses on environmental and personal habits of the patient that may influence his or her general state of health. A complete current health status may not be obtained on each patient because of time constraints; however, certain aspects of the current health status may be relevant to the problem your patient is experiencing. Following are items that should be included in a complete current health status:

- *Current medications:* Discuss all current medications, including dosage and frequency of administration. Ask whether the patient is taking his or her medications as prescribed. If possible, collect all medication containers to verify medications reported

by the patient. Also ask specifically about over-the-counter medications, herbal remedies, vitamins, and other alternative therapies the patient may be using.
- *Allergies:* Ask about any drug to which the patient may be allergic; also include the type of reaction the patient experienced.
- *Tobacco use:* Ask the patient if he or she currently or in the past has used any tobacco products. Make sure to include a discussion of cigarettes as well as pipes, cigars, chewing tobacco, and dip. Try to quantify how much tobacco the patient uses and estimate the length of time the patient has been using the product.
- *Alcohol, drugs, and other related substances:* Asking about alcohol and drug-related substances can be a sensitive subject to approach with patients. To ensure your patient does not feel singled out, reassure the patient that you ask these questions of every patient. In a nonjudgmental way, ask about the type of substance used and the frequency with which it is used. Be sure to avoid questions such as "Do you drink alcohol?" This question can be answered with a "yes" or "no" answer without any elaboration. Also avoid questions that can be answered with a vague "I drink socially." Instead, attempt to quantify amounts and frequency. Is "a beer" 12 oz or 24 oz? How large is "a bottle"—a pint or a fifth? Is socially once a month with dinner or two to three nights each weekend? These questions provide more valuable information. Pay close attention to the patient's responses. An answer of "I have not had a drink [or used drugs] in years" is significant because it indicates the possibility of past substance abuse problems as well as a major decision point in the patient's life. However, these types of questions can miss several people with substance abuse problems, and many people underreport their use of substances. One tool that can be used for inquiry into alcohol use and is easily adapted to other substances is the CAGE questionnaire (Box 16-2).
- *Diet:* Ask about any specific dietary requirements or food allergies in addition to information about what foods are consumed in a typical day.
- *Screening tests:* Ask about recent screening tests that are gender and age appropriate. Examples of screening tests for all patients include measurement of blood pressure, colonoscopies, and checks of cholesterol levels. Screening tests specific for men include prostate and testicular examinations. Female-specific screening tests include Pap smears, breast examinations, and mammograms. Unless part of a routine physical, a history of a screening test often indicates a physician was suspicious for a specific disease process.
- *Immunizations:* Ask about any recent immunizations, including flu vaccinations during the fall and winter

months and tetanus boosters in patients who have sustained trauma.
- *Sleep patterns:* Ask about any changes in sleep patterns such as difficulty falling asleep or excessive drowsiness during the daytime hours.
- *Exercise and leisure activities:* Try to get an idea of what type of physical activity the patient routinely performs.
- *Environmental hazards:* Ask about specific hazards that may be present at home or at a worksite that would make the patient more vulnerable to injury or illness.
- *Safety measures:* Ask about use of safety belts, protective eyewear, bicycle helmet use, gun locks, medication lockboxes, outlet covers if small children are present in the home, and so forth.

Family History

Ask about general medical illnesses that affect other members of the patient's family, including all first-degree relatives. Also ask about the age and cause of death of immediate family members. Conditions that should be evaluated in family members include the following:

- Alcoholism
- Anemia
- Arthritis
- Cancer
- Diabetes
- Drug addiction
- Epilepsy
- Headaches
- Heart disease
- High blood pressure (hypertension)
- Kidney disease
- Mental illness
- Stroke
- Tuberculosis

Psychosocial History

- *Home situation and significant other:* Ask about home life to identify sources of support or stress. Be mindful of alternative lifestyles and make sure you ask about significant others with respect.
- *Daily life:* Get an idea of what the patient does on a daily basis, which may help assess the patient's ability to function independently in society.
- *Important experiences:* Ask about any recent significant life experiences such as divorce, job changes, or a move to a new home. Even some of the positive experiences in life such as weddings can be some of the most stressful to patients.
- *Religious beliefs:* Asking about religious preference is important to ensure you are respectful of the patient's personal belief systems. For example, Jehovah's Witnesses may not want a blood transfusion. Many view religious friends as a main system of support.
- *Patient's outlook:* In general, ask about the patient's mood and outlook on life to screen for depression or other psychiatric conditions.

Prehospital professionals often use the SAMPLE mnemonic to recall information to ask about the patient's current and past medical history (Box 16-3).

Case Scenario CONCLUSION

The patient's family informs you that the last similar episode resulted in 1 to 2 days of intensive care unit stay with no complications. The patient's SpO$_2$ on room air is 86%. The patient and family request that you delay intubation until he can be evaluated by his primary care physician. The patient's family requests transport to a hospital that is 7 minutes away. You begin assisted ventilation with a bag-mask device with 100% oxygen. Your partner starts an intravenous line and prepares the patient for transport. During transport the patient's SpO$_2$ improves to 95%, and he nods affirmatively when you ask if he is feeling better. On arrival at the emergency department, the patient's color is greatly improved and his pulse is 104 beats/min, blood pressure is 148/88 mm Hg, and respiratory rate is 30 breaths/min. The patient is diagnosed with a myasthenic crisis and is intubated, placed on a ventilator, and admitted to intensive care unit.

Looking Back

10. How helpful was the information from the family regarding prior episodes? Did it affect your treatment decisions? How?
11. Given the patient's final disposition, was your treatment appropriate? Why or why not?

Review of Systems

A comprehensive **review of systems** can be defined as a review of each organ system to screen for symptoms that may not have been mentioned in the history of current illness. For example, questions pertaining to the ear may include the following: "Have you experienced any change in your hearing?" "Have you had any ringing in your ears?" "Have you experienced any pain in your ear?" "Have you had any drainage from your ear?" Questions should be asked to determine the following:

- *General:* Fever, chills, cough, temperature intolerance, weakness, fatigue, recent weight change, changes in the way clothes fit
- *Diet:* Changes (increase, decrease, frequency) in eating, dietary restrictions, supplements, caffeine intake
- *Skin, hair, and nails:* Rashes, itching, lumps, sores, color changes, dryness, unusual changes
- *Head:* Headache (location, quality, character, pattern, prior episodes), dizziness, syncope, loss of consciousness, past or recent head injury
- *Eyes:* Visual changes (diplopia, blurred, scotomata, hemianopias), use of corrective devices (glasses or contact lenses), photophobia, excessive tearing, pain, redness, glaucoma, retinal degeneration, cataracts, use of eye medications
- *Ears:* Changes in hearing, use of assistive devices, ringing in the ears, earaches, vertigo, discharge, infection
- *Nose:* Sense of smell, obstruction, stuffiness, discharge, itching, bleeding, sinus infections, frequent colds
- *Throat and mouth:* Hoarseness, changes in voice, sore throat or tongue, oral ulcers, condition of teeth and gums, bleeding gums, use of dentures, dry mouth, dental procedures, taste disturbances
- *Neck:* Pain, stiffness, decreased mobility, goiter, lumps, swollen glands
- *Respiratory:* Cough, sputum (amount, color, quantity), respiratory distress, pain on respiration, dyspnea, orthopnea, cyanosis, night sweats, wheezing, past respiratory diseases, pleurisy, chest wall dysfunction, prior chest radiographs
- *Cardiac:* Chest pain (precipitating causes, timing, duration, quality, aggravating and mitigating factors), existing cardiac history, hypertension, palpitations, history of rheumatic fever, heart murmurs, peripheral edema, dyspnea, orthopnea, paroxysmal nocturnal dyspnea, previous electrocardiogram or other cardiac testing
- *Gastrointestinal:* Trouble swallowing, appetite changes, digestion troubles, nausea, vomiting, heartburn, intolerance of specific foods, regurgitation, vomiting of blood, changes in bowel habits, frequency of bowel movements, character of stool (color; size; consistency; presence of blood, mucus, or undigested food), rectal bleeding, hemorrhoids, abdominal pain, excessive belching or flatulence, jaundice, liver or gallbladder trouble
- *Genitourinary:* Frequency (polyuria, anuria, oliguria, nocturia), pain or other sensations with urination, flank or suprapubic pain, difficulty in starting flow or reduced force of stream, presence of blood, change in color, unusual odor, urgency, incontinence, presence of or history of stones or infections, history of micturition syncope
- *Male genitalia:* Emissions, pain, hernias, masses, sores
- *Female genitalia:*
  - *Menses:* Age at onset, regularity, frequency, duration, flow, amount, bleeding (between

periods, after intercourse), last menstrual period, dysmenorrhea, premenstrual tension

- *Menopause:* Age at onset, signs and symptoms, postmenopausal bleeding, discharge, itching, sores
- *Obstetric:* Number of fetuses (if currently pregnant), number of pregnancies, number of deliveries, types of deliveries, complications, abortions (natural or induced), prenatal care, birth control methods
- *Breasts:* Pain, lumps, sores, discharge, past mammograms
- *Peripheral vascular system:* Cramps, deep vein thrombosis or other clots, varicose veins, edema
- *Musculoskeletal:* Stiffness of the joints, pain, restricted movement, arthritis, gout, back pain, decreased range of motion, swelling, redness, increased temperature, deformity, sensations when moving a joint, weakness, tenderness
- *Neurologic:* Syncope, seizures, blackouts, weakness, paralysis, numbness or tingling, tremors, involuntary movements, loss of sensation or coordination, memory loss
- *Hematologic:* Anemia, easy bruising or bleeding, past transfusions and reactions
- *Endocrine:* Hyperthyroidism, hypothyroidism, changes in metabolism, skin changes, intolerance of heat or cold, unexplained weight change, excessive sweating, diabetes, changes in urination, changes in skin color, changes in thirst or appetite
- *Psychiatric:* Depression, mood changes, nervousness, tension, memory changes, difficulty concentrating, irritability, sleep disturbances, suicidal thoughts

Unique Components of a Pediatric History

[OBJECTIVE 4]

The caregivers of pediatric patients need to answer additional questions to complete important aspects of the child's medical history. Asking about the birth history is particularly important in infants, toddlers, and children with special health needs. Ask questions about the prenatal history to determine if the mother had routine prenatal checkups or any complications during pregnancy that required the use of medications. Find out about any prenatal blood work to assess risk of infection transmission to the child, in particular the group B streptococcal status of the mother.

Ask about any problems that may have surfaced during the delivery of the child. What was the method of delivery—vaginal or cesarean section? If the mother had a cesarean section, why did she need one? Did the child require any special treatment in the delivery room or in the nursery? How long did the infant stay in the hospital before discharge home?

Ask about any problems that may have surfaced in the first few weeks of life, known as the neonatal period. Did the infant have jaundice or any signs of infection? Did the child have any problems gaining weight or feeding? A detailed nutritional history, including amounts, frequency, and type of feedings, is important. A review of growth parameters and developmental skills achieved helps identify children who may have special needs. Finally, ask about the child's immunization status regarding diphtheria, tetanus, pertussis, and varicella.

Comprehensive versus Targeted History

As a medical professional, the paramedic must be familiar with the entire comprehensive history. As more and more paramedics are being employed in healthcare outside the emergency setting, this skill is being used on a more regular basis. However, in the emergency setting the comprehensive history is rarely performed as has been described; rather, a history targeted to the patient's chief complaint and presentation is used. In these situations the paramedic uses the knowledge of the comprehensive examination to choose the components appropriate to the specific patient and situation.

Confidentiality

The information you receive from the patient during the medical history should be treated as confidential and privileged information. Doing all you can to maintain the privacy of your patients is expected. However, several circumstances dictate when privacy rules should be violated. If a patient states he intends to harm himself or someone else, this information must be reported to potential victims and other members of the healthcare team to ensure the safety of everyone involved.

Adolescents in most states can seek treatment for substance abuse, sexually transmitted disease, contraception, and pregnancy-related issues without the consent of a parent or caregiver. Always encourage adolescent patients to have an open dialogue with family members. Be willing to help the teen talk with his or her parents about sensitive issues if asked.

Case Scenario SUMMARY

1. *What is your general impression of this patient?* The combination of color, posture, and respiratory distress makes this patient a high priority.

2. *What questions are important to ask to understand the nature of this episode better?* One of the most important history questions to ask in situations in which the patient is conscious and/or family members are available is, "has this ever happened before?" A significant number of EMS cases involve exacerbations of previous medical problems. This single question is vital and, if the answer is yes, opens the door to further questions about diagnosis, medications, and so forth. The symptom itself (shortness of breath) also should be evaluated by using the OPQRST mnemonic: *o*nset, *p*rovoking/*p*alliative/*p*ositional factors, *q*uality of symptoms, *r*egion/*r*adiation, *s*everity, and *t*iming. This evaluation provides additional information to help identify this episode as related to a preexisting condition.

3. *What additional assessment will be important in the evaluation of this patient?* After completing the primary survey, the focus of the examination should be respiratory: chest wall examination, breath sounds, assessment for retractions, vital signs, and oxygen saturation.

4. *What intervention should you initiate at this time?* Because this patient is both hypoxic (gray color) and probably hypoventilating (two- to three-word dyspnea, quiet voice), initial treatment should include high-flow oxygen and assisted ventilations with a bag-mask device.

5. *Does this patient require emergent transport? Why or why not?* The rapid respiratory rate and minimal air movement confirm this patient as high priority. You should keep your scene time to a minimum and expedite treatment and transport.

6. *What is the significance of the history of myasthenia gravis? Is it related to this episode?* Expecting paramedics to be familiar with the names and symptoms of all diseases is unrealistic. You may know that myasthenia gravis is a neuromuscular disease that could cause hypoventilation. However, the best source of information about myasthenia gravis in this case is the family, who would have told you that this episode was virtually identical to a prior exacerbation of his disease.

7. *What additional information could the family and/or patient provide?* Quite a bit. You want to know pertinent medical history, what medications the patient takes, how this episode compares to previous ones, what happened the last time an episode was this bad, and what treatment has been successful in the past. You should also determine the name of the patient's physician and his or her hospital affiliation.

8. *In a case such as this, what role does prior history and patient/family information play in your decision making? Why?* The history of previous episodes is a key fact when evaluating a patient with a chronic condition. Research has proven that the family and patient are quite accurate in their assessment of the situation's severity. In this case, the family's information regarding the severity of this attack and its relation to the patient's underlying myasthenia gravis was a crucial fact that helped guide appropriate decisions.

9. *What destination is most appropriate for this patient? Should you transport to the hospital with lights and siren? Why or why not?* Unless it dramatically prolongs transport time, this patient should be taken to the facility where his physician practices and where he has been seen before. Having a familiar physician coordinate his care and having access to prior hospitalization records are both important to provide the best care possible. Assuming that the patient can be stabilized with manual ventilation and oxygenation, transport with lights and siren is unnecessary.

10. *How helpful was the information from the family regarding prior episodes? Did it affect your treatment decisions? How?* It was very helpful. The family helped frame this episode as not too bad. Their request that you delay intubation until the patient was evaluated by his primary care physician was reasonable because your transport time was short and you could maintain ventilation and oxygenation by using manual methods. Had the family responded differently, stating that prior similar episodes were quite difficult and that they had been unable to ventilate the patient's lungs until he was intubated, considering providing prehospital intubation and transporting with lights and siren would have been prudent.

11. *Given the patient's final disposition, was your treatment appropriate? Why or why not?* The patient's improved condition on arrival in the emergency department (improved color, lowered pulse and respiratory rate, adequate SpO_2) validates the appropriateness of prehospital care.

Chapter Summary

- The medical interview is designed to gather information about the patient's past and present medical conditions and establish rapport with the patient.
- The technique of active listening and knowledge of when to use open-ended versus direct questions allow you to obtain an accurate history from your patients in an efficient manner.
- Understand that the components of a comprehensive medical history include the chief complaint, history of present illness, past medical history, current health status, and review of systems.
- Recognize that special challenges to obtaining the medical history require changing your standard approach to the medical interview to accommodate the issues facing the patient.

REFERENCES

Bates, B., Bickley, L. S., & Hoekelman, R. A. (2003). *A guide to physical examination and history taking* (8th ed.). Philadelphia: J.B. Lippincott.

Feldman, M. D., & Christensen, J. F. (1997). *Behavioral medicine in primary care: A practical guide.* Stamford, CT: Appleton and Lange.

Ramsey, P. G., Curtis J. R., Paauw D. S., Carline J. D., & Wenrich M. D. (1998). History-taking and preventive medicine skills among primary care physicians: An assessment using standardized patients. *The American Journal of Medicine, 104,* 152-158.

Seidel, H. M., Ball, J. W., Dains, J. E., & Benedict, G. W. (1999). *Mosby's guide to physical examination* (4th ed.). St. Louis: Mosby.

Willett, R. (2005). *Syllabus: Foundations for clinical medicine.* Richmond, VA: Virginia Commonwealth University.

SUGGESTED RESOURCES

National Highway Traffic Safety Administration. (1998). *Emergency medical technician paramedic: National standard curriculum (EMT-P).* Retrieved May 29, 2008, from http://www.nhtsa.gov.

Chapter Quiz

1. List three examples of resources that could be used as a source of a patient's medical history.

   _____
   _____
   _____

2. List three pieces of information that describe a patient's current health status.

   _____
   _____
   _____

3. Unique components of the pediatric history include _____.
   a. childhood illnesses
   b. developmental assessment
   c. review of systems
   d. tobacco product use

4. The best way to deal with a patient who is intoxicated is to
   a. ask the patient what substance(s) he or she took.
   b. ask an on-scene relative for pertinent medical history.
   c. assume the patient is suicidal.
   d. tell the patient to be quiet.

5. When is it acceptable to break patient confidentiality?
   a. When the patient admits to using birth control
   b. When the patient expresses the intention to commit suicide
   c. When the patient has recently used cocaine
   d. When the patient is at fault in a minor motor vehicle crash

Terminology

Chief complaint The reason the patient has sought medical attention.

Current health status Focus on the environmental and personal habits of the patient that may influence the patient's general state of health.

Differential diagnosis The list of problems that could produce the patient's chief complaint.

History of present illness A narrative detail of the symptoms the patient is experiencing.

Past medical history A summary of all past health-related events.

Review of systems A review of symptoms for each organ system.

Patient Assessment

Objectives *After completing this chapter, you will be able to:*

1. Explain the rationale for the use of an otoscope.
2. Explain the rationale for the use of an ophthalmoscope.
3. Define the terms inspection, palpation, percussion, and auscultation.
4. Describe the techniques of inspection, palpation, percussion, and auscultation.
5. Discuss medical identification devices and systems.
6. Describe trending of assessment components and explain the value of trending assessment components to other health professionals who assume care of the patient.
7. Describe the methods used to locate and assess a pulse.
8. Differentiate locating and assessing a pulse in an adult, child, and infant patient.
9. Distinguish among methods of assessing breathing in the adult, child, and infant patient.
10. Differentiate a patient with adequate and inadequate minute ventilation.
11. Discuss methods of assessing mental status and differentiate assessing altered mental status in the adult, child, and infant patient.
12. Categorize levels of consciousness in the adult, infant, and child.
13. Recognize hazards and potential hazards.
14. Determine and describe common hazards found at the scene of a traumatic event and at the scene of a medical patient.
15. Differentiate safe from unsafe scenes.
16. Describe methods of making an unsafe scene safe.
17. Discuss common mechanisms of injury and nature of illness.
18. Predict patterns of injury based on mechanism of injury.
19. Discuss the reason for identifying the total number of patients at the scene.
20. Organize the management of a scene after size-up.
21. Explain the reasons for identifying the need for additional help or assistance.
22. Summarize the reasons for forming a general impression of the patient.
23. Explain the value of performing an initial assessment.
24. State reasons for management of the cervical spine once the patient has been determined to be a trauma patient.
25. Discuss methods of assessing the airway in the adult, child, and infant patient.
26. Describe methods used for assessing whether a patient is breathing.
27. Discuss the need for assessing the patient for external bleeding.
28. Describe normal and abnormal findings when assessing skin color, temperature, and condition.
29. Describe the evaluation of a patient's perfusion status based on findings in the primary survey.
30. Discuss the reasons for reconsidering the mechanism of injury.
31. Analyze a scene to determine if spinal precautions are required.
32. Explain the reason for prioritizing a patient for care and transport.
33. Identify patients who require expeditious transport.
34. Differentiate the assessment performed for a patient who is unresponsive or has an altered mental status and other medical patients requiring assessment.
35. Apply the techniques of physical examination to the medical patient.
36. State the reasons for performing a rapid trauma assessment.
37. Cite examples and explain why patients should receive a rapid trauma assessment.
38. Apply the techniques of physical examination to the trauma patient.
39. Describe the areas included in the rapid trauma assessment and discuss what should be evaluated.
40. Discuss the reason for performing a focused history and physical examination.
41. Describe when and why a detailed physical examination is necessary.
42. Discuss the components of the detailed physical examination in relation to the techniques of examination.
43. State the areas of the body that are evaluated during the detailed physical examination.
44. Explain what additional care should be provided while performing the detailed physical examination.
45. Distinguish between the detailed physical examination performed on a trauma patient and that of the medical patient.
46. Differentiate patients requiring a detailed physical examination from those who do not.
47. Differentiate normal and abnormal findings of the assessment of the skin, hair, and nails.
48. Distinguish the importance of abnormal findings of the assessment of the skin.
49. Describe the examination of the head and neck.
50. Differentiate normal and abnormal findings of the scalp examination.
51. Describe the normal and abnormal assessment findings of the skull.
52. Describe the assessment of visual acuity.
53. Describe the examination of the eyes.
54. Distinguish between normal and abnormal assessment findings of the eyes.

55. Describe the examination of the ears.
56. Differentiate normal and abnormal assessment findings of the ears.
57. Describe the examination of the nose.
58. Differentiate normal and abnormal assessment findings of the nose.
59. Describe the examination of the mouth and pharynx.
60. Describe the examination of the neck.
61. Differentiate normal and abnormal assessment findings of the neck.
62. Describe the assessment of jugular venous pressure and pulsations.
63. Differentiate normal and abnormal assessment findings of the chest examination.
64. Describe the examination of the anterior and posterior chest.
65. Differentiate the characteristics of breath sounds.
66. Describe the examination of the heart and blood vessels.
67. Differentiate normal and abnormal assessment findings of the heart and blood vessels.
68. Describe auscultation of the heart.
69. Differentiate the characteristics of normal and abnormal findings associated with auscultation of the heart.
70. Describe special examination techniques of the cardiovascular examination.
71. Describe the examination of the abdomen.

72. Differentiate normal and abnormal assessment findings of the abdomen.
73. Describe auscultation of the abdomen.
74. Distinguish normal and abnormal findings of the auscultation of the abdomen.
75. Describe the examination of the female genitalia.
76. Differentiate normal and abnormal assessment findings of the female genitalia.
77. Describe the examination of the male genitalia.
78. Differentiate normal and abnormal findings of the male genitalia.
79. Describe the examination of the anus and rectum.
80. Distinguish between normal and abnormal findings of the anus and rectum.
81. Describe the examination of the musculoskeletal system.
82. Differentiate normal and abnormal findings of the musculoskeletal system.
83. Describe the examination of the nervous system.
84. Differentiate normal and abnormal findings of the nervous system.
85. Discuss the considerations of examination of an infant or child.
86. Discuss the reasons for repeating the primary survey as part of the reassessment.
87. Describe the components of the reassessment.
88. Describe the general guidelines of recording examination information.

Chapter Outline

Introduction to Patient Assessment
Comprehensive Patient Assessment System

Documentation
Chapter Summary

Case Scenario

You and your partner respond to a private residence for a "woman with pneumonia." On arrival, you find a 51-year-old, moderately obese woman reporting acute shortness of breath. She is in obvious respiratory distress with 1- to 2-word dyspnea. Her skin is pale and diaphoretic with cyanotic nail beds and lips. She informs you that she has had self-diagnosed, untreated pneumonia for the past month as well as asthma and hypertension (she does not take her medications). Her pulse is strong and rapid.

Questions
1. *What is your general impression of this patient?*
2. *What are some possible causes of this patient's respiratory distress and cyanosis?*
3. *What history questions or physical assessment procedures would be most useful in differentiating the conditions you listed in question 2 above?*
4. *What intervention should you initiate at this time?*

INTRODUCTION TO PATIENT ASSESSMENT

Arguably, the most important tool any paramedic possesses is the ability to perform a thorough and accurate patient assessment. Every patient encountered receives one. Patient assessment begins with the scene size-up and continues as you enter the scene, noting the mechanism of injury or nature of the patient's illness, smells, and noises. When you first lay eyes on your patient, you form a general impression by observing how he or she is positioned, listening to the patient speak (or not speak), noting skin color and condition, and watching facial expressions. A good patient assessment is not a separate skill performed at only one point during an emergency call. It is an ongoing assessment that is continuously being performed, often in conjunction with the history.

Several reasons exist for performing a physical examination. It allows further investigation of a patient's complaint, discovers hidden and underlying problems, and anticipates problems that may arise in the future.

Physical Examination

Taking a good history is essential in an alert, stable patient. Important historical information can also be obtained from family members, bystanders, and observations of the scene. As a paramedic, you must also perform a thorough physical examination to confirm or refute your first impression of the patient. Because the physical examination may be the only tool you have to assess the unresponsive and/or unstable medical or trauma patient, an understanding of the techniques of physical examination is essential to paramedic practice.

Tools

Several tools enhance patient assessment. These tools and their results are not stand-alone devices. Instead, they help complete the picture of your patient's illness or injury. As you use these tools, remember to keep their results in context of the patient's presentation and general condition.

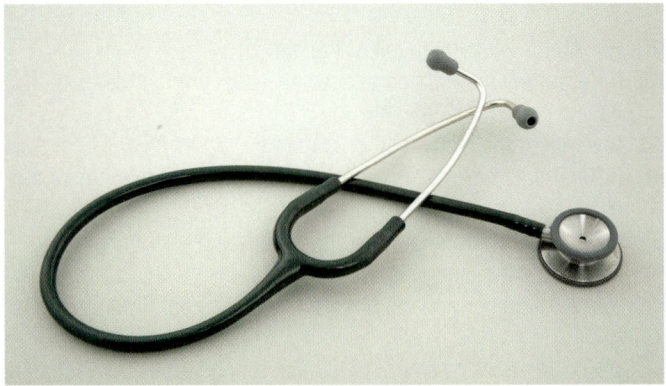

Figure 17-1 Stethoscope.

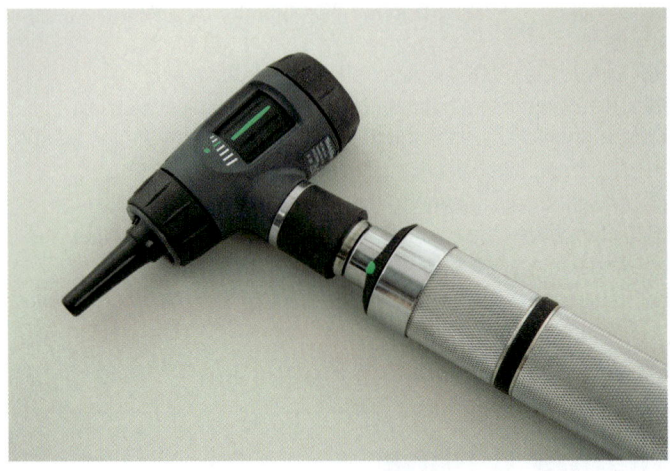

Figure 17-2 Otoscope.

PARAMEDIC*Pearl*

Keep in mind that the pieces of equipment used during a patient assessment are simply tools. They can be wrong. If something seems off, it may be.

Stethoscope. Used to auscultate sound and vibrations, the stethoscope is one of the most useful tools a paramedic possesses (Figure 17-1). The stethoscope transmits sound waves from its source through a hollow tube to the ears. Most stethoscopes have a bell and diaphragm on the functional end. The diaphragm is used for listening to high-pitched sounds such as lung sounds (other than the low-pitched vesicular sounds), the S1 and S2 heart tones, high-pitched murmurs, and ejection clicks; it also screens out lower pitched sounds. The bell is designed to amplify low-pitched sounds when applied to the patient with light pressure, making it ideal to listen to the Korotkoff sounds of blood pressure; the S3 and S4 heart tones; as well as gallops, rubs, diastolic rumbles, low-pitched murmurs, vesicular breath sounds, and most bowel sounds. If you push firmly with the bell, it functions nearly identically to the diaphragm. A stethoscope equipped with both a diaphragm and bell has a closure

valve so that only one end piece (the diaphragm or bell) is functional at any one time.

Finding a stethoscope that is functional and works for you is important. A good stethoscope has the following features:

- A rigid diaphragm cover
- A bell of sufficient size to span an intercostal space in an adult
- Thick tubing made of either rubber or neoprene that is no more than 18 inches (40 cm) long
- Properly fitting earpieces to reduce extraneous noise

Otoscope
[OBJECTIVE 1]
You occasionally may use an otoscope to visualize the inner ear and tympanic membrane (eardrum) (Figure 17-2). The otoscope uses a light and magnifier glass to illuminate the ear canal. Functionally, the otoscope is a good way to assess for cerebrospinal fluid in the ear and nose after a traumatic brain injury. It also is used to determine if the eardrum is inflamed, infected, or ruptured.

Sphygmomanometer. As a paramedic, you will see many devices used to assess blood pressure. Most cardiac monitors include a noninvasive blood pressure monitoring system. Although these pieces of advanced equipment may be commonplace in your system, they are no replacement for manually determining a blood pressure with a sphygmomanometer. Automatic devices are prone to failure and can be wrong. Always manually assess a blood pressure before relying on mechanical monitoring. The aneroid sphygmomanometer is the blood pressure cuff most EMS professionals recognize. It is used with a stethoscope to auscultate the sound of blood movement through the brachial artery.

The three key parts on the sphygmomanometer are the bulb, cuff, and manometer (Figure 17-3). Enclosed in the fabric cuff is an airtight rubber bladder, which is inflated to increase pressure on the brachial artery. Cuffs come in predetermined sizes ranging from infant to adult to extra large for obese patients or use on the adult thigh (Figure 17-4). Air is added to the bladder

from a rubber bulb attached by a piece of tubing. A manual control valve allows you to adjust it to either pump air into, or slowly allow air out of, the bladder. Also attached to the blood pressure cuff is a carefully calibrated scale called a *manometer*. The manometer measures pressure in millimeters of mercury (mm Hg). Aneroid sphygmomanometers are scaled so that each line of the dial denotes 2 mm Hg, with numbers every 10 mm Hg. When applied snuggly to the upper arm, the manometer measures the air pressure inside the rubber bladder, rising as you squeeze air in and lowering as you let it out.

2/3 size of arm

Ophthalmoscope
[OBJECTIVE 2]

An ophthalmoscope is used to examine the inside of an eye (Figure 17-5). It uses a series of mirrors and lenses and a light to illuminate the eye's interior. Although still generally used in facility examinations, ophthalmoscopes are used in the prehospital setting in some areas. The paramedic working in the emergency department may be expected to use this device.

Using an ophthalmoscope takes practice. Remember that the pupil is simply a hole in the eye that you look through to evaluate the retina. The retina should have a yellow-orange or creamy pink appearance, and you should be able to see its vasculature. Start the examination by evaluating the overall appearance of the retina, its coloration, and the presence of any spots (areas of abnormal coloration) or hemorrhages. These findings can indicate conditions such as diabetes, hypertension, or retinal ischemia. Next evaluate the vasculature of the retina, paying particular attention to the arteriovenous crossing(s). Note whether the veins appear to taper, abruptly stop, or twist as they approach the arterioles. An overabundance of vessels may be visible in diabetic retinopathy. Finally, trace the vessels inward to locate the optic disc. The margins of the optic disc should be sharp and crisp on the temporal border. Although the nasal border is generally sharp as well, slight blurring may be

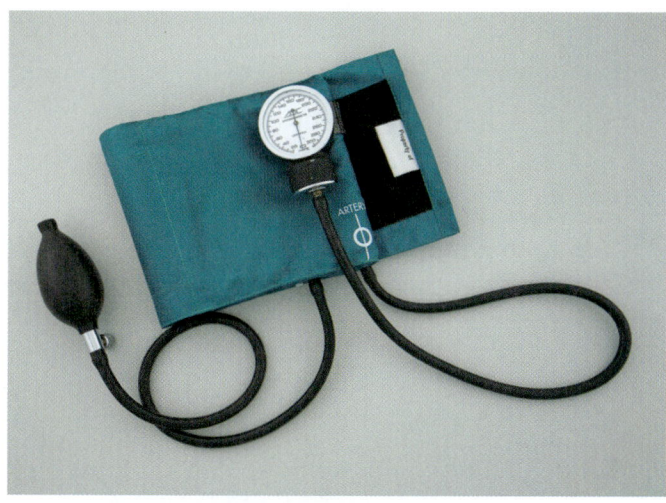

Figure 17-3 Sphygmomanometer.

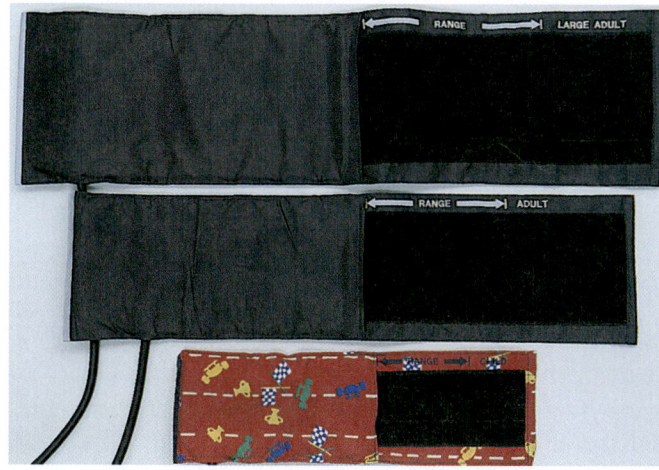

Figure 17-4 *From top,* Large adult, adult, and child blood pressure cuffs.

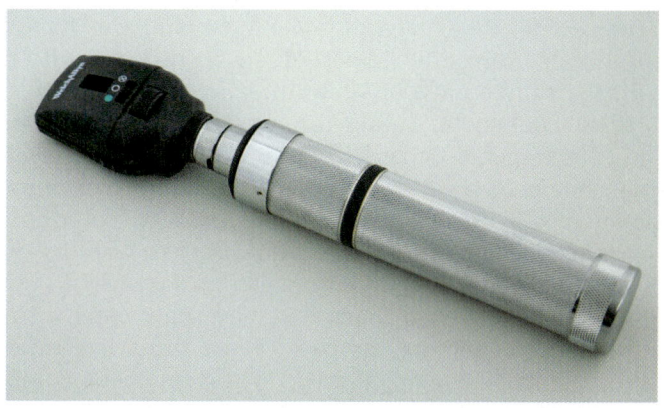

Figure 17-5 Ophthalmoscope.

normal in some individuals. Papilledema (blurring of the optic disc) can occur as a result of increased intracranial pressure.

When using the ophthalmoscope, be sure to examine the patient's eye with your corresponding eye. In other words, use your right eye to look in the patient's right eye and your left eye to look in the patient's left eye. Hold the instrument in the same hand as the eye you are using. This avoids a nose-to-nose situation that could cause discomfort for both the patient and paramedic.

In most situations setting the ophthalmoscope to zero diopters is fine. However, if your patient is hyperopic (farsighted), you may need to adjust the lens to a positive diopter (the black numbers); if the patient is myopic (nearsighted), you may need to adjust the lens to a negative diopter (the red numbers).

Ask your patient to fixate on a distant object. Then place the ophthalmoscope against your eye and your other hand on the patient's forehead for depth reference. Approach the patient's eye with the light directed away from the nasal border. This will keep the light from focusing on the fovea centralis, which may be painful. As you approach the pupil, you may see a red reflection (the red reflex). As you near the patient, continue to look through the pupil and the retina will become visible. Evaluate the retina as described above, noting any normal and abnormal findings.

Thermometer. Differential diagnosis can often be difficult without a thermometer. The thermometer measures a patient's core body temperature in either degrees of Celsius (C) or degrees of Fahrenheit (F). Core body temperature is important when evaluating any patient with an environmental emergency or when trying to differentiate pneumonia and congestive heart failure.

Thermometers come in many forms: glass (mercury), electronic, and colorimetric. Some thermometers are designed to be used on specific parts of the body, such as orally, in the ear canal, and rectally (Figure 17-6). Because not all thermometers take temperature readings below 35° C (95° F), be sure to have both a normothermic and hypothermic thermometer.

Penlights. A penlight has a variety of functions. It allows you to assess pupillary response and illuminate openings such as the ear, nasopharynx, and oropharynx to inspect for fluids (Figure 17-7). Most penlights have a pupil scale along the side. They are turned on and off with the simple press of a button.

Other Equipment. Paramedics working in urgent care clinics, emergency departments, and in nonemergent settings may need a variety of other equipment to examine a patient (Figure 17-8). Scales are used to determine patient weight. Some scales also have the ability to measure height at the same time. Reflex hammers to test tendon reflexes, vision charts to test eyesight, and tongue depressors to examine the back of the throat are other tools that may be used. Because of the emergent nature of a paramedic's work, these tools generally are not used during the patient assessment in the field.

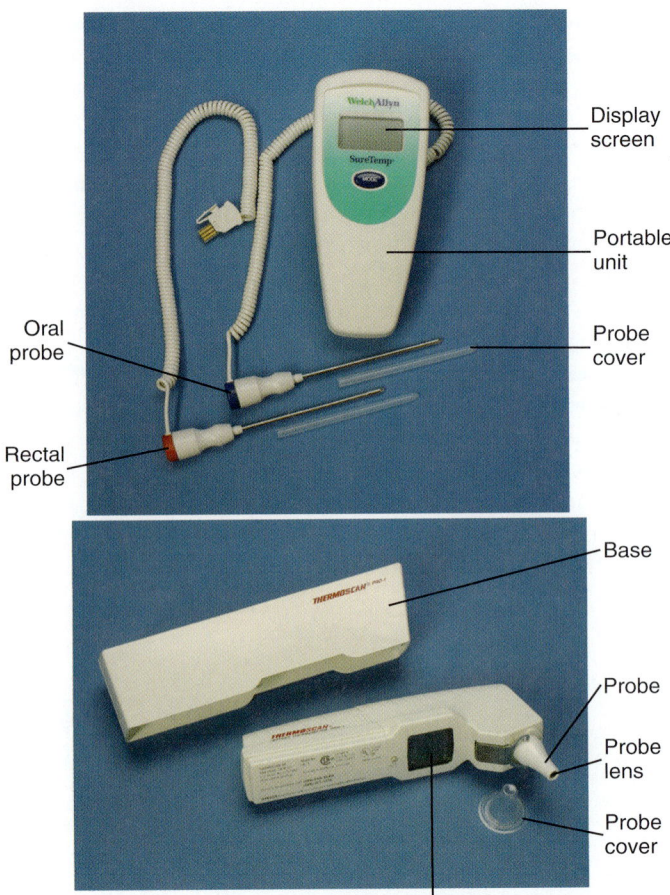

Figure 17-6 Thermometers.

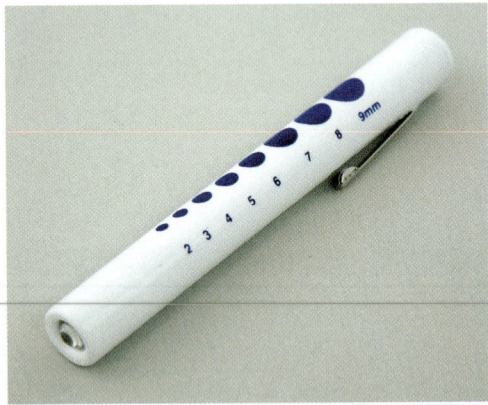

Figure 17-7 Penlight.

Examination Techniques

[OBJECTIVES 3, 4]

Every paramedic approaches patient assessment in a slightly different manner. However you choose to approach your assessment, you will use four basic examination techniques: inspection, auscultation, percussion, and palpation. All four examination techniques provide

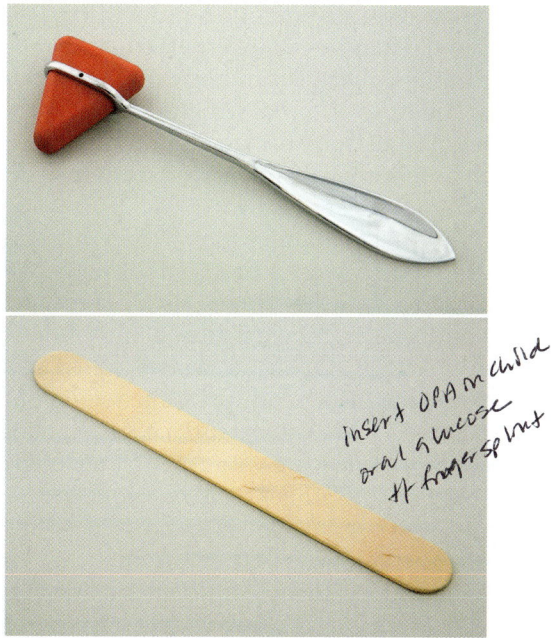

(handwritten note beside image: insert OPA in child oral glucose if finger splint)

Figure 17-8 Paramedics who work in urgent care clinics, emergency departments, and in nonemergent settings may need additional equipment to examine a patient.

unique information essential to performing a thorough and complete assessment.

These techniques are generally performed in the order listed from least to most invasive: Look, listen, feel, inspect, auscultate, percuss, palpate. Another reason for the order listed is that during examination of the abdomen, performance of palpation and/or percussion alters the bowel sounds.

Inspection
[OBJECTIVE 5]

Inspection is the visual observation of the patient seeking physical signs. The eyes are the most sensitive tool the paramedic has to gather data about the patient. Observe a patient with pneumonia and you may see flushed skin from a fever, nasal flaring and intercostal retractions from increased work of breathing, and a frequent cough producing yellow sputum, all without laying a stethoscope on the patient. The surrounding environment should be noted. Is evidence of trauma or a recent fire visible? Are any unusual odors present? Are empty pill bottles present? Do the medications present on scene belong to the patient? Is the patient on home oxygen? Be sure to note any medical alert tags that may indicate preexisting medical problems, such as diabetes mellitus or allergies to any medications.

Remember that you cannot see a finding covered by clothing, so the area of interest must be exposed. Although completely undressing every medical patient is not necessary, all clothing should be lifted and the skin underneath inspected. In general, all trauma patients should be completely undressed. Poor lighting may cause subtle skin findings to be missed, so move to an area of adequate lighting if necessary.

Inspection is an ongoing process and continues from the moment you first see the patient until the time the patient is delivered to the next higher level of care. Many practitioners are tempted to abbreviate the inspection phase and get straight to the more tactile portions of the physical examination. This desire may persist from infancy, when human beings explore the environment through touch and taste. You must make a conscious effort to concentrate on inspection. Visual observation is not an inborn skill; it must be learned. The well-known puzzle that follows illustrates this point well. Read the following sentence and count the number of times the letter *F* appears:

FINISHED FILES ARE THE RESULT OF YEARS OF SCIENTIFIC STUDY COMBINED WITH THE EXPERIENCE OF YEARS.

You probably counted three *F*'s, but the sentence contains six. The average person counts three because the brain tends to ignore conjunctions, and the word *of* has the sound of "V" instead of "F." The point is, we must train our eyes to see.

Auscultation. Literal interpretation of the term **auscultation** implies using the sense of hearing to obtain physical signs, but common use is restricted to hearing with the aid of a stethoscope. One commonly thinks of auscultation of the lungs, heart, and abdomen, but any region of the body can be auscultated, including the head, neck, and extremities. The head and neck may *(handwritten: bruée)* be examined for bruits in the intracranial, carotid, and vertebrobasilar arteries as well as over the thyroid gland. One may also hear a bruit over an injured blood vessel in penetrating trauma. Subcutaneous emphysema may be heard over the chest, and the heart and lungs are examined for various characteristics of the breath and heart sounds and the presence of extra sounds. Auscultation of the abdomen may reveal bruits from an aneurysm associated with hypotension or a stenotic renal artery associated with hypertension. Bowel sounds may be heard in the scrotum in the presence of a hernia.

(handwritten: vesicular sounds - normal breathing (bronchioles) tracheal sounds - higher pitched)

PARAMEDIC*Pearl*

Proper auscultation requires a quiet environment and a relaxed patient—two things paramedics rarely have. Do your best to eliminate extraneous sounds, such as talking and sirens.

(handwritten: wheezes - inspiratory or expiratory or both head bobbing + silent chest - nearing resp. failure)

Before listening, explain to the patient what you are about to do. Remember that stethoscopes always feel cold to the patient even if the surrounding environment is warm, so always warm the diaphragm of the stethoscope before you examine the patient. Applying a cold stethoscope against the skin tends to startle the patient, which increases anxiety.

(handwritten: coarse rales - crackles fine rales - lower levels of lungs)

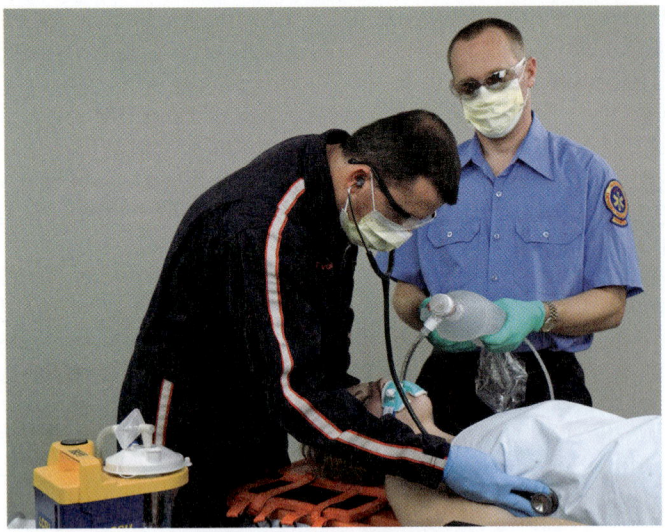

Figure 17-9 Auscultation.

heart sounds
1st - mitral & tricuspid valves close
2nd - aortic & pulmonic valves close

Accurate auscultation requires hours of practice and a quiet environment. Whenever listening, ask the patient to be quiet, refrain from talking yourself, and be patient. Do not rush yourself; good auscultation skills require taking your time. You are listening to the sound's intensity, pitch, duration, quality, and sometimes rhythm. When listening to lung sounds, check for bilateral equality (Figure 17-9). When assessing the chest and abdomen, auscultate before percussing and/or palpating.

Percussion. **Percussion** consists of striking the surface of the body, thereby emitting sounds of varying pitch depending on the density of the underlying tissues. The middle finger of the nondominant hand is laid on the body surface. A sharp blow is delivered to the distal interphalangeal joint of the nondominant hand by the tip of the middle finger of the dominant hand. The most common notes of percussion are tympany, resonance, hyperresonance, dull, and flat. Tympany is the sound heard when you percuss over an empty air-filled stomach. Resonance is the sound heard when the lung is percussed. Percussion over a tension pneumothorax sounds like hitting a drum and is hyperresonant to percussion. Dullness is the note obtained when percussing over the heart and flatness when percussing the thigh. Percussion can be used to determine the size of an organ (e.g., heart, liver), detect abnormal collections of fluid (e.g., pleural effusions, distended bladder) or air (e.g., tension pneumothorax, perforated viscus), and detect localized tenderness in the abdomen. Accurate percussion requires a quiet environment and much practice.

Palpation. **Palpation** is the act of feeling with the hand by the sense of touch, but information is also gathered from the ability to sense temperature and vibration. Palpation discriminates consistency, texture (skin and hair), shape, temperature, and moisture as well as events such as pulsation, movement, crepitus, and pulses. Palpation is used to examine all external structures such as the skin (including collections of body fluids, pus, or blood); hair; ears; and nose; internal structures such as the tongue accessible through body orifices; and other internal structures such as tendons, ligaments, arteries, muscles, joints, and abdominal viscera.

Sensitivity of the hand varies by region, so different parts of the hand are used for different tasks. The fingertips are used to detect textures, such as very small skin papules, and consistency, such as a fluid-filled versus a solid mass. Several fingers or even both hands may be used to detect shape depending on the region of the body being palpated. The palmar surface of the fingers and hand is best at detecting movement and crepitus. The ulnar surface of the fingers and hand is used to detect vibration. The dorsum of the hand, where the skin is thinnest, is used to detect temperature.

Palpation of the skin and soft tissues can reveal various pathologic conditions. **Induration** is a feeling of firmness in the subcutaneous tissue and may occur after trauma associated with hemorrhage in the soft tissues or may be seen with the presence of infection or inflammation. **Fluctuance** is a wavelike motion felt between two fingertips when palpating a fluid-filled structure, such as a subcutaneous abscess. Palpation of various bony structures may reveal crepitus associated with fracture fragments rubbing against each other or step-offs associated with displaced fractures.

Localized tenderness may also be discovered by palpation. Pain is the subjective sensation a patient experiences before examination, whereas tenderness is the pain a patient experiences during palpation. This technique is especially useful in examination of the abdomen, where localized right lower quadrant tenderness is associated with appendicitis and right upper quadrant tenderness is associated with gallstones or cholecystitis (infection of the gallbladder). Light palpation of the abdomen in all four quadrants should first be done as a general survey to detect the area of maximal tenderness. This is a one-handed technique and should be performed very gently. Deep palpation is a two-handed technique used to examine structures deeper in the abdomen, such as the aorta. The dominant hand is placed on top of the nondominant hand touching the abdominal wall. The dominant hand is used to apply pressure to and guide the nondominant hand to accomplish deep palpation. Remember to warm your hands before palpating the patient and always begin palpation at the most distant site from the area of maximal pain. If you start palpation at the most tender site, the patient is likely to have **voluntary guarding** (conscious contraction of the abdominal muscles in an attempt to prevent painful palpation) for the rest of the examination. Involuntary guarding is subconscious contraction of the abdominal muscles, which may be seen overlying areas of infection such as appendicitis. Palpation is also useful to check for local

SQ emphysema - air under skin

Rebound tenderness - painful when you let up pressure at end of palpation

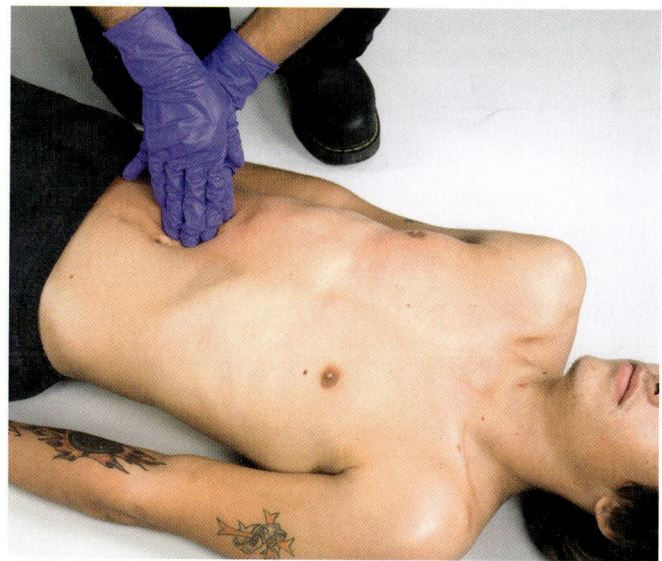

Figure 17-10 Palpation.

areas of tenderness associated with fracture sites or areas of infection in the skull, facial bones, spine, hands, feet, and long bones (Figure 17-10).

> **PARAMEDIC***Pearl*
>
> Tenderness exists when palpation causes discomfort. Pain is felt without any external pressure.

Vital Signs

Initial assessment - don't take rates yet - check for yes or no

[OBJECTIVE 6]

Performance of the physical examination usually begins with the assessment of the vital signs, including pulse, respirations, blood pressure, temperature, skin, and mental status (Table 17-1). Taking accurate and complete vital signs is extremely important. Often in EMS, EMTs and paramedics alike call the hospital and say, "The patient's vitals are stable," when they have only taken one full set of vital signs. In this situation, the EMT or paramedic is incorrect. One set of vitals tells nothing. Two complete sets of vital signs are a starting point. Once three or more sets of vitals have been taken, trends can be observed. Vital sign trends are the key to patient monitoring. Consider a pulse of 46 beats/min. By itself, this number means nothing. It must be put in context with the patient's normal vital signs and what all other vitals are like. A marathon runner may have a normal resting pulse in the low 40s. If the pulse is 46 beats/min, all other vitals are within normal limits, and everything remains unchanged over 30 or 40 minutes, then the patient's vital signs truly are stable.

TABLE 17-1	Normal Adult Vital Signs
Measurement	**Normal Range**
Mental status (AVPU)	Alert and oriented to person, place, time, and event
Pulse rate	60-100 beats/min
Ventilatory rate	12-20 breaths/min
Blood pressure	Systolic, 110-140 mm Hg Diastolic, 60-90 mm Hg
Core temperature	98.6° F (37° C)
Skin	Pink, warm, dry

AVPU, Alert, verbal, pain, unresponsive.   *Pulse OX 95% or greater*

> **PARAMEDIC***Pearl*
>
> How often then should you take vital signs to observe trends? That depends; you must use your judgment. Stable patients with minor injuries may only need vital signs taken every 15 minutes. More seriously ill or injured patients need vital signs taken every 5 minutes or even more frequently.

Always be sure to note the time when vital sign sets are taken. The exact minute is not as important as being able to look back and see how quickly vital signs are changing. Did the pulse rise 10 points over 5 minutes, or over 30? The implications are huge if the cause is internal bleeding.

> **PARAMEDIC***Pearl*
>
> Think of vital signs as a "six pack": pulse, respirations, blood pressure, temperature, skin, and mental status. Always complete the entire set of vital signs together. This is important because vitals change together in many conditions. For example, a rising blood pressure and a rising pulse may suggest a drug overdose, whereas a rising blood pressure and a decreasing pulse suggest increasing intracranial pressure.

Pulse

[OBJECTIVES 7,8]

Assess the rate and quality of central and peripheral pulses. When you feel a patient's pulse, you are feeling the movement of blood past a point in the artery. Each time blood is ejected from the heart it is sent out in a wavelike fashion. You feel the expansion and contraction of the arterial wall as blood moves past. Assess the carotid and radial pulses simultaneously to help determine perfusion status. Assess the rate (in beats per minute) by counting for 30 seconds, then multiplying by 2. Observe if the pulse feels like **bradycardia** (less than 60 beats/min) or **tachycardia** (more than 100 beats/min) (Figure 17-11).

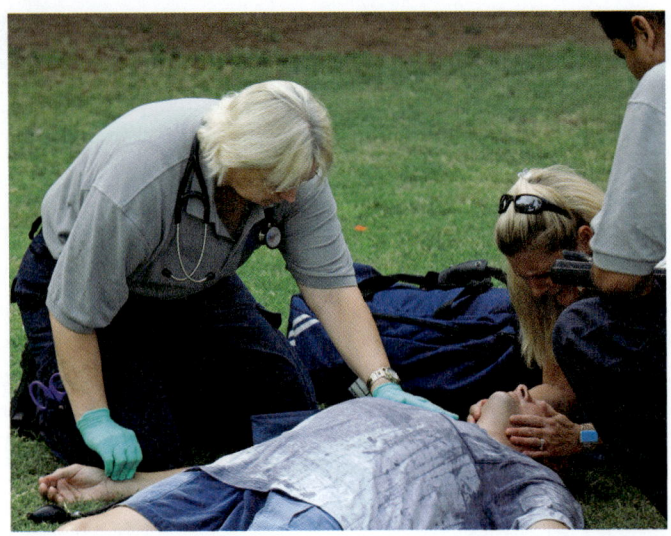

Figure 17-11 Palpate the carotid and radial pulses.

TABLE 17-2	Common Breathing Patterns
Name	**Pattern**
Normal	
Kussmaul respirations *Diabetes - deep "sighing" breaths*	
Biot's respirations	
Cheyne-Stokes respirations	

Also note the rhythm of the pulse. Is it regular or irregular? Does it follow a general pattern? Slower irregular pulses should be checked for 60 seconds to ensure accuracy. Additionally, pay attention to the strength, or quality, of the pulse. Strength indicates pulse pressure. Is it easy to feel, weak, or bounding? A bounding pulse reflects a wide pulse pressure. A weak pulse reflects a narrow pulse pressure. Document the rate and quality of the pulse.

In the newly born, assess the strength and quality of a central pulse by palpating the base of the umbilical cord between your thumb and index finger. In an infant, assess the brachial or femoral pulse. Assess the carotid pulse in any unresponsive patient older than 1 year.

Respirations

[OBJECTIVES 9, 10]

Assess the rate and quality of the patient's breathing. You will recall that respiration is the exchange of carbon dioxide and oxygen between the alveoli and blood vessels. It cannot be seen. What is known is that respiration is and must be continuous. Respiration keeps the body properly oxygenated and also balances the body's pH. Ventilation is the inhalation and exhalation of air. Each ventilation (counted as 1) requires both inhalation and exhalation. Although *counting respirations* is technically a misnomer, this terminology persists because when we count ventilation, we assume that respiration is taking place.

Accurately determine the patient's rate of breathing. **Tachypnea** is a rapid rate of breathing. It may be an abnormal finding because of a disease process or a compensatory response caused by excitement, anxiety, fever, or pain, among other causes. **Bradypnea** (an abnormally slow rate of breathing) is usually a red flag. It may be caused by fatigue, hypothermia, or central nervous system depression, among other causes. If the patient is breathing too quickly or too slowly, emergency interventions are usually indicated.

Assess whether the patient's ventilatory effort (also called the *work of breathing*) is normal, meaning that the patient is breathing adequately with minimal effort. If the patient is using accessory muscles to breathe, respiratory distress is likely present. Exhalation is normally a passive process. This means that a person does not need to work to get air out of the lungs. If you notice a patient is working to exhale air, this finding suggests the presence of bronchoconstriction from asthma, bronchitis, or other illness.

Respirations in infants and children younger than 6 or 7 years primarily are abdominal (diaphragmatic) because the intercostal muscles of the chest wall are not well developed and fatigue easily from the work of breathing. Effective breathing may be jeopardized when diaphragmatic movement is compromised (such as gastric or abdominal distention or backboard straps over the lower chest) because the chest wall cannot compensate. As the child grows older, the chest muscles strengthen and chest expansion becomes more noticeable.

Assess the quality of the patient's ventilations. Notice the depth and pattern of respirations (Table 17-2). **Tidal volume** is the volume of air moved into or out of the lungs during a normal breath. Normal ventilations at rest are regular and have a tidal volume of approximately 5 to 7 mL/kg. **Minute volume** is the amount of air moved in and out of the lungs in 1 minute and is determined by multiplying the tidal volume by the respiratory rate. Thus a change in either the tidal volume *or* respiratory rate will affect minute volume. Although physically measuring tidal volume is impractical, you can indirectly evaluate it by observing the amount of rise and fall of the patient's chest and abdomen.

Breathing patterns often are easily determined by palpating the chest for 30 seconds or 1 minute or by simply observing. Recognition of specific patterns, such as Kuss-

Capnography - CO₂ (35-45) normal   *CO₂ is potent vasodilator - don't let it build up when intracranial bleed - relative hyperventilation* maul's respirations, helps identify specific underlying problems.

Blood Pressure

Inside vessels, blood is kept under pressure. The cardiovascular system's pressure at rest is the **diastolic blood pressure.** When the ventricles of the heart contract, more blood is forced into and through the system. This causes an increase in pressure, which is measured as the **systolic blood pressure.** The more blood ejected from the ventricles, the higher the systolic blood pressure is relative to the diastolic. Because the ventricles eject blood in boluses with each contraction, the blood moves through the cardiovascular system at an inconsistent rate. Blood moves during a contraction, when the system is at higher pressure **(systole).** Blood flow slows when the ventricles relax **(diastole).** When the blood moves quickly through the arterial system, it rubs against the arterial walls. This movement can be heard in some of the larger vessels. It is called **Korotkoff sounds.**

Blood pressure within the body is constantly changing. It increases during exercise, with caffeine ingestion, during stress, and while smoking. Loss of fluids, relaxation, medications, and a reclined position may decrease blood pressure. This helps illustrate why sets of vital signs are taken; blood pressure values must be used in comparison with their trend over time as well as compared with other vital signs. Look to see how blood pressure changes compared with pulse and respirations. The goal of maintaining blood pressure is to maintain end-tissue perfusion. End-tissue perfusion is most easily monitored by watching the skin and the mental status. The skin is the first organ to have blood shunted away; thus changes in skin color, condition (moisture), and temperature are early signs of blood pressure changes affecting tissue perfusion. Mental status changes can signify failure to perfuse enough blood to the brain.

Cardiologists frequently disagree on what numbers signal a normal blood pressure. Traditionally this number has been 120/80 mm Hg for a healthy adult man. Women tend to run a little bit lower. Notice that the difference between the two numbers is 40 mm Hg. The **pulse pressure** is the difference between the systolic and diastolic pressures and typically is between 30 and 40 mm Hg. It may be higher, however; if you notice a decreasing (narrowing) pulse pressure, it can signal that the heart is not functioning properly. During cases of trauma to the chest, it may suggest that the pericardial sac is filling with fluid. During increases in intracranial pressure, the pulse pressure increases (widens). So the question remains regarding what is a normal blood pressure. In general, any systolic blood pressure between 100 and 140 and diastolic pressure less than 90 are considered normal. Mild **hypertension** exists when the systolic blood pressure is between 140 and 160; any systolic pressure greater than 160 or diastolic above 90 is

considered severely hypertensive. **Hypotension** is low blood pressure and is more relative to a patient. A blood pressure of 90/60 mm Hg may be normal for one patient but abnormal for another. Patients often know their own normal blood pressure range and will tell you if you ask.

Body Temperature

Although often skipped by many EMS providers, body temperature is an important vital sign. The average **core body temperature** is 98.6° F (37° C), and the human body strives to keep the core within a few tenths of a degree. Normal temperatures vary among individuals. Body temperature is affected by perfusion, environmental exposure, pregnancy, time of day, and the patient's level of activity.

The body maintains heat through thermoregulation. Heat is produced through muscle movement, which requires energy. However, bodies lose heat through evaporation, radiation, conduction, and convection. The body controls loss by limiting the amount of blood that reaches the skin in cool and cold environments.

Many physiologic conditions, diseases, and medicines affect core body temperature. Core temperatures that are too low or too high impair the body's ability to function. **Hypothermia** occurs when the core temperature falls below normal, usually below 95° F (35° C), and **hyperthermia** is a higher than normal body temperature. High core body temperatures can lead to problems such as heat stroke and febrile seizures.

To obtain a true core body temperature requires use of an esophageal probe. Esophageal probes are out of the scope of practice of paramedics. However, many services do carry rectal thermometers, which closely approximate core body temperature. Rectal thermometers must be lubricated before insertion and should be single patient use only. If your local medical direction does not allow rectal temperatures to be taken, obtain either an oral, tympanic (ear), or axillary (armpit) temperature (Figure 17-12). When interpreting a temperature measurement, you must know the range of normal values at the site used (Table 17-3).

When taking an axillary temperature, place the thermometer into the center of the patient's armpit. Then lower the patient's arm over the axilla and place the arm across the patient's chest. Temperatures measured in the axillae are approximately 1° F lower than those measured orally. Even when performed properly, axillary measurement is the most inaccurate method of determining a patient's temperature.

Mental Status
[OBJECTIVES 11, 12]

A patient's mental status is initially assessed with the **AVPU** scale (Table 17-4). A patient's mental status is the best measurement of the body's homeostasis and

If pulse pressure getting wider but pulse ↓, sign of intracranial pressure/bleed

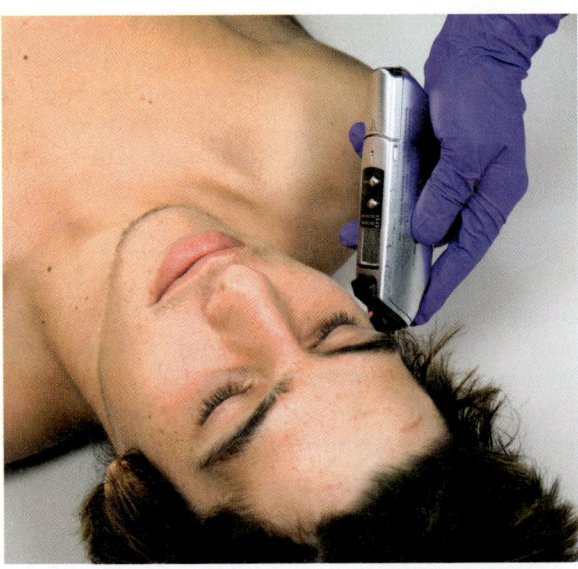

Figure 17-12 Taking a patient's tympanic temperature.

TABLE 17-3 Temperature Measurement Variances

Location	Temperature (°F)	Temperature (°C)
Actual core temperature	97.5-100.2	36.4-37.9
Esophageal probe	97.5-100.2	36.4-37.9
Rectal	97.8-100.2	36.6-37.9
Oral	95.9-99.9	35.5-37.7
Tympanic (ear)	96.3-99.5	35.7-37.5

TABLE 17-4 Mental Status and AVPU

AVPU Level	Assessment Findings	
Alert	Responds spontaneously; further define mental status	
	Alert and oriented ×4	Person, place, time, and event
	Alert and oriented ×3	Person, place, and time
	Alert and oriented ×2	Person and place
	Alert and oriented ×1	Person only
Verbal	Responds to verbal stimuli	
Pain	Responds to painful stimuli	
Unresponsive	Does not responds to stimuli	

systemic perfusion. A patient who is awake, alert, and has no mental status changes is considered "Awake and Oriented ×4" (A&O×4). It is written as "×4" for person, place, time, and event. When patients exhibit mental status changes, they remain awake but become disoriented. Patients generally become disoriented first to events. They then forget the time and then where they are. Who they are is the last point of orientation lost.

Describing how a patient is acting is more helpful than simply documenting level of responsiveness. For example, you may describe a patient as "alert and cooperative," or "awake and combative," or even "awake but slow to respond to questions."

Another useful assessment tool is the Glasgow Coma Scale (GCS) (Table 17-5). The GCS may be used to establish a baseline for comparison in later assessments. For example, in the setting of head trauma an increasing GCS may result in the patient being discharged from the hospital. A static GCS may result in admission and observation, and a decrease in the GCS by 2 or more points may result in surgery. If a change in the GCS occurs in the prehospital setting but is not reported, the baseline falsely becomes the first evaluation of the receiving facility staff. Because a change of as little as 2 points makes a difference in patient management, an unreported change of 1 point in the EMS setting and a reported change of 1 point in the emergency department will give the false impression that the change was only 1 point, resulting in possible mismanagement because of lost data.

Additional "Vital Signs"

While performing advanced life support monitoring, other values and assessments may be monitored along with vital signs (Box 17-1). **Pulse oximetry** can be constantly monitored (see Chapter 13). A pulse oximeter gives a reading in percent of hemoglobin saturated and is written as SpO_2. This value should be documented on room air before oxygen administration with the patient's respiratory rate. An SpO_2 of 96 means that 96% of the hemoglobin is saturated. Normally only oxygen is binding with hemoglobin, so a pulse oximetry reading is an accurate assessment. However, when a patient is exposed to carbon monoxide, a pulse oximeter essentially becomes useless. The carbon monoxide bonds with hemoglobin better than oxygen and therefore displaces the oxygen. This means that although the reading will still state 96%

BOX 17-1 Additional "Vital Signs"

- Pulse oximetry
- End-tidal carbon dioxide
- Glucometry
- Pain level

TABLE 17-5 Adult, Child, and Infant Glasgow Coma Scale

Glasgow Coma Scale	Adult/Child	Score	Infant
Eye opening	Spontaneous	4	Spontaneous
	To verbal	3	To verbal
	To pain	2	To pain
	No response	1	No response
Best verbal response	Oriented	5	Coos, babbles
	Disoriented	4	Irritable cry
	Inappropriate words	3	Cries only to pain
	Incomprehensible sounds	2	Moans to pain
	No response	1	No response
Best motor response	Obeys commands	6	Spontaneous
	Localizes pain	5	Withdraws from touch
	Withdraws from pain	4	Withdraws from pain
	Abnormal flexion (decorticate)	3	Abnormal flexion (decorticate)
	Abnormal extension (decerebrate)	2	Abnormal extension (decerebrate)
	No response	1	No response
Total = E + V + M		3 to 15	

Know GCS - will have scenarios

of the hemoglobin is saturated, how much of that percent is oxygen and how much is carbon monoxide cannot be determined in the field.

Another respiratory rate–related value is end-tidal carbon dioxide level ($ETCO_2$). This often is monitored in intubated patients but frequently is used for non-intubated patient monitoring as well. Pulse oximetry measures the amount of molecules on the hemoglobin, which can be oxygen or carbon monoxide molecules. End-tidal carbon dioxide levels allow monitoring of how well patients are exhaling, which is critical in acid-base balance. Patients with low $ETCO_2$ may have a problem with oxygen/carbon dioxide exchange at the alveolar level. Although not a true vital sign, consider assessing a blood glucose level with vital signs (see Chapter 33).

Some medical services also have begun measuring pain level as a vital sign, asking for a numeric value of the patient's pain on a scale of 0 to 10. Zero means no pain, and 10 is the worst pain ever felt. If your patient is in pain, reevaluate the pain level each time you assess vital signs to determine whether your pain management is working.

General Approach

A thorough and complete patient assessment is not a free-for-all investigation. You must have a systematic, organized approach. When assessing a patient, consider the patient's privacy needs as well as comfort. Patients in an emergency setting often are anxious, especially if they have never required emergency medical assistance before. If you start examining and poking with equipment they have never seen before, anxiety will increase. Explain to your patient what you are about to do. Act in a calm, professional, and confident manner. Advise the patient that you are investigating their problems and, by finding what is wrong, you can work to correct the problem.

PARAMEDIC Pearl

Remember to communicate with the patient throughout your assessment. Make him or her feel a part of your team, not just an object of your work.

Keep your examination efficient and focused without being so focused that essential associated findings are missed. Work through each assessment skill quickly. Do not spend too much time on any one skill. Without neglecting to investigate for additional problems, focus on the patient's primary complaint(s) as much as possible to make him or her feel you are doing as much as you possibly can.

Case Scenario—continued

The patient is alert but has difficulty following commands, attempts to get up off your stretcher, and repeatedly pulls off the nonrebreather oxygen mask you have provided. On examination, you find retractions and the use of accessory muscles of respiration. You observe no jugular venous distension while she is sitting upright. Auscultation of the lungs reveals loud crackles (rales) in all fields, no pedal edema, and strong peripheral pulses. Vital signs are pulse, 130 beats/min; blood pressure, 230/120 mm Hg; respirations, 28 breaths/min; and SpO_2, 80%. Her electrocardiogram demonstrates sinus tachycardia without ectopy.

Questions

5. *Is this patient high priority? Why or why not?*
6. *How does the history of untreated pneumonia, asthma, and untreated hypertension fit into the clinical picture?*
7. *What conditions are consistent with retractions and use of the accessory muscles? What is the significance of the absence of jugular venous distension or pedal edema? What conditions cause crackles (rales)? What do the vital signs contribute to the picture?*
8. *Given the information from the previous question, what provisional diagnoses do you have in mind? Why?*
9. *Do you need additional history or assessment information to determine how you will manage this patient? Why or why not?*
10. *What treatment will you initiate at this time?*

COMPREHENSIVE PATIENT ASSESSMENT SYSTEM

This patient assessment system is designed to be an organized and systematic assessment for any situation you may encounter, whether involving one patient or 100. The assessment has three main sections: the scene size-up, the initial assessment, and the reassessment (Figure 17-13). Complete each part of the assessment before moving to the next part of the system. Each portion of the patient assessment system has equal importance.

Scene Size-Up

[OBJECTIVES 13 to 22]

The scene size-up begins at dispatch as you gather information. Observe the scene as you arrive and begin to take in information. As the paramedic, you are the highest level of care on scene and are responsible for the overall scene management. During the scene size-up, the goal is to take in the whole picture (Figure 17-14). First consider scene safety. Make sure the scene is safe for you and your partner. Your safety is a priority because you must go home at the end of your shift. Do not become another patient. Determine whether any hazards are present or if

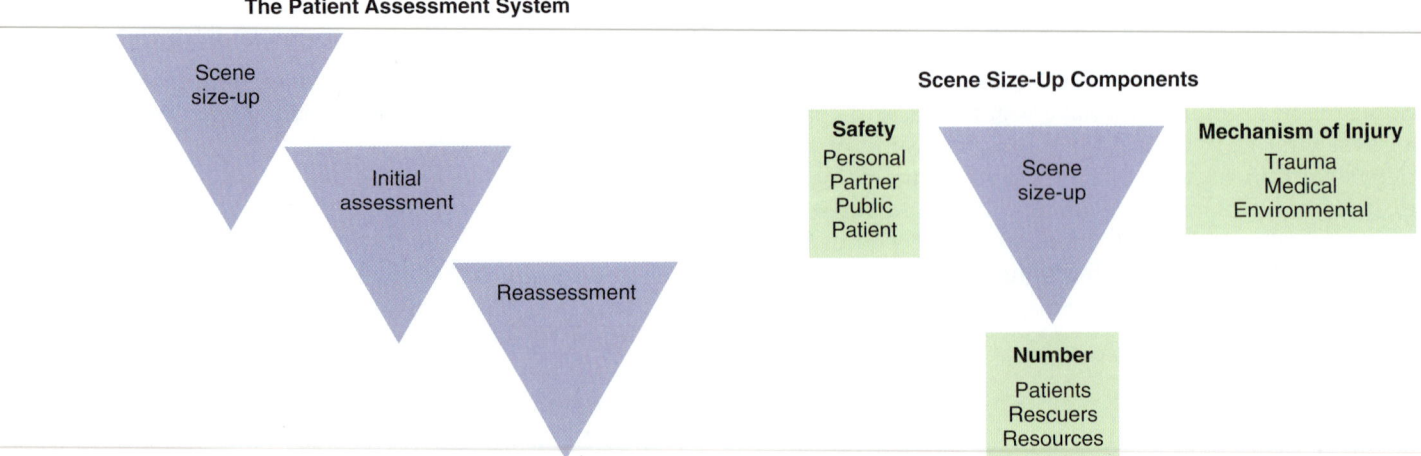

Figure 17-13 Patient assessment overview.

Figure 17-14 Scene size-up.

anything may become a hazard. Assess for any hazards to the public and, finally, assess what hazards the patient faces. If you can do anything to improve scene safety without compromising your own safety, do it. If you can move the patient somewhere to improve his or her safety, do so. Anticipate how the scene may change.

Next, consider your numbers. How many patients are there? How many rescuers do you have? What additional resources may you need? Start thinking early about these resources and ask dispatch for them. Do you need a helicopter, a second ambulance, or an extrication team? Also start to think about what hospitals are local to your area. Will you need to transport your patient to a hospital with specialized care such as a trauma, cardiac, stroke, burn, or pediatric center?

The third side of the scene size-up triangle is evaluation of the mechanism of injury or illness (MOI). Is the mechanism traumatic, medical, or environmental? Is it a mix? For example, a diabetic emergency may have lead to a motor vehicle collision. Your scene size-up also includes the following, all before you may even see the patient (Table 17-6):

- Time of year
- Time of day
- Physical location of the scene
- "Track record" of other calls to the location
- General appearance of the environment while approaching the scene
- Apparent attitudes and movements of all those in the general vicinity while approaching
- Presence of hazards as well as any potential hazards near the scene
- Physical layout of the environment
- The most likely egress route as well as alternate quick egress routes
- Presence of physical clues about the reason for the emergency call
- Information that can be gleaned from all those present on arrival
- Physical barriers to patient movement
- Ambient temperature, ventilation, sounds, odors
- Physical condition of the setting where the patient is located

TABLE 17-6 Data Collection at Dispatch and en Route to the Scene	
Cue	**Considerations**
Seasonal events	Heat illnesses occur more commonly in the summer; hypothermia and upper respiratory illnesses are more common in the winter. Allergies are worse in the spring; holidays, especially late December to early January, are the worst for depression.
Time of day	5-6 AM: frequent serious medical emergency dispatches 2-3 AM: frequent alcohol-related motor vehicle crashes
Environmental conditions	Is the scene safe? Are any potential hazards present? What type of neighborhood is it? Are any signs of violence or violent people in the area?
Egress routes	Always determine your exit route and options as you enter the scene.
Physical clues	Are signs of vehicular collisions visible in cars parked in front of the houses? Is any physical damage to property or furniture visible? What is the condition of the residence, vehicle, or office? Is it clean, neat, and free of obnoxious odors? Is it unkempt and strewn with trash or garbage? Does it appear that no one has cleaned the area in recent weeks or months?
Bystanders	Can family, friends, acquaintances, or witnesses provide helpful and meaningful information? Can you begin gathering information about the patient and what equipment you might need as you step out of your vehicle and before entering the home or building?
Barriers	Are any barriers present to accessing or removing the patient? Do you need to look for an alternate route in or out of the scene?
Ambient temperature	Is the temperature too hot or cold? Too windy or wet? Is the heating system or air conditioner working?
Ventilation	Is enough air circulating?
Odors	Do you smell foul odors indicative of incontinence, disease, poor hygiene, spoiled food, or other conditions or possible hazards?
Sounds	Can you hear the sound of a ventilator or oxygen system, people fighting behind a door, or the sound of a gun being cocked?
Physical condition	Is the structure sound? Is it clean, neat, and well maintained, or is it messy, damaged, and in poor repair?

Initial Assessment

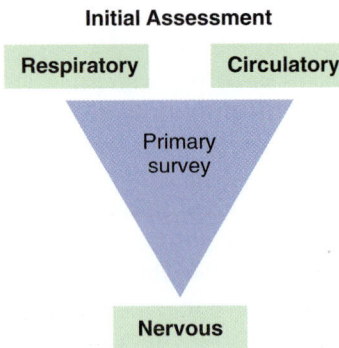

Figure 17-15 The purpose of the primary survey is to find life-threatening conditions and fix them. The focus for life-threatening conditions is on the critical body systems: the respiratory, circulatory, and nervous systems.

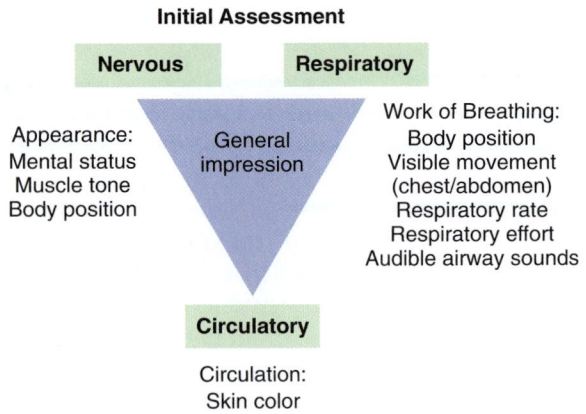

Figure 17-16 General impression components.

Initial Assessment

Primary Survey

[OBJECTIVE 23]

The purpose of the primary survey is to find **life-threatening conditions** and fix them. The focus for life-threatening conditions is on the critical body systems: the respiratory, circulatory, and nervous system (Isaac, 1998) (Figure 17-15). These three critical systems balance the body like a three-legged stool. Together they support the body. However, if you kick out one leg (such as the respiratory system), the other two will only momentarily support the body before the whole thing collapses.

The primary survey begins with your general impression of the patient, a quick hands-on assessment for life threats, and then a determination of whether you have a priority (critical patient). When you identify any potentially life-threatening condition, you need to stop and fix it. If a problem is identified with one of the critical body systems, give necessary care: "treat as you find." Priority is given to the respiratory system because without oxygen, life cannot be sustained for more than approximately 6 minutes.

General Impression. Once you come into view of the patient, immediately begin to form a general impression, which is an impression of the severity of the patient's condition. Your general impression should initially focus on three main areas that can be remembered by the mnemonic ABC: *a*ppearance, (work of) *b*reathing, and *c*irculation (Figure 17-16). As you finish forming your general impression, you will have a good idea if the patient is sick (unstable) or not sick (stable).

- *Appearance.* The patient's appearance reflects the adequacy of oxygenation, ventilation, brain perfusion, homeostasis, and central nervous system function. When forming a general impression, *appearance* refers to the patient's mental status, muscle tone, and body position. Is the patient's condition life threatening? Can you tell if the patient is in severe distress, moderate distress, mild distress, or no apparent distress?

- You can assess the patient's level of apparent distress by the presence or absence of spontaneous writhing, grimacing, crying out for help, and other overt signs. However, you also need to observe for subtle, or covert, signs of distress and reasons the call for help was placed. Covert signs include furtive behaviors (sneaky, suspicious), such as hiding medicines or alcohol or denying that anything is wrong when the patient's appearance leads you to believe that something must be wrong.

- Assess the patient's general posture. Is the patient lying unnaturally on the ground or comfortably in bed? Is the patient sitting comfortably in a living room chair or leaning over a bucket vomiting? Abnormal body positions may include a **sniffing position**, **tripod position**, or **head bobbing**. In a sniffing position, the patient sits upright and leans forward with the chin slightly raised. In this position, the axes of the mouth, pharynx, and trachea are aligned and open the airway, increasing airflow. In a tripod position, the patient sits upright and leans forward, supported by his or her arms, with the neck slightly extended, chin projected, and mouth open. This position is used to maintain an open airway. Head bobbing is an indicator of increased work of breathing in infants. The head falls forward with exhalation and comes up with expansion of the chest on inhalation.

- *Breathing.* When forming a general impression, *breathing* refers to the presence or absence of visible movement of the chest or abdomen, signs of breathing effort, and the presence of audible airway sounds. Breathing reflects the adequacy of the patient's airway, oxygenation, and ventilation. Abnormal findings include **nasal flaring; retractions;** muffled or hoarse speech; a respiratory rate outside the normal range for the patient's age; use of accessory muscles to breathe; and abnormal respiratory sounds such as **stridor, grunting, gasping, gurgling,** or **wheezing.**

- *Circulation.* Circulation reflects the adequacy of cardiac output and perfusion of vital organs (core perfusion). When forming a general impression, circulation refers to skin color. Skin color normally is some shade of pink. Even patients of African descent, who have heavy pigmentation, have an underlying pink color to the skin. Abnormal findings include pallor, mottling, and cyanosis.

PARAMEDIC*Pearl*

Primary Survey Components

- General impression
  - Appearance
  - (Work of) breathing
  - Circulation
- **A**irway, level of responsiveness, cervical spine protection
- **B**reathing (ventilation)
- **C**irculation (perfusion)
- **D**isability (mini-neurologic examination)
- **E**xpose
- Identify priority patients and transport decision

Establishing Rapport with the Patient. When approaching the patient, consider the affect, or emotional state, of the patient and family. If the patient is alert and responsive, you must establish rapport before beginning a series of questions (Table 17-7). However, if the patient is lying unconscious or in extremis (near death or at the extreme stage of a disease), you must rapidly begin your physical examination while attempting to elicit a patient history.

At this early stage of patient contact you are beginning the physical examination, obtaining the history, and establishing the patient's mental status. Your initial assessment of the patient's mental status should include the patient's responsiveness on the AVPU scale. Start by asking "What's your name?" If the patient is responsive, your mental status examination might also include a brief impression of the muscle tone and voluntary muscle responses to commands, including whether movements and strength are equal on the right and left sides.

Respiratory System
[OBJECTIVES 24, 25, 26]
Evaluate the respiratory system by checking for an open airway and adequate breathing. If cervical spine injury is suspected (by examination, history, or mechanism of injury), ask a member of your crew to manually stabilize the head and neck in a neutral, inline position or maintain spinal stabilization if already completed. If the patient is responsive and the airway is open, assess breathing. If the patient is responsive but cannot talk or cough forcefully, assess for possible airway obstruction. If the patient is unresponsive, the head tilt/chin lift maneuver is typically used to open the airway. If trauma is suspected, the jaw thrust without head tilt maneuver is pre-

---

TABLE 17-7	Establishing Rapport with the Patient
Goal	**Example**
Identify yourself by name and title.	"Hello, I'm Tricia. We are paramedics with Central EMS."
Position yourself at the patient's eye level if the patient is sitting in a chair or upright on the ground.	Pull up a chair next to the patient or kneel down at the patient's side.
Ask appropriate initial questions to discern the patient's level of responsiveness and distress.	"Can you tell me what happened today?" "Where do you hurt the most?" "Can you take a deep breath?"
Touch the patient appropriately.	"Shake and shout" when patients appear to be unconscious; a painful stimulus should be used if the patient is unresponsive to verbal and tactile stimuli. Begin to take the radial pulse of a conscious patient who is sitting up. Take a carotid and radial pulse on a patient more than 1 year old who is supine and unresponsive.

ferred. If trauma is suspected but the airway cannot be opened with the jaw thrust without head tilt maneuver, use a head tilt/chin lift.

Assess the patient's airway for the following immediate life threats: the tongue, foreign body airway obstruction, liquids, and anatomic (crush/swelling) obstruction. If the airway is clear of debris and obstruction, evaluate the patient's breathing. If the airway is not open, assess for sounds of airway compromise (**snoring,** gurgling, or stridor). Gurgling is an indication for immediate suctioning. Look in the mouth for blood, broken teeth, loose dentures, gastric contents, and foreign objects. If you see blood, vomitus, or other secretions, suction the mouth and throat with a rigid (tonsil tip) suction catheter while manually opening the airway. Orotracheal or nasotracheal intubation or insertion of another advanced airway (such as a Combitube or laryngeal mask airway) may be indicated (see Chapter 13).

The next step is to check for breathing life threats, which include open pneumothorax, tension pneumothorax, flail chest, and inadequate minute volume. Start by looking for chest or stomach rise and fall. Assessment of breathing should take no more than 10 seconds. If the patient is breathing, determine if breathing is adequate or inadequate.

Count the respiratory rate, assess the depth and pattern of the patient's breathing, check the color of the lips and tongue, and look for chest trauma. A patient with breathing difficulty often has a respiratory rate outside the normal limits for his or her age. Note the rhythm of respirations (regular, irregular, periodic).

Listen for air movement through the patient's mouth or nose. Note whether respirations are quiet, absent, or noisy. With the soft hairs on the side of your face, feel for moisture condensation on exhalation. Listen for breath sounds (Figure 17-17). Breath sounds should be clear and equal. Listen under each armpit and in the midclavicular line under each clavicle. Alternate from side to side and compare your findings. During the primary survey, the type of lung sounds a patient has is

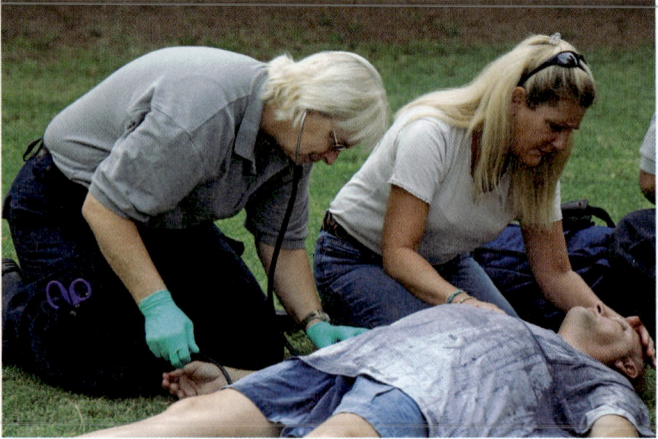

Figure 17-17 Listen to breath sounds.

as important as noting whether they are present and equal.

If the patient has signs of mild to moderate respiratory distress, help the patient into a position of comfort and give oxygen. If the patient is having breathing difficulty and the rate is too slow or too fast, give oxygen and positive-pressure ventilation if necessary. If breathing is absent, insert an airway adjunct (if not previously done) and begin positive-pressure ventilation with supplemental oxygen. If an open wound is present on the torso, cover it with an airtight dressing taped on three sides. If a patient shows signs of respiratory failure or shock and has diminished or absent breath sounds on one side of the chest, consider the possibility of a tension pneumothorax. Needle decompression of the chest should be performed, if indicated. If breathing is adequate, move on to assessment of circulation.

Circulatory System
[OBJECTIVES 27, 28]

BP: at least 80 rad(c)
 " 70 femoral
 " 60 carotid

Assess the integrity of the circulatory system by checking for a pulse and looking for severe bleeding. If no pulse is present, cardiopulmonary resuscitation may be indicated. Control severe bleeding if present. Severe bleeding is generally found below the chin down to the knees and out to the mid-upper arm. Control severe external bleeding with well-aimed direct pressure. Well-aimed direct pressure means applying pressure directly on the bleeding site, not just the general area. Consider possible areas of major internal bleeding. Significant internal bleeding may occur in the chest, abdomen, pelvis, retroperitoneum, and femoral areas. Pain or swelling in any of these areas may signal possible internal bleeding. Definitive care for internal bleeding requires a surgeon. If you suspect internal bleeding, begin rapid transport.

Determine whether the patient's heart rate is within normal limits for age. Compare the strength and quality of central and peripheral pulses. A weak central pulse may indicate decompensated shock (see Chapter 21). A peripheral pulse that is difficult to find, weak, or irregular suggests poor peripheral perfusion and may be a sign of **shock,** hemorrhage, or a cardiac dysrhythmia. If signs of shock are present, give oxygen (if not already done), initiate intravenous access (usually en route to the hospital), and keep the patient warm.

Assess the patient's skin color, temperature, and moisture. Decreased skin perfusion is an early sign of shock. Skin color is most reliably evaluated in the sclera, conjunctiva, nail beds, tongue, oral mucosa, palms, and soles. Use the dorsal surfaces of your hands and fingers to assess the moisture of the skin.

In a child younger than 6 years, assess capillary refill by firmly pressing the skin over the warmest point on the child's body and release. Observe the time necessary for the blanched tissue to return to its original color. If the ambient temperature is warm, color should return within 2 seconds. Capillary refill time of 3 to 5 seconds is delayed and may indicate poor perfusion or exposure to cool

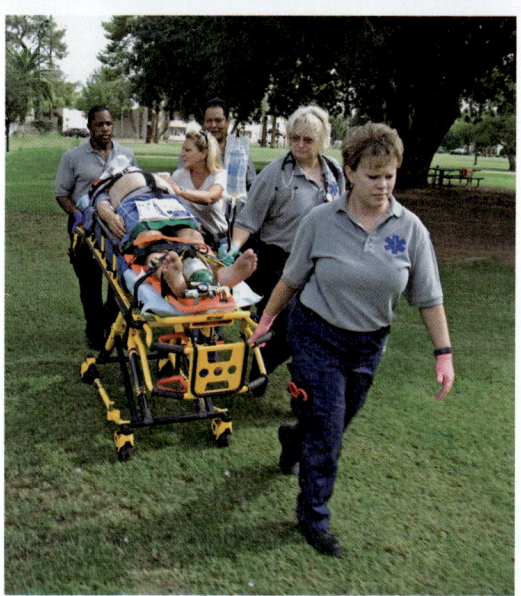

ambient temperatures. Capillary refill time more than 5 seconds is markedly delayed and suggests shock.

Nervous System
[OBJECTIVES 29, 30, 31, 32, 33]

One life-threatening condition in the nervous system is the presence of a mechanism of injury for a spinal injury. If a traumatic mechanism exists in which the spine could have been hurt, assume an injury exists and take spinal precautions. This is one reason the MOI is assessed during the scene size-up. A spine injury is a life threat because the loss of nervous system function can lead to respiratory arrest, digestive problems, and vasculature size control problems.

Spinal precautions mean assuming hands-on (manual) stabilization of the spine and preparing to restrict the motion of the patient fully with a cervical collar and long spine board. You do not need to fully spinally restrict the patient during the primary survey. This can wait until you have treated all life threats. Recognize the need for manual stabilization, however, and begin it early.

Potentially life-threatening problems with the nervous system are manifested with a decreased level of consciousness. A GCS score is assessed during the disability phase of the primary survey to obtain a more detailed assessment of the patient's neurologic status.

The assessment goal of the patient with a decreased level of consciousness is to identify the cause. Is the patient diabetic? Has a traumatic brain injury occurred? Inspect the patient for medical alert tags for guidance. Focus your time on identifying and correcting the cause of impaired brain function. Further assessment often can wait until the brain-based problem is corrected.

Figure 17-18 After controlling immediate life threats, make a transport decision.

PARAMEDIC*Pearl*

Possible causes of a loss of consciousness can be remembered by the mnemonic STOPEATS: **s**ugar, **t**emperature, **o**xygen deprivation (hypoxia), increased intracranial **p**ressure, **e**lectricity, **a**lcohol, **t**oxins, and **s**alts.

BOX 17-2 Priority Patients

- Poor general impression
- Unresponsive patients—no gag or cough reflex
- Responsive, not following commands
- Difficulty breathing
- Shock (hypoperfusion)
- Complicated childbirth
- Chest pain with blood pressure <100 mm Hg systolic
- Uncontrolled bleeding
- Severe pain anywhere
- Multiple injuries

At the end of the primary survey you must have evaluated for the six immediate life threats: uncontrolled airway, inadequate breathing, pulselessness, severe bleeding (internal and external), decreased level of consciousness, and potential spinal injury. After controlling these problems, make a transport decision. Do you need to begin rapid transport to the most appropriate facility at this time, or can you continue with your assessment on scene (Figure 17-18)? Examples of priority patients requiring expedited transport are listed in Box 17-2.

Secondary Survey
[OBJECTIVES 34 to 46]

As you transition into the secondary survey, take a breath. The secondary survey has three parts: a physical examination, vital signs, and SAMPLE history (Figure 17-19).

Regardless of your transport decision, all three corners of the triangle must be completed. They can be done on scene or en route to the hospital.

Before you begin, make a decision on how to focus your examination. Are you focusing on a medical condition, for which time should be spent on a detailed history and an abbreviated physical examination, or is this trauma? Trauma examinations are either rapidly performed or focused. A **rapid trauma assessment** is a quick head-to-toe assessment of a trauma patient with a significant mechanism of injury. It focuses on identifying major injuries such as fractures and dislocations or other injuries that could produce significant morbidity if not corrected. If the patient's MOI is not significant, perform a focused physical examination of the injured body part and other body areas as needed.

A **rapid medical assessment** is a quick head-to-toe assessment of a medical patient who is unresponsive or has an altered mental status. If the patient is responsive and has a medical condition, time should be spent on

Initial Assessment

Physical exam	SAMPLE history

Secondary survey

Vital signs

Figure 17-19 Components of the secondary survey.

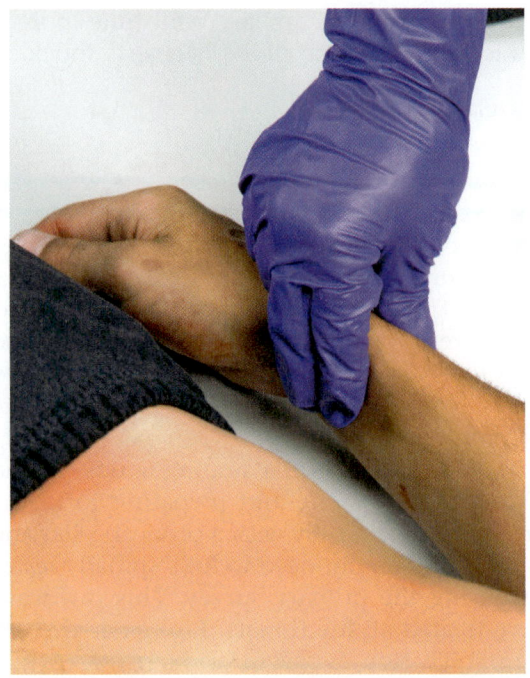

Figure 17-20 In a responsive patient older than 1 year, check the pulse first at the radial artery.

obtaining a detailed history and then performing a focused physical examination based on the patient's symptoms.

In general, which portion of the secondary survey is performed first does not matter as long as all three—physical examination, vital signs, and SAMPLE history—are completed at some point. Do not provide nonemergency treatments during the secondary survey. Use this time to fully explore all the patient's symptoms and problems. Develop a complete list of every problem the patient has. Use the list to anticipate what problems may arise later. Then prioritize which problems to manage first, creating a treatment plan for managing the problems. Only treat non–life-threatening problems after you have completed the secondary survey.

Vital Signs. Take the six vital signs: pulse, respirations, blood pressure, temperature, mental status/AVPU, and skin. Always be sure to note the time.

Pulse. In a *responsive* patient older than 1 year, check a pulse first at the radial artery. With two pads of your fingers, press the radial artery against the radius on the inside of the forearm just proximal to the wrist (Figure 17-20). Count for 30 seconds and multiply by 2. If the pulse is slow or irregular, count for 60 seconds to obtain an accurate rate. If you cannot feel the radial pulse, check the femoral artery. The femoral pulse can be located at the fold of the groin (Figure 17-21). To locate the carotid artery, find the patient's Adam's apple, place two fingers on it, and slide your fingers laterally against the trachea, following down into the groove against the soft tissues alongside the trachea (Figure 17-22). Between the trachea and soft tissues you will feel the carotid artery. Be sure to document quality and rhythm also. Note the pulse check site as well.

Respirations. Counting breaths per minute can be difficult. If you tell a patient you are counting breaths, he or she becomes conscious of breathing and stops breathing normally. A good technique is to count the radial pulse first, then without saying anything place the patient's arm against the chest, continue to hold the wrist, and watch and feel as the arm rises and falls with the chest. Either count for 30 seconds and multiply by 2

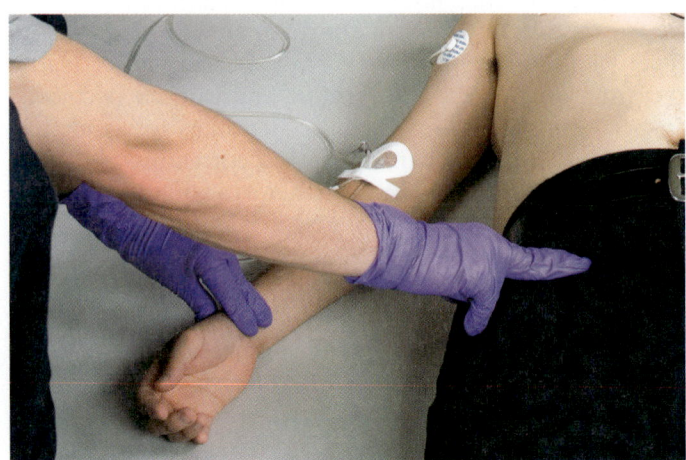

Figure 17-21 Palpation of the femoral artery.

or count for a full minute. If the patient has a decreased level of consciousness, simply place your hand against the chest and count. Note the patient's breathing rate, effort, and quality. Differentiate actual ventilatory effort from any rescue breaths and artificial ventilations you are providing.

Blood Pressure. Begin blood pressure assessment by getting down to bare skin on the arm and place the blood pressure cuff snugly against it. If you observe any sort of dialysis shunt, or central line, use the other arm. Instruct the conscious patient to relax the arm; if the patient holds the arm up or locks the elbow straight, blood pressure in the arm changes (Figure 17-23).

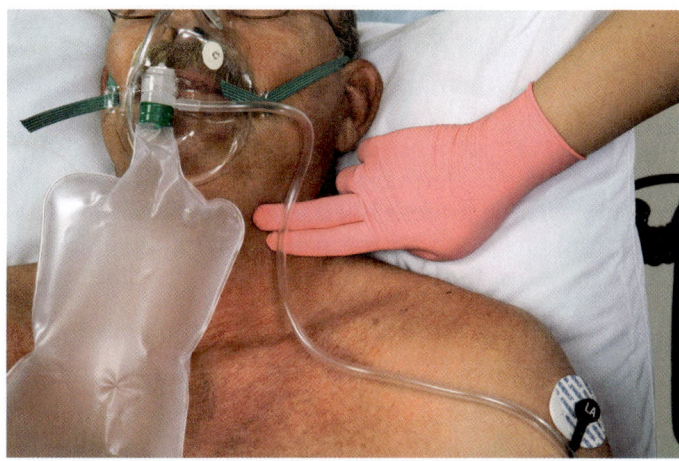

Figure 17-22 Palpation of the carotid artery.

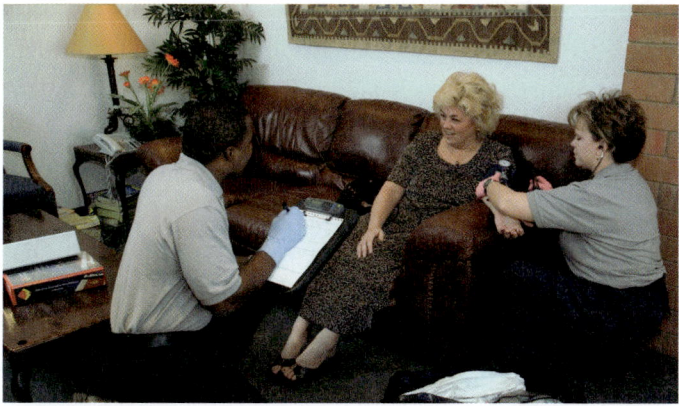

Figure 17-23 Auscultating a blood pressure.

Be sure to use a properly sized blood pressure cuff. Using the incorrect size produces an incorrect value. A correctly sized cuff has a width between one half and one third the length of the patient's arm. The blood pressure cuff should not come down onto the elbow. If it does, it is too low and you need to readjust the cuff. Locate the patient's radial artery. Rapidly inflate the cuff until you can no longer feel the radial pulse. Inflate the cuff 30 mm Hg beyond the point at which you last felt the pulse. Place the bell side of your stethoscope against the medial side of the elbow. Slowly allow the cuff to deflate at a rate approximately 2 to 3 mm Hg/sec. Watch the manometer as the pressure releases. Note the systolic blood pressure when you first hear the blood pressure. Continue listening until the sound disappears; this is the diastolic pressure.

You will encounter problems if you allow the tubes on the blood pressure cuff to become twisted or bounce against one another or the stethoscope while you evaluate the blood pressure. Auscultation difficulties also can be caused by pressing too hard or not hard enough with the stethoscope or by using your thumb to hold the stethoscope in place. Document the systolic and diastolic blood pressure (e.g., 142/84 mm Hg). Also document the arm it was taken from and the patient's position (supine, sitting, or standing).

Body Temperature. Obtain the patient's temperature. Electronic thermometers, whether placed orally or rectally, require as little as 20 seconds to obtain an accurate number. Tympanic thermometers now take relatively accurate readings in just a few moments. Whatever model thermometer you decide to use, make sure you learn how to use it first. Always follow the manufacturer's instructions. Replace thermometers meant for single-patient use after each patient contact or properly decontaminate reusable models. Document the type of temperature taken (e.g., oral, rectal, tympanic, axillary).

Mental Status/AVPU. Determine exactly where patients are on the AVPU scale. A patient who knows who he or she is (oriented to person), where he or she is (oriented to place), the time and date (oriented time), and what has happened (oriented to event) is A&O×4. Subtract 1 point for each item for which the patient is not oriented.

A patient can be awake but completely disoriented. Verbally responsive patients respond to a **verbal stimulus,** such as a shout or hearing their name, with some action. The patient may only respond with an arm movement, a groan or moan, or grimace. Document what kind of stimuli the patient does respond to. If the patient only responds when you illicit pain, such as pressing on a nail bed, then the patient is P on the AVPU scale (responsive to **painful stimulus**). If the patient does not respond to verbal or painful stimuli, the rating is U on AVPU, which means unresponsive. Document to which stimulus the patient responded and what the response was.

Assessment of mental status is only one component of evaluating the integrity of the brain and spinal cord. The AVPU scale allows assessment of a patient's responsiveness and pieces of memory. In a responsive patient, assess both short- and long-term memory because they represent two distinctly different portions of the brain. Short-term memory lapses could be common for your patient or may indicate a more serious problem. For example, after a traumatic brain injury, a patient who cannot remember information after the event has **antegrade amnesia.** Antegrade amnesia is a warning sign that the patient is likely to have brain swelling and increased intracranial pressure. Patients who have forgotten more long-term events, such as where they live, who they are, or what they have done until a given point in time (e.g., falling on the head) have **retrograde amnesia.** Some degree of retrograde amnesia is common after a concussion.

Pay attention to a patient's attention span. It is appropriate? The inability to focus on your conversation may be driven by pain or impaired brain function. Attention deficit disorders are becoming more common in today's society. People often are too easily distracted from important events around them. An acute onset of attention loss, or patients who are unexplainably daydreaming, should be evaluated for hypoglycemia and proper hydration. On the opposite side of the spectrum, be prepared to encounter patients who obsessively focus on a single, individual detail. This obsessive focus may signal a mental disorder, such as obsessive-compulsive disorder.

Skin Condition. Although you noted the skin during the primary survey, thoroughly assess it again. Check color, condition, and temperature. The skin temperature is different from core body temperature; do not confuse the two. Note whether the skin is red, pink (normal), gray, or cyanotic. Is the patient sweating or extremely dry, or does the skin tent? Does the skin feel very warm or cold to the touch? Cool, gray, or pale, moist skin suggests blood has been shunted away from the skin to another organ.

SAMPLE History. Obtain a SAMPLE history (Box 17-3). Investigate the patient's **signs and symptoms** with the OPQRST mnemonic (Box 17-4). Determine allergies to medications, foods, and the environment. Ask the patient what medications he or she is taking, should be taking, and if the patient is compliant with medicines. Inquire about both prescription and over-the-counter medicines. A *pertinent* medical history must be obtained. Remember, the patient's broken hand at age 10 years does not affect chest pain today. Keep it limited to what could affect the presenting problem. Determine what the patient ate and drank last. This information is important if the patient may go into surgery. Finally, ask about what led up to the patient calling 9-1-1.

Obtaining history information from unreliable and unresponsive patients can be difficult. Begin by questioning those around the patient, particularly family members, whenever possible. Carefully examine the patient for any clues that may help identify the patient's problem. In particular, check the patient's wrists and neck for medical alert tags. Patients with diabetes or Alzheimer's disease often wear medic alert tags. Also look for insulin pumps, a small device that looks like a pager but provides a constant flow of insulin to the patient. Insulin pumps are common. Use the best information available when attempting to complete a SAMPLE history; if you simply cannot obtain the information, explain why in your report.

PARAMEDIC*Pearl*

Take advantage of information obtained from family members and bystanders. When someone says a patient is acting differently than normal, take it as a sign of an underlying illness or injury until proven otherwise.

Throughout patient contact time, make an effort to notice how the patient acts. Ask yourself whether your patient's actions are appropriate for age, sex, and general condition. When gathering the patient's history, note the patient's posture and body language. Crossed arms signal a defensive nature. Making an effort to stand above another, or approaching with an outwardly puffed chest are signs of aggressiveness. At the same time, inferiority is established by having to look up toward another person. A patient who shifts position often or shows signs of restlessness may be in pain. Be aware of the body language you and your team are conveying as well.

Note your patient's general attitude. Determine whether the patient is calm, sad, pessimistic, optimistic, scared, nervous, or anxious. To the best of your ability, try to keep patients calm and comfortable. Attitude concerns and changes often provide insight to a patient's underlying problem.

Physical Examination. A comprehensive physical examination can be performed in many ways. However, the two most common methods are the head-to-toe approach and the body systems approach. During the head-to-toe approach, begin examining the patient at the head and inspect each region of the body, moving down toward the feet, then coming back up to the arms and back last. A physical examination that uses the body systems approach examines each system in detail one at a time. You may choose to evaluate the cardiac system, then the gastrointestinal, musculoskeletal, and then nervous. Whichever format selected, the goal is the same: evaluate the entire body for anything that is abnormal. As a general rule, follow the DCAPBTLS mnemonic as a guide of what to inspect (Box 17-5). Practice your physical examination so it is organized and efficient. Working in an emergency setting requires that you approach the examination professionally and are proficient.

BOX 17-3   SAMPLE History Mnemonic

Signs and symptoms
Allergies
Medicines
Past (pertinent) medical history
Last oral intake and output (urination and bowel movements)
Events prior

BOX 17-4   OPQRST Mnemonic

Onset
Provocation, **p**alliation, **p**osition
Quality
Region, **r**adiation
Severity
Timing (duration)

BOX 17-5	DCAPBTLS Mnemonic

Deformities
Contusions
Abrasions
Punctures
Bruises
Tenderness
Lacerations
Swelling

Skin

[OBJECTIVES 47, 48]

Even though you have already assessed the skin several times for color, condition, and temperature in a general context, the skin still requires its own detailed examination. The skin can reveal information about many disorders and other body systems. Although the patient's skin baseline is a function of heredity, age, sex, and family background, you can still perform the same basic examination.

Examine all patients for skin color in the fingernail beds, palms, soles, mucous membranes of the mouth, and inner surface of the eyelids. The skin's pinkness results from well-oxygenated hemoglobin in the blood. When the skin appears pale, blood has been shunted away to other, more vital, organs. This could be a result of hypovolemia from dehydration, hypovolemic shock, or hypothermia. If only one limb has pale skin, suspect that circulation has been significantly reduced or cut off to the entire limb because of a vascular injury or occlusion. Pale skin also may result from decreased hemoglobin, which may occur from blood loss or nutritional factors such as inadequate intake.

Cyanosis, or blueness, in the skin results when the blood is deoxygenated. Work to correct the underlying respiratory problem when you see cyanosis. Pale, gray skin tends to be widespread in appearance, whereas cyanosis first manifests in the most distal portions of the skin—fingernail beds, lips, and ears—before becoming generalized. Remember, even though cyanosis only manifests in local areas, it is a very serious systemic problem and needs to be aggressively treated.

Hyperpigmentation is a manifestation of increased melanin in the skin. It is diffuse in appearance but may be especially noticeable over the knuckles, knees, and palmar creases and as dark patches on the buccal mucosa of the mouth. A patient in shock with hyperpigmentation should raise the suspicion for **Addison's disease** (adrenal insufficiency), which requires aggressive fluid resuscitation and treatment with steroids.

Evaluate the moisture content of the skin. Is the patient sweating profusely? Is the skin dry and cracking? As people age, the skin loses elasticity and becomes more brittle. Expect older adults to have more sensitive skin with less water and oil content.

The skin can be a good indicator of dehydration. Check the mucous membranes (inside of eyelids, gums, tongue). Dry mucous membranes suggest dehydration. **Skin turgor** is the skin's resistance to deformation when pinched or depressed. Pinch the skin over the forehead or sternum and release. Loss of skin turgor, one of the signs of dehydration, will cause the skin to remain tented for some period after it is released, although poor skin turgor may be seen in the normal elderly patient as a result of age-related loss of elasticity.

With the back side of your hand, note the skin temperature. Whether warm, hot, or cold, the temperature should feel the same throughout the body. Localized temperature increases suggest increased vascularity from inflammation or infection, whereas diffuse increase in skin temperature suggests the presence of a fever. Temperature decreases in a localized area suggest decreased circulation.

Assess the texture of the skin. The skin is normally soft and has a very slight texture to it from hair follicles. Does it feel smooth or rough? Note if it appears thicker in some areas. Inspect for any **lesions.** A skin lesion is any disruption in the structure of the skin. Lesions result from many causes that are often difficult to ascertain for any particular lesion. An accurate description of skin lesions is essential. They may be elevated, flat, or depressed. Lesions also may be categorized as vascular (associated with a blood vessel), primary, or secondary. Primary skin lesions are directly caused by the disease process. Secondary skin lesions are primary lesions that have undergone evolution from external trauma, such as scratching or infection. Grouping of the lesions is important to note. In particular, a linear grouping of lesions may indicate exposure to poison ivy, oak, sumac, or shingles. Lesions that conform to the distribution of clothing, have the shape of a piece of jewelry the patient wears, or in general have a geometric shape may be caused by a contact (allergic) dermatitis. Lesions are discussed in more detail in Chapter 29.

Hair. The hair should be inspected for texture, quantity, distribution, and color. Many of these qualities vary according to genetic makeup. **Hirsutism** is the term for male-pattern hair growth (face, chest) in women and often is associated with an endocrine disorder.

Nails. The nails should be inspected for the presence of pallor or cyanosis. **Clubbing** is the flattening of the nail base angle to greater than the normal 160 degrees and is associated with chronic hypoxia from long-term smoking or a number of cardiorespiratory disorders (see Chapter 22).

Head

[OBJECTIVES 49, 50, 51]

Begin assessment of the head by palpating its structural integrity (Figure 17-24). Feel for any crepitus or deformities in the cranial and facial bones (Figure 17-25). The skull acts as a vault protecting the brain. Any destruction to its protective properties can be disastrous. A soft spot

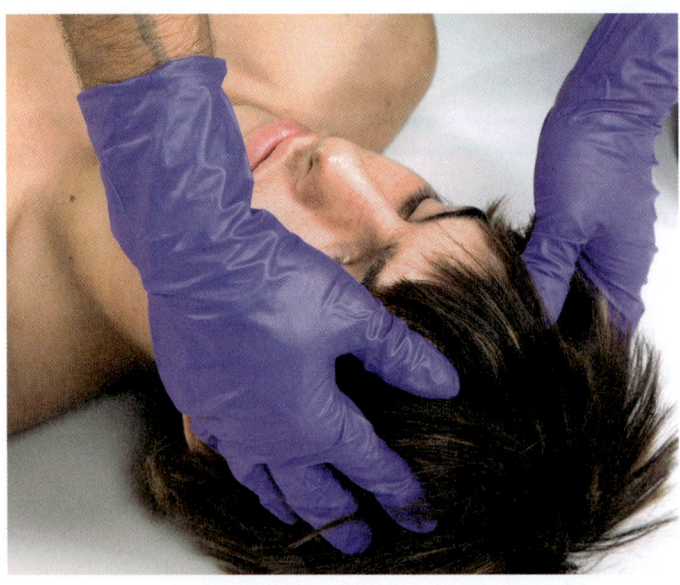

Figure 17-24 Palpate the head for structural integrity.

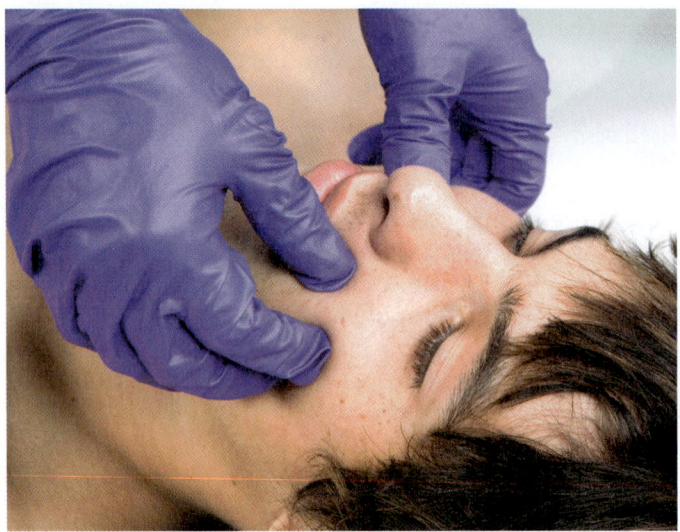

Figure 17-25 Palpation of the facial bones.

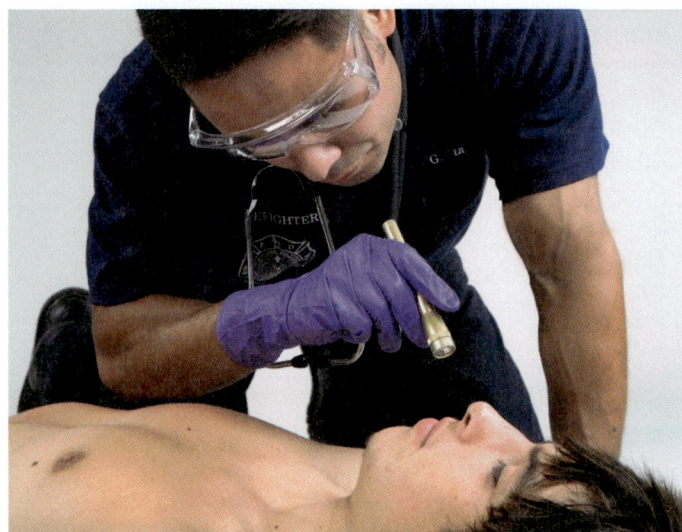

Figure 17-26 Inspect the mouth and nose for any objects that are loose or out of place.

Blood from ear - differentiate from CSF by putting drop on gauze - CSF separates from blood - looks like halo

Compare one side of the face to the other, checking for symmetry. Observe the patient's face for symmetry while he or she smiles and frowns, raises the eyebrows, and speaks. Does everything look "right"? Any indication of asymmetric facial movement indicates the facial nerve is impaired. This is most commonly seen during a stroke in the prehospital setting. Palpate both sides of the face at the same time for any step-offs indicative of fracture. Although deformity in the facial bones often is obvious, it may be subtle, so be sure to palpate carefully. The bones of the face should be palpated sequentially, including the frontal bones, supraorbital, lateral orbital and infraorbital ridges, zygomatic arches (cheek bones), maxilla (upper lip below the nose), and mandible. Significant bruising around the mastoid process (behind the ears) is called **Battle's sign.** Bruising around the orbits of the eyes is called **raccoon eyes**. If present, these signs suggest a basilar skull fracture. *old trauma*

Inspect the mouth and nose for any objects that are loose or out of place (Figure 17-26). Clear any potential airway obstructions. Have the patient run the tongue around the teeth; ask whether anything feels loose or rough, which could be indicative of a fracture. Instruct the patient to bite down on the teeth and ask whether the teeth fit together correctly—a sensitive indicator of proper alignment of the teeth. Often with a mandible fracture a subtle displacement of the jaw may be present that the patient may notice because of the teeth being misaligned. Check the integrity of the lower jaw. Ask the patient to squeeze the upper and lower jaws together while monitoring for pain. Have the patient open and close the mouth as much as possible. Ask the patient to bite down on a tongue blade. Twist the tongue blade from side to side and ask about location of pain.

or deformity in the cranium suggests a depressed skull fracture, meaning the skull may be pressing inward on the brain. Lacerations of the scalp often are obscured by large amounts of bloody, matted hair. The best way to locate a laceration of the scalp is through careful palpation of the skin. The fingertip will drop into any laceration that is present. Remember that scalp abrasions cause large amounts of bleeding. If a large amount of blood is in the hair or on the ground under the head, a scalp laceration is present; you just need to find it. Cranial nerve dysfunction often is one of the first outward signs when the central nervous system is impaired. Cranial nerve assessment is discussed in Chapter 23.

Pain on either side usually indicates a fracture on that side.

Note whether the patient's breath has a particular odor. Has the patient been drinking? An extremely fruity breath suggests diabetic ketoacidosis. Ask the patient to stick out his or her tongue. Then ask the patient to move the tongue from side to side. The inability to stick out the tongue or move it to either side may indicate damage to the hypoglossal cranial nerve.

Note the general appearance of the face. A rounded, swollen appearance to the face may occur with **Cushing's syndrome** or other chronic steroid excess (steroid facies), hypothyroidism, or **nephrotic syndrome.** A "bug-eyed" (exophthalmia) appearance may be seen in hyperthyroidism (Grave's disease). The patient who appears markedly underweight or malnourished may have cancer or severe pulmonary disease or be unable to take care of his or her own nutritional needs.

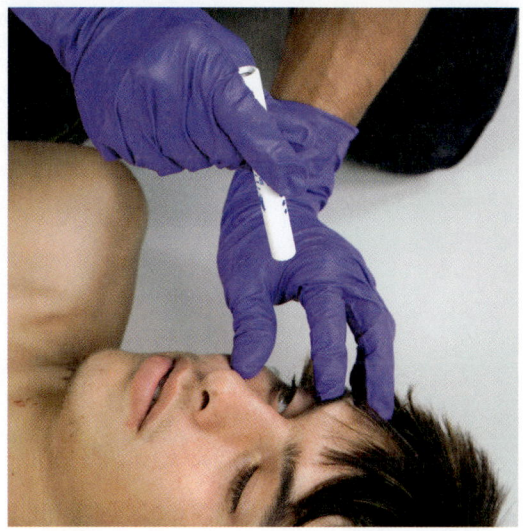

Figure 17-27 Assess the pupils for reactivity.

Eyes

[OBJECTIVES 52, 53, 54]

Begin evaluating the eyes by looking at their general appearance. Do they look symmetric? Inspect the physical shape of the eyes. Look to see whether the sclera (white of the eye) is intact and free of debris. Carefully flush out any debris. Is the sclera discolored? Patients with liver failure may have yellowing of the sclera (jaundice). Evaluate the position of the eyelids, checking for lesions, edema, and inflammation. The underside of both eyelids should be moist and pink in color. Note any discoloration. Be sure no debris is caught between an eyelid and the eye as well. Ask the patient to close the eyes. Watch to see if both eyes close completely. If the eyelashes are flipped inward or outward, they will obstruct the eyelid's ability to close. Look for discharge. If discharge is present, note its color and consistency. Blood from inside the eye is a serious emergency and may require surgery.

The pupil size in millimeters as well as shape and reaction to light should be tested in all patients. Shine a penlight into one eye and note whether the pupil constricts (Figure 17-27). The opposite pupil should constrict simultaneously with the examined pupil. This is called a *consensual light response.* Repeat the test by shining the penlight in the opposite eye. This test evaluates the oculomotor cranial nerve, which controls pupil dilation. Document a sluggish pupil response or whether the pupils are unequal. An irregular pupil may occur from prior surgery or remote trauma but also may be seen in acute blunt or penetrating trauma with rupture of the iris. Usually the patient will be able to relate a previous history of irregular pupil. Physiologic **anisocoria** (difference in pupil size) is one cause of asymmetrical pupils. The difference in size is usually less than 1 mm, and both pupils react normally by constricting to light and dilating in darkness. A single dilated pupil may represent impending uncal herniation (from pressure on the third nerve),

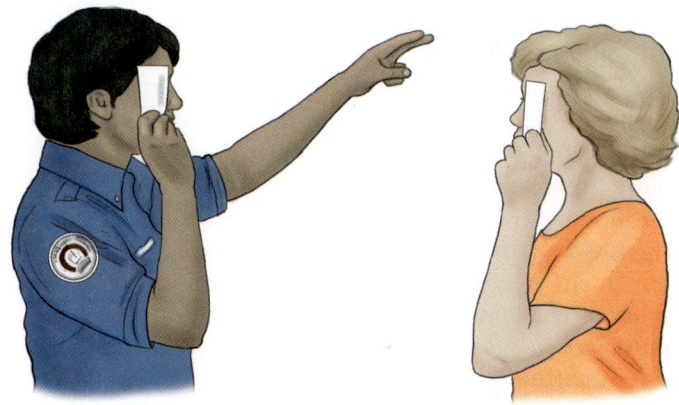

Figure 17-28 Testing the fields of vision.

but these patients most always have a depressed level of consciousness and abnormal neurologic examination. A single dilated pupil also may be seen when the patient is using prescribed eye drops that cause pupil dilation or if an anticholinergic medication (such as ipratropium from a nebulization treatment for bronchospasm) is splashed into the eye. Note whether the patient is extremely sensitive to the bright light. Patients with **photosensitivity,** a fever, and neck stiffness may have meningitis.

Test all four quadrants of the visual field by having the patient cover one eye and look at your nose (Figure 17-28). Close your opposite eye and hold a finger halfway between the patient and yourself. Wiggle your finger as you move it toward the patient. The patient typically should see movement at approximately the same time as you do. A visual field defect may represent a pathologic condition anywhere from the occipital cortex to the optic nerve.

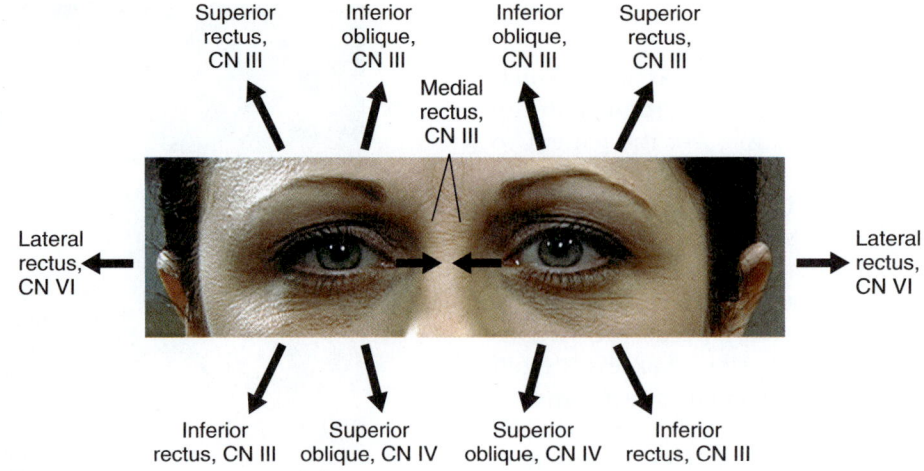

Figure 17-29 The six cardinal fields of vision with their associated cranial nerves and extraocular muscles. *CN*, Cranial nerve.

Assess the patient's ability to move the eyes. A patient can typically move the eye through six cardinal positions of gaze (Figure 17-29). Both eyes should always move together in unison. Have the patient follow your finger from center, to the left and right, upward and downward, making an H motion. The patient should be able to follow in all directions (extraocular movements). Failure to follow your finger to any one position suggests one of the muscles attached to the eye is damaged. Extraocular movement may be impaired by direct muscle irritation, injury or entrapment from orbital cellulitis, direct muscle trauma, or blowout fractures. In addition, central nervous system pathology may interrupt nervous impulses to the extraocular muscles, affecting extraocular movement. Document any extraocular muscle motions or abnormal pauses in eye motion, known as **nystagmus.** Nystagmus is most often observed when a patient looks to the side or downward. A common cause of this phenomenon is drug or alcohol overdose, particularly barbiturates.

Always check for the presence of diplopia, or double vision, which may be a subtle sign of problems with extraocular movement. Patients with diplopia should be asked if it persists when one eye is covered. Resolution of diplopia when one eye is covered represents pathology of an extraocular muscle or its innervation. Looking in the direction of the involved muscle usually exaggerates the diplopia. Patients with lesions of the superior oblique muscle or the fourth cranial nerve may tilt the head to compensate for the diplopia.

If you have time, consider performing a vision test with a **visual acuity card.** Visual acuity should be tested with contact lenses or glasses in place. If the patient's glasses or contacts are unavailable, pinhole testing of the visual acuity should be performed. A commercial pinhole occluder may be used (Figure 17-30), although a perforated metal eye shield or a note card perforated with an 18-gauge needle is an acceptable sub-

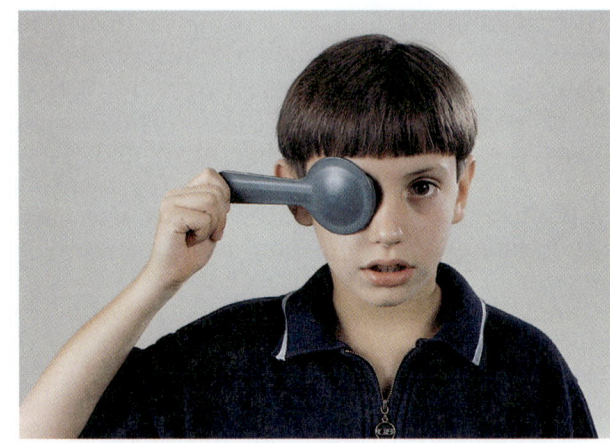

Figure 17-30 When testing a patient's visual acuity, an eye occluder is used to cover the eye that is not being tested.

stitute. Testing is ideally done with a standard wall-mounted visual acuity chart (Snellen chart) with the patient at a distance of 20 feet (Figure 17-31). The visual acuity is recorded as 20/x, with the numerator being the distance from which the patient can read the line (always 20); the denominator is the distance from which a person with normal vision can read the same line. The visual acuity is determined by the smallest line a patient can read with half of the letters correct. The number of incorrect letters is listed after the visual acuity as follows: 20/x – y, such as 20/40 – 2. If necessary because of immobility of the patient, visual acuity can be tested with a near card (Rosenbaum chart) held 14 inches from the patient. An example of a near visual acuity card is shown in Figure 17-32. For patients with visual acuity less than 20/200, figure counting at a distance (such as figure counting at 3 feet), perception of hand motion, and ulti-

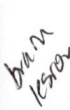

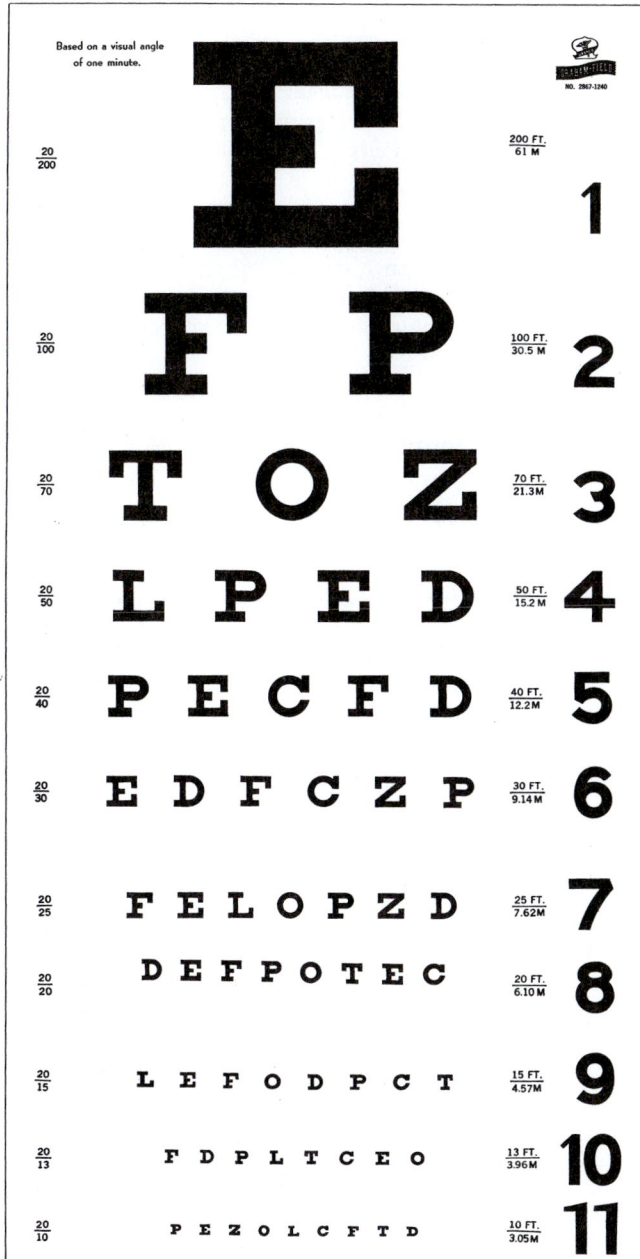

Figure 17-31 A Snellen eye chart is used to measure distance visual acuity.

mately light perception can be used for progressively worse visual acuity. A verbal child or illiterate patient can be tested by using the direction of the letter E on the chart (Figure 17-33).

A visual acuity test requires several minutes to set up and run, so it is usually impractical in the field setting. Rather, hold up several fingers a few feet from the patient's face and ask how many fingers you are holding up. If the patient can see the proper number, double vision is ruled out. Then ask whether the patient sees your fingers clearly or if they are blurred. Determine whether any

blurred vision is new or whether the patient always has blurred vision.

If you work in an emergency department, you may become trained to inspect the inside of the eye with an ophthalmoscope (Figure 17-34). Direct ophthalmoscopy may be used to examine the cornea, lens, vitreous, and retina. The positive numbered lenses (black) may be used to examine the cornea. Progressing to more negative numbered lenses (red) allows visualization deeper into the eye through the anterior chamber, lens, vitreous, and finally the retina. Opacities of the lens may obscure the view of the retina and appear as black spots of various shapes. Vitreous hemorrhage also obscures the view of the retina, has an irregular shape, and may have a reddish hue. The optic disc should be examined for shape, size of the optic cup, and blurring of the edges. The relative size of the arteries and veins should be noted, as should the presence of spontaneous venous pulsations. The macula should be examined for presence of edema, hemorrhages, and exudates. Abnormalities on funduscopic examination may represent primary ocular disease (e.g., glaucoma, retinal detachment, direct trauma), systemic disease, or retinopathy (e.g., diabetes mellitus, hypertension).

Ears
[OBJECTIVES 55, 56]

An ear examination is generally limited in the emergency setting, except when the ear is a portion of the patient's complaint. Inspect the outer ear for signs of trauma such as swelling and bleeding and for infection (Figure 17-35). An infected ear looks red and is warm to the touch. If the patient has experienced head trauma, look for cerebrospinal fluid coming from the ear canal.

Inspection of the inside of the ear requires the use of an otoscope (Figure 17-36). Pull the ear posteriorly to straighten the ear canal and place the otoscope inside with the light illuminated. The ear canal will point toward the eyes. With the otoscope you can inspect inner ear inflammation, any foreign bodies, and the integrity of the eardrum. Loud percussive noises, such as a nearby lightning strike, can rupture the eardrum, causing temporary deafness and bleeding. Do not attempt to remove foreign bodies from the ear.

No. 1.
.37M

In the second century of the Christian era, the empire of Rome comprehended the fairest part of the earth, and the most civilized portion of mankind. The frontiers of that extensive monarchy were guarded by ancient renown and disciplined valor. The gentle but powerful influence of laws and manners had gradually cemented the union of the provinces. Their peaceful inhabitants enjoyed and abused the advantages of wealth.

No. 2.
.50M

fourscore years, the public administration was conducted by the virtue and abilities of Nerva, Trajan, Hadrian, and the two Antonines. It is the design of this, and of the two succeeding chapters, to describe the prosperous condition of their empire; and afterwards, from the death of Marcus Antoninus, to deduce the most important circumstances of its decline and fall; a revolution which will ever be remembered, and is still felt by

No. 3.
.62M

the nations of the earth. The principal conquests of the Romans were achieved under the republic; and the emperors, for the most part, were satisfied with preserving those dominions which had been acquired by the policy of the senate, the active emulations of the consuls, and the martial enthusiasm of the people. The seven first centuries were filled with a rapid succession of triumphs; but it was

No. 4.
.75M

reserved for Augustus to relinquish the ambitious design of subduing the whole earth, and to introduce a spirit of moderation into the public councils. Inclined to peace by his temper and situation, it was very easy for him to discover that Rome, in her present exalted situation, had much less to hope than to fear from the chance of arms; and that, in the prosecution of

No. 5.
1.00M

the undertaking became every day more difficult, the event more doubtful, and the possession more precarious, and less beneficial. The experience of Augustus added weight to these salutary reflections, and effectually convinced him that, by the prudent vigor of

No. 6.
1.25M

his counsels, it would be easy to secure every concession which the safety or the dignity of Rome might require from the most formidable barbarians. Instead of exposing his person or his legions to the arrows of the Parthinians, he obtained, by an honor-

No. 7.
1.50M

able treaty, the restitution of the standards and prisoners which had been taken in the defeat of Crassus. His generals, in the early part of his reign, attempted the reduction of Ethiopia and Arabia Felix. They marched near a thou-

No. 8.
1.75M

sand miles to the south of the tropic; but the heat of the climate soon repelled the invaders, and protected the unwarlike natives of those sequestered regions

No. 9.
2.00M

The northern countries of Europe scarcely deserved the expense and labor of conquest. The forests and morasses of Germany were

No. 10.
2.25M

filled with a hardy race of barbarians who despised life when it was separated from freedom; and though, on the first

No. 11.
2.50M

attack, they seemed to yield to the weight of the Roman power, they soon, by a signal

Figure 17-32 An example of a near visual acuity card.

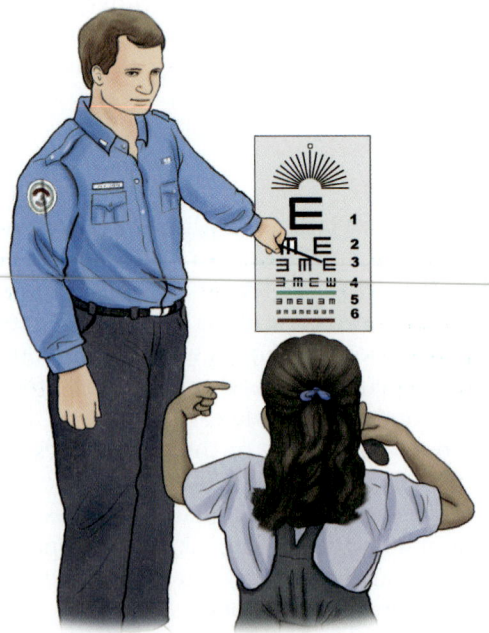

Figure 17-33 When a Snellen E chart is used to test visual acuity, the patient is asked to point in the direction of the open part of the capital letter E.

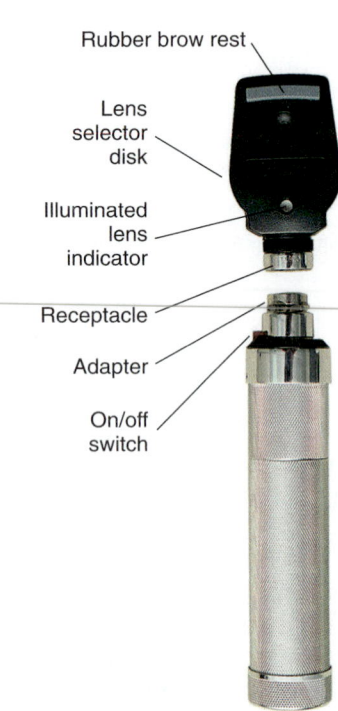

Figure 17-34 Use of an ophthalmoscope requires practice.

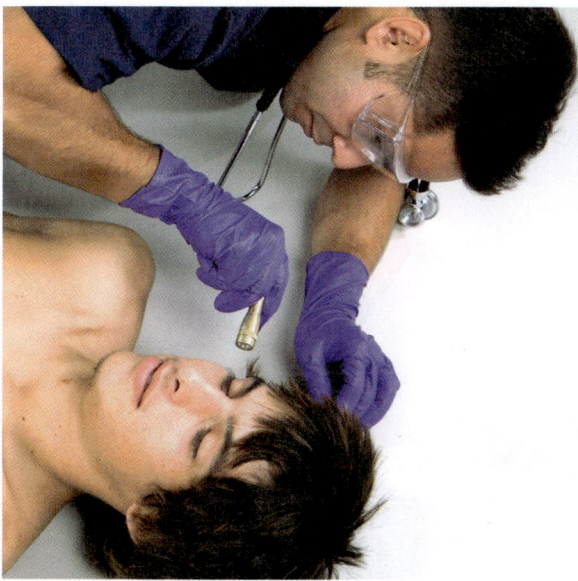

Figure 17-35 Inspection of the outer ear.

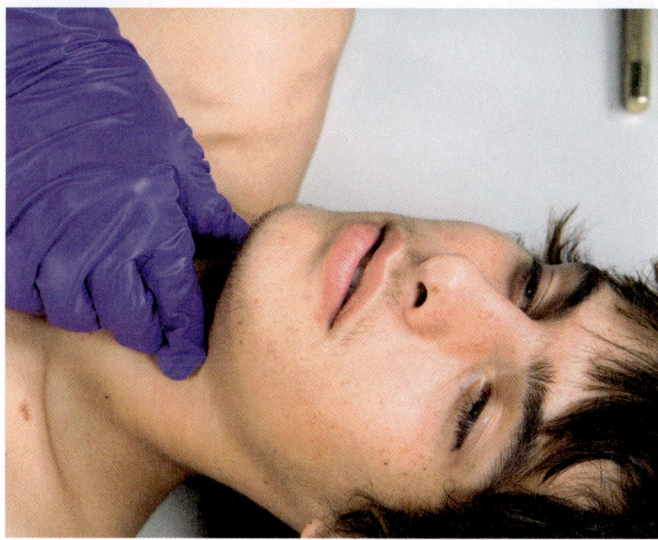

Figure 17-37 Palpate the trachea for midline position.

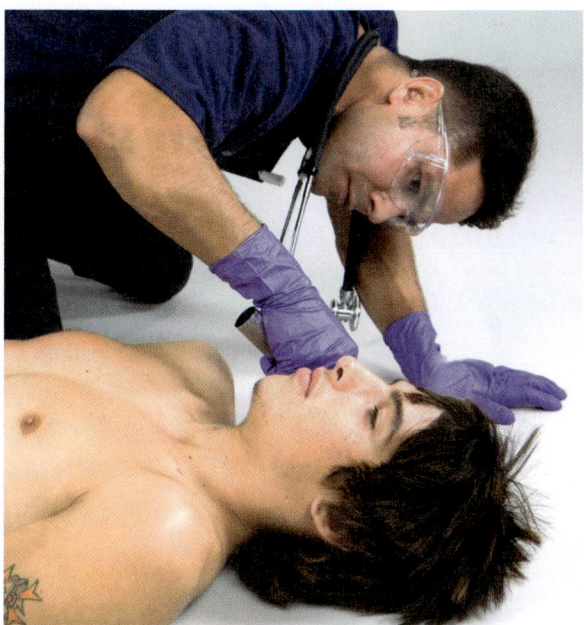

Figure 17-36 Inspection of the inner ear requires the use of an otoscope.

Nose

[OBJECTIVES 57, 58]

Look at the shape and positioning of the nose. If it is deformed, ask the patient about it because some patients have misshapen noses. A bloody nose after trauma does not mean it is broken; however, a broken nose does bleed. Test any blood from the nose for signs of cerebrospinal fluid by catching some of the fluid on a gauze pad. After several minutes the lighter cerebrospinal fluid will form a halo around the blood, if present.

Mouth/Pharynx

[OBJECTIVE 59]

Inspect the mouth and pharynx for DCAPBTLS, blood, absent or broken teeth, gastric contents, foreign objects, or an injured or swollen tongue. Assess the color of the mucous membranes of the mouth. Note the presence and character of vomitus and any fluids. If sputum is present, note its color, amount, and consistency. Listen for hoarseness and note any unusual odors.

Neck

[OBJECTIVES 60, 61, 62]

Visualize the neck. Inspect for any swelling, bruising, or inflammation. Ask the patient to swallow; determine whether any difficulty occurs. Palpate the trachea to determine whether it is in a midline position (Figure 17-37). Tracheal deviation toward an injured lung (a late sign) suggests a simple pneumothorax. Tracheal deviation away from an injured lung (a late sign) suggests a tension pneumothorax. Inspect the neck for jugular venous distention (JVD). When a patient is lying supine and the upper torso is raised at less than 45 degrees, the jugular veins are naturally distended in a patient with an adequate blood volume (Figure 17-38). If JVD is present when the patient's upper torso is raised at a 45-degree angle, it is a sign of venous system overload or hypertension. Report JVD in finger widths above the clavicle.

Palpate the soft tissues of the neck and each of the cervical vertebrae for tenderness (Figure 17-39). A broken vertebra will not cause further injury when palpated. Finally, palpate for swollen lymph nodes, which are a sign of infection (Figure 17-40). Lymph nodes normally are approximately the size of peas. When full of infectious material, they can increase to the size of a grape.

In older adults, consider auscultating for **bruits** in the carotid arteries (Figure 17-41). A bruit is a sound made when blood in an artery passes over built-up plaque.

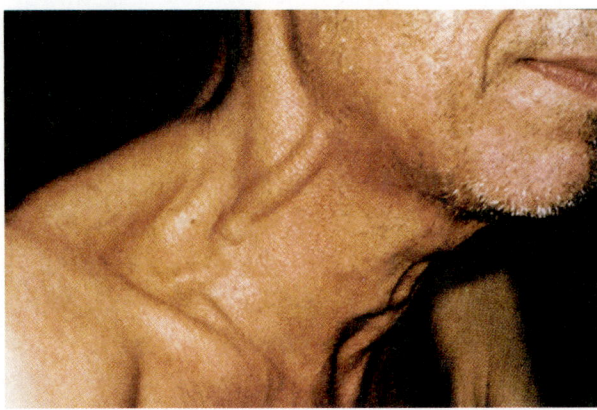

Figure 17-38 Inspect the neck for jugular venous distention (JVD). If it is present when the patient is sitting up at more than 45 degrees, it is a sign of venous system overload or hypertension.

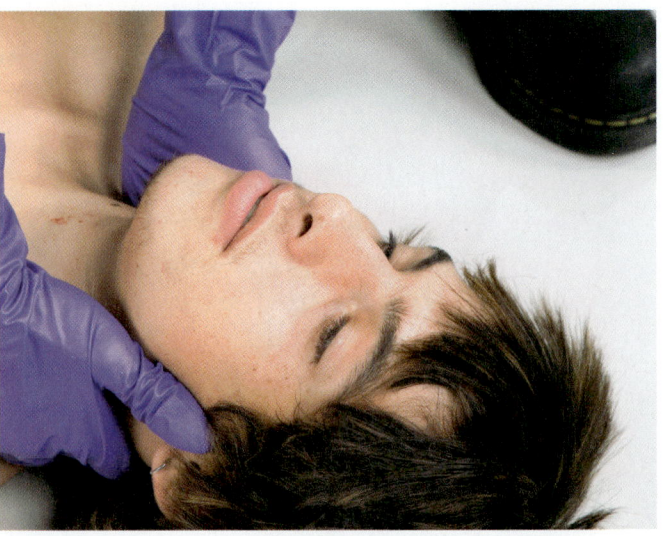

Figure 17-39 Palpate the soft tissues of the neck and each of the cervical vertebrae for tenderness.

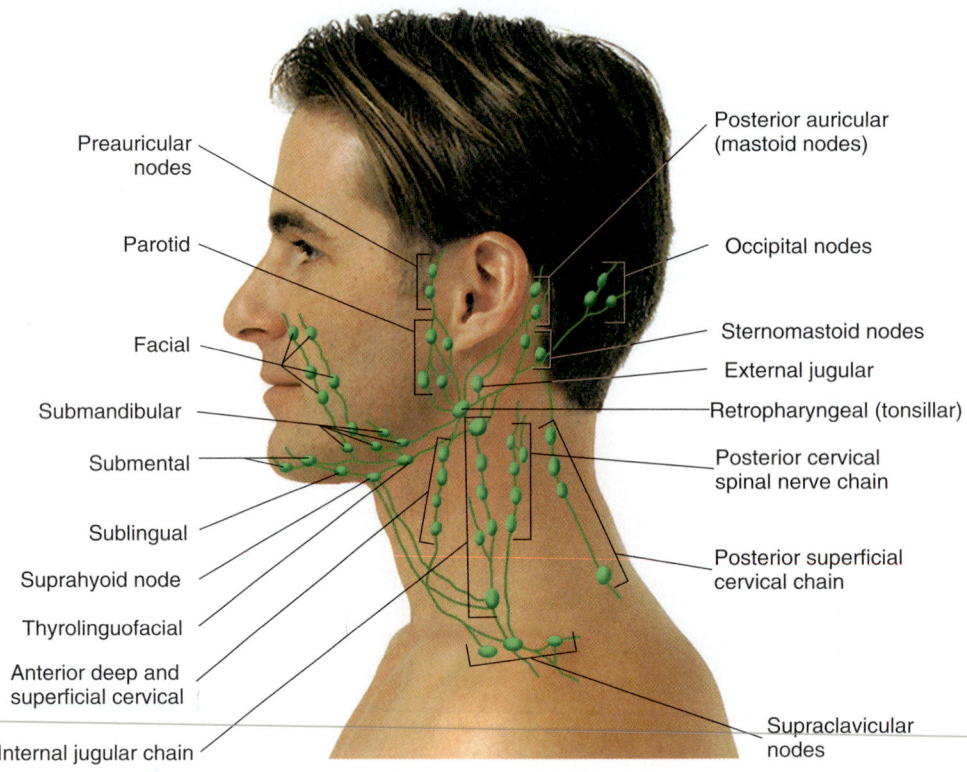

Preauricular nodes
Parotid
Facial
Submandibular
Submental
Sublingual
Suprahyoid node
Thyrolinguofacial
Anterior deep and superficial cervical
Internal jugular chain

Posterior auricular (mastoid nodes)
Occipital nodes
Sternomastoid nodes
External jugular
Retropharyngeal (tonsillar)
Posterior cervical spinal nerve chain
Posterior superficial cervical chain
Supraclavicular nodes

Figure 17-40 Lymph nodes of the head and neck.

Listen to both carotid arteries, especially if you are considering performing carotid massage to treat a tachycardia (see Chapter 22). The presence of a **carotid bruit** is a contraindication for carotid massage.

Chest
[OBJECTIVES 63, 64, 65]

Expose the chest and watch the patient breathe. Look for signs of accessory muscle use, including the neck and intercostal muscles. Accessory muscle use suggests respi-

ratory distress. Inspect the chest for bruising, redness, and deformity. Evaluate both the anterior and posterior chest walls. Watch the chest rise and fall. The entire chest cavity normally moves in unison. If a portion appears to be moving in the opposite direction of the rest of the chest, that is, it moves inward while the rest of the chest is expanding (called *paradoxic motion*), this is a flail chest segment caused by multiple broken ribs.

After inspection, auscultate lung sounds. Lung sounds can be obtained in more than 20 places, but auscultating

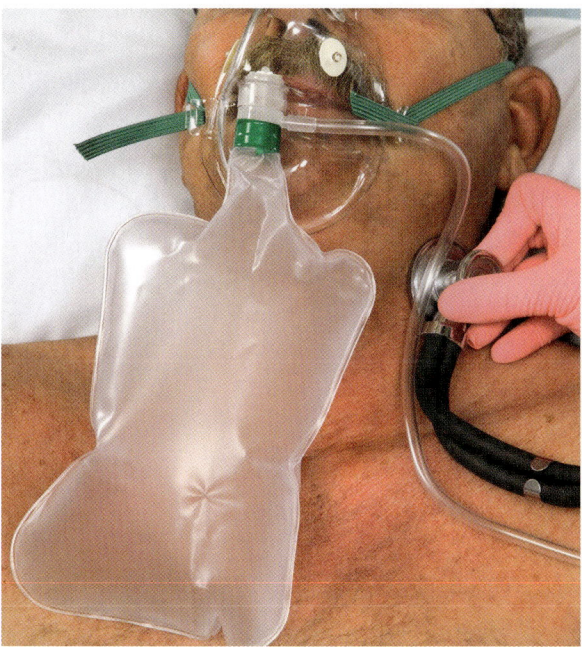

Figure 17-41 Auscultate for carotid bruits in older adults.

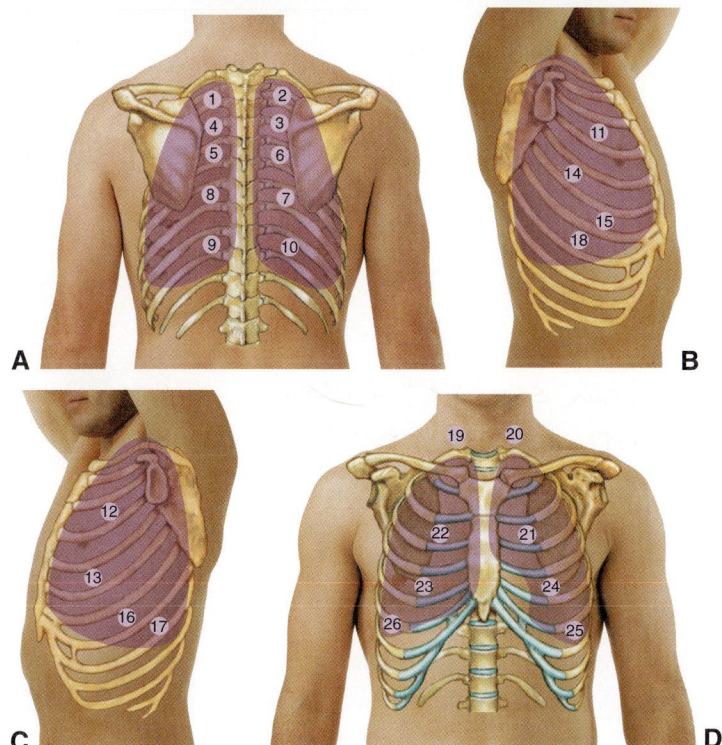

Figure 17-42 When listening to lung sounds, listen to one lung and then at the same place on the other lung. Listen to at least one full inhalation and exhalation at each location. **A,** Posterior chest. **B,** Right lateral chest. **C,** Left lateral chest. **D,** Anterior chest.

all of them during emergency care is not possible (Figure 17-42). At a minimum, be sure to auscultate all five lung lobes—three of the right lung and two of the left lung. As you listen, auscultate bilaterally, which means listen to one lung and then the same place on the other lung. With each stethoscope placement, listen to at least one full inhalation and exhalation. If the patient is able to cooperate, have him or her breathe through an open mouth to help emphasize the breath sounds. Begin on the anterior chest, placing your stethoscope just inferior to the clavicle on the midclavicular line to listen to the apices of the lungs. Next place your stethoscope at the third intercostal space just lateral to the sternum. Listen first to one lung, then the other. The last place to obtain lung sounds on the anterior chest is along the fifth intercostal space along the midaxillary line.

Lung sound auscultation on the posterior chest follows the shape of the scapula. Begin just superior to the center of the scapula and move medially, following the scapula as it curves along the chest wall. Listen along the posterior chest in at least six spots, listening first to one lung and then the other.

Lung sounds are classified as vesicular, bronchovesicular, and bronchial (Figure 17-43). Vesicular lung sounds are soft, low-pitched sounds heard over healthy lung tissue. Bronchovesicular lung sounds are of medium pitch and heard mainly over the major bronchi. Bronchial lung sounds are high pitched and heard only over the trachea (Table 17-8). Normal lung sounds sound like air passing through hollow tubes. Listening bilaterally allows you to compare lungs for equality. Listen for equal lung sounds that have an equal volume, duration, and pitch in both lungs. Identifying abnormal lung sounds

TABLE 17-8	Normal Lung Sounds
Sound	**Description/Characteristics**
Vesicular	Soft, low-pitched sounds heard over healthy lung tissue
Bronchovesicular	Medium-pitched sounds heard mainly over the major bronchi
Bronchial	High-pitched sounds normally heard only over the trachea/manubrium

and considering their cause is an important action (Figure 17-44, Table 17-9). Muffled sounds appear distant. Muffled lung sounds can be caused by a hemothorax, which is blood in the chest cavity. Absent lung sounds mean no air flows in that lung lobe. Lack of air flow may be caused by a collapsed lung, fluid within the chest cavity, or bronchioles so constricted that no air can pass through them. Severe bronchoconstriction is a major problem in cases of severe asthma and anaphylaxis.

Another test you can perform while assessing the lungs is listening to the patient speak. Ask the patient to say "ninety-nine" while auscultating the lungs. The words

lungs- 4 areas front 6 areas back   *Listen to each area for one inspir. + one expir.*

KEY:

■ Bronchovesicular over main bronchi

■ Vesicular over lesser bronchi, bronchioles, and lobes

■ Bronchial over trachea

[handwritten] Have person say "e" & listen to lungs. If it sounds like "a", there is consolidation on lung (pneumonia)

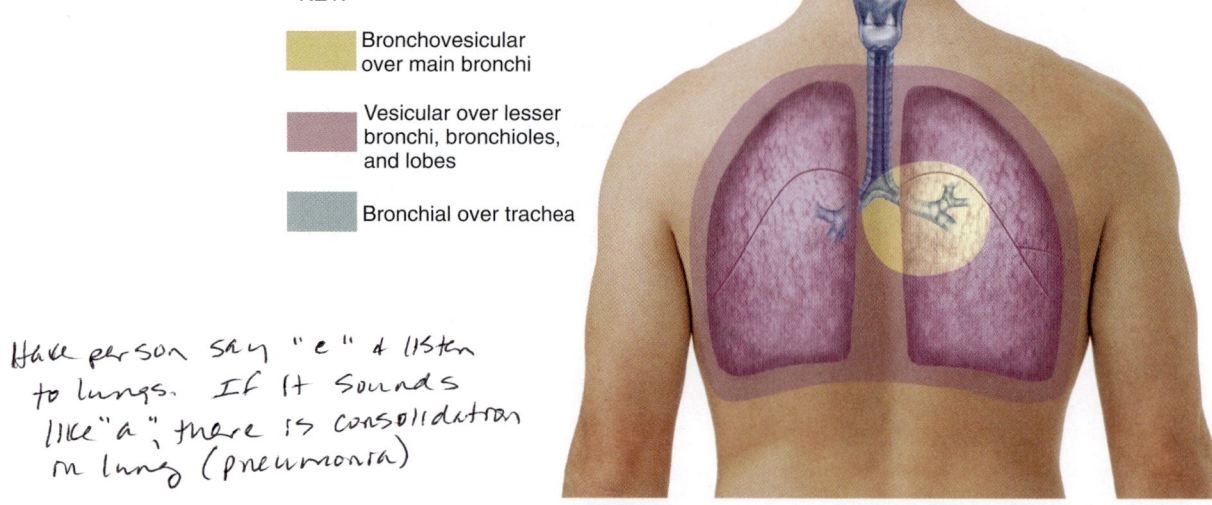

Figure 17-43 Lung sounds are classified as vesicular, bronchovesicular, and bronchial.

TABLE 17-9	Abnormal Lung Sounds	
Sound	**Characteristics**	**Possible Cause**
Crackles (rales)	High-pitched crackling sounds that do not clear with coughing; caused by air passing through moisture	Congestive heart failure Pneumonia Chronic obstructive pulmonary disease
Rhonchi	Loud, low, coarse sounds that resemble snoring and often clear with coughing; caused by a buildup of mucus or fluid in the trachea or large bronchi	Asthma Upper respiratory tract infection
Wheezes	High-pitched whistling sounds caused by air moving through passages narrowed by mucus or bronchospasm	Asthma Chronic bronchitis Anaphylaxis
Friction rub	Scratchy, high-pitched sound (like two pieces of sandpaper rubbing together) caused by inflamed pleural surfaces rubbing against each other	Pleurisy Pneumonia

[handwritten] Tactile fremesis feel vibration on person when they talk.
If not there, may have asthma

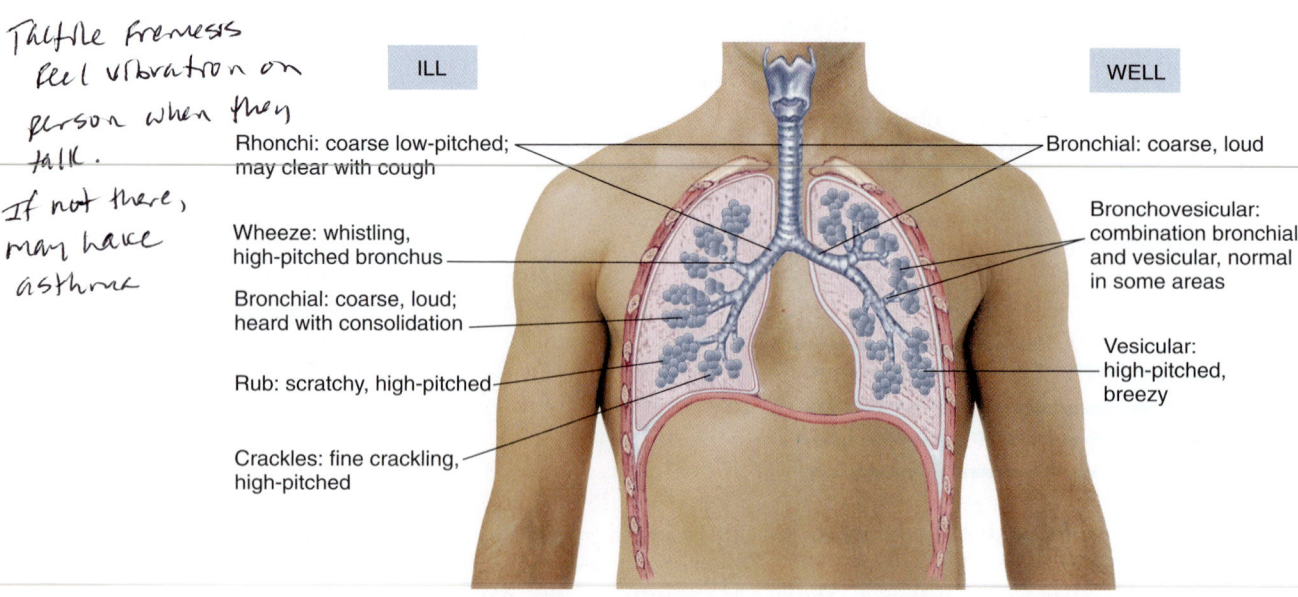

Figure 17-44 Lung sounds that may be heard in an ill patient *(left)* and a well patient *(right)*.

normally sound dense and slightly muffled throughout the chest cavity. You also may notice that the words echo as though the patient is speaking through several socks; it sounds muted and distant. When "ninety-nine" sounds high pitched and clear, the lung lobe you are listening to is obstructed in some way. The obstruction could be a mucus plug or fluid, or that lobe may be collapsed.

> ### PARAMEDIC*Pearl*
>
> When auscultating lung sounds, avoid placing the stethoscope directly over large tissues, such as breast tissue, and avoid bones, such as the scapula. These tissues disrupt the ability to auscultate lung sounds by muffling the sounds you are listening for.

Evaluate the integrity of the sternum by placing your hand's medial edge vertically along the sternum and have the patient breathe. Assess the integrity of the lateral chest wall by pressing medially with your hands against the lateral rib cage while the patient breathes (Figure 17-45). Distinguish if the patient has chest pain, tenderness, or both. Cardiac chest pain generally has no associated tenderness and does not change with respirations. Musculoskeletal chest wall pain typically has both tenderness and pain on palpation. Ask the patient to point with one finger to the location of the discomfort (point tenderness). Remember to use the OPQRST memory aid when assessing a report of pain or discomfort. In cases of major trauma or chest wall trauma, be sure to palpate each individual rib for tenderness.

If the patient complains of any point pain or tenderness that worsens on inspiration, auscultate that point. Listen for what sounds like two pieces of sandpaper rubbing together. This is a **pleural friction rub,** which is the sound of the visceral and parietal pleura rubbing together. Pleural friction rubs also may make squeaking noises or a grating sound. Many causes exist for multiple pleural rubs, but they most often are triggered by pneumonia or inflammation of the pleura (pleurisy).

Cardiovascular System
[OBJECTIVES 66 to 70]

Perform a cardiovascular system assessment. Start by comparing bilateral peripheral pulse points (Figure 17-46). Compare both radial and pedal pulses. Consider comparing femoral and carotid pulses. Pulses are rated for their strength from 0, for no pulse present, to 3+, for a bounding pulse (Table 17-10). Unilateral pulse point weaknesses suggest vascular impairment or vascular disease.

While assessing pulses, also evaluate peripheral edema. Edema, which is excessive fluid that shifts out of the vascular space and into the interstitial spaces, may be a sign of heart failure, hypothyroidism, or liver failure.

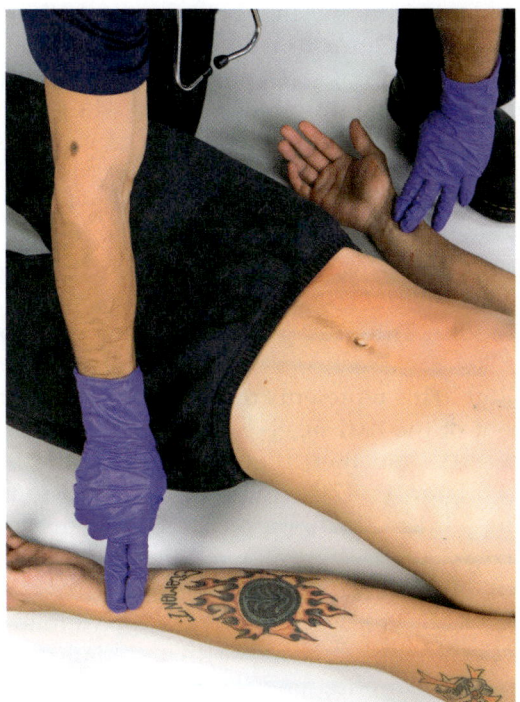

Figure 17-46 Compare bilateral peripheral pulses.

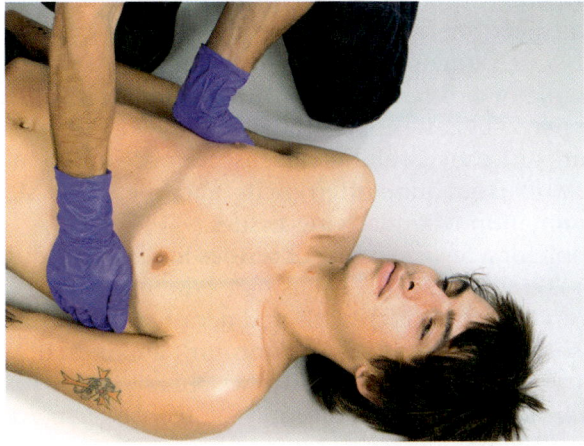

Figure 17-45 Evaluate the integrity of the patient's lateral chest wall by pressing your hands against the lateral rib cage.

TABLE 17-10	Pulse Strength
Grade	**Quality**
0	No pulse felt
1+	Weak, thready pulse
2+	Normal pulse
3+	Bounding pulse

TABLE 17-11	Documenting Edema
Grade	**Condition**
0	No edema
1+	Edema pits for 1 second
2+	Edema pits for 2 seconds
3+	Edema pits for 3 seconds
4+	Edema pits for ≥4 seconds

During right ventricular failure, edema builds up in the peripheral tissues. In left ventricular failure, edema builds up in the lungs. Edema collects in body areas with gravity, building up at the lowest point on the body. Thus if a patient commonly sits in a recliner or wheelchair, fluid will build up in the lower extremities. Patients who lie supine in bed for long periods often have edema build up in the sacral region of the back and in the arms. Edema is rated according to its severity (Table 17-11). No edema is denoted with 0+. When you compress edema-filled tissues, count the number of seconds that elapse before the skin returns to its original shape. If 1 second elapses before return, the patient has 1+ edema, 2 seconds is 2+, and so forth. Pitting edema occurs when more than 4 seconds is necessary for the tissue to return to its original shape. Inspect all extremities, the sacrum, and buttocks for edema. Document edema with its location and severity (such as 3+ pedal edema).

Next auscultate heart sounds. Begin by palpating along the fifth intercostal space where you can feel the heart's apical impulse. This is the **point of maximum impulse (PMI).** The PMI is normally just lateral to the midclavicular line. This represents the heart's apex. Lateral displacement of the PMI suggests heart enlargement. Listen over the atria and then the ventricles for the heart to contract (Figure 17-47). The contraction will sound like "lubb dupp." The "lubb," also called **S1**, is the sound of the tricuspid and mitral valves closing at the beginning of systole. After approximately a quarter of a second pause (silence), you will hear the "dupp" sound, called **S2,** which signals the closing of the pulmonic and aortic valves at the beginning of diastole. Both the "lubb" and "dupp" are normally concise and clear sounds. In addition to listening for the S1 and S2 heart tones, listen for sounds that should not be there. A heart murmur is a whooshing heart sound that usually follows S2. This may be a sign that a heart valve is not completely closing. This backflow may reduce cardiac output. By listening over each valve you may be able to determine which valve is leaking. The location where the sound is the loudest is the leak. Locate the aortic valve by listening in the second intercostal space right parasternal border. The pulmonic valve is heard over the second intercostal space left parasternal boarder. The mitral valve is heard over the fourth or fifth intercostal spaces left parasternal boarder, and the tricuspid valve is best heard just beneath the xiphoid

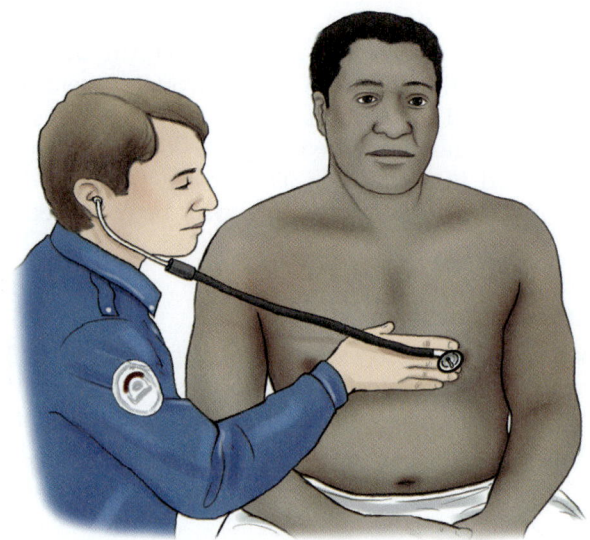

Figure 17-47 Auscultate heart sounds.

process. A gallop occurs when an extra heart sound called S3 or S4 is heard either between S1 and S2 or after S2. It may be an early sign of heart failure or cardiac overload. Heart sounds are discussed further in Chapter 22.

Abdomen
[OBJECTIVES 71, 72, 73, 74]
Begin an abdominal assessment by asking the patient about any recent abdominal pain. If the patient has any discomfort, investigate it further with the OPQRST mnemonic. Determine whether the pain is localized in one particular part of the abdomen or generalized across the entire body region. Ask if it is constant or if it comes and goes. If possible, have the patient point to the abdominal quadrant where the pain is. Mentally divide the abdomen into four quadrants along the midline—vertically and horizontally at the umbilicus. The abdominal quadrants are referred to as the right upper quadrant, left upper quadrant, right lower quadrant, and left lower quadrant (Figure 17-48).

Visualize the abdomen by lifting the patient's clothing and inspect for any discoloration, bruising, or swelling. Note which quadrant is discolored and if pain is felt in the same or a different quadrant. **Ecchymosis,** or bruising, may suggest internal bleeding. Redness is often accompanied by swelling and discomfort. Palpation of a red, swollen quadrant often elicits tenderness. This signals inflammation of underlying tissues.

Look for a few key signs of serious medical conditions. **Grey-Turner's sign** is bruising of the flanks. This may be seen in acute pancreatitis and occasionally in trauma. It also can be caused by a rupturing abdominal aortic aneurysm. **Cullen's sign** is yellow-blue bruising of the umbilical region. This sign may be seen in pancreatitis and, in women, also can indicate ectopic pregnancy.

Next auscultate each quadrant for bowel sounds (Figure 17-49). **Bowel sounds** are the noises made by the intes-

*Kehr's sign - @shoulder pain ⊙/@M)
bladder disease*

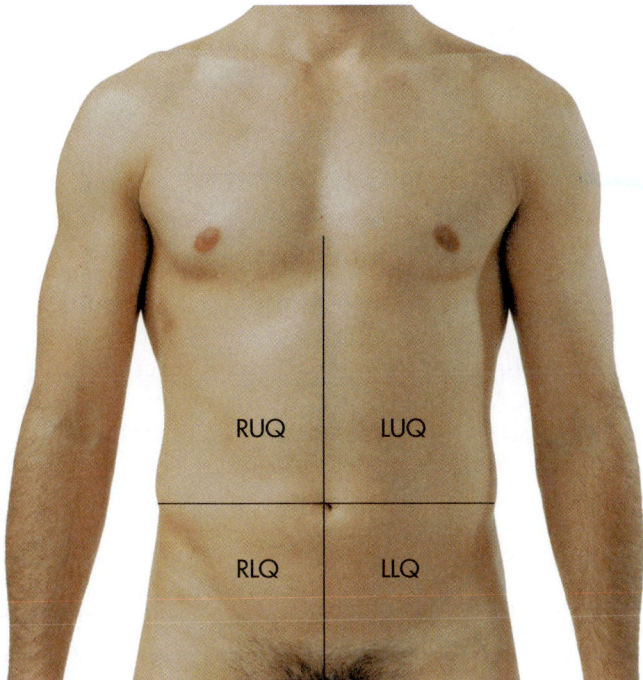

Figure 17-48 The abdominal quadrants are referred to as the right upper quadrant (RUQ), left upper quadrant (LUQ), right lower quadrant (RLQ), and left lower quadrant (LLQ).

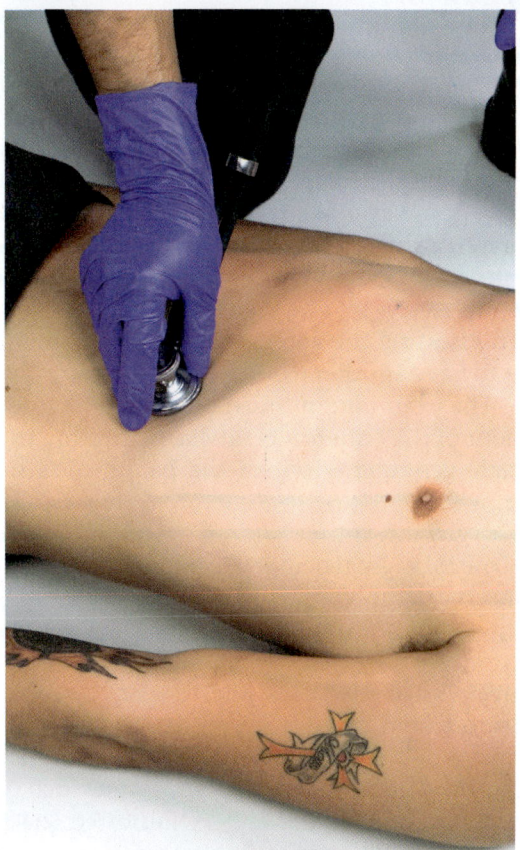

Figure 17-49 Auscultate each abdominal quadrant for bowel sounds.

tinal smooth muscles as they squeeze fluids and food products through the digestive tract. Because bowel sounds are not constant, be prepared to listen for as long as 30 seconds per quadrant. Bowel sounds generally mimic the noise made by water tumbling through pipes. **Borborygmus** is the hyperactivity of bowel sounds and is commonly associated with gastroenteritis. It is also an early indicator of a bowel obstruction if hyperactive sounds are present in one quadrant and silence (ileus) is present in another.

After auscultating bowel sounds, palpate the abdomen for tenderness. Listen before palpating because palpation creates a natural ileus of the bowel for a short time. Begin by palpating the quadrant diagonal from where any pain is located. If the patient indicates pain is localized to one quadrant, palpate that area last. To properly palpate the abdomen, lay one hand on top of the quadrant, place your other hand directly on top of your first hand, and push down with the top hand (Figure 17-50). This increases the bottom hand's sensitivity when feeling for masses within the abdomen. Monitor the patient's facial expressions for signs of discomfort. Observe for tenderness on palpation as well as rebound tenderness. **Rebound tenderness** is tenderness that occurs when pressure is released during palpation.

Genitalia
[OBJECTIVES 75, 76, 77, 78]
Often there is no need to examine the genitalia in the field setting. Whether the patient is male or female, this examination is embarrassing for the patient. Inspection

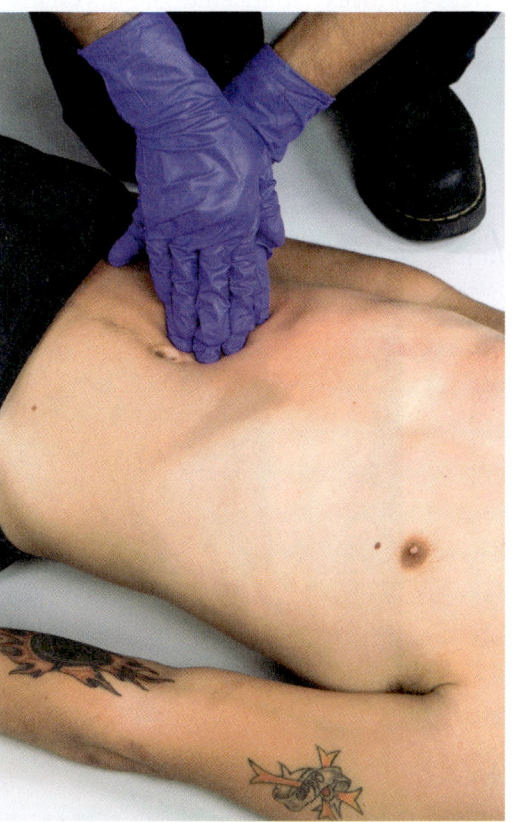

Figure 17-50 Palpate the abdomen.

witness for exam

of the male genitalia should be limited to check for priapism during trauma and when the genitalia have taken a direct blow. If the male is conscious, try asking him to perform his own examination. He will likely tell you if something is not right. If you need to expose the genitalia, do so in a respectful manner, maintaining the patient's privacy as much as possible. Try to have at least two rescuers present; this protects you. Other reasons to assess the genitalia include uncontrolled bleeding and severe pain in the area.

When assessing the genitalia of a woman, make every attempt to have another woman present during the examination. The examination must be limited to an external assessment of the patient's genitalia. Inspecting the internal female genitalia is out of the paramedic's scope of practice. If the patient reports severe uncontrolled bleeding or if childbirth is imminent, inspection becomes necessary. Control vaginal hemorrhage with external padding; never insert anything into the vagina.

Anus
[OBJECTIVES 79, 80]

During most field physical examinations, the anus will not be examined by a paramedic. However, if a patient is complaining of rectal bleeding or severe anal pain, a visual examination of the area is indicated. Be sure to obtain the patient's permission for the examination very carefully and respect his or her privacy. Look for outward signs of trauma. Patients reporting burning, itching, and bright red blood when wiping likely have a hemorrhoid. If the patient has an external hemorrhoid, you may notice this as a thin sac of tissue along the edge of the anus.

Because scope of practice varies from state to state, find out whether an internal rectal examination is within your scope. A number of states include a Hemoccult test as a part of the paramedic scope of practice, particularly in the setting of determining possible contraindications for fibrinolytic therapy.

Pelvis
[OBJECTIVES 81, 82]

Evaluate the pelvis and hip joint for instability and deformity. The neurovascular bundle following the femoral artery runs directly through the pelvis and the hip joints. Damage to any of the bones in these areas puts the neurovascular bundle at risk for damage. Inspect for bruising and redness. Assess the integrity of the pelvis by pressing the iliac crests of the pelvis inward toward each other and posteriorly toward the back (Figure 17-51). Instability indicates an unstable pelvis fracture. Anticipate internal bleeding in these patients.

Locate the greater trochanter. It is the bony prominence felt just before the femur curves into the hip joint. Compress both trochanters medially, palpating to elicit tenderness and feeling for instability (Figure 17-52). Look for hip deformity. Hip dislocations also present with shortening of one leg and sometimes inward or outward rotation of the affected leg. Distinguishing a hip dislocation from a hip fracture may be impossible, so assume they are both present.

Extremities. Evaluate extremities in pairs—both upper extremities and then both lower extremities. This allows you to take advantage of the human body's bilateral symmetry. When assessing an injured limb, compare the injured limb to the opposite and uninjured limb. Compare stability, size, strength, and **range of motion.** Evaluate any obviously injured extremity last. Be sure to question your patient about any natural limb deformities

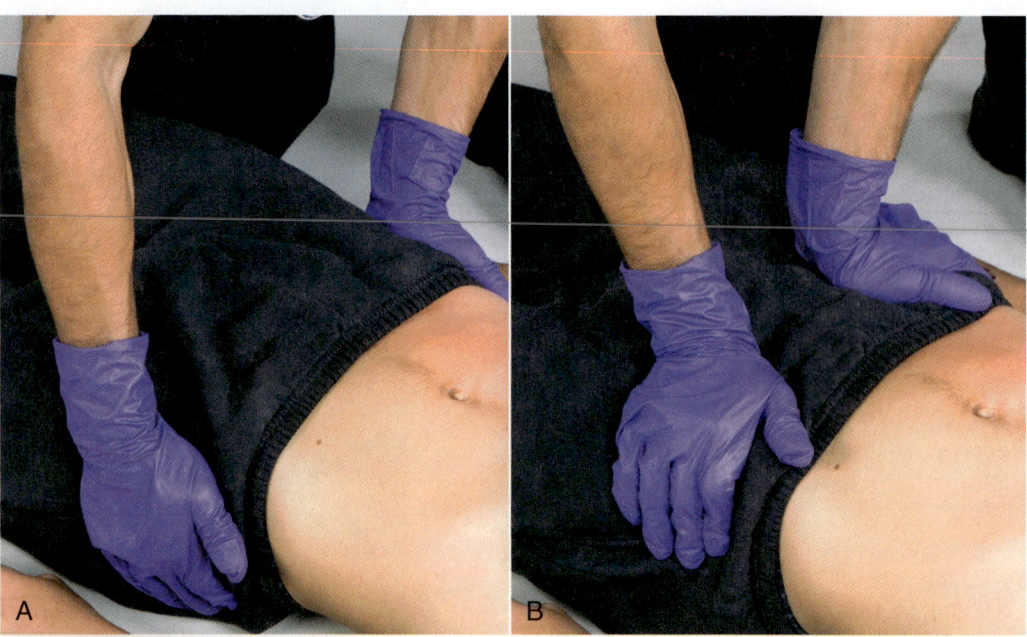

A   B

Figure 17-51 A, Press the iliac crests medially. **B,** Press the iliac crests posteriorly.

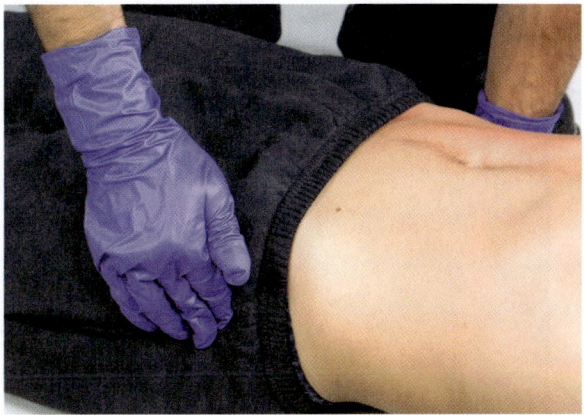

Figure 17-52 Palpate the greater trochanter.

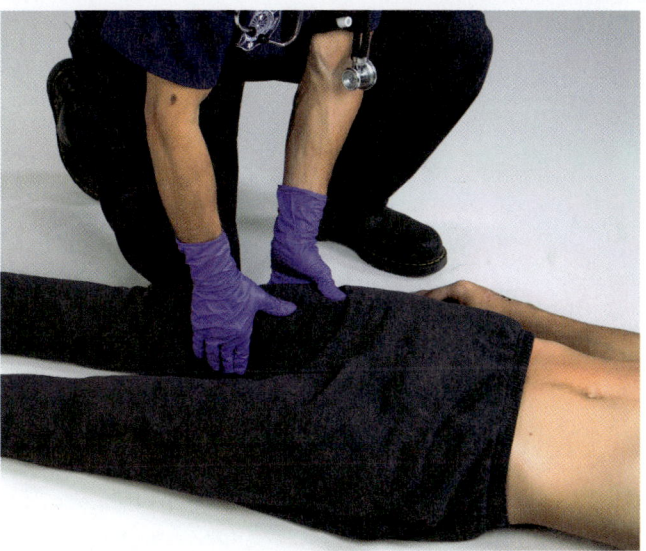

Figure 17-53 Palpate the femur.

or decreased range of motion. Consider any new decreased range of motion as a sign of an injured joint. Begin by visualizing both upper or lower extremities, looking for swelling, discoloration, minor bleeding and abrasions as well as obvious deformities. Test muscle strength and range of motion at each joint of all extremities. Pay attention to determine whether one body region is noticeably weaker. Attempt to determine whether a weakness is caused by an underlying condition such as arthritis, or if the weakness is of acute onset.

After assessment of the pelvis, evaluate the hips next. If you suspect a hip injury, visually inspect the injured leg for a shortened appearance (compared with the unaffected leg) and rotation of the entire leg. Palpate the head of the femur and press inward to assess structural strength. Visualize and inspect the upper leg. Femur injuries are not always obvious even though they are commonly associated with significant pain. Palpate the upper leg (Figure 17-53). Instability or deformity suggests a femur fracture, which is a life-threatening condition.

Move distally to the knee. Inspect and palpate both the knee and the kneecap (Figure 17-54). A kneecap most often dislocates laterally. It often is reduced by straightening the leg. Knee joint dislocations frequently lead to significant circulation, sensory, and motor (CSM) impairment and may require surgical repair. Palpate the lower leg as you did the upper leg (Figure 17-55). Remember to palpate both bones of the lower leg.

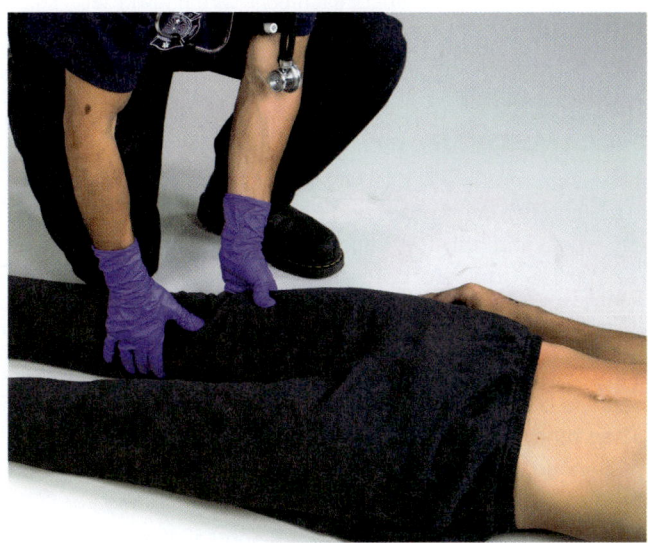

Figure 17-54 Palpate the knee and knee cap.

The ankle and foot can be assessed together. Note any crepitus and instability. The ankle's range of motion should be tested with resistance. Ask the patient to move both ankles together while you apply moderate pressure. Monitor for identical movement. Ankle movement includes both extension and flexion. Do not prevent movement; simply apply resistance (Figure 17-56). Suspect ligament and tendon damage if the patient cannot move the ankle against resistance. Evaluate the foot for crepitus and instability in the metatarsals and phalanges (digits). Foot dislocations are uncommon; however, if you notice obvious deformity anticipate the patient will require surgery.

Complete the lower extremity assessment by evaluating CSM. Lower leg circulation can be evaluated by palpating the dorsalis pedis or posterior tibialis pulse (Figure 17-57).

PARAMEDIC*Pearl*

The goal of a CSM assessment is to evaluate the integrity of the neurovascular bundle running through the limb, particularly when a segment of the limb is injured. Impaired, or decreased, CSM on an injured limb is generally indicated by a decrease in all three components and indicates the neurovascular bundle is damaged at the injury site. Common causes of decreased CSM are crush injuries and skeletal injuries with deformity.

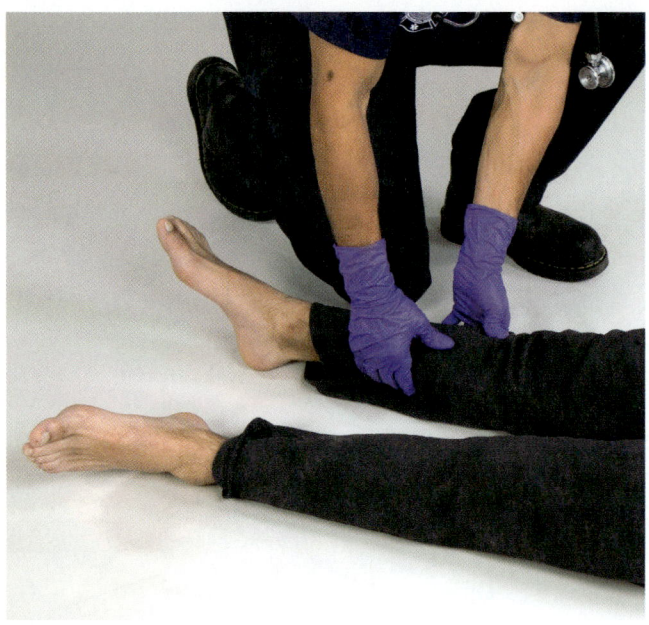

Figure 17-55 Palpate each bone of the lower leg.

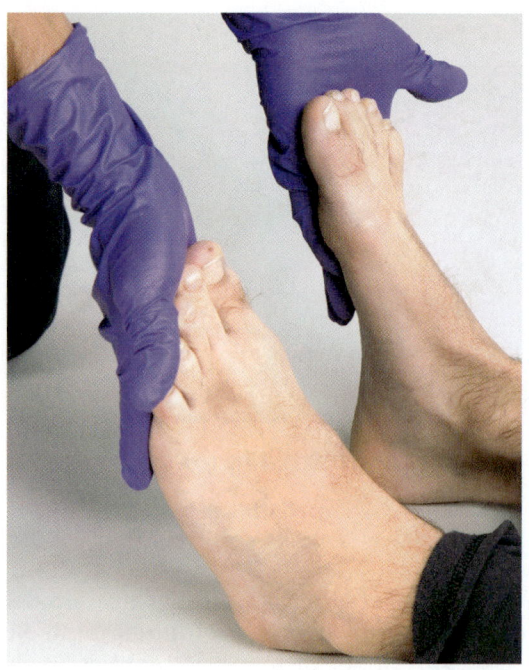

Figure 17-56 Ask the patient to move both ankles while you apply moderate resistance.

PARAMEDIC*Pearl*

Assessing motor skill integrity when the patient has a spine injury is a two-step process. First, assess the hands. Isolate the wrist, and ask the patient to extend the wrist against resistance. Compare both sides to ensure equal strength. When the wrist is injured, this test can be performed with finger extension only. Grip strength is an inaccurate assessment of motor skill integrity for spine injuries. Because this nerve is buried deep within the spinal cord, it often is intact when other spine injuries are present.

Second, isolate the ankles and ask your patient to extend and flex them against pressure. Be sure to monitory carefully for one-sided weakness. When the ankle is injured, ask the patient to flex and extend the great toe against pressure.

Palpate and compare both shoulders and clavicles (Figures 17-58 and 17-59). A step-off deformity, or anterior displacement of the humoral head, indicates a dislocation. However, superior displacement of the clavicle suggests shoulder separation.

Palpate the upper arm firmly (Figure 17-60). Pay special attention for crepitus or instability of the humerus. After inspecting the elbow for deformity and crepitus, continue your examination through the forearm and then to the wrist (Figure 17-61). Remember to compare the wrists to each other. Although deformity in the hand is usually obvious, do not forget to assess for crepitus and tenderness along all the metacarpals and phalanges (digits).

Complete the upper extremity examination by assessing CSM (Figure 17-62). Circulation can be assessed by palpating a radial pulse and noting that the extremity is

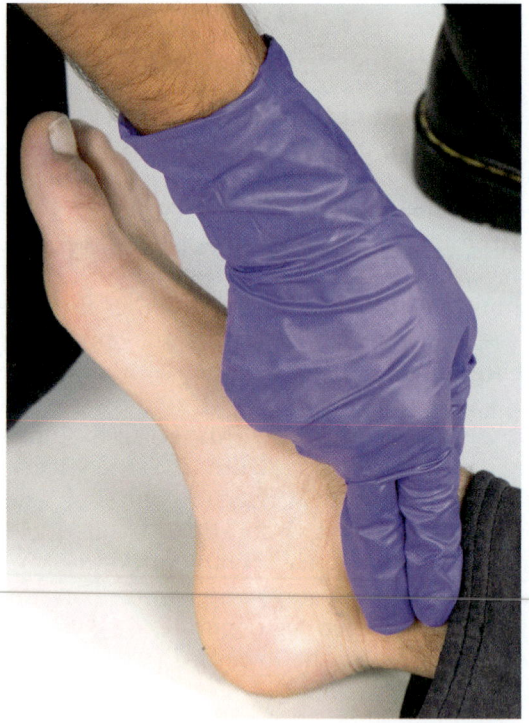

Figure 17-57 Palpation of the posterior tibialis pulse.

entirely pink and warm. Sensation can be verified by assessing whether the patient can distinguish which finger you are holding or by having the patient acknowledge he or she can feel your touch. Motion compares grip strength between hands, finger movement, or wrist movement.

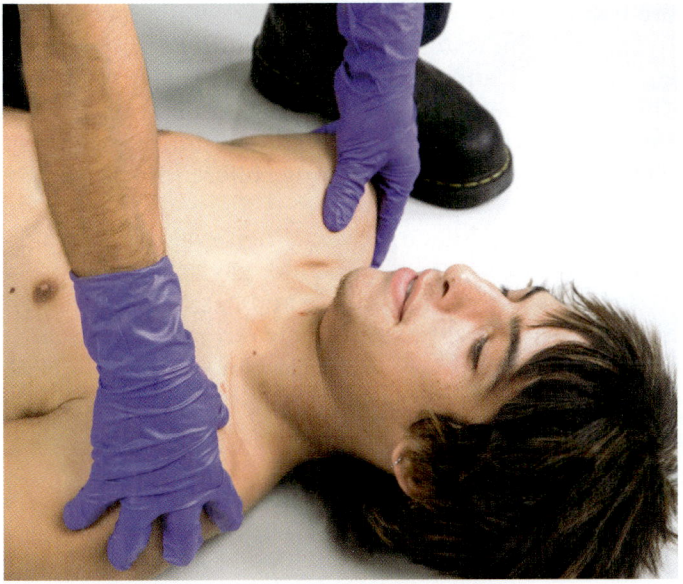

Figure 17-58 Palpate and compare both shoulders.

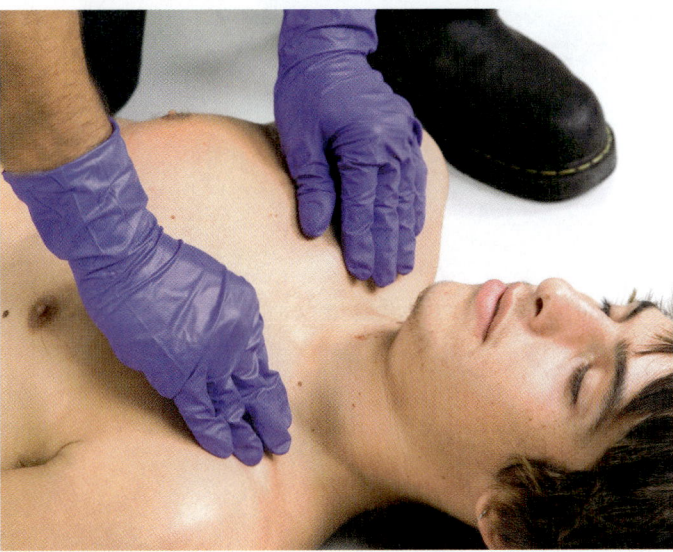

Figure 17-59 Palpate and compare both clavicles.

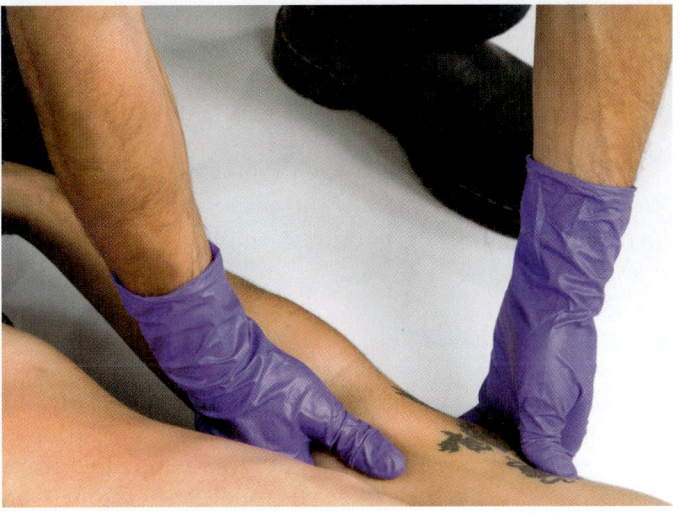

Figure 17-60 Palpate the humerus and elbow.

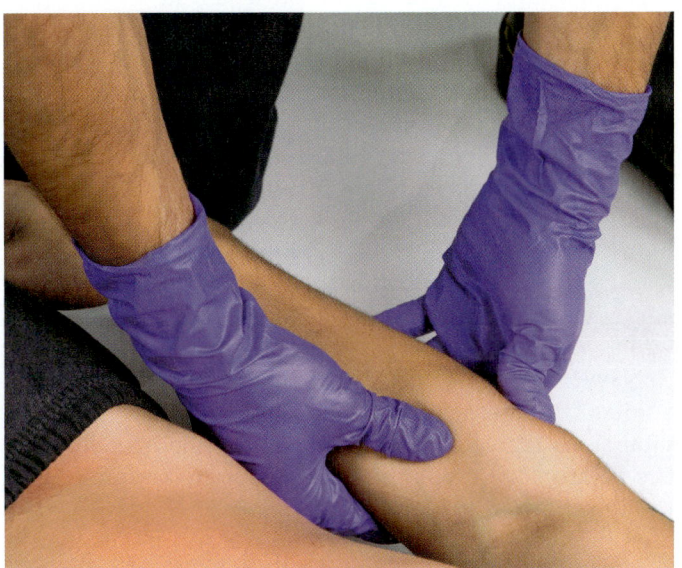

Figure 17-61 Palpate the lower arm and then the wrist.

Nervous System
[OBJECTIVES 83, 84]

Although you have been monitoring and evaluating portions of the nervous system throughout your examination, dedicate some time to focus directly on the nervous system as a whole. The nervous system examination requires assessment of both the central and the peripheral nervous systems. Central nervous system dysfunction can be a life-threatening condition and must be corrected. On the other hand, peripheral nervous system impairment may indicate a spinal cord injury, a musculoskeletal injury, or both. However, no peripheral nervous system impairment will quickly cause your patient to die. You should perform a full neurologic assessment if your patient has or has had the following:

- Altered mental status
- A loss of consciousness (for any length of time)

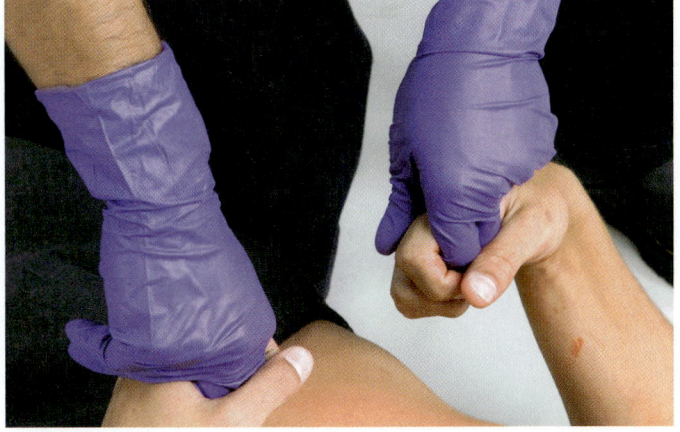

Figure 17-62 Check circulation, sensation, and movement (CSM) in each upper extremity.

- A loss or alteration of strength or sensation
- A loss of function of an extremity

A full neurologic assessment is explained in detail in Chapter 23.

Physical Examination Special Considerations. Not all patients can be examined in the same way. Infants, children, and older adults require a modified approach to assessment style.

Infants and Children
[OBJECTIVE 85]

One of the biggest challenges to assessing infants and children is gaining trust. Begin by speaking to the patient's caregiver. Obtain as much information as possible from that person. Stay calm and professional. The child will be able to tell if the caregiver trusts you. The caregiver's trust often transfers to the patient. At the same time, never ignore the patient. Children hate being invisible. Speak to a child directly and be honest. If you lie to the child (e.g., saying that a finger stick to determine blood sugar will not hurt, and then it does), the patient will not trust you again and other caregivers will have difficulty gaining cooperation.

Infants and children often cower from strangers. Rushing in to assess lung sounds on a patient who is not acutely ill puts the child on the defensive. One technique many paramedics use is a toe-to-head examination, leaving any area of obvious pain or injury to last. This allows you an opportunity to build trust with your patient while you explain what you are doing along the way.

Never forget that infants and children are not small adults. This is especially apparent when taking pediatric vital signs (Table 17-12). As a general rule, the younger the patient, the faster the respiratory rate and pulse and the lower the blood pressure. In a young child, the pulse and mental status are better indicators of circulatory status than is blood pressure. As long as a patient is awake, you know the brain is receiving adequate perfusion. Mental status changes indicate the outer layers of

the brain are receiving less blood, whereas a drop in the AVPU scale indicates the brain is no longer receiving enough blood and oxygen to support proper function. The brachial pulse should be assessed in infants because their radial and carotid pulses are too difficult to detect (Figure 17-63). Infants and young children are inherently belly breathers. Respiratory rate is assessed by counting the times the abdomen moves. When evaluating respiratory effort of the infant and child, pay special attention to signs of accessory muscle use and heart rate. Although an adult's heart rate usually increases with hypoxemia, an infant's decreases. Bradycardia in a young child is an ominous sign of impending respiratory failure. Assessment of the pediatric patient is discussed in detail in Chapter 37.

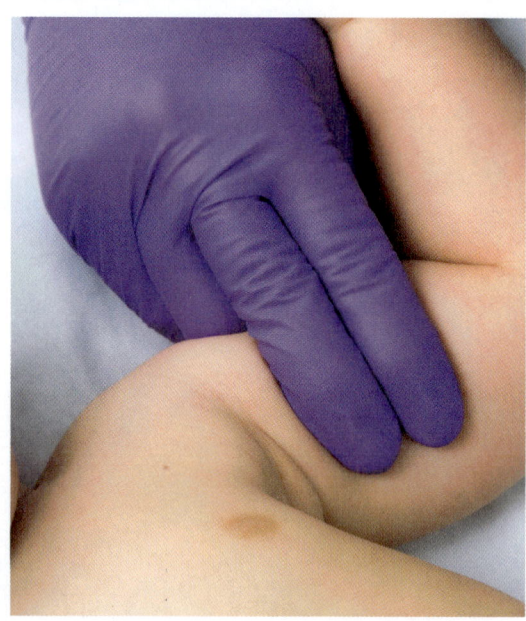

Figure 17-63 Palpate the brachial artery to assess a pulse in an infant.

TABLE 17-12 Pediatric Vital Signs							
Age	**Premature**	**Newborn**	**1-12 Mo**	**1-3 Yr**	**3-5 Yr**	**6-12 Yr**	**13+ Yr**
Weight	1-2 kg	2-3 kg	4-10 kg	10-14 kg	14-18 kg	20-42 kg	>50 kg
Pulse (beats/min)	140+	120-160	80-140	80-130	80-120	70-110	60-90
Respirations (breaths/min)	30-40	30-50	30-60	20-40	20-30	20-30	12-20
Systolic blood pressure (mm Hg)	40±10	60±10	85±15	90±15	95±15	100±15	115±15
Skin			←Pink, warm, moist→				
Temperature			←98.6° F→				
AVPU			←Alert→				

AVPU, Alert, verbal, pain, unresponsive.

Older Adults. In most EMS systems, an overwhelming majority of emergency calls are for older adults. One reason for this is that as the body ages the body systems become less efficient. Like a machine, they begin to wear and break down over time. Eventually, most people reach a point when help is needed to complete the activities of daily living. This comes with an incredible loss of independence. Independence is one of the most personal and valuable beliefs human beings hold, and the thought of giving it up is devastating. Because of this, many older adults wait as long as possible before calling for help. The patient may believe he or she is being bothersome by calling at 2 AM, so they wait until 7 AM to call about chest discomfort or difficulty breathing. When caring for an older adult, reassure them that it is okay to call for help. Remind them that EMS is there to provide a service.

Another important concern that arises with older adults is their sense of fear. Older adults may fear not returning home to the life they know. Many believe that if medical professionals discover a serious medical condition, they may not be able to return home and/or their independence will be taken away. This leads patients to be hesitant to reveal all their problems and symptoms and an even bigger mistrust of emergency care providers develops. Take the extra time to really talk to your older patients. Make them know you care. Speak on their level by sitting next to patients rather than standing over them (Figure 17-64). In most cultures, sitting or squatting and looking into a patient's eyes invites conversation. Consider spending extra time on scene, as the patient's condition allows, securing their home so they are comfortable receiving transport.

As already mentioned, older adults experience many physical changes as they age (Figure 17-65). Body systems tire and become less efficient. Cells break down and body size decreases. Particularly when people become sedentary or inactive, they develop either an obese or an extremely frail appearance. Physical examinations can become much more difficult and important in these patients.

One of the most important reasons for performing a careful physical examination is the neurologic changes that occur with age. Over time the peripheral nervous system deteriorates, which causes the body to respond more slowly to external and internal stimuli. For example, sensory nerves become less responsive. As a result, older adults do not sense pain and pressure as well. Patients may not sense the discomfort from soft tissue inflammation, bone fractures, or even cuts and scrapes as well as they once did. A patient may not realize he or she has an abdominal problem until you palpate it and discover rigidity or tenderness. The timing of motor signals also decreases with time. This leads to a decrease in agility and movement speed. Consequently, patients may be exposed to hazardous conditions for longer periods, such as placing the hand on a hot surface. The decrease in motor signals can lead to patients losing balance more often, sometimes resulting in fall injuries.

Another neurologic change occurs within the central nervous system. Brain cells begin to tire and wear down, which often manifests in the loss of some memory or cognitive skills. When this problem becomes serious enough, it often is diagnosed as dementia. However, understanding when patients cannot remember simple items, such as where they placed their keys, is extremely important. Many patients often keep pads of paper with them to write down this simple information. Another aid patients often use is organizers, such as pill dispensers and routines.

Dynamic changes occur within the cardiovascular system over time. As the body ages, blood vessels do not constrict and dilate as efficiently. As a result, an older adult compensates for shorter periods before experiencing cardiovascular collapse. This is compounded by arteriosclerosis, or hardening of the arteries. Decreased peripheral circulation leads to lengthened healing time for wounds and injuries. The body of an older adult becomes less efficient in shunting blood to the periphery to cool the body's core. Similarly, an older adult's body is less efficient at diverting blood from the periphery to the core when blood volume decreases to maintain adequate perfusion to the critical organs.

Older adults undergo age-related changes within the heart as well. Dysrhythmias such as atrial fibrillation and premature ventricular complexes are common. The coronary arteries often are plagued by the buildup of plaque within the arterial walls (atherosclerosis). Atherosclerosis leads to a decrease in blood supply and oxygen to the heart, which requires a constant supply of oxygen to function properly. Also remember that the heart has been beating since before the patient was born. As a muscle, it is beginning to tire and wear thin. The heart will not pump as hard or as well as it once did. This can manifest itself as a decreased blood pressure and/or heart failure.

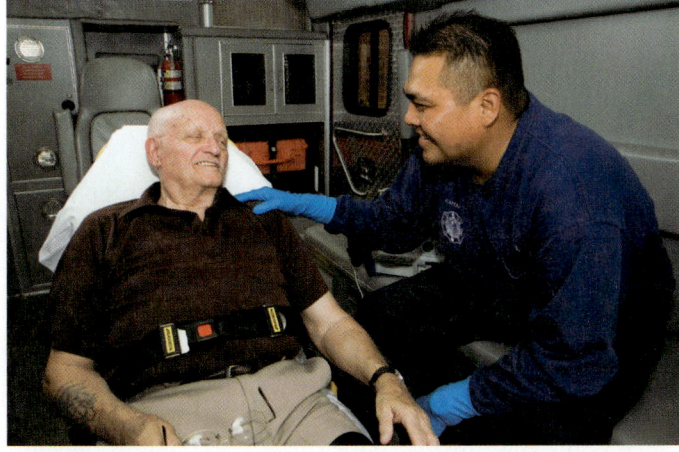

Figure 17-64 When speaking with an older adult, take the extra time to really talk to the patient. Make him or her know you care.

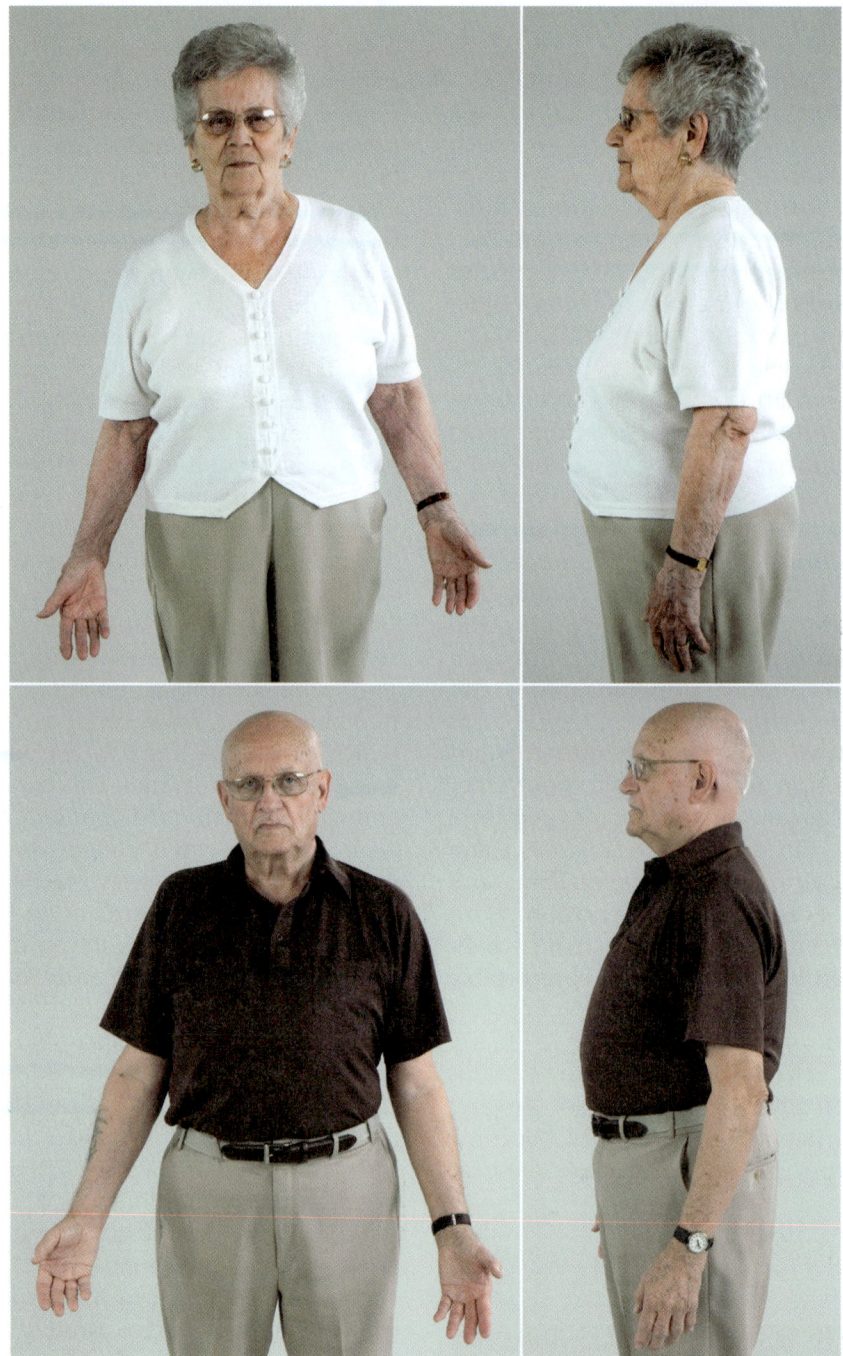

Figure 17-65 Older adults experience many physical changes as they age.

Several important changes occur within the musculo-skeletal system as people age. As physical activity decreases, so does muscle density. Muscles become more frail and offer less protection. This exposes an older adult's internal organs to a greater risk of damage from trauma. Bone density also decreases, which increases the risk of fracture from falls. The bones of an infant are like fresh, green saplings with great flexibility, and an older adult's bones are those same pieces of wood—but similar to dry kindling for the fireplace. Dried-out wood snaps very easily; a similar transition takes place in the bones of older adults. Once broken, the bones of an older adult do not heal as easily because of the decreased efficiency of the circulatory system.

Reassessment

[OBJECTIVES 86, 87]

Once you have finished your initial assessment, develop a treatment plan to care for all the identified problems. An important step in providing emergency care is continuing your assessment, called *reassessment.* Remember that a single set of vital signs is simply meaningless; it is only a snapshot of time. Developing a full picture of the patient's condition requires trending vital signs over time. Stable patients, such as those with a sprained ankle, may only require vital signs every 15 minutes. Unstable patients (such as an injured patient or those with respiratory distress, chest pain, or seizures) require more frequent reassessment of vital signs, at least every 5 minutes. Vitals also must be taken shortly after giving any medication to a patient.

Anytime the patient's condition changes, such as noticeable mental status changes (increase or decrease), vomiting, or additional symptoms, repeat the primary survey and vital signs. This will help identify any life-threatening conditions or new problems. In addition, perform a focused examination, concentrating attention on the portion of the body where the change took place. Another time to repeat portions of the physical examination is after any treatment or intervention. For example, whenever you provide care for fracture you need to reassess CSM distal to the injury site. A prudent paramedic also assesses the patient's pain level and vital signs after performing such a skill.

An injury occasionally may be extremely distracting, such as a traumatic amputation. After managing life threats, perform (or repeat) the physical examination. Significant new injuries occasionally may be found.

Case Scenario CONCLUSION

Your partner starts an intravenous (IV) line as you contact medical direction. The emergency department physician denies your request to administer IV morphine and furosemide. As you load her into the ambulance, she becomes combative and pulls the IV out of her arm. You restart the IV and transport the patient to the nearest hospital. When you arrive, her condition is essentially unchanged, with the following vital signs: pulse, 140 beats/min; blood pressure, 234/132 mm Hg; respirations, 40 breaths/min; SpO$_2$, 74%. Twenty minutes after your arrival she is diagnosed with acute pulmonary edema and treated with morphine and furosemide before intubation.

Looking Back

11. *What is the significance of the patient's increasing disorientation and vital signs changes?*
12. *Given the patient's final disposition, would your proposed treatment have been helpful or harmful? Why?*

DOCUMENTATION

[OBJECTIVE 88]

A good prehospital care report is thorough, accurate, and consistent. Get in the habit early in your career of detailing every portion of your assessment. Identify all the normal and abnormal findings to demonstrate you assessed that portion of the body. Document all your pertinent assessment findings as well as the pertinent negatives. For example, as you discuss the patient's chest discomfort, pertinent negatives would include an absence of nausea or vomiting and lack of relief with nitroglycerin. The more you write, the better picture you create for the physician and possibly an attorney reading your report later. A run report is a legal document. Falsifying or making up any information is morally wrong as well as illegal. Do not document a portion of the physical examination you did not complete or a finding that was not there. Consider having your partner review your report for accuracy after each call.

Patient assessment and treatment can be documented in many ways. No one way is necessarily better than the other. Most EMS systems have a basic run report format with ample space in the paperwork for your own narration. However you choose to document your assessment is fine as long as you do it the same every time. Writing a report in the same format each time keeps your documentation consistent and reduces your chances of making an error. Documentation is discussed in more detail in Chapter 19.

PARAMEDIC Pearl

Remember, your skills and abilities as a paramedic often are interpreted through your documentation. This means that if you write a poor report, those reading it may think you are a poor paramedic. Make writing a thorough, accurate, and consistent report a habit.

Case Scenario SUMMARY

1. *What is your general impression of this patient?* High priority based on her skin color, obvious respiratory distress, one- to two-word dyspnea, and cyanosis.

2. *What are some possible causes of this patient's respiratory distress and cyanosis?* At this stage you do not have enough information to narrow down the possible causes, which may include ventilation problems (upper or lower airway compromise, asthma, chronic obstructive pulmonary disease), oxygenation problems (pulmonary edema or pneumonia with hypoxia), or perfusion problems (pulmonary embolus).

3. *What history questions or physical assessment procedures would be most useful in differentiating the conditions you listed in question 2 above?* History questions include finding out whether she has had these symptoms before (she has not), any other medications she takes, and what she was doing at the time the episode began. Does she have a cough (is it productive, and what is the color of the sputum)? Does she feel feverish with chills? What makes her breathing better and what makes it worse? Does she have any pain with the shortness of breath? Has she smoked in the past (how much and for how long)? What medical problems has she had in the past? Does she have any allergies? Physical assessment procedures include evaluating ventilation (chest wall excursion, breath sounds, feeling air movement at the mouth, and SpO_2 and $ETCO_2$ evaluation), oxygenation (evaluation for signs of congestive heart failure [CHF], including crackles [rales], JVD, pedal edema, and prior history), and pulmonary perfusion (evaluation of blood pressure, skin color, and JVD) as well as obtaining her temperature.

4. *What intervention should you initiate at this time?* High-flow oxygen, assisted ventilation if air movement is poor, rapid transport, and IV.

5. *Is this patient high priority? Why or why not?* Yes. In addition to the findings on the initial survey, she is becoming anxious and combative. Her vital signs are abnormal, and her oxygen saturation is quite low.

6. *How does the history of untreated pneumonia, asthma, and untreated hypertension fit into the clinical picture?* They provide more confusion than clarity. The history of pneumonia could help explain her shortness of breath, although she does not have several key signs of pneumonia, including sputum production or fever. Asthma also may play a role, but her breath sounds (crackles) are inconsistent with asthma. Her untreated hypertension (and current high blood pressure) is consistent with CHF, which may lead to pulmonary edema and hypoxia. This seems to be the most likely problem.

7. *What conditions are consistent with retractions and use of the accessory muscles? What is the significance of the absence of JVD or pedal edema? What conditions cause crackles (rales)? What do the vital signs contribute to the clinical picture?* These questions highlight the potential differential process for causes of dyspnea. Retractions and use of accessory muscles confirm respiratory distress and impaired airflow. JVD and pedal edema are typically signs found with CHF and pulmonary edema. Their absence in this case may lessen the likelihood that CHF is the cause of this patient's symptoms or may be hidden by the patient's obesity. Crackles and rales are associated with small airway obstructions often found with pulmonary edema or congestion. However, crackles frequently are mistaken for rhonchi, the most common breath sound of patients with pneumonia. All these findings narrow the likely causes to congestive heart failure and pulmonary edema or pneumonia. The vital signs make diagnosis much simpler: tachycardia, tachypnea, and a low SpO_2 signal hypoxia. This patient needs rapid intervention and transport.

8. *Given the information from the previous question, what provisional diagnoses do you have in mind? Why?* This patient presents with one of the more difficult assessments in the field: differentiating pneumonia from CHF with pulmonary edema. The relevance is that the treatment for each is quite different. Given the history of hypertension and the absence of sputum production and fever, CHF is probably the more likely cause.

9. *Do you need additional history or assessment information to determine how you will manage this patient? Why or why not?* No. Continuing the evaluation in an effort to lock the decision between CHF and pneumonia is tempting. However, the patient's confusion, tachycardia, and low SpO_2 clearly communicate the need to treat and transport rather than continue the assessment.

10. *What treatment will you initiate at this time?* Continued efforts to administer high-flow oxygen, consider supplemental ventilation, initiate transport, start an IV, and consider medication therapy depending on transport time and patient condition.

11. *What is the significance of the patient's increasing disorientation and vital signs changes?* Worsening hypoxia.

12. *Given the patient's final disposition, would your proposed treatment have been helpful or harmful? Why?* This question has no easy answer. The ultimate diagnosis of CHF and pulmonary edema suggests that your proposed treatment (morphine and furosemide) was appropriate. However, data are equivocal regarding the value of morphine in the prehospital management of CHF and, if you had been incorrect in your assessment (and the patient had pneumonia), morphine and furosemide would have been inappropriate. As previously noted, this differential is one of the hardest in prehospital medicine, and you will learn more about it in subsequent chapters. Remember the basics; ensure that the patient is adequately ventilated, oxygenated, and rapidly transported to a facility where a more definitive diagnosis can be made.

Chapter Summary

- A thorough and complete patient assessment is the paramedic's most important tool. To provide a thorough examination, the paramedic must have his or her equipment prepared and be familiar with how to use all the tools.

- A well-organized format to patient assessment is critical; it helps address higher priority problems earlier. First identify and manage any scene-related problems. Second, identify and stabilize critical body system problems. Finally, perform a thorough examination to identify and manage all the patient's noncritical problems.

- Organize your physical examination in a logical pattern that makes sense for you. During the detailed examination, completely assess each anatomic region before moving on to another portion of the body.

- Remember, children are not small adults. Anytime a child is sick or injured, you have multiple patients—the child and his or her parents. Keep the immaturity of the child's organ systems in mind while performing an examination, and attempt to earn the patient's trust before trying to examine his or her body.

- As patients age, so do their organ systems. Anticipate multiple and more complicated problems in older adults. Also remember that older adults cannot compensate as well or as long as they once did. Intervene on seemingly minor problems early before they become life-threatening conditions.

- Never assume a patient is completely stable until you have the continued assessment evidence to back up your analysis. A single set of vital signs is only a place to start; two sets are merely interesting. Once you have three sets of vital signs you can begin to observe trends over time. These trends offer great insight into underlying conditions.

- Quite simply, if you do not write it down, you have not done it. Completely and thoroughly document all parts of your assessment. Do not simply document the interesting problems and conditions found; also remember to note normal findings and identify pertinent negatives. Select a documenting format that works for you and use it consistently to decrease your chances of forgetting to write that critical information down.

REFERENCE

Isaac, J. (1998). *The Outward Bound wilderness first-aid handbook*. Guilford, CT: Lyons Press.

SUGGESTED RESOURCES

WebMD. *Emergency medicine medical reference*, www.emedicine.com/emerg.

Gondim, F. de A. A., & Thomas, F. P. (2005). *Spinal cord, topographical and functional anatomy*. Retrieved May 5, 2006, from http://www.emedicine.com.

Issac, J., & Johnson, D. (2006). *Wilderness and rescue medicine: a practical guide for the basic and advanced practitioner*, Portland, ME: Wilderness Medical Associates.

University of California San Diego. *A practical guide to clinical medicine*. Retrieved February 15, 2008, from http://medicine.ucsd.edu.

Singh, J., & Stock, A. (2004). *Head trauma*. Retrieved March 21, 2006, from http://www.emedicine.com.

Wilderness Medical Associates, http://www.wildmed.com.

Chapter Quiz

1. Palpating with fingertips allows the paramedic to _____.
   a. detect fine sensations
   b. discriminate deep vibrations in the intestinal tract
   c. identify a hemothorax
   d. provide support for broken bones while evaluating them

2. During the primary survey, the paramedic's goal is to _____.
   a. ensure the scene is safe
   b. establish a baseline set of vitals
   c. identify and treat immediate life threats
   d. perform a head-to-toe examination

3. A full set of vital signs includes _____.
   a. pulse, respirations, and blood pressure
   b. pulse, respirations, blood pressure, AVPU, CSM, and pain level
   c. pulse, respirations, blood pressure, pulse oximetry, and blood glucose level
   d. pulse, respirations, blood pressure, skin, AVPU, core temperature

Chapter Quiz—continued

4. The difference between pain and tenderness is _____.
   a. pain is more serious than tenderness
   b. pain is sharp and intense, whereas tenderness is more of a dull ache
   c. the patient feels pain; you discover tenderness on palpation
   d. the patient feels tenderness; you discover pain on palpation

5. When evaluating a 6-month-old child in respiratory distress ___.
   a. bradycardia is an ominous sign of impending respiratory failure
   b. crying is always an indication of adequate respirations
   c. cyanosis will not appear until very late
   d. the infant's heart rate will continue to increase until the problem is corrected

6. When would you not stabilize a primary survey problem before continuing with your assessment?
   a. Primary survey problems are not corrected until after the secondary survey is completed.
   b. No reason exists to *not* stabilize a primary survey problem before continuing with your assessment.
   c. When you cannot identify a cause for a decreased level of consciousness and need the physical examination, SAMPLE history, and vital signs to aid you in making a differential diagnosis.
   d. You do not need to stabilize primary survey problems when you provide rapid transport to the hospital.

7. The skilled paramedic should be competent at auscultating:

   _____

   _____

   _____

8. What is the difference between sensory and motor examinations and checking CSM?
   a. Sensory and motor examinations are part of a CSM check; the last part is pulse detection.
   b. Sensory and motor examinations test spine and nerve integrity; CSM checks evaluate neurovascular bundle integrity in an extremity.
   c. Sensory examinations test the spine; CSM checks are the motor tests for the spine.
   d. They test the same thing and thus are redundant examinations.

9. Which of the following is the term used to describe short-term memory loss of information after a head injury?
   a. Antegrade amnesia
   b. Amnesia
   c. Partial amnesia
   d. Retrograde amnesia

10. What is the correct term used to describe hyperactivity of bowel sounds?
    a. Borborygmus
    b. Hyperperistalsis
    c. Korotkoff
    d. Peristalsis

Terminology

Antegrade amnesia The inability to remember short-term memory information after an event during which the head was struck.

Auscultation The process of listening to body noises with a stethoscope.

AVPU Mnemonic for *a*wake, *v*erbal, *p*ain, *u*nresponsive; used to evaluate a patient's mental status.

Battle's sign Significant bruising around the mastoid process (behind the ears).

Borborygmus Hyperactivity of bowel sounds.

Bowel sounds The noises made by the intestinal smooth muscles as they squeeze fluids and food products through the digestive tract.

Bradycardia Heart rate slower than 60 beats/min (from *brady*, meaning slow).

Bradypnea A respiratory rate less than 12 breaths/min.

Bruit The blowing or swishing sound created by the turbulence within a blood vessel.

Carotid bruit The noise made when blood in the carotid arteries passes over plaque buildups.

Core body temperature The measured body temperature within the core of the body; generally measured with an esophageal probe; normal is 98.6° F.

CSM *C*irculation, *s*ensation, and *m*ovement.

Cullen's sign Yellow-blue ecchymosis surrounding the umbilicus.

Cyanosis A bluish coloration of the skin as a result of hypoxemia, or deoxygenation of hemoglobin.

Diastole The period when the ventricles are relaxed and filling with blood.

Diastolic blood pressure The pressure exerted against the walls of the large arteries during ventricular relaxation.

Ecchymosis Collection of blood within the skin that appears blue-black, eventually fading to a greenish-brown and yellow; commonly called a bruise.

Fluctuance A wavelike motion felt between two fingertips when palpating a fluid-filled structure such as a subcutaneous abscess.

Gasping Inhaling and exhaling with quick, difficult breaths.

Grey-Turner's sign Bruising along the flanks that may indicate pancreatitis or intraabdominal hemorrhage.

Grunting A short, low-pitched sound heard at the end of exhalation that represents an attempt to generate positive end-expiratory pressure by exhaling against a closed glottis, prolonging the period of oxygen and carbon dioxide exchange across the alveolar-capillary membrane; a compensatory mechanism to help maintain patency of small airways and prevent atelectasis.

Gurgling Abnormal respiratory sound associated with collection of liquid or semisolid material in the patient's upper airway.

Head bobbing Indicator of increased work of breathing in infants; the head falls forward with exhalation and comes up with expansion of the chest on inhalation.

Hypertension Elevated blood pressure.

Hyperthermia A core body temperature greater than 98.6° F.

Hypotension Low blood pressure significant enough to cause inadequate perfusion.

Hypothermia A core body temperature below 95° F (35° C).

Induration Hardened mass within the tissue typically associated with inflammation.

Korotkoff sounds The noise made by blood under pressure tumbling through the arteries.

Lesions A wound, injury, or pathologic change in body tissue; any visible, local abnormality of the tissues of the skin, such as a wound, sore, rash, or boil.

Life-threatening conditions A problem of the circulatory, respiratory, or nervous system that will kill a patient within minutes if not properly managed.

Minute volume The amount of air moved in and out of the lungs in 1 minute; determined by multiplying the tidal volume by the respiratory rate.

Nasal flaring Widening of the nostrils on inhalation; an attempt to increase the size of the airway and increase the amount of available oxygen.

Nystagmus Involuntary rapid movement of the eyes in the horizontal, vertical, or rotary planes of the eyeball.

Painful stimulus Any stimulus that causes discomfort to the patient, triggering some sort of response.

Palpation The process of applying pressure against the body with the intent of gathering information.

Percussion A diagnostic technique that uses tapping on the body to differentiate air, solids, and fluids.

Photosensitivity A condition in which the patient's eyes are sensitive or feel pain when exposed to bright light.

Pleural friction rub Noise made when the visceral and parietal pleura rub together.

Point of maximum impulse (PMI) The apical impulse; the site where the heartbeat is most strongly felt.

Pulse oximetry A measured percent of saturated hemoglobin.

Pulse pressure The difference between the systolic and diastolic blood pressures.

Raccoon eyes Bruising around the orbits of the eyes.

Range of motion The full and natural range of a joint's movement.

Rapid medical assessment A quick head-to-toe assessment of a medical patient who is unresponsive or has an altered mental status.

Rapid trauma assessment A quick head-to-toe assessment of a trauma patient with a significant mechanism of injury.

Rebound tenderness Discomfort experienced by the patient that occurs when the pressure from palpation is released.

Retractions Sinking in of the soft tissues above the sternum or clavicle or between or below the ribs during inhalation.

Retrograde amnesia The inability to remember events or recall memories from before an event in which the head was struck.

S1 The sound of the tricuspid and mitral valves closing.

S2 The sound of the closing of the pulmonary and aortic valves.

Signs and symptoms Signs are a medical or trauma condition of the patient that can be seen, heard, smelled, measured, or felt during the examination; symptoms are conditions described by the patient, such as shortness of breath, or pieces of information bystanders tell you about the patient's chief complaint.

Shock Inadequate systemic perfusion.

Skin turgor The elasticity of the skin; good skin turgor returns the skin's natural shape within 2 seconds.

Sniffing position Neck flexion at the fifth and sixth cervical vertebrae, with the head extended at the first and second cervical vertebrae. This position aligns the axes of the mouth, pharynx, and trachea, opening the airway and increasing airflow.

Snoring Noisy breathing through the mouth and nose during sleep; caused by air passing through a narrowed upper airway.

Terminology—continued

Stridor A harsh, high-pitched sound heard on inspiration associated with upper airway obstruction; often described as a high-pitched crowing or "seal bark" sound.

Systole The period when the ventricles are contracting.

Systolic blood pressure The pressure exerted against the walls of the large arteries at the peak of ventricular contraction.

Tachycardia A heart rate grater than 100 beats/min.

Tachypnea An increased respiratory rate, usually greater than 30 breaths/min.

Tidal volume The volume of air moved into or out of the lungs during a normal breath; can be indirectly evaluated by observing the rise and fall of the patient's chest and abdomen.

Tripod position Position used to maintain an open airway that involves sitting upright and leaning forward with the neck slightly extended, chin projected, and mouth open and supported by the arms.

Verbal stimulus Any noise that elicits some sort of response from the patient.

Visual acuity card A standardized board used to test vision.

Voluntary guarding Conscious contraction of the abdominal muscles in an attempt to prevent painful palpation.

Wheezes High-pitched whistling sounds produced by air moving through narrowed airway passages.

Communication

Objectives *After completing this chapter, you will be able to:*

1. Identify why good communication skills are important when providing EMS.
2. Identify the roles of verbal, written, and electronic communication in providing EMS.
3. Identify why you should use the proper terminology when communicating during an EMS event.
4. Identify why you should use proper verbal communication during an EMS event.
5. List factors that enhance and hinder effective verbal communication.
6. Identify why you should use proper written communication during an EMS event.
7. List factors that enhance and hinder effective written communication.
8. Recognize the legal status of your written communication documenting an EMS event.
9. State why you should collect data during an EMS event.
10. Identify technology that you can use to collect and exchange patient and/or scene information electronically.
11. Recognize the legal status of any patient medical information that has been exchanged electronically.
12. Identify ways you use the following communication equipment:
    - Digital communications
    - Fax machine
    - Computer

13. Describe the phases of communication you will use to complete a typical EMS event.
14. Identify the various parts of a typical EMS communications system and describe their function and use.
15. Describe the functions and responsibilities of the Federal Communications Commission.
16. Identify and distinguish the following communications systems:
    - Simplex
    - Multiplex
    - Duplex
    - Half duplex
    - Trunked
17. Describe how an EMS dispatcher functions as an integral member of the EMS team.
18. Identify the role of emergency medical dispatch in a typical EMS event.
19. Identify the importance of prearrival instructions in a typical EMS event.
20. Describe the purpose or reason that you verbally communicate the patient's information to the hospital.
21. Describe any information that you should include in the patient assessment information that you verbally report to medical direction.

Chapter Outline

Process of Communication
Modes of EMS Communication
Phases of EMS Communication
EMS Communication Systems

Dispatch Centers
Relaying Patient Information
Chapter Summary

Case Scenario

A young mother finds her 11-month-old son unconscious in her hot tub. She pulls him out and picks up the phone to call 9-1-1. She is sobbing to the 9-1-1 operator as she describes how she "just left him alone for a minute" and then found him unresponsive and limp.

Questions

1. *What is the most important information the operator needs to get from this woman at this time?*
2. *What barriers stand in the way of the operator getting this information?*
3. *What information does the young mother need to get from the 911 operator? How can this information help the mother?*
4. *What barriers hinder the operator from effectively communicating this information to the mother?*

[OBJECTIVE 1]

Communication is the exchange of information between two or more individuals. It is essential in almost every area of life. Consider how poor communication can lead to disaster when you are trying to talk with your parents, your spouse, your boss—even the Internal Revenue Service. But regarding EMS, poor communication can cost lives. As a paramedic, you must be able to communicate with the dispatch center to receive the information you need to respond to a call. You must also be able to communicate effectively with the patients, family members, bystanders, other resource agencies, and the hospital. Someday you may even have to use your communication skills in court. Consequently, you must be proficient in all forms of communication.

PROCESS OF COMMUNICATION

The process of communication—or the act of communicating—involves an idea being relayed from one person to another. Methods of communicating include speaking, listening, reading, writing, and using gestures or body language. The person relaying the idea is the *sender*. The sender must express his or her idea in the form of a message. A message consists of the signs and symbols transmitted by the sender. The person receiving the idea or message is the *receiver*.

These messages are carried by a medium or channel. A *channel* refers to messages sent that correspond to the senses, such as the auditory (sound) channel. *Medium* refers to sending messages using a combination of different communication channels. For example, standard telephone communication is a channel because it involves only sound. Face-to-face communication is a medium because it may involve the use of the auditory channel (sound), visual channel (sight), tactile channel (touch) and, in some cases, the olfactory channel (smell). For a message to be understood, it must be in the appropriate medium. For example, a visual means of communicating would not be appropriate when communicating with a blind patient. An auditory means of communicating

would not be useful when communicating with a deaf patient.

During face-to-face communication, the sender creates (encodes) a message through the use of symbols (such as words) and signs (such as facial expressions, tone of voice, and body movements). During radio or telephone communication, the radio or telephone encodes the sounds of the sender's voice and transmits these sounds in electrical impulses.

Once the message has been sent, the receiver must interpret (decode) the signs and symbols of the message. The response from the receiver that allows the sender to know how his or her message is being received is called *feedback*. Feedback may be verbal or nonverbal, such as "Yes, I understand," or a nod, smile, frown, or a change in posture or gaze (Box 18-1).

MODES OF EMS COMMUNICATION

[OBJECTIVE 2]

Three basic modes of communication are used in EMS: verbal, written, and electronic. These methods are used in a typical EMS call in the following ways:

- Communication between the party requesting help and the dispatcher
- Communication between the dispatcher and the paramedic
- Communication between the paramedic, patient, receiving facility, and/or medical direction physician
- Communication with receiving facility personnel (on arrival)

BOX 18-1 | **Elements of Communication**

- Source/idea
- Sender/encoder
- Message
- Medium/channel
- Receiver/decoder
- Feedback

Verbal Communication

[OBJECTIVES 3, 4, 5]
Your command of verbal communication skills is important. You often will communicate verbally during an EMS event. This form of communication is used to exchange information with the patient, EMS personnel on the scene, dispatch, medical direction, and staff at the receiving facility.

As a paramedic, your use of verbal (and nonverbal) communication must be professional. Your ability to communicate effectively with others is affected by several factors, including your knowledge level, communication skills (e.g., grammar, vocabulary), life experience, and prejudices. When speaking to others, keep in mind that your words and actions affect the message that others receive. Attempt to minimize any barriers to communication. For example, when you are speaking to the patient, family members, and bystanders, use terms that are easily understood. Avoid the use of medical terms. On the other hand, when you are speaking with other members of the healthcare team, use proper terminology. When relaying patient information, make sure that your verbal report is accurate and concise.

When speaking to others, the words you choose to relay your message can affect the message that is received. For instance, if you are speaking with a Spanish-speaking patient and have only a limited number of Spanish phrases in your vocabulary, using the wrong word can be insulting to the receiver. Your attitude toward the receiver also can affect the message received. For example, the message that you send (intentionally or unintentionally) when caring for a homeless patient may be different from the message you send to a patient who is not homeless. You should treat each patient you encounter professionally and to the best of your ability, regardless of his or her circumstances. Also remember not to make assumptions about others when you are speaking to them. For instance, do not assume that all older adults have difficulty hearing or that a 6-year-old will not understand you. Therapeutic communication is covered in more detail in Chapter 15.

PARAMEDIC Pearl
As a paramedic, you can be your own worst enemy regarding communication. Paramedics sometimes use big words to try to impress the person listening to or reading their reports. However, some of these words can be misunderstood, especially over a radio or telephone. Words that contain *hyper-*, *hypo-*, *inter-*, or *intra-* tend to sound the same when a person is excited or in a hurry. As a result, orders for medications or procedures can be incorrect. In some cases, the orders may not be received at all. To avoid errors, remember to keep your communication simple and to the point. Moreover, make sure you use proper terminology, grammar, and spelling.

Written Communication

[OBJECTIVES 6, 7, 8, 9]
As a paramedic, you will write many reports. In fact, written reports are an important part of the prehospital care that you provide. A patient care report (PCR) is the record you write after each patient encounter. The PCR has many functions. For one, it is a legal record of the EMS call. It also ensures the continuity of patient care and is available for medical audits, quality management, billing and reimbursement, and research and data collection purposes.

A common phrase states, "If it is not documented, then it did not happen." Incomplete, inaccurate, or illegible documentation implies that the care provided also was inappropriate or inadequate. Therefore your PCR must be complete, accurate, and legible and contain all the information pertinent to the patient encounter. The report must contain the patient's location; the reason you were called; the reasons the patient required 9-1-1 assistance; the time the incident occurred; the people involved in the incident; the number of patients; and the patient's physical findings, vital signs, and medical history; as well as all patient information pertaining to what you saw and found. Include your treatment of the patient, the patient's response, your re-evaluation and subsequent treatment, and to whom you transferred the patient (and patient's belongings).

When the call is completed and before you turn in the report, check your PCR to verify that you have accurately documented the events of the call. Consider any problems en route to the call. Document any factors that affected your response, such as adverse weather conditions, mechanical problems, or crowd control. Also consider and document what the scene size-up indicated. Document whether any other resources were called for and what they were. Be sure to document all pertinent patient information and the treatments you performed. Document any and all orders requested and received from medical direction. In addition, submit all supporting information with your PCR, including copies of electrocardiographic (ECG) strips and interpretation of the ECG rhythm, rate, regularity, ectopic beats, and abnormalities. Additional supporting documentation may include a list of medications taken by the patient (see Chapter 19).

PARAMEDIC Pearl
Sometime in your career you may be called to court to testify about an EMS call, your report, and patient care issues. This will most likely occur years after a call. Your PCR must contain enough detail to paint a picture of the scene, the patient, and your findings. That way, when you are called to court your report will stir your memory and you will be able to recall what occurred. Your PCR should contain the five *W*'s and one *H*: *w*ho, *w*hat, *w*here, *w*hy, *w*hen, and *h*ow. Remember: the details will save you.

Quality Management Process

Another form of written communication is the quality management process. EMS agencies have a quality management process in place that evaluates the appropriateness and effectiveness of the prehospital care its personnel provides. PCRs are checked for thoroughness and completeness as well as adherence to existing patient care protocols.

Electronic Communication

[OBJECTIVES 10, 11, 12]
In addition to verbal and written communication, you also engage in electronic communication as a paramedic. Electronic communication allows you to transmit PCRs, 12-lead ECGs, and billing reports generated from PCRs to various facilities and persons. Many forms of equipment allow the paramedic to transmit this information. The most popular form of electronic communication is the computer-generated report. These reports allow you to

incorporate ECG strips, pictures of the scene or patient, patient information, patient treatment issues, and an inventory of supplies, among other things. With computer-generated reports, you can use tools such as spell check and grammar check, and you can check for missing required information within the report. You can use desktop computers at the station or ones that are as small as a personal digital assistant. In some EMS systems, laptop computers in vehicles allow wireless connection with dispatch. These systems allow instant messaging, can show the identical information on the dispatcher's screen, and allow use of global positioning mapping systems to aid in appropriate dispatch and response.

One of the most-used electronic devices in EMS is the fax machine. It can be used to send copies of a PCR and an ECG strip to the hospital. Some dispatch centers send trip information and report numbers along with the unit's times without having to tie up the radio system or give this information over the telephone. In some EMS systems, wireless transceivers are used to transmit data, such as ECGs, over a cellular phone to the hospital.

Case Scenario—continued

After speaking with the mother, the dispatcher notifies an ambulance, a fire unit, and a police cruiser to respond to the scene. The call taker also maintains telephone contact with the mother, who waits with her son in her arms.

Questions

5. What is the most critical information for the dispatcher to convey to responding units? How will they use this information to provide better service to the mother?
6. What are the benefits of having the operator remain in contact with the mother while the ambulance is responding?
7. Imagine yourself as this mother; think how you might feel holding your limp son in your arms. What would you need the operator to communicate to you?
8. When you (the paramedic) arrive on the scene, what information do you need to get from the mother? What do you need to communicate to her?

PHASES OF EMS COMMUNICATION

[OBJECTIVE 13]
Five main phases of communication occur during a typical EMS call (Box 18-2). The first phase involves the occurrence of the emergency. Remember, all calls are an emergency to the caller. The second phase is detecting that an emergency has occurred. In the third phase, the EMS dispatcher determines what resources are needed to respond to the call and sends them to the scene. The patient is treated and prepared for transport during the fourth phase. During the fifth phase, communication occurs on the scene with other healthcare professionals and the patient.

BOX 18-2 Phases of Communication Necessary to Complete a Typical EMS Call

- Occurrence
- Detection
- Notification and response
- Treatment and preparation for transport
- Preparation for next event

EMS COMMUNICATION SYSTEMS

Radio Communication

[OBJECTIVE 14]

The communication system widely used within EMS is the two-way radio. A base station is a radio used by dispatch to contact and send units to emergency and nonemergency calls (Figure 18-1). These radios are generally stationary units and transmit from a large tower or a series of towers with a trunk system or a repeater system (covered later in this chapter). The calls are transmitted to either a mobile radio or a portable radio.

The **mobile radio** is a fixed unit within the emergency vehicle (Figure 18-2). Most mobile units transmit at 50 to 100 W. Most mobile radios can only transmit efficiently over less than a 20-mile radius. Because of the limited power and limited transmitting distance, tower repeaters may be used throughout an area to help increase the distance a mobile unit can transmit.

Portable radios also are referred to as *handheld units* (Figure 18-3). They are typically used when the crew is away from the emergency vehicle. The portable radio's power output is minimal, approximately 1 to 5 W. These radios are limited to very short distances. They are used to talk to personnel on the scene, request additional resources, and request help in dangerous situations. To increase the **range** of these radios, a vehicular repeater can be installed, a high-gain antenna can be used, or you can stand on top of a tall building. Vehicular repeaters take the transmission of the portable radio, send the transmission through the mobile radio, and increase the output to 50 to 100 W. This allows you to transmit at a higher output and over a longer distance and provides a safer working environment by allowing you to call for help directly from dispatch.

Radio Frequencies

[OBJECTIVE 15]

A radio wave is an invisible electromagnetic wave. When the current is supplied to an antenna, the electromagnetic field propagates through space. Radio waves have different frequencies. A range of radio frequencies is called a **band.** A radio frequency can be picked up by tuning a receiver to a specific frequency.

Ultra-high-frequency (UHF) radio waves have a radio frequency between 300 MHz and 3 GHz. Frequencies used by EMS are typically in the 450 to 470 MHz range. UHF frequencies are advantageous because they have high penetrating power and can easily pass through

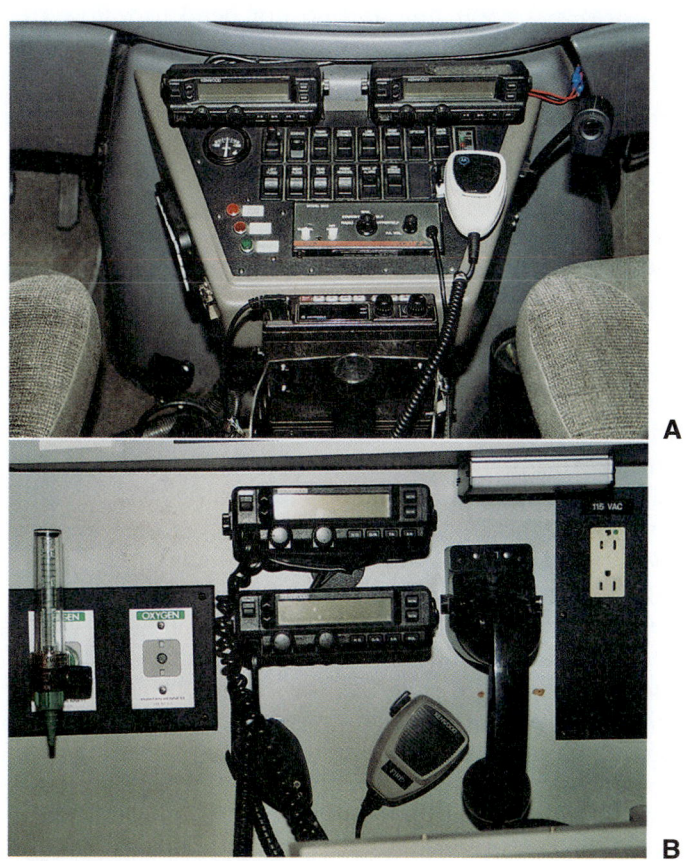

Figure 18-2 A, Mobile radio in the cab. **B,** Mobile radio in the patient care compartment.

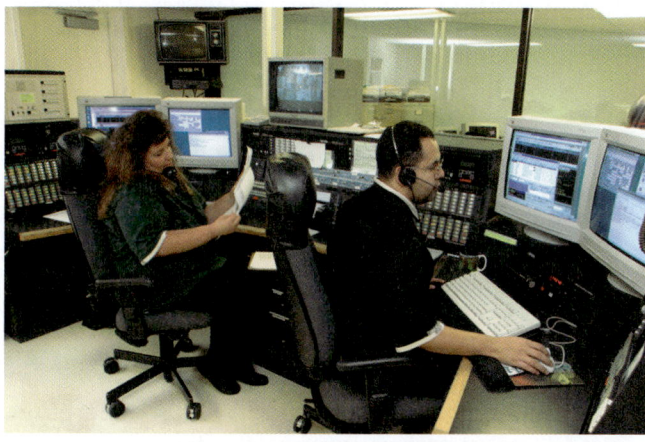

Figure 18-1 9-1-1 dispatch center.

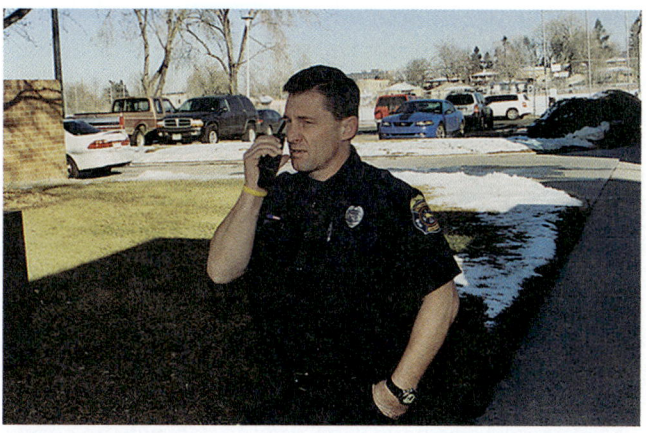

Figure 18-3 Handheld radios are low power with limited transmission distance.

buildings. Disadvantages are that they only travel a short distance and are limited to line of sight. This generally makes these frequencies more applicable to urban areas.

Very-high-frequency (VHF) is the radio frequency range from 30 to 300 MHz. The VHF low-band frequencies range from 32 to 50 MHz. VHF low-band radio waves are able to curve and follow the shape of the earth or move around other obstacles. This enables communication over long distances. VHF high-band frequencies range from 150 to 174 MHz. VHF high-band radio waves travel in a straight line and do not bend to follow the curve of the earth or around obstacles. Although they are limited to line of site, they are less susceptible to interference than VHF low-band frequencies. The main advantage of VHF frequencies is the distance they can travel; however, these frequencies are susceptible to interference from buildings, electrical equipment, and weather. This frequency range is generally more advantageous for rural areas, where there are great distances with minimal physical structures to block the waves.

Over the last several years the 800-MHz band has been widely used by emergency services. Within this spectrum the frequencies from 821 to 824 MHz and 866 to 869 MHz have been allocated exclusively for public safety systems. This spectrum allows traditional radio functions to work with the capabilities of a computer. Rather than having a single frequency that all radios operate on, such as in the UHF and VHF ranges, a "bank" of frequencies is allocated to an agency. When a radio is activated the computer searches for an open frequency to allow the user to communicate with someone else. This often is called a *trunking system*. Meanwhile, the computer can assign other frequencies in the bank to other users at the same time. This has helped reduce frequency congestion. The downside to this system has been interference from commercial radio carriers such as cellular telephone companies, which also use the 800-MHz band. The frequencies they use are close to the range used by public safety systems. To resolve this conflict, the 800-MHz spectrum is currently undergoing "rebanding" to increase the space between frequencies for these two groups.

Radio frequencies are assigned and licensed by the **Federal Communications Commission (FCC).** One of the main challenges of the advancement of technology is that radio frequencies have become extremely congested. One concern of the FCC is that a shortage of available frequencies will occur as demand potentially surpasses supply. In 1996 more than 1 million licensed stations were authorized to operate 12 million transmitters in the Private Land Mobile Radio Services (FCC, 2006). This number is expected to double by 2010. In comparison, only 600 available frequencies are in the VHF high band; the UHF band has only 302 primary frequencies. The portion of the 800-MHz band allocated for emergency services has only 240 primary frequencies.

Many programs have been used to combat the congestion problem. Most frequencies licensed by the FCC are shared frequencies, meaning multiple entities may be assigned the same frequency. To reduce interference both geographic separation and continuous-tone coded squelch systems are used. These often are referred to by their trade names, such as Private Line (Motorola Inc., Schaumburg, Ill.) or Channel Guard (General Electric, Fairfield, Conn.).

To further control congestion, the FCC combined radio frequencies into two pools in 1997: the public safety radio pool and the industrial/business radio pool. To obtain a license in the public safety radio pool an entity must meet certain criteria in the provision of public safety services. However, although this has decreased interference from other types of radio transmissions, it did not reduce the number of entities using two-way radios.

In an attempt to increase the number of available frequencies and reduce congestion, the FCC is working to reclaim a number of current frequencies in the 700-MHz range (it has already reclaimed several). These currently are being used for commercial television broadcasts. As these broadcasts are being moved to other frequencies to meet the requirements of high-definition television, part of the frequencies they are vacating will be allocated to the public safety radio pool. The remainder will be allocated to the industrial/business radio pool.

In addition to assigning and licensing radio frequencies, the FCC also monitors radio operations in the United States. In EMS, frequencies are used for dispatch to communicate with fire, ground, mutual aid, and general communications from unit to unit. The language of a radio license issued in the public safety radio pool includes wording that states the radio frequency must only be used for communications relevant to the provision of public safety services. To the paramedic this means that any communication on the radio must fall within this requirement. This includes any communications on what an EMS agency may consider a "talk around" channel. The single most important thing the individual paramedic can do to reduce radio congestion is to keep transmissions relevant and appropriate to the provision of emergency services. Another aspect about the FCC that must be appreciated is that they only regulate transmission on licensed radio frequencies. They do not regulate or control reception of these frequencies. This means that anyone can monitor radio transmissions in the United States through the use of a scanner or the Internet. Although more difficult, even the 800 MHz frequencies can be monitored. The paramedic must assume that someone is listening to every transmission being made; as a result, you must ensure you are professional and do not transmit any personally identifiable information pertaining to yourself or the patient.

Cellular and Satellite Telephones

Cellular phone use is widespread in EMS. These phones are used to relay patient information to receiving facilities and speak with medical direction. However, cellular phones are an unreliable mode of communication because of the dead areas in which the phones cannot transmit or receive. Mobile or portable radios have the same issue—dead spots. As you drive the roadways, you drive through areas where the phone drops the call or the signal fades in and out. If you are trying to get orders for treatment or trying to give patient care, reporting it by a cellular telephone may complicate patient care.

> **PARAMEDIC Pearl**
>
> An essential part of the quality management process involves recording conversations between medical direction and the EMS crew and the receiving facility and the EMS crew. This information can be used in legal proceedings to determine what was ordered for the patient and what you did.

Satellite phones are more reliable than cellular phones because few obstructions, such as inclement weather, interfere with the signal. The major downfall is the cost to operate a satellite telephone. Purchase cost is only a little more expensive than a cellular phone, but the cost of operation is much more per minute.

> **PARAMEDIC Pearl**
>
> During a major incident, cellular phones and land lines may be so congested that getting an open line is impossible. However, satellite telephones will work as long as the lines they are trying to reach are open. Satellite telephones have proved to be invaluable during major incidents that taxed the normal telephone and cellular phone systems.

Repeater Systems

A **repeater** system is a device that receives transmissions from a low-wattage radio and rebroadcasts the signal at a higher wattage and perhaps a different frequency. As previously mentioned, a typical base and mobile radio system has a range of 50 to 110 W and a typical portable radio transmits at a range of 1 to 5 W. The farther the mobile radio is from the dispatch center, the weaker the signal. To make sure that the signal remains strong enough to give a clear transmission, the signal must be boosted so that the watts can be maintained. This is done by setting up a series of repeaters along the path of the transmission. This allows the transmission to be rebroadcast and maintain the high level of wattage. With the portable radio, this can be accomplished by using a vehicular repeater that rebroadcasts the signal through the mobile radio at the same wattage as the mobile unit. Once you leave the emergency vehicle, you rely on the portable radio for constant communication with dispatch. Without a repeater system, you will be out of communication range if you are a significant distance from dispatch or in rough terrain.

Radio Systems

[OBJECTIVE 16]

Simplex

one frequency

A **simplex** system is the most common type of radio system. It allows one-at-a-time communication. When the dispatch center is dispatching a call on a simplex system, the receiving unit must wait for the communication to finish before it can reply. If multiple agencies use one frequency, someone may have to wait to finish a transmission.

Duplex

A **duplex** system allows transmitting and receiving at the same time through two different frequencies. A telephone is an example of a duplex system. One frequency is used for transmission and a different frequency is used for reception. A duplex system allows both parties to speak at the same time.

Half Duplex

A **half-duplex** system is commonly used in conjunction with repeaters. In this system two frequencies are used: one to transmit and one to receive (as in a duplex system). But like a simplex system, only one person can transmit at a time.

Multiplex

Multiplex systems allow transmission of voice and data at the same time. This allows you to send an ECG to the hospital while continuing to give the patient report. This technology is now placed into the ECG monitor and can be set up with hard-line telephone systems as well as over a cellular telephone with a wireless transceiver. This technology is available through several different manufacturers.

> **PARAMEDIC Pearl**
>
> A multiplex system is like a stereo in which the frequency band is split into two parts, such as the right and left speakers. With a multiplex system, the medical radio has one part for voice and the other part for data.

Digital Equipment

Digital communication equipment generally encodes information into binary, a computer language composed of the numbers 0 and 1. Digital technology has the following advantages:

- Better security
- Voice and data transmission
- Signal that does not degrade

Because all computer systems use binary language, the signal from digital communication equipment may cause interference with other devices, such as medical equipment.

Carefully monitor your medical equipment to ensure it is working correctly while using digital communication equipment. If it does not appear to be functioning correctly, discontinue use of the digital equipment and switch to analog devices if available.

Analog communication equipment transmits data through a continuously varying signal. The primary disadvantage of an analog signal is that noise (random variation in the signal) can cause distortion and signal loss. Although the quality of an analog signal is not as a good as that of digital, it is less likely to interfere with your equipment.

Telematic

Telematic is new technology that is also called a *mayday call reporting system*. This is the system placed in cars through services such as On Star and Tele-aid. These systems automatically detect when the vehicle is involved in an accident and then contact a dispatcher from one of these services. The service verifies that the vehicle was involved in an accident and also detects whether the air bags have been deployed. The service then locates the position of the vehicle by using a global positioning system and contacts the local dispatch center to have law enforcement, fire, and EMS respond (Bass, 2004).

Trunking System

In a **trunking system** all repeaters and frequencies are in one system, and a computer chooses the frequency that is open and uses that frequency to make the transmission. As other calls come in, the system picks the next frequency to be used in the bank of frequencies. This system is usually associated with the 800-MHz systems and typically has a clearer signal. The trunk system eliminates the need for manual searching and choosing of frequencies. As frequencies become clear, they go into the bank of frequencies available.

PARAMEDIC*Pearl*

Interoperability is the ability for all communication equipment to work during any incident anywhere in the United States. The U.S. government set this up to avoid communication problems during major incidents, such as those that occurred on September 11, 2001, and during Hurricane Katrina. Interoperability mandates that all communication equipment must meet certain standards so that the equipment can be used at any scene. These standards were enacted by the U.S. Department of Homeland Security.

Case Scenario CONCLUSION

You and your partner arrive and meet the mother at her front door. The mother started airway maneuvers and mouth-to-mouth resuscitation following the instructions provided by the 9-1-1 operator. When you arrive, her baby is conscious, breathing spontaneously, and crying. His vital signs are within acceptable limits. You and your partner place the boy on oxygen, start an intravenous line and cardiac monitoring, and transport him to the hospital without incident.

Looking Back

9. What information is essential for you to communicate to the hospital en route? Is information needed from the hospital during that conversation? How will the hospital use the information you provide to take better care of the patient?
10. In addition to the information you conveyed in your radio/telephone report to the hospital, what else will you communicate during your bedside report to the receiving physician? Who will benefit from this communication?

DISPATCH CENTERS

Dispatch centers use **computer-aided dispatch (CAD).** CAD is a computer system that has automated dispatching by enhanced data collection, rapid recall of information, and dispatch mapping. It can track emergency units and the resources allocated to a particular call or calls. By tracking the equipment in use on one or several calls at a time, the dispatcher knows what units are available for calls and what units already are on a call. The dispatcher uses CAD to send the proper equipment to the proper location. This ensures that the closest appropriate unit will be sent to the appropriate call. The system gives the dispatcher all the necessary information he or she needs when making decisions.

Public Safety Answering Point

A **public safety answering point (PSAP)** is the point at which the dispatch center receives the call from the public. Multiple PSAPs may be available within the same exchange, or a PSAP may cover multiple exchanges. This system allows the dispatcher to isolate the call to a street map location. With a cellular phone, the PSAP identifies the location as a coordinate.

9-1-1/Enhanced 9-1-1

A **9-1-1** system was developed for communities to gain quicker access to the necessary services. The system uses a three-digit access number. This number is routed directly to the appropriate dispatch center. This system has been adopted nationwide, but some areas still do not use this system. **Enhanced 9-1-1** is the next generation of the 9-1-1 system. It allows dispatch to pinpoint the address from which the call originated.

EMS Dispatchers

[OBJECTIVES 17, 18, 19]
An EMS dispatcher is a trained professional and an important member of the EMS team. The dispatcher's responsibilities include the following:

- Call taking
- Alerting and directing response
- Monitoring and coordinating communications
- Giving prearrival instructions
- Maintaining incident records

With the assistance of CAD, the EMS dispatcher determines the closest units to the call and sends the appropriate resources. Large calls may involve multiple agencies, including the fire department, law enforcement, air ambulances, and specialized teams. An EMS dispatcher is trained to give prearrival instructions to the calling party. Prearrival instructions have the following benefits:

- Provides the caller with immediate assistance
- Complements call screening
- Provides updated information to the responding unit(s)
- May be life sustaining in critical incidents
- Provides emotional support for caller, bystanders, or victim

After asking the appropriate questions of the caller, the dispatcher can give the patient, family, or bystanders the information needed to assist the patient before EMS personnel arrive on the scene. For example, the dispatcher may instruct the caller how to control minor bleeding or perform cardiopulmonary resuscitation. Prearrival instructions also have been called *dispatch life support*. Dispatch activities are covered in more detail in Chapter 60.

The dispatcher communicates with the units while they are en route to the scene. First the units go en route, at which time the dispatcher gives the unit its en route time and any additional patient or scene information. This is important because it provides the crew with information about possible scene hazards, patient status, and other details that help determine a course of action. The crew notifies dispatch when they arrive on the scene. Then they perform a scene size-up to determine if any other resources are needed. The crew provides dispatch with any critical information that will help incoming crews stage (await further instruction), properly position their vehicles, or be aware of any dangerous situations that may be present at the scene.

After crew members have treated the patient and begin transport, they contact dispatch and inform them that they are en route to a receiving facility. Their destination could be the closest appropriate facility, or it could be a landing zone to meet an incoming helicopter for transport to a specialty facility. Dispatch then gives the crew an en route time. The crew then contacts the hospital and gives the receiving facility a brief patient report with an estimated time of arrival at the facility. During this communication, the crew may ask for orders for specialty care procedures or simply inform the facility what has been done and that the patient is en route. When the crew arrives at the receiving facility, dispatch is notified. The dispatcher notes their time of arrival. When patient care is complete (and the vehicle has been readied for the next call), the crew notifies dispatch and advises that the unit is in service and available for another call.

RELAYING PATIENT INFORMATION

[OBJECTIVES 20, 21]
Relaying information to medical direction or the receiving facility is a critical and essential part of ensuring the continuity of patient care. Radio use is a fairly simple and straightforward skill to master. To ensure clear radio transmissions, always speak at a normal rate and in a normal voice without wide fluctuations in tone. Clearly state your request or intentions in a professional manner without slang, ambiguous terms, or profanity. The following principles apply whenever using the radio:

- Protect the privacy of the patient.
- Ensure the radio is on and the volume is properly adjusted.
- Make sure the frequency is clear before beginning your transmission.
- Press the microphone key or "push to talk" key and wait 1 or 2 seconds before speaking. This allows the circuitry of the radio to engage and ensures the beginning of your transmission is heard.
- Speak in a normal tone of voice, at a normal rate, with the microphone 2 to 3 inches from your mouth.
- Identify whom you are calling followed by who you are. Use the proper unit numbers, hospital numbers, and names and titles.
- Wait for a response from the party you are calling indicating you can go ahead with your transmission.
- Unless codes are standard for your EMS system, use plain English or clear text.
- Do not use slang or profanity.
- Keep transmissions brief and avoid meaningless phrases; however, ensure your complete message is received and understood.

- Clarify sound-alike phrases to avoid confusion. Names such as "Brandy Wine Road" and "Branding Iron Road" may not be distinguishable on the radio. Numbers also often sound familiar. The receiving facility may not be sure if your estimated time of arrival is 4 to 5 minutes or 45 minutes. When needed, state the individual digits of the number.
- Use words that are easy to hear, such as "affirmative" and "negative" rather than "yes" or "no."
- Use the "echo" procedure (repeat the information heard) when receiving directions from the dispatcher or physician orders.
- Use standard formats for transmission.
- Obtain a confirmation that the message was received.

A standardized reporting format allows efficient use of the communications system, assists medical direction, and helps ensure that no significant information is omitted. One possible reporting format is as follows:

- Unit identification and provider identification
- Description of scene
- Patient's age, gender, and approximate weight (for medication orders)
- Patient's chief complaint
- Associated symptoms
- Brief, pertinent history of the present illness or injury
- Pertinent medical history, medications, and allergies

- Pertinent physical examination findings
- Treatment given so far and patient response
- Estimated time of arrival at the receiving facility
- Other pertinent information

When you arrive at the receiving facility, the legal transfer of care must include a verbal report, also called a *hand-off report*. During this report you will have the opportunity to give a more comprehensive description of the patient's complaint and conditions and provide any assessment and treatment information not included in the radio report or any findings or changes after you made initial radio contact.

If you are giving the report to a person who did not receive your radio report, you must include all the information from your radio report as well as this additional information. If you are giving the report to the same person you spoke with on the radio, the verbal report will only include additional information not transmitted or found after transmission.

In addition to the information from the radio report, the following information is always included in the verbal report:

- The patient's name
- Description of the patient's complaint(s) and condition
- History that was not provided over the radio
- Treatment and response to treatment administered after radio contact
- Vital signs taken after radio contact

Case Scenario SUMMARY

1. *What is the most important information the operator needs to get from this woman at this time?* Her location and callback number are the most critical pieces of information. They are vital to getting help to her.

2. *What barriers stand in the way of the operator getting this information?* Multiple barriers exist to adequate communication at this stage. Because the operator cannot see the mother, he or she must completely rely on verbal communication, which is much less effective than a combination of verbal and nonverbal communication. The mother's fear and panic also may create barriers because she may scream, be difficult to understand, or even stop speaking to the operator (especially because the caller is the mother of this unconscious infant). Individuals in a critical stress situation often are unable to focus on cognitive functions and may not be able to provide the operator with complete or accurate information.

3. *What information does the young mother need to get from the 9-1-1 operator? How can this information help the mother?* The mother needs to know that help is on the way. This information may help calm her and help her understand that she is not alone and will be helped soon. In a less life-threatening situation, she would probably receive additional instructions to facilitate care, such as to turn on an outside light, unlock her door, or put her dog in a fenced yard. These instructions and information would make it easier for the responding units to find and access her. Depending on the dispatch center, the mother may also receive specific medical advice on how to help her son while waiting for the paramedics.

4. *What barriers hinder the operator from effectively communicating this information to the mother?* Once again, this line of communication can be hindered because of its reliance on verbal communication—reassurance

often is communicated primarily through nonverbal methods. Psychomotor skills (how to open an airway) are difficult to teach verbally (over the phone) without a demonstration. A final barrier remains—the mother's panic.

5. *What is the most critical information for the dispatcher to convey to responding units? How will they use this information to provide better service to the mother?* Most critical is the physical location of the mother along with any routing information needed to find it. In addition, they may need the nature of the call; they will use this information to prepare for the call mentally and select the best equipment to take to the scene.

6. *What are the benefits of having the operator remain in contact with the mother while the ambulance is responding?* The mother benefits by having verbal contact with someone during this frightening experience as well as by receiving any advice the operator may provide. The operator also benefits because he or she can be made aware of any changes in the patient's condition and can pass that information to the responding units.

7. *Imagine yourself as this mother; think how you might feel holding your limp son in your arms. What would you need the operator to communicate to you?* Considering the possibility that your son might be gravely ill or even dead is terrifying. That terror would undoubtedly be magnified by possible guilt related to having left him alone. It would help to have the operator be a calm presence to keep the mother focused on the current episode (her child is sick) and not on the unknown future (her child has died, her family is angry because she left him alone). Knowing what will happen next, how long it will take, and what to expect would also be beneficial.

8. *When you (the paramedic) arrive on the scene, what information do you need to get from the mother? What do you need to communicate to her?* The paramedic primarily needs information about the episode itself:

how long the child was alone, how long he may have been in the tub, any medical history, and any interventions the mother performed in an attempt to revive the child. The paramedic needs to communicate a sense of calm and complete competence to the mother. Both of these are much easier to communicate by verbal and nonverbal methods.

9. *What information is essential for you to communicate to the hospital en route? Do you need information from the hospital during that conversation? How will the hospital use the information you provide to take better care of the patient?* You should communicate the patient's initial condition, the interventions the mother provided, the patient's condition when you arrived, any additional interventions provided, the patient's current condition, and the estimated time of arrival to the hospital. The hospital will use this information to organize the resources necessary to take care of the baby (and his mother); these resources could include equipment, rooms, or staff. You would need any additional instructions deemed necessary by the hospital staff. The information you have provided will help the hospital staff better prepare for the child's arrival and the expectant care necessary based on your assessment findings and prehospital interventions.

10. *In addition to the information you conveyed in your radio/telephone report to the hospital, what else will you communicate during your bedside report to the receiving physician? Who will benefit from this communication?* In addition to transfer of medical condition, the bedside report provides the perfect chance to introduce the mother and child to the emergency department (ED) staff. By introducing the ED staff to the mother, you provide reassurance and information the mother needs to stay calm. By introducing the mother to the staff, you "hand off" communication and reassurance to the ED staff and ensure that the mother's needs are understood and met. It is a critical step, especially in an emotionally charged situation such as this one.

Chapter Summary

- Each phase of an emergency requires good, effective communication.
- Accurate communication of every type—verbal, written, and electronic—is essential for the patient's health and documentation.
- Quality management is essential to the overall improvement of communication and patient care.
- A good knowledge of terminology helps eliminate communication problems.

- Radios are the backbone of the communication system in EMS.
- Repeater systems are essential to ensuring quality radio communication over extreme distances and rough terrain.
- Radio systems vary depending on the local EMS system and the type of equipment used.
- CAD systems send and receive numerous types of data quickly and accurately.

REFERENCES

Bass, R. (2004). Surveying emerging trends in emergency-related information for the EMS profession. *Top Emergency Medicine, 26,* 93-102.

Federal Communications Commission. (2006). Retrieved May 29, 2008, from http://wireless.fcc.gov.

SUGGESTED RESOURCES

Federal Communications Commission
445 12th Street SW
Washington, DC 20554
Phone: 1-888-CALL-FCC (1-888-225-5322)
Website: http://www.fcc.gov

Metropolitan Coordination Association, Inc.
Church Street Station
P.O. Box 107
New York, NY 10008-0107
Website: http://www.metrocor.net

Chapter Quiz

1. A system that allows one-at-a-time communication on the same frequency is a _____ system.
   a. duplex
   b. multiplex
   c. simplex
   d. telematic

2. A radio carried by an individual that has a low output is a _____ radio.
   a. base
   b. mobile
   c. portable
   d. portable repeater

3. A system that receives transmissions from a low output and rebroadcasts the signal at a higher output is called a _____.
   a. PSAP
   b. receiver
   c. repeater
   d. transponder

4. _____ describes a system that allows components of different radio systems to communicate on a scene.
   a. CAD
   b. Interoperability
   c. Multiplexing
   d. Repeating

5. A radio system that allows transmitting and receiving at the same time through two different frequencies is a _____.
   a. duplex system
   b. multiplex system
   c. simplex system
   d. trunking system

6. A radio system that uses multiple repeaters so that the computer searches for an open channel and transmits on that channel is called a(n) _____.
   a. interoperability system
   b. telematic system
   c. transmitter
   d. trunking system
   e. private line

7. A radio installed in a fixed unit that transmits at a higher wattage is a _____ radio.
   a. fixed
   b. mobile
   c. portable
   d. repeater

8. The federal organization that regulates interstate and international communications through radio, television, wire, and satellite is the _____.
   a. DEA
   b. FAA
   c. FCC
   d. FFA

9. What are the three primary modes of EMS communication?
   a. Electronic, verbal, dispatched
   b. Verbal, written, electronic
   c. Verbal, written, telephone
   d. Written, transmitted, e-mail

10. List three reasons why good communication is important.

    _____

    _____

    _____

Terminology

9-1-1/Enhanced 9-1-1 A set of three numbers that automatically sends the call to the emergency dispatch center. Enhanced 9-1-1 gives the dispatcher the ability to determine the caller's location by routing the call through several CAD systems.

Band A range of radio frequencies.

Computer-aided dispatch (CAD) A computer-aided system that automates dispatching by enhanced data collection, rapid recall of information, dispatch mapping, as well as unit tracking and the ability to track and dispatch resources.

Communication The exchange of information between two or more individuals.

Dispatch A central location that receives information and collects, disseminates, and transmits the information to the proper resources.

Duplex A radio system that allows transmitting and receiving at the same time through two different frequencies.

Federal Communications Commission (FCC) An independent U.S. government agency, directly responsible to Congress, established by the Communications Act of 1934; it regulates interstate and international communications by radio, television, wire, satellite, and cable. The FCC's jurisdiction covers the 50 states, the District of Columbia, and U.S. possessions.

Half duplex A radio system that uses two frequencies: one to transmit and one to receive; however, like a simplex system, only one person at a time can transmit.

Interoperability Describes a radio system that can use the components of several different systems; it can use specialized equipment to connect several different radio systems and components together and have them communicate with each other.

Mobile radio A radio installed in an emergency vehicle. A mobile radio usually transmits by higher wattage than a portable radio.

Multiplex A system that allows the crew to transmit voice and data at the same time, enabling the crew to call in a patient report while transmitting an ECG strip to the hospital.

Portable radio Also referred to as a *walkie-talkie*. These radios are carried by emergency personnel and have a lower wattage output than the mobile or base unit. To use these portable radios with a higher watt output, the units can be connected through a repeater system to increase their output, which increases range.

Public Safety Answering Point (PSAP) A dispatch center that is set up to receive and dispatch 9-1-1 calls.

Radio frequency Radio frequencies are channels that allow communication from one specific user to another. For simple communication, both users must be on the same frequency or channel.

Repeater A system that receives transmissions from a low-wattage radio and rebroadcasts the signal at a higher wattage to the dispatch center.

Simplex A system that allows only one-at-a-time communication. The transmission cannot be interrupted; both operators use the same frequency.

Telematic A system setup as mayday call reporting, such as On-Star and Tele-aid. This system can send information from an automobile that has been involved in an accident directly to an emergency dispatch center with the exact location and the amount of damage that may have occurred.

Trunking system A system that uses multiple repeaters (five or more) so that the computer can search for an open channel to transmit by.

Documentation

Objectives *After completing this chapter, you will be able to:*

1. Describe the potential consequences of illegible, incomplete, or inaccurate documentation.
2. Explain the role and importance of documentation as it pertains to the following:
   - Continuity of patient care
   - Quality management
   - Data collection
   - Research
   - Billing and reimbursement
3. Explain how to document information received from bystanders and other third-party sources.
4. Explain how to document scene assessment findings.
5. Discuss the importance of documenting pertinent positive and pertinent negative findings.
6. Explain the importance of using medical terminology appropriately.
7. Discuss the importance of using only locally approved medical abbreviations.
8. Discuss the importance of timely report writing and submission.
9. Be familiar with the different methods used to document, including the following:

- Handwritten documentation
- Electronic or computer-based documentation
- Dictation
10. Discuss the importance of documenting with a consistent narrative style, as identified by local protocol.
11. Describe the differences between subjective and objective elements of documentation.
12. Identify irrelevant or unprofessional information.
13. Describe the special considerations for documenting a patient refusal of care or transport.
14. Describe the special considerations for documenting a multiple-casualty incident.
15. Evaluate a completed prehospital care report for the following:
   - Completeness
   - Thoroughness
   - Accuracy
   - Spelling
   - Grammar
   - Use of medical terminology
   - Use of approved abbreviations

Chapter Outline

Functions of Documentation
Components of the Prehospital Care Report
Medical Terminology
Medical Abbreviations
Errors
Timeliness
Addendums

Methods of Documentation
Documentation Formats
Special Situations
Documentation Essentials
Quality Management Process
Chapter Summary

Case Scenario

You and your partner respond to a skilled nursing facility to evaluate a "woman who has fallen." On arrival, you find a 93-year-old woman who has a 1- to 2-inch laceration on the right side of her forehead. According to a facility staff member, the patient was walking to the dining room when she stumbled in a doorway. She struck her head on the door, gripped the door handle, lowered herself to the ground, and sat down. According to the staff member, the patient did not lose consciousness. At this time, the patient is pale, in no apparent distress, and sitting on the floor. She is conscious; alert; and oriented to person, place, time, and event. Her only complaint is a headache.

Questions

1. After you complete and submit the prehospital care report (PCR) for this case, what potential functions will it fulfill?
2. Given these functions, when should the PCR be completed and submitted?
3. Much of the information about the accident itself came from the nursing staff member. Because you did not observe it, can you document this information on the PCR? How?

[OBJECTIVE 1]

The **prehospital care report (PCR)** is the document written after a call has been completed. This report outlines what you saw, what you heard, and what you did. This report is read and used by many different people. Long after a call is over, the report will remain as a record of what transpired on the scene and in the ambulance. In many instances the report you write will be the only record of the events that occurred during the prehospital care and transport of the patient. As a result, documentation is one of the most important tasks you will perform as a paramedic. Your PCRs must be complete, thorough, accurate, and legible. Incomplete, inaccurate, or illegible documentation can have immediate and long-term ramifications. You can help establish yourself as a medical professional by using and practicing good documentation skills (Cohn & Azarra, 1998).

PARAMEDIC Pearl

One of the most important, yet most neglected, skills of a paramedic is documentation. Many outstanding paramedics poorly document even the most serious patients. No legitimate or good reason exists for this. When documenting your care, assessment, and treatment for any patient, follow a simple rule: If it is not on the report, you did not ask it, assess it, check it, or perform it.

FUNCTIONS OF DOCUMENTATION

[OBJECTIVE 2]

Continuity of Care

First and foremost, documentation is used to provide patients with continuity of care. When paramedics first arrive on the scene, they perform a scene size-up. They evaluate things such as the mechanisms involved in traumatic events, the presence of home oxygen, and any concerns of abuse. They perform a physical examination and then establish and execute a treatment plan. During the course of care the patient's condition may remain unchanged, but it is likely to improve or worsen. The paramedics transport the patient to an appropriate facility, give a verbal report to the receiving facility staff, and transfer patient care. As the patient is cared for in the emergency department (ED), questions about the scene may arise: What did the automobile look like after the crash? How did the patient look when the symptoms first appeared? What treatment was given on the scene, and how did the patient respond? What is the condition of the patient's living environment? Healthcare professionals caring for the patient will look to the PCR you have written to find this information. If the information on the PCR is wrong, the patient may receive inappropriate care, such as no medications or the wrong medication. If the PCR is incomplete, the patient may be subjected to unnecessary tests or procedures. Your physical examination findings or any statements the patient made on the scene (or during transport) may help the physician make an accurate diagnosis.

Legal

The prehospital care report is a legal document. The legal uses or functions of the PCR fall into two categories; one involves legal questions that may arise about the scene, and the other involves legal questions that may arise about the actions of the paramedic. The PCR plays a large role in both cases.

You will often respond to calls that involve an infraction of the law. These infractions can range from a minor traffic collision to a homicide. During the legal investigation the PCR written by the paramedic may be subpoenaed. Information on the PCR may be used to help establish blame, such as for a motor vehicle crash or in cases of nonaccidental trauma, such as child abuse or elder abuse. Information on the PCR also may be used in sentencing convicted persons. The severity of injury, the patient's affect, and the condition of the scene, to name only a few examples, can play a role in how or whether a person accused of committing a crime is punished.

The PCR is a legal document. When the PCR is subpoenaed, any information in it is considered admissible and evaluated. If the PCR is incomplete or additional questions arise about the call, the paramedic may be subpoenaed to testify. In addition, court cases may be initiated years after a call took place. As a result, you may not clearly remember details of the call. The PCR you wrote must function as your memory; you should therefore ensure that the information is complete and correct (Lee, 2001).

When the care a paramedic provides is questioned, the PCR acts as a legal document. As a paramedic, you are always responsible for your acts and omissions. Doing a good job does not free you from having your acts questioned. If a call ends with patient disability or patient death, the patient care may be questioned as a causative factor. In other words, the call may be evaluated to see if your acts or omissions contributed to the patient's death or disability. The paramedic's PCR often is an important part of the investigation. Thus the PCR must clearly state what was done, why it was done, and the patient's response. If an indicated procedure was not performed, the PCR should make clear why it was not done. For example, nitroglycerin is usually indicated for a patient with cardiac chest pain. However, if the patient's blood pressure is too low, nitroglycerin is contraindicated. Facts such as these must be documented. The PCR should leave no room for reader interpretation.

Legislative

Your documentation may be used to justify a request for a change in laws or statutes or requests for grants or governmental funding. If the change would benefit EMS practice, EMS may be asked to justify the request. PCRs completed over a specified period may be evaluated to see if the request is justified. For example, past reports may be used to evaluate the need for a new or different medication (e.g., lorazepam for seizures or midazolam for chemical restraint) or procedure (e.g., adult intraosseous infusion).

Research

Your documentation can and does aid research. EMS has dramatically changed over the last several decades. The role of EMS has grown from a mode of rapid transport to a hospital to an essential component of the healthcare system. The paramedic **scope of practice** continues to expand. In fact, some recent research projects include prehospital ultrasound, artificial blood products, and prehospital laboratory tests. As research progresses, data are collected from the PCR. As a result, the data must be clear and accurate.

Retrospective research is occasionally conducted. In this type of research, reports from months to years earlier are evaluated. In many studies reports must be thrown out of the study because they are incomplete or unclear. Whether or not you are participating in an active research study, you must write your PCR as though it were going to be reviewed in an effort to collect detailed information.

Quality Management

As a paramedic, you are expected to maintain proficiency in your practice. Paramedic reports are read and evaluated to ensure paramedics are performing up to standard. If a paramedic is consistently unable to establish a successful intravenous line, is not routinely obtaining two sets of vital signs, fails to use pulse oximetry or capnography when indicated, or is not recognizing patient signs and symptoms (resulting in misdiagnoses), the paramedic deserves the chance for remediation to improve his or her performance. These trends can be recognized during a review of PCRs, and the paramedic can be offered educational opportunities. Topics for an EMS agency's continuing education classes are often driven by trends identified from the review of PCRs. These trends help individual paramedics as well as the entire department or agency improve patient care.

Billing and Reimbursement

Finally, your documentation is used for billing and reimbursement purposes. Many EMS organizations bill for the services they provide. Billing provides salaries, training, supplies, and equipment. Insurance companies, Medicare, and Medicaid review the bills they receive for the necessity of the service provided. If the description of the patient's injury or illness does not support the treatment received, then the bill may be rejected. ICD-9 codes are used in billing to describe injury and illness. These codes are based on the patient's presentation and affect how the agency is reimbursed. Some EMS services require their paramedics to do their own ICD-9 coding, and some have other staff read the PCR and assign the codes. Codes are assigned on the basis of what the paramedic has written. If an EMS service is found to be applying the wrong codes, it may be investigated for insurance fraud. Even if miscoding is unintentional, the EMS agency could be found guilty and fined. The PCRs you write should not leave room for speculation on a patient's presentation or why treatment was performed.

COMPONENTS OF THE PREHOSPITAL CARE REPORT

Identifying Data

A key component of the PCR is the *identifying data* (Figure 19-1). Identifying data is the information unique to the patient. Examples include the patient's name, address, Social Security number, and birth date. This information is usually required by EMS agencies and is necessary for billing. This information is protected by the **Health Insurance Portability and Accountability Act (HIPAA).** Agencies should give patients HIPAA disclosure forms when they collect this information (Lee, 2001).

Source of Information

[OBJECTIVE 3]

In the PCR, the *source of information* is where the patient information originated, or where it came from. Patients do not always make the call to EMS. Sometimes family members, law enforcement personnel, or others initiate the call. This information should be identified in the PCR. Assessment findings and patient-related medical information received from sources other than the patient should be identified as well (e.g., "The patient's spouse stated . . . "). If the source is not identified, the information documented is typically assumed to have come from the patient or was witnessed by you, the paramedic. You should use quotation marks to quote a patient or bystander exactly.

Location of the Call

[OBJECTIVE 4]

In the PCR, the *location of the call* is where the call took place. You should identify if it was in a house, store, park, and so forth. The address, cross streets, and business names all help identify the location of the call. At indefinite locations, use specifics if possible, such as "the southwest corner of Main and Vine" or "in the kitchen of XYZ Restaurant."

Times

In the PCR you must record and document all *times* throughout the call, including, at a minimum, the following times:

- Dispatch
- En route
- On scene
- Transport
- Hospital arrival
- Back in service

You must record treatment times, such as each time you perform a skill or each time you give a drug. Some cases under review do not question whether the paramedic performed a procedure, but rather *when* the procedure was performed. Unclear times are subjective and difficult to confirm.

Assessment

[OBJECTIVE 5]

On most PCRs, the largest portion of documentation involves the physical examination findings. In the *assessment* section of the report, you have an opportunity to document all pertinent findings on the scene and with the patient. Your documentation should include a description of the scene. This should include specifics such as damage to vehicles, location of the patient, living conditions, and presence of bystanders. Your patient assessment should include the patient's chief complaint followed by your initial findings involving life-threatening injuries or conditions and the status of the patient's airway, breathing, and circulation. This should be followed by a description of the focused assessment based on the patient's chief complaint and a detailed assessment as appropriate for the situation.

Your documentation should include **pertinent positive** findings and **pertinent negative** findings. A pertinent positive finding is a sign or symptom significant to the field impression. For example, circumoral cyanosis in a patient with an asthma attack is a pertinent positive finding. A pertinent negative finding is a sign or symptom significant to the working field impression that is not seen. For example, no circumoral cyanosis in an asthmatic patient would be a pertinent negative finding. The presence and absence of signs and symptoms help establish a field impression. You must evaluate and document these findings and include all diagnostic tests, such as blood glucose, capnography, and 12-lead ECG findings. If an assessment is not documented, it is assumed to have not been performed. If a good assessment is not documented, justifying treatment or lack of treatment may be difficult.

Past Medical History

You must discover and document the patient's *past medical history* on the PCR. The patient's past medical problems have a large impact on treatment and diagnosis of new complaints or findings. This information should include the following:

- Allergies
- Medications
- Previous diagnoses
- Previous surgeries
- Previous similar episodes
- Family medical history
- Social history

PREHOSPITAL CARE REPORT PCR# _____

Call Date	Provider Number	Unit Number	Incident Number	Interfacility Transfer Number	Call Disposition
__/__/__					

Response	Transport	Time of Call	Time Enroute	Time First ALS on Scene	Time Arrived on Scene	Time Left Scn / Call Canceled	Time Arrived at Destination	Contact Made with:	Time of Contact
☐ 1 Code	☐ 1							☐ Base Hospital	
☐ 2	☐ 2							☐ Receiving Facility	
☐ 3	☐ 3 :	:	:	:	:	:	:	☐ Control Facility ☐ None	:

Patient Name (Last, First, Mi) _____ **Patient Address** _____ **Incident Location** _____

Patient Age	Patient DOB	Patient Gender	Est. Patient Weight	County	Map Zone	No. Pts. At Scene
Mos / Yrs	__/__/__	☐ Male ☐ Female	___ kg			

Chief Complaint _____ Pain Level: ___ **Allergies** _____

Medical History _____ **Medications** _____

Initial Physical Examination

Unremarkable

		GCS			Mechanism of Injury
Head	☐				
Neck	☐	Eye	Verbal	Motor	
Chest	☐	4 spont	5 oriented	6 obeys	Types of Illness/Injury
Abdomen	☐	3 voice	4 confused	5 localizes	
Back	☐	2 pain	3 inapprop	4 withdrwl	
Pelvis	☐	1 none	2 incompr	3 flexion	
Limbs	☐		1 none	2 extensn	
Neuro	☐			1 none	
Skin Signs	☐				

Time E V M Total
: __+__+__ =
: __+__+__ =
: __+__+__ =

Field Clinical Impression:

Care Giver FD/PD/BS/PH	Time	Procedure / Medication (with dose, route) CODE / DESCRIPTION	Response / Comments / ECG (MD Signature: Base Order)	Resp Rate	Blood Pressure	Pulse Rate	Pain Level
	:				/		
	:				/		
	:				/		
	:				/		
	:				/		
	:				/		
	:				/		
	:				/		
	:				/		
	:				/		
	:				/		

☐ Medication Wasted: Time: Signature: Witness Signature:

Special Scene Conditions:
☐ ALS w/o base contact ☐ MCI
☐ Complicated extrication ☐ Multiple EMS providers
☐ DNR ☐ Possible provider exposure
☐ Drug use suspected ☐ Unsafe scene
☐ ETOH use suspected ☐ Other:
☐ Hazardous materials

Safety Eq Used:
☐ Lap Restraint
☐ Lap/Shoulder restraint
☐ Child Safety seat
☐ Airbag
☐ Helmet
☐ Protective Clothing

MVA Conditions:
☐ Bent steering wheel
☐ Death in same vehicle
☐ Ejection
☐ Passenger comptmnt intrusn
☐ Rollover

Destination Decision Reason
☐ Nearest Rec. Facility ☐ Triage to trauma center
☐ MCI/DCF ☐ Triage to other specialty center
☐ Physician request ☐ Other
☐ Pt/Family request _____

Receiving Hosp

Base Hospital

Tier I Trauma Triage:
☐ GCS Motor Score < 5
☐ Systolic BP < 85
☐ Penetrating Trauma: Head, Neck, Chest, Torso
☐ Paramedic Judgement

Tier II Trauma Triage
☐ Flail Chest
☐ Combo Burn/Trauma
☐ 2 or more long bone fx.
☐ Pelvic fracture
☐ pedestrian thrown/run over
☐ Judgement of the paramedic or flight nurse
☐ Open/depress, skull fx
☐ Paralysis
☐ Amput. Prox. wrist/ankle
☐ Fall > 20 ft.
☐ Pregnancy

Pediatric Trauma Triage
☐ Glasgow Coma Score Motor Component < 5 AND
☐ BP < 80 if patient over age 6; < 70 if under 6
☐ Advanced airway or continuous support of airway
☐ Penetrating trauma: head, neck, chest, torso or proximal to elbow/knee with vascular compromise
☐ Flail Chest ☐ Pelvis Fracture
☐ Amput. Prox. wrist/ankle ☐ Traumatic paralysis

Base MD

MICN

Care Transferred To		Cert. Number	Name (print)	Signature
Agency	Time :	A)		
Name		B)		
		C)		

☐ Continuation form used

Figure 19-1 Prehospital care report (PCR).

PREHOSPITAL CARE REPORT CONTINUATION

PCR NUMBER

Page ___ of ___

Care Giver	Time	Procedure / Medication (with dose, route) CODE — DESCRIPTION	Response / Comments / ECG (MD Signature: Base Order)	Pain Level	Blood Pressure	Pulse Rate	Resp Rate
	:				/		
	:				/		
	:				/		
	:				/		
	:				/		
	:				/		
	:				/		
	:				/		
	:				/		
	:				/		
	:				/		
	:				/		
	:				/		
	:				/		
	:				/		
	:				/		
	:				/		
	:				/		
	:				/		
	:				/		
	:				/		
	:				/		
	:				/		
	:				/		

Care Giver	Time	Comments
	:	
	:	
	:	
	:	
	:	
	:	
	:	
	:	
	:	
	:	
	:	
	:	
	:	
	:	
	:	

Figure 19-1, cont'd

History of the Present Illness

The PCR also must include the patient's *history of the present illness*. In addition to establishing the patient's medical history and overall health status, you must obtain a history of the current event. In other words, find out as much as possible about the patient's current chief complaint. This information should include the following:

- Time of onset of illness or time of injury
- Patient's activity when the injury or illness occurred
- Level of pain or discomfort
- Description of pain or discomfort
- Provoking or palliative measures (does anything make it better or worse?)
- Any treatment done before the arrival of EMS

Treatment

You must document all *treatment* on the PCR. Your documentation must reflect the patient's signs and symptoms that warranted the treatment, including specific descriptions for the skills you performed. Do not simply write that you started an intravenous line. Document where, how many attempts, the size of the needle, the fluid type, and total fluid given while the patient was in your care. If you attempted a skill but were unsuccessful, document the number of attempts. Your documentation of the skills you performed, such as endotracheal intubation, also must include the methods used to confirm proper placement of the tube. You must document the presence or absence of breath sounds and epigastric sounds. If you used capnography, the results must be documented. If you did not provide treatment, then you must include the reason in the PCR (e.g., "the patient refused medications" or "unable to establish IV after three attempts").

Response to Treatment

Your PCR also must include the patient's *response to treatment*. After the patient has received treatment, document the patient's response to the care you have given, including desired outcome, undesirable outcome, and any side effects. If you performed a procedure, document how the patient tolerated the procedure and his or her behavior afterward. For example, if you temporarily restrained an extremity to start an intravenous line, be sure to document if the patient is able to move the extremity after the procedure (as well as circulation and sensation checks in that extremity).

Transport

You must include all *transport*-related information in your PCR. This information should identify the patient's transport destination and the mode of transport. Clearly outline any information or finding influencing transport decisions, such as patient severity, weather conditions, traffic patterns, and patient request. When transferring patient care, document the facility name, room number, the patient's condition at transfer, the transfer of any patient belongings in your possession, and who received the patient and belongings (with signature).

MEDICAL TERMINOLOGY

[OBJECTIVE 6]

The common language of medical professionals uses **medical terminology,** which are words often derived from Greek and Latin terms. The **root word** identifies the primary meaning of the word. A **prefix** can be added to the beginning of a word to add information such as frequency or location. A **suffix** can be added to the end of a word to add information such as the condition of or status of the root word (Leonard, 2007). As a paramedic, you must be proficient with medical terminology.

When writing a PCR, you must use appropriate medical terminology. Your use of medical terms helps others understand what you are trying to express. For example, a "3-mm superficial laceration" is more specific than "a little cut that is not that deep." The appropriate use of medical terms also adds credibility and professionalism to your report. On the other hand, using the wrong words distracts from your professionalism and can make the PCR unclear (Gylys, 2005).

MEDICAL ABBREVIATIONS

[OBJECTIVE 7]

Medical abbreviations can save time and space on the report form. The use of abbreviations is widely accepted in the medical community; however, abbreviations can vary from region to region. You must use abbreviations that are accepted by your service and local hospital. Moreover, the meaning of an abbreviation can change based on whether it is uppercase or lowercase. For example, "CC" commonly means chief complaint, whereas "cc" means cubic centimeter. A list of common abbreviations is shown in Table 19-1.

PARAMEDIC *Pearl*

Making up abbreviations is never a good idea. Remember that the purpose of the PCR is to communicate information to other healthcare professionals who will care for the patient. If the paramedic has made up his or her own abbreviations, the reader is left to guess what is trying to be conveyed.

ERRORS

[OBJECTIVE 1]

Paramedics should ensure that the PCR is free of errors. If you make an error, cross out the error with a single line, write the correction, and then initial the correction

Text continued on p. 659

TABLE 19-1	Commonly Accepted Abbreviations for Field Use			

<	Less than	Bld	Blood
>	More than	BLS	Basic life support
=	Equal	BM	Bowel movement
↑	Increased	BMR	Basal metabolic rate
↓	Decreased	BOW	Bag of waters
→	Going to or leading to	BP, B/P	Blood pressure
♀ or F	Female	BPH	Benign prostatic hypertrophy
♂ or M	Male	bpm	Beats per minute
2°	Secondary, second degree	BS	Breath sounds, blood sugar
@	At	BSA	Body surface area
ā	Before	BVM	Bag-valve-mask
A&O	Alert and oriented	BW	Birth weight
A&O×4	Alert and oriented to person, place, time, and event	BX, Bx	Biopsy
A&P	Anterior and posterior; anatomy and physiology	c̄	With
AAA	Abdominal aortic aneurysm	Ca++	Calcium
AB	Abortion	CA, Ca, ca	Cancer, carcinoma
ABD, abd	Abdomen	CABG	Coronary artery bypass graft
a.c.	Before meals	CAD	Coronary artery disease
AC	Antecubital (vein)	cath	Catheter, catheterization
ACE	Angiotensin-converting enzyme	CBC	Complete blood count
ACS	Acute coronary syndrome	cc	Cubic centimeter
ADL	Activities of daily living	CC	Chief complaint
ad lib	As desired	CCU	Coronary care unit
adm.	Admission	CHF	Congestive heart failure
Afib	Atrial fibrillation	CHI	Closed head injury
AIDS	Acquired immunodeficiency syndrome	Clr	Clear
AMA	Against medical advice	cm	Centimeter
AMI	Acute myocardial infarction	c/m	Cool and moist
Amt	Amount	CMS	Circulation, motor, sensory; circulation, movement, sensation
Ant, ant.	Anterior	CN	Courtesy notification
approx	Approximately	CNS	Central nervous system
ARDS	Adult respiratory distress syndrome	CO	Carbon monoxide, cardiac output
ASA	Aspirin	C/O	Complains of
ASHD	Atherosclerotic heart disease	CO₂	Carbon dioxide
ass't	Assisted/assist	Conc	Conscious
AV	Arteriovenous, atrioventricular	Cond	Condition
BBB	Bundle branch block	COPD	Chronic obstructive pulmonary disease
BBO₂	Blow-by oxygen	CP	Chest pain
BCP	Birth control pills	CPh	Cellular phone
b.i.d.	Twice a day	CPR	Cardiopulmonary resuscitation
Bilat	Bilateral	C-section	Cesarean section

Continued

TABLE 19-1 **Commonly Accepted Abbreviations for Field Use**—continued

CSF	Cerebrospinal fluid	fl	Fluid
C-spine	Cervical spine	FSI	Full spinal immobilization
CT	Computed tomography	FUO	Fever of undetermined origin
CTS	Carpal tunnel syndrome	Fx	Fracture
CVA	Cerebrovascular accident	g, gm, G	Gram
D50	50% dextrose	GB	Gallbladder
D5W	5% dextrose in water	GI	Gastrointestinal
D&C	Dilatation and curettage	GLF	Ground level fall
D/C	Discontinue	gr	Grain
DCAP-BTLS	Deformities, contusions, abrasions, punctures, burns, tenderness, lacerations, swelling	gravida	Number of pregnancies
Defib	Defibrillation	GSW	Gunshot wound
detox	Detoxification	gtt	Drops
DNP	Did not patch	GU	Genitourinary
DO	Doctor of osteopathy	GYN, gyn	Gynecology
DOA	Dead on arrival	H&P	History and physical
DOS	Dead on scene in field	H/A, HA	Headache
DPT	Diphtheria, pertussis, and tetanus	Hb, hgb	Hemoglobin
Dr.	Doctor	Hct	Hematocrit
DT	Delirium tremens	h/d	Hot/dry
D/T	Dispatched to	h/m	Hot/moist
DX, Dx, dx	Diagnosis	HEENT	Head, eyes, ears, nose, throat
ea	Each	Hg	Mercury
ECF	Extended care facility	HIV	Human immunodeficiency virus
ECG or EKG	Electrocardiogram	HPI	History of present illness
ED	Emergency department	Hr	Hour
EDC	Expected date of confinement (due date)	HR	Heart rate
EEG	Electroencephalogram	h.s.	At bedtime, hour of sleep
EENT	Eye, ear, nose, and throat	HTN	Hypertension
ENT	Ear, nose, and throat	Hx	History
EOM	Extraocular movement	H2O	Water
Epi	Epinephrine	ICS	Intercostal space, incident command system
ER	Emergency room	ICU	Intensive care unit
et	And	IDDM	Insulin-dependent diabetes mellitus
ETA	Estimated time of arrival	inf	Inferior
etc.	And so on	inj	Injection
ETOH	Ethyl alcohol	IM	Intramuscular
exam	Examination	IU	International unit
exc	Excision	IUD	Intrauterine device
Ext	Extremities	IV	Intravenous
F	Fahrenheit	JVD	Jugular venous distention
F/U	Follow-up	K+	Potassium
FHT	Fetal heart tones	kg	kilogram

TABLE 19-1 **Commonly Accepted Abbreviations for Field Use**—continued

KO	Keep open	neuro	Neurology
KVO	Keep vein open	NFO	No further orders
L	Left	NG, N/G	Nasogastric
lat.	Lateral	noc., noct.	Night
lb.	Pound	NPA	Nasal airway, nasopharyngeal airway
lg	Large	NPO	Nothing by mouth
LBBB	Left bundle branch block	NSR	Normal sinus rhythm
LLL	Left lower lobe	NTG	Nitroglycerin
LLQ	Left lower quadrant	n/v	Nausea/vomiting
LMP	Last menstrual period	n/v/d	Nausea/vomiting/diarrhea
LOC	Loss of consciousness, level of consciousness	O2	Oxygen
LPM	Liters per minute	OB	Obstetrics
LR	Lactated Ringer's	OB/GYN	Obstetrics and gynecology
L-spine	Lumbar spine	occ.	Occasional
lt	Left	OD	Overdose
LUQ	Left upper quadrant	OPA	Oral airway, oropharyngeal airway
LV	Left ventricle	ophth.	Ophthalmology
MAE	Moves all extremities	O.R.	Operating room
mcg, μg	Microgram	Orth.	Orthopedics
MD	Medical doctor, muscular dystrophy	OTC	Over the counter
MDI	Metered-dose inhaler	oz.	Ounce
meds	Medications	p̄	After
mEq	Milliequivalent	P	Pulse
mg	Milligram	PAC	Premature atrial complex
ml, mL	Milliliter	para	Number of births
MI, M.I.	Myocardial infarction	PAT	Paroxysmal atrial tachycardia
misc	Miscellaneous	path.	Pathology
mm	Millimeter	p.c.	After meals
MOE	Movement of extremities	PCN	Penicillin
MOI	Mechanism of injury	PE	Physical examination, pulmonary edema, or pulmonary embolism
MRI	Magnetic resonance imaging	PEA	Pulseless electrical activity
MS	Multiple sclerosis, morphine sulfate (MSO_4)	peds	Pediatrics
MVC	Motor vehicle crash	per	By or through
N/A	Not applicable	PERL	Pupils equal and reactive to light
NaCl or NS	Normal saline	PERRLA	Pupils equal, round, reactive to light and accommodation
NaHCO3	Sodium bicarbonate	pH	Hydrogen ion concentration
N/C	Nasal cannula	PG	Pregnant
NKA	No known allergies	P.I.	Present illness
NKDA	No known drug allergies	P.I.D.	Pelvic inflammatory disease
neg., −	Negative	PJC	Premature junctional complex

Continued

TABLE 19-1 **Commonly Accepted Abbreviations for Field Use**—continued

PMH	Past medical history	sm.	Small
PMS	Premenstrual syndrome; pulses, motor, sensory; pulses, movement, sensation	Stat	At once
PND	Paroxysmal nocturnal dyspnea	sup.	Superior
p.o.	By mouth	Sx	Sign or symptom
pos, +	Positive	surg.	Surgery
post	Posterior	Sz	Seizure
POV	Privately owned vehicle	T	Temperature
p.r.n.	As needed, as necessary	Tabs	Tablets
PSVT	Paroxysmal supraventricular tachycardia	TB	Tuberculosis
psych.	Psychiatric	temp.	Temperature
pt	Patient	TIA	Transient ischemic attack
PT	Physical therapy	t.i.d.	Three times a day
PTA	Prior to arrival	TKO	To keep open
PVC	Premature ventricular complex, premature ventricular contraction	TM	Tympanic membrane
q	Every	TMJ	Temporomandibular joint
q.d.	Every day	tol.	Tolerated
®, R	Right	TPR	Temperature, pulse, respirations
RBBB	Right bundle branch block	TRX, x-port	Transport
RBC	Red blood cell	TV	Tidal volume
R, resp	Respirations	Tx	Treatment
RHD	Rheumatic heart disease	U/A	Upon arrival
RLQ	Right lower quadrant	URI	Upper respiratory infection
R/O	Rule out	UTI	Urinary tract infection
ROM	Range of motion	vag	Vaginal
ROS	Review of systems, rate of speed	via	By way of
RP	Reporting or responsible party	VF	Ventricular fibrillation
RSR	Regular sinus rhythm	VS	Vital signs
R/T	Respond to	VT	Ventricular tachycardia
RUQ	Right upper quadrant	vol.	Volume
Rx	Prescription	WBC	White blood cell
S&S, S/S	Signs and symptoms	w/d	Warm/dry
SQ, SubQ	Subcutaneous	w/d/p	Warm/dry/pink
sec	Second	w/m	Warm/moist
SIDS	Sudden infant death syndrome	WNL	Within normal limits
SL	Sublingual	wt.	Weight
SNT	Soft, nontender	×	Times
SO	Standing order	x-fer	Transfer
SOB	Shortness of breath	y.o./YO	Year old
sol.	Solution		

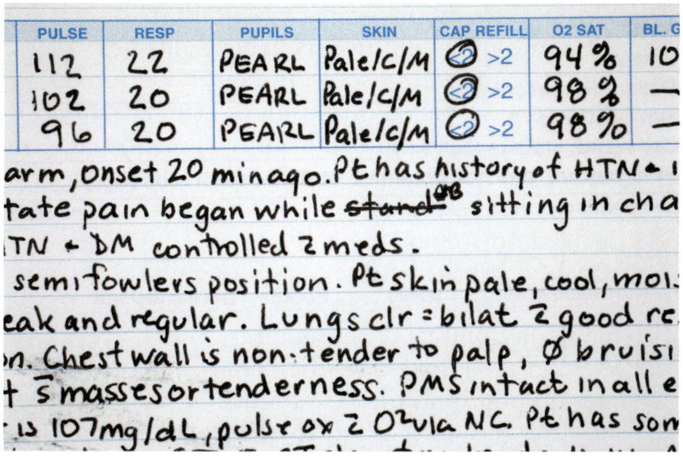

PULSE	RESP	PUPILS	SKIN	CAP REFILL	O2 SAT	BL. G
112	22	PEARL	Pale/C/M	⊘ >2	94%	10
102	20	PEARL	Pale/C/M	⊘ >2	98%	—
96	20	PEARL	Pale/C/M	⊘ >2	98%	—

arm, onset 20 min ago. Pt has history of HTN + I
tate pain began while ~~stand~~ sitting in cha
TN + DM controlled 2 meds.
semi fowlers position. Pt skin pale, cool, moi.
eak and regular. Lungs clr = bilat 2 good re.
n. Chest wall is non-tender to palp, ∅ bruisi
+ s̄ masses or tenderness. PMS intact in all e
is 107mg/dL, pulse ox 2 O2 via NC. Pt has son

Figure 19-2 Corrections should be made by striking through the error with a single line and then initialing the change.

(Figure 19-2). If several errors appear in a report, begin again. Remember that a sloppy report looks unprofessional.

TIMELINESS

[OBJECTIVE 8]

Time is of the essence with documentation. A copy of your PCR should be included in the patient's records at the hospital where you take the patient. Optimally, you should leave a copy of the report before you leave the hospital. In busy systems that is not always possible. Many agencies and hospitals accept a 24-hour time frame to have the PCR completed and delivered to the receiving hospital.

Time also benefits you, the author of the PCR. The more time that passes from the call to when you write the report, the more details can be lost. Write the PCR as soon after a call as possible while the details are still fresh in your mind.

ADDENDUMS

A paramedic occasionally may find an error in a report that has already been completed or want to add information to a report that has already been completed. These situations should be rare because they can raise questions regarding why the document was modified at a later date.

Although agency policies regarding addendums may vary, certain general procedures should be followed when adding or correcting information in a completed report. The original author should write the addendum as soon as the need is realized, indicate the reason for the addendum, and record the date it was written.

Ideally, addendums should be completed on a separate form rather than squeezing in the information on the original report. Most often this is done on a form attached to the original report, and both are filed. In some instances

a completely new report may be written. If this is done, ensure the new report indicates that it is a rewrite. In this situation both the old and new report often are filed together.

METHODS OF DOCUMENTATION

[OBJECTIVE 9]

You can use several different methods of documentation. EMS agencies select a method of documentation on the basis of a number of variables, including cost, call volume, and paramedic preference. The method of documentation is not as important as the content of the report. Regardless of the method used, the report must be complete and not contain any unprofessional jargon, slang, bias, or subjective opinions. The document also must be free of any unsubstantiated claims or libelous statements. Some of the more common methods are described below.

Handwritten Documentation

The handwritten method is the original method of EMS reporting and is still used by many agencies. This method begins with a blank report form. These reports commonly come as a multiple-copy NCR ("no carbon required") form. That way a copy can be left with the hospital and other copies kept with the agency for billing and quality management purposes. This form usually has blank boxes to be filled in with identified criteria. Typically a large section is provided in which to write the narrative.

These reports should be written in pen, not pencil. Pencil can be erased and changed. The PCR is designed to be a permanent record. Penmanship must be legible, and you should print rather than write in script, which can be difficult to read. Some agencies require a specific color of ink (such as black) when documenting on a PCR.

Computer-Based Documentation

Computer-based reporting is becoming more popular in the EMS community. This method allows the paramedic to use an electronic report form with a series of data collection boxes to be checked or left unchecked. This method of reporting also has a section for a narrative. The narrative must be complete. Some computer programs create a template report based on the data points checked. This feature can be convenient, but you must review the report and make corrections as necessary to ensure that the computer has not generated a report with unclear, incomplete, or inaccurate information.

Computer-based reporting allows easy data collection. The reports can be linked to a database to track patient types, paramedic skills, response times, and any other data an agency wishes to evaluate and track. Computer-based reports can be easily sent to hospitals and downloaded to the hospital's electronic patient files (Marx et al., 2006).

Dictation

Dictation is a less-common method of reporting in EMS. With dictation, the paramedic calls a designated number and records his or her report over the telephone. A paid dictation company then transcribes the report and sends it to the paramedic. The paramedic must then proofread and sign the report. This method is commonly used by physicians and can be expensive.

DOCUMENTATION FORMATS

[OBJECTIVE 10]

Several different documentation formats are commonly used by paramedics. The format used is largely up to the paramedic writing the report as long as all the required information is included. Some agencies or hospitals mandate the format to use; the more common formats are covered below.

CHART

The mnemonic <u>CHART</u> stands for *c*hief complaint, *h*istory, *a*ssessment, *R*x (treatment), and *t*ransport. This model is designed to help you remember what needs to be documented. It also organizes the PCR (Figure 19-3).

The CHART mnemonic for documentation has its benefits and drawbacks. The main benefit is the standard template to follow, which helps ensure that no information is left out of the report. This template also helps the reader extract information from the report, and the report can be easier to read. The drawbacks are that the template works best for stable patients who are transported with minimal treatment required. For patients who are dynamic in presentation and receive several treatments, making everything "fit" may be difficult. This commonly results in confusing phrases such as "O_2-IV-monitor-nitro $\times$ 3-defibrillation $\times$ 4" (i.e., oxygen, intravenous line, monitor, three doses of nitroglycerin, four defibrillations). This leaves many questions about what took place, and when. Strict following of the CHART format often results in the description of the scene being omitted, which is another drawback.

Chief Complaint

The chief complaint is the reason the patient called EMS. The chief complaint is usually identified as a report of pain or discomfort, a weird feeling, or a strange sensation. This information should come directly from the patient. Quoting the patient is appropriate. With patients who have an altered level of consciousness, you can obtain information from bystanders or by evaluating the scene.

History

You must obtain two histories from the patient, the first being the history of the present illness. The following mnemonic, OPQRST, can be helpful here:

- **O**nset: Identify the events or conditions surrounding when the chief complaint (e.g., pain, sensation) began or when the injury occurred.
- **P**rovocation/palliation/position: Does anything make the chief complaint improve or worsen (e.g., moving, changing position)? What did the patient do to address the chief complaint before you arrived on scene?
- **Q**uality: What does the pain, discomfort, or sensation feel like? Can the patient describe the pain, discomfort, or sensation?
- **R**egion/radiation: Does the pain or discomfort stay in one spot, or does it move or radiate to another location? Referred pain is pain in an area different from the injury or illness.
- **S**everity: On a scale of 0 to 10 (0 being none and 10 being worst), how bad is the chief complaint?
- **T**iming: When did the chief complaint begin?

The second history to obtain is the medical history. The following mnemonic, AMPLE, can be helpful here:

- **A**llergies: What is the patient allergic to (e.g., plants, medications, foods)?
- **M**edication: What medications is the patient taking? Are they new or changed medications? Is the patient taking the medications as prescribed? What medications is he or she supposed to be taking? Why did he or she stop taking them? What over-the-counter medications has the patient taken? What herbal medications is the patient using?
- **P**ast medical history: What is the patient's medical history? How does the patient's previous pain or discomfort compare with this current event? Does the patient have a history of surgeries or hospitalizations?
- **L**ast oral intake: When was the last time the patient had anything to eat or drink? What was it?
- **E**vents prior: What were the events leading up to this current chief complaint?

Other histories to consider are the family history and social history. These can be indicators of potential disease processes. The history you obtain must be complete. When the patient's condition worsens during transport or in the ED, the only history available to the physician may be what you documented in your report.

Assessment

[OBJECTIVES 11, 12]

Your objective findings are documented in the assessment section. Your assessments of the patient can be documented by a system approach or a head-to-toe approach. One approach is not necessarily better than the other, but you should select one method you are

Southwest Ambulance - Arizona   **Patient Care Record**   PT# 1 of 1

INCIDENT INFO

DISPATCH DATE	RUN NUMBER	UNIT REPORTING	COM/DISP CTR	OTHER UNIT	INV
070506	06142713	AP19	0140	——	

INCIDENT LOCATION: 71642 N Pin Lane   DESTINATION: Groves Hosp

BEGIN MILES	END MILES	DISPATCH TIME	SCENE TIME	TRANSPORT TIME	AT HOSP TIME	2ND ALS ON SCN	ZIP CODE / PICK UP
6527	6628	0907	0915	0928	0940	——	74298

PATIENT INFO

PATIENT LAST NAME	PATIENT FIRST NAME	MI	GENDER
Smith	Gary	A	☐ FEMALE ☑ MALE

PATIENT MAILING ADDRESS DIRECTION: N STREET NAME: Pin Lane   71642   APT.# ——

CITY	STATE	ZIP CODE	WEIGHT (kg)
Seminary	NV	80741	084

BIRTH DATE	AGE	SOCIAL SECURITY NUMBER	PHONE NUMBER
070456	050 ☐M ☐D	123-45-6789	297-643-1856

CLINICAL

DISPATCHED FOR: Chest Pain   CHIEF COMPLAINT: Chest Pain - poss MI   PATIENT CODES: Dun   PT. PHYSICIAN:

PRE-EXISTING CONDITIONS: ☐ Unk ☐ Denied ☑ HTN ☐ MI ☐ CVA ☑ DM ☐ CHF ☐ ASTHMA ☐ SZ ☐ List:

MEDICATIONS: ☐ Unk ☐ Denied ☑ List: Norvasc, Insulin

ALLERGIES: ☐ Unk ☑ Denied ☐ List:

TIME	GCS	LOC	ORIENT	B/P	POS.	EKG	PULSE	RESP	PUPILS	SKIN	CAP REFILL	O2 SAT	BL. GLU.	BY
0921	15	(A)VPU	⬤⬤⬤⬤	196/100	⟋⟍	ST	112	22	PEARL	Pale/c/M	⬤ >2	94%	107	1
0932	15	AVPU	⬤⬤⬤⬤	178/92	⟋⟍	ST	102	20	PEARL	Pale/c/M	⬤ >2	98%	—	1
0937	15	AVPU	⬤⬤⬤⬤	154/86	⟋⟍	SR	96	20	PEARL	Pale/c/M	⬤ >2	98%	—	1

Chief Complaint —— Pt ℅ CP c̄ radiation to neck and Ⓛ arm, onset 40 min ago

History —— Pt states a history of HTN and IDDM. Father had MI at age 50. Pt feels he is in good health c̄ HTN and IDDM controlled c̄ meds

Assessment —— Pt V/s are listed above c̄ pt in semifowlers position. Pt skin is pale, cool, moist c̄ cap refill < 2 sec. Radial pulses are weak and regular. Lungs alr = bilat c̄ good resp effort & adequate chest expansion. Chest wall is non-tender to palp, ∅ bruising or deformity noted, ∅ scars. Abd soft s̄ masses or tenderness, PMS intact in all extremities s̄ edema. Blood glucose level via lancett is 107 mg/dl, pulse ox c̄ O2 via NC. Pt has some mild nausea c̄ vomiting. Cardiac monitor shows SR c̄ ST elevation in leads II, III, AVF c̄ depression in AVL. Patient rating pain at "9" on 1-10 scale. Pt appears to have ⅗ MI.

Rx (Treatment) —— O2 via NC @ 3Lpm, IVNS, Cardiac monitor, NTG, ASA, Morphine, reassessment

Transport —— Pt responded c̄ NTG SL X 3 and Morphine IVP, rating pain @ "2" on same scale upon hosp arrival. Pt ground transport immediate c̄ contact c̄ Dr. Happy, ∅ additional orders. Pt monitored throughout transport c̄ improvement.

TIME	TREATMENT, MEDICATION, DOSE, ROUTE, & RESPONSE	BY	TIME	TREATMENT, MEDICATION, DOSE, ROUTE, & RESPONSE	BY
IV: Fluid NS cc 1000 ga 18 site Ⓡ Forearm	attempt 1 S/U S gtts/min —— total infused 20 cc				
0918	Pt contact	1,2	0932	NTG SL 0.4mg	1
0919	O2 via NC @ 3Lpm	2	0937	NTG SL 0.4mg	1
0921	V/S + pulse ox, Blood glucose check	1	0940	12-lead - poss Inferior MI	1
0922	Cardiac monitor	1	0946	Morphine Sulfate 4mg IVP	1
0924	IVNS c̄ 18g Ⓡ forearm, ∅ complications	1	0947	Hospital Report	1
0927	NTG SL 0.4mg	1	0953	Transport to hospital, care by staff	1,2

MEDIC/EMT/RN SIGNATURE COMPLETING REPORT ☑ EMT-P ☐ EMT-B ☐ RN: *Susri Seas*
TELEMETRY HOSP/MD: Oscar Dun / Dr Happy
RECEIVING FAC. SIGNATURE: *Megan RN*

| 1 | PRINT NAME & CERT # OF ABOVE MEDIC/EMT/RN: S. Seas 1234 | 2 | PRINT NAME & CERT # OF OTHER MEDIC/EMT: O. Oter 5678 | 3 | PRINT NAME & CERT # OF OTHER MEDIC/EMT |

ADDITIONAL FORMS: ☐ Continuation ☐ Refusal ☐ Sec. Clinical ☐ Attachments

Morphine 6mg waste

Narcotic Waste Witnessed By: *Megan RN*

P52-131 (Rev. 7/03)   ADMINISTRATION/BILLING

Figure 19-3 CHART (chief complaint, history, assessment, Rx [treatment], transportation) example.

comfortable with and use it consistently. Consistency helps avoid errors and omissions.

Your assessment should be documented in detail. Statements such as "physical assessment unremarkable" are not acceptable. This statement does not tell the reader what assessment was performed. It also leaves room for interpretation and assumption, which increases your liability. You should document what was assessed and any pertinent positive findings and negative findings. Remember, if it was not documented, it was not assessed.

The assessment must be objective. You must document what you see and hear. Opinions have no place in a PCR. "The patient presented with slurred speech and staggered gait" is appropriate. It documents what you see. "The patient is intoxicated" is inappropriate. This statement makes an assumptive leap. Slurred speech and staggered gait could be caused by several medical or traumatic causes. The assumption that the patient is intoxicated is merely an opinion.

Treatment

In the treatment section of the PCR, you must clearly document the treatment you provided to the patient. The treatment you document here should be supported by the chief complaint and the assessment findings. The description of the treatment must be detailed. Do not simply document that the patient was intubated. Document the number of attempts, the tube size used, the depth of the tube, how the proper tube position was confirmed, and how the tube was secured. Recheck (and document) the position of the tube every time the patient is moved, such as from his or her bed at home to the EMS stretcher, from the EMS stretcher to the hospital stretcher, and so forth. You must also document the patient's response to the treatment.

Transport

In the transport section of the PCR, document where the patient was transported and why. You should include hospital diversion status, patient severity, and patient request. If a patient is not transported to the closest hospital—the hospital the reader of the report would expect—you must justify this in the report. No justification allows the reader to make assumptions.

SOAP

The mnemonic SOAP stands for **s**ubjective findings, **o**bjective findings, **a**ssessment of the condition, and **p**lan for treatment and transport (Figure 19-4). As with the CHART mnemonic, the SOAP mnemonic has benefits and drawbacks. It does provide a standard template to follow, which helps ensure that information is not omitted. This template also helps the reader extract information from the report, and it can be easier to read. A drawback is that the template works best for stable patients who are transported with minimal treatment required. For patients whose presentation is dynamic and who receive several treatments, making everything fit into the format may be difficult. Be sure to avoid creating one phrase that is supposed to describe and justify all treatment. Strict following of this format often results in the description of the scene being omitted, which is another drawback.

Subjective

The **subjective information** section of the PCR is reserved for information that has been told to you. This should include the patient's chief complaint. Place any additional information the patient gives you here as well. You must include information such as additional sensations (e.g., shortness of breath or dizziness). You should also include your impression of the scene and statements from bystanders here.

Objective

The **objective information** section of the PCR is reserved for verifiable findings, including information you have seen, felt, or heard. Record physical examination findings here along with electrocardiographic interpretations, capnography readings, and any other assessment values.

Assessment

The assessment section is where you record your assessment of the patient. For example, "The patient's signs and symptoms and ECG findings are consistent with an inferior wall MI." The information in this section must be supported by the information documented in the two previous sections.

Plan

This section documents your treatment plan. Use caution here; a one-word treatment plan may not be defendable. All treatment must be justified by a reassessment. Be aware that effectively documenting the treatment of dynamic patients is difficult to do in this section.

Narrative

The narrative portion of the PCR is written exactly as it sounds—in a storytelling format. This format works well to document the flow of a call. It easily allows you to document procedures, followed by treatment, followed by patient response, and so forth (Figure 19-5). The pitfalls of this format are that details are easy to miss. If several events occur at the same time on the scene, fitting them all in the report may be difficult. Another downfall is that information is difficult to extract. If the reader is looking for a single assessment finding, he or she will have to read the entire report instead of simply going to the section where the assessment is documented.

Southwest Ambulance - Arizona — **Patient Care Record**

PT# ___ of ___

INCIDENT INFO

DISPATCH DATE	RUN NUMBER	UNIT REPORTING	COM/DISP CTR	OTHER UNIT	INV
070506	06142713	AP19	0140	——	

INCIDENT LOCATION: 71642 N Pin Lane
DESTINATION: Groves Hosp

BEGIN MILES	END MILES	DISPATCH TIME	SCENE TIME	TRANSPORT TIME	AT HOSP TIME	2ND ALS ON SCN	ZIP CODE / PICK UP
6527	6628	0907	0915	0928	0940	——	74298

PATIENT INFO

PATIENT LAST NAME: Smith
PATIENT FIRST NAME: Gary
MI: C
GENDER: ☐ FEMALE ☑ MALE

PATIENT MAILING ADDRESS: 71642
DIRECTION: N
STREET NAME: Pin Lane
APT.#: ——

CITY: Seminary
STATE: NV
ZIP CODE: 74298
WEIGHT (kg): 084

BIRTH DATE: 070456
AGE: 050 ☐M ☐D
SOCIAL SECURITY NUMBER: 123-45-6789
PHONE NUMBER: 297-643-1856

CLINICAL

DISPATCHED FOR: Chest Pain
CHIEF COMPLAINT: Chest Pain - poss MI
PATIENT CODES:
PT. PHYSICIAN: Don

PRE-EXISTING CONDITIONS: ☐ Unk ☐ Denied ☑ HTN ☐ MI ☐ CVA ☑ DM ☐ CHF ☐ ASTHMA ☐ SZ ☐ List:

MEDICATIONS: ☐ Unk ☐ Denied ☐ List: Norvasc, Insulin

ALLERGIES: ☐ Unk ☑ Denied ☐ List:

TIME	GCS	LOC	ORIENT	B/P	POS.	EKG	PULSE	RESP	PUPILS	SKIN	CAP REFILL	O2 SAT	BL. GLU.	BY
0921	15	Ⓐ VPU	⊙⊙⊙⊙	196/100	⚬-●	ST	112	22	PEARL	Pale/c/M	Ⓒ >2	94%	107	1
0932	15	Ⓐ VPU	⊙⊙⊙⊙	178/92	⚬-●	ST	102	20	PEARL	Pale/c/M	Ⓒ >2	98%	—	1
0937	15	Ⓐ VPU	⊙⊙⊙⊙	154/86	⚬-●	SR	96	20	PEARL	Pale/c/M	Ⓒ >2	98%	—	1

Subjective — Pt c/c CP c̄ radiation to neck + Ⓛ arm, onset 20 min ago. Pt has history of HTN + IDDM. Pt father had MI at age 50. Pt state pain began while standing sitting in chair. Pt feels he is in good health c̄ HTN + DM controlled c̄ meds.

Objective — Pt vital signs are above c̄ pt in semi fowlers position. Pt skin pale, cool, moist c̄ cap refill < 2 sec. Radial pulses weak and regular. Lungs clr = bilat c̄ good resp effort and adequate chest expansion. Chest wall is non-tender to palp, Ø bruising or deformity noted, Ø scars. Abd soft s̄ masses or tenderness. PMS intact in all extremities, Ø edema. Blood glucose via lancet is 107 mg/dL, pulse ox c̄ O2 via NC. Pt has some mild nausea s̄ vomiting. Cardiac monitor shows ST c̄ ST elevation leads II, III, AVF c̄ depression AVL. Pt rates pain @ "9" on 1-10 scale.

Assessment — Poss Inferior MI

Plan — O2 via NC @ 3 Lpm (pt c̄ nausea), IV NS, Cardiac monitor, NTG, ASA, Morphine, Reassessment — Pt rating pain @ "2" on same scale upon hosp arrival. Pt transported ground immediate. Contacted c̄ Dr Happy @ hosp, Ø additional orders. Pt condition improved upon hospital arrival. Pt transferred to hosp, report to RN, care by staff

TIME	TREATMENT, MEDICATION, DOSE, ROUTE, & RESPONSE	BY	TIME	TREATMENT, MEDICATION, DOSE, ROUTE, & RESPONSE	BY
IV: Fluid NS cc 1000 ga 18 site Ⓡ Forearm #attempt 1 S/U S gtts/min ___ total infused 20 cc					
0918	Pt contact	1,2	0932	NTG SL 0.4 mg	1
0919	O2 via NC @ 3 Lpm	2	0937	NTG SL 0.4 mg	1
0921	vls + pulse ox, blood glucose check	1	0940	12-lead - poss inferior MI	1
0922	Cardiac Monitor	1	0946	Morphine Sulfate 4 mg IVP	1
0924	IV NS c̄ 18 g Ⓡ Forearm, Ø complications	1	0947	Hospital report	1
0927	NTG SL 0.4 mg	1	0953	Transfer to hosp, care by staff	1,2

MEDIC/EMT/RN SIGNATURE COMPLETING REPORT: ☑ EMT-P ☐ EMT-B ☐ RN
Susu Seas
TELEMETRY HOSP/MD: Dr Happy
RECEIVING FAC. SIGNATURE: M___ RN

1 — PRINT NAME & CERT # OF ABOVE MEDIC/EMT/RN: S. Seas 1234
2 — PRINT NAME & CERT # OF OTHER MEDIC/EMT: O. Other 5678
3 — PRINT NAME & CERT # OF OTHER MEDIC/EMT:

ADDITIONAL FORMS: ☐ Continuation ☐ Refusal ☐ Sec. Clinical ☐ Attachments
morphine 6mg waste

Narcotic Waste Witnessed By: M___ RN

P52-131 (Rev. 7/03)
ADMINISTRATION/BILLING

Figure 19-4 SOAP (**s**ubjective, **o**bjective, **a**ssessment, **p**lan) example.

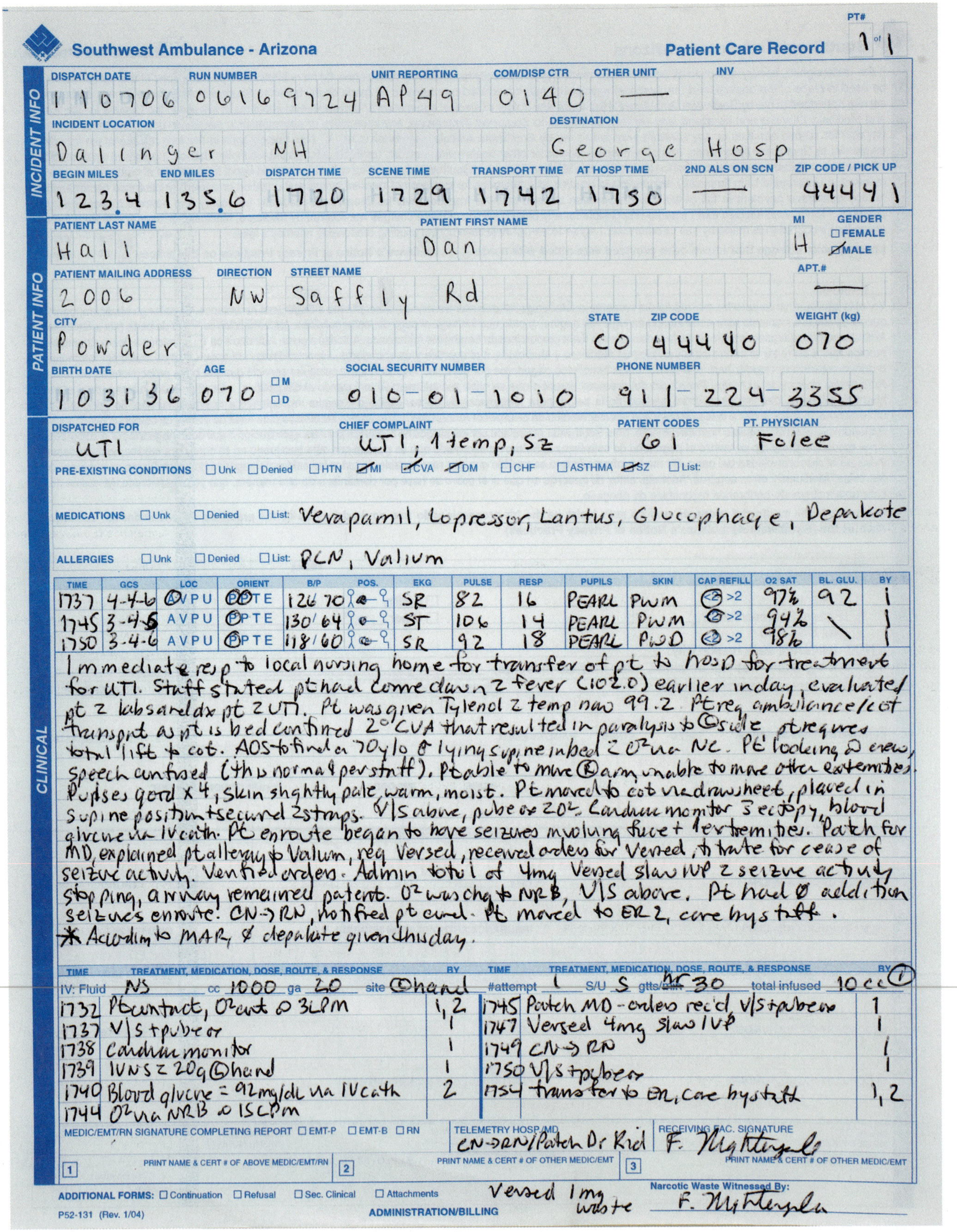

Figure 19-5 Narrative example.

Case Scenario—continued

The patient is sitting on the ground near where her incident occurred. You can see a loose flap of carpet in the doorway. The patient reports that she tripped on the carpet and fell forward. As you begin to evaluate the patient, you discover a significant amount of swelling surrounding the laceration on the forehead and note that the woman's pupils are unequal. The patient informs you that she has diabetes and needs to get to dinner right away. She also tells you that in addition to her headache she also feels a little dizzy. Her vital signs are pulse, 90 beats/min; blood pressure, 144/76 mm Hg; and respirations, 18 breaths/min.

Questions

4. *What part of this information is subjective in nature?*
5. *What part of this information is objective in nature?*
6. *Given this patient's mechanism of injury and presentation, what information would be appropriate as a pertinent negative? What would be a pertinent positive?*
7. *Name at least two different ways of organizing your narrative on the PCR. How should you decide which method to follow?*
8. *You have the patient sign the PCR on the signature line. Depending on your system, what may this signature document?*

SPECIAL SITUATIONS

[OBJECTIVES 13, 14]

On occasion, you will be faced with a call that adds another dimension to the process of documentation. Some types of calls deserve special consideration, including calls with more than one patient, calls for multiple casualty situations, and calls that do not result in patient transport.

Multiple Patients

On occasion, you will have a call that is not a multiple casualty incident but does involve more than one patient. Examples include a mother who has delivered a baby, a motor vehicle crash with multiple patients in one car, and a family in a house with a carbon monoxide leak. You must remember that each patient requires a separate PCR. You may be tempted to include more than one patient involved in the same event on a single PCR. However, avoid this short cut. Each patient report should be a stand-alone document.

Refusals

[OBJECTIVE 13]

At some point you will be called to evaluate and treat a patient who does not wish to be transported to the ED. If you have determined the patient is awake, alert, and oriented; free of mind-altering substances; and of legal age, then he or she has the right to refuse transport. You are obligated to inform the patient of the potential risks involved with refusing transport. You must be sure to document the events of the call thoroughly. Stating that "the patient was informed of the risks of refusing care" is not sufficient. You must document the specific information you told the patient, how you confirmed the patient understood those risks, and the follow-up instructions you gave the patient. Many agencies carry preprinted refusal documents. These documents list the risks of refusal for a variety of complaints. These documents help ensure the consistency of the information disseminated in a refusal. When a patient refuses transport, if possible have the patient and a bystander sign a refusal acknowledging that the patient was informed of the risks of refusal (Figure 19-6) (Lee, 2001; Marx et al., 2006).

Cancellations

Several situations exist in which you may be dispatched to a call and then cancelled either en route or on arrival at the scene. Policies for these situations vary from agency to agency; however, you will generally need to document your response, who cancelled you and, if on scene, your general impression of the scene and circumstances surrounding the cancellation.

GCH EMS RELEASE FORM

I, THE UNDERSIGNED, DO AGREE THAT THE GREATER COMMUNITY HOSPITAL AMBULANCE SERVICE ANSWERED MY CALL FOR ASSISTANCE TO MY SATISFACTION. THROUGH MY OWN FREE WILL, (OR SOMEONE RESPONSIBLE), I AT THIS TIME REFUSE THE SERVICE OF THE AFOREMENTIONED ORGANIZATION AND RELEASE GCH EMS AND ANYONE AFFILIATED WITH IT OF ANY RESPONSIBILITY FOR MY HEALTH AND WELL BEING.

THE POSSIBLE CONSEQUENCES OF MY REFUSING MEDICAL TREATMENT AND NECESSARY PRECAUTIONS LISTED BELOW, WERE EXPLAINED TO ME AND I UNDERSTAND COMPLETELY:

HEAD INJURY

_____ Hard to wake up
_____ Change in usual behavior
_____ Can't walk or talk right
_____ Vomits more than once
_____ Headache that worsens over 24 hours
_____ Blurred vision, double vision, or unequal pupils

SPRAIN INJURY

_____ Elevate injured part above the level of chest
_____ Use cold packs while swollen, for 20 min., several times/day.

INFECTIONS/LACERATIONS

_____ Keep area clean and dry
_____ Call your Dr. if you have any of the following:
Pus, red streaking, worse pain, fever, or chills.

SPECIAL INSTRUCTIONS

_____
_____
_____
_____
_____

VITAL SIGNS

BP _____ PULSE _____ RESP. _____

_____ Pt. refuses to allow vital signs to be taken.

_____ Pt. refuses the recommended immobilization, but does agree to be transported.

I was advised to, and will seek further medical care as needed, if any of the above or other symptoms develop or worsen.

_____   _____
Witness   Name (Print)

_____   _____
Witness   Address

_____   _____
Driver   Date of Birth   Age

_____   _____
Attendant   Signature

_____   _____
Date   Time   Relationship to Patient

Figure 19-6 Refusal forms should be completed on any patient who does not want to be transported by EMS.

Case Scenario CONCLUSION

Your examination reveals no abnormalities other than the laceration. The patient is alert and oriented to person, place, time, and event. She requests that you put a bandage on her laceration and "get the hell out" so that she can go to dinner. She refuses transportation to the hospital and informs you and the nursing center staff that she is going to "sue you for all you're worth" for letting her fall in the hall. After bandaging her laceration, you assist the nurse in guiding the patient to the dining room and go back into service.

Looking Back

9. In your PCR, do you document the loose flap of carpet? Why or why not?
10. The patient is refusing transport. What information must be included in your PCR related to her refusal? Why?
11. In your PCR, you decide to include the patient's statement that you should "get the hell out." How should you document this statement?

Multiple-Casualty Incidents

[OBJECTIVE 14]

Multiple-casualty incidents allow only brief contact with patients. Commonly, all you will do in these situations is a primary survey. In these events, you can use an abbreviated report form, such as a triage tag. An example of a triage tag is shown in Figure 19-7.

DOCUMENTATION ESSENTIALS

[OBJECTIVE 15]

Following are essential characteristics of all documentation:

Objective: State what you see, hear, feel, and do. Opinions do not belong.
Thorough: Document everything completely. Avoid shortcuts.
Legible: Print legibly; type or print reports.
Timely: Turn in the patient's report as soon as possible.
Free of errors: Check misspellings and misused words.

The perfect report should leave no questions in the reader's mind.

QUALITY MANAGEMENT PROCESS

PCRs play a large role in an agency's quality management process. EMS agencies must have a process of evaluating what is and is not working in their systems. Moreover,

paramedics must be individually monitored for skill proficiency. A great gauge of how a system is doing in the patient care arena is the reports written by its paramedics.

Some agencies have a person or a department whose sole job is to read reports and review calls. Other agencies use a peer approach. With a peer approach, paramedics read and review one another's reports.

Depending on the call volume of an agency a 100% **trip audit,** in which every PCR is read and reviewed, may occur. In busier systems a selected trip audit may be more effective. With these, each month a different call type is selected for review. As data are collected, the agency must review those data. If a paramedic has problems with a skill, the agency can offer remediation to help the paramedic improve. If paramedics across the board are having difficulties with a specific call type, the agency can build a continuing education program to help them improve.

These reviews can help guide staffing and posting. If a specific call type increases, this may highlight the need to purchase additional or different equipment.

PARAMEDIC Pearl

"It is important to review where we have been to help us see where we need to go" (Hamilton et al., 2003).

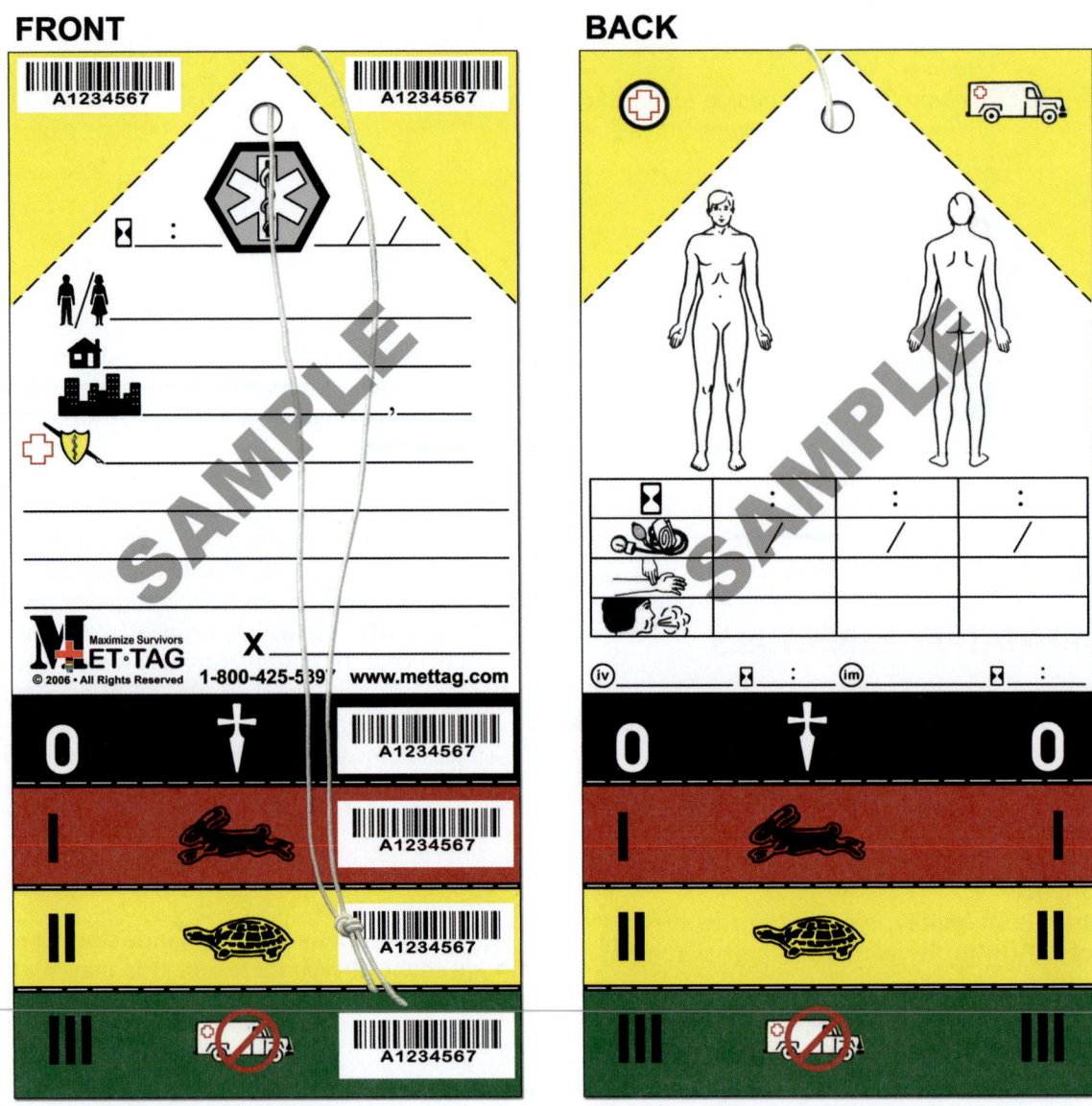

Figure 19-7 An abbreviated report form, such as a triage tag, is typically used in a multiple-casualty incident.

Case Scenario SUMMARY

1. *After you complete and submit the PCR for this case, what potential functions will it fulfill?* The PCR may be used in the ED and hospital to ensure continuity of care. It may be reviewed as part of a quality management program and, in many cases, will play a role in billing and reimbursement. PCRs also may be reviewed to justify or expand paramedic scope of practice. They also are an important component of EMS research. The PCR occasionally serves as a legal document.

2. *Given these functions, when should the PCR be completed and submitted?* To ensure continuity of care, the PCR should be submitted to the ED at the time patient care is transferred. For all other purposes, the PCR should be submitted by the end of the paramedic's shift.

3. *Much of the information about the accident itself came from the nursing staff member. Because you did not observe it, can you document this information on the PCR? How?* Yes. Information from bystanders or others on the scene can be simply recorded as, "According to the nurse who witnessed the fall . . . " Be sure to clarify that these observations occurred before EMS arrival.

4. *What part of this information is subjective in nature?* Subjective information comes from the patient and/or others on the scene. In this case, the nurse's description of the event, the reported "no loss of consciousness," the patient's report of head pain and dizziness, the patient's description of the event, and the patient's statement that she has diabetes are all subjective.

5. *What part of this information is objective in nature?* Objective information includes *your* observations. In this case, the patient's skin color, general appearance, mental status, laceration, pupillary status, and swelling are all objective data.

6. *Given this patient's mechanism of injury and presentation, what information would be appropriate as a pertinent negative? What would be a pertinent positive?* Given her age, a distinct possibility exists that the patient's fall was the result of a medical event, such as syncope or a stroke. Therefore pertinent negatives could include the patient's denial that she was dizzy before falling and denial of a loss of consciousness. Because the patient's injuries appear to be primarily to her head, additional pertinent negatives could be her normal mental status and the absence of any abnormalities in motor or sensory status. Pertinent positives related to the patient's head injury include her head pain, dizziness, laceration, and uneven pupils.

7. *Name at least two different ways of organizing your narrative on the PCR. How should you decide which method to follow?* SOAP and CHART are two of many different methods for organizing a PCR narrative. In most cases local protocols will dictate what format to use.

8. *You have the patient sign the PCR on the signature line. Depending on your system, what may this signature document?* In many cases, the signature includes acknowledgement of HIPAA rules and consent to treat and/or transport.

9. *In your PCR, do you document the loose flap of carpet? Why or why not?* Although the loose flap of carpet may be the cause of the patient's fall, documenting it in the PCR is not necessary. The PCR should include information about how the patient fell (she tripped) and her mechanism of injury (she fell against the door and lowered herself to the floor). However, the information about what she tripped on is irrelevant to her medical condition. If you are concerned about unsafe conditions at the nursing facility, communicate your concerns through an incident report or other avenue that is focused on issues other than the specific condition of the patient you are evaluating or treating. The presence of irrelevant data in the PCR confuses the presentation of appropriate information, makes your assessment and care appear distracted or even inflammatory, and serves no useful purpose related to evaluation and management of your patient.

10. *The patient is refusing transport. What information must be included in your PCR regarding her refusal? Why?* Your documentation of a patient's refusal of treatment or transport must include the patient's mental status (to demonstrate that she is alert, oriented, and legally capable of making a decision), your evaluation and *communication to the patient* of potential injuries and the benefits of treatment for those injuries, your assessment and communication to the patient of the risks of failure to get treatment, and the patient's acknowledgement of understanding those potential benefits and risks.

11. *In your PCR, you decide to include the patient's statement that you should "get the hell out." How should you document this statement?* Document any specific statements that the patient (or others on scene) makes by placing them in quotes: "The patient told me to 'get the hell out.'"

Chapter Summary

- Documentation is one of the most important parts of a paramedic's job.
- The report written by the paramedic is commonly the only documentation of the medical events on scene and during transport.
- Documentation can affect the following:
  - Patient care
  - Legal proceedings
  - Scope of practice
  - Education and training
  - Agency reimbursement
- The report written by the paramedic must be timely, complete, accurate, legible, objective, and free of errors.
- The report written by the paramedic should attempt to leave no questions in the reader's mind.
- The report written by the paramedic should leave no room for reader interpretation.
- Reports should be written in a set format, such as following the mnemonics CHART or SOAP or a narrative structure.
- Reports can be written by hand, entered in a computer-based system, or completed by dictation.
- All interactions with a patient should result in a written report.

REFERENCES

Cohn, B., & Azarra, A. (1998). *Legal aspects of emergency medical services*. Philadelphia: Elsevier.

Gylys, B. A. (2005). *Masters medical terminology simplified: A programmed learning approach by body systems* (3rd ed.). Philadelphia: F. A. Davis.

Hamilton, G., Sanders, A., Strange, G., & Trott, A. (2003). *Emergency medicine: An approach to clinical problem-solving* (2nd ed.). Philadelphia: Saunders.

Lee, N. G. (2001). *Legal aspects of emergency care*. Philadelphia: Elsevier.

Leonard, P. (2007). *Quick & easy medical terminology*, Philadelphia: Elsevier.

Marx, J., Hockberger, R., & Walls, R. (2006). *Rosen's emergency medicine: Concepts and clinical practice* (6th ed.). Philadelphia: Mosby.

Chapter Quiz

1. Which of the following statements would be inappropriate to include in a PCR?
   a. The patient had a staggered gait.
   b. The patient admits to drinking two beers.
   c. The patient was intoxicated.
   d. The patient had slurred speech.

2. List three reasons why statements such as "physical assessment unremarkable" should be avoided in a PCR.

   _____

   _____

   _____

3. Your patient is a 5-year-old girl who may have been physically abused. Which of the following would be inappropriate in a PCR?
   a. Document that the father beat the child.
   b. Document injuries found.
   c. Document statements made by the patient.
   d. Document vital signs.

4. Your patient is a 25-year-old man with an allergic reaction. Which of the following would be a pertinent positive finding?
   a. Patient has an allergy to peanuts.
   b. Patient has circumoral cyanosis.
   c. Patient breath sounds were clear.
   d. Patient denies a loss of consciousness.

5. True or False: Only patients who are transported require a PCR.

6. True or False: When a patient refuses transport, having that patient sign a refusal form clears the paramedic from any legal action against him or her.

7. Which of the following regulates how a paramedic must protect a patient's personal information?
   a. COBRA
   b. OSHA
   c. HIPAA
   d. DOT

8. Which of the following is an appropriate way to correct an error on a printed form?
   a. "White out" the error completely.
   b. Mark out with a single line, then initial.
   c. Cross out multiple times with a pen and then initial.
   d. Cross out with a black marker.

9. Which of the following is true regarding the use of abbreviations?
   a. Use only abbreviations approved for use in your agency.
   b. Never use abbreviations.
   c. Made-up abbreviations are fine as long as they are logical.
   d. Abbreviate using the first, third, and last letter of the word.

10. Which of the following is not an accepted use of a PCR?
    a. Billing for services
    b. Maintaining continuity of care
    c. Addressing quality management issues
    d. Notifying patient's friends

Terminology

Health Insurance Portability and Accountability Act (HIPAA) Rules governing the protection of a patient's identifiable information.

Medical terminology Greek- and Latin-based words (typically) that function as a common language for the medical community.

Objective information Verifiable findings, such as information seen, felt, or heard by the paramedic.

Pertinent negative In a patient assessment, the signs and symptoms found not to be present that support a working diagnosis.

Pertinent positive In a patient assessment, the signs and symptoms found to be present that support a working diagnosis.

Prefix Added to the beginning of a root word to alter the meaning. Usually identifies location or frequency.

Prehospital care report (PCR) The report written by the paramedic after the call has been completed. The report becomes part of the patient's permanent medical record.

Root word In medical terminology, the part of the word that gives the primary meaning.

Scope of practice The set of procedures a paramedic is allowed and expected to perform.

Subjective information Information told to the paramedic.

Suffix Added to the end of a root word to change the meaning. Usually identifies the condition of the root word.

Trip audit The review of a PCR written by a paramedic by a peer or a third party.

DIVISION 5

MEDICAL

Head, Ear, Eye, Nose, and Throat Disorders

Objectives *After completing this chapter, you will be able to:*

1. Describe the etiology, demographics, history, and physical findings for the following conditions:
- Lice
- Impetigo
- Lesions
- Headache
- Bell's palsy
- Ludwig's angina

2. By using the patient history and physical examination findings, develop a treatment plan for patients with the following conditions:
- Lice
- Impetigo
- Lesions
- Headache
- Bell's palsy
- Ludwig's angina

3. Describe the etiology, demographics, history, and physical findings for the following conditions:
- Conjunctivitis
- Inflammation of the eyelids
- Glaucoma
- Central retinal artery occlusion
- Retinal detachment

4. By using the patient history and physical examination findings, develop a treatment plan for patients with the following conditions:
- Conjunctivitis
- Inflammation of the eyelids
- Glaucoma
- Central retinal artery occlusion
- Retinal detachment

5. Describe the etiology, demographics, history, and physical findings for the following conditions:
- Ear foreign bodies
- Vertigo
- Tinnitus
- Otitis externa

6. By using the patient history and physical examination findings, develop a treatment plan for patients with the following conditions:
- Ear foreign bodies
- Vertigo
- Tinnitus
- Otitis externa

7. Describe the etiology, demographics, history, and physical findings for the following conditions:
- Epistaxis
- Nose foreign bodies
- Piercing
- Rhinitis

8. By using the patient history and physical examination findings, develop a treatment plan for patients with the following conditions:
- Epistaxis
- Nose foreign bodies
- Piercing
- Rhinitis

9. Describe the etiology, demographics, history, and physical findings for the following conditions:
- Thrush
- Broken, missing, or loose teeth
- Sore throat
- Epiglottitis
- Peritonsillar abscess

10. By using the patient history and physical examination findings, develop a treatment plan for patients with the following conditions:
- Thrush
- Broken, missing, or loose teeth
- Sore throat
- Epiglottitis
- Peritonsillar abscess

Chapter Outline

Specific Head and Face Disorders
Specific Eye Disorders
Specific Ear Disorders

Specific Nose Disorders
Specific Mouth Disorders
Chapter Summary

Case Scenario

You and your partner respond to an employee clinic at a large company for a "possible stroke." When you arrive, you find a 36-year-old woman lying in a darkened examination room. The nurse who called 9-1-1 informs you that the patient's chief complaint is severe headache, but that she had become concerned that the problem could be more serious when her assessment revealed that the patient was having difficulty speaking and said that her right arm and leg felt "numb." As you approach the patient, you note that she is alert, oriented, has no visible difficulty breathing, and has normal skin color. Her pulse is strong and regular. She tells you that her chief complaint is "the worst headache I've ever had" for 3 days. You also observe that she has difficulty forming sentences and has slightly slurred speech.

Questions

1. *What is your general impression of this patient?*
2. *What conditions might cause these symptoms?*
3. *What treatment should be immediately initiated?*

The head is composed of the skull, eyes, ears, nose, and mouth. Each of these structures has distinct properties, specific assessment concerns, and unique disorders to be aware of while you perform a patient evaluation. The head contains four of the five senses: eyes, ears, nose, and mouth. It also is the start of the airway, is the start of the digestive tract, and contains one of the primary ways human beings maintain balance, the inner ear.

SPECIFIC HEAD AND FACE DISORDERS

[OBJECTIVES 1, 2]

Lice

Etiology and Demographics

Lice (pediculosis) are wingless insects that live in human hair. They are highly transmittable from person to person through close contact or sharing personal grooming items. The most commonly infected group is children from 4 to 10 years of age because they tend to play closely together in small groups. Other potential hosts include the homeless and nursing home patients who receive substandard care.

History and Physical Findings

Lice appear as small white clusters (nits) around the root of the hair. This can be helpful in differentiating lice from dandruff, which typically is more diffuse throughout the hair (Figure 20-1). To evaluate for the presence of lice, part the hair in several locations around the head and observe for tiny white, shiny clusters that do not readily fall off near hair roots. Dry scalp or dandruff will appear as flakes on the scalp and will fall off when the hair is parted.

Therapeutic Interventions

If lice clusters are found, consider covering the head during transport and notifying the receiving facility on arrival.

Patient and Family Education

The treatment for lice consists of washing the hair multiple times with a specific lice shampoo and using a fine-toothed comb to remove any remnants. Because lice lay eggs while in the hair, this procedure must be continued for several days to kill newly hatched lice. Lice-killing shampoo is available over the counter at most major drug stores or pharmacies. Families should be instructed to keep the infected person's personal care items, such as combs and brushes, separate from the rest of the family's until they can be thoroughly cleaned. Consideration should be given to discarding these items as soon as possible once treatment has been initiated.

Impetigo

Etiology and Demographics

Impetigo is a highly contagious infection caused by staphylococcal or streptococcal bacteria. It is most commonly seen in young children, especially those in group care settings such as day care. However, anyone around an individual with impetigo can contract the infection and pass it to others.

History and Physical Findings

Impetigo is typically seen on the face and extremities. Patients with impetigo may report itching and/or burning before eruption of the lesions. These symptoms may continue once lesions are visible. The honey-colored crusts that form from the **exudate** of the vesicles as they rupture distinguish it from other lesions on the face (Figure 20-2). Impetigo initially appears as pustules and vesicles that can be differentiated from chickenpox by the lack of systemic symptoms (no fever) and a reaction to poison oak or poison ivy by the typical pattern of infection on the face.

Therapeutic Interventions

Because impetigo is contagious, be sure to use standard precautions. To reduce the risk of spreading the infection,

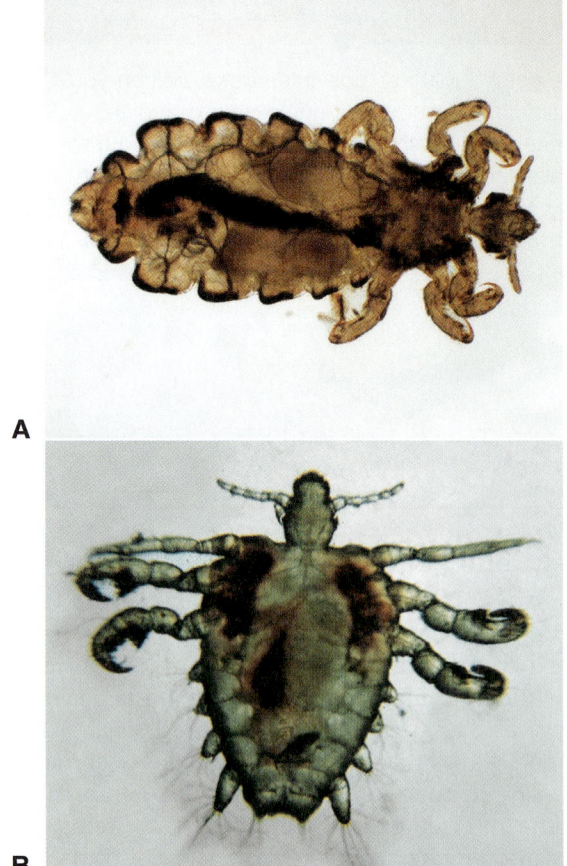

Figure 20-1 A, Head louse. **B,** Pubic louse.

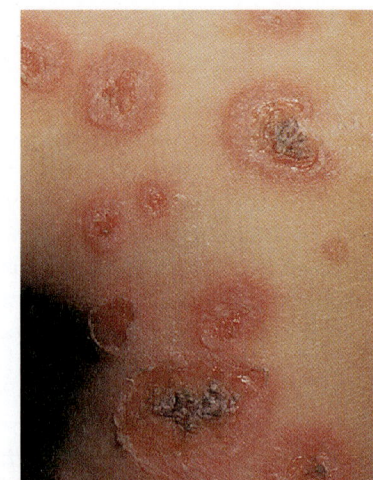

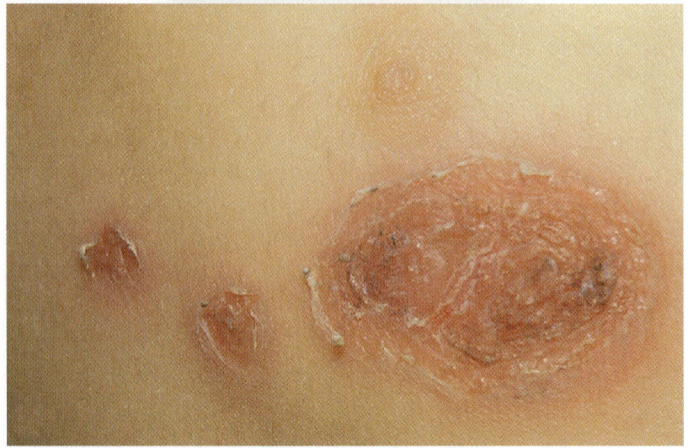

Figure 20-2 Impetigo.

instruct the patient not to scratch the infected area. Consider covering the lesions with a nonstick dressing.

Patient and Family Education

Handwashing is the most effective way to reduce the spread of impetigo in a household or day care center. Families must be instructed to keep all items used by the infected individual separate. This includes clothes, towels, washcloths, cups, glasses, silverware, and plates until they are thoroughly washed with soap and water. Once the condition is diagnosed by a physician, the infected individual is treated with antibiotics.

Lesions

Etiology

Lesions on the face can be the result of many conditions, including chickenpox, measles, acne, cancers, or allergic reactions.

History and Physical Findings

To rule out infectious causes check for fever, general **malaise,** and nausea and vomiting. To determine if the lesion may be from an allergic reaction, ask about any recent changes in diet, medication, or personal care products. Note the color, texture, size, and shape of the erup-

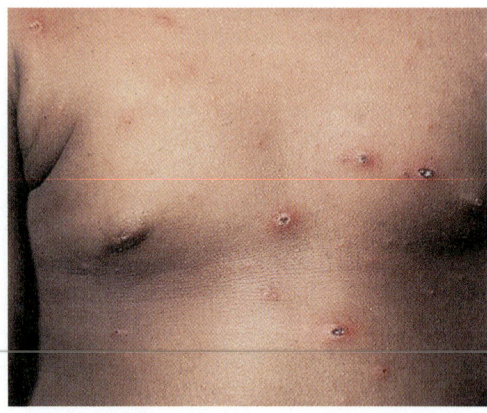

Figure 20-3 Chickenpox.

tions. Documenting any redness, itchiness, drainage, and the pattern of distribution of the lesions is important. All these characteristics can be helpful in determining the field impression and treatment (Figure 20-3).

Therapeutic Interventions

Use standard precautions. Consider covering the lesions with a nonstick dressing. No ointments or creams should be applied to the area unless ordered by medical direction.

Case Scenario—continued

You and your partner administer oxygen (2 L by nasal cannula) as you continue your evaluation. The patient informs you that she has had severe head pain for the past 2 days. Yesterday she believed she was having difficulty concentrating and frequently saw bright flashes of light. This morning her headache was "much better," but she felt like she had a "fuzzy head" and her right hand was so weak that she needed to use her left hand to fix breakfast. Her speech is slow and disjointed, and on several occasions she becomes frustrated because she used the wrong word or mixed her word sequence in a sentence. On examination you find equal and reactive pupils and a noticeably weak right hand grip. Her Cincinnati Stroke Scale score is normal with the exception of her speech difficulty. Vital signs are pulse, 104 beats/min; blood pressure, 128/80 mm Hg; and respirations, 12 breaths/min.

Questions

4. *Has your general impression of this patient changed after a more complete examination? Why or why not?*
5. *This patient is reporting headache and "bright flashes of light." What condition(s) frequently present in this way?*
6. *How does the Cincinnati Stroke Scale influence your treatment plan for this patient?*
7. *This woman is 36 years old and is experiencing dysphasia and one-sided weakness. What do you think her fears might be? How could you help?*
8. *What additional treatment should be provided?*

Patient and Family Education

Instruct patients and families to keep the area of the lesion clean and dry.

Headache

Etiology and Demographics

Headaches are probably one of the most common complaints. Some headaches can be extreme and require immediate assistance. **Migraine headaches** are more commonly found in women and often can be associated with the hormonal cycle; however, migraines can affect both genders and often run in families. **Cluster headaches** are found predominately in the male population and can be precipitated by alcohol consumption (Seidel et al., 2003). Other possible causes of headaches are listed in Box 20-1.

History and Physical Findings

Patients with a history of persistent headaches, or who describe them as severe and recurring, should be medically evaluated. Table 20-1 compares several of the most common types of headaches. Although not all headaches require medical attention, a physician should evaluate persistent or recurring headaches. Headaches can be classified as life-threatening or non–life-threatening. Life-threatening causes of headaches include expanding intracranial masses, such as hemorrhages and tumors, and meningeal irritation. Non–life-threatening causes of headaches include tension headaches; migraine headaches; cluster headaches; and headaches associated with disorders of the eyes, facial nerve, sinuses, and cranial

BOX 20-1	**Headache: Possible Causes**

- Migraine headache
- Muscle tension
- Stress
- Subarachnoid hemorrhage
- Ear or tooth infection
- Vigorous exercise
- Meningitis
- Hypertensive emergency
- Sinusitis
- Foods (nuts, caffeine, chocolate)
- Toxic exposure
- Preeclampsia

arteries. When presented with a patient reporting a headache, the paramedic must determine whether it is life threatening or benign. When assessing a patient with a headache, determine the following:

- When was the onset? Is it new or of recent origin?

Headaches with acute or sudden onset, headaches in patients without a history of headaches, or headaches that differ from prior headaches may indicate a life-threatening condition.

- What is the location and quality of the headache?

These factors can provide clues to the cause of the headache. Headaches caused by mass lesions often are focal

TABLE 20-1	Headache Types					
Type of Headache	Age at Onset	Location	Duration	Pain Quality	Prodromal Event	Typical Gender
Classic migraine	Childhood	One side	Hours to days	Pulsating or throbbing	Well defined	Female
Common migraine	Childhood	Generalized	Hours to days	Pulsating or throbbing	Vague symptoms	Female
Cluster	Adulthood	One side	1-2 hours	Intense, burning, stabbing	Personality changes	Male
Muscular tension	Adulthood	Either side or occipital	Hours	Throbbing	None	Both equally

Modified from Seidel, H. M. (2003). *Mosby's guide to physical assessment* (5th ed.) (p. 269). St. Louis: Mosby.

in nature. Determine whether the pain is throbbing, constant, stabbing, or shooting.

- Were precipitating factors present?

Certain activities may precipitate headaches, such as stress, certain foods and beverages, or activities. Patients with a history of headaches may be able to provide past associations and patterns.

- What time of day did the headache occur?

Certain headaches occur at specific times of day. If the patient has a history of headaches, determine if this presentation follows his or her normal pattern. Variations in this pattern may indicate a new cause of the headache and warrant further evaluation and may be indicative of a life-threatening condition.

- Do any factors mitigate or worsen the headache?

Headaches caused by increasing intracranial masses often worsen with sneezing, coughing, or other activities that increase intracranial pressure. Migraine and cluster headaches often decrease with exposure to darkness or pressure application to the temporal artery. They may increase in intensity with exposure to bright light (photophobia) or loud noises. Photophobia also may be present in headaches caused by meningitis.

- Does the patient have a history of head trauma?

Cranial hemorrhages can occur months after seemingly minor head trauma.

- Does the patient have associated seizures, altered mental status, confusion, coma, or focal motor abnormalities?

Headaches associated with seizures, changes in mental status, or focal motor findings strongly indicate the presence of increased intracranial pressure or meningitis. Patients with increased intracranial pressure also may have ipsilateral pupil dilation.

- Does the patient show signs of meningeal irritation?

Headaches caused by meningitis are acute and often associated with a stiff neck, fever, and rash. Subarachnoid hemorrhages are sudden in onset, unique to the patient (i.e., they are unlike any headache the patient has ever had), and often are associated with signs of meningeal irritation.

Therapeutic Interventions

Prehospital care for headaches primarily is supportive and limited to the prompt recognition and appropriate transport of patients with headaches attributable to a life-threatening condition.

Patient and Family Education

Patients with frequent headaches should consider keeping a headache log, noting the date and time of each headache, precipitating factors, length of the headache, and any treatment that helped. This type of information can be useful during the diagnostic process.

Bell's Palsy

Etiology and Demographics

Bell's palsy is an inflammation of the facial nerve (cranial nerve VII) and is thought to be caused by the herpes simplex virus, although research has implicated other viruses including cytomegalovirus, Epstein-Barr virus, rubella, and mumps. This condition can affect an individual at any age; no one segment of the population is at higher risk than another.

History and Physical Findings

Bell's palsy has a strokelike appearance because of the marked facial drooping on the affected side. Pain may or may not be present, increasing the difficulty in differentiating it from a stroke. Bell's palsy can be differentiated from a stroke by asking the patient to talk, wrinkle the forehead, and/or evaluate the movement and strength in the extremities. Patients who have had a stroke may or may not be able to talk, they will be able to wrinkle their forehead, and they will have marked differences in the movement and strength of their extremities on one side (Figure 20-4).

Therapeutic Interventions

All patients should be sent to the hospital for further evaluation and appropriate medication. Treatment for Bell's palsy includes physical therapy, possible steroids to reduce inflammation, and antiviral medication.

Patient and Family Education

Families need to understand that recovery from this condition can be slow, and some patients may never regain complete use of the affected side of the face.

Ludwig's Angina

Etiology and Demographics

Ludwig's angina is a bacterial infection of the floor of the mouth resulting from an infection in the root of the teeth, an abscessed tooth, or an injury to the mouth. This condition is uncommon in children.

History and Physical Findings

Ludwig's angina is a marked redness and swelling of one side of the face, beginning near the base of the ear and extending down into the neck and up under the chin. Because the infection is under the tongue, swelling can push the tongue up and back, covering the airway.

Therapeutic Interventions

Ludwig's angina is a potentially life-threatening emergency and should be immediately treated in an emergency department. Treatment consists of maintaining the airway and administering antibiotics.

Patient and Family Education

Patients and families should be instructed to have their teeth checked at least annually and have all painful teeth evaluated as soon as possible by a dentist.

SPECIFIC EYE DISORDERS

[OBJECTIVES 3, 4]

Conjunctivitis

Etiology and Demographics

Conjunctivitis is the inflammation of the conjunctiva, the continuous, usually transparent tissue that extends from the inside of the upper eyelid across the eye to the lower lid. Conjunctivitis can be the result of irritation caused by debris that was inadvertently rubbed into the eye, an allergic response to pollen in the air, or an infection such as pink eye. Anyone is at risk for conjunctivitis; however, individuals who wear contact lenses may be at a slightly higher risk because of the ability of objects to get trapped under and around the lens.

History and Physical Findings

One of the first indications of conjunctivitis often is the presence of thick, sticky drainage, especially on awakening in the morning. To inspect the conjunctiva, gently pull the lower lid forward. Normal conjunctiva should appear pink and moist. With conjunctivitis, the conjunctival space appears bright red and swollen and may contain purulent drainage (Figure 20-5). Redness and swelling involving the conjunctiva are not usually associated with any other eye condition.

Therapeutic Interventions

Conjunctivitis from an infection is highly contagious. Be sure to use standard precautions. All items coming in contact with the eye should be handled carefully until washed with soap and water. The cause of the conjunctivitis dictates the type of treatment.

Patient and Family Education

Patients should be instructed to keep their hands away from the face until the condition has been diagnosed and treatment initiated.

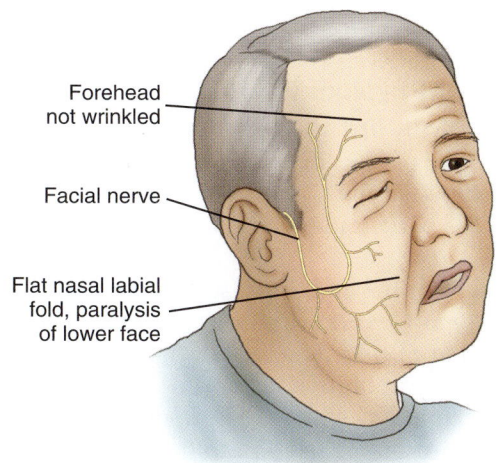

Forehead not wrinkled

Facial nerve

Flat nasal labial fold, paralysis of lower face

Figure 20-4 Bell's palsy (facial palsy).

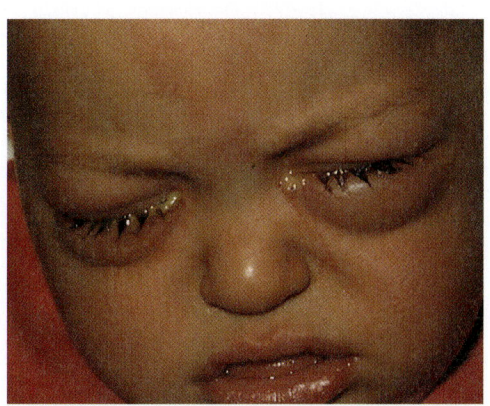

Figure 20-5 Acute bacterial conjunctivitis.

Inflammation of the Eyelids

Etiology and Demographics

Most infections of the eyelid result from bacteria. A **chalazion** is a small bump on the eyelid that results from a blocked oil gland. A **hordeolum** is a common acute infection of the glands of the eyelids. It may be internal or external. An external hordeolum is commonly called a **stye.**

History and Physical Findings

A chalazion appears red and swollen but is not usually painful unless it becomes infected (Figure 20-6). Hordeola are usually recognized as raised pustules that are often associated with swelling of the eyelid, redness, and tenderness (Figure 20-7).

Therapeutic Interventions

The patient must be seen by a physician. Warm compresses are usually applied for 10 to 15 minutes several times a day to help relieve the pain. Topical antibiotics may be prescribed. The infected gland may burst on its own, drain, and then heal.

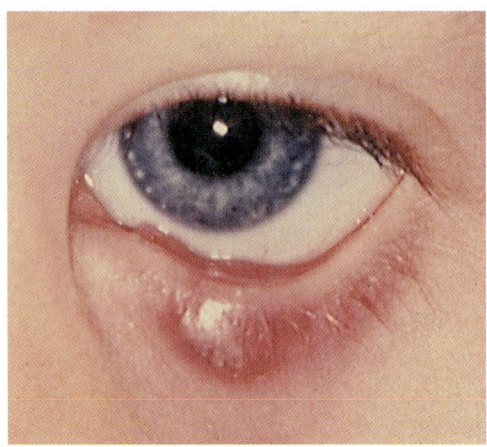

Figure 20-6 Chalazion.

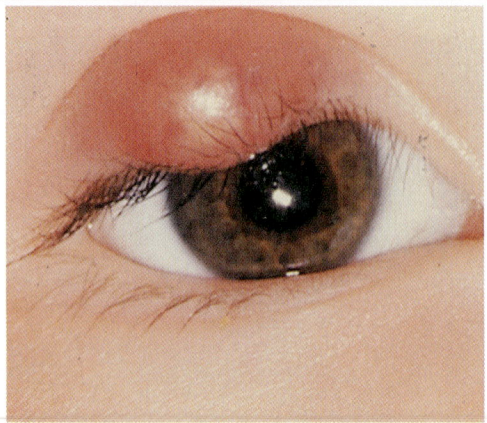

Figure 20-7 Hordeolum.

Patient and Family Education

The patient should be taught not to squeeze the lesion. Some patients may be affected by recurring hordeola. Frequent face and handwashing is helpful.

Glaucoma

Etiology and Demographics

Glaucoma is an eye disease that may cause blindness. Several types of glaucoma have been described. According to The Glaucoma Foundation, risk factors for glaucoma include the following:

- Family history
- Nearsightedness
- Previous eye injury
- Low blood pressure
- African descent
- Diabetes
- Long-term exposure to cortisone

Aqueous humor is a watery fluid produced by the eye that fills the eye's anterior chamber. This fluid normally drains through a meshlike network in the eye, through a drainage channel with a one-way valve, and then into the bloodstream. In chronic glaucoma (also called *open-angle glaucoma*), the aqueous fluid drains too slowly. Over time, pressure builds up within the eye (intraocular pressure) and damages the optic nerve. This is the most common type of glaucoma. Normal-tension glaucoma (also called *normal-pressure glaucoma*) is a type of open-angle glaucoma that can cause vision changes with no increase in intraocular pressure. In narrow-angle glaucoma (also called *angle-closure glaucoma*), access to the meshwork and drainage channel is narrowed. This prevents proper drainage of aqueous fluid. Pressure builds up in the posterior chamber of the eye, which pushes the lens forward. The lens pushes the iris into the drainage channel, completely blocking it. Secondary glaucoma occurs as a result of conditions that damage the drainage channel in the eye. Examples of these conditions include diabetes, eye injuries, leukemia, sickle cell anemia, some types of arthritis, and cataracts.

History and Physical Findings

Glaucoma usually first affects a person's peripheral vision. Eventually the patient develops tunnel vision, in which he or she can see only what is directly ahead. In chronic glaucoma the patient may have no symptoms until vision loss occurs.

A patient who has an acute attack of narrow-angle glaucoma may report severe eye pain, headache, photophobia, nausea, and vomiting. The cornea may look cloudy. The patient may report blurred vision and halos around lights because of corneal swelling. The pupils often have irregular margins and can be fixed in mid-position and dilated. An attack may be triggered by pupil dilation, such as eye drops given during an eye examination or dim lighting.

The paramedic must be familiar with these signs and symptoms because narrow-angle glaucoma is a contraindication for the administration of atropine.

Therapeutic Interventions

Acute narrow-angle glaucoma is a medical emergency. The patient needs evaluation by a physician. If intraocular pressure is not reduced, permanent vision loss can occur.

Patient and Family Education

Patients should be encouraged to have regular eye examinations. Early detection and treatment can prevent blindness.

Central Retinal Artery Occlusion

Etiology

Central retinal artery occlusion (CRAO) is a condition in which the blood supply to the retina is blocked because of a clot or embolus in the central retinal artery or one of its branches (Box 20-2). The most common cause is an embolus from the carotid artery or heart. CRAO may cause partial blindness, which may be temporary or permanent.

History and Physical Findings

The patient usually seeks medical assistance because of a sudden, painless loss of vision in one eye. If the central retinal artery is blocked, complete loss of vision in one eye usually occurs. If a branch of the central retinal artery is blocked, partial loss of vision in one eye usually occurs. In some patients symptoms may be preceded by flickering or a transient loss of vision weeks or months before the acute event.

Therapeutic Interventions

A situation involving a rapid loss of vision is an emergency. Retinal damage begins within 30 to 60 minutes of the cessation of blood flow, which can lead to permanent visual deficits. Immediately transport to the closest appropriate facility and provide supportive care en route.

Patient and Family Education

The prognosis for the return of vision is poor. Because high blood pressure can increase the risk of problems that may affect the vessels of the eye, patients must be taught to take their blood pressure medications as prescribed to keep their blood pressure under control.

Retinal Detachment

Retinal detachment is a condition in which the retina is lifted or pulled from its normal position, resulting in a loss of vision. It is a serious eye emergency that requires immediate medical attention and surgery. Three types of retinal detachment occur: rhegmatogenous, tractional, and exudative.

Rhegmatogenous retinal detachment is the most common type. It occurs when a tear or break develops in the sensory layer of the retina, allowing fluid to seep under the retina (Figure 20-8). When fluid seeps under the retina, it becomes separated from the layer of cells that provide the retina nourishment.

Tractional retinal detachment is a less-common type. It happens when scar tissue on the surface of the retina contracts, pulling it loose. This causes the retina to separate from the layer of cells that provide it nourishment.

Exudative retinal detachment occurs when no tear in the retina is present, but a tumor, injury, or disease process causes swelling or bleeding, which causes the retina to elevate. Elevation of the retina allows fluid to leak into the area underneath the retinal layers, causing the retina to separate from the back wall of the eye.

Etiology and Demographics

Nearsightedness and cataract removal surgery are the most common predisposing causes of rhegmatogenous retinal detachment. The eyes of nearsighted individuals are longer than average from front to back. This causes the retina to be thinner and more fragile, predisposing those with myopia to this type of retinal detachment. Spontaneous detachment, which is most common in patients older than 50 years, also can occur. Spontaneous detachment may be caused by changes in the vitreous humor or a result of trauma.

Patients with diabetes or sickle cell disease are more likely to experience tractional retinal detachment. Exudative retinal detachment usually occurs in individuals who have other eye diseases or disorders.

BOX 20-2	Central Retinal Artery Occlusion: Possible Causes

- Carotid artery embolus
- Valvular heart disease
- Drug abuse
- Fat emboli
- Arterial spasm
- Oral contraceptives

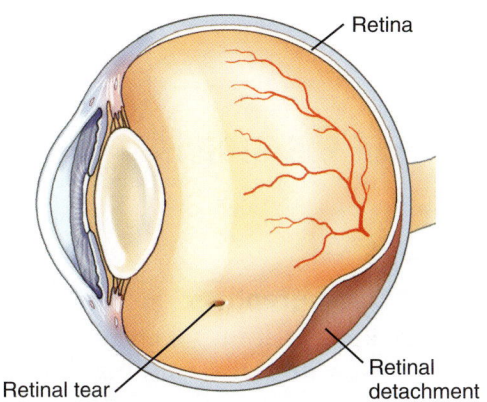

Figure 20-8 Retinal detachment.

BOX 20-3	**Retinal Detachment: Possible Signs and Symptoms**

- "Veil," "curtain," or dark shadow obstructing peripheral vision
- Blurred vision in the affected eye
- Flashes of light and "floaters" in the affected eye
- No pain or redness

History and Physical Findings

Visual changes associated with retinal detachment may be sudden or gradual. Patients usually complain of a "veil," "curtain," or dark shadow obstructing their peripheral vision. These symptoms occur because most retinal tears occur in the peripheral portion of the retina. As the detachment enlarges and extends toward the macula, the veil or curtain also enlarges and affects the patient's central vision. The patient also may complain of flashes of light or "floaters" that resemble bugs, spider webs, or spots in the affected eye. Signs and symptoms of retinal detachment are given in Box 20-3.

Therapeutic Interventions

Retinal detachment is an emergency. Although retinal reattachment is successful in 80% of cases, prolonged detachment can cause permanent visual deficits. Immediately transport the patient to the closest appropriate facility. Alert the hospital of the patient's signs and symptoms. Provide supportive care en route. On arrival at the hospital, the emergency department staff will arrange to have the patient seen by an ophthalmologist.

Patient and Family Education

The earlier the treatment of retinal detachment, the greater the chances of restoring vision. Patients at high risk of retinal detachment, such as those who are diabetic or nearsighted, should be particularly alert for visual changes. If a tear has occurred in the retina but it has not detached, a laser is sometimes used to treat the tear. The laser creates a series of burns around the tear. Scar tissue from the burns seals the retina to the underlying layers of tissue. Surgery is usually required to repair a detached retina.

SPECIFIC EAR DISORDERS

[OBJECTIVES 5, 6]

Foreign Bodies

Etiology and Demographics

The ear canal is a potential site for any number of different types of **foreign bodies**. Beans, peas, rocks, insects, screws, bolts, sticks, and packed **cerumen** (ear wax) are just a few examples of things that can be found in the ear canal.

History and Physical Findings

When evaluating patient complaints that involve a change in hearing, begin with a visual inspection of the auricle. Look for clues that might provide more information about the ear problem, such as redness, swelling, and signs of trauma. Next, move your attention to the external auditory canal. To visualize the canal better, take a pen light and gently pull the ear back to expose the front part of the canal; this will make looking for foreign or impacted objects easier.

Therapeutic Interventions

Never put anything into the ear and do not attempt to extract the foreign material. If you visualize something in the ear, instruct the patient to seek medical attention to have the ear examined.

Patient and Family Education

Parents and caregivers should be instructed to teach children to keep things away from their ears. Nothing should go in the ear smaller than an elbow.

Vertigo

Etiology and Demographics

Vertigo is as an out-of-control spinning sensation not relieved by lying down and that may get worse when the eyes are closed. Vertigo is a serious medical condition that requires evaluation and treatment. Although the exact cause of vertigo is unknown, the bones in the middle ear or the fluid in the inner ear are believed to be subjected to continuous vibrations from an unknown source. Because vertigo often comes without an associated cause, it can occur in any segment of the population.

Menière's disease and **labyrinthitis** are two possible causes of vertigo. Labyrinthitis is an inflammation in the labyrinth of the middle ear. Menière's disease is a progressive condition with an unknown etiology. Approximately 100,000 people develop Menière's disease each year (Campellone, 2004). It is a disease that damages the balance and hearing parts of the inner ear (Osborne, 2005). This disease mainly affects the white segment of the population and both males and females equally. It can occur at all ages and most frequently starts between ages of 20 and 50 years. Approximately 7% to 10% of patients with Menière's have a family history of the disease (Joseph, 2004).

History and Physical Findings

Vertigo is debilitating to those who have it. Individuals with vertigo find activities of daily living difficult to carry out; most find walking across the room or standing for prolonged periods to be difficult. Many have bouts of nausea and vomiting, and some report associated headaches. Because of the association with the inner and middle ear, vertigo has no obvious physical findings except for an inability to ambulate without assistance and nausea and vomiting. Patients with Menière's disease report progressive deafness, ringing in the ears, vertigo, and pressure in the ears.

Therapeutic Interventions

Treatment for labyrinthitis is primarily antihistamines and bed rest until the inflammation subsides. Treatment for Menière's disease usually consists of antihistamines and bed rest.

Patient and Family Education

Most people who have vertigo know what to do when they have an attack; however, for patients who have never had vertigo the situation can be frightening. Instruct families to allow the patient to lie down, keep lights off or very dim, take any prescribed medications as ordered, and be patient. Most bouts of vertigo pass within 24 hours.

Tinnitus

Etiology and Demographics

Tinnitus is described by patients as a quiet humming sound that never stops. It can be caused by allergic reactions, medications, Lyme disease, tumors or growths in the head, foreign bodies in the ear, or diseases that affect any part of the ear. As many as one in five people are affected to some degree by tinnitus. The problem is most often found in middle-aged to older patients, primarily because of their reliance on prescription and over-the-counter medications, which can combine to create the problem.

History and Physical Findings

Patients with tinnitus complain of an unrelenting ringing in one or both ears, sometimes worsening enough to cause hearing loss. As with vertigo, little or no physical findings are revealed during a patient assessment—only the symptoms presented by the patient. Most patients with vertigo also report associated tinnitus.

Therapeutic Interventions

No definitive treatment exists for tinnitus except to remove the source, if it is related to medications or a foreign body, or manage the vertigo if the conditions occur in conjunction with each other. Patients whose tinnitus is caused by a foreign body notice improvement as soon as the debris is removed. Much like vertigo, little can be done during a bout of tinnitus except to reduce auditory stress, rest, and take medications as prescribed.

Patient and Family Education

Salicylate toxicity is a common cause of tinnitus. Patients frequently do not realize the variety of medications that contain salicylate, which when used in combination can quickly reach the toxic level. In addition to aspirin and other pain relievers containing aspirin, salicylates are found in cough and cold medications, antacids, topical creams, rubbing alcohols, and many herbal remedies.

Otitis Externa

Etiology and Demographics

Otitis externa (swimmer's ear) is a condition manifested by redness and irritation of the external auditory canal. The most common time for otitis externa is the summer, when children spend many hours in swimming pools, irrigation canals, or other bodies of water. Otitis externa is not limited to children; anyone who spends time in water is at risk.

History and Physical Findings

The patient usually reports pain in the ear and may have an associated tinnitus. Examination of the ear reveals visible redness to the external canal. Patient history is consistent with recent exposure to polluted water, continuous exposure to water without drying the ear, or recent use of an object to reach into the canal.

Therapeutic Interventions

No specific treatment exists for otitis externa other than antibiotic and analgesic drops to the ear canal after otoscopic evaluation by a physician.

Patient and Family Education

Parents should be instructed to dry the auricle and external auditory canal thoroughly after each swim and avoid contact with potentially polluted water.

Case Scenario CONCLUSION

You and your partner start an intravenous line. The patient's blood glucose level is 145 mg/dL and her SpO₂ is 97% on oxygen. The cardiac monitor shows a sinus tachycardia. During transport to the hospital you learn that the patient has been in the emergency department (at a different hospital than you are transporting to) twice during the past 2 days for her severe head pain. In both cases she received pain medications (she could not remember the name) and was discharged. After clearing from the call, you and your partner consider the case and how young the patient is to have a stroke. You later learn that she was treated and released with a diagnosis of complicated migraine.

Looking Back

9. *Is evaluating this patient's blood glucose level important? Why or why not?*
10. *Given the patient's final diagnosis and disposition, was your treatment appropriate? Why or why not?*

SPECIFIC NOSE DISORDERS

[OBJECTIVES 7, 8]

Epistaxis

Etiology and Demographics

A nosebleed, or **epistaxis,** can be one of the most challenging conditions to treat. The highly vascular nature of the nose puts it at risk for a bleed after trauma, high-force sneezing, use of recreational drugs, or seemingly no reason at all. Recall from Chapter 7 the vascular nature of the turbinates. Rupture of these structures can lead to significant hemorrhage and may require posterior packing at the emergency department.

History and Physical Findings

Patients with a nosebleed may be able to relate a recent incident that initiated the epistaxis; others may not. When children present with epistaxis, consider the possibility of a foreign body in the nose, recent trauma, or nose picking. For adults the epistaxis may be related to a change in climate or medication that has severely dried the nasal passages, making them more susceptible to bleeding.

Therapeutic Interventions

To stop a nosebleed, have the patient sit down, lean forward, and spit out any blood that drains into the mouth. Pinch the nose firmly about halfway between the tip and the face for approximately 5 minutes. Repeat this process four or five times. Hospital evaluation and treatment are required for epistaxis that exceeds 15 minutes or is associated with changes in the patient's condition.

Patient and Family Education

Families can be taught this method for stopping a nosebleed but should be instructed to seek medical attention if the bleeding does not stop in 15 minutes or the patient feels worse.

Foreign Bodies

Etiology and Demographics

As with the ears, the nose is a great location to put stuff. Young children have been known to insert rocks, marbles, beans, screws, beads, and other small objects into the nose.

History and Physical Findings

Sometimes these objects can be in place for several days before someone realizes something is wrong; by then the drainage and smell have become significant.

Therapeutic Interventions

Do not remove foreign objects from the nose in the prehospital environment. Instruct the patient or guardian to take the child to the hospital, urgent care clinic, or physician's office for treatment.

Patient and Family Education

Families and care providers should be instructed to watch small children at play and teach older children that the nose and ears are not safe places to put objects of any kind.

Piercing

Etiology

Nose piercings in the lower third of the nose probably do not result in a significant problem other than a potential for infection. Piercings in the respiratory region of the nose put the patient at risk for significant bleeding if one of the turbinates is pierced during the procedure.

History and Physical Findings

When assessing the patient, be sure to look at all piercing sites to make sure the skin is healthy and no redness, drainage, or bleeding is present. When not inserted under proper conditions or appropriately cared for, piercings can become a source of serious infection or abscess.

Therapeutic Interventions

Patients with an infected piercing site should receive supportive care during transport. Definitive care consists of removal of the jewelry, a tetanus shot if indicated, and antibiotics.

Patient and Family Education

Families and friends should encourage anyone interested in having body piercing to have it done at a licensed jewelry store, tattoo shop, or clinic; this should help avoid the possibility of improper technique.

Rhinitis

Etiology and Demographics

Rhinitis (runny nose) is the fate of anyone with environmental allergies. Under most circumstances this type of drainage should be clear. If the drainage is laced with blood or discolored in any way, it can be a sign of a more serious problem that requires an evaluation by a physician.

History and Physical Findings

Initial assessment of these patients should include a history of recent environmental exposures, changes in talc or powder used on the body, or exposures in the workplace to toxic materials. In young children rhinitis often precedes tooth eruption and may be associated with a slight fever. In school-age children, it is usually a combination of environmental allergies and an ongoing viral infection. In children always consider the possibility of a foreign body in the nose if the rhinitis has been continuous for more than 2 days and occasionally contains a small amount of blood.

Therapeutic Interventions

Prehospital care for rhinitis is primarily supportive.

Patient and Family Education

Educating children regarding the insertion of objects into the nose should be the focus of discussion with parents and care providers.

SPECIFIC MOUTH DISORDERS

[OBJECTIVES 9, 10]

Thrush

Etiology and Demographics

Newborns and very young children are susceptible to a variety of infections that do not normally affect an older child or adult. One of these infections is **thrush,** a fungal infection of the mouth.

History and Physical Findings

Thrush is characterized by white, scaly patches on the tongue and inside the mouth and throat that can become ulcers if left untreated. A fever and nausea, vomiting, and diarrhea can be associated with this infection. Thrush can be differentiated from milk residue by scraping lightly on the patch. Milk will scrape away easily, and thrush will remain.

Therapeutic Interventions

Once confirmed by the physician, treatment for thrush includes an antifungal medication.

Patient and Family Education

If an infant has thrush and is breastfeeding, the infant and mother will most likely be treated with antifungal medications by a physician. In this way, the likelihood of passing the infection back and forth is decreased. If an infant has thrush and is being fed from a bottle, the caregivers should be taught to wash and rinse nipples and pacifiers every day until the infection is gone.

Broken, Missing, or Lost Teeth

Etiology and Demographics

Children are by far the most likely group to have lost, broken, or missing teeth because of their active lifestyle, but tooth conditions can occur at any age and under a variety of circumstances.

History and Physical Findings

During the examination of the mouth, if a tooth is found broken or unexpectedly missing, ask the patient how the incident occurred. Determine whether the tooth could have been aspirated into the lung. Patients who present with a tooth that has unexpectedly fallen out, usually because of trauma, should first be assessed for injury to the face, jaw, or head. Once the face has been determined to be intact or that no immediate emergency exists, then evaluate the tooth and tooth socket.

Therapeutic Interventions

The best treatment for teeth that have fallen out is to rinse the tooth in clean water and reinsert it into the socket. This should be done under the instructions of medical direction and only if the patient is alert. Replacing the tooth helps preserve the tooth, and it may heal over time. If it is not possible to put the tooth back into the socket, then place the tooth in milk or an appropriate "tooth saver" solution as quickly as possible. Transport the avulsed tooth and solution in an appropriate container to the hospital with the patient.

Patient and Family Education

Parents or care providers should be instructed in how to clean and salvage a tooth as well as to monitor their children's activities to reduce traumatic injuries.

Sore Throat

Etiology and Demographics

Viral infections, bacterial infections, breathing through the mouth, and moderate drainage from the nose are only a few of the potential causes of a **sore throat.** For the most part, a sore throat is not an emergent situation. With patience, rest, and plenty of fluids it will resolve over time.

History and Physical Findings

When assessing a patient with a sore throat, begin by evaluating his or her general condition and look for signs of a systemic infection, which usually include fever, general malaise, poor appetite, and possibly a runny nose. Evaluate the degree of discomfort that accompanies swallowing. Examining the throat is not necessary in the prehospital environment.

Therapeutic Interventions

The complaint of sore throat in conjunction with the presentation of a systemic infection and difficulty swallowing is sufficient to warrant an evaluation by a physician at a hospital or clinic.

Patient and Family Education

Instruct patients or families to encourage fluids, whatever the individual will tolerate, and complete all medication provided by the physician.

Epiglottitis

Etiology and Demographics

At the extreme end of the sore throat range is **epiglottitis,** an inflammation of the epiglottis. This is a true emergency that requires immediate transport, in the position of comfort, to the closest facility. The epiglottis is the leaflet-like structure that sits at the opening of the trachea. When it becomes infected and swollen, it can block the airway and result in death. Epiglottitis occurs most frequently in the winter months during cold and flu season, and the most common age group affected is children. However, it can be seen in adults as well.

History and Physical Findings

Patients with epiglottitis have a high-pitched, croupy cough, drool excessively, and sit in a tripod position. Assessment of a suspected case of epiglottitis should begin with a general assessment of the patient. These patients appear acutely ill ("toxic appearance") and sit in the classic tripod position. The history of the present illness will reveal a sudden onset of a high fever and cold or flulike symptoms with coughing and drooling (Figure 20-9).

Therapeutic Interventions

No prehospital treatment is available for epiglottitis except supportive measures during transport. Take care not to agitate these patients. Under no circumstances does a paramedic need to look in the mouth or throat of an individual with a suspected case of epiglottitis. Placing anything in the mouth will result in spasm and total occlusion of the airway. Because of the inflammation of the epiglottis, obtaining an airway will be extremely difficult, if not impossible. Many patients with epiglottitis are taken to the operating room for placement of a temporary tracheostomy to prevent loss of the airway. Once the diagnosis is made, often with a soft tissue radiograph of the neck, patients are started on appropriate antibiotics.

Patient and Family Education

Parents and care providers can do little to prevent epiglottitis except to understand the need for immediate medical care if it occurs again. Calm reassurance is needed.

Peritonsillar Abscess

Because the role of the tonsils is to collect bacteria for destruction by the body, they can easily become a potential source of significant infection. The result of a significant infection in the tonsils is called a **peritonsillar abscess.**

Etiology and Demographics

This condition occurs in children but is more common in adults, especially persons with a history of recurrent tonsillitis.

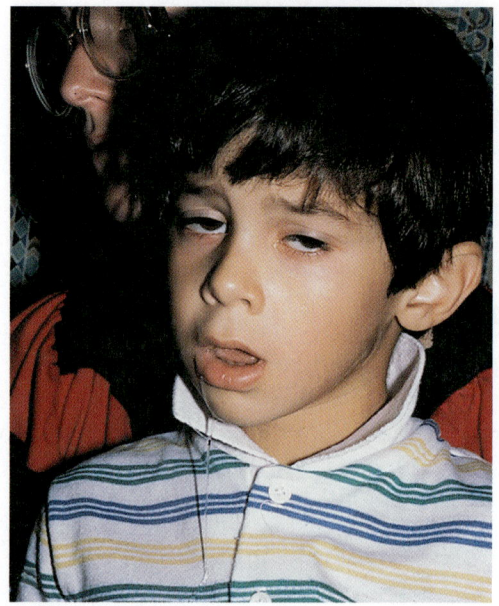

Figure 20-9 Epiglottitis. This 5 year old has been symptomatic for hours. Note the head held forward, mouth breathing, and drooling.

History and Physical Findings

Patients with a peritonsillar abscess describe a sore throat that continued to worsen until swallowing became quite difficult. Differentiating a peritonsillar abscess from epiglottitis is not easy. Both manifest with drooling and general malaise, but patients with epiglottitis have a cough and sit in the classic tripod position. Looking at the back of the throat is not necessary.

Therapeutic Interventions

Although these patients will not develop a potentially life-threatening airway occlusion, they can easily gag or choke, rupturing the abscess and aspirating infected material into the lungs. Allow these patients to assume a position of comfort for transport. Treatment includes opening and draining the abscess and administering antibiotic therapy by hospital personnel.

Patient and Family Education

As with epiglottitis, little can be done to prevent the development of a peritonsillar abscess, but parents and family members can be advised to watch children and young adults for early signs of infection.

Case Scenario SUMMARY

1. *What is your general impression of this patient?* Although this patient clearly merits treatment and transport, her mental status, respiratory effort, and cardiovascular system appear stable. However, cerebral ischemia is a time-sensitive condition, so her evaluation, treatment, and transportation should be rapid.

2. *What conditions might cause these symptoms?* Several conditions come to mind, including migraine headache,

cerebrovascular accident, transient ischemic attack, or cerebral aneurysm. Differentiation among these conditions, although not essential to initial treatment, can primarily be made through the history and neurologic examination.

3. *What treatment should be immediately initiated?* Oxygen is important because several of the conditions under consideration are primarily hypoxic events.

4. *Has your general impression of this patient changed after a more complete examination? Why or why not?* The general impression that the patient is stable has not changed. However, additional information has provided insight about potential causes of the patient's condition.

5. *This patient is reporting a headache and "bright flashes of light." What condition(s) frequently present in this way?* These symptoms are fairly classic for migraine headache. Unfortunately, they do not enable you to rule out any of the more serious causes, such as cerebrovascular accident or aneurysm, so treatment still must be based on the more severe conditions.

6. *How does the Cincinnati Stroke Scale influence your treatment plan for this patient?* Her abnormal Cincinnati Stroke Scale score does not directly affect prehospital treatment. However, because 72% of patients with an abnormal Cincinnati Stroke Scale score are having a cerebrovascular accident, it should drive you to keep your scene time short. In addition, in some communities patients with abnormal stroke scale scores are transported to designated hospitals.

7. *This woman is 36 years old and is experiencing dysphasia and one-sided weakness. What do you think her fears might be? How could you help?* Most people have seen depictions of strokes on television or have had a family member who has had a stroke that may have included dysphasia and/or motor impairment. She may fear she is having a stroke and is considering her life with permanent neurologic impairment. You can provide reassurance by keeping her informed about what you are doing and what will happen next. In addition, you can assure her that these symptoms have causes other than stroke.

8. *What additional treatment should be provided?* In addition to oxygen, this patient should receive intravenous access, cardiac monitoring, and rapid transport to an appropriate facility.

9. *Is evaluating this patient's blood glucose level important? Why or why not?* Yes. Hypoglycemia can sometimes cause focal neurologic findings such as those experienced by this patient. However, blood glucose levels above normal also are associated with a poor outcome from stroke or head trauma. You should evaluate the patient's blood glucose level and, if it is below normal, consider administration of IV glucose. Do not give glucose if the level is normal or elevated.

10. *Given the patient's final diagnosis and disposition, was your treatment appropriate? Why or why not?* The paramedics in this case had never encountered a patient with migraine headaches who had focal neurologic deficits (complicated migraine) and assumed the patient was having a transient ischemic attack or cerebrovascular accident. Despite their "wrong" field impression, their treatment was perfect: oxygen, intravenous access, cardiac monitoring, evaluation of the blood sugar level, and rapid transport to an appropriate facility.

Chapter Summary

Head

- Inspection and palpation are the primary ways to evaluate the structures of the head. Because of the vascular nature of this area, bleeding may be greater than the seriousness of the wound. Evaluate and reassure as needed. Both sides of the face should appear somewhat symmetric on inspection. Gross deformities or a droop on one side should be further evaluated. Gross deformities of the face are typically the result of trauma. A droop on one side of the face, however, can be caused by several different illnesses. Elicit a good history to assist in the decision-making process.

Eyes

- The oval-shaped eyeballs sit in bony orbital cavities. The bones of the orbits are thin and susceptible to fracture from blunt force trauma. Assessment of the eye should primarily consist of inspection. Look for drainage, redness, movement through the fields of gaze, pupil size, and response to light. Whenever something being splashed into the eye is suspected, immediately begin flushing the eye and continue flushing until instructed to stop by medical staff.

Chapter Summary—continued

Ears

- The external auditory canal should always be dry; any signs of drainage should be referred for further medical care. The tympanic membrane is located at the end of the auditory canal and serves as a barrier between the external and internal ear.

Nose

- The primary function of the nose is to filter, warm, and humidify incoming air before it gets to the lungs. The nose also houses the nerves that allow smell. Common problems with the nose usually involve foreign objects. Patient should be referred for removal and further medical care.

Mouth

- Assessment of the mouth requires visualization of the internal structures. Having the patient open the mouth should be adequate. Never put anything in the mouth.
- Patients with hoarseness, stridor on inspiration or expiration, or drooling should be kept quiet and allowed to assume a position that facilitates breathing during transport. These signs suggest a possible life-threatening condition.

REFERENCES

Campellone, J. (2004). *Menière's disease*. Retrieved November 29, 2007, from http://www.nlm.nih.gov.

Osborne, G. (2005). *About Menière's disease*. Retrieved November 7, 2005, from http://www.menieres.org.uk.

Seidel, H. M., Ball, J. W., Dains, J. E., & Benedict, G. W. (2003). *Mosby's guide to physical examination* (5th ed.) (pp. 251-355). St. Louis: Mosby.

SUGGESTED RESOURCES

American Academy of Ophthalmology. (2002). *Important facts about eye injuries*. Retrieved November 29, 2007, from http://www.medem.com.

Drake, R. L., Vogl, W., & Mitchell, A. W. M. (2005). *Gray's anatomy for students* (pp. 747-1030). Philadelphia: Elsevier.

Feinberg, E. B. (2004). *Retinal detachment*. Retrived November 29, 2007, from http://www.nlm.nih.gov.

Sherwood, L. (2004). *Human physiology: From cells to systems* (5th ed.). Belmont, CA: Brooks/Cole.

The Glaucoma Foundation
80 Maiden Lane, Suite 1206
New York, NY 10038
Phone: 212-285-0080
Website: http://www.glaucomafoundation.org

Mayo Clinic
4500 San Pablo Road
Jacksonville, FL 32224
Phone: 904-953-2000
Website: http://www.mayoclinic.com

Medline Plus
U.S. National Library of Medicine
8600 Rockville Pike
Bethesda, MD 20894
Website: http://www.medlineplus.gov

Chapter Quiz

1. The aqueous humor _____.
   a. cannot be replaced if lost
   b. fills the anterior chamber of the eye
   c. flows between the anterior and posterior cavity
   d. is a thick, jellylike substance

2. A constant humming in the ears is called _____.
   a. epistaxis
   b. labyrinthitis
   c. tinnitus
   d. tympani

3. With this infectious process the airway can quickly become occluded by the tongue.
   a. Ludwig's angina
   b. Menière's disease
   c. Otitis externa
   d. Peritonsillar abscess

4. Which of the following statements about lice is correct?
   a. Lice most commonly infect adults of middle age.
   b. Lice are highly transmittable from person to person through close contact.
   c. Lice appear as flakes on the scalp and fall off when the hair is parted.
   d. A patient who has lice should wear a mask to prevent transmission of the insects to health care personnel.

5. Bell's palsy _____.
   a. is an inflammation of the optic nerve
   b. often is preceded by a viral upper respiratory tract infection
   c. may lead to blindness if it is not rapidly treated
   d. requires long-term hospitalization and antibiotic therapy

6. Which of the following is the most accurate statement regarding impetigo?
   a. It causes systemic effects.
   b. It is caused by a virus.
   c. It is not easily spread.
   d. It is treated with antibiotics.

7. List at least three risk factors for glaucoma.

_____

_____

_____

8. Which type of retinal detachment is most commonly associated with a tumor or trauma?
   a. Exudative
   b. Occlusive
   c. Rhegmatogenous
   d. Tractional

9. Which of the following is true regarding thrush?
   a. It is a fungal infection.
   c. It often affects the elderly.
   b. It is treated with antibiotics.
   d. It produces no systemic response.

10. Which of the following also is referred to as "swimmer's ear"?
   a. Labyrinthitis
   b. Otitis externa
   c. Rhinitis
   d. Tinnitus

Terminology

Bell's palsy An inflammation of the facial nerve (cranial nerve VII) that is thought to be caused by the herpes simplex virus.

Central retinal artery occlusion (CRAO) A condition in which the blood supply to the retina is blocked because of a clot or embolus in the central retinal artery or one of its branches.

Cerumen Earwax.

Cluster headache A migraine-like condition characterized by attacks of intense unilateral pain. The pain occurs most often over the eye and forehead and is accompanied by flushing and watering of the eyes and nose. The attacks occur in groups, with a duration of several hours.

Chalazion A small bump on the eyelid caused by a blocked oil gland.

Conjunctivitis Inflammation of the conjunctiva.

Epiglottitis An inflammation of the epiglottis.

Epistaxis Bloody nose.

Exudate Drainage from a vesicle or pustule.

Foreign body Any object or substance found in an organ or tissue where it does not belong under normal circumstances.

Glaucoma Increased intraocular pressure caused by a disruption in the normal production and drainage of aqueous humor; causes are often unknown.

Headache A pain in the head from any cause.

Hordeolum A common acute infection of the glands of the eyelids.

Impetigo A highly contagious infection caused by staphylococcal or streptococcal bacteria.

Labyrinthitis An inflammation of the structures in the inner ear.

Lesions A wound, injury, or pathologic change in body tissue; any visible, local abnormality of the tissues of the skin, such as a wound, sore, rash, or boil.

Lice Wingless insects that live in human hair.

Ludwig's angina A bacterial infection of the floor of the mouth resulting from an infection in the root of the teeth, an abscessed tooth, or an injury to the mouth.

Malaise General feeling of illness without any specific symptoms.

Migraine headache A recurring vascular headache characterized by unilateral onset, severe pain, sensitivity to light, and autonomic disturbances during the acute phase, which may last for hours or days.

Otitis externa A condition manifested by redness and irritation of the external auditory canal. Also called *swimmer's ear*.

Peritonsillar abscess An infection of tissue between the tonsil and pharynx, usually the result of a significant infection in the tonsils.

Retinal detachment A condition in which the retina is lifted or pulled from its normal position, resulting in a loss of vision.

Rhinitis Runny nose; inflammation of the mucous membranes of the nose, usually accompanied by swelling of the mucosa and nasal discharge.

Sore throat Any inflammation of the larynx, pharynx, or tonsils.

Stye An external hordeolum.

Swimmer's ear See *Otitis externa*.

Thrush A fungal infection of the mouth.

Tinnitus Ringing in the ears.

Vertigo An out-of-control spinning sensation not relieved by lying down that may get worse when the eyes are closed.

Pulmonology

Objectives *After completing this chapter, you will be able to:*

1. Explain the importance of the respiratory tract and the prevalence of pulmonary disease.
2. Explain the basic role of pulmonary diagnostic testing in medical care.
3. Identify the anatomy of the upper airway.
4. Describe the etiology, epidemiology, history, and physical findings, and develop a treatment plan for a patient having any of the following upper airway disorders: upper respiratory tract infection, epiglottitis, croup, bacterial tracheitis, and peritonsillar abscess.
5. Describe the etiology, epidemiology, history, and physical findings, and develop a treatment plan for a patient having any of the following situations: upper airway obstruction, trauma, and tracheostomy.
6. Describe the etiology, epidemiology, history, and physical findings, and develop a treatment plan for a patient having any of the following disorders of the pleura, mediastinum, lung, and chest wall: costochondritis, pleurisy, pneumomediastinum, pneumothorax, pleural effusion,

noncardiogenic pulmonary edema, and acute respiratory distress syndrome.
7. Identify the anatomy of the lower airway.
8. Describe the etiology, epidemiology, history, and physical findings, and develop a treatment plan for a patient having any of the following lower airway disorders: asthma, bronchiolitis, bronchopulmonary dysplasia, chronic obstructive pulmonary disease, cystic fibrosis, pneumonia, lung abscess, pulmonary thromboembolism, hyperventilation syndrome, atelectasis, and tumors.
9. Describe the etiology, epidemiology, history, and physical findings, and develop a treatment plan for a patient having a pulmonary infection such as pneumonia, tuberculosis, or aspiration pneumonia.
10. Describe the etiology, epidemiology, history, and physical findings, and develop a treatment plan for environmental and occupational exposure to inhaled agents and irritants, gases, fumes, and vapors.

Chapter Outline

Approach to the Patient
The Upper Airway
Disorders of the Pleura, Mediastinum, and
   Chest Wall

The Lower Airway
Nontraumatic Diseases of the Lung
Ventilator Management
Chapter Summary

Case Scenario

You and your partner are called to a trailer park for a "woman who has fallen." On arrival you find a conscious and alert 68-year-old woman who fell in the bathroom 24 hours before your arrival and was found by her daughter-in-law who came to pick her up for church. The patient informs you that she has had diarrhea for the past 3 days and apologizes for her (significant) incontinence of stool. She is oriented and is pale and warm to the touch with cyanotic nail beds. Her respiratory rate is rapid and deep, although she has no visible respiratory distress, and her pulse is rapid and thready.

Questions

1. What is your general impression of this patient?
2. What are some possible causes of this patient's pallor, cyanosis, and tachypnea?
3. What history questions or physical assessment procedures would be most useful in differentiating between the conditions you listed in question 2?
4. What intervention should you initiate at this time?

[OBJECTIVE 1]

The respiratory tract is the primary means of gaseous exchange for the body. It is also a means to expel waste and balance blood and body chemistry. Respiratory

diseases, including chronic disease, were the fourth leading cause of death in the United States in 2002. Respiratory disease was exceeded only by heart disease, cancer, and stroke and accounted for almost 123,000 deaths in 1 year alone (National Vital Statistics Report, 2005).

One of the most important skills you can provide as a paramedic is to establish and maintain the patient's airway to provide ventilation. Your mastery of these skills can mean the difference between life and death for your patients. You must be able to recognize life-threatening illnesses rapidly. Moreover, you must be able to manage the airway and pulmonary functions expediently.

Diseases of the respiratory tract can be divided into two broad categories: those that affect the upper airway and those that affect the lower airway. Problems with the upper airway often involve obstruction of delivery of air to the lungs. Examples of diseases that affect the upper airway include epiglottitis, croup, and bacterial tracheitis. Below the glottis is the lower airway. Diseases of the lower airway often involve impairment of the ability to deliver oxygen to the bloodstream by either preventing sufficient oxygen from reaching the alveoli or by disrupting oxygen movement across the alveolar membrane. Examples include pneumonia, pneumothorax, and pulmonary edema. Regardless of the location of the disorder, pulmonary dysfunction is generally the result of interference with ventilation, diffusion, perfusion, or a combination of these conditions. Interference with ventilation can result from obstruction of the upper airway or lower airway, impairment of the chest wall, or interference with the neurologic control of respiration. Interference with diffusion of oxygen and carbon dioxide to and from the bloodstream can result from insufficient atmospheric oxygen, destruction of the alveoli, destruction of the capillary beds, or pulmonary edema. Interference in perfusion can be caused by hypovolemia, anemia, or impaired circulation.

Many causes of disease in the pulmonary tract exist, and all can have potentially life-threatening consequences. The initial management of more severe cases frequently falls to EMS. EMTs and paramedics often are the first skilled medical professionals to encounter and assess the patient. Thus aggressive airway management and support can reduce long-term complications and avoid catastrophic injuries or death.

APPROACH TO THE PATIENT

The overall approach to the patient with respiratory symptoms is much like the approach to any patient with a medical complaint. As with any scene the safety of responding personnel is paramount. Respiratory emergencies can be caused by a lack of oxygen or presence of toxins in the atmosphere. The paramedic must ensure the environment is safe and call specialized teams as necessary to make this determination and/or make the scene safe for entry.

Primary Assessment

After ensuring an open airway, immediately treat any existing life threats involving the respiratory system before performing additional assessments. Indicators of life-threatening respiratory distress include alterations in mental status, dyspnea at rest, severe cyanosis, absent breath sounds, audible stridor or other adventitious breath sounds, severe difficulty in speaking, tachycardia, pallor and diaphoresis, the presence of **retractions,** or the use of accessory muscles.

History

Once any life threats have been addressed, the focus shifts to the chief complaint, history, and physical examination. The chief complaint often includes dyspnea, an abnormal awareness of one's breathing, and chest pain. A thorough history of the complaint is necessary to determine the cause of the respiratory distress so appropriate treatment can be performed. Determine when the event started; activities at the onset; prior episodes and diagnoses; comparison of this episode to prior episodes; past treatments, including intubation; medical history; medications and compliance; allergies; and the presence of associated signs and symptoms. Ask about episodes of orthopnea or paroxysmal nocturnal dyspnea. Assess for the presence of signs of infection such as fever, chills, or a cough. If a cough is present, determine whether it is productive or nonproductive. If productive, determine the color and consistency of the sputum. Thick green or brown sputum suggests infection and/or pneumonia, whereas yellow or pale-gray sputum may be related to an allergic or inflammatory response. Frank hemoptysis indicates tuberculosis or carcinoma, and pink frothy sputum is associated with severe pulmonary edema. Disease-specific findings are presented later in this chapter.

Physical Examination

Perform an overall evaluation of the patient. The position of the patient can provide valuable clues to the cause of the respiratory distress. Patients with reactive airway disease often sit in a tripod position to maximize airflow through the lower airways, whereas patients with pulmonary edema typically sit straight up with their feet dangling. Assess the patient's mental status. Hypoxia and/or hypercarbia can cause confusion, restlessness, irritability, lethargy, or coma. Indicators of respiratory compromise include the inability to complete sentences, the use of accessory muscles in the respiratory effort, and pursed lips on exhalation. Exaggerated chest movement with minimal air movement and tracheal tugging suggests an upper airway obstruction. Make note of the color and condition of the patient's skin. Cyanosis, pallor, and diaphoresis are indicators of respiratory distress.

Evaluate the patient's vital signs. Patients in respiratory distress are often tachycardic; however, bradycardia is associated with severe hypoxia and may indicate imminent cardiac arrest. In general, the blood pressure remains unchanged in respiratory distress; however, associated diseases may cause an increase or decrease in blood pressure. For example, patients with respiratory distress from congestive heart failure are often hypertensive. The respiratory rate must be closely monitored. Slowing respirations may be a sign of improvement or a sign of fatigue and respiratory failure. A decreased respiratory rate associated with an increased mental status, increased ability to speak, or other improvement in the patient's presentation indicates an improvement in the patient's overall condition. Conversely, slowing respirations in the setting of decreased mental status, absence of breath sounds, increased difficulty in speaking, and worsening skin color indicate decompensation and require prompt intervention and treatment.

In addition to the respiratory rate, also evaluate the quality and pattern of the respirations. Respirations may be regular, irregular, shallow, deep, fast, slow, or absent.

Evaluate the shape of the chest. An increased antero-posterior diameter indicates chronic obstructive pulmonary disease. Further evaluate for signs of trauma, retractions, expansion, effort, and symmetry. Auscultate breath sounds, making note of both normal and adventitious breathing as described in Chapter 17.

In addition to assessing skin color, evaluate the extremities for clubbing, carpopedal spasms, and edema. Clubbing is the result of chronic hypoxia and is considered present when the angle at which the fingernail meets the eponychium (cuticle) is greater than 180 degrees. Hypocapnia can cause spasms of the hands, fingers, feet, and toes, which are referred to as *carpopedal spasms*. Edema of the extremities and jugular venous distension are evidence of venous engorgement with blood that cannot return to the right heart. This can be caused by a failing right ventricle or compression of the heart, such as occurs with a mediastinal shift in a **tension pneumothorax.** The presence of dependent edema depends on the position of the patient and which parts of the body are dependent. Patients who are primarily upright exhibit edema in the lower extremities; patients who are primarily supine exhibit edema in the lower back and buttocks.

Diagnostic Testing

[OBJECTIVE 2]
A variety of diagnostic tools are available to the paramedic to evaluate the patient in respiratory distress as well as the effectiveness of treatment. These tools include pulse oximetry, peak flow meters, and capnography.

Pulse Oximetry

The concepts of pulse oximetry were introduced in Chapter 14. Recall that the normal partial pressure of oxygen (PaO_2) of the arterial blood is 80 to 100 mm Hg, representing the pressure exerted by oxygen in the blood. However, this is not what is represented by the pulse oximeter reading. Pulse oximetry is a reflection of the percentage of bound hemoglobin and, as a result, cannot be greater than 100%. Typical values are between 95% and 100%. Because PaO_2 is a measurement of the pressure exerted by the oxygen in the blood (measured in millimeters of mercury [mm Hg]), it can be greater than 100.

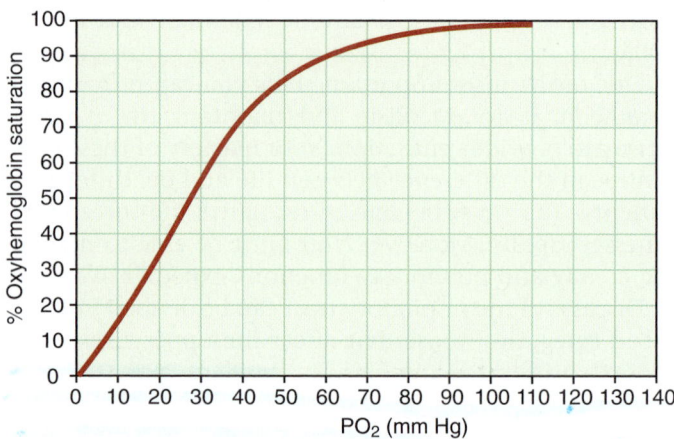

Figure 21-1 Oxyhemoglobin dissociation curve.

The oxyhemoglobin dissociation curve represents the relation between these two factors (Figure 21-1). Venous blood has a PaO_2 of 40 mm Hg, and when the PaO_2 is between 10 and 60 mm Hg oxygen readily binds with hemoglobin. This accounts for the steep climb in oxygen saturation. However, once the PaO_2 reaches 60 mm Hg the hemoglobin is approximately 90% saturated. Further increases in the PaO_2 have minimal effect on oxygen saturation past this point, accounting for the plateau on the curve. Recall from Chapter 7 that left, or alkalotic, shifts in the curve cause an increased affinity of hemoglobin for oxygen, whereas right, or acidotic, shifts cause a decrease in the affinity of hemoglobin for oxygen. These normal shifts are responsible for the efficient diffusion of oxygen from the lungs to the blood and from the blood to the cells.

Peak Flow Meters

Pulmonary function testing determines the amount of air a person can move with each breath after maximal inhalation and maximal exhalation. Several measurements can be made during this process, one of which is maximal expiratory flow. The maximal expiratory flow is a function of lung elasticity, lung volume, and bronchial resistance to airflow. As the lungs empty the maximal expiratory flow will decrease until only the residual volume is left in the lungs and the flow of air stops. The highest flow rate reached during this process is the peak expiratory flow rate (PEFR), which can be measured in liters per minute with a peak expiratory flow meter. In reactive airway diseases the maximal expiratory flow rate, as a result the PEFR, is significantly reduced from increased resistance on exhalation. Knowing the pretreatment PEFR can help the paramedic determine improvement or decompensation of the patient after treatment is administered.

Measurement of PEFR requires a patient who is capable of performing a maximal inhalation followed by a maximal exhalation. Ask the patient to inhale as deeply as possible and then exhale, as though inflating a balloon through the peak flow meter. This action causes an indicator on the device to move upward, showing the peak flow during the exhalation. Note this result, which is provided in liters per minute. The test is performed three times and the highest peak flow is recorded. Several charts, tables, and formulas are available to determine normal PEFR for the patient. These values are based on combinations of height, age, and gender. However, several studies have shown that abnormalities of the PEFR do not necessarily correlate to the severity of the reactive airway disease exacerbation. Therefore their use is most beneficial in determining a baseline for the individual patient and for comparing subsequent posttreatment results. Increases in PEFR indicate an improvement in the patient's condition, whereas decreases in PEFR indicate a worsening condition.

Capnography

Capnography is an adjunct for confirming the placement of advanced airway devices (see Chapter 14). However, this function is only a small portion of the benefits of continually monitoring exhaled carbon dioxide (CO_2).

The production and exhalation of CO_2 are functions of both ventilation and perfusion. In brief, ventilation must be adequate to allow the inhalation of adequate amounts of oxygen, which ultimately is diffused to the red blood cells. Perfusion must be adequate to deliver the oxygen to the cells and return CO_2 to the lungs, where ventilation again must be adequate to allow exhalation of CO_2. Although the pulse oximeter measurements provide information regarding oxygenation, capnography provides information about ventilation and perfusion. When changes occur in exhaled CO_2 levels the paramedic must first ensure ventilations are adequate. If impaired ventilation is not the cause of the change, then the status of the patient's perfusion must be investigated.

Recall that the waveform associated with capnography is divided into four phases. Phase I of the waveform occurs during the beginning of exhalation when air from the anatomic dead space is being exhaled. Because this air contains undetectable amounts of CO_2, the wave does not move from the baseline. During phase II, CO_2 from the larger bronchi begins to pass the sensor, resulting in the expiratory upslope. This represents a sharp increase in the concentration of CO_2 passing the sensor and results in a rapid departure of the waveform from the baseline. Phase III, or the alveolar plateau, results from CO_2-rich alveolar air passing the sensor. Phase 0 indicates the end of exhalation and the beginning of inhalation in which the levels of CO_2 passing the sensor quickly drop to zero, resulting in a quick return of the waveform to the baseline.

Changes in the morphologic features of any of these phases or in the end-tidal CO_2 ($ETCO_2$) occur when the respiratory system is impaired. The vertical axis of the waveform represents the amount of CO_2 exhaled with each breath (measured in millimeters of mercury [mm Hg]), and the horizontal axis represents the time of the exhalation. Use a methodical approach when interpreting the CO_2 waveform. Determine the presence of CO_2, the morphologic features of the waveform, and the $ETCO_2$ (Figure 21-2).

Phase II should depart rapidly from the baseline (phase I) and essentially be a vertical line. The junction of phase II and phase III should be roughly a 90-degree angle, and phase III should be a flat line that may be straight or angled slightly upward. The junction of phase III and phase 0 should essentially be a 90-degree angle, and phase 0 should be a straight line that rapidly returns to the baseline.

Variations in the capnogram can exist with normal alterations in respiration or by speaking, which causes slight changes in inhalation and exhalation with the formation of words. Alterations that are repetitive and consistent—that is, they appear in the same place in every waveform—require investigation.

Prolongation of the expiratory phase, such as in bronchoconstriction, causes phase III to become lengthened. In this situation the angle between phase II and phase III is lost, resulting in a combination of the two phases on the waveform. Often referred to as a *shark fin waveform* because of the similarity to the dorsal fin of a shark, this is the result of the constant increase in the amount of exhaled CO_2 rather than a constant level being increased. The $ETCO_2$ can help determine if the bronchoconstriction is acute or chronic. In an acute setting the $ETCO_2$ level will be normal or near normal; however, as the condition progresses, this level will increase as a result of retention of CO_2. In the setting of chronic bronchoconstriction CO_2 levels generally are increased as a result of longstanding CO_2 retention.

Several other variations in morphologic characteristics of the capnogram are possible. A CO_2-rich environment can cause a baseline that does not begin and end at 0 mm Hg, and an elevating baseline and $ETCO_2$ can indicate the rebreathing of CO_2. Abnormalities of phase 0 indicate problems with inhalation. Any consistent variation in the morphologic features of the capnogram should be investigated.

In addition to the features of the capnogram, the $ETCO_2$ can provide valuable information to the paramedic. Normal $ETCO_2$ levels are 33 to 43 mm Hg and in most cases are direct reflections of $PaCO_2$ levels, which are normally 35 to 45 mm Hg. The difference of 2 mm Hg is attributable to gas exchange laws and the presence of atmospheric CO_2. Causes of a decreased CO_2 include hyperventilation, hypoperfusion, metabolic acidosis, decreased metabolism, pulmonary embolism, or any other condition that causes an increase in ventilations, a decrease in the ability of CO_2 to enter the alveoli, or decreases in perfusion. Increased CO_2 levels are generally the result of a state of hypoventilation but also may be caused by hypermetabolic states.

THE UPPER AIRWAY

[OBJECTIVE 3]

Anatomy of the Upper Airway

The pulmonary tree is typically divided into two broad categories: the upper airway and lower airway. The upper airway is composed of the nasopharynx and oropharynx

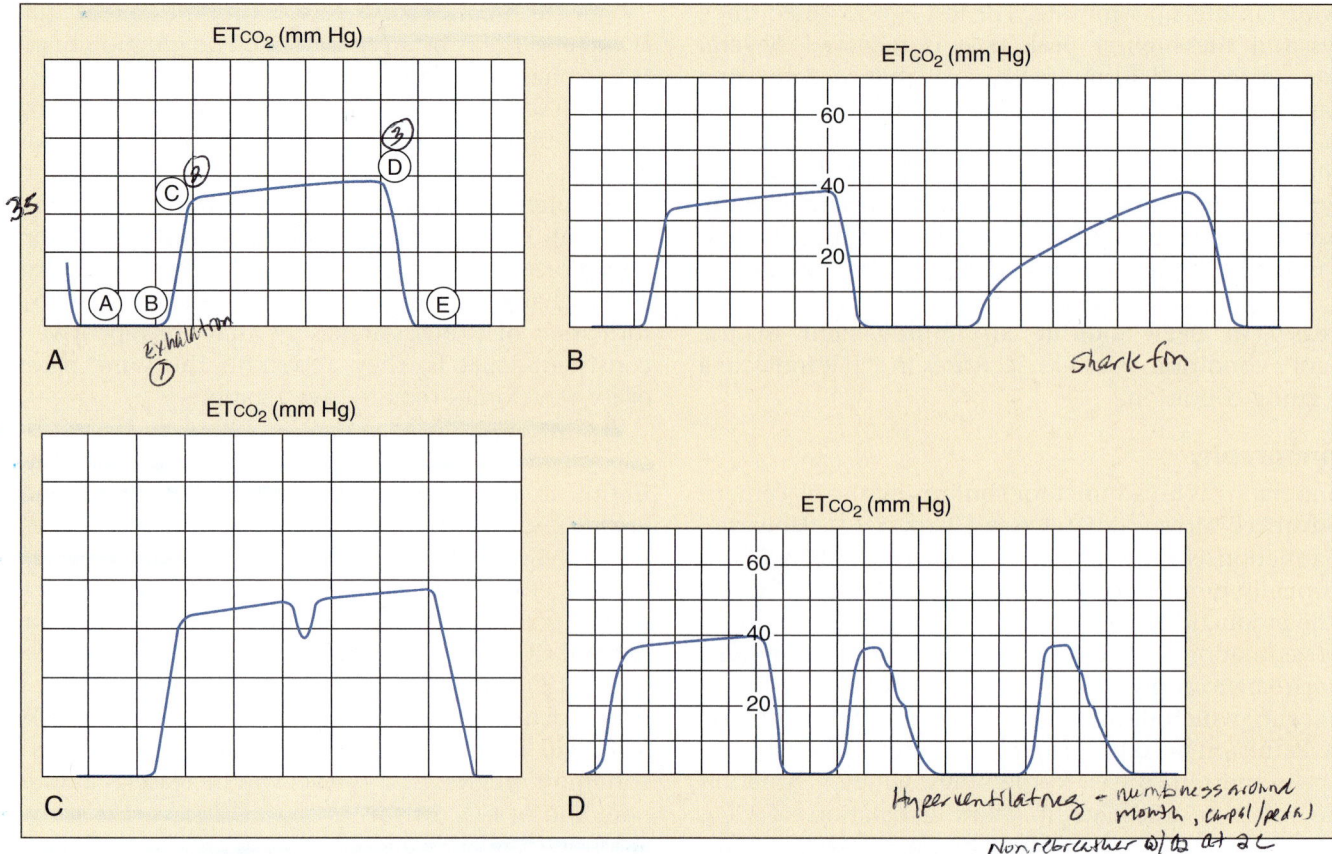

Handwritten annotations on figure:
- 35
- Exhalation
- Shark fin
- Hyperventilating - numbness around mouth, carpal/pedal
- Nonrebreather @ O2 at 2L

Figure 21-2 Four phases of a normal capnogram. *A-B,* The carbon dioxide–free portion of the respiratory cycle. *B-C,* The rapid upstroke of the curve, representing the transition from inspiration to expiration and the mixing of dead space and alveolar gas. *C-D,* The alveolar plateau, representing the alveolar gas rich in carbon dioxide and tending to slope gently upward with the uneven emptying of the alveoli. *D-E,* The respiratory downstroke, which is a nearly vertical drop to baseline. *ETCO₂,* End-tidal carbon dioxide.

Handwritten margin notes:
- Trachea - cilia + goblet cells (mucus)
- Smokers - smooth cells change to squamous - ↓ cilia
- MV = 6L air (500ml × 12 breaths/min)
- Speaking in sentences - no accessory muscle use

(Figure 21-3). The primary functions of the upper airway are to humidify and clean the air entering the lower respiratory tract. This reduces the chances of infection or foreign objects entering an environment that is ideal for pathogen growth. In contrast to the lower airway, the upper airway is not sterile. It is suited for handling potential airborne infections. Mucus is secreted by specialized epithelial cells in the sinuses, nasopharynx, and oropharynx. This mucus helps trap airborne particles and pathogens, allowing expectoration. However, long-term tobacco abuse can overstimulate these cells, increasing mucus production and clogging the upper and lower airways.

Assessment of the Upper Airway

Evaluation of the upper airway centers on ensuring airway patency (Figure 21-4). Observe the quality and frequency of the patient's respirations. Be watchful for very low respiratory rates (6 breaths/min and less for adults) and very high rates (more than 20 breaths/min for adults). As patients age, elasticity of the chest wall is lost, resulting in a decreased ability for chest expansion and therefore decreased tidal volume. Effective respiration largely depends on the amount of air moved in and out of the lungs each minute, known as *minute volume.* This is a function of the tidal volume and respiratory rate (see Chapter 6). To compensate for the decreased tidal volume, elderly patients normally have an increased respiratory rate. Respiratory rates for children vary and depend on age (Table 21-1). Examination of the patient's oropharynx should include looking for obstructing foreign objects, assessing the mucous membranes and tongue for the degree of hydration, and evaluating the potential for aspiration if vomiting occurs. Examine the neck and spaces above the clavicles for retractions. Retractions involve the use of accessory muscles, indicating respiratory distress (Figure 21-5). Palpate the trachea for signs of deviation, which is a possible indicator of pneumothorax (Figure 21-6). By placing a stethoscope over the trachea, you can reveal upper airway stridor as well as airway noises transmitted from other places in the airways.

Acute Upper Airway Disorders

Upper Respiratory Tract Infection

[OBJECTIVE 4]

Description. Upper respiratory tract infection (URI) is an infection of any of the structures of the upper airway, such as sinusitis, pharyngitis, laryngitis, or

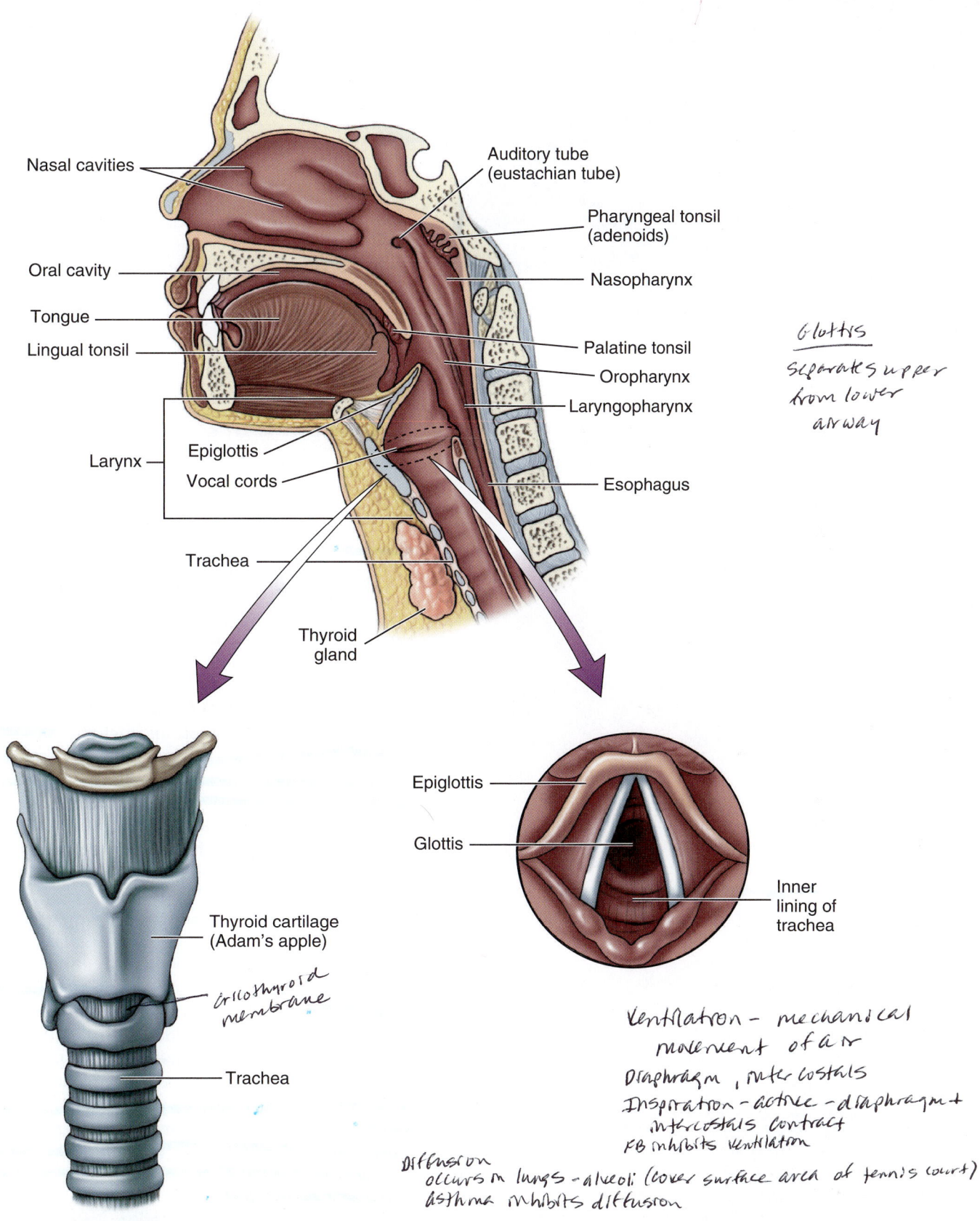

Glottis
separates upper
from lower
airway

cricothyroid
membrane

Ventilation - mechanical
movement of air
Diaphragm, intercostals
Inspiration - active - diaphragm +
intercostals contract
FB inhibits ventilation

Diffusion
occurs in lungs - alveoli (cover surface area of tennis court)
Asthma inhibits diffusion

Figure 21-3 Airway anatomy. Structures above the glottis compose the upper airway. Below the glottis is the lower airway. The structures of the lower airway include the trachea, bronchial tree, alveoli, and lungs.

Perfusion
Blood flow to lungs
P.E. inhibits perfusion - hear all lung sounds still
PE stops blood flow

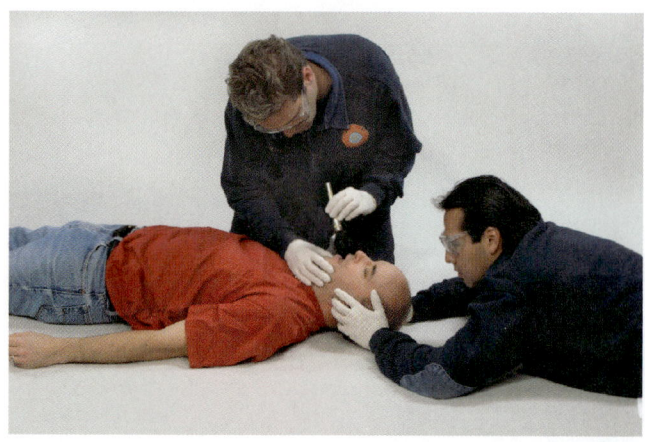

Figure 21-4 Assessment of the upper airway centers on ensuring airway patency.

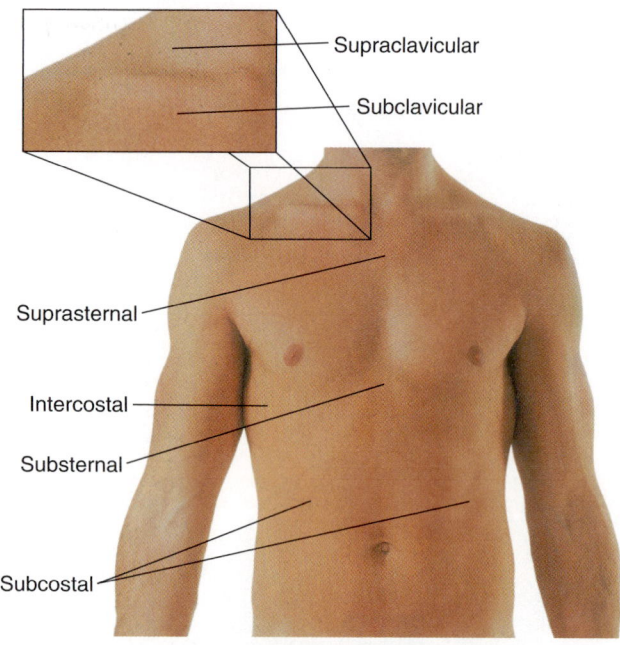

Figure 21-5 Retractions are an indicator of dyspnea. The *lead lines* indicate the areas of the chest to look for retractions.

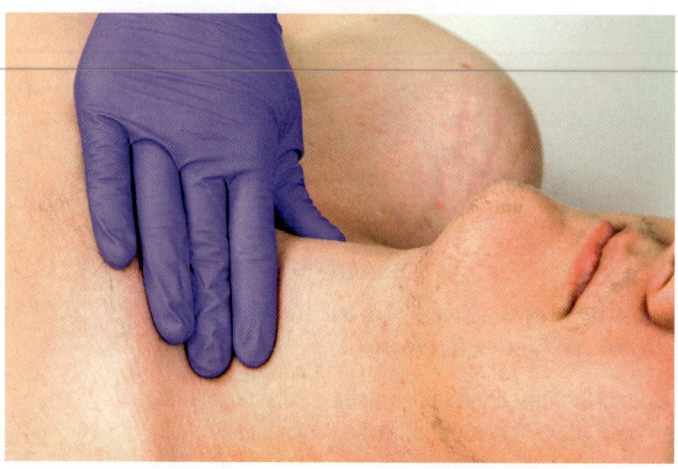

Figure 21-6 Feel for any deviation of the trachea from the midline.

TABLE 21-1	Normal Respiratory Rates for Children
Age	**Rate (Breaths/Min)**
Newborn	35
1-11 months	30
2 years	25
4 years	23
6 years	21
8 years	20
10 years	19
12 years	19
14 years	18
16 years	17
18 years	16-18

Reprinted from Hockenberry, M. J., & Wilson, D. (2007). *Wong's nursing care of infants and children* (8th ed.). St. Louis: Elsevier.

tonsillitis. It is one of the most frequent reasons patients seek care in emergency departments (EDs).

Etiology and Demographics. Children younger than 1 year average six to eight URIs per year, and adults average three to four URIs per year. Thousands of viruses can cause a URI. However, 66% to 75% are attributable to 200 genetically different viruses (Rajnik, 2006).

History and Physical Findings. URIs can cause a wide array of respiratory symptoms, including headache, nasal congestion, nasal drainage, nasal inflammation, sore throat, cough, mucus production with cough, fever, chills, and muscle aches. Fortunately, once a person is infected by a specific virus and recovers, a lifelong immunity to that virus is established. Unfortunately, immunity to one virus does not provide immunity to the many other viruses that cause URIs.

Differential Diagnosis. URIs are implicated in a wide variety of illnesses, both respiratory and systemic. URIs may often precede a more serious infection. Examples of these infections include meningitis, sinusitis, and pneumonia. Differentiating more complex illnesses from the routine cough and cold often is a challenging task.

Therapeutic Interventions. The care you provide for a URI is mainly supportive. Allow the patient to assume a position of comfort, give oxygen, and apply a pulse oximeter. Maintain oxygen saturation at greater than 95%. If the patient shows signs of respiratory distress, establish an intravenous line (IV) and apply a cardiac monitor, including capnography.

Patient and Family Education. You can instruct the patient and family to use proper hygiene, including frequent handwashing, not eating or drinking after the affected person, covering the nose and mouth while sneezing or coughing, and disposing of used tissues in the proper receptacles.

Epiglottitis

Description. **Epiglottitis** is a potentially life-threatening infection of the supraglottic structures of the airway. This results in inflammation of the base of the tongue, aryepiglottic folds, arytenoids, tonsils, and the epiglottis (Figure 21-7). However, some adult patients with severe epiglottitis do not have an inflamed epiglottis.

Etiology and Demographics. In the past, epiglottitis more frequently affected young children, but immunizations against the bacteria *Haemophilus influenzae* (commonly called *H. flu*) have reduced the rate of epiglottitis to 0.4 per every adult case (Bowman, 2006). Children are commonly affected at approximately 3 years of age, but this can range from 1 year to 6 years. Adults often are affected in the fourth or fifth decade of life. The mortality rate in adults can be as high as 7%, but in children it is approximately 1%. The male:female ratio is approximately 3:1 (Bowman, 2006), and there is no seasonal distribution of incidence. The disease has changed significantly since the introduction of the *Haemophilus influenzae* type B (also known as *Hib*) vaccine because *H. influenzae* was the primary cause of epiglottitis (Khan, 2006). Other causes of epiglottitis include *Streptococcus* species, *Klebsiella* species, and *Candida* species (a yeast) (Khan, 2006).

History and Physical Findings. Although strictly defined as inflammation caused by bacterial infection of the epiglottis, epiglottitis often involves surrounding tissues of the trachea and **supraglottic** areas (Figure 21-8). This edema often can result in narrowing, or even closure, of the airway. Obviously this condition requires rapid treatment to avoid airway compromise.

The history and physical signs and symptoms associated with epiglottitis differ slightly between adult and pediatric patients. In the adult patient, signs and symptoms of an upper respiratory infection typically precede the onset of epiglottitis. These symptoms usually last 1 to 2 days but can exist for 7 days before epiglottitis occurs. Fevers associated with the condition occur in only 50% of patients. Acute onset is possible in this population, and in this setting airway intervention is more likely to be required. Patients may experience difficult swallowing, painful swallowing, sore throat, a muffled voice, and tachycardia. Pain on palpation of the anterior neck or when moving the larynx is a common finding. Stridor, drooling, and respiratory distress are uncommon in the adult patient. However, adults who are in a sniffing position, are unable to speak, have respiratory distress, are drooling, or have stridor are in extreme danger of complete airway obstruction.

Pediatric epiglottitis is usually acute without preceding signs and symptoms, and it is almost always associated

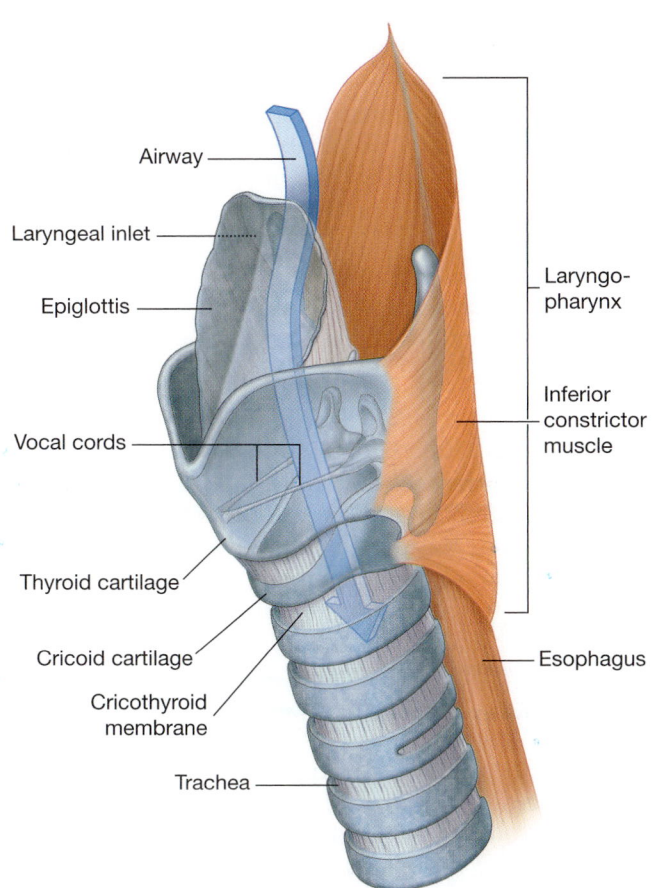

Figure 21-7 Structures of the hypopharynx.

Airway
Laryngeal inlet
Epiglottis
Vocal cords
Thyroid cartilage
Cricoid cartilage
Cricothyroid membrane
Trachea
Laryngopharynx
Inferior constrictor muscle
Esophagus

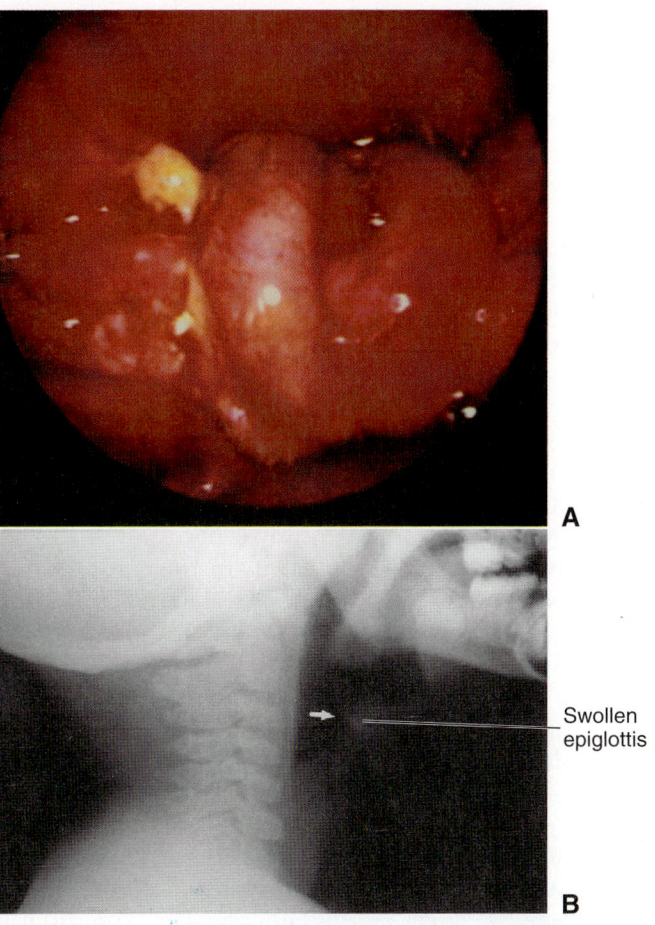

A

B

Swollen epiglottis

Figure 21-8 A, Epiglottitis. **B,** This radiograph is from a 5-year-old child who has epiglottitis. The *arrow* points to diffuse supraglottic swelling.

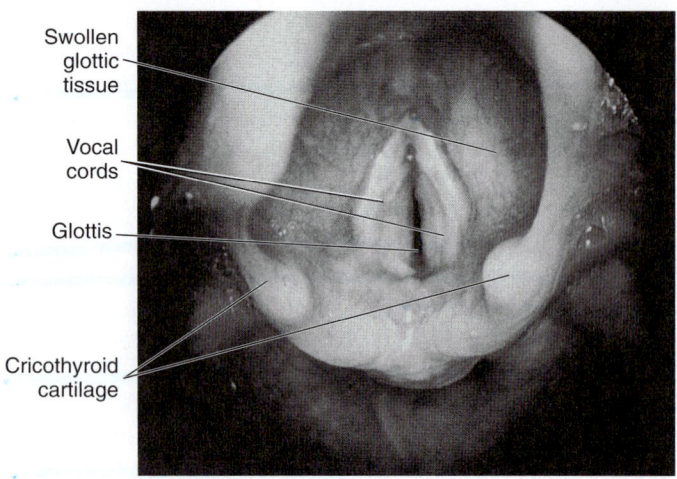

Swollen glottic tissue

Vocal cords

Glottis

Cricothyroid cartilage

Figure 21-9 Severe vocal fold and subglottic edema from viral croup.

with a high fever. The patient is anxious and generally in the sniffing position to maximize airflow. Difficulty breathing, stridor, changes in or the absence of the voice (or cry), drooling, and difficulty swallowing are classically present.

Therapeutic Interventions. Manipulation of an inflamed and irritated epiglottis can cause further edema and possible airway occlusion. Therefore care for the patient with epiglottitis is limited to supplemental oxygen and rapid transport. You must recognize this potentially disastrous diagnosis in the prehospital setting. This will allow you to notify the receiving facility and mobilize the expertise necessary to manage such a perilous scenario. You should obtain IV access only if possible without agitating the patient. Your airway equipment should be nearby, but aggressive intervention should be limited to impending respiratory failure, and blind nasotracheal intubation is contraindicated. If intubation becomes necessary, tubes smaller than would normally be used must be immediately accessible, as should surgical airway equipment. Epiglottitis is best handled in the ED or operating room with multiple specialists, including emergency medicine physicians, anesthesiologists, and surgeons, who can provide a surgical airway if necessary.

Patient and Family Education. Instruct the patient and family to observe proper hygiene. In addition, educate them about why the patient is having trouble swallowing and controlling secretions. You may even want to educate them about bacterial infections. Your instruction should be limited because of the urgent nature of this disease.

Croup

Description. Croup (laryngotracheobronchitis) is manifested by infection of the upper airways. The area below the glottis is most commonly affected, resulting in swollen, inflamed mucosa (Figure 21-9).

Etiology and Demographics. Croup is a respiratory virus. Parainfluenza type 1 is the most common cause, but it may also result from parainfluenza types 2 or 3,

influenza A and B, respiratory syncytial virus, echovirus, rhinovirus, and mycoplasma (infrequently). Croup affects young children and is the most common pediatric infection causing stridor, accounting for approximately 15% of all clinic and ED visits for respiratory infections (Molodow, 2006). The peak incidence is 2 years of age, although it can occur between the ages of 6 months and 6 years. The male:female ratio is approximately 1.5:1.

History and Physical Findings. This condition tends to affect children late at night or early in the morning. Croup often produces a characteristic "seal bark" sound when the patient coughs. This sound, along with a hoarse voice and inspiratory stridor, characterizes the classic presentation of croup. **Stridor** often sounds like a whistling noise and is caused by narrowing of the subglottic trachea at the narrowest portion of the child's airway. Unlike patients with epiglottitis, croup patients do not have difficulty swallowing, do not drool, and usually do not look acutely ill. A fever may be present and, if present is low grade, unlike the high fever associated with epiglottitis. The traditional bark often is preceded by the signs and symptoms of an upper respiratory infection. This can last from 1 to 5 days. The barking cough then typically lasts 3 to 4 days. A patient who has croup typically has clear lung sounds. Clinically, croup can be divided into the following three categories.

- Children with minor croup have minimal distress, a normal mental status, and are well hydrated. They do not have stridor at rest but may when agitated, and the cough is intermittent. They may have mild tachycardia and mild tachypnea.
- Children with moderate croup are alert and interactive but may be irritable. Stridor is present at rest and worsens with agitation; they have a classic cough as well as tachypnea, tachycardia, and retractions.
- Children with severe croup are at risk for respiratory failure and complete obstruction. Signs and symptoms include fatigue, altered mental status, hypoxia and hypercarbia, severe respiratory distress, and stridor.

Therapeutic Interventions. Care includes keeping the patient calm and comfortable. Allow the patient to assume a position of comfort, give oxygen, and apply a pulse oximeter. Maintain oxygen saturation at greater than 95%. Because the illness often manifests in the late winter or early spring, many patients improve during transport to the hospital because cold air reduces airway edema. Humidified oxygen and nebulized saline soothe inflamed tissues and often are effective in the setting of mild croup. However, these treatments do not reduce edema. If the patient continues to be in distress or have moderate croup symptoms, administer nebulized epinephrine. Either racemic epinephrine or L-epinephrine is acceptable; both are effective at reducing airway edema. The alpha$_1$ agonist actions of these medications reduce edema, thereby increasing airflow. The administration of nebulized epinephrine plays no role in the decision to admit or discharge the patient; therefore patient disposition should not be a consideration in the decision to provide this treatment. If local protocols provide for fever management, you can give antipyretics in appropriate dosages. Transport the patient in a position of comfort and provide supportive care. If signs of severe croup, such as respiratory failure or respiratory arrest, are present assist the patient's breathing with a bag-mask device and 100% oxygen. Management in the ED includes inhaled or intramuscular steroids. Steroids reduce the inflammatory component of croup and reduce the need for intubation and admission.

Patient and Family Education. Instruct the patient and family about the cause of the disease, why not to use a hot vaporizer or steam, and proper hygiene. Cool mist vaporizers, if available, may be of benefit. The combination of cool vapor and moisture can help reduce edema in the airways. Hot vaporizers should not be used because of the risk of increasing upper airway edema. Your instruction should not delay transport of the patient.

Bacterial Tracheitis

Description. **Bacterial tracheitis** is a potentially serious bacterial infection of the trachea (Figure 21-10). The seriousness of bacterial tracheitis can be described as intermediate between epiglottitis and croup.

Etiology and Demographics. Bacterial tracheitis most commonly involves infection with *Staphylococcus aureus*, *Haemophilus influenzae*, and *Corynebacterium diphtheriae*, but parainfluenza virus type 1, *Moraxella catarrhalis*, and anaerobic organisms have also been identified. This disease can affect any age group. However, it predominates in children around the age of 4 years. A small portion of children hospitalized for croup in fact have bacterial tracheitis (Clark, 2003). The majority of deaths and morbidity from bacterial tracheitis come from acute

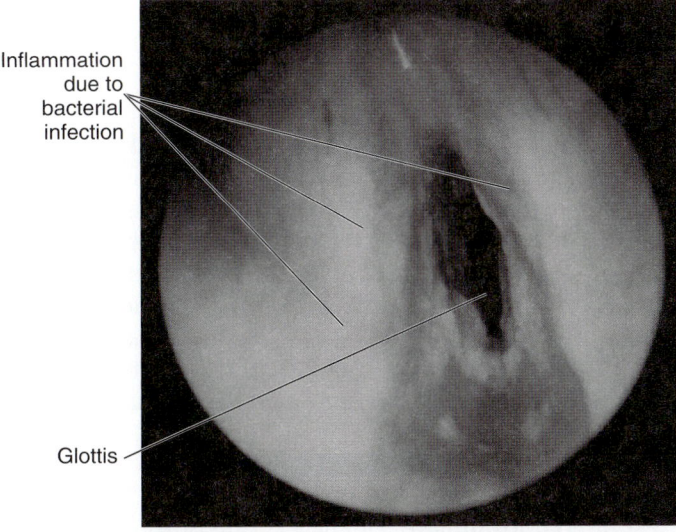

Figure 21-10 This 22-month-old boy has bacterial tracheitis caused by *Staphylococcus aureus*. This view of the trachea shows debris in the tracheal lumen and purulent laryngotracheal secretions.

airway obstruction. Males have bacterial tracheitis approximately twice as often as females.

History and Physical Findings. Bacterial tracheitis often results in fever, chills, inspiratory stridor, barking or brassy cough, hoarseness, and occasionally degrees of dyspnea. It has features of both croup and epiglottitis. Thus differentiation may be difficult in the prehospital setting. Unlike epiglottitis, drooling is often absent.

Therapeutic Interventions. Tracheitis can be caused by a range of bacteria and requires treatment with antibiotics. The care you provide depends on supporting and maintaining the airway and obtaining IV access if it will not overly upset the patient. If protocols provide for fever management, give antipyretics in appropriate dosages. Rapid transport to a facility where definitive airway management can be obtained should take priority over establishing IV access. Supplemental humidified oxygen may be helpful. If intubation is necessary, use an endotracheal tube 0.5 or 1.0 mm smaller than normal to help compensate for the tracheal edema. However, intubating the patient in this instance may prove challenging. It may best be achieved by an experienced practitioner.

Peritonsillar Abscess

Peritonsillar abscess (PTA) is an extremely painful and frightening illness. In rare instances it may compromise the upper airway. The abscess begins when a bacterial infection forms on the back of the oropharynx, rooted in the richly vascular tissues of the adenoid tonsils.

Etiology and Demographics. The genus *Streptococcus* is one of the most frequent causative bacteria, similar to strep throat. Rare cases of streptococcal tonsillar infection result in abscess, most frequently on one side. PTA rarely affects both sides of the pharynx at the same time. The frequency of PTA is approximately 30 cases per 100,000 persons, or approximately 45,000 cases each year. The highest incidence is in patients aged 30 to 50 years (Kazzi, 2004).

History and Physical Findings. The patient with PTA is often febrile and has notable difficulty swallowing (dysphagia). You often will see headache, malaise, neck pain, and a "hot potato voice" (the patient speaking as though hot food were in the mouth). In the hospital setting, examination of the throat shows unilateral swelling of the posterior throat occasionally deviating the uvula to the opposite side (Figure 21-11).

Therapeutic Interventions. Care includes keeping the patient calm and comfortable. Allow the patient to assume a position of comfort, then give oxygen and apply a pulse oximeter. Maintain oxygen saturation at greater than 95%. If signs of respiratory failure or respiratory arrest are present, assist the patient's breathing with a bag-mask device and 100% oxygen. Although the patient is usually well hydrated, you can provide supplemental IV fluids, which may increase comfort. If your protocols provide for fever management, give antipyretics in appropriate dosages. In the hospital, definitive treatment will include surgical drainage and frequently antibiotics.

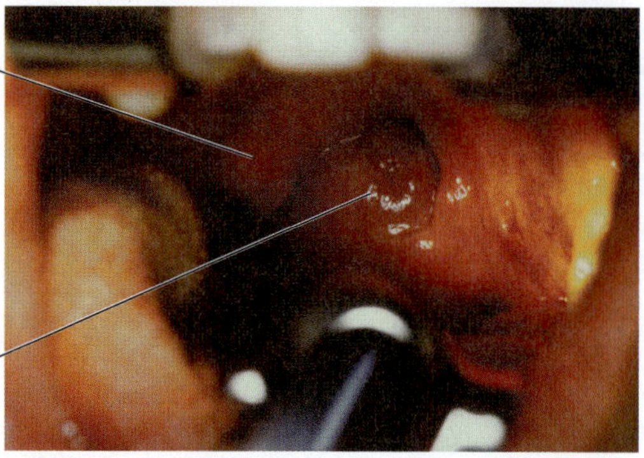

Uvula, deviated to patient's right

Peritonsillar abscess

Figure 21-11 Peritonsillar abscess with displacement of the uvula to the right.

| BOX 21-1 | Factors for Airway Foreign Objects or Aspiration |

- Seizures
- Intoxication by alcohol or drugs
- Decreased mental status
- Chronic medical conditions such as paraplegia or quadriplegia
- Transient ischemic attack or cerebrovascular accident
- Respiratory distress
- Feeding tubes (Dobhoff tubes)
- Bowel strictures

Patient and Family Education. Instruct the patient and family about how peritonsillar infections start as strep throat as well as the importance of early treatment, fever control, and proper hygiene.

Foreign Body Airway Obstruction
[OBJECTIVE 4]
Description. A foreign body airway obstruction is a blockage of the upper airway by a foreign object. Foreign objects can range from pins and needles to toys. Nearly anything that can fit in the airway has been put there, as well as some things that cannot fit.

Etiology and Demographics. Although the majority of patients are young children, some are adults. Factors for airway foreign objects or aspiration are shown in Box 21-1. The primary danger of inhaled foreign objects is an airway obstruction, most often of the upper airway. The most common offenders are foods such as nuts, hot dogs, sausages, and grapes. These items can be both round and small. They can cause an obstruction at a lower level such as the trachea, mainstem bronchi, or midlevel bronchi. In 2000 a total of 4313 deaths (1.6 per 100,000 population) occurred from unintentional ingestion or inhalation of food or other objects resulting in airway obstruction (Warshawsky, 2006).

History and Physical Findings. Maintain suspicion for foreign body aspiration in patients who exhibit sudden and severe coughing, wheezing with no asthmatic history, inability to speak, or unexplained dyspnea. Auscultation

of the patient's lung may reveal unilateral wheezing, rhonchi, or crackles (rales). You also may see retractions with exaggerated attempts of ventilation, drooling, and the patient assuming a tripod position in an effort to relieve the obstruction.

PARAMEDIC *Pearl*
By cutting the round end off a soft suction catheter, you may be able to remove a foreign object with suction. The new flat end can grip objects, particularly round objects, much easier than forceps can.

Therapeutic Interventions. Care of the patient involves paying careful attention to the airway and maintaining oxygenation. Give supplemental oxygen. In the setting of partial airway obstruction the patient may be able to speak, cough, and ventilate. In this situation the patient should be encouraged to cough to dislodge the object. Be prepared for more aggressive airway management if the obstruction is or becomes complete, or if ventilation becomes inadequate (evidenced by the inability to speak, ineffective cough, worsening stridor and altered mental status or cyanosis). In these settings immediate basic life support intervention is needed to maintain a patent airway. Basic life support procedures include abdominal or chest thrusts and visual inspection of the airway for the foreign object. If these maneuvers are unsuccessful, Magill forceps can be instrumental in removing foreign objects under direct visualization. Have suction ready because of the tendency for foreign objects to stimulate the salivary system. You must balance the need for immediate direct laryngoscopy with the effectiveness of basic life support procedures. This will often be a judgment call on your part. Factors favoring immediate removal include the following:

- Total or near-total airway obstruction
- Oxygen saturations below 80% to 85%
- Cyanosis
- Inability to ventilate the patient

If the airway is completely obstructed and cannot be cleared, consider performing a cricothyrotomy if trained and authorized to do so by your local medical director.

Patient and Family Education. Instruction of the patient and family includes emphasizing careful supervision of children, those with impaired mentation (including intoxication), and those with impaired oral sensation (such as dentures) as well as teaching about signs that may indicate possible foreign objects in the airway.

Trauma   Jaw Thrust
[OBJECTIVE 5]
Description. Trauma to the neck is one of the most challenging situations you can encounter in the prehospital setting. Many large vessels and the trachea are relatively close to the surface. The cervical spine may not be close

to the surface, but damage to the spinal cord at this level can be fatal. Penetrating and blunt trauma have the potential to generate life-threatening injuries.

Etiology and Demographics. The majority (>95%) of penetrating trauma to the neck is the result of knife or gunshot wounds. Gunshot wounds, with significantly more kinetic energy, have the potential to generate more devastating wounds. Even small-caliber projectiles, such as .22- or .25-caliber bullets, have the potential to generate tremendous damage if they encounter critical vessels or structures. Vascular injuries may be seen in as many as 40% of gunshot wounds to the neck. Major nerve injury only occurs in approximately 3% to 8% of injuries (Levy, 2006).

History and Physical Findings. Blunt force trauma, on the other hand, is more frequently seen in motor vehicle crashes. Although the risk of severing vital vessels is less, resultant edema to both the airway and vessels is a potential avenue of injury. The airway often is the site of blunt force trauma because the cricoid cartilage and associated structures are positioned anteriorly. Direct-force blunt trauma to the cricoid cartilage is capable of crushing the cartilage and creating an airway obstruction. The tracheal rings also may be bruised, possibly causing edema that may threaten airway stability.

Therapeutic Interventions. Management of these potentially serious injuries involves paying close attention to the airway and providing ventilation if necessary. You must maintain cervical spine precautions at all times in the setting of trauma to the neck. Moreover, be alert to changes in vital signs, dyspnea, changes in voice, hoarseness, upper airway stridor, or accessory muscle use. Bleeding in the airway should prompt aggressive airway management to ensure ventilation.

You must maintain in-line cervical spine stabilization during any intubation attempt (Figure 21-12). Suction and

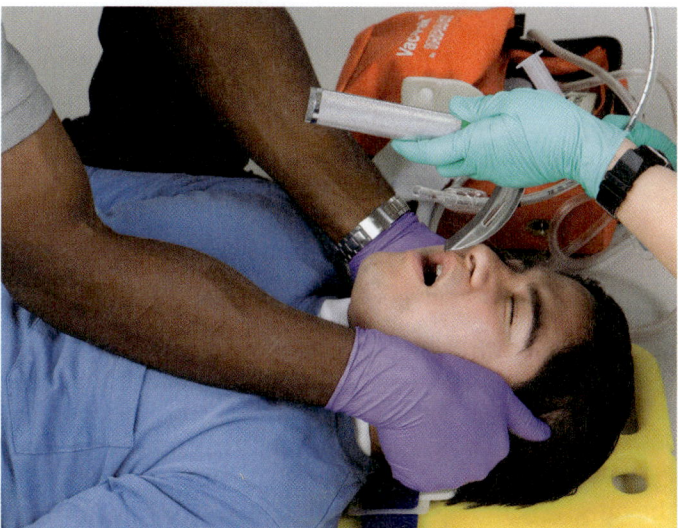

Figure 21-12 In-line cervical spine stabilization is critical in potential cervical spine injuries. This may make orotracheal intubation extremely challenging.

oxygenation must be available. Patient survival depends on your rapid recognition of the serious nature of these injuries and transport of the patient to a trauma center.

Tracheostomy

[OBJECTIVE 5]

Description. In some chronic medical conditions a hole must be surgically placed in the trachea to support respiration. This hole is called a **tracheostomy.** A tracheostomy can be used to provide ventilation, if necessary, by connecting the tracheostomy tube to a ventilator. A tracheostomy can be performed for many reasons, including the following:

- Obstructive sleep apnea
- Pickwickian syndrome
- Upper airway obstruction or cancer
- Laryngeal cancer
- Need for ventilator support for more than 2 weeks

You will not place tracheostomies emergently. Rather, they are placed under controlled conditions in the operating room. A tracheostomy is performed below the cricoid cartilage. A short tube is placed in the opening created by the procedure (Figure 21-13). Some of these tubes have a cuff, much like an endotracheal tube. Some tracheostomy tubes are made of metal, with a central obturator that can be placed into the tube to allow speaking. In both cases a standard endotracheal tube ring on the outside of the tracheal tube allows a bag-mask device to be attached so that ventilation can take place if respiratory distress or failure occurs.

Although helpful in certain situations, tracheostomies have several drawbacks. When the upper respiratory tract is bypassed, many of the cleaning and humidifying functions are bypassed, increasing the chance of infections in the lungs, such as pneumonia. Patients who require tracheostomies often have other medical problems. These problems can include chronic obstructive pulmonary disease, diabetes, heart problems, or circulatory problems. These patients spend more time in the hospital, allowing them to develop infections quite different from those in the community at large. Many of these infections are resistant to common antibiotics (such as **methicillin-resistant Staphylococcus aureus [MRSA]** or **vancomycin-resistant Enterococcus spp. [VRE]**). Patients with tracheostomies often are carriers of *Pseudomonas*, a bacterium that can cause severe pneumonia.

Therapeutic Interventions. In the prehospital setting, patients with difficulties involving tracheostomies often call EMS for dyspnea. Although these patients could have dyspnea for several reasons, many benefit from additional oxygen administration. Patients who do not respond to an initial trial of oxygenation can be assisted with a bag-mask device by connecting the bag-mask directly to the tracheostomy hub and gently assisting ventilations.

Some patients accidentally displace the tracheostomy, often pulling it out entirely. In general, you should trans-

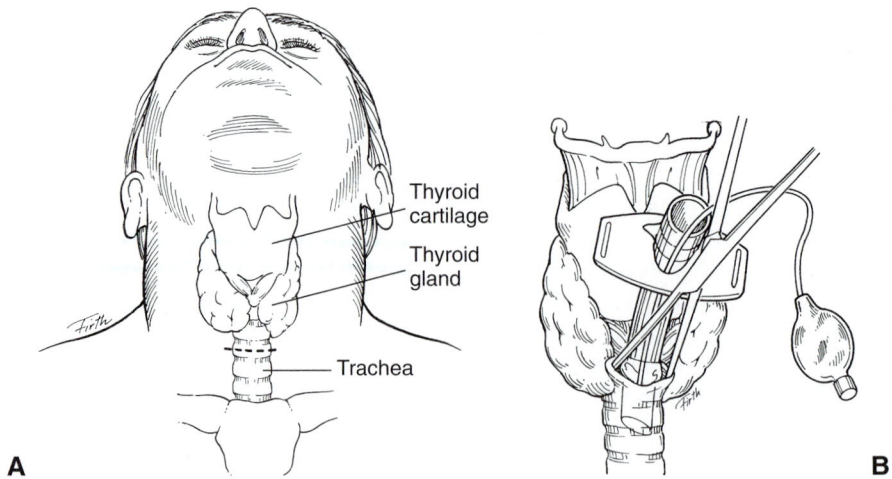

Thyroid cartilage

Thyroid gland

Trachea

A

B

Figure 21-13 A, Site for a tracheostomy incision. **B,** Placement of a tracheostomy tube.

port these patients to the ED rather than replace the tracheostomy in the field. In these patients dyspnea initially can be treated with oxygen. If orotracheal intubation becomes necessary, it can be extremely difficult. If oxygen administration does not relieve the patient's symptoms, you can intubate the patient through the **ostomy** hole. It may be necessary to select a tube size at least 0.5 mm smaller than the tracheostomy tube to pass through the tracheostomy hole. Generous lubrication is key. Gentle introduction of the tube into the ostomy hole may be somewhat painful and upsetting to the patient. Under no circumstances should you force the tube into the tracheostomy. If resistance is encountered, use a smaller tube size. Few patients should need this degree of intervention. Contact medical control early if any questions arise.

Patient and Family Education. Instruction of the patient and family includes reinforcing education by the attending physician, including proper tracheostomy care and hygiene, and discussing the potential development of antibiotic-resistant infections.

Case Scenario—continued

You administer 4 L of oxygen by nasal cannula as you continue your assessment. The patient reports focal right chest pain that she believes is related to her fall. She also states that she is dizzy, especially when she sits up. For the past 1 to 2 weeks she has also had a cough that is producing thick, green mucus. Chest wall movement is normal and her breath sounds are diminished, with coarse rhonchi in both lungs. Medical history includes what she refers to as "mild COPD" related to her 50-year habit of smoking 2 packs of cigarettes per day. Vital signs are pulse, 128 beats/min; blood pressure, 90/60 mm Hg; respirations, 40 breaths/min; temperature, 101.4° F; and SpO$_2$, 74%.

Questions

5. *Is this patient high priority? Why or why not?*
6. *What conditions are consistent with a productive cough, fever, tachycardia and hypotension, and hypoxia? What do the vital signs contribute to the picture?*
7. *How does the history of COPD, cough, fever, and 24 hours on the floor fit into the clinical picture?*
8. *What treatment will you initiate at this time?*

DISORDERS OF THE PLEURA, MEDIASTINUM, AND CHEST WALL

Anatomy and Physiology

The chest wall is composed of multiple layers of skin, bone, muscle, and connective tissue. The bones of the rib cage and thoracic spine protect the important structures in the thorax (Figures 21-14 to 21-16).

Respiration is a complex sequence of events that requires the participation of several components of the body. Inspiration begins with the signal passed from the brain to inhale. The diaphragm, the principal muscle of breathing, begins to contract. This contraction causes the thoracic cavity to increase in size. This increase in size creates a negative pressure in the chest, drawing air into the lungs to fill the void created by the negative pressure. Assistance may be added by the intercostal muscles, which are the muscles that connect the ribs in the rib cage. Intercostal muscles allow the ribs to move apart, further increasing the size of the chest and thus increasing negative pressure.

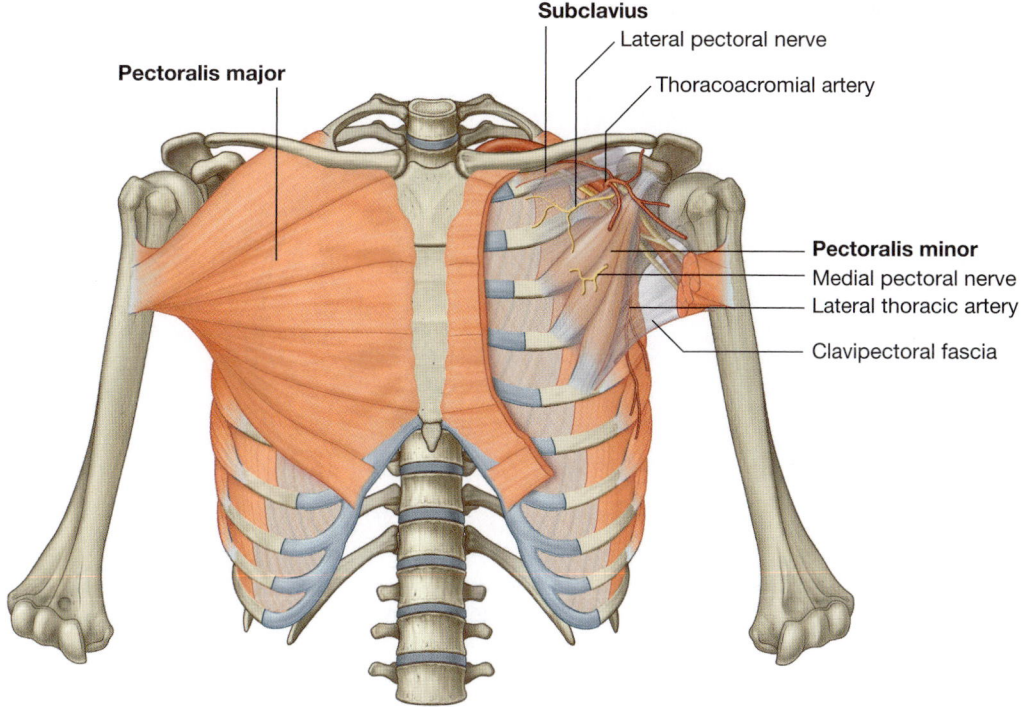

Figure 21-14 Bones and muscles of the thorax, which protect the mediastinum against damage and allow the muscles to function.

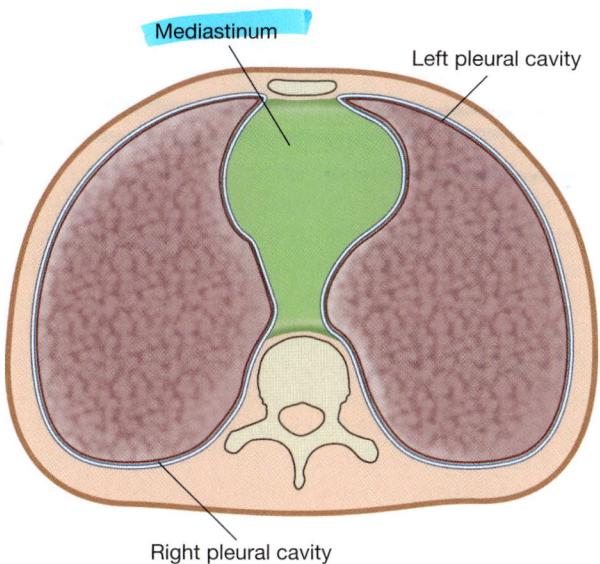

Figure 21-15 Cross-section of the thorax showing the position of the mediastinum.

During exhalation the diaphragm and the accessory muscles of respiration relax, enabling the intrathoracic pressure to increase above the air pressure outside the body. This positive pressure forces air out of the lungs and into the environment. Intercostal muscles may assist by pulling the ribs together and increasing lung pressures. The abdominal muscles may contribute but function to increase pressure in the chest cavity and force air out. Normally abdominal muscles rarely assist in inspiration.

The mediastinum is the area between the lungs. It contains many important structures, including the heart,

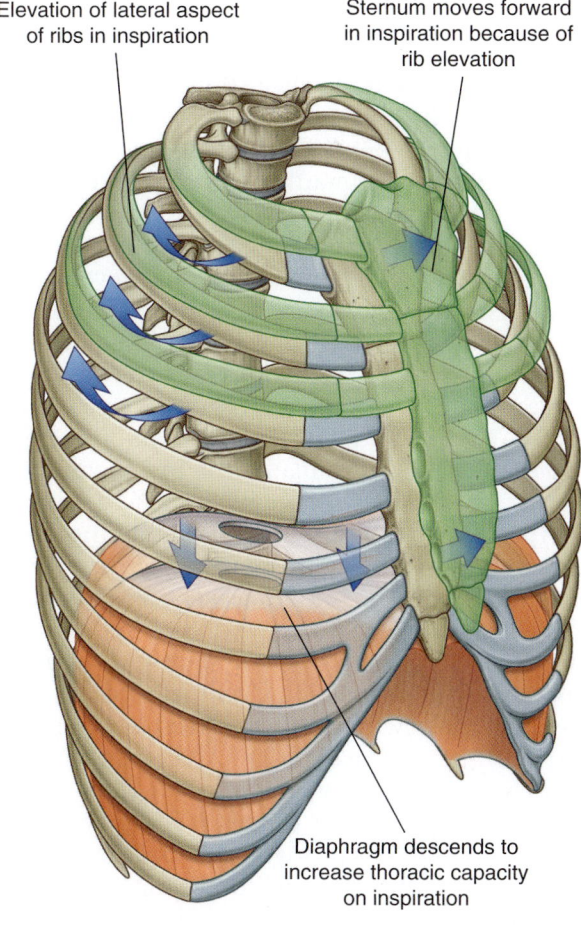

Figure 21-16 Motions of the chest wall in inspiration and expiration.

"Blue bloater" cyanotic & fat

Bronchitis - coughing for 3 months out of year for 2 consecutive years

Fewer alveoli over time, more scar tissue (↓ diffusion) COPD, emphysema

"pink puffer" - ↑ RBCs (polycythemia) to make up for ↓ diffusion

* 1° Drive to breathe = ↑ CO_2

* Hypoxic drive - back up system ↓ O_2 levels

If give too much O_2, will breathe more slowly

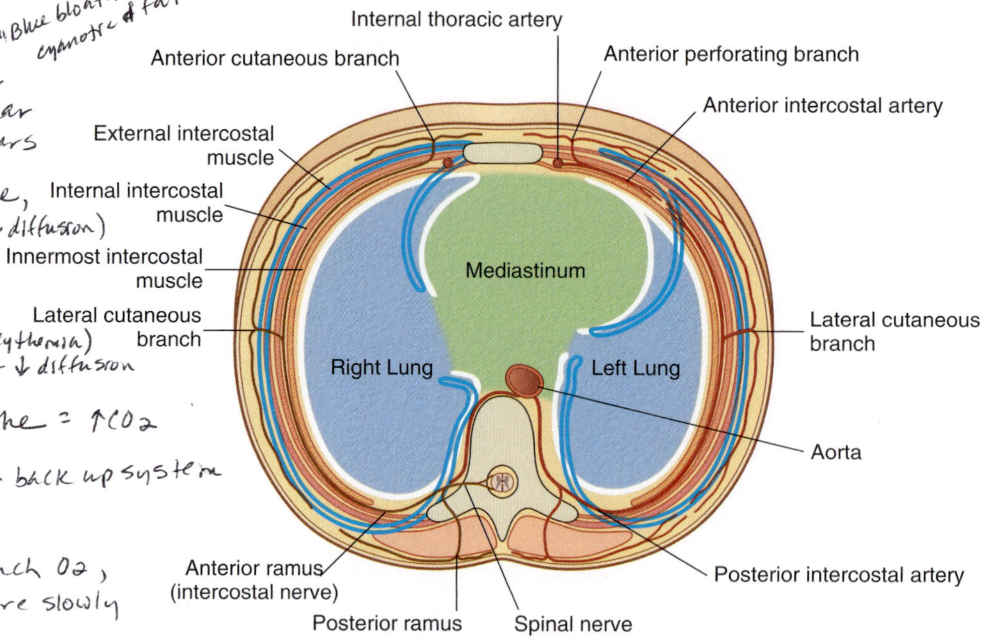
Internal thoracic artery
Anterior cutaneous branch
Anterior perforating branch
Anterior intercostal artery
External intercostal muscle
Internal intercostal muscle
Innermost intercostal muscle
Mediastinum
Lateral cutaneous branch
Right Lung
Left Lung
Lateral cutaneous branch
Aorta
Anterior ramus (intercostal nerve)
Posterior ramus
Spinal nerve
Posterior intercostal artery

Figure 21-17 The mediastinum.

aorta, inferior and superior venae cavae, the trachea, and main bronchi (Figure 21-17). The mediastinum does not directly contribute to respiration. It is a place where important structures are sheltered by the ribs and chest wall. It plays an important part in respiration, not by oxygenation but by allowing return of the deoxygenated blood and circulation of the oxygenated blood.

Adjacent to the respiratory center in the brain is a chemosensitive area that, when stimulated by changes in hydrogen ions (H^+), excites or depresses the respiratory center. Because H^+ cannot effectively cross the blood-brain barrier, this is primarily controlled by the levels of CO_2 in the blood. CO_2 can cross this barrier and then dissociate into carbonic acid and H^+ in the area surrounding the chemosensitive center. When CO_2 levels increase, a greater amount of carbonic acid and H^+ is produced, which results in greater stimulation of the chemosensitive area and ultimately the respiratory center, causing an increase in respirations. The inverse is true when CO_2 levels fall. Because of the reduced amount of H^+ from the dissociation of CO_2, stimulation of the chemosensitive area is decreased and respirations ultimately decrease.

This process is highly effective in maintaining an appropriate amount of CO_2, and therefore oxygen, in the system to meet metabolic demands. However, this system is only effective for acute changes in CO_2 levels. In the setting of chronically increased CO_2 levels, such as in COPD, the chemosensitive area will adjust to these increased levels and establish a new baseline, or effectively become less sensitive to the presence of CO_2. As a result, changes in CO_2 levels no longer drive respirations.

As discussed previously, oxygen levels play no role in the primary respiratory drive. In fact, the respiratory center of the brain has no ability to respond directly to oxygen levels. However, chemoreceptors in the carotid and aortic bodies do respond to oxygen levels and, to a lesser extent, CO_2 and H^+ levels. When the primary drive for respiration fails, this acts as a redundant system to drive respirations. This is often referred to as the *hypoxic drive* because the patient now breathes in response to decreased oxygen levels rather than increased CO_2 levels. The exact mechanism by which the chemoreceptors stimulate the respiratory center is not fully understood. As patients with COPD become increasingly tolerant to hypercapnia, the primary respiratory drive shifts to the hypoxic drive mechanism. Because the level of oxygen in the blood drives the stimulus to breathe, there is a theoretical possibility that an increased oxygen level will decrease the respiratory drive. This has led to the ill-founded and dangerous practice of withholding oxygen from these patients. The likelihood of depressing a patient's respirations in the prehospital setting with the administration of oxygen is essentially nonexistent. In addition, patients rarely depend purely on the hypoxic drive. Although the hypoxic drive provides the main stimulus to breathe, some component of the primary (CO_2) respiratory drive exists. Therefore the paramedic must never withhold oxygen from any patient in respiratory distress.

Costochondritis

[OBJECTIVE 6]

Description

Of the many causes for chest pain, **costochondritis** is among the more benign.

History and Physical Findings

Inflammation of the cartilage connecting the ribs to the sternum can produce chest pain that can startle a patient. The patient may worry that the heart may be causing the pain. Any of the several joints can be affected. In more than 90% of cases, more than one joint is involved. The exact prevalence of costochondritis is not well known (Flowers, 2005). This inflammation can come from many causes, including infection, strain, or sprain. Although this diagnosis can be difficult to make, suspicion is raised when a patient has chest pain that is worse with deep breathing and has a specific point on the chest that exactly reproduces the pain when palpated.

Therapeutic Interventions

Costochondritis is often treated by antiinflammatory medications after other, more life-threatening illnesses are ruled out. Care includes administering oxygen; establishing IV access; and using pulse oximetry, capnography, and ECG monitoring. If the patient is hypoventilating or becoming hypoxic as a result of pain on respiration, pain relief can be considered.

Patient and Family Education

You can educate the patient and family about the potential causes of costochondritis, including trauma and infection. Because this is a diagnosis of exclusion, no therapy should be recommended until other, more serious causes are ruled out.

Pleurisy

Description

Pleurisy is painful rubbing of the pleural lining. ✳

Etiology. The pleural space is lined by two tough connective tissue linings: the visceral pleura and the parietal pleura. These linings allow rubbing between the lungs and the chest wall to occur without causing extensive tissue damage. A small amount of pleural fluid (usually only a few milliliters) acts as a lubricant, reducing friction. A small area of either pleura occasionally may become inflamed and cause chest pain. The cause of the inflammation often is unknown. Trauma and viral infection have been suggested as possible causes but have not been proven.

History and Physical Findings

A small area of inflammation often causes pain on inspiration, usually at a specific point on the chest or upper back. The pain is worsened by breathing ("pleuritic pain") and sometimes lessened when the patient takes shallow breaths. Nausea, vomiting, diaphoresis, and radiation to the extremities are rare. If present, these signs and symptoms should prompt you to consider other problems. Your auscultation of the patient's lungs may reveal a "rub," which is a rubbing sound in a specific area of inflammation. A rub may be quite difficult to hear. The diagnosis of pleurisy does not require you to hear the rub. Although the patient may have subjective dyspnea, it is usually related to a reluctance to take a deep breath, not true dyspnea. In severe cases the patient may become hypoxic simply from decreased respirations in an effort to avoid pain. However, any degree of hypoxia should prompt you to search for another disease.

Therapeutic Interventions

Treatment of the patient includes checking oxygen saturation, monitoring capnography, providing reassurance, applying ECG monitoring, and establishing IV access in more severe cases. If the patient is hypoventilating or becoming hypoxic as a result of pain on respiration, pain relief can be considered.

Patient and Family Education

Educate the patient and family about the potential causes of pleurisy and the need to rule out other, more serious diseases such as pneumonia and pulmonary embolus, if indicated.

Pneumomediastinum

[OBJECTIVE 6]

Description

The presence of air in the mediastinum is called **pneumomediastinum.** ✳

Etiology. Pneumomediastinum may occur spontaneously or as a result of trauma to the chest, mechanical ventilation, asthma, emphysema, lung or chest tumors, cocaine use, violent emesis or coughing, or childbirth. These conditions are associated with increased pressure within the conducting airways or alveoli, causing them to rupture. This results in the escape of air into surrounding structures. Pneumomediastinum may also occur during medical procedures such as **esophagoduodenoscopy** or **mediastinoscopy.** Air in the mediastinum is a worrisome condition because air often carries bacteria, and infection in the mediastinum (called **mediastinitis**) is a serious infection that often requires prolonged hospitalization.

History and Physical Findings

Pneumomediastinum is difficult to detect in the field. Some patients may only have indistinct chest pain or mild dyspnea. The physical examination may reveal **subcutaneous emphysema.** Your auscultation of the patient's heart may reveal a "crunching" sound, called **Hamman's sign** (Tintinalli et al., 2004).

Therapeutic Interventions

You must ensure oxygenation and ventilation, establish IV access, and apply ECG monitoring. Patients with suspected pneumomediastinum should be rapidly transported.

THE LOWER AIRWAY

[OBJECTIVE 7]

Anatomy of the Lower Airway

The lower airway is composed of the trachea, bronchi, bronchioles, and alveoli in each lung (Figure 21-18). The trachea is the main passageway for air. It splits into two

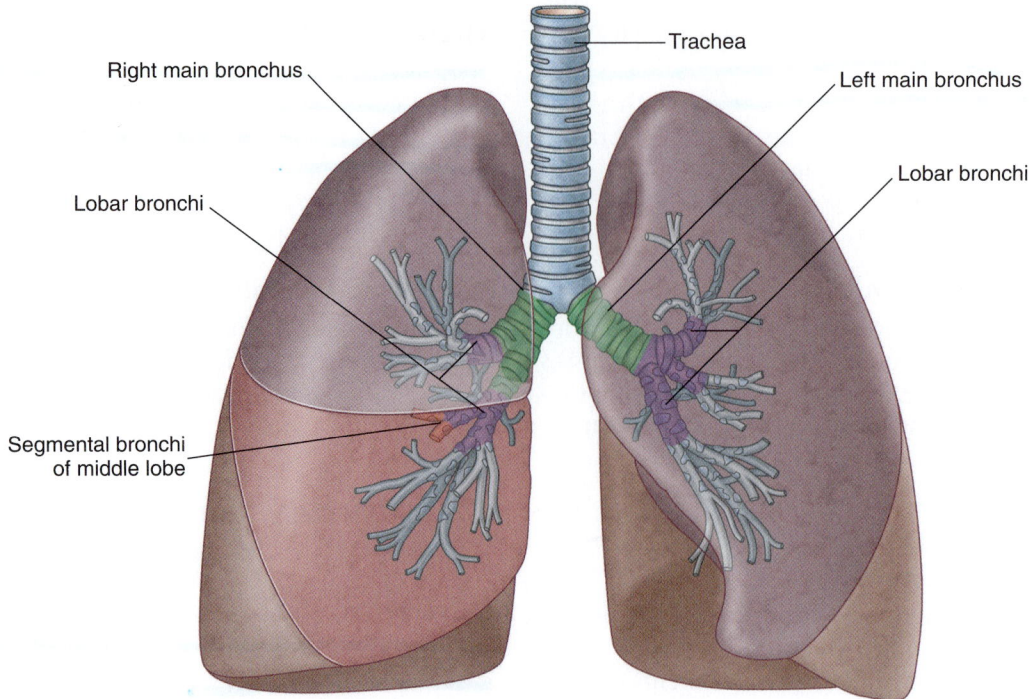

Figure 21-18 Lower airway structures.

main bronchi, the **right** and **left mainstem bronchi.** These mainstem bronchi feed directly into one lung each. The left mainstem bronchus feeds into the left lung and the right feeds into the right. The mainstem bronchi each divide further into segmental bronchi, then into bronchioles. Bronchioles further split into smaller bronchioles and terminate in **alveoli.** The alveoli are the tiny breathing spaces where gas transfer takes place (Figure 21-19).

The lower airways traditionally are sterile but also have the capacity for mucus production. Thus they serve as an additional line of defense against airborne pathogens. Air passes into successively smaller diameter airways, distributing the inhaled air to the alveoli, the air sacs that allow gaseous transfer. At the lowest level the single cell–layer alveoli work to transfer oxygen to hemoglobin, an essential component of the red blood cell, as well as extract CO_2 from the venous blood. Other byproducts of metabolism may be excreted from the respiratory system as well. These byproducts include acetones in the case of diabetic ketoacidosis, acids in the case of metabolic or renal failure, and carbon monoxide in the case of poisoning.

Assessment of the Lower Airway

Auscultate the lungs in a systematic fashion, ensuring that all areas of the lung are examined. Many paramedics start with the front of the patient, auscultating both upper lobes, progressing to both middle-lung areas and then both lower lobes (Figure 21-20). After having the patient sit up, auscultate the posterior of each lung, progressing from top to bottom. This ensures that all lobes

of each lung are evaluated. Figure 21-21 shows a diagram of the lobes of each lung.

Pay careful attention to determining unusual breath sounds. Abnormal breath sounds can be grouped into typical descriptions: stridor, crackles (rales), rhonchi, and wheezing. They can also be described as continuous or discontinuous. Continuous breath sounds can be present during any phase of the respiratory cycle, whereas discontinuous breath sounds are heard only during inhalation. Stridor is a harsh, high-pitched inspiratory sound heard best over the neck. It is the result of restricted air movement through large central airways, usually in the upper airway. It is caused by obstruction of the larynx or trachea, such as in epiglottitis, laryngospasm, or foreign body aspiration.

Crackles, sometimes called *rales* or *wet lung* sounds, indicate the presence of fluid in the smaller airways. Crackles are similar to the sound made when hair is rolled between two fingers and are common in pneumonia and pulmonary edema. Crackles are heard during inhalation and are therefore discontinuous breath sounds. Fine crackles are normally heard late in inspiration, are high pitched, have a short duration, and are not cleared by a cough. Medium crackles are heard midway through inspiration. They are lower pitched and have a longer duration than fine crackles and also are not cleared by a cough. Course crackles also are heard midway through inspiration but are louder than fine or medium crackles and may have a "bubbly" quality to them. The pitch is lower and the duration is longer than medium crackles but, like fine and medium crackles, they are not cleared by a cough.

Rhonchi are more varied in description. They are most commonly described as rattling or rumbling in the

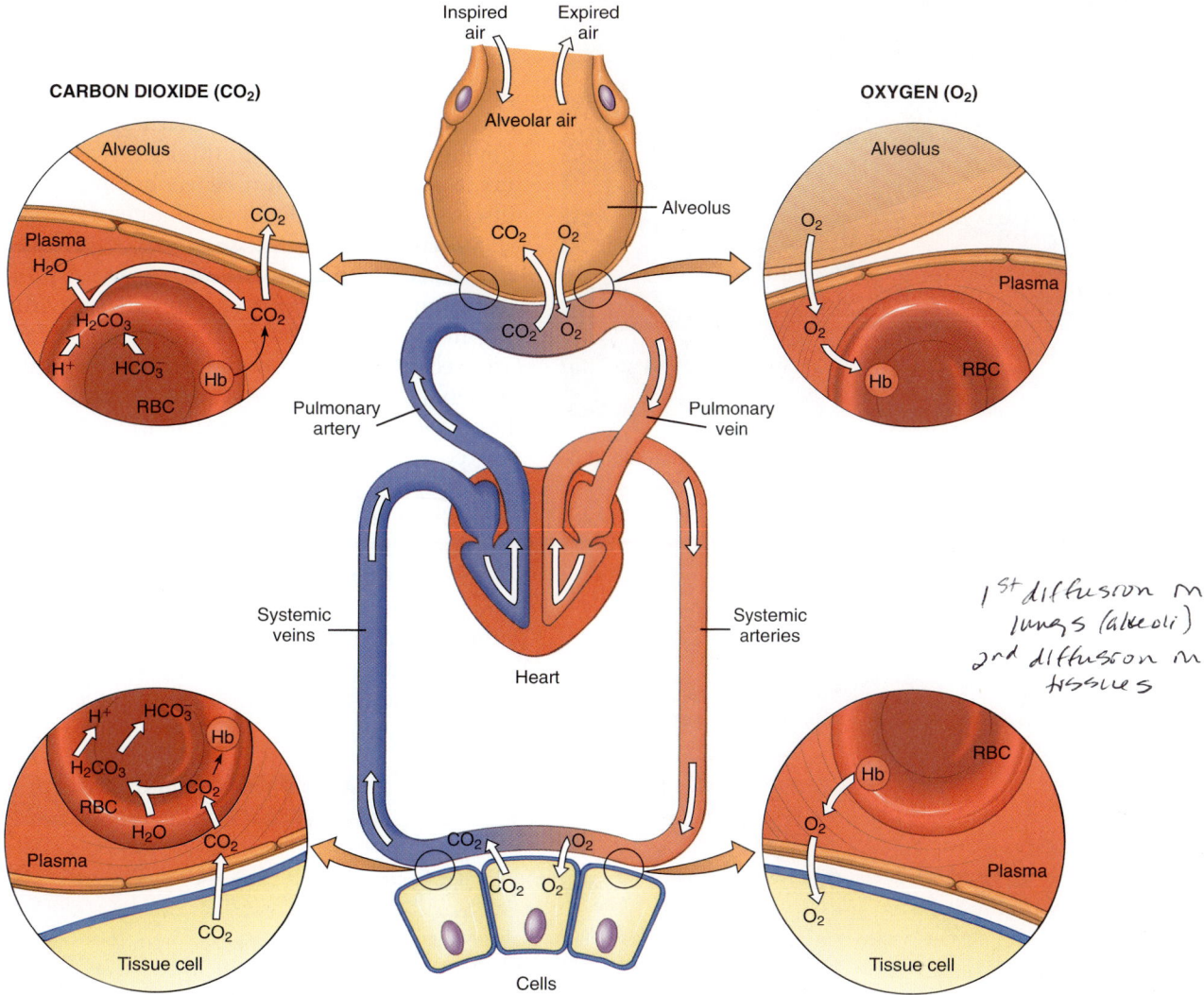

Figure 21-19 Exchange of gases in lung and tissue capillaries. The right insets show oxygen diffusing out of alveolar air into blood and associating with hemoglobin (Hb) in lung capillaries to form oxyhemoglobin. In tissue capillaries, oxyhemoglobin dissociates, releasing oxygen, which diffuses from the red blood cells (RBCs) and then crosses the capillary wall to reach the tissue cells. As the left insets show, carbon dioxide (CO_2) diffuses in the opposite direction (into RBCs), and some of it associates with Hb to form carbaminohemoglobin. However, most CO_2 combines with water to form carbonic acid (H_2CO_3), which dissociates to form hydrogen (H^+) and bicarbonate (HCO_3^-) ions. Back in the lung capillaries, CO_2 dissociates from the HCO_3^- and carbaminohemoglobin molecules and diffuses out of the blood into alveolar air.

lungs. Rhonchi are continuous breath sounds and can be heard on inspiration or expiration; however, they are often louder during exhalation. Rhonchi are the result of fluid in the larger airways and may be cleared by coughing. This sound can be heard in patients with pneumonia, congestion from URIs, or chronic obstructive pulmonary disease (COPD).

Wheezing is a musical whistling sound caused by turbulent movement of air through constricted bronchioles. Wheezes may be heard on inhalation or exhalation but often are more prominent on exhalation, which is the phase of respiration when the smaller airways tend to collapse in reactive airway diseases. The pitch of wheezes may be singular or variable. Wheezing often occurs as the result of asthma or COPD. Possible causes of wheezing are shown in Box 21-2. See Table 21-2 for a comparison of the different breath sounds.

Traumatic Pleural and Pulmonary Injuries

Additional information about thoracic trauma is located in Chapter 49.

Pneumothorax

Description

[OBJECTIVE 6]

Partial or full collapse of a lung is referred to as **pneumothorax.**

Etiology. Trauma is one of the more dramatic causes of pneumothorax, including both blunt and penetrating

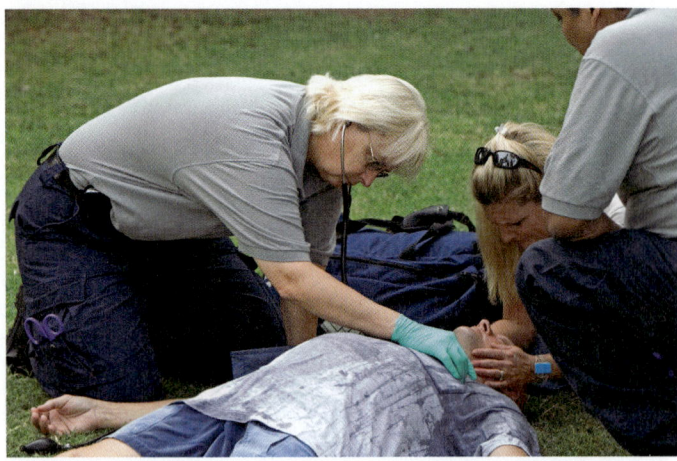

Figure 21-20 Auscultation of the lungs should be performed in a systematic fashion, ensuring that all areas of the lung are examined.

trauma (see Chapter 49). Rib fractures may produce sharp, bony fragments that can pierce the pleura or lung itself, allowing the lung to collapse. Penetrating trauma may pierce the chest wall, allowing atmospheric air to enter and the lung to collapse. In these cases the reason is obvious, but in other, nontraumatic cases of pneumothorax, the reason may not be as obvious. Pneumothorax is discussed in more detail in Chapter 49.

Spontaneous pneumothorax is a pneumothorax that occurs in the absence of trauma. A primary spontaneous pneumothorax occurs in patients without underlying lung disease. Young, thin, tall males are frequently affected by primary spontaneous pneumothorax, which presents with sudden dyspnea. These patients may also have tachypnea, tachycardia and, depending on the degree of collapse of the lung, hypoxia. A secondary spontaneous pneumothorax occurs in patients with an underlying lung disease. Patients with emphysema are at risk for a secondary spontaneous pneumothorax because of the destruction of the alveoli and formation of blebs, which are large cavities that may rupture and cause pneumothorax (Chang, 2006) (Figure 21-22).

Mechanical ventilation may also cause pneumothorax. Another term used in this instance is **barotrauma.**

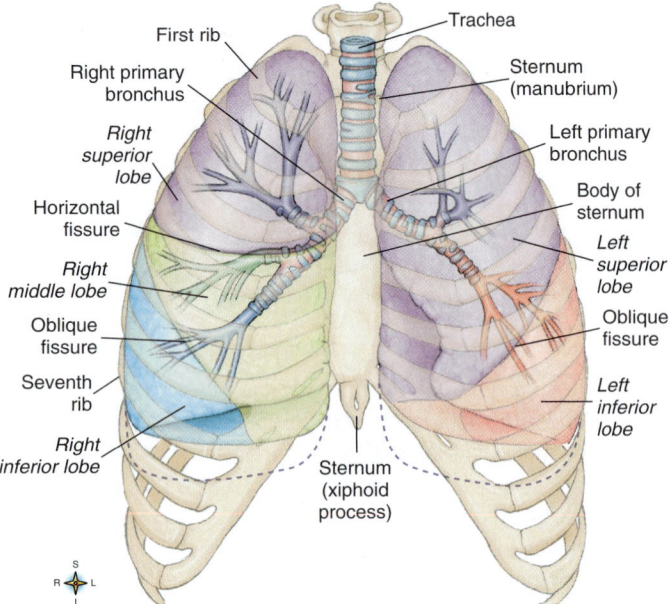

Figure 21-21 Lobes of the lung.

BOX 21-2	Possible Causes of Wheezing

- Asthma
- Toxic inhalation
- Bronchospasm
- Congestive heart failure
- Pulmonary embolism
- Chronic bronchitis
- Emphysema
- Croup
- Pneumothorax
- Pneumonia
- Anaphylaxis
- Obstruction by foreign body or tumor
- Pulmonary edema

TABLE 21-2	Abnormal Breath Sounds		
Sound or Symptom	**Normal?**	**Usual Source**	**Possible Conditions**
Tachypnea	No	Systemic	Hyperventilation, pulmonary embolus
Bradypnea	No*	Systemic	Brain injury, narcotic overdose
Stridor	No	Upper airway	Croup, foreign object in airway
Rhonchi	No†	Upper or lower airway	Bronchitis, pneumonia, pulmonary edema
Crackles (rales)	No	Lower airway or alveoli	Pneumonia, pulmonary edema
Wheezing	No†	Middle or terminal airways	Asthma, foreign object

*Physically fit patients may exhibit mild bradypnea and bradycardia as normal vital signs.
†Patients with chronic lung disease may exhibit some degree of rhonchi or wheezing at all times as a result of their disease process.

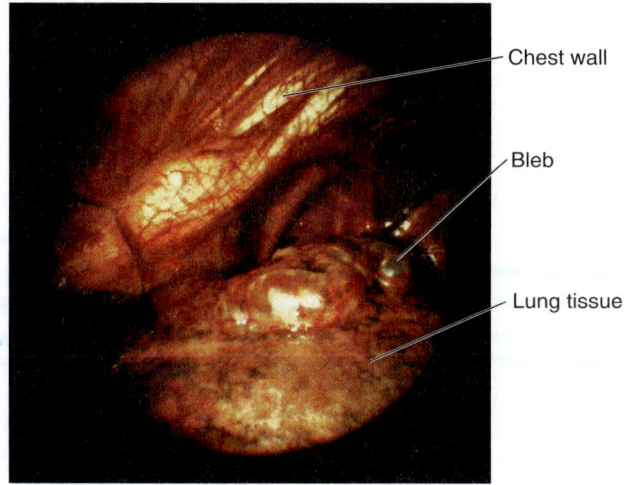

Figure 21-22 This patient has a spontaneous pneumothorax. In this view through a thoracoscope, large apical blebs can be seen on the surface of the lung (lower part of photo).

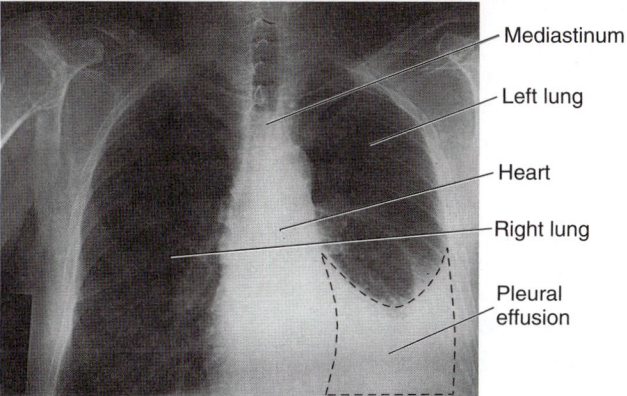

Figure 21-23 Chest radiograph showing a left pleural effusion. Fluid appears as *white areas*.

Patients who have respiratory failure and require ventilatory assistance or intubation are at risk for barotrauma. Patients who require more pressure to ventilate, such as patients with asthma or airway blockage, are at higher risk for barotrauma.

History and Physical Findings. A 15% to 20% pneumothorax is generally well tolerated and may have minimal, if any, signs and symptoms. When signs and symptoms are present patients typically experience a sudden onset of dyspnea, occasionally chest pain, tachycardia, hypoxia, **hyperpnea** (deep respirations), and cough. Many of these may occur while at rest. More severe signs include diaphoresis, altered mentation, cyanosis, and subcutaneous emphysema. Assessment of the patient may reveal decreased breath sounds on the affected side and good breath sounds on the opposite side. The differential diagnosis can be difficult in a patient with underlying lung disease because the symptoms of the disease and the pneumothorax can overlap. A pulmonary embolus also can present similarly to a spontaneous pneumothorax. Whenever a patient with a history of underlying lung disease has atypical acute dyspnea, consider a spontaneous pneumothorax as a possible cause.

Therapeutic Interventions. Treatment of pneumothorax involves the basics: providing oxygenation and ventilation; obtaining IV access; and using pulse oximetry, capnography, and ECG monitoring. The patient should be transported in a position of comfort. Because a spontaneous pneumothorax rarely causes a mediastinal shift, thoracic decompression is seldom considered. However, the paramedic should be alert to the possibility of the development of a tension pneumothorax. Rarely you may have to intubate the patient, which can increase the pneumothorax.

Patient and Family Education. Instruction of the patient and family can include drawing a diagram of a **collapsed lung.** This will help the patient understand his or her injury and the importance of treatment.

NONTRAUMATIC DISEASES OF THE LUNG
Pleural Effusion

Description

Fluid that collects in the pleural cavity is referred to as a **pleural effusion.** This fluid is composed of water, proteins, often white blood cells, and components of plasma. Normally a very small amount of fluid (approximately 3 to 5 mL) is present in the space between the visceral and parietal pleurae. In pleural effusion, much more fluid collects, sometimes as much as several liters (Figure 21-23). Accumulation of this much fluid is a sign of some type of disease, whether old or new.

Etiology and Demographics

An estimated 1.3 million people each year have pulmonary effusion. Some major causes of effusion include congestive heart failure, bacterial pneumonia, cancer, pulmonary embolus, advanced liver disease (cirrhosis), pancreatitis, vascular disease, and tuberculosis (Abrahamian, 2005). A pulmonary embolism is a common cause of pleural effusion in patients younger than 40 years; therefore the presence of a coexisting embolus must be considered in these patients. Because the fluid is not bound in the pleural space, it can shift depending on the position of the patient. When the patient is lying flat, the fluid covers the entire back side of the lung. However, when the patient is sitting up, the fluid pools in the bottom of the pleural space. Many patients are more comfortable sitting up than lying down.

History and Physical Findings

The patient's history of risk factors for a pleural effusion often is helpful in determining the likelihood of its development. Physical findings may be obscured by the underlying disease process, making recognition difficult. Pleural effusion often presents with dyspnea and tachypnea with exertion, but in the setting of a large effusion these can occur at rest. The patient may have chest pain and low oxygen saturation. Patients who have coexisting pneu-

[handwritten:] Salt water drowning - hypertonic solution pulls water into lungs - pulmonary edema

monia also may have a fever and productive cough. Patients with tuberculosis also may have night sweats, fever, hemoptysis, and weight loss. Physical examination may reveal no breath sounds in the lower parts of one or both lungs in patients sitting up and the presence of a pleural friction rub. Indicators of the presence of fluid, such as tactile fremitus, egophony, and bronchophony, may be present. Accessory muscles may be used to assist breathing.

Therapeutic Interventions

Care of the patient includes ensuring oxygenation and ventilation; establishing IV access; and using pulse oximetry, capnography, and ECG monitoring.

Noncardiogenic Pulmonary Edema

[handwritten:] #1 in field

Description

Noncardiogenic pulmonary edema (NCPE) is not a disease, but rather a condition in which fluid builds up in the alveoli in the absence of heart failure (Figure 21-24).

Etiology. This NCPE is the result of a condition of high permeability in the capillary beds in which fluid leaks into the interstitial space and alveoli. In addition, plasma proteins leave the capillary beds, causing an increase in the oncotic pressure in the interstitial space and promoting further escape of fluid from the capillary beds. Surfactant production decreases and alveolar collapse

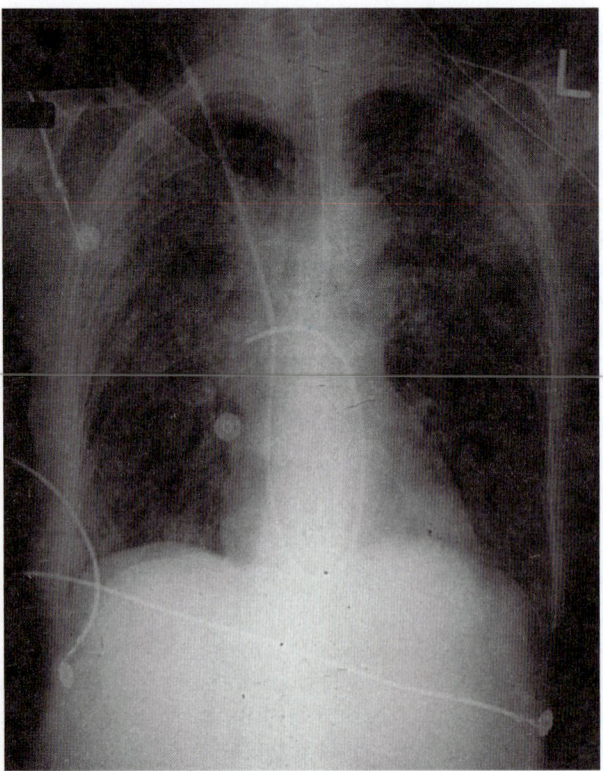

Figure 21-24 Chest radiograph showing noncardiogenic pulmonary edema (NCPE) caused by salicylate use.

(atelectasis) ultimately occurs. Recall that surfactant is the fluid produced within the alveoli that lines its walls to prevent atelectasis. The widened interstitial space between the capillary beds and alveoli interferes with diffusion of oxygen and CO_2.

Demographics

Several reasons for NCPE exist, including exposure to high altitude, pulmonary embolus, drowning, acute glomerulonephritis, fluid overload, aspiration, inhalation injury, neurogenic pulmonary edema, allergic reaction, and acute respiratory distress syndrome (Tintinalli et al., 2004). The cause of neurogenic pulmonary edema is not well understood; however, a strong association exists with increased intracranial pressure and instigation of a sympathetic nervous response. NCPE also has been noted in overdoses of opioids, salicylates, cyclic antidepressants, and other medications. The cause in opioid overdose is unknown.

History and Physical Findings

In the prehospital setting, distinguishing heart failure from NCPE can be difficult. A few clues exist, including a lack of jugular venous distention; a lack of peripheral edema; evidence of adequate cardiac output and end-organ perfusion; and the presence of an initial insult, such as drowning, allergic reaction, shock, high altitude, renal failure, or fluid overload. NCPE can manifest with varying degrees of respiratory distress that may progress to respiratory failure. The primary findings include dyspnea, orthopnea, crackles, rales, tachypnea, tachycardia, hypoxemia or hypoxia, and anxiety.

Therapeutic Interventions

Management of the patient is the same as management of other pulmonary diseases: ensuring oxygenation and ventilation; establishing IV access; and applying pulse oximetry, capnography, and ECG monitoring. Continuous positive airway pressure can be extremely beneficial in these patients and can lessen the incident's severity or the need for intubation. Elevating the patient's upper body and dangling the feet (if possible) may provide some relief. If the incident was induced by high altitude, the patient must be brought to a lower altitude. Placing the patient in an inflatable pressure bag (e.g., a Gamow bag) is beneficial while descending to a lower altitude. Typical management of cardiac-induced pulmonary edema may not provide sufficient relief because nitroglycerin may provide venous relaxation but does not reverse fluid buildup in the alveoli. The same is true for morphine. The judicious use of diuretics can be considered. Although the cause of NCPE is not high capillary pressures, small reductions in circulating volume can cause significant reduction in alveolar extracellular edema. Take caution to avoid extreme diuresis, which can lead to decreased cardiac output and decreased organ perfusion. Cornerstones in management of this patient include providing supplemental oxygen and assisting with ventilation. In severe cases you may have to intubate the patient.

Patient and Family Education

Educate the patient and family about the potential causes of pulmonary edema and possible treatment with diuretics and supplemental oxygen.

usually adults - rarely kids

Acute Respiratory Distress Syndrome

Takes weeks to develop

Acute respiratory distress syndrome (ARDS) is a clinical syndrome in which alveoli are damaged because of significant illness or injury. Some alveoli collapse and others fill with fluid, impairing the exchange of oxygen and carbon dioxide. As the syndrome progresses, more alveoli are affected, gas exchange is further impaired, and respiratory failure ensues, resulting in dyspnea, hypoxia, and pulmonary edema. Conditions such as volume overload or ventricular dysfunction (such as congestive heart failure) do not qualify as ARDS. Possible triggers for ARDS are shown in Box 21-3. Mortality rates range as high as 30% to 40% (Rothenhaus, 2005).

History and Physical Findings

ARDS is often preceded by another massive insult to the body, as previously mentioned. Signs and symptoms include shortness of breath, rapid breathing, inadequate oxygenation, and decreased lung compliance.

noncardiogenic pulmonary edema

Therapeutic Interventions

Management of the patient often is dictated by the nature of the preceding insult. Administer oxygen and apply a pulse oximeter, capnography, and ECG monitor. The patient in moderate to severe respiratory distress typically requires mechanical ventilation to maintain adequate gas exchange. This may include **positive end-expiratory pressure (PEEP)** or continuous positive airway pressure (CPAP). CPAP is discussed later in this chapter.

Self PEEP - blow through pursed lips

Patient and Family Education

keeps alveoli open

Educate the patient and family about the potential causes of ARDS, focusing on the possible causes in each individual patient.

Have other underlying conditions (diabetes, HTN) then something else happens (below) - ok for 2-3 weeks then deteriorate

BOX 21-3 ARDS: Possible Triggers

- Aspiration (near drowning, aspiration of gastric contents) *acid*
- Cardiopulmonary bypass surgery
- Sepsis
- Multiple blood transfusions
- Oxygen toxicity
- Trauma, burns
- Pneumonia, tuberculosis

ARDS, Acute respiratory distress syndrome.

Obstructive and Restrictive Pulmonary Diseases

Asthma
[OBJECTIVE 8]

Histamine → vasodilation (capillary leakage) bronchoconstriction

Description. **Asthma** is most simply defined as a type I allergic reaction associated with an inflammatory response that is expressed in the lower airways. Asthma is classified as a reactive airway disease. All reactive airway diseases lead to air trapping, CO_2 retention, and the eventual development of respiratory acidosis. Unlike chronic reactive airway diseases, in which the patient is in a chronic state of respiratory acidosis, the patient with asthma maintains a normal acid-base balance early in an attack. If the attack is prolonged, respiratory acidosis occurs. The classic components of asthma are bronchospasm, bronchial edema, and excessive mucus production.

Etiology and Demographics. Asthma is estimated to be responsible for as many as 2 million ED visits (Camargo & Brenner, 2006) and 5000 deaths per year. The prevalence of asthma has been increasing over recent years, as have associated healthcare costs. It is the most common chronic disease of childhood, with a prevalence of 5% to 10%. However, asthma is not limited to the pediatric population. It occurs in adults as well and has a prevalence in the elderly of 7% to 10%. Half of all cases develop by the age of 10 years, and another third develop by the age of 30 years. The 2:1 male-to-female ratio equalizes by the age of 30 years. As with any manifestation, allergies may be in response to any substance, such as airborne pollen, mold, dust, mildew, or animal dander. When these allergens initiate an allergic response, middle and lower airways develop edema. This results in narrowed airways, which in turn result in the characteristic wheezing. An additional component contributing to the narrowed airways is the constriction of bronchial smooth muscle. This element also is mediated by a complex interaction of chemical mediators of allergic reaction, as described in Chapter 8. In addition, the goblet cells become hyperactive, producing large amounts of mucus. This further adds to obstruction of the lower airways. The characteristic components of asthma are smooth muscle contraction, vascular congestion, bronchial wall edema and thickening, and the presence of thick secretions. As with many other respiratory diseases, an asthma exacerbation may be concurrent with, or preceded by, a URI.

History and Physical Findings. Patients typically have a history of asthma and describe exposure to a trigger that causes an acute onset of respiratory distress. Bronchial collapse is more prevalent during exhalation, air trapping resulting in hyperinflation of the lungs, and complaints of chest tightness. As this process continues it can interfere with the ability to inhale as the functional capacity of the lungs continues to decrease.

Symptoms vary with the severity of the episode. Because differences exist among patients and their perception of, and response to, bronchoconstriction, correlating signs and symptoms with the degree of airway obstruction is difficult. The paramedic must evaluate each patient individually and compare the current episode to past episodes, including perception, successful and unsuccessful therapies, and disposition. Inquire about increased use of prescribed inhalers, which may indicate an increase in asthma attacks as well as a tolerance to the medication, resulting in decreased effectiveness of treatments. Assess for a history that may affect treatment, such as a medical condition that would be worsened by, or a contraindication for, the administration of corticosteroids. Finally, ask about other medications recently taken that may have caused the attack or would inhibit treatment, such as aspirin or beta-blockers.

The patient is almost always found in the tripod position unless his or her mental status does not allow an upright position. The classic triad of asthma—dyspnea, wheezing, and cough—will be present. In patients with severe cases of asthma, auscultation may reveal few to no breath sounds because the severely restricted air movement through the bronchioles results in insufficient air movement to produce wheezing. This is an ominous finding and is indicative of impending respiratory failure. The paramedic must be able to discern the difference between clear lung sounds and absent lung sounds.

> **PARAMEDIC*Pearl***
>
> Beware a quiet asthmatic. Lack of breath sounds in an asthmatic patient can signal impending respiratory failure.

Additional physical findings may include anxiety, agitation, tachypnea, tachycardia, difficulty completing sentences, prolonged expiration, pallor or cyanosis, decreased muscle tone, attempts to increase positive end-expiratory pressure, and the use of accessory muscles. Accessory muscles of respiration include the suprasternal notch muscles, supraclavicular muscles, and the intercostal muscles. Although the use of accessory muscles may indicate severe distress, it is not prognostic of outcome. The paramedic must thoroughly evaluate the use of accessory muscles and any change that takes place during treatment. Decreased use can occur with improvement in the patient's status or if the patient becomes fatigued from the respiratory effort. Patient fatigue, absent breath sounds, profound diaphoresis, and altered mental status are signs of impending respiratory failure.

You can partially assess the severity of asthma episodes and subsequent improvement or decompensation by using a **peak flow meter,** as previously described (Figure 21-25). Asthma limits the amount of air that can be exhaled in 1 second. Therefore patients with asthma episodes can have peak flows as low as 100 L/min.

As previously described, capnography also is a valuable assessment tool for both the severity of the episode and the patient's response to treatment. Evidence of bronchoconstriction and prolonged expiration appears before the shark-fin waveform. $ETCO_2$ levels are typically

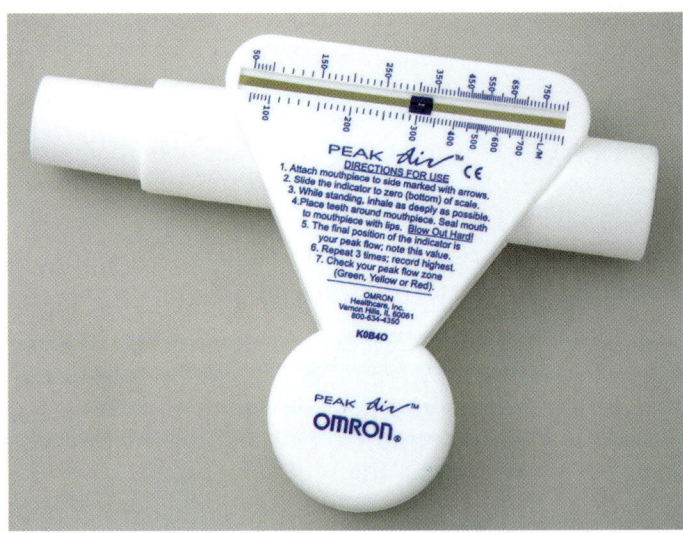

Figure 21-25 Peak flow meter.

normal or only slightly elevated because this is an acute disease process. Elevated $ETCO_2$ levels indicate a prolonged episode. If treatment is effective, the waveform will migrate toward a normal morphologic appearance and $ETCO_2$ levels will remain at or return to normal. If treatment is ineffective, the morphologic features of the waveform will indicate continued or increased bronchoconstriction, and $ETCO_2$ levels will elevate and can be an indication of impending respiratory failure.

> **PARAMEDIC*Pearl***
>
> Ask a patient with asthma whether he or she has been intubated for asthma. This gives you a clue regarding the severity of the patient's disease. Asking how many ED visits and hospital admissions the patient has had is also helpful.

CPAP ↑PEEP

Therapeutic Interventions. Treatment of the asthmatic patient hinges on ensuring adequate ventilation and oxygenation. Place the patient in a position of comfort and administer oxygen. Humidified oxygen is preferred to avoid drying of respiratory secretions, which could lead to an increase in airway obstruction. CPAP is beneficial in reactive airway diseases and may prevent the need for advanced airway management and manual ventilation. Apply a pulse oximeter, capnography, and cardiac monitor. You may need to provide IV therapy to improve hydration and thin and loosen mucus.

Use of inhaled medications such as albuterol can reverse the symptoms of asthma and reduce the need for mechanical ventilation. Albuterol is an inhaled beta$_2$ agonist, acting on beta receptors to dilate airways, reducing the symptoms of wheezing. Ipratropium bromide is an anticholinergic medication that has slower acting bronchodilation effects than albuterol and also reduces airway secretions. Both medications are administered in

↳ works on edema of lower airways

nebulized form, which is a suspension of small particles of medication in air or oxygen. This method encourages delivery of the medication to the affected bronchioles, reducing the loss of the medication in the pharynx. In the setting of respiratory acidosis the effectiveness of these medications is reduced; they work better in the setting of a normal pH.

If the patient is unable to comply with nebulizer therapy because of an altered level of consciousness or inadequate ventilatory effort, the subcutaneous or IV administration of terbutaline may be considered. As a longer acting beta$_2$ agonist, this medication is similar to epinephrine in its ability to cause bronchodilation. Terbutaline also may be nebulized. *If pt. on steroids, is severe asthma*

The administration of IV corticosteroids (e.g., Solu-Medrol) is a frequent adjunct to inhaled beta agonists. Although much slower in onset, corticosteroids can help reduce the allergic response and start the resolution of the airway swelling that precipitated the episode. Corticosteroids reach peak effectiveness approximately 6 to 8 hours after administration. However, their effects may be seen as early as 1 to 2 hours.

Theophylline is a medication that can be used in addition to inhaled beta agonists. It often is taken as a pill in a maintenance dose. You can also administer it IV or rectally. Before the arrival of more specific medications such as inhaled albuterol, theophylline was widely used to treat asthma and lung disease. Theophylline currently is used only as an adjunct to other, more specific medications because of its potential side effects. Theophylline, unlike most of the medications used to treat asthma, must be monitored to avoid toxicity such as agitation, hypertension, and heart dysrhythmias. *O Brou Im if at least 66#*

Patients who are in severe distress, have impending respiratory failure, or are in respiratory failure should be considered candidates for the administration of epinephrine. In the past this has been done by the subcutaneous administration of 1:1000 epinephrine. However, new evidence indicates intramuscular injection is more beneficial. Epinephrine is not specific to the beta$_2$ receptors, but rather has general alpha and beta effects. Therefore many more cardiac effects and potential risks exist when administering this medication. Careful consideration must be made regarding alternative treatment decisions and the patient's response to prior treatments. However, if other treatments are ineffective and the patient is approaching respiratory failure, epinephrine administration is indicated. *30 mm. or more - not responding to tx*

Patients who do not respond to initial treatment **(status asthmaticus)** or those already in respiratory failure before your arrival may require intubation and mechanical ventilation. These patients often benefit from preintubation sedation with benzodiazepines (or similar medications) if available. Once you have secured the patient's airway, you must note that ventilating the asthmatic patient's lungs may be more difficult than for other patients, mostly because of the increased resistance to air movement. Because intubation does not have any effect

on bronchoconstriction, the patient may still remain hypoxic despite mechanical ventilation. The treatment for status asthmaticus is the same as for asthma. Attempts at reversing the underlying bronchoconstriction must continue even in the intubated patient and may include the use of an inline nebulizer to administer bronchodilators and continued use of injected beta agonists.

Patient and Family Education. Educate the patient and family about the mechanism of asthma. This may allow the patient to understand effects of the disease. Emphasize that avoiding potential allergens is key in avoiding exacerbations of asthma. Exposure to any potential allergen can initiate an asthma episode. Active or passive smoke exposure is a major contributor to asthmatic disease. Thus educating the patient about avoiding tobacco exposure may help reduce future episodes. Some asthma medications are preventative only; therefore taking them when an episode flares up is not as effective. Medications such as inhaled steroids have little or no efficacy during an acute episode. Stress to the patient and family that medication compliance is important in minimizing the effects that asthma has on the patient's life.

Bronchiolitis

Description. Wheezing is caused by many things in an infant. However, **bronchiolitis** is one of the more frequently encountered conditions. Bronchiolitis is an acute, infectious, inflammatory disease of the upper and lower respiratory tracts that results in obstruction of the small airways. Although it may occur in all age groups, the larger airways of older children and adults tolerate the infection better than infants. Severe respiratory problems usually are limited to young infants.

Etiology and Demographics. Bronchiolitis is estimated to affect more than 1.5 million infants each year, primarily children younger than 2 years. Patients younger than 1 year account for 80% of those with bronchiolitis, with a peak incidence at age 2 to 6 months. It accounts for an estimated 90,000 hospitalizations each year and 4500 deaths annually. The condition is seasonal and generally occurs from mid-winter to mid-spring. Those born within 6 months of the typical season have an increased likelihood of contracting bronchiolitis. It is slightly more common in males, with approximately 1.25 males affected for each female. Risk factors include low birth weight, crowded living conditions, daycare exposure, smoking exposure, and chronic heart and lung conditions (Louden, 2006). **Respiratory syncytial virus** is the primary cause of bronchiolitis and pneumonia in children younger than 1 year.

History and Physical Findings. Infection results in obstruction of bronchioles from inflammation and edema. This obstruction leads to hyperinflation of the lungs, increased wheezing, course crackles, and atelectasis. This makes differentiating it from asthma difficult. Bronchiolitis frequently starts much the same as a URI, including cough, runny nose, low-grade fever (temperature below 101° F), and decreased appetite. Parents may describe the patient as "fussy" and not eating well. This can lead to signs of dehydration such as dry mucous membranes, depressed fontanels, a decrease in wet diapers, crying without tear production, and signs of poor perfusion. The dehydration can be severe in some cases. The presence of dehydration can assist in the differentiation from asthma. More severe cases can cause tachypnea, tachycardia, accessory muscle use, nasal flaring, grunting, cyanosis, crackles, wheezing and, rarely, apnea. Severe symptoms are more frequently seen in young infants or those with preexisting pulmonary problems (Krilov, 2006).

Therapeutic Interventions. In the prehospital setting, primary intervention includes supportive care; treatment is similar to the treatment of asthma. Assist the patient into a position of comfort. Keep him or her calm and comfortable. Apply a pulse oximeter and capnography. Give oxygen in a manner that does not agitate the patient. Keep the oxygen saturation above 95%. Nebulized beta agonists may be administered for bronchoconstriction. There is conflicting evidence regarding the efficacy of anticholinergic bronchodilator therapy. Support hydration as necessary. If signs of respiratory failure or respiratory arrest are present, assist ventilation with a bag-mask device with 100% oxygen. Closely coordinate more aggressive intervention, such as the use of bronchodilators, with medical control.

Patient and Family Education. Educate the patient and family about the cause of the disease. Respiratory syncytial virus is spread by direct or indirect contact with infected nasal secretions. Individuals may transmit the virus by hand-to-hand (sneezing into the hand) or hand-to-nose contact for 1 to 2 days before and 1 to 2 weeks after symptoms begin. Diligent handwashing and good hygiene are necessary to avoid spreading the disease. Also discuss appropriate methods of fever control.

Bronchopulmonary Dysplasia (NO)

Description. Preterm infants (less than 36 weeks' gestation) may have more difficulties than term infants. One of the more common problems with very early infants is an immature pulmonary system. **Bronchopulmonary dysplasia (BPD)** is defined as any child needing oxygen supplementation at 28 days to maintain a PO_2 of 50 mm Hg. In BPD, inflammation and scarring of the smaller airways and alveoli make breathing difficult and impair gas exchange.

Etiology and Demographics. Prolonged treatment with positive-pressure ventilation and high oxygen concentrations are among the causes of BPD. Children with severe BPD are at higher risk of death or disability in the first 2 years of life (Driscoll, 2006).

History and Physical Findings. Infants with BPD are usually premature and of very low birth weight. Signs and symptoms include tachypnea, tachycardia, retractions, and nasal flaring. On auscultation, patients may show decreased breath sounds, rhonchi, fine crackles, or wheezing.

Therapeutic Interventions. You may provide supplemental oxygen in the prehospital setting, but in careful amounts. High levels of oxygenation can be damaging to the patient with BPD. Maintain oxygen saturation in the 90% to 95% range and provide supportive care.

Patient and Family Education. Educate the family about possible causes of BPD and encourage medical compliance during treatment.

Chronic Obstructive Pulmonary Disease

Description. **Chronic obstructive pulmonary disease (COPD)** is a catchall term that may include varying degrees of bronchitis, emphysema, and asthma. Often occurring in combination, these diseases often are initiated or perpetuated by long-term tobacco abuse or other long-term exposure to inhaled toxins. Other examples include cotton dust (brown lung), coal dust (black lung), sawdust, and dust from grains.

Each of these disease processes is slightly different and bears consideration separately, then together as the collective condition COPD.

Etiology and Demographics. An estimated 32 million people have COPD. It is the fourth leading cause of death in the United States (Kleinschmidt, 2005) and the only leading cause of death that has increased in prevalence. Patients diagnosed with COPD are almost always age 40 years or older. However, the consideration of COPD should not be limited to this age group. A genetic condition called *alpha₁ antitrypsin deficiency* is a cause of early-onset emphysema. This can occur in the absence of smoking or exposure to other inhaled toxins. COPD is the result of a combination of emphysema, chronic bronchitis, and asthma. Some patients have bronchitis predominant; others may have the emphysematous portion predominant (Figure 21-26). Either patient may have fea-

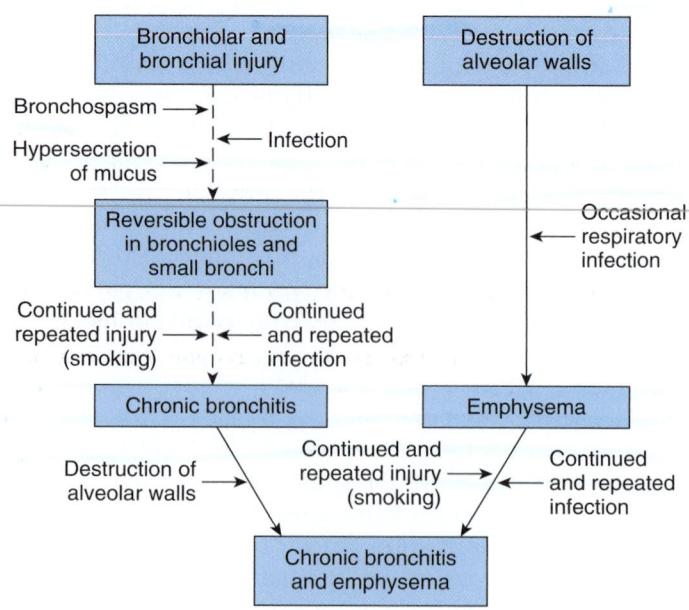

Figure 21-26 Algorithm for chronic obstructive pulmonary disease (COPD).

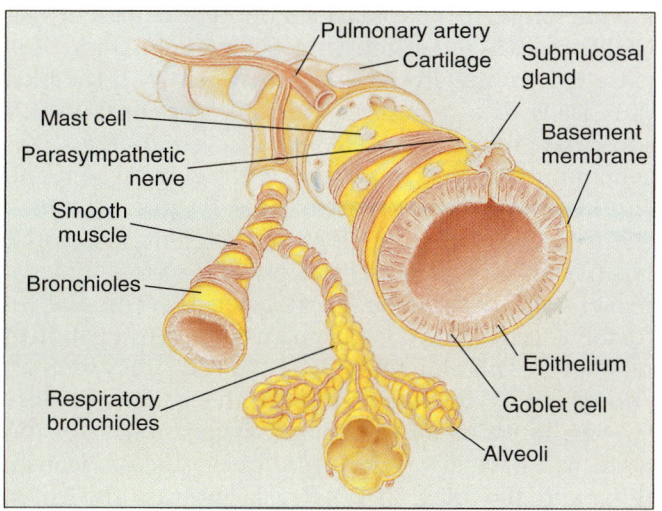

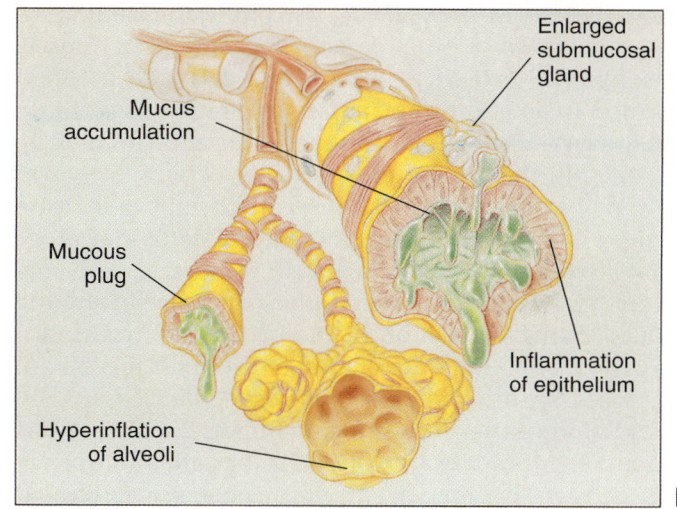

A   **B**

Figure 21-27 A, Normal lung. **B,** Chronic bronchitis: inflammation and thickening of mucous membrane with accumulation of mucus and pus leading to obstruction; characterized by cough.

tures of asthma superimposed. All varieties of COPD are heavily affected by smoking.

History and Physical Findings

CO$_2$ 44-45

[OBJECTIVE 8]

Those with **bronchitis**-predominant COPD have an overproduction of mucus and enlargement of the cells in the lungs and airways that make mucus and cause congestion and blockage of the airways (Figure 21-27). Unlike emphysema, chronic bronchitis does not involve extensive damage to the alveoli. Therefore it is defined in clinical terms rather than terms of anatomic pathology. A productive cough for 3 months or longer, occurring for 2 or more consecutive years and without an identifiable cause, leads to the diagnosis of chronic bronchitis. This condition is caused by hypertrophy of the goblet cells and an increase in mucus production. It results in hypoventilation of the alveoli, dropping the oxygen level in the blood. CO$_2$ is retained in the blood for the same reason. Acidosis develops as a result of the hypoventilation. The body responds by increasing cardiac output and increasing red blood cell production in an effort to get sufficient oxygen into the tissues (Rosen & Barkin, 1998).

Emphysema, in contrast to bronchitis, does involve the alveoli (Figure 21-28). Long-term damage by either tobacco or inhaled agents causes alveolar destruction, alveolar coalescence, and destruction of the elastin fibers surrounding the alveoli. These pathologic changes are permanent and lead to a decrease in alveolar surface area, a decrease in elasticity of the alveoli, right-to-left shunting, a ventilation-perfusion mismatch, an increase in the residual volume of the lung, a decrease in the expiratory reserve capacity, and a decrease in vital capacity of the lung. Combined, these factors cause chronic hypoxia and chronic hypercarbia. Blebs, or weakened areas of large alveoli, are often present on the surface of the lungs, are

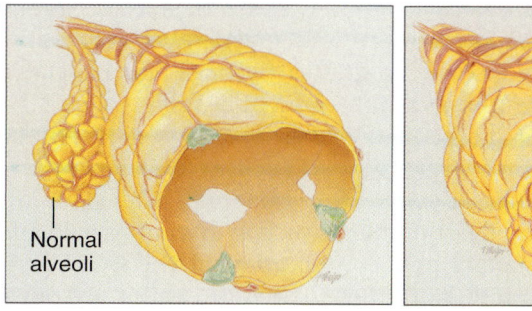

Normal alveoli

Figure 21-28 Enlargement and destruction of alveolar walls caused by emphysema.

vulnerable to spontaneous rupture, and can lead to a possible pneumothorax. The increased work of breathing as a result of hypoxia affects the entire body. Polycythemia eventually occurs in all patients with COPD in an attempt to increase oxygen delivery to the cells. This progresses more slowly in the patient with emphysema than in the patient with chronic bronchitis. Muscle wasting occurs because of the increased caloric requirement of the work of breathing. The presence of muscle wasting gives the patient a thin and almost malnourished appearance. The increased residual volume results in physical changes of the thoracic cage as the anteroposterior diameter becomes larger than the lateral diameter. This is commonly referred to as a *barrel chest.* *over inflation + weak muscles*

Asthma in the setting of COPD is similar to purely asthmatic patients. Hyperstimulation and constriction of the bronchioles result in wheezing and dyspnea, which can occur with varying degrees of either bronchitis, emphysema, or both. However, the combination of asthma with the other disease processes can make management much more difficult.

Patients with emphysema-predominant COPD may exhibit increasing chronic dyspnea, little or no cough,

↑ RBC

pink puffer

No goblet cells

and little mucus production. The physical examination typically shows a thin patient as a result of muscle wasting. The patient may be bent forward in a tripod position in an effort to maximize respiration. Dyspnea is the universal finding, and the accessory muscles may be recruited in the respiratory effort. The patient likely will have pursed lips on exhalation in an attempt to increase positive end-expiratory pressure. Mental status may range from alert and anxious to agitated, combative, or comatose. Both hypoxia and hypercarbia play a role in altering mental status. Evaluation of the hands may reveal cyanosis and clubbing. Auscultation of the chest may reveal decreased breath sounds or a hyperresonant chest from destruction of the alveoli (Kleinschmidt, 2006). If this is the first significant exacerbation for the patient, he or she may deny the presence of emphysema because the patient is unaware it exists. Because the onset of emphysema is gradual, patients often attribute decreased respiratory function to the aging process and reduce physical activity to match respiratory abilities. Not until an acute episode during exertion, generally in the fifth or sixth decade of life, does the patient receive an actual diagnosis of emphysema. As the diseases progresses, dyspnea and associated signs and symptoms will be present at rest.

Bronchitis-predominant patients also exhibit chronic dyspnea, are frequently obese, have a chronic, productive cough, and have progressive weight gain. These patients often develop heart problems such as cor pulmonale and ventricular failure as a complication of the COPD. On physical examination these patients exhibit dyspnea, cough, accessory muscle use, prolonged exhalation, and low oxygen levels. You can obtain a history of chronic lung infections from the patient. On auscultation of the chest, you can hear coarse rhonchi and wheezing. The patient may show signs of right ventricular failure, such as edema in the legs. As with emphysema the patient may be unaware of the presence of chronic bronchitis early in the course of the disease process. Early symptoms are subtle and include an intermittent cough that eventually progresses to a more constant productive cough, increased frequency in chest colds, and eventually hypoxemia associated with dyspnea on exertion.

Therapeutic Interventions. Management of patients with COPD hinges on rapid assessment of oxygenation and supplementation of both oxygenation and ventilation. Initial steps should include providing oxygen sufficient to relieve symptoms of dyspnea or at least raise saturations to 90%. Several modalities exist for this. You can choose a nasal cannula, Venturi mask, or nonrebreather mask according to oxygen delivery need and patient comfort. As previously described, compare and contrast the current episode with past episodes, evaluate attempts at medication, and determine medication use and compliance. Because the underlying lung disease places these patients at risk for other conditions, the paramedic should be alert for other causes of the respiratory distress such as pulmonary embolus or a spontaneous pneumothorax.

One problem you may encounter in patients with COPD is CO_2 retention. Insufficient ventilation leaves extra CO_2 in the alveoli and subsequently in the blood. This leads to a condition known as **carbon dioxide narcosis.** You may see PCO_2 levels as high as 80, 90, or even more than 100 in patients with severe exacerbation. High CO_2 levels result in increased sleepiness and sedation. CPAP is beneficial for these patients because the positive pressure prevents collapse of the bronchioles and makes exhalation easier. CPAP often prevents the need for advanced airway management such as intubation and manual ventilation. However, the CO_2 may rise high enough that you must intubate the patient to ensure airway protection and adequate oxygenation. The capnogram will have a waveform indicating bronchoconstriction, and the high $ETCO_2$ levels indicate the chronic nature of the illness. The effectiveness of treatment can be monitored by changes in $ETCO_2$ levels. A decreasing $ETCO_2$ level indicates improvement, whereas an increasing level indicates decompensation. Unlike acute asthma, the waveform will not likely return to normal in these patients because some degree of bronchoconstriction is always present.

As with asthma, COPD is a reactive airway disease. Therefore treatment is directed at reducing bronchoconstriction and airway secretions. Nebulized beta agonists often are beneficial in patients with COPD, including albuterol and ipratropium bromide. Injected beta agonists such as terbutaline and epinephrine can also be considered. However, extreme caution must be observed with the administration of epinephrine in these patients because of its cardiovascular side effects; it should be considered only in the setting of impending respiratory failure. Solu-Medrol may also be considered for the same reasons. Obtain IV access and initiate ECG monitoring, pulse oximetry, capnography, and peak expiratory flow testing. During transport, pay careful attention to reassessment, ensuring that ventilation does not deteriorate into a situation requiring intubation.

Patient and Family Education. Educate the patient and family about avoiding cigarette smoke exposure, whether active or passive. Patients may have had many years of tobacco abuse, and nicotine addiction can be challenging to overcome. Encourage routine follow-up with the patient's physician. These follow-ups will help reduce current episodes and the recurrence rate.

Cystic Fibrosis
Skin is salty

[OBJECTIVE 8] *Lots of mucus in lungs*

Cystic fibrosis (CF) is a genetic disease that has multiple complications. The most relevant complication for EMS professionals is pulmonary distress.

Etiology and Demographics. Changes in the functioning of the chemistry of the glands create thicker than normal secretions. These thicker secretions cause chronic infections, resulting in the most common complication of the disease—pulmonary infections. Most fatalities from the disease result from progressive lung disease. CF also can affect the liver and pancreas, but symptoms predominate in the respiratory tract. CF is the most common inherited disorder in whites, with one in 25 people carrying the genes and almost one in 3200 people contracting the condition. The median life span of a patient with clinical CF is 36.8 years (Sharma, 2006).

History and Physical Findings. Other than a history of CF, many patients may present similar to those with COPD or pneumonia. You may see cough, chest wall pain, dyspnea, or fever. Physical examination may reveal crackles on close auscultation. The chest wall may be tender on palpation.

Therapeutic Interventions. As with the other pulmonary disease processes, management hinges on supplemental oxygen, ventilation, and monitoring of oxygenation and ventilatory and cardiac function.

Patient and Family Education. Instruct the patient and family about symptomatic relief by controlling fever and avoiding passive tobacco smoke exposure. Also encourage close supervision by a physician specializing in CF.

Pneumonia

[OBJECTIVE 9]

Pneumonia is classically interpreted as an infection in the terminal breathing spaces, specifically the alveoli (Figure 21-29). Overall, pneumonia is the sixth leading cause of death in the United States and the leading cause of death from infectious disease. Of the 2 to 4 million cases per year, approximately 500,000 are admitted to the hospital. This disease is particularly deadly in the elderly population.

Etiology and Demographics. Pneumonia can be caused by a wide variety of pathogens, ranging from bacteria to funguses to viruses. The responsible organism is not definitively identified in 20% to 60% of pneumonia cases. The more common pathogens include the following:

- Virus—respiratory syncytial virus, parainfluenza, influenza, adenovirus

↳ most common cause of pneumonia in children (handwritten)

- Bacteria—Common: *H. influenzae, Streptococcus pneumoniae* (Figure 21-30), *Mycoplasma* spp., *Klebsiella* spp., *Pseudomonas* spp. Uncommon: *Pneumocystis carinii, Mycobacterium tuberculosis, Acinetobacter* spp., *Enterococcus* spp.
- Fungi

Influenza is a common viral URI that may result in a viral pneumonia. Pneumonia caused by influenza is one of the leading causes of morbidity from influenza infections (Tintinalli et al., 2004).

Pneumonia may occur as a primary infection or secondary to another illness or infection. It often is classified in the following manner by anatomic location:

- *Lobar pneumonia:* localized to one or more lobes of the lung
- *Bronchopneumonia:* inflammation around medium-sized airways, which causes patchy consolidation of parts of the lobes
- *Interstitial pneumonia:* inflammation of lung tissue between the air sacs

Pneumonia often is classified as community acquired or hospital acquired. Although the latter term seems to specify a hospital, the location can be any health care facility. In general, community-acquired pneumonia is managed in the outpatient setting and has a low mortality rate. However, its incidence is increasing. Infections acquired in a healthcare setting have a higher mortality rate because they tend to be more virulent strains of infectious organisms that may be resistant to medications.

History and Physical Findings. Possible signs and symptoms of pneumonia are shown in Box 21-4 and largely depend on the causative organism. The history

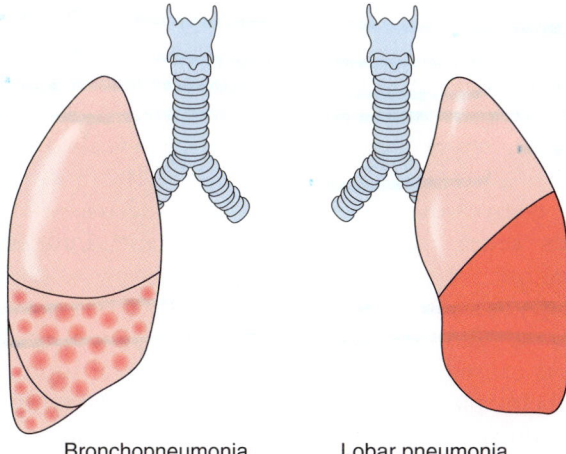

Bronchopneumonia   Lobar pneumonia

Figure 21-29 Pneumonia.

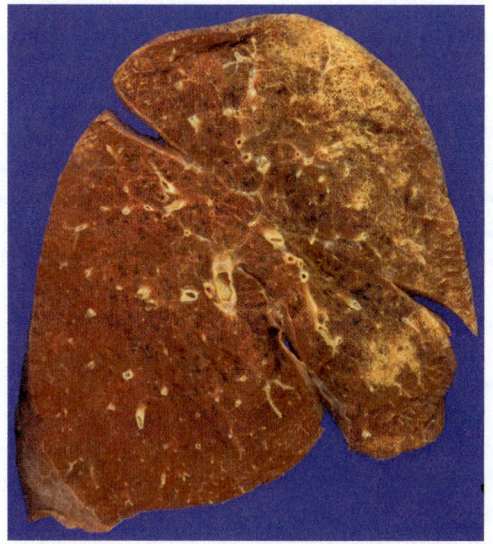

Figure 21-30 Lobar pneumonia caused by *Streptococcus pneumoniae.* Note the involvement of the entire lower lobe and portions of the upper and middle lobes of the right lung.

BOX 21-4 Signs and Symptoms of Pneumonia

Typical Pneumonia

- Acute onset of fever and chills
- Productive cough with purulent sputum - *yellow*
- Pleuritic chest pain (in some cases)
- Pulmonary consolidation on auscultation - *agophany*
- Location of bronchial breath sounds
- Crackles
- Lethargy
- Anorexia
- Tachypnea
- Tachycardia
- Chest, side, or back pain

Atypical Pneumonia - *older people*

- Nonproductive cough
- Extrapulmonary symptoms
- Headache
- Myalgias
- Fatigue
- Sore throat
- Nausea, vomiting, diarrhea
- Fever and chills
  ↳ lower grade

often includes the abrupt onset of chills, pleuritic chest pain, and a purulent, productive cough with sputum that may be green, yellow, or rust in color. Physical examination of the patient may reveal varying degrees of respiratory distress, fever, tachycardia, tachypnea, and potentially low oxygen saturation. Crackles may be present over affected lobes (with other lobes normal) in lobar pneumonia, scattered crackles in bronchopneumonia, and scattered crackles and wheezes in interstitial pneumonia. In the elderly pneumonia often presents with nonspecific complaints such as acute confusion or changes in the normal ability to function. Often by the time pneumonia is recognized in these patients, it may be severe and the patient may be septic without prior indicators of an infection. Certain agents cause atypical pneumonia. In these cases the patient may have a gradual onset of the disease, a nonproductive cough, and a low-grade fever or the absence of fever. Although the determination of typical or atypical pneumonia is unnecessary in the prehospital setting, the paramedic must be aware of its presence so as not to miss the diagnosis of pneumonia in the absence of a productive cough and fever.

Complicating factors may make pneumonia more severe, including advanced age and underlying medical problems such as COPD, heart disease, alcoholism, or diabetes. AIDS or other immunocompromised conditions open the door for a wide variety of unusual infections, including fungi and viruses.

Therapeutic Interventions. Care of the patient hinges on optimizing oxygenation. Supplemental oxygen is the starting point, whether by nasal cannula or nonrebreather

mask for more severely ill patients, along with standard monitoring of respiratory status (pulse oximetry, capnography, and ECG monitoring). The use of bronchodilators is generally avoided in these patients. However, if the patient has a history of COPD and evidence of bronchoconstriction is present, these may be considered. Severely ill patients may require endotracheal intubation. Obtain IV access after securing the airway. Patients who are hypovolemic or in septic shock should be treated for these conditions. In many cases antibiotic therapy is required, but this often is reserved for in-hospital management. The paramedic must take all possible precautions for personal protection and respect the fact that pneumonia is an infectious disease. The increase in drug-resistant tuberculosis has received large amounts of media attention, but the incidence of drug-resistant pneumonia also is on the rise.

Patient and Family Education. Instruct the patient and family about proper hygiene. Also educate them about reducing communicability by reducing spread by respiratory droplets. Emphasize to the patient and family that good hygiene may not prevent transmission, and that some bacteria commonly live in the respiratory tract. Also emphasize preventive care, including avoiding tobacco use, getting regular exercise, and following the primary care physician's instructions.

Lung Abscess

Description. In some cases pneumonia may involve an abscess, called a **pulmonary abscess.** Pulmonary abscesses are collections of pus in the lung tissue itself (Figure 21-31). They often are the result of aspiration of gastric contents. An abscess develops more slowly than pneumonia. It can take several weeks for clinical signs to develop.

Etiology and Demographics. Patients who are intoxicated, under the influence of drugs, or have an impaired gag reflex are at higher risk of aspiration and development of pulmonary abscess. Pulmonary abscesses have a mortality rate of 4% to 20% or higher depending on the cause.

History and Physical Findings. Patients may already have been diagnosed with pneumonia and on physical examination show a productive cough of sputum with unusual odors, dyspnea, fever, night sweats, decreased appetite or weight loss, and occasionally chest or chest wall pain. Physical examination often reveals a patient who has a low-grade fever (100.5° F to 102.0° F), tachypnea, tachycardia, crackles, rhonchi, decreased breath sounds often in the lower lobes, and dullness to percussion.

Empyema, in contrast to pulmonary abscess, is a collection of pus outside the lung in the pleural space. It often is caused by chest trauma, esophageal rupture, or tubes being placed into the chest. The physical symptoms and findings are quite similar to pulmonary abscess.

Therapeutic Interventions. These patients often benefit from supplemental oxygen and supportive care. Rarely

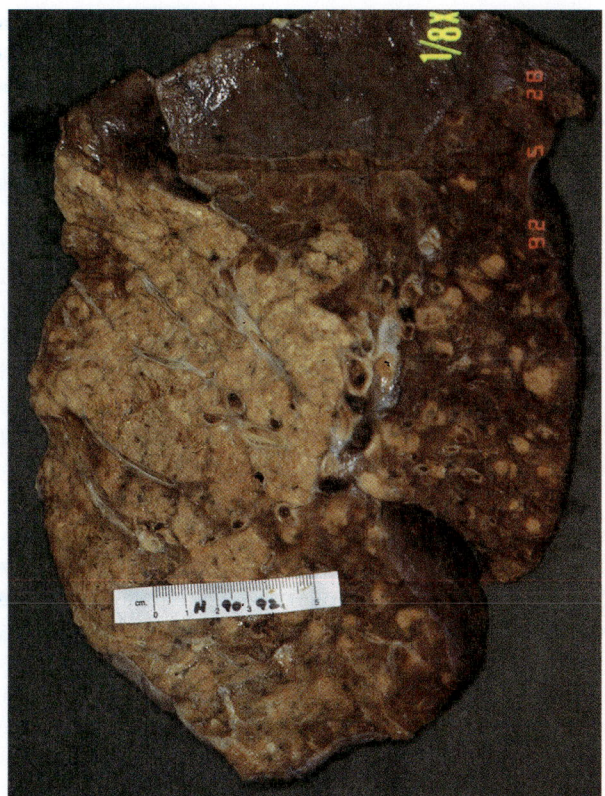

Figure 21-31 Multiple lung abscesses seen at autopsy of a patient with acute pneumonia.

you may be required to intubate to protect the airway from further aspiration, but this is caused by conditions other than the pulmonary abscess. These patients require antibiotics and possible surgical drainage of the abscess (Zwanger, 2006).

Patient and Family Education. Instruct the patient and family about the basics of abscess and the need for intervention, including possibly surgery. You may emphasize that abscesses are not contagious, but they do require proper evaluation and treatment to avoid complications.

Aspiration Pneumonia and Pneumonitis

Description. The inspiration of fluids not intended for the lungs is termed **aspiration.** A small amount of saliva may be aspirated each day. This only amounts to a few milliliters and rarely creates problems. However, aspiration of gastric acid or food from the upper airway or stomach can cause an inflammatory response that can lead to hypoxia and respiratory failure.

Etiology and Demographics. Aspiration is a significant problem for patients who have an altered mental status. Patients who are intoxicated or who have chronic disability, feeding tubes, a history of strokes, head trauma, or problems controlling the airway are at increased risk for aspiration.

Two injuries may occur with aspiration. **Aspiration pneumonitis** is lung and bronchoalveolar irritation caused by aspirated stomach acid. It produces swelling and occasionally fluid collection in the alveoli. Patients who aspirate pure stomach acid are at most risk of pneumonitis. Recent meals, acid-blocking medications, and decreased stomach emptying decrease the risk of pneumonitis. Aspiration pneumonitis may take several hours to develop, but the risk decreases significantly several days after the insult.

However, those who inhale stomach contents or food are more at risk for developing aspiration pneumonia. The food particles clog the airways and bring bacteria to the lower parts of the lungs. These parts of the lungs are prime locations for pneumonia. Pneumonia, frequently bacterial, often takes several hours to days to develop after aspiration. Because of the types of bacteria, patients with aspiration pneumonia are at higher risk for developing pulmonary abscesses (Swaminathan, 2006). Distinguishing aspiration pneumonia and aspiration pneumonitis is extremely difficult. However, several studies suggest that 5% to 15% of the 4.5 million cases of community-acquired pneumonia result from aspiration pneumonia. Approximately 10% of patients who are hospitalized after drug overdoses have aspiration pneumonitis (Swaminathan, 2006).

History and Physical Findings. Patients with either aspiration pneumonitis or pneumonia often have dyspnea and occasional airway obstruction with aspirated gastric or oropharyngeal contents. Conducting a careful history frequently reveals some decrease in mental status, either acute or chronic. Patients also may have fever, chills, dyspnea on exertion, orthopnea (which often occurs during sleep and may be referred to as *paroxysmal nocturnal dyspnea* or *supine dyspnea*), pleuritic chest pain, and a productive cough that may or may not contain food particles.

Physical examination of the patient may reveal any degree of respiratory distress from mild to severe. Signs of typical pneumonia may or may not be present. You may see altered mental status, possibly as a result of hypoxia.

Therapeutic Interventions. You must consider aggressive airway control in any patient who may have aspirated. Consider intubating any patient with altered mental status, but this should be guided by patient presentation as well as oxygenation and ability to control the airway. Initiate IV access and apply standard monitoring. For patients with chronic illness, determine do not intubate status with the family or caregivers, if possible. If a do not resuscitate order does not exist, your local protocols may dictate intubation. Follow your local protocols.

Patient and Family Education. Educate the patient and family about recognizing possible opportunities for aspiration and point out avenues for reducing the exposure to potential aspiration. Under the care of a physician, various dietary changes can be explored, including thickened liquids and solids, nutrition by means other than oral ingestion, or assistance in feeding.

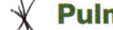

Pulmonary Tuberculosis

Night sweats
Homeless, prisons

Description. **Tuberculosis (TB)** is a pulmonary disease caused by the bacterium *Mycobacterium tuberculosis*. It is transmitted by airborne droplets.

Etiology and Demographics. According to the World Health Organization, tuberculosis is the primary health problem in the world today. An estimated nearly 3 million people die each year of TB infections. Worldwide, an estimated 10 to 12 million people harbor TB and are potentially infectious or may eventually develop the disease (Herchline, 2006). In 2004 the national active TB case rate was 4.9 cases per 100,000 persons, representing 14,511 reported cases and a decline of 3% from 2003. The majority of cases reported (60%) came from seven states: California, Florida, Illinois, New York, New Jersey, Georgia, and Texas (Li, 2006).

TB bacteria are inhaled into the lungs and produce disease either immediately or in the future. Among immigrants to the United States, the top three countries of incidence are Vietnam, The Philippines, and India. In the United States more than 60% of cases were in patients aged 25 to 64 years old. TB can affect many organs, including the lungs, bones, skin, urinary tract, gastrointestinal tract, or lymphatic system. A single cough can generate 3000 infective droplets. Fewer than 10 mycobacterial bacilli may initiate a pulmonary infection (Li, 2006).

Tuberculosis evolves through four distinct stages in the human body. In the first stage the bacterium is inhaled into the lungs and standard inflammatory and immune responses are triggered. If the body's defenses are able to contain and eradicate the bacteria, the infection does not progress. If the body is not able to fend off the infection, stage two begins. In this stage, although the inflammatory and immune responses continue, they are ineffective and the bacteria multiply rapidly. An infected area of the lung, called a *tubercle,* is formed in this stage. Also during this stage the infection can spread through the lymphatic system and eventually into the vascular system and throughout the body, possibly causing extrapulmonary tuberculosis. This condition can affect the lymphatic system, renal system, central nervous system, skeletal system, and the genitals. Pericarditis, peritonitis, and gastrointestinal disease also can result from extrapulmonary tuberculosis.

The third stage begins 2 to 3 weeks after the first stage. During this stage the inflammatory and immune responses are finally able to contain the spread of the infectious organisms. As part of this stage granulomas are formed and tissue destruction occurs. However, the bacteria can survive in a dormant state in the body for years. Depending on the function of the host defenses, the bacteria may remain dormant or progress to an active TB infection. The first three stages represent the processes that take place in primary TB. Unless the patient is unable to contain the infection and develops active TB, these stages often occur without signs and symptoms, and the patient is unaware of the infection until a TB skin test result is positive. The fourth and final stage of TB can occur months, years, or decades after the initial infection. During this stage the dormant bacteria reactivate as a result of the tubercle eroding and releasing the contained bacteria back into the lung. This can result in bronchopneumonia or an active case of TB, often called *reactivation TB* or *postprimary TB.*

History and Physical Findings. As stated previously, the initial infection often results in few, if any, signs and symptoms. If signs and symptoms do develop, they typically show up 4 to 6 weeks after the initial infection and are nonspecific. These symptoms are often a result of the immune response, such as a low-grade fever and malaise. This is of particular concern to the paramedic and the general population because a patient may carry the bacteria unbeknownst to others.

Active TB is characterized by a productive cough, fever, and weight loss. Symptoms include hemoptysis, chest or chest wall pain, weight or appetite loss, fatigue, irritability, weakness, headache, chills, fever, and night sweats. Elderly patients often have an atypical presentation of TB and have a chronic cough, failure to thrive, and fewer respiratory symptoms. Physical examination of these patients is often similar to that for patients with pneumonia. You may see fever, occasionally dyspnea, and rhonchi or rales. Unlike most types of pneumonia, TB shows an affinity for the upper lobes. Thus the respiratory sounds of the upper lobes may be more notable (Figure 21-32).

Therapeutic Interventions. Treatment hinges on identifying patients at risk for TB so that respiratory isolation may be initiated. Obtain a detailed history regarding TB exposure or treatment if possible. If you suspect this diagnosis, initiate respiratory isolation with masks, as described below, and notify the receiving ED. Failure to notify the ED as soon as possible carries the risk of expos-

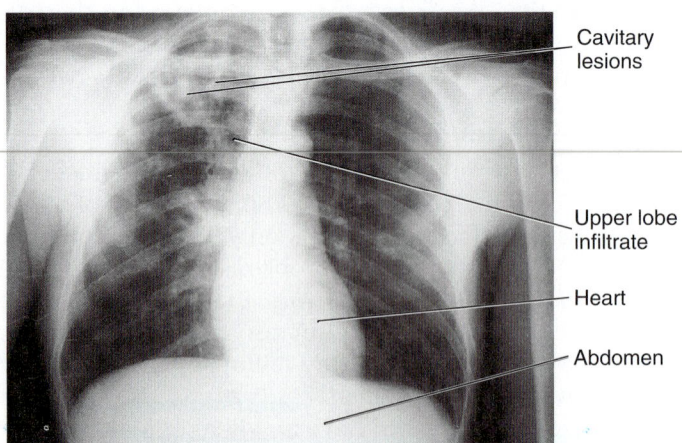

Figure 21-32 Radiograph showing pulmonary tuberculosis caused by *Mycobacterium tuberculosis*. The patient is a 38-year-old man with a 3-month history of cough, hemoptysis, fever, and a 30-pound weight loss. He had been incarcerated recently for 6 months.

ing the entire staff and all patients in the ED to TB and may result in a negative pressure room being unavailable on your arrival. The most significant emergent risk for patients with active TB is aspiration of blood from hemoptysis. Be prepared to take precautions against this, including securing the airway through advanced airway management.

Finally, the paramedic should consider personal protection as part of treatment to prevent infection. Place a surgical mask on the patient and a high-efficiency particulate air (HEPA) or N-95 mask on yourself. The HEPA or N-95 mask should never be placed on the patient because it will be ineffective and may increase respiratory distress. With the increased incidence of drug-resistant TB the paramedic should take every precaution to avoid exposure and infection. If you suspect you have been exposed to any form of TB, immediately notify your infection control officer and follow your agency's policies regarding testing and treatment.

Patient and Family Education. Instruction of the patient and family should focus on isolating those suspected of having TB and medical evaluation of those possibly exposed to infected individuals. Antibiotic therapy may be indicated for patients diagnosed with TB as well as close family members who may have preclinical disease. Antibiotics may be taken for longer periods than with normal pneumonia, possibly 6 months to 1 year. Discuss the appropriate use of antibiotics and the relation of inappropriate use to the development of drug-resistant TB.

Pulmonary Thromboembolism

Description. A **pulmonary embolus (PE),** or pulmonary thromboembolism, occurs when a thrombus (clot) becomes dislodged and travels through the bloodstream. The travelling clot whether a blood clot, fat, or air, is now an embolus and lodges in a pulmonary artery, obstructing blood flow to a portion of the lung (Figure 21-33).

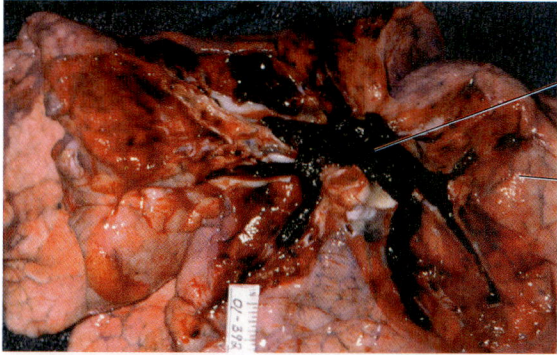

Figure 21-33 A massive pulmonary embolism observed on autopsy. This man had vague respiratory symptoms for 2 weeks. A physician diagnosed bronchitis. The patient died as a result of a large clot that plugged the distal lobar arterial branches. The clot eventually produced nearly complete obstruction of blood flow and resulted in cardiac arrest.

The more vessels that are blocked, the more severe the condition. Often these are blood clots that originate in the legs, traveling through the inferior vena cava, to the right ventricle, and into the pulmonary artery. PEs also may originate from the right atrium in the case of atrial fibrillation. The fibrillation pattern and subsequent ineffective blood flow may allow blood to clot in the heart, and these clots often pass to the lungs.

Etiology and Demographics. PE is a unique pathology that has proven elusive in many cases. For most diagnoses, physicians look for a few unique clinical criteria that narrow down of a list of differential diagnoses. For example, in pneumonia physicians look for fever, dyspnea, and rales. Unfortunately, PE has proven difficult to distill to a narrow set of clinical signs.

Patients with PE may have a wide range of clinical signs, ranging from no clinical signs to sudden death. Perhaps one of the reasons that PEs are so hard to identify clinically is the variability of the size, number, and placement of the clot in the lungs. Larger clots theoretically make for a higher chance of detectable clinical signs. However, sometimes smaller clots also can create clinical signs. Patients who have a PE with few or no clinical signs often are young, with a notable amount of pulmonary reserve and in good physical condition with no comorbid conditions. Those with larger clots or patients who have comorbid conditions such as heart problems, diabetes, congestive heart failure, COPD, or hypertension certainly are at more risk than healthy persons. In patients with comorbid conditions, even small clots are likely to cause symptoms.

History and Physical Findings. As previously described, the detection of a PE can be difficult and may depend on the paramedic's index of suspicion. The three factors that lead to the development of a PE include local trauma to a vessel wall, stasis of the blood, and hypercoagulability of the blood. These factors collectively are referred to as *Virchow's triad.* The paramedic should obtain a history to determine the presence of these factors as well as other risk factors for a PE. These may include a sedentary lifestyle, smoking, a history of deep vein thrombosis, long-bone fractures, pregnancy or recent pregnancy, recent leg or hip surgery, the use of contraceptive medications and stasis of position, such as long periods of air or ground travel.

Signs and symptoms are a direct result of the effects of the PE, including a right-to-left shunt, atelectasis, hypoxemia, pulmonary hypertension, right heart strain, and possibly hypotension. The most common finding is the acute onset of dyspnea, often without explanation. The second most common finding is pleuritic chest pain at the onset, which often is fleeting. Of note, one third of patients with a PE do not have chest pain, and half do not describe the onset of dyspnea and chest pain as sudden. Additional signs include anxiety, tachycardia, fever, cough, chills, mucus production, and tachypnea. The skin may be cool, pale, diaphoretic, or cyanotic. If hypotensive the patient may have a shock index (systolic

Acute onset dyspnea (50%)
Pleuritic chest pain (2/3 of people)

blood pressure/pulse rate) of greater than 1, which may be a preterminal finding. Because of the effect on the right heart, changes in the ECG are possible. The classic change associated with a PE is referred to as the S1/Q3/T3 pattern (Figure 21-34). This situation is defined by abnormally large S waves in lead I and Q waves in lead III and an absent or very small T wave in lead III. Although this finding should be noted, it also must be understood that it is both insensitive and nonspecific to the presence of a PE. Its presence or absence should have no effect on the paramedic's differential diagnosis. The most effective use of the cardiac monitor is in the assessment for other causes of chest pain and respiratory distress. Breath sounds typically are clear, although localized wheezing or a pleural friction rub may be present. This may sound like two dry pieces of leather being rubbed together. If capnography is used in the assessment, the waveform will have normal morphologic features with a low ETCO$_2$. This can be the result of reduced air exchange in the lungs and circulating volume.

Unfortunately, a PE may be present without showing any of these clinical signs and, as previously mentioned, it often is one of the most challenging diagnoses to make in the emergency setting. Sadly it often is misdiagnosed for a more benign process such as anxiety or hyperventilation, especially in younger patients; this can lead to disastrous results.

In the ED, PE often is diagnosed after an extensive workup, including complete blood count, electrolytes, arterial blood gasses, chest radiograph, a CT scan of the chest, a ventilation/perfusion scan, and a pulmonary angiogram. Even after such an extensive workup a PE may not be detected, and the patient will be admitted for observation.

Therapeutic Interventions. Care of the patient with PE, as with other patients with pulmonary diseases, hinges on ensuring adequate oxygenation and ventilation. Supplemental oxygen by nasal cannula or nonrebreather mask is the starting point. PEs rarely require intubation in the prehospital setting, but these patients often benefit

from application of oxygen. You should establish IV access at the first opportunity, but do not delay transport for definitive evaluation. ECG monitoring en route may show mild to moderate tachycardia (100 to 130 beats/min). Oxygen saturation often correlates with the severity of dyspnea.

Patient and Family Education. Educate the patient and family about how clots form and how they are spread through the vascular system to lodge eventually in the lungs. You may discuss risk factors such as tobacco use, sedentary lifestyle, obesity, and clotting disorders.

Hyperventilation Syndrome

Description. Hyperventilation, strictly defined, is excess ventilation. It may take the form of **tachypnea** (rapid respirations) or hyperpnea but most often involves both simultaneously. This condition results in respiratory alkalosis caused by the increased elimination of CO$_2$.

Etiology and Demographics. Exact numbers are not available, but a transient condition of hyperventilation syndrome is relatively common. It often occurs in association with panic attacks or other anxiety-causing conditions, including stress. It affects males and females equally. Psychogenic hyperventilation is a diagnosis of exclusion and can only be considered after all other causes of respiratory distress have been ruled out.

History and Physical Findings. An identifiable event typically precedes hyperventilation syndrome, and the patient may report a particularly stressful or emotional event before the onset of signs and symptoms. The patient may complain of "not getting enough air"; tingling in the tips of the fingers, toes, or around the mouth (called **circumoral paresthesia**); and chest pain or neurologic symptoms such as dizziness or lightheadedness. Physical findings include agitation, anxiety, tachypnea, tachycardia, generalized weakness, and possibly syncope. Hyperventilation causes hypocalcemia in the muscles, thus causing cramping in the extremities. This phenomenon is called **carpopedal spasm.** Paresthesia and carpopedal spasms are more common in the upper extremities than

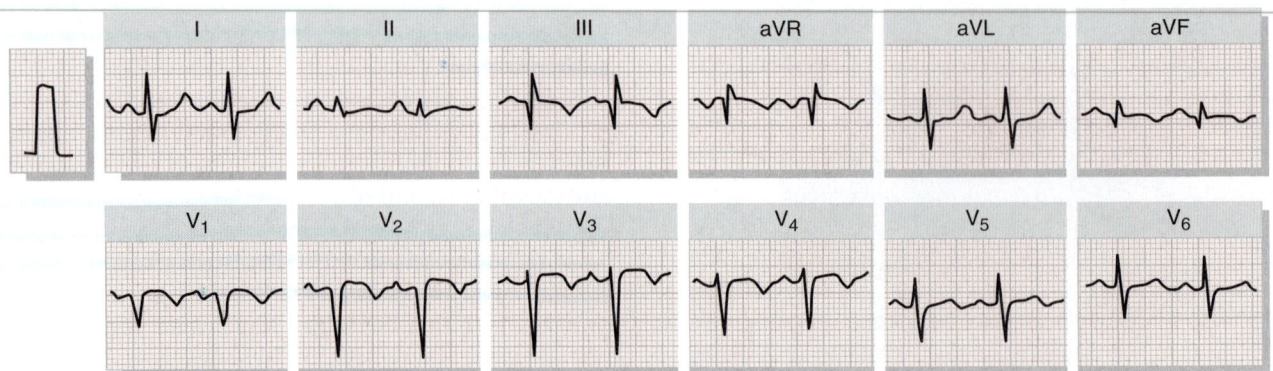

Figure 21-34 The electrocardiogram (ECG) in pulmonary embolism (PE). In 12-lead ECGs, the trilogy of S waves in lead I, Q waves in lead III, and ST-wave changes in lead III may suggest a PE.

the lower extremities and generally are bilateral when present. If a unilateral presentation occurs it is commonly in the left arm. An additional finding related to hypocalcemia is Trousseau's sign. To illicit this sign, inflate the blood pressure cuff above the systolic pressure and observe for cramping of the hand. This cramping is the result of the hypocalcemia and the reduced blood flow causing ischemia of the ulnar and median nerve.

Physical examination is usually notable only for simultaneous hyperpnea and tachypnea. Lung sounds are clear, air movement is good, and oxygen saturations are 100% or almost 100%. Capnography shows a normal waveform with a reduced $ETCO_2$. *Nonrebreather at 2L/min*

Therapeutic Interventions. Care of the hyperventilating patient includes reassurance and coaching to slow the respiratory rate. Because hyperventilation syndrome is a diagnosis of exclusion, administer oxygen and initiate IV access and ECG monitoring. Remember that a few respiratory conditions (including a potentially deadly pulmonary embolus) and compensation for metabolic acidosis can be confused with hyperventilation syndrome. Assuming hyperventilation syndrome in these patients and treating by increasing inspired CO_2 can be deadly. Thus hyperventilating patients should be given the benefit of full care.

Induced controlled hyperventilation does have a role in medical care. It can be used in certain cases to help reduce intracranial pressure in head injuries. Because it reduces cerebral blood flow, it is only used transiently until the cause of the increased pressure can be evaluated and treated. In these circumstances hyperventilation can be life saving and can temporarily reduce intracranial pressure until more definitive treatment of the intracranial hypertension can be undertaken (Robertson, 2004). Further discussion of this concept can be found in Chapter 47.

Patient and Family Education. Help the patient and family understand why the patient is hyperventilating and ways to manage stress.

Atelectasis

Description. Partial or full physical collapse of the alveoli in parts of the lungs is called **atelectasis.** This condition is not like pneumothorax. In pneumothorax, the lung is partially or fully collapsed in the chest cavity. In atelectasis, the lung is fully expanded, but collections of alveoli are collapsed, inhibiting oxygenation.

Etiology and Demographics. Atelectasis may have many causes. However, one of the most frequent is failure to take deep breaths regularly. Periodic yawning often serves to reduce atelectasis. Rib fractures or chest wall trauma often are causes of atelectasis because the pain of full inspiration prevents regular expansion of the alveoli. This condition often is seen after surgery, particularly of the chest or abdomen. Atelectasis is a risk factor for developing pneumonia because of the closed alveoli. Atelectasis can be prevented by regular coughing and deep breathing.

History and Physical Findings. The diagnosis of atelectasis usually requires a chest radiograph. Thus it is rarely diagnosed in the field. Symptoms that may cause the patient with atelectasis to call EMS are chest wall pain, dyspnea, coughing, or fever. Breath sounds may reveal a "snapping" noise on inhalation as collapsed alveoli open. $ETCO_2$ may be decreased because of the reduced ability for gas exchange in the lungs.

Therapeutic Interventions. The mainstays of treatment involve ensuring oxygenation, establishing IV access, and applying standard monitoring for the respiratory patient.

Patient and Family Education. Instruction of the patient includes stressing an activity level suggested by his or her physician and emphasizing avoiding a sedentary lifestyle. Also emphasize the importance of avoiding tobacco products.

Tumors

Description. Pulmonary tumors have two varieties: **benign** (noncancerous) and **malignant** (cancerous). Malignant tumors may originate in the lung (called **primary tumors**) or may have spread from some other location, such as the liver, stomach, or pancreas (called **secondary tumors**).

Etiology and Demographics. Benign tumors compose only a small amount of lung tumors, an estimated 2% to 5% of all pulmonary tumors. Even though benign tumors may not spread and cause further cancer, they may still cause problems on the basis of their location—blockage of airways, atelectasis, or hemoptysis in certain cases. A few examples of benign tumors are hamartomas, bronchial adenomas, and fibromas (Perez, 2005).

Malignant tumors are tumors that most people refer to as *lung cancer.* Many different types of malignant tumors exist, as do many degrees of aggressiveness. In the United States, deaths from primary lung cancer (cancer that originates in the lungs) account for one third of all cancer deaths, with approximately 170,000 new cases of lung cancer diagnosed each year (Figure 21-35). This is one of the few cancers whose mortality rate is increasing and accounts for more years of productive life lost than any other cancer. The onset of the disease is generally between ages 50 and 70 years and has a male predominance; smoking is responsible for 90% of cases. The 5-year survival rate is approximately 14%. At initial diagnosis, 20% of these patients have cancer localized to the affected areas of the lungs, 25% have cancer that has spread to the lymphatic system, and 55% have cancer that has metastasized from other areas of the body. Metastatic lung cancer (cancer that originated elsewhere in the body) often originates in the breast, colon, prostate, or kidneys.

History and Physical Findings. Although you rarely will be able to suspect cancer as the reason for dyspnea, most patients with undiagnosed cancer may present with malaise, dyspnea on exertion, hemoptysis, weight loss,

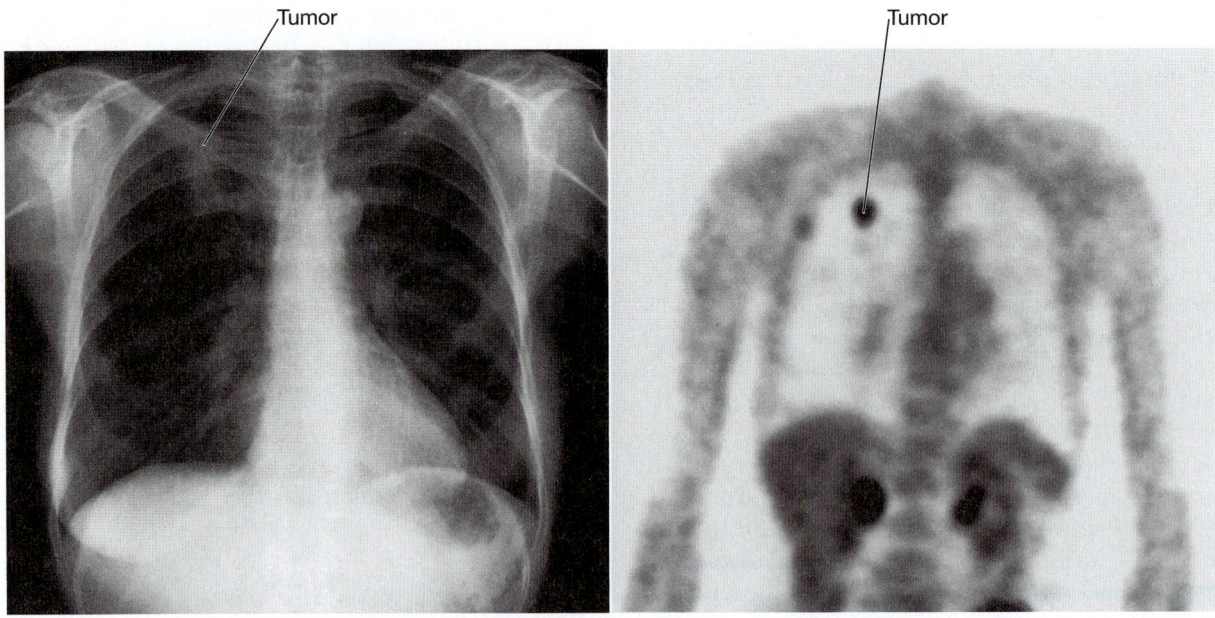

Tumor   Tumor

Figure 21-35 Lung cancer shown on chest radiograph, confirmed on bone scan.

or a long history of cigarette smoking. Patients may provide a history of bronchitis or nonspecific lung disease. Physical examination of the patient may be entirely normal or show a thin patient with **pallor** (lack of color), cough, hemoptysis, fever, stridor, wheezing, rhonchi, crackles, dyspnea, chest pain, or low oxygen saturation. In the case of advanced cancer, pulmonary effusions may develop in the lungs and limit expansion of the lungs and cause dyspnea. Auscultation of the lungs, in this case, may reveal absent breath sounds in the lower parts of the lung because of the effusion and solidness to percussion of the chest.

Therapeutic Interventions. Care of the patient with new-onset or existing lung cancer centers on providing oxygen to maintain sufficient saturation and assisting respirations if necessary. Before you attempt aggressive airway interventions, seek family assistance in determining the presence or absence of an advance directive regarding intubation or cardiopulmonary resuscitation. Additional treatment may include bronchodilators if bronchoconstriction is present, circulatory support if evidence of hypovolemia exists or to thin pulmonary secretions, and pain relief.

Patient and Family Education. Instruction of the patient can focus on encouraging physician-suggested therapy and activity level. Specific therapies can be difficult to discuss because the extent of the tumor cannot be predicted reliably in the prehospital setting.

Environmental and Occupational Inhalation Exposures

chlorine gas
ammonia gas - refrigerant

[OBJECTIVE 10]

Description. Environmental chemical exposures often are the result of mixing chemicals, usually cleaning products, or the use of solvent-based chemicals in enclosed spaces. These scenarios often present more of a challenge for you than occupational exposures because many more chemicals and combinations are available to the average homeowner. Mixing chemicals can give rise to unpredicted consequences or byproducts. Even worse, many of these exposures occur indoors, where limited fresh air and circulation are available, worsening the symptoms.

History and Physical Findings. The respiratory symptoms you see may be similar to asthma, even in patients with no clinical history of the disease. These symptoms include dyspnea, wheezing, tachypnea, anxiety, coughing (sometimes productive), tearing, or drooling.

Therapeutic Interventions. Removal of the offending substance is the first and most important step in recovery. Remove patients from the house if this has not already been done. Remember, the safety of the responding crew must remain a priority. If the safety of the atmosphere cannot be determined, the paramedic should not enter the environment until it is absolutely safe or appropriate personal protection, such as a self-contained breathing apparatus, is available. Ventilation of the house to eliminate the offending agent(s) is a secondary priority. Provide supportive care and assess vital signs, including oxygen saturation. Provide humidified supplemental oxygen as needed to maintain saturation greater than 90%. Inhaled beta agonists such as albuterol may be of benefit in reversing bronchoconstriction and wheezing if present. Establish IV access and begin ECG monitoring. Medical direction can provide assistance in early treatment.

Occupational exposures, in contrast to home exposures, usually occur with agents that are identified and for which materials safety data sheets (MSDSs) as well as individuals familiar with the specific agents are available. The offending agent must be identified to plan treatment. However, this identification should come second

Throat burning - consider intubation early (give Versed)

only to removing the patient from the area and ensuring the airway and ventilation are patent. The initial steps you should take are supportive: checking vital signs and oxygen saturation. Supplemental oxygen should be available if needed and humidified. When possible, obtain an MSDS to accompany the patient or have co-workers locate a copy and fax it to the ED. Do not delay transport waiting for an MSDS. Keep in mind a possible need for decontamination with certain industrial chemicals. In addition, use local procedures to enable decontamination of both the responding medical team and any affected patients.

Long-term occupational exposures often are already diagnosed. You can obtain further history from the patient. Conditions such as asbestosis or silicosis, both chronic occupational exposure respiratory diseases, often are quite familiar to the patient. The patient in a chronic situation may be relatively asymptomatic or show mild asthmatic or COPD symptoms (Amanullah, 2005). Most patients are familiar with beta agonists and whether they are beneficial. Provide supportive care while transporting the patient and carefully monitor his or her vital signs.

Patient and Family Education. Instruction of the patient centers on the acuity of the exposure and nature of the chemical. Mixing chemicals, even seemingly benign ones such as house cleaners, is highly discouraged because of possible inhalation risks. Discuss following the employer's safety routines in dealing with possible hazards in the workplace.

VENTILATOR MANAGEMENT

When endotracheal or nasotracheal intubation becomes necessary in the field, you will greatly appreciate the assistance of a mechanical ventilator. A wide variety of ventilators exist. Oxygen-powered ventilators allow you to determine inspiratory time and therefore inspired volume (Figure 21-36). Highly complex yet portable ventilators are available that control every aspect of ventilation. Exploring the intricacies of such units is beyond the scope of this chapter, but understanding the basics of mechanical ventilation can help you understand how these machines operate.

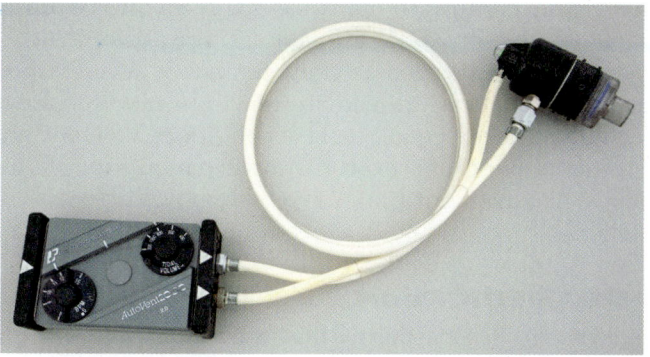

Figure 21-36 Automatic transport ventilator.

Most machines require setting a mode, such as assist control (A/C) or **synchronous intermittent mandatory ventilation (SIMV).** Some machines allow only A/C, a setting at which the ventilator always gives a full breath regardless of whether the machine or the patient triggered the breath. These machines allow you to set a base rate, the rate if the patient does not breathe at all. A/C is often used in patients who have virtually no respiratory drive. These include patients who are extremely intoxicated, those with severe head injury, and those with total respiratory failure.

SIMV is a more varied setting. It generally allows the patient to inspire at will and to the depth that he or she desires. It also has a default rate that is used if the patient is apneic or is in respiratory failure. SIMV is a common setting for patients who are partially or mostly awake during ventilator use. Patients who have a moderate respiratory drive do well with SIMV. These include patients with COPD who tire from the work of breathing and patients with moderate head injuries.

Noninvasive Mechanical Ventilation

Continuous Positive Airway Pressure

Continuous positive airway pressure (CPAP) is the delivery of slight positive pressure (such as blowing through a straw) to prevent airway collapse and improve oxygenation and ventilation in spontaneously breathing patients. The introduction of this technology to the prehospital setting has significantly reduced the need for intubation in patients with severe respiratory distress. When using CPAP, the patient wears a mask that covers the mouth and nose, providing continuous increased airway pressure throughout the respiratory cycle as the patient breathes (Figure 21-37). CPAP may be used to assist ventilation in patients with neuromuscular weakness, chronic pulmonary edema, or obstructive sleep apnea. Some patients use the device continuously, whereas others require it only at night when airway obstruction is most likely.

> **PARAMEDIC*Pearl***
>
> CPAP and BiPAP are noninvasive methods of ventilatory assistance used in spontaneously breathing patients. They do not require a tracheal tube or tracheostomy.

Bilevel Positive Airway Pressure *Easier for pts.*

Bilevel positive airway pressure (BiPAP) is delivered through a tight-fitting mask. The mask fits over either the patient's nose or the mouth and nose (Figure 21-38). In BiPAP therapy, two (bi) levels of positive pressure are delivered. One is delivered during inspiration to keep the airway open as the patient inhales and the other (lower) pressure is delivered during expiration to reduce the work of exhalation. The BiPAP device can be set to deliver pressure at a set rate or sense when an inspiratory

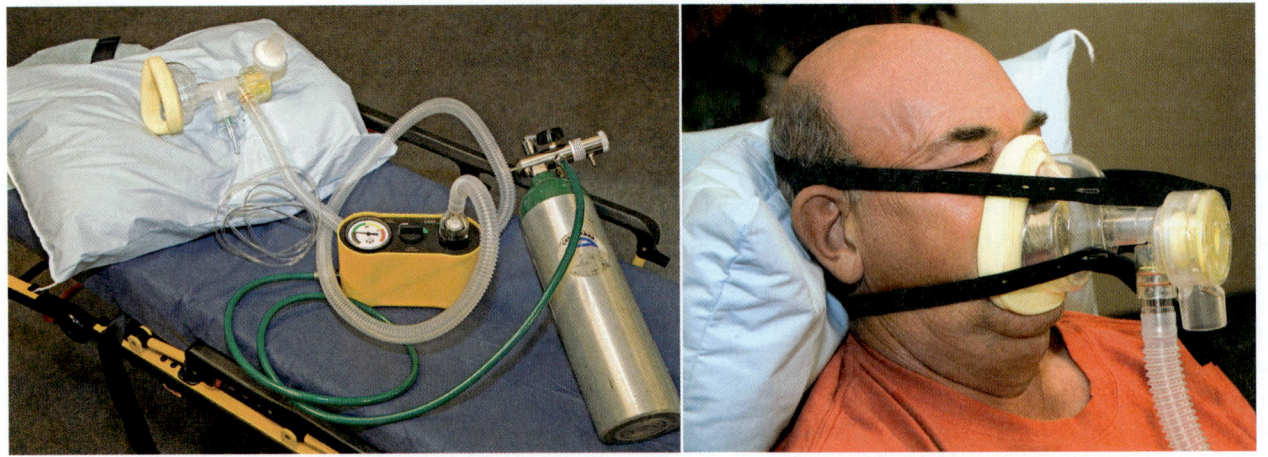

A

B

Figure 21-37 A, Equipment used for continuous positive airway pressure (CPAP). **B,** CPAP applied to a patient.

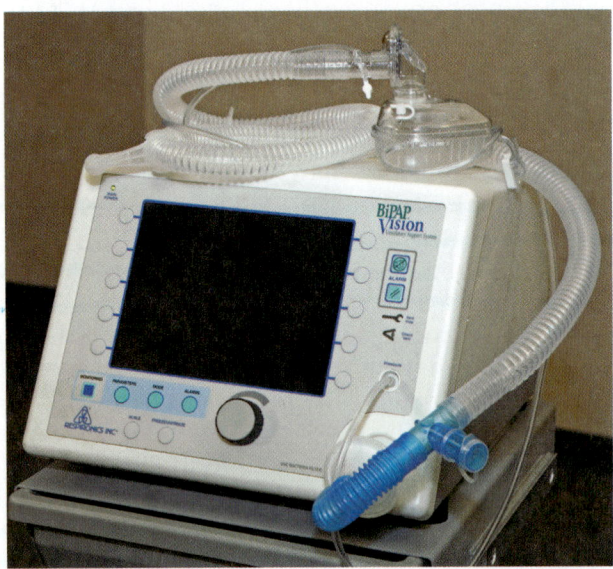

Figure 21-38 A bilevel positive airway pressure (BiPAP) machine.

BOX 21-5	Common Causes of Respiratory Failure

- Chest trauma
- Head trauma
- Transient ischemic attack or cerebrovascular accident
- COPD
- Status asthmaticus
- Status epilepticus
- Severe pneumonia
- Intracranial hemorrhage
- Drug or alcohol intoxication
- Tension pneumothorax
- Severe aspiration
- Congestive heart failure

COPD, Chronic obstructive pulmonary disease.

effort is being made by the patient and deliver a higher pressure during inspiration. BiPAP is used in the treatment of patients with chronic respiratory failure. It may be helpful in the transition from invasive to noninvasive respiratory support.

Respiratory Failure

All patients with dyspnea are at risk for **respiratory failure.** Strictly defined, respiratory failure is the inadequacy of ventilation or oxygenation. Respiratory failure is often preceded by respiratory distress in which the patient's work of breathing is increased in an attempt to compensate for hypoxia. Signs of impending respiratory failure include the following:

- Sleepy, intermittently combative, or agitated
- Decreased muscle tone
- Decreased level of responsiveness or response to pain
- Inadequate respiratory rate, effort, or chest excursion
- Tachypnea with periods of bradypnea; slowing to bradypnea/agonal breathing

Even though respiratory failure arises from a wide variety of clinical conditions, management of it is clear: aggressive airway control. In many cases this involves endotracheal intubation and mechanical ventilation. Acute, severe conditions such as chest trauma or severe aspiration can create an immediate need for airway control. Less-dramatic but equally severe conditions such as status asthmaticus or COPD exacerbation can require aggressive airway management (Box 21-5).

PARAMEDIC*Pearl*

A common misconception is that respiratory failure requires apnea. Respiratory failure includes apnea, but it may also be present with spontaneous and insufficient respirations.

Case Scenario CONCLUSION

Your partner initiates an IV as you complete your assessment and prepare for transport. En route you administer high-flow oxygen by nonrebreather mask and infuse 1 L of normal saline because of her significant dehydration and hypotension. Her vital signs upon arrival at the hospital are pulse, 116 beats/min, blood pressure, 88/58 mm Hg; respirations, 30 breaths/min; temperature, 102.5°F; and SpO_2, 84% on 15 L of oxygen. The patient remains conscious, but is irritable, anxious, and restless when you transfer her to the ED. Her chest radiograph shows right middle lobe pneumonia. While in the ED she receives an additional 500 mL normal saline. She was admitted to the intensive care unit with a diagnosis of pneumonia and septic shock. You later learn that she required intubation 2 hours after arriving at the intensive care unit and died of shock 3 days after admission.

Looking Back

9. *What is the significance of the patient's vital sign changes during transport?*

This patient's condition, including her profound hypoxia, required high-flow oxygen, and her significant dehydration and hypotension warranted infusion of 1 to 2 L normal saline.

Case Scenario SUMMARY

1. *What is your general impression of this patient?* This patient's presentation is deceiving. She is alert, oriented, and in no apparent distress with a primary complaint of diarrhea and having fallen. These factors create an illusion of stability. However, the presence of pallor and peripheral cyanosis, coupled with a thready pulse and rapid, deep respiratory distress signal a significant underlying problem for this elderly woman. You should assume that she is high priority as you continue your evaluation.

2. *What are some possible causes of this patient's pallor, cyanosis, and tachypnea?* Pallor typically is associated with poor perfusion; possible causes in this situation could include dehydration (related to the history of diarrhea) or septic shock (related to the warm skin). Cyanosis indicates hypoxemia; a broad variety of conditions may result in hypoxia, including respiratory compromise (caused by COPD, asthma, pneumonia, or pneumothorax) or a reduction in cardiac output (caused by shock or congestive heart failure). Tachypnea is a compensatory response that may be seen in either respiratory or cardiac compromise.

3. *What history questions or physical assessment procedures would be most useful in differentiating between the conditions you listed in question 2?* To evaluate potential causes of poor perfusion, the skin should be examined for signs of dehydration, the body temperature should be measured, and a full set of vital signs should be performed. In addition, potential sites of infection should be considered related to the potential for septic shock. The patient's medical history should be evaluated for potential respiratory or cardiac conditions that might result in hypoxia, and a respiratory and cardiac examination (including chest examination, breath sounds, evaluation of peripheral pulses, cardiac sounds) should be performed. The SpO_2 and ECG also should be evaluated.

4. *What intervention should you initiate at this time?* High-flow oxygen is appropriate for both shock and hypoxia.

5. *Is this patient high priority? Why or why not?* Yes. Her vital signs and SpO_2 have confirmed the nature of her initial shock and hypoxia; she is in decompensatory shock and has significant hypoxia. She requires aggressive therapy and rapid transport to the appropriate facility.

6. *What conditions are consistent with a productive cough, fever, tachycardia and hypotension, and hypoxia? What do the vital signs contribute to the picture?* Cough, fever, and hypoxia are consistent with pneumonia, bronchitis, or a URI. The vital signs establish shock (tachycardia and hypotension), probably infection (fever), and significant hypoxemia.

7. *How does the history of COPD, cough, fever, and 24 hours on the floor fit into the clinical picture?* This patient's smoking history and COPD make her high risk for the development of pneumonia. Her productive cough and fever make it even more likely. Immobility is a prime risk factor for the development of pneumonia, even more likely for this patient.

8. *What treatment will you initiate at this time?* Her two primary problems are shock and hypoxia. Treatment should include high-flow oxygen and infusion of a significant amount of IV fluids (10 to 20 mL/kg). Although fluid infusion is controversial in cases of hemorrhage, no questions exist about its efficacy in dehydration and septic shock.

9. *What is the significance of the patient's vital sign changes during transport?* They are ominous. The reduction of pulse and respiratory rate in the face of worsening hypoxia suggests that the patient is becoming fatigued and may require assisted ventilation and possible airway control. Monitor carefully and be prepared to intervene.

Chapter Summary

- Pulmonary dysfunction is generally the result of interference with ventilation, interference with diffusion, interference with perfusion, or combinations of any of these factors.
- Indicators of life-threatening respiratory distress include alterations in mental status, dyspnea at rest, severe cyanosis, absent breath sounds, audible stridor or other adventitious breath sounds, severe difficulty in speaking, tachycardia, pallor and diaphoresis, the presence of retractions, or the use of the accessory muscles.
- Hypoxia and/or hypercarbia can cause confusion, restlessness, irritability, lethargy, or coma.
- Indicators of respiratory compromise include the inability to complete sentences, the use of accessory muscles in the respiratory effort, or pursed lips on exhalation.
- Patients in respiratory distress are often tachycardic. However, bradycardia is associated with severe hypoxia and may indicate imminent cardiac arrest.
- Diagnostic tools available to the paramedic for evaluation of the patient in respiratory distress and the effectiveness of treatment include pulse oximetry, peak flow meters, and capnography.
- Respiratory diseases are categorized as two major varieties: upper respiratory conditions and lower respiratory conditions.
- Upper respiratory diseases tend to affect or limit inspired or expired air. An upper respiratory infection can cause a wide array of respiratory symptoms, including headache, nasal congestion, nasal drainage, nasal inflammation, sore throat, coughing, muscle aches, and mucus production with cough, fever, or chills.
- Epiglottitis is a potentially life-threatening infection of the supraglottic structures of the airway. It results in inflammation of the base of the tongue, aryepiglottic folds, arytenoids, tonsils, and the epiglottis itself. The patient with epiglottitis requires rapid transport and specialty care.
- Croup (laryngotracheobronchitis) affects young children and is manifested by infection of the upper airways. The area below the glottis is most commonly affected, resulting in swollen, inflamed mucosa.
- Bacterial tracheitis is a serious infection of the trachea, often requiring hospitalization.
- Peritonsillar abscess is a painful and frightening illness. The abscess begins when a bacterial infection forms on the back of the oropharynx, rooted in the richly vascular tissues of the adenoid tonsils. In rare instances it may compromise the upper airway.
- Foreign bodies in the airway can range from pins and needles to toys. Although the majority of patients are young children, some are adults.
- Penetrating and blunt trauma to the neck have the potential to generate life-threatening injuries. Most penetrating trauma to the neck is the result of knife or gunshot wounds. Blunt trauma is more frequently seen in motor vehicle crashes. Direct-force blunt trauma to the cricoid cartilage is capable of crushing the cartilage and creating an airway obstruction.
- In some chronic medical conditions, a tracheostomy must be surgically performed to support respiration.
- Costochondritis is inflammation of the cartilage in the anterior chest that causes chest pain.
- Pleurisy is painful rubbing of the pleural lining. The cause of the inflammation is often unknown.
- The presence of air in the mediastinum is called *pneumomediastinum*, which may occur spontaneously or as a result of trauma to the chest, mechanical ventilation, asthma, emphysema, lung or chest tumors, cocaine use, violent emesis or coughing, or childbirth, among other causes.
- Lower respiratory diseases limit the ability of the body to oxygenate the blood.
- A pneumothorax is a collection of air in the pleural space. Spontaneous pneumothorax is a pneumothorax that occurs in the absence of trauma. A primary spontaneous pneumothorax occurs in patients without underlying lung disease. A secondary spontaneous pneumothorax occurs in patients with an underlying lung disease.
- Fluid that collects in the pleural cavity is referred to as a *pleural effusion*. A pulmonary embolism is a common cause of pleural effusions in patients less than 40 years of age; therefore the presence of a coexisting embolus must be considered in these patients.
- Noncardiogenic pulmonary edema (NCPE) is a condition in which fluid accumulates in the alveoli in the absence of heart failure. NCPE has been noted in overdoses secondary to opioids, salicylates, cyclic antidepressants, and other medications.
- Acute respiratory distress syndrome is a clinical syndrome in which alveoli are damaged because of significant illness or injury. Some alveoli collapse and others fill with fluid, impairing the exchange of oxygen and carbon dioxide. As the syndrome progresses, more alveoli are affected, gas exchange is further impaired, and respiratory failure ensues, resulting in dyspnea, hypoxia, and pulmonary edema.
- Asthma is a type I allergic reaction associated with an inflammatory response that is expressed in the lower airways. Asthma is a reactive airway disease that many people underestimate.
- Bronchiolitis is an acute, infectious, inflammatory disease of the upper and lower respiratory tracts that results in obstruction of the small airways. Although it may occur in all age groups, the larger airways of

older children and adults tolerate the respiratory syncytial virus infection better than infants.

- Bronchopulmonary dysplasia may occur in preterm infants as a result of prolonged treatment with positive-pressure ventilation and high oxygen concentrations.
- COPD may include varying degrees of bronchitis, emphysema, and asthma and is usually caused or worsened by tobacco abuse.
- Cystic fibrosis (CF) is a genetic disease in which glands create thicker-than-normal secretions. These thicker secretions cause chronic infections, resulting in the most common complication of the disease—pulmonary infections. Most fatalities from the disease result from progressive lung disease.
- Pneumonia is an infection in the alveoli and is particularly deadly in the elderly population. It can be caused by a wide variety of pathogens, ranging from bacteria to fungi to viruses. Pneumonia, regardless of cause, can prevent oxygenation. Thus it requires aggressive medical treatment.
- Pulmonary abscesses are collections of pus in the lung tissue itself. They are often the result of aspiration of gastric contents. It can take several weeks to develop clinical signs. Empyema is a collection of pus outside the lung in the pleural space.
- The inspiration of fluids not intended for the lungs is termed *aspiration*. Aspiration of gastric acid or food from the upper airway or stomach can cause an inflammatory response that can lead to hypoxia and respiratory failure. Aspiration pneumonitis is lung and bronchoalveolar irritation caused by aspirated stomach acid.
- Tuberculosis (TB) is a pulmonary disease caused by the bacterium *Mycobacterium tuberculosis*. It is transmitted by airborne droplets. Active TB is characterized by a productive cough, fever, and weight loss. Symptoms include hemoptysis, chest or chest wall pain, weight or appetite loss, fatigue, irritability, weakness, headache, chills, fever, and night sweats. TB requires respiratory isolation.
- A pulmonary embolus (PE) occurs when a thrombus (clot) becomes dislodged and travels (the clot is now an embolus), lodging in a pulmonary artery and obstructs blood flow to a portion of the lung. The clot may consist of blood, fat, or air. PE is often difficult to diagnose and can be a potentially fatal condition.
- Hyperventilation, strictly defined, is excess ventilation. This condition results in a respiratory alkalosis secondary to the increased elimination of carbon dioxide. Psychogenic hyperventilation is a diagnosis of exclusion and can be considered only after all other causes of respiratory distress have been ruled out.
- Partial or full physical collapse of the alveoli in parts of the lungs is called *atelectasis*. In atelectasis, the lung is fully expanded, but collections of alveoli are collapsed, inhibiting oxygenation.
- Pulmonary tumors have two varieties: benign (noncancerous) and malignant (cancerous). Malignant tumors may originate in the lung (called *primary tumors*) or may have spread from some other location, such as the liver, stomach, or pancreas (called *secondary tumors*).
- Environmental chemical exposures are often the result of mixing chemicals, usually cleaning products, or the use of solvent-based chemicals in enclosed spaces. Respiratory symptoms include dyspnea, wheezing, tachypnea, anxiety, coughing, and sometimes coughing mucus, tearing, or drooling. Exposure to inhaled toxins is immediately managed by removal of the patient and medical team to a safe area.
- Continuous positive airway pressure (CPAP) is the delivery of slight positive pressure to prevent airway collapse and improve oxygenation and ventilation in spontaneously breathing patients. The patient wears a mask that covers the mouth and nose, providing continuous increased airway pressure throughout the respiratory cycle as the patient breathes. CPAP may be used to assist ventilation in patients with neuromuscular weakness, chronic pulmonary edema, or obstructive sleep apnea.
- Bilevel positive airway pressure (BiPAP) is delivered through a tight-fitting mask. In BiPAP therapy, two levels of positive pressure are delivered. One is delivered during inspiration to keep the airway open as the patient inhales, and the other (lower) pressure is delivered during expiration to reduce the work of exhalation.
- Care should be used when mechanically ventilating patients' lungs to avoid pneumothorax.

REFERENCES

Abrahamian, F. M. *Pleural effusion.* Retrieved June 24, 2006, from http://www.emedicine.com.

Amanullah, S. *Chemical worker's lung.* Retrieved June 28, 2006, from http://www.emedicine.com.

Bowman, J. G. *Epiglottis, adult.* Retrieved September 10, 2006, from http://www.emedicine.com.

Bowling, W. M., Wilson, R. F., Kelen, G. B., & Buchman, T. G. (2004). *Thoracic trauma in emergency medicine: A comprehensive study guide* (pp. 1595-1613). New York: McGraw-Hill.

Camargo, C. A., & Brenner, B. *Asthma.* Retrieved October 1, 2006, from http://www.emedicine.com.

Chang, A. K. *Pneumothorax, iatrogenic, spontaneous, and pneumomediastinum.* Retrieved June 21, 2006, from http://www.emedicine.com.

Clark, K. *Bacterial tracheitis.* Retrieved October 1, 2006, from http://www.emedicine.com.

Driscoll, W. *Bronchopulmonary dysplasia.* Retrieved June 27, 2006, from http://www.emedicine.com.

Eggerstedt, J. M. *Carcinoid lung tumors.* Retrieved June 29, 2006, from http://www.emedicine.com.

Flowers, L. K. *Costochondritis.* Retrieved June 18, 2006, from www.emedicine.com.

Green, S. M. (2005). *Tarascon pocket pharmacopeia* (p. 7). Lompoc, CA: Tarascon Publishing.

Herchline, T. *Tuberculosis.* Retrieved June 28, 2006, from http://www.emedicine.com.

Kazzi, A. *Peritonsillar abscess.* Retrieved October 3, 2006, from http://www.emedicine.com.

Khan, F. H. *Pediatrics, epiglottitis.* Retrieved September 10, 2006, from http://www.emedicine.com.

Kleinschmidt, P. *Chronic obstructive pulmonary disease and emphysema.* Retrieved June 19, 2006, from http://www.emedicine.com.

Krilov, L. R. *Respiratory syncytial virus,* Retrieved June 26, 2006, from http://www.emedicine.com.

Levy, D. *Neck trauma.* Retrieved June 28, 2006, from http://www.emedicine.com.

Li, J. *Tuberculosis.* Retrieved September 29, 2006, from http://www.emedicine.com.

Louden, M. *Pediatrics, bronchiolitis.* Retrieved September 20, 2006, from http://www.emedicine.com.

Molodow, R. E. *Croup.* Retrieved October 1, 2006, from http://www.emedicine.com.

Anderson, R. N., & Smith, B. L. (2005). *National Vital Statistics Reports: Deaths: Leading causes for 2002 (vol. 53, no. 17) (p. 7).* Atlanta, GA: Centers for Disease Control and Prevention.

Perez, N. *Benign lung tumors.* Retrieved June 29, 2006, from http://www.emedicine.com.

Perina, D. G. (2003). Noncardiogenic pulmonary edema. *Emergency Medicine Clinics of North America, 21,* 385-393.

Rajnik, M. *Rhinoviruses.* Retrieved September 10, 2006, from http://www.emedicine.com.

Robertson, C. (2004). Every breath you take: Hyperventilation and intracranial pressure. *Cleveland Clinic Journal of Medicine, 71,* Suppl 1, S14-S15.

Rosen, P., & Barkin, R. (Eds.). (1998). *Emergency medicine: Concepts and clinical practice* (4th ed.). St. Louis: Mosby.

Rothenhaus, T. *Adult respiratory distress syndrome.* Retrieved June 22, 2006, from http://www.emedicine.com.

Sharma, G. *Cystic fibrosis.* Retrieved September 30, 2006, from http://www.emedicine.com.

Swaminathan, A. *Pneumonia, aspiration.* Retrieved June 22, 2006, from http://www.emedicine.com.

Tintinalli, J., Kelen, G., & Stapczynski, J. (2004). *Emergency medicine: A comprehensive study guide* (6th ed.). New York: McGraw-Hill.

Warshawsky, M. E. *Foreign body aspiration.* Retrieved October 1, 2006, from http://www.emedicine.com.

Zwanger, M. *Pneumonia, empyema, and abscess.* Retrieved June 27, 2006, from http://www.emedicine.com.

Chapter Quiz

1. Name three URIs that can require medical treatment.

   _____

   _____

2. Describe the treatment of URIs such as croup.

   _____

   _____

3. Describe the management of a tracheostomy patient who called EMS for dyspnea.

   _____

   _____

4. Describe the clinical findings of pneumothorax.

   _____

   _____

5. Describe the prehospital management of pneumothorax.

   _____

6. What are the clinical signs of pneumonia?

   _____

   _____

7. How can EMS help patients with COPD exacerbations?

   _____

   _____

8. How are inhaled irritants treated by EMS?

   _____

   _____

9. Define respiratory failure and some conditions that cause it.

   _____

   _____

10. Define TB and how it is spread.

    _____

Terminology

Acute respiratory distress syndrome (ARDS) Collection of fluid in the alveoli of the lung, usually as a result of trauma or serious illness.

Alveoli Functional units of the respiratory system; area in the lungs where the majority of gas exchange takes place; singular form is *alveolus*.

Aspiration Inhalation of foreign contents into the lungs.

Aspiration pneumonitis Inflammation of the bronchi and alveoli caused by inhaled foreign objects, usually acids such as stomach acid.

Asthma Allergic response of the airways causing wheezing and dyspnea.

Atelectasis Partial or full collapse of the alveoli in the lung.

Bacterial tracheitis A potentially serious bacterial infection of the trachea.

Barotrauma An injury that results from rapid or extreme changes in pressure.

Bilevel positive airway pressure (BiPAP) device Breathing device that can be set at one pressure for inhaling and a different pressure for exhaling.

Bronchiolitis An acute, infectious, inflammatory disease of the upper and lower respiratory tracts that results in obstruction of the small airways.

Bronchitis Inflammation of the lower airways, usually with mucus production. Often chronic and related to tobacco abuse.

Bronchopulmonary dysplasia (BPD) Respiratory condition in infants usually arising from preterm birth.

Carbon dioxide narcosis Condition mostly seen in patients with COPD, in whom CO_2 is excessively retained, causing mental status changes and decreased respirations.

Carpopedal spasm Cramping of the extremities secondary to hyperventilation-induced hypocalcemia.

Chronic obstructive pulmonary disease (COPD) Collection of pulmonary diseases that cause dyspnea, coughing, and occasionally sputum production.

Circumoral paresthesia A feeling of tingling around the lips and mouth caused by hyperventilation.

Collapsed lung See *Pneumothorax*.

Continuous positive airway pressure (CPAP) device Breathing device that allows the delivery of slight positive pressure to prevent airway collapse and improve oxygenation and ventilation in spontaneously breathing patients.

Costochondritis Inflammation of the cartilage in the anterior chest that causes chest pain.

Crackles A lung sound that indicates the presence of fluid in the smaller airways; sometimes called *rales*.

Croup A viral infection of the upper airway that is notorious for causing a "seal bark" cough.

Cystic fibrosis (CF) Genetic disease marked by hypersecretion of glands, including mucous glands in the lungs.

Emphysema Lung disease in which destruction of the alveoli creates dyspnea; often associated with tobacco abuse.

Empyema A collection of pus in the pleural cavity.

Epiglottitis An inflammation of the epiglottis.

Esophagoduodenoscopy Medical procedure in which an endoscope is used to look at the esophagus, stomach, and duodenum.

Hamman's sign A crunching sound occasionally heard on auscultation of the heart when air is in the mediastinum.

Hyperpnea A respiratory pattern characterized by rapid, deep breathing. Also called *hyperventilation*.

Mainstem bronchi Each of two main breathing tubes that lead from the trachea into the lungs. There is one right mainstem bronchus and one left mainstem bronchus.

Mediastinitis Infection of the mediastinum; a serious medical condition.

Mediastinoscopy Surgical procedure of looking into the mediastinum with an endoscope.

Methicillin-resistant *Staphylococcus aureus* (MRSA) Any of several bacterial strains of *S. aureus* resistant to methicillin (a penicillin) and related drugs; typically acquired in the hospital.

Noncardiogenic pulmonary edema (NCPE) Fluid collection in the alveoli of the lung that does not result from heart failure.

Ostomy A hole, usually referring to a surgically made hole in some part of the body. Examples include tracheostomy, gastrostomy, and colostomy.

Pallor Pale, washed-out coloration of skin; often a result of extreme anemia or chronic illness. A patient with pallor can be referred to as *pallid*.

Peak flow meter A device used to assess severity of respiratory distress.

Peritonsillar abscess (PTA) An infection of tissue between the tonsil and pharynx, usually the result of a significant infection in the tonsils.

Pleural effusion Collection of fluid in the pleural space, usually fluid that has seeped through the lung or chest wall tissue.

Pleurisy Painful rubbing of the pleural lining.

Pneumomediastinum Air entrapped within the mediastinum; a serious medical condition.

Pneumonia Infection of the lungs.

Pneumothorax A collection of air in the pleural space, usually from either a hole in the lung or a hole in the chest wall.

Positive end-expiratory pressure (PPEP) The amount of pressure above atmospheric pressure present in the airway at the end of the expiratory cyle; when forcing air into the lungs (positive-pressure ventilation), airway pressure is maintained above atmospheric pressure at the end of exhalation by means of a mechanical device, such as a PEEP valve.

Primary tumor A collection of cells that grow out of control, far in excess of normal rates. A primary tumor is a tumor that develops in one tissue only (e.g., a primary liver tumor originates in the liver).

Pulmonary abscess A collection of pus within the lung itself.

Pulmonary bleb Cavity in the lung much like a balloon; may rupture to create a pneumothorax.

Pulmonary embolus (PE) A blood clot that has lodged in the pulmonary artery, causing shortness of breath and hypoxia.

Respiratory failure A clinical condition in which there is inadequate blood oxygenation and/or ventilation to meet the metabolic demands of body tissues.

Respiratory syncytial virus (RSV) A virus linked to bronchiolitis in infants and children.

Terminology—continued

Retractions Use of accessory muscles of respiration to assist in ventilation during times of distress; sinking in of the soft tissues above the sternum or clavicle or between or below the ribs during inhalation.

Rhonchi Rattling or rumbling in the lungs.

Sepsis Body-wide infection regardless of source; common causes include pneumonia and urinary tract infections.

Spontaneous pneumothorax Pneumothorax occurring without trauma, usually by rupture of a pulmonary bleb.

Status asthmaticus Condition of severe asthma that is minimally responsive to therapy; a serious condition.

Stridor Harsh, high-pitched inspiratory sound best heard over the neck.

Subcutaneous emphysema Air entrapped beneath the skin; feels like crackling when palpated.

Supraglottic Any airway structure above the vocal cords (e.g., the epiglottis).

Synchronized intermittent mandatory ventilation (SIMV) A ventilator setting that generally allows the patient to inspire at will and to the depth that he or she desires.

Tachypnea Rapid respirations.

Tension pneumothorax Life-threatening injury in which air enters the space between the lungs and the chest wall but cannot exit. With each breath, the pressure increases until it prevents ventilation and causes death.

Tracheostomy A surgically created hole in the anterior trachea for breathing.

Tuberculosis (TB) A highly contagious bacterial infection known for causing pneumonia and infecting other parts of the body.

Tumor, benign An abnormal growth of cells or tissue that is not malignant (i.e., is not known for spreading and growing aggressively).

Tumor, malignant An abnormal growth of cells or tissue that is known for being aggressive and spreading to other parts of the body.

Tumor, primary A tumor in the location where it originates.

Tumor, secondary A tumor that has spread from its original location (e.g., lung tumor that spreads to the brain); also called metastasis.

Upper respiratory tract infection (URI) Viral syndrome causing nasal congestion, coughing, fever, and runny nose.

Vancomycin-resistant *Enterococcus* (VRE) Bacteria resistant to vancomycin (a potent antibiotic); commonly acquired by patients in the hospital or patients who have indwelling catheters.

Wheezing A musical whistling sound caused by turbulent movement of air through constricted bronchioles.

Cardiovascular Disorders

Objectives *After completing this chapter, you will be able to:*

1. Describe the epidemiology of cardiovascular disease.
2. Identify the risk factors most predisposing to coronary heart disease.
3. Discuss prevention strategies that may reduce the morbidity and mortality rates of coronary heart disease.
4. Identify the major structures of the vascular system.
5. Describe the anatomy of the heart, including the position in the thoracic cavity, layers of the heart, chambers of the heart, and location and function of cardiac valves.
6. Identify the normal characteristics of the point of maximal impulse.
7. Identify phases of the cardiac cycle.
8. Identify the arterial blood supply to any given area of the myocardium.
9. Compare the coronary arterial distribution with the major portions of the cardiac conduction system.
10. Identify the structures of the autonomic nervous system and their effect on heart rate, rhythm, and contractility.
11. Define and give examples of positive and negative inotropism, chronotropism, and dromotropism.
12. Identify and define the components of cardiac output and the factors affecting venous return.
13. Define *preload, afterload,* and *left ventricular end-diastolic pressure* and relate each to the pathophysiology of heart failure.
14. Describe the clinical significance of Starling's law.
15. Define the functional properties of cardiac muscle.
16. List the most important ions involved in cardiac action potential and their primary function in this process.
17. Describe the events involved in the steps from excitation to contraction of cardiac muscle fibers.
18. Define the events composing the cardiac action potential.
19. Correlate the electrophysiologic and hemodynamic events occurring throughout the entire cardiac cycle with the various ECG waveforms, segments, and intervals.
20. Identify the structure and course of all divisions and subdivisions of the cardiac conduction system.
21. Identify and describe how the heart's pacemaking control, rate, and rhythm are determined.
22. Explain the physiologic basis of conduction delay in the atrioventricular node.
23. Differentiate the primary mechanisms responsible for producing cardiac dysrhythmias.
24. Describe reentry.
25. Explain the purpose of ECG monitoring.
26. Identify the limitations of the ECG.
27. Relate the cardiac surfaces or areas represented by the ECG leads.
28. Describe correct anatomic placement of the chest leads.
29. Identify how heart rates, durations, and amplitudes may be determined from ECG recordings.
30. Describe how ECG waveforms are produced.
31. Recognize the changes on the ECG that may reflect evidence of myocardial ischemia and injury.
32. Describe a systematic approach to the analysis and interpretation of cardiac dysrhythmias.
33. Describe the ECG characteristics, possible causes, signs and symptoms, and initial emergency care for dysrhythmias originating in the sinus node.
34. Describe the ECG characteristics, possible causes, signs and symptoms, and initial emergency care for dysrhythmias originating in the atria.
35. Describe aberrant conduction.
36. Define *synchronized cardioversion* and discuss the indications and methods for this procedure.
37. Describe the significance of accessory pathways.
38. Describe the ECG characteristics, possible causes, signs and symptoms, and initial emergency care for dysrhythmias originating in the atrioventricular junction.
39. Describe the electrocardiographic characteristics, possible causes, signs and symptoms, and initial emergency care for dysrhythmias originating in the ventricles.
40. Describe the conditions of pulseless electrical activity.
41. Describe the process and pitfalls in the differentiation of wide QRS complex tachycardias.
42. Describe the dysrhythmias seen in cardiac arrest.
43. Define *defibrillation* and discuss the indications and methods for this procedure.
44. Describe the electrocardiographic characteristics, possible causes, signs and symptoms, and initial emergency care of atrioventricular blocks.
45. Describe the characteristics of an implanted pacemaking system.
46. List the causes and implications of pacemaker failure.
47. Recognize the complications of artificial pacemakers as evidenced on electrocardiogram.
48. Identify additional hazards that interfere with artificial pacemaker function.
49. Describe artifacts that may cause confusion when evaluating the ECG of a patient with a pacemaker.
50. Describe the components and the functions of a transcutaneous pacing system.

Objectives—continued

51. Identify the indications for transcutaneous cardiac pacing.
52. Describe the technique of applying a transcutaneous pacing system.
53. Explain what each setting and indicator on a transcutaneous pacing system represents and how the settings may be adjusted.
54. List the possible complications of transcutaneous pacing.
55. Based on the pathophysiology and clinical evaluation of the patient with a suspected acute myocardial infarction, list the anticipated clinical problems according to their life-threatening potential.
56. Identify the ECG changes characteristically seen during evolution of an acute myocardial infarction.
57. Recognize the limitations of the ECG in reflecting evidence of myocardial ischemia and injury.
58. Describe the abnormalities originating within the bundle branch system.
59. Identify the ECG changes characteristically produced by electrolyte imbalances.
60. Identify and describe the components of the focused history as it relates to the patient with cardiovascular compromise.
61. Identify what is meant by the OPQRST of chest pain assessment.
62. Explain the clinical significance of paroxysmal nocturnal dyspnea.
63. Identify patient situations for which ECG rhythm analysis is indicated.
64. Identify and describe the details of inspection, auscultation, and palpation specific to the cardiovascular system.
65. Identify and define the heart sounds.
66. Relate heart sounds to hemodynamic events in the cardiac cycle.
67. Describe the differences between normal and abnormal heart sounds.
68. Define pulse deficit, pulsus paradoxus, and pulsus alternans.
69. Describe how to determine if pulsus paradoxus, pulsus alternans, or electrical alternans is present.
70. Describe the clinical significance of unequal arterial blood pressure readings in the arms.
71. Describe the etiology, epidemiology, history, and physical findings of acute coronary syndromes.
72. Using the patient history, physical examination findings, and ECG analysis, develop a treatment plan for a patient with an acute coronary syndrome.
73. Describe the incidence of myocardial conduction defects.
74. List other clinical conditions that may mimic signs and symptoms of acute coronary syndromes.
75. Describe the etiology, epidemiology, history, and physical findings of heart failure.
76. Using the patient history, physical examination findings, and ECG analysis, develop a treatment plan for a patient in heart failure.
77. Describe the etiology, epidemiology, history, and physical findings of myocarditis.
78. Using the patient history, physical examination findings, and ECG analysis, develop a treatment plan for a patient with myocarditis.
79. Describe the etiology, epidemiology, history, and physical findings of cardiogenic shock.
80. Using the patient history, physical examination findings, and ECG analysis, develop a treatment plan for a patient in cardiogenic shock.
81. Describe the etiology, epidemiology, history, and physical findings of cardiac arrest.
82. Using the patient history, physical examination findings, and ECG analysis, develop a treatment plan for a patient in cardiac arrest.
83. Assess and manage an adult immediately after resuscitation from a cardiac arrest.
84. Identify and list the inclusion and exclusion criteria for termination of resuscitation efforts.
85. Identify communication and documentation protocols with medical direction and law enforcement used for termination of resuscitation efforts.
86. Describe the etiology, epidemiology, history, and physical findings of a hypertensive emergency.
87. Using the patient history, physical examination findings, and ECG analysis, develop a treatment plan for a patient with a hypertensive emergency.
88. Describe the etiology, epidemiology, history, and physical findings of endocarditis.
89. Using the patient history, physical examination findings, and ECG analysis, develop a treatment plan for a patient with endocarditis.
90. Describe the etiology, epidemiology, history, and physical findings of pericarditis.
91. Using the patient history, physical examination findings, and ECG analysis, develop a treatment plan for a patient with pericarditis.
92. Describe the etiology, epidemiology, history, and physical findings of pericardial tamponade.
93. Using the patient history, physical examination findings, and ECG analysis, develop a treatment plan for a patient with pericardial tamponade.
94. Describe the etiology, epidemiology, history, and physical findings of an aortic aneurysm.
95. Using the patient history, physical examination findings, and ECG analysis, develop a treatment plan for a patient with an aortic aneurysm.
96. Describe the etiology, epidemiology, history, and physical findings of vascular disorders.
97. Using the patient history, physical examination findings, and ECG analysis, develop a treatment plan for a patient with a vascular disorder.

Chapter Outline

Case Scenario

You and your partner are called to a private residence for a "man complaining of chest pain." When you arrive, you find a 32-year-old man reporting severe crushing chest pain that has been present for the past 1 to 2 hours. He informs you that the pain came on at rest, has steadily increased in intensity, and is now accompanied by shortness of breath. The patient denies any prior cardiac history. He is conscious, alert, and oriented with pale, diaphoretic skin and he is in visible respiratory distress. His initial vital signs are pulse, 150 beats/min; blood pressure, 96/40 mm Hg; respirations, 20 breaths/min and deep. The patient denies any recent surgery or trauma.

Questions

1. *What is your general impression of this patient?*
2. *What are some possible causes of this patient's symptoms?*
3. *This patient is fairly young to have a myocardial infarction (MI). What factors might be associated with a cardiac event in a patient this age?*
4. *What additional assessment will be important in the evaluation of this patient?*
5. *What intervention should you initiate at this time?*

During your career as a paramedic, you will care for patients experiencing a cardiovascular emergency. Because the term "cardiovascular" is sometimes used incorrectly, this study of the cardiovascular system begins by clarifying terms. **Cardiovascular disorders** are diseases and conditions that involve the heart (cardio) and blood vessels (vascular). **Heart disease** is a broad term that refers to conditions affecting the heart. **Coronary heart disease** refers to disease of the coronary arteries and their resulting complications, such as angina pectoris or acute MI. The most common cause of cardiovascular disease death is coronary heart disease. **Coronary artery disease** affects the arteries that supply the heart muscle with blood.

RISK FACTORS AND PREVENTION STRATEGIES

[OBJECTIVE 1]

Heart disease is the leading cause of death in the United States. Approximately 950,000 Americans die of cardiovascular disease each year. This amounts to about one death every 33 seconds. Approximately 400,000 to 460,000 Americans die of heart disease in an emergency department or before reaching a hospital each year (*Morbidity and Mortality Weekly Report*, 2002). Almost one fourth of the American population has some form of cardiovascular disease. Coronary heart disease is a leading cause of premature, permanent disability among working adults.

According to the National Center for Chronic Disease Prevention and Health Promotion (NCCDPHP), heart disease death rates per 100,000 population for the five largest U.S. racial or ethnic groups are as follows: blacks, 300; whites, 228; Hispanics, 173; American Indian or Alaskan Natives, 160; and Asian and Pacific Islanders, 128 (U.S. Department of Health and Human Services, 2006).

Risk Factors

[OBJECTIVE 2]

Prevention of cardiovascular disease requires managing risk factors. **Risk factors** are traits and lifestyle habits that may increase a person's chance of developing a disease. More than 300 risk factors have been associated with coronary heart disease and stroke. Some risk factors can be modified. Risk factors that cannot be modified are called nonmodifiable, or fixed, risk factors. Modifiable risk factors can be changed or treated. Contributing risk factors are thought to lead to an increased risk of heart disease, but their exact role has not been defined.

Nonmodifiable (Fixed) Risk Factors

Heredity plays an important part in the development of cardiovascular disease. It also affects some of the modifiable risk factors. The younger the onset in a first-degree relative, the greater the risk of cardiovascular disease. First-degree relatives include parents, children, and siblings.

Race, gender, and age also play a part in the development of cardiovascular disease (Box 22-1). Heart disease

is the leading cause of death for American Indians and Alaska Natives, blacks, Hispanics, and whites (NCCDPHP, 2006). The incidence of cardiovascular disease increases sharply with age. Men develop coronary heart disease approximately 10 years earlier than women (Castelli, 1984). However, this difference is less pronounced after menopause.

> ### Did you know?
>
> Each year, the number of women who die from cardiovascular disease is more than 10 times the number of women who die from breast cancer.

Modifiable Risk Factors

[OBJECTIVE 3]

High Blood Pressure. High blood pressure is a major risk factor for heart disease, stroke, and end-stage renal disease. According to the World Health Organization, the risk of cardiovascular disease doubles for every 10-point increase in diastolic blood pressure or every 20-point increase in systolic blood pressure (Mackay & Mensah, 2004). Medications to control blood pressure decrease coronary heart disease in men and women (Chobanian et al, 2003).

Elevated Serum Cholesterol Levels. A direct link exists between increased serum cholesterol levels and coronary heart disease. Lipoproteins consist of lipids, such as cholesterol, and water-soluble proteins. Lipids are not soluble in water-based substances, such as blood. Lipoproteins enable water-insoluble materials to be transported in the bloodstream. The human body needs only a small amount of cholesterol, from which it makes substances such as vitamin D and hormones.

Low-density lipoproteins (LDLs) move cholesterol from the liver through the blood to other parts of the body where it can be used. LDLs carry most of the cholesterol in the blood. They are often called *bad cholesterol.* If these lipoproteins are not removed from the blood, excess cholesterol builds up in the arteries. The buildup of cholesterol along the arterial walls narrows the size of the vessel and contributes to atherosclerosis. In general, the higher the LDL level, the greater the risk of developing heart disease. Lowering total cholesterol and LDL levels significantly reduces the risk of coronary heart disease.

High-density lipoproteins (HDLs) move cholesterol from body tissues and organs through the blood and back to the liver, where it is broken down or recycled. Because this helps prevent a buildup of cholesterol in the arterial walls, HDLs are often called *good cholesterol.* Increases in physical activity, regular exercise, and weight loss have been shown to increase the concentration of HDL in the blood.

Tobacco Use. Smoking greatly increases the risk of heart disease and peripheral vascular disease (disease in the vessels that supply blood to the arms and legs). The likelihood of a heart attack is increased sixfold in women and threefold in men who smoke at least 20 cigarettes

---

BOX 22-1	Cardiovascular Disease Risk Factors

Nonmodifiable (Fixed)

- Heredity
- Race
- Gender ~ *female* [handwritten]
- Advancing age

Prior MI [handwritten]

Modifiable

- High blood pressure
- Elevated serum cholesterol levels
- Tobacco use
- Diabetes
- Physical inactivity
- Obesity
- Metabolic syndrome

oral contraceptive use [handwritten]

Contributing Factors

- Stress
- Inflammatory markers
- Psychosocial factors
- Alcohol intake

Type A personality [handwritten]

per day compared with persons who have never smoked (Prescott et al, 1998).

Research has shown that smoking damages the inner lining of blood vessels and speeds up the process of atherosclerosis. The chemicals in cigarettes affect levels of fibrinogen, increasing clotting. Nicotine increases heart rate and blood pressure. Smoking also promotes coronary artery spasm (Mackay & Mensah, 2004). Quitting smoking reduces the risk of heart disease by 50% after only 1 year. Within 2 to 6 years, the risk of developing coronary heart disease is similar to that of a nonsmoker.

Diabetes. Diabetes increases the risks of coronary heart disease, cerebrovascular disease, peripheral vascular disease, and heart failure. Coronary heart disease occurs more often in diabetic patients than in the general population, affecting approximately 55% of patients (Fodor & Tzerovska, 2004). Adult-onset, or type 2, diabetes (also known as non-insulin-dependent diabetes) is largely preventable because it is related to physical inactivity, excess calorie intake, and obesity. Persons with type 2 diabetes have a twofold to fourfold increased risk of coronary heart disease and a fourfold increase in death from coronary heart disease (Haffner & Cassells, 2003).

Physical Inactivity. Sedentary death syndrome is a term used by researchers to represent the growing number of health conditions caused or worsened by a lack of adequate physical activity. People who are not active have a greater risk of cardiovascular disease than do people who exercise regularly. Physical activity reduces the risk of coronary heart disease, diabetes, high blood pressure, and obesity. It also can help reduce stress. According to the World Health Organization, doing more than 150 minutes of moderate physical activity or 60 minutes of vigorous physical activity a week can reduce the risk of coronary heart disease by approximately 30% (Mackay & Mensah, 2004).

Obesity and Body Fat Distribution. Obesity is associated with an increased risk of heart disease. It also increases the likelihood of developing other coronary heart disease risk factors, including high blood pressure, diabetes, and high cholesterol. Body mass index (BMI) is formula used to assess body weight in relation to body height. This formula, used for adult men and women, has been shown to be an effective estimate of body fat (Table 22-1). Studies have shown that even a 10% reduction in body weight can help reduce the risks associated with obesity.

Body fat distribution appears to be an important factor in determining the risk of coronary heart disease. Persons who have abdominal (central) obesity are referred to as *apple shaped*. In "apple type" obesity, fat is distributed more on the upper body than around the hips. This type of fat distribution is more common in men. In pear-shaped or "pear type" obesity, fat distribution is more around the hips. This type of distribution is more common in women. Individuals who have abdominal obesity are at greatest risk of coronary heart disease. An increased waist circumference (more than 40 inches in men and more than 35 inches in women) is a stronger predictor of cardiovascular risk in both genders than is BMI (Fodor & Tzerovska, 2004).

Metabolic Syndrome. Metabolic syndrome (sometimes called syndrome X, the deadly quartet, or insulin resistance syndrome) is a group of disorders related to body metabolism. The disorders include high blood pressure, elevated insulin levels, excess body weight (particularly around the abdomen), and one or more abnormal cholesterol levels. An estimated one in four adults in the United States meets the criteria for metabolic syndrome (Ford et al, 2002). In the United States the frequency with which this syndrome occurs appears to be increasing as the incidence of obesity and sedentary lifestyle is increasing.

One of the main features of this syndrome is insulin resistance. Insulin resistance is a condition in which the normal amount of insulin secreted by the pancreas is not enough to cause an effect in body cells. The pancreas responds by secreting even more insulin so insulin has an effect. As a result, insulin levels rise. Blood glucose levels also begin to rise when the pancreas is no longer able to produce enough insulin.

Insulin resistance is aggravated by obesity and physical inactivity. Some patients eventually develop type 2 diabetes, further increasing their risk of cardiovascular disease. In many cases metabolic syndrome can be prevented with weight loss and increased physical activity.

Contributing Risk Factors

Stress. Because every person deals with stress differently, researchers are not sure how stress increases the risk of heart disease. What is known is that hormones such as epinephrine are released during times of stress. The release of epinephrine results in an increase in heart rate, blood pressure, and the body's need for oxygen. Chronic stress exposes the body to persistent levels of epinephrine and increased blood pressure.

During stress, hormones are released that increase the amount of clotting factors in the blood. This increases the risk of a clot lodging in an artery, which increases the risk of a heart attack.

The body's response to stress can worsen other risk factors. For example, a person who is stressed may exercise less, overeat, start smoking, or smoke more than usual.

Inflammatory Markers. C-reactive protein is a protein produced by the liver and released into the bloodstream

TABLE 22-1 Body Mass Index	
Body Mass Index Category	**Value**
Underweight	<18.5
Normal weight	18.5-24.9
Overweight	25.0-29.9
Obese	30 or greater

when active inflammation is present in the body. Atherosclerosis is an inflammatory disease. An elevated level of C-reactive protein in the bloodstream suggests persistent inflammation is present. High blood levels of C-reactive protein can be used to predict serious events such as heart attack, stroke, peripheral vascular disease, and sudden cardiac death.

Fibrinogen is a protein produced by the liver that is necessary for normal blood clotting. High blood levels of fibrinogen increase the thickness (viscosity) of the blood and may play a direct role in the clumping (aggregation) of platelets. Several studies have shown that fibrinogen levels can be used to predict the future risk of heart attack and stroke.

Psychosocial Factors. People with depression are at greater risk for developing heart disease than are those who are otherwise healthy (Nemeroff et al, 1998). Depression is common in people with coronary heart disease and indicates a poor prognosis for patients after a heart attack (Shimbo et al, 2005; Rowan et al, 2005).

Matters such as education, family income, and employment affect risk factors for heart disease and stroke (Centers for Disease Control and Prevention, 2005). People from lower socioeconomic groups may not have easy access to health care, are more likely to smoke, and are less likely to eat a healthy diet. For those who do have access to health care, they may be less likely to report warning signs of coronary heart disease, such as chest discomfort, to their physician.

Alcohol Intake. Heavy alcohol intake (three or more drinks per day) is associated with an increased risk of death from several causes, including stroke, several kinds of cancer, cirrhosis, and pancreatitis as well as accidents, suicide, and homicide (Friedman & Klatsky, 1993; Pearson, 1996). However, several studies have shown that light to moderate alcohol intake (one drink per day for women and two drinks for men) has a protective effect for coronary disease in both men and women. Alcohol intake increases HDL levels and may protect against coronary heart disease through an antiinflammatory mechanism (Zairis et al, 2004). Alcohol also may reduce fibrinogen and hinder platelet clumping.

SECTION 1: CARDIOVASCULAR ANATOMY AND PHYSIOLOGY
ANATOMY REVIEW

Blood Vessels

[OBJECTIVE 4]

Arteries are conductance vessels. The main function of the large arteries is to carry blood from the heart to the arterioles. Arteries are designed to carry blood under high pressure. Arterioles are the smallest branches of the arteries; they connect arteries and capillaries. Capillaries are the smallest and most numerous of the blood vessels.

They connect arterioles and venules and function as exchange vessels. Venules are the smallest branches of veins; they connect capillaries and veins. Veins are capacitance vessels. They carry deoxygenated (oxygen-poor) blood from the body to the right side of the heart. The walls of veins are thinner than arteries. Valves in the larger veins of the extremities and neck are arranged to allow blood flow in one direction, toward the heart.

Anatomy of the Heart
Location of the Heart

[OBJECTIVE 5]

The heart lies in the space between the lungs (**mediastinum**) in the middle of the chest. The heart sits behind the sternum and just above the diaphragm (Figure 22-1). Approximately two thirds of the heart lies to the left of the midline of the sternum. The remaining third lies to the right of the sternum. The **base** of the heart is its upper portion. It lies at approximately the level of the second rib. The heart's **apex,** or lower portion, is formed by the tip of the left ventricle. The apex lies just above the diaphragm, between the fifth and sixth ribs, in the midclavicular line. The heart is tilted slightly toward the left in the chest. Thus the anterior surface of the heart is composed mostly of the right ventricle. The heart's inferior surface is formed by both the right and left ventricles.

Heart Chambers

[OBJECTIVE 6]

The heart has four chambers. The two upper chambers are the right and left **atria.** The atria have thin walls. The right atrium receives blood low in oxygen from the superior vena cava, inferior vena cava, and the coronary sinus, which is the largest vein that drains the heart. The left atrium receives freshly oxygenated blood from the lungs by way of the right and left pulmonary veins.

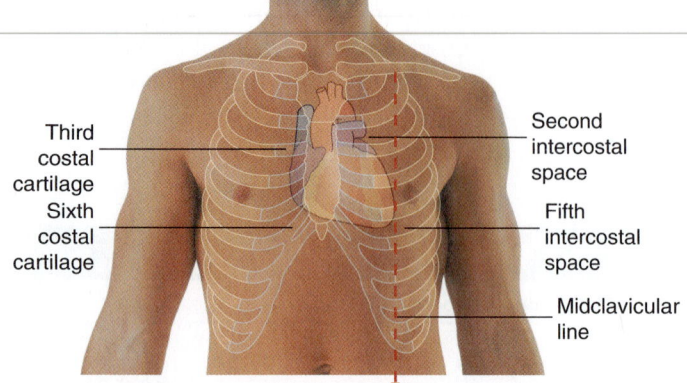

Third costal cartilage

Sixth costal cartilage

Second intercostal space

Fifth intercostal space

Midclavicular line

Figure 22-1 The heart lies in the middle of the thoracic cavity behind the sternum and between the lungs.

When the atria contract, blood is pumped through a valve into the ventricles.

The heart's two lower chambers are the right and left **ventricles.** The walls of the ventricles are much thicker than those of the atria. The right ventricle pumps blood to the lungs. The left ventricle pumps blood out to the body. When the left ventricle contracts, it normally produces an impulse that can be felt at the apex of the heart (apical impulse). This occurs because as the left ventricle contracts, it rotates forward. In a normal heart, this causes the apex of the left ventricle to hit the chest wall. You may be able to see the apical impulse in thin individuals. The apical impulse is also called the **point of maximal impulse** because it is the site where the heartbeat is most strongly felt.

The right and left sides of the heart are separated by an internal wall of connective tissue called a **septum.** The *interatrial septum* separates the right and left atria. The *interventricular septum* separates the right and left ventricles (Figure 22-2, *A*). The septa separate the heart

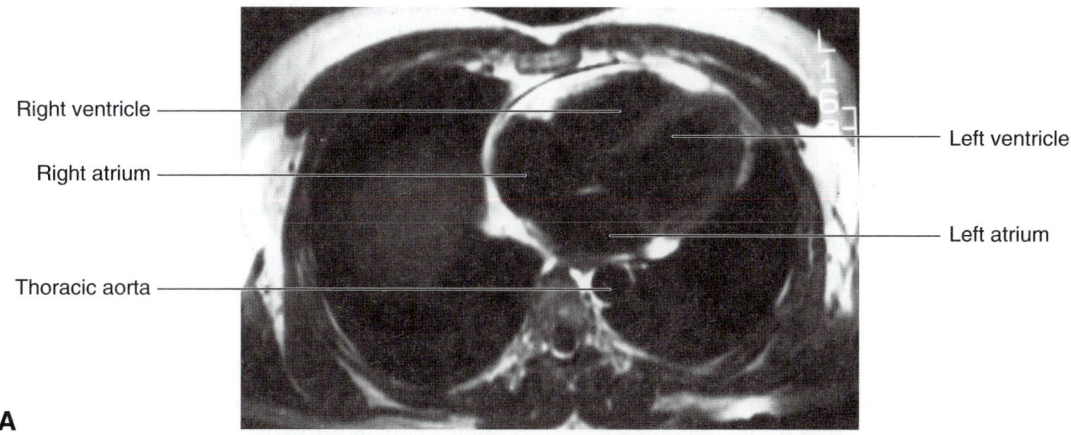

A

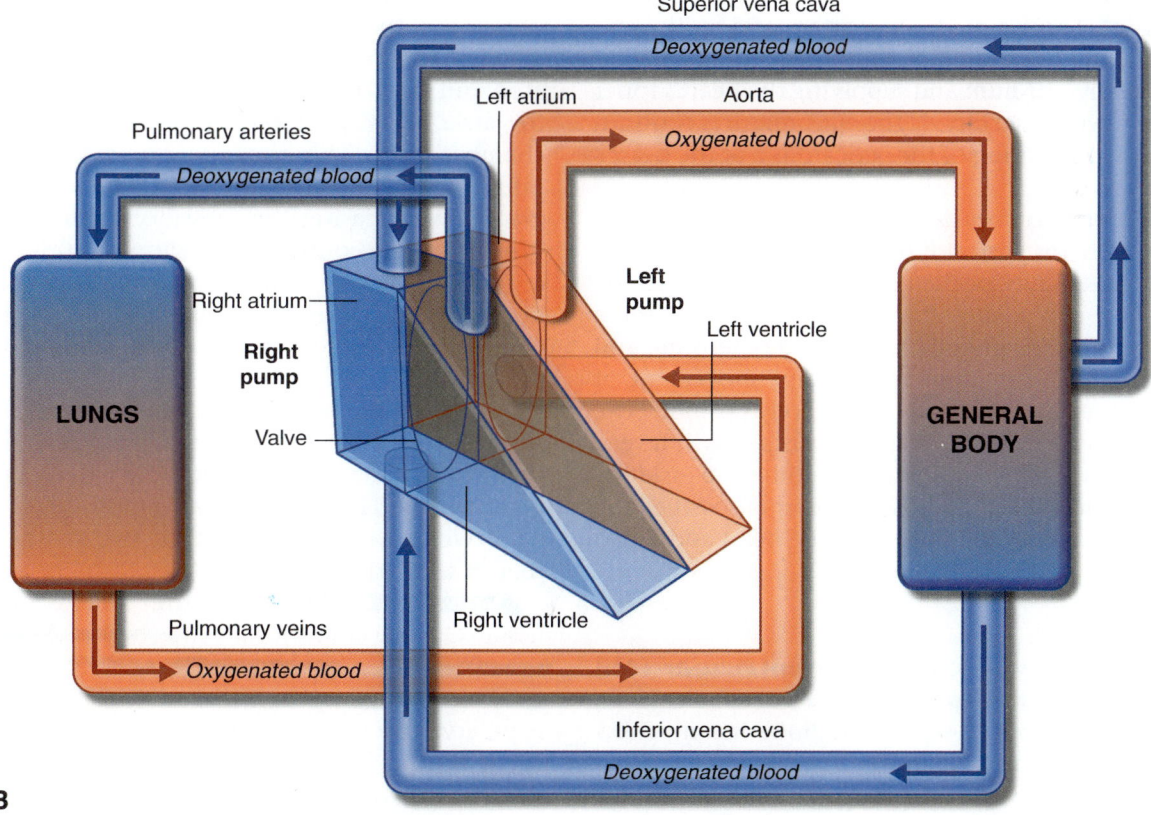

B

Figure 22-2 A, Magnetic resonance image of the mid-thorax, showing the heart's chambers and septa. **B**, The heart has two functional pumps.

into two functional pumps. The right atrium and right ventricle comprise one pump. The left atrium and left ventricle comprise the other (Figure 22-2, *B*). The right side of the heart is a low-pressure system. It pumps unoxygenated blood to and through the lungs to the left side of the heart. This is called the *pulmonary circulation.* The left side of the heart is a high-pressure pump. The left heart receives oxygenated blood and pumps it out to the rest of the body. This is called the *systemic circulation.* Blood is carried from the heart to the organs of the body through arteries, arterioles, and capillaries. Blood is returned to the right heart through venules and veins.

Layers of the Heart

The walls of the heart are composed of three tissue layers: the endocardium, myocardium, and epicardium. The heart's innermost layer, the **endocardium,** is a thin, smooth layer of epithelium and connective tissue that lines the heart's inner chambers, valves, chordae tendineae, and papillary muscles. It is continuous with the innermost layer of the arteries, veins, and capillaries of the body. This creates a continuous, closed circulatory system.

The **myocardium** (middle layer) is a thick, muscular layer that consists of cardiac muscle fibers (cells) responsible for the pumping action of the heart. The heart's outermost layer is called the **epicardium.** The epicardium contains blood capillaries, lymph capillaries, nerve fibers, and fat. The main coronary arteries lie on the epicardial surface of the heart. They feed this area first before entering the myocardium and supplying the heart's inner layers with oxygenated blood. The epicardium is continuous with the inner lining of the pericardium at the heart's apex.

The **pericardium** is a double-walled sac that encloses the heart and helps protect it from trauma and infection. The rough outer layer of the pericardial sac is called the *fibrous parietal pericardium.* It anchors the heart to some of the structures around it, such as the sternum and diaphragm. This helps prevent excessive movement of the heart in the chest with changes in body position. The inner layer, the *serous pericardium,* consists of two layers: parietal and visceral. The parietal layer lines the inside of the fibrous pericardium. The visceral layer (also called the *epicardium*) adheres to the outside of the heart and forms the outer layer of the heart muscle.

Heart Valves

The heart has four valves: two **atrioventricular (AV) valves** and two **semilunar (SL) valves** (Table 22-2). Their purpose is to make sure blood flows in one direction through the heart's chambers and prevent the backflow of blood. AV valves separate the atria from the ventricles. The tricuspid valve is the AV valve that lies between the right atrium and right ventricle. It consists of three separate cusps or flaps. The mitral (or bicuspid) valve has only two cusps. It lies between the left atrium

TABLE 22-2	Heart Valves		
Valve Type	**Name**	**Side of Heart**	**Location**
AV	Tricuspid	Right	Separates right atrium and right ventricle
	Mitral (bicuspid)	Left	Separates left atrium and left ventricle
SL	Pulmonic	Right	Between right ventricle and pulmonary artery
	Aortic	Left	Between left ventricle and aorta

AV, Atrioventricular; *SL,* semilunar.

and left ventricle. The AV valves open when a forward pressure gradient forces blood in a forward direction. They close when a backward pressure gradient pushes blood backward. The AV valves require almost no backflow to cause closure (Guyton & Hall, 1996).

The flow of blood from the superior and inferior venae cavae into the atria is normally continuous. Approximately 70% of this blood flows directly through the atria and into the ventricles before the atria contract. As the atria fill with blood, the pressure within the atrial chamber rises. This pressure forces the tricuspid and mitral valves open and the ventricles begin to fill, gradually increasing the pressure within the ventricles. When the atria contract, an additional 30% of the returning blood is added to filling of the ventricles. This additional contribution of blood resulting from atrial contraction is called **atrial kick.** On the right side of the heart, blood low in oxygen empties into the right ventricle. On the left side of the heart, freshly oxygenated blood empties into the left ventricle. When the ventricles then contract (systole), the pressure within the ventricles rises sharply. The tricuspid and mitral valves completely close when the pressure within the ventricles exceeds that of the atria.

Chordae tendineae are thin strands of connective tissue. On one end, they are attached to the underside of the AV valves. On the other end, they are attached to small mounds of myocardium called **papillary muscles.** Papillary muscles project inward from the lower portion of the ventricular walls. When the ventricles contract and relax, so do the papillary muscles. The papillary muscles adjust their tension on the chordae tendineae, preventing them from bulging too far into the atria.

The pulmonic and aortic valves are SL valves. The SL valves prevent backflow of blood from the aorta and pulmonary arteries into the ventricles. When the ventricles contract, the SL valves open, allowing blood to flow out of the ventricles. When the right ventricle contracts, blood low in oxygen flows through the pulmonic valve into the right and left pulmonary arteries. When the left ventricle contracts, freshly oxygenated blood flows through the **aortic valve** into the aorta and out to the body. The SL valves close as ventricular contraction ends and the pressure in the pulmonary artery and aorta exceeds that of the ventricles. Closure of the SL valves prevents the backflow of blood into the ventricles.

Blood Flow through the Heart

The right atrium receives blood low in oxygen and high in carbon dioxide from the superior and inferior venae cavae and the coronary sinus. Blood flows from the right atrium through the tricuspid valve into the right ventricle. When the right ventricle contracts, the tricuspid valve closes. The right ventricle expels the blood through the pulmonic valve into the pulmonary trunk. The pulmonary trunk divides into a right and left pulmonary artery, each of which carries blood to one lung (pulmonary circuit).

Blood flows through the pulmonary arteries to the lungs. Blood low in oxygen passes through the pulmonary capillaries. There it comes in direct contact with the alveolar-capillary membrane, where oxygen and carbon dioxide are exchanged. Blood then flows into the pulmonary veins. Carbon dioxide is exhaled as the left atrium receives oxygenated blood from the lungs by the four pulmonary veins (two from the right lung and two from the left lung). Blood flows from the left atrium through the mitral (bicuspid) valve into the left ventricle. When the left ventricle contracts, the mitral valve closes. Blood leaves the left ventricle through the aortic valve to the aorta. Blood is distributed throughout the body (systemic circuit) through the aorta and its branches.

Blood from the tissues of the head, neck, and upper extremities is emptied into the superior vena cava. Blood from the lower body is emptied into the inferior vena cava. The superior and inferior venae cavae carry their contents into the right atrium.

Cardiac Cycle

[OBJECTIVE 7]

The cardiac cycle refers to a repetitive pumping process that includes all the events associated with blood flow through the heart. The cycle has two phases for each heart chamber: systole and diastole. **Systole** is the period during which the chamber is contracting and blood is being ejected. Both the atria and ventricles have a systolic phase. **Diastole** is the period of relaxation during which the chambers are allowed to fill. Both the atria and ventricles have a diastolic phase. The myocardium receives its fresh supply of oxygenated blood from the coronary arteries during ventricular diastole. The cardiac cycle depends on the ability of the cardiac muscle to contract and on the condition of the heart's conduction system. The efficiency of the heart as a pump may be affected by abnormalities of the cardiac muscle, the valves, or the conduction system.

During the cardiac cycle, the pressure within each chamber of the heart rises in systole and falls in diastole. The heart's valves make sure that blood flows in the proper direction. Blood flows from one heart chamber to another if the pressure in the chamber is more than the pressure in the next. This pressure relationship depends on the careful timing of contractions. The heart's conduction system provides the necessary timing of events between atrial and ventricular systole.

Coronary Arteries

[OBJECTIVES 8, 9]

The heart provides itself with a fresh supply of oxygenated blood before supplying the rest of the body to ensure it has an adequate blood supply. This freshly oxygenated blood is mainly supplied by the branches of two vessels: the right and left coronary arteries. The right and left coronary arteries are the first branches off the proximal aorta. The openings to these vessels are just beyond the cusps of the aortic SL valve. When the ventricles contract, blood flow to the tissues of the heart is significantly reduced because the heart's blood vessels are compressed. Thus the coronary arteries fill when the ventricles are relaxed (diastole).

The main coronary arteries lie on the outer (epicardial) surface of the heart. Branches of the main coronary arteries penetrate the heart's muscle mass and supply the endocardium and myocardium with blood. The three major coronary arteries are the left anterior descending (LAD), left circumflex (LCX), and right coronary artery (RCA) (Figure 22-3).

> **PARAMEDIC Pearl**
>
> A person is said to have coronary artery disease if more than 50% diameter stenosis is present in one or more of the coronary arteries. Coronary artery disease is classified as one-, two-, or three-vessel disease.

Coronary Veins

The coronary (cardiac) veins travel alongside the arteries. The coronary sinus is the largest vein that drains the heart. It lies in the groove that separates the atria from the ventricles. Blood that has passed through the myocardial capillaries is drained by branches of the cardiac veins that join the coronary sinus. The coronary sinus drains into the right atrium.

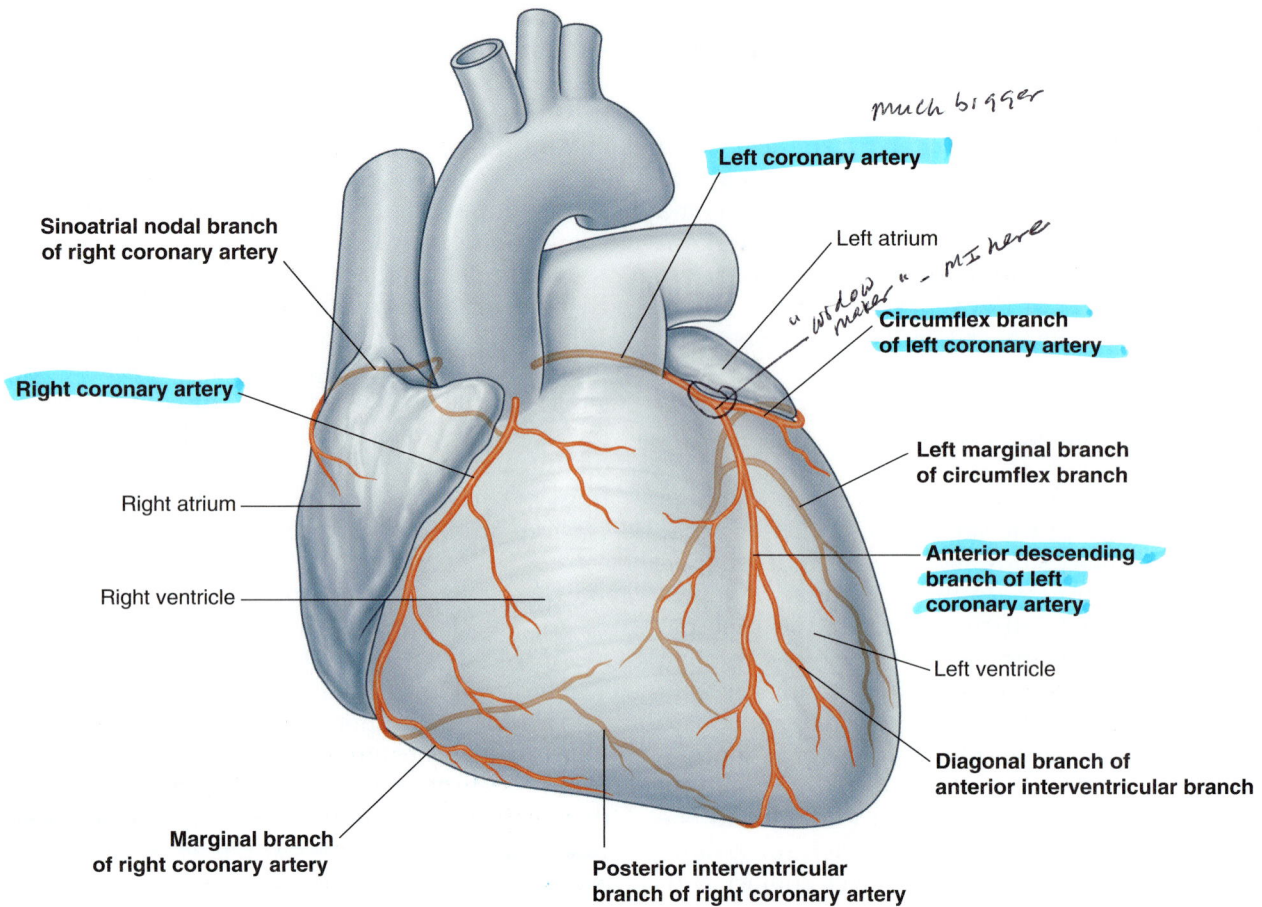

much bigger (handwritten)

Left coronary artery

Left atrium

"widow maker" - MI here (handwritten)

Circumflex branch of left coronary artery

Sinoatrial nodal branch of right coronary artery

Right coronary artery

Left marginal branch of circumflex branch

Right atrium

Anterior descending branch of left coronary artery

Right ventricle

Left ventricle

Diagonal branch of anterior interventricular branch

Marginal branch of right coronary artery

Posterior interventricular branch of right coronary artery

Figure 22-3 The three major coronary arteries are the left anterior descending (LAD; also called the anterior intraventricular artery), left circumflex (LCX), and right coronary artery (RCA).

Heart Rate

[OBJECTIVES 10, 11]

The heart is affected by both the sympathetic and parasympathetic divisions of the autonomic nervous system. The sympathetic division prepares the body to function under stress (fight-or-flight response). The parasympathetic division conserves and restores body resources (feed-and-breed or rest-and-digest response).

Chronotropy, inotropy, and dromotropy are terms used to describe effects on heart rate, myocardial contractility, and speed of conduction through the AV node. These terms are explained in Box 22-2.

Baroreceptors and Chemoreceptors

Baroreceptors (pressoreceptors) are specialized nerve tissue (sensors). They are found in the internal carotid arteries and the aortic arch. These sensory receptors detect changes in blood pressure. When they are stimulated, they cause a reflex response in either the sympathetic or the parasympathetic divisions of the autonomic nervous system. For example, if the blood pressure decreases, the body will attempt to compensate by the following actions:

- Constricting peripheral blood vessels
- Increasing heart rate
- Increasing the force of myocardial contraction

These compensatory responses occur because of a response by the sympathetic division. This is called a *sympathetic* or *adrenergic* response. If the blood pressure increases, the body will decrease sympathetic stimulation and increase the response by the parasympathetic division. This is called a *parasympathetic* or **cholinergic** response. The baroreceptors will be "reset" to a new "normal" after a few days of exposure to a specific pressure.

Chemoreceptors in the internal carotid arteries, aortic arch, and medulla detect changes in the concentration of hydrogen ions (pH), oxygen, and carbon dioxide in the blood. The response to these changes by the autonomic nervous system can be sympathetic or parasympathetic.

Parasympathetic Stimulation

Parasympathetic (inhibitory) nerve fibers supply the sinoatrial node, atrial muscle, and the AV junction of the heart by the vagus nerves. Acetylcholine is a chemical messenger (neurotransmitter) released when parasympathetic nerves are stimulated. Acetylcholine binds to parasympathetic receptors. Parasympathetic stimulation has the following actions:

- Slows the rate of discharge of the sinoatrial node
- Slows conduction through the AV node
- Decreases the strength of atrial contraction
- Can cause a small decrease in the force of ventricular contraction

Sympathetic Stimulation

Sympathetic (accelerator) nerves supply specific areas of the heart's electrical system, atrial muscle, and the ventricular myocardium. When sympathetic nerves are stimulated, norepinephrine is released. Remember: the sympathetic division of the autonomic nervous system prepares the body for emergency or stressful situations. So the release of norepinephrine results in the following predictable results:

- Increased force of contraction
- Increased heart rate
- Increased blood pressure

Increases in heart rate shorten all phases of the cardiac cycle. When the length of time for ventricular relaxation is shortened, less time is available for them to fill adequately with blood. If the ventricles do not have time to fill, the following occur:

- The amount of blood sent to the coronary arteries is reduced
- The amount of blood pumped out of the ventricles decreases (cardiac output)
- Signs of myocardial **ischemia** may be seen

Other factors that influence heart rate include electrolyte and hormone levels, medications, stress, anxiety, fear, and body temperature. Heart rate increases when body temperature increases and decreases when body temperature decreases.

THE HEART AS A PUMP

[OBJECTIVES 12, 13, 14]

Venous Return

The heart functions as a pump to propel blood through the systemic and pulmonary circulations. As the heart chambers fill with blood, the heart muscle is stretched. The most important factor determining the amount of blood pumped out by the heart is the amount of blood flowing into the right heart from the systemic circulation (venous return). *Preload*

Cardiac Output

Cardiac output is the amount of blood pumped into the aorta each minute by the heart. It is defined as the **stroke volume** (amount of blood ejected from a ventricle with each heartbeat) multiplied by the heart rate. In the average adult, normal cardiac output is between 4 and 8 L/min. The cardiac output at rest is approximately 5 L/min (stroke volume of 70 mL multiplied by a heart rate of 70 beats/min). Cardiac output may be increased by an increase in heart rate or stroke volume. Stroke volume is determined by the following:

- The degree of ventricular filling when the heart is relaxed (preload)
- The pressure against which the ventricle must pump (afterload)
- The myocardium's contractile state (contracting or relaxing)

Preload (end-diastolic volume) is the force exerted on the walls of the ventricles at the end of diastole. The volume of blood returning to the heart influences preload. More blood returning to the right atrium increases preload. Less blood returning decreases preload. **Afterload** is the pressure or resistance against which the ventricles must pump to eject blood. Afterload is influenced by the following:

- Arterial blood pressure
- The ability of the arteries to become stretched (arterial distensibility)
- Arterial resistance

The lower the resistance (lower afterload), the more easily blood can be ejected. Increased afterload (increased resistance) increases the heart's workload. Conditions that contribute to increased afterload include increased thickness of the blood (viscosity) and high blood pressure.

Now that cardiac output and stroke volume have been discussed, consider this example. A patient has a stroke volume of 80 mL/beat. His heart rate is 70 beats/min. Is his cardiac output normal, decreased, or increased? Substitute numbers into the formula already presented (CO = SV × HR): 5600 mL/min = 80 mL/beat × 70 beats/min. Cardiac output normally is between 4 and 8 L/min. This patient's cardiac output is within normal limits.

According to Frank–Starling's law of the heart, the greater the volume of blood in the heart during diastole (preload), the more forceful the cardiac contraction and the more blood the ventricle will pump (stroke volume)—to a point. This is important so that the heart can adjust its pumping capacity in response to changes in venous return. For example, during exercise, the heart muscle fibers stretch in response to increased volume (preload) before contracting. Stretching of the muscle fibers allows the heart to eject the additional volume with increased force, thereby increasing stroke volume and cardiac output.

Cardiac output varies depending on hormone balance, an individual's activity level and body size, and the body's metabolic needs. Factors that increase cardiac output include increased body metabolism, exercise, and the age and size of the body. Factors that may decrease cardiac output include **shock,** hypovolemia, and heart failure. Signs and symptoms of decreased cardiac output appear in Box 22-3. Heart failure may result from any condition that impairs preload, afterload, cardiac contractility, or heart rate. As the heart begins to fail, the body's compensatory mechanisms attempt to improve cardiac output by manipulating one or more of these factors.

BOX 22-3	**Signs and Symptoms of Decreased Cardiac Output**

- Cold, clammy skin
- Color changes in the skin and mucous membranes
- Dyspnea
- Orthopnea
- Crackles (rales)
- Changes in mental status
- Changes in blood pressure
- Dysrhythmias
- Fatigue
- Restlessness

SECTION 2: ELECTROPHYSIOLOGY OF THE HEART

CARDIAC CELLS

Types of Cardiac Cells

In general, cardiac cells have either a mechanical (contractile) or an electrical (pacemaker) function. **Myocardial cells** (working or mechanical cells) contain contractile filaments. When these cells are electrically stimulated, the contractile filaments slide together and the myocardial cell contracts. These myocardial cells form the thin muscular layer of the atrial walls and the thicker muscular layer of the ventricular walls (the myocardium). These cells do not normally generate electrical impulses on their own. They rely on pacemaker cells for this purpose.

Pacemaker cells are specialized cells of the heart's electrical system. Pacemaker cells also are referred to as *conducting cells* or *automatic cells.* They are responsible for spontaneously generating and conducting electrical impulses.

Properties of Cardiac Cells

[OBJECTIVE 15]

When a nerve is stimulated, a chemical (neurotransmitter) is released. The chemical crosses the space between the end of the nerve and the muscle membrane (neuromuscular junction). The chemical binds to receptor sites on the muscle membrane and stimulates the receptors. An electrical impulse develops and travels along the muscle membrane, resulting in contraction. Thus a skeletal muscle contracts only after it is stimulated by a nerve.

The heart is unique because it has pacemaker cells that can generate an electrical impulse without being stimulated by a nerve. The ability of cardiac pacemaker cells to create an electrical impulse without being stimulated from another source is called **automaticity.** The heart's normal pacemaker (the sinoatrial node) usually prevents other areas of the heart from assuming this function because its cells depolarize more rapidly than other pacemaker cells. **Excitability** (irritability) refers to the ability of cardiac muscle cells to respond to an outside stimulus. The stimulus may be from a chemical, mechanical, or electrical source. **Conductivity** refers to the ability of a cardiac cell to receive an electrical impulse and conduct it to an adjoining cardiac cell. All cardiac cells possess this characteristic. **Contractility** refers to the ability of myocardial cells to shorten in response to an impulse, which results in contraction. The heart normally contracts in response to an impulse that begins in the sinoatrial (SA) node.

The properties of cardiac cells are:

- Automaticity
- Excitability (irritability)
- Conductivity
- Contractility

CARDIAC ACTION POTENTIAL

[OBJECTIVE 16]

Before the following discussion of the cardiac action potential, think about how a battery releases energy. A battery has two terminals: one terminal is positive and the other is negative. Charged particles exert forces on each other, and opposite charges attract. Electrons (negatively charged particles) are produced by a chemical reaction inside the battery. If a wire is connected between the two terminals, the circuit is completed and the stored energy is released. This allows electrons to flow quickly from the negative terminal along the wire to the positive terminal. If no wire is connected between the terminals, the chemical reaction does not take place and no current flow occurs. **Current** is the flow of electrical charge from one point to another.

Separated electrical charges of opposite polarity (positive versus negative) have potential energy. The measurement of this potential energy is called **voltage.** Voltage is measured between two points. In the battery example, the current flow is caused by the voltage, or potential difference, between the two terminals. Voltage is measured in units of volts or millivolts.

In the normal heart, electrical activity occurs because of changes that occur in the body's cells. Human body fluids contain **electrolytes,** which are elements or compounds that break into charged particles **(ions)** when melted or dissolved in water or another solvent. The main electrolytes that affect the function of the heart are sodium ($Na+$), potassium ($K+$), calcium ($Ca++$), and chloride (Cl^-). Body fluids that contain electrolytes conduct an electric current in much the same way as the wire in the battery example. Electrolytes move about in body fluids and carry a charge, just as electrons moving along a wire conduct a current. The **action potential** is a five-phase cycle that reflects the difference in the concentration of these charged particles across the cell membrane at any given time.

Polarization

In the body, cells spend a lot of time moving ions back and forth across their membranes. As a result, a slight difference in the concentrations of charged particles across the membranes of cells is normal. Thus potential energy (voltage) exists because of the imbalance of charged particles. This imbalance makes the cells excitable.

Cell membranes contain pores or channels through which specific electrolytes and other small, water-soluble molecules can cross the cell membrane from outside to inside. When a cell is at rest, $K+$ leaks out of it. Large molecules such as proteins and phosphates remain inside the cell because they are too big to pass easily through the cell membrane. These large molecules carry a negative charge. This results in more negatively charged ions on the inside of the cell. When the inside of a cell is more negative than the outside, it is said to be in a **polarized state** (Figure 22-4). The voltage (difference in electrical charges) across the cell membrane is the **membrane potential.** Electrolytes are quickly moved from one side of the cell membrane to the other by means of pumps.

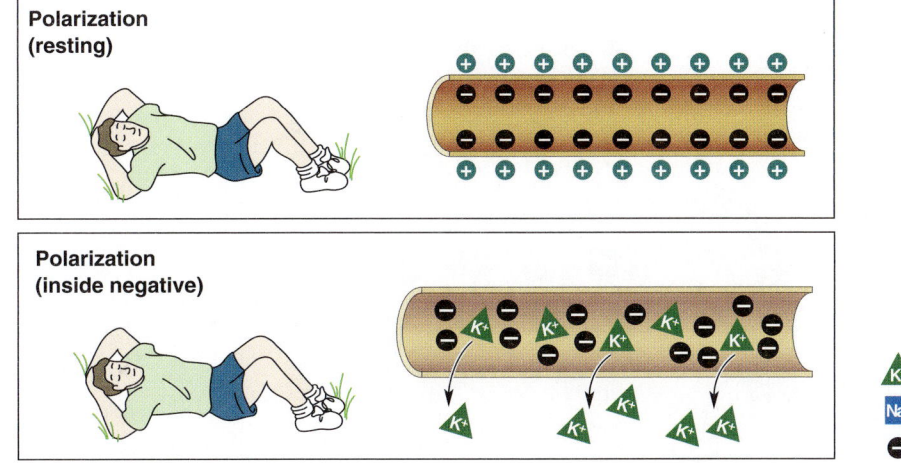

Potassium (K^+)
Sodium (Na^+)
Anions

Figure 22-4 Polarization. When the inside of a cell is more negative than the outside it is said to be polarized.

These pumps require energy (adenosine triphosphate) when movement occurs against a concentration gradient. The energy expended by the cells to move electrolytes across the cell membrane creates a flow of current. This flow of current is expressed in volts. Voltage appears on an electrocardiogram (ECG) as spikes or waveforms. Thus an ECG is actually a sophisticated voltmeter.

Depolarization

[OBJECTIVE 17]

For a pacemaker cell to "fire" (produce an impulse), a flow of electrolytes across the cell membrane must exist. When a cell is stimulated, the cell membrane changes and becomes **permeable** to Na+ and K+. Permeability refers to the ability of a membrane channel to allow passage of electrolytes once it is open. Na+ rushes into the cell through Na+ channels. This causes the inside of the cell to become more positive. A spike (waveform) is then recorded on the ECG. Threshold is the membrane potential at which the cell membrane becomes more positive. The stimulus that alters the electrical charges across the cell membrane may be electrical, mechanical, or chemical.

As described in the battery example, when opposite charges come together, energy is released. When the movement of electrolytes changes the electrical charge of the inside of the cell from negative to positive, an impulse is generated. The impulse causes channels to open in the next cell membrane and then the next. The movement of charged particles across a cell membrane causing the inside of the cell to become positive is called **depolarization** (Figure 22-5). Depolarization must take place before the heart can mechanically contract and pump blood. Depolarization occurs because of the movement of Na+ into the cell. Depolarization proceeds from the innermost layer of the heart (endocardium) to the outermost layer (epicardium).

An impulse normally begins in the pacemaker cells found in the SA node of the heart. A chain reaction occurs from cell to cell in the heart's electrical conduction system until all the cells have been stimulated and depolarized. This chain reaction is a wave of depolarization. The chain reaction is made possible because of gap junctions that exist between the cells. Eventually the impulse is spread from the pacemaker cells to the working myocardial cells. The working myocardial cells contract when they are stimulated. When the atria are stimulated, a P wave is recorded on the ECG. Thus the P wave represents atrial depolarization. When the ventricles are stimulated, a QRS complex is recorded on the ECG. Thus the QRS complex represents ventricular depolarization.

Be sure to note that depolarization is *not* the same as contraction. Depolarization (an electrical event) is expected to result in contraction (a mechanical event). Organized electrical activity on the cardiac monitor may still be seen when assessment of the patient reveals no palpable pulse. This clinical situation is called pulseless electrical activity.

Repolarization

After the cell depolarizes, it quickly begins to recover and restore its electrical charges to normal. The movement of charged particles across a cell membrane in which the inside of the cell is restored to its negative charge is called **repolarization.** The cell stops the flow of Na+ into the cell and allows K+ to leave it. Negatively charged particles are left inside the cell. Thus the cell is returned to its resting state (Figure 22-6). This causes contractile proteins in the working myocardial cells to separate (relax). The

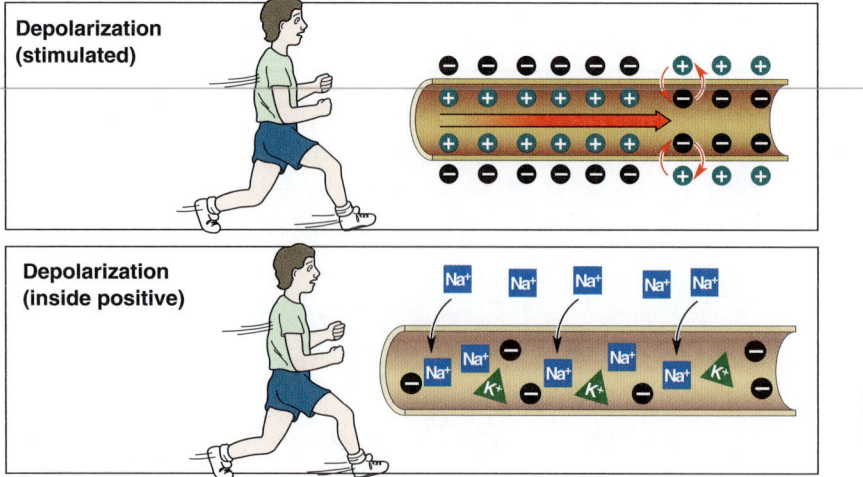

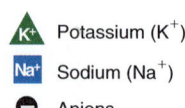

Figure 22-5 Depolarization is the movement of ions across a cell membrane, causing the inside of the cell to become more positive.

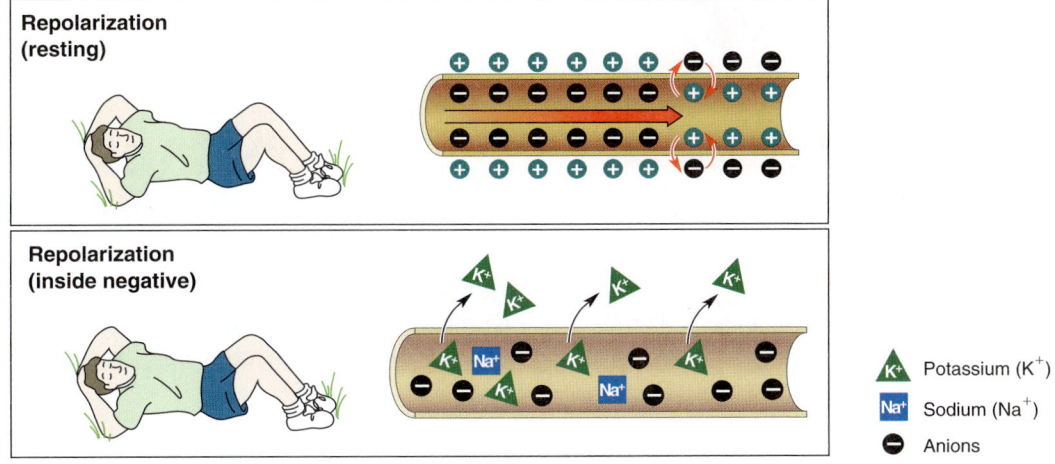

Figure 22-6 Repolarization is the movement of charged particles across a cell membrane in which the inside of the cell is restored to its negative charge.

cell can be stimulated again if another electrical impulse arrives at the cell membrane. Repolarization proceeds from the epicardium to the endocardium. On the ECG, the ST segment and T wave represent ventricular repolarization.

Phases of the Cardiac Action Potential

[OBJECTIVE 18]
The action potential of a cardiac cell consists of five phases labeled 0 to 4:

- Phase 0: rapid depolarization
- Phase 1: early rapid repolarization
- Phase 2: plateau

- Phase 3: final rapid repolarization
- Phase 4: resting membrane potential

These phases reflect the rapid sequence of voltage changes that occur across the cell membrane during the electrical cardiac cycle. Phases 1, 2, and 3 have been referred to as *electrical systole*. Phase 4 has been referred to as *electrical diastole*. The configuration of the action potential varies depending on the location, size, and function of the cardiac cell. Figure 22-7 shows the action potential of a normal ventricular muscle cell.

Phase 0: Depolarization

[OBJECTIVE 19]
The rapid entry of Na+ into the cell is largely responsible for phase 0 of the cardiac action potential. Phase 0

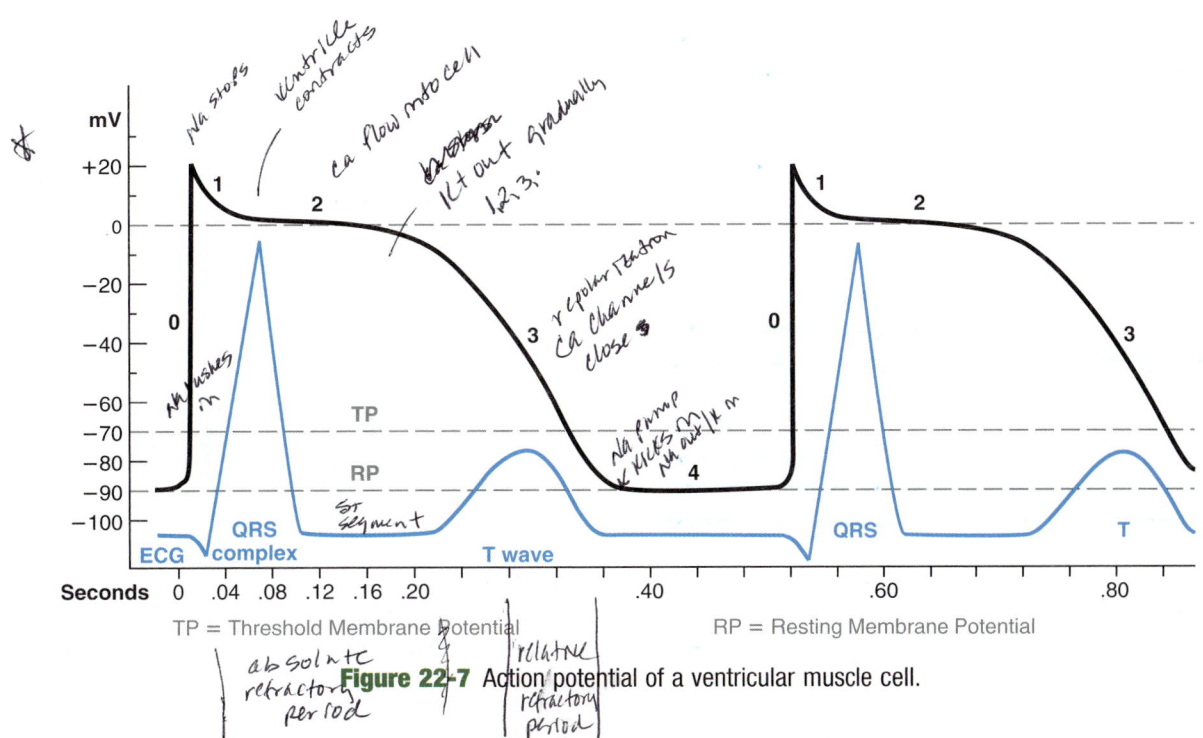

Figure 22-7 Action potential of a ventricular muscle cell.

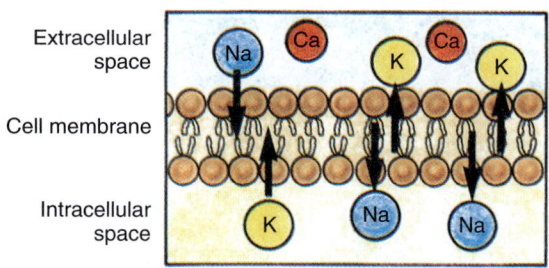

Figure 22-8 Phase 0 of the cardiac action potential represents depolarization. Na+ moves rapidly into the cell through Na+ channels. K+ leaves the cell and Ca++ moves slowly into the cell through Ca++ channels.

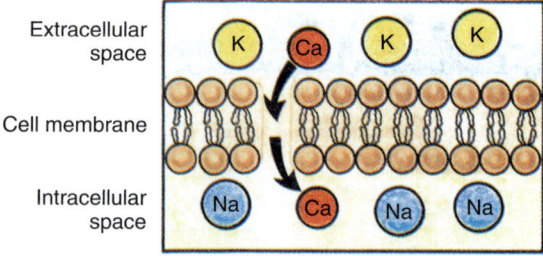

Figure 22-9 Phase 2 (plateau phase) of the cardiac action potential is caused by the slow inward movement of Ca++ and slow outward movement of K+ from the cell.

represents depolarization (Figure 22-8) and is called the rapid depolarization phase. Phase 0 also is called the *upstroke*, *spike*, or *overshoot*. Phase 0 begins when the cell receives an impulse. Na+ moves rapidly into the cell through the Na+ channels, K+ leaves the cell, and Ca++ moves slowly into the cell through Ca++ channels. The cell depolarizes and cardiac contraction begins. Phase 0 is represented on the ECG by the QRS complex.

The cells of the atria, ventricles, and the Purkinje fibers of the conduction system have many sodium channels. The SA and AV nodes of the heart have relatively few sodium channels. If the flow of sodium through the sodium channels is slowed or blocked, the heart rate slows, the cells become less excitable, and the speed of conduction decreases. Phase 0 of the cardiac action potential is immediately followed by repolarization, which is divided into three phases.

Phase 1: Early Repolarization

During phase 1 of the cardiac action potential, the Na+ channels partially close, slowing the flow of Na+ into the cell. At the same time, Cl⁻ enters the cell and K+ leaves it through K+ channels. The result is a decrease in the number of positive electrical charges within the cell. This produces a small negative deflection in the action potential.

Phase 2: Plateau Phase

Phase 2 is the plateau phase of the action potential (Figure 22-9). During this phase, Ca++ slowly enters the cell through Ca++ channels. The cells of the atria, ventricles, and the Purkinje fibers of the conduction system have many calcium channels. K+ continues to leave the cell slowly through K+ channels. The plateau phase allows cardiac muscle to sustain an increased period of contraction. The cells of the atria, ventricles, and Purkinje fibers spend less time in phase 2 if the flow of calcium through calcium channels is slowed or blocked. Phase 2 is responsible for the ST segment on the ECG. The ST segment reflects the early part of repolarization of the right and left ventricles.

Phase 3: Final Rapid Repolarization

Phase 3 begins with the downslope of the action potential. The cell rapidly completes repolarization as K+

quickly flows out of the cell. Na+ and Ca++ channels close, stopping the entry of Na+ and Ca++. The rapid movement of K+ out of the cell causes the inside to become progressively more electrically negative. The cell gradually becomes more sensitive to external stimuli until its original sensitivity is restored. Phase 3 of the action potential corresponds with the T wave (ventricular repolarization) on the ECG. Repolarization is complete by the end of phase 3. If potassium channels are blocked, the result is a longer action potential.

Phase 4: Resting Membrane Potential

Phase 4 is the resting membrane potential (return to resting state) (Figure 22-10). During phase 4, an excess of Na+ is inside the cell and an excess of K+ is outside the cell. The Na+/K+ pump is activated to move Na+ out of the cell and K+ back into the cell. The heart is polarized during this phase (i.e., ready for discharge). The cell will remain in this state until the cell membrane is reactivated by another stimulus.

The heart typically beats at a regular rate and rhythm. If this pattern is interrupted, an abnormal heart rhythm can result. Health care professionals use the terms **arrhythmia** and **dysrhythmia** interchangeably to refer to an abnormal heart rhythm. Medications used to correct irregular heartbeats and slow down hearts that beat too fast are called **antiarrhythmics.** Antiarrhythmic medications are classified by their effects on the cardiac action potential.

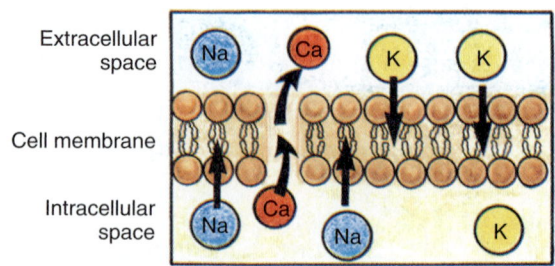

Figure 22-10 During phase 4, an excess of Na+ is inside the cell and an excess of K+ is outside the cell. The Na+/K+ pump is activated to move Na+ out of the cell and move K+ back into the cell.

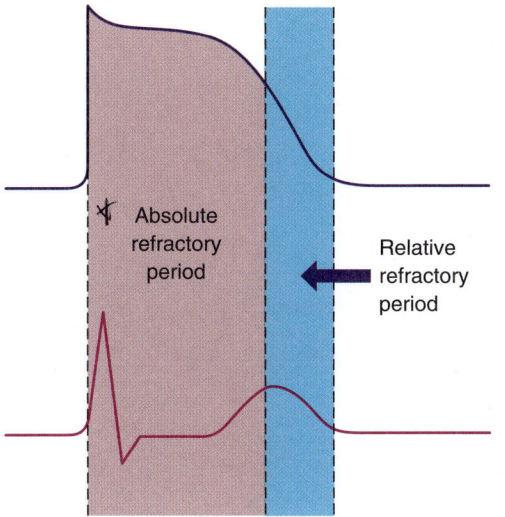

Figure 22-11 The absolute and relative refractory periods correlate with the action potential of a cardiac muscle cell and an ECG tracing.

REFRACTORY PERIODS ✻ *Need to know*

Refractoriness is a term used to describe the period of recovery that cells need after being discharged before they are able to respond to a stimulus. In the heart, the refractory period is longer than the contraction itself.

During the **absolute refractory period** (also known as the *effective refractory period*), the cell will not respond to further stimulation. This means that the myocardial working cells cannot contract and the cells of the electrical conduction system cannot conduct an electrical impulse—no matter how strong the stimulus. On the ECG, the absolute refractory period corresponds with the onset of the QRS complex to the peak of the T wave (Figure 22-11). It includes phases 0, 1, 2, and part of phase 3 of the cardiac action potential.

During the **relative refractory period** (also known as the *vulnerable period*), some cardiac cells have repolarized to their threshold potential and can be stimulated to respond (depolarize) to a stronger than normal stimulus (Figure 22-12). This period corresponds with the downslope of the T wave on the ECG.

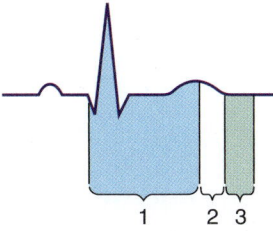

Figure 22-12 *1*, The absolute refractory period; *2*, relative refractory period; and *3*, supernormal period.

After the relative refractory period is a **supernormal period.** A weaker than normal stimulus can cause cardiac cells to depolarize during this period. The supernormal period extends from the end of phase 3 to the beginning of phase 4 of the cardiac action potential. On the ECG, this corresponds with the end of the T wave. Dysrhythmias can develop during this period.

CONDUCTION SYSTEM

[OBJECTIVE 20]

The specialized electrical (pacemaker) cells in the heart are arranged in a system of pathways called the **conduction system.** In the normal heart, the cells of the conduction system are interconnected. The conduction system makes sure that the chambers of the heart contract in a coordinated fashion. The pacemaker site with the fastest firing rate typically controls the heart.

Sinoatrial Node   *P wave*

[OBJECTIVE 21]

The normal heartbeat is the result of an electrical impulse that begins in the SA node. The SA node is normally the primary pacemaker of the heart because it has the fastest firing rate of all of the heart's normal pacemaker sites (Figure 22-13). The built-in (intrinsic) rate of the SA node is 60 to 100 beats/min.

The SA node is located in the upper posterior part of the right atrium where the superior vena cava and the right atrium meet. The fibers of the SA node directly connect with the fibers of the atria. As the impulse leaves the SA node, it is spread from cell to cell in wavelike form across the atrial muscle. As the impulse spreads, it stimulates the right atrium, the interatrial septum, and then the left atrium. This results in contraction of the right and left atria at almost the same time.

Conduction through the AV node begins before atrial depolarization is completed. The impulse is spread to the AV node by three internodal pathways. These pathways consist of a mixture of working myocardial cells and specialized conducting fibers.

Atrioventricular Junction

The internodal pathways merge gradually with the cells of the AV node. Depolarization and repolarization are slow in the AV node, making this area vulnerable to blocks in conduction (AV blocks). The **AV junction** is the AV node and the nonbranching portion of the bundle of His. This area consists of specialized conduction tissue that provides the electrical links between the atria and ventricles. When the AV junction is bypassed by an abnormal pathway, the abnormal route is called an **accessory pathway.** An accessory pathway is an extra bundle of working myocardial tissue that forms a connection between the atria and ventricles outside the normal conduction system.

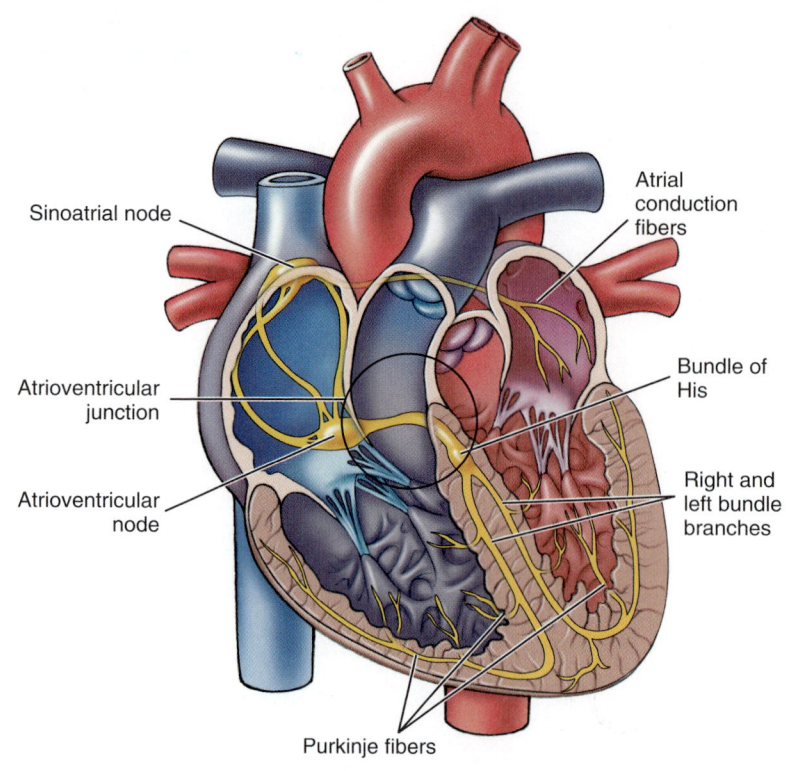

Figure 22-13 The conduction system.

[handwritten left margin:] Depolarization from endocardium out repolarization from epicardium in

[handwritten below figure:] Narrow QRS - originating above Bundle of His
Wide QRS - Originating below Bundle of His - impulse has to go back up one sided down the other - ventricles don't contract at exactly same time

Atrioventricular Node

[OBJECTIVE 22]

The **AV node** is a group of cells located in the floor of the right atrium immediately behind the tricuspid valve and near the opening of the coronary sinus. The AV node is supplied by the RCA in 85% to 90% of the population. In the remainder, the LCX provides the blood supply. The AV node is supplied by both sympathetic and parasympathetic nerve fibers.

As the impulse from the atria enters the AV node, a delay occurs in conduction of the impulse to the ventricles. This delay allows the atria to empty blood into the ventricles before the next ventricular contraction begins. This increases the amount of blood in the ventricles, increasing stroke volume.

Bundle of His

The AV junction is composed of the AV node (the upper portion of the AV junction) and the nonbranching portion of the bundle of His (the lower portion of the AV junction). The bundle of His is also called the *common bundle,* or the *atrioventricular bundle,* and is located in the upper portion of interventricular septum. The AV junction has pacemaker cells that are capable of firing at a rate of 40 to 60 beats/min. The bundle of His conducts the electrical impulse to the right and left bundle branches.

The bundle of His receives a dual blood supply from the branches of the left anterior and posterior descending coronary arteries. Because of this dual blood supply, the bundle of His is less vulnerable to ischemia. The term **His-Purkinje system** or *His-Purkinje network* refers to the bundle of His, bundle branches, and Purkinje fibers.

Right and Left Bundle Branches

The right bundle branch innervates the right ventricle. The left bundle branch spreads the electrical impulse to the interventricular septum and left ventricle, which is thicker and more muscular than the right ventricle. The left bundle branch divides into three divisions called **fascicles,** which are small bundles of nerve fibers. The three fascicles are called the *anterior fascicle, posterior fascicle,* and the *septal fascicle.* The anterior fascicle spreads the electrical impulse to the anterior portions of the left ventricle. The posterior fascicle relays the impulse to the posterior portions of the left ventricle, and the septal fascicle relays the impulse to the mid-septum.

Purkinje Fibers

The right and left bundle branches divide into smaller and smaller branches and then into a special network of fibers called the **Purkinje fibers.** These fibers spread from the interventricular septum into the papillary muscles. They continue downward to the apex of the heart, comprising an elaborate web that penetrates

TABLE 22-3	Normal Pacemaker Sites	
Order	Pacemaker	Beats/Min
1	SA node (primary pacemaker)	60-100
2	AV junction	40-60
3	Purkinje fibers	20-40

SA, Sinoatrial; *AV*, atrioventricular.

approximately one third of the way into the ventricular muscle mass. The fibers then become continuous with the muscle cells of the right and left ventricles. The Purkinje fibers have pacemaker cells capable of firing at a rate of 20 to 40 beats/min (Table 22-3). The electrical impulse spreads rapidly through the right and left bundle branches and the Purkinje fibers to reach the ventricular muscle. The electrical impulse spreads from the endocardium to the myocardium, finally reaching the epicardial surface. The ventricular walls are stimulated to contract in a twisting motion that wrings blood out of the ventricular chambers and forces it into arteries.

Did you know?

An escape pacemaker is a pacemaker site other than the SA node, such as the AV junction and ventricles. If the SA node fails to fire, the escape pacemaker sites serve as a fail-safe mechanism to make sure another site steps in and assumes pacing responsibility.

CAUSES OF DYSRHYTHMIAS

[OBJECTIVE 23]

Enhanced Automaticity

Enhanced automaticity is an abnormal condition in which one of the following occurs:

- Cardiac cells that are not normally associated with a pacemaker function begin to depolarize spontaneously, *or*
- A pacemaker site other than the SA node increases its firing rate beyond that which is considered normal.

Possible reasons for enhanced automaticity are shown in Box 22-4. Examples of rhythms associated with enhanced automaticity include atrial flutter; atrial fibrillation; supraventricular tachycardia; premature atrial, junctional, or ventricular complexes; ventricular tachycardia or ventricular fibrillation; junctional tachycardia; accelerated idioventricular rhythm; and accelerated junctional rhythm.

BOX 22-4	Possible Causes of Enhanced Automaticity

- Catecholamines, such as epinephrine
- Administration of atropine sulfate
- Digitalis toxicity
- Acidosis
- Alkalosis
- Hypoxia
- Myocardial ischemia or myocardial infarction
- Electrolyte disturbances such as hypokalemia, hyperkalemia, or hypocalcemia

Triggered Activity

Triggered activity results from abnormal electrical impulses that sometimes occur during repolarization, when cells are normally quiet. These abnormal electrical impulses are called afterdepolarizations. Triggered activity requires a stimulus to begin depolarization. It occurs when pacemaker cells from a site other than the SA node and myocardial working cells depolarize more than once after being stimulated by a single impulse.

Causes of triggered activity include:

- Hypoxia
- Increase in catecholamines
- Hypomagnesemia
- Myocardial ischemia or injury
- Medications that prolong repolarization (such as quinidine)

Triggered activity can result in atrial or ventricular beats that occur alone, in pairs, in runs (three or more beats), or as a sustained ectopic rhythm. **Ectopic** refers to an impulse originating from a source other than the SA node.

Reentry

[OBJECTIVE 24]

An impulse normally spreads through the heart only once after it is initiated by pacemaker cells. **Reentry** is the spread of an impulse through tissue already stimulated by that same impulse. An electrical impulse is delayed or blocked (or both) in one or more areas of the conduction system while the impulse is conducted normally through the rest of the conduction system. This results in the delayed electrical impulse entering cardiac cells that have just been depolarized by the normally conducted impulse. Reentry requires the following three conditions (Figure 22-14):

- A potential conduction circuit or circular conduction pathway
- A block within part of the circuit
- Delayed conduction with the remainder of the circuit

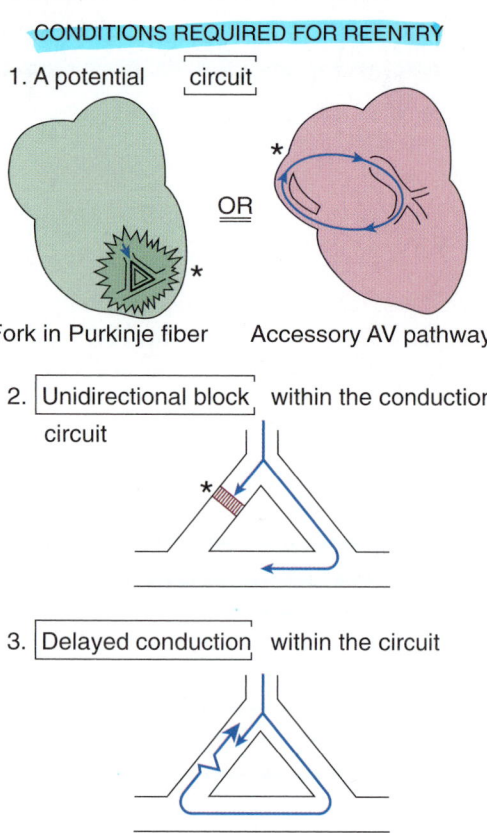

CONDITIONS REQUIRED FOR REENTRY

1. A potential [circuit]

OR

Fork in Purkinje fiber   Accessory AV pathway

2. [Unidirectional block] within the conduction circuit

3. [Delayed conduction] within the circuit

Figure 22-14 Reentry requires (1) a potential conduction circuit or circular conduction pathway, (2) a block within part of the circuit, and (3) delayed conduction with the remainder of the circuit.

If the area the delayed impulse stimulates is relatively refractory, the impulse can cause depolarization of those cells, producing a single premature beat or repetitive electrical impulses. This can result in short periods of an abnormally fast heart rate. Common causes of reentry include:

- Hyperkalemia
- Myocardial ischemia
- Some antiarrhythmic medications

Examples of rhythms associated with reentry are paroxysmal supraventricular tachycardia; ventricular tachycardia; and premature atrial, junctional, or ventricular complexes.

Escape Beats or Rhythms

Escape is the term used when the SA node slows or fails to initiate depolarization and a lower site spontaneously produces electrical impulses, assuming responsibility for pacing the heart. Escape beats or rhythms are protective mechanisms to maintain cardiac output. They begin in the AV junction or the ventricles. Examples of escape beats or rhythms include junctional escape beats, junctional rhythm, idioventricular rhythm (also known as a ventricular escape rhythm), and ventricular escape beats.

Conduction Disturbances

Conduction disturbances may occur because of trauma, drug toxicity, electrolyte disturbances, myocardial ischemia, or infarction. Conduction may be too rapid or too slow. Examples of rhythms associated with disturbances in conduction include AV blocks.

THE ELECTROCARDIOGRAM

[OBJECTIVES 25, 26]

The ECG records the electrical activity of a large mass of atrial and ventricular cells as specific waveforms and complexes. The electrical activity within the heart can be observed by electrodes connected by cables to an ECG machine. Think of the ECG as a voltmeter that records the electrical voltages (potentials) generated by depolarization of the heart's cells. The basic function of the ECG is to detect current flow as measured on the patient's skin.

ECG monitoring may be used to:

- Monitor a patient's heart rate
- Evaluate the effects of disease or injury on heart function
- Evaluate pacemaker function
- Evaluate the response to medications (e.g., antiarrhythmics)
- Obtain a baseline recording before, during, and after a medical procedure

The ECG *can* provide information about the following:

- The orientation of the heart in the chest
- Conduction disturbances
- Electrical effects of medications and electrolytes
- The mass of cardiac muscle
- The presence of ischemic damage

The ECG does *not* provide information about the mechanical (contractile) condition of the myocardium. To evaluate the effectiveness of the heart's mechanical activity, the patient's pulse and blood pressure are assessed.

Electrodes   Reads from neg to pos.

Electrode refers to the paper, plastic, or metal device that contains conductive media and is applied to the patient's skin. Electrodes are applied at specific locations on the patient's chest wall and extremities to view the heart's electrical activity from different angles and planes. To minimize distortion (artifact), be sure the conductive jelly in the center of the electrode is not dry, and avoid placing the electrodes directly over bony areas (Skill 22-1).

One end of a monitoring cable is attached to the electrode and the other end to an ECG machine. The cable is a wire that attaches to the electrode and conducts current back to the cardiac monitor.

SKILL 22-1   ECG MONITORING

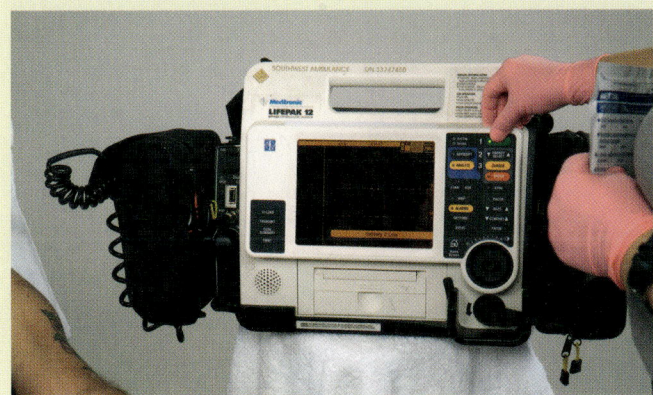

Step 1 Explain the procedure to the patient while checking your equipment. Make sure no loose pins are in the end of the ECG cable and that cable or lead wires are not frayed or broken. Make sure the monitor has an adequate paper supply. Connect the ECG cable to the machine. Connect the lead wires to the ECG cable (if not already connected). Turn the power on to the monitor. Adjust the contrast on the screen if necessary.

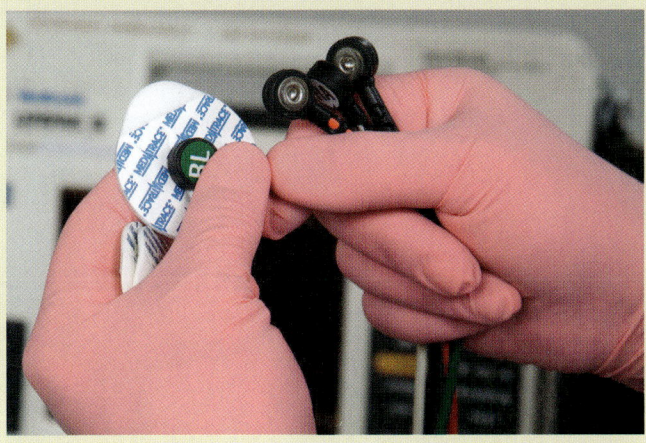

Step 2 Open a package of ECG electrodes. Make sure the electrode gel in the electrodes to be used is moist. Attach an electrode to each lead wire.

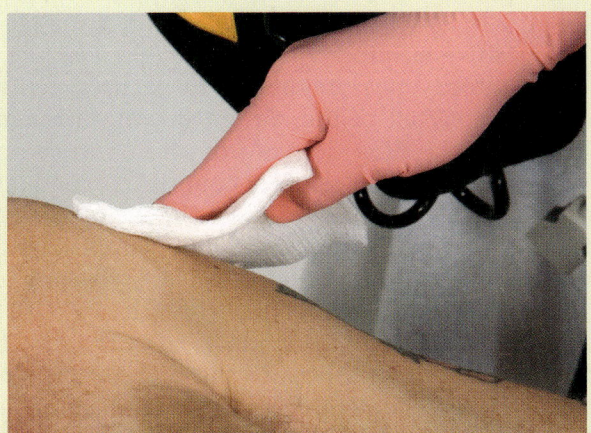

Step 3 Prepare the patient's skin to minimize distortion of the ECG tracing. Do this by briskly rubbing the skin with a dry gauze pad. Do not use alcohol, tincture of benzoin, or antiperspirant when preparing the skin. If electrodes will be applied to the patient's chest instead of limbs, shave small amounts of chest hair if needed before applying electrodes to ensure good contact.

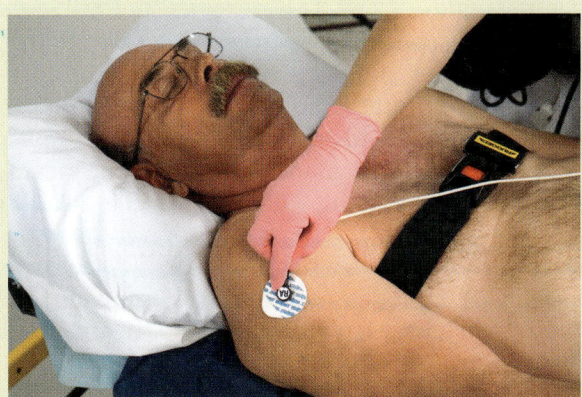

Step 4 One at a time, remove the backing from each electrode and apply them to the patient. Limb lead electrodes usually are placed on the wrists and ankles but may be positioned anywhere on the appropriate limb. To reduce muscle tension, make sure the patient's limbs are resting on a supportive surface. Do not apply electrodes over bony areas, broken skin, joints, skin creases, scar tissue, burns, or rashes. Connect the lead wires to the electrodes.

Continued

SKILL 22-1 ECG MONITORING—continued

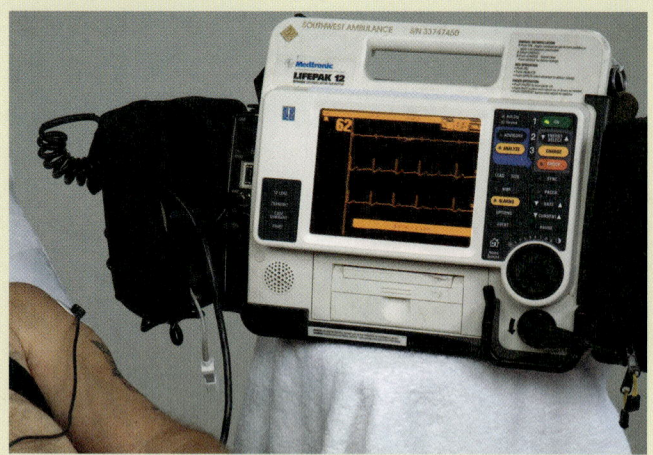

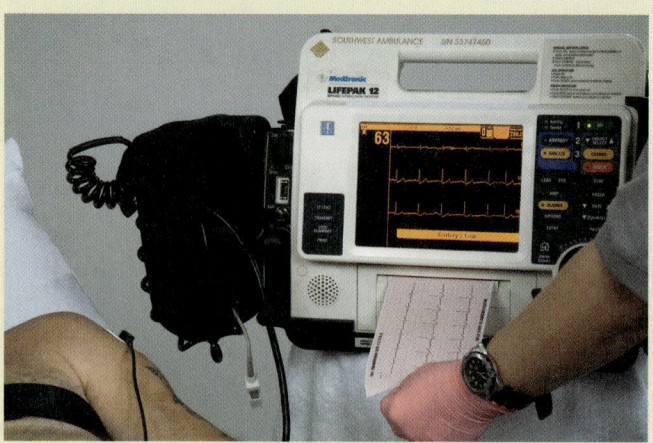

Step 5 Coach the patient to relax. Select the desired lead on the cardiac monitor. Adjust the ECG size if necessary. If the ECG size is set too low, the monitor will not detect QRS complexes and the heart rate display will be incorrect. Feel the patient's pulse and compare it with the heart rate indicator on the monitor. If not already preset, set the heart rate alarms on the monitor according to your agency's policy.

Step 6 Select the print or record button to obtain a copy of the patient's ECG. Interpret the ECG rhythm. Assess the patient to find out how he is tolerating the rate and rhythm. Attach the rhythm strip to the prehospital care report. Continue emergency care.

Reads from neg → pos.

I, II, III – bipolar

Leads

aVR, aVF, aVL – augmented (unipolar)
& chest leads (V₁-V₆)

A lead is a record (tracing) of electrical activity between two electrodes (Box 22-5). Each lead records the *average* current flow at a specific time in a portion of the heart. Leads allow viewing the heart's electrical activity in two different planes: frontal (coronal) and horizontal (transverse). Frontal plane leads view the heart from the front of the body. Horizontal plane leads view the heart as if the body were sliced in half horizontally. A 12-lead ECG provides views of the heart in both the frontal and horizontal planes and views the surfaces of the left ventricle from 12 different angles. From this, ischemic injury and infarct affecting any wall of the heart can be identified.

Three types of leads are used: standard limb leads, augmented limb leads, and chest (precordial) leads. Each lead has a positive electrode (pole). Think of the positive electrode as an eye looking at the heart. The particular portion of the heart that each lead "sees" is determined

ECG machine picks out Wilson's point at center of heart – then reads out from those to unipolar leads

by two factors. The first factor is the dominance of the left ventricle on the ECG, and the second is the position of the positive electrode on the body. Because the ECG does not directly measure the heart's electrical activity, it does not detect all of the current flowing through the heart. What the ECG detects from its position on the body surface is the net result of countless individual currents competing in a "tug-of-war." For example, the QRS complex, which represents ventricular depolarization, is not a display of all the electrical activity occurring in the right and left ventricles; it is the net result of a tug-of-war produced by the many individual currents in both the right and left ventricles. Because the left ventricle is much larger than the right, the left ventricle exerts more power. What is seen in the QRS complex is the additional electrical activity of the left ventricle—that is, the portion that exceeds the activity of the right ventricle. Therefore, in a normally conducted beat, the QRS complex primarily represents the electrical activity occurring in the left ventricle. The second factor—position of the positive electrode on the body—determines which portion of the left ventricle is detected by each lead. You can commit the view of each lead to memory, or you can easily reason it by remembering where the positive electrode is located (Phalen & Aehlert, 2006).

When electrical activity is not detected, a straight line is recorded. This line is called the **baseline** or **isoelectric line.** A **waveform** (deflection) is movement away from the baseline in a positive (upward) or negative (downward) direction. Each waveform seen on the ECG

BOX 22-5 | "Lead"

In this text, the word *lead* is used in two ways. *Lead* refers to both the actual tracing obtained and the position of the electrode. For example, the term *V₁ position* represents its proper location on the chest wall, and *lead V₁* refers to the tracing obtained from that position (Phalen & Aehlert, 2006).

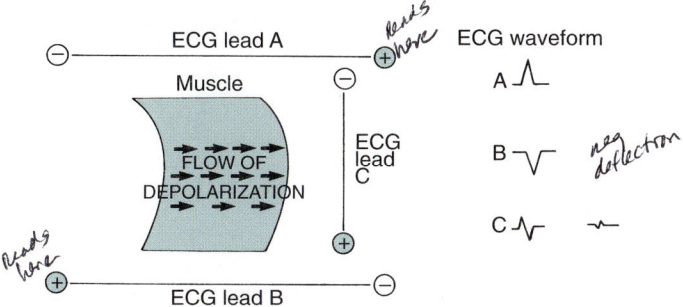

Figure 22-15 A, If the wave of depolarization moves toward the *positive* electrode, the waveform recorded on the ECG graph paper will be upright. **B,** If the wave of depolarization moves toward the *negative* electrode, the waveform produced will be inverted. **C,** A biphasic (partly positive, partly negative) waveform is recorded when the wave of depolarization moves perpendicularly to the positive electrode.

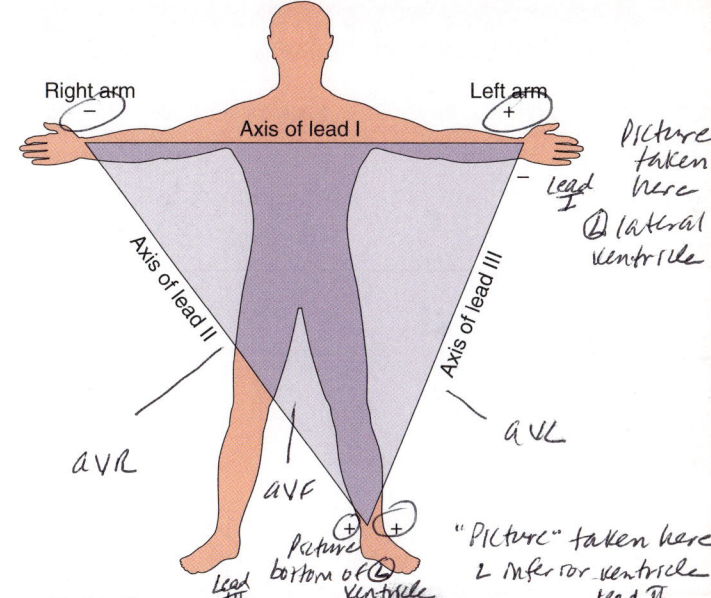

Figure 22-16 The axes of the standard limb leads form an equilateral triangle with the heart at the center (Einthoven's triangle).

is related to a specific electrical event in the heart. If the wave of depolarization (electrical impulse) moves toward the positive electrode, the waveform recorded on ECG graph paper will be upright (positive deflection). If the wave of depolarization moves away from the positive electrode, the waveform recorded will be inverted (downward or negative deflection). A **biphasic** (partly positive, partly negative) waveform or a straight line is recorded when the wave of depolarization moves perpendicularly to the positive electrode (Figure 22-15).

> **PARAMEDIC*Pearl***
>
> Although not immediately obvious, your patient's position can have an effect on the ECG. One reason for differences between tracings obtained in various positions is that although the electrode does not move when the patient changes position, the position of the heart does move relative to that electrode (Phalen & Aehlert, 2006).

Standard Limb Leads

[OBJECTIVE 27]

Leads I, II, and III are the standard limb leads. If an electrode is placed on the right arm, left arm, and left leg, three leads are formed. A bipolar lead is an ECG lead that has a positive and negative electrode. Each lead records the difference in electrical potential (voltage) between two selected electrodes. Although all ECG leads are bipolar, Leads I, II, and III use two distinct electrodes, one of which is connected to the positive input of the ECG machine and the other to the negative input. The positive electrode is located at the left wrist in lead I, and leads II and III both have their positive electrode located at the left foot. Proper electrode positioning for leads I, II, and III includes placement on the patient's *extremities*, not the chest. Where the electrodes are placed on the

extremity does not matter as long as bony prominences are avoided.

An imaginary line joining the positive and negative electrodes of a lead is called the **axis** of the lead. The axes of these three limb leads form an equilateral triangle with the heart at the center (Einthoven's triangle) (Figure 22-16). Einthoven's triangle is a way of showing that the two arms and the left leg form apexes of a triangle surrounding the heart.

Lead I records the difference in electrical potential between the left arm (+) and right arm (−) electrodes. The positive electrode is placed on the left arm and the negative electrode is placed on the right arm. The third electrode is a ground that minimizes electrical activity from other sources. Lead II records the difference in electrical potential between the left leg (+) and right arm (−) electrodes. The positive electrode is placed on the left leg and the negative electrode is placed on the right arm. This lead is commonly used for cardiac monitoring because positioning of the positive and negative electrodes in this lead most closely resembles the normal pathway of current flow in the heart. Lead III records the difference in electrical potential between the left leg (+) and left arm (−) electrodes. In lead III the positive electrode is placed on the left leg and the negative electrode is placed on the left arm. A summary of the standard limb leads is given in Table 22-4.

Augmented Limb Leads

Leads aVR, aVL, and aVF are **augmented limb leads** that record measurements at a specific electrode with respect to a reference electrode. Frank Norman Wilson and colleagues used the term *central terminal* to describe a reference point that is the average of the limb lead

TABLE 22-4	Standard Limb Leads		
Lead	Positive Electrode	Negative Electrode	Heart Surface Viewed
I	Left arm	Right arm	Lateral
II	Left leg	Right arm	Inferior
III	Left leg	Left arm	Inferior

TABLE 22-5	Augmented Leads	
Lead	Positive Electrode	Heart Surface Viewed
aVR	Right arm	None
aVL	Left arm	Lateral
aVF	Left leg	Inferior

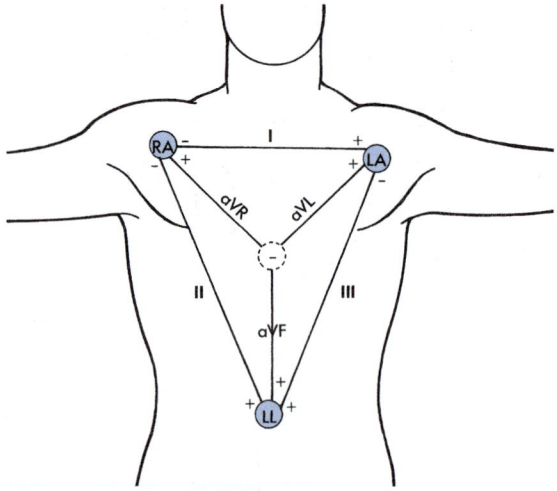

Figure 22-17 View of the standard limb leads and augmented leads.

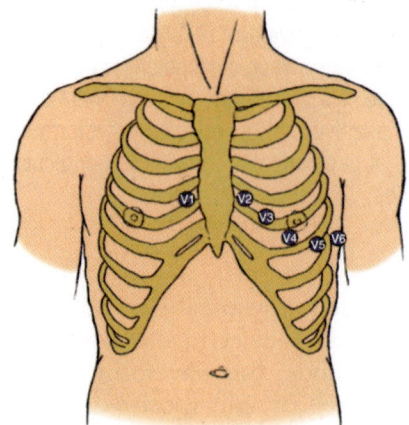

Figure 22-18 The position of the six chest leads.

electrical potentials. In the augmented leads, the Wilson central terminal (WCT) is calculated by the ECG machine's computer as an average potential of the electrical currents from the two electrodes other than the one being used as the positive electrode. For example, in lead aVL the positive electrode is located on the patient's left arm. The ECG machine's computer calculates the central terminal by joining the electrical currents obtained from the electrodes on the patient's right arm and left leg. Lead aVL therefore represents the difference in electrical potential between the left arm and the central terminal. The electrical potential of the central terminal is essentially zero." (Figure 22-17).

The electrical potential produced by the augmented leads normally is relatively small. The ECG augments (magnifies) the amplitude of the electrical potentials detected at each extremity by approximately 50% over those recorded at the standard limb leads. The *a* in aVR, aVL, and aVF refers to augmented. The *V* refers to voltage, the *R* refers to right arm, the *L* to left arm, and the *F* to left foot (leg). The position of the positive electrode corresponds to the last letter in each of these leads. The positive electrode in aVR is located on the right arm, aVL has a positive electrode at the left arm, and aVF has a positive electrode positioned on the left leg.

A summary of augmented leads is provided in Table 22-5.

Chest Leads

[OBJECTIVE 28]

The six chest leads view the heart in the horizontal plane. The chest leads are identified as V_1, V_2, V_3, V_4, V_5, and V_6. Each electrode placed in a V position is a positive electrode, measuring electrical potential with respect to the Wilson Central Terminal. The positive electrode for each lead is placed at a specific location on the chest (Figure 22-18).

The wave of ventricular depolarization normally moves from right to left. In the right chest leads (V_1 and V_2), the QRS deflection is mostly negative (moving away from the positive chest electrode). As the chest electrode is placed further left, the wave of depolarization (R wave progression) is moving toward the positive electrode. Thus the QRS deflection recorded as the electrode is moved to the left becomes more and more positive. A summary of the chest leads is given in Table 22-6.

PARAMEDIC *Pearl*

Because their location varies, do not use the nipples as landmarks for electrode placement in men or women. If your patient is a woman, place the electrodes for leads V_3-V_6 *under* the breast, rather than *on* the breast.

Right Chest Leads

Other chest leads that are not part of a standard 12-lead ECG may be used to view specific surfaces of the heart.

TABLE 22-6	Chest Leads	
Lead	**Positive Electrode Position**	**Heart Surface Viewed**
V_1	Right side of sternum, fourth intercostal space	Septum
V_2	Left side of sternum, fourth intercostal space	Septum
V_3	Midway between V_2 and V_4	Anterior
V_4	Left midclavicular line, fifth intercostal space	Anterior
V_5	Left anterior axillary line at same level as V_4	Lateral
V_6	Left midaxillary line at same level as V_4	Lateral

TABLE 22-7	Right Chest Leads and Their Placement
Lead	**Placement**
V_1R	Lead V_2
V_2R	Lead V_1
V_3R	Midway between V_2R and V_4R
V_4R	Right midclavicular line, fifth intercostal space
V_5R	Right anterior axillary line at same level as V_4R
V_6R	Right midaxillary line at same level as V_4R

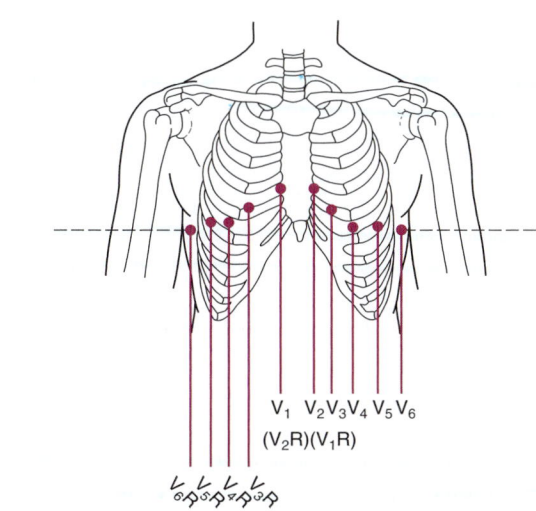

Figure 22-19 Placement of the left and right chest leads.

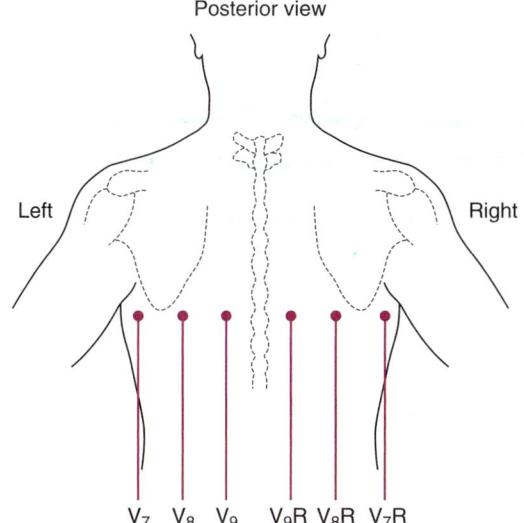

Figure 22-20 Posterior chest lead placement.

When a right ventricular MI is suspected, right chest leads are used. Placement of right chest leads is identical to placement of the standard chest leads except they are on the right side of the chest (Figure 22-19). If time does not permit obtaining all of the right chest leads, the lead of choice is V_4R. The right chest leads and their placement are listed in Table 22-7.

Posterior Chest Leads

On a standard 12-lead ECG, no leads look directly at the posterior surface of the heart. Additional chest leads may be used for this purpose. These leads are placed further left and toward the back. All the leads are placed on the same horizontal line as V_4 to V_6. Lead V_7 is placed at the posterior axillary line. Lead V_8 is placed at the angle of the scapula (posterior scapular line), and lead V_9 is placed over the left border of spine (Figure 22-20).

PARAMEDIC*Pearl*

Fifteen- and 18-lead ECGs are being used with increasing frequency to help spot infarctions of the right ventricle and the posterior wall of the left ventricle. The 15-lead ECG uses all leads of a standard 12-lead plus leads V_4R, V_8, and V_9. An 18-lead ECG uses the 15-lead ECG plus leads V_5R, V_6R, and V_7.

ECG Paper

[OBJECTIVE 29]

The ECG is a graphical representation of the heart's electrical activity. When electrodes are placed on the patient's body and connected to an ECG, the machine records the voltage (potential difference) between the electrodes. The needle (or pen) of the ECG moves a specific distance depending on the voltage measured. This recording is made on ECG paper.

ECG paper is graph paper composed of small and large boxes measured in millimeters. The smallest boxes are

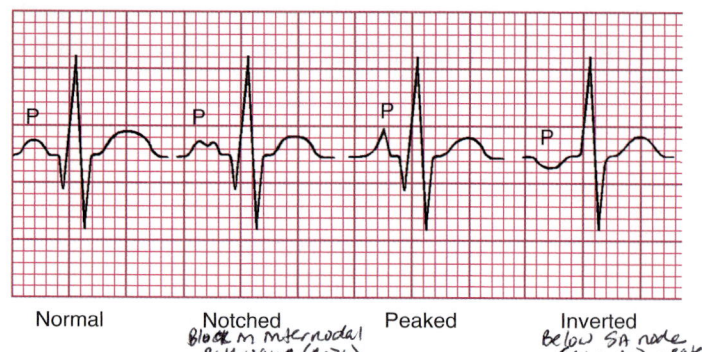

Normal   Notched   Peaked   Inverted

[handwritten annotations:] Block in internodal Pathways (R→L)   Below SA node (AV node) → rate 40-60

Figure 22-21 A normal P wave is smooth and rounded. Abnormal P waves may be notched, tall and pointed (peaked), or inverted (negative).

[handwritten annotation:] ↓ going against normal electrical flow

[handwritten annotation:] Notched P wave - bundle branch block

1 mm wide and 1 mm high (Figure 22-21). The horizontal axis of the paper corresponds with time. Time is used to measure the interval between or duration of specific cardiac events and is stated in seconds.

The rate at which ECG paper goes through the printer is adjustable. ECG paper normally records at a constant speed of 25 mm/sec. Thus each horizontal 1-mm box represents 0.04 seconds (25 mm/sec × 0.04 sec = 1 mm). Look closely at the boxes in Figure 22-21. You can see that the lines after every five small boxes on the paper are heavier. The heavier lines indicate one large box. Because each large box is the width of five small boxes, a large box represents 0.20 seconds. Five large boxes, each consisting of five small boxes, represent 1 second. Fifteen large boxes equal an interval of 3 seconds. Thirty large boxes represent 6 seconds.

The vertical axis of the ECG paper measures the *voltage*, or *amplitude*, of a waveform. Voltage is measured in millivolts (mV). Voltage may be a positive or negative value. Amplitude is measured in millimeters. The ECG machine's sensitivity must be calibrated so that a 1-mV electrical signal will produce a deflection measuring exactly 10 mm tall. When properly calibrated, a small box is 1 mm high (0.1 mV) and a large box (equal to five small boxes) is 5 mm high (0.5 mV). Clinically the height of a waveform usually is stated in millimeters, not millivolts.

Waveforms

[OBJECTIVE 30]

A **waveform** is movement away from the baseline in either a positive (upward) or negative (downward) direction (Box 22-6). Waveforms are named alphabetically, beginning with P, QRS, T, and U.

P Wave

The first waveform in the cardiac cycle is the P wave (Box 22-7). The beginning of the P wave is recognized as the first abrupt or gradual movement away from the baseline; its end is the point at which the waveform returns to the baseline (see Figure 22-21). The P wave represents atrial

depolarization and the spread of the electrical impulse throughout the right and left atria. A waveform representing atrial repolarization usually is not seen on the ECG because it is small and buried in the QRS complex. A P wave normally precedes each QRS complex. Normal P waves are smooth and rounded, no more than 2.5 mm in height, and no more than 0.11 seconds in duration.

[handwritten annotation:] Q: old MI - wider than 1 small box larger than 1/3 of R

QRS Complex

A **complex** consists of several waveforms. The QRS complex consists of the Q wave (Figure 22-22), R wave, and S wave. It represents the spread of the electrical impulse through the ventricles (ventricular depolarization). Depolarization normally triggers contraction of ventricular tissue. Thus shortly after the QRS complex begins, the ventricles contract. A QRS complex normally follows each P wave.

Although the term *QRS complex* is used, not every QRS complex contains a Q wave, R wave, and S wave. When the first deflection of the QRS complex is negative (below the baseline), the waveform is called a *Q wave*. A Q wave

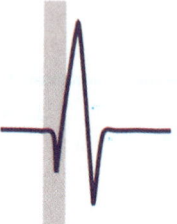

Figure 22-22 The Q wave is a negative deflection preceding an R wave.

[handwritten annotation:] first neg deflection after P wave

is **always** a negative waveform and is the first negative waveform following the P wave. The Q wave represents depolarization of the interventricular septum, which is activated from left to right. An abnormal (pathologic) Q wave is more than 0.04 seconds in duration or more than one third the height of the following R wave in that lead.

The QRS complex continues as a large, upright, triangular waveform known as the *R wave*. The R wave is the first positive deflection (above the baseline) in the QRS complex. A negative deflection following the R wave is called an *S wave*. The R and S waves represent simultaneous depolarization of the right and left ventricles. If the QRS complex consists entirely of a positive waveform, it is called an *R wave*. If the complex consists entirely of a negative waveform, it is called a *QS wave*. If two positive deflections are present in the same complex, the second is called *R prime* and is written *R'*. If two negative deflections follow an R wave, the second is called *S prime* and is written *S'*. Uppercase letters are used to designate waveforms of relatively large amplitude, and lowercase letters are used to label relatively small waveforms (Figure 22-23).

The QRS duration is a measurement of the time required for ventricular depolarization (Box 22-8). The beginning of the QRS complex is measured from the point where the first wave of the complex begins to move away from the baseline. The point at which the last wave of the complex begins to level out or distinctly change direction at, above, or below the baseline marks the end of the QRS complex. In adults, the normal duration of the QRS complex is 0.11 seconds or less. (Surawicz, 2009). If an electrical impulse does not follow the normal ventricular conduction pathway, it will take longer to depolarize the myocardium. This delay in conduction through the ventricles produces a wider QRS complex.

T Wave

Ventricular repolarization is represented on the ECG by the T wave (Box 22-9, Figure 22-24). The beginning of the T wave is identified as the point where the slope of the ST segment appears to become abruptly or gradually steeper. The T wave ends when it returns to the baseline. T waves usually are 5 mm or less in height in any limb lead or 10 mm or less in any chest lead; T waves usually are 0.5 mm or more in height in leads I and II.

A T wave following an abnormal QRS complex usually is opposite in direction of the QRS. In other words, when the QRS complex points down, the T wave points up, and vice versa. This may be seen with ventricular beats or rhythms and in bundle branch block. Tall, pointed

---

BOX 22-8	Normal Characteristics of the QRS Complex

- Normal duration of the QRS complex in an adult is 0.11 second or less   ⟨.06-.10⟩
- A normal Q wave is less than 0.04 seconds in duration and less than one third of the amplitude of the R wave in that lead

---

BOX 22-9	Normal Characteristics of the T Wave

- Slightly asymmetric
- Usually 5 mm or less in height in any limb lead or 10 mm in any chest lead and 0.5 mm or more in height in leads I and II

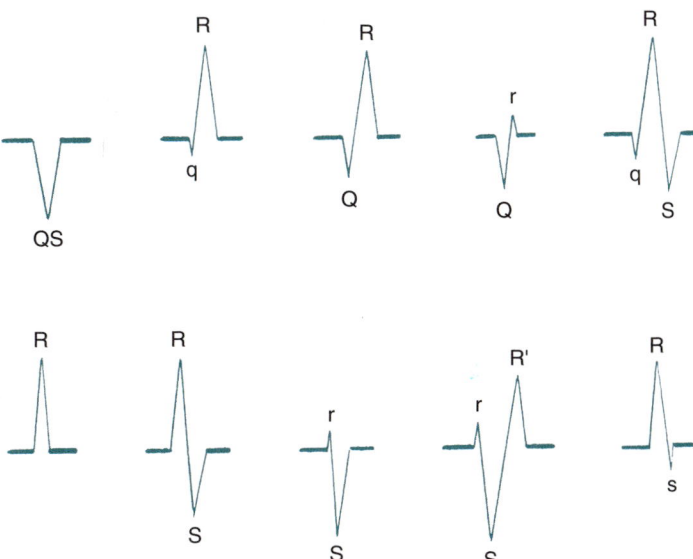

Figure 22-23 QRS complexes may appear in various forms.

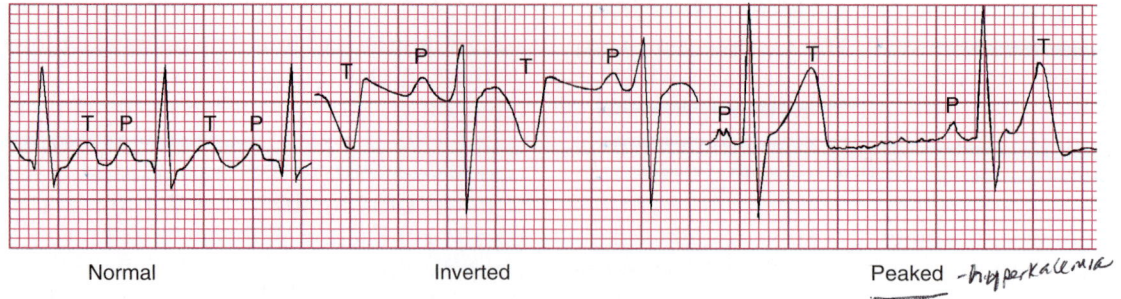

Figure 22-24 Examples of normal and abnormal T waves.

(peaked) T waves are commonly seen in hyperkalemia. Low-amplitude T waves may be seen in hypokalemia.

U Wave (NO)

A U wave is a small waveform that, when seen, follows the T wave (Box 22-10). The mechanism of the U wave is not definitively known. One theory suggests that it represents repolarization of the Purkinje fibers. U waves are most easily seen when the heart rate is slow and are difficult to identify when the rate exceeds 90 beats/min. When seen, they normally are tallest in leads V_2 and V_3 (Figure 22-25). U waves typically appear in the same direction as the T wave that precedes it.

Segments

A **segment** is a line between waveforms. It is named by the waveform that precedes and follows it.

BOX 22-10	Characteristics of the U Wave

- Rounded and symmetric
- Usually less than 1.5 mm in height and smaller than that of the preceding T wave
- In general, a U wave more than 1.5 mm in height in any lead is considered abnormal

PR Segment

The PR segment is part of the PR interval. The PR segment is the horizontal line between the end of the P wave and the beginning of the QRS complex (Figure 22-26). It represents activation of the AV node, the bundle of His, the bundle branches, and the Purkinje fibers. Atrial repolarization also occurs during this period.

TP Segment

[OBJECTIVE 31]

The TP segment is the portion of the ECG tracing between the end of the T wave and the beginning of the following P wave. When the heart rate is within normal limits, the TP segment usually is isoelectric. With rapid heart rates, the TP segment is often unrecognizable because the P wave encroaches on the preceding T wave.

PR interval .12–.20 (3-5 small boxes)

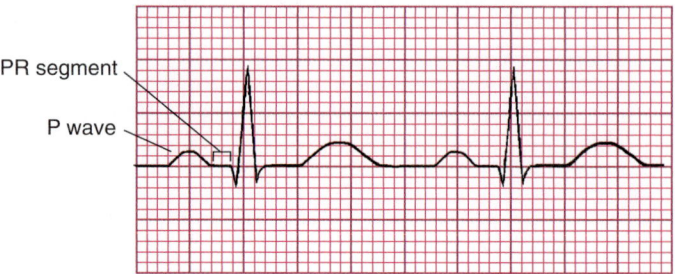

Figure 22-26 The P wave and PR segment.

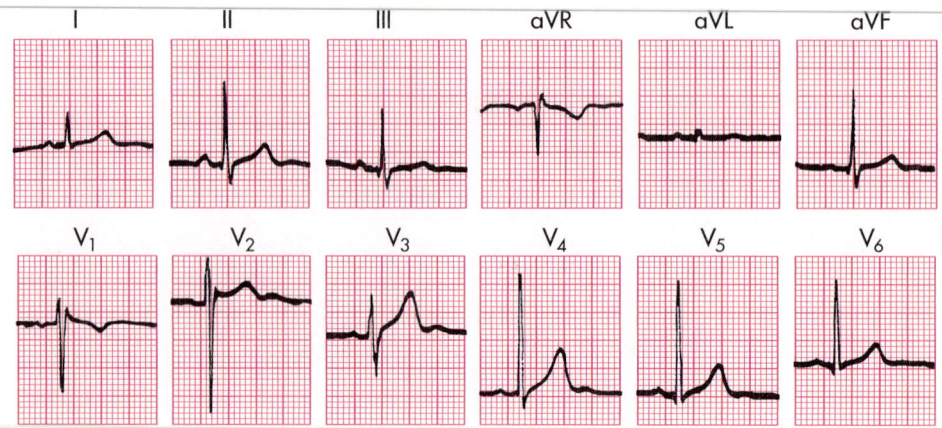

Figure 22-25 Normal U waves (best viewed in leads V_2 through V_4) in a 22-year-old man.

ST Segment

The portion of the ECG tracing between the QRS complex and the T wave is the ST segment (Box 22-11, Figure 22-27). The term *ST segment* is used regardless of whether the final wave of the QRS complex is an R or an S wave. The ST segment represents the early part of repolarization of the right and left ventricles. The normal ST segment begins at the isoelectric line, extends from the end of the S wave, and curves gradually upward to the beginning of the T wave.

The point where the QRS complex and the ST segment meet is called the *ST-junction* or *J-point*. It may be difficult to determine the J-point clearly in patients with rapid heart rates or hyperkalemia. Various conditions may cause displacement of the ST segment from the isoelectric line in either a positive or negative direction. Myocardial ischemia, injury, and infarction are among the causes of ST segment displacement. The ST segment is considered elevated if the segment is deviated above the baseline. It is considered depressed if the segment is deviated below it.

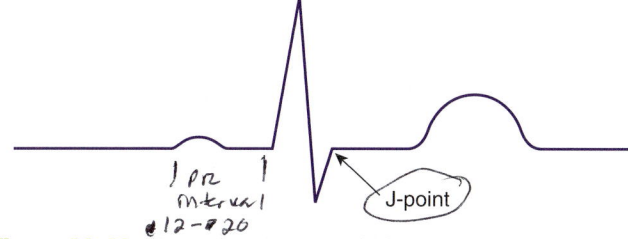

Figure 22-28 The point where the QRS complex and the ST segment meet is called the *ST-junction* or *J-point*.

When looking for ST-segment displacement, the topic of interest is the *early* portion of the ST segment. First locate the J-point. Next use the TP segment and the PR segment to estimate the position of the isoelectric line. Then compare the level of the ST segment to the isoelectric line (Figure 22-28). Some displacement of the ST-segment from the isoelectric line is normal and dependent on age, gender, and ECG lead. For men 40 years of age and older, the threshold value for abnormal J-point elevation is 2 mm in leads V_2 and V_3 and 1 mm in all other leads. For men less than 40 years of age, the threshold value for abnormal J-point elevation in leads V_2 and V_3 is 2.5 mm. For women, the threshold value for abnormal J-point elevation is 1.5 mm in leads V_2 and V_3 and greater than 1 mm in all other leads. For men and women, the threshold for abnormal J-point elevation in V_3R and V_4R is 0.5 mm, except for males less than 30 years of age, for whom 1 mm is more appropriate. For men and women, the threshold value for abnormal J-point elevation in leads V_7 through V_9 is 0.5 mm. For men and women of all ages, ST-segment depression of more than 0.5 mm in leads V_2 and V_3 and more than 1 mm in all other leads suggests myocardial ischemia. (Rautaharju 2009, Wagner 2009).

Intervals

PR Interval

An **interval** is a waveform and a segment. The P wave plus the PR segment equals the PR interval (Figure 22-29, Box 22-12). The PR interval is measured from the point where the P wave leaves the baseline to the beginning of the QRS complex. The term PQ interval is preferred by some because it is the period actually measured unless a Q wave is absent.

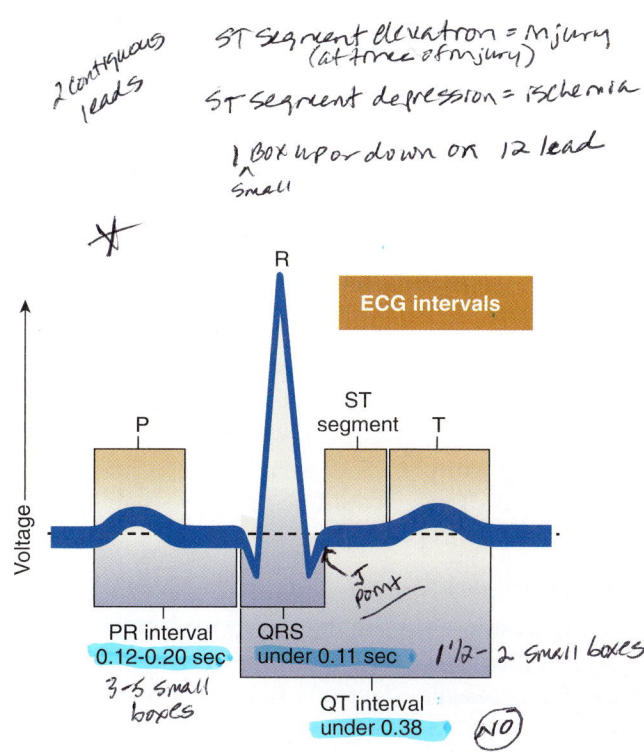

Figure 22-27 The ST segment is the line between the QRS complex and the T wave.

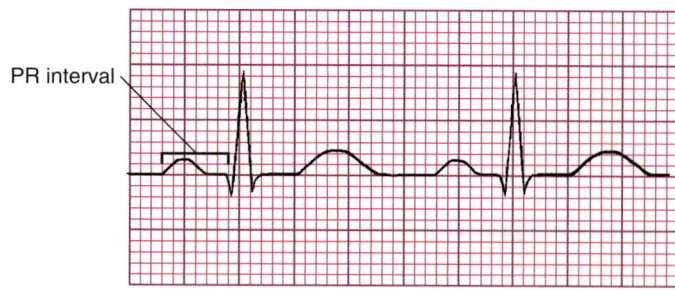

Figure 22-29 The P wave plus the PR segment equals the PR interval.

BOX 22-12	Normal Characteristics of the PR Interval

- Measures 0.12 to 0.20 seconds in adults; may be shorter in children and longer in older persons
- Shortens as heart rate increases
- Lengthens as heart rate decreases

Remember that the P wave reflects depolarization of the right and left atria. The PR segment represents the spread of the impulse through the AV node, bundle of His, right and left bundle branches, and the Purkinje fibers. The PR interval changes with heart rate but normally measures 0.12 to 0.20 seconds in adults.

QT Interval

The QT interval represents the time from ventricular depolarization (activation) to repolarization (recovery). It is measured from the beginning of the QRS complex to the end of the T wave. In the absence of a Q wave, the QT interval is measured from the beginning of the R wave to the end of the T wave. The duration of the QT interval varies according to age, gender, and heart rate. As the heart rate increases, the QT interval shortens (decreases). As the heart rate decreases, the QT interval lengthens (increases). Because of the variability of the QT interval with the heart rate, it can be measured more accurately if it is corrected (adjusted) for the patient's heart rate. The corrected QT interval is noted as QTc. Many clinicians do not consider the QT interval abnormally long unless the QT interval corrected for the heart rate exceeds 0.44 seconds.

To determine the QT interval quickly, measure the interval between two consecutive R waves (R-R interval) and divide the number by two. Measure the QT interval. If the measured QT interval is less than half the R-R interval, it probably is normal. A QT interval that is approximately half the R-R interval is considered borderline. A QT interval that is more than half the R-R interval is considered prolonged.

R-R and P-P Intervals

The R-R (R wave to R wave) and P-P (P wave to P wave) intervals are used to determine the rate and regularity of a cardiac rhythm. To evaluate the regularity of the ventricular rhythm on a rhythm strip, the interval between two consecutive R-R waves is measured. The distance between succeeding R-R intervals is measured and compared. If the ventricular rhythm is regular, the R-R intervals will measure the same. To evaluate the regularity of the atrial rhythm, the same procedure is used but the interval between two consecutive P-P waves is measured and compared to succeeding P-P intervals.

Artifact

Accurate ECG rhythm recognition requires a tracing in which the waveforms and intervals are free of distortion. Distortion of an ECG tracing by electrical activity that is noncardiac in origin is called **artifact.** Because artifact can mimic various cardiac dysrhythmias, including ventricular fibrillation, you must assess the patient before beginning any medical intervention.

Artifact may be caused by loose electrodes, broken ECG cables or wires, muscle tremor, patient movement, external chest compressions, and 60-cycle interference. Proper preparation of the patient's skin and evaluation of the monitoring equipment (electrodes, wires) before use can reduce the problems associated with artifact.

ANALYZING A RHYTHM STRIP

[OBJECTIVE 32]

A systematic approach to rhythm analysis that is consistently applied when analyzing a rhythm strip is essential. If you do not develop such an approach, you are more likely to miss something important. Begin analyzing the rhythm strip from left to right.

Assess Rhythm and Regularity R-R

The term *rhythm* is used to indicate the site of origin of an electrical impulse (e.g., sinus rhythm, junctional rhythm) and describe the regularity or irregularity of waveforms. The waveforms on an ECG strip are evaluated for regularity by measuring the distance between the P waves and QRS complexes. If the rhythm is regular, the R-R intervals (or P-P intervals, if assessing atrial rhythm) are the same. In general, a variation of ±10% is acceptable. For example, if 10 small boxes comprise an R-R interval, an R wave could be off by 1 small box and still be considered regular.

Ventricular Rhythm

To determine whether the ventricular rhythm is regular or irregular, measure the distance between two consecutive R-R intervals. Place one point of a pair of calipers (or make a mark on a piece of paper) on the beginning of an R wave. Place the other point of the calipers (or make a second mark on the paper) on the beginning of the R wave of the next QRS complex. Without adjusting the calipers, evaluate each succeeding R-R interval. (If paper

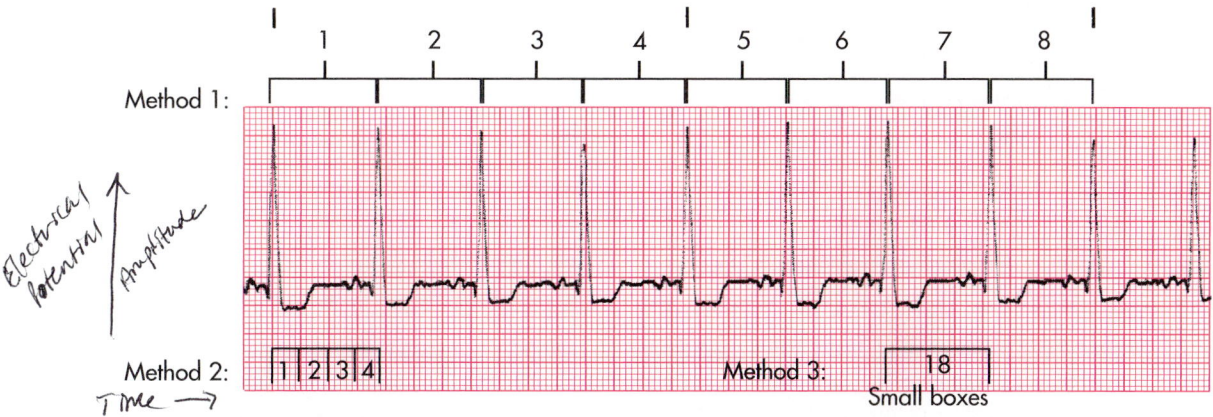

Figure 22-30 Calculating heart rate. Method 1: Number of R-R intervals in 6 seconds × 10 (e.g., 8 × 10 = 80 beats/min). Method 2: Number of large boxes between QRS complexes divided into 300 (e.g., 300/4 = 75 beats/min). Method 3: Number of small boxes between QRS complexes divided into 1500 (e.g., 1500/18 = 84 beats/min).

TABLE 22-8	Heart Rate Determination Based on the Number of Large Boxes		
Number of Large Boxes	**Heart Rate (beats/min)**	**Number of Large Boxes**	**Heart Rate (beats/min)**
1	300	6	50
2	150	7	43
3	100	8	38
4	75	9	33
5	60	10	30

is used, lift the paper and move it across the rhythm strip.) Compare the distance measured with the other R-R intervals. If the ventricular rhythm is regular, the R-R intervals will measure the same. Rhythm and regularity also may be determined by counting the small squares between intervals and comparing the intervals.

Atrial Rhythm

To determine if the atrial rhythm is regular or irregular, follow the same procedure previously described for evaluation of ventricular rhythm but measure the distance between two consecutive P-P intervals (instead of R-R intervals) and compare that distance with the other P-P intervals. The P-P intervals will measure the same if the atrial rhythm is regular. For accuracy, the R-R or P-P intervals should be evaluated across an entire 6-second rhythm strip.

Assess the Rate

Several methods are used to calculate heart rate. A discussion of each method follows.

Method 1: 6-Second Method

Most ECG paper is printed with 1-second or 3-second markers on the top or bottom of the paper. To determine

the ventricular rate, count the number of complete QRS complexes within a period of 6 seconds and multiply that number by 10 to find the number of complexes in 1 minute (Figure 22-30). This method may be used for regular and irregular rhythms. This is the simplest, quickest, and most commonly used method of rate measurement, but it also is the most inaccurate.

Method 2: Large Boxes

To determine the ventricular rate, count the number of large boxes between the R-R interval and divide into 300. To determine the atrial rate, count the number of large boxes between the P-P interval and divide into 300 (Table 22-8). This method is best used if the rhythm is regular; however, it may be used if the rhythm is irregular and a rate range (slowest [longest R-R interval] and fastest [shortest R-R interval] rate) is given.

Method 3: Small Boxes

Each 1-mm box on the graph paper represents 0.04 seconds. A total of 1500 boxes represents 1 minute (60 sec/min divided by 0.04 sec/box = 1500 boxes/min). To calculate the ventricular rate, count the number of small boxes between the R-R interval and divide

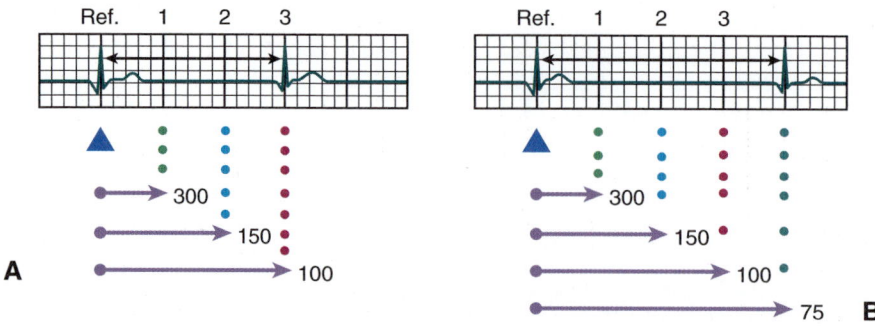

Figure 22-31 Determining heart rate by the sequence method. To measure the ventricular rate, find a QRS complex that falls on a heavy, dark line. Count 300, 150, 100, 75, 60, and 50 until a second QRS complex occurs. This will be the heart rate. **A**, Heart rate = 100. **B**, Heart rate = 75.

into 1500. To determine the atrial rate, count the number of small boxes between the P-P interval and divide into 1500. This method is time consuming but accurate. If the rhythm is irregular, a rate range should be given.

Method 4: Sequence Method *"Triplicet"*

To determine ventricular rate, select an R wave that falls on a dark vertical line. Number the next six consecutive dark vertical lines as follows: 300, 150, 100, 75, 60, and 50 (Figure 22-31). Note where the next R wave falls in relation to the six dark vertical lines already marked. This is the heart rate.

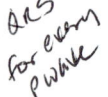 ③ *Identify and Examine P Waves* *upright & rounded PR interval*

To locate P waves, look to the left of each QRS complex. Normally one P wave precedes each QRS complex; they occur regularly; and they look similar in size, shape, and position. If no P wave is present, the rhythm originated in the AV junction or the ventricles.

If one P wave is present before each QRS and the QRS is *narrow* consider the following:

QRS for every P wave

- Is the P wave positive? If so, the rhythm probably began in the SA node.
- Is the P wave negative or absent? If so, and the QRS complexes occur regularly, the rhythm probably started in the AV junction.

Assess Intervals (Evaluate Conduction)

PR Interval

Measure the PR interval. The PR interval is measured from the point where the P wave leaves the baseline to the beginning of the QRS complex. The normal PR interval is 0.12 to 0.20 seconds. If the PR intervals are the same, they are said to be constant. If the PR intervals are different, is a pattern present? In some dysrhythmias, the

duration of the PR interval will increase until a P wave appears with no QRS after it. This is referred to as lengthening of the PR interval. PR intervals that vary in duration and have no pattern are said to be variable.

⑤ QRS Duration

Identify the QRS complexes and measure their duration. The beginning of the QRS is measured from the point where the first wave of the complex begins to deviate from the baseline. The point at which the last wave of the complex begins to level out at, above, or below the baseline marks the end of the QRS complex. The QRS is considered narrow (normal) if it measures 0.11 seconds or less and wide if it measures more than 0.11 seconds. A QRS complex of 0.11 seconds or less (narrow) is presumed to be **supraventricular** in origin.

QT Interval

Measure the QT interval in the leads that show the largest amplitude T waves. The QT interval is measured from the beginning of the QRS complex to the end of the T wave. If no Q wave is present, measure the QT interval from the beginning of the R wave to the end of the T wave. If the measured QT interval is less than half the R-R interval, it is probably normal. This method of QT interval measurement works well as a general guideline until the ventricular rate exceeds 100 beats/min.

Evaluate the Overall Appearance of the Rhythm

ST Segment

Determine the presence of ST-segment elevation or depression. The TP and PR segments are used as the baseline from which to evaluate the degree of displacement of the ST segment from the isoelectric line. The ST segment is considered elevated if the segment is deviated above the baseline and is considered depressed if the segment deviates below it.

T Wave

Evaluate the T waves. Are the T waves upright and of normal height? The T wave following an abnormal QRS complex is usually opposite in direction of the QRS. Negative T waves may be an indicator of myocardial ischemia. Tall, pointed (peaked) T waves are commonly seen in hyperkalemia.

Interpret the Rhythm and Evaluate Its Clinical Significance

Interpret the rhythm, specifying the site of origin (pacemaker site) of the rhythm (sinus), the mechanism (bradycardia), and the ventricular rate. For example, "sinus bradycardia at 38 beats/min." Assess the patient to find out how he or she is tolerating the rate and rhythm.

SECTION 3: CARDIAC DYSRHYTHMIAS
SINUS MECHANISMS

[OBJECTIVE 33]

The normal heartbeat is the result of an electrical impulse that starts in the SA node. A rhythm that begins in the SA node has the following characteristics:

- A positive (upright) P wave before each QRS complex
- P waves that look alike
- A constant PR interval
- A regular atrial and ventricular rhythm (usually)

An electrical impulse that begins in the SA node may be affected by the following:

- Medications
- Diseases or conditions that cause the heart rate to speed up, slow down, or beat irregularly
- Diseases or conditions that delay or block the impulse from leaving the SA node
- Diseases or conditions that prevent an impulse from being generated in the SA node

Sinus Rhythm

Sinus rhythm is the name given to a normal heart rhythm. Sinus rhythm is sometimes called a *regular sinus rhythm* (RSR) or *normal sinus rhythm* (NSR). Sinus rhythm reflects normal electrical activity; that is, the rhythm starts in the SA node and then heads down the normal conduction pathway through the atria, AV junction, bundle branches, and ventricles. This results in depolarization of the atria and ventricles. The SA node normally produces electrical impulses faster than any other part of

TABLE 22-9   Normal Heart Rates by Age

Age	Beats/min*
Infant (1-12 months)	100-160
Toddler (1-3 years)	90-150
Preschooler (4-5 years)	80-140
School-age (6-12 years)	70-120
Adolescent (13-18 years)	60-100
Adult	60-100

*Pulse rates for a sleeping child may be 10% lower than the low rate listed in age group.

the heart's conduction system. As a result, the SA node is normally the heart's primary pacemaker. A person's heart rate varies with age (Table 22-9). In adults and adolescents, the SA node normally fires at a regular rate of 60 to 100 beats/min. An example of a sinus rhythm is shown in Figure 22-32. A summary of the ECG characteristics of a sinus rhythm is shown in Table 22-10.

Sinus Bradycardia

If the SA node fires at a rate slower than normal for the patient's age, the rhythm is called sinus **bradycardia** (see Figure 22-32). In adults and adolescents, a sinus bradycardia has a heart rate of less than 60 beats/min. The term *severe sinus bradycardia* is sometimes used to describe a sinus bradycardia with a rate of less than 40 beats/min.

Assess how the patient tolerates the rhythm at rest and with activity. If the patient has no symptoms, no treatment is necessary. If the patient has serious signs and symptoms because of the slow rate, emergency care may include oxygen, IV access, atropine, and/or transcutaneous pacing. In the setting of a heart attack, sinus bradycardia is often short lived. A slow heart rate can be beneficial in the patient who has had a heart attack (and has no symptoms

TABLE 22-10   Characteristics of Sinus Rhythm

Rate	60-100 beats/min
Rhythm	P-P interval regular, R-R interval regular
P waves	Positive (upright) in lead II, one precedes each QRS complex, P waves look alike
PR interval	0.12-0.20 sec and constant from beat to beat
QRS duration	0.11 sec or less unless an intraventricular conduction delay exists

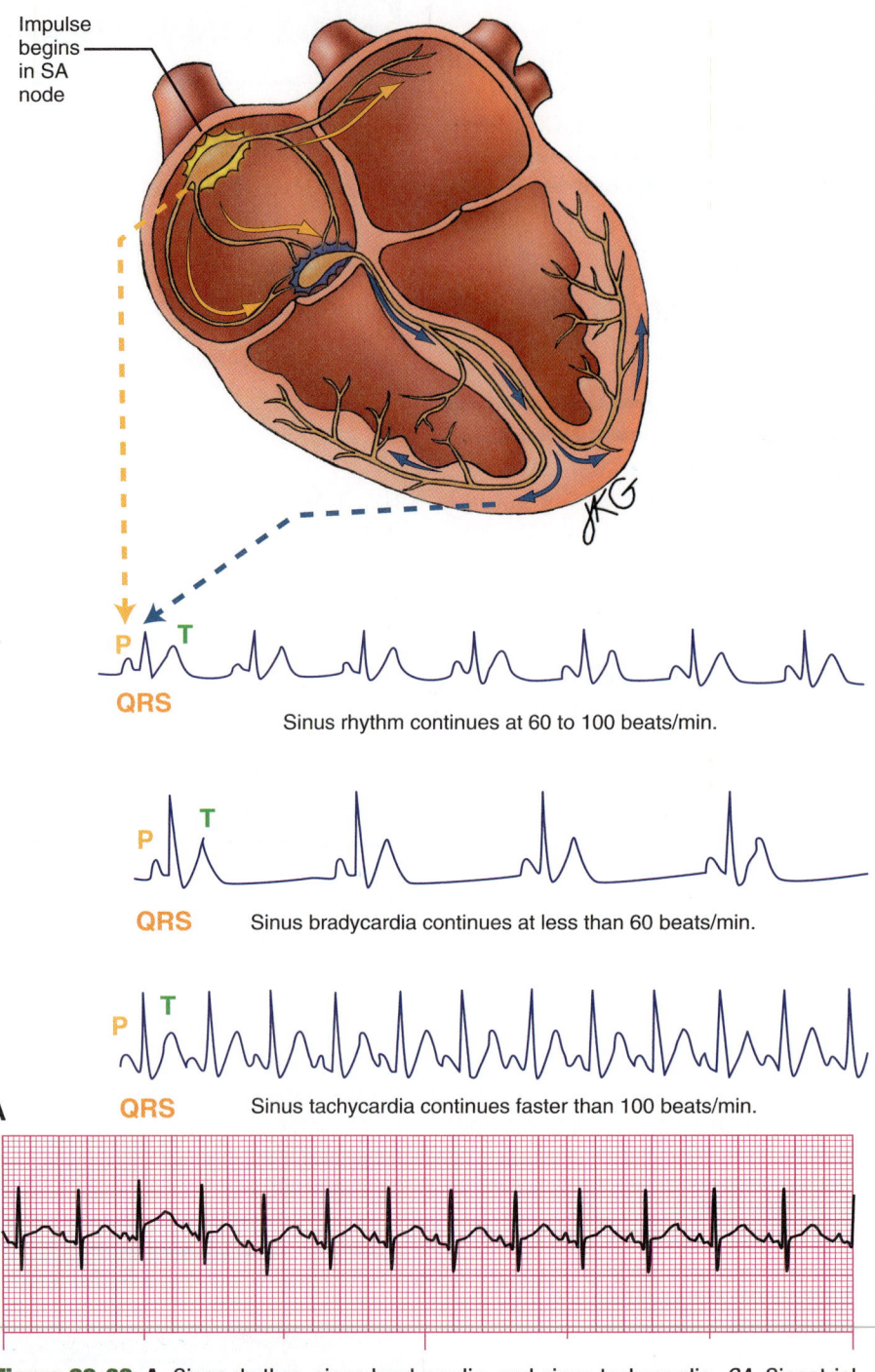

Impulse begins in SA node

P   T

QRS

Sinus rhythm continues at 60 to 100 beats/min.

P   T

QRS   Sinus bradycardia continues at less than 60 beats/min.

P   T

A   QRS   Sinus tachycardia continues faster than 100 beats/min.

Figure 22-32 A, Sinus rhythm, sinus bradycardia, and sinus tachycardia. *SA,* Sinoatrial.

because of the slow rate). This is because the heart's demand for oxygen is lower when the heart rate is slow. Recommended treatment guidelines for a symptomatic bradycardia are shown in Figure 22-33. The ECG characteristics of sinus bradycardia are shown in Table 22-11.

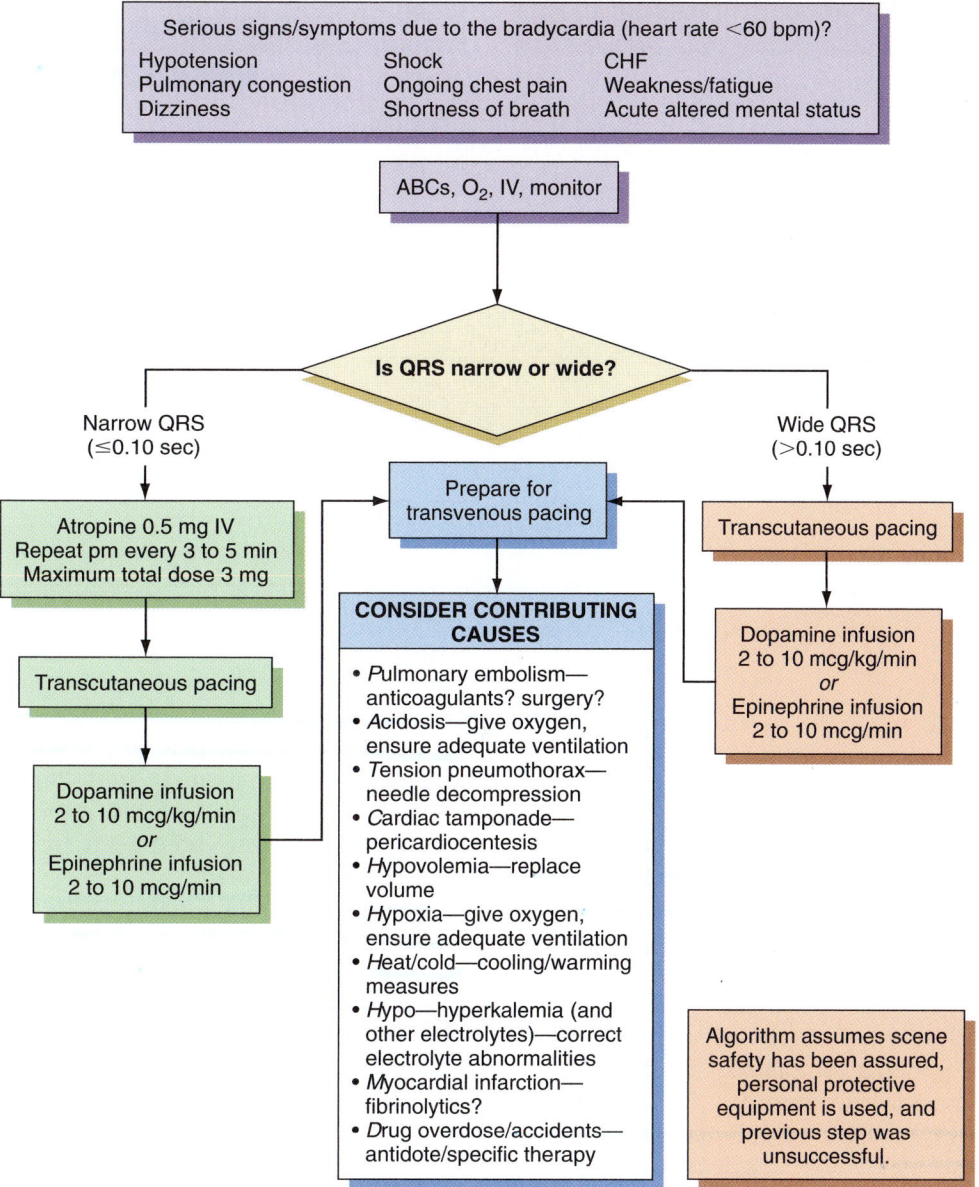

Figure 22-33 Symptomatic bradycardia algorithm.

Bradydysrhythmias: Too-Slow Rhythms

In infants and children, a bradycardia is present if the heart rate is slower than the lower limit of normal for the patient's age. In the pediatric patient, most slow rhythms occur as a result of hypoxia and acidosis.

A bradycardia can produce significant symptoms unless stroke volume increases to compensate for the decrease in heart rate. Unless corrected promptly, decreasing cardiac output will eventually produce serious signs and symptoms.

TABLE 22-11	Characteristics of Sinus Bradycardia
Rate	Less than 60 beats/min
Rhythm	P-P interval regular, R-R interval regular
P waves	Positive (upright) in lead II, one precedes each QRS complex, P waves look alike
PR interval	0.12-0.20 sec and constant from beat to beat
QRS duration	0.11 sec or less unless an intraventricular conduction delay exists

BOX 22-13 Causes of Sinus Tachycardia

- Exercise
- Fever
- Pain
- Fear and anxiety
- Hypoxia
- Congestive heart failure
- Acute myocardial infarction
- Infection
- Sympathetic stimulation
- Shock
- Dehydration, hypovolemia
- Pulmonary embolism
- Hyperthyroidism
- Medications such as epinephrine, atropine, dopamine, and dobutamine
- Caffeine-containing beverages
- Nicotine
- Drugs such as cocaine, amphetamines, "ecstasy," and cannabis

TABLE 22-12 Characteristics of Sinus Tachycardia

Rate	101-180 beats/min
Rhythm	P-P interval regular, R-R interval regular
P waves	Positive (upright) in lead II, one precedes each QRS complex, P waves look alike
	At very fast rates, differentiating a P wave from a T wave may be difficult
PR interval	0.12-0.20 sec (may shorten with faster rates) and constant from beat to beat
QRS duration	0.11 sec or less unless an intraventricular conduction delay exists

Sinus Tachycardia

If the SA node fires at a rate faster than normal for the patient's age, the rhythm is called *sinus tachycardia* (see Figure 22-32). Sinus tachycardia begins and ends gradually. Sinus tachycardia is a normal response to the body's demand for increased oxygen because of many conditions (Box 22-13). The patient is often aware of an increase in heart rate. Some patients complain of a "racing heart" or pounding sensation in the chest.

In a patient with coronary artery disease, sinus tachycardia can cause problems. The heart's demand for oxygen increases as the heart rate increases. As the heart rate increases, less time is available for the ventricles to fill and less blood is available for the ventricles to pump out with each contraction. This can lead to decreased cardiac output. Because the coronary arteries fill when the ventricles are at rest, rapid heart rates decrease the time for coronary artery filling. This decreases the heart's blood supply. Chest discomfort can result if the supply of blood and oxygen to the heart is inadequate. Sinus tachycardia in a patient who is having a heart attack may be an early warning signal for heart failure, cardiogenic shock, and more serious dysrhythmias.

Treatment for sinus tachycardia is directed at correcting the underlying cause, that is, fluid replacement and relief of pain and/or anxiety. The ECG characteristics of sinus tachycardia are shown in Table 22-12.

Sinus Arrhythmia

When the SA node fires irregularly, the resulting rhythm is called *sinus arrhythmia*. Sinus arrhythmia associated with the phases of respiration and changes in intrathoracic pressure is called *respiratory sinus arrhythmia*. Respiratory sinus arrhythmia is a normal phenomenon that occurs with changes in intrathoracic pressure. The heart rate increases with inspiration (R-R intervals shorten) and decreases with expiration (R-R intervals lengthen). Sinus arrhythmia is most often seen in children and adults younger than 30 years.

Sinus arrhythmia usually does not require treatment unless it is accompanied by a slow heart rate that causes serious signs and symptoms (hemodynamic compromise). If hemodynamic compromise is present, IV atropine may be indicated. An example of sinus arrhythmia is shown in Figure 22-34. The characteristics of sinus arrhythmia are shown in Table 22-13.

TABLE 22-13 Characteristics of Sinus Arrhythmia

Rate	Usually 60-100 beats/min but may be slower or faster
Rhythm	Irregular, phasic with respiration; heart rate increases gradually during inspiration (R-R intervals shorten) and decreases with expiration (R-R intervals lengthen)
P waves	Positive (upright) in lead II, one precedes each QRS complex, P waves look alike
PR interval	0.12-0.20 sec and constant from beat to beat
QRS duration	0.11 sec or less unless an intraventricular conduction delay exists

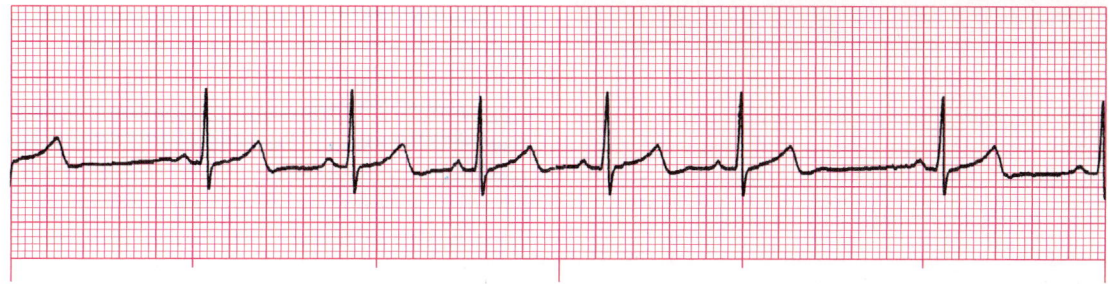

Figure 22-34 Sinus arrhythmia at 54 to 88 beats/min.

Sinoatrial Block *stops temporarily then restarts*

In SA block, the pacemaker cells within the SA node initiate an impulse, but it is blocked as it exits the SA node. This is thought to occur because of failure of cells in the SA node to conduct the impulse from the pacemaker cells to the surrounding atrium. The SA node generally falls back into rhythm after one skipped beat. SA block is rather uncommon. Causes of SA block are provided in Box 22-14.

If episodes of SA block are frequent and/or accompanied by a slow heart rate, the patient may show signs and symptoms of hemodynamic compromise. If episodes of SA block are frequent and signs of hemodynamic compromise are present, IV atropine or pacing may be needed. An example of SA block is shown in Figure 22-35. The ECG characteristics of SA block are shown in Table 22-14.

Sinus Arrest *Looks like SA block but longer pause*

In sinus arrest, the pacemaker cells of the SA node fail to initiate an electrical impulse for more than one beat.

When the SA node fails to initiate an impulse, an escape pacemaker site (the AV junction or ventricles) should assume responsibility for pacing the heart. If it does not, you will see absent PQRST complexes on the ECG. Causes of sinus arrest are shown in Box 22-15.

If serious signs or symptoms are present, IV atropine may be indicated. If the episodes of sinus arrest are frequent and/or prolonged (more than 3 seconds), pacing may be warranted. An example of sinus arrest is shown in Figure 22-36. The ECG characteristics of sinus arrest are shown in Table 22-15.

BOX 22-14 Causes of Sinoatrial Block

- Acute coronary syndromes
- Medications such as digitalis, quinidine, procainamide, or salicylates
- Coronary artery disease
- Myocarditis
- Heart failure
- Carotid sinus sensitivity
- Increased vagal tone

TABLE 22-14 Characteristics of Sinoatrial Block

Rate	Usually normal but varies because of the pause
Rhythm	Irregular because of the pause(s) caused by the SA block; the pause is the same as (or an exact multiple of) the distance between two other P-P intervals
P waves	Positive (upright) in lead II, P waves look alike; when present, one precedes each QRS complex.
PR interval	0.12-0.20 sec and constant from beat to beat
QRS duration	0.11 sec or less unless an intraventricular conduction delay exists

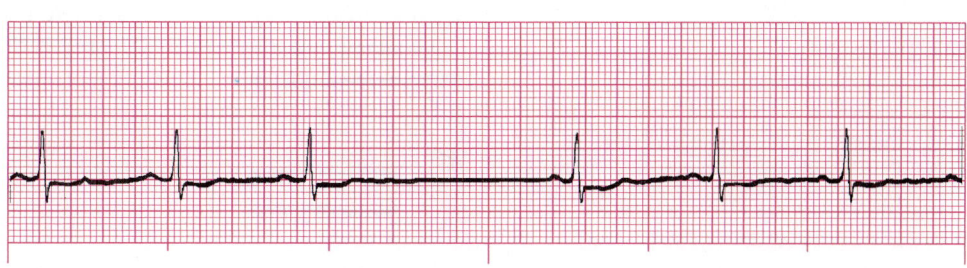

Figure 22-35 Sinus rhythm at a rate of 36 to 71 beats/min with an episode of sinoatrial (SA) block.

BOX 22-15 Causes of Sinus Arrest

- Hypoxia
- Acute coronary syndrome
- Hyperkalemia
- Digitalis toxicity
- Reactions to medications such as beta-blockers and calcium channel blockers
- Carotid sinus sensitivity
- Increased vagal tone

Atrial dysrhythmias reflect abnormal electrical impulse formation and conduction in the atria. They result from altered automaticity, triggered activity, or reentry. Altered automaticity and triggered activity are disorders in impulse *formation*. Reentry is a disorder in impulse *conduction*. Dysrhythmias that result from disorders of impulse formation often are referred to as automatic. Dysrhythmias that result from a disorder in impulse conduction are referred to as reentrant.

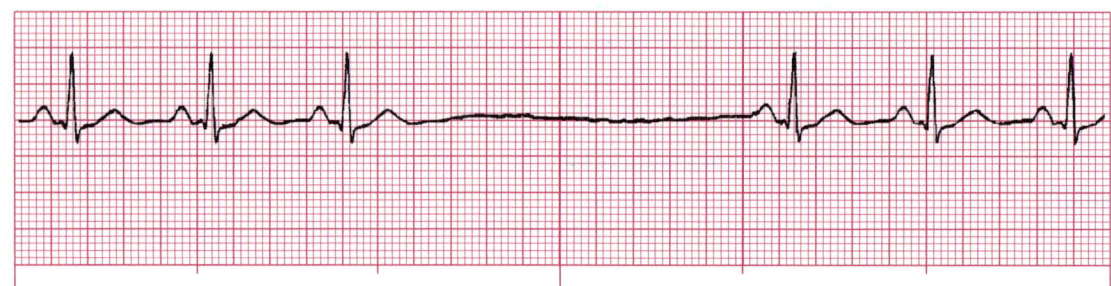

Figure 22-36 Sinus rhythm at a rate of 24 to 81 beats/min with an episode of sinus arrest.

TABLE 22-15 Characteristics of Sinus Arrest

Rate	Usually normal but varies because of the pause
Rhythm	Irregular; the pause is of undetermined length (more than one PQRST complex is missing) and is not the same distance as other P-P intervals
P waves	Positive (upright) in lead II, P waves look alike; when present, one precedes each QRS complex
PR interval	0.12-0.20 sec and constant from beat to beat
QRS duration	0.11 sec or less unless an intraventricular conduction delay exists

ATRIAL DYSRHYTHMIAS

[OBJECTIVE 34]

P waves reflect atrial depolarization. A rhythm that begins in the atria has a positive P wave shaped differently than P waves that begin in the SA node. This difference in P-wave configuration occurs because the impulse begins in the atria and follows a different conduction pathway to the AV node.

PARAMEDIC *Pearl*

Premature beats appear early; that is, they occur before the next expected beat. Premature beats are identified by their site of origin:

- Premature atrial complexes (PACs)
- Premature junctional complexes (PJCs)
- Premature ventricular complexes (PVCs)

Premature Atrial Complexes

(handwritten: Sinus beat early in rhythm Non lethal)

A premature atrial complex (PAC) occurs when an irritable site (focus) within the atria fires before the next SA node impulse is due to fire (Figure 22-37). This interrupts the sinus rhythm. If the irritable site is close to the SA node, the atrial P wave will look very similar to the P waves initiated by the SA node. The P wave of a PAC may be biphasic (partly positive, partly negative), flattened, notched, or pointed. Ectopic complexes, such as PACs, may occur in patterns:

- *Pairs (coupled):* two ectopic complexes in a row
- *Runs or bursts:* three or more ectopic complexes in a row
- *Bigeminy:* every other beat is an ectopic complex
- *Trigeminy:* every third beat is an ectopic complex

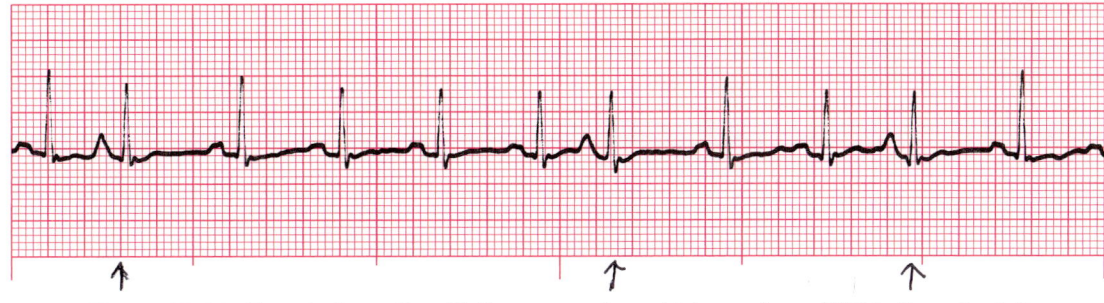

Figure 22-37 Sinus tachycardia with three premature atrial complexes (PACs). *From the left,* beats 2, 7, and 10 are PACs.

- *Quadrigeminy*: every fourth beat is an ectopic complex

The ECG characteristics of PACs are shown in Table 22-16.

occurs during relative refractory phase of preceding complex

TABLE 22-16	Characteristics of PACs
Rate	Usually within normal range but depends on underlying rhythm
Rhythm	Regular with premature beats
P waves	Premature (occurring earlier than the next expected sinus P wave), positive (upright) in lead II, one before each QRS complex, often differ in shape from sinus P waves; may be flattened, notched, pointed, biphasic, or lost in the preceding T wave
PR interval	May be normal or prolonged depending on the prematurity of the beat
QRS duration	Usually 0.11 sec or less but may be wide **(aberrant)** or absent, depending on the prematurity of the beat; the QRS of the PAC is similar in shape to those of the underlying rhythm unless the PAC is abnormally conducted

Aberrantly Conducted Premature Atrial Complexes

Don't really need to know

[OBJECTIVE 35]

If a PAC occurs early, the right bundle branch can be slow to respond to the impulse (refractory). The impulse travels down the left bundle branch with no problem. Stimulation of the left bundle branch subsequently results in stimulation of the right bundle branch. The QRS will appear wide (greater than 0.11 seconds) because of this delay in ventricular depolarization. PACs associated with a wide QRS complex are called *aberrantly conducted PACs.* This indicates that conduction through the ventricles is abnormal. Figure 22-38 shows a rhythm strip with two PACs. The first PAC was conducted abnormally, producing a wide QRS complex. The second PAC was conducted normally. Compare the T waves before each PAC with those of the underlying sinus bradycardia.

Nonconducted Premature Atrial Complexes

Sometimes, when a PAC occurs early and close to the T wave of the preceding beat, only a P wave may be seen with no QRS after it (appearing as a pause) (Figure 22-39). This type of PAC is called a *nonconducted* or **blocked PAC** because the P wave occurred too early to be conducted.

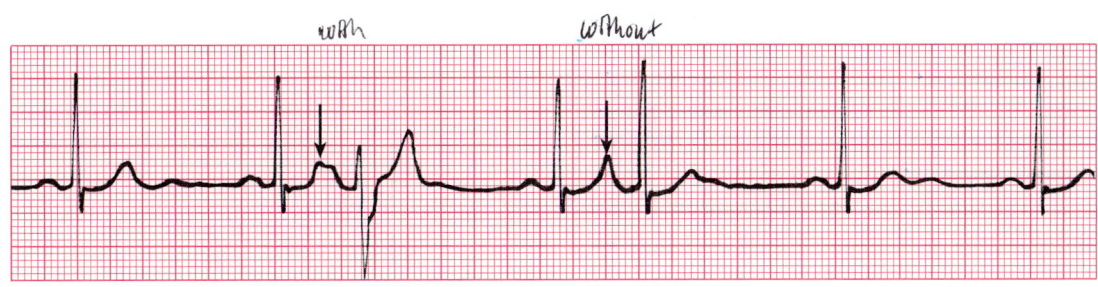

with   *without*

Figure 22-38 PACs with and without abnormal conduction (aberrancy).

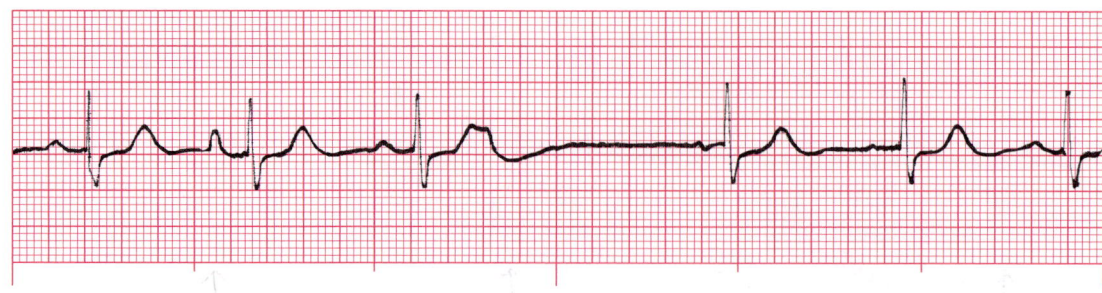

Figure 22-39 Sinus rhythm with a nonconducted (blocked) premature atrial complex (PAC).

PACs are quite common and can occur at any age. Their presence does not necessarily imply underlying cardiac disease. Causes of PACs include the following:

- Emotional stress
- Heart failure
- Acute coronary syndromes
- Mental and physical fatigue
- Atrial **enlargement**
- Valvular heart disease
- Digitalis toxicity
- Electrolyte imbalance
- Hyperthyroidism
- Stimulants (caffeine, tobacco, cocaine)

PACs do not usually require treatment if they are infrequent. The patient may complain of a "skipped beat" or "racing heart" (if PACs are frequent) or may be unaware of them. In susceptible individuals, frequent PACs may trigger episodes of atrial fibrillation, atrial flutter, or paroxysmal supraventricular tachycardia (PSVT). Frequent PACs are treated by correcting the underlying cause such as reducing stress, reducing or eliminating stimulants, or treating heart failure.

Wandering Atrial Pacemaker

Multiformed atrial rhythm is an updated term for the rhythm formerly known as *wandering atrial pacemaker*. With this rhythm the size, shape, and direction of the P waves vary, sometimes from beat to beat. The difference in the look of the P waves is a result of the gradual shifting of the dominant pacemaker between the SA node, the atria, and/or the AV junction (Figure 22-40). At least three different P-wave configurations seen in the same lead are required for a diagnosis of wandering atrial pacemaker or multifocal atrial tachycardia (discussed below). Multiformed atrial rhythm may be seen in patients with healthy hearts (particularly in athletes) and during sleep. It also may occur with some types of underlying heart disease and with digitalis toxicity. This dysrhythmia usually produces no signs and symptoms unless it is associated with a slow rate.

Multiformed atrial rhythm is usually a short-lived rhythm that resolves on its own when the firing rate of the SA node increases and the sinus resumes pacing responsibility. The ECG characteristics of multiformed atrial rhythm are shown in Table 22-17.

PARAMEDIC*Pearl*

At least three different P-wave configurations, seen in the same lead, are required for a diagnosis of wandering atrial pacemaker or multifocal atrial tachycardia.

TABLE 22-17	Characteristics of Wandering Atrial Pacemaker
Rate	Usually 60-100 beats/min but may be slow; if the rate is greater than 100 beats/min, the rhythm is termed *multifocal* (or *chaotic*) AT
Rhythm	May be irregular as the pacemaker site shifts from the SA node to ectopic atrial locations and the AV junction
P waves	Size, shape, and direction may change from beat to beat; at least three different P-wave configurations (seen in the same lead) are required for a diagnosis of wandering atrial pacemaker or MAT
PR interval	Variable
QRS duration	0.11 sec or less unless an intraventricular conduction delay exists

AT, Atrial tachycardia; *SA*, sinoatrial; *AV*, atrioventricular; multifocal atrial tachycardia.

[handwritten annotation: usually pretty regular]

Lead II (continuous)

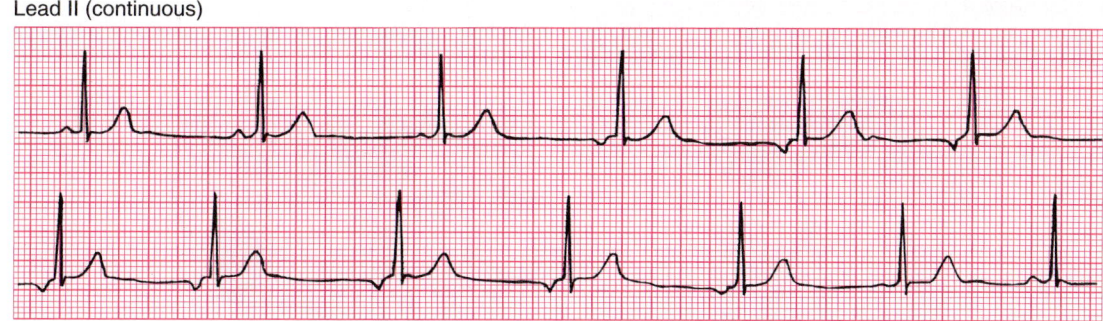

Figure 22-40 Wandering atrial pacemaker. Continuous strip (lead II).

Multifocal Atrial Tachycardia

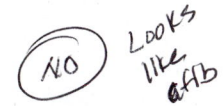

NO — LOOKS like afib

When multiformed atrial rhythm is associated with a ventricular rate greater than 100 beats/min, the rhythm is called *multifocal atrial tachycardia* (MAT) (Figure 22-41). MAT also is called *chaotic atrial tachycardia*. In MAT, multiple ectopic sites stimulate the atria. MAT is most often seen in the following conditions:

- Severe chronic obstructive pulmonary disease
- Hypoxia
- Acute coronary syndromes
- Digoxin toxicity
- Rheumatic heart disease

- Theophylline toxicity
- Electrolyte imbalances

Treatment of MAT is directed at the underlying cause. If the patient is stable and symptomatic but you are uncertain if the rhythm is MAT, you can try a vagal maneuver (Skill 22-2, Box 22-16) if no contraindications exist. If vagal maneuvers are ineffective, you can try adenosine IV. Because MAT does not involve reentry through the AV node, it is unlikely that vagal maneuvers or adenosine administration will stop the rhythm. However, these treatments may temporarily slow the rate enough so that you can look at the P waves and determine the specific type of tachycardia. By determining the type of tachycardia, treatment specific to that rhythm can be given.

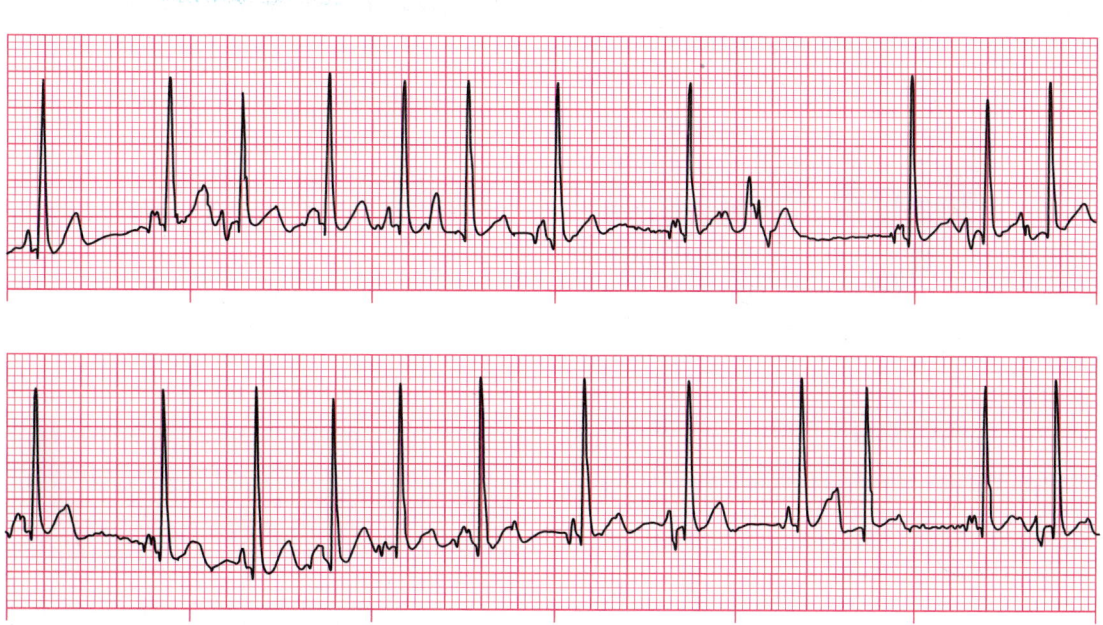

Figure 22-41 Multifocal atrial tachycardia, also known as chaotic atrial tachycardia. Premature atrial complexes occur at varying cycle lengths and with differing shapes.

SKILL 22-2 CAROTID SINUS MASSAGE

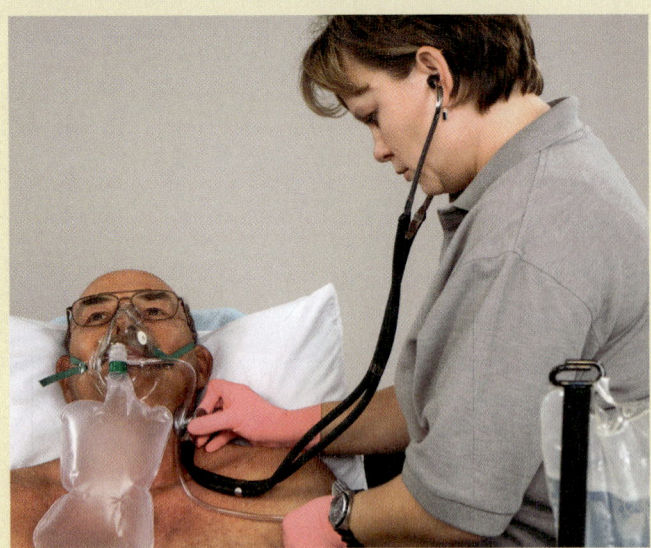

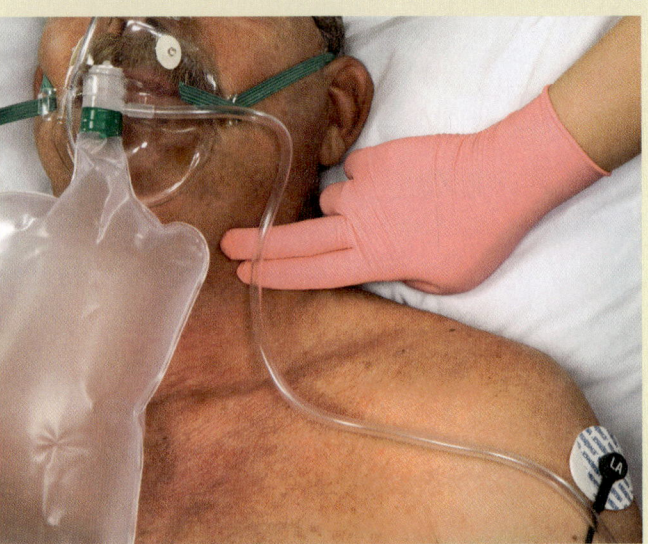

Step 1 Before performing this procedure, take appropriate standard precautions. Make sure suction, a defibrillator, and emergency medications are available. Place the patient on oxygen, assess the patient's vital signs, establish IV access, and apply ECG electrodes. Explain the procedure to the patient. Gently palpate each carotid artery separately to assess pulse quality. If the pulses are markedly unequal, consult medical direction before performing the procedure. Check for carotid bruits by listening to each carotid artery with a stethoscope. A bruit is a blowing or swishing sound created by the turbulence within the vessel. If a bruit is heard, do *not* perform this procedure.

Step 2 If no bruit is heard and no contraindications are present, turn the patient's head to one side. Press print or record on the cardiac monitor to run a continuous ECG strip during the procedure. With two fingers, locate the carotid pulse just underneath the angle of the jaw. With firm pressure, press the carotid artery toward the cervical vertebrae. Begin an up-and-down motion for *no longer* than 10 seconds. *Never* massage both carotid arteries at the same time.

Visually monitor the patient and ECG throughout the procedure. Note the onset and end of the vagal maneuver on the rhythm strip.

Not done in region XI

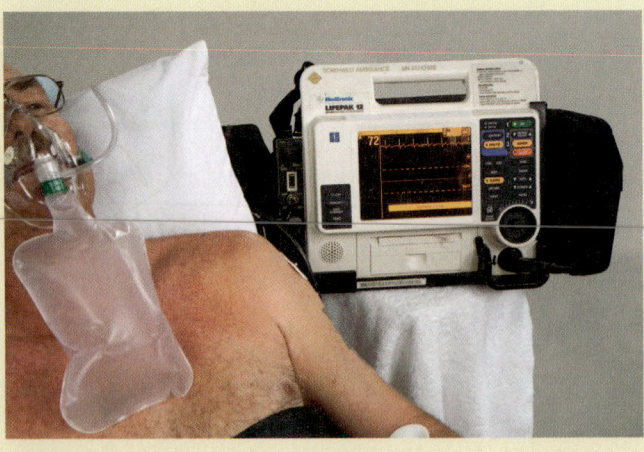

Step 3 After the procedure, reassess the patient's vital signs and the ECG rhythm.

BOX 22-16 | Vagal Maneuvers

Vagal maneuvers are methods used to stimulate baroreceptors located in the internal carotid arteries and the aortic arch. Stimulation of these receptors results in reflex stimulation of the vagus nerve and release of acetylcholine. Acetylcholine slows conduction through the AV node, resulting in slowing of the heart rate. Although the right and left vagus nerves overlap somewhat, the right vagus nerve is believed to have more fibers to the SA node and atrial muscle and the left vagus more fibers to the AV node and some ventricular muscle.

Examples of vagal maneuvers include the following:

- Coughing
- Squatting
- Breath holding
- Carotid sinus massage (see Skill 22-2). Carotid massage is less effective in children than in adults and is not recommended. Carotid massage should be avoided in older patients. This procedure has been associated with a number of complications, including stroke, syncope, and dysrhythmias (including asystole).
- Application of a cold stimulus to the face (such as a washcloth soaked in iced water, cold pack, or crushed ice mixed with water in a plastic bag or glove) for up to 10 seconds. This technique often is effective in infants and young children. When using this method, do not obstruct the patient's mouth or nose or apply pressure to the eyes.
- Valsalva's maneuver. Instruct the patient to blow through an occluded straw or take a deep breath and bear down as if having a bowel movement for up to 10 seconds. This strains the abdominal muscles and increases intrathoracic pressure.

When using vagal maneuvers, keep the following points in mind:

- Before performing a vagal maneuver, make sure suction, a defibrillator, and emergency medications are available.
- Place the patient on oxygen, assess the patient's vital signs, establish IV access, and apply ECG electrodes.
- Continuous visual monitoring of the patient's ECG is *essential*. Run a continuous ECG when performing any vagal maneuver. Note the onset and end of the vagal maneuver on the ECG rhythm strip. A 12-lead ECG recording is desirable when a vagal maneuver is performed.
- In general, a vagal maneuver should not be continued for more than 10 seconds.

AV, Atrioventricular.

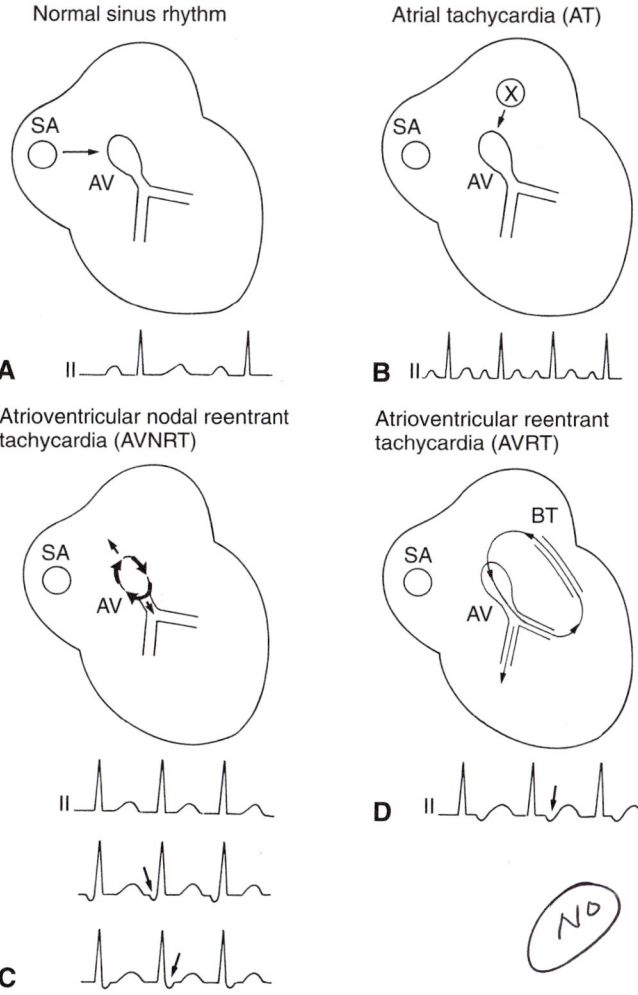

Figure 22-42 Types of supraventricular tachycardia (SVT). **A**, Normal sinus rhythm is presented here as a reference. **B**, Atrial tachycardia (AT). **C**, Atrioventricular nodal reentrant tachycardia (AVNRT). **D**, Atrioventricular reentrant tachycardia (AVRT).

Supraventricular Tachycardia

Supraventricular dysrhythmias begin above the bifurcation of the bundle of His. This means that supraventricular dysrhythmias include rhythms that begin in the SA node, atrial tissue, or the AV junction. The term *supraventricular tachycardia* (SVT) includes the following three main types of fast rhythms (Figure 22-42):

- Atrial tachycardia (AT). In AT, an irritable site in the atria automatically fires at a rapid rate.
- AV nodal reentrant tachycardia (AVNRT). In AVNRT, fast and slow pathways in the AV node form an electrical circuit or loop. The impulse spins around the AV nodal (junctional) area.
- AV reentrant tachycardia (AVRT). In AVRT, the impulse begins above the ventricles but travels by a pathway other than the AV node and bundle of His.

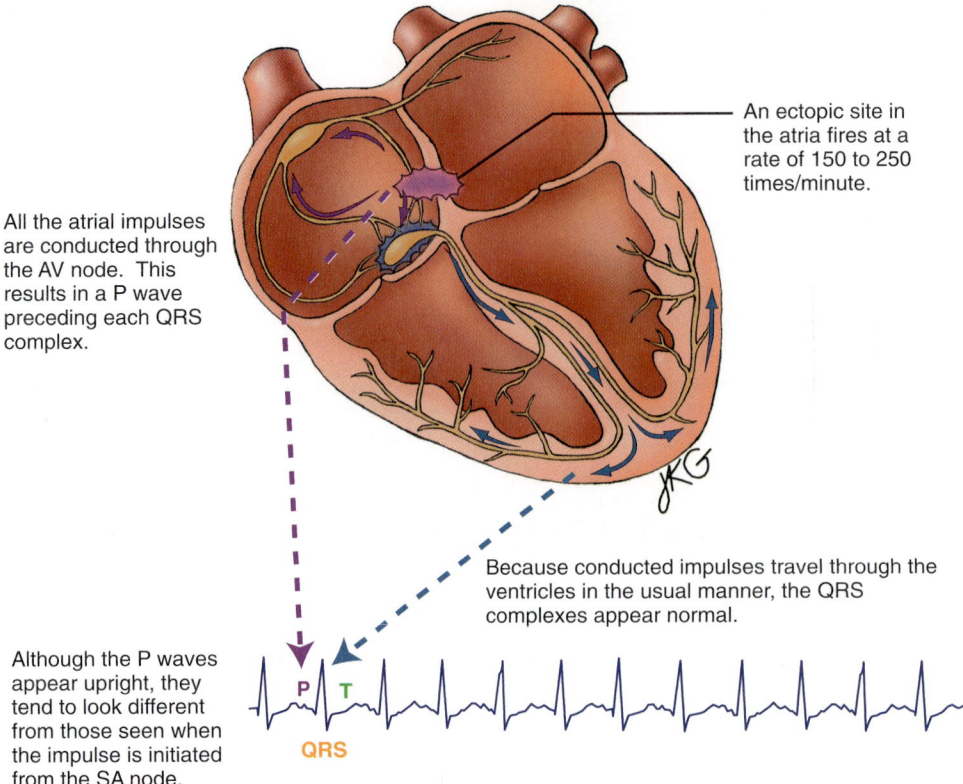

An ectopic site in the atria fires at a rate of 150 to 250 times/minute.

All the atrial impulses are conducted through the AV node. This results in a P wave preceding each QRS complex.

Because conducted impulses travel through the ventricles in the usual manner, the QRS complexes appear normal.

Although the P waves appear upright, they tend to look different from those seen when the impulse is initiated from the SA node.

Figure 22-43 Atrial tachycardia (AT).

Atrial Tachycardia

AT consists of a series of rapid beats from an irritable site in the atria. This rapid atrial rate overrides the SA node and becomes the pacemaker. Conduction of the atrial impulse to the ventricles is often 1:1. This means that every atrial impulse is conducted to the ventricles. AT looks similar to sinus tachycardia, but atrial P waves differ in shape from sinus P waves. An example of AT is shown in Figure 22-43.

AT that suddenly starts or ends is called **paroxysmal atrial tachycardia.** With extremely rapid atrial rates, the AV node begins to filter some of the impulses coming to it. By doing so, it protects the ventricles from excessively rapid rates. When the AV node selectively filters conduction of some of these impulses, the rhythm is called paroxysmal atrial tachycardia with block. The ECG characteristics of AT are shown in Table 22-18.

AT can occur in persons with normal hearts or in patients with organic heart disease. AT associated with automaticity or triggered activity is often related to an acute event, including the following:

- Stimulant use (e.g., caffeine, albuterol, theophylline, cocaine)
- Infection
- Electrolyte imbalance
- Acute illness with excessive catecholamine release
- MI

If episodes of AT are short, the patient may be asymptomatic. If AT is sustained (lasting more than 30 seconds) and the patient is symptomatic because of the rapid rate, treatment usually includes oxygen, IV access, and vagal maneuvers. Although AT rarely stops with vagal maneuvers, they are attempted to try to stop the rhythm to slow conduction through the AV node. If this fails, antiarrhythmic medications should be tried.

TABLE 22-18	Characteristics of Atrial Tachycardia
Rate	100-250 beats/min
Rhythm	Regular
P waves	One positive P wave precedes each QRS complex in lead II; P waves differ in shape from sinus P waves; an isoelectric baseline is usually present between P waves
PR interval	May be shorter or longer than normal
QRS duration	0.11 sec or less unless an intraventricular conduction delay exists

BOX 22-17 **AVNRT: Possible Triggers**

- Hypoxia
- Stress
- Overexertion
- Anxiety
- Caffeine
- Smoking
- Sleep deprivation
- Medications

AVNRT, Atrioventricular nodal reentrant tachycardia.

Atrioventricular Nodal Reentrant Tachycardia (NO)

[OBJECTIVE 36]

AVNRT is the most common type of SVT. It is caused by reentry in the area of the AV node. In the normal AV node, only one pathway exists through which an electrical impulse is conducted from the SA node to the ventricles. Patients with AVNRT have two conduction pathways within the AV node that conduct impulses at different speeds and recover at different rates. The fast pathway conducts impulses rapidly but has a long refractory period (slow recovery time). The slow pathway conducts impulses slowly but has a short refractory period (fast recovery time). Under the right conditions, the fast and slow pathways can form an electrical circuit, or loop. As one side of the loop is recovering, the other is firing.

AVNRT is usually caused by a PAC that is spread by the electrical circuit (Box 22-17). This allows the impulse to spin around in a circle indefinitely, reentering the normal electrical pathway with each pass around the circuit. The result is a very rapid and regular rhythm that ranges from 150 to 250 beats/min. An example of AVNRT is shown in Figure 22-44.

A regular, narrow-QRS tachycardia that starts or ends suddenly is called **paroxysmal supraventricular tachycardia (PSVT)** (Figure 22-45). P waves are seldom seen because they are hidden in T waves of preceding beats. The QRS is narrow unless a problem occurs with conduction of the impulse through the ventricles, as in a bundle branch block.

AVNRT can occur at any age. Whether a person is born with a tendency to have AVNRT or whether it develops later in life for an unknown reason has not been clearly determined. AVNRT is common in young, healthy persons with no structural heart disease. It occurs more often in women than in men. AVNRT also occurs in persons with chronic obstructive pulmonary disease, coronary artery disease, valvular heart disease, heart failure, and digitalis toxicity. AVNRT can cause angina or MI in patients with coronary artery disease.

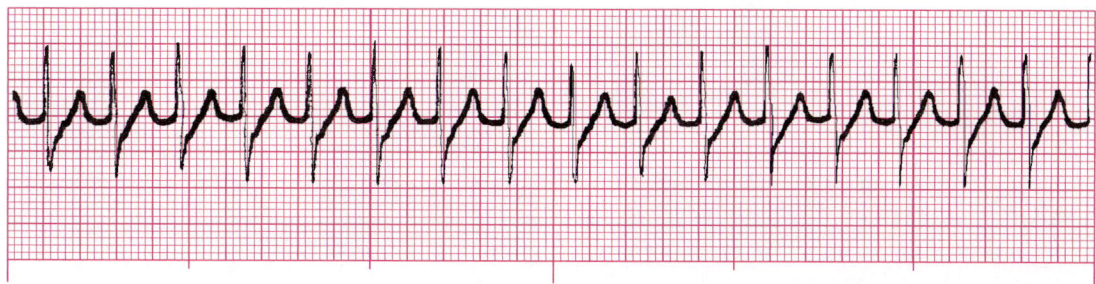

Figure 22-44 Atrioventricular nodal reentrant tachycardia (AVNRT).

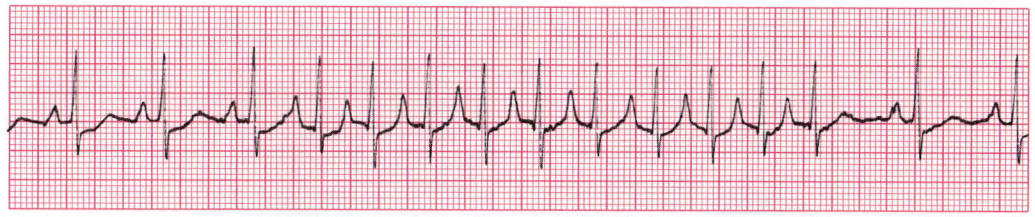

Figure 22-45 Paroxysmal supraventricular tachycardia (PSVT).

Treatment depends on the severity of the patient's signs and symptoms. If the patient is stable but symptomatic (and symptoms are caused by the rapid heart rate), treatment usually includes oxygen, IV access, and vagal maneuvers. If vagal maneuvers do not slow the rate or cause conversion of the tachycardia to a sinus rhythm, the first medication given is usually adenosine. If the patient is unstable, treatment typically includes oxygen, IV access, sedation (if the patient is awake and time permits), followed by synchronized cardioversion (Box 22-18, Skill 22-3). The ECG characteristics of AVNRT are summarized in Table 22-19. The narrow QRS tachycardia treatment algorithm is shown in Figure 22-46.

[Handwritten margin notes:]

Right AC

Biphasic monitor — Impulse goes from each pad to heart (lighter monitor, less damage to heart)

Cardioversion
Atria — start at 50J
Ventricles — start at 100J
Repeat 1X at 200J
5mg Valium
2 mg Morphine } Premed
Shock at peak of T wave

Pacing — shock every beat to maintain. See end of chp.

---

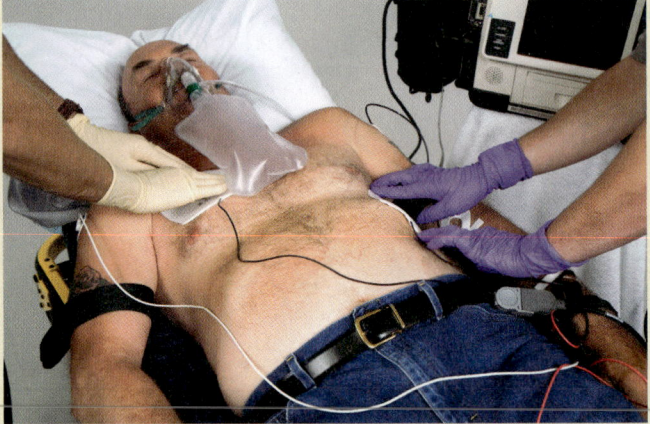

BOX 22-18 — Electrical Therapy: Synchronized Cardioversion

Synchronized cardioversion is the timed delivery of a shock during the QRS complex. A synchronized shock means the shock is timed to avoid the vulnerable period during the cardiac cycle. On the ECG, this period occurs during the peak of the T wave to approximately the end of the T wave. When the "sync" control is pressed, the machine searches for the highest (R wave deflection) or deepest (QS deflection) part of the QRS complex. When a QRS complex is detected, the monitor places a flag or sync marker on that complex that may appear as an oval, square, line, or highlighted triangle on the ECG display, depending on the monitor and defibrillator used. When the shock controls are pressed while the defibrillator is charged in "sync" mode, the machine will discharge energy only if both discharge buttons are pushed and the monitor tells the defibrillator that a QRS complex has been detected.

Indications (Unstable Patient)

- Tachycardias (except sinus tachycardia) with a ventricular rate greater than 150 beats/min that have a clearly identifiable QRS complex (such as some narrow QRS tachycardias and VT)

SKILL 22-3 SYNCHRONIZED CARDIOVERSION

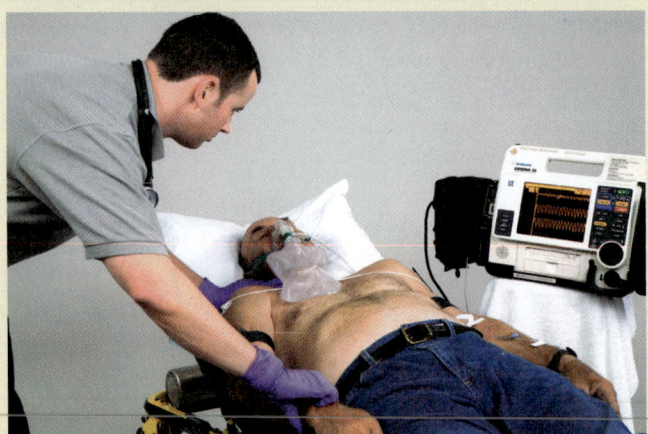

Step 1 Before performing synchronized cardioversion, take appropriate standard precautions and verify that the procedure is indicated. Identify the rhythm on the cardiac monitor. Print an ECG strip to document the patient's rhythm. Assess the patient for serious signs and symptoms from the tachycardia. Make sure suction and emergency medications are available. Give oxygen and start an IV. If the patient is awake, explain the procedure.

Step 2 Remove clothing from the patient's upper body. With gloves, remove NTG paste or patches from the patient's chest if present and quickly wipe away any medication residue. If present, remove excessive hair from the sites where the paddles or electrodes will be placed. Shave hair if necessary (and if time permits). Avoid cutting the skin. Do not apply alcohol, tincture of benzoin, or antiperspirant to the skin.

Turn the power on to the defibrillator. If using standard paddles, you must use defibrillation gel or defibrillation gel pads between the paddle electrode surface and the patient's skin. Place pregelled defibrillation pads on the patient's chest at this time. If using multipurpose adhesive electrodes, place them in proper position on the patient's bare chest.

SKILL 22-3 SYNCHRONIZED CARDIOVERSION—continued

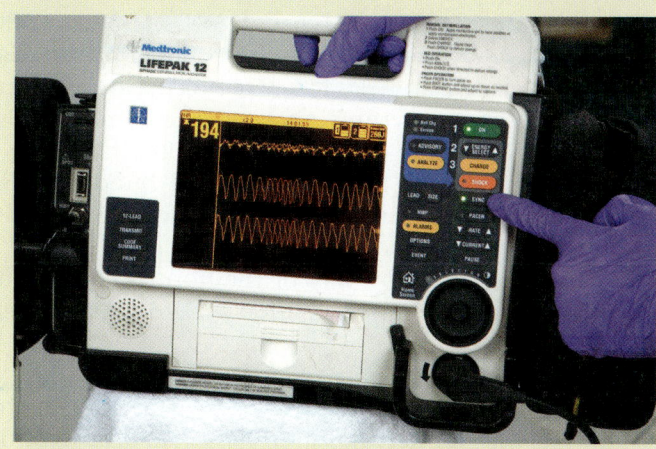

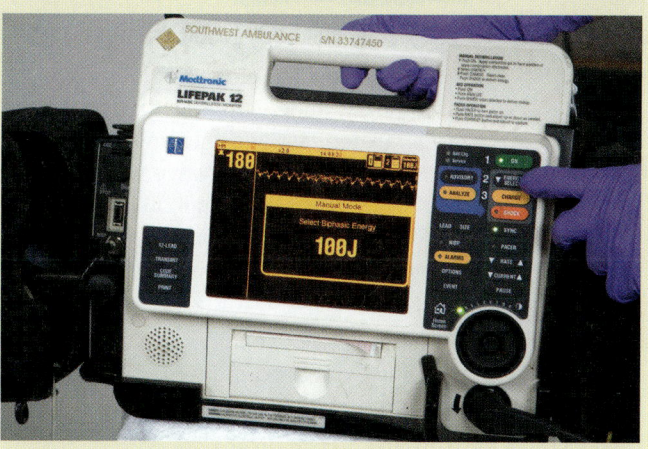

Step 3 Press the "sync" control on the defibrillator. Select a lead with an optimum QRS complex amplitude (positive or negative) and no artifact. If using adhesive electrodes, select the "paddles" lead. Make sure the machine is marking or flagging each QRS complex and no artifact is present. The sense marker should appear near the middle of each QRS complex. If sense markers do not appear or are seen in the wrong place (such as on a T wave), adjust the ECG size or select another lead.

Step 4 If the patient is awake and time permits, administer sedation per local protocol or instructions from medical direction unless contraindicated. Make sure the machine is in "sync" mode and then select the appropriate energy level on the defibrillator.

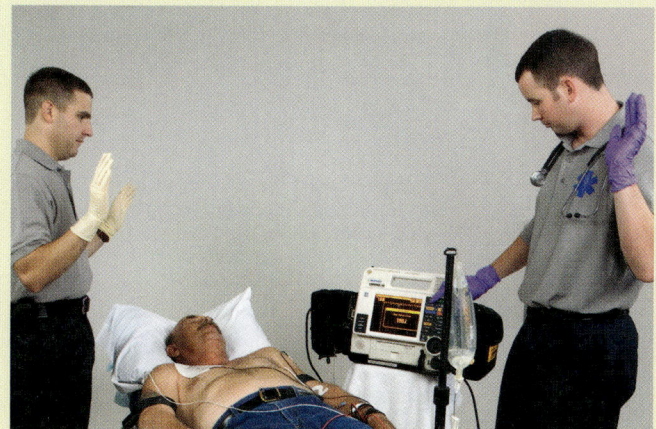

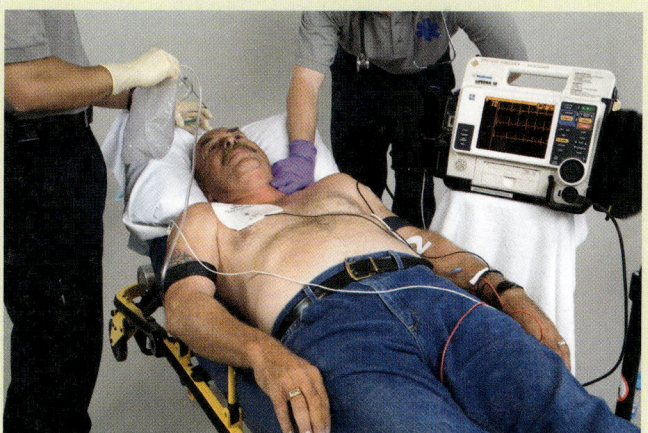

Step 5 Charge the defibrillator and recheck the ECG rhythm. If using standard paddles, place the paddles on the pre-gelled defibrillator pads on the patient's chest and apply firm pressure. If the rhythm is unchanged, call "Clear!" and look around you. Make sure everyone is clear of the patient, bed, and any equipment connected to the patient. Make sure oxygen is not flowing over the patient's chest.

Step 6 If the area is clear, press and hold both discharge buttons at the same time until the shock is delivered. A slight delay may occur while the machine detects the next QRS complex. Release the shock controls after the shock has been delivered. Reassess the rhythm and the patient. If tachycardia persists, make sure the machine is in sync mode before delivering another shock. If the rhythm changes to VF, make sure the patient has no pulse. If no pulse is present, make sure the sync control is off and defibrillate.

Goes back to defib by default

TABLE 22-19	Characteristics of AVNRT
Rate	150-250 beats/min
Rhythm	Ventricular rhythm is usually very regular
P waves	P waves are often hidden in the QRS complex. If the ventricles are stimulated first and then the atria, a negative (inverted) P wave will appear after the QRS in leads II, III, and aVF. When the atria are depolarized after the ventricles, the P wave typically distorts the end of the QRS complex.
PR interval	P waves are not seen before the QRS complex; therefore the PR interval is not measurable
QRS duration	0.11 sec or less unless an intraventricular conduction delay exists

AVNRT, Atrioventricular nodal reentrant tachycardia.

Atrioventricular Reentrant Tachycardia

[OBJECTIVE 37]

The next most common type of SVT is AVRT. AVRT involves a pathway of impulse conduction outside the AV node and bundle of His. **Preexcitation** is a term used to describe rhythms that originate from above the ventricles but in which the impulse travels by a pathway other than the AV node and bundle of His (Figure 22-47). As a result, the supraventricular impulse excites the ventricles earlier than would be expected if the impulse traveled by way of the normal conduction system. Patients with preexcitation syndromes are prone to AVRT.

Wolff-Parkinson-White (WPW) syndrome is the most common type of preexcitation syndrome. In this syndrome, the PR interval is short (less than 0.12 seconds) because the impulse travels very quickly across the accessory pathway, bypassing the normal delay in the AV node (Figure 22-48). As the impulse crosses the insertion point

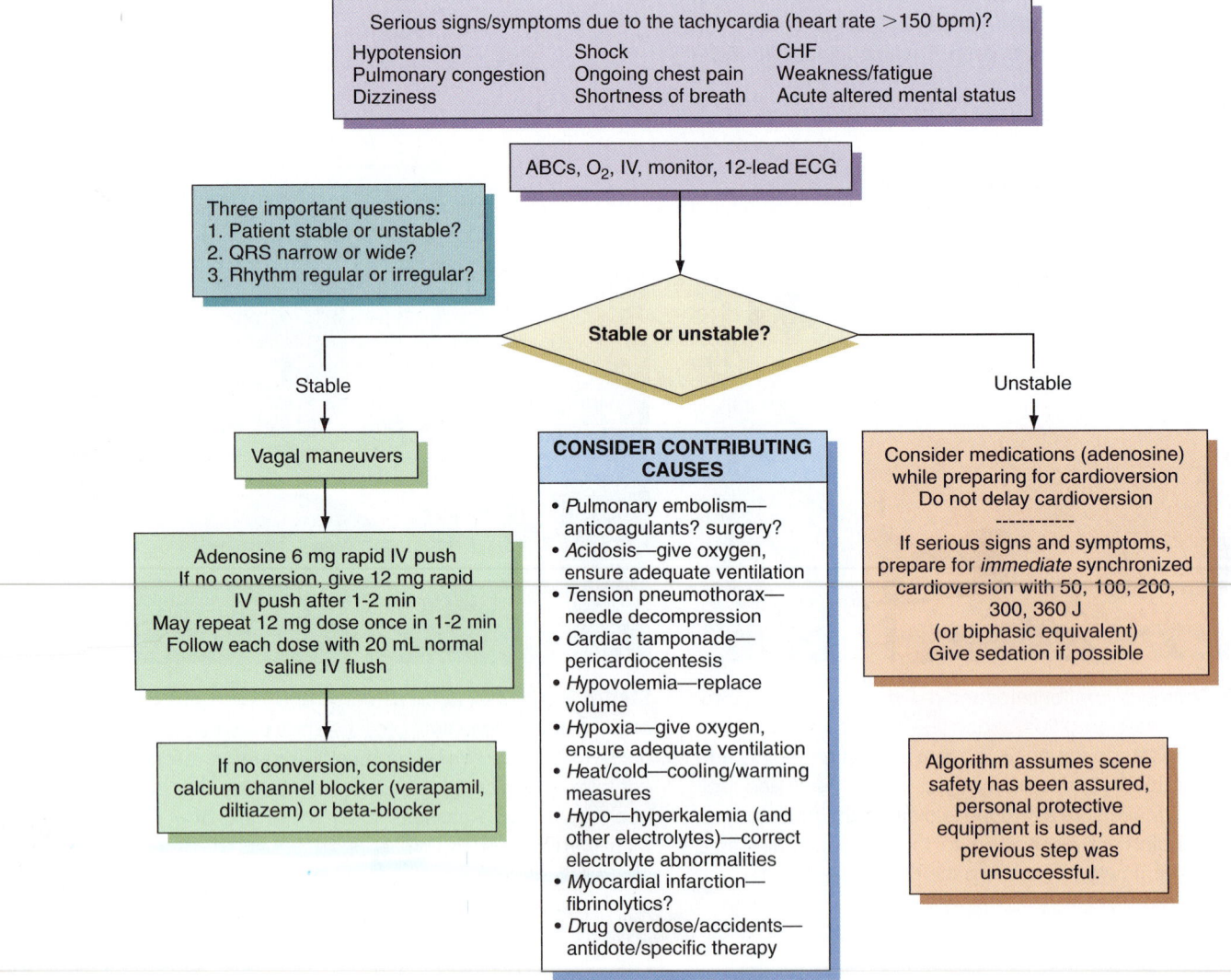

Figure 22-46 Narrow-QRS tachycardia algorithm.

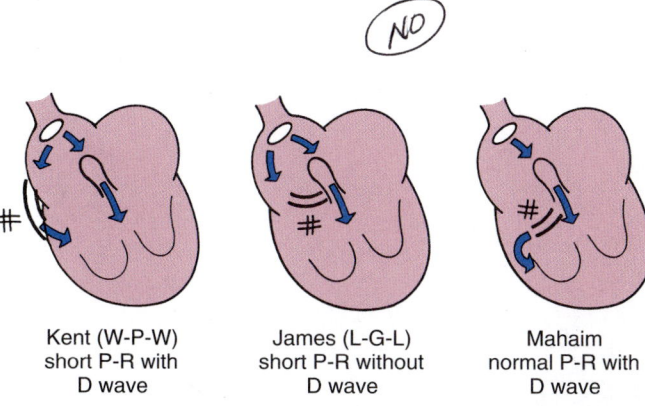

NO

Kent (W-P-W)
short P-R with
D wave

James (L-G-L)
short P-R without
D wave

Mahaim
normal P-R with
D wave

Figure 22-47 The three major forms of preexcitation. Location of the accessory pathways and corresponding ECG characteristics.

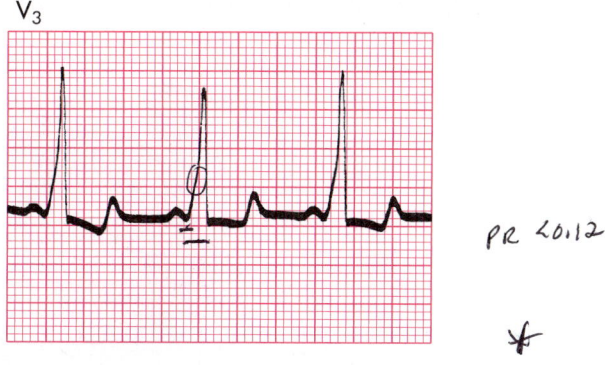

V_3

PR <0.12

Figure 22-48 Lead V_3. Typical Wolff-Parkinson-White syndrome pattern showing the short PR interval, delta wave, wide QRS complex, and secondary ST-segment and T-wave changes.

of the accessory pathway in the ventricular muscle, that part of the ventricle is stimulated earlier (preexcited) than if the impulse had followed the normal conduction pathway through the bundle of His and Purkinje fibers. On the ECG, preexcitation of the ventricles can be seen as a **delta wave** in some leads. A delta wave is an initial slurring of the QRS complex. The direction of the ST segment and T-wave changes are usually opposite the direction of the delta wave and QRS complex.

If the patient is symptomatic because of the rapid ventricular rate, treatment will depend on how unstable the patient is, the width of the QRS complex, and the regularity of the ventricular rhythm. A stable but symptomatic patient with narrow-QRS AVRT is usually treated with oxygen, IV access, and attempts to slow or convert the rhythm with vagal maneuvers. If vagal maneuvers fail, IV medications such as amiodarone may be used. Do not give drugs that slow or block conduction through the AV node, such as adenosine, digoxin, diltiazem, or verapamil. They may speed up conduction through the accessory pathway, which can result in a further increase in heart rate. The ECG characteristics of WPW syndrome are summarized in Table 22-20.

Atrial Flutter

saw tooth flutter waves

Atrial flutter has been classified into two types. Type I atrial flutter is caused by reentry. In this type of atrial flutter, an impulse circles around a large area of tissue, such as the entire right atrium. Type I atrial flutter is also called *typical* or *classic atrial flutter*. In type I atrial flutter, the atrial rate ranges from 250 to 350 beats/min. Type II atrial flutter is called *atypical* or *very rapid atrial flutter*. The precise mechanism of type II atrial flutter has not been defined. Patients with this type of atrial flutter often develop atrial fibrillation. In type II atrial flutter, the atrial rate ranges from 350 to 450 beats/min. If the AV node blocks the impulses coming to it at a regular rate, the resulting ventricular rhythm will be regular. If the AV node blocks the impulses at an irregular rate, the resulting ventricular rhythm will be irregular.

The severity of signs and symptoms associated with atrial flutter vary depending on the ventricular rate, how long the rhythm has been present, and the patient's cardiovascular status (Box 22-19). The patient may be asymptomatic and not require treatment or may have serious signs and symptoms. Patients with atrial flutter

TABLE 22-20	Characteristics of Wolff-Parkinson-White Syndrome
Rate	Usually 60-100 beats/min if the underlying rhythm is sinus in origin
Rhythm	Regular unless associated with AFib
P waves	Normal and positive in lead II unless WPW syndrome is associated with AFib
PR interval	If P waves are observed, less than 0.12 sec
QRS duration	Usually greater than 0.12 sec; slurred upstroke of the QRS complex (delta wave) may be seen in one or more leads

AFib, Atrial fibrillation; *WPW*, Wolff-Parkinson-White.

BOX 22-19	Conditions Associated with Atrial Flutter

- Hypoxia
- Pulmonary embolism
- Chronic lung disease
- Mitral or tricuspid valve stenosis or regurgitation
- Pneumonia
- Ischemic heart disease
- Complication of myocardial infarction
- Cardiomyopathy
- Hyperthyroidism
- Digitalis or quinidine toxicity
- Cardiac surgery
- Pericarditis or myocarditis

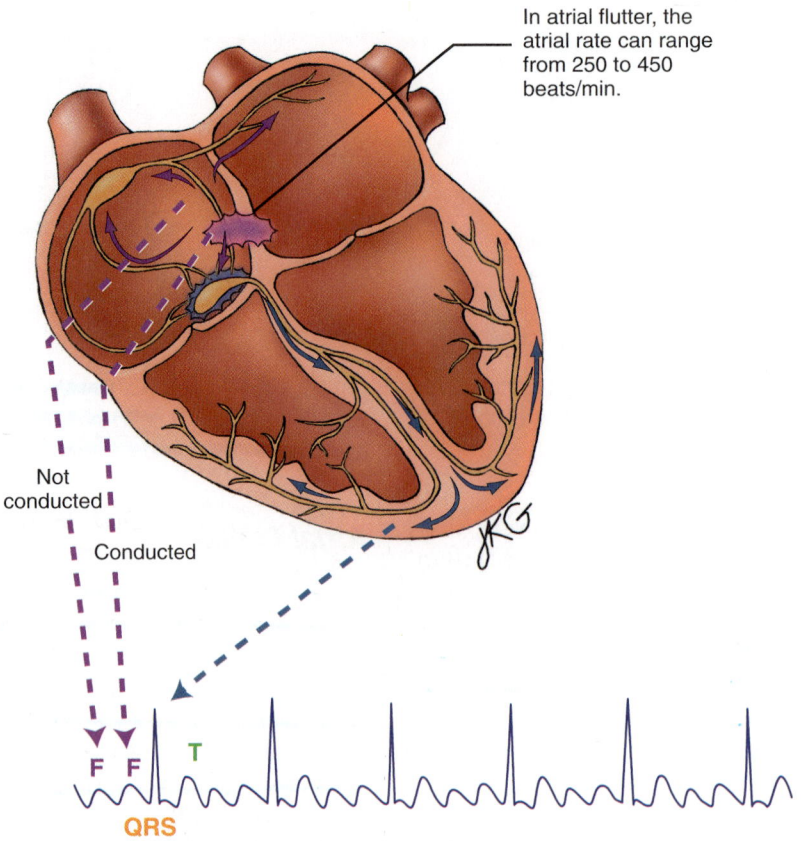

In atrial flutter, the atrial rate can range from 250 to 450 beats/min.

Not conducted

Conducted

F F T QRS

Figure 22-49 Atrial flutter. *F*, Flutter wave.

commonly have palpitations, difficulty breathing, fatigue, or chest discomfort.

Prehospital care for a patient in atrial flutter who has serious signs and symptoms because of a *rapid* ventricular rate is usually aimed at controlling the ventricular rate. An example of atrial flutter is shown in Figure 22-49. The ECG characteristics of atrial flutter are shown in Table 22-21. The irregular tachycardia treatment algorithm is shown in Figure 22-50.

PARAMEDIC*Pearl*

Atrial flutter or AFib with a ventricular rate of more than 100 beats/min is described as *uncontrolled*. The ventricular rate is considered *rapid* when it is 150 beats/min or more. Atrial flutter or AFib with a rapid ventricular response is commonly called *Aflutter with RVR* or *AFib with RVR*.

Atrial flutter or AFib with a ventricular rate of less than 100 beats/min is described as *controlled*. A controlled ventricular rate may be the result of the following:

- A healthy AV node protecting the ventricles from very fast atrial impulses
- Medications used to control (block) conduction through the AV node, decreasing the number of impulses reaching the ventricles

Regularly irregular

TABLE 22-21	Characteristics of Atrial Flutter
Rate	Atrial rate 250-450 beats/min, typically 300 beats/min; ventricular rate variable—determined by AV blockade; the ventricular rate will not usually exceed 180 beats/min because of the intrinsic conduction rate of the AV junction
Rhythm	Atrial regular, ventricular regular or irregular depending on AV conduction or blockade
P Waves	No identifiable P waves; saw-toothed "flutter" waves are present
PR Interval	Not measurable
QRS Duration	0.11 sec or less but may be widened if flutter waves are buried in the QRS complex or an intraventricular conduction delay exists

AV, Atrioventricular.

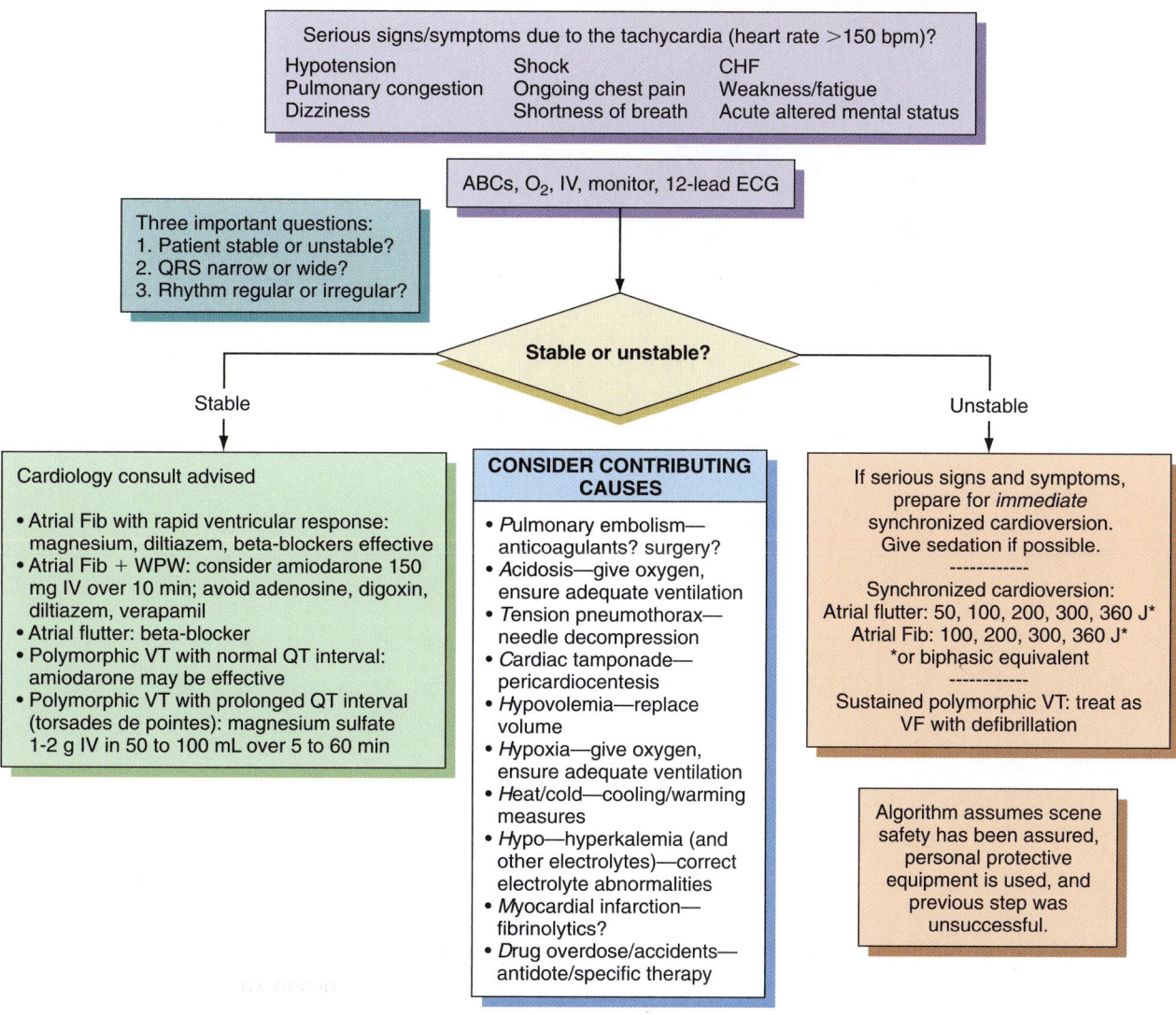

Figure 22-50 Irregular tachycardia treatment algorithm.

Atrial Fibrillation

Irregularly irregular
Risk of microemboli

Atrial fibrillation (AFib) occurs because of irritable sites in the atria firing at a rate of 400 to 600 times per minute. These rapid impulses cause the muscles of the atria to quiver (fibrillate). This results in ineffectual atrial contraction, decreased stroke volume, a subsequent decrease in cardiac output, and loss of atrial kick. AFib can occur in patients with or without detectable heart disease or related symptoms. Conditions associated with AFib are shown in Box 22-20.

Patients with AFib are at increased risk of having a stroke. Because the atria do not contract effectively and expel all the blood within them, blood may pool within them and form clots. A stroke can result if a clot moves from the atria and lodges in an artery in the brain.

BOX 22-20	**Conditions Associated with Atrial Fibrillation**

- Idiopathic (no clear cause)
- Hypertension
- Ischemic heart disease
- Advanced age
- Rheumatic heart disease
- Cardiomyopathy
- Heart failure
- Congenital heart disease
- Sick sinus syndrome
- Wolff-Parkinson-White syndrome
- Pericarditis
- Pulmonary embolism
- Chronic lung disease
- After surgery
- Diabetes
- Stress
- Sympathomimetics
- Excessive caffeine
- Hypoxia
- Hypokalemia
- Hypoglycemia
- Systemic infection
- Hyperthyroidism
- Electrocution

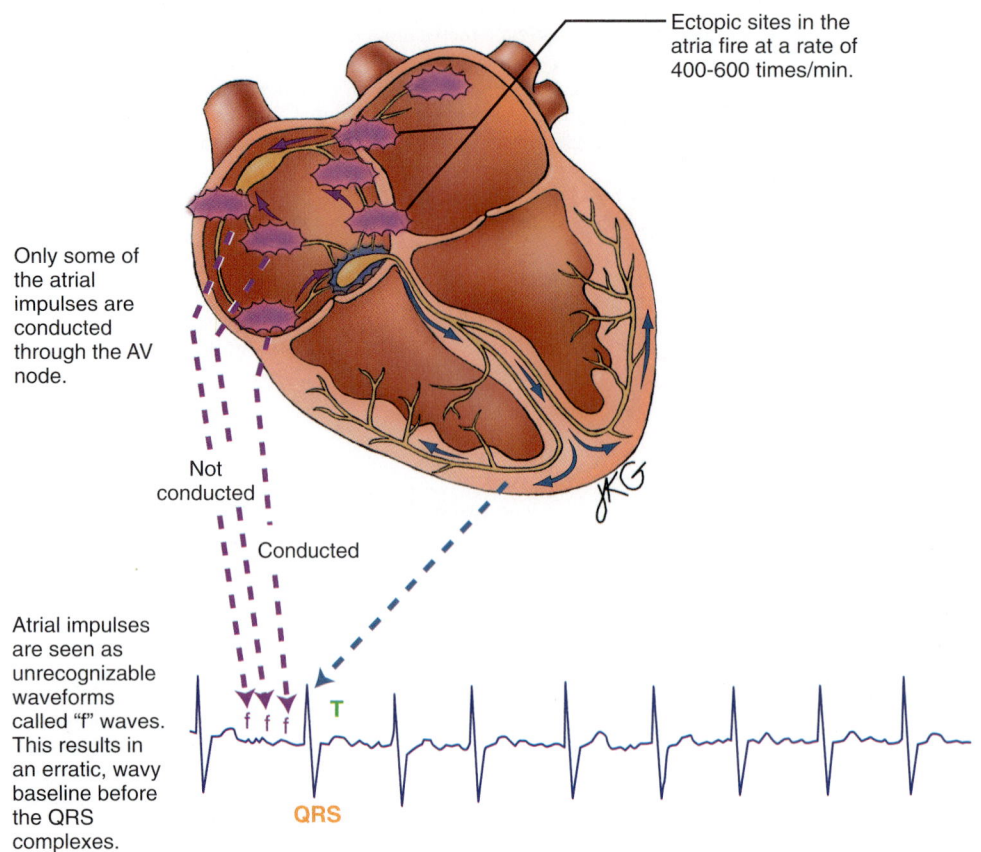

Ectopic sites in the atria fire at a rate of 400-600 times/min.

Only some of the atrial impulses are conducted through the AV node.

Not conducted

Conducted

Atrial impulses are seen as unrecognizable waveforms called "f" waves. This results in an erratic, wavy baseline before the QRS complexes.

T

QRS

Figure 22-51 Atrial fibrillation. *AV*, Atrioventricular; *f*, fibrillatory wave.

Treatment decisions are based on the ventricular rate, the duration of the rhythm, the patient's general health, and how he or she is tolerating the rhythm. AFib with a rapid ventricular response may produce signs and symptoms that include lightheadedness, palpitations, dyspnea, chest discomfort, and low blood pressure. If AFib is associated with a rapid ventricular rate and the patient has serious signs and symptoms, prehospital treatment is usually aimed at controlling the ventricular rate. An example of AFib is shown in Figure 22-51. The ECG characteristics of AFib are shown in Table 22-22.

JUNCTIONAL DYSRHYTHMIAS

[OBJECTIVE 38]

The AV junction may assume responsibility for pacing the heart if the following occur:

- The SA node fails to discharge (such as sinus arrest)
- An impulse from the SA node is generated but blocked as it exits the SA node (such as SA block)
- The rate of discharge of the SA node is slower than that of the AV junction (such as a sinus bradycardia or the slower phase of a sinus arrhythmia)
- An impulse from the SA node is generated and is conducted through the atria but is not conducted to the ventricles (such as an AV block)

If the AV junction paces the heart, the electrical impulse must travel in a backward (retrograde) direction to activate the atria (Figure 22-52). If a P wave is seen, it will be inverted in leads II, III, and aVF because the impulse is traveling away from the positive electrode. If the atria depolarize before the ventricles, an inverted P wave will be seen *before* the QRS complex and the PR interval will usually measure 0.12 seconds or less. The PR interval is shorter than usual because an impulse that

TABLE 22-22	Characteristics of Atrial Fibrillation
Rate	Atrial rate usually 400-600 beats/min; ventricular rate variable
Rhythm	Ventricular rhythm usually irregularly irregular
P waves	No identifiable P waves, fibrillatory waves present; erratic, wavy baseline
PR interval	Not measurable
QRS duration	0.11 sec or less but may be widened if an intraventricular conduction delay exists

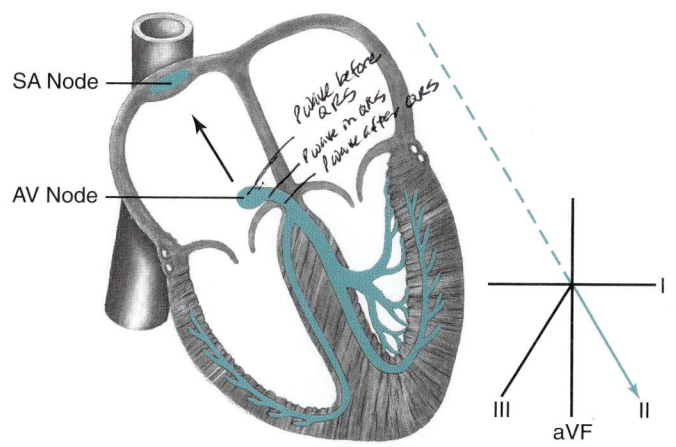

Figure 22-52 If the atrioventricular (AV) junction paces the heart, the electrical impulse must travel in a backward (retrograde) direction to activate the atria. If a P wave is seen, it will be inverted in leads II, III, and aVF because the impulse is traveling away from the positive electrode. *SA,* Sinoatrial.

begins in the AV junction does not have to travel as far to stimulate the ventricles. If the atria and ventricles depolarize at the same time, a P wave will not be visible because it will be hidden in the QRS complex. If the atria depolarize after the ventricles, an inverted P wave will appear *after* the QRS complex.

Premature Junctional Complexes

A premature junctional complex (PJC) occurs when an irritable site (focus) within the AV junction fires before the next SA node impulse is due to fire. This interrupts the sinus rhythm. Because the impulse is conducted through the ventricles in the usual manner, the QRS complex will usually measure 0.11 seconds or less. A noncompensatory (incomplete) pause often follows a PJC. This pause represents the delay during which the SA node resets its rhythm for the next beat.

Junctional complexes may come early (before the next expected sinus beat) or late (after the next expected sinus beat). If the complex is *early* it is called a *PJC*. If the

complex is *late* it is called a *junctional escape beat*. To determine whether a complex is early or late, you need to see at least two sinus beats in a row to establish the regularity of the underlying rhythm.

PJCs are less common than either PACs or premature ventricular contractions. Causes of PJCs include the following:

- Heart failure
- Acute coronary syndromes
- Mental and physical fatigue
- Valvular heart disease
- Digitalis toxicity
- Electrolyte imbalance
- Rheumatic heart disease
- Stimulants (e.g., caffeine, tobacco)

PJCs normally do not require treatment because most individuals who have PJCs are asymptomatic. However, PJCs may lead to the feeling of skipped beats. Lightheadedness, dizziness, and other signs of decreased cardiac output can occur if PJCs are frequent. Examples of PJCs are shown in Figure 22-53. The ECG characteristics of PJCs are shown in Table 22-23.

TABLE 22-23	Characteristics of PJCs
Rate	Usually within normal range but depends on underlying rhythm
Rhythm	Regular with premature beats
P waves	May occur before, during, or after the QRS; if visible, the P wave is inverted in leads II, III, and aVF
PR interval	If a P wave occurs before the QRS, the PR interval will usually be 0.12 sec or less; if no P wave occurs before the QRS, no PR interval will be present
QRS duration	Usually 0.11 sec or less unless it is aberrantly conducted or an intraventricular conduction delay exists

PJC, Premature junctional complex.

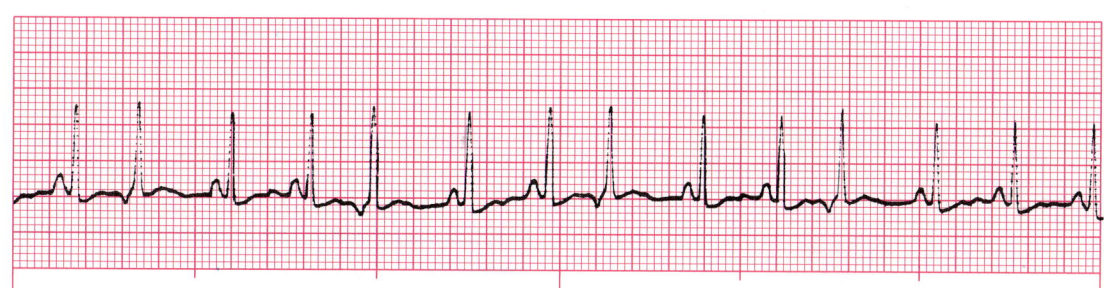

Figure 22-53 Sinus tachycardia at 136 beats/min with frequent premature junctional complexes (PJCs).

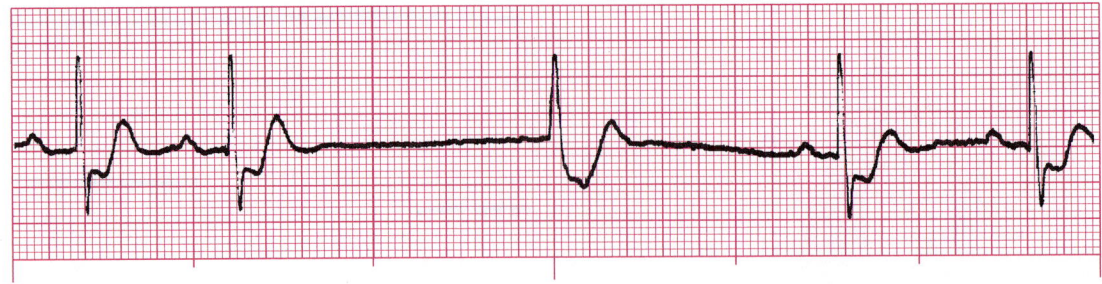

Figure 22-54 Sinus rhythm at 71 beats/min with a prolonged PR interval (0.24 seconds), an episode of sinus arrest, a junctional escape beat, and ST-segment depression.

Junctional Escape Beats or Rhythm

A junctional escape beat begins in the AV junction and appears *late* (after the next expected sinus beat). Junctional escape beats frequently occur during episodes of sinus arrest or follow pauses of nonconducted PACs. An example of a junctional escape beat is shown in Figure 22-54. The ECG characteristics of junctional escape beats are shown in Table 22-24.

A junctional *rhythm* is several sequential junctional escape beats. Remember that the built-in rate of the AV junction is 40 to 60 beats/min. Because a junctional rhythm starts from above the ventricles, the QRS complex is usually narrow and its rhythm is quite regular. If the AV junction paces the heart at a rate slower than 40 beats/min, the resulting rhythm is called a **junctional bradycardia.** This may seem confusing because the AV junction's normal pacing rate (40 to 60 beats/min) *is* bradycardic. However, the term *junctional bradycardia* refers to a rate slower than normal for the AV junction.

Junctional escape beats frequently occur during episodes of sinus arrest or following pauses of nonconducted PACs. Junctional escape beats also may be observed in healthy individuals during sinus bradycardia. Causes of a junctional rhythm include the following:

- Acute coronary syndromes (particularly inferior wall MI)
- Hypoxia
- Rheumatic heart disease
- Valvular disease
- SA node disease
- Increased parasympathetic tone
- Cardiac surgery (can occur immediately after)
- Effects of medications, including digitalis, quinidine, beta-blockers, and calcium channel blockers

Treatment depends on the cause of the dysrhythmia and the patient's presenting signs and symptoms. If the patient's signs and symptoms are related to the slow heart rate, consider atropine and/or transcutaneous pacing. Examples of junctional rhythms are shown in Figure 22-55. The ECG characteristics of a junctional rhythm are shown in Table 22-25.

Accelerated Junctional Rhythm

If the AV junction speeds up and fires at a rate of 60 to 100 beats/min, the resulting rhythm is called an *accelerated junctional rhythm*. The only ECG difference between a junctional rhythm and an accelerated junctional rhythm is the increase in the ventricular rate.

Causes of this dysrhythmia include digitalis toxicity, acute MI, cardiac surgery, rheumatic fever, chronic obstructive pulmonary disease, and hypokalemia. The patient usually is asymptomatic because the ventricular rate is 61 to 100 beats/min; however, the patient should be closely monitored. An example of an accelerated junctional rhythm is shown in Figure 22-55. The ECG characteristics of this rhythm are shown in Table 22-26.

TABLE 22-24	Characteristics of Junctional Escape Beats
Rate	Usually within normal range but depends on underlying rhythm
Rhythm	Regular with *late* beats
P waves	May occur before, during, or after the QRS; if visible, the P wave is inverted in leads II, III, and aVF
PR interval	If a P wave occurs before the QRS, the PR interval will usually be 0.12 sec or less; if no P wave occurs before the QRS, no PR interval will be present
QRS duration	Usually 0.11 sec or less unless it is aberrantly conducted or an intraventricular conduction delay exists

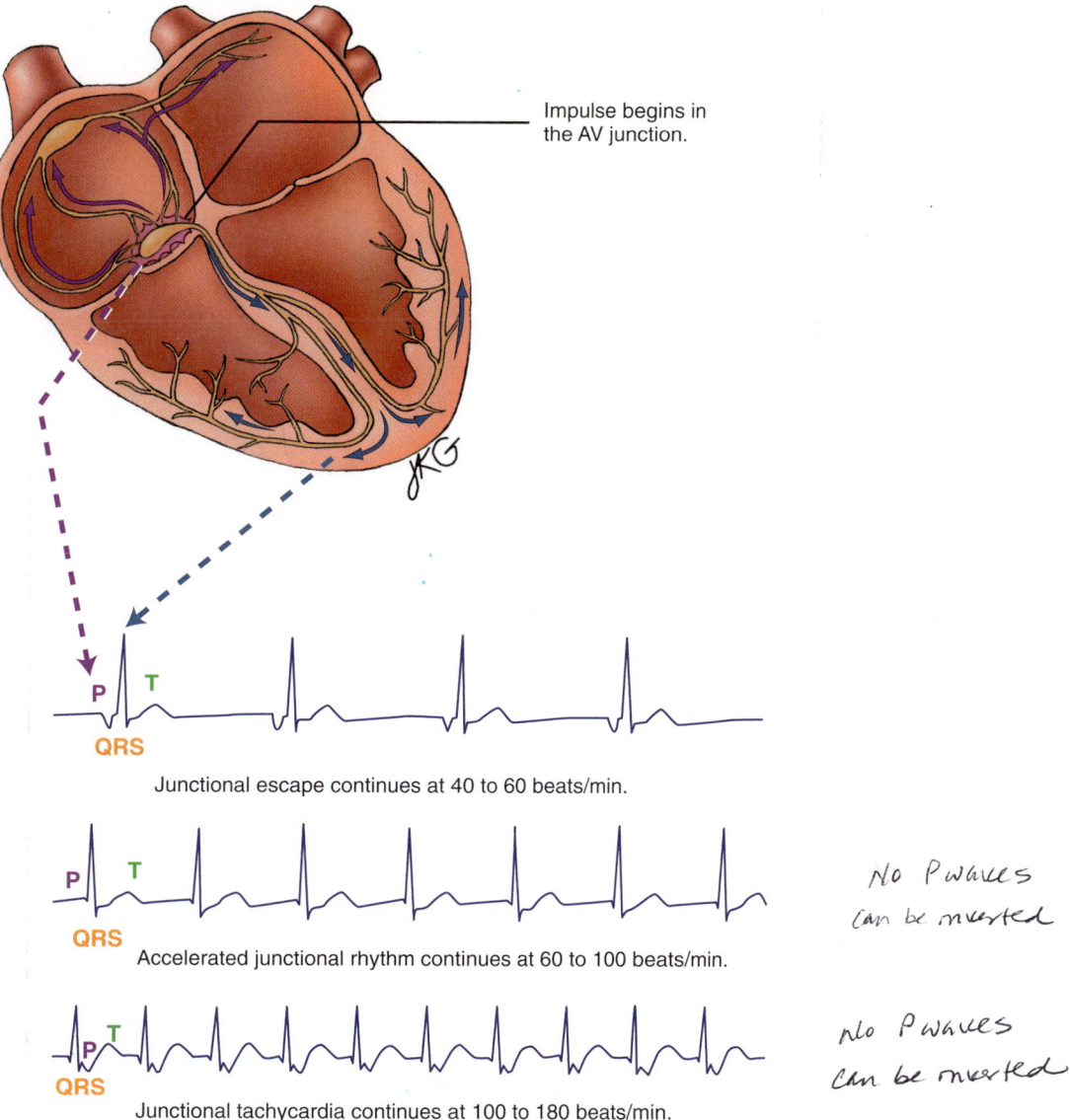

Impulse begins in the AV junction.

Junctional escape continues at 40 to 60 beats/min.

Accelerated junctional rhythm continues at 60 to 100 beats/min.

No P waves can be inverted

Junctional tachycardia continues at 100 to 180 beats/min.

no P waves can be inverted

Figure 22-55 Junctional rhythms. *AV,* Atrioventricular.

TABLE 22-25	Characteristics of Junctional Escape Rhythm
Rate	40-60 beats/min
Rhythm	Very regular
P waves	May occur before, during, or after the QRS; if visible, the P wave is inverted in leads II, III, and aVF
PR interval	If a P wave occurs before the QRS, the PR interval will usually be 0.12 sec or less; if no P wave occurs before the QRS, no PR interval will be present
QRS duration	Usually 0.11 sec or less unless it is aberrantly conducted or an intraventricular conduction delay exists

TABLE 22-26	Characteristics of Accelerated Junctional Rhythm
Rate	61-100 beats/min
Rhythm	Very regular
P waves	May occur before, during, or after the QRS; if visible, the P wave is inverted in leads II, III, and aVF
PR interval	If a P wave occurs before the QRS, the PR interval will usually be 0.12 sec or less; if no P wave occurs before the QRS, no PR interval will be present
QRS duration	0.11 sec or less unless it is aberrantly conducted or an intraventricular conduction delay exists

Junctional Tachycardia

Junctional tachycardia is an ectopic rhythm that begins in the pacemaker cells found in the bundle of His. When three or more sequential PJCs occur at a rate of more than 100 beats/min, junctional tachycardia exists. Nonparoxysmal (gradual onset) junctional tachycardia usually starts as an accelerated junctional rhythm, but the heart rate gradually increases to more than 100 beats/min. The usual ventricular rate for nonparoxysmal junctional tachycardia is 101 to 140 beats/min. Paroxysmal junctional tachycardia starts and ends suddenly and often is precipitated by a PJC. The ventricular rate for paroxysmal junctional tachycardia generally is faster, at 140 beats/min or more.

PARAMEDIC*Pearl*

When the ventricular rate is greater than 150 beats/min, distinguishing junctional tachycardia from AVNRT and AVRT is difficult. *SVT*

Junctional tachycardia may occur as a result of an acute coronary syndrome, heart failure, theophylline administration, or digitalis toxicity. With sustained ventricular rates of 150 beats/min or more, the patient may complain of a "racing heart" and severe anxiety. Because of the fast ventricular rate, the ventricles may be unable to fill completely, resulting in decreased cardiac output.

Treatment depends on the severity of the patient's signs and symptoms. If the patient tolerates the rhythm, observation is often all that is needed. If the patient is symptomatic because of the rapid rate, initial treatment should include oxygen and IV access. Because distinguishing junctional tachycardia from other narrow-QRS tachycardias is often difficult, vagal maneuvers and, if necessary, IV adenosine may be used to help determine the origin of the rhythm. A beta-blocker or calcium channel blocker may be ordered (if no contraindications exist). An example of junctional tachycardia is shown in Figure 22-55. The ECG characteristics of this rhythm are shown in Table 22-27.

VENTRICULAR DYSRHYTHMIAS *Wide QRS*

[OBJECTIVE 39]

The ventricles are the heart's least efficient pacemaker. If the ventricles function as the heart's pacemaker, they normally generate impulses at a rate of 20 to 40 beats/min. The ventricles may assume responsibility for pacing the heart if the following occur:

- SA node fails to discharge
- Impulse from the SA node is generated but blocked as it exits the SA node

TABLE 22-27	Characteristics of Junctional Tachycardia
Rate	101-180 beats/min
Rhythm	Very regular
P waves	May occur before, during, or after the QRS; if visible, the P wave is inverted in leads II, III, and aVF
PR interval	If a P wave occurs before the QRS, the PR interval will usually be 0.12 sec or less; if no P wave occurs before the QRS, no PR interval will be present
QRS duration	0.11 sec or less unless it is aberrantly conducted or an intraventricular conduction delay exists

- Rate of discharge of the SA node is slower than that of the ventricles
- Irritable site in either ventricle produces an early beat or rapid rhythm

If an area of either ventricle becomes ischemic or injured, it can become irritable. This irritability affects the manner in which impulses are conducted. Ventricular beats and rhythms can start in any part of the ventricles. When an ectopic site within a ventricle assumes responsibility for pacing the heart, the electrical impulse bypasses the normal intraventricular conduction pathway. This results in stimulation of the ventricles at slightly different times. As a result, ventricular beats and rhythms usually have QRS complexes that are abnormally shaped and longer than normal. *Wide QRS*

Premature Ventricular Complexes

A **premature ventricular complex (PVC)** arises from an irritable site within either ventricle. By definition, a PVC is *premature*, occurring earlier than the next expected sinus beat. The QRS of a PVC is typically equal to or greater than 0.12 seconds because the PVC causes the ventricles to fire prematurely and in an abnormal manner (Figure 22-56). The T wave is usually in the opposite direction of the QRS complex.

Types of PVCs

Premature ventricular beats that look the same in the same lead and begin from the same anatomic site (focus) are called uniform PVCs. PVCs that look different from one another in the same lead are called *multiform PVCs*. A PVC may occur without interfering with the normal cardiac cycle. An interpolated PVC is squeezed between two regular complexes and does not disturb the underlying rhythm. R-on-T PVCs occur when the R wave of a PVC falls on the T wave of the preceding beat (Figure 22-57). Two PVCs in a row are called a *couplet* or *paired*

Ron T not tx in field now.

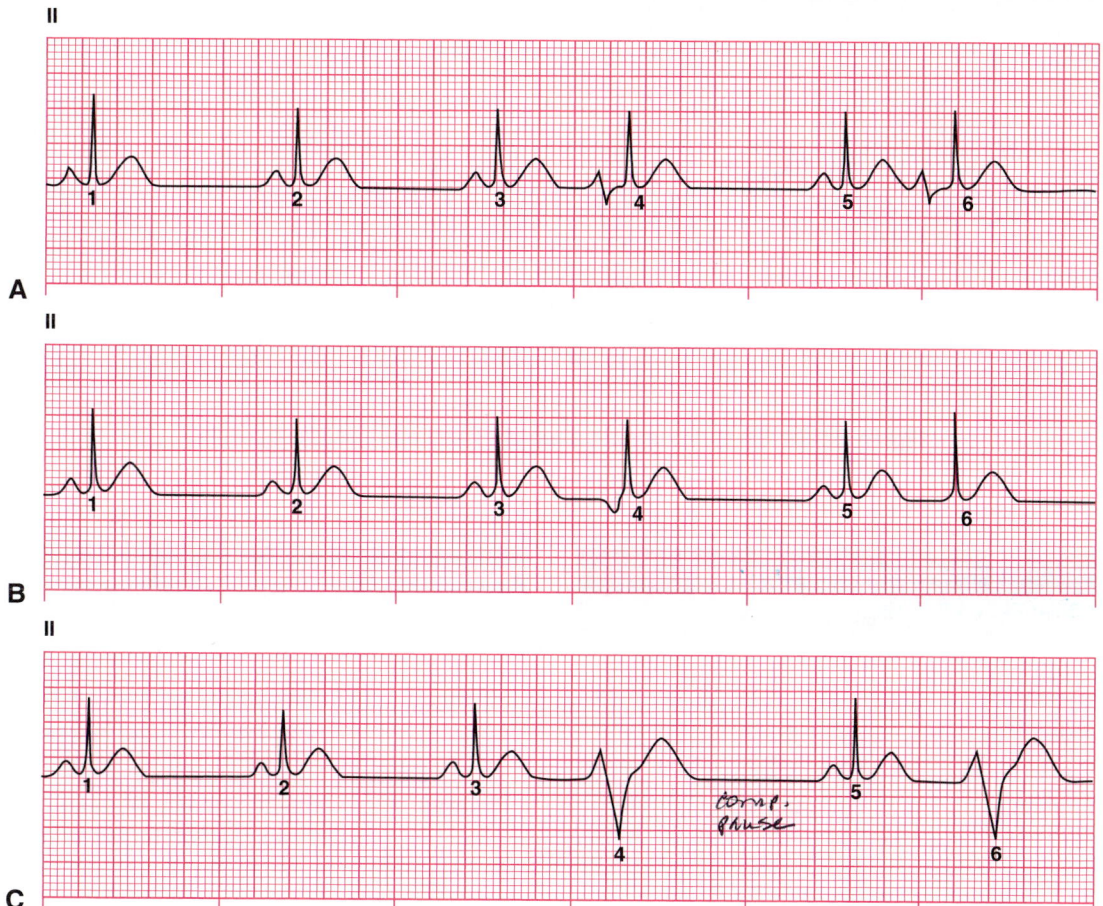

Figure 22-56 Premature beats. **A**, Sinus rhythm with premature atrial complexes (PACs). The fourth and sixth beats are preceded by premature P waves that look different from the normally conducted sinus beats. Note that the QRS complex that follows each of these PACs is narrow and identical in appearance to that of the sinus-conducted beats. **B**, Sinus rhythm with premature junctional complexes (PJCs). The fourth and sixth beats are PJCs. Beat 4 is preceded by an inverted P wave with a short PR interval. No identifiable atrial activity is associated with beat 6. **C**, Sinus rhythm with premature ventricular complexes (PVCs). The fourth and sixth beats are quite different in appearance from the normally conducted sinus beats. Beats 4 and 6 are PVCs. They are not preceded by P waves.

Unifocal PVC - same site

multifocal PVCs - different sites
worse because more irritable tissue

Interpolated PVC - squeezed between 2 regular complexes.
Does not disturb underlying rhythm (rare)

☆ Compensatory pause - 2x distance of normal R-R
occurs with most PVCs (not PACs or PJCs)

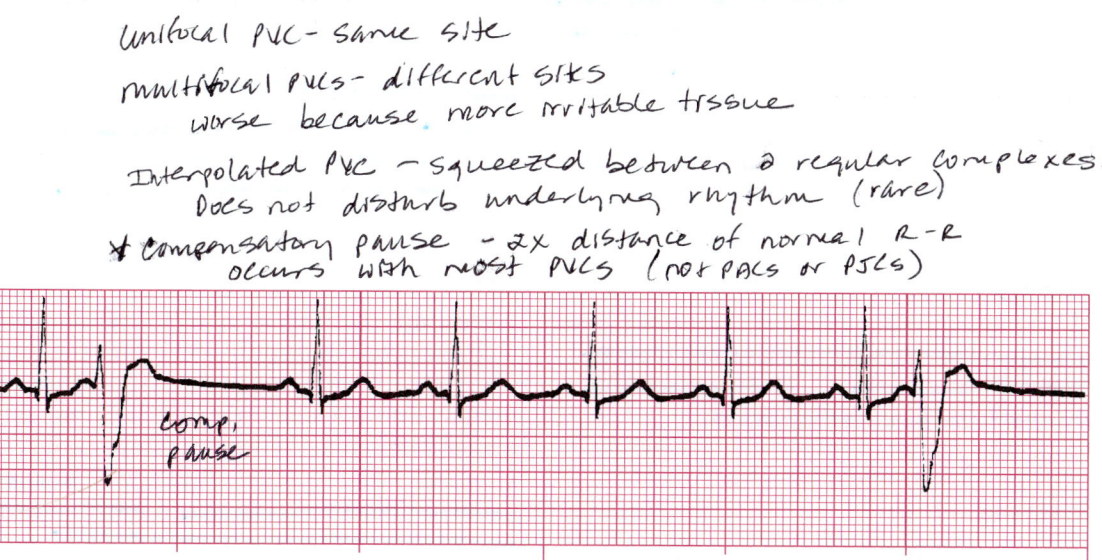

Figure 22-57 Sinus rhythm with two R-on-T premature ventricular complexes (PVCs).

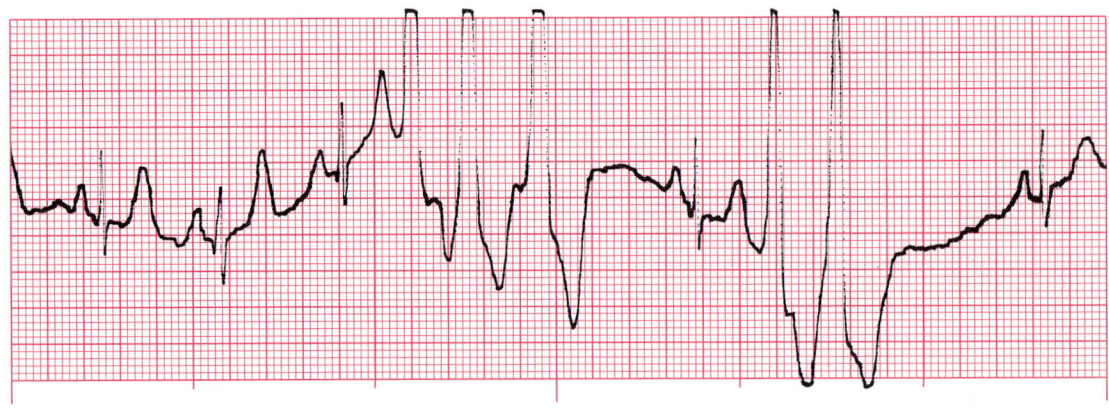

Figure 22-58 Sinus rhythm with a run of VT and one episode of couplets.

BOX 22-21	Common Causes of Premature Ventricular Complexes

- Normal variant
- Hypoxia
- Stress, anxiety
- Exercise
- Digitalis toxicity
- Acid-base imbalance
- Myocardial ischemia
- Electrolyte imbalance
- Heart failure
- Increased sympathetic tone
- ACS
- Stimulants (caffeine, tobacco) *cocaine*
- Medications (sympathomimetics, cyclic antidepressants, phenothiazines)

TABLE 22-28	Characteristics of PVCs
Rate	Usually within normal range but depends on underlying rhythm
Rhythm	Essentially regular with premature beats; if the PVC is an interpolated PVC, the rhythm will be regular
P waves	Usually absent or, with retrograde conduction to the atria, may appear after the QRS (usually upright in the ST segment or T wave)
PR interval	None with the PVC because the ectopic originates in the ventricles
QRS duration	Greater than 0.12 sec, wide and bizarre; T wave usually in opposite direction of the QRS complex

PVC, Premature ventricular complex.

PVCs. The appearance of couplets indicates the ventricular ectopic site is quite irritable. Three or more PVCs in a row at a rate of more than 100 beats/min is considered a salvo, run, or burst of ventricular tachycardia (Figure 22-58). *will go into V fib soon*

PVCs may or may not produce palpable pulses. Patients with PVCs may be asymptomatic or complain of palpitations, a "racing heart," skipped beats, or chest or neck discomfort. Common causes of PVCs are shown in Box 22-21. The general characteristics of PVCs are shown in Table 22-28. Treatment of PVCs depends on the cause, patient's signs and symptoms, and on the clinical situation. Most patients with PVCs do not require treatment with antiarrhythmic medications. Treatment of PVCs focuses on treatment of the underlying cause.

Ventricular Escape Beats or Rhythm

[OBJECTIVE 40]

Remember that premature beats are *early* and escape beats are *late*. To determine whether a complex is early or late, you must see at least two sinus beats in a row to establish the regularity of the underlying rhythm. Although ventricular escape beats share some of the same physical characteristics as PVCs (wide QRS complexes, T waves deflected in a direction opposite the QRS), they differ in some important areas. A PVC appears *early*, before the next expected sinus beat. PVCs often reflect irritability in some area of the ventricles. A ventricular escape beat occurs after a pause in which a supraventricular pacemaker failed to fire. Thus the escape beat is *late*, appearing after the next expected sinus beat. A ventricular escape beat is a *protective* mechanism. It protects the heart from more extreme slowing or even asystole. Because it is protective, you should not administer any medication that would wipe out the escape beat. An example of a ven-

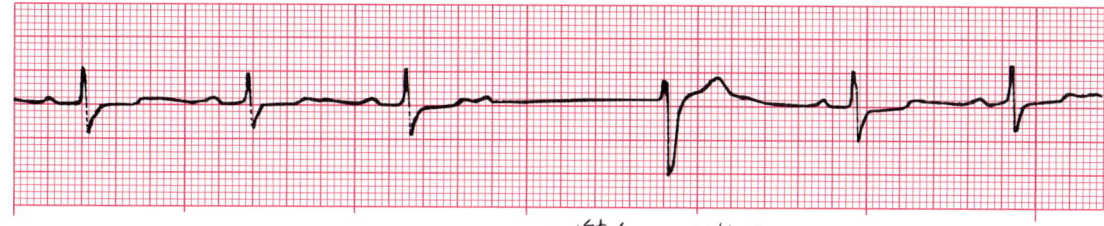

→ 1st degree AV block

Figure 22-59 Sinus rhythm with a prolonged PR interval and ST-segment depression. Note the ventricular escape beat following nonconducted premature atrial complex.

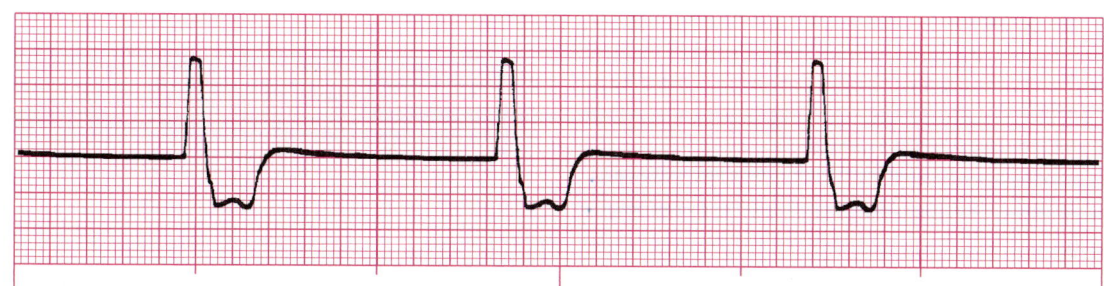

Figure 22-60 Idioventricular rhythm (IVR) at 35 beats/min.

may or may not have pulse

PEA - 5 Hs, 5Ts
H - hypotension, hypovolemia hypoglycemia
T - tension pneumo, tamponade

tricular escape beat is shown in Figure 22-59. The ECG characteristics of ventricular escape beats are shown in Table 22-29.

A ventricular escape or idioventricular rhythm (IVR) exists when three or more ventricular escape beats occur in a row at a rate of 20 to 40 beats/min. This rate is the built-in firing rate of the ventricles. The QRS complexes seen in IVR are wide and bizarre because the impulses begin in the ventricles, bypassing the normal conduction pathway. When the ventricular rate slows to a rate of less than 20 beats/min, some refer to the rhythm as an *agonal rhythm* or dying heart. IVR may occur when the following occur:

- The SA node and the AV junction fail to initiate an electrical impulse
- The rate of discharge of the SA node or AV junction becomes less than the intrinsic rate of the ventricles
- Impulses generated by a supraventricular pacemaker site are blocked

IVR also may occur because of MI, digitalis toxicity, or metabolic imbalances.

Because the ventricular rate associated with IVR is slow (20 to 40 beats/min) with a loss of atrial kick, the patient may have serious signs and symptoms because of decreased cardiac output. If the patient has a pulse and is symptomatic because of the slow rate, transcutaneous

pacing may be attempted. If the patient is not breathing and has no pulse despite the appearance of organized electrical activity on the cardiac monitor, a clinical situation called **pulseless electrical activity (PEA)** exists. An example of IVR is shown in Figure 22-60. The ECG characteristics of this rhythm are described in Table 22-30.

TABLE 22-29	Characteristics of Ventricular Escape Beats
Rate	Usually within normal range but depends on underlying rhythm
Rhythm	Essentially regular with late beats; the ventricular escape beat occurs *after* the next expected sinus beat
P waves	Usually absent or, with retrograde conduction to the atria, may appear after the QRS (usually upright in the ST segment or T wave)
PR interval	None with the ventricular escape beat because the ectopic beat originates in the ventricles
QRS duration	Greater than 0.12 sec, wide and bizarre; T wave frequently in opposite direction of the QRS complex

Accelerated Idioventricular Rhythm

An *accelerated idioventricular rhythm (AIVR)* exists when three or more ventricular escape beats occur in a row at a rate of 41 to 100 beats/min (Figure 22-61). Some cardiologists consider the upper end of the rate range to be approximately 120 beats/min. Because AIVR usually begins and ends gradually, it is also called nonparoxysmal VT. AIVR is usually considered a benign escape rhythm that appears when the sinus rate slows and disappears when the sinus rate speeds up. Episodes of AIVR usually last a few seconds to a minute.

AIVR is often seen during the first 12 hours of MI. It is particularly common after successful reperfusion therapy. AIVR generally requires no treatment because the rhythm is protective and often transient, spontaneously resolving on its own. However, possible dizziness, lightheadedness, or other signs of hemodynamic compromise may occur because of the loss of atrial kick. Atropine may be ordered in an attempt to block the vagus nerve and stimulate the SA node to overdrive the ventricular rhythm. The ECG characteristics of AIVR are shown in Table 22-31.

TABLE 22-30	Characteristics of IVR
Rate	20-40 beats/min
Rhythm	Essentially regular
P waves	Usually absent or, with retrograde conduction to the atria, may appear after the QRS (usually upright in the ST segment or T wave)
PR interval	None
QRS duration	Greater than 0.12 second; T wave frequently in opposite direction of the QRS complex

IVR, Idioventricular rhythm.

TABLE 22-31	Characteristics of Accelerated Idioventricular Rhythm
Rate	41-100 beats/min
Rhythm	Essentially regular
P waves	Usually absent or, with retrograde conduction to the atria, may appear after the QRS (usually upright in the ST segment or T wave)
PR interval	None
QRS duration	Greater than 0.12 sec; T wave frequently in opposite direction of the QRS complex

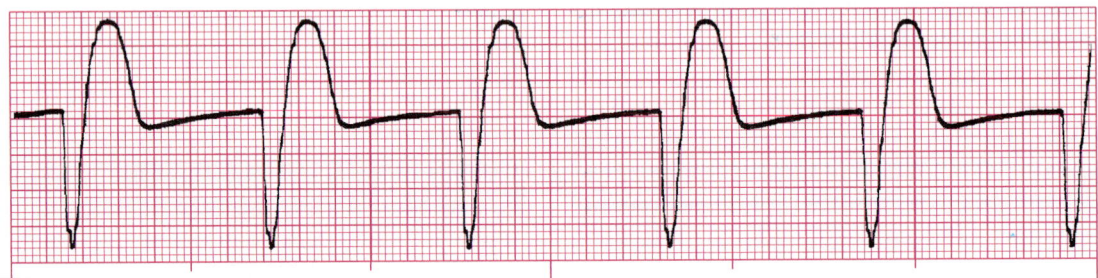

Figure 22-61 Accelerated idioventricular rhythm at 56 beats/min.

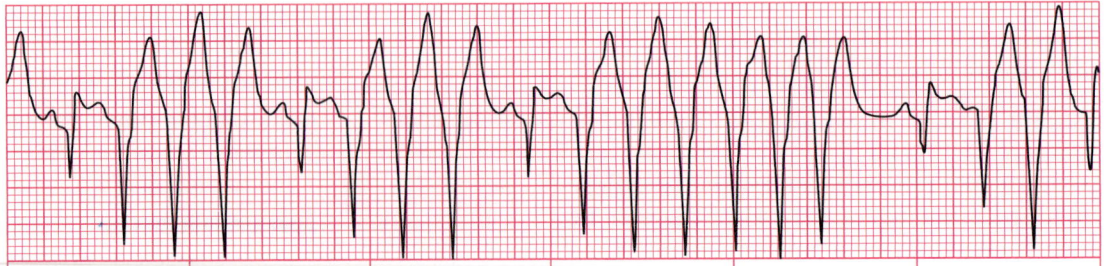

Figure 22-62 Nonsustained ventricular tachycardia.

Ventricular Tachycardia

Ventricular tachycardia (VT) exists when three or more PVCs occur in a row at a rate greater than 100 beats/min. If VT occurs as a short run lasting less than 30 seconds, it is called *nonsustained VT* (Figure 22-62). When VT persists for more than 30 seconds it is called *sustained VT*.

> **PARAMEDIC***Pearl*
>
> **Tachydysrhythmias: Too-Fast Rhythms**
>
> A tachycardia is present if a patient's heart rate is faster than the upper limit of normal for his or her age. Tachycardia may represent either a normal compensatory response to the need for increased cardiac output or oxygen delivery or an unstable dysrhythmia.
>
> Three types of tachycardia generally are seen in children: sinus tachycardia, SVT, and VT with a pulse. Sinus tachycardia is the most common of these rhythms.

Monomorphic Ventricular Tachycardia

[OBJECTIVE 41]

VTs, like PVCs, may originate from an ectopic focus in either ventricle. When the QRS complexes of VT are of the same shape and amplitude, the rhythm is called *monomorphic VT* (Figure 22-63). Monomorphic VT with a ventricular rate greater than 200 beats/min is called *ventricular flutter* by some cardiologists. Sustained monomorphic VT is often associated with underlying heart disease, particularly myocardial ischemia. It rarely occurs in patients without underlying heart disease. The ECG characteristics of monomorphic VT are shown in Table 22-32.

Common causes of VT include the following:

- Acute coronary syndromes
- Cardiomyopathy
- Tricyclic antidepressant overdose
- Digitalis toxicity
- Valvular heart disease
- Cocaine abuse

TABLE 22-32	Characteristics of Monomorphic Ventricular Tachycardia
Rate	101-250 beats/min *(usually 160-240)*
Rhythm	Essentially regular
P waves	May be present or absent; if present, they have no set relation to the QRS complexes appearing between the QRSs at a rate different from that of the VT
PR interval	None
QRS duration	Greater than 0.12 sec; often difficult to differentiate between the QRS and T wave

- Mitral valve prolapse
- Acid-base imbalance
- Trauma (e.g., myocardial contusion, invasive cardiac procedures)
- Electrolyte imbalance (e.g., hypokalemia, hyperkalemia, hypomagnesemia)

Signs and symptoms associated with VT vary. VT may occur with or without pulses. The patient in sustained monomorphic VT may be stable for long periods. However, when the ventricular rate is quite fast or when myocardial ischemia is present, monomorphic VT can degenerate to polymorphic VT or ventricular fibrillation.

> **PARAMEDIC***Pearl*
>
> Signs and symptoms of hemodynamic instability related to VT may include the following:
>
> - Altered mental status
> - Shock
> - Chest pain
> - Hypotension
> - Shortness of breath
> - Pulmonary congestion

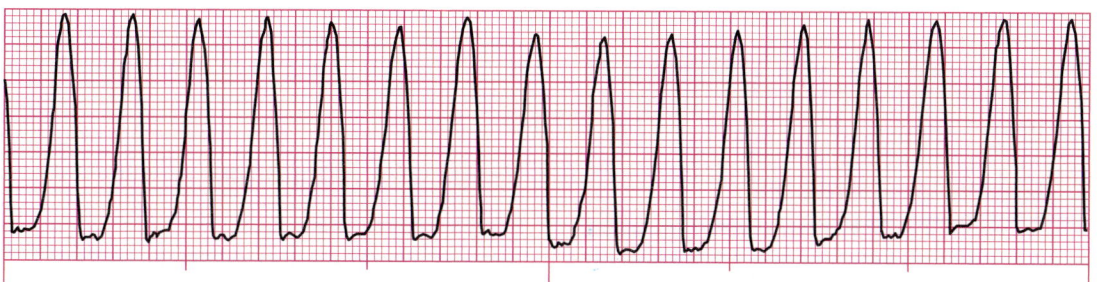

Figure 22-63 Monomorphic ventricular tachycardia (VT).

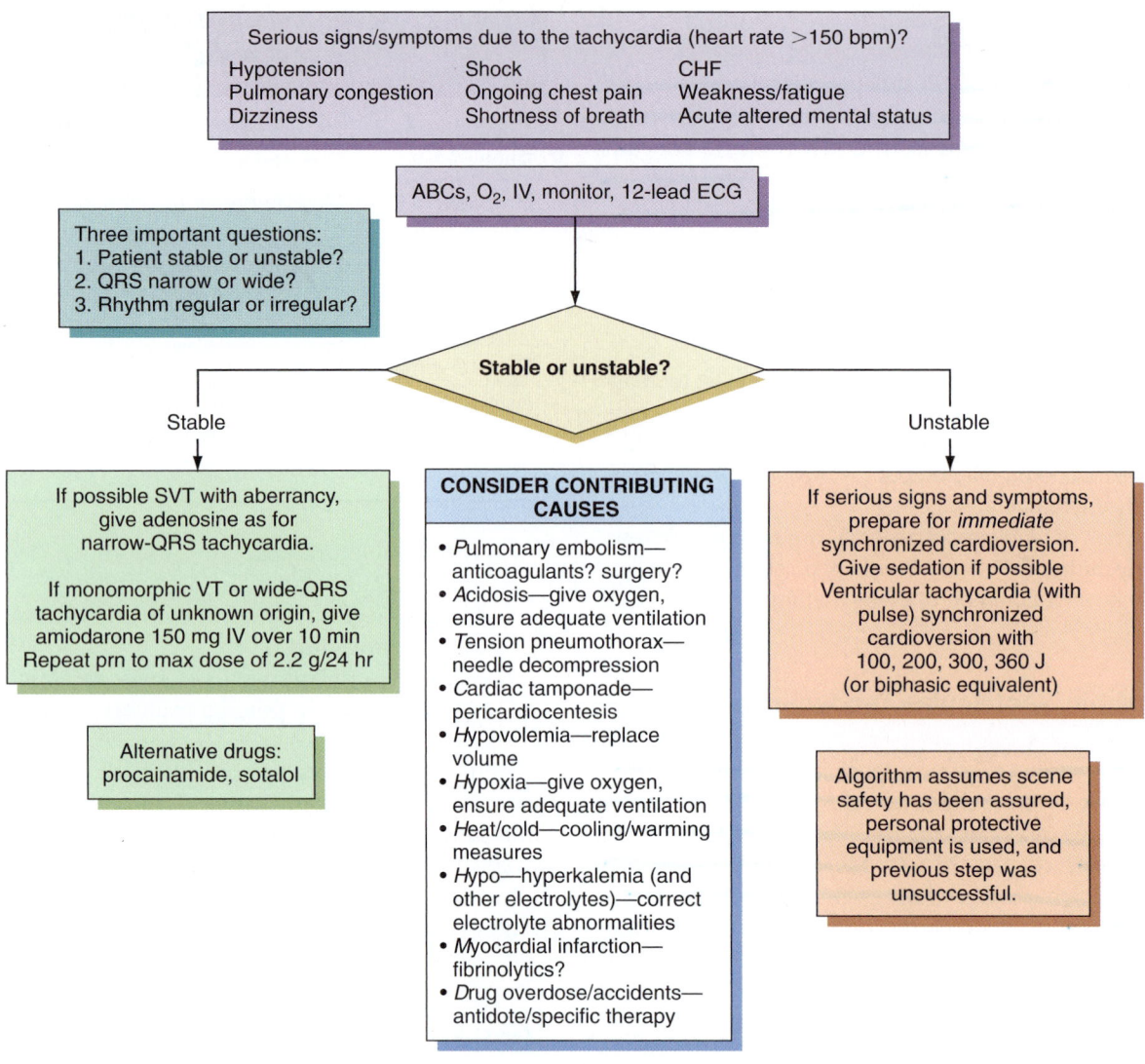

Figure 22-64 Wide QRS tachycardia treatment algorithm.

During VT, the severity of the patient's symptoms depend on how rapid the ventricular rate is, how long the tachycardia has been present, and the presence and extent of underlying heart disease. Treatment is based on the patient's signs, symptoms, and the type of VT (see Figures 22-50 and 22-64).

An SVT with an intraventricular conduction delay may be difficult to distinguish from VT. Keep in mind that VT is a potentially life-threatening dysrhythmia. If you are unsure whether a regular, wide-QRS tachycardia is VT or SVT with an intraventricular conduction delay, treat the rhythm as VT until proven otherwise. Obtaining a 12-lead ECG may help differentiate VT from SVT, but do not delay treatment if the patient is symptomatic.

Polymorphic Ventricular Tachycardia

When the QRS complexes of VT vary in shape and amplitude from beat to beat, the rhythm is called *polymorphic VT* (Figure 22-65). In polymorphic VT, the QRS complexes appear to twist from upright to negative or negative to upright and back. Polymorphic VT is divided into two classifications on the basis of its association with a normal or prolonged QT interval. Polymorphic VT that occurs in the presence of a long QT interval is called *torsades de pointes*. Torsades de pointes is French for "twisting of the points," which describes the QRS that changes in shape, amplitude, and width and appears to twist around the isoelectric line, resembling a spindle. Polymorphic VT that occurs in the presence of a normal QT interval is simply referred to as *polymorphic VT* or *polymorphic VT resembling torsades de pointes*. The ECG characteristics of polymorphic VT are shown in Table 22-33.

Ventricular Fibrillation

[OBJECTIVES 42, 43]

Ventricular fibrillation (VF) is a chaotic rhythm that begins in the ventricles. In VF, no organized depolarization of the ventricles occurs. The ventricular muscle

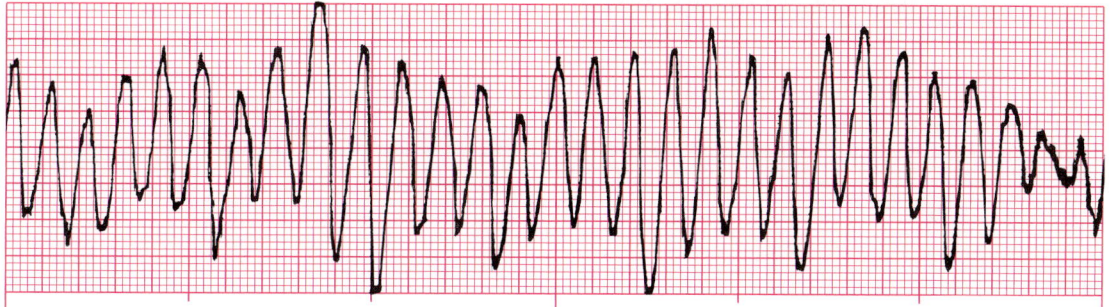

Figure 22-65 Polymorphic ventricular tachycardia. This rhythm strip is from a 77-year-old man 3 days after a myocardial infarction (MI). His chief complaint at the onset of this episode was chest pain. He had a medical history of a previous MI and an abdominal aortic aneurysm repair. The patient was given lidocaine and defibrillated several times without success. Lab work revealed a serum K+ level of 2.0. IV K+ was given and the patient converted to a sinus rhythm with the next defibrillation.

Like Cheyne Stokes resp.

Torsades de pointes

Drug of choice mg SO4 (national)

TABLE 22-33	Characteristics of Polymorphic Ventricular Tachycardia
Rate	150-300 beats/min, typically 200-250 beats/min
Rhythm	May be regular or irregular
P waves	None
PR interval	None
QRS duration	Greater than 0.12 sec; gradual alteration in amplitude and direction of the QRS complexes; a typical cycle consists of five to 20 QRS complexes

quivers. As a result, no effective myocardial contraction occurs. A patient who is unresponsive, not breathing, and has no pulse is in cardiopulmonary, or cardiac, arrest. Rhythms that may be seen in cardiac arrest include VT, VF, and asystole. PEA also may be observed.

In VF the ECG rhythm looks chaotic, with deflections that vary in shape and amplitude. No normal-looking waveforms are visible. VF with waves that are 3 mm or more high is called *coarse* VF (Figure 22-66). VF with low amplitude waves (less than 3 mm) is called **fine VF** (Figure 22-67).

> **PARAMEDIC***Pearl*
>
> Because artifact can mimic VF, *always* check the patient's pulse before beginning treatment for VF.

Factors that increase the susceptibility of the heart muscle to fibrillate include the following:

- Acute coronary syndromes
- Heart failure
- Dysrhythmias
- Vagal stimulation
- Electrolyte imbalance
- Antiarrhythmics and other medications
- Increased sympathetic nervous system activity
- Environmental factors (such as electrocution)
- Hypertrophy

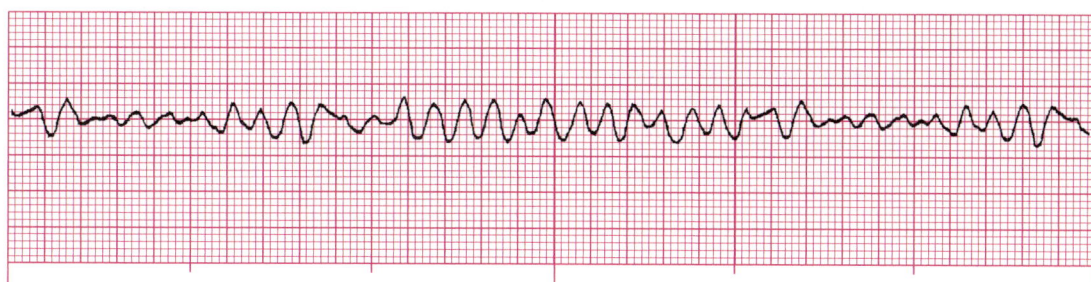

Figure 22-66 Coarse ventricular fibrillation.

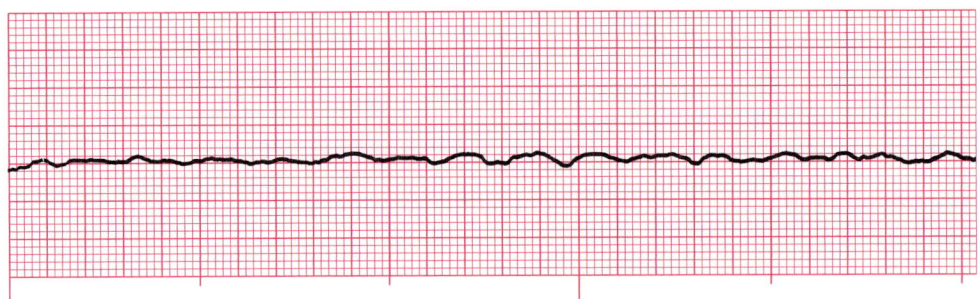

Figure 22-67 Fine ventricular fibrillation.

The ECG characteristics of VF are shown in Table 22-34. Current recommendations for the treatment of pulseless VT and VF are shown in Figure 22-68. Defibrillation is explained in Box 22-22 and shown in Skill 22-4.

TABLE 22-34	Characteristics of Ventricular Fibrillation
Rate	Cannot be determined because no waves or complexes are discernible to measure
Rhythm	Rapid and chaotic with no pattern or regularity
P waves	Not discernible
PR interval	Not discernible
QRS duration	Not discernible

PARAMEDIC*Pearl*

Absent or Pulseless Rhythms

In cardiopulmonary arrest, breathing and central pulses are absent and the patient is unresponsive. Absent or pulseless rhythms include the following:

- Pulseless VT, in which the ECG displays a wide QRS complex at a rate usually faster than 150 beats/min
- VF, in which irregular chaotic deflections that vary in shape and amplitude are observed on the ECG but no coordinated ventricular contraction occurs
- Asystole, in which no ventricular electrical activity is present
- PEA, in which electrical activity is visible on the ECG but c1entral pulses are absent

---

BOX 22-22	Electrical Therapy: Defibrillation

Defibrillation is delivery of an electrical current across the heart muscle over a brief period to terminate an abnormal heart rhythm. Defibrillation also is called unsynchronized countershock or asynchronous countershock because the delivery of current has no relation to the cardiac cycle. Indications for defibrillation include sustained polymorphic VT, pulseless VT, and VF.

Defibrillation does not "jump start" the heart. The shock attempts to deliver a uniform electrical current of sufficient intensity to depolarize ventricular cells (including fibrillating cells) at the same time, causing momentary asystole. This provides an opportunity for the heart's natural pacemakers to resume normal activity. When the cells repolarize, the pacemaker with the highest degree of automaticity should assume responsibility for pacing the heart.

VT, Ventricular tachycardia; *VF*, ventricular fibrillation.

PARAMEDIC*Pearl*

Factors Known to Affect Defibrillation Success
- Paddle or electrode size
- Paddle or electrode position
- Use of conductive material (when using hand-held paddles)
- Phase of patient's respiration
- Paddle pressure (when using hand-held paddles)
- Selected energy

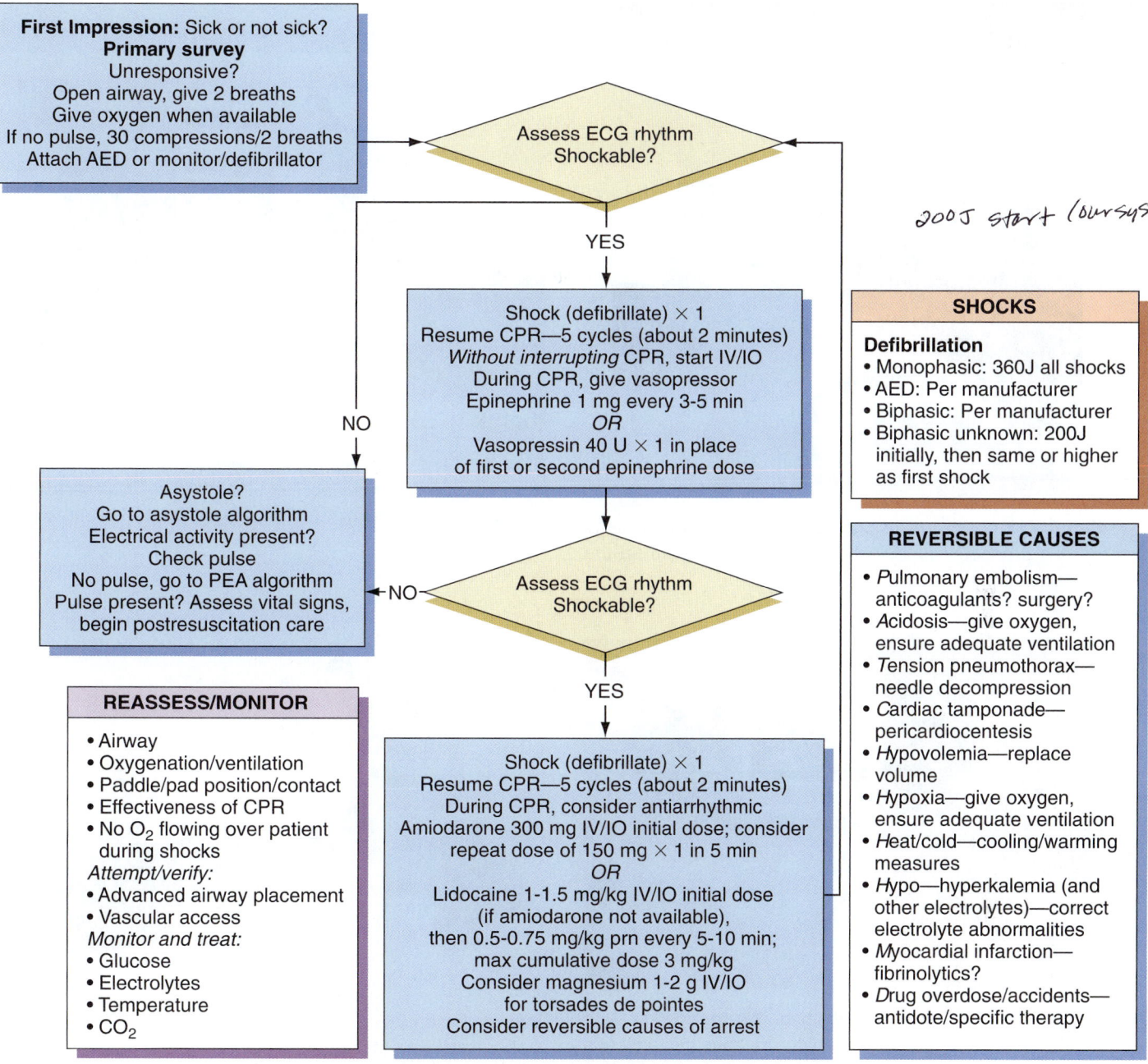

First Impression: Sick or not sick?
Primary survey
Unresponsive?
Open airway, give 2 breaths
Give oxygen when available
If no pulse, 30 compressions/2 breaths
Attach AED or monitor/defibrillator

Assess ECG rhythm
Shockable?

200J start (our system)

YES

Shock (defibrillate) × 1
Resume CPR—5 cycles (about 2 minutes)
Without interrupting CPR, start IV/IO
During CPR, give vasopressor
Epinephrine 1 mg every 3-5 min
OR
Vasopressin 40 U × 1 in place
of first or second epinephrine dose

SHOCKS

Defibrillation
• Monophasic: 360J all shocks
• AED: Per manufacturer
• Biphasic: Per manufacturer
• Biphasic unknown: 200J
  initially, then same or higher
  as first shock

NO

Asystole?
Go to asystole algorithm
Electrical activity present?
Check pulse
No pulse, go to PEA algorithm
Pulse present? Assess vital signs,
begin postresuscitation care

Assess ECG rhythm
Shockable?

NO

REVERSIBLE CAUSES
• *P*ulmonary embolism—
  anticoagulants? surgery?
• *A*cidosis—give oxygen,
  ensure adequate ventilation
• *T*ension pneumothorax—
  needle decompression
• *C*ardiac tamponade—
  pericardiocentesis
• *H*ypovolemia—replace
  volume
• *H*ypoxia—give oxygen,
  ensure adequate ventilation
• *H*eat/cold—cooling/warming
  measures
• *H*ypo—hyperkalemia (and
  other electrolytes)—correct
  electrolyte abnormalities
• *M*yocardial infarction—
  fibrinolytics?
• *D*rug overdose/accidents—
  antidote/specific therapy

YES

REASSESS/MONITOR

• Airway
• Oxygenation/ventilation
• Paddle/pad position/contact
• Effectiveness of CPR
• No O_2 flowing over patient
  during shocks
Attempt/verify:
• Advanced airway placement
• Vascular access
Monitor and treat:
• Glucose
• Electrolytes
• Temperature
• CO_2

Shock (defibrillate) × 1
Resume CPR—5 cycles (about 2 minutes)
During CPR, consider antiarrhythmic
Amiodarone 300 mg IV/IO initial dose; consider
repeat dose of 150 mg × 1 in 5 min
OR
Lidocaine 1-1.5 mg/kg IV/IO initial dose
(if amiodarone not available),
then 0.5-0.75 mg/kg prn every 5-10 min;
max cumulative dose 3 mg/kg
Consider magnesium 1-2 g IV/IO
for torsades de pointes
Consider reversible causes of arrest

Algorithm assumes scene safety has been assured, personal protective
equipment is used, no signs of obvious death or presence
of do not resuscitate order, and previous step was unsuccessful

Figure 22-68 Pulseless ventricular tachycardia/fibrillation (VT/VF) treatment algorithm. *PEA*,
Pulseless electrical activity.

SKILL 22-4 DEFIBRILLATION

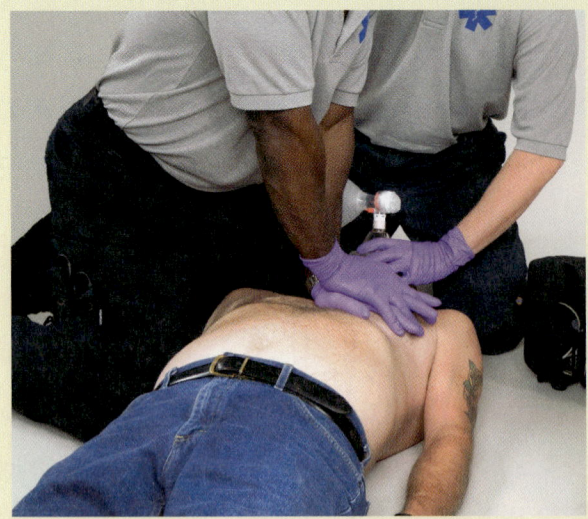

Step 1 Take appropriate standard precautions and verify that the procedure is indicated. Identify the rhythm on the cardiac monitor.

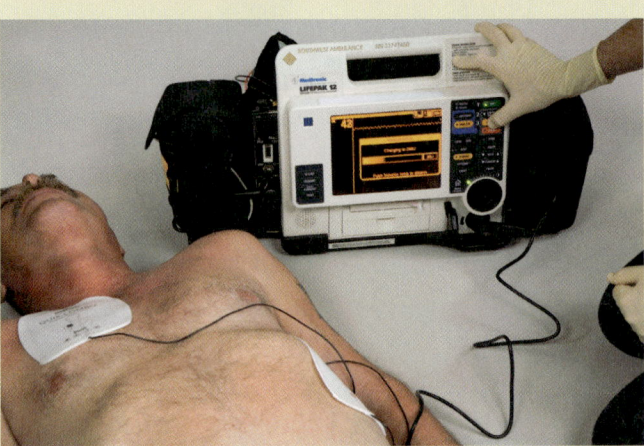

Step 3 Charge the defibrillator. Because oxygen flow over the patient's chest during electrical therapy increases the risk of spark or fire, make sure oxygen is not flowing over the patient's chest.

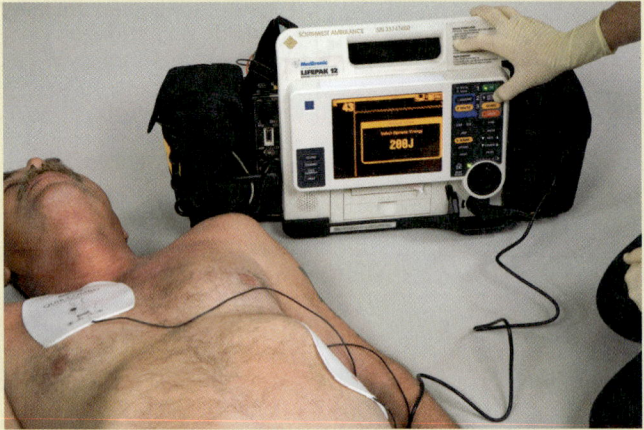

Step 2 Remove clothing from the patient's upper body. With gloves, remove NTG paste or patches from the patient's chest if present and quickly wipe away any medication residue. Do not apply alcohol, tincture of benzoin, or antiperspirant to the skin.

If using multipurpose adhesive electrodes, place them in proper position on the patient's bare chest. If excessive hair is present in the areas where the paddles or electrodes will be placed, quickly check to see if you have two pairs of adhesive electrodes available. If so, quickly apply and then immediately remove the first set of electrodes. This will remove some of the chest hair, allowing better contact when you apply the second set. If using standard paddles, you must use defibrillation gel or defibrillation gel pads between the paddle electrode surface and the patient's skin. Place pregelled defibrillator pads on the patient's chest (or apply defibrillator gel to the electrode surface of the paddles).

Once the pads are in place, recheck the ECG rhythm and then select the appropriate energy level.

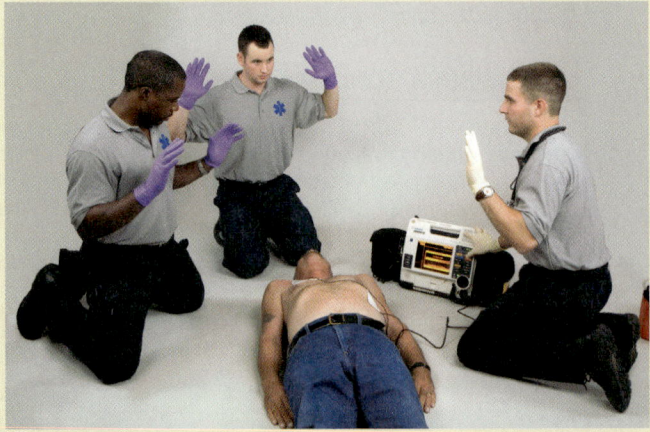

Step 4 If the ECG rhythm is unchanged, call "Clear!" and look around you. Make sure everyone is clear of the patient, bed, and any equipment connected to the patient. If CPR is in progress, all team members with the exception of the person performing chest compressions should immediately clear the patient. Once the defibrillator is charged, the chest compressor should clear the patient and a shock should immediately be delivered to the patient.

If the area is clear, press the shock control. If using standard paddles, depress the shock control on both paddles at the same time. Release the shock controls after the shock has been delivered. Resume CPR.

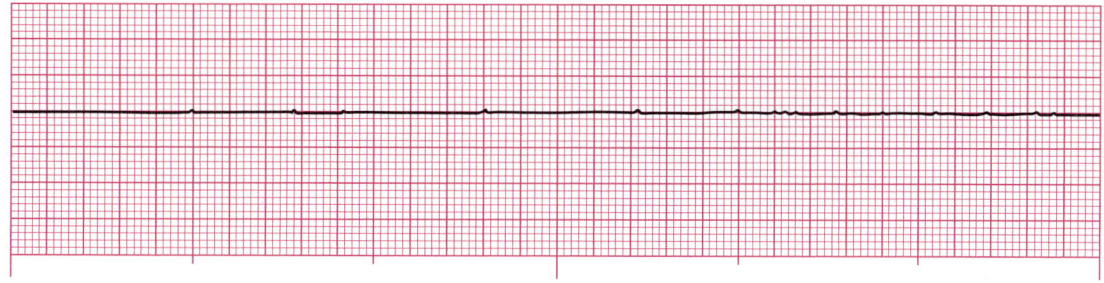

Figure 22-69 Asystole.

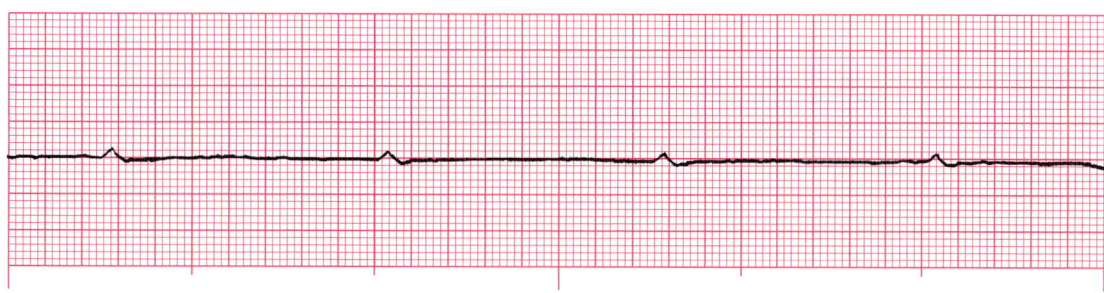

Figure 22-70 P-wave asystole (also known as ventricular standstill).

Asystole (Cardiac Standstill)

Asystole is a total absence of ventricular electrical activity (Figure 22-69). No ventricular rate or rhythm, pulse, or cardiac output is present. Some atrial electrical activity may be evident. If atrial electrical activity is present, the rhythm is called *P-wave asystole* (Figure 22-70). The causes of asystole are the same as those for PEA. In addition, ventricular asystole may temporarily occur after termination of a tachycardia with medications, defibrillation, or synchronized cardioversion. The ECG characteristics of asystole are shown in Table 22-35. Current recommendations for the treatment of asystole and PEA are shown in Figure 22-71.

TABLE 22-35	Characteristics of Asystole
Rate	Ventricular usually not discernible but atrial activity may be seen (P-wave asystole)
Rhythm	Ventricular not discernible, atrial may be discernible
P waves	Usually not discernible
PR interval	Not measurable
QRS duration	Absent

ATRIOVENTRICULAR BLOCKS

The AV junction is an area of specialized conduction tissue that provides the electrical links between the atrium and ventricle. If a delay or interruption in impulse conduction occurs within the AV node, bundle of His, or His-Purkinje system, the resulting dysrhythmia is called an **AV block** (Figure 22-72). The PR interval is the key to differentiating the type of AV block. The key to differentiating the level (location) of the block is the width of the QRS complex and, in second- and third-degree AV blocks, the rate of the escape rhythm.

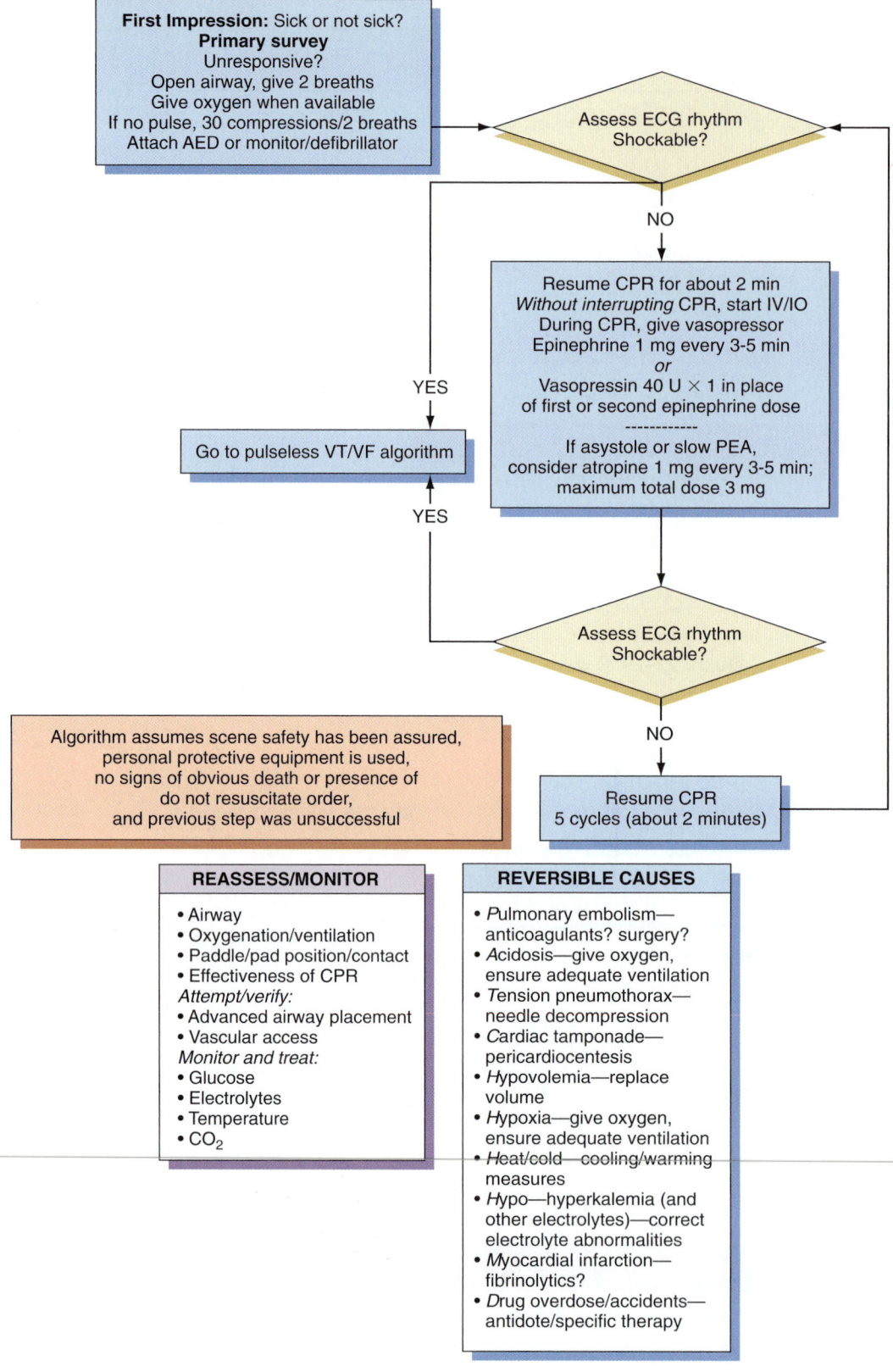

First Impression: Sick or not sick?
Primary survey
Unresponsive?
Open airway, give 2 breaths
Give oxygen when available
If no pulse, 30 compressions/2 breaths
Attach AED or monitor/defibrillator

Assess ECG rhythm
Shockable?

NO

Resume CPR for about 2 min
Without interrupting CPR, start IV/IO
During CPR, give vasopressor
Epinephrine 1 mg every 3-5 min
or
Vasopressin 40 U × 1 in place
of first or second epinephrine dose

If asystole or slow PEA,
consider atropine 1 mg every 3-5 min;
maximum total dose 3 mg

YES

Go to pulseless VT/VF algorithm

YES

Assess ECG rhythm
Shockable?

NO

Algorithm assumes scene safety has been assured,
personal protective equipment is used,
no signs of obvious death or presence of
do not resuscitate order,
and previous step was unsuccessful

Resume CPR
5 cycles (about 2 minutes)

REASSESS/MONITOR

- Airway
- Oxygenation/ventilation
- Paddle/pad position/contact
- Effectiveness of CPR
Attempt/verify:
- Advanced airway placement
- Vascular access
Monitor and treat:
- Glucose
- Electrolytes
- Temperature
- CO_2

REVERSIBLE CAUSES

- *P*ulmonary embolism—
anticoagulants? surgery?
- *A*cidosis—give oxygen,
ensure adequate ventilation
- *T*ension pneumothorax—
needle decompression
- *C*ardiac tamponade—
pericardiocentesis
- *H*ypovolemia—replace
volume
- *H*ypoxia—give oxygen,
ensure adequate ventilation
- *H*eat/cold—cooling/warming
measures
- *H*ypo—hyperkalemia (and
other electrolytes)—correct
electrolyte abnormalities
- *M*yocardial infarction—
fibrinolytics?
- *D*rug overdose/accidents—
antidote/specific therapy

Figure 22-71 Asystole/pulseless electrical activity (PEA) treatment algorithm.

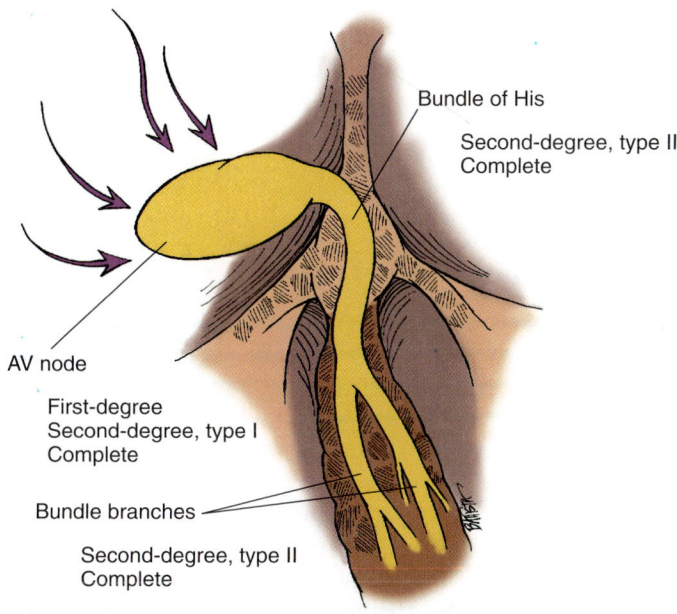

Figure 22-72 Locations of atrioventricular (AV) block.

First-Degree Block

[OBJECTIVE 44]

In first-degree AV block, all components of the ECG tracing usually are within normal limits except the PR interval. This is because electrical impulses travel normally from the SA node through the atria, but a delay in impulse conduction occurs, usually at the level of the AV node. This delay in AV conduction results in a PR interval that is longer than normal (more than 0.20 seconds in duration) and constant (Figure 22-73).

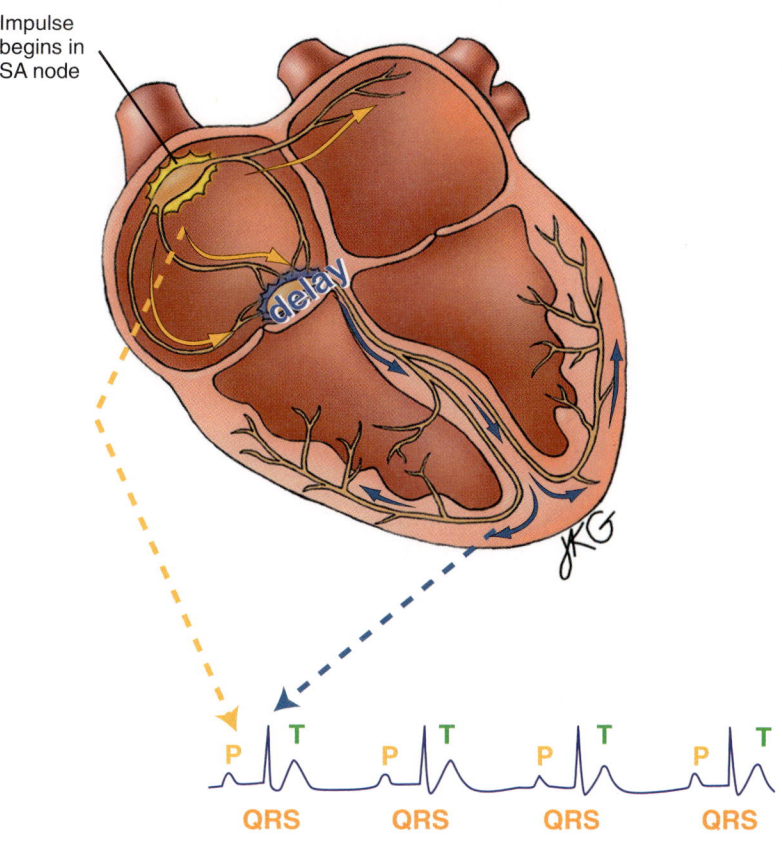

Figure 22-73 First-degree atrioventricular (AV) block. *SA,* Sinoatrial.

TABLE 22-36	Characteristics of First-Degree AV Block
Rate	Usually within normal range but depends on underlying rhythm
Rhythm	Regular
P waves	Normal in size and shape, one positive (upright) P wave before each QRS in leads II, III, and aVF
PR interval	Prolonged (Greater than 0.20 second) but constant
QRS duration	Usually 0.11 sec or less unless an intraventricular conduction delay exists

AV, Atrioventricular.

First-degree AV block may be a normal finding in individuals with no history of cardiac disease, especially in athletes. In some people mild prolongation of the PR interval may be normal, especially with sinus bradycardia during rest or sleep. First-degree AV block also may occur because of the following:

- Ischemia or injury to the AV node or junction
- Medications such as amiodarone, procainamide, beta-blockers
- Rheumatic heart disease
- Hyperkalemia
- Acute MI (often inferior wall MI)
- Increased vagal tone

The patient with a first-degree AV block often has no symptoms. First-degree AV block that occurs with acute MI should be closely monitored. The ECG characteristics of first-degree AV block are shown in Table 22-36.

Second-Degree Block, Type I (Wenckebach, Mobitz Type I)

Second-degree AV block type I is also known as *Mobitz type I* or *Wenckebach.* The Wenckebach pattern is the progressive lengthening of the PR interval followed by a P wave with no QRS complex. The conduction delay in second-degree AV block type I usually occurs at the level of the AV node. Remember that the RCA supplies the AV node in approximately 90% of the population. Thus RCA occlusions are associated with AV block occurring in the AV node.

The patient with this type of AV block is usually asymptomatic because the ventricular rate often remains nearly normal and cardiac output is not significantly affected. If the heart rate is slow and serious signs and symptoms occur because of the slow rate, atropine and/or transcutaneous pacing should be considered. When this rhythm occurs in conjunction with acute MI, the patient should be observed for increasing AV block. An example of this type of AV block is shown in Figure 22-74. ECG characteristics of second-degree AV block type I are shown in Table 22-37.

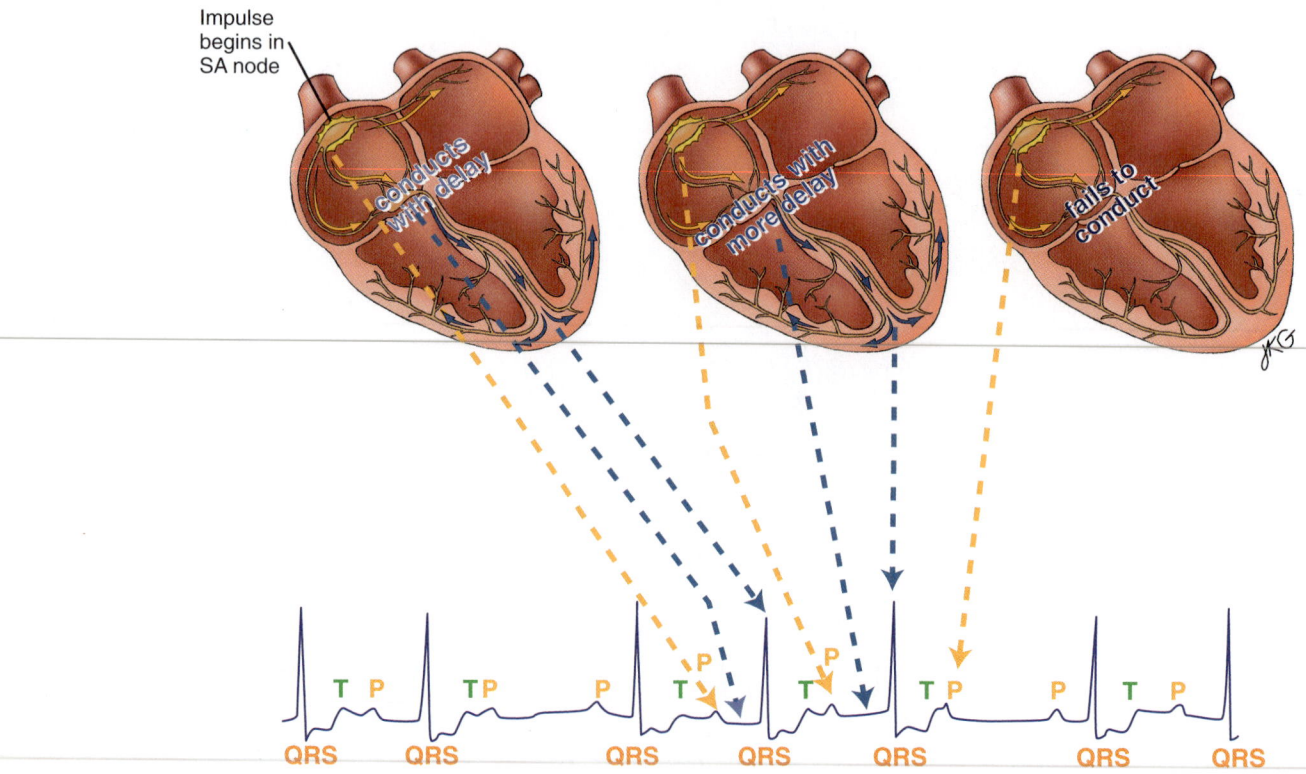

Figure 22-74 Second-degree atrioventricular (AV) block type I. *SA,* Sinoatrial.

TABLE 22-37	Characteristics of Second-Degree AV Block Type I
Rate	Atrial rate is greater than the ventricular rate
Rhythm	Atrial regular (P waves plot through on time); ventricular irregular
P waves	Normal in size and shape; some P waves are not followed by a QRS complex (more P waves than QRSs)
PR interval	Lengthens with each cycle (although lengthening may be very slight), until a P wave appears without a QRS complex; the PR interval *after* the nonconducted beat is shorter than the interval preceding the nonconducted beat
QRS duration	Usually 0.11 sec or less but is periodically dropped

AV, Atrioventricular.

Regularly Irregular

TABLE 22-38	Characteristics of Second-Degree AV Block Type II
Rate	Atrial rate is greater than the ventricular rate; ventricular rate often is slow
Rhythm	Atrial regular (P waves plot through on time), ventricular irregular
P waves	Normal in size and shape; some P waves are not followed by a QRS complex (more P waves than QRSs)
PR interval	Within normal limits or slightly prolonged but constant for the conducted beats; some shortening of the PR interval may follow a nonconducted P wave
QRS duration	Usually 0.11 sec or greater, periodically absent after P waves

AV, Atrioventricular.

Regularly Irregular

PARAMEDIC*Pearl*

AV blocks that occur in the AV node usually produce a narrow QRS complex (just as a junctional rhythm does), and an AV block in the bundle branches usually produces a wide QRS complex (just as a ventricular rhythm does). Although this rule is not absolute, it is another useful clue in determining the site of an AV block (Phalen & Aehlert, 2006).

Second-Degree Block, Type II (Mobitz Type II)

The conduction delay in second-degree AV block type II occurs below the AV node, either at the bundle of His or, more commonly, at the level of the bundle branches. This type of block is more serious than second-degree AV block type I and frequently progresses to third-degree AV block.

The bundle branches receive their primary blood supply from the left coronary artery. Thus disease of the left coronary artery or an anterior MI is usually associated with blocks that occur within the bundle branches. Second-degree AV block type II may also occur because of acute myocarditis or other types of organic heart disease. Second-degree AV block type II may rapidly progress to third-degree AV block without warning.

The patient's response to this rhythm is usually related to the ventricular rate. If the ventricular rate is within normal limits, the patient may be asymptomatic. More commonly, the ventricular rate is significantly slowed and serious signs and symptoms result because of the slow rate and decreased cardiac output. Preparations should be made for pacing when this rhythm is recognized. Avoid administering atropine. An example of second-degree AV block type II is shown in Figure 22-75. The ECG characteristics of second-degree AV block type II are shown in Table 22-38.

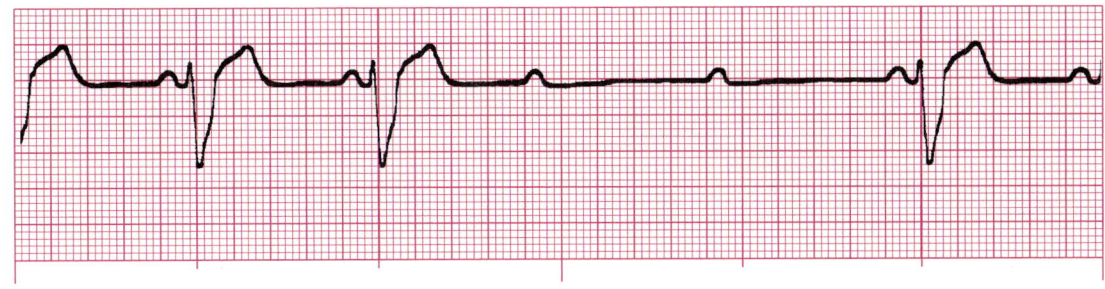

Figure 22-75 Second-degree atrioventricular block type II at 20 to 60 beats/min, ST-segment elevation.

P-R prolonged but constant

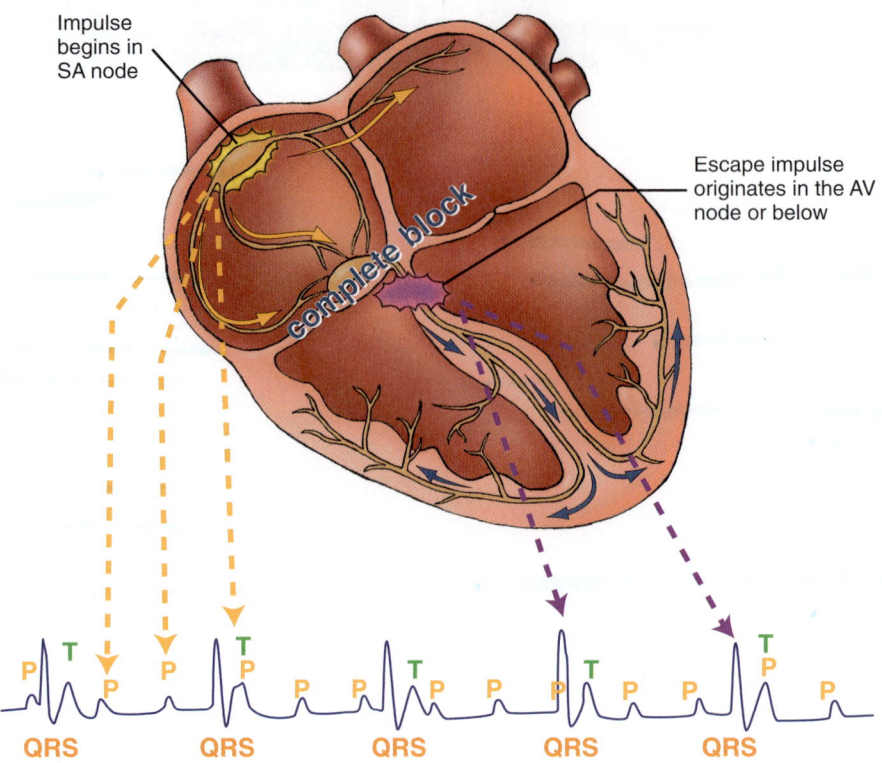

Figure 22-76 Third-degree atrioventricular (AV) block. *SA,* Sinoatrial.

Third-Degree Block

Second-degree AV blocks are types of incomplete blocks because the AV junction conducts at least some impulses to the ventricles. In third-degree AV block, impulses generated by the SA node are blocked before reaching the ventricles, so no P waves are conducted (Figure 22-76). The atria and ventricles beat independently of each other. Thus third-degree AV block is also called *complete* AV block. The block may occur at the AV node, bundle of His, or bundle branches. A secondary pacemaker (either junctional or ventricular) stimulates the ventricles; therefore the QRS may be narrow or wide, depending on the location of the escape pacemaker and the condition of the intraventricular conduction system.

Third-degree AV block associated with an inferior MI is thought to be the result of a block above the bundle of His. It often occurs after progression from first-degree AV block or second-degree AV block type I. The resulting rhythm is usually stable because the escape pacemaker is typically junctional (narrow QRS complexes), with a ventricular rate of more than 40 beats/min. Third-degree AV block associated with an anterior MI is usually preceded by second-degree AV block type II or an intraventricular conduction delay (right or left bundle branch block). The resulting rhythm is usually unstable because the escape pacemaker is typically ventricular (wide QRS complexes), with a ventricular rate of less than 40 beats/min.

complete block

TABLE 22-39	Characteristics of Third-Degree AV Block
Rate	Atrial rate is greater than the ventricular rate; ventricular rate determined by origin of the escape rhythm
Rhythm	Atrial regular (P waves plot through on time), ventricular regular; no relation between the atrial and ventricular rhythms
P waves	Normal in size and shape
PR interval	None; the atria and ventricles beat independently of each other, thus no true PR interval
QRS duration	Narrow or wide depending on the location of the escape pacemaker and the condition of the intraventricular conduction system; narrow = junctional pacemaker, wide = ventricular pacemaker

AV, Atrioventricular.

The patient's signs and symptoms depend on the origin of the escape pacemaker (junctional versus ventricular) and the patient's response to a slower ventricular rate (see Figure 22-33). The ECG characteristics of third-degree AV block are shown in Table 22-39.

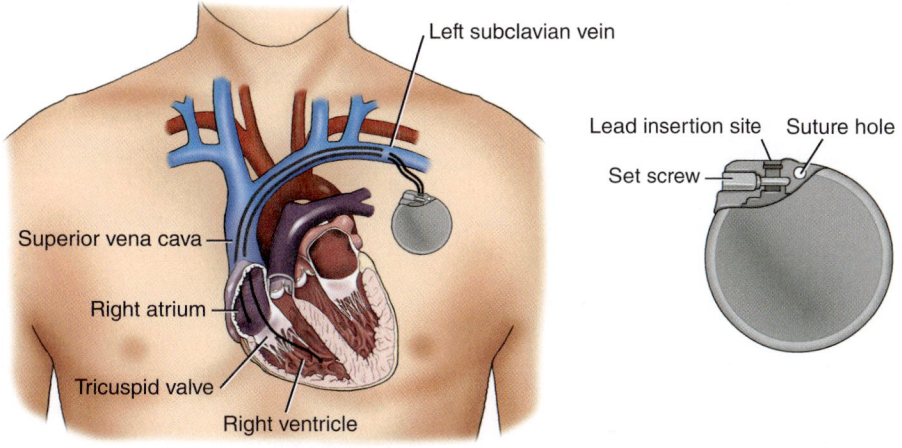

Dual Chamber Pacemaker

Figure 22-77 Permanent pacemaker.

Pace when symptomatic bradycardia unresponsive to atropine

PACEMAKER RHYTHMS

A **pacemaker** is an artificial pulse generator that delivers an electrical current to the heart to stimulate depolarization. Pacemaker systems are usually named according to where the electrodes are located and the route the electrical current takes to the heart. A pacemaker system consists of a pulse generator (power source) and pacing lead(s) (Figure 22-77). The pulse generator houses a battery and electronic circuitry. The circuitry works like a computer, converting energy from the battery into electrical pulses. A pacing lead is an insulated wire used to carry an electrical impulse from the pacemaker to the patient's heart. It also carries information about the heart's electrical activity back to the pacemaker. The exposed portion of the pacing lead is called an *electrode*, which is placed in direct contact with the heart.

Permanent Pacemakers

[OBJECTIVE 45]
A permanent pacemaker is implanted in the body, usually under local anesthesia. Pacemaker wires are surrounded by plastic catheters. The pacemaker's circuitry is housed in a hermetically sealed case made of titanium that is airtight and impermeable to fluid.

Temporary Pacemakers

Temporary pacing can be accomplished through transvenous, epicardial, or transcutaneous means.

- Transvenous pacemakers stimulate the endocardium of the right atrium or ventricle (or both) by an electrode introduced into a central vein, such as the subclavian or cephalic vein.

- Epicardial pacing is the placement of pacing leads directly onto or through the epicardium. Epicardial leads may be used when a patient is undergoing surgery and the outer surface of the heart is easy to reach. They are frequently used in neonates, children, and adolescents because of cardiac anatomy, small body size, and/or difficulty accessing the superior vena cava.

- Transcutaneous pacing delivers pacing impulses to the heart using electrodes placed on the patient's thorax. Transcutaneous pacing is also called *temporary external pacing* or *noninvasive pacing* and is covered later in this chapter.

Pacemaker Modes

Fixed-Rate (Asynchronous) Pacemakers

A **fixed-rate pacemaker** continuously discharges at a preset rate (usually 70 to 80 beats/min) regardless of the patient's heart rate. An advantage of the fixed-rate pacemaker is its simple circuitry, which reduces the risk of pacemaker failure. However, this type of pacemaker does not sense the patient's own cardiac rhythm. This may result in competition between the patient's cardiac rhythm and that of the pacemaker. VT or VF may be induced if the pacemaker were to fire during the T wave (vulnerable period) of a preceding patient beat. Fixed-rate pacemakers are not often used today.

Demand (Synchronous, Noncompetitive) Pacemakers

A **demand pacemaker** discharges only when the patient's heart rate drops below the pacemaker's preset (base) rate. For example, if the demand pacemaker was

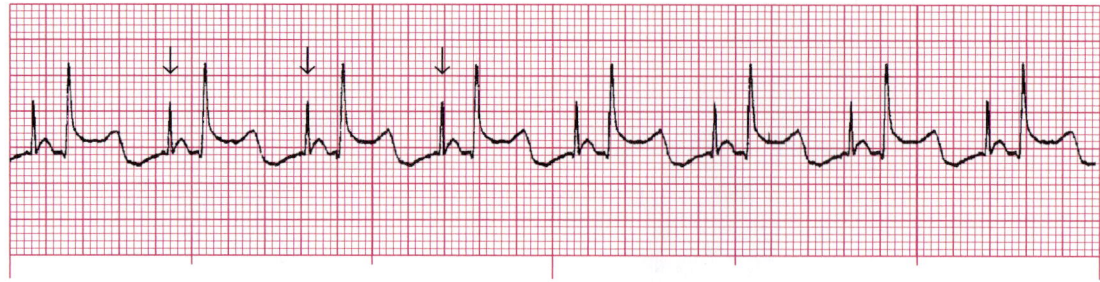

Figure 22-78 Atrial pacing.

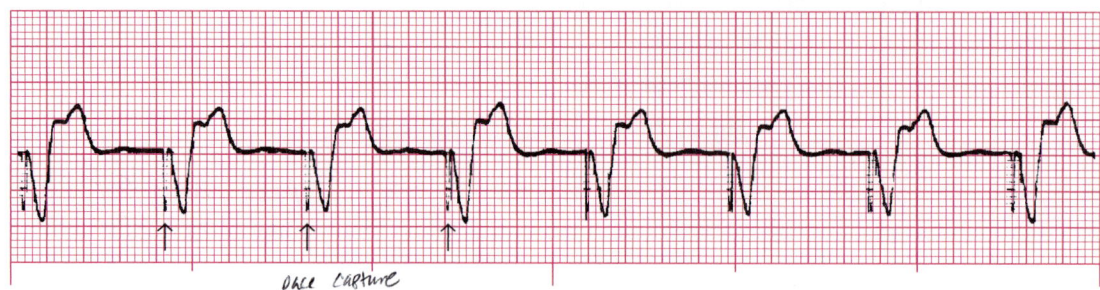

pace capture

Figure 22-79 Ventricular pacing.

preset at a rate of 70 impulses per minute, it would sense the patient's heart rate and allow electrical impulses to flow from the pacemaker through the pacing lead to stimulate the heart only when the rate fell below 70 beats/min. Demand pacemakers can be programmable or nonprogrammable. The voltage level and impulse rate are preset at the time of manufacture in nonprogrammable pacemakers.

Single-Chamber Pacemakers

A pacemaker that paces a single heart chamber (either the atrium or ventricle) has one lead placed in the heart. Atrial pacing is achieved by placing the pacing electrode in the right atrium. Stimulation of the atria produces a pacemaker spike on the ECG, followed by a P wave (Figure 22-78). Atrial pacing may be used when the SA node is diseased or damaged but conduction through the AV junction and ventricles is normal. This type of pacemaker is ineffective if an AV block develops because it cannot pace the ventricles.

Ventricular pacing is accomplished by placing the pacing electrode in the right ventricle. Stimulation of the ventricles produces a pacemaker spike on the ECG followed by a wide QRS, resembling a ventricular ectopic beat (Figure 22-79). The QRS complex is wide because a paced impulse does not follow the normal conduction pathway in the heart.

Dual-Chamber Pacemakers

A pacemaker that paces both the atrium and ventricle has a two-lead system placed in the heart; one lead is placed in the right atrium, the other in the right ventricle. This type of pacemaker is called a *dual-chamber pacemaker*. An **AV sequential pacemaker** is an example of a dual-chamber pacemaker. The AV sequential pacemaker stimulates the right atrium and right ventricle sequentially (stimulating first the atrium, then the ventricle), mimicking normal cardiac physiology and thus preserving the atrial contribution to ventricular filling (atrial kick) (Figure 22-80).

Implanted Pacemaker Malfunction

[OBJECTIVES 46, 47, 48]

Failure to Pace

Failure to pace is a pacemaker malfunction that occurs when the pacemaker fails to deliver an electrical stimulus or when it fails to deliver the correct number of electrical stimulations per minute. Failure to pace is recognized on the ECG as an absence of pacemaker spikes (even though the patient's intrinsic rate is less than that of the pacemaker) and a return of the underlying rhythm for which the pacemaker was implanted. Patient signs and symptoms may include syncope, chest pain, bradycardia, and hypotension.

Causes of failure to pace include battery failure, fracture of the pacing lead wire, displacement of the electrode tip, pulse generator failure, a broken or loose connection between the pacing lead and the pulse generator, electromagnetic interference, and/or the sensitivity setting set too high.

Treatment may include adjusting the sensitivity setting, replacing the pulse generator battery, replacing the pacing lead, replacing the pulse generator unit, tight-

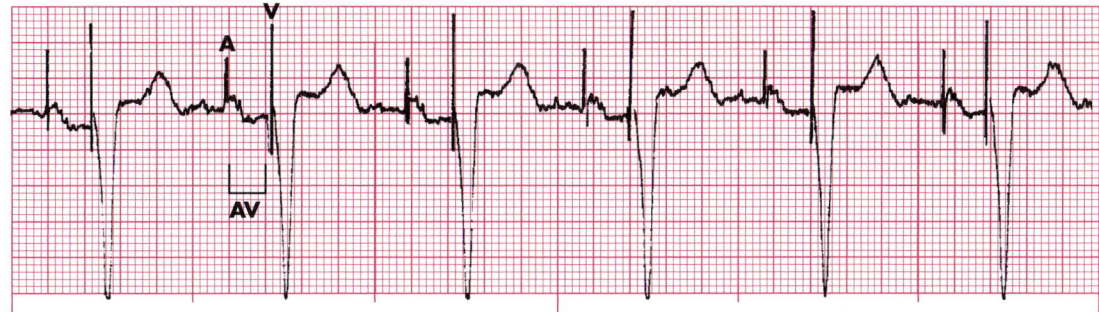

Figure 22-80 Atrioventricular sequential pacing. *A,* Atrial pacing; *V,* ventricular pacing; *AV,* AV interval.

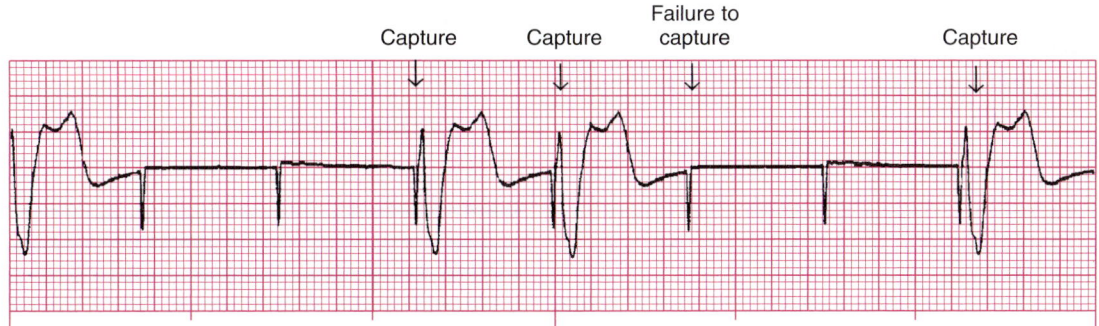

Figure 22-81 Failure to capture.

ening connections between the pacing lead and pulse generator, performing an electrical check, or removing the source of electromagnetic interference.

Failure to Capture

Capture is successful depolarization of the atria and/or ventricles by an artificial pacemaker. Failure to capture is the inability of the pacemaker stimulus to depolarize the myocardium. It is recognized on the ECG by visible pacemaker spikes not followed by P waves (atrial pacing) or QRS complexes (ventricular pacing) (Figure 22-81).

Causes of failure to capture include recent defibrillation, battery failure, fracture of the pacing lead wire, displacement of pacing lead wire (common cause), perforation of the myocardium by a lead wire, swelling or scar tissue formation at the electrode tip, or output energy (in milliamperes) set too low (a common cause). Treatment may include repositioning the patient, slowly increasing the output setting until capture occurs or the maximal setting is reached, replacing the pulse generator battery, replacing or repositioning of the pacing lead, or performing surgery.

Failure to Sense (Undersensing)

Sensitivity is the extent to which a pacemaker recognizes intrinsic electrical activity. Failure to sense occurs when the pacemaker fails to recognize the patient's ECG wave-forms (Figure 22-82). This pacemaker malfunction is recognized on the ECG by pacemaker spikes that follow too closely behind the patient's QRS complexes. Because pacemaker spikes occur when they should not, this type of pacemaker malfunction may result in pacemaker spikes that fall on T waves (R-on-T phenomenon) and/or competition between the pacemaker and the patient's own cardiac rhythm. The patient may complain of palpitations or skipped beats. R-on-T phenomenon may cause VT or VF.

Causes of failure to sense include battery failure, fracture of the pacing lead wire, displacement of the electrode tip (most common cause), loose connections, recent defibrillation, decreased P wave or QRS voltage, circuitry dysfunction (generator unable to process QRS signal), antiarrhythmic medications, and severe electrolyte disturbances. Treatment may include increasing the sensitivity setting, replacing the pulse generator battery, or replacing or repositioning the pacing lead.

Oversensing

Oversensing is a pacemaker malfunction that results from inappropriate sensing of unrelated electrical signals. Atrial sensing pacemakers may inappropriately sense ventricular activity; ventricular sensing pacemakers may misidentify a tall, peaked T wave as a QRS complex.

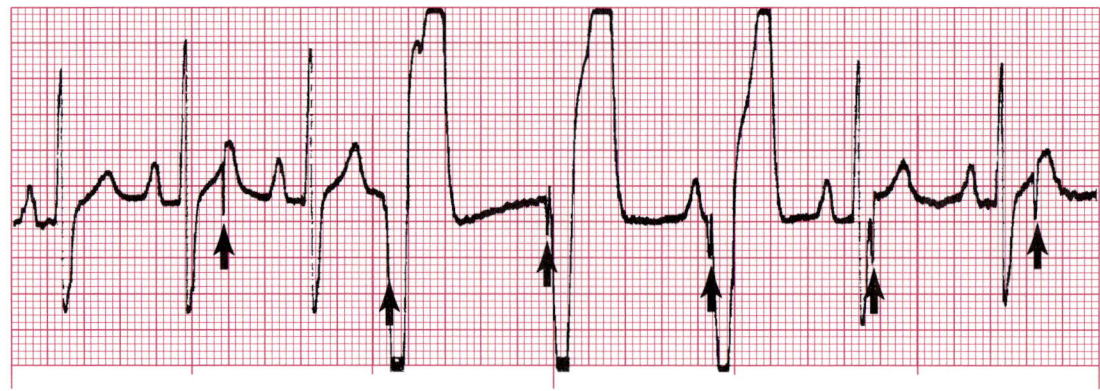

Figure 22-82 Failure to sense.

Oversensing is recognized on the ECG as pacemaker spikes at a rate slower than the pacemaker's preset rate or no paced beats even though the pacemaker's preset rate is greater than the patient's own rate.

The patient with a pacemaker should avoid strong electromagnetic fields such as those associated with welding equipment or a magnetic resonance imaging machine. Treatment includes adjustment of the pacemaker's sensitivity setting.

Pacemaker-Induced Tachycardia

Pacemaker-induced tachycardia is an uncommon pacer malfunction. It is seen in patients who have a dual-chamber pacemaker as the result of a PVC or depolarization that is conducted backward through the AV node to the atrium. This depolarizes the atrium before the next atrial-paced beat. The atrial depolarization is detected by the pacemaker. In response, the pacemaker generates a ventricular depolarization and paces the ventricle. The ventricular depolarization is conducted back to the atrium and the cycle self-perpetuates. Because of the increased rate, the patient may complain of a "racing heart," light-headedness, syncope, or chest discomfort. Treatment usually includes the application of a magnet over the device and reprogramming the pacemaker.

Pacemaker Artifact

[OBJECTIVE 49]

Do not rely on the cardiac monitor's heart rate display for an accurate reading when caring for a patient with an implanted pacemaker or when using a transcutaneous pacemaker. The cardiac monitor may not accurately count the patient's own QRS complexes or paced complexes during pacing. The cardiac monitor also may mistakenly count pacemaker artifact as beats and display an inaccurate heart rate.

Some newer monitors and defibrillators are equipped with an internal pacemaker pulse detector. When this handy feature is turned on, internal pacemaker pulses are identified by the machine with an arrow or similar mark. However, the machine can mistake ECG artifact as internal pacer pulses.

Transcutaneous Pacing

[OBJECTIVES 50, 51, 52, 53]

Transcutaneous pacing (TCP) is the use of electrical stimulation through pacing pads positioned on a patient's torso to stimulate contraction of the heart. Although TCP is a type of electrical therapy, the current delivered is considerably less than that used for cardioversion or defibrillation. The energy levels selected for cardioversion or defibrillation are indicated in joules. The stimulating current selected for TCP is measured in **milliamperes** (mA). The range of output current of a transcutaneous pacemaker varies depending on the manufacturer. For example, the range of output current for one brand of transcutaneous pacemaker is 0 to 140 mA. The range for another brand is 0 to 200 mA. Most transcutaneous pacemakers have a heart rate selection that ranges from 30 to 180 beats/min. You must be familiar with your equipment before you need to use it.

TCP requires attaching two pacing electrodes to the skin surface of the patient's outer chest wall. The pacing pads used during TCP function as a bipolar pacing system. The electrical signal exits from the negative terminal on the machine (and subsequently the negative electrode) and passes through the chest wall to the heart. Small or medium pediatric electrodes should be used for a child weighing less than 15 kg. Adult electrodes should be used for a child weighing more than 15 kg.

Indications

TCP is effective, quick, safe, and the least invasive pacing technique currently available. TCP is indicated for significant bradycardias unresponsive to atropine therapy or when atropine is not immediately available or indicated. It may also be used as a bridge until transvenous pacing can be accomplished or the cause of the bradycardia is reversed (as in cases of drug overdose or hyperkalemia). The steps to perform TCP are shown in Skill 22-5.

SKILL 22-5 TRANSCUTANEOUS PACING

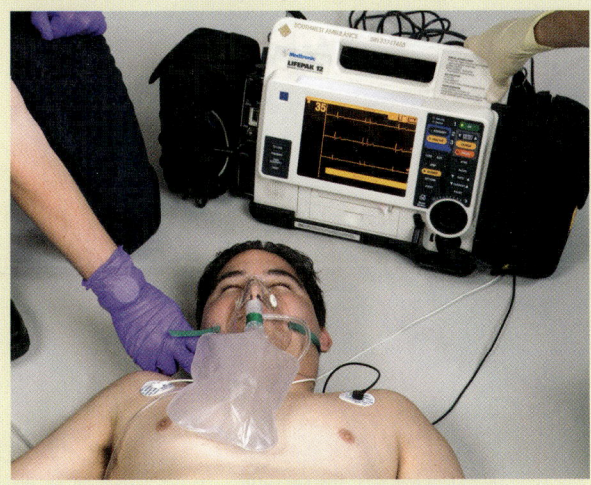

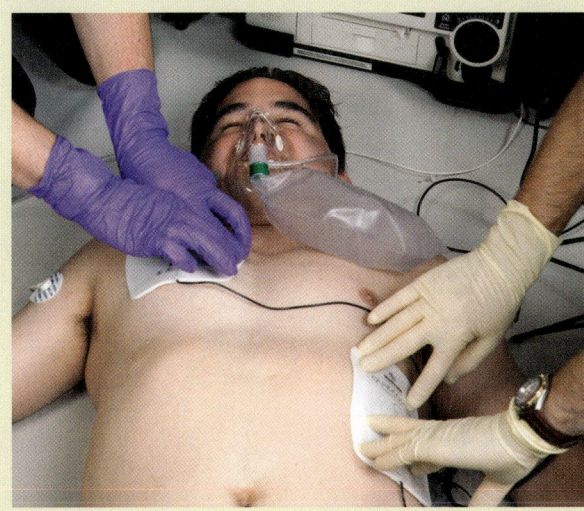

Step 1 Take appropriate standard precautions and verify that the procedure is indicated.

Place the patient on oxygen, assess the patient's vital signs, establish IV access, and apply ECG electrodes. Identify the rhythm on the cardiac monitor. Record a rhythm strip and verify the presence of a paceable rhythm. Continuous monitoring of the patient's ECG is *essential* throughout the procedure.

Step 2 Apply adhesive pacing pads to the patient according to the manufacturer's recommendations. Do not place the pads over open cuts, sores, or metal objects. The pacing pads should fit completely on the patient's chest; have a minimum of 1 to 2 inches of space between electrodes (pads); and not overlap bony areas of the sternum, spine, or scapula.

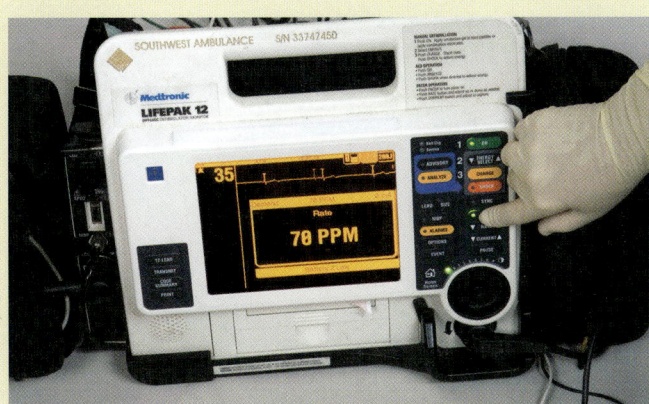

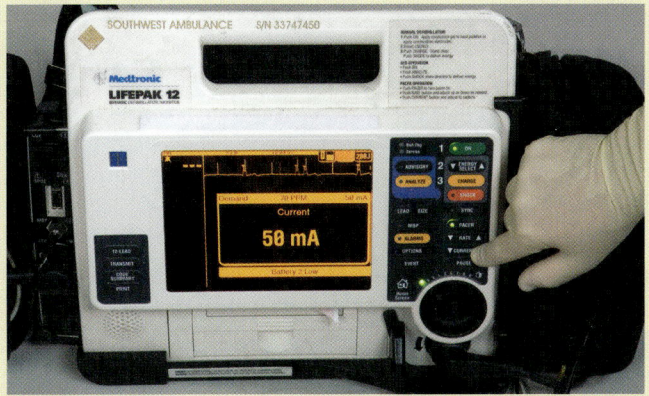

Step 3 Connect the pacing cable to the pacemaker and to the adhesive pads on the patient. Turn the power on to the pacemaker. Set the pacing rate to the desired number of paced pulses per minute (ppm). In an adult, set the initial rate at a nonbradycardic rate between 60 and 80 beats/min.

Step 4 After the rate has been regulated, start the pacemaker. Increase the stimulating current (output or milliamperes) until pacer spikes are visible before each QRS complex. Increase the current slowly but steadily until capture is achieved. Sedation or analgesia may be needed to minimize the discomfort associated with this procedure (common with currents of 50 mA or more). Give medications according to local protocol or medical direction instructions.

Continued

SKILL 22-5 TRANSCUTANEOUS PACING—continued

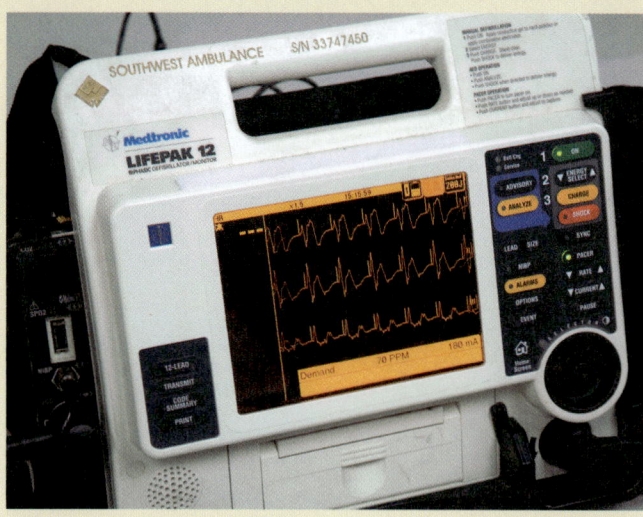

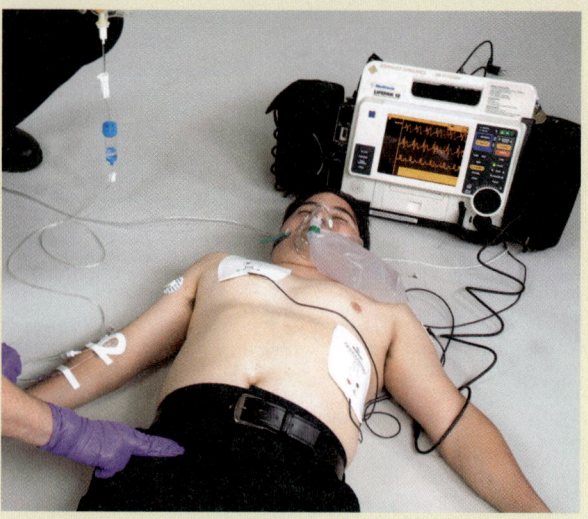

Step 5 Watch the cardiac monitor closely for *electrical* capture. This usually is seen by a wide QRS and broad T wave. In some patients electrical capture is less obvious—indicated only as a change in the shape of the QRS.

Step 6 Assess *mechanical* capture. Mechanical capture occurs when pacing produces a response that can be measured, such as a palpable pulse and blood pressure. Assess mechanical capture by assessing the patient's right upper extremity or right femoral pulses. Once capture is achieved, continue pacing at an output level slightly higher (approximately 2 mA) than the threshold of initial electrical capture. For example, if the monitor reveals 100% capture when you reached 80 mA, your final setting would be 82 mA.

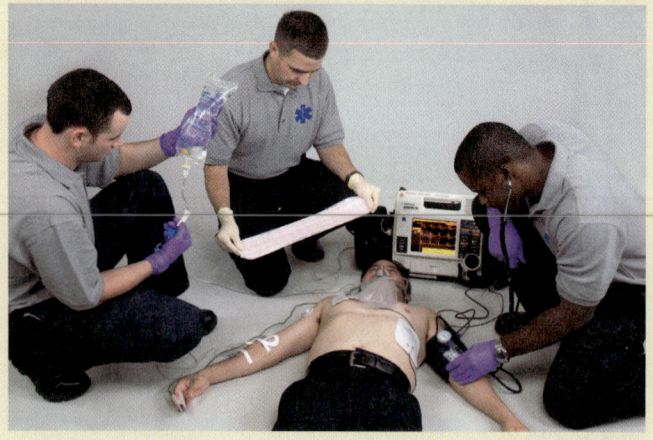

Step 7 Assess the patient's blood pressure, SpO$_2$, and level of responsiveness. Closely monitor the patient, including assessment of the skin for irritation where the pacing pads have been applied. Document and record the ECG rhythm. Documentation should include the date and time pacing was initiated (including baseline and pacing rhythm strips), the current required to obtain capture, the pacing rate selected, the patient's responses to electrical and mechanical capture, medications administered during the procedure, and the date and time pacing was terminated (if applicable).

Complications

[OBJECTIVE 54]

Complications of TCP include the following:

- Coughing
- Skin burns
- Interference with sensing from patient agitation or muscle contractions
- Pain from electrical stimulation of the skin and muscles
- Failure to recognize that the pacemaker is not capturing
- Failure to recognize the presence of underlying treatable VF
- Tissue damage, including third-degree burns (reported in pediatric patients with improper or prolonged TCP)
- When pacing is prolonged, pacing threshold changes, leading to capture failure

OVERVIEW OF THE 12-LEAD ECG

A standard 12-lead ECG provides views of the heart in both the frontal and horizontal planes and views the surfaces of the left ventricle from 12 different angles. Multiple views of the heart can provide useful information, including the following:

- Recognition of bundle branch blocks
- Identification of ST-segment and T-wave changes associated with myocardial ischemia, injury, and infarction
- Identification of ECG changes associated with certain medications and electrolyte imbalances

Indications

Indications for using a 12-lead ECG include the following:

- Chest pain or discomfort
- Assisting in dysrhythmia interpretation
- Right and/or left ventricular failure
- Status before and after electrical therapy (defibrillation, cardioversion, pacing)
- Syncope or near syncope
- Electrical injuries
- Stroke
- Known or suspected medication overdoses
- Known or suspected electrolyte imbalances

The procedures for standard chest lead placement, right chest lead placement, and posterior chest lead placement are shown in Skills 22-6 to 22-8.

Text continued on p. 817.

J point : where baseline stops going N↓S ↓ starts going E↑W (after QRS) [handwritten annotation]

SKILL 22-6   CHEST LEAD PLACEMENT

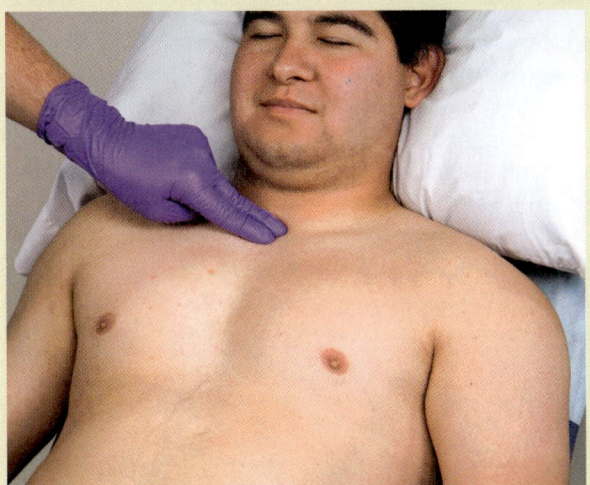

Step 1 An accurate 12-lead ECG requires correctly placing the electrodes. Begin positioning of the chest leads by placing your finger at the notch at the top of the sternum.

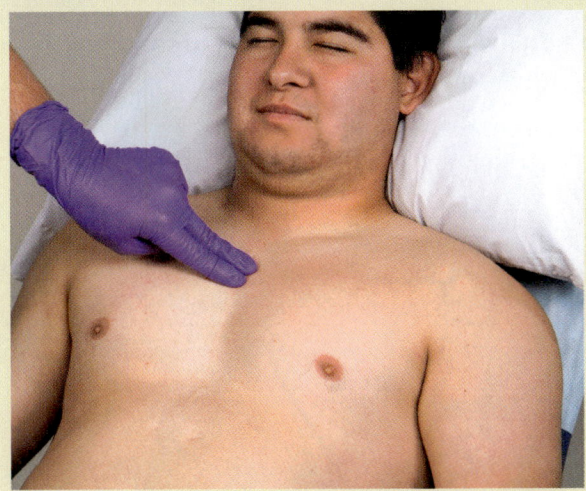

Step 2 Move your finger slowly downward until you feel a slight horizontal ridge or elevation. This is the angle of Louis (sternal angle), where the manubrium joins the body of the sternum.

Continued

SKILL 22-6 CHEST LEAD PLACEMENT—continued

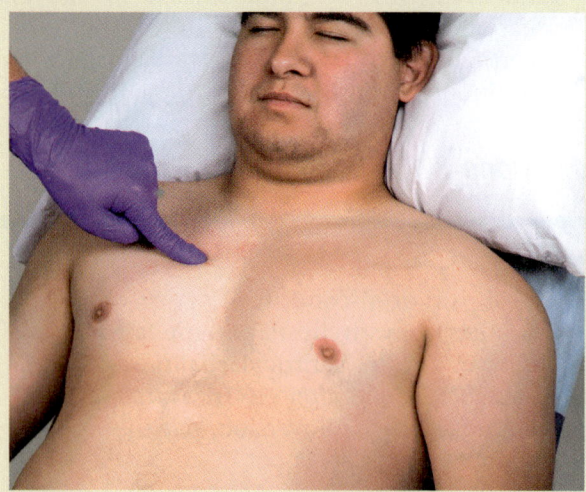

Step 3 Follow the angle of Louis to the patient's right until it articulates with the second rib.

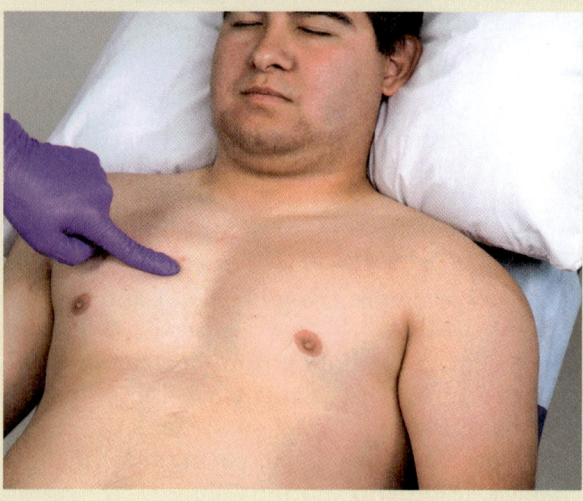

Step 4 Locate the second intercostal space (immediately below the second rib).

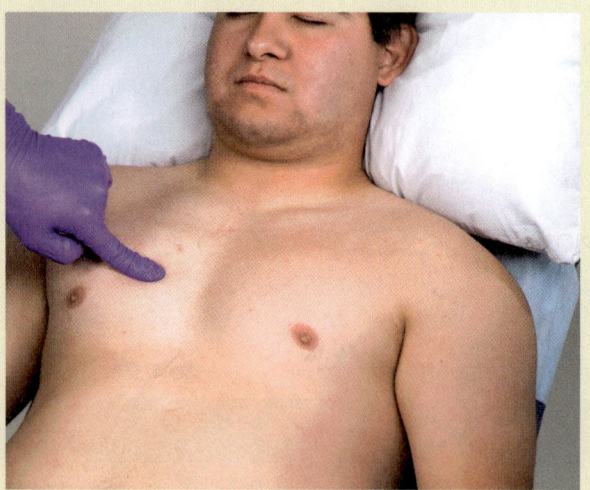

Step 5 From the second intercostal space, the third and fourth intercostal spaces can be found.

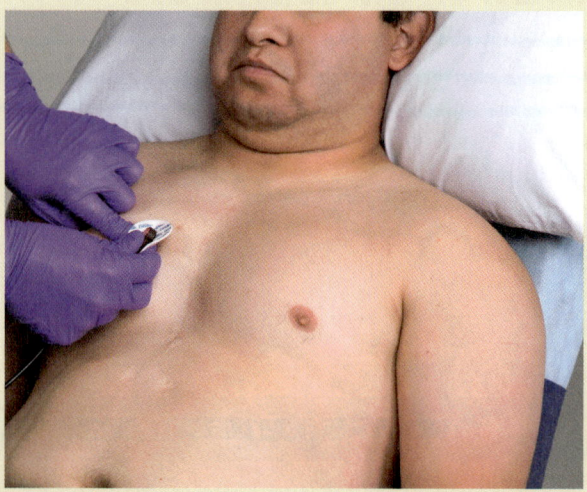

Step 6 V$_1$ is positioned in the fourth intercostal space just to the right of the sternum. Note: All the electrode positions refer to the location of the gel. For example, the gel of the V$_1$ electrode, not the entire adhesive patch, is positioned in the fourth intercostal space, just to the right of the sternum.

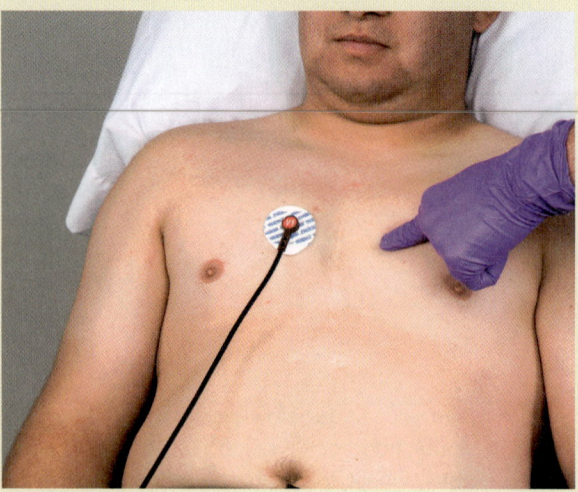

Step 7 From the V$_1$ position, find the corresponding intercostal space on the left side of the sternum.

SKILL 22-6   CHEST LEAD PLACEMENT—continued

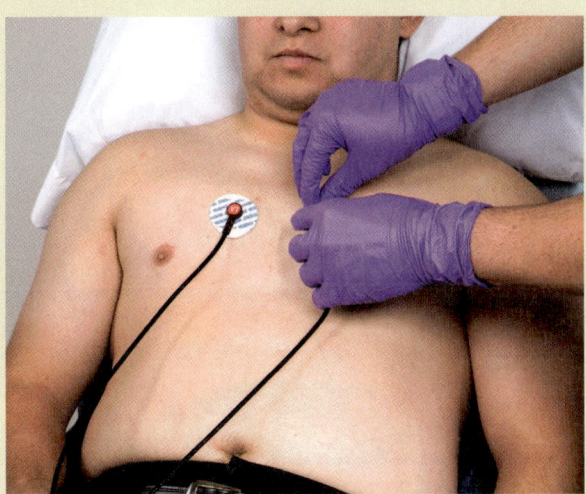

Step 8 Place the V₂ electrode in the fourth intercostal space just to the left of the sternum.

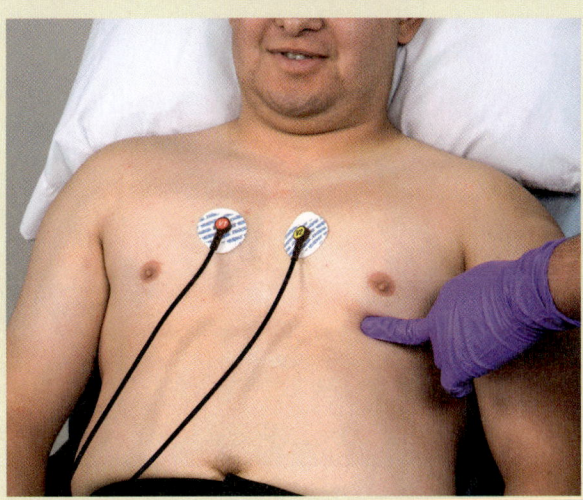

Step 9 From the V₂ position, locate the fifth intercostal space and follow it to the midclavicular line.

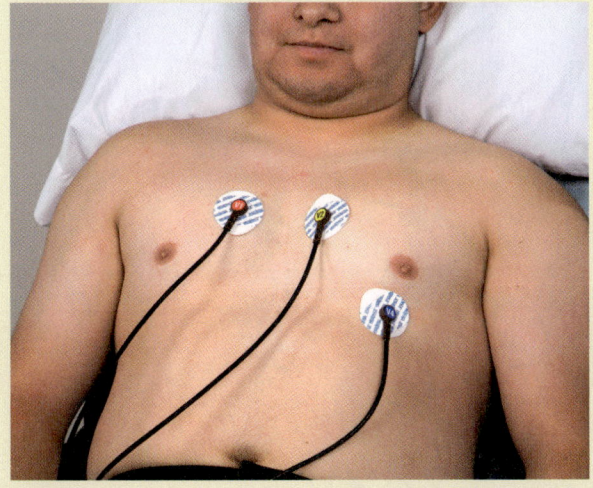

Step 10 Position the V₄ electrode in the fifth intercostal space in the midclavicular line.

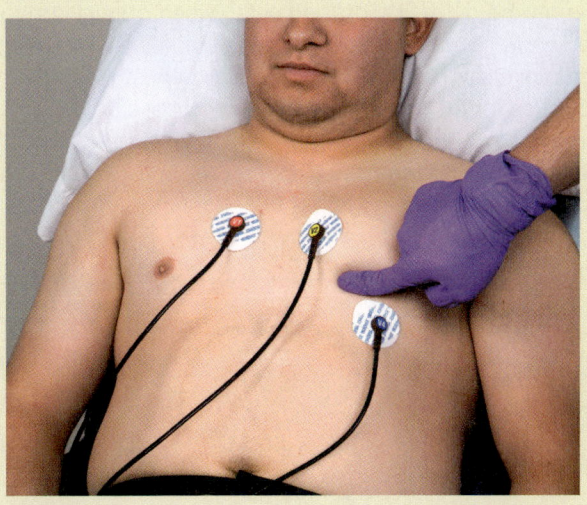

Step 11 V₃ is positioned halfway between V₂ and V₄.

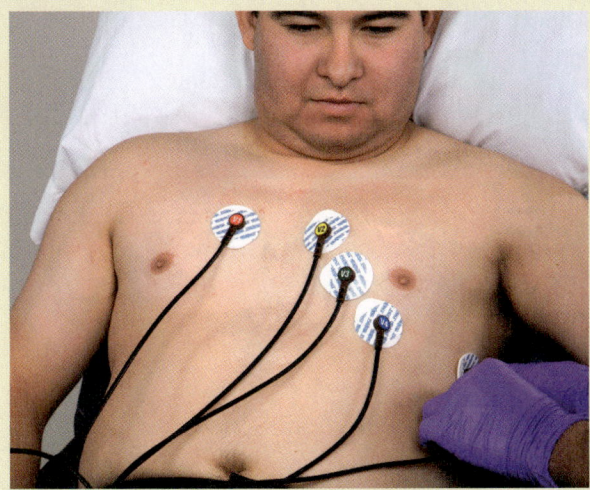

Step 12 V₆ is positioned in the midaxillary line, level with V₄.

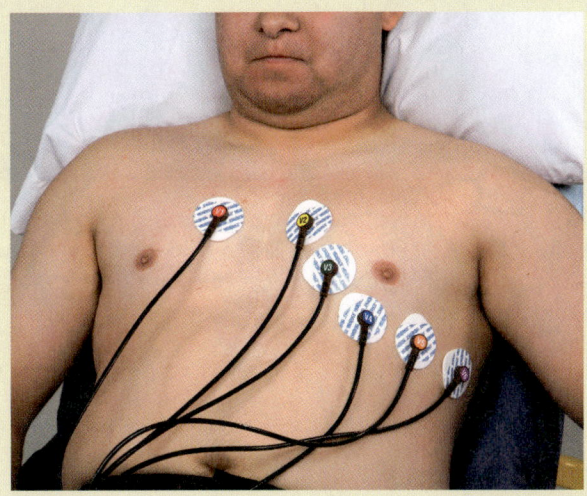

Step 13 V₅ is positioned in the anterior axillary line, level with V₄.

SKILL 22-7 RIGHT CHEST LEAD PLACEMENT

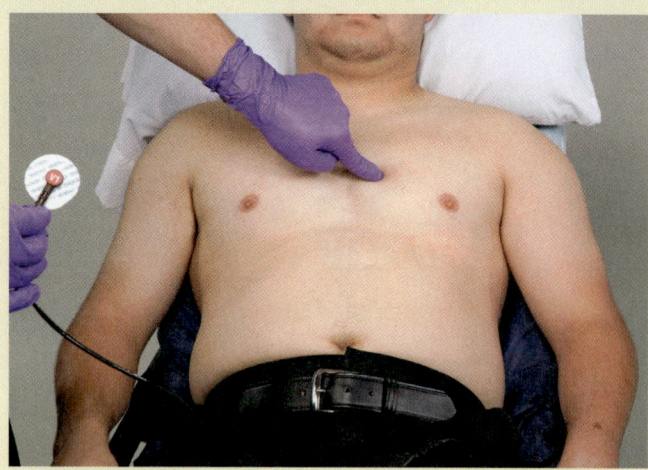

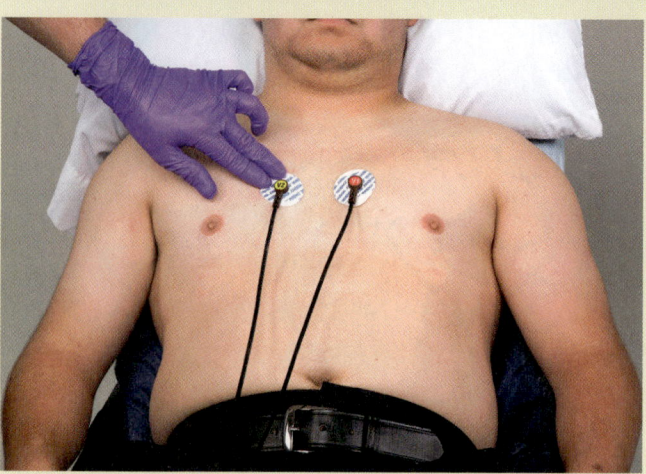

Step 1 A right-sided 12-lead ECG should be obtained when an RVI is suspected. Placement of right chest leads is identical to placement of the standard chest leads except it is done on the right side of the chest. When obtaining right-sided and/or posterior leads, obtain a standard 12-lead first. Then move the cables for the standard chest leads to the electrodes for the additional leads. Any chest lead cable can be moved to obtain the right and/or posterior leads.

Begin by placing the electrode for V_1R in the fourth intercostal space, just to the left of the sternum.

Step 2 From the V_1R position, find the corresponding intercostal space on the right side of the sternum. This is V_2R. Place the V_2R electrode in the fourth intercostal space, just to the right of the sternum.

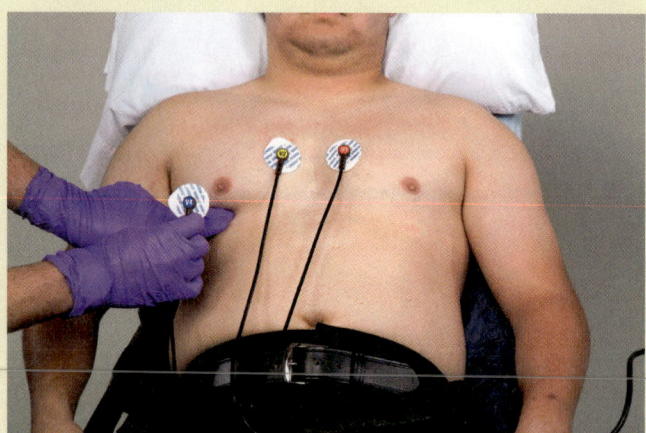

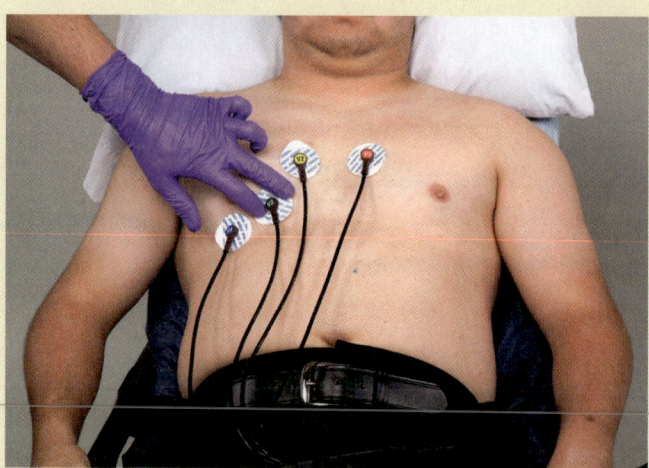

Step 3 From the V_2R position, move your fingers down, find the fifth intercostal space, and follow it to the midclavicular line. Place the V_4R electrode in the fifth intercostal space in the midclavicular line.

Step 4 Imagine a line between V_2R and V_4R. Position the V_3R electrode halfway between V_2R and V_4R on the imaginary line.

SKILL 22-7 RIGHT CHEST LEAD PLACEMENT—continued

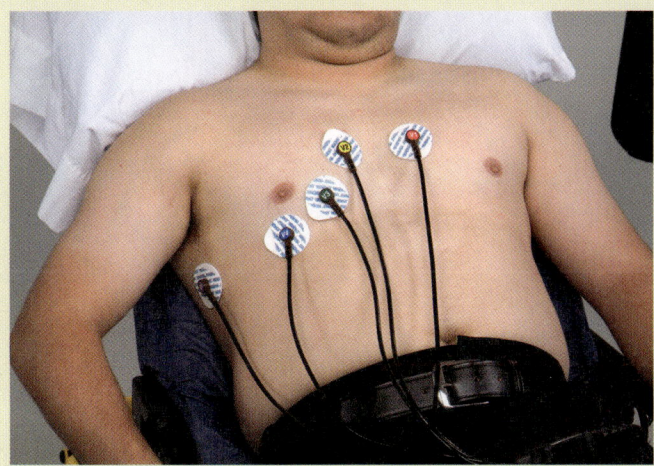

Step 5 The electrode for V_6R is positioned in the right midaxillary line, level with V_4R.

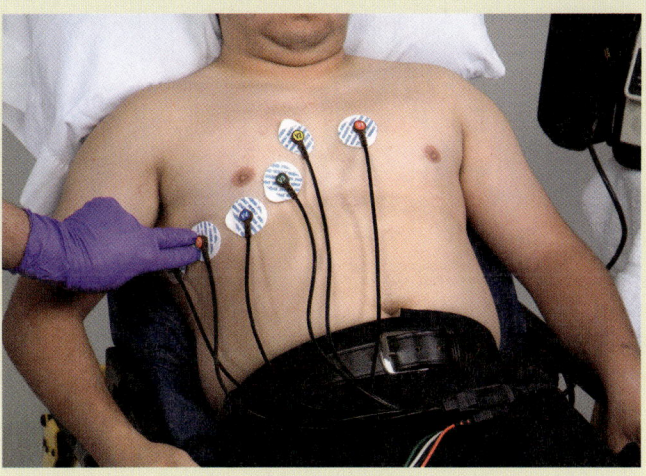

Step 6 Position V_5R in the right anterior axillary line, level with V_4R.

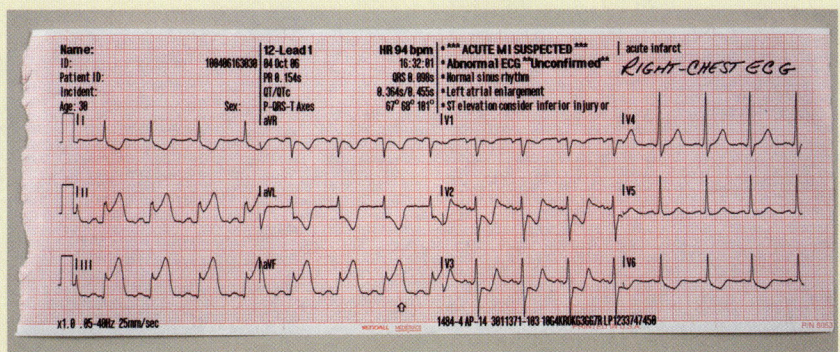

Step 7 Once these leads are printed, the correct lead must be handwritten onto the ECG to indicate the origin of the tracing. Clearly label the upper portion of the ECG tracing "right chest ECG." The computer-generated interpretation also must be disregarded in the event that the cables have been moved.

SKILL 22-8 POSTERIOR CHEST LEAD PLACEMENT

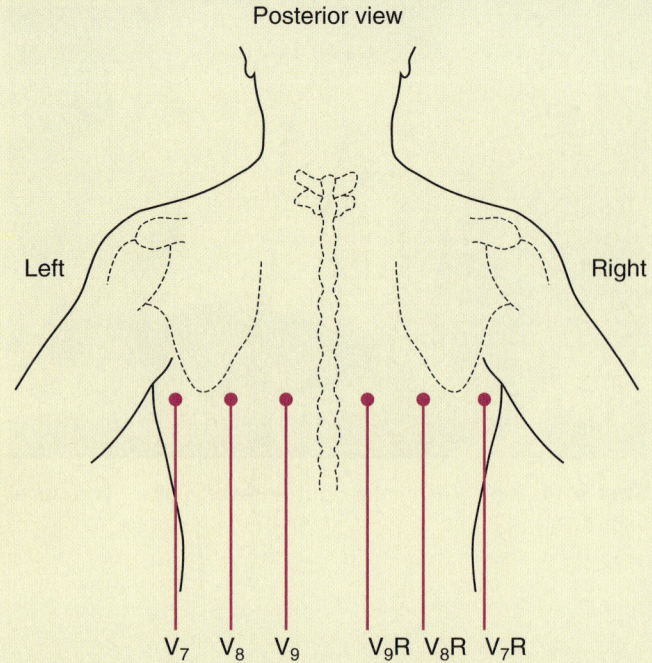

Posterior view

Left | Right

V₇ V₈ V₉ V₉R V₈R V₇R

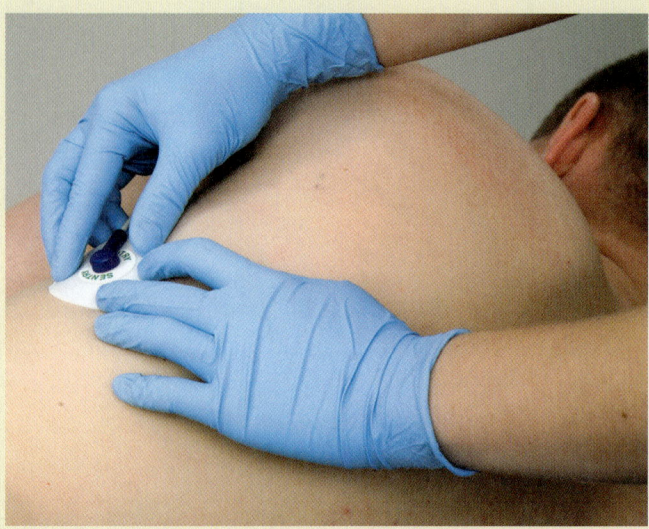

Step 1 Posterior chest leads are used when a posterior infarction is suspected. First obtain and print a standard 12-lead ECG. Then locate the landmarks for the posterior leads: posterior axillary line, midscapular line, and left border of the spine. Leads V_7, V_8, and V_9 are on the same horizontal line as leads V_4, V_5, and V_6 on the front of the chest.

Step 2 Position the patient on his or her side. Find the posterior axillary line. Now locate the fifth intercostal space and place the V_7 electrode. Attach the V_4 lead wire to the V_7 electrode.

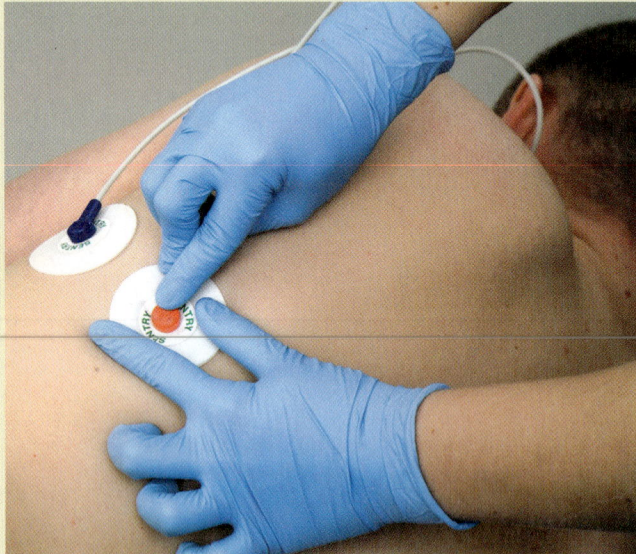

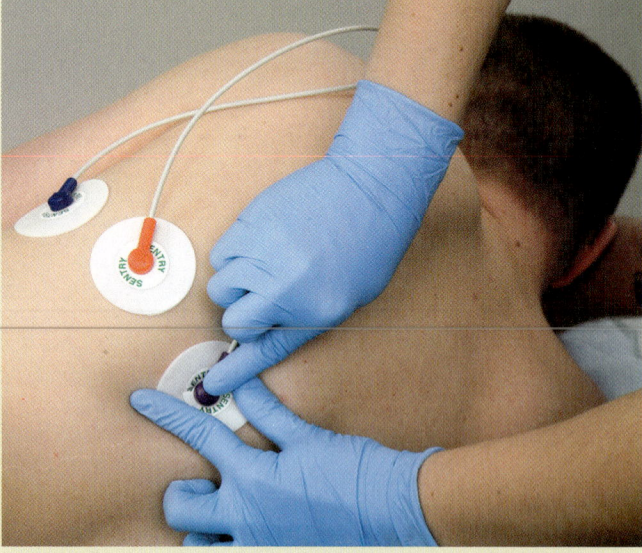

Step 3 Find the left midscapular line and fifth intercostal space. Place the V_8 electrode here. Attach the V_5 lead wire to the V_8 electrode.

Step 4 Place the electrode for V_9 just left of the spinal column at the fifth intercostal space. Attach the V_6 lead wire to the V_9 electrode.

SKILL 22-8 POSTERIOR CHEST LEAD PLACEMENT—continued

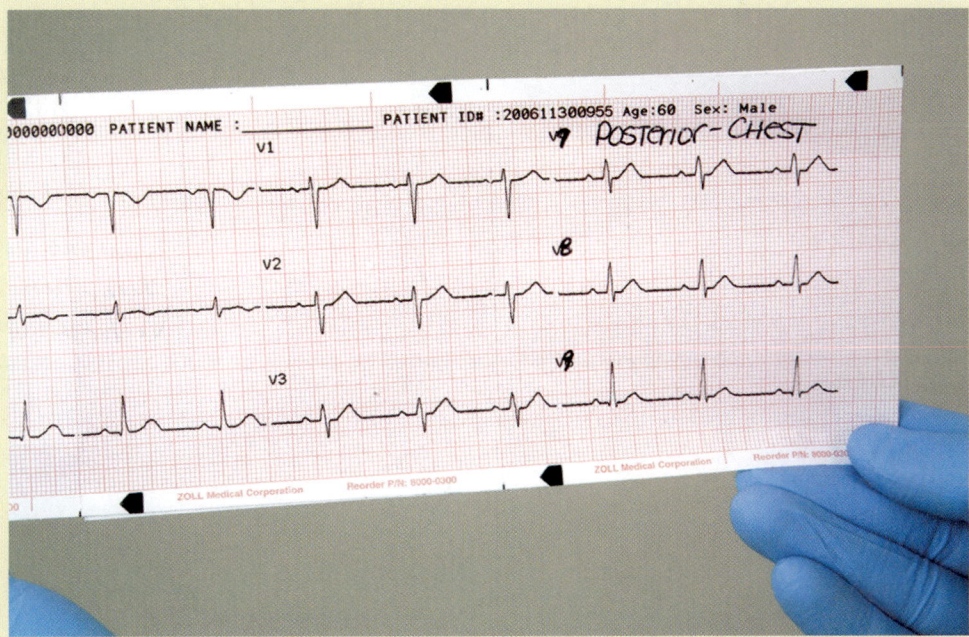

Step 5 Obtain and print the 12-lead ECG. Clearly label the upper portion of the ECG tracing "posterior chest ECG." Remember to relabel lead V_4 on the printout V_7, relabel V_5 to V_8, and V_6 to V_9.

Axis determination
Lead I & aVF
If both point up= correct axis
If I up & aVF down = LAD
(pregnant? or left vent hypertrophy)

If I down & aVF up = RAD (lung dz)
If I down & aVF down = Indeterminate

Axis

The axes of leads I, II, and III form an equilateral triangle with the heart at the center. If the augmented limb leads are added to this configuration and the axes of the six leads moved in a way in which they bisect each other, the result is the hexaxial reference system (Figure 22-83). The hexaxial reference system represents all the frontal plane (limb) leads, with the heart in the center, and is the means used to express the location of the frontal plane axis. This system forms a 360-degree circle surrounding the heart. The positive end of lead I is designated at 0 degrees. The six frontal plane leads divide the circle into segments, each representing 30 degrees. All degrees in the upper hemisphere are labeled as negative degrees, and all degrees in the lower hemisphere are labeled as positive degrees.

In adults, the normal QRS axis is considered to be between −30° and +90° in the frontal plane. Current flow to the right of normal is called right axis deviation (between +90° and ±180° degrees). Current flow in the direction opposite of normal is called *indeterminate, no*

man's land, northwest, or extreme right axis deviation (−90° and ±180° degrees). Current flow to the left of normal is called left axis deviation (between −30° and −90° degrees).

Leads I and aVF divide the heart into four quadrants. These two leads can be used to estimate electrical axis quickly. In leads I and aVF, the QRS complex normally is positive. If the QRS complex in either or both of these leads is negative, axis deviation is present (Table 22-40).

Analyzing the 12-Lead ECG

When analyzing a 12-lead ECG, a systematic method is necessary. See Box 22-23 for the step-by-step procedure.

Localization of Infarctions

Contiguous Leads

[OBJECTIVE 56]

When ECG changes of myocardial ischemia, injury, or infarction occur, they are not found in every lead of the ECG. Findings are considered significant if viewed in two

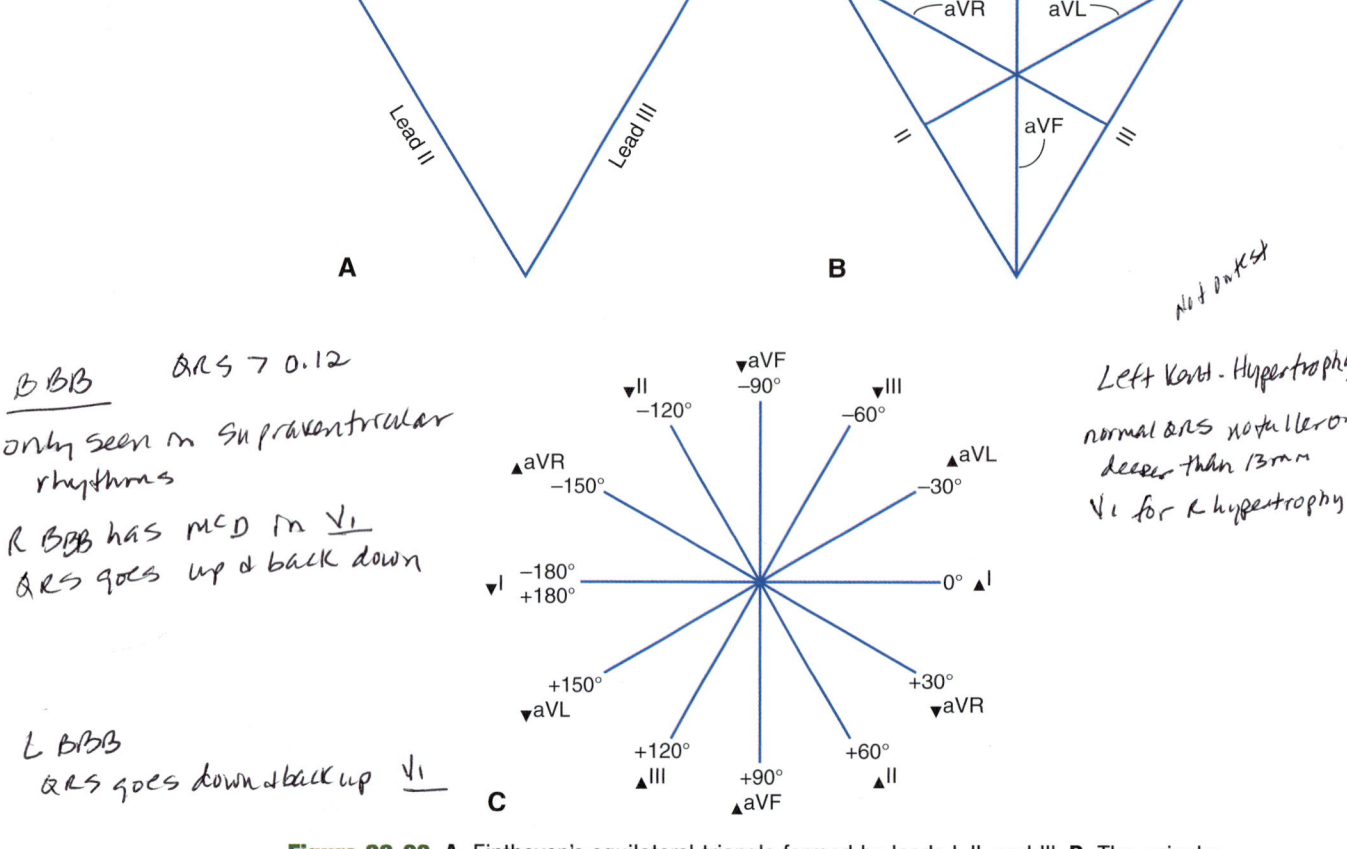

Handwritten notes (left):

BBB   QRS > 0.12

only seen in Supraventricular rhythms

R BBB has mcD in V1
QRS goes up & back down

L BBB
QRS goes down & back up V1

Handwritten notes (right):

Not onKst

Left Vent - Hypertrophy

normal QRS notaller or deeper than 13mm
V1 for R hypertrophy

Figure 22-83 A, Einthoven's equilateral triangle formed by leads I, II, and III. **B,** The unipolar leads are added to the equilateral triangle. **C,** The hexaxial reference system derived from **B.**

TABLE 22-40	Two-Lead Method of Axis Determination			
Axis	Normal	Left	Right	Indeterminate (No Man's Land)
Lead I: QRS direction	Positive	Positive	Negative	Negative
Lead aVF: QRS direction	Positive	Negative	Positive	Negative

BOX 22-23	Analyzing a 12-Lead ECG

1. Assess the quality of the tracing. If baseline wander or artifact is present to any significant degree, note it. If the presence of either of these conditions interferes with the assessment of any lead, use a modifier such as "possible" or "apparent" in your interpretation.
2. Identify the rate and underlying rhythm.
3. Evaluate intervals: PR interval, QRS duration, QT interval
4. Evaluate waveforms: P waves, Q waves, R waves (R-wave progression), T waves, U waves. If a Q wave is present, express the duration in milliseconds.
5. Examine each lead for the presence of ST-segment displacement (elevation or depression). If ST-segment eleva-

tion is present, express it in millimeters. Assess the areas of ischemia or injury by assessing lead groupings. Examine the T waves for any changes in orientation, shape, and size.
6. Determine axis.
7. Look for evidence of hypertrophy or chamber enlargement (this topic is beyond the scope of this text. Consult a 12-lead ECG text for more information).
8. Look for effects of medications and electrolyte imbalances.
9. Interpret your findings.

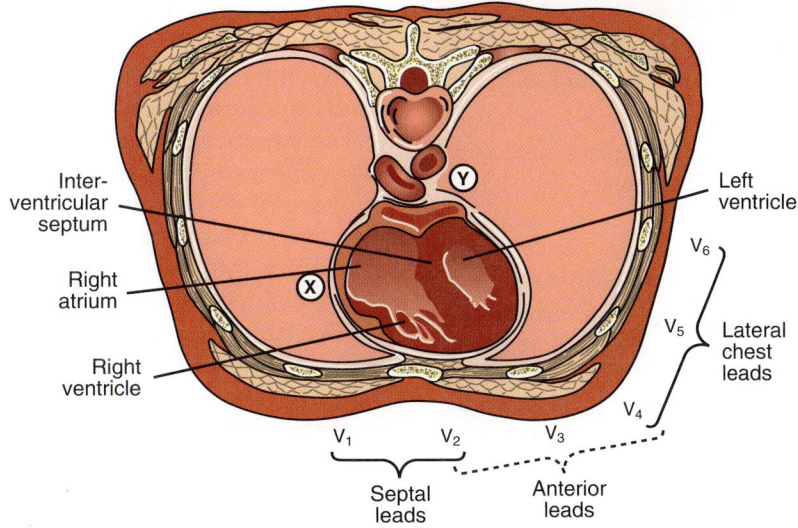

Figure 22-84 The areas of the heart as seen by the chest leads. Leads V_1, V_2, and V_3 are contiguous. Leads V_3, V_4, and V_5 are contiguous as well as V_4, V_5, and V_6. Note that neither the right ventricular wall *(X)* nor the posterior wall of the LV *(Y)* is well visualized by any of the usual six chest leads.

or more leads looking at the same area of the heart. If these findings are seen in leads that look directly at the affected area, they are called **indicative changes.** If findings are seen in leads opposite the affected area, they are called **reciprocal changes.** Of the indicative changes, ST-segment elevation provides the strongest evidence for the early recognition of MI.

Indicative changes are significant when they are seen in two *anatomically contiguous* leads. Two leads are contiguous if they look at the same area of the heart or they are numerically consecutive chest leads (Figure 22-84). Consider the following examples:

- Leads II, III, and aVF are anatomically contiguous because they all look at adjoining tissue in the inferior area of the left ventricle (Table 22-41).
- Leads V_2 and V_3 are anatomically contiguous, being next to each other on the patient's chest. When their "eyes" or "cameras" look in at tissue, they see adjoining tissue in the heart as well.
- Leads II and V_2 are not contiguous. Remember: two leads are anatomically contiguous if they look at the same area of the heart or they are numerically consecutive *chest* leads. Lead II is a limb lead that looks at the inferior wall. V_2 is a chest lead that looks at the septum.

Predicting the Site and Extent of Coronary Artery Occlusion

[OBJECTIVE 57]

In the standard 12-lead ECG, leads II, III, and aVF examine at tissue supplied by the RCA and eight leads evaluate tissue supplied by the left coronary artery: leads I, aVL, V_1, V_2, V_3, V_4, V_5, and V_6. When evaluating the extent of infarction produced by a left coronary artery occlusion, determine how many of these leads are showing changes consistent with an acute infarction (Phalen & Aehlert, 2006). The more of these eight leads demonstrating acute changes, the larger the infarction is presumed to be.

To recognize signs of ischemia, injury, and infarction, knowing which portion of the heart each lead is viewing is necessary. To localize the site, note which leads display that evidence and consider which part of the heart that those leads "see." If an ECG shows changes in leads II, III, and aVF, the inferior wall is affected. Because the inferior wall of the left ventricle is supplied by the RCA in most people, assuming that these ECG changes are from partial or complete blockage of the RCA is reasonable. When indicative changes are seen in the leads viewing the septal, anterior, and/or lateral walls of the left ventricle (V_1 to V_6, I, and aVL), suspecting that these ECG changes are from partial or complete blockage of the left coronary artery is reasonable.

TABLE 22-41	Localizing ECG Changes									
Lead	**View**	**Lead**	**View**	**Lead**	**View**	**Lead**	**View**	**Lead**	**View**
I	Lateral	aVR	—	V_1	Septum	V_4	Anterior	V_4R	Right ventricle
II	Inferior	aVL	Lateral	V_2	Septum	V_5	Lateral	V_5R	Right ventricle
III	Inferior	aVF	Inferior	V_3	Anterior	V_6	Lateral	V_6R	Right ventricle

Although ECG localization of the infarct site is possible, it is not perfect. For example, what appears to be a lateral wall infarction on the ECG may actually be an anterior wall infarction. This can occur with any location of infarction and is because the ECG is simply a measure-ment of current flow on the patient's skin. Factors including anatomic variations, patient position, and other underlying conditions may affect the perceived locations versus the actual location.

The patient's unique pattern of coronary artery distribution also can affect the location of infarct, as can the presence of collateral circulation. For these reasons, you may occasionally encounter infarctions that are difficult to localize into the previously mentioned regions (Box 22-24, Figure 22-85). Table 22-42 summarizes the pattern in which coronary arteries most commonly supply the myocardium.

Anterior Wall Infarctions

[OBJECTIVE 55]

Leads V_3 and V_4 face the anterior wall of the left ventricle. The left main coronary artery supplies the LAD artery and the LCX artery. Blockage of the left main coronary artery (the "widow maker") often leads to cardiogenic shock and death without prompt reperfusion (Figure 22-86). Because the LAD artery supplies approximately 40% of the heart's blood and a critical section of the left ventricle, a blockage in this area can lead to complications such as left ventricular dysfunction, including heart failure and cardiogenic shock. Increased sympathetic nervous system activity is common with anterior MIs with resulting sinus tachycardia and/or high blood pressure.

An anterior wall MI may cause dysrhythmias including PVCs, atrial flutter, or AFib. Although some portions of the bundle branches are supplied by the RCA, the left coronary artery supplies most of the bundle branch tissue. Thus bundle branch blocks may occur if the left coronary artery is blocked. An example of an anterior wall infarction is shown in Figure 22-87.

Inferior Wall Infarctions

Leads II, III, and aVF view the inferior surface of the left ventricle. In most individuals the inferior wall of the left ventricle is supplied by the posterior descending branch of the RCA (Figure 22-88). Increased parasympathetic

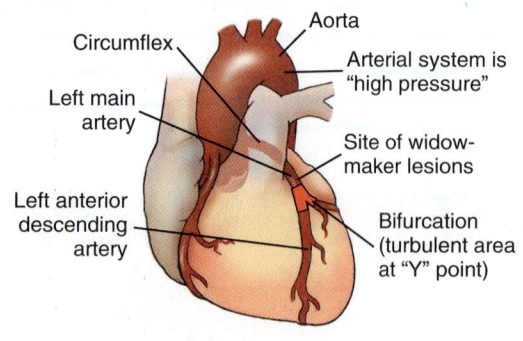
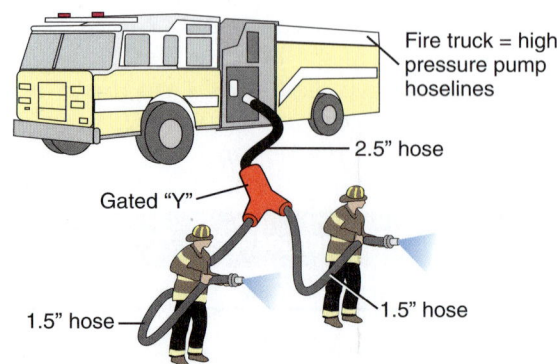

Figure 22-85 The epicardial coronary arteries can be compared to a high-pressure hose used by firefighters.

TABLE 22-42 | Localization of a Myocardial Infarction

Location of MI	Indicative Changes (Leads Facing Affected Area)	Reciprocal Changes (Leads Opposite Affected Area)	Affected (Culprit) Coronary Artery
Anterior	V_3, V_4	V_7, V_8, V_9	Left coronary artery • LAD, diagonal branch
Anteroseptal	V_1, V_2, V_3, V_4	V_7, V_8, V_9	Left coronary artery • LAD, diagonal branch • LAD, septal branch
Anterolateral	I, aVL, V_3, V_4, V_5, V_6	II, III, aVF, V_7, V_8, V_9	Left coronary artery • LAD, diagonal branch and/or circumflex branch
Inferior	II, III, aVF	I, aVL	RCA (most common), posterior descending branch or Left coronary artery, circumflex branch
Lateral	I, aVL, V_5, V_6	II, III, aVF	Left coronary artery • LAD, diagonal branch and/or circumflex branch RCA
Septum	V_1, V_2	V_7, V_8, V_9	Left coronary artery • LAD, septal branch
Posterior	V_7, V_8, V_9	V_1, V_2, V_3	RCA or left circumflex artery
Right ventricle	V_1R-V_6R	I, aVL	RCA, proximal branches

MI, Myocardial infarction; *LAD*, left anterior descending; *RCA*, right coronary artery.

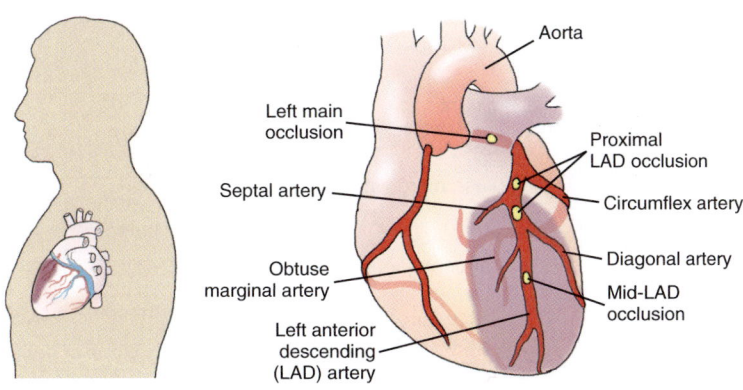

Figure 22-86 Anterior wall infarction. Occlusion of the mid-portion of the left anterior descending (LAD) artery results in an anterior infarction. Proximal occlusion of the LAD may become an anteroseptal infarction if the septal branch is involved or an anterolateral infarction if the marginal branch is involved. If the occlusion occurs proximal to both the septal and diagonal branches, an extensive anterior infarction (anteroseptal-lateral myocardial infarction) will result.

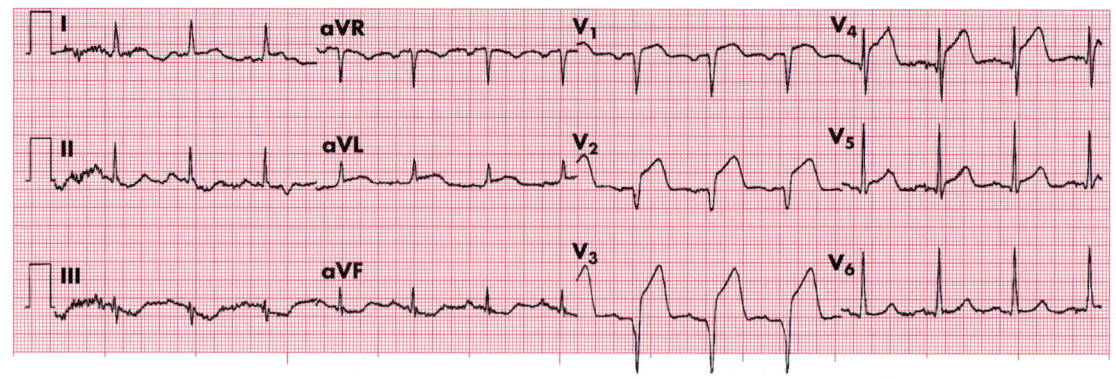

Figure 22-87 Extensive anterior infarction.

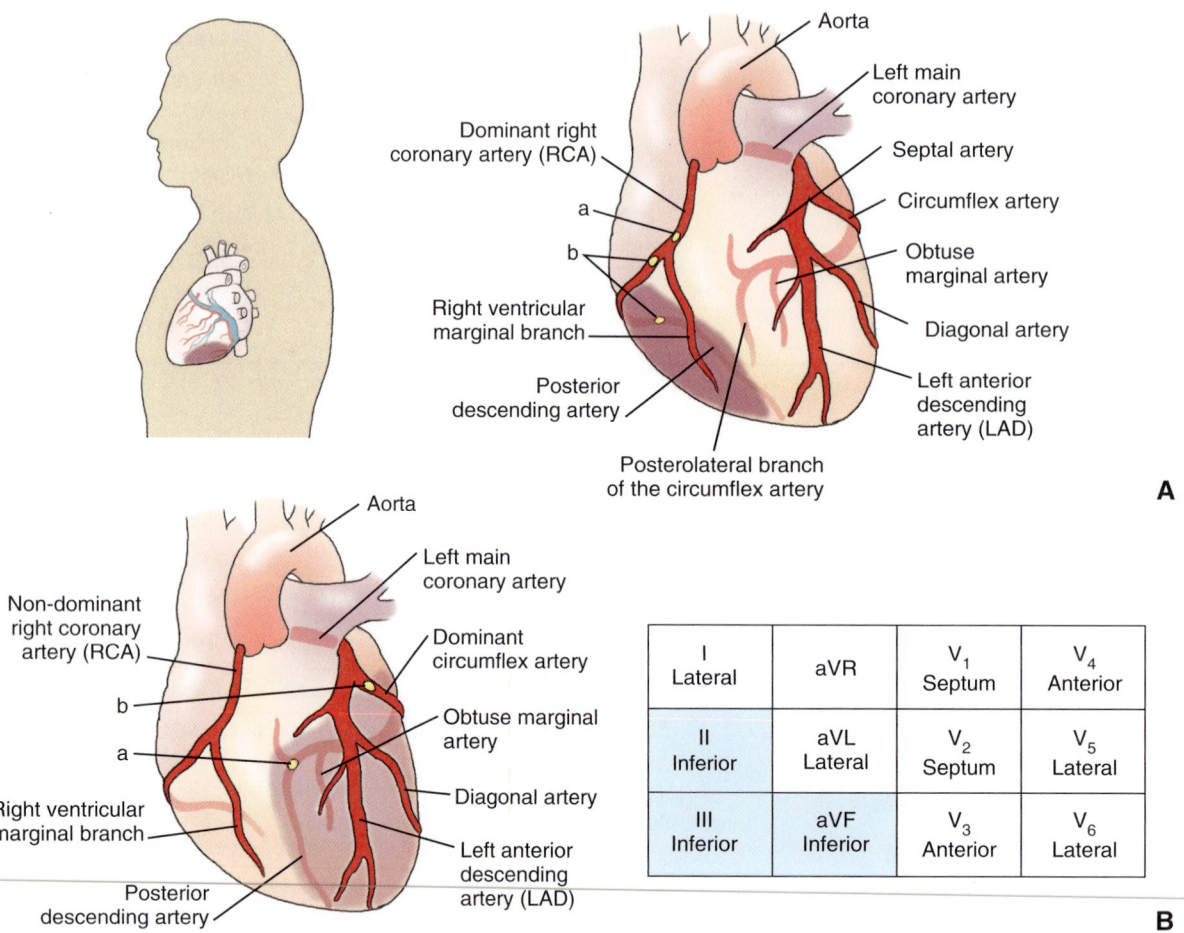

I Lateral	aVR	V₁ Septum	V₄ Anterior
II Inferior	aVL Lateral	V₂ Septum	V₅ Lateral
III Inferior	aVF Inferior	V₃ Anterior	V₆ Lateral

Figure 22-88 A, Inferior wall infarction. Coronary anatomy shows a dominant right coronary artery (RCA). Occlusion at point *a* results in an inferior and right ventricular infarction. Occlusion at point *b* is limited to the inferior wall, sparing the right ventricle. **B**, Inferior wall infarction. Coronary anatomy shows a dominant left circumflex (LCX). Occlusion at point *a* results in an inferior infarction. An occlusion at *b* may result in infarction in the lateral and posterior walls.

nervous system activity is common with inferior wall MIs, resulting in bradydysrhythmias. Conduction delays such as first-degree AV block and second-degree AV block type I are common and usually transient. An example of an infarction involving the inferior wall is shown in Figure 22-89.

Lateral Wall Infarctions

Leads I, aVL, V₅, and V₆ view the lateral wall of the left ventricle. The lateral wall of the left ventricle may be supplied by the LCX artery, the LAD artery, or a branch of the RCA (Figure 22-90).

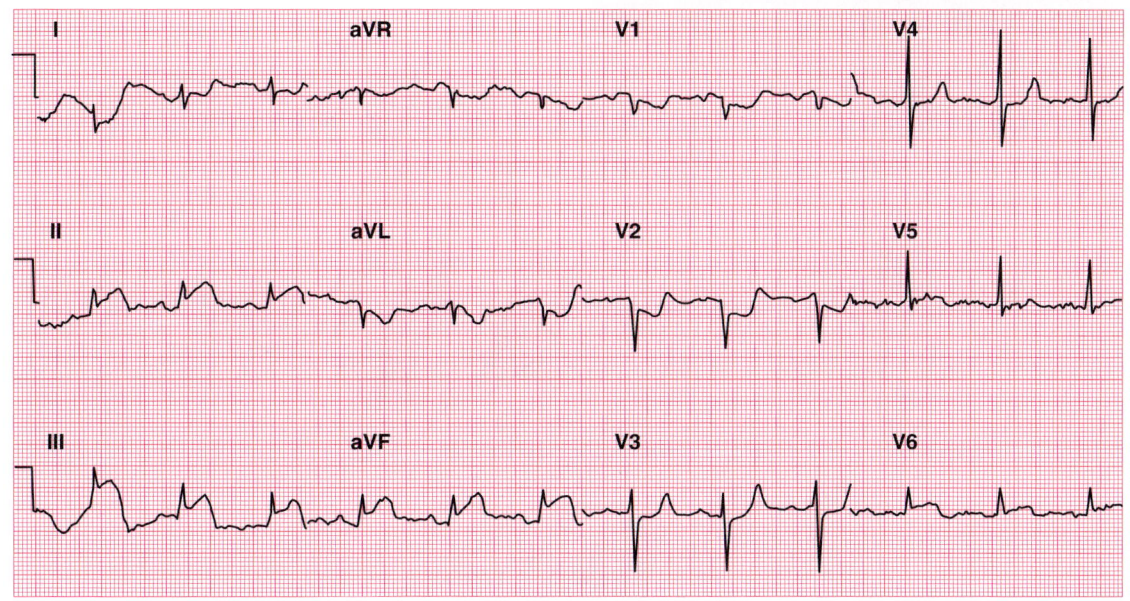

Figure 22-89 Inferior wall infarction. Reciprocal changes are present in leads I and aVL.

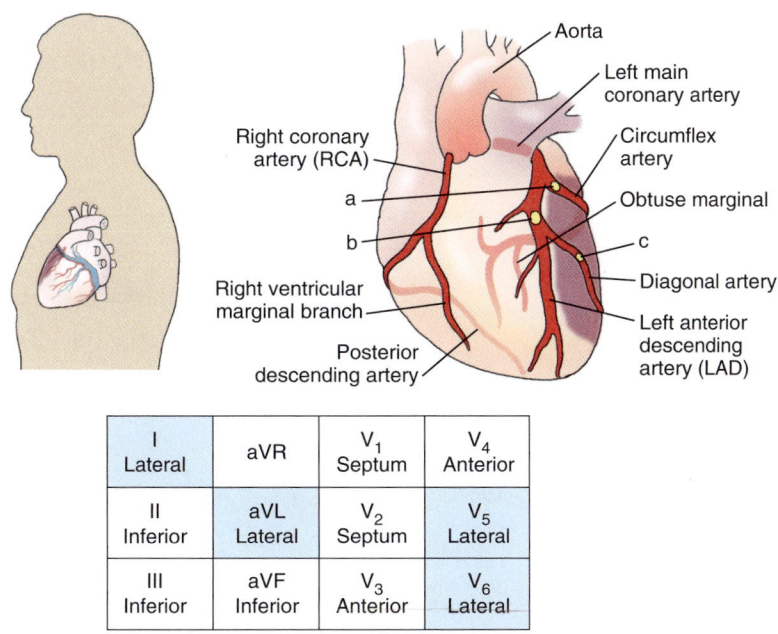

I Lateral	aVR	V₁ Septum	V₄ Anterior
II Inferior	aVL Lateral	V₂ Septum	V₅ Lateral
III Inferior	aVF Inferior	V₃ Anterior	V₆ Lateral

Figure 22-90 Lateral wall infarction. Coronary artery anatomy shows *a* occlusion of the left circumflex (LCX), *b* occlusion of the proximal LAD artery, and *c* occlusion of the diagonal artery.

Septal Infarctions

Leads V_1 and V_2 face the septal area of the left ventricle. The septum, which contains the bundle of His and bundle branches, is normally supplied by the LAD artery (Figure 22-91). If the site of infarction is limited to the septum, ECG changes are seen in V_1 and V_2. If the entire anterior wall is involved, ECG changes will be visible in V_1, V_2, V_3, and V_4. A blockage in this area may result in both right and left (more common) bundle branch blocks, second-degree AV block type II, and complete AV block.

Posterior Wall Infarctions

The posterior wall of the left ventricle is supplied by the LCX artery in most patients; however, in some patients it is supplied by the RCA (Figure 22-92). Because no leads of a standard 12-lead ECG directly view the posterior wall of the left ventricle, additional chest leads (V_7 to V_9) may be used to view the heart's posterior surface. Indicative changes of a posterior wall infarction include ST-segment elevation in these leads. Complications of a posterior wall MI may include left ventricular dysfunction. If the

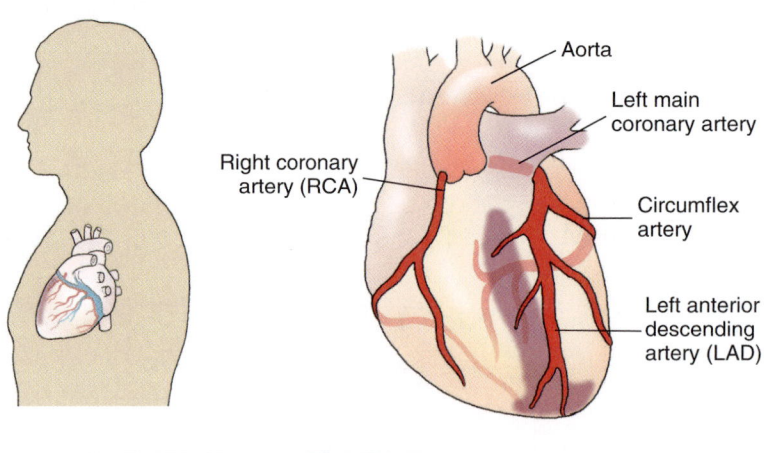

I Lateral	aVR	V₁ Septum	V₄ Anterior
II Inferior	aVL Lateral	V₂ Septum	V₅ Lateral
III Inferior	aVF Inferior	V₃ Anterior	V₆ Lateral

Figure 22-91 Septal infarction.

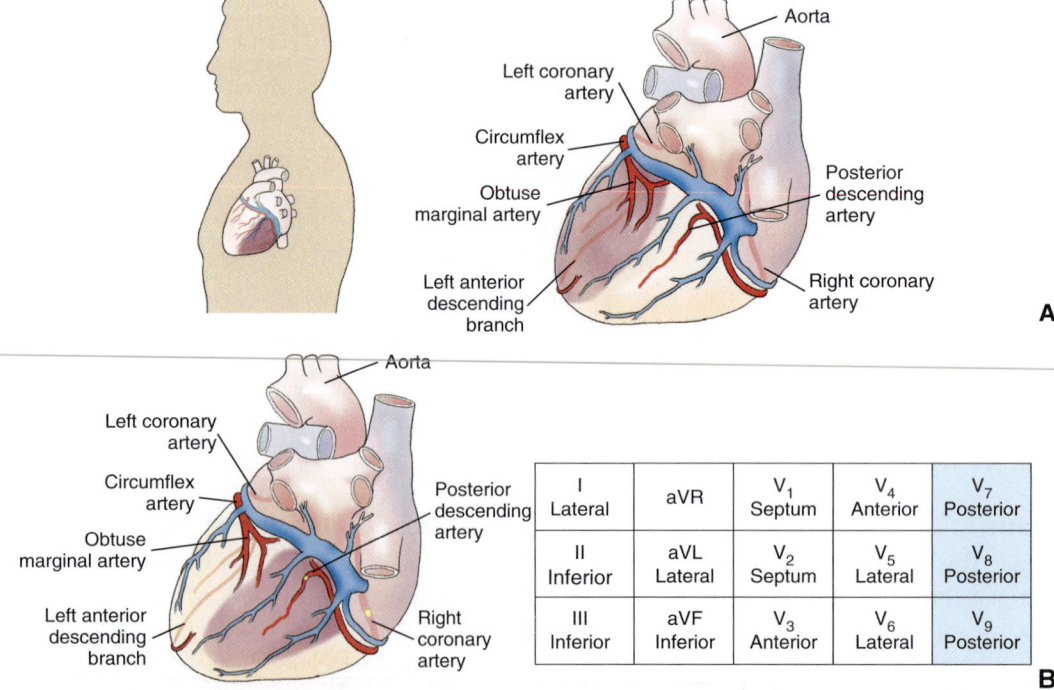

I Lateral	aVR	V₁ Septum	V₄ Anterior	V₇ Posterior
II Inferior	aVL Lateral	V₂ Septum	V₅ Lateral	V₈ Posterior
III Inferior	aVF Inferior	V₃ Anterior	V₆ Lateral	V₉ Posterior

Figure 22-92 A, Posterior infarction. Coronary anatomy shows a dominant right coronary artery (RCA). Occlusion of the RCA commonly results in an inferior and posterior infarction. **B**, Coronary anatomy shows a dominant left circumflex (LCX) artery. Occlusion of a marginal branch is the cause of most isolated posterior infarctions.

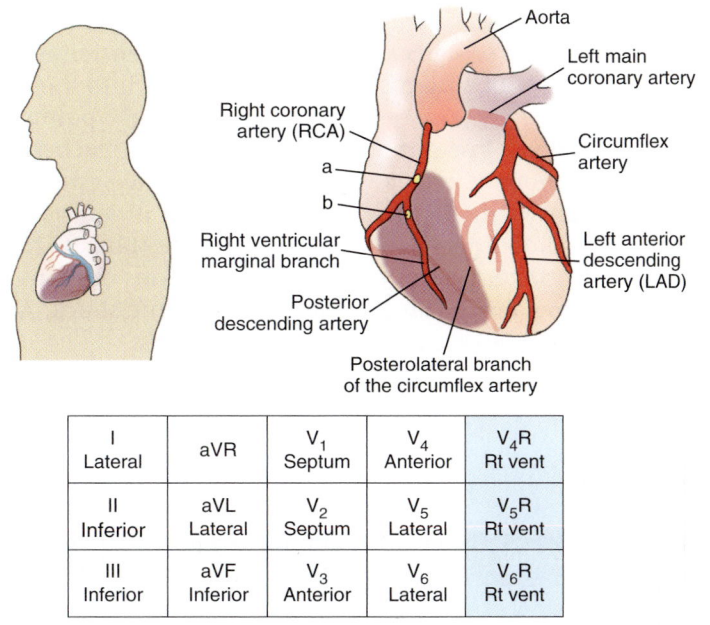

I Lateral	aVR	V$_1$ Septum	V$_4$ Anterior	V$_4$R Rt vent
II Inferior	aVL Lateral	V$_2$ Septum	V$_5$ Lateral	V$_5$R Rt vent
III Inferior	aVF Inferior	V$_3$ Anterior	V$_6$ Lateral	V$_6$R Rt vent

Figure 22-93 Right ventricular infarction (RVI). Occlusion of the right coronary artery (RCA) proximal to the right ventricular marginal branch results in an inferior and right VI. An occlusion of the right ventricular marginal branch results in an isolated RVI.

posterior wall is supplied by the RCA, complications may include dysrhythmias involving the SA node, AV node, and bundle of His.

Right Ventricular Infarctions

Approximately 50% of patients with inferior infarction have some involvement of the right ventricle (Phalen & Aehlert, 2006). The right ventricle is supplied by the right ventricular marginal branch of the RCA (Figure 22-93). An occlusion of the right ventricular marginal branch results in an isolated right ventricular infarction (RVI). Occlusion of the RCA proximal to the right ventricular marginal branch results in an inferior and right ventricular infarction. RVI should be suspected when ECG changes suggesting an inferior infarction (ST-segment elevation in leads II, III, and/or aVF) are seen. An example of an infarction involving the right ventricle is shown in Figure 22-94.

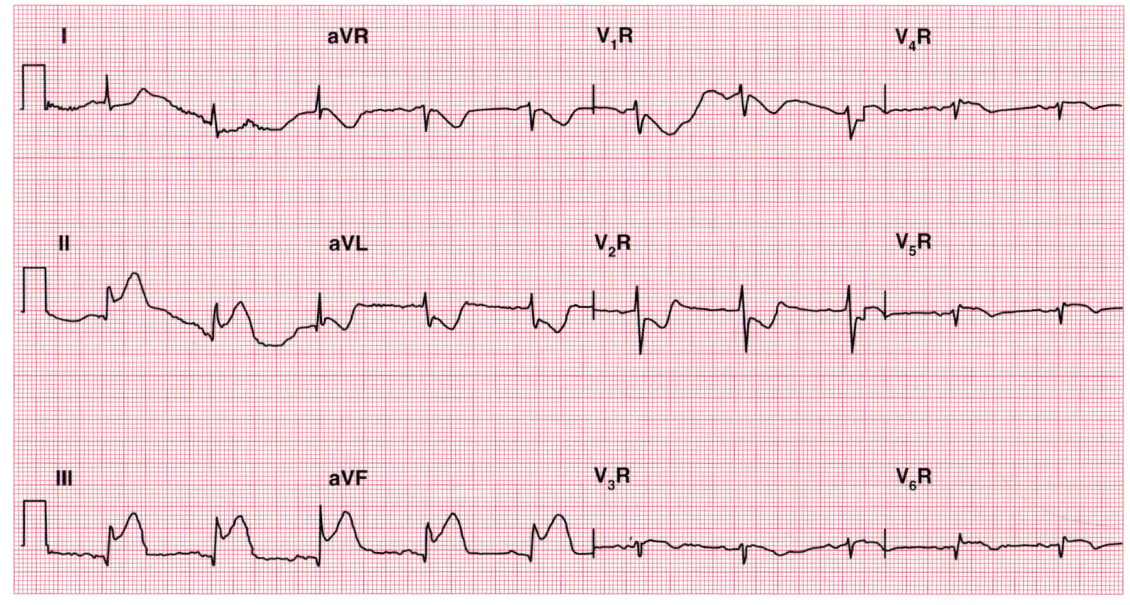

Figure 22-94 Inferior infarction, right ventricular infarction (RVI).

In addition to ECG evidence, certain clinical signs also support the suspicion of RVI. The clinical evidence of RVI involves three main areas: hypotension, jugular venous distention, and clear breath sounds. This triad of signs is estimated to be present in only 10% to 15% of patients with RVI.

In the setting of RVI, the right ventricle may lose some of its ability to pump blood into the pulmonary circuit. When this happens, blood stalls in the right ventricle and may begin to back up. (Technically, the blood does not back up; the venous return exceeds ventricular output and blood begins to build up). This stalling and backing up produce the hypotension, jugular venous distention, and absence of **pulmonary edema** (clear lung sounds) considered the clinical triad of RVI. As blood backs up from the right ventricle, the jugular veins become enlarged. Hypotension results from the decrease in blood volume moving into the lungs and left ventricle. The left ventricle can only pump as much blood as it receives, and if less blood reaches the left ventricle, less blood is pumped into the systemic circulation. The net effect of this reduction in left ventricular output is a decrease in blood pressure (Box 22-25).

Complications associated with RVI include hypotension, cardiogenic shock, AV blocks, atrial flutter or fibrillation, and PACs.

BOX 22-25 | Right Ventricular Infarction: Another Point of View

A fire pump and the human heart function similarly. To better understand what happens in the setting of RVI, compare the two. When an increase in demand is needed at the end of a hose line, more gallons per minute are needed to go out. This increase in demand must be met by the fire pump: a sufficient amount of water must be going through the pump to meet the demand. If an inadequate amount of water is coming into the pump to meet the required discharge pressures, the pump will cavitate and cease to function effectively. Once the pump loses effectiveness, discharge pressures fall and pressures are lost at the end of the hose lines.

In RVI, the right ventricle becomes stunned (dyskinetic) because of myocardial ischemia. The effectiveness of the right ventricle decreases, and the right heart becomes more preload dependent. If preload is further decreased, the systolic pressure drops, resulting in hypotension. This occurs because an inadequate volume of fluid is leaving the right ventricle to satisfy the increasing demand from the left ventricle. In both situations (fire pump and human pump), the pump must be fed more fluid (increased preload) to meet the demand and sustain vital functions.

Modified from Phalen, T., & Aehlert, B. (2006). *The 12-lead ECG in acute coronary syndromes*, St. Louis: Elsevier.
RVI, Right ventricular infarction.

Case Scenario—continued

You apply high-flow oxygen by nonrebreather mask and prepare the patient for transfer into the ambulance for further assessment and transport. As you lift the stretcher into the ambulance, the patient experiences a grand mal seizure lasting 30 to 45 seconds, followed by agonal respirations at a rate of 4 to 6 breaths/min. He is unresponsive. Your partner attaches the patient to the monitor as a first responder ventilates the patient and you insert an endotracheal tube. The cardiac monitor shows a wide QRS complete heart block with a ventricular rate of 36 beats/min. Before departing for the hospital, your partner establishes an IV and gets a second set of vital signs: pulse, 36 beats/min; blood pressure, 62/40 mm Hg; respirations, 6 breaths/min; SpO$_2$, 97%.

Questions

6. Is this patient high priority? Why or why not?
7. Given what you know at this time, what is the most likely cause of the seizure activity?
8. What is this patient's greatest life threat at this time? How will you treat it?
9. How will you manage the cardiac rhythm?

INTRAVENTRICULAR CONDUCTION DELAYS

[OBJECTIVE 58]

Bundle Branch Activation

During normal ventricular depolarization, the left side of the interventricular septum (stimulated by the left posterior fascicle) is stimulated first. The electrical impulse (wave of depolarization) then traverses the septum to stimulate the right side. The right bundle branch conducts the impulse to the right ventricle and the left bundle branch conducts the impulse to the left ventricle. The left and right ventricles are then depolarized at the same time. If a delay or block occurs in one of the bundle branches, the ventricles will not be depolarized at the same time. The impulse first travels down the unblocked branch and stimulates that ventricle. Because of the block, the impulse must then travel from cell to cell through the myocardium (rather than through the normal conduction pathway) to stimulate the other ventricle. This means of conduction is slower than normal, and the QRS complex appears widened on the ECG. The ventricle with the blocked bundle branch is the last to be depolarized.

ECG Criteria

Following are ECG criteria for identification of a right or left bundle branch block (BBB):

- QRS duration measuring more than or equal to 0.12 second (if a complete BBB)
- QRS complexes produced by supraventricular activity (i.e., the QRS complex is not a paced beat, and it did not originate in the ventricles)

When measuring for BBB, select the widest QRS complex with a discernible beginning and end. Lead V_1 is probably the single best lead to use when differentiating between right and left BBB.

A QRS duration between 0.10 and 0.12 second in adults is called an *incomplete* right or left BBB. In adults, a QRS measuring more than or equal to 0.12 second is called a *complete* right or left BBB. If the QRS is wide but no BBB pattern is discernible, the term *wide QRS* or *intraventricular conduction delay* is used to describe the QRS.

In right BBB, the electrical impulse travels through the AV node and down the left bundle branch into the interventricular septum. The septum is activated by the left posterior fascicle and is depolarized in a left-to-right direction. Thus septal depolarization moves in a left-to-right direction, which is toward V_1, and produces an initial small R wave. As the left bundle continues to conduct impulses, the entire left ventricle is depolarized from right to left. This produces movement away from

V_1 and results in a negative deflection (S wave). The impulses that depolarized the left ventricle conduct through the myocardial cells and depolarize the right ventricle. This depolarization creates a movement of electrical activity in the direction of V_1, and so a second positive deflection is recorded (R'). The RSR' pattern is characteristic of right BBB. Whenever the two criteria for BBB have been met, and V_1 displays an RSR' pattern, right BBB is suspected. The RSR' pattern is sometimes referred to as an M or "rabbit ear" pattern.

In left BBB, the septum is depolarized by the right bundle branch, as is the right ventricle. The septum is part of the left ventricle, and thus the wave of depolarization has begun with the net movement of current going away from V_1. This movement of current continues to move away from V_1 as the rest of the left ventricle is depolarized, and the QRS complex continues in its negative direction. Thus left BBB produces a QS pattern in V_1. When BBB is known to exist and a QS pattern is seen in V_1, left BBB is suspected.

Unfortunately, not every BBB presents with a clear RSR' or QS pattern in V_1. Often the pattern more closely resembles a qR pattern or an rS pattern, making the differentiation less clear. When this occurs, focus should be on the terminal force of the QRS complex. Examination of the terminal force (final portion) of the QRS complex reveals the ventricle that was depolarized last, and therefore the bundle that was blocked. To identify the terminal force, first look at lead V_1 and locate the J-point. Move from the J-point backward into the QRS complex and determine if the terminal portion (last 0.04 second) of the QRS complex is a positive (upright) or negative (downward) deflection (Figure 22-95). If it is directed upward, a right BBB is present (the current is

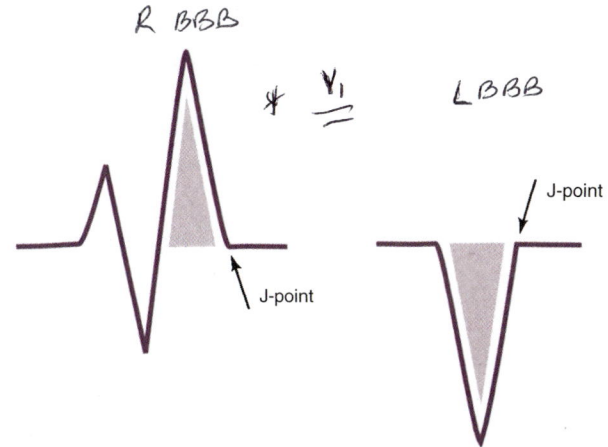

Figure 22-95 Determining the direction of the terminal force. Move from the J-point into the QRS complex and determine if the terminal portion (last 0.04 second) of the QRS complex is a positive or negative deflation. If the two criteria for bundle branch block (BBB) are met and the terminal portion of the QRS is positive, right BBB is most likely present. If the terminal portion of the QRS is negative, left BBB is most likely present.

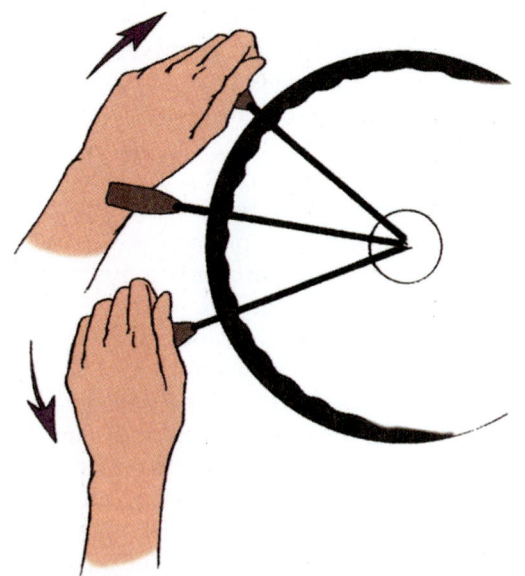

Figure 22-96 Differentiating between right and left bundle branch block (BBB). The turn signal theory—right is up, left is down.

moving toward the right ventricle and toward V_1). A left BBB is present when the terminal force of the QRS complex is directed downward (the current is moving away from V_1 and toward the left ventricle). A simple way to remember this rule is demonstrated in Figure 22-96. As shown in the figure, this rule is similar to the turn indicator on a vehicle. When a right turn is made, the turn indicator is lifted up. Likewise, when a right BBB is present, the terminal force of the QRS complex points up. Conversely, left turns and left BBB are directed downward.

ECG CHANGES ASSOCIATED WITH ELECTROLYTE DISTURBANCES AND HYPOTHERMIA

Electrolyte Disturbances

[OBJECTIVE 59]

A summary of the ECG changes associated with electrolyte disturbances can be found in Table 22-43.

Hypothermia

Dysrhythmias are common in patients who have moderate to severe hypothermia. Worsening hypothermia is associated with prolongation of the PR interval, then the QRS duration, and finally the QT interval (Danzl, 2002). AFib often occurs when the core body temperature is less than 32° C (89.6° F) (Danzl, 1998). When core body temperature falls below 25° C (77° F), asystole and VF often spontaneously occur.

Patients with a temperature less than 32° C (89.6° F) may develop a unique ECG pattern in which a hump is seen at the J-point (the junction of the QRS complex and ST segment). This hump is called a *J wave* or an *Osborn wave* (Figure 22-97). It increases in size with temperature depression and disappears with rewarming.

TABLE 22-43	ECG Changes Associated with Electrolyte Disturbances						
Electrolyte Disturbance	P Wave	PR Interval	QRS Complex	ST Segment	T Wave	QT Interval	Heart Rate
Hypocalcemia				Long, flattened		Prolonged	
Hypercalcemia		Prolonged		Shortened		Shortened	
Hypokalemia			Widen as level decreases	Depressed	Flattened; U wave present	Prolonged	
Hyperkalemia	Disappear as level increases	Normal or prolonged	Widen as level increases	Disappear as level increases	Tall, peaked or tented		Slows
Hypomagnesemia	Diminished voltage (amplitude)		Widen as level decreases; diminished voltage	Depressed	Flattened; U wave present	Prolonged	
Hypermagnesemia		Prolonged	Widened		Tall or elevated		

Systemic Hypothermia

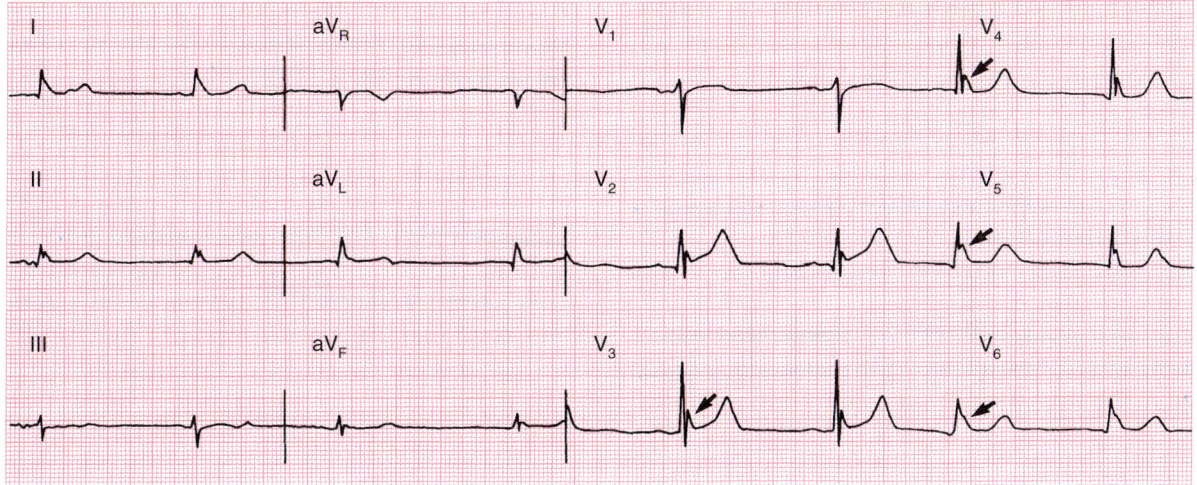

Figure 22-97 The *arrows* in this 12-lead ECG point to J waves, which are sometimes called *Osborn waves.*

SECTION 4: CARDIOVASCULAR ASSESSMENT

A cardiac-related complaint is a common reason a person seeks medical care. A patient with cardiovascular-related symptoms may be a young, middle-aged, or older adult. He or she may be unresponsive, awake and alert, or have an altered mental status. The patient may be stable or unstable and may or may not have a pulse. Regardless of the situation, a systematic approach to assessment of the patient is important. When used consistently, this type of approach will help ensure that you do not overlook physical findings or important questions pertinent to the treatment plan for your patient.

INITIAL ASSESSMENT

After making sure the scene is safe to enter, survey the area for hazards or potential hazards. Quickly determine the number of patients and decide if additional resources will be needed. While looking at the patient's environment, make a mental note of the interaction between the patient and others who may be present. Does the interaction demonstrate concern, or is it angry or indifferent? Quickly note the patient's environment. Does the patient's home appear clean and orderly? Does the patient appear well cared for? Are any medical devices present? For example, is a hospital bed, wheelchair, walker, or home oxygen bottle visible?

Primary Survey

Next form a general impression of the patient. As you approach him or her, use your senses of sight and hearing (look and listen) to find out quickly if a life-threatening problem exists that requires immediate care. Assess the following three main areas: appearance, (work of) breathing, and circulation (the ABCs):

- *Appearance.* Is the patient aware of your presence? Is he or she in pain and moving about as though trying to find a comfortable position? Altered mental status or unresponsiveness indicates a need for immediate care.
- *(Work of) breathing.* Is the patient breathing? Is respiratory effort normal, or does he or she appear to have difficulty breathing? Is the respiratory rate fast, slow, or normal for the patient's age? Is the patient's breathing noisy? An absence of chest wall movement or labored or noisy breathing indicates a need for immediate care.
- *Circulation.* Does the patient's skin appear pale, mottled, or cyanotic? Abnormal skin color indicates a need for immediate care.

Continue the primary survey, treating life-threatening problems as you find them, then perform a secondary survey (physical examination, vital signs, and patient history).

BP ↑, skin pale, cool & diaphoretic = pain & SNS stim.

Airway and Cervical Spine Protection

As you approach the patient, identify yourself and ask, "How can I help you?" or "Can you tell me what is bothering you today?" The patient's answer will quickly tell you about the condition of the airway and mental status.

If the patient is responsive and the airway is open, evaluate his or her breathing. If the patient is responsive but cannot talk, cry, or cough forcefully, assess for a possible airway obstruction.

If the patient is unresponsive and trauma is suspected, use the jaw thrust without head tilt maneuver to open the airway. Assess for sounds of airway compromise such as snoring, gurgling, or stridor. Make sure the airway is clear of blood, broken teeth or loose dentures, gastric contents, and foreign objects. Suction as needed. If a foreign body airway obstruction is suspected but not visualized, clear the obstruction per current resuscitation guidelines. Insert an oral or nasal airway as needed to help keep the airway open.

Breathing and Ventilation

If the patient is breathing, determine whether breathing is adequate or inadequate. Look at the rise and fall of the patient's chest. Chest expansion should be equal with enough tidal volume to make the chest rise. Excessive use of accessory muscles should not occur during inspiration or expiration. A patient who has difficulty breathing often has inadequate or shallow respirations. Shallow respirations, even in the presence of an increased respiratory rate, may not be enough to ventilate the patient adequately. The patient with inadequate breathing may need positive-pressure ventilation with 100% oxygen.

Estimate the patient's respiratory rate. Is he or she breathing at an age-appropriate rate? An increase in respiratory rate is an early sign of respiratory distress. A patient who has breathing difficulty often has a respiratory rate outside the normal limits for age. Note the patient's respiratory effort (work of breathing). Signs of increased work of breathing include nasal flaring, pursed-lip breathing, use of accessory muscles, a leaning forward position to inhale, and/or retractions.

Before using a stethoscope, note whether the patient's breathing is quiet, absent, or noisy. Examples of noisy breathing include stridor, wheezing, snoring, and gurgling. Listen for the presence or absence of breath sounds. Breath sounds should be clear and equal bilaterally. Listen closely for crackles (rales) that may indicate pulmonary congestion.

If breathing is adequate, ask your partner to give the patient oxygen, then move on to assessment of circulation. If breathing is difficult and the rate is too slow or too fast, give oxygen and, if necessary, positive-pressure ventilation. If breathing is absent, begin rescue breathing and make sure the patient's chest rises with each breath.

Circulation with Bleeding Control

Begin assessment of the patient's circulation by looking for visible external hemorrhage. Control major bleeding if present. Check for the presence of a pulse. While your hands are in contact with the patient's skin, assess skin color, temperature, moisture, turgor (elasticity), and mobility. Note whether edema is present. If a pulse is present, quickly estimate its rate and quality. Is it weak or strong, fast or slow, regular or irregular? If no pulse is detected, begin cardiopulmonary resuscitation (CPR) (and defibrillation if needed) according to current resuscitation guidelines.

> ### PEDIATRIC *Pearl*
> - Assess capillary refill if the patient is younger than 6 years. If capillary refill initially is assessed in the hand or fingers and it is delayed, recheck it in a more central location, such as the chest.
> - Keep in mind that a positive finding is more helpful than a negative one. Never assume a child is well perfused on the basis of a good capillary refill time.

Disability (Mental Status)

Although you will most likely have a good idea of the patient's mental status by this point in your assessment, use the Glasgow Coma Scale to establish a baseline and for comparison in later, serial observations.

Expose/Environment

While preserving body heat, undress the patient as needed for further assessment. Respect the patient's modesty and replace clothing promptly after examining each body area.

When you have completed the primary survey, you should have enough information to determine if the patient is sick (unstable) or not sick (stable). With the information available to you, make a decision regarding patient transport and destination. Remember: your patient's condition can change at any time. A patient that initially appears stable may rapidly get worse and become unstable. Reassess frequently.

> ### PEDIATRIC *Pearl*
> Maintaining appropriate temperature is particularly important in the pediatric patient because children have a large body surface area/weight ratio, providing a greater area for heat loss.

Secondary Survey

[OBJECTIVES 60, 61, 62]

Obtain the patient's focused history by the SAMPLE format. This information is often obtained simultaneously while assessing vital signs, performing the physical examination, and providing emergency care. While assessing the patient, keep in mind that other body systems affect or may be affected by a cardiovascular disorder.

CULTURAL *Considerations*

When talking with patients, try to avoid using medical terms. Ask the patient questions and explain what you are going to do to help by using words that are easy to understand. This is important when communicating with any patient, but it is particularly important when speaking with patients for whom English is a second language.

Signs/Symptoms

Determining what prompted the patient's call for medical help is important. Be sure to document the patient's chief complaint in his or her own words. Some patients may have more than one chief complaint. For example, a patient may complain of chest pain and difficulty breathing or palpitations and chest pain. If this occurs, ask the patient which symptom started first and which bothers him or her the most. For example, with further questioning of the patient complaining of palpitations and chest pain, you may learn that the patient felt his or her heart racing for a few minutes and then began having chest pain. Common chief complaints in patients who have heart disease include:

- Chest pain or discomfort
- Shoulder, arm, neck, or jaw pain or discomfort
- Dyspnea
- Cough
- Fainting (syncope)
- Abnormal heartbeat or palpitations
- Fatigue

PEDIATRIC *Pearl*

Chest pain is a relatively infrequent chief complaint in a young child, but increases in frequency as the child ages. Following are the three most common causes of pediatric chest pain:

- A pathologic condition of the chest wall (trauma or muscle strain)
- Costochondritis (an inflammation of the cartilage that connects the inner end of each rib to the sternum)
- Respiratory diseases, especially those associated with coughing

These three conditions account for 45% to 65% of chest pain in children.

Chest Pain or Discomfort. Chest pain or discomfort is a common symptom in a patient with an acute coronary syndrome. Because many causes of chest discomfort exist other than a cardiac disorder, you must gather as much information as possible from the patient related to the current complaint. Use the OPQRST memory aid to recall appropriate questions to ask.

Onset. *When did the discomfort begin? Did it begin suddenly or gradually? Have you ever had this discomfort before? When? How long did it last? Were you seen, evaluated, or treated for it? If so, what was the diagnosis? How does the discomfort you are feeling right now compare with that?*

Establishing when the patient's symptoms began is quite important—particularly if the patient is a candidate for clot-busting drug therapy.

Provocation/Palliation/Position. *What were you doing when your symptoms started? What makes the discomfort better or worse? Before we arrived, what did you try to relieve the problem? Does a change in position, such as leaning forward, lessen the discomfort?*

Angina pectoris is chest discomfort that occurs when the heart muscle does not receive enough oxygen (myocardial ischemia). Examples of activities that increase the heart's demand for oxygen include undergoing emotional upset, cigarette smoking, eating a heavy meal, walking up an incline or against a wind, working with the arms over the head, or being exposed to cold weather. A heart attack (MI) may occur when a patient is at rest, after a serious illness or unusually vigorous exercise, in conjunction with severe emotional stress, or without warning.

The circumstances that provoke the patient's symptoms can provide a clue to the cause of the pain or discomfort. For example, pain that worsens with exertion and resolves with rest is probably related to myocardial ischemia. Pain that worsens after a meal may be from a gastrointestinal cause. Pain that worsens when the patient takes a deep breath may be attributable to a respiratory or musculoskeletal cause.

Find out what the patient has done to try to relieve the symptoms before you arrived. Ask if rest has relieved or lessened discomfort. If the patient has taken any medication, find out what it was, how much was taken and when, and if the symptoms have changed since taking it.

Quality. *What does your discomfort feel like?* Document the words the patient uses to describe discomfort. Note that the word *discomfort* is used in these questions instead of *pain*. Although many patients having a cardiac-related event will tell you they have chest pain, some will not feel true pain. Some patients having a cardiac-related event present with signs and symptoms other than chest pain or discomfort, such as generalized weakness, sweating, lightheadedness, shortness of breath, back pain, or nausea and vomiting.

Region/Radiation. *Where is your discomfort? Does it stay in one area or does it move?* Chest discomfort associated with myocardial ischemia usually begins in the central or left chest and then radiates to the arm (especially the little finger [ulnar] side of the left arm), wrist, jaw, epigastrium, left shoulder, or between the shoulder blades. A similar pattern also may occur in pericarditis. Severe ischemia may result in radiation to the right chest, right arm, and/or back.

A patient having a cardiac-related event who has epigastric pain, nausea, and vomiting may be confused with one who has a gastrointestinal disorder, such as a peptic ulcer. Aortic dissection or enlargement of an aortic aneurysm may produce pain that begins in the center of the chest and radiates to the back.

Severity. *On a scale of 0 to 10, with 0 being the least and 10 being the worst, what number would you assign your discomfort?* Because no individual can feel another's pain, "pain is whatever the experiencing person says it is, existing whenever [he or she] says it does" (McCaffery & Pasero, 1998). Although physical signs of pain may be obvious in many patients, some may feel severe pain and not show visible signs of discomfort. Remember that the patient is the authority regarding his or her pain. A pain scale will allow you to evaluate the effectiveness of the emergency care you provide. Document the patient's initial rating of his pain or discomfort. Reassess (and document) the degree of discomfort after each treatment you perform and before transferring care at the receiving facility.

Time. *Is your discomfort still present? Is it getting better, worse, or staying about the same? Does it come and go or is it constant?* Myocardial ischemia is usually associated with symptoms that gradually intensify over a period of minutes. Chest pain or discomfort that comes and goes is called recurrent, or stuttering, chest pain.

Determine how long the patient's discomfort has been present. Anginal symptoms usually last fewer than 15 minutes. Chest discomfort associated with a heart attack often lasts 20 minutes to several hours. Chest discomfort that lasts for hours also may be seen with pericarditis and aortic dissection.

PARAMEDIC*Pearl*

Pain is underestimated and inadequately treated by many health care professionals despite the availability of effective medications and other therapies. Some do not view pain relief as important or do not want to "waste time" assessing pain. The safe and effective relief of pain should be a priority in the management of a patient of any age.

Shoulder, Arm, Neck, or Jaw Pain or Discomfort. Pain or discomfort in the shoulder, arm, neck, or jaw may occur with or without chest discomfort. The patient may describe numbness or tingling in these areas instead of pain. To assess the patient's chief complaint, use the same OPQRST questions asked of patients who have chest discomfort.

Dyspnea. Dyspnea is an uncomfortable awareness of one's breathing. Dyspnea is associated with many conditions affecting the heart, lungs, and respiratory muscles. Dyspnea may occur in healthy persons after strenuous exercise. It also is common during the later months of pregnancy and in obese patients. Dyspnea may occur after moderate exertion in healthy persons who are not physically conditioned. Dyspnea should be regarded as abnormal only when it occurs at rest or at a level of physical activity not expected to cause this symptom (Braunwald, 2001).

To help determine the cause of the patient's breathing difficulty, find out whether the patient has any associated symptoms such as a headache, fever, chills, chest pain, pain or swelling in the lower legs, or tightness in the throat. Dyspnea that occurs with inspiration suggests obstruction of the upper airway. Examples of conditions that may compromise the upper airway include an allergic reaction, foreign body, laryngeal infection, or chemical or thermal injury. Dyspnea that occurs on expiration suggests lower airway obstruction. Examples of conditions that may compromise the lower airway include pulmonary embolism, pneumothorax, acute pulmonary edema, pneumonia, asthma, and emphysema.

Dyspnea may vary in intensity from simply being aware of one's breathing to severe respiratory distress. Because dyspnea is not a sign but a symptom, assessing its severity is difficult. Ask the patient to rate the severity of his or her breathing difficulty on a scale of 0 to 10.

Dyspnea that occurs on exertion or at rest suggests the presence of left ventricular failure or chronic obstructive pulmonary disease. Dyspnea that suddenly develops suggests pulmonary embolism, pneumothorax, acute pulmonary edema, pneumonia, or airway obstruction. Dyspnea also may be an associated symptom of MI. Dyspnea relieved by squatting is most often caused by tetralogy of Fallot, a congenital heart condition.

Dyspnea may be a sign of a failing pump. Left ventricular failure (LVF) causes blood to build up in the lungs. In patients who have chronic LVF, dyspnea often develops slowly over weeks or months. Patients who have chronic heart failure may have dyspnea when resting in a horizontal position. This occurs because blood pools in the lungs when the patient lies down. Dyspnea that is relieved by a change in position (either sitting upright or standing) is called **orthopnea.** To avoid this symptom, patients with orthopnea often sleep on two or more pillows to achieve an upright or semi-upright position.

Paroxysmal nocturnal dyspnea (PND) is a sudden onset of difficulty breathing in which the patient suddenly awakens from sleep. PND often is associated with LVF. PND usually begins 2 to 4 hours after the onset of sleep. It often is accompanied by coughing, wheezing, and sweating. The patient may awaken with a feeling of suffocation. The patient's condition usually improves after sitting up or standing for 15 to 30 minutes.

Cough. Cough is one of the most common symptoms for which a patient seeks medical care. Coughing may be a result of the common cold or other infection, chronic bronchitis, emphysema, or environmental allergies. Coughing also may be an early symptom of a potentially life-threatening condition such as asthma, heart failure, pneumonia, pulmonary embolism, and aspiration syndromes. Although definitions differ, a chronic cough is generally defined as a cough that has persisted for 3 weeks or more. A chronic cough may be the result of a throat infection, cancer, gastroesophageal reflux disease, chronic sinus infection, chronic bronchitis, asthma, or the use medications for high blood pressure, such as angiotensin-converting enzyme inhibitors.

A vigorous cough has been estimated to generate 1 to 25 J of energy (Irwin et al, 1998; Wei et al, 1980). Vigorous coughing can produce complications such as:

- Fast or slow heart rate
- Headache
- Rib fractures
- Urinary incontinence
- Laryngeal trauma
- Hoarseness
- Pneumothorax
- Dizziness
- Inguinal hernia
- Disruption of surgical wounds
- Bronchial rupture

If your patient has a cough, find out whether it is dry or productive. A dry cough is a nonproductive cough. A productive (or wet) cough clears the airway of mucus (sputum) and foreign material. The characteristics of the sputum produced may be helpful in determining the cause of the cough. For example, pulmonary edema often is accompanied by frothy, pink-tinged sputum. Blood-streaked sputum may be associated with conditions such as tuberculosis or lung cancer. Pneumonia may produce sputum that is rusty, green, or blood tinged.

Fainting. **Fainting** (syncope) is a brief loss of consciousness caused by a temporary decrease in blood flow to the brain. Fainting may occur while sitting, standing, walking, and occasionally during exercise. Fainting has many possible causes, including prolonged standing, cardiac dysrhythmias, seizure disorder, hyperventilation, gastrointestinal bleeding, and ruptured ectopic pregnancy. Fainting also may occur when experiencing or anticipating an unpleasant situation, such as seeing blood, feeling pain, or being pricked with a needle. Consider a cardiac cause if fainting occurs in a recumbent position, is provoked by exercise, is associated with chest pain, or if a family history of fainting or sudden death is present.

In near syncope (also called *presyncope*) signs and symptoms of impending syncope occur, including dizziness with or without blackout (called a *gray-out*), anxiety, pale skin, sweating, thready pulse, and low blood pressure.

In addition to a SAMPLE history, find out the patient's position and level of activity before the incident. Were any symptoms present before the event, such as weakness, lightheadedness, sweating, dizziness, visual disturbances, headache, chest pain, or palpitations? If the patient's episode of fainting was witnessed, try to determine the following:

- Duration of unresponsiveness
- Occurrence of any involuntary movements
- Duration of any confusion or disorientation after awakening
- Possibility of a fall or other trauma
- Patient's medical history, including medications and previous episodes of fainting
- Medical identification for conditions such as diabetes or seizures

Abnormal Heartbeat or Palpitations. Palpitations are an unpleasant awareness of one's heartbeat. Common descriptions patients use to describe palpitations are shown in Box 22-26. Palpitations can be caused by anxiety, lack of sleep, certain medicines, caffeine, stress, cocaine or amphetamine use, heavy cigarette smoking, or metabolic conditions such as hyperthyroidism. They also may be caused by changes in the heart's rhythm or rate, including tachycardias, premature beats, and **compensatory pauses.**

Try to determine when the palpitations began, how often they occur, and how long they last. Ask the patient to describe the palpitations and document the patient's

---

BOX 22-26 Common Patient Descriptions of Palpitations

- Skipping beats
- Flip-flopping
- Fluttering in the chest
- Pounding in the neck
- Running away
- Going too fast or too slow
- Jumping
- Racing
- Stopping

words, such as "skipping beats." Be sure to ask about associated symptoms such as chest discomfort, dyspnea, or syncope.

Fatigue. Fatigue is a common complaint in patients with impaired cardiovascular function. It also is one of the vaguest of all symptoms. Fatigue may be caused by many conditions. Electrolyte disorders, such as an unusually high or low potassium level, are a common cause of generalized weakness and fatigue. Fatigue may precede or accompany other symptoms associated with a heart attack. It also may be caused by medications, such as beta-blockers, diuretics, or antihypertensives.

Try to determine when the patient's fatigue began and how long it has been present. Ask about associated symptoms such as chest discomfort, nausea, dyspnea, syncope, or palpitations.

CULTURAL*Considerations*

When speaking with patients, understand that people from Asian, Middle Eastern, Native American, or possibly Hispanic cultures may not maintain direct eye contact with you out of respect. People from some Middle Eastern cultures view direct eye contact as sexually suggestive. Most Native Americans avoid direct eye contact out of respect and/or because they believe the eyes are a window to the soul. Looking at you directly in the eye might permit you to steal their soul.

Allergies

Ask the patient about allergies to medications, food, environmental elements (e.g., pollen), and products (e.g., latex).

Medications

What prescription and over-the-counter medications is the patient currently taking? Find out the name of the medication, dose, and indication for the medication. Be sure to document this information. If possible, bring the medication containers with you to the receiving facility. Ask the patient if he takes his medicine as prescribed. Has he missed any doses or taken extra doses of any medicine? Common cardiac medications include the following:

- Antiarrhythmics, such as digitalis (Lanoxin), procainamide (Procan, Pronestyl), amiodarone (Cordarone), and verapamil (Calan, Isoptin, Verelan)
- Anticoagulants, such as enoxaparin (Lovenox), clopidogrel (Plavix), and warfarin (Coumadin)
- Angiotensin-converting enzyme inhibitors, such as captopril (Capoten), enalapril (Vasotec), and lisinopril (Prinivil, Zestril)

- Beta-blockers, such as atenolol (Tenormin), metoprolol (Lopressor), and propranolol (Inderal)
- Lipid-lowering agents, such as gemfibrozil (Lopid), atorvastatin (Lipitor), fluvastatin (Lescol), lovastatin (Mevacor), pravastatin (Pravachol), rosuvastatin calcium (Crestor), and simvastatin (Zocor)
- Diuretics, such as furosemide (Lasix)
- Vasodilators, such as nitroglycerin (Nitrostat)

Ask whether the patient takes any herbal supplements or uses recreational drugs such as cocaine. Herbal supplements can cause serious, and even fatal, interactions when taken with certain cardiac medicines. Cocaine constricts blood vessels and can cause a sudden rise in blood pressure and heart rate.

Ask the patient whether he or she has taken sildenafil (Viagra), Cialis, Levitra, or similar medication in the last 24 to 48 hours. Although you may be uncomfortable asking the question, the patient's response is important and may affect the care you provide. For example, these medications should not be taken with drugs such as nitroglycerin.

Has the patient taken any medications that were not prescribed for him or her? Sometimes well-meaning family members or neighbors recognize a patient's signs and symptoms as being similar to, or the same as, a condition for which they are being treated. They may offer the patient a dose of their own medication in an effort to relieve the patient's symptoms. This unsafe practice is particularly common with diuretics (water pills), nitroglycerin, and blood pressure medications.

(Pertinent) *Past Medical History*

If time and the patient's condition permits, try to find out the answers to the following questions.

- *Are you currently under a physician's care?*
- *Do you have a history of a heart attack, angina, heart failure, high blood pressure, or abnormal heart rhythm?* If the patient answers yes to this question, ask him how his current symptoms compare to his previous episode.
- *Have you ever had a heart-related medical procedure such as a bypass (open-heart surgery), angioplasty, transplant, valve replacement, or pacemaker?*
- *Do you have a history of stroke; diabetes; lung, liver, or kidney disease; or other medical condition?*
- Find out the patient's risk factors for heart disease. Ask the patient if he or she smokes. If the answer is yes, ask how many packs per day. Ask the patient if a history of heart disease is in the family. If the answer is yes, ask whether anyone died of heart disease and at what age. Ask about a family history of high blood pressure, diabetes, and high cholesterol.
- *Have you been hospitalized recently? Any recent surgery?*

Cardiogenic Shock = poor prognosis

Last Oral Intake

Ask the patient when he or she last had anything to eat or drink and if any recent changes in eating patterns or fluid intake (or output) have occurred.

Events Leading to the Incident

Try to find out what precipitated the patient's current symptoms. For example, did an event or activity cause the patient's symptoms, such as strenuous exercise, sexual activity, or unusual stress?

Vital Signs and Physical Examination

[OBJECTIVE 63]

After completing the primary survey and managing any immediate life threats, assess the patient's vital signs, including pulse oximetry.

Assess the patient's respiratory rate and effort. Signs of respiratory compromise include the use of accessory muscles of respiration and the presence of retractions.

A pulse that is rapid (more than 150 beats/min), very slow (less than 40 beats/min), or irregular may be one of the first indicators of a cardiac dysrhythmia and requires further evaluation by ECG. Any patient who has a cardiac-related symptom should be placed on a cardiac monitor. Document the initial rhythm strip and any changes in the patient's rhythm. Each rhythm strip should be at least 6 seconds in duration. Attach the rhythm strips to the prehospital care report. Obtain a 12-lead ECG if indicated. Examples of indications for a 12-lead ECG include the following:

- Cardiac-related symptom, including chest discomfort or anginal equivalents (generalized weakness, difficulty breathing, excessive sweating, unexplained nausea and vomiting, dizziness, syncope or near-syncope, palpitations, isolated arm or jaw pain, fatigue, dysrhythmias)
- Stroke
- Respiratory failure
- Congestive heart failure
- Suspected electrolyte disturbances
- Overdose of unknown etiology
- Known or suspected tricyclic antidepressant overdose
- Blunt chest trauma
- Electrical injuries
- Before and after transcutaneous pacing or synchronized cardioversion
- After defibrillation

PARAMEDIC*Pearl*

A patient complaining of chest pain or discomfort should *immediately* be placed on a cardiac monitor.

In most patients a systolic blood pressure of less than 90 mm Hg is considered low blood pressure. In a patient with a cardiac-related problem, low blood pressure may indicate cardiogenic shock. Markedly elevated blood pressures may contribute to aortic dissection, heart failure, or stroke.

If the patient is unresponsive, perform a detailed (head to toes) physical examination if time and the patient's condition permit. If the patient is responsive, perform a focused examination.

Look (Inspection)

[OBJECTIVE 64]

Low cardiac output results in inadequate tissue perfusion. This often results in pale, mottled, or cyanotic skin. The skin of a patient having a heart attack may be cool and sweaty. The skin of a patient in cardiogenic shock may be cold and sweaty. This finding is a sympathetic response in which the blood within peripheral vessels is shunted to the vital organs to maintain adequate perfusion. Flushed, warm skin may be a sign of infection, such as pericarditis. Note that the body's response to pain may include restlessness, flushed skin, increased heart rate, increased respiratory rate, and/or elevated blood pressure.

Look at the patient's neck veins for jugular venous distention (JVD) (Figure 22-98). The patient should be sitting at a 45-degree angle with the head turned slightly away from you. The neck veins normally are flat when a patient is sitting or standing. They normally are mildly distended when the patient is supine. Thus the presence of JVD with the patient sitting at a 45-degree angle is abnormal. The jugular veins reflect the activity of the right side of the heart. Venous pressure rises with a significant increase in blood volume when the right ventricle fails or when increased pressure in the pericardial sac hinders the return of blood to the right atrium. Venous pressure falls when blood volume is significantly decreased or ejection of blood occurs from the left ventricle.

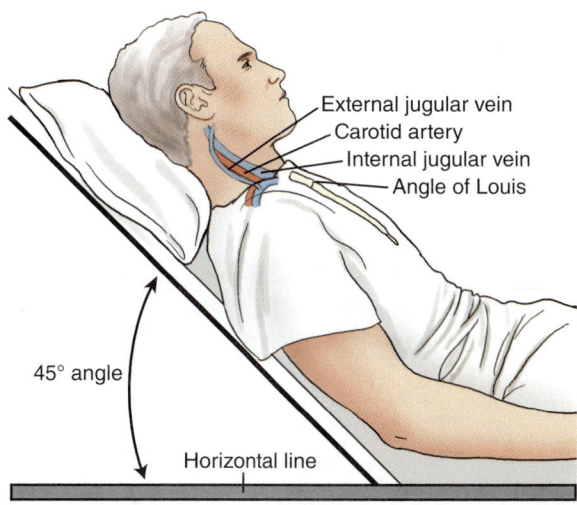

Figure 22-98 Look for jugular venous distention (JVD) with the patient sitting at a 45-degree angle.

Look at the patient's chest. A scar in the center of the patient's sternum suggests previous heart surgery. Look at the shape of the patient's chest. An expanded chest that resembles the shape of a barrel is called barrel chest. This finding may be seen in patients with chronic obstructive pulmonary disease. Look for signs of increased respiratory effort, such as retractions and the use of accessory muscles during breathing.

Look at the patient's abdomen for pulsations. Strong pulsations in the epigastric area may be a sign of an aortic aneurysm. Look for abdominal distention. Abdominal distention has many possible causes, including a tumor, fluid (ascites), gas, pregnancy, or fat.

Look at the patient's arms, hands, legs, feet, and ankles for swelling (edema). Because swelling occurs in the most dependent body areas, check for swelling in the lower back (sacral) area if the patient has been confined to bed. Determine if the swelling is pitting or nonpitting by pressing your thumb or finger to the skin over a bony area for 5 seconds. Edema is nonpitting if minimal or no depression is seen when pressure is removed. Pitting edema is present if an impression is left in the skin. Bilateral pitting edema may be a sign of right ventricular failure. Pitting edema limited to one side of the body suggests a blockage in a major vein. Pitting edema severity is rated on a scale ranging from 0 to 4+ (Table 22-44).

Look for other signs that suggest the patient has a history of cardiac disease. For example, the presence of a nitroglycerin patch on the patient's skin suggests a history of angina. A slight bulge under the skin of the patient's upper right or left chest or abdominal wall is probably a pacemaker or implantable defibrillator. Clubbing of the nails is associated with a variety of respiratory and cardiovascular conditions, including cyanotic congenital heart disease and pulmonary disease with hypoxia (Figure 22-99).

Listen (Auscultation)

[OBJECTIVES 65, 66, 67]

Listen to breath sounds. Remember to listen to the apexes and bases, comparing side to side. Determine whether breath sounds are present, diminished, or absent; equal or unequal; clear or noisy. Note the presence of crackles (rales), rhonchi, wheezes, or other abnormal sounds,

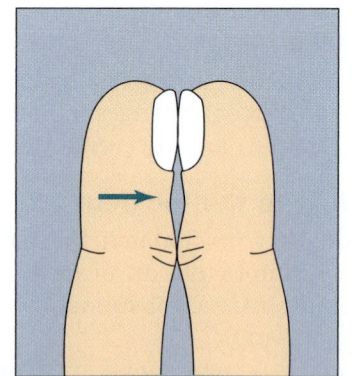

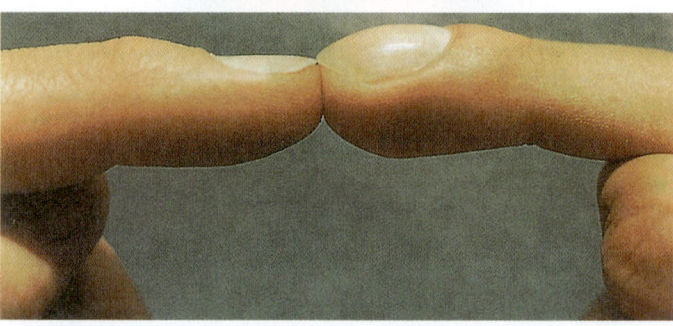

Figure 22-99 A, A patient who has healthy nails has a diamond-shaped window at the base of the nails when the corresponding fingers from the right and left hands are placed together. When nail clubbing is present, the diamond-shaped window is lost. **B**, Nail clubbing *(right)* and a normal nail *(left)*.

Kids - cystic fibrosis

such as gurgling. A patient who has pulmonary edema may have foamy, blood-tinged sputum present in the mouth or nose.

Assessment of heart sounds requires a relatively quiet environment. As a result, detailed assessment of heart sounds is usually not practical in the prehospital setting. However, the ability to recognize normal heart sounds can be useful. Heart sounds occur because of vibrations in the tissues of the heart caused by the closing of the heart's valves (Figure 22-100). Vibrations are created as blood flow is suddenly increased or slowed with the contraction and relaxation of the heart chambers and with the opening and closing of the heart's valves. Heart

TABLE 22-44	Degrees of Pitting Edema		
Description	Depth (inches)	Degree	Notes
Nonpitting	0	0	No pitting or swelling
Mild	0 to ¼	1+	Slight pitting, disappears quickly, no obvious swelling
Moderate	¼ to ½	2+	Pitting disappears in 10-15 sec, no obvious swelling
Severe	½ to 1	3+	Pitting may last more than 1 min, affected area appears swollen
Extreme	>1	4+	Pit lasts 2-5 min, affected area appears grossly distorted

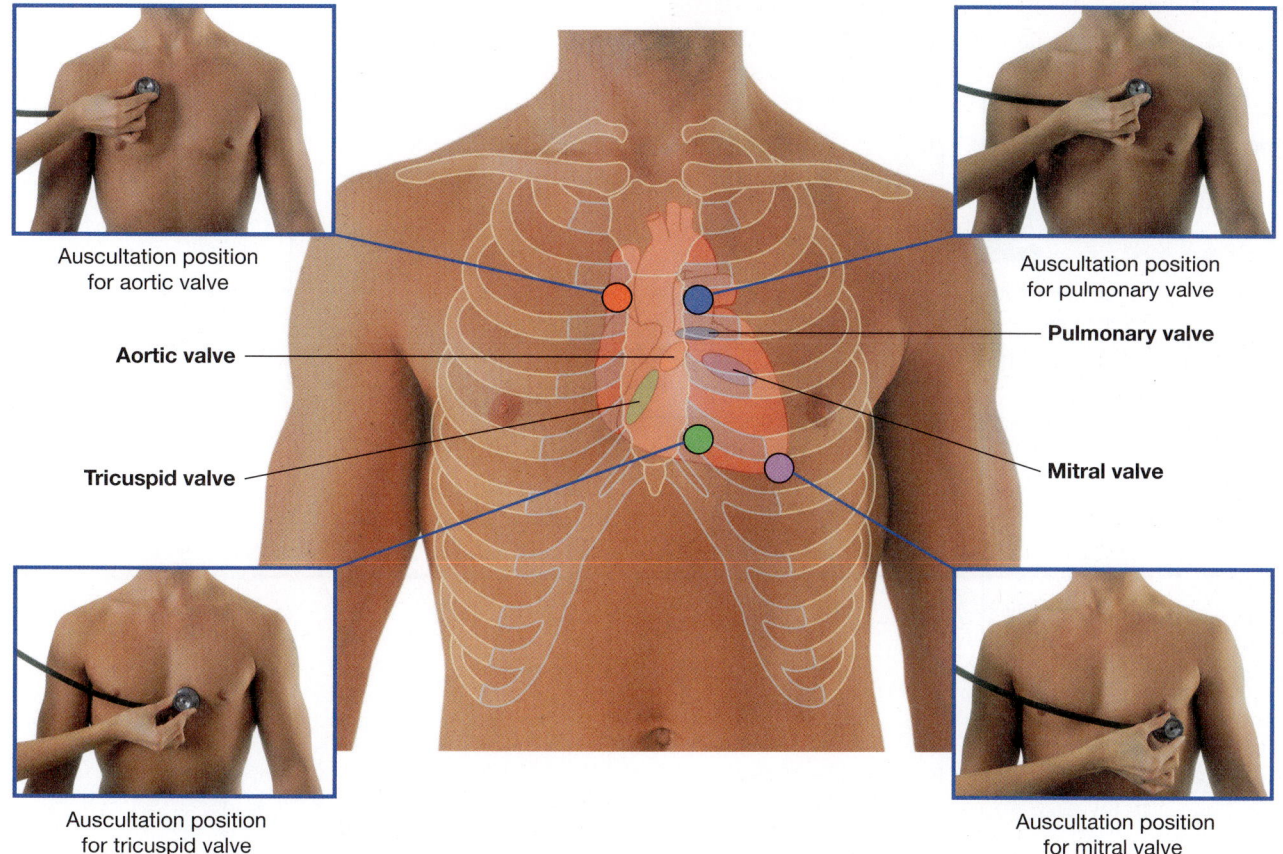

Auscultation position
for aortic valve

Auscultation position
for pulmonary valve

Pulmonary valve

Aortic valve

Mitral valve

Tricuspid valve

Auscultation position
for tricuspid valve

Auscultation position
for mitral valve

Figure 22-100 Anterior view of the chest showing the heart, location of the heart's valves, and where to listen to heart sounds.

sounds may be difficult to hear in obese individuals and may be quite loud in patients with thin chests.

S_1 and S_2 (S_1 = sound one; S_2 = sound two) are normal heart sounds. The first heart sound ("lubb") is low pitched and dull. It occurs during ventricular contraction when the tricuspid and mitral valves are closing. The second heart sound ("dupp") is shorter, higher-pitched, and louder than S_1. It occurs during ventricular relaxation when the pulmonic and aortic valves are closing.

A third heart sound is normal in children and young adults. When an S_1, S_2, S_3 sequence is heard in adults, it is called a ventricular gallop or gallop rhythm because it sounds like a horse galloping. A sound like "Ken (S_1) – tuck (S_2) – y (S_3)" is audible. S_3 is heard in early ventricular diastole. It is caused by vibration of the ventricular walls during rapid ventricular filling and often is associated with heart failure.

Applying carotid sinus massage may be warranted in the treatment of specific dysrhythmias. Before performing this procedure, you first must listen to the patient's carotid arteries for bruits with a stethoscope. If an artery is narrowed, blood flowing through the affected portion of the vessel creates turbulence. A **bruit** is the blowing or swishing sound created by the turbulence within the vessel. Narrowing of the vessel is often caused by atherosclerosis. Carotid sinus massage is contraindicated if a bruit is present. Applying pressure or massaging the vessel may loosen plaque, potentially causing a stroke.

Feel (Palpation)

[OBJECTIVES 68, 69, 70]

Palpation of the chest may reveal areas of tenderness or crepitus. For example, costochondritis is a condition that may cause chest pain from inflammation of the cartilage and bones in the chest wall. Lightly palpate the abdomen for pulsations and distention. These findings may be a sign of an abdominal aortic aneurysm.

Assess the rate, rhythm, strength, and equality of peripheral pulses (Figure 22-101, Table 22-45). Assess an apical pulse before giving medications that can alter heart rate or rhythm, when a child's peripheral pulse is too fast to count, or if a patient's heart rate is irregular. An apical pulse is assessed with a stethoscope. Place the stethoscope over the heart's apex, which is between the fifth and sixth ribs on the left side of the chest in adults. Count the apical pulse with each "lubb" sound that is heard for one full minute. Normally the apical pulse rate is the same as the pulse rate in a peripheral location, such as the radial pulse. A **pulse deficit** exists if a difference is found between the apical pulse and the peripheral pulse. For example, if a patient's apical pulse rate is 100 beats/min and the radial pulse rate is 75 beats/min, a pulse deficit

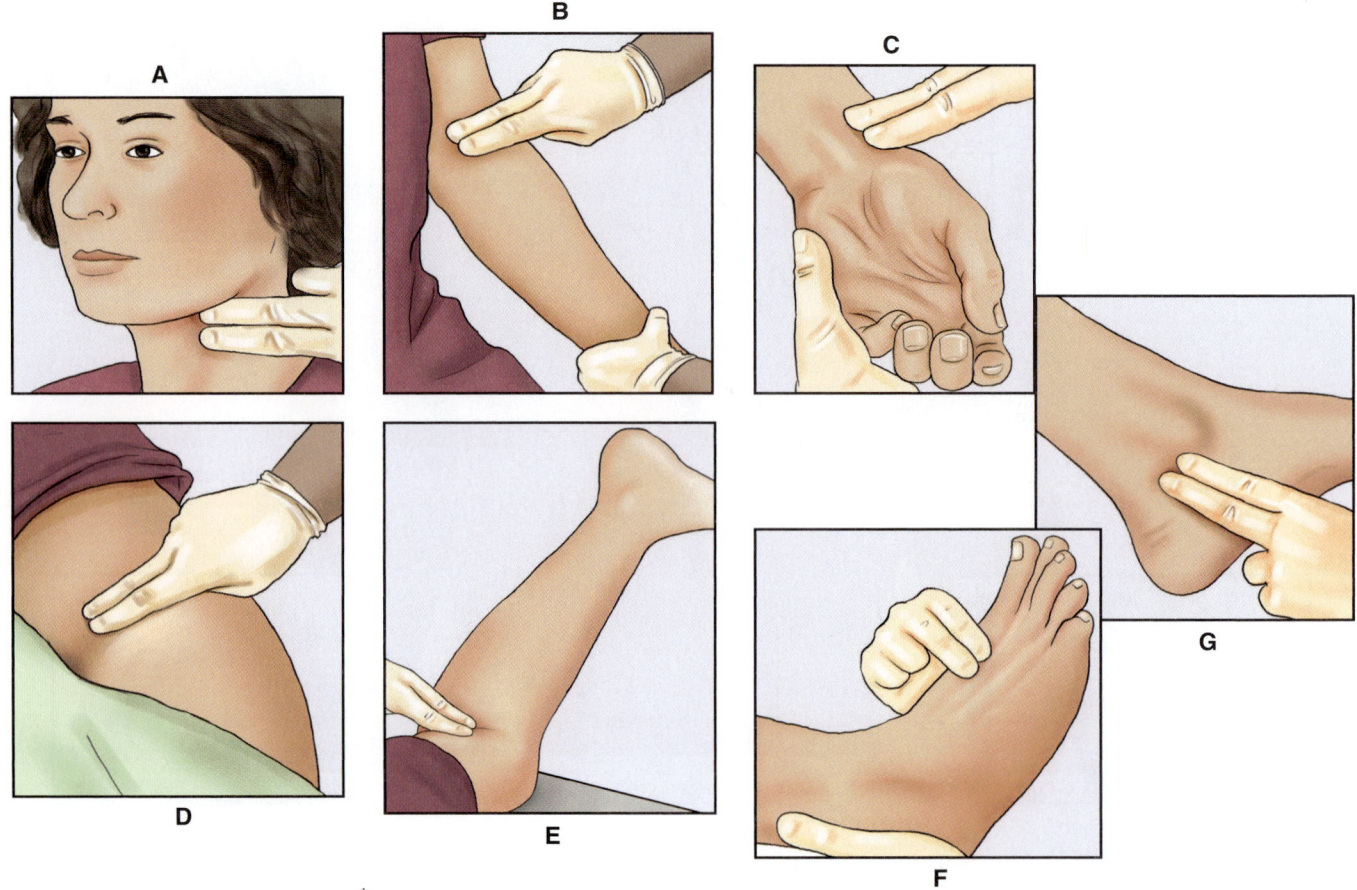

Figure 22-101 Palpation of arterial pulses. **A**, Carotid. **B**, Brachial. **C**, Radial. **D**, Femoral. **E**, Popliteal. **F**, Dorsalis pedis. **G**, Posterior tibial.

TABLE 22-45	Location of Palpable Arterial Pulses
Pulse	**Location**
Carotid	In the neck, medial to and below the angle of the jaw (do *not* palpate both sides of the neck at the same time)
Brachial	Just medial to the biceps tendon
Radial	Thumb side of the wrist (use gentle pressure)
Popliteal	Behind the knee; assess with knee flexed (press firmly)
Dorsalis pedis	Medial side of dorsum of foot (may be hard to feel and may not be felt in some well persons)
Posterior tibial	Behind and slightly inferior to the medial malleolus of the ankle (may be hard to feel and may not be felt in some well persons)

Modified from Seidel, H. M. (2003). *Mosby's guide to physical examination* (5th ed.) (p. 471), St. Louis: Mosby.

of 25 beats/min is present. A pulse deficit may occur with many abnormal heart rhythms or when the heart's contractions are too weak to propel blood through the peripheral arteries.

A beat-to-beat difference in the strength of a pulse is called **pulsus alternans** (also called *mechanical alternans*) (Figure 22-102). The difference in the beats is best detected by palpating femoral pulses rather than the brachial, radial, or carotid pulses (Weber, 2003). Pulsus alternans may be a sign of severe ventricular failure. The beat-to-beat changes in pulse strength are believed to be the result of a decrease in the number of myocardial cells contracting during alternate beats, resulting in decreased myocardial contractility. Pulsus alternans is not the same as electrical alternans, although they may coexist. **Electrical alternans** is a beat-to-beat change in waveform amplitude on the ECG. Changes in QRS amplitude may be seen in conditions such as LVF, myocardial ischemia, AFib, WPW syndrome, pulmonary embolism, and myocardial contusion. ST-segment and T-wave changes are common in patients at increased risk for ventricular dysrhythmias. Changes may be seen after cardiac resuscitation and in conditions such as angina pectoris, acute MI, electrolyte

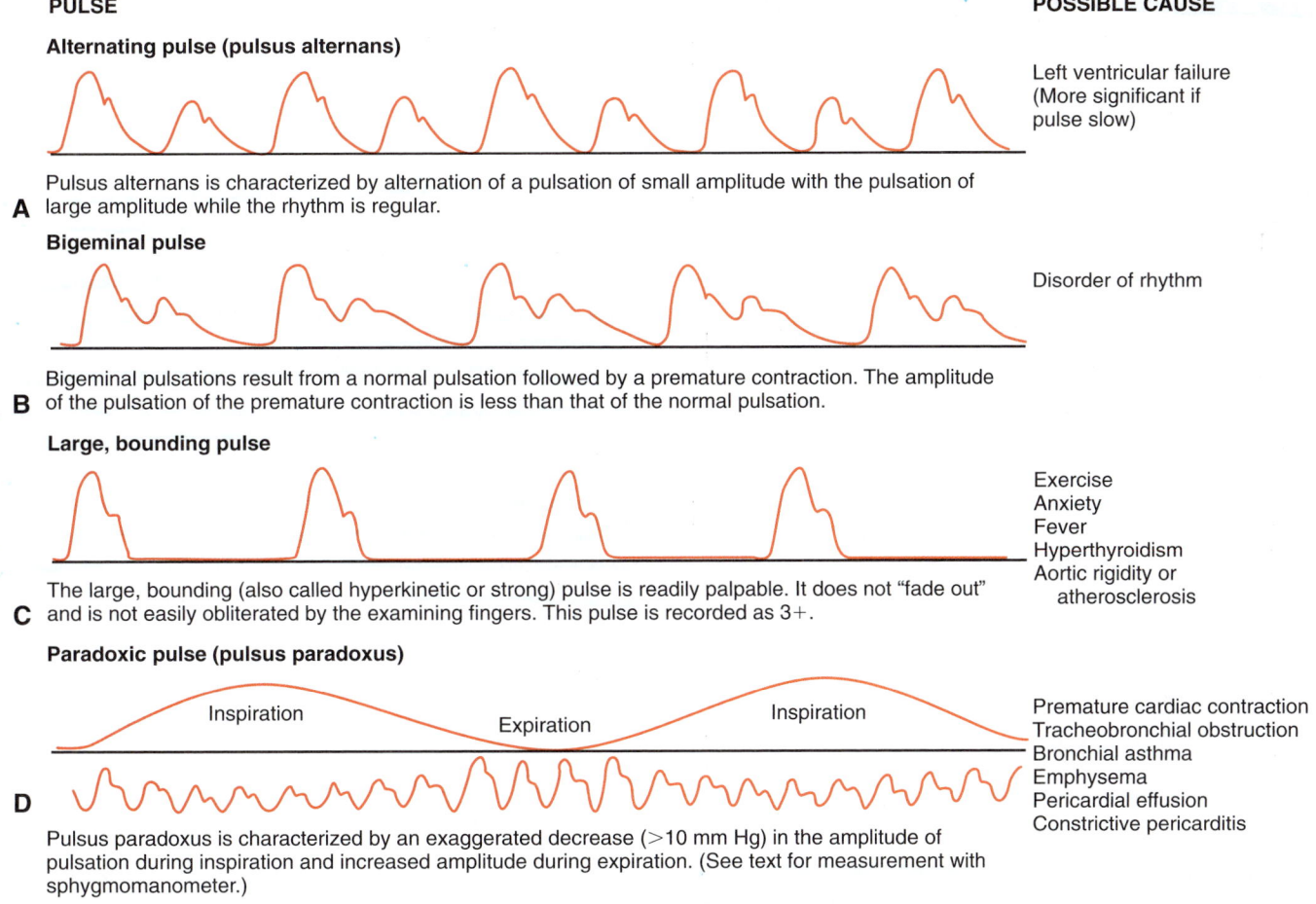

PULSE	POSSIBLE CAUSE

Alternating pulse (pulsus alternans)

Left ventricular failure (More significant if pulse slow)

A Pulsus alternans is characterized by alternation of a pulsation of small amplitude with the pulsation of large amplitude while the rhythm is regular.

Bigeminal pulse

Disorder of rhythm

B Bigeminal pulsations result from a normal pulsation followed by a premature contraction. The amplitude of the pulsation of the premature contraction is less than that of the normal pulsation.

Large, bounding pulse

Exercise
Anxiety
Fever
Hyperthyroidism
Aortic rigidity or atherosclerosis

C The large, bounding (also called hyperkinetic or strong) pulse is readily palpable. It does not "fade out" and is not easily obliterated by the examining fingers. This pulse is recorded as 3+.

Paradoxic pulse (pulsus paradoxus)

Inspiration   Expiration   Inspiration

Premature cardiac contraction
Tracheobronchial obstruction
Bronchial asthma
Emphysema
Pericardial effusion
Constrictive pericarditis

D Pulsus paradoxus is characterized by an exaggerated decrease (>10 mm Hg) in the amplitude of pulsation during inspiration and increased amplitude during expiration. (See text for measurement with sphygmomanometer.)

Figure 22-102 Pulse abnormalities.

disturbances, heart failure, and pulmonary embolism. Electrical alternans also may occur from changes in the position or motion of the heart, such as in cardiac tamponade and cardiomyopathy.

While at rest blood pressure normally fluctuates during the respiratory cycle, falling with inspiration and rising with expiration. The accepted upper limit for a fall in systolic blood pressure with inspiration is 10 mm Hg. **Pulsus paradoxus** (also called *paradoxic pulse*) occurs when the systolic blood pressure falls more than 10 mm Hg with inspiration. This may occur because of the following mechanisms, alone or in combination (Khasnis & Lokhandwala, 2002):

- Decreased blood flow to the right ventricle and pulmonary artery during inspiration
- Greater than normal pooling of blood in the pulmonary circulation
- Wide changes in intrathoracic pressure during inspiration and expiration
- Interference with venous return to either atrium, especially during inspiration

Conditions in which pulsus paradoxus may be present include the following:

- Cardiac tamponade
- Constrictive pericarditis
- Pulmonary embolism
- Acute MI
- Emphysema
- Cardiogenic shock
- Severe bronchial asthma
- Tension pneumothorax
- Hypovolemia

When dissection of the thoracic aorta occurs, a difference in blood pressure measurements may be detectable in the arms. This discrepancy occurs when one of the vessels to the arm is blocked by the dissection. A difference of more than 10 mm Hg is highly suggestive of dissection.

Pulse pressure reflects stroke volume and arterial elasticity. **Pulse pressure** is the difference between the systolic and diastolic blood pressure. For example, if the systolic blood pressure is 120 mm Hg and the diastolic blood pressure is 80 mm Hg, the pulse pressure is 40 mm Hg. Normal pulse pressure is 30 to 40 mm Hg. A widened (high) pulse pressure (more than 40 mm Hg) may be seen in conditions such as the later stages of shock. A narrowed pulse pressure (less than 30 mm Hg) may be seen in conditions such as tachycardia and cardiac tamponade.

REASSESSMENT

In most cases, you will reassess the patient en route to the receiving facility. If the patient's chief complaint was pain or discomfort when you arrived, be sure to reassess the patient's pain intensity, location, and duration frequently while he or she is in your care. If medications were given, monitor the patient's response to them. Frequently reassess the patient's breath sounds, ECG, and vital signs. Compare these findings to the baseline information obtained during the physical examination. Adjust the treatment plan accordingly.

SECTION 5: CARDIOVASCULAR DISORDERS
ACQUIRED DISEASES OF THE MYOCARDIUM
Acute Coronary Syndromes

[OBJECTIVES 71, 72, 73]

When a temporary or permanent blockage occurs in a coronary artery, the blood supply to the heart muscle is impaired. An impaired blood supply results in a decreased supply of oxygen to the myocardium. When the heart's demand for oxygen exceeds its supply from the coronary circulation, chest discomfort or related symptoms often occur. A decreased supply of oxygenated blood to a body part or organ is called **ischemia**.

Description and Definition

Acute coronary syndromes (ACS) are conditions caused by a similar sequence of pathologic events—a temporary or permanent blockage of a coronary artery. This sequence of events results in conditions ranging from myocardial ischemia or injury to death (necrosis) of heart muscle. ACS include unstable angina, non-ST-segment elevation MI (NSTEMI), and ST-segment elevation MI (STEMI). Sudden cardiac death can occur with any of these conditions.

Etiology

The usual cause of an ACS is the rupture of an atherosclerotic plaque. To understand this process, some anatomy must be reviewed quickly.

Arteries consist of three layers. The outermost layer is the tunica adventitia. It consists of flexible connective tissue and helps hold the vessel open. The middle layer is the tunica media. It consists of smooth muscle tissue and elastic connective tissue. This layer is encircled by smooth muscle and innervated by fibers of the auto-

nomic nervous system that allows constriction and dilation of the vessel. Smooth muscle cells function to maintain vascular tone and regulate local blood flow depending on the body's metabolic needs. These cells also are capable of producing collagen, elastin, and other substances important in the formation of atherosclerotic plaques. The innermost layer of an artery is the tunica intima. It is composed of endothelium that lines the vascular system. Endothelium is a single layer of cells in direct contact with the blood. The intima is at risk of damage from conditions such as hypertension, high cholesterol, smoking, and diabetes.

Arteriosclerosis is a chronic disease of the arterial system characterized by abnormal thickening and hardening of the vessel walls. **Atherosclerosis** (from *athero*, meaning gruel or paste, and *sclerosis*, meaning hardness) is a form of arteriosclerosis in which the thickening and hardening of the vessel walls are caused by a buildup of fatty deposits in the inner lining of large and middle-sized muscular arteries (Figure 22-103). As the fatty deposits build up, the opening of the artery slowly narrows and blood flow to the muscle decreases.

Any artery in the body can develop atherosclerosis. If the coronary arteries are involved (coronary artery disease) and blood flow to the heart is decreased, angina or more serious signs and symptoms may result. If the arteries in the leg are involved (peripheral vascular disease), leg pain (claudication) may result. If the arteries supplying the brain are involved (carotid artery disease), a stroke or transient ischemic attack may result.

Atherosclerotic plaques differ in their makeup, vulnerability to rupture, and tendency to make blood clots. Stable plaques are unlikely to rupture. They consist mainly of collagen-rich tissue that has hardened. They have a thick, fibrous cap over the fatty center that separates it from contact with the blood, making them less likely to rupture (Figure 22-104). As these plaques increase in size, the artery can become severely narrowed. Plaques prone to rupture are called vulnerable plaques. They are soft and have a thin cap of fibrous tissue over the fatty center that separates it from the opening of the artery. If the fibrous cap tears or ruptures, the contents of the plaque are exposed to flowing blood. Platelets stick to the damaged lining of the vessel and to each other and form a plug. Sticky platelets secrete several chemicals, including thromboxane A_2. These substances stimulate vasoconstriction, reducing blood flow at the site. Aspirin blocks the production of thromboxane A_2, slowing the clumping (aggregation) of platelets.

Once platelets are activated, glycoprotein IIb/IIIa receptors needed for platelet clumping appear on the surface of the platelet. Fibrinogen molecules bind to these receptors to form bridges (cross links) between nearby platelets, allowing them to clump. Medications called glycoprotein IIb/IIIa receptor inhibitors prevent fibrinogen binding and platelet clumping.

As the process continues, thrombin is made and fibrin is formed, ultimately producing a clot. Clots can be

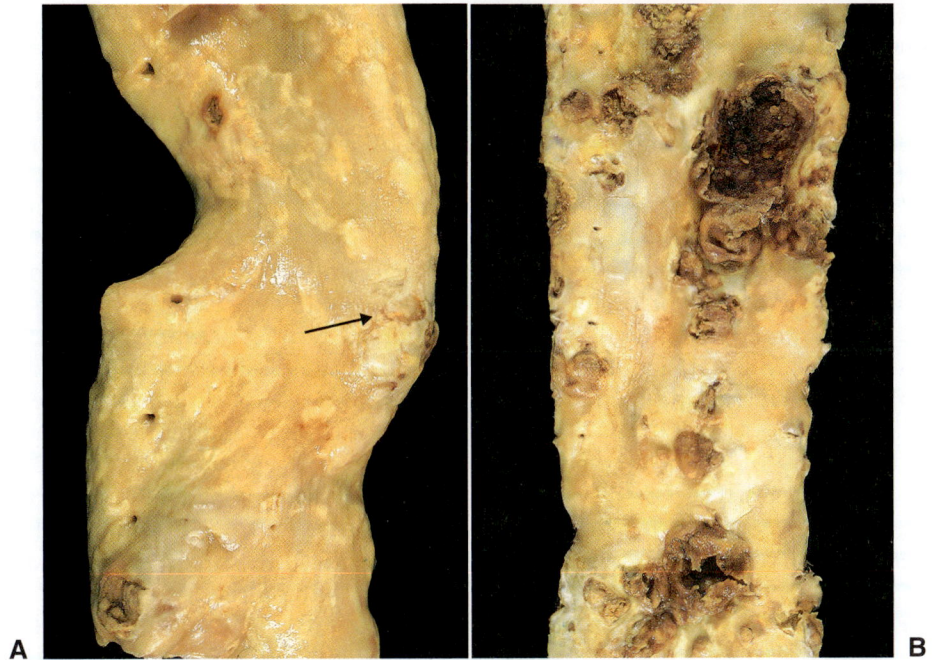

Figure 22-103 Atherosclerosis in the aorta. **A**, Mild atherosclerosis composed of fibrous plaques, one of which is denoted by the *arrow*. **B**, Severe disease with diffuse and complicated lesions.

Artery has to be 50% occluded to have coronary artery disease

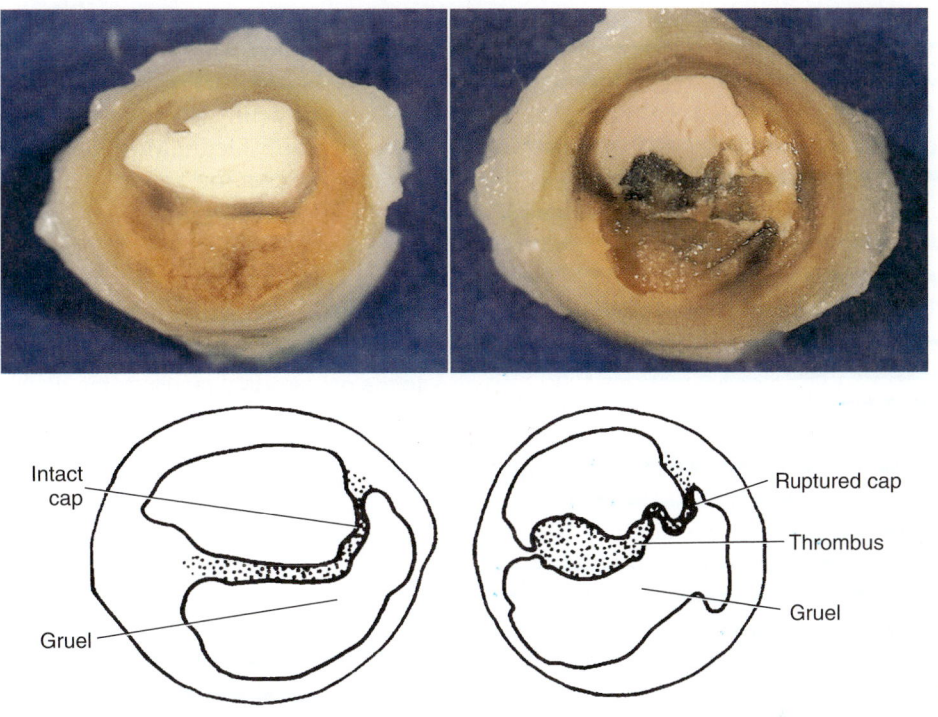

Figure 22-104 View of a vulnerable plaque. **A**, The yellow, soft atheromatous material (gruel) is separated from the opening of the vessel only by a thin, but intact, fibrous cap. The vessel opening contains white radiographic contrast medium. **B**, This specimen was just a few millimeters distal to the one shown in **A**. Here the thin fibrous cap is ruptured, a big cap fragment and some of the soft atheromatous gruel are missing (from downstream embolization), and a clot has evolved where the gruel has been exposed. White contrast medium has penetrated the soft gruel through the ruptured cap.

[handwritten top margin: NSR 1st → ST segment depression ischemia → ST segment elevation injury → elevation + Q wave infarct]

dissolved by a process called **fibrinolysis.** Fibrinolytics (clot busters) are medications that stimulate the conversion of plasminogen to plasmin, which dissolves the clot.

Rupture of a vulnerable plaque may follow extreme physical activity (especially in someone unaccustomed to regular exercise), severe emotional trauma, sexual activity, exposure to illicit drugs (cocaine, marijuana, or amphetamines), exposure to cold, or acute infection (Shah, 2003). Contributing factors to plaque rupture include the frictional force from blood flow, coronary spasm at the site of the plaque, internal plaque changes, and the effects of risk factors, such as high blood pressure and high cholesterol.

Blockage of a coronary artery by a clot may be complete or incomplete. Complete blockage of a coronary artery may result in STEMI or sudden death. Partial (incomplete) blockage of a coronary artery by a clot may result in no clinical signs and symptoms (silent MI), unstable angina, NSTEMI, or possibly sudden death.

Angina Pectoris. Angina pectoris is chest discomfort that occurs when the heart muscle does not receive enough oxygen (myocardial ischemia). Ischemia can occur because of increased myocardial oxygen demand (demand ischemia), reduced myocardial oxygen supply (supply ischemia), or both. If the cause of the ischemia is not reversed and blood flow restored to the affected area of the heart muscle, ischemia may lead to cellular injury and ultimately infarction.

Angina most often occurs in patients with coronary artery disease involving at least one coronary artery. However, it can be present in patients with normal coronary arteries. Angina also occurs in persons with uncontrolled high blood pressure or valvular heart disease.

Stable Angina. Stable (classic) angina remains relatively constant and predictable in terms of severity, signs and symptoms, precipitating events, and response to treatment. It is characterized by brief episodes of chest discomfort related to activities that increase the heart's need for oxygen, such as emotional upset, exercise or exertion, and exposure to cold weather. Related symptoms include shortness of breath, palpitations, sweating, nausea, or vomiting. Symptoms typically last 2 to 5 minutes and occasionally 5 to 15 minutes. Prolonged discomfort (more than 30 minutes) is uncommon in stable angina.

[handwritten left margin: Nitro responsive]

Unstable Angina. Unstable angina (also known as preinfarction angina) is a condition of intermediate severity between stable angina and acute MI. Unstable angina is characterized by one or more of the following:

[handwritten left margin: can be Nitro responsive but not completely / others longer]

- Symptoms that occur at rest (or minimal exertion) and usually last more than 20 minutes
- Symptoms that are severe and/or of new onset (i.e., within 2 months)
- Symptoms that are increasing in intensity, duration, and/or frequency in a patient with a history of stable angina

Unlike stable angina, the discomfort associated with unstable angina may be described as painful. Patients with untreated unstable angina are at high risk of a heart attack or death. Early assessment and emergency care are essential to prevent worsening ischemia.

Prinzmetal's Angina. Prinzmetal's angina (also called Prinzmetal's variant angina, variant angina, or vasospastic angina) is a form of unstable angina. Patients with Prinzmetal's angina often have coronary artery plaques (Braunwald et al, 2002), but some patients have normal coronary arteries. This uncommon type of angina is the result of intense spasm of a segment of a coronary artery. The spasm occurs almost exclusively at rest, often occurs at night or in the early morning hours, and may awaken the patient from sleep. It is usually not brought on by physical exertion or emotional stress. Chest discomfort may be accompanied by difficulty breathing and/or palpitations. Episodes usually last only a few minutes, but this may be long enough to produce serious dysrhythmias, including AV block and VT, as well as sudden death.

Myocardial Infarction. Ischemia prolonged more than just a few minutes results in myocardial *injury*. Injured myocardial cells are still alive but will die (infarct) if the ischemia is not quickly corrected. If blood flow is quickly restored, no tissue death occurs. Methods to restore blood flow include administration of fibrinolytic agents, coronary angioplasty, or a coronary artery bypass graft, among others.

A **myocardial infarction (MI)** occurs when blood flow to the heart muscle stops or is suddenly decreased long enough to cause cell death (Box 22-27, Figure 22-105). An acute MI usually results from a thrombus. Less commonly, acute MI may occur because of coronary spasm (as in cocaine abuse) or coronary embolism (rare).

PARAMEDIC *Pearl*

In the strictest sense, the term *MI* relates to dead heart muscle tissue. In a practical sense, the term *MI* is applied to the process that results in the death of myocardial tissue. Think of the process of MI as a continuum rather than the presence of dead heart tissue. If efforts are made to recognize the process of MI, patients may be identified earlier. If they are promptly treated, the loss of heart tissue may be avoided (Phalen & Aehlert, 2006).

Patients with a STEMI show evidence of ST-segment elevation on their ECG. As its name implies, patients with an NSTEMI do not show signs of myocardial injury (ST-segment elevation) on their ECG. Distinguishing patients with unstable angina from those with acute MI may be impossible during initial presentation because their signs, symptoms, and ECG findings may be identical. The diagnosis of infarction is made on the basis of the patient's signs and symptoms, ECG findings, history,

[handwritten bottom margin left: Nitro-dilates coronary + peripheral vessels / ↓ preload → ↓ HR - more O₂ to myocardium]

[handwritten bottom margin right: After 1 hr, infarcted area 50% dead / After 6 hrs, " " 100% dead]

Terminology

- Acute MI = 6 hours to 7 days
- Healing MI = 7 to 28 days
- Healed MI = 29 days or more

Classification by Size

- Microscopic: focal necrosis
- Small: <10% of the left ventricle
- Medium: 10% to 30% of the left ventricle
- Large: >30% of the left ventricle

MI, Myocardial infarction.

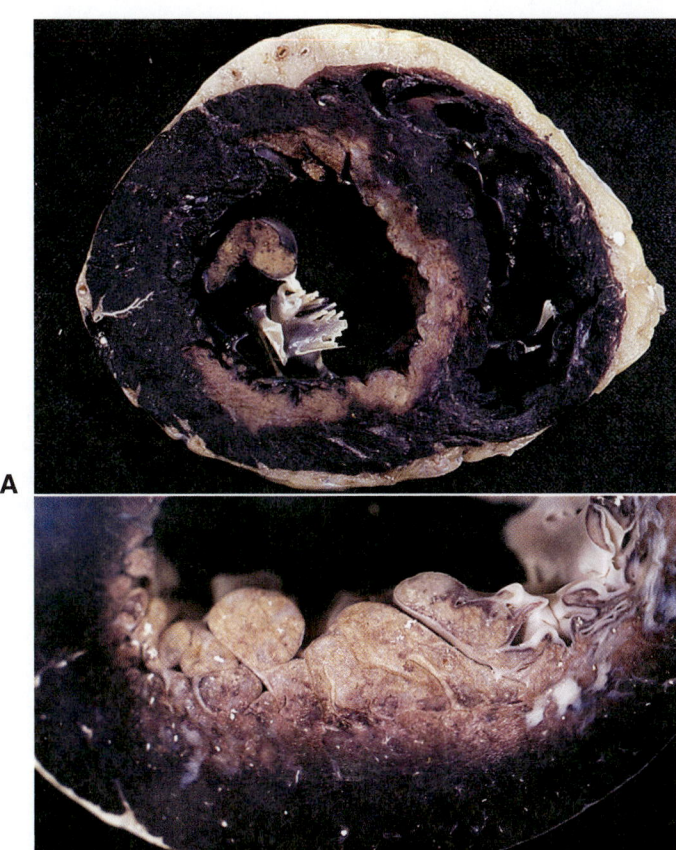

A

B

Figure 22-105 Myocardial infarction. **A**, Massive infarction caused by blockage of three coronary arteries; **B**, Local infarction confined to one area of the heart.

and blood test results that confirm the presence of an infarction (cardiac biomarkers).

Myocardial Infarction and Trauma. Although uncommon, MI may occur from blunt chest trauma. Injury to the heart may occur when the chest wall strikes the steering wheel, as in high-speed motor vehicle crashes. Other causes include sports injuries, falls from heights, crushing injuries, blast injuries, and direct blows.

Blunt injury to the chest may result in a myocardial concussion. Commotio cordis is a type of myocardial concussion caused by a sharp, direct blow to the chest, such as by a baseball. If the blow occurs during a vulnerable portion of the T wave, the victim may develop VF.

Bruising of the heart muscle occurs with a myocardial contusion. Although permanent myocardial damage is rare, a myocardial contusion may cause atrial and ventricular dysrhythmias, bradydysrhythmias, and BBBs. A widespread myocardial contusion can cause a significant decrease in cardiac output, heart failure, and cardiogenic shock. A traumatic MI may occur because of a severe myocardial contusion or direct trauma to the coronary arteries. The severest form of blunt cardiac injury is cardiac rupture.

Complications of Myocardial Infarction. Dysrhythmias are the most common complication in the first few hours after MI (Box 22-28). Most deaths from STEMI occur within the first 1 to 2 hours after the onset of symptoms, usually from VF (Antman et al, 2004).

An AIVR is often seen during the first 12 hours of acute MI. PVCs may accompany sinus tachycardia early in the course of MI, possibly because of increased sympathetic nervous system activity. Most instances of VT and VF after STEMI occur within the first 48 hours. AFib is more common than atrial flutter or PSVT in patients with STEMI (Antman et al, 2004). Sinus bradycardia occurs often in MI (30% to 40%), particularly with inferior and posterior infarction. An accelerated junctional rhythm is more common with inferior STEMI than with anterior STEMI. AV blocks may develop in approximately 6% to 14% and BBBs may occur in approximately 10% to 20% of patients with STEMI (Antman et al, 2004).

Remember that infarcted tissue is dead tissue. Because dead tissue cannot contract, a large infarction can result

- Dysrhythmias (most common)
- Heart failure, pulmonary edema
- Cardiogenic shock : *BP <100 — fluid challenge if no pulmonary edema — next is Dopamine*
- Systemic or pulmonary thromboembolism
- Papillary muscle rupture, mitral valve insufficiency
- Dressler's syndrome (pericarditis occurring 2 to 4 weeks after MI)
- Ventricular aneurysm or rupture — *occurs ~2 weeks after MI*
- Ventricular septal defect

MI, Myocardial infarction.

MI usually starts in smaller vessels in endocardium

in pump failure and pulmonary congestion. If the pump continues to fail, cardiac output will decrease and cardiogenic shock will result. Complications of acute MI are listed in Box 22-34.

Epidemiology and Demographics

- Each year, approximately 1.1 million Americans have a heart attack. Approximately 460,000 of these events are fatal, and about half of these deaths occur within 1 hour of the onset of symptoms and before the person reaches the hospital (Greenlund et al, 2004).
- In 2001 the number of premature deaths (age younger than 65 years) from diseases of the heart was greatest among American Indians and Alaska Natives (36%) and blacks (31.5%) and lowest among whites (14.7%) (American Heart Association, 2005a).
- An estimated 30 patients with stable angina exist for every patient with infarction who is hospitalized (Gibbons et al, 2002).
- Unstable angina occurs most often in men and women aged 60 to 80 years who have one or more of the major risk factors for coronary artery disease.
- Between the ages of 40 and 60 years, the incidence of MI increases fivefold (Schoen, 2005a).
- Nearly 10% of MIs occur in people younger than 40 years, and 45% occur in people younger than age 65 years (Schoen, 2005b).
- In a 2000 study, 33% of patients admitted to a hospital with a MI did not have chest pain on presentation to the hospital. MI patients without chest pain had a longer delay before hospital presentation; were less likely to be diagnosed as having confirmed MI at the time of hospital admission; and were less likely to receive fibrinolytics, angioplasty, aspirin, beta-blockers, or heparin (Canto et al, 2000).

History

Not all chest pain is cardiac related. Obtaining an accurate history is important to help determine if the patient's signs and symptoms are most likely related to ischemia caused by coronary artery disease. Following are the five most important historical factors, ranked in order of importance (Braunwald et al, 2002):

1. The nature of the anginal symptoms
2. Previous history of CAD
3. Gender
4. Age
5. The number of risk factors present

Angina means squeezing or tightening, not pain. Chest discomfort associated with myocardial ischemia usually begins in the central or left chest and then radiates to the arm (especially the little finger [ulnar] side of the left

arm), wrist, jaw, epigastrium, left shoulder, or between the shoulder blades. Ischemic chest discomfort is usually not sharp, worsened by deep inspiration, affected by moving muscles in the area where the discomfort is localized, or positional in nature.

Chest discomfort is the most common symptom of infarction. It is present in 75% to 80% of patients with acute MI. Patients having a heart attack may describe the sensation they are feeling as similar to angina, or use words such as "heartburn," "indigestion," "dull," "squeezing," "gnawing," "aching," "tightness," or "pressure." The patient may describe discomfort with a clenched fist held against the sternum (Levine's sign). The discomfort typically lasts longer than 30 minutes. It may be constant or come and go and occasionally may be relieved with belching (Antman et al, 2004). Common cardiac-related symptoms include:

- Altered mental status
- Restlessness, anxiety
- Feeling of impending doom
- Anguished facial expression
- Nausea and vomiting
- Profuse sweating
- Fatigue
- Palpitations
- Edema of extremities, sacral area
- Headache
- Syncope
- Activity limitations

Anginal equivalent symptoms are symptoms of myocardial ischemia other than chest pain or discomfort. Examples of anginal equivalents include the following:

- Generalized weakness
- Difficulty breathing
- Excessive sweating
- Unexplained nausea and vomiting
- Dizziness
- Syncope or near syncope
- Palpitations
- Isolated arm or jaw pain
- Fatigue
- Dysrhythmias

Chest discomfort is absent in approximately 20% of patients having an infarction. Patients more likely to appear atypical include older adults, diabetic individuals, and women. Older adults may have atypical symptoms such as a change in mental status, generalized weakness, syncope, shortness of breath, fatigue, unexplained nausea, and abdominal or epigastric discomfort. Diabetic patients may present atypically with generalized weakness, syncope, lightheadedness, or a change in mental status. Women with an ACS often describe their discomfort as aching, tightness, pressure, sharpness, burning, fullness, or tingling. The location of the discomfort often is in the back, shoulder, or neck. Some women have

---

BOX 22-29 **Common Reasons for Delays in Seeking Medical Care for Ischemic-Type Chest Discomfort**

- Unaware of the importance of calling EMS or 911 for symptoms
- Unaware of the need for rapid treatment
- Mild discomfort began slowly, not abruptly, and with severe pain as depicted on television or in the movies ("Hollywood heart attack")
- Believed symptoms would go away or were not serious
- Believed symptoms were caused by another chronic condition, such as arthritis, muscle strain, or "the flu"

- Did not want to "bother" EMS personnel or their physician
- Afraid of embarrassment if symptoms turned out to be a false alarm
- Wanted family approval before seeking medical care
- Believed they were not at risk for a heart attack (especially women or young, healthy men)

Data from Antman, E. M., Anbe, D. T., Armstrong, P. W., Bates, E. R., Green, L., et al. (2004). *ACC/AHA guidelines for the management of patients with ST-elevation myocardial infarction: A report of the American College of Cardiology/American Heart Association Task Force on Practice Guidelines (Committee to Revise the 1999 Guidelines for the Management of Patients With Acute Myocardial Infarction).* Retrieved April 25, 2008, from http://www.acc.org/qualityandscience/clinical/guidelines/stemi/Guideline1/index.htm.

measure BP in both arms — pulses deficit

---

vague chest discomfort that tends to come and go with no known aggravating factors. Frequent acute symptoms include shortness of breath, weakness, unusual fatigue, cold sweats, dizziness, and nausea or vomiting.

A precipitating factor is present in approximately 50% of patients having an MI. Examples include unusually vigorous exercise, severe emotional stress, or serious illness. Approximately two thirds of patients describe the new onset of angina or a change in their anginal pattern in the month preceding infarction. Cocaine use may be a factor, particularly in patients older than 40 years.

After the onset of ischemic chest pain symptoms, most patients do not seek medical care for 2 hours or more. Women often delay longer than men do in seeking medical help. Common reasons for the delay in seeking medical care are shown in Box 22-29. The likelihood of death from acute MI decreases as the interval between symptom onset and initiation of treatment decreases. According to the National Heart Attack Alert Program, each hour of delay equals a 1% increase in the likelihood of death.

PARAMEDIC *Pearl*

"Although typical characteristics substantially raise the probability of [coronary artery disease], features not characteristic of chest pain, such as sharp stabbing pain or reproduction of pain on palpation, **do not exclude** the possibility of ACS" (Braunwald et al., 2000).

Physical Findings

The physical examination is important in patients with a possible ACS. The patient's physical findings may help identify potential causes of myocardial ischemia, such as

uncontrolled high blood pressure. The physical examination also allows you to assess the impact of the ischemic event on the patient's cardiovascular system. Physical findings may vary from few abnormalities to many depending on the site and extent of ischemia, injury, or infarction.

The patient may appear restless, anxious, or frightened. Breath sounds may be clear or reveal congestion in the bases. Labored breathing may or may not be present. Patients who present with crackles have a higher likelihood of severe underlying CAD. The patient's skin may be cool, clammy, pale, or ashen. The heart rate may be within normal limits, fast, or slow. A rapid heart rate and high blood pressure may be a result of the sympathetic nervous system's response to the ischemic event. These findings may be seen in patients experiencing an anterior MI. A slow heart rate and low blood pressure may be a result of the parasympathetic nervous system's response to the ischemic event. These findings may be seen in patients experiencing an inferior and/or posterior MI. The cardiac rhythm may be regular or irregular. A fast, slow, or irregular pulse may be due to atrial or ventricular dysrhythmias, or a heart block. Pulses that are difficult to feel may be due to low cardiac output or vascular disease. When possible, measure the patient's blood pressure in both arms. The presence of a pulse deficit suggests vascular disease and a higher likelihood of significant coronary artery disease. Altered mental status; hypotension; and cool, clammy, pale, or cyanotic skin in a patient with an ACS may be signs of cardiogenic shock. The combination of hypotension (of varying degrees), clear lung sounds, and JVD in a patient with inferior MI suggests RVI.

Ischemia affects the heart's cells responsible for contraction as well as those responsible for generation and conduction of electrical impulses. These effects can be viewed on the ECG as brief changes in ST segments and T waves in the leads facing the affected area of the ventricle. ST-segment *depression* is suggestive of myocardial ischemia. It is considered significant when the ST segment is 0.5 mm or more below the baseline. Negative (inverted) T waves also may be present. T-wave inversion is significant if it is new and the T waves are 3 mm or more. These ECG changes, and the chest discomfort that accompanies myocardial ischemia, usually resolve when the following occur:

- The demand for oxygen is reduced (by resting or slowing the heart rate with medications such as beta-blockers) to a level that can be supplied by the coronary artery
- Blood flow is increased by dilating the coronary arteries with medications such as nitroglycerin

✗ Although typical angina produces ST-segment *depression,* Prinzmetal's angina produces ST-segment *elevation.* After the episode of chest pain is resolved, ST segments usually return to the baseline. Because nitroglycerin is effective at relieving the coronary spasm, ECG evidence of Prinzmetal's angina may be lost if no pretreatment ECG is obtained (Phalen & Aehlert, 2006).

PARAMEDIC*Pearl*

In a patient with an ACS, keep in mind that myocardial injury refers to myocardial tissue that has been cut off from or experienced a severe reduction in its blood and oxygen supply. The tissue is not yet dead and may be salvageable if the blocked vessel can be quickly opened, restoring blood flow and oxygen to the injured area.

PARAMEDIC*Pearl*

A completely normal ECG in a patient with chest pain or discomfort does not exclude the possibility of an ACS. From 1% to 6% of such patients eventually are proved to have had an acute MI. A total of 4% or more will be found to have unstable angina (Braunwald et al, 2002).

Differential Diagnosis

[OBJECTIVE 74]

For chest pain and discomfort, a variety of differential diagnoses exist:

- Cardiovascular causes
  - Aneurysm
  - Aortic dissection
  - Microvascular disease (syndrome X)
  - Myocardial ischemia
  - Myocarditis
  - Pericarditis
- Respiratory causes
  - Pleurisy
  - Pneumothorax
  - Pulmonary embolism
  - Respiratory infections
- Gastrointestinal causes
  - Cholecystitis
  - Dyspepsia
  - Esophageal spasm
  - Gastroesophageal reflux disease
  - Hiatal hernia
  - Pancreatitis
  - Peptic ulcer disease
- Musculoskeletal causes
  - Acromioclavicular disease
  - Chest wall syndrome
  - Chest wall tumors
  - Chest wall trauma
  - Costochondritis
  - Intercostal muscle cramps
- Other causes
  - Herpes zoster (shingles)
  - Panic attack

Therapeutic Interventions

The goals in the immediate management of ACS include:

- Minimize infarct size
- Save ischemic heart muscle
- Lessen vasoconstriction
- Reduce myocardial oxygen demand
- Prevent and manage complications
- Improve chances of survival

As previously mentioned, many conditions other than a cardiac-related problem can cause chest discomfort. Because determining the exact cause of chest discomfort (or anginal equivalents) in the field is difficult, suspect an ACS until it is ruled out.

In canine studies, an estimated 50% of tissue loss occurs within 2 hours of coronary artery blockage. Tissue death may be noted as early as the first 20 minutes of infarction, and studies estimate that approximately 90% of tissue loss occurs within the first 6 hours. Therefore, if heart muscle is to be saved, the blockage must be removed before irreversible tissue death occurs. Several factors contribute to the value of reperfusion therapy, but probably the most significant is the duration from symptom onset to treatment. The benefits of reperfusion therapy often are time dependent. Remember: time is muscle. Work quickly and efficiently when providing emergency care.

Begin by placing the patient in a position of comfort and giving oxygen (Figure 22-106). Most patients prefer a semi-Fowler's position. To decrease the heart's workload, do not allow the patient to perform any activity, such as walking to the stretcher.

Continuously monitor the patient's vital signs, pulse oximetry, and ECG. For the patient with a possible ACS, obtain a 12-lead ECG within 10 minutes of patient contact. Repeat the 12-lead ECG with each set of vital signs, when the patient's symptoms change, and as often as necessary. This is important because the patient's ECG may be normal between episodes of discomfort but show signs of ischemia, injury, or infarction during episodes of discomfort. However, keep in mind that the patient may be having an ACS and have a completely normal ECG.

Establish IV access. While providing care, ask the patient specific questions to help determine his or her eligibility for reperfusion therapy (Table 22-46). Scene time should not be delayed, and completion of the checklist should not interfere with other patient care.

If no contraindications are present, ask the patient to chew aspirin (Box 22-30). Give nitroglycerin (NTG) sublingually or by spray if no contraindications are present. For example, if there are indications of right ventricular involvement, NTG may be contraindicated and fluid administration may be indicated. NTG relaxes vascular smooth muscle, increasing coronary artery blood flow. It also decreases the heart's workload and oxygen demand by decreasing the amount of blood returned to the heart (preload) and the resistance the heart must pump against (afterload). Before giving NTG, ensure the following:

- An IV is in place
- The patient's systolic blood pressure is greater than 90 mm Hg

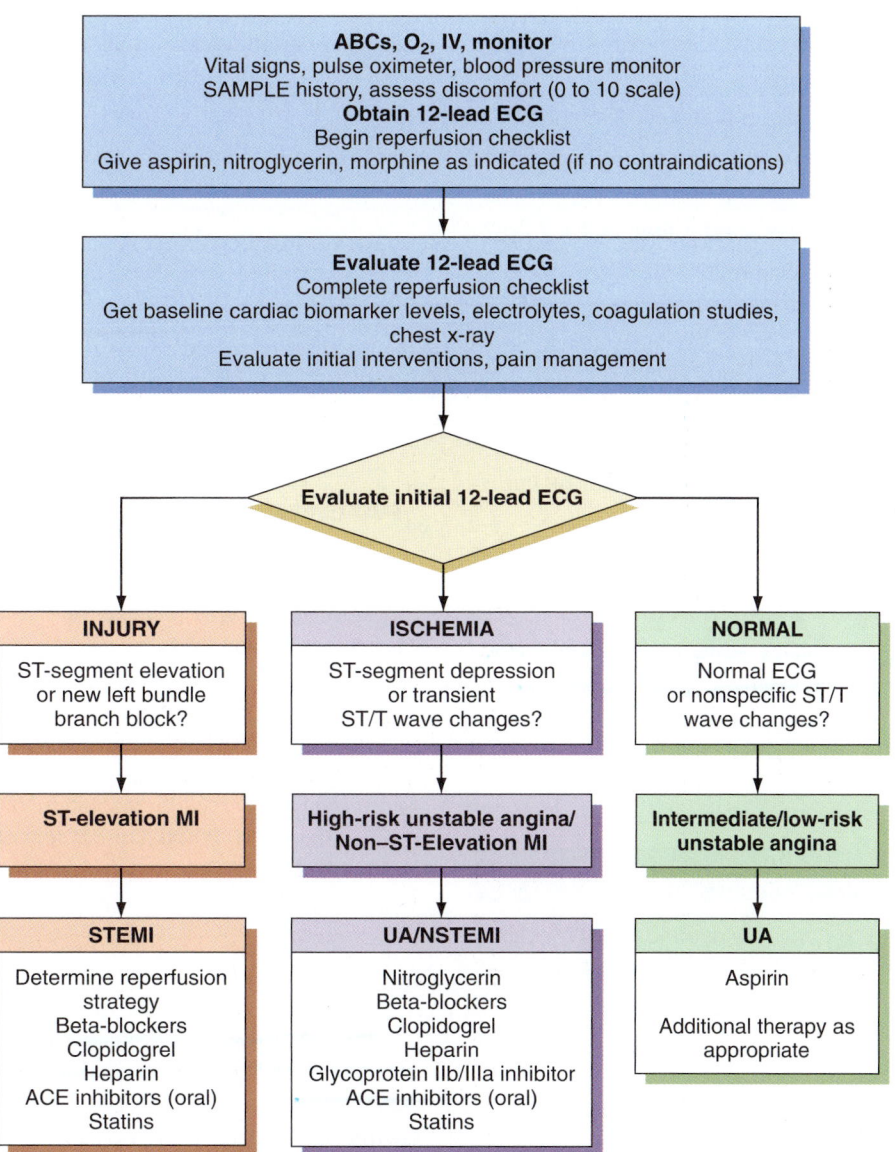

Figure 22-106 Ischemic chest pain algorithm.

TABLE 22-46	Reperfusion Checklist		

Date _____ Time _____

Duration of Chest Pain/Discomfort: _____ Hours _____ Minutes (>15 min and <6 hr)

Time 12-lead ECG obtained _____ Results _____

If any of the following boxes are checked "yes," fibrinolysis may be contraindicated	Yes	No
Is patient taking any blood thinners?	☐	☐
Any known bleeding or clotting disorders?	☐	☐
Recent surgery (including laser eye surgery) within last 6 weeks?	☐	☐
Recent major trauma within last 6 weeks?	☐	☐
Any gastrointestinal or genitourinary bleeding within last 6 weeks?	☐	☐
Is systolic blood pressure >180 mm Hg?	☐	☐
Is diastolic blood pressure >110 mm Hg?	☐	☐
Pregnant?	☐	☐
Any history of advanced/terminal cancer, kidney, or liver disease?	☐	☐
CPR >10 min?	☐	☐
Significant closed head/facial trauma within last 3 months?	☐	☐
History of structural central nervous system disease (intracranial neoplasm, arteriovenous malformation, or aneurysm)?	☐	☐
Right versus left arm systolic blood pressure difference >15 mm Hg	☐	☐
Does the patient have severe heart failure or cardiogenic shock such that percutaneous coronary intervention is preferable?		
Pulmonary edema (crackles/rales greater than halfway up)?	☐	☐
Signs of hypoperfusion (cool, clammy)?	☐	☐

Modified from Antman, E. M., Anbe, D. T., Armstrong, P. W., Bates, E. R., Green, L. A., Hand, M., et al. (2004). *ACC/AHA guidelines for the management of patients with ST-elevation myocardial infarction: A report of the American College of Cardiology/American Heart Association Task Force on Practice Guidelines (Committee to Revise the 1999 Guidelines for the Management of Patients With Acute Myocardial Infarction)*. Retrieved April 25, 2008, from http://www.acc.org/qualityandscience/clinical/guidelines/stemi/Guideline1/index.htm.

- The patient's heart rate is greater than 50 beats/min but less than 100 beats/min
- No signs of RVI are present
- The patient has not used Viagra, Cialis, or similar medication in the last 24 to 48 hours

NTG can be repeated every 5 minutes up to 3 tablets or sprays, provided the patient's vital signs remain stable. Recheck (and document) the patient's rating of discomfort and vital signs after each dose.

BOX 22-30	"MONA"

MONA is a memory aid that may be used to recall medications used in the management of ACS (although not in the order they are given):

Morphine
Oxygen
NTG
Aspirin

ACS, Acute coronary syndrome; *NTG,* nitroglycerin.

PARAMEDIC*Pearl*

In the past, the relief of chest discomfort with the use of NTG was one criteria used to distinguish angina and MI. If the discomfort was relieved with NTG, the patient's symptoms were assumed to be caused by angina. If not relieved with NTG, the patient's symptoms were thought to be from an infarction. This practice is not accurate. A 2002 study showed that 70% of patients with cardiac-related chest discomfort and 73% of patients with noncardiac chest discomfort had complete resolution of their discomfort with NTG (Shry et al, 2002). Do not rely on a patient's response to sublingual NTG to determine the cause of the patient's chest discomfort and the seriousness of the condition.

Relief of cardiac-related discomfort often requires a combination of oxygen, NTG, narcotic analgesics, and beta-blockers. Relief of pain must be a priority when caring for a patient with an ACS. Relief of pain decreases anxiety, myocardial oxygen demand, and the risk of dysrhythmias. Morphine sulfate is the analgesic of choice for chest discomfort associated with MI, except in cases of morphine sensitivity (Antman et al, 2004). Morphine is usually given in small IV doses and repeated every 5 minutes, provided the patient's vital signs remain stable. Several doses may be required for adequate pain relief. Be sure to watch the patient's blood pressure and respiratory rate closely because morphine can cause hypotension and respiratory depression.

Remember: dysrhythmias are common in the first few hours of an infarction. Be prepared to give antiarrhythmics or perform TCP, synchronized cardioversion, or defibrillation. If the patient's condition is stable, transport without lights and sirens. Rapid transport is warranted if the patient has had no relief of symptoms after your initial care, signs and symptoms of shock are present, or significant changes are seen in the patient's ECG. Significant ECG changes may include the development of a dysrhythmia, changes in ST segments, or the development of pathologic Q waves.

You will encounter patients who refuse treatment or transport, but have signs and symptoms consistent with an ACS. A patient with chest discomfort and refuses care is an example of a high-risk refusal. This means a high risk of legal liability exists. Try to persuade the patient calmly and carefully to accept the care you wish to provide, including transport. If you believe the patient may be having an MI, explain that to him in words he can easily understand. For example, use the phrase "heart attack" instead of MI. Let him know what emergency care you need to provide and the benefits of doing so. Explain the risks of not providing the care you have described. Because an MI may result in death, this possible outcome must be explained to the patient. Do not deliberately scare the patient. However, he or she must clearly understand the dangers of refusing treatment, including transport. In these situations contacting medical direction may be helpful. In some cases the physician may ask to speak directly to the patient and may be successful in convincing him or her to accept treatment and transport. If you are unable to convince the patient to receive care, carefully document the patient's refusal.

Patient and Family Education

The time from symptom onset to emergency care can be shortened if patients, families, and bystanders are taught to recognize symptoms early and activate the EMS system. Teach your patients and their families how to recognize the signs and symptoms of a heart attack. They should be taught to call 911 within 5 minutes of symptom onset. Let them know that not all heart attacks are accompanied by sudden, crushing chest pain and a loss of responsiveness. Symptoms may begin gradually or may come and go. Patients who have had a previous heart attack should be taught that the signs and symptoms of a second one may differ from those of the first.

Delays in calling 911 can occur because patients take an aspirin in response to their symptoms. Teach your patients to call 911 first. If no contraindications are present, emergency medical dispatchers may advise the patient to chew aspirin while EMS personnel are en route; aspirin may be given during EMS care or on arrival at the hospital if it was not given in the prehospital setting.

PARAMEDICPearl

Approximately 1 in every 300 patients with chest pain or discomfort transported to the emergency department by private vehicle goes into cardiac arrest en route (Becker et al, 1996).

Heart Failure

[OBJECTIVES 75, 76]

[handwritten: Myocardial damage of 40% or greater
See in lungs first]

Description and Definition

Heart failure is a condition in which the heart is unable to pump enough blood to meet the metabolic needs of the body. Heart failure is a syndrome, not a disease, that can result from disorders that impair the ability of the ventricle to fill with or eject blood.

Heart failure can be defined on the basis of symptom onset (acute versus chronic) and the ventricle initially involved (left versus right). In acute heart failure, symptoms suddenly occur. In chronic heart failure, symptoms develop more slowly. A person with chronic heart failure can develop acute heart failure. Although failure of either ventricle can occur by itself, they often occur together. Right ventricular failure (RVF) is often a result of LVF.

Etiology

Heart failure may result from disorders of the pericardium, myocardium, endocardium, or great vessels. Examples of these disorders include coronary artery disease, valvular heart disease, dysrhythmias, cardiomyopathy, and long-standing high blood pressure. Coronary artery disease, with or without MI, is the most common cause of heart failure.

Regardless of the cause, most patients with heart failure have symptoms because of the left ventricle's inability to pump blood effectively. To understand what happens in heart failure, a quick review the physiology of the normal heart is helpful. Remember that cardiac output is equal to stroke volume multiplied by the heart rate. Three main factors affect stroke volume: preload, afterload, and cardiac contractility. Thus heart failure may result from any condition that impairs preload, afterload, cardiac contractility, or heart rate.

According to Starling's law of the heart, increased venous return increases preload. Heart muscle fibers stretch in response to the increased volume (preload) before contracting. Stretching of the muscle fibers allows the heart to eject the additional volume with increased force, thereby increasing stroke volume. So in the normal heart, the greater the preload, the greater the force of ventricular contraction and the greater the stroke volume, resulting in increased cardiac output.

The heart's normal workload can prove to be too much if the left ventricle is damaged. When LVF develops, the left ventricle has trouble pumping all its blood out to the body. Common causes of the left ventricle's reduced pumping ability are a faulty heart valve, MI, and cardiomyopathy (Box 22-31). Heart failure also can result from increased demands made on the heart because of excessive volume or pressure. For example, giving a large volume of IV fluid over a short period (as in a runaway IV) in a patient with a weakened left ventricle can result in volume overload. Pressure overload can occur if a heart valve becomes thickened or narrowed, obstructing blood flow through it.

Acute

Left Ventricular Failure and Pulmonary Edema. When the left ventricle fails, blood backs up behind it, causing a chain reaction (Figure 22-107). Blood builds up in the lungs because the left ventricle is unable to eject all the blood within its walls. The left atrium swells with blood because it cannot empty the blood within its walls into the left ventricle. Stretching of the atrial muscle fibers may result in atrial dysrhythmias. The pulmonary veins cannot empty the blood from the pulmonary arteries into the left atrium because it already is full. Pressure within the pulmonary vessels increases, forcing fluid from the pulmonary capillaries across the alveolar walls into the alveoli of the lungs. This results in pulmonary edema. The congestion heard in the lungs is the reason

heart failure often is called congestive heart failure. The buildup of fluid widens the gap between the alveoli/capillary membrane, impairing the diffusion of oxygen and carbon dioxide.

BOX 22-31 **Cardiomyopathy**

Cardiomyopathy is a disease of the heart muscle. The main types of cardiomyopathy are dilated, hypertrophic, and restrictive—named by the type of muscle damage they cause. In dilated cardiomyopathy (also called congestive cardiomyopathy), the heart muscle weakens, decreasing its ability to pump enough blood to the rest of the body. The pressure of the blood within the left ventricle causes the heart to enlarge and stretch.

In hypertrophic cardiomyopathy, the growth and arrangement of muscle fibers is abnormal. Individual heart muscle cells enlarge, leading to thickened heart walls. The greatest thickening tends to occur in the left ventricle. The thickened heart walls are stiff, resulting in impaired ventricular filling. This can lead to left atrial enlargement and pulmonary congestion. Most cases of hypertrophic cardiomyopathy are inherited. In other cases, no clear cause can be found.

In restrictive cardiomyopathy, the walls of the ventricles stiffen because of abnormal substances deposited throughout the heart between heart muscle cells or because the inner surface of the heart is coated with a layer of scar tissue. The rigid ventricular walls hinder ventricular filling and the heart eventually loses its ability to pump properly.

CHF - Chronic
Seen w/ R sided failure too
Can develop pulmonary edema
long term

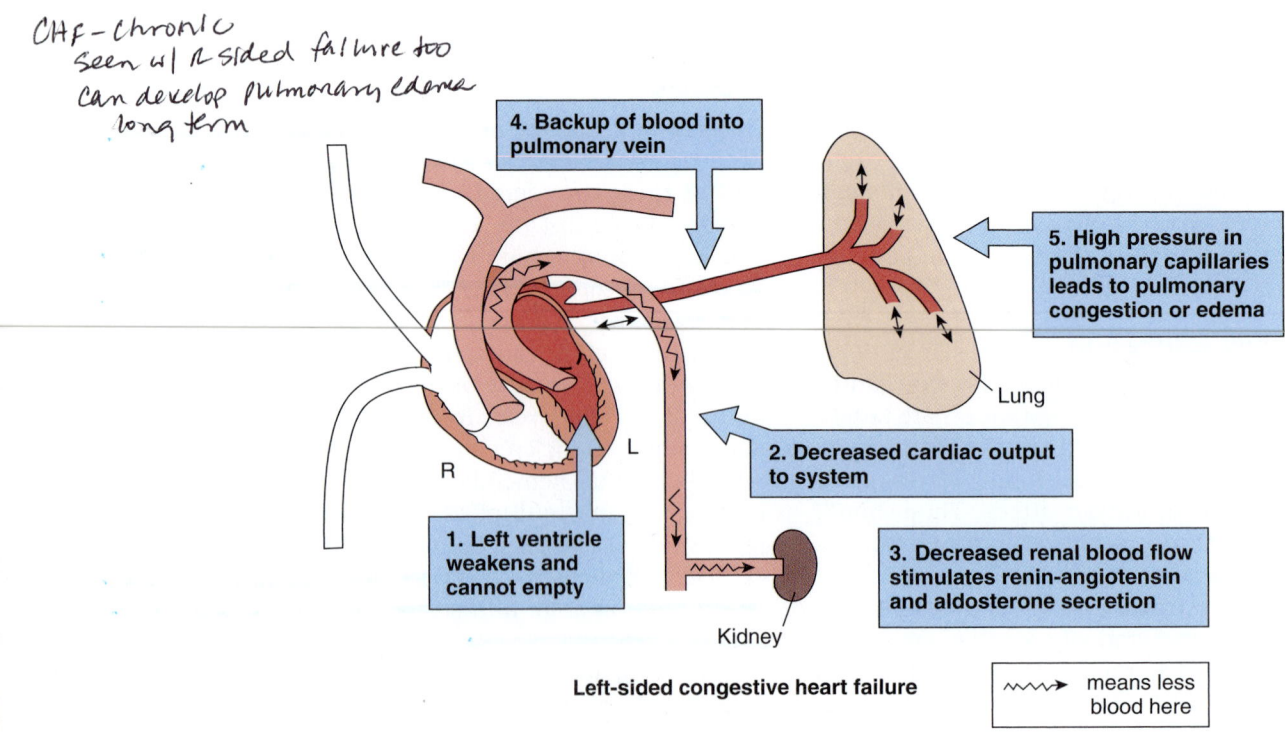

Figure 22-107 Left-sided heart failure.

4. **Backup of blood into pulmonary vein**

5. **High pressure in pulmonary capillaries leads to pulmonary congestion or edema**

Lung

2. **Decreased cardiac output to system**

1. **Left ventricle weakens and cannot empty**

3. **Decreased renal blood flow stimulates renin-angiotensin and aldosterone secretion**

Kidney

Left-sided congestive heart failure

means less blood here

Right Ventricular Failure. To eject the blood within its walls, the right ventricle must work harder to overcome the high pressure and congestion within the pulmonary vessels. When it cannot keep up with the increased workload, the right ventricle fails (Figure 22-108). Blood backs up behind the right ventricle, increasing the pressure in the right atrium. If the right atrium is unable to eject the blood within its walls, blood backs up into the superior and inferior venae cavae. Veins become congested with blood because the superior and inferior venae cavae cannot drain into an already full right atrium. Because venous return is delayed, organs become congested with blood. For example, the liver enlarges (hepatomegaly) and becomes tender because of increased pressure in the hepatic veins. As venous congestion worsens, increased pressure within the veins forces serous fluid through capillary walls and into body tissues, producing edema. Peripheral edema is most easily seen in dependent areas of the body, such as the feet and ankles. Serous fluid may build up in the abdomen (ascites), pleural cavity (pleural effusion), and/or pericardial cavity (pericardial effusion). As RVF worsens, generalized edema of the entire body may be seen. This is called **anasarca.**

Cor Pulmonale. RVF may occur by itself (without LVF) in conditions such as RVI, pulmonary embolism, or pulmonary hypertension. Pulmonary hypertension is a disorder in which the pressure in the pulmonary arteries is higher than normal. The right ventricle must work quite hard to overcome this increased resistance and eject blood. Over time, the right ventricle enlarges and eventually fails. Right-sided heart failure caused by pulmonary disease is called **cor pulmonale** (Figure 22-109). Cor pulmonale usually is the result of chronic obstructive pulmonary disease. *& chronic pulmonary hypertension*

Compensatory Mechanisms. As the heart begins to fail, the body's compensatory mechanisms attempt to improve cardiac output by manipulating preload, afterload, cardiac contractility, and/or heart rate. Ultimately, compensatory mechanisms may actually worsen heart failure. For example, the sympathetic nervous system increases heart rate and force of contraction and constricts blood vessels. The increase in heart rate and force

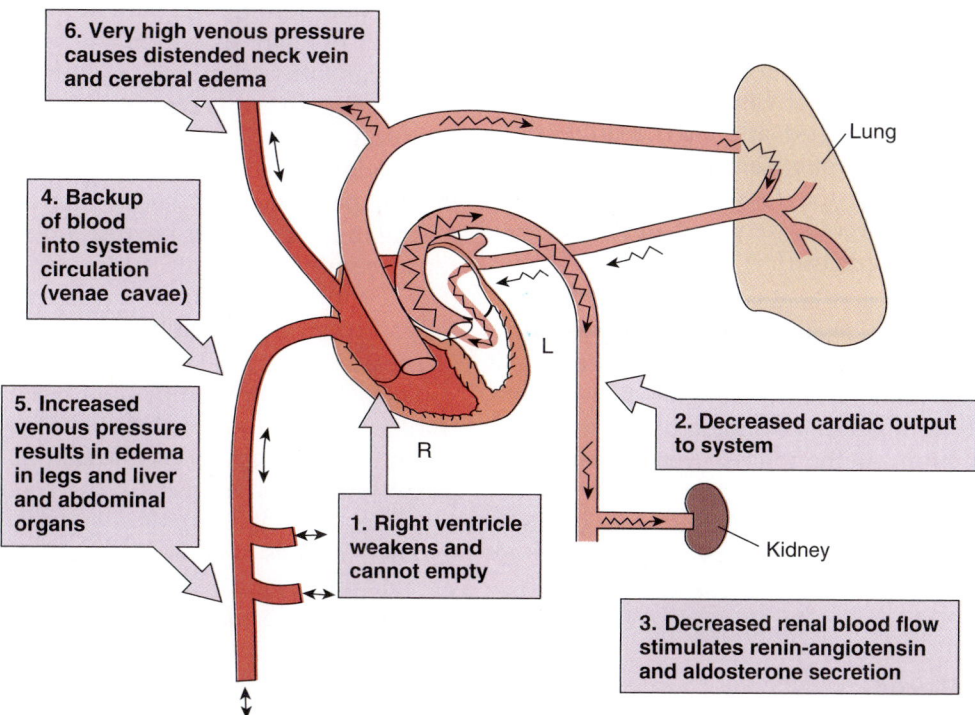

6. Very high venous pressure causes distended neck vein and cerebral edema

4. Backup of blood into systemic circulation (venae cavae)

5. Increased venous pressure results in edema in legs and liver and abdominal organs

1. Right ventricle weakens and cannot empty

2. Decreased cardiac output to system

3. Decreased renal blood flow stimulates renin-angiotensin and aldosterone secretion

Lung

Kidney

L

R

Right-sided congestive heart failure

Figure 22-108 Right-sided heart failure.

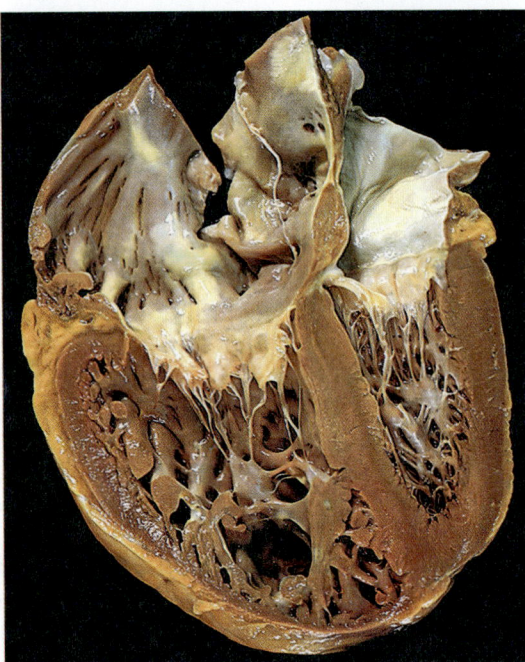

Figure 22-109 Chronic cor pulmonale. Notice the markedly dilated and enlarged right ventricle *(left)*. The shape of the left ventricle *(right)* has been altered because of the enlarged right ventricle.

of contraction increases the heart's demand for oxygen, decreases the amount of time the ventricles have to fill, and decreases time for coronary artery perfusion. Decreased blood flow to the kidneys stimulates the renin-angiotensin-aldosterone system. Angiotensin I forms angiotensin II, resulting in more vasoconstriction. Constricted blood vessels (increased afterload) require the heart to work even harder to pump against high pressure. Angiotensin II encourages the release of aldosterone, which leads to sodium and water retention and increased blood volume (increased preload).

These compensatory mechanisms are effective in increasing cardiac output for a time but eventually worsen heart failure. Sodium and water retention leads to enlargement of the heart's chambers, thickening of the walls of the ventricles and, ultimately, a decrease in the force of ventricular contraction. As the force of ventricular contraction decreases, the weakened heart muscle is unable to handle the increased volume of fluid and cardiac output falls.

PARAMEDIC*Pearl*

Physicians may prescribe angiotensin-converting enzyme inhibitors to patients with heart failure. These medications block the conversion of angiotensin I to angiotensin II, a powerful vasoconstrictor.

Epidemiology and Demographics

Approximately 5 million patients in the United States have heart failure, and nearly 500,000 patients are initially diagnosed each year (Hunt et al., 2005). Approximately 6% to 10% of the population older than 65 years has heart failure (Kannel, 2004).

Heart failure increases dramatically with age. It occurs in 1% to 2% of patients aged 50 to 59 years and up to 10% of patients older than 75 years. Once heart failure is diagnosed, the prognosis is poor. The overall 5-year mortality rate for all patients with heart failure is approximately 50%, and the 1-year mortality rate in patients with severe heart failure may be as high as 35% to 40% (Givertz & Colucci, 2001).

History

The patient with heart failure may complain of a sudden onset of shortness of breath or shortness of breath that has worsened over a period of hours or days. At first, the patient may have difficulty breathing only with activity or when lying down for a while. As LVF worsens, signs and symptoms also become present at rest. Difficulty breathing with activity and orthopnea can occur because of respiratory disorders as well as cardiac disorders. The likelihood that these symptoms are from a cardiac cause is increased if the patient tells you he has a history of a previous heart attack, high blood pressure, valvular disease, or other cardiovascular condition.

The patient may complain of difficulty sleeping. On further questioning, the patient will most likely describe episodes of PND in which he or she awakens with a feeling of suffocation and coughing. In LVF, this occurs because the patient is literally drowning in his or her own secretions.

In addition to difficulty breathing or shortness of breath, patients with heart failure often complain of feeling tired or weak or having "no energy." These symptoms, combined with a history of recent weight gain over a short period and/or progressive swelling of the lower extremities, should be a red flag for heart failure (Table 22-47).

The patient may complain of recent difficulty concentrating. This symptom may be the result of hypoxia. The patient may complain of nausea and a loss of appetite. These symptoms are usually the result of congestion of the liver and abdominal organs. Some patients may describe feelings of faintness, palpitations, or an irregular or rapid pulse. Find out about the medications the patient is taking. For example, whether the patient is taking calcium channel blockers is important because these medications can affect the force with which the heart contracts.

Although an accurate medical history is important, the patient who has heart failure is often too short of breath to supply the answers to your questions. While providing emergency care for the patient, you may need

TABLE 22-47 Signs and Symptoms of Heart Failure

Left Ventricular Failure	Right Ventricular Failure
Signs	
Restlessness, anxiety	Weight gain
Respiratory rate above normal for age	Dependent edema
Heart rate above normal for age	Ascites
Pulsus alternans	Anasarca
Crackles	JVD
Cough with frothy sputum	Liver enlargement (hepatomegaly)
Third heart sound	Spleen enlargement (splenomegaly)
Retractions	
Accessory muscle use	
Labored breathing	
Sweating	
Unable to speak in sentences, speech limited to phrases or words	
Symptoms	
Fatigue	Fatigue
Difficulty breathing	Nausea
Orthopnea	Loss of appetite
Paroxysmal nocturnal dyspnea	Upper abdominal quadrant pain

to obtain the patient's history from a family member or neighbor if someone is available at the scene.

PEDIATRIC *Pearl*

Signs of heart failure in an infant or child may include rapid breathing, grunting respirations, tachycardia, diminished pulses, and fatigue and/or sweating with feeding.

Physical Findings

When either side of the heart fails, blood supply to the body's tissues decreases and oxygenation is impaired. Signs of hypoxia may appear as restlessness, anxiety, or unexplained confusion (especially in older adults). When talking with the patient, notice if he or she is able to speak in complete sentences. As heart failure worsens, the patient's shortness of breath will limit speech from sentences to phrases and then only to words. Because keeping the upper body elevated improves breathing (orthopnea), the patient may instinctively assume a tripod position.

The patient's respiratory rate and heart rate are often rapid. The skin may be pale and feel cool. Peripheral pulses may be diminished. These signs are a result of the sympathetic nervous system's response to hypoxia and

an attempt to maintain cardiac output. You may see signs of increased work of breathing, including retractions and the use of accessory muscles.

As hypoxia worsens, the patient may become cyanotic. The patient may frequently cough because the fluid in the airways is an irritant. Coughing may produce pink, frothy sputum. As compensatory mechanisms fail, crackles (rales) that do not clear with coughing can be heard because of the progressive buildup fluid in the lungs. Crackles may be accompanied by wheezing if bronchospasm is present. Crackles are heard first in the bases of the lungs. As the buildup of fluid increases, you will hear crackles further up the chest. Pulsus paradoxus, pulsus alternans, and a third heart sound may be present. The apical pulse may be displaced because enlargement of the left ventricle displaces the cardiac apex.

If right ventricular failure accompanies LVF, JVD will be visible as the venous system becomes congested. Swelling of the ankles, feet, calves, or legs will be present in patients who are able to walk. Swelling of the sacral area may be present in patients confined to bed. If edema is present, note (and document) if it is pitting or nonpitting and localized in the ankles, to the mid-calf, or to the knees. **Ascites** may be seen because of a buildup of fluid in the peritoneal cavity. As the liver and spleen swell, the patient may complain of upper abdominal quadrant pain.

As the pump continues to fail, the heart rate begins to slow, blood pressure falls, and cardiac output decreases. Heart failure accompanied by hypotension is cardiogenic shock.

PARAMEDIC*Pearl*

JVD may be present in conditions other than RVF. Listening to breath sounds and heart sounds can help differentiate the patient's underlying problem. For example, JVD in a patient with cardiac tamponade usually reveals clear lung sounds but muffled heart sounds. JVD in a patient who has a tension pneumothorax usually reveals diminished or absent lung sounds on the affected side. JVD in a patient who has RVF because of LVF will usually have crackles in the lungs. In these patients, fluid administration is usually limited and closely monitored. JVD in a patient who has RVF because of RVI usually has clear lung sounds. A patient with an RVI often requires IV fluid boluses to increase preload.

Differential Diagnosis

Differential diagnoses for heart failure include:

- Cardiovascular Causes
  - Cardiogenic shock
  - Myocardial infarction
  - Myocardial ischemia
  - Cardiogenic pulmonary edema
  - High-altitude pulmonary edema
  - Noncardiogenic pulmonary edema
  - Pulmonary embolism
- Respiratory Causes
  - Acute respiratory distress syndrome
  - Chronic bronchitis
  - Chronic obstructive pulmonary disease
  - Emphysema
  - Pneumonia
  - Pneumothorax
  - Reactive airway disease
  - Respiratory failure

Therapeutic Interventions

A patient who has difficulty breathing is usually quite anxious. Begin emergency care by providing reassurance. Treatment of heart failure focuses on correcting hypoxia, reducing preload, reducing afterload, and improving myocardial contractility. You will need to work quickly to help relieve the patient's symptoms.

Place the patient in a position of comfort. If pulmonary congestion is present and the patient's blood pressure will tolerate it, place him or her in a sitting position with the feet dangling. This will help decrease venous return and decrease the work of breathing. Administer high-concentration oxygen. If breathing is adequate, give oxygen by mask if the patient will tolerate it. Some patients will feel they are suffocating if a mask in used.

You may need to reassure the patient that the oxygen mask is necessary and will help breathing. If you are unable to convince the patient to accept the mask, you may have to resort to using blow-by oxygen or a nasal cannula. If the patient is unresponsive or his breathing is inadequate, administer oxygen by positive-pressure ventilation. Apply a pulse oximeter. Maintain the patient's oxygen saturation at greater than 95%.

Limit the patient's physical activity. Do not allow walking up or down stairs or to the stretcher. Place the patient on a cardiac monitor and obtain a 12-lead ECG. Heart failure may occur because of a dysrhythmia. On the other hand, hypoxia and acidosis predispose patients with heart failure to dysrhythmias. Dysrhythmias may range from tachycardias to bradycardias.

Establish IV access. To help ensure that the patient in heart failure does not receive too much IV fluid, the use of a heparin lock or saline lock is preferred. If local protocols require you to use an IV bag and tubing, infuse the fluid at a to-keep-open rate (30 mL/hr). Check and recheck the volume of fluid in the bag while the patient is in your care. Be certain to document the amount of fluid in the bag when you started the IV and the amount of fluid remaining in the bag when you transfer patient care at the receiving facility.

Give medications as requested by medical direction or according to local protocol. Medications used in the treatment of heart failure may include the following:

- Antiarrhythmics to treat dysrhythmias
- Analgesics to treat pain, if present
- Diuretics, such as furosemide, to reduce preload
- Venodilators, such as morphine sulfate and NTG, to reduce preload
- Positive inotropic agents, such as dopamine and dobutamine, to increase myocardial contractility
- Angiotensin-converting enzyme inhibitors, angiotensin receptor blockers, and/or beta-blockers to reduce afterload

When preparing to transport the patient, keep in mind that the use of lights and sirens may increase the patient's anxiety, heart rate, and blood pressure. This response increases the heart's workload and demand for oxygen and should be avoided. If the patient's condition is stable, transport without lights and sirens. Rapid transport is warranted if the patient's breathing worsens, signs and symptoms of shock are present, or life-threatening dysrhythmias develop.

Patient and Family Education

A patient with heart failure should weigh himself or herself every day because an increase in weight may reflect fluid retention. The patient should call his or her physician if gaining more than 2 pounds in 1 day or 5 pounds over a 3- to 4-day period. He or she should avoid salt and salty foods and talk with a physician before using salt substitutes. Because salt substitutes contain potassium, the patient's kidney function and the medications being taken must be considered.

To avoid respiratory infections, patients should keep up-to-date on vaccinations for influenza and pneumococcal pneumonia. Patients with chronic heart failure should be reminded to take their medicines as prescribed, even when they are without symptoms. Nonsteroidal antiinflammatory drugs should be avoided because they can cause sodium retention and blood vessel constriction.

Patients are encouraged to exercise regularly. Before beginning an exercise program, the patient should meet with his or her physician to determine appropriate types of exercise, how long to exercise, and how often.

Myocarditis

Description and Definition

[OBJECTIVES 77, 78] *usually viral*

Myocarditis is an inflammation of the middle and thickest layer of the heart, the myocardium. The myocardium contains the conduction system and the cardiac muscle fibers that cause contraction of the heart. Myocarditis may occur with or without involvement of the endocardium or pericardium.

Myocarditis is usually benign and self-limiting. However, if the inflammation is widespread in the heart muscle, the destruction of too many heart muscle cells will affect the heart's ability to pump. This can result in RVF and LVF, dysrhythmias, and death. In some cases, myocarditis may lead to dilated cardiomyopathy.

Etiology

Myocarditis can be caused by many different pathogens, including bacteria, viruses, and parasites. The most common cause of myocarditis is a viral infection. Other causes of myocarditis include rheumatic fever, exposure to chemical poisons such as chronic alcoholism, and a side effect of radiation therapy for cancer, especially with large doses to the chest. In many cases the cause of myocarditis is unknown.

Epidemiology and Demographics

Myocarditis is uncommon in the United States because many patients are not symptomatic with this disease. The frequency with which it occurs is unknown.

History

Most cases of myocarditis are associated with flulike symptoms for which the patient does not seek medical care. The patient may have fatigue, decreased appetite, mild shortness of breath, and joint and muscle aches and pains. Fever is present in approximately 20% of patients. Cardiac-related symptoms usually appear 10 to 14 days after the initial onset of symptoms, at which time the patient seeks medical attention. Complaints of palpitations are common. Some patients complain of chest discomfort and describe it as a sharp, stabbing pain in the center of the chest. If the patient describes squeezing chest discomfort, myocarditis is difficult to distinguish from an ACS in the field.

Physical Findings

The patient's physical examination may range from mild or no signs to severe heart failure. Tachycardia and tachypnea are common. The ECG may show low-voltage QRS complexes and/or ST-segment elevation. Atrial or ventricular dysrhythmias are common. Although sinus tachycardia is probably the most common rhythm seen, approximately 20% of patients will have a second- or third-degree AV block. Left or right BBB also may be seen. JVD, crackles, ascites, and peripheral edema may be seen if heart failure is present. Signs and symptoms of myocarditis are shown in Box 22-32.

BOX 22-32	Signs and Symptoms of Myocarditis

Newborns and Infants

- Fever
- Irritability or listlessness
- Periodic episodes of pallor that precede tachypnea or respiratory distress
- Diaphoresis
- Poor feeding; sweating while feeding if heart failure is present
- Mild cyanosis
- Cool, mottled skin from decreased cardiac output
- Rapid, labored respirations; grunting
- Crackles (uncommon)
- Heart failure (tachycardia, gallop rhythm)

Older Children, Adolescents, Adults

- Low-grade fever
- Fatigue, exhaustion
- Pallor
- Decreased appetite
- Muscle aches and pain
- Chest pain (usually described as sharp, stabbing)
- Dyspnea with activity
- Orthopnea and shortness of breath at rest
- Palpitations (common)
- Heart failure (tachycardia, gallop rhythm, muffled heart sounds [especially in the presence of pericarditis])

Differential Diagnosis

The differential diagnoses for myocarditis include:

- Acute coronary syndrome
- Heart failure
- Aortic dissection
- Pneumonia
- Pulmonary embolism
- Esophageal perforation, rupture, or tear
- Kawasaki disease

Therapeutic Interventions   *Rruc → transport*

Any patient complaining of chest discomfort or shortness of breath should receive oxygen and be placed on a cardiac monitor. Make sure oxygenation and ventilation are effective. If the patient's breathing is inadequate, administer oxygen with positive-pressure ventilation. Apply a pulse oximeter. Maintain the patient's oxygen saturation at greater than 95%. Establish IV access. Be prepared to treat heart failure and dysrhythmias according to local protocol or instructions from medical direction.

Patient and Family Education

To reduce the heart's workload, patients recovering from myocarditis should have limited activity for approximately 6 months. Patients who have second-degree AV block type II or third-degree AV block may need a permanent pacemaker.

CARDIOGENIC SHOCK   * Know Smo *

[OBJECTIVES 79, 80]

Description and Definition

Cardiogenic shock is a condition in which heart muscle function is severely impaired, leading to decreased cardiac output and inadequate tissue perfusion. The most common cause of cardiogenic shock is MI.

Etiology

Cardiogenic shock may occur as a complication of shock of any cause. Cardiogenic shock also can occur if myocardial contractility is decreased because of prolonged cardiac surgery, ventricular aneurysm, cardiac arrest, or rupture of the ventricular wall. Cardiogenic shock caused by rupture of the ventricular wall may account for 10% to 30% of all deaths from a heart attack (Timm, 2003). Although rare, this complication usually occurs 4 to 7 days after an MI. When the ventricular wall ruptures, blood leaks into the pericardial space and quickly leads to cardiac tamponade and cardiovascular collapse.

Other causes of cardiogenic shock include cardiac dysrhythmias, rupture of the ventricular septum, myocarditis, cardiomyopathy, myocardial trauma, heart failure, hypothermia, severe electrolyte or acid-base imbalances, and severe congenital heart disease.

Epidemiology and Demographics

Cardiogenic shock occurs in approximately 7% to 10% of patients with an acute MI. Eighty percent of patients who have cardiogenic shock have had a large infarction involving 40% or more of the left ventricle. A recent RVI is present in 10%, and mechanical complications (such as cardiac tamponade or papillary muscle rupture) occur in 10% of patients with cardiogenic shock.

At autopsy, more than two thirds of patients with cardiogenic shock have 75% or more narrowing of the three major coronary arteries (Webb et al, 2003).

History

A patient in cardiogenic shock may be too ill to provide a medical history. If family members are present, they may be able to tell you whether the patient has a history of heart disease. They also may be able to describe the patient's signs and symptoms that prompted a call to 911.

The patient's history often includes cardiomyopathy, congenital heart disease, or a recent MI. Patients with cardiogenic shock who have had a recent MI are more likely to be older, have had an STEMI, have a history of a previous MI or heart failure, and have had an anterior infarction at the time shock develops.

Mechanical problems from a recent MI often occur several days to a week after the infarction. If a dysrhythmia is associated with the patient's symptoms, the patient may describe recent episodes of palpitations, fainting, or lightheadedness.

Physical Findings

In compensated cardiogenic shock, the patient's mental status initially may be normal. As perfusion to the brain decreases, the patient becomes restless, agitated, and confused. Breath sounds reveal crackles in most patients. However, patients with RVI or those who are hypovolemic may have less evidence of pulmonary congestion. JVD, indicating RVF, may be present. If the patient is hypovolemic, JVD will be absent. Peripheral pulses often are weak and rapid. However, pulses may be weak and slow if an AV block is present. The patient's skin is usually pale or mottled. The extremities often feel cool and moist. This finding is a sympathetic response in which the blood within peripheral vessels is shunted to the vital organs to maintain adequate perfusion. The ECG may show evidence of both old and new infarctions. RVI can be detected by right-sided chest leads. Initially the patient's systolic blood pressure may be normal, but pulse pressure is usually narrowed. If cardiogenic shock is associated with cardiac tamponade, heart sounds may be muffled.

In decompensated cardiogenic shock, the patient usually has an altered mental status or may be unresponsive. Breathing is often rapid and shallow. Breath sounds usually reveal increasing pulmonary congestion and crackles. Peripheral pulses may be absent. Central pulses are often weak and rapid. The patient's skin is usually pale, mottled, or cyanotic. The extremities feel cold and sweaty. As ventricular function worsens and cardiac output falls, the systolic blood pressure progressively decreases.

Differential Diagnosis

The most common cause of cardiogenic shock is MI. Cardiogenic shock caused by rupture of the ventricular wall may account for 10% to 30% of all deaths from a heart attack (Timm, 2003). Other differential diagnoses include:

- Cardiovascular Causes
  - Acute coronary syndrome
  - Aortic dissection
  - Myocardial rupture
  - Myocarditis
- Respiratory Cause
  - Pulmonary embolism
- Other Causes
  - Hypovolemic shock
  - Sepsis, septic shock

Therapeutic Interventions

Dopamine
No atropine

The treatment of cardiogenic shock is generally based on increasing contractility without significant increases in heart rate, altering preload and afterload, and controlling dysrhythmias if they are present and contributing to shock.

Give high-concentration oxygen. Make sure oxygenation and ventilation are effective. Apply a pulse oximeter. Maintain the patient's oxygen saturation at greater than 95%. Place the patient in a position of comfort. If pulmonary congestion is present and the patient's blood pressure will tolerate it, place the patient in a sitting position with the feet dangling. Be sure to limit the patient's physical activity while in your care. This includes making sure that the patient does not walk up or down stairs or to the stretcher.

Place the patient on a cardiac monitor and establish IV access. Obtain a 12-lead ECG. Maintain normal

---

BOX 22-33 Patient Management: Cardiogenic Shock

- ABCs, O_2 (endotracheal intubation if needed), IV, monitor
- Vital signs, pulse oximetry
- Treat dysrhythmias if they are present and contributing to shock
- Check blood pressure
  - If the systolic blood pressure (SBP) is >100 mm Hg, give NTG IV
  - If the SBP is 70 to 100 mm Hg with *no* signs or symptoms of shock, give dobutamine IV
  - If the SBP is 70 to 100 mm Hg *with* signs and symptoms of shock, give dopamine IV
  - If the SBP is <70 mm Hg, give norepinephrine IV
- Check patient's response; assess mental status, heart rate, respiratory effort, breath sounds, and blood pressure
- Complete reperfusion checklist

NTG, nitroglycerin.

---

body temperature. Give IV fluids and medications per local protocol or medical direction instructions. IV medications often used to treat cardiogenic shock include NTG, dobutamine, dopamine, and norepinephrine (Box 22-33). The choice of medication depends on the patient's systolic blood pressure. If you are instructed to give dopamine or norepinephrine, be sure to check the IV site often during administration. These medications can cause significant vasoconstriction. If the IV fluid leaks out of a vein and into the patient's tissues, considerable tissue damage can result. Check the patient's response to the medication given by assessing his mental status, heart rate, respiratory effort, breath sounds, and blood pressure. If no improvement occurs, give additional emergency care as instructed by medical direction. Treat dysrhythmias if they are present and contributing to shock.

A patient with signs and symptoms of shock requires rapid transport to the closest appropriate facility. En route to the hospital, complete a reperfusion checklist. Although cardiogenic shock is associated with a high mortality rate, patients who are candidates for reperfusion therapy and receive prompt treatment may have an increased chance of survival. If the patient refuses care, repeatedly try to persuade him or her to accept the care you wish to provide, including transport. Explain to the patient that if his or her condition is not treated, symptoms may worsen and could result in death. Consider contacting medical direction for advice. If you are unable to convince the patient to receive care, carefully document the patient's refusal.

Patient and Family Education

In many cases cardiogenic shock cannot be prevented. Provide emotional support to the patient and family.

CARDIOPULMONARY ARREST

Description and Definition

[OBJECTIVES 81, 82]

Cardiac arrest is the absence of cardiac pump function confirmed by the absence of a detectable pulse, unresponsiveness, and apnea or agonal, gasping respirations. Cardiac arrest may be reversible but will lead to death without prompt emergency care. **Sudden cardiac death (SCD)** is an unexpected death from a cardiac cause that either occurs immediately or within 1 hour of the onset of symptoms. Some victims of SCD have no warning signs of the impending event. For others, warning signs may be present up to 1 hour before the actual arrest.

Etiology

In Western cultures, most cases of SCD in adults are caused by underlying coronary artery disease. Coronary atherosclerosis with significant (more than 75%) narrowing involving one or more of the three major coronary arteries is present in 80% to 90% of victims of SCD (Schoen, 2005b). A healed MI is present in approximately 40% of patients, but in those who were successfully resuscitated from sudden cardiac arrest a new MI is found in only 25% or less (Schoen, 2005b).

In the United States, hypertrophic cardiomyopathy and congenital coronary artery anomalies account for more than 50% of all cases of SCD in young athletes (Hosey & Armsey, 2003). In children, cardiopulmonary arrest usually is the result of respiratory failure or shock that progresses to cardiopulmonary failure, with profound hypoxemia and acidosis and eventually cardiopulmonary arrest.

SCD may result from commotio cordis, in which a mechanical stimulus is delivered to the heart by a nonpenetrating blow to the chest. Commotio cordis is most common in young children and has been associated with a wide range of activities, with sporting activities the most common (Box 22-34).

The period of 1 hour or less between sudden changes in the patient's cardiovascular status and the cardiac arrest itself is called the "onset of the terminal event" (Myerburg & Castellanos, 2005). In an arrhythmic death, the victim abruptly collapses and the pulse stops without prior circulatory collapse. In deaths from circulatory failure, the victim's pulse stops only after peripheral circulation has collapsed (Hinkle & Thaler, 1982). Although SCD may be the result of dysrhythmias or circulatory failure, most deaths are the result of dysrhythmias.

Epidemiology and Demographics

Following are important facts about SCD:

- An estimated 50% of all coronary heart disease deaths are sudden and unexpected (Saxon, 2005).
- A total of 50% of men and 64% of women who die suddenly of coronary heart disease have no previous symptoms of this disease (AHA, 2005a).
- People who have had a heart attack have a sudden death rate that is four to six times that of the general population (AHA, 2005a).
- SCD occurs in two age ranges of peak incidence: between birth and 6 months of age (sudden infant death syndrome) and between 45 and 75 years of age (Myerburg & Castellanos, 2005).
- SCD accounts for 19% of sudden deaths in children between ages 1 and 13 years and 30% between ages 14 and 21 years (AHA, 2005a).

History

Patients at risk for SCD may have signs and symptoms such as chest discomfort, dyspnea, weakness or fatigue,

---

BOX 22-34 | **Sources of Blunt Trauma to the Chest Resulting in Commotio Cordis**

- Baseballs, softballs, lacrosse balls, cricket balls, soccer balls
- Tennis balls filled with coins for training pitchers
- Hockey pucks, hockey sticks
- Play (shadow boxing)
- Parent-to-child discipline
- Gang rituals
- Scuffle
- Plastic sledding saucers
- Plastic (hollow) toy bats
- Snowballs
- Playground swing carriages
- Charging pet dog head blows
- Hiccup remedy
- Falls from a playground apparatus (monkey bars)
- Knees, feet, elbows, forearms, shoulders, fists, heads (football helmet)
- Goalposts

Modified from Geddes, L. A., & Roeder, R. A. (2005). Evolution of our knowledge of sudden death due to commotio cordis. *American Journal of Emergency Medicine*, 23(1), 67-75; and Maron, B. J., Gohman, T. E., Kyle, S. B., Estes, N. A. III, & Link, M. S. (2002). Clinical profile and spectrum of commotio cordis. *Journal of the American Medical Association*, 287(9), 1142-1146.

palpitations, syncope, or nonspecific complaints before an MI or SCD.

If you arrive on the scene of a patient in cardiac arrest, find out the answers to the following questions while performing emergency care:

- *Did anyone see the patient collapse? Can you describe what happened? What time did the patient collapse?* Family members often do not know the exact time the event occurred. If this is the case, ask when the patient was last seen without symptoms. Keep in mind that even if family members are able to give you an idea of when the collapse occurred, the information received is often inaccurate.
- Did anyone begin CPR? If so, how long was the period from the time the patient was found until the time CPR was started?
- How long was the period before a call was made to 911?
- Was an automated external defibrillator used?
- Does the patient have a do not attempt resuscitate (DNAR) order?

If the patient collapses after you arrive on the scene, be sure to note the time this occurred when you document the events of the call.

Physical Findings

In cardiopulmonary arrest, central pulses and the work of breathing are absent and the patient is unresponsive. Absent or pulseless rhythms include pulseless VT, VF, asystole, and PEA. Cardiac arrest is usually associated with a poor outcome. Less than 2% of all arrests and just over 6% of patients with witnessed VF arrest survive neurologically intact to hospital discharge (Eckstein et al, 2005). The pulseless patient in VT on EMS arrival has the greatest likelihood of survival. Patients who have a bradydysrhythmia or asystole at initial contact have the worst prognosis. The outcome of patients in whom VF is the initial rhythm recorded is in between the outcomes associated with sustained VT and bradydysrhythmias or asystole (Myerburg & Castellanos, 2005).

Differential Diagnosis

Differential diagnoses for cardiopulmonary arrest include:

- Cardiovascular causes
  - Acute coronary syndrome
  - Cardiac tamponade
  - Cardiomyopathy
  - Congenital heart disease
  - Hypovolemia

- Myocardial infarction
- Wolff-Parkinson-White syndrome
- Respiratory causes
  - Hypoxia
  - Pulmonary embolism
  - Tension pneumothorax
- Other causes
  - Preexisting acidosis (renal failure or dialysis, aspirin overdose, methanol ingestion)
  - Drug overdose (tricyclic antidepressants, narcotics, beta or calcium channel blockers)
  - Hypoglycemia
  - Hyperkalemia
  - Hypokalemia
  - Hyperthermia
  - Hypothermia

BOX 22-35 Four Critical Tasks of Resuscitation

1. Airway management
2. Chest compressions
3. Monitoring and defibrillation
4. Vascular access and medication administration

Therapeutic Interventions

En route to a call for a patient who has had a cardiac arrest, determine which members of your team will perform the critical tasks of resuscitation (Box 22-35). Some tasks can be performed by personnel with basic life support training, whereas others require advanced training. One person must be designated as the team leader. The team leader will direct the members of the team and oversee the resuscitation effort, making sure each member of the team performs the tasks safely and correctly.

As the team leader, you will need to make decisions based on your knowledge of current resuscitation guidelines, local protocols, and the patient's condition. Act professionally throughout the resuscitation effort. Speak in a firm, confident tone to the members of your team. Be open to and actively seek suggestions from team members. Ask your team members to relay the patient's vital signs every 3 to 5 minutes or when any change in the patient's ABCs occurs. Also ask that they tell you when procedures are completed and drugs are given. For example, if you instructed a team member to establish an IV or give a drug, he or she should respond by saying something like, "IV started, left antecubital vein" or "1 mg 1:10,000 epinephrine given IV" when the task is completed. Team members should be instructed to ask you for clarification if your instructions are unclear.

Because perfusion of the heart muscle falls dramatically when chest compressions are stopped, begin care where the patient is found unless you do not have enough space in which to resuscitate the patient or conditions exist that may be hazardous to you, your crew, or the patient.

On arrival at the scene, quickly assess the patient's ABCs. Check for signs of obvious death such as dependent lividity, rigor mortis, or decomposition. If obvious signs of death are present, do not begin CPR. If no signs of obvious death are present and the patient is unresponsive, not breathing, and has no central pulse, make sure the patient is on a firm surface while a member of your crew quickly checks for documentation or other evidence of a DNAR order. If a properly completed DNAR form exists, do not begin CPR. If a DNAR order exists but its validity is questionable, place the patient on a cardiac monitor and immediately contact medical direction for instructions about how to proceed. Follow your local protocol about what should be done on the scene in these situations while waiting to talk with medical direction. Note that a person in cardiac arrest may have no pulse, yet gasping may be present and last from 2 to 4 minutes after the arrest (Ewy, 2005).

If no DNAR exists, quickly apply the cardiac monitor. The rhythm present on the cardiac monitor will guide the sequence of procedures that need to be done. For example, if the patient is in cardiac arrest and the cardiac monitor shows no ventricular electrical activity, asystole is present. If the monitor shows an organized rhythm despite no central pulse when you assess the patient, PEA is present. Defibrillation is not indicated for asystole or PEA. If the monitor shows VF or VT, defibrillation is indicated.

CPR 30:2
Advanced airway M: 100 comp/min
breaths q. 6-8 sec.

Pulseless Ventricular Tachycardia or Ventricular Fibrillation

If you observed the patient's collapse and the monitor shows VT or VF, defibrillation should be performed immediately. If applying the cardiac monitor or preparing the defibrillator is delayed, begin CPR. If you did not witness the patient's collapse and the monitor shows VT or VF, begin CPR. After five cycles of CPR (approximately 2 minutes), defibrillate once using the energy levels recommended by the defibrillator's manufacturer. When defibrillation is indicated, all team members with the exception of the person performing chest compressions should immediately clear the patient. The team member responsible for airway management must make sure that oxygen is not flowing over the patient's chest during defibrillation. Once the defibrillator is charged, the chest compressor should clear the patient and a shock should be delivered immediately to the patient. In this way, chest compressions are interrupted for the least amount of time possible during the resuscitation effort.

Ventilate the patient's lungs with a bag-valve-mask device and 100% oxygen at a rate of 1 breath every 5 to 6 seconds. Apply an endotracheal CO_2 monitor. Establish vascular access with normal saline or lactated Ringer's solution. If IV access can be obtained, use the antecubital or external jugular vein. If IV access is unsuccessful, establish intraosseous access. Give medications according to current resuscitation guidelines (see Figure 22-68). Follow each medication with a 20-mL flush of IV fluid to speed delivery of the drug to the central circulation. Use a smaller volume, such as 5 mL, for infants and children.

Consider placement of an advanced airway (endotracheal tube, laryngeal mask airway, or Combitube) if time permits. Make sure suction equipment is within arm's reach. Confirm proper position of the tube. Remember to minimize interruptions of chest compressions during these procedures.

Look for and treat possible reversible causes of the arrest. If the patient's rhythm changes, run a rhythm strip for placement in the patient's medical record. If the rhythm on the monitor changes (is not VT or VF) or any question exists about the rhythm displayed, assess the patient's pulse. If defibrillation terminates pulseless VT or VF and then recurs, begin defibrillation at the last energy setting that resulted in an ECG rhythm change.

Pulseless Electrical Activity and Asystole

In asystole, no ventricular activity is present on the cardiac monitor. To confirm that the rhythm is asystole on the monitor, check the lead and cable connections and make sure the power to the monitor is on, the correct lead is selected, the gain (ECG size) is turned up, and the same rhythm is present when checked in a second lead. PEA exists when organized electrical activity (other than VT) *or VF* is seen on the cardiac monitor but the patient *pulseless* is unresponsive, is not breathing, and a central pulse cannot be felt. Asystole and PEA have a poor prognosis unless the underlying cause can be rapidly identified and appropriately managed. Current treatment recommendations for asystole and PEA are shown in Figure 22-71.

PARAMEDIC Pearl

PATCH-4-MD can be used as an aid in memorizing some of the possible causes of a cardiac emergency:

- **P**ulmonary embolism
- **A**cidosis (preexisting)
- **T**ension pneumothorax
- **C**ardiac tamponade
- **H**ypovolemia
- **H**ypoxia, hypoglycemia
- **H**ypothermia, hyperthermia
- **H**yperkalemia (and other electrolytes)
- **M**yocardial infarction
- **D**rug overdose or acciden1ts

National Standards: use epi then
1mg atropine if pt changes to bradycardia
(3 rounds each)
Chicago: epi only - after 3 rounds, if
still asystole, can stop CPR

Although the prognosis for a massive pulmonary embolism or massive MI is poor, definitive treatment for these conditions is usually done in the hospital. Preexisting acidosis may be seen in conditions such as renal failure, methanol ingestion, and aspirin overdose. Sodium bicarbonate may be considered. A tension pneumothorax requires immediate needle decompression. Cardiac tamponade requires temporizing measures in the field, such as an IV fluid challenge, then pericardiocentesis (usually performed in the hospital). Hypovolemia is a common cause of PEA and requires IV fluid replacement. Normal saline or lactated Ringer's solution is usually infused in 250- to 500-mL boluses up to 1000 mL. Further fluid replacement is guided by instructions from medical direction. To correct hypoxia, ventilate the patient with 100% oxygen. If the patient is intubated, confirm the position of the tracheal tube with capnography. Be careful not to ventilate the patient at too fast a rate. Generally no more than 12 breaths/min is appropriate. If the patient's blood glucose level is less than 60 mg/dL, dextrose should be given IV push. If hypothermia is likely, the patient should be moved to a warm environment and protected from further cooling. Follow local protocol and instructions from medical direction for the hypothermic patient. Hyperkalemia may be seen in patients with renal failure. Sodium bicarbonate may be ordered to correct hyperkalemia. Tricyclic antidepressant overdose may require treatment with sodium bicarbonate. Naloxone may be ordered for a narcotic overdose. Glucagon may be ordered for beta-blocker overdose.

Postresuscitation Care

[OBJECTIVE 83]

The interval between restoration of spontaneous circulation and transfer to an intensive care unit is called the postresuscitation period. The immediate goals of postresuscitation care include the following (AHA, 2005b):

- Providing cardiorespiratory support to optimize tissue perfusion, especially to the heart, brain, and lungs (the organs most affected by cardiac arrest)
- Transporting to the emergency department and then to an appropriately equipped critical care unit
- Attempting to identify the precipitating cause of the arrest and start specific treatment if necessary
- Taking actions to prevent recurrence
- Taking actions to improve long-term, neurologically intact survival

Immediate Postresuscitation Care. Reassess the following ABCDs:

- Airway
  - Reassess the effectiveness of initial airway maneuvers and interventions
  - If not already done, perform endotracheal intubation if needed
- Breathing
  - Assess the adequacy of ventilations
  - Confirm advanced airway placement
  - Provide positive-pressure ventilation with oxygen
  - Assess the effectiveness of ventilations with capnography
  - Apply pulse oximeter and assess oxygen saturation
  - Rule out potential breathing complications from resuscitation (such as pneumothorax, rib fractures, sternal fractures, misplaced endotracheal tube)
  - Positive-pressure ventilation may be necessary for absent or inadequate spontaneous respirations
- Circulation
  - Reassess vital signs, skin color, mental status
  - Establish IV access with normal saline or lactated Ringer's solution if not already done
  - ECG monitoring; obtain 12-lead ECG
  - If the arrest rhythm was VF or VT, continuing an infusion of the antiarrhythmic associated with a return of spontaneous circulation is reasonable
  - Use of beta-blockers in the postresuscitation setting may be considered if no contraindications and approved by medical direction
- Differential diagnosis
  - Consider possible causes of the arrest
    - MI
    - Primary dysrhythmias
    - Electrolyte disturbances (such as tall T waves on the monitor)
    - Aortic aneurysm (brachial pulses present, femoral pulses absent)
- Additional actions
  - Assess for complications that may have occurred during resuscitation (such as rib fracture, pneumothorax, pericardial tamponade, misplaced endotracheal tube)
  - Evaluate IV infusions used during the resuscitation effort. Are the infusions currently running? Are they still needed?

- Ensure family has been updated regarding events
- Finish documentation as needed
- Acknowledge the efforts of the resuscitation team
- Postresuscitation critique

Temperature Regulation. Monitor the patient's body temperature closely. Fever can impair brain recovery by creating an imbalance between oxygen supply and demand; avoid hyperthermia. Do not actively rewarm stable patients who spontaneously develop mild hypothermia after resuscitation from cardiac arrest (AHA, 2005c). Mild hypothermia may be beneficial to neurologic outcome and may be well tolerated without significant risk of complications.

After prehospital cardiac arrest, unresponsive adults who have a return of spontaneous circulation should be cooled to 32° to 34° C (89.6° to 93.2° F) for 12 to 24 hours when the initial rhythm was VF. Similar therapy may be beneficial for prehospital patients with cardiac arrest caused by other rhythms or for in-hospital arrest (AHA, 2005c).

Glucose Control. Closely monitor serum glucose levels. Signs of hypoglycemia often are not obvious in comatose patients. Studies have documented poor neurologic outcomes in patients who have high blood glucose levels after resuscitation from cardiac arrest.

Field Termination of Resuscitation

[OBJECTIVES 84, 85]

In some cases the patient in cardiac arrest will not respond despite appropriate basic and advanced life support care. Some EMS systems have developed protocols that allow field termination of resuscitation efforts in specific circumstances. The National Association of EMS Physicians (NAEMSP) has recommended factors that should be considered when establishing termination of resuscitation protocols (Bailey et al, 2000). Following are the NAEMSP recommendations with explanations:

- Termination of resuscitation may be considered for any adult (18 years of age or older) patient who sustains SCD that is likely to be medical and is not associated with a condition potentially responsive to hospital treatment. Examples include hypothermia, cold water drowning, drug overdose, and toxic exposure. These patients generally should not be considered candidates for field termination of resuscitation.
- Unwitnessed cardiac arrest with a delayed start of CPR beyond 6 minutes and delayed defibrillation beyond 8 minutes has a poor prognosis.
- In the absence of do not resuscitate or advanced directives, a full resuscitative effort—including CPR, definitive airway management, medication administration, defibrillation if necessary, and 20 to 30 minutes of treatment following advanced cardiac life support guidelines and/or local protocols—should be performed before declaring the patient dead.

- A patient whose rhythm changes to, or remains in, VF or VT should have continued resuscitative efforts. Patients in asystole or PEA are considered to be in terminal rhythms, and termination of resuscitation should be considered.
- Logistics should be considered, such as collapse in a public place, family wishes, and safety of the EMS crew and public. If the family wants resuscitation continued, or if the family's wishes are unclear, particularly if a communication barrier exists, continuing resuscitation may be beneficial.
- Online medical direction should be established before termination of resuscitation. The decision to terminate efforts should be an agreement between the on-scene paramedic and the online physician. When speaking with medical direction, be sure to relay the following information:
  - Medical condition of the patient
  - Circumstances surrounding the arrest, if known
  - Emergency care provided and the patient's response to that care
  - Family present and made aware of the situation
  - Any resistance or uncertainty on the part of the family
- On-scene EMS professionals and the family should have access to resources such as clergy, crisis counselors, and social workers. EMS systems that have a field termination protocol must ensure their EMS personnel are trained in grief counseling and providing support to family members of the deceased.
- Maintain continuous documentation of the events of the call, including continuous ECG monitoring. After the call, the documentation will be reviewed as part of the quality management process. The quality management review is necessary to ensure the protocol was appropriately applied, law enforcement personnel were notified, the medical examiner or coroner was involved, and support services were available for the family.

At the scene, law enforcement personnel may need to communicate with the patient's physician for the death certificate. They also may determine if the event or patient requires assignment to the medical examiner. This may occur if any suspicion exists about the nature of the death or if the patient's physician refuses or hesitates to sign the death certificate. If the patient does not have a personal physician, the patient will be assigned to the medical examiner.

Patient and Family Education

Although all persons can benefit from learning CPR, family members of patients who have coronary heart disease should be taught how to do CPR and learn how to use an automated external defibrillator.

TABLE 22-48	Blood Pressure Values in Adults*	
Category	Systolic Blood Pressure (mm Hg)	Diastolic Blood Pressure (mm Hg)
Normal	<120	<80
Prehypertension	120-139	80-89
Stage 1 high BP	140-159	90-99
Stage 2 high BP	≥160	≥100

Modified from National Heart, Lung, and Blood Institute. (2005). *High blood pressure*. Retrieved May 15, 2005, from http://www.nhlbi.nih.gov/health/dci/Diseases/Hbp/HBP_WhatIs.html.
BP, Blood pressure.
*For adults 18 and older who are not on medicine for high blood pressure, are not having a short-term serious illness, and do not have other conditions such as diabetes and kidney disease.

HYPERTENSION

Description and Definition

[OBJECTIVES 86, 87]

According to the National Heart, Lung, and Blood Institute, an adult's normal blood pressure is a systolic blood pressure less than 120 mm Hg and a diastolic blood pressure less than 80 mm Hg (Table 22-48). A person who has a systolic blood pressure of 120 to 139 mm Hg or diastolic blood pressure of 80 to 89 mm Hg is considered to have prehypertension. For adults 18 and older, high blood pressure (hypertension) exists if they have a systolic blood pressure of 140 mm Hg or higher or a diastolic blood pressure of 90 mm Hg or higher measured on two or more occasions and the following conditions exist:

- They are not taking medicine for high blood pressure
- They do not have a short-term serious illness
- They do not have other conditions, such as diabetes and kidney disease.

One important exception exists to the definition of high blood pressure; a person who has diabetes or chronic kidney disease has high blood pressure if his or her blood pressure is 130/80 mm Hg or higher.

Etiology

High blood pressure has been called the silent killer because it usually has no signs or symptoms yet it silently causes damage to the heart, brain, eyes, blood vessels, and kidneys. A person can have it for years without knowing it. Uncontrolled high blood pressure can lead to vision problems and increases the risk of serious health problems such as stroke, heart attack, heart failure, or kidney failure (Figure 22-110).

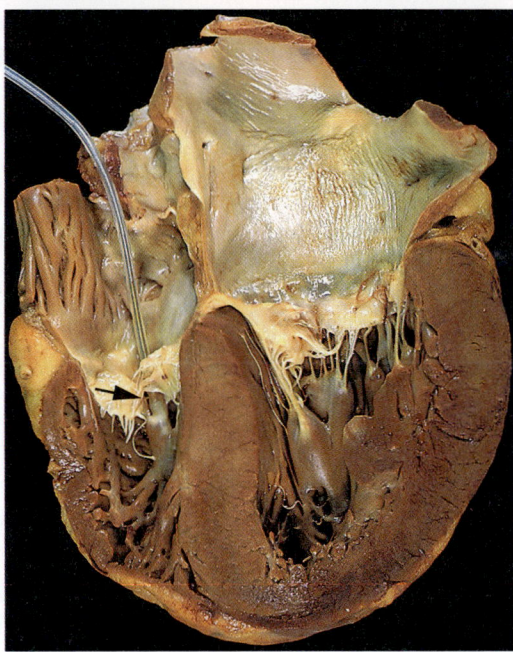

Figure 22-110 Hypertensive heart disease with marked thickening of the left ventricular wall, causing reduction in lumen size. The left ventricle is on the right in this view of the heart. A pacemaker is present in the right ventricle *(arrow)*.

Stage 2
160/100

diastolic >130 = hypertensive crisis

23-25% of blood in arterial system at any one time
65-70% of blood in venous system at any one time
5%   "   capillaries   "

In 90% to 95% of cases high blood pressure has no identifiable cause. This type of high blood pressure is called **essential hypertension** or **primary hypertension.** Behaviors such as not exercising and excessive intake of calories, salt, or alcohol contribute to high blood pressure. Essential hypertension tends to develop gradually over many years. Because it tends to occur in families, researchers believe that heredity is a factor in essential hypertension.

In the other 5% to 10% of cases, high blood pressure has an identifiable cause, such as medications or an underlying disease or condition (Box 22-36). This type of high blood pressure is called **secondary hypertension**.

Blood pressure is equal to cardiac output multiplied by peripheral vascular resistance. Therefore blood pressure is affected by any condition that affects peripheral resistance or cardiac output (Box 22-37). Blood pressure also is affected by the condition of the heart, arteries, kidneys, and nervous system. For example, if blood vessels are narrowed from atherosclerosis, blood pressure may increase as the heart attempts to pump blood through constricted passageways. An excessive amount of sodium intake may cause the kidneys to retain too much water and sodium. This can increase blood volume and subsequently increase blood pressure.

BOX 22-36	Possible Causes of Secondary Hypertension

Medications

- Amphetamines
- Anabolic steroids
- Antidepressants such as desipramine (Norpramin), phenelzine (Nardil), bupropion (Wellbutrin, Zyban), venlafaxine (Effexor)
- Appetite suppressants
- Cocaine
- Cold medicines and nasal decongestants
- Ephedra (ma-huang)
- Herbal supplements such as ginkgo, ginseng, licorice, St. John's wort
- Immunosuppressants such as corticosteroids (Medrol), cyclosporine (Neoral, Sandimmune), tacrolimus (Prograf, Protropic)
- NSAIDs such as ibuprofen (Advil, Motrin), meloxicam (Mobic), naproxen (Naprosyn), naproxen sodium (Aleve)
- Oral contraceptives
- Phencyclidine (PCP, "angel dust")

Disease or Condition

- Abnormal blood vessels
- Adrenal disease
- Coarctation of the aorta
- Cushing syndrome's
- Hyperaldosteronism
- Hyperparathyroidism
- Hyperthyroidism
- Kidney disease
- Lead poisoning
- Pheochromocytoma
- Preeclampsia
- Quadriplegia
- Sleep apnea

NSAID, Nonsteroidal antiinflammatory drug.

BOX 22-37	Medications and Conditions That Affect Blood Pressure

Increase Peripheral Resistance

- Atherosclerosis
- Pheochromocytoma
- Cushing's syndrome
- Stress
- Hyperthyroidism
- Diabetes
- Cold medicines and nasal decongestants
- Amphetamines, anabolic steroids, cocaine, pseudoephedrine, phencyclidine
- Tobacco use

Increase Cardiac Output

- Excessive sodium intake
- Pheochromocytoma
- Preeclampsia
- Stress
- Hyperthyroidism
- Kidney disease
- Hyperaldosteronism

Hypertensive Emergencies

[OBJECTIVES 86, 87]

Some patients have transient hypertension related to anxiety or their chief complaint. **Hypertensive urgencies** are significant elevations in blood pressure with nonspecific symptoms that should be corrected within 24 hours. **Hypertensive emergencies** are situations that require rapid (within 1 hour) lowering of blood pressure to prevent or limit organ damage. Evidence of end-organ failure secondary to the hypertension is necessary for these conditions to exist. **Malignant hypertension** is one type of hypertensive emergency. Malignant hyper-

---

Case Scenario CONCLUSION

You maintain positive-pressure ventilation with high-flow oxygen and begin TCP with capture verified by peripheral pulses. On arrival in the emergency department, the patient remains unresponsive with a pulse of 70 beats/min by the pacemaker, blood pressure 100/70 mm Hg, and respirations, 0. The patient's wife informs the physician that her husband has been smoking crack cocaine on a regular basis for the past year, with increasing use during the last 2 months. The physician inserts a temporary pacemaker. The patient's mental status improves and he is admitted to the ICU. Seven days after placement of a permanent pacemaker, the patient is discharged from the hospital.

Looking Back

10. *Assume that the patient remained unconscious with an unacceptably low blood pressure despite pacing. What treatment would be appropriate at that time?*
11. *Given the patient's final disposition, was your treatment appropriate? Why or why not?*

tension is a medical emergency that occurs because of a rapid rise in blood pressure with signs of acute and progressive damage to end organs, such as the heart, brain, and kidneys. The increase in blood pressure damages blood vessels, causing them to become inflamed. Inflamed blood vessels may leak fluid or blood. If untreated, malignant hypertension may result in acute renal failure, MI, stroke, or hypertensive encephalopathy. Hypertensive encephalopathy is a combination of signs and symptoms that occur with malignant hypertension. Signs and symptoms of hypertensive encephalopathy include severe hypertension, headache, vomiting, visual disturbances, mental status changes, seizures, and abnormalities of the retina of the eye (retinopathy). If untreated, death may result within a few hours.

Epidemiology and Demographics

Hypertensive emergencies usually occur in patients with a history of hypertension. Failure to take blood pressure medications or other treatments as prescribed is a common cause of the emergency. A hypertensive emergency also may occur as a result of toxemia of pregnancy.

History   #1 the headache (pounding)

Hypertensive emergencies often develop rapidly. The patient is usually quite anxious and may present with a severe headache, blurred vision, dizziness, ringing in the ears (tinnitus), dyspnea, chest pain or tightness, nosebleed, muscle cramps, weakness, or palpitations. The patient may describe symptoms of PND and orthopnea.

Be sure to ask the patient about the medications he or she is taking (prescription and over the counter). Because noncompliance with blood pressure medication is a common cause of malignant hypertension, find out if the patient has been prescribed blood pressure medication and if he or she takes it as prescribed. Ask the patient about the use of recreational drugs such as amphetamines, cocaine, or other sympathomimetic agents. Effects of these drugs can cause severe hypertension.

Physical Findings

Patients having a hypertensive emergency look sick. The patient's mental status may range from responsive to altered or unresponsive. The patient's skin may be pale, flushed, or normal and feel dry or moist, warm or cool. Peripheral pulses may feel strong or bounding. Be sure to check (and document) the patient's blood pressure in both arms in case aortic dissection is present. The patient's diastolic blood pressure usually is higher than 130 mm Hg. The patient may have seizures, signs of heart failure such as crackles in the lungs, or signs consistent with a

heart attack. Ischemic changes may be seen on the 12-lead ECG.

Differential Diagnosis

Differential diagnoses for hypertension include:

- Cardiovascular causes
  - Aortic dissection
- Neurological causes
  - Epilepsy or postictal state
  - Head injury
  - Intracranial mass
  - Stroke
  - Subarachnoid hemorrhage
- Genitourinary causes
  - Pheochromocytoma
  - Renal failure
  - Toxemia of pregnancy
- Other causes
  - Acute anxiety
  - Cocaine or amphetamine use
  - Connective tissue disease
  - Drug overdose or withdrawal

Therapeutic Interventions

Emergency care for hypertensive emergencies involves careful lowering of the patient's blood pressure with continuous monitoring with IV medications such as nitroprusside or labetalol. This is usually done in the hospital because these medications typically are not available in the prehospital setting. Prehospital care for hypertensive emergencies includes supportive care. Give oxygen, establish an IV, and apply the cardiac monitor and a pulse oximeter. Maintain oxygen saturation at greater than 95%. Avoid performing additional procedures on the scene that will delay transport to the hospital.

If the conditions are present, provide care for heart failure or chest discomfort from myocardial ischemia according to local protocols or instructions from medical direction. If vasodilators are given for these conditions, be sure to monitor the patient's blood pressure closely. Treat seizures if present. Provide reassurance to the patient and family while providing care at the scene and during rapid transport to the hospital.

A patient with a hypertensive emergency requires rapid transport to the closest appropriate facility. If the patient refuses care, repeatedly try to persuade him or her to accept the care you wish to provide, including transport. Explain to the patient that if his or her condition is not treated, symptoms may worsen and could result in death. Consider contacting medical direction for advice. If you are unable to convince the patient to receive care, carefully document the patient's refusal.

Patient and Family Education

Patients with hypertension should be taught methods to help control blood pressure. They should be taught how to take and record blood pressure measurements. If the patient smokes, he or she should quit. If the patient is overweight, he or she should lose weight, eat a diet low in salt, and ingest appropriate amounts of vitamins and minerals. The patient should exercise regularly and take steps to reduce stress. If the patient is prescribed blood pressure medication, teach the importance of taking the medication as prescribed, even when the patient is feeling well.

ENDOCARDITIS

Description and Definition

[OBJECTIVES 88, 89]

Infective endocarditis is an infection of the innermost surface of the heart, which may include the heart's chambers, one or more heart valves, or the septum.

Etiology

 Endocarditis occurs when bacteria in the bloodstream lodge and begin to multiply on a heart valve or other damaged tissue in the heart (Figure 22-111). If untreated, the bacteria can damage the heart valve, causing it to malfunction (Box 22-38).

Endocarditis occurs most often in people with preexisting valvular disease such as mitral or aortic valve disease or in individuals with mechanical (prosthetic) heart valves. It can also occur in people with congenital heart disease. Right-sided endocarditis is a type of infective endocarditis that affects the tricuspid and pulmonary valves. This type of endocarditis is most often seen in IV drug users, patients who have infected central venous catheters, dialysis shunts, or transvenous pacing wires.

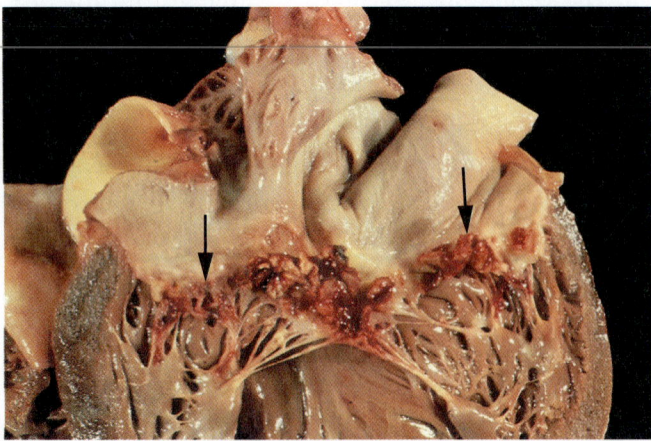

Figure 22-111 Infective (bacterial) endocarditis. Endocarditis of mitral valve denoted by *arrows*.

BOX 22-38	Valvular Disorders

The heart's valves open and close in a specific sequence. This ensures a smooth flow of blood through the heart's chambers. Blood flow through the heart can be hampered if a valve does not function properly. Valvular heart disease is the term used to describe a malfunctioning heart valve. Types of valvular heart disease include the following:

- *Valvular stenosis*. If a valve narrows, stiffens, or thickens, the valve is said to be stenosed. The heart must work harder to pump blood through a stenosed valve.
- *Valve prolapse*. If a valve flap inverts, it is said to prolapse. Prolapse can occur if one valve flap is larger than the other. It can also occur if the chordae tendineae stretch markedly or rupture.
- *Valvular regurgitation*. Blood can flow backward, or regurgitate, if one or more of the heart's valves does not close properly. Valvular regurgitation is also known as valvular incompetence or valvular insufficiency.

Think about what might happen if a papillary muscle in the left ventricle were to tear or rupture. The flaps of the mitral valve may not completely close and the valve flap may invert (prolapse). This may result in blood leaking from the left ventricle into the left atrium (regurgitation) during ventricular contraction. Blood flow to the body (cardiac output) would probably be decreased as a result.

Endocarditis may be caused by a variety of different organisms. Most organisms originate from the skin, upper airway, or genitourinary or gastrointestinal tract. The organism may gain access to the body in many ways, including a minor skin infection, dental cleaning, upper respiratory infection, or major surgery. Body piercing and tattooing also have been associated with endocarditis.

The severity of the patient's illness is often a reflection of the virulence of the infecting organism. Less-virulent organisms cause a low-grade temperature and symptoms that usually develop over several weeks to months. Organisms that are more virulent cause high-grade fevers and signs of serious illness that develop over days to weeks.

Epidemiology and Demographics

Most cases of endocarditis are caused by a bacterial infection. More than half of all cases in the United States occur in patients older than 60 years (Cantrell & Yoshikawa, 1984). Predisposing factors include the following:

- Artificial heart valve
- Previous history of endocarditis
- Heart valves damaged by rheumatic fever
- Congenital heart or heart valve defects
- Hypertrophic cardiomyopathy
- Intravascular (i.e., arterial or venous) catheter

History

The most common symptoms of endocarditis are fever and chills. The patient may also complain headache, loss of appetite, weight loss, muscle and joint aches and pains, night sweats, shortness of breath, or cough.

The patient may describe recent dental work in the previous 1 to 2 months; IV drug use; recent valvular surgery; or a history of rheumatic fever, valvular heart disease, or endocarditis.

Physical Findings

A new or significantly changed heart murmur is common. Central nervous system involvement occurs in 30% to 40% of patients, with symptoms ranging from transient ischemic attacks to subarachnoid hemorrhage. Signs of heart failure may be present because of progressive destruction of the heart's valves. If infective endocarditis invades the heart's conduction system, ECG changes may be seen, including a prolonged PR interval, complete heart block, or left BBB. Flat, painless, red-to-blue lesions (Janeway lesions) may be present on the palms and soles. Some patients develop small, tender nodules on the pads of the fingers or toes (Osler's nodes).

Differential Diagnosis

Differential diagnoses for endocarditis include:

- Neurologic causes
  - Encephalitis
  - Meningitis
- Respiratory causes
  - Lung abscess
  - Pneumonia
  - Pulmonary emboli
- Other causes
  - Acute rheumatic fever
  - Systemic lupus erythematosus

Therapeutic Interventions

Prehospital care for endocarditis is mainly supportive. Allow the patient to assume a position of comfort, give oxygen, establish an IV, and apply the cardiac monitor. Apply a pulse oximeter. Maintain oxygen saturation at greater than 95%. If present, provide care for heart failure according to local protocols or instructions from medical direction. The patient will usually receive IV antibiotics in the hospital. If a prosthetic valve is the site of infection, surgery may be necessary.

Most patients with endocarditis can be transported to the closest appropriate facility without lights and sirens. If the patient refuses care, repeatedly try to persuade him or her to accept the care you wish to provide, including transport. Consider contacting medical direction for advice. If you are unable to convince the patient to receive care, carefully document the patient's refusal.

Patient and Family Education

Patients with a history of endocarditis should carry a wallet card to alert health care professionals about their needs. Patients at high risk for endocarditis should receive prophylactic antibiotics before undergoing dental, surgical, or other invasive procedures. Examples include prostate surgery, tonsillectomy and/or adenoidectomy, and dental procedures such as prophylactic cleaning of teeth or implants or a tooth extraction.

DISEASES OF THE PERICARDIUM

Pericarditis

Description and Definition

[OBJECTIVES 90, 91]

Pericarditis is an inflammation of the double-walled sac (pericardium) that encloses the heart. The pericardium helps anchor the heart in place, preventing excessive movement of the heart in the chest when body position changes, and protecting it from trauma and infection.

Etiology

Pericarditis is usually the result of an infection that may be viral (most common), bacterial or, occasionally, fungal. Pericarditis may develop days or weeks after a patient has a heart attack (Figure 22-112). It also may develop after blunt or penetrating chest trauma, open-heart surgery, or procedures such as coronary angioplasty or insertion of an implantable defibrillator or pacemaker. Drugs such as

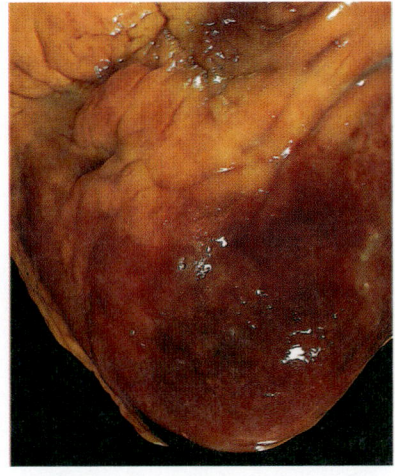

Figure 22-112 Pericarditis shown as a dark, roughened epicardial surface over an acute infarction.

procainamide and hydralazine and radiation therapy also can cause pericarditis. It can develop in patients with kidney failure or inflammatory disorders such as rheumatoid arthritis and lupus. It can also develop as a result of breast or lung cancer, lymphomas, or leukemia. In many cases no cause for pericarditis is identified (idiopathic pericarditis).

Epidemiology and Demographics

Pericarditis most often occurs in men between the ages of 20 and 50 years. Most cases of pericarditis are from a virus or the cause is unknown.

History

Ask the patient about recent flulike signs and symptoms. Patients with pericarditis may relay a history of a recent upper respiratory infection. The patient may describe a recent fever with shaking chills, shortness of breath, coughing, skin rash, or weight loss. The patient may have a history of a recent MI, leukemia, Hodgkin's disease, lymphoma, lupus, kidney disease, chest trauma, or heart surgery.

Physical Findings

Chest discomfort is the most common symptom of pericarditis. The patient usually describes it as a sharp, stabbing pain, but sometimes it is a steady, constricting pain that radiates to the shoulder and either arm or both arms, mimicking the discomfort of a heart attack. However, unlike the pain of a heart attack, the discomfort associated with pericarditis is commonly made worse by deep inspiration, coughing, or lying flat. The discomfort often improves when the patient sits up and leans forward.

The patient's chest discomfort is most often located under the sternum but may be centered in the left anterior chest or the epigastrium. The discomfort may persist for days. Listening to heart sounds may reveal a pericardial friction rub, although this sign is not always present. A pericardial friction rub is a scratchy or grating sound caused by contact between the visceral and parietal pericardium. It is best heard with the patient leaning forward and listening at the third to fifth intercostal space to the left of the sternum. Ask the patient to hold his or her breath while you listen. If you hear a sound like two pieces of dried leather rubbing together or the sound made when walking on crunchy snow, pericarditis is the likely cause.

The patient often has a fever, tachycardia, and tachypnea. He or she may look pale, and JVD may or may not be present. If JVD is present, it may indicate pericardial effusion (a buildup of fluid in the pericardial space) resulting from the infection. Breath sounds are usually normal unless another condition exists, such as heart failure. The ECG often reveals ST-segment elevation in multiple leads (Figure 22-113). PR-segment depression may be present (except in lead aVR) and can be the initial ECG sign of acute pericarditis (Baljepally & Spodick, 1998).

Differential Diagnosis

Differential diagnoses for pericarditis include:

- Cardiovascular causes
  - Aortic dissection
  - Cardiomyopathy
  - Myocardial infarction

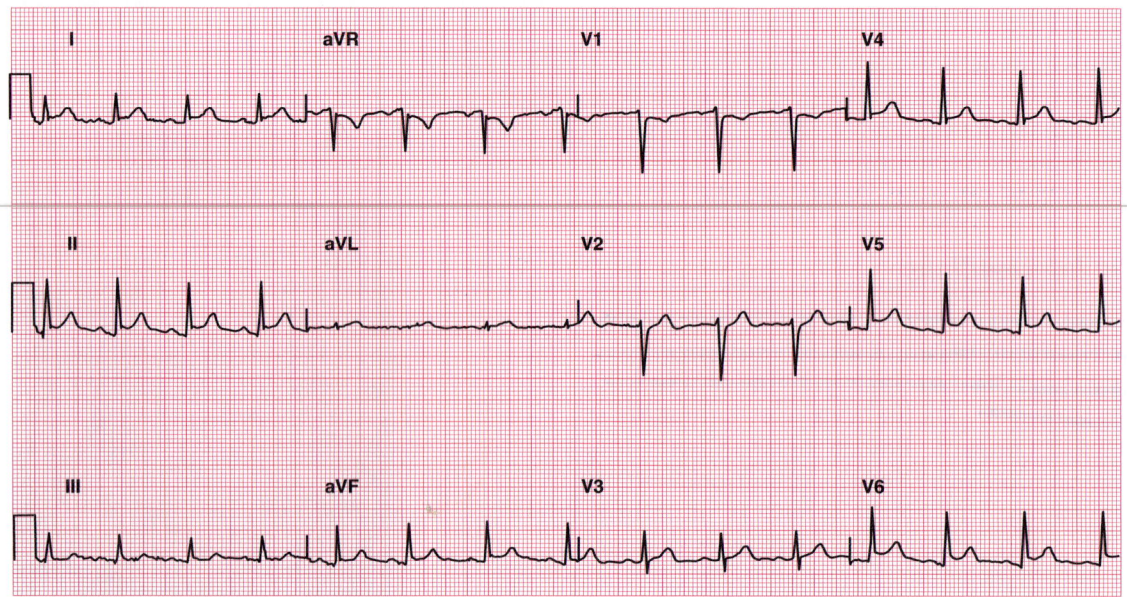

Figure 22-113 The ECG pattern of pericarditis. Note the diffuse pattern of ST-segment elevation; PR-segment depression in lead II; and J-point notching in leads II, V_5, and V_6.

- Respiratory causes
  - Pleurisy
  - Pneumothorax
  - Pulmonary embolism
- Other causes
  - Costochondritis
  - Gastroesophageal reflux disease
  - Lupus

Therapeutic Interventions

Prehospital care for pericarditis is mainly supportive. Allow the patient to assume a position of comfort, give oxygen, establish an IV, and apply the cardiac monitor. Apply a pulse oximeter. Maintain oxygen saturation at greater than 95%. Pericarditis is usually treated with nonsteroidal antiinflammatory drugs such as aspirin and ibuprofen. Viral pericarditis usually resolves on its own. Bacterial pericarditis is treated with antibiotics, and fungal pericarditis is treated with antifungal medications.

Most patients with pericarditis can be transported to the closest appropriate facility without lights and sirens. If the patient refuses care, repeatedly try to persuade him or to accept the care you wish to provide, including transport. Consider contacting medical direction for advice. If you are unable to convince the patient to receive care, carefully document the patient's refusal.

Patient and Family Education

Patients with pericarditis should avoid strenuous activity if they have a fever greater than 37.8° C (100° F). If the patient has been diagnosed with bacterial pericarditis, he or she must take the antibiotics as prescribed—even if beginning to feel better before the medication is gone. Pericarditis can recur depending on the cause.

Pericardial Tamponade

Description and Definition

[OBJECTIVES 92, 93]

A **pericardial effusion** is an increase in the volume and/or character of pericardial fluid that surrounds the heart (Figure 22-114). The pressure within the pericardium increases as pericardial fluid builds up. The amount of blood or fluid in the pericardial space needed to impair the heart's ability to fill depends on the following:

- The rate at which the buildup of blood or fluid occurs
- The ability of the pericardium to stretch and make room for the increased volume of fluid

If excess fluid builds up slowly, the pericardium will gradually expand and make room for a large volume before signs and symptoms appear. If the fluid builds up rapidly, the pressure within the pericardium significantly increases with a smaller volume of fluid.

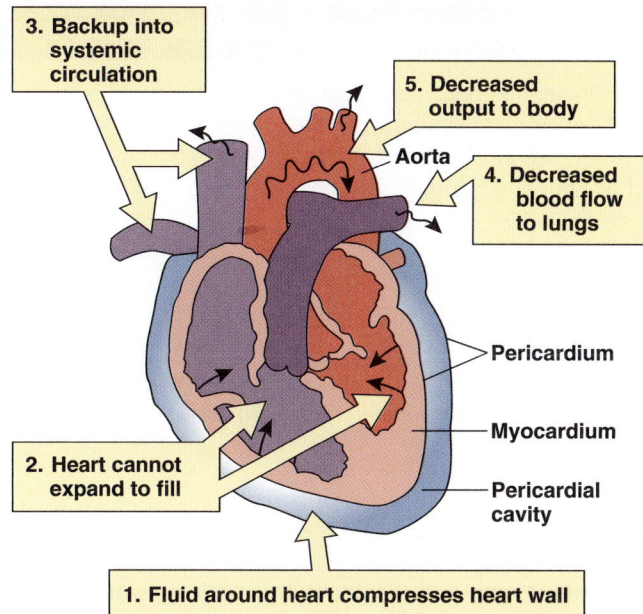

Figure 22-114 Effects of pericardial effusion and cardiac tamponade.

Cardiac tamponade occurs when the buildup of pericardial fluid compresses the heart and impairs contraction and ventricular filling. Limited ventricular filling results in decreased stroke volume, decreased cardiac output, and signs of shock.

> **PARAMEDIC Pearl**
>
> **Three Main Features of Cardiac Tamponade**
> 1. Increased intracardiac pressure
> 2. Limited ventricular filling
> 3. Reduced cardiac output

Etiology

Cardiac tamponade may be caused by the same conditions that cause pericarditis. It may develop gradually if caused by an infection or tumor. It can develop rapidly when caused by heart surgery, insertion of a pacemaker or central venous catheter, or trauma to the heart, such as a stab wound or gunshot wound. Some of the possible causes of cardiac tamponade are shown in Box 22-39.

Epidemiology and Demographics

- Cardiac tamponade reportedly occurs in approximately 2 out of 10,000 people.
- From 60% to 80% of patients with stab wounds involving the heart develop cardiac tamponade (Harris et al, 1999).

BOX 22-39	Possible Causes of Cardiac Tamponade

- Pericarditis, pericardial effusion
- Cardiac rupture after myocardial infarction
- Blunt trauma (including CPR)
- Penetrating trauma
- Result of renal disease
- Hypothyroidism
- Aortic dissection
- Radiation induced (cancer treatment)
- Heart surgery
- Hospital procedures (angioplasty, central venous catheter insertion, pacemaker wire insertion)

History

The patient who has cardiac tamponade is usually too ill to answer questions pertaining to medical history. The patient likely is anxious and restless and complains of shortness of breath, chest tightness, and/or dizziness. Family members may tell you of a recent invasive procedure, heart attack, chronic illness, or medications that the patient is taking that may provide clues regarding the reason cardiac tamponade may have developed. Although tension pneumothorax is more common, suspect cardiac tamponade in any patient who has sustained a penetrating wound of the chest or upper abdomen. If the tamponade is not from trauma, the patient may relay a history of a medical illness such as pericarditis or end-stage renal disease.

Physical Findings

Signs of injury to the chest wall are usually present if cardiac tamponade is from trauma. Classic signs of cardiac tamponade include JVD, hypotension, and muffled heart sounds (Beck's triad), but these signs are present in less than half of all patients with cardiac tamponade. JVD may be absent if the patient is hypovolemic. Heart sounds may be normal early on, becoming progressively faint or muffled as the condition worsens. Other signs include cold, pale, mottled, or cyanotic skin; tachycardia; weak or absent peripheral pulses; narrowing pulse pressure; and pulsus paradoxus. Pulsus paradoxus is a late sign and may be absent if the patient has severe hypotension. If cardiac tamponade develops slowly, the patient's signs and symptoms may resemble those of heart failure, including dyspnea, orthopnea, and JVD.

ECG changes often show low-voltage QRS and T waves. ST-segment elevation (caused by inflammation of the epicardium) or nonspecific T-wave changes also may be seen. Changing levels of the ECG voltage of the P wave, QRS complex, and T wave (electrical alternans) may be seen.

Differential Diagnosis

Differential diagnoses for pericardial tamponade include:

- Cardiovascular causes
  - RVF
  - RVI
- Respiratory causes
  - Pulmonary embolism
  - Tension pneumothorax

Therapeutic Interventions

If trauma is the source of the patient's signs and symptoms, stabilize the cervical spine as needed. Make sure the patient's airway is open. Give high-concentration oxygen. Make sure ventilation and oxygenation are effective. Apply a pulse oximeter. Maintain oxygen saturation at greater than 95%. Suction as needed. Control life-threatening bleeding if present. Apply the cardiac monitor. Maintain normal body temperature. Avoid performing additional procedures on the scene that will delay transport to the hospital.

Establish IV access en route to definitive care. Give IV fluids and medications per local protocol or medical direction instructions. If no signs of heart failure are present, an IV fluid challenge of normal saline or lactated Ringer's solution is usually given to maintain circulating blood volume. Check the patient's response by assessing mental status, heart rate, respiratory effort, breath sounds, and blood pressure.

The definitive treatment for cardiac tamponade is in-hospital pericardiocentesis. **Pericardiocentesis** is a procedure in which a needle is inserted into the pericardial space and the excess fluid is drained (aspirated) through the needle. If scarring is the cause of the tamponade, surgery may be necessary to remove the affected area of the pericardium.

Giving IV fluids is a temporizing measure and should not delay transport of the patient for definitive care.

A patient who has signs and symptoms of shock requires rapid transport to the closest appropriate facility. If the patient refuses care, repeatedly try to persuade him or her to accept the care you wish to provide, including transport. Explain to the patient that if the condition is not treated, the symptoms may worsen and could result in death. Consider contacting medical direction for advice. If you are unable to convince the patient to receive care, carefully document the patient's refusal.

Patient and Family Education

Explain all procedures to the patient and provide emotional support to the patient and family.

CONGENITAL ABNORMALITIES OF THE CARDIOVASCULAR SYSTEM

Congenital cardiovascular defects are present in approximately 1% of live births. Heart defects may obstruct blood flow in the heart or the vessels near it or cause an alteration in the normal pattern of blood flow through the heart. Although rare, defects may occur in which only one ventricle exists (single ventricle), both the pulmonary artery and aorta arise from the same ventricle (double-outlet ventricle), or the right or left side of the heart is incompletely formed (hypoplastic right or left heart).

Because of the number of congenital abnormalities presented here, the epidemiology, history, physical findings, and therapeutic interventions are briefly discussed with each condition.

Acyanotic Heart Defects

Acyanotic heart defects (are also called pink defects) are congenital abnormalities in which oxygenated blood is shunted from the left (systemic) side of the heart to the right (pulmonary) side. This defect is called a *left-to-right shunt*. Acyanotic defects may be classified according to their hemodynamic effects (Table 22-49).

Atrial Septal Defect

With an atrial septal defect (ASD), an abnormal opening (hole or defect) exists in the wall (septum) separating the atrial chambers of the heart (Figure 22-115). This opening allows some of the oxygenated blood from the left atrium (at higher pressure) to flow through the hole to the right atrium (at lower pressure) instead of flowing through the left ventricle, out the aorta, and to the body. The increased volume of blood flowing to the right atrium and ventricle causes enlargement of these chambers. If the defect is not repaired, pulmonary hypertension usually develops in adult life.

ASD is more common in females than males and accounts for 5% to 10% of all congenital heart defects. Infants and children with ASD are usually asymptomatic, although height and weight are often below normal and endurance may be limited. A characteristic murmur is

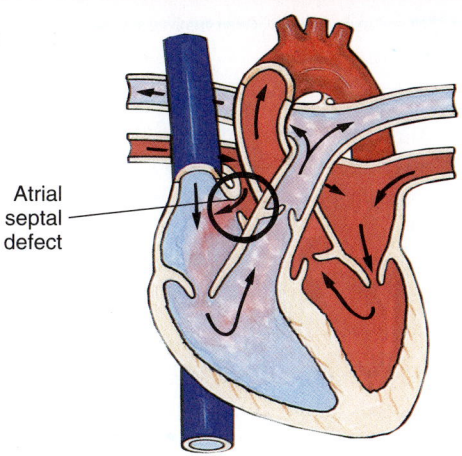

Figure 22-115 Atrial septal defect.

present with ASD. Patients are at risk for atrial dysrhythmias, probably from atrial enlargement and stretching of conduction fibers. Small ASDs (less than 8 mm) often close on their own by 18 months of age. Large defects often require surgery, usually before school age.

Ventricular Septal Defect

In a ventricular septal defect (VSD), an abnormal opening exists in the wall separating the right and left ventricles (Figure 22-116). This opening allows some of the oxygenated blood to flow from the left ventricle through the hole to the right ventricle and pulmonary artery instead of being pumped into the aorta. Because less blood is pumped out of the left ventricle, stroke volume is reduced, affecting cardiac output. Because the right ventricle is under greater pressure and must pump extra blood, it may enlarge. If the right ventricle is unable to accommodate the increased workload, the right atrium also may enlarge.

VSD is the most common (15% to 20%) congenital heart defect. If the opening is small, the patient usually is asymptomatic and growth and development are unaf-

TABLE 22-49	Acyanotic Heart Defects
Blood Flow	**Defect**
Increased pulmonary blood flow	Atrial septal defect
	Ventricular septal defect
	Patent ductus arteriosus
Obstruction to blood flow from the ventricles	Coarction of the aorta
	Aortic stenosis
	Pulmonary stenosis

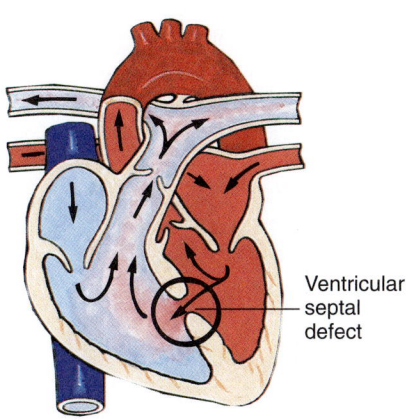

Figure 22-116 Ventricular septal defect.

fected. If the opening is of moderate to large size, the following occur:

- Delayed growth and development (height usually is normal but weight may be decreased)
- Decreased exercise tolerance
- Repeated pulmonary infections
- Signs of congestive heart failure (e.g., tachypnea, grunting respirations, tachycardia, diminished pulses, fatigue with feeding, and diaphoresis)
- A characteristic murmur

Infants and children with a VSD are at risk for bacterial endocarditis and must take antibiotics before certain dental and surgical procedures. Many small defects close on their own during the first year of life. Moderate and large defects may require surgical closure.

Patent Ductus Arteriosus

Patent ductus arteriosus (PDA) occurs when the ductus arteriosus, a blood vessel present during fetal development that connects the pulmonary artery to the descending aorta, fails to close after birth (Figure 22-117). The ductus arteriosus normally closes within a few hours of birth. Persistence of the ductus arteriosus beyond 10 days of life is considered abnormal. PDA is common in premature infants. An increased incidence of PDA exists with maternal rubella infection. PDA is more common in patients born at a high altitude. The consequences of PDA are determined by the diameter and length of the ductus and the level of peripheral vascular resistance.

In PDA, oxygenated blood traveling through the aorta is shunted from the aorta, across the duct, to the pulmonary artery (instead of flowing from the aorta and on to the body), where it mixes with deoxygenated blood. The workload of the left atrium and ventricle is increased because of the additional blood that is recirculated through the lungs to these heart chambers. At the same time, less blood is delivered to the lungs to be oxygenated.

Patient signs and symptoms depend on the size of the ductus and how much blood flow it carries. The patient with a small shunt may be asymptomatic. Signs and symptoms associated with a large shunt include the following:

- Wide pulse pressure
- Bounding peripheral pulses
- A characteristic murmur
- Rapid breathing, increased work of breathing
- Frequent respiratory infections
- Fatigue and/or poor growth

In term infants, surgical tying of the patent ductus is recommended if heart failure develops. If the infant is asymptomatic, surgery is postponed until 6 months to 3 years of age unless the infant develops symptoms. A small PDA may be closed by using plugs or coils positioned by a catheter inserted in an artery in the groin during cardiac catheterization.

Coarctation of the Aorta

In coarctation (narrowing, constriction) of the aorta (COA), the aorta is pinched or constricted in the area of the ductus arteriosus, just beyond the aorta's branching vessels to the head and arms (Figure 22-118). Because a segment of the aorta is narrowed, the left ventricle must work harder to force blood through the narrowed area to the lower part of the body. This results in increased blood pressure proximal to the defect (head and arms) and decreased blood flow distal to it (the body and legs). In cases of severe narrowing, the left ventricle may not be strong enough to perform this extra work, resulting in heart failure or poor perfusion.

COA occurs in 8% to 10% of all cases of congenital heart defects. It affects males twice as often as females. COA may be associated with other cardiac defects, typically those involving the left side of the heart.

Most patients with COA are asymptomatic until later in childhood, at which time the child presents with a heart murmur or systolic hypertension. Physical findings may include the following:

- Dyspnea, poor feeding, poor weight gain, and signs of shock may develop in the first 6 weeks of life.
- High blood pressure and bounding pulses in the arms.
- Lower blood pressure with weak or absent femoral pulses and cool lower extremities; differential cyanosis may be present (e.g., the lower half of the body is cyanotic).
- Infants may show signs of heart failure. From 20% to 30% of patients with COA develop heart failure by 3 months of age.
- Dizziness, frequent headaches, fainting, and nosebleeds may be present in the older child as a result of hypertension.

Patients with COA are at risk for hypertension, ruptured aorta, aortic aneurysm, or stroke. Surgical repair is

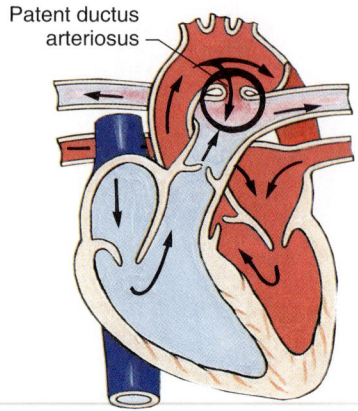

Figure 22-117 Patent ductus arteriosus.

that are thick and stiff. The thick and stiffened valve does not open freely, causing the left ventricle to work harder to eject blood into the aorta. Over time, the muscle of the left ventricle thickens (hypertrophies) to compensate for the increased workload.

Aortic stenosis occurs in 3% to 6% of all cases of congenital heart defects and is four times more common in males than in females. Most children with mild to moderate aortic stenosis have no symptoms. Some children may experience chest pain, dizziness, fainting, or unusual tiring with severe aortic stenosis. A characteristic murmur is present. Blood pressure is usually normal, but a narrow pulse pressure may be present in cases of severe stenos. Exercise restriction against sustained strenuous activity is recommended in children with moderate to severe stenosis. The need for surgical intervention depends on the severity of the stenosis.

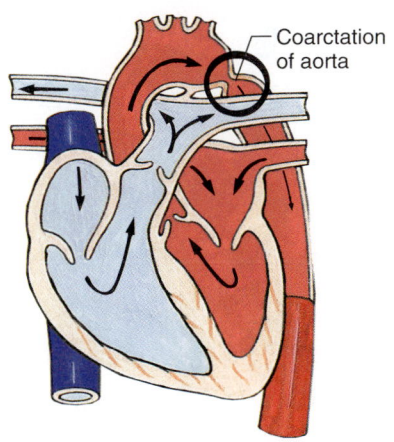

Figure 22-118 Coarctation of the aorta (COA).

recommended within the first 2 years of life. COA has a 15% to 30% risk of recurrence in patients who undergo surgical repair as infants. Some of these cases can be treated by balloon angioplasty. The long-term results of this procedure are being studied. Before and after treatment, infants and children with COA are at risk for bacterial endocarditis and must take antibiotics before certain dental and surgical procedures.

Aortic Stenosis

In aortic stenosis the aortic valve (located between the left ventricle and the aorta) is narrowed (Figure 22-119). Narrowing may occur below the aortic valve, at the valve itself, or immediately above the valve. The most common form of aortic stenosis is obstruction at the valve itself.

A normal aortic valve consists of three cusps (valve leaflets) that spread apart when the left ventricle ejects blood into the aorta. In aortic stenosis, the valve may have only one cusp (unicuspid) or two cusps (bicuspid)

Pulmonary Stenosis

In pulmonary stenosis the pulmonic valve (located between the right ventricle and pulmonary artery) is narrowed (Figure 22-120). Narrowing may occur below the pulmonic valve, at the valve itself, or immediately above the valve. The most common form of pulmonary stenosis is obstruction at the valve itself.

A normal pulmonic valve consists of three cusps that spread apart when the right ventricle ejects blood into the pulmonary artery. In pulmonary stenosis, the valve cusps are thickened and stiff, hindering blood flow from the right ventricle. The right ventricle must overcome increased resistance to eject blood into the pulmonary artery and gradually hypertrophies because of its increased workload.

Pulmonary stenosis occurs in 8% to 12% of all cases of congenital heart defects. Most children with mild pulmonary stenosis have no symptoms. Children with moderate or severe pulmonary stenosis may experience shortness of breath and chest pain or epigastric pain with exertion and diminished exercise tolerance. A characteristic murmur is present. Cyanosis and signs of congestive

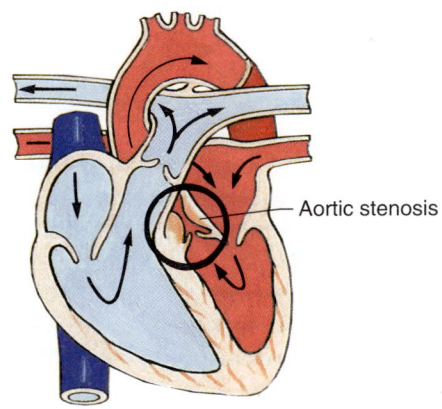

Figure 22-119 Aortic stenosis.

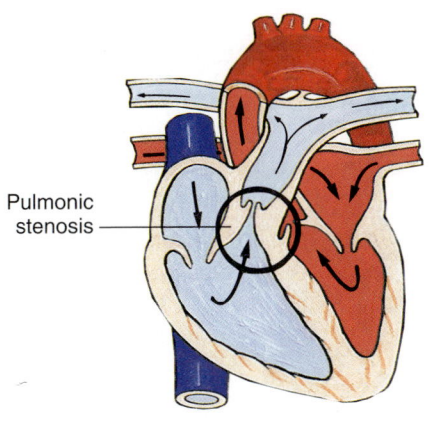

Figure 22-120 Pulmonic stenosis.

heart failure may be present in infants with severe pulmonary stenosis. Sudden death is possible during heavy physical activity in a child with severe stenosis.

Mild pulmonary stenosis rarely requires treatment. Moderate to severe pulmonary stenosis usually requires treatment that may involve balloon dilation or open-heart surgery, depending on the type of valve abnormality present. Before and after treatment, infants and children with pulmonary stenosis are at risk for bacterial endocarditis and must take antibiotics before certain dental and surgical procedures.

Cyanotic Heart Defects

Cyanotic heart defects (also called *blue defects*) are congenital abnormalities in which deoxygenated blood from the right (pulmonary) side of the heart mixes with oxygenated blood from the left (systemic) side and enters the systemic circulation, bypassing the pulmonary circulation. This defect is called a *right-to-left shunt*. Cyanotic defects may be classified according to their hemodynamic effects (Table 22-50).

Tetralogy of Fallot

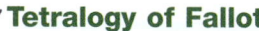

Tetralogy of Fallot (TOF) occurs in 10% of all congenital heart defects and is the most common cyanotic heart defect seen in children beyond infancy. Following are the four (tetra) elements of TOF:

1. A large ventricular septal defect (Figure 22-121). The defect allows blood to pass from the right ventricle to the left ventricle without going through the lungs.
2. Narrowing (stenosis) at or just below the pulmonary valve (pulmonary stenosis). This narrowing partially obstructs the flow of blood from the right ventricle to the lungs.
3. A right ventricle that is more muscular than normal (right ventricular hypertrophy). Right ventricular hypertrophy occurs because the right ventricle is pumping at high pressure.
4. The aorta lies directly over the ventricular septal defect (overriding aorta).

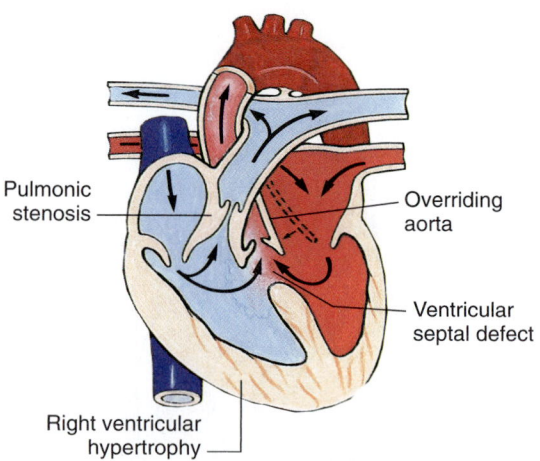

Figure 22-121 Tetralogy of Fallot.

Most infants with TOF are pink at birth because they usually have a patent ductus arteriosus that provides additional pulmonary blood flow. However, as the ductus closes in the first hours or days of life, cyanosis may develop or become more severe. Clubbing occurs as pulmonary stenosis becomes more significant, reducing blood flow to the lungs. A characteristic murmur is present after the first few days of life.

When arterial oxygen saturation suddenly decreases, an infant or child may experience a tetralogy spell. Tetralogy spells also are called *tet spells, hypoxic spells, hypercyanotic spells,* or *blue spells.* A hypoxic spell usually results from sudden, increased constriction of the outflow tract to the lungs, further restricting pulmonary blood flow. During a hypoxic spell, the child becomes increasingly cyanotic and irritable in response to hypoxemia and breathes quite deeply and rapidly (hyperpnea). If left untreated, a severe spell may result in syncope, seizures, stroke, or death. In infants, a hypoxic spell often occurs in the morning after crying, feeding, or a bowel movement.

Emergency care for a hypoxic spell includes keeping the infant or child as calm as possible. An infant having a hypoxic spell should be picked up and held in a knee-chest position (i.e., place the infant on the caregiver's shoulder with the knees tucked up underneath) (Figure 22-122). This provides a calming effect and reduces venous return. The older child having a hypoxic spell often squats to recover. Squatting compresses the superior vena cava and increases systemic vascular resistance, directing blood through the pulmonary stenosis and into the lungs (rather than across the ventricular septal defect). Give oxygen, IV fluids, and medications as ordered by medical direction. Morphine may be ordered to suppress the respiratory center and resolve the hyperpnea. A normal saline fluid bolus may be ordered to counteract morphine's vasodilating effects and ensure adequate preload. Sodium bicarbonate may be ordered

TABLE 22-50	Cyanotic Heart Defects
Blood Flow	**Defect**
Decreased pulmonary blood flow	Tetralogy of Fallot (TOF)
	Tricuspid atresia
Mixed blood flow	Transposition of the great vessels (TGV)
	Total anomalous pulmonary venous return or communication
	Truncus arteriosus
	Hypoplastic heart syndrome

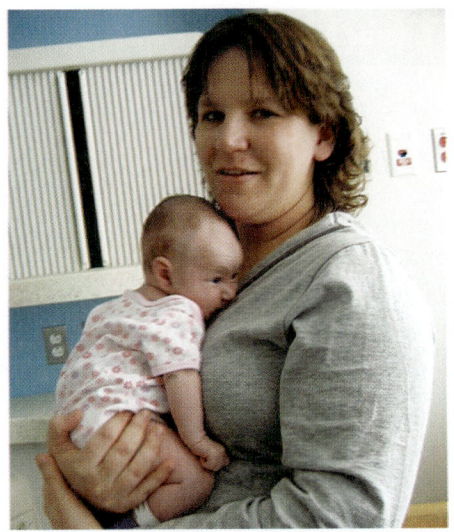

Figure 22-122 Infant held in knee-chest position.

to reduce the respiratory center–stimulating effect of acidosis.

Infants with TOF usually need surgery. A temporary shunt procedure may be used to allow more blood to reach the lungs until the defects can be completely corrected with surgery when the child is older.

Transposition of the Great Vessels

Transposition of the great vessels (TGV) is also called *transposition of the great arteries*. In this condition, the positions of the pulmonary artery and the aorta are reversed (Figure 22-123).

The aorta is connected to the right ventricle, so deoxygenated blood returning to the right atrium from the body is pumped out to the aorta and back to the body without first going to the lungs for oxygenation. The pulmonary artery is connected to the left ventricle, so oxygenated blood returning from the lungs to the left

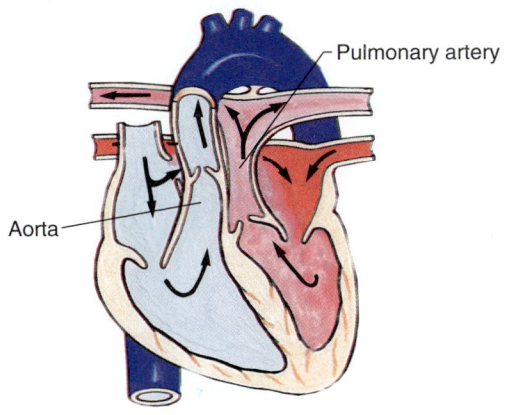

Figure 22-123 Transposition of the great vessels.

atrium goes back to the lungs by the pulmonary artery without being sent to the body.

TGV occurs in approximately 5% of all congenital heart defects and is three times more common in males than in females. An infant born with TGV can survive only if one or more associated defects permits oxygenated blood to reach the systemic circulation, such as an atrial septal defect, ventricular septal defect, or patent ductus arteriosus that allows mixing of oxygenated and deoxygenated blood.

Cyanosis is usually present soon after birth. At birth, a patent ductus arteriosus may permit sufficient mixing of oxygenated and deoxygenated blood to prevent severe cyanosis. However, as the ductus closes in the first hours or days of life, cyanosis becomes increasingly severe. A murmur may be present depending on the type of associated cardiac defects, but many infants do not have a murmur. Signs of heart failure and hypoglycemia may be present. Without surgery, death occurs in 90% of patients before 6 months of age.

DISORDERS OF CIRCULATION (VASCULAR DISORDERS)

Aortic Aneurysm and Dissecting Aneurysm

Description and Definition
[OBJECTIVES 94, 95]

Like other arteries, the aorta is composed of three layers. The adventitia is the thin outer layer, the media is the thick, elastic middle layer, and the intima is the thin innermost layer. The elastic tissue of the aorta's middle layer stretches when blood is forcefully ejected from the left ventricle and recoils when the heart relaxes. These efficient movements keep blood moving in a forward direction throughout the cardiac cycle.

The ability of the arteries to stretch and recoil declines with aging. These changes occur even in healthy adults. In some people the constant stress on the wall of the aorta causes it to weaken and gradually swell (dilate). This localized dilation or bulging of a blood vessel wall (or wall of a heart chamber) is called an **aneurysm.** The dilated area may leak or rupture if it stretches too far.

Aortic dissection is thought to begin with a tear in the inner lining of the aorta. Blood flows through the tear, exposing the middle layer of the vessel to blood under high pressure. Blood present between the layers of the vessel causes them to separate (dissect). Because blood in the aorta is constantly under high pressure, the separation begins to extend along the wall of the aorta. Although an aortic dissection may begin anywhere along the aorta, most begin in the ascending aorta within 5 cm of the aortic valve or the descending thoracic aorta just beyond the origin of the left subclavian artery at the site of the ligamentum arteriosum. From 65% to 75% of patients with untreated aortic dissection die within the first 2 weeks after the onset of symptoms (Finkelmeier & Marolda, 2001).

Etiology

Coronary heart disease, high blood cholesterol, and hypertension are conditions that cause the arteries to lose their elasticity prematurely. Atherosclerosis is the most common cause of aneurysms. The buildup of plaque in the innermost lining of the vessel eventually weakens and erodes the middle (medial) layer.

Aneurysms of the ascending thoracic aorta usually result from **cystic medial degeneration** (formerly called *cystic medial necrosis*), a connective tissue disease in which the elastic tissue and smooth muscle fibers of the middle layer of large arteries degenerates. The area of the vessel that was previously filled with normal elastic tissue is replaced with connective tissue resembling cysts. A mild form of medial degeneration is often present in the aortas of older adults and is thought to occur as a normal consequence of aging. In younger persons, medial degeneration of the aorta frequently accompanies Marfan syndrome (Figure 22-124). Marfan syndrome is an inherited connective tissue disease that causes severe elastic tissue degeneration and increased stiffness of the aortic wall.

Aortic aneurysms also can be congenital or caused by trauma (usually deceleration injuries in motor vehicle crashes), syphilis, infective endocarditis, or other infection (Box 22-40).

BOX 22-40 Aortic Aneurysm Risk Factors

- Age
- Gender
- Family history of aortic aneurysm
- Smoking
- Atherosclerosis
- Hypertension
- Hyperlipidemia
- Pregnancy
- Crack cocaine use
- Trauma
- Inflammatory diseases that cause vasculitis
- Connective tissue disorders (Marfan syndrome)
- Congenital cardiovascular abnormalities (coarctation of the aorta, patent ductus arteriosus)

Epidemiology and Demographics

Following are facts about aortic aneurysms:

- Up to 13% of patients who have an aortic aneurysm have multiple aneurysms. From 25% to 28% of those with thoracic aortic aneurysms also have an abdominal aortic aneurysm (Isselbacher, 2005).

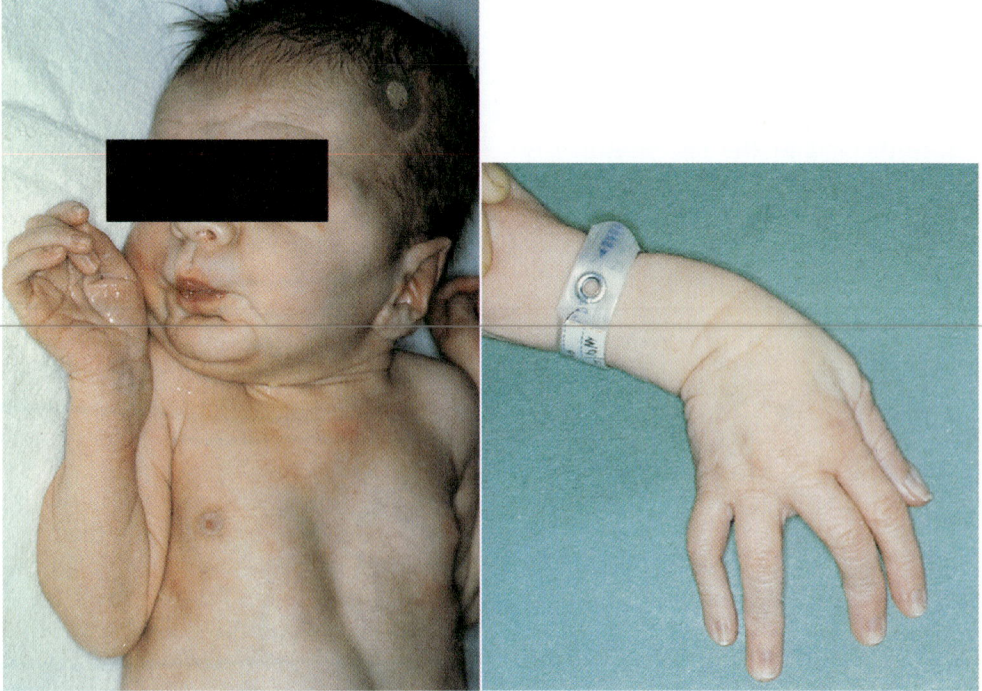

A   **B**

Figure 22-124 Infant with Marfan syndrome. **A,** Note the narrow elongated face, sunken chest (pectus excavatum), and long arms and fingers. **B,** A close-up view of the infant's hand.

- Three fourths of aneurysms occur in the abdominal aorta.
- Abdominal aortic aneurysms occur five to 10 times more often in men than in women.
- The frequency with which abdominal aortic aneurysms occur increases rapidly after 55 years of age in men and 70 years of age in women (Isselbacher, 2005).
- Women who have an abdominal aneurysm have a risk of rupture three times higher than men and at a smaller aortic diameter (Isselbacher, 2005).
- Persons with a family history (first-degree relative) of abdominal aortic aneurysm have an increased risk of 13% to 32% compared with the 2% to 5% risk in the general population (Isselbacher, 2005).
- Dissection of the thoracic aorta has been associated with crack cocaine use and hospital procedures such as cardiac catheterization.
- Most aortic dissections occur in men between ages 60 and 70 years. Men are affected twice as often as women. Approximately three quarters of patients with aortic dissection have a history of hypertension (Isselbacher, 2005).
- Approximately half of all aortic dissections in women younger than 40 years occur during pregnancy, usually in the third trimester, and occasionally in the early postpartum period (Isselbacher, 2005).

History

An aneurysm does not always cause symptoms. If it does, the patient's signs and symptoms will depend on where the aneurysm is located. As an aneurysm increases in size, stretching of the aortic wall produces pain. Symptoms may result because of the pressure of a large amount of blood on surrounding organs. For example, difficulty swallowing (dysphagia) may be present as a result of compression of the esophagus. Hoarseness may be present from laryngeal nerve compression. Difficulty breathing may be present and caused by heart failure or tracheal or bronchial compression. The sudden development of new or worsening pain may be a sign of impending aneurysm rupture.

The location and description of the pain may provide clues about the location of the dissection. When the aorta dissects, almost all patients will complain of pain that begins abruptly and is constant and unbearable. The pain may last for hours to days. It is described as tearing or ripping and sharp, stabbing, or knifelike. Common phrases used to describe the pain include "it feels like someone stabbed me in the chest with a knife" or "hit me in the back with an axe" (Isselbacher, 2005). Dissection of the ascending aorta is usually associated with pain that is substernal or located in the neck, throat, jaw, or face. The pain associated with dissection of the descending aorta is usually between the shoulder blades, back, abdomen, flank, or lower extremities. No matter where

the pain begins, it may move as the dissection extends along the aorta. Approximately 10% of patients with aortic dissection do not have pain. This finding is more common in patients with neurologic complications from the dissection and those with Marfan syndrome (Isselbacher, 2005).

The patient is usually anxious and may describe a feeling of impending doom. He or she may complain of pain, weakness, or numbness and tingling in the extremities because of peripheral nerve ischemia. Signs of myocardial ischemia may be present because of coronary artery compression. Less-common symptoms that may occur with or without chest pain include symptoms of heart failure, altered mental status, stroke, paraplegia, cardiac arrest, or sudden death. Syncope is present in some patients and may be caused by increased vagal tone, hypovolemia, or dysrhythmias.

Physical Findings

The patient who has a dissecting thoracic aneurysm often has variations in blood pressure measurements taken in the upper extremities. A dissecting abdominal aneurysm usually reveals variations in blood pressure measurements in the lower extremities. The patient's blood pressure may be elevated or decreased. Hypotension may be present because of increased vagal tone, cardiac tamponade, or hypovolemia from rupture of the dissection. Hypertension may result from an increase in circulating catecholamines or underlying high blood pressure. Peripheral pulses may be hard to feel. Pulse deficits may come and go and are present in approximately two thirds of patients. The patient's skin is usually pale and diaphoretic. Tracheal or bronchial compression can result in tracheal deviation, wheezing, coughing, dyspnea, or hemoptysis.

Rupture of a thoracic aneurysm usually occurs into the left intrapleural space or mediastinum or less commonly into the esophagus. Signs of a hemothorax may be present if the dissection ruptures into the pleural cavity. Signs of cardiac tamponade may be present if the dissection ruptures into the pericardial cavity. Rupture of an abdominal aortic aneurysm usually is associated with sudden back pain with abdominal pain and tenderness (Figure 22-125). The patient may be hypotensive and have a pulsating abdominal mass of varying size between the xiphoid process and umbilicus. However, the triad of abdominal and back pain, a pulsating abdominal mass, and hypotension because of a ruptured abdominal aortic aneurysm is only seen in approximately one third of patients (Kiell & Ernst, 1993). An aneurysm is often sensitive to palpation and may be quite tender if it is rapidly expanding or about to rupture (Isselbacher, 2005). Use caution when palpating the abdomen of a patient with a possible abdominal aortic aneurysm, although palpation appears to be safe and has not been reported to cause rupture (Lederle & Simel, 1999). When rupture of an abdominal aortic aneurysm does occur, rupture into the

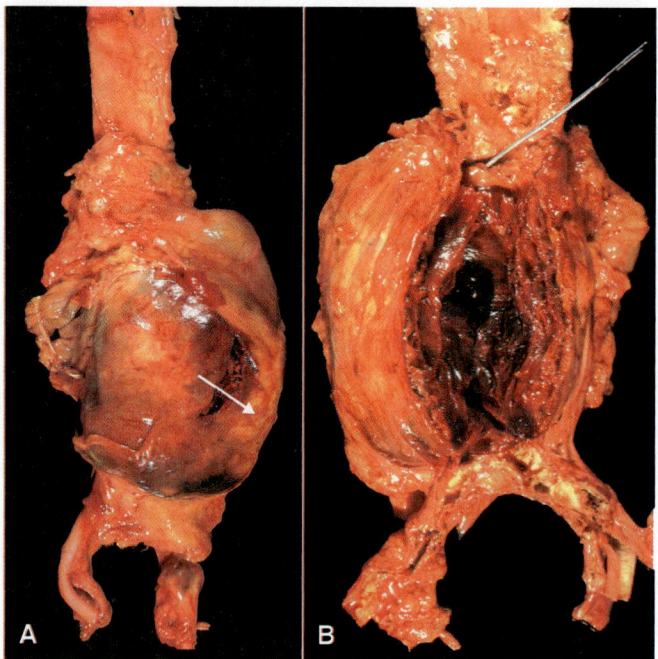

Figure 22-125 Abdominal aortic aneurysm. **A**, External view of a large aortic aneurysm that ruptured; the rupture site is indicated by the *arrow*. **B**, Opened view, with the location of the rupture tract indicated by a probe. The wall of the aneurysm is very thin. The vessel lumen is filled with a large number of layered clots.

abdominal cavity usually results in abdominal distention. Massive gastrointestinal hemorrhage may be present if rupture occurs into the duodenum.

Differential Diagnosis

Differential diagnoses for aortic and dissecting aneurysms include:

- Cardiovascular Causes
  - Cardiac tamponade
  - Cardiogenic, hypovolemic, hemorrhagic shock
  - Cardiomyopathy
  - Hypertensive emergencies
  - Myocardial infarction
  - Myocarditis
  - Pericarditis
- Respiratory Causes
  - Pleural effusion
  - Pulmonary embolism
- Musculoskeletal Causes
  - Back pain
  - Costochondritis
- Gastrointestinal Causes
  - Diverticulitis
  - Gastroenteritis
  - Gastrointestinal bleeding
- Other Causes
  - Hernia
  - Kidney stone

Therapeutic Interventions   *usually no IV fluids*

Aortic dissection is a medical emergency. Give high-concentration oxygen. Make sure ventilation and oxygenation are effective. Apply a pulse oximeter. Maintain oxygen saturation at greater than 95%. Apply the cardiac monitor. Maintain normal body temperature. Avoid performing additional procedures on the scene that will delay transport to the hospital. Establish IV access with two large-bore catheters en route to definitive care. Give IV fluids and medications per local protocol or medical direction instructions. If the patient's blood pressure can tolerate it, narcotics may be ordered for pain control. However, narcotics may not be strong enough to relieve the patient's pain.

Be sure to contact medical direction as soon as you suspect the patient has a dissecting aneurysm. Relaying this information to the receiving facility will allow staff time to gather necessary resources for the patient while you are en route. En route to the hospital, reassess the patient at least every 5 minutes. A patient who has signs and symptoms of a dissecting aortic aneurysm requires rapid transport to the closest appropriate facility.

Patient and Family Education

If the patient has a history of high blood pressure, teach the importance of following his or her physician's instructions for keeping it under control. This includes taking blood pressure medications as prescribed, avoiding salty foods, and not adding salt to food. Patients with Marfan syndrome are often prescribed beta-blockers to decrease the heart's workload. These patients also should be taught to take their medications as prescribed. If the patient smokes, he or she should stop. If the patient is overweight, he or she should strive to lose weight and work toward maintaining an ideal weight.

Acute Arterial Occlusion and Acute Limb Ischemia

Description and Definition
[OBJECTIVES 96, 97]

An **acute arterial occlusion** is a sudden disruption of arterial blood flow that occurs because of a thrombus, embolus, tumor, direct trauma to an artery, or an unknown cause. Acute limb (extremity) ischemia results when an arterial occlusion suddenly reduces blood flow to an arm or leg.

Etiology

Most acute arterial occlusions are caused by an embolus that begins in the heart and travels to the extremities. Conditions that may be responsible for an embolus originating in the heart include AFib, a clot that forms in the left ventricle after a heart attack, rheumatic or prosthetic heart valves, or left ventricular aneurysm. Arterial emboli can travel to a variety of sites in the body but most lodge in the femoral artery. When this occurs, circulation to the lower extremities is affected. Arterial emboli may also lodge in the brain, intestines, kidneys, spleen, and upper extremities, but to a lesser extent. Most emboli occur in patients who have significant underlying heart disease.

Blockage of an artery from a thrombus usually occurs in an artery that was previously open but narrowed by atherosclerosis. The area distal to the blockage becomes ischemic. When the blockage affects an extremity, blood flow is limited to the muscle. During exercise, blood flow to the area decreases further and muscle contraction may actually stop blood flow. However, some patients may notice few symptoms because the process occurs gradually, allowing the development of collateral circulation as the major vessel becomes narrowed from atherosclerosis. If the patient has an extensive collateral circulation in the extremity, he or she may notice no change or only a mild increase in symptoms when a major atherosclerotic vessel becomes blocked. Patients who have peripheral arterial disease often have **intermittent claudication,** or pain, cramping, muscle tightness, fatigue, or weakness of the legs when walking or during exercise. These symptoms occur because tissues demand more oxygen with these activities. Increased blood flow to the area is not possible because the arteries supplying the muscles of the calves, hips, or buttocks are narrowed or blocked. Symptoms disappear within a few minutes after a brief rest and the patient can resume activity until the pain recurs.

Direct trauma to an artery may occur because of an extremity injury or diagnostic procedures such as cardiac catheterization. Less-common causes of acute arterial occlusion include dissecting aneurysms, vasospasm (usually attributable to IV drug use), and blockage of vascular grafts.

Epidemiology and Demographics

Smoking is one of the most important risk factors for peripheral arterial disease. From 84% to 90% of patients with claudication are current or former smokers (Lu & Creager, 2004).

Within 10 years of the onset of intermittent claudication, 43% develop coronary heart disease, 21% strokes, and 24% heart failure (Kannel, 1996).

History

An accurate history must be gathered from a patient with acute limb ischemia. If the patient tells you symptoms began suddenly, an embolus is the likely cause of the ischemia. If the patient tells you symptoms have gradually worsened, a thrombus is the more likely cause. Ask the patient whether he or she has ever experienced this problem before. If the answer is yes, find out if the episodes are increasing in frequency and how long each event lasts.

Keep in mind the five *P*'s of acute arterial occlusion when obtaining the patient's history and performing the physical examination: *p*ain, *p*ulselessness, *p*allor, *p*aresthesias, and *p*aralysis. Pain associated with acute limb ischemia usually begins distal to the site of obstruction and gradually increases in severity. Ischemia of peripheral nerves in the affected limb causes motor impairment and sensory loss. The patient may complain of a decrease in pain as sensory loss progresses. Paralysis and paresthesias are signs and symptoms of limb-threatening ischemia.

Find out whether the patient has any risk factors for the development of a blood clot, such as a recent extremity injury, IV drug use, heart surgery or heart attack, a history of a clotting disorder, pulmonary embolism, irregular heart beat (AFib), or rheumatic heart disease.

> **PARAMEDIC Pearl**
>
> **The Five *P*'s of Acute Arterial Occlusion**
> - *P*ain
> - *P*allor
> - *P*ulselessness
> - *P*aralysis
> - *P*aresthesia

Venous occlusion warm, swollen, has pulses, pain out of proportion

Physical Findings

Assessment of the patient with acute limb ischemia should include feeling for arterial pulses. Feel the brachial, radial, femoral, posterior tibial, and dorsalis pedis arteries in pairs and document your findings. Normally, approximately 10% of the population does not have one of the dorsalis pedis pulses (Aufderheide, 2002). The skin color of the affected limb usually appears pale or mottled distal to or over the affected area. If arterial blood flow to the limb is severely restricted, the foot will turn chalk white when it is raised and very red after 1 minute of placing it at a level lower than the heart. The skin of the affected limb may feel cool and be moist or dry.

Because advanced limb ischemia affects motor and sensory function, be sure to assess movement and sensation in all extremities. Sensory deficits over the dorsum of the foot are often an early sign of vascular compromise.

Breath sounds are usually clear. Changes in heart rate and rhythm may occur. Peripheral pulses may be absent or diminished in the affected limb. Be sure to check the patient's blood pressure in both arms. Unequal blood pressure readings in each arm may indicate a thoracic aneurysm. Listen for a bruit over the affected vessel(s). In general, the patient's ECG does not contribute significant information related to emergency care of this condition.

If the patient has had symptoms of peripheral arterial disease for some time, signs of chronic limb ischemia may be present. These signs include muscle wasting with shiny, scaly skin on the affected limb; loss of hair growth over the dorsum of the toes and foot, and thickening of the toenails.

Differential Diagnosis

The differential diagnoses for acute arterial occlusion and acute limb ischemia include:

- Abdominal aneurysm
- Arthritis
- Deep vein thrombosis
- Scleroderma
- Soft tissue injury
- Systemic lupus erythematosus

Therapeutic Interventions

Allow the patient to assume a position of comfort. If limb ischemia affects a lower extremity, place the patient im a sitting position if no contraindications are present. By placing the patient's feet lower than the chest, gravity may help perfuse the limb. Give oxygen, establish an IV, and apply the cardiac monitor. Apply a pulse oximeter. Maintain oxygen saturation at greater than 95%. Give medications as instructed by medical direction. Medications to reduce pain may be ordered. Keep the patient compartment of the ambulance warm to avoid cold-induced vasoconstriction of the skin. Do not apply heat or cold to the affected limb. Ischemic tissue burns at lower temperatures and is more susceptible to frostbite.

The patient with acute limb ischemia requires rapid transport to the closest appropriate facility. Reassess the patient's condition frequently en route. Monitor the five *P*'s.

If the patient refuses care, repeatedly try to persuade him or her to accept the care you wish to provide, including transport. Consider contacting medical direction for advice. If you are unable to convince the patient to receive care, carefully document the patient's refusal.

Patient and Family Education

Patients who have peripheral arterial disease should be taught how to avoid situations that may cause blood pooling or interrupt blood flow to the extremities. For example, the patient should avoid crossing the legs, smoking, or sitting or standing for long periods. If the disease affects the patient's lower extremities, he or she should be taught to keep the feet warm, clean, and dry and cut the toenails straight across. If a cut or sore develops on the affected limb, the wound will be prone to infection. Poor circulation to the area slows the body's normal processes to fight infection (Box 22-41). Explain the importance of follow-up care with a physician.

Acute Deep Vein Thrombosis

Description and Definition

Thrombophlebitis is the development of a clot in a vein in which inflammation is present. Although the terms thrombophlebitis, phlebothrombosis, and phlebitis often are used interchangeably, the difference in terms is used to point out whether the main condition is caused by clot formation or inflammation.

Superficial thrombophlebitis occurs when a clot develops in a vein near the skin surface (Figure 22-126). If a clot develops in the deep veins of the extremities, **deep vein thrombosis (DVT)** is present. DVT is associated with an increased risk of pulmonary embolism.

Etiology

Three important factors (Virchow's triad) predispose a person to developing a thrombus (Box 22-42). Risk factors for thrombophlebitis include the following.

1. Venous stasis or sluggish blood flow. This risk factor is present in those who are pregnant, obese, have heart failure, or are immobile for long periods.

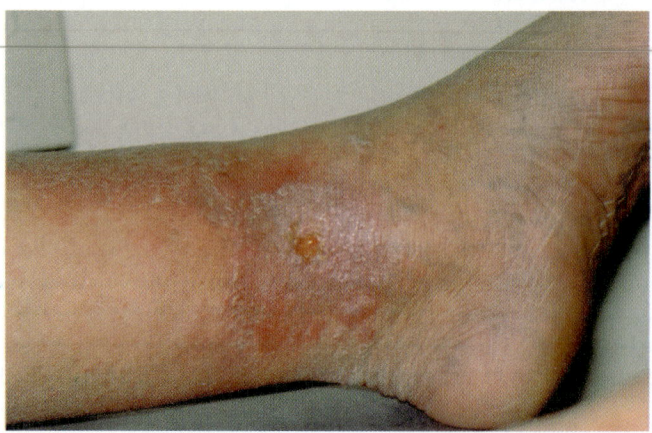

Figure 22-126 Venous stasis ulcer.

BOX 22-42 Thrombophlebitis: Risk Factors

- Increasing age
- Recent direct trauma to a vein
- Recent prolonged inactivity, such as from sitting in a car or an airplane
- Recent prolonged bed rest, such as after surgery, a heart attack, spinal cord injury, or a leg fracture
- Certain types of cancer, such as cancer of the pancreas, colon, or lung
- Obesity
- Central venous catheterization
- Pregnancy and postpartum period
- Stroke with paralysis
- Family history of a clotting disorder
- History of DVT, pulmonary embolism
- Heart failure
- Use of oral contraceptives or hormone replacement therapy

DVT, Deep vein thrombosis.

2. Damage to the inner lining of the vessel. This can occur because of trauma, inflammation, when a venipuncture is performed, or as a result of substances given during IV therapy.
3. Blood clotting disorders. Conditions that increase blood clotting include dehydration, certain types of cancer, and use of oral contraceptives or hormone replacement therapy.

Epidemiology and Demographics

- The exact incidence of DVT is unknown because of variations in patient signs and symptoms and the accuracy of the patient's diagnosis.
- DVT of the lower extremities is the most common cause of pulmonary embolism.

History

The patient with DVT may seek medical care because of swelling, pain, or tenderness in a limb. In some cases, the patient will seek help because of the onset of symptoms from a pulmonary embolus. Ask the patient questions to find out if he or she has risk factors for DVT.

Physical Findings

Assess the patient's upper and lower extremities carefully. Compare the extremities in pairs. Classic signs of DVT include swelling of the affected limb with pain or tenderness. However, these findings are only present in approximately 50% of patients with DVT. Look for signs of inflammation, such as redness and warmth of the skin over the affected vein. A positive Homan's sign (pain and

tenderness in the calf muscle on dorsiflexion of the foot) is present in fewer than 40% of patients with DVT. When assessing the patient, be careful not to rub or massage the affected limb. Such action could dislodge a clot.

Differential Diagnosis

The differential diagnoses for DVT include:

- Arthritis
- Cellulitis
- Muscle or soft tissue injury
- Pulmonary embolism
- Superficial thrombophlebitis

Therapeutic Interventions

Prehospital care for DVT is mainly supportive. Allow the patient to assume a position of comfort, give oxygen, establish an IV, and apply the cardiac monitor. Apply a pulse oximeter. Maintain oxygen saturation at greater than 95%. Monitor the patient closely for development of a pulmonary embolism. Signs and symptoms of a pulmonary embolism are shown in Box 22-43.

Most patients with DVT can be transported to the closest appropriate facility without lights and sirens. If the patient refuses care, repeatedly try to persuade him or her to accept the care you wish to provide, including transport. Consider contacting medical direction for advice. If you are unable to convince the patient to receive care, carefully document the patient's refusal.

Patient and Family Education

Teach the patient ways to reduce risk of thrombophlebitis in the veins of the legs, including avoiding dehydration by drinking plenty of fluids. Teach the patient to avoid wearing constrictive clothing around the arms, waist, and

BOX 22-43 Signs and Symptoms of Pulmonary Embolism

Signs

- Tachypnea
- Tachycardia
- Crackles
- Fever

Symptoms

- Dyspnea
- Chest discomfort
- Anxiety
- Cough

legs. When traveling, instruct to walk around roughly every hour. If that is not possible, tell him or her to keep the blood moving in the legs by pointing the toes and feet down and up in succession several times. If the patient's occupation requires standing for long periods, explain the importance of frequent rest periods with the legs raised.

Some patients at risk for DVT are instructed to wear compression stockings (Box 22-44). Compression stockings are thought to work by preventing backward flow through the veins of the legs. They are available in various lengths, including knee high, thigh high, and pantyhose. Compression stockings should not be used if the patient has peripheral arterial disease.

If the patient is taking blood thinners, he or she should wear a medical identification bracelet or other emblem indicating the name of the medication and the reason for its use. While taking blood thinners, the patient will need to have blood drawn regularly to check and monitor blood-clotting times.

BOX 22-44 | **Varicose Veins**

Varicose means twisted. Varicose veins are vessels that have become gnarled and stretched. Any vein can become varicose. For example, hemorrhoids are varicose veins located in and around the anus. Esophageal varices are varicose veins in the esophagus. The most common site of varicose veins is the superficial veins of the upper and lower legs.

Normally valves in the veins direct blood flow from the superficial tissues of the legs to the deep veins and back to the heart. If the valves are faulty, injured, or weakened due to aging, blood can flow backward in the veins and pool in the legs. Increased pressure in the leg veins can cause damage to the valves and stretch the vessel. Pregnancy, obesity, and standing for long periods increase the pressure in the veins of the legs. This can lead to pooling of blood in the legs, lower leg swelling, and varicosities. Long-term increases in pressure in the legs can result in painful ulcers. These ulcers are called venous stasis ulcers (see Figure 22-126). They form on the skin near varicose veins, mainly near the ankles. Venous stasis ulcers can result in significant bleeding if they rupture. Bleeding can usually be controlled with direct pressure.

Case Scenario SUMMARY

1. *What is your general impression of this patient?* High priority for several reasons. First, he is pale and diaphoretic with tachycardia and hypotension. Together these signs suggest poor cellular perfusion, shock, and increased oxygen demand. The symptoms sound cardiac in nature, and their onset at rest suggests an unstable origin. You should expedite evaluation, stabilization, and transport to an appropriate facility.

2. *What are some possible causes of this patient's symptoms?* Given the description of the pain (crushing), a cardiac cause must be considered. Other possible causes of chest pain may include trauma, pneumothorax, or pneumonia.

3. *This patient is fairly young to have an MI. What factors might be associated with a cardiac event in a patient this age?* Although an MI is not impossible for a young person, especially with a family history, stimulant drugs (cocaine or methamphetamine) are commonly associated with acute MI in young people. However, initial management remains the same, so do not waste valuable time trying to identify a drug cause.

4. *What additional assessment will be important in the evaluation of this patient?* Evaluation of the skin and vital signs (to assess cardiac output), the heart and lungs (to look for other causes and signs of congestive heart failure), and the prior medical history. The ECG will also play an important role in the evaluation of this patient.

5. *What intervention should you initiate at this time?* High-flow oxygen, IV access, and evaluation of the ECG all should be performed rapidly in this case.

6. *Is this patient high priority? Why or why not?* He was high priority before the seizure, and he is very high priority now. In addition to having a grand mal seizure, the patient has compromised airway and ventilation, bradycardia, and decreased cardiac output.

7. *Given what you know at this time, what is the most likely cause of the seizure activity?* In the absence of other information, the two most likely causes of seizure are hypoxia (caused by a sudden drop in the pulse rate and cerebral perfusion) or stimulant drug use (given the risk for stimulant use related to cardiac symptoms in young people).

8. *What is this patient's greatest life threat at this time? How will you treat it?* Shock. His sudden drop in cardiac rate has resulted in a dramatic decrease in blood pressure. Overall, the strategy for treating this patient should be to first attempt to restore a normal cardiac rhythm and rate, then to improve cardiac output and blood pressure.

Case Scenario SUMMARY—continued

9. *How will you manage the cardiac rhythm?* The treatment of choice for a symptomatic wide-QRS bradycardia is TCP.

10. *Assume that the patient remained unconscious with an unacceptably low blood pressure despite pacing. What treatment would be appropriate at this time?* Once the pulse rate is normalized, several strategies may be used to improve blood pressure depending on local protocols. If the patient's breath sounds remain clear, a fluid challenge (usually 250 mL) may be used to increase preload and attempt to improve cardiac contractility and output. Dopamine also may be considered to improve contractility and, depending on the dose, increase afterload. A disadvantage of dopamine is that it increases myocardial oxygen demand, which may increase the size and severity of infarction.

11. *Given the patient's final disposition, was your treatment appropriate? Why or why not?* Consider two things when answering this question. First, a better choice may have been to attach the patient to the cardiac monitor *before* preparing for transfer to the ambulance. Although this may have increased scene time, it has the potential to allow identification of a lethal dysrhythmia (we do not know what the preseizure rhythm was). Early recognition and treatment *may have* prevented the onset of complete heart block.

Chapter Summary

- Cardiovascular disorders are diseases and conditions that involve the heart and blood vessels. Heart disease refers to conditions affecting the heart. Heart disease is the leading cause of death in the United States. Coronary heart disease refers to disease of the coronary arteries and their resulting complications, such as angina pectoris or acute MI. Coronary artery disease affects the arteries that supply the heart muscle with blood.

- Risk factors are traits and lifestyle habits that may increase a person's chance of developing a disease. Some risk factors associated with coronary heart disease can be modified. Risk factors that cannot be modified are called nonmodifiable or fixed risk factors. Contributing risk factors are thought to lead to an increased risk of heart disease, but their exact role has not been defined.

- Arteries are conductance vessels that carry blood from the heart under high pressure. Arterioles are the smallest branches of the arteries. They are called *resistance vessels* because they have smooth muscle in their walls that allows the vessel to adjust its diameter, controlling the amount of blood flow to specific tissues. Capillaries are the smallest blood vessels. They connect arterioles and venules and function as exchange vessels. Venules connect capillaries and veins. Veins carry oxygen-poor blood from the body to the right side of the heart. Because most of the body's blood is located in them at any one time, veins are called capacitance (storage) vessels.

- The heart has four chambers that function as two functional pumps. The right atrium and right ventricle comprise one pump. The left atrium and left ventricle comprise the other. The right side of the heart is a low-pressure system (pulmonary circulation). The left side of the heart is a high-pressure pump (systemic circulation). The walls of the heart are composed of the endocardium, myocardium, and epicardium. Four valves in the heart (two AV valves and two SL valves) ensure blood flows in one direction through the heart's chambers and prevent the backflow of blood. The heart has three major coronary arteries: the LAD, LCX, and RCA.

- Parasympathetic stimulation of the heart slows the firing rate of the SA node, slows conduction through the AV node, decreases the strength of atrial contraction, and can cause a small decrease in the force of ventricular contraction. Sympathetic stimulation of the heart results in increased force of contraction, increased heart rate, and increased blood pressure.

- Cardiac output is the amount of blood pumped into the aorta each minute by the heart. It is defined as the stroke volume (amount of blood ejected from a ventricle with each heartbeat) multiplied by the heart rate. Stroke volume is determined by the degree of ventricular filling when the heart is relaxed (preload), the pressure against which the ventricle must pump (afterload), and the myocardium's contractile state (contracting or relaxing).

Chapter Summary—continued

- The cardiac action potential is a five-phase cycle that reflects the difference in the concentration of charged particles across the cell membrane at any given time. The polarized state is the period after repolarization of a myocardial cell (also called the *resting state*) when the outside of the cell is positive and the interior of the cell is negative. Depolarization is movement of ions across a cell membrane, causing the inside of the cell to become more positive. It is an electrical event expected to result in contraction. Repolarization is movement of ions across a cell membrane in which the inside of the cell is restored to its negative charge.

- The SA node is the heart's normal pacemaker. The built-in (intrinsic) rate of the SA node is 60 to 100 beats/min. The AV junction is the AV node and the nonbranching portion of the bundle of His. The bundle of His has pacemaker cells capable of discharging at a rate of 40 to 60 beats/min. The Purkinje fibers have pacemaker cells capable of firing at a rate of 20 to 40 beats/min.

- The ECG records the electrical activity of a large mass of atrial and ventricular cells as specific waveforms and complexes. Three types of leads are used: standard limb leads, augmented limb leads, and chest (precordial) leads. The position of the positive electrode on the body determines which portion of the left ventricle is seen by each lead. Leads I, II, and III are the standard limb leads. Leads aVR, aVL, and aVF are augmented limb leads. The chest leads are identified as V_1, V_2, V_3, V_4, V_5, and V_6.

- ECG paper is graph paper composed of small and large boxes measured in millimeters. The horizontal axis of the paper corresponds with time. The vertical axis of the ECG paper measures the voltage or amplitude of a waveform. Voltage is measured in millivolts (mV).

- A waveform is movement away from the baseline in either a positive (upward) or negative (downward) direction. Waveforms are named alphabetically, beginning with P, QRS, T, and U. A segment is a line between waveforms. It is named by the waveform that precedes or follows it. An interval is a waveform and a segment. A complex is several waveforms.

- The P wave represents atrial depolarization and the spread of the electrical impulse throughout the right and left atria. The QRS complex consists of the Q wave, R wave, and S wave. It represents the spread of the electrical impulse through the ventricles (ventricular depolarization). The T wave represents ventricular repolarization.

- The PR interval represents the interval between the onset of atrial depolarization and ventricular depolarization. The ST segment represents the early part of repolarization of the right and left ventricles. The

point where the QRS complex and the ST segment meet is called the junction, or J-point. The TP segment is the portion of the ECG tracing between the end of the T wave and the beginning of the next P wave.

- A rhythm that begins in the SA node has a positive (upright) P wave before each QRS complex, P waves that look alike, a constant PR interval, and (usually) a regular atrial and ventricular rhythm. A rhythm that begins in the atria has a positive P wave shaped differently than P waves that begin in the SA node.

- A rhythm that begins in the atria has a positive P wave shaped differently than P waves that begin in the SA node. This difference in P-wave configuration occurs because the impulse begins in the atria and follows a different conduction pathway to the AV node.

- If the AV junction paces the heart, the electrical impulse must travel in a backward (retrograde) direction to activate the atria. If a P wave is seen, it will be inverted in leads II, III, and aVF because the impulse is traveling away from the positive electrode. If the atria depolarize before the ventricles, an inverted P wave will be seen before the QRS complex. If the atria and ventricles depolarize at the same time, a P wave will not be visible because it will be hidden in the QRS complex. If the atria depolarize after the ventricles, an inverted P wave will appear after the QRS complex.

- When an ectopic site within a ventricle assumes responsibility for pacing the heart, the electrical impulse bypasses the normal intraventricular conduction pathway. This results in stimulation of the ventricles at slightly different times. As a result, ventricular beats and rhythms usually have QRS complexes that are abnormally shaped and longer than normal (greater than 0.12 seconds).

- In first-degree AV block, all components of the ECG tracing are usually within normal limits except the PR interval. This is because electrical impulses normally travel from the SA node through the atria, but a delay occurs in impulse conduction, usually at the level of the AV node. Second-degree AV blocks are types of incomplete blocks because the AV junction conducts at least some impulses to the ventricles. In third-degree AV block, impulses generated by the SA node are blocked before reaching the ventricles, so no P waves are conducted. Third-degree AV block also is called complete AV block. The block may occur at the AV node, bundle of His, or bundle branches.

- A pacemaker is an artificial pulse generator that delivers an electrical current to the heart to stimulate depolarization. Pacemaker systems usually are named according to where the electrodes are located and the route the electrical current takes to the heart.

- In right BBB, the last portion of the QRS complex points up. In left BBB, the last portion of the QRS complex is directed downward. Patients with a temperature less than 32° C (89.6° F) may develop a unique ECG pattern called a J wave (also called an *Osborn wave*), which is seen at the J-point.

- A systematic approach to the assessment of the cardiac patient is important so that you do not overlook physical findings or important information that is pertinent to the treatment plan for your patient.

- ACSs are conditions caused by a similar sequence of pathologic events—a temporary or permanent blockage of a coronary artery. This sequence of events results in conditions ranging from myocardial ischemia or injury to death (necrosis) of heart muscle. ACSs include unstable angina, NSTEMI, and STEMI. SCD can occur with any of these conditions.

- Heart failure is a condition in which the heart is unable to pump enough blood to meet the metabolic needs of the body. Heart failure is a syndrome, not a disease, that can result from disorders that impair the ability of the ventricle to fill with or eject blood. In acute heart failure, symptoms occur suddenly. In chronic heart failure, symptoms develop more slowly. Although failure of either ventricle can occur by itself, they often fail together. RVF often is a result of LVF.

- Shock is inadequate tissue perfusion that results from the failure of the cardiovascular system to deliver sufficient oxygen and nutrients to sustain vital organ function. The underlying cause must be recognized and treated promptly or cell and organ dysfunction and death may result.

- Cardiac arrest is the absence of cardiac pump function, confirmed by the absence of a detectable pulse, unresponsiveness, and apnea or agonal, gasping respirations. Cardiac arrest may be reversible but will lead to death without prompt emergency care. SCD is an unexpected death from a cardiac cause that either occurs immediately or within 1 hour of the onset of symptoms. In some cases the patient in cardiac arrest will not respond despite appropriate basic and advanced life support care. Some EMS systems have developed protocols that allow field termination of resuscitation efforts in specific circumstances.

- Uncontrolled high blood pressure can lead to vision problems and increases the risk of serious health problems such as stroke, heart attack, heart failure, or kidney failure. Hypertensive urgencies are significant elevations in blood pressure with nonspecific symptoms that should be corrected within 24 hours. Hypertensive emergencies are situations that require rapid (within 1 hour) lowering of blood pressure to prevent or limit organ damage.

- Endocarditis occurs when bacteria in the bloodstream lodge and begin to multiply on a heart valve or other damaged tissue in the heart. If untreated, the bacteria can damage the heart valve, causing it to malfunction. Pericarditis is an inflammation of the double-walled sac (pericardium) that encloses the heart. A pericardial effusion is an increase in the volume and/or character of pericardial fluid that surrounds the heart. Cardiac tamponade occurs when the buildup of pericardial fluid compresses the heart and impairs contraction and ventricular filling.

- Congenital heart defects may obstruct blood flow in the heart or the vessels near it or cause an alteration in the normal pattern of blood flow through the heart.

- An aneurysm is a localized dilation or bulging of a blood vessel wall (or wall of a heart chamber). The dilated area may leak or rupture if it stretches too far. Dissection or rupture of the aorta is a medical emergency.

- An acute arterial occlusion is a sudden disruption of arterial blood flow that occurs because of a thrombus, embolus, tumor, direct trauma to an artery, or an unknown cause. Acute limb (extremity) ischemia results when an arterial occlusion suddenly reduces blood flow to an arm or leg. Intermittent claudication is pain, cramping, muscle tightness, fatigue, or weakness of the legs when walking or during exercise.

- Vasculitis is an inflammation of blood vessels. This disorder can affect vessels of any type in any organ. Thrombophlebitis is the development of a clot in a vein in which inflammation is present. Superficial thrombophlebitis occurs when a clot develops in a vein near the skin surface. If a clot develops in the deep veins of the extremities, DVT is present. DVT is associated with an increased risk of pulmonary embolism.

REFERENCES

American Heart Association. (2005a). *Heart disease and stroke statistics—2005 update*. Dallas: American Heart Association.

American Heart Association. (2005b). American Heart Association guidelines for cardiopulmonary resuscitation and emergency cardiovascular care, part 7.5: Postresuscitation support. *Circulation, 112*(suppl IV), IV-84-IV-85.

Antman, E. M., Anbe, D. T., Armstrong, P. W., Bates, E. R., Green, L. A., Hand, M., et al. (2004). *ACC/AHA guidelines for the management of patients with ST-elevation myocardial infarction: A report of the American College of Cardiology/American Heart Association Task Force on Practice Guidelines (Committee to Revise the 1999 Guidelines for the Management of Patients With Acute Myocardial Infarction)*. Retrieved December 21, 2007, from http://www.acc.org.

Aufderheide, T. P. (2002). Peripheral arteriovascular disease. In J. A. Marx (Ed.), *Rosen's emergency medicine: Concepts and clinical practice* (5th ed.) (p. 1190). St. Louis: Mosby.

Bailey, E. D., Wydro, G. C., Cone, D. C. (2000). Termination of resuscitation in the prehospital setting for adult patients suffering nontraumatic cardiac arrest. National Association of EMS Physicians Standards and Clinical Practice Committee. *Prehospital Emergency Care, 4*(2), 190-195.

Baljepally, R., & Spodick, D. H. (1998). PR-segment deviation as the initial electrocardiographic response in acute pericarditis. *American Journal of Cardiology, 81*(12), 1505-1506.

Becker, L., Larsen, M. P., & Eisenberg, M. S. (1996). Incidence of cardiac arrest during self-transport for chest pain. *Annals of Emergency Medicine, 28*, 612-616.

Braunwald, E. (2001). The history. In E. Braunwald, D. P. Zipes, & P. Libby (Eds.). *Heart disease: A textbook of cardiovascular medicine* (6th ed.) (p. 28), Philadelphia: Saunders.

Braunwald, E., Antman, E. M., Beasley, J. W., Califf, R. M., Cheitlin, M. D., Hochman, J. S., et al. (2000). ACC/AHA guidelines for the management of patients with unstable angina and non–ST-segment elevation myocardial infarction: A report of the American College of Cardiology/American Heart Association Task Force on Practice Guidelines (Committee on the Management of Patients With Unstable Angina). *Journal of the American College of Cardiology, 36*, 970-1062.

Braunwald, E., Antman, E. M., Beasley, J. W., Califf, R. M., Cheitlin, M. D., Hochman, J. S., et al. (2002). *ACC/AHA 2002 guideline update for the management of patients with unstable angina and non–ST-segment elevation myocardial infarction: a report of the American College of Cardiology/American Heart Association Task Force on Practice Guidelines (Committee on the Management of Patients With Unstable Angina).* Retrieved on June 9, 2006 from http://www.acc.org.

Canto, J. G., Shlipak, M. G., Rogers, W. J., Malmgren, J. A., Frederick, P. D., Lambrew, C. T., et al. (2000). Prevalence, clinical characteristics, and mortality among patients with myocardial infarction presenting without chest pain. *Journal of the American Medical Association, 283*(24), 3223-3229.

Cantrell, M., & Yoshikawa, T. T. (1984). Infective endocarditis in the aging patient. *Gerontology, 30*(5), 316-326.

Castelli, W. P. (1984). Epidemiology of coronary heart disease: The Framingham study. *American Journal of Medicine, 76*(2A), 4-12.

Centers for Disease Control and Prevention. (2005). Racial/ethnic and socioeconomic disparities in multiple risk factors for heart disease and stroke—United States, 2003. *Morbidity and Mortality Weekly Report, 54*(5), 113-117.

Chobanian, A. V., Bakris, G. L., Black, H. R., Cushman, W. C., Green, L. A., Izzo, J. L. Jr., et al. (2003). Joint National Committee on Prevention, Detection, Evaluation, and Treatment of High Blood Pressure. National Heart, Lung, and Blood Institute; National High Blood Pressure Education Program Coordinating Committee. Seventh report of the Joint National Committee on prevention, detection, evaluation, and treatment of high blood pressure. *Hypertension, 42*(6), 1206-1252.

Danzl, D. F. (1998). Accidental hypothermia. In P. Rosen, et al. (Eds.). *Emergency medicine: Concepts and clinical practice* (4th ed.). St. Louis: Mosby.

Danzl, D. F. (2002). Accidental hypothermia. In J. A. Marx (Ed.). *Rosen's emergency medicine: Concepts and clinical practice* (5th ed.) (p. 1981). St. Louis: Mosby.

Eckstein, M., Stratton, S. J., & Chan, L. S. (2005). Cardiac arrest resuscitation evaluation in Los Angeles: CARE-LA. *Annals of Emergency Medicine, 45*(5), 504-509.

Eftestol, T., Wik, L., Sunde, K., & Steen, P. A. (2004). Effects of cardiopulmonary resuscitation on predictors of ventricular fibrillation defibrillation success during out-of-hospital cardiac arrest. *Circulation, 110*(1), 10-15.

Ewy, G. A. (2005). Cardiocerebral resuscitation: The new cardiopulmonary resuscitation. *Circulation, 111*(16), 2134-2142.

Finkelmeier, B. A., & Marolda, D. (2001). Aortic dissection. *Journal of Cardiovascular Nursing, 15*(4), 15-24.

Fodor, J., & Tzerovska, R. (2004). Coronary heart disease: is gender important? *Journal of Men's Health and Gender, 1*(1), 32.

Ford, E. S., Giles, W. H., & Dietz, W. H. (2002). Prevalence of the metabolic syndrome among US adults: Findings from the third National Health and Nutrition Examination Survey. *Journal of the American Medical Association, 287*(3), 356-359.

Friedman, G. D., & Klatsky, A. L. (1993). Is alcohol good for your health? *New England Journal of Medicine, 329*(25), 1882-1883.

Gibbons, R. J., Abrams, J., Chatterjee, K., Daley, J., Deedwania, P. C., Douglas, J. S., et al. (2002). *ACC/AHA 2002 guideline update for the management of patients with chronic stable angina: A report of the American College of Cardiology/American Heart Association Task Force on Practice Guidelines (Committee to Update the 1999 Guidelines for the Management of Patients with Chronic Stable Angina).* Retrieved December 21, 2007 from http://www.acc.org.

Givertz, M. M., & Colucci, W. S. (2001). Heart failure. In J. Noble (Ed.). *Textbook of primary care medicine* (3rd ed.). St. Louis: Mosby.

Greenlund, K. J., Keenan, N. L., Giles, W. H., Zheng, Z. J., Neff, L. J., Croft, J. B., & Mensah, G. A. (2004). Public recognition of major signs and symptoms of heart attack: Seventeen states and the US Virgin Islands, 2001. *American Heart Journal, 147*(6), 1010-1016.

Guyton, A. C., & Hall, J. E. (1996). Heart muscle: the heart as a pump. In *Textbook of medical physiology* (9th ed.). Philadelphia: W. B. Saunders.

Haffner, S. J., & Cassells, H. (2003). Hyperglycemia as a cardiovascular risk factor. *American Journal of Medicine, 115*(Suppl 8A), 6S-11S.

Harris, D. G., Papagiannopoulos, K. A., Pretorius, J., Van Rooyen, T., & Rossouw, G. J. (1999). Current evaluation of cardiac stab wounds. *Annals of Thoracic Surgery, 68*(6), 2119-2122.

Hinkle, L. E. Jr., & Thaler, H. T. (1982). Clinical classification of cardiac deaths. *Circulation, 65*(3), 457-464.

Hosey, R. G., & Armsey, T. D. (2003). Sudden cardiac death. *Clinical Sports Medicine, 22*(1), 51-66.

Hunt, S. A., Abraham W. T., Chin, M. H., Feldman, A. M., Francis, G. S., Ganiats, T. G., et al. (2005). *ACC/AHA guidelines for the evaluation and management of chronic heart failure in the adult: A report of the American College of Cardiology/American Heart Association Task Force on Practice Guidelines (Writing Committee to Update the 2001 Guidelines for the Evaluation and Management of Heart Failure).* Retrieved December 21, 2007 from http://www.acc.org.

Irwin, R. S., Boulet, L. P., Cloutier, M. M., Fuller, R., Gold, P. M., Hoffstein, V., et al. (1998). Managing cough as a defense mechanism and as a symptom. A consensus panel report of the American College of Chest Physicians. *Chest, 114*(2 Suppl), 133S-181S.

Isselbacher, E. M. (2005). Diseases of the aorta. In D. P. Zipes, P. Libby, R. O. Bonow, & E. B. Braunwald (Eds.). *Braunwald's heart disease: A textbook of cardiovascular medicine* (7th ed.) (pp. 1403-1436). St. Louis: Elsevier-Saunders.

Kannel, W. B. (1996). The demographics of claudication and the aging of the American population. *Vascular Medicine, 1*(1), 60-64.

Kannel, W. B. (2004). Lessons from curbing the coronary artery disease epidemic for confronting the impending epidemic of heart failure. *Medical Clinics of North America, 88*(5), 1129-1133, ix.

Khasnis, A., & Lokhandwala, Y. (2002). Clinical signs in medicine: Pulsus paradoxus. *Journal of Postgraduate Medicine, 48*, 46-49.

Kiell, C. S., & Ernst, C. B. (1993). Advances in management of abdominal aortic aneurysm. *Advances in Surgery, 26*, 73-98.

Lederle, F. A., & Simel, D. L. (1999). The rational clinical examination. Does this patient have abdominal aortic aneurysm? *Journal of the American Medical Association, 281*(1), 77-82.

Lu, J. T., & Creager, M. A. (2004). The relationship of cigarette smoking to peripheral arterial disease. *Review of Cardiovascular Medicine, 5*(4), 189-193.

Mackay, J., & Mensah, G. A. (2004). *Atlas of heart disease and stroke,* Geneva: World Health Organization.

McCaffery, M., & Pasero, C. L. (1998). When the physician prescribes a placebo. *American Journal of Nursing, 98*, 52-53.

Myerburg, R. J., & Castellanos, A. (2005). Cardiac arrest and sudden cardiac death. In D. P. Zipes, P. Libby, R. O. Bonow, & E. B. Braunwald (Eds.). *Braunwald's heart disease: A textbook of cardiovascular medicine,* (7th ed.) (pp. 868-869). St. Louis: Elsevier-Saunders.

National Center for Chronic Disease Prevention and Health Promotion, Cardiovascular Health. (2006). Heart disease fact sheet. Retrieved September 21, 2006 from http://www.cdc.gov.

Nemeroff, C. B., Musselman, D. L., & Evans, D. L. (1998). Depression and cardiac disease. *Depression and Anxiety, 8*(Suppl 1), 71-79.

Pearson, T. A. (1996). Alcohol and heart disease. *Circulation, 94*(11), 3023-3025.

Phalen, T., & Aehlert, B. (2006). *The 12-lead ECG in acute coronary syndromes.* St. Louis: Elsevier.

Prescott, E., Hippe, M., Schnohr, P., Hein, H. O., & Vestbo, J. (1998). Smoking and risk of myocardial infarction in women and men: Longitudinal population study. *British Medical Journal, 316*(7137), 1043-1047.

Rowan, P. J., Haas, D., Campbell, J. A., Maclean, D. R., & Davidson, K. W. (2005). Depressive symptoms have an independent, gradient risk for coronary heart disease incidence in a random, population-based sample. *Annals of Epidemiology, 15*(4), 316-320.

Saxon, L. A. (2005). Sudden cardiac death: Epidemiology and temporal trends. *Review of Cardiovascular Medicine, 6*(Suppl 2), S12-S20.

Schoen, F. J. (2005a). Blood vessels. In V. Kumar, A. K. Abbas, & N. Fausto (Eds.). *Robbins and Cotran pathologic basis of disease* (7th ed.). Philadelphia: Elsevier.

Schoen, F. J. (2005b). The heart. In V. Kumar, A. K. Abbas, & N. Fausto (Eds.). *Robbins and Cotran pathologic basis of disease* (7th ed.). Philadelphia: Elsevier.

Shah, P. K. (2003). Mechanisms of plaque vulnerability and rupture. *Journal of the American College of Cardiology, 41*(4 Suppl S), 15S-22S.

Shimbo, D., Davidson, K. W., Haas, D. C., Fuster, V., & Badimon, J. J. (2005). Negative impact of depression on outcomes in patients with coronary artery disease: mechanisms, treatment considerations, and future directions. *Journal of Thrombosis and Haemostasis, 3*(5), 897-908.

Shry, E. A., Dacus, J., Van De Graaff, E., Hjelkrem, M., Stajduhar, K. C., & Steinhubl, S. R. (2002). Usefulness of the response to sublingual nitroglycerin as a predictor of ischemic chest pain in the emergency department. *American Journal of Cardiology, 90*(11), 1264-1266.

State-specific mortality from sudden cardiac death—United States, 1999. (2002). *Morbidity and Mortality Weekly Report, 51*(6), 123-126.

Timm, C. (2003). Cardiogenic shock. In M. H. Crawford (Ed.). *Current diagnosis & treatment in cardiology* (2nd ed.). New York: McGraw-Hill Companies.

U. S. Department of Health and Human Services. (2006). *Heart disease fact sheet.* Retrieved October 9, 2006 from http://www.cdc.gov.

Webb, J. G., Lowe, A. M., Sanborn, T. A., White, H. D., Sleeper, L. A., Carere, R. G., et al. (2003). Percutaneous shock intervention for cardiogenic shock in the SHOCK Trial. *Journal of the American College of Cardiology, 42,* 1380.

Weber, M. (2003). Pulsus alternans. A case study. *Critical Care Nurse, 23*(3), 51-54.

Wei, J. Y., Greene, H. L., & Weisfeldt, M. L. (1980). Cough-facilitated conversion of ventricular tachycardia. *American Journal of Cardiology, 45*(1), 174-176.

Zairis, M. N., Ambrose, J. A., Lyras, A. G., Thoma, M. A., Psarogianni, P. K., Psaltiras, P. G., et al. (2004). GENERATION Study Group. C Reactive protein, moderate alcohol consumption, and long term prognosis after successful coronary stenting: Four year results from the GENERATION study. *Heart, 90*(4), 419-424.

SUGGESTED RESOURCES

Aehlert, B. (2007). *ACLS study guide* (3rd ed.). St. Louis: Elsevier.

Aehlert, B. (2007). *ECGs made easy* (3rd ed.). St. Louis: Elsevier.

National Heart, Lung, and Blood Institute: www.nhlbi.nih.gov.

National Library of Medicine: www.nlm.nih.gov/medlineplus.

Phalen, T., & Aehlert, B. (2006). *The 12-lead ECG in acute coronary syndromes,* St. Louis: Elsevier.

Chapter Quiz

1. Explain the difference between the terms *coronary heart disease* and *coronary artery disease.*

2. Traits and lifestyle habits that may increase a person's chance of developing a disease are called _____ _____.

3. List the three major coronary arteries.

4. List three factors that determine stroke volume.

5. What are the four properties of cardiac cells?

6. List the intrinsic rates for each of the heart's normal pacemaker sites.

7. List three characteristics of an ECG rhythm that begins in the SA node.

8. Name the three main types of SVT.

9. List the five *P*'s of acute arterial occlusion.

10. What is an aneurysm?

11. What is the most common congenital heart defect?

12. List the classic signs of cardiac tamponade.

Terminology

Aberrant Abnormal.

Absolute refractory period Corresponds with the onset of the QRS complex to approximately the peak of the T wave; cardiac cells cannot be stimulated to conduct an electrical impulse, no matter how strong the stimulus.

Accessory pathway An extra bundle of working myocardial tissue that forms a connection between the atria and ventricles outside the normal conduction system.

Action potential A five-phase cycle that reflects the difference in the concentration of these charged particles across the cell membrane at any given time.

Acute arterial occlusion A sudden blockage of arterial blood flow that occurs because of a thrombus, embolus, tumor, direct trauma to an artery, or an unknown cause.

Acute coronary syndrome (ACS) A term used to describe ischemic chest discomfort. ACSs consist of three major syndromes: unstable angina, NSTEMI, and STEMI.

Afterload Pressure or resistance against which the ventricles must pump to eject blood.

Amplitude Height (voltage) of a waveform on the ECG.

Anasarca Massive generalized body edema.

Aneurysm Localized dilation or bulging of a blood vessel wall or wall of a heart chamber.

Anginal equivalents Symptoms of myocardial ischemia other than chest pain or discomfort.

Angina pectoris Chest discomfort or other related symptoms of sudden onset that may occur because the increased oxygen demand of the heart temporarily exceeds the blood supply.

Antiarrhythmic Medications used to correct irregular heartbeats and slow hearts that beat too fast.

Aortic valve SL valve on the left of the heart; separates the left ventricle from the aorta.

Apex of the heart Lower portion of the heart, tip of the ventricles (approximately the level of the fifth left intercostal space); points leftward, downward, and forward.

Arrhythmia Term often used interchangeably with dysrhythmia; any disturbance or abnormality in a normal rhythmic pattern; any cardiac rhythm other than a sinus rhythm.

Arteriosclerosis A chronic disease of the arterial system characterized by abnormal thickening and hardening of the vessel walls.

Asystole A total absence of ventricular electrical activity.

Atherosclerosis A form of arteriosclerosis in which the thickening and hardening of the vessel walls are caused by a buildup of fatty deposits in the inner lining of large and middle-sized muscular arteries

(from *athero*, meaning gruel or paste, and *sclerosis*, meaning hardness).

Artifact Distortion of an ECG tracing by electrical activity that is noncardiac in origin (e.g., electrical interference, poor electrical conduction, patient movement).

Ascites Marked abdominal swelling from a buildup of fluid in the peritoneal cavity.

Asynchronous pacemaker Fixed-rate pacemaker that continuously discharges at a preset rate regardless of the patient's intrinsic activity.

Atria Two upper chambers of the heart (singular, *atrium*)

Atrioventricular junction The AV node and the nonbranching portion of the bundle of His.

Atrioventricular node A group of cells that conduct an electrical impulse through the heart; located in the floor of the right atrium immediately behind the tricuspid valve and near the opening of the coronary sinus.

Atrioventricular sequential pacemaker Type of dual-chamber pacemaker that stimulates first the atrium, then the ventricle, mimicking normal cardiac physiology.

Atrioventricular valve Valve located between each atrium and ventricle; the tricuspid separates the right atrium from the right ventricle, and the mitral (bicuspid) separates the left atrium from the left ventricle.

Augmented limb lead Leads aVR, aVL, and aVF; these leads record the difference in electrical potential at one location relative to zero potential rather than relative to the electrical potential of another extremity, as in the bipolar leads.

Automaticity Ability of cardiac pacemaker cells to initiate an electrical impulse spontaneously without being stimulated from another source (such as a nerve).

Axis Imaginary line joining the positive and negative electrodes of a lead.

Baseline Straight line recorded on ECG graph paper when no electrical activity is detected.

Base of the heart Top of the heart; located at approximately the level of the second intercostal space.

Biphasic Waveform that is partly positive and partly negative.

Bipolar limb lead ECG lead consisting of a positive and negative electrode; a pacing lead with two electrical poles that are external from the pulse generator; the negative pole is located at the extreme distal tip of the pacing lead, and the positive pole is located several millimeters proximal to the negative electrode. The stimulating pulse is delivered through the negative electrode.

Blocked premature atrial complex PAC not followed by a QRS complex.

Blood pressure Force exerted by the blood against the walls of the arteries as the ventricles of the heart contract and relax.

Bradycardia Heart rate slower than 60 beats/min (from *brady*, meaning "slow")

Bruit Blowing or swishing sound created by the turbulence within a blood vessel.

Bundle branch block (BBB) Abnormal conduction of an electrical impulse through either the right or left bundle branches.

Bundle of His Fibers located in the upper portion of the interventricular septum that conduct an electrical impulse through the heart.

Burst Three or more sequential ectopic beats; also referred to as a salvo or run.

Calibration Regulation of an ECG machine's stylus sensitivity so that a 1 mV electrical signal will produce a deflection measuring exactly 10 mm.

Capture Ability of a pacing stimulus to depolarize successfully the cardiac chamber being paced; with one-to-one capture, each pacing stimulus results in depolarization of the appropriate chamber.

Cardiac arrest Absence of cardiac mechanical activity, confirmed by the absence of a detectable pulse, unresponsiveness, and apnea or agonal, gasping respirations.

Cardiac cycle Period from the beginning of one heart-beat to the beginning of the next; normally consisting of PQRST waves, complexes, and intervals.

Cardiac output (CO) Amount of blood pumped into the aorta each minute by the heart.

Cardiogenic shock A condition in which heart muscle function is severely impaired, leading to decreased cardiac output and inadequate tissue perfusion.

Cardiomyopathy A disease of the heart muscle.

Cardiovascular disorders A collection of diseases and conditions that involve the heart (cardio) and blood vessels (vascular).

Cholinergic Having the characteristics of the parasympathetic division of the autonomic nervous system.

Chordae tendineae Thin strands of fibrous connective tissue that extend from the AV valves to the papillary muscles that prevent the AV valves from bulging back into the atria during ventricular systole (contraction).

Chronotropism A change in heart rate.

Circumflex artery Division of the left coronary artery.

Compensatory pause Pause for which the normal beat after a premature complex occurs when expected; also called a complete pause.

Complex Several waveforms.

Conduction system A system of pathways in the heart composed of specialized electrical (pacemaker) cells.

Conductivity Ability of a cardiac cell to receive an electrical stimulus and conduct that impulse to an adjacent cardiac cell.

Contractility Ability of cardiac cells to shorten, causing cardiac muscle contraction in response to an electrical stimulus.

Coronary artery disease Disease of the arteries that supply the heart muscle with blood.

Coronary heart disease Disease of the coronary arteries and their resulting complications, such as angina pectoris or acute myocardial infarction.

Coronary sinus Venous drain for the coronary circulation into the right atrium.

Cor pulmonale Right-sided heart failure caused by pulmonary disease.

Couplet Two consecutive premature complexes.

Current Flow of electrical charge from one point to another.

Cystic medial degeneration A connective tissue disease in which the elastic tissue and smooth muscle fibers of the middle arterial layer degenerate.

Cytokines Protein molecules produced by white blood cells that act as chemical messengers between cells.

Deep vein thrombosis (DVT) Presence of a clot in the deep veins of the extremities.

Defibrillation Therapeutic use of electric current to terminate lethal cardiac dysrhythmias.

Delta wave Slurring of the beginning portion of the QRS complex caused by preexcitation.

Demand pacemaker Synchronous pacemaker that discharges only when the patient's heart rate drops below the preset rate for the pacemaker.

Depolarization Movement of ions across a cell membrane, causing the inside of the cell to become more positive; an electrical event expected to result in contraction.

Diastole Phase of the cardiac cycle in which the atria and ventricles relax between contractions and blood enters these chambers; when the term is used without reference to a specific chamber of the heart, the term implies ventricular diastole.

Diastolic blood pressure Pressure exerted against the walls of the large arteries during ventricular relaxation.

Dromotropism The speed of conduction through the AV junction.

Dual-chamber pacemaker Pacemaker that stimulates the atrium and ventricle.

Terminology—continued

Dyspnea An uncomfortable awareness of one's breathing; shortness of breath or difficulty breathing.

Dysrhythmia Any disturbance or abnormality in a normal rhythmic pattern; any cardiac rhythm other than a sinus rhythm.

Ectopic Impulse(s) originating from a source other than the SA node.

Electrical alternans A beat-to-beat change in waveform amplitude on the ECG.

Electrodes Adhesive pads that contain a conductive gel and are applied at specific locations on the patient's chest wall and extremities and connected by cables to an ECG machine.

Electrolytes Elements or compounds that break into charged particles (ions) when melted or dissolved in water or another solvent.

Endocardium Innermost layer of the heart that lines the inside of the myocardium and covers the heart valves.

Enlargement Implies the presence of dilatation or hypertrophy or both.

Epicardium Also known as the visceral pericardium; the external layer of the heart wall that covers the heart muscle.

Escape Term used when the sinus node slows or fails to initiate depolarization and a lower pacemaker site spontaneously produces electrical impulses, assuming responsibility for pacing the heart.

Essential hypertension High blood pressure for which there no cause is identifiable; also called primary hypertension.

Excitability Ability of cardiac muscle cells to respond to an outside stimulus.

Fainting A brief loss of consciousness caused by a temporary decrease in blood flow to the brain.

Fascicle Small bundle of nerve fibers.

Fibrinolysis The breakdown of fibrin, the main component of blood clots.

Fine ventricular fibrillation VF with fibrillatory waves less than 3 mm in height.

Fixed-rate pacemaker Asynchronous pacemaker that continuously discharges at a preset rate regardless of the patient's heart rate.

Focal atrial tachycardia AT that begins in a small area (focus) within the heart.

Great vessels Large vessels that carry blood to and from the heart: superior and inferior venae cavae, pulmonary veins, aorta, and pulmonary trunk.

Ground electrode Third ECG electrode (the first and second are the positive and negative electrodes), which minimizes electrical activity from other sources.

Heart disease A broad term referring to conditions affecting the heart.

Heart failure A condition in which the heart is unable to pump enough blood to meet the metabolic needs of the body.

His-Purkinje system Portion of the conduction system consisting of the bundle of His, bundle branches, and Purkinje fibers.

Homan's sign Pain and tenderness in the calf muscle on dorsiflexion of the foot.

Hypertensive emergencies Situations that require rapid (within 1 hour) lowering of blood pressure to prevent or limit organ damage.

Hypertensive urgencies Significant elevations in blood pressure with nonspecific symptoms that should be corrected within 24 hours.

Hypertrophy Increase in the thickness of a heart chamber because of chronic pressure overload.

Hypovolemic shock Inadequate tissue perfusion caused by inadequate vascular volume.

Indicative change ECG changes seen in leads looking directly at the wall of the heart in an infarction.

Infarction Death of tissue because of an inadequate blood supply.

Inotropism A change in myocardial contractility.

Intermittent claudication Pain, cramping, muscle tightness, fatigue, or weakness of the legs when walking or during exercise.

Interval Waveform and a segment; in pacing, the period, measured in milliseconds, between any two designated cardiac events.

Intrinsic rate Rate at which a pacemaker of the heart normally generates impulses.

Ion Electrically charged particle.

Ischemia Decreased supply of oxygenated blood to a body part or organ.

Isoelectric line Absence of electrical activity; observed on the ECG as a straight line.

J-point Point where the QRS complex and ST segment meet.

Junctional bradycardia A rhythm that begins in the AV junction with a rate of less than 40 beats/min.

Lead Electrical connection attached to the body to record electrical activity.

Malignant hypertension Severe hypertension with signs of acute and progressive damage to end organs such as the heart, brain, and kidneys.

Mediastinum Located in the middle of the thoracic cavity; contains the heart, great vessels, trachea, and esophagus, among other structures; extends from the sternum to the vertebral column.

Membrane potential Difference in electrical charge across the cell membrane.

Milliampere (mA) Unit of measure of electrical current needed to elicit depolarization of the myocardium.

Millivolt (mV) Difference in electrical charge between two points in a circuit.

Monomorphic Having the same shape.

Multiformed atrial rhythm Cardiac dysrhythmia that occurs because of impulses originating from various sites, including the SA node, the atria, and/or the AV junction; requires at least three different P waves, seen in the same lead, for proper diagnosis.

Myocardial cells Working cells of the myocardium that contain contractile filaments and form the muscular layer of the atrial walls and the thicker muscular layer of the ventricular walls.

Myocardial infarction (MI) Necrosis of some mass of the heart muscle caused by an inadequate blood supply.

Myocarditis Inflammation of the middle and thickest layer of the heart, the myocardium.

Myocardium Middle and thickest layer of the heart; contains the cardiac muscle fibers that cause contraction of the heart as well as the conduction system and blood supply.

Neurotransmitter A chemical released from one nerve that crosses the synaptic cleft to reach a receptor.

Orthopnea Dyspnea relieved by a change in position (either sitting upright or standing).

Oxidation A normal chemical process in the body caused by the release of oxygen atoms created during normal cell metabolism.

Pacemaker Artificial pulse generator that delivers an electrical current to the heart to stimulate depolarization.

Pacemaker cells Specialized cells of the heart's electrical conduction system capable of spontaneously generating and conducting electrical impulses.

Palpitations An unpleasant awareness of one's heartbeat.

Papillary muscles Muscles attached to the chordae tendineae of the heart valves and the ventricular muscle of the heart.

Paroxysmal atrial tachycardia AT that starts or ends suddenly.

Paroxysmal nocturnal dyspnea (PND) A sudden onset of difficulty breathing that awakens the patient from sleep.

Paroxysmal supraventricular tachycardia (PSVT) A regular, narrow-QRS tachycardia that starts or ends suddenly.

Pericardial effusion An increase in the volume and/or character of pericardial fluid that surrounds the heart.

Pericardiocentesis A procedure in which a needle is inserted into the pericardial space and the excess fluid is drawn out (aspirated) through the needle.

Pericarditis Inflammation of the double-walled sac (pericardium) that encloses the heart.

Pericardium Protective sac that surrounds the heart.

Permeability Ability of a membrane channel to allow passage of electrolytes once it is open.

Point of maximal impulse (PMI) Apical impulse; the site where the heartbeat is most strongly felt.

Polarized state Period after repolarization of a myocardial cell (also called the resting state) when the outside of the cell is positive and the interior of the cell is negative.

Polymorphic Varying in shape.

Potential difference Difference in electrical charge between two points in a circuit; expressed in volts or millivolts.

Preexcitation Term used to describe rhythms that originate from above the ventricles but in which the impulse travels by a pathway other than the AV node and bundle of His; thus the supraventricular impulse excites the ventricles earlier than normal.

Preload Force exerted by the blood on the walls of the ventricles at the end of diastole.

Premature complex Early beat occurring before the next expected beat; can be atrial, junctional, or ventricular.

Primary hypertension High blood pressure for which no cause is identifiable; also called *essential hypertension*.

Pulmonary circulation Blood from the right ventricle is pumped directly to the lungs for oxygenation through the pulmonary trunk; blood becomes oxygenated and is then delivered through the pulmonary arteries for the left atrium.

Pulmonary edema A buildup of fluid in the lungs, usually a complication of LVF.

Pulse deficit A difference between the apical pulse and the peripheral pulse rates.

Pulse generator Power source that houses the battery and controls for regulating a pacemaker.

Pulseless electrical activity (PEA) Organized electrical activity observed on a cardiac monitor (other than VT) without the patient having a palpable pulse.

Pulse pressure Difference between the systolic and diastolic blood pressures.

Pulsus alternans A beat-to-beat difference in the strength of a pulse (also called mechanical alternans).

Pulsus paradoxus A fall in systolic blood pressure of more than 10 mm Hg during inspiration (also called paradoxical pulse).

Purkinje fibers Fibers found in both ventricles that conduct an electrical impulse through the heart.

Terminology—continued

P wave First wave in the cardiac cycle; represents atrial depolarization and the spread of the electrical impulse throughout the right and left atria.

QRS complex Several waveforms (Q wave, R wave, and S wave) that represent the spread of an electrical impulse through the ventricles (ventricular depolarization).

Reciprocal change Mirror image ECG changes seen in the wall of the heart opposite the location of an infarction.

Reentry Spread of an impulse through tissue already stimulated by that same impulse.

Refractoriness Period of recovery that cells need after being discharged before they are able to respond to a stimulus.

Relative refractory period Corresponds with the downslope of the T wave; cardiac cells can be stimulated to depolarize if the stimulus is strong enough.

Repolarization Movement of ions across a cell membrane in which the inside of the cell is restored to its negative charge.

Retrograde Moving backward or moving in the opposite direction to that which is considered normal.

Risk factors Traits and lifestyle habits that may increase a person's chance of developing a disease.

R wave On an EGG, the first positive deflection in the QRS complex, representing ventricular depolarization.

Secondary hypertension High blood pressure that has an identifiable cause, such as medications or an underlying disease or condition.

Segment Line between waveforms; named by the waveform that precedes and follows it.

Semilunar (SL) valves Valves shaped like half moons that separate the ventricles from the aorta and pulmonary artery.

Sensing Ability of a pacemaker to recognize and respond to intrinsic electrical activity.

Septum Partition.

Shock Inadequate tissue perfusion that results from the failure of the cardiovascular system to deliver sufficient oxygen and nutrients to sustain vital organ function.

Sinus rhythm A normal heart rhythm.

Stroke volume Amount of blood ejected by either ventricle during one contraction; can be calculated as cardiac output divided by heart rate.

Sudden cardiac death (SCD) An unexpected death from a cardiac cause that either occurs immediately or within 1 hour of the onset of symptoms.

Supernormal period Period during the cardiac cycle when a weaker than normal stimulus can cause cardiac cells to depolarize; extends from the end of phase 3 to the beginning of phase 4 of the cardiac action potential.

Supraventricular Originating from a site above the bifurcation of the bundle of His, such as the SA node, atria, or AV junction.

Supraventricular dysrhythmias Rhythms that begin in the SA node, atrial tissue, or the AV junction.

Syncope A brief loss of consciousness caused by a temporary decrease in blood flow to the brain.

Systole Contraction of the heart (usually referring to ventricular contraction) during which blood is propelled into the pulmonary artery and aorta; when the term is used without reference to a specific chamber of the heart, the term implies ventricular systole.

Systolic blood pressure Pressure exerted against the walls of the large arteries at the peak of ventricular contraction.

Thrombophlebitis Development of a clot in a vein in which inflammation is present.

Thrombus Blood clot.

TP segment Interval between two successive PQRST complexes during which electrical activity of the heart is absent; begins with the end of the T wave through the onset of the following P wave and represents the period from the end of ventricular repolarization to the onset of atrial depolarization.

Unipolar lead A pacing lead with a single electrical pole at the distal tip of the pacing lead (negative pole) through which the stimulating pulse is delivered. In a permanent pacemaker with a unipolar lead, the positive pole is the pulse generator case.

Vascular resistance Amount of opposition that the blood vessels give to the flow of blood.

Venous return Amount of blood flowing into the right atrium each minute from the systemic circulation.

Ventricle Either of the two lower chambers of the heart.

Voltage Difference in electrical charge between two points.

Waveform Movement away from the baseline in either a positive or negative direction.

Wolff-Parkinson-White syndrome Type of pre-excitation syndrome characterized by a slurred upstroke of the QRS complex (delta wave) and wide QRS.

CHAPTER 23

Disorders of the Nervous System

Objectives *After completing this chapter, you will be able to:*

1. Discuss the anatomy and physiology of the organs and structures related to the nervous system.
2. Discuss indications for a neurologic assessment.
3. Discuss and practice the components of the neurologic assessment, including the following:
   - Posture and gait
   - Mental status
   - Examination of the cranial nerves
   - Sensory examination
   - Motor examination
   - Deep tendon reflexes
   - Meningeal examination
   - Glasgow Coma Scale
4. Describe the etiology, epidemiology, history, and physical findings for the following neurologic conditions or situations:
   - Altered mental status
   - Delirium
   - Dementia
   - Seizures
   - Status epilepticus
   - Syncope
   - Headache
   - Brain tumor
   - Brain abscess
   - Stroke
   - Transient ischemic attack
5. With the patient history and physical examination findings, develop a treatment plan for a patient having any of the following neurologic conditions or situations:
   - Altered mental status
   - Delirium
   - Dementia
   - Seizures
   - Status epilepticus
   - Syncope
   - Headache
   - Brain tumor
   - Brain abscess
   - Stroke
   - Transient ischemic attack
6. Identify risk factors that may affect the nervous system.
7. Describe the etiology, epidemiology, history, and physical findings for the following infectious neurologic diseases:
   - Meningitis
   - Encephalitis
   - Shingles
   - Poliomyelitis
8. With the patient history and physical examination findings, develop a treatment plan for a patient having any of the following infectious neurologic diseases:
   - Meningitis
   - Encephalitis
   - Shingles
   - Poliomyelitis
9. Describe the etiology, epidemiology, history, and physical findings for the following degenerative neurologic diseases:
   - Alzheimer's disease
   - Parkinson's disease
   - Amyotrophic lateral sclerosis
   - Multiple sclerosis
   - Guillain-Barré syndrome
   - Myasthenia gravis
   - Huntington's disease
10. With the patient history and physical examination findings, develop a treatment plan for a patient having any of the following degenerative neurologic diseases:
    - Alzheimer's disease
    - Parkinson's disease
    - Amyotrophic lateral sclerosis
    - Multiple sclerosis
    - Guillain-Barré syndrome
    - Myasthenia gravis
    - Huntington's disease
11. Describe the etiology, epidemiology, history, physical findings, and management of spinal cord disorders.
12. Describe the etiology, epidemiology, history, physical findings, and management of autonomic dysreflexia.
13. Describe the etiology, epidemiology, history, physical findings, and management of hydrocephalus.
14. Describe the etiology, epidemiology, history, physical findings, and management of spina bifida.
15. Define the following:
    - Muscular dystrophy
    - Dystonia
    - Trigeminal neuralgia
    - Bell's palsy

Chapter Outline

Case Scenario

You are called to the scene of a motor vehicle crash. The dispatch report provides information on a rollover personal injury accident with multiple victims ejected from the vehicle. You arrive on scene to find a vehicle with significant front, rear, and hood damage. You notice five bodies, each at least 50 yards from the vehicle. No one is moving and no sound is being made. You approach a patient and notice that she is moaning softly and lying on her back. Multiple EMS professionals have arrived on the scene and have assumed care of the other patients. You begin your assessment.

Questions

1. What is critical in the assessment of this scene?
2. What should be the initial actions?
3. What is the mechanism of injury and how does this affect the assessment?

Normal axons impulse travel 2½-3 miles/hr
myelinated axons, travel 20+ miles/hr
impulse

Partnered with the endocrine system, the nervous system controls almost every function of the body. Everything that human beings do, from maintaining homeostasis within the body's tissues, to walking down the street, to calculating drug dosages, happens by way of the nervous system.

In your career as a paramedic, proper assessment and management of neurologic emergencies are essential skills. You will respond to many patients with problems originating in the nervous system, such as seizures and stroke, as well as illnesses and injuries to other body systems that may have neurologic symptoms. To function properly, the brain needs a steady flow of blood rich in oxygen and nutrients. If blood flow to the brain decreases, the patient may have an altered mental status or become unresponsive. If the decrease is prolonged, the patient can sustain permanent brain damage. When responding to patients such as these, you often will not know the cause of these symptoms. A thorough assessment of the nervous system will help point you in the right direction.

ANATOMY AND PHYSIOLOGY OF THE NERVOUS SYSTEM

The Neuron

[OBJECTIVE 1]

The most basic part of the nervous system is the nerve cell, or **neuron** (Figure 23-1). Nerve cells are present throughout the body. Most of the body's nerve cells are found in the brain and spinal cord. When connected, neurons act as conduits, sending signals to and from other neurons, muscles, and glands and receiving sensory information from the outside world.

PARAMEDIC*Pearl*

Although they share some of the same characteristics as other cells of the body, nerve cells are unique in their ability to receive, store, and transmit information (Frosh et al., 2005).

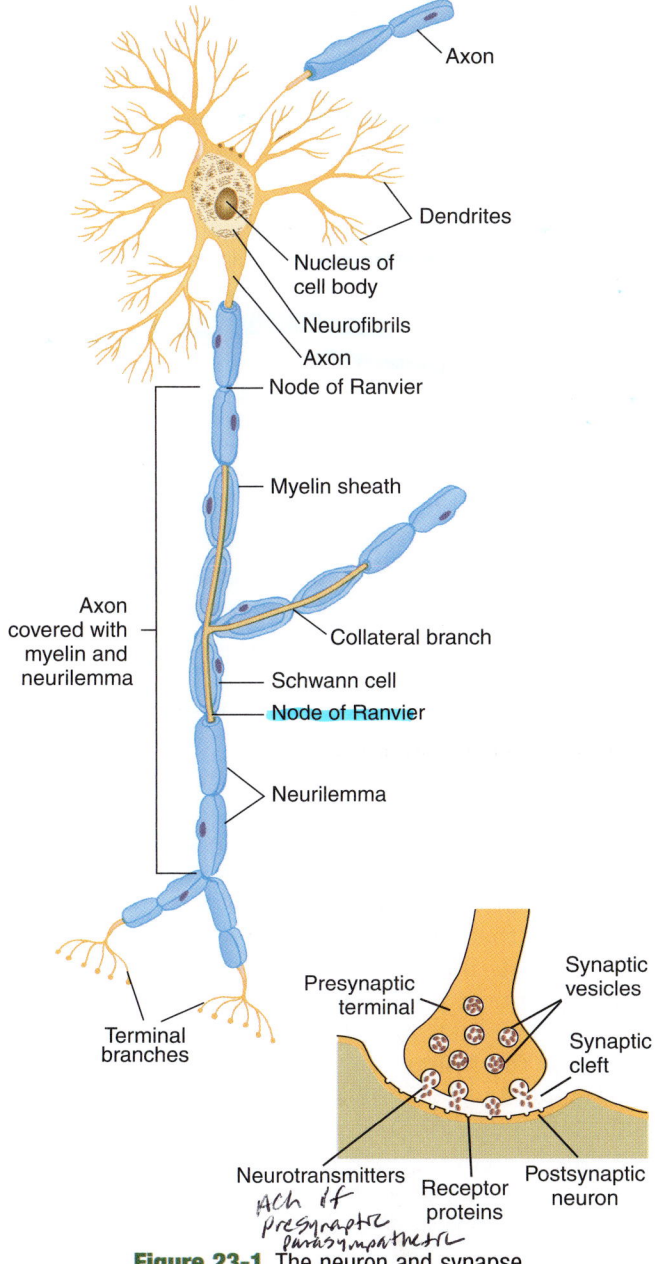

Figure 23-1 The neuron and synapse.

surrounded by a myelin sheath with gaps in the sheath called *nodes of Ranvier*. As the impulse skips from node to node, the speed of transmission is increased compared with traveling the entire axon, as it does in unmyelinated axons, or gray matter.

Nerve cells are classified by the direction in which they transmit impulses. Sensory (afferent) nerves carry impulses from sensory receptors in the internal organs and skin to the brain and spinal cord. Motor (efferent) nerves carry impulses from the central nervous system (CNS) to the viscera, muscles, and glands. Interneurons carry impulses from sensory neurons to motor neurons.

Nerves

Nerves are composed of several neurons bundled within connective tissue. The neurons that compose a nerve are supplied with oxygen and nutrients from the bloodstream by blood vessels also contained in the nerve. Nerves are information highways. Impulses travel to and from the brain and spinal cord along these highways. One such nerve, the sciatic, descends from the lower part of the sacral spinal cord and continues through the muscles of the thigh, leg and foot, with many branches along the way (Anderson & Anderson, 1994).

Nerve Conduction and Neurotransmitters

The end of an axon and the receptors of the target tissue together comprise the **neuroeffector junction.** Nerve cells do not physically touch or connect to each other. Instead, they are separated by a microscopic space called the **synapse** (see Figure 23-1). The neuron sending the impulse is called the *presynaptic neuron.* The target cell receives the signal on the postsynaptic membrane.

Impulses travel through the neuron as electrical energy. Electrical energy is created by the shift of potassium and sodium concentrations within and surrounding the cell. When the impulse reaches the synapse, the presynaptic neuron releases neurotransmitters. A **neurotransmitter** is a chemical that crosses the synapse and attaches to receptor sites on the postsynaptic membrane. Once stimulated, these receptors cause the target tissue to carry out the intended function. Many neurotransmitters are found throughout the body. Table 23-1 lists several common neurotransmitters, their locations, and function. Once the target receptors have been stimulated, the neurotransmitter is released back into the synapse and is usually pulled back into the presynaptic cell to be degraded or reused. This is known as the **reuptake** of neurotransmitters.

Nervous System

The nervous system is composed of two primary divisions: the central and the peripheral nervous systems (Figure 23-2). The central nervous system is composed of

Neurons have three basic parts: dendrites, the cell body, and the axon. **Dendrites** are short, branchlike projections that conduct impulses from nearby cells toward the **cell body.** Essential cell functions, such as energy production and waste removal, are performed within the nucleus of the cell body. Cell bodies form the gray matter in the brain, brainstem, and spinal cord. After being conducted through the cell body, the impulse exits the neuron through the axon. An **axon** is another projection that sends the signal to target tissues or other neurons. Neurons may have dozens of dendrites but usually only one axon. An axon is long and highly branched, allowing it to link with many other cells. Myelinated axons form the white matter in the brain, brainstem, and spinal cord. Recall that these axons are

TABLE 23-1	Neurotransmitters, Locations, and Functions	
Neurotransmitter	**Locations**	**Functions**
Dopamine	CNS: Brain, extrapyramidal system	Brain "reward" system; may play a role in certain mental illnesses and drug addictions
Norepinephrine	CNS: Brain, particularly the reticular activating system PNS: postganglionic sympathetic system	Almost identical in structure to epinephrine; may play a role in certain mental illnesses
Acetylcholine	CNS: motor cortex of brain PNS: all skeletal muscle neuroeffector junctions, preganglionic sympathetic system, entire parasympathetic system	Effects prolonged by organophosphates and nerve gas; receptors destroyed in myasthenia gravis
Gamma-aminobutyric acid (GABA)	CNS only	Mostly inhibitory; hyperpolarizes neurons to prevent them from firing; efficacy increased by benzodiazepines and decreased by alcohol
Glutamate	CNS	Mostly excitatory; widespread in the brain
Serotonin	CNS	May play a role in sleep, appetite, mood regulation

CNS, Central nervous system; *PNS*, peripheral nervous system.

[handwritten notes] Nicotinic—skeletal muscles muscarinic—organs   MAOIs inhibit epi, norepi, serotonin

Central Nervous System

Brain. The brain is the primary organ of the nervous system. It is the control center for nearly all the body's functions. The brain is fully enclosed and well protected by the cranium. The **cranium** is the vaultlike portion of the skull behind and above the face. Although the brain only comprises 2% of the body's weight, it uses almost 20% of the body's cardiac output at any given time. The brain is supplied with blood by the carotid and vertebral arteries, which are primarily joined at the circle of Willis. In this area a dense network of capillaries allows only certain molecules into the brain's blood circulation, forming the **blood-brain barrier.** This filter prevents most drugs from acting directly on brain neurons.

At birth the typical brain contains approximately 100 billion nerve cells. This number declines with age. Each neuron may have thousands or tens of thousands of synapses, making the brain a highly complex organ (Ramachandran, 1998). It is divided according to structure and function into three main regions: the cerebrum, the brainstem (composed of the diencephalon, mesencephalon, pons, and medulla oblongata), and the cerebellum (Figure 23-3).

Cerebrum (Telencephalon). The outermost portion of the brain is called the **cerebrum.** Gray in appearance, it is approximately 2 to 6 mm thick. The cerebrum is rich with neurons. The tissue of the cerebrum folds onto itself and forms elevations (gyri) and depressions (sulci) to maximize surface area. The cerebrum is divided by a deep groove called the longitudinal fissure. This division runs down the center of the brain, from anterior to posterior, and divides the cerebrum into the left and right hemispheres (Weiderholt, 2000).

The outermost portion of the cerebrum is called the *cerebral cortex.* Each hemisphere is further divided into four lobes: the frontal, temporal, parietal, and occipital (see Figure 23-3, *A*). The lobes are named for the cranial bones that cover them. The **frontal lobe** extends from the anterior cerebrum and continues roughly halfway to the rear of the brain. This area regulates many important functions, including speech, abstract thinking, and personality. The **sensory cortex** is a narrow strip of the frontal lobe where tactile (touch) information from the body is received and processed. Directly beside it lies the **motor cortex,** which controls much of the voluntary muscle movement of the body. The right cortex controls the left half of the body and vice versa as a result of the path that the signals follow when exiting the brain.

Behind and inferior to the frontal lobe lies the **temporal lobe.** Here impulses from the ears are received and then processed into sounds. One portion of the temporal lobe, Wernicke's area, is the brain's center for understanding speech.

Directly above the temporal lobe lies the **parietal lobe.** This area also contains functions related to speech. In addition, the sense of body positioning (proprioception) is regulated within the parietal lobe. When you raise your arm above your head, you know the location of your arm because of parietal lobe activity.

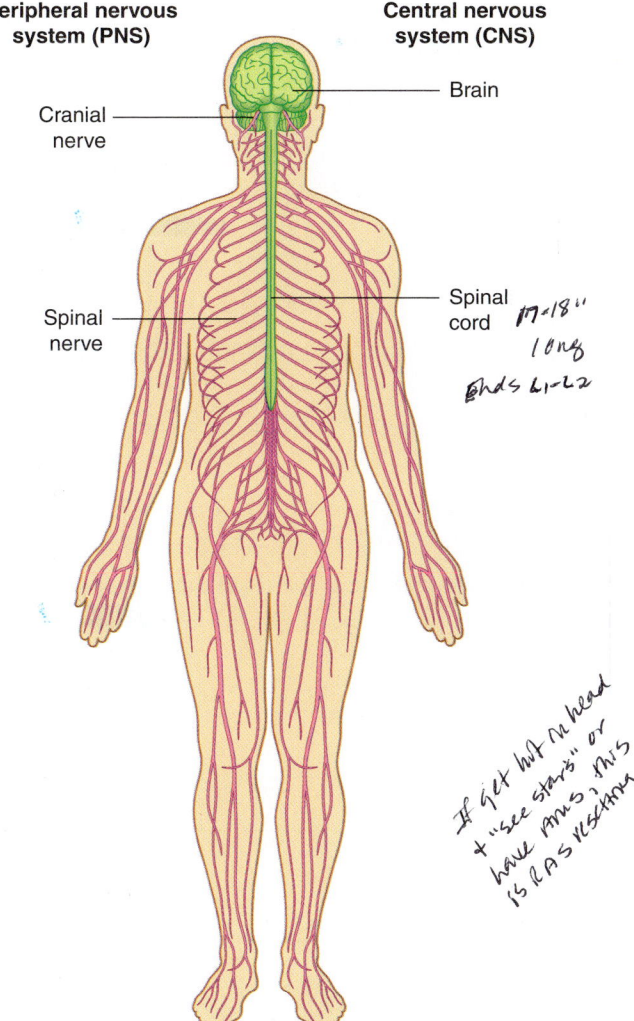

Peripheral nervous
system (PNS)

Central nervous
system (CNS)

Cranial
nerve

Brain

Spinal
nerve

Spinal
cord 17-18"
long
Ends L1-L2

If get hit in head
+ "see stars" or
have PNS, this
is RAS resetting

Figure 23-2 The central and peripheral nervous systems.

Body to brain → afferent (Sensory)
Brain to body → efferent

The most posterior portion of the cerebrum is the **occipital lobe.** The primary function of this lobe is to process information from the optic nerve (cranial nerve [CN] II) and form the sense of sight.

Brainstem. The **brainstem** is composed of the diencephalon, midbrain, pons, and medulla oblongata (see Figure 23-3, *B*). The **diencephalon** is the uppermost portion of the brainstem. It is hidden from view beneath the cerebrum and contains the thalamus and hypothalamus. The **thalamus,** found at the anterior portion of the diencephalon, is the sensory switchboard. All sensory information (except the sense of smell) is routed through here to the sensory cortex. Below the thalamus is the **hypothalamus,** which regulates much of the body's vital functions, including core temperature and hormone release. This part of the brain plays a large role in regulating the pituitary gland, which is attached to the hypothalamus and releases hormones that control much of the endocrine system. Because of its numerous regulatory functions, the hypothalamus often is called the seat of the autonomic nervous system and is further discussed

later in this chapter. By using the endocrine and nervous systems, the hypothalamus is the primary mechanism maintaining homeostasis in the body (Weiderholt, 2000). These structures and others in this portion of the brain form the limbic system, which has a significant role in emotions and psychiatric illness.

Residing below the diencephalon are the **midbrain (mesencephalon)** and the **pons (metencephalon).** This area acts as a bridge between the brainstem and the upper portions of the brain. In addition, many of the cranial nerves terminate within the midbrain.

The most inferior portion of the brain is known as the **medulla oblongata (myelencephalon).** Although it appears to be part of the spinal cord, it is structurally different and ends at the **foramen magnum.** Basic regulation of essential life functions occurs here, including heart rate, breathing, and blood pressure.

Reticular Formation. No single place in the brain is responsible for maintaining consciousness. This function is performed by a group of approximately 100 neuronal nuclei scattered throughout the midbrain and hindbrain. These nuclei collectively are called the **reticular formation,** or the reticular activating system. Sensory axons from many different sources, particularly the cranial nerves, send impulses into the reticular formation. The reticular formation filters and then sends impulses that excite the cerebrum and keep the body awake (Ramachandran, 1998). Consciousness is maintained by the interaction of the reticular formation and the cerebral cortex. Disruption of either of these causes an altered level of consciousness. Disruptions in both, or a loss of connection between the two, results in unconsciousness.

Cerebellum. The lower, most posterior portion of the brain is called the **cerebellum** (see Figure 23-3). Similar in size and shape to two large walnuts, the cerebellum fine tunes motor control, allowing movements to be smooth and flowing. The jerky tremors of patients with Parkinson's disease are an example of dysfunction within this area.

Spinal Cord. Roughly cylindrical in shape, the **spinal cord** runs from the foramen magnum, at the base of the skull, to the level of the first or second lumbar vertebra. It is housed within the vertebral canal, a tunnel formed down the centers of the bony vertebrae that protect the cord and provide support for the spinal arteries that supply the neurons of the cord.

Impulses travel up and down the spinal cord in a line. Any injury to the cord disrupts transmission and may completely block all impulses traveling to or from nerves below the injury. Once spinal tissue is damaged, the body cannot repair it. Therefore most spinal cord injuries are devastating and permanent. All impulses to and from the brain must travel through the spinal cord, except those transmitted by the cranial nerves (Weiderholt, 2000).

Meninges. The **meninges** are three layered connective tissue coverings that surround, protect, and suspend the brain and spinal cord in the cranium and spinal canal

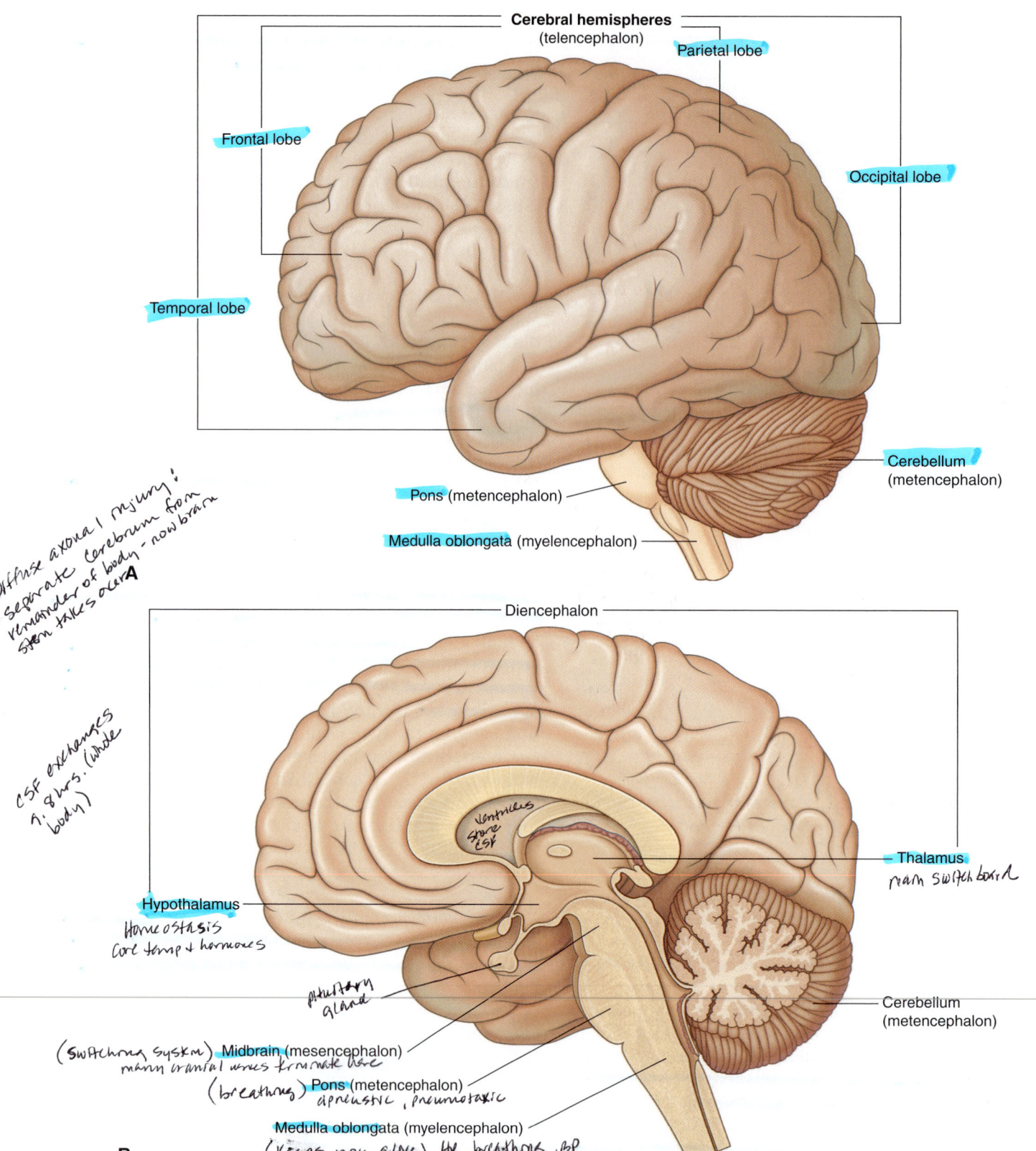

Handwritten notes (left margin, top):
Diffuse axonal injury:
- Separate cerebrum from remainder of body - now brain stem takes over

Handwritten notes (left margin, middle):
CSF exchanges
~ 8 hrs. (whole body)

Handwritten notes near Hypothalamus:
Homeostasis
Core temp + hormones

Handwritten note near ventricles:
Ventricles store CSF

Handwritten note near Thalamus:
main switchboard

Handwritten note near pituitary:
Pituitary gland

Handwritten notes near Midbrain:
(switching system)
many cranial nerves terminate here

Handwritten notes near Pons:
(breathing)
apneustic, pneumotaxic

Handwritten notes near Medulla:
(keeps you alive) HR, breathing, BP

Figure 23-3 The brain. **A,** Each hemisphere is further divided into four lobes: the frontal, temporal, parietal, and occipital. **B,** The brainstem is composed of the diencephalon, midbrain, pons, and medulla oblongata.

Handwritten notes (bottom):
Brain takes 20% of O2 output, uses 15% of glucose
Is only 2-3% of BW

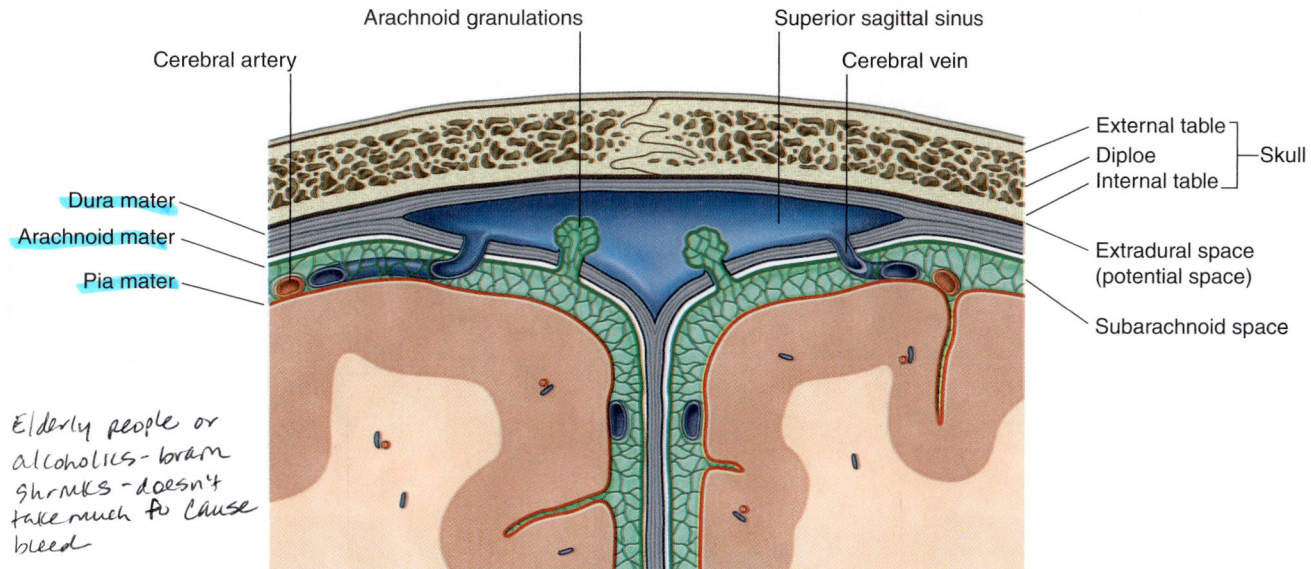

Cerebral artery

Arachnoid granulations

Superior sagittal sinus

Cerebral vein

External table
Diploe
Internal table
Skull

Dura mater

Arachnoid mater

Pia mater

Extradural space
(potential space)

Subarachnoid space

[handwritten note: Elderly people or alcoholics - brain shrinks - doesn't take much to cause bleed]

Figure 23-4 The meninges.

(Drake, 2005). The outermost layer is the dura mater, which is on top of the arachnoid membrane, which is above the pia mater (Figure 23-4).

The **dura mater** is the thickest of the meninges. It is fused to the inside of the cranium, but once inside the vertebral canal it is detached and flexible. This prevents injury to the dura mater when the spine moves.

Beneath the dura mater is the **arachnoid membrane,** a thin, delicate, weblike tissue. This web runs between the dura mater and the pia mater and forms the subarachnoid space. **Cerebrospinal fluid (CSF)** is a clear, watery fluid that circulates beneath the arachnoid membrane and bathes the brain and spinal cord. This bath of CSF cushions and provides some nutrients to the CNS. Large blood vessels supplying the CNS also run through this space, and bleeding into this area can be rapidly fatal.

Below the subarachnoid space is the **pia mater,** a thin, vascular membrane that firmly attaches to the brain and spinal cord (Drake, 2005).

Peripheral Nervous System

Any nervous tissue not part of the brain or spinal cord is considered part of the **peripheral nervous system.** The nerves of the peripheral nervous system can be divided by function into two categories: somatic nerves and visceral nerves.

Somatic Nerves. The **somatic** *[handwritten: voluntary]* (from the Greek *soma,* meaning *body*) part of the nervous system innervates the skin and most of the skeletal muscle. It is mainly involved with sensing and responding to information from the external environment. Most somatic nerves in the body originate at the spinal cord and are therefore called **spinal nerves** (Figure 23-5). Each spinal nerve is formed from the spinal cord by two roots. The posterior root contains the sensory (afferent) processes. These are impulses travel-

ing from the body to the CNS. The anterior root carries motor (efferent) processes. These are impulses traveling from the central nervous system to muscles and glands. The following 31 pairs of spinal nerves are named for their position in relation to the vertebrae:

- Eight cervical nerves: C1 to C8
- Twelve thoracic nerves: T1 to T12
- Five lumbar nerves: L1 to L5
- Five sacral nerves: S1 to S5
- One coccygeal nerve: Co

Each sensory spinal nerve carries sensory information from a specific area of skin on the surface of the body. These areas, known as **dermatomes,** correspond to specific spinal nerves at various levels (Figure 23-6). Testing sensation of the dermatomes can be useful when assessing a spinal cord injury (discussed in depth later in this chapter). In the same manner, **myotomes** are portions of muscle tissue controlled by their corresponding spinal nerves. Myotomes are more difficult to assess because many muscles are controlled by more than one spinal nerve.

Visceral Nerves. The body's internal environment is monitored and controlled by the **visceral** (from the Greek *viscera,* meaning *guts*) portion of the peripheral nervous system. These nerves innervate the organ systems and other related elements, such as smooth muscle and glands. Unlike somatic nerves, visceral nerves often follow indirect paths to the CNS, which is why pain originating from organs often is felt in other locations throughout the body.

Some visceral nerves play roles in the **autonomic nervous system (ANS),** which controls many of the automatic functions of the body. These functions include heart rate, blood pressure, and digestion. The ANS is divided into two opposing parts: the sympathetic and the parasympathetic divisions.

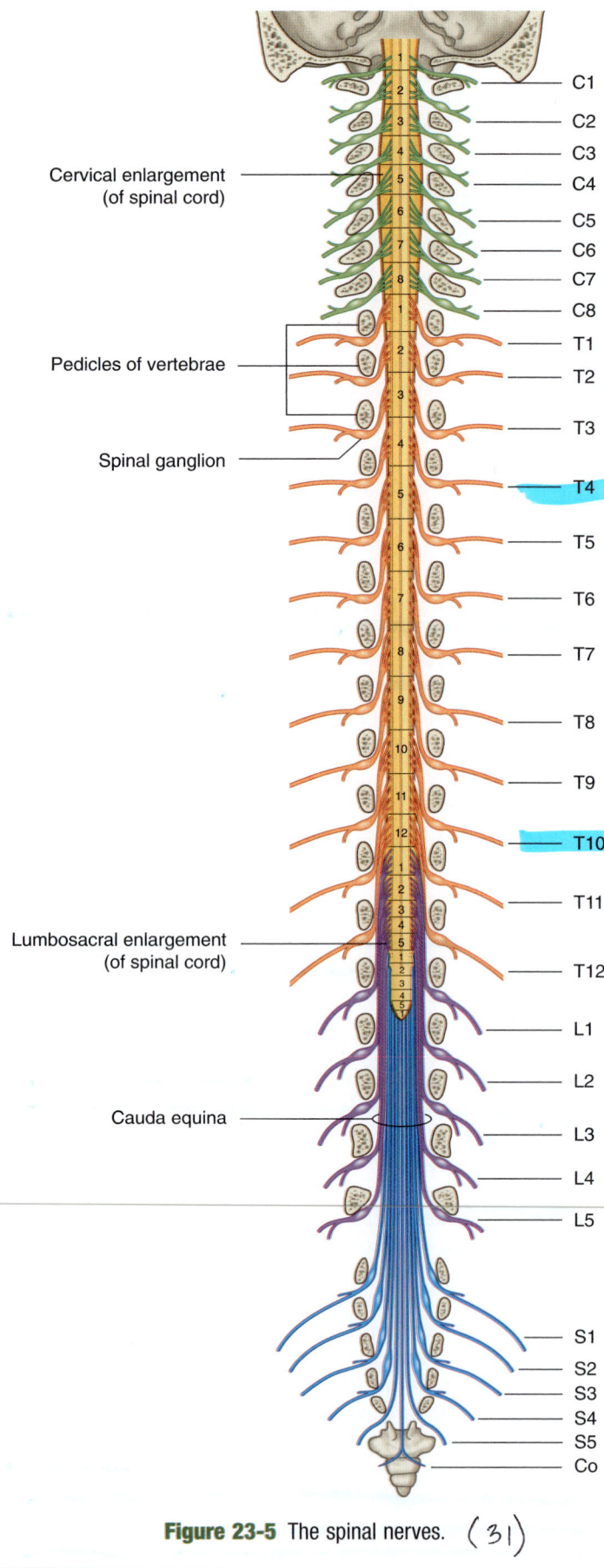

Cervical enlargement
(of spinal cord)

Pedicles of vertebrae

Spinal ganglion

Lumbosacral enlargement
(of spinal cord)

Cauda equina

C1
C2
C3
C4
C5
C6
C7
C8
T1
T2
T3
T4 — *Nipple line*
T5
T6
T7
T8
T9
T10 — *Belly button*
T11
T12
L1
L2
L3
L4
L5
S1
S2
S3
S4
S5
Co

Figure 23-5 The spinal nerves. (31)

Figure 23-6 Map of the dermatomes.

Stimulation of the **sympathetic division** of the ANS results in the fight-or-flight response designed to prepare the body for stress, such as running away or fighting with an enemy (Figure 23-7). During the fight-or-flight response heart rate increases, blood is shunted from the skin to the muscles, and the bronchi and pupils dilate. Most of the sympathetic division originates from the thoracic spinal nerves, between T1 and L2 (Weiderholt, 2000).

The **parasympathetic division** causes responses opposite those of the sympathetic division (Figure 23-8). These include decreased heart rate, bronchoconstriction, and increased blood flow to the gastrointestinal tract. This often is known as the "rest and digest" response. The parasympathetic division is composed of several cranial nerves (CN III, VII, IX, and X, discussed below) and some of the spinal nerves (S2 to S4) that exit the sacrum (Weiderholt, 2000).

Cranial Nerves. Exiting the cranium through small holes (fissures) are 12 pairs of **cranial nerves.** Although they are considered part of the peripheral nervous system, all but one of these nerves (CN XI) originates from the brain itself. The cranial nerves demonstrate somatic and visceral properties similar to the spinal nerves. However, they also must transmit some special sensory information, such as the senses of sight, hearing, balance, smell,

Peripheral

Organs

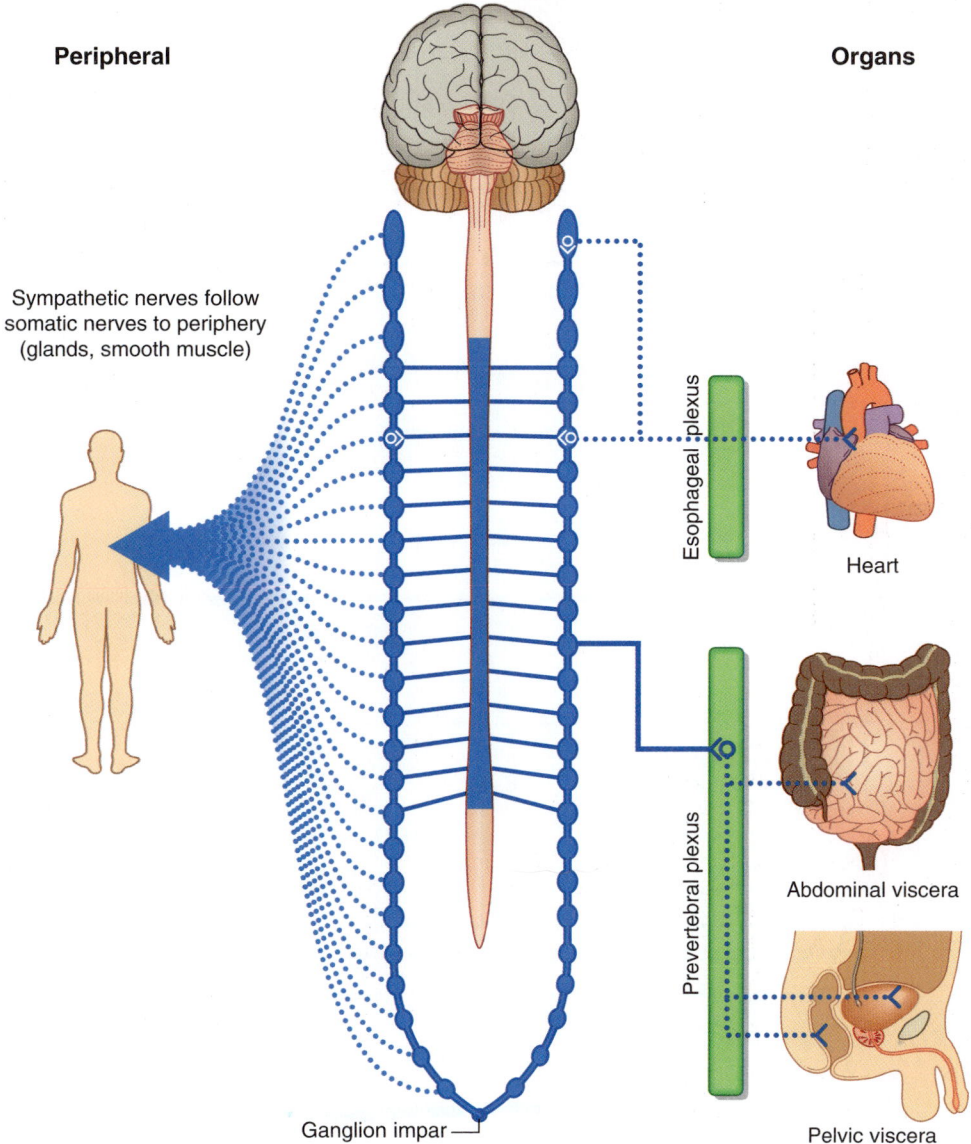

Sympathetic nerves follow somatic nerves to periphery (glands, smooth muscle)

Esophageal plexus

Heart

Prevertebral plexus

Abdominal viscera

Pelvic viscera

Ganglion impar

Figure 23-7 Sympathetic nerve roots.

and taste. These nerves also innervate the muscles of the eye, face, neck, shoulders, tongue, and pharynx. Unlike spinal nerves, some of the cranial nerves have sensory and motor function. Table 23-2 lists the 12 cranial nerves and their functions.

PARAMEDIC *Pearl*

Cranial nerves exit the skull through the TOES bones:

Temporal
Occipital
Ethmoid
Sphenoid

Reprinted from Schulte, J. L. (2005). *Easy memory system for EMS.* Taneytown, MD: Emergency Publishers.

ASSESSMENT OF THE NEUROLOGIC SYSTEM

[OBJECTIVE 2]

Careful assessment of the neurologic system is essential to recognize subtle presentations of potentially serious conditions. Perform the full neurologic assessment if your patient has or has had the following:

- Altered mental status
- A loss of consciousness (for any length of time)
- A loss or alteration of strength or sensation
- A loss of function of an extremity

The neurologic examination has the following components:

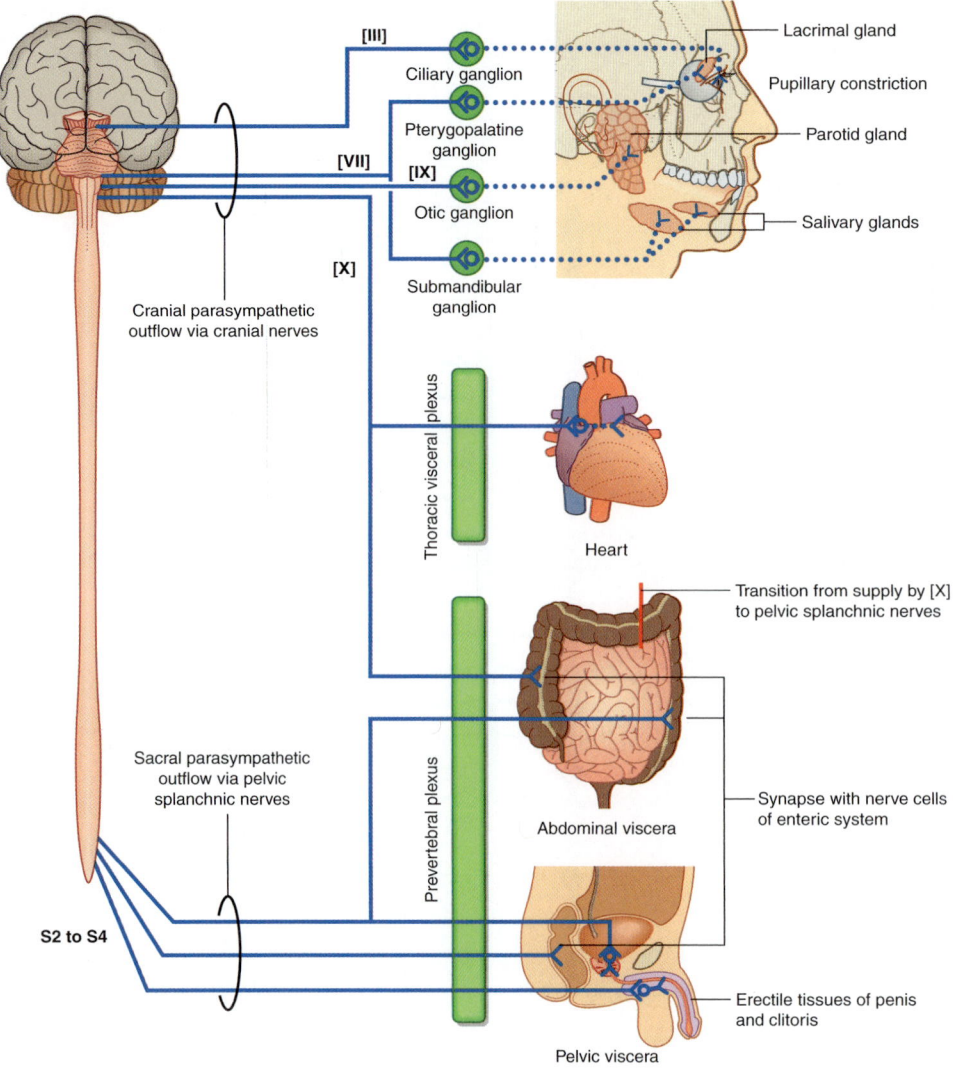

Figure 23-8 Parasympathetic nerve roots.

- Posture and gait
- Mental status
- Cranial nerves examination
- Spinal nerves examination
- Deep tendon reflexes
- Meningeal examination
- Glasgow Coma Scale

As you perform a neurologic examination, remember that your main goal is to find focal deficits. **Focal deficits** are absent or altered functions or sensations in a part of the body. They suggest damage or injury to a part of the nervous system. Pinpointing the locations of these deficits is vital to determining the causes of a patient's symptoms.

Posture and Gait

[OBJECTIVE 3]
Assessment begins as you approach the patient. Note the position in which the patient is sitting or lying. Is the patient able to sit up straight without leaning or falling?

Does he or she appear to have any involuntary movements or tremors? Observe the patient's muscle tone in the face and arms. Does one side appear to lack muscle tone? Are the normal creases (forehead and upper lip) of the face present (Boskeret et al., 1996)?

If feasible, have the patient walk across a room. This should *not* be attempted if the patient has a gross neurologic deficit, in cases of trauma, if the patient is in respiratory distress or has chest discomfort, or if the patient cannot or has trouble walking normally. Watch the patient's gait. Note whether the patient favors one leg, has an odd or wide-based stance, or appears to walk with a limp.

Patients with severe neurologic injury and dysfunction may exhibit posturing (abnormal positioning). The two types of posturing are flexion and extension. **Flexion posturing (decorticate)** occurs when an injury to the cerebrum has occurred. It manifests as a bending of the arms at the elbow, with the patient's arms pulled upward to the chest and hands turned downward at the wrists (Figure 23-9). Injury to the brainstem often presents with

TABLE 23-2 Cranial Nerve Functions

	Nerve	Function
I	Olfactory	(S) Sense of smell
II	Optic	(S) Sense of sight
III	Oculomotor	(M) Eye movement, pupil constriction
IV	Trochlear	(M) Downward gaze
V	Trigeminal	(S) Facial sensation, branching to the forehead (ophthalmic), cheek (maxillary division), and lower jaw (mandibular division) (M) Chewing
VI	Abducens	(M) Lateral eye movement
VII	Facial	(M) Secretion of saliva, facial expressions (S) Taste
VIII	Acoustic	(S) Senses of hearing and balance
IX	Glossopharyngeal	(M) Muscles of swallowing and gag reflex (S) Taste and sensation from posterior tongue and pharynx
X	Vagus	(M) Decreases heart rate, increases peristalsis, contracts muscles for voice production (S) Receives taste information, sensation from the back of the throat, sensation in the larynx and trachea, and stretch receptors in the gut
XI	Spinal accessory	(M) Shoulder movements, turning movements of head, movements of viscera
XII	Hypoglossal	(M) Tongue movements

Inferior MI ↓HR, nausea [handwritten]

M, Motor; *S,* sensory.

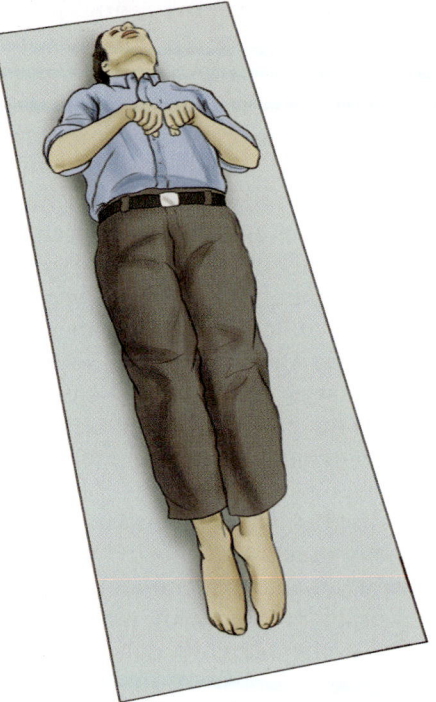

Figure 23-9 Flexion (decorticate) posturing.

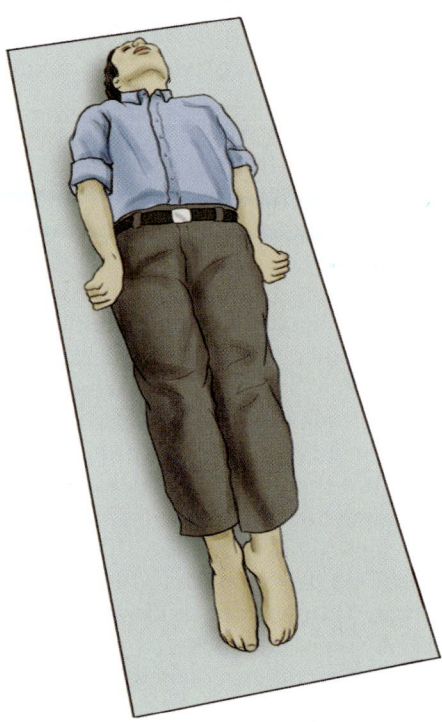

Figure 23-10 Extension (decerebrate) posturing.

extension posturing (decerebrate), in which the patient's arms are at the side, with the wrists turned outward (Figure 23-10). Both types of posturing show downward pointing of the feet and toes and hyperextension of the neck.

Mental Status *1st thing you see if conscious* [handwritten]

[OBJECTIVE 3]

Assessing a patient's mental status includes examining the patient's mental state as well as level of consciousness. The AVPU scale is useful for quickly determining a

✳

patient's level of responsiveness during the initial assessment. After the initial assessment, a more global survey of the patient's mental status should be performed and then summarized with the Glasgow Coma Scale.

First look at the patient's general appearance, including hygiene, clothing, and dress. Given the patient's living arrangements, is the patient's presentation normal and appropriate? Does the patient appear to be able to care for himself or herself? Why or why not?

While you ask the patient about the present illness, note the patient's speech. Does the patient speak slowly and with difficulty? Or is the patient's speech rapid and pressured, as if the patient believes he or she must continue talking? Is the patient's speech clear and coherent? Patients with previous neurologic problems, such as a stroke, may have some residual neurologic deficit. Thus be sure to ask the patient or the patient's family how the patient normally speaks and acts.

Remember that many neurologic and psychiatric emergencies often present with similar symptoms. In these situations, the patient's emotional state should be assessed. **Affect** is the combination of facial and body expressions of a patient's mood as judged by you, the healthcare professional. Does the patient appear elated, smiling, and filled with joyful energy? Or perhaps the patient appears depressed—talking very little, not making eye contact, and speaking in a monotone voice. You do not need to go into much depth when assessing a patient's affect. A one- or two-word description will suffice.

Flat affect

While asking the patient questions about the current illness or injury, you have an opportunity to assess **form of thought.** Do the patient's ideas and thoughts seem logical, or does the patient make jumps in thought that do not make sense? Can the patient organize his or her thoughts into a logical structure that you can understand? Does the patient answer the questions you ask, or does he or she often stray off the topic?

What is the patient's **thought content?** Is the patient having hallucinations or delusions? **Hallucinations** are false sensory perceptions, such as hearing voices or seeing things that are not there. **Delusions** are false ideas about situations. A man who believes he is from another planet and has been sent here to study Earthlings is delusional. A woman who sees flying saucers when no one else does is hallucinating. Thought content also includes any preoccupations. A **preoccupation** is a recurrent idea or thought that comes up in conversation over and over again.

Is the patient oriented? You often will hear that a patient is "alert and oriented times four," meaning that the patient is oriented to person, place, time, and event. Assess orientation to person by asking the patient for his or her full name. Orientation to place is best determined by asking specific questions, such as "What city are we in right now?" or "What state is this?" Avoid being too general by asking "Where are you right now?" because this can yield many nonspecific answers and often is a

waste of time. Assess the patient's orientation to time. Start specific and ask the patient if he or she knows the current date. Bear in mind, however, that many people do not keep track of the date or day of the week and may not be able to give a correct answer even though they are neurologically intact. If not, ask what the current month or season is, either of which most people should readily know. Assess the patient's orientation to the event by asking him or her to tell you what happened.

Briefly assess the patient's memory. Attempt to test three different types of memory: hold-function, recent, and remote. These terms are relative, which can lead to some confusion. No clear definition exists to describe when hold-function memory becomes recent memory, or when recent becomes remote. In general, hold-function memory is considered to be events that just happened within the past few seconds. This can be tested by telling the patient three words (e.g., dog, cucumber, house) and then having the patient immediately repeat those words back to you. Recent memory is of events that happened within an hour or two. This can be tested easily by waiting 5 minutes or so after testing hold-function memory and then asking the patient to repeat those same three words back to you. Patients often have some trouble doing this, but if given choices of words, the patient is usually able to choose the correct ones quickly. Finally, remote memory is anything in the more distant past, including the events of the previous day to childhood memories. This is best assessed by asking the patient about significant national and international events that may have occurred in the past few years. Loss of remote memory indicates widespread and severe brain dysfunction (Weiderholt, 2000).

Examination of the Cranial Nerves

[OBJECTIVE 3]

At first, the cranial nerve examination may seem cumbersome and time consuming. With a little practice, however, it is a quick and easy tool that can provide a great deal of information about the patient's brain function. Although 12 pairs of cranial nerves are present in the body, many of them are tested simultaneously. Be sure to test the left and right sides separately when possible so a comparison of the two can be made.

ammonia

The olfactory nerve, or CN I, transmits the sense of smell to the brain. To test CN I, simply ask the patient to close their eyes. Then take an alcohol wipe and hold it approximately 1 to 2 inches (3 to 5 cm) from the patient's face (Figure 23-11). Wait for several seconds, then ask what the patient smells. This test should not be performed if the patient is taking disulfiram (Antabuse). Be aware that the patient may normally have a poor sense of smell, particularly if he or she is elderly or a tobacco smoker. Inability to smell is most often caused by blockage of the nasal passages, not nerve dysfunction (Weiderholt, 2000). The olfactory nerve often is not tested in the prehospital environment.

CN II, the optic nerve, carries only the sense of sight. To test CN II, ask the patient to cover one eye with the hand (Figure 23-12). Then hold up two fingers and ask the patient how many he or she sees. Repeat with the other eye. Ask about and note findings such as blindness, blurry vision, or double vision.

CN III, IV, and VI can be assessed simultaneously because they work together to control the movements of the eye (Figure 23-13). Hold your index finger upright approximately 4 inches (10 cm) in front of the patient's face. Instruct the patient to follow your finger using only his or her eyes. The patient must not move the head during the examination. Slowly move your finger right to left and up and down in an H pattern, making sure to include the far corners of the patient's eyes. Then come back to the center of the H and slowly move your finger toward the patient's nose. Both eyes should begin to look toward each other. Look for any asymmetry in the movement of the eyes. Also note any sluggish or delayed movements.

CN III, the oculomotor nerve, also is responsible for pupillary constriction and movement of the eye. Try to minimize any bright environmental lights, such as the lights inside the ambulance, then ask the patient to stare directly at your nose. Bring a penlight toward the eye from the patient's side and watch the pupil constrict as the light shines on the eye. If you are in a bright environment, try shading the patient's eyes with your hand and look for the pupils to dilate. Test each side individually and then compare the two. Pupil size ranges from 1 to 6 mm. Normal pupil constriction should be brisk and

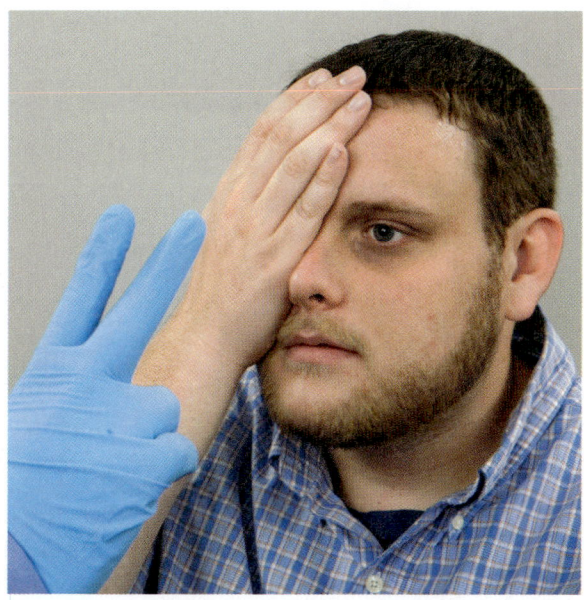

Figure 23-12 Test cranial nerve II by assessing the extent of the patient's peripheral vision.

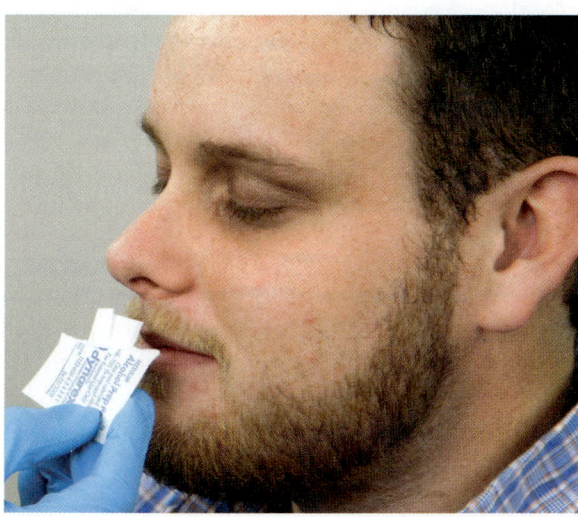

Figure 23-11 Test cranial nerve I by evaluating the patient's sense of smell.

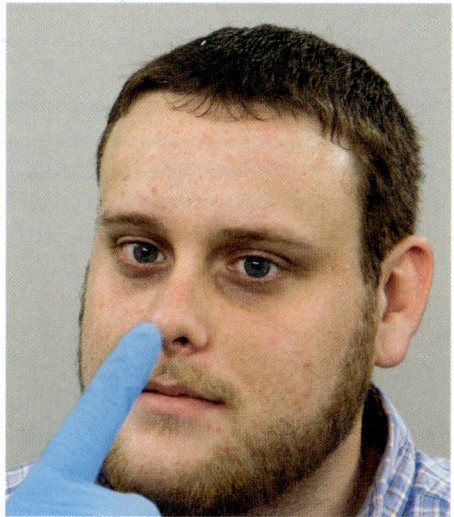

Figure 23-13 Monitoring eye movement evaluates cranial nerves III, IV, and VI.

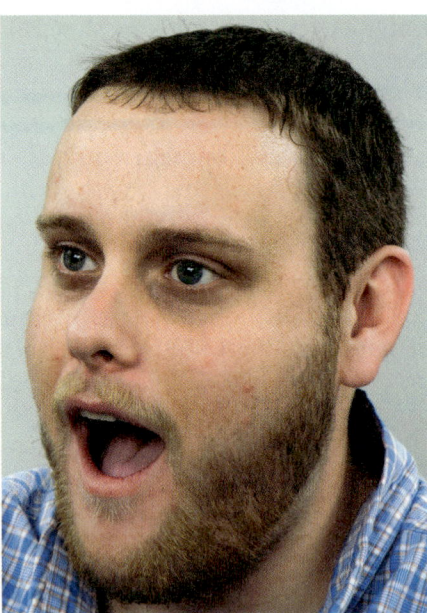

Figure 23-14 Test motor function of cranial nerve V by asking the patient to open and close the mouth.

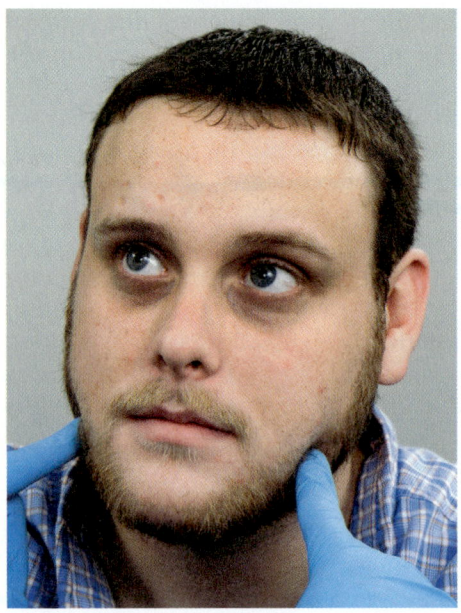

Figure 23-15 Asking the patient to discriminate between sharp and dull sensation on the face evaluates sensation in cranial nerve V.

VII - affected by Bell's Palsy - can wrinkle forehead - If can't wrinkle it → Stroke

equal. When the light is shined on one pupil, the other pupil should constrict at the same time (consensual response). Abnormal findings include a pupil that is dilated, constricted, sluggish, or fixed (does not constrict). Bear in mind, however, that a small percentage of the population normally has unequal pupils (anisocoria), though the difference should be less than 1 mm and the patient most likely will be aware of this condition before-hand. Constricted, pinpoint pupils may indicate an over-dose of opiate drugs or damage to the pons. Dilated pupils may be caused by panic or anxiety, seizures, or the use of stimulant drugs such as cocaine or methamphet-amines. A sluggish or fixed pupil often is seen in the patient with brain injury or swelling. This is typically caused by compression of the oculomotor nerve, which runs along the floor of the cranium.

The trigeminal nerve, CN V, has both motor and sensory components. It provides motor control of the muscles of the lower jaw, which you can test simply by asking the patient to open and close the mouth (Figure 23-14). The patient should be able to do this without difficulty. The trigeminal nerve also provides most of the sensation for the face and has three branches that inner-vate the forehead (ophthalmic), the upper lip (maxillary), and the lower jaw (mandibular). Apply a light touch with your fingers on both sides of the patient's face at the same time, moving through each of those areas (Figure 23-15). The patient should feel your touch equally on both sides.

CN VII, the facial nerve, provides most of the motor control of the facial muscles. You can assess this while interviewing the patient. Observe the patient's facial

muscles while he or she is speaking. Are facial move-ments asymmetric? Does one side droop? Ask the patient to smile and raise the eyebrows, then puff out the cheeks like a blowfish. Any asymmetry should be considered abnormal. Impairment of the facial nerve often is a sign of a stroke at the middle cerebral artery.

Place both of your hands approximately $1^1/_2$ inches (4 cm) away from each of the patient's ears. Gently rub together your index finger and thumb on one hand and then the other. Ask the patient to say "right" or "left," depending on which side he or she hears the rubbing (Figure 23-16). This tests the acoustic nerve, CN VIII, which is responsible for the sense of hearing.

Cranial nerves IX and X, the glossopharyngeal and vagus nerves, respectively, control the muscles of the pharynx, soft palate, and larynx. Ask the patient to open the mouth; while looking inside with a penlight, ask the patient to say "ah" (Figure 23-17). Observe the muscles of the pharynx. The soft palate should move upward symmetrically and the uvula should remain midline. The muscles on either side of the pharynx should constrict medially, like a curtain. If CN IX is not functioning nor-mally, the uvula will be pulled to the side opposite the affected area. For example, a stroke affecting CN IX on the left side will cause the uvula to be pulled to the right.

Gag reflex tests also can be used to evaluate the func-tion of CN X. However, on a conscious patient this is painful and unnecessary. Also note that a significant portion of the population normally has a diminished or absent gag reflex. If done, use a tongue depressor to stimulate the posterior portion of the tongue gently. Do

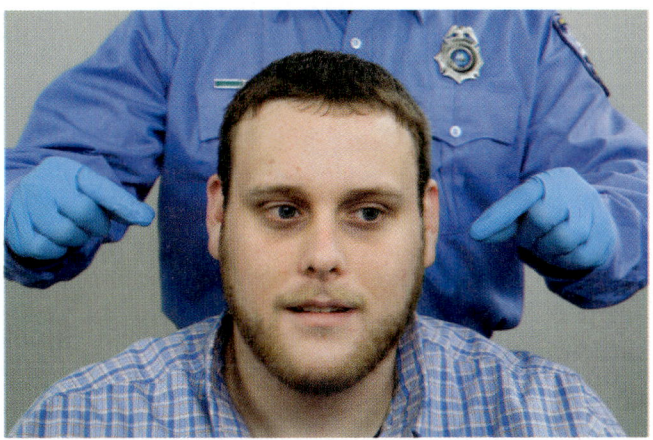

Figure 23-16 To test cranial nerve VIII, gently rub your index finger and thumb of one hand together, then the other, in front of the patient's ears. Ask the patient to say "right" or "left," depending on which side he hears the rubbing.

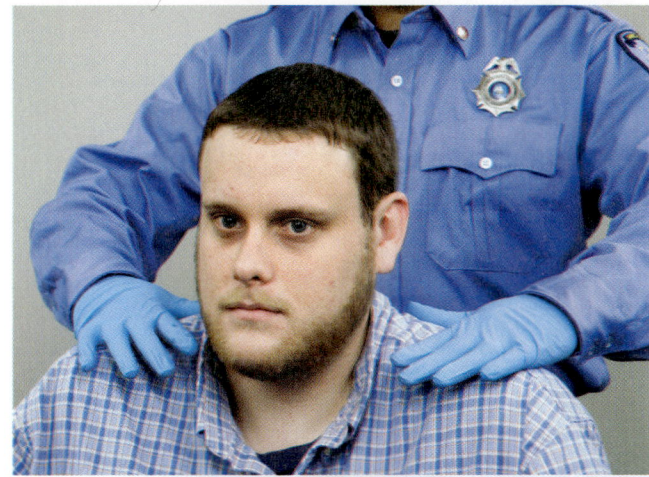

A

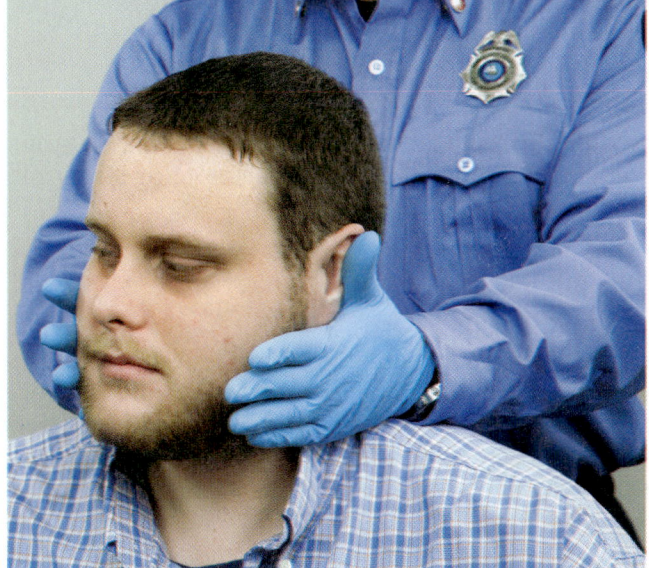

B

Figure 23-18 To evaluate cranial nerve XI, place your hand on top of the patient's shoulder and apply gentle resistance as the patient shrugs the shoulders upward. Then have the patient turn his head to one side and then back toward the center against gentle resistance.

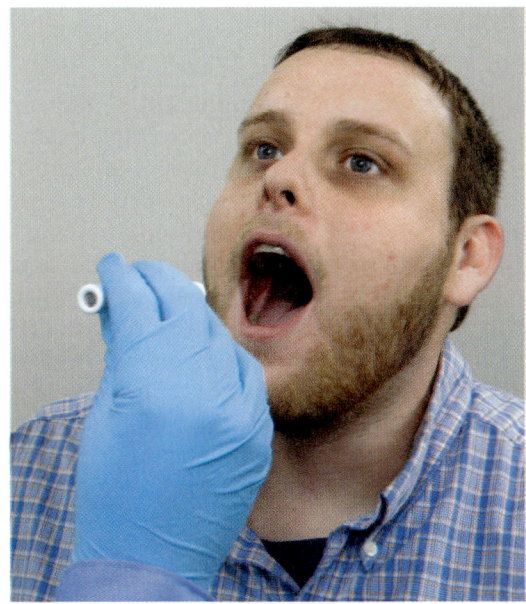

Figure 23-17 To test cranial nerves IX and X, ask the patient to open the mouth; while looking inside with a penlight, ask the patient to say "ah." Observe the muscles of the pharynx.

not attempt to place anything past this point because you may cause pharyngeal trauma or a choking hazard. Remember that the physiologic purpose of the gag reflex is to induce vomiting. If you decide to test the gag reflex, be prepared for the result.

The spinal accessory nerve, CN XI, controls the trapezius muscles of the shoulders and the sternocleidomastoid muscles of the neck. To assess, place your hand on top of the patient's shoulder and apply gentle resistance as the patient shrugs the shoulders upward. Then have the patient turn his or her head to one side and then back

toward the center against gentle resistance. Evaluate for equal strength in these muscles on both sides (Figure 23-18).

Finally, assess CN XII, the hypoglossal nerve, which controls most of the movement of the tongue. Have the patient open the mouth and stick out the tongue, then move it from side to side and up and down (Figure 23-19). Note if the tongue seems to pull to one side or does not demonstrate smooth, fluid movement.

Sensory Examination

[OBJECTIVE 3]

Palpate down the body, checking the patient's dermatomes bilaterally at the same time. Verify that the patient can feel your touch at each point. Anytime you discover

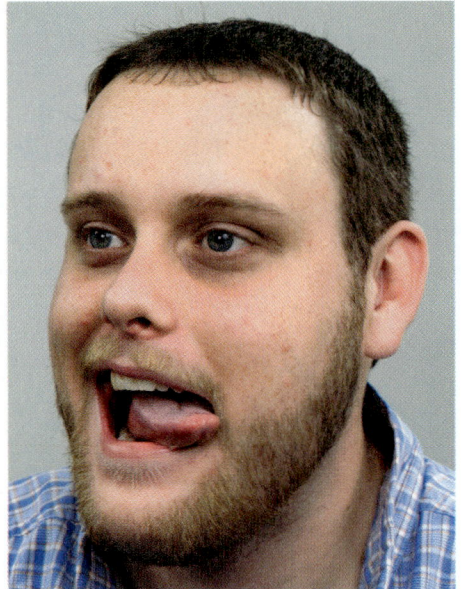

Figure 23-19 To assess cranial nerve XII, have the patient open the mouth and stick out his tongue, then move it from side to side and then up and down.

Look back at C spine notes

an area of decreased sensation, evaluate each side separately to determine if the problem is on one or both sides. The patient may report a complete lack of sensation **(anesthesia)** or a "pins and needles" sensation **(paresthesia).**

PARAMEDIC*Pearl*

You should be familiar with the chart of dermatomes, although a few shortcuts can help you quickly remember certain areas:

- Nipple line (male): T5
- Umbilicus: T10
- Great toe: L5

Motor Examination

[OBJECTIVE 3]

Check all the major muscle groups for strength, testing both sides at the same time for comparison. Weakness on one side may be caused by a problem with the brain, the spinal nerve, or the muscle itself, but it should be noted. Perform strength tests at the shoulders (covered under the cranial nerve examination), elbows, wrists, hands, hips, knees, and ankles. The term *weakness* means a lack of muscle strength. However, patients often use this word to describe lethargy, fatigue, or a general lack of energy. Be aware of this when assessing a patient's symptoms. Ask specific questions such as, "Can you stand up from

TABLE 23-3	Deep Tendon Reflexes
Area Assessed	**Expected Response**
Biceps	The arm should flex slightly
Brachioradialis tendon	The palm should turn upward as the forearm rotates laterally
Triceps	The arm should extend at the elbow
Patellar tendon	The leg should extend at the knee
Ankle or Achilles tendon	The foot should plantar flex

a chair without using your arms?" and "Are you able to climb stairs without difficulty and without using the railing?"

Deep Tendon Reflexes

[OBJECTIVE 3]

With a reflex hammer or stethoscope, test the deep tendon reflexes as part of the neurologic examination, particularly in patients with changes in sensation or strength. Remember that the reflex response does not come from the brain. Instead, the impulse travels to the spinal cord along the sensory spinal nerve. The response is immediately sent back along the motor spinal nerve to move the body away from danger quickly. Each deep tendon reflex corresponds to a different level of spinal cord function. Test deep tendon reflexes at the biceps (C5, C6), the brachioradialis muscle (C5, C6), the triceps (C6, C7), the knee (L2, L3, and L4), and the ankle (L5, S1, and S2). Reflexes are rated on a 5-point scale:

0 = Absent
$1+$ = Sluggish
$2+$ = Normal
$3+$ = Normal to hyperactive
$4+$ = Hyperactive

Expected reflex responses are shown in Table 23-3. Absent reflexes may indicate a problem with the spinal nerve or the spinal cord itself. Hyperactive reflexes usually originate within the brain, as is the case for seizures.

Meningeal Examination

[OBJECTIVE 3]

Recall that the meninges are the coverings of the entire CNS. If infection or hemorrhage in the CSF, cranium, or vertebral canal is present, the meninges often become irritated. When stretched or moved, they become further irritated and produce pain. Two simple tests assess for irritation of the meninges.

First, test for the Brudzinski sign. Have the patient sit on a table or chair, with their legs hanging off the end. Then ask the patient to flex the neck forward and touch his or her chin to the chest while sitting up straight. Someone with meningeal irritation only will be able to do this with pain and may try and lift the leg to reduce the strain on the meninges. This test may also be performed with the patient lying in a recumbent position. In this case place your hands behind the patient's head and flex his or her neck forward. As before, observe for flexion of the hips and knees.

Second, test for the Kernig sign. Have the patient lie flat on a bed or table and lift one of the patient's upper legs so that the thigh is perpendicular to the bed. Slowly extend the patient's lower leg at the knee. This normally may be uncomfortable, because of muscle tension, but will produce extreme pain in a patient with meningeal irritation.

The presence of pain when performing either of these tests should be a warning sign to the possibility of meningitis, subarachnoid hemorrhage, or another serious condition in the central nervous system. However, the absence of pain should never be used to rule out meningitis or any other condition because meningeal pain is not always present in these cases. The meningeal examination should never be performed in cases of trauma because it requires manipulation of the cervical spine.

Glasgow Coma Scale

[OBJECTIVE 3]

Accurately assessing and communicating a patient's level of consciousness to others can be difficult. Words such as *stupor, coma, lethargic,* and *semiconscious* are general and often mean different things to different healthcare professionals. Many agencies and facilities have adopted the

Glasgow Coma Scale (GCS) as the standard for describing a patient's level of consciousness. This scoring system was specifically designed for the evaluation of the acutely ill or injured patient whose status may change rapidly (Table 23-4).

TABLE 23-4	Glasgow Coma Scale
Score	
	Best Eye Opening Response
4	Spontaneous
3	To verbal stimuli
2	To painful stimuli
1	No response
	Best Verbal Response
5	Converses, oriented (A&O×4)
4	Converses, disoriented (A&O×4)
3	Inappropriate words
2	Incomprehensible words
1	No response
	Best Motor Response
6	Obeys simple commands
5	Localizes to pain
4	Withdraws from pain
3	Flexion posturing
2	Extension posturing
1	No response
Total =	E + V + M

A&O×4, Alert and oriented to person, time, place, and event.

Case Scenario—continued

The volunteer fire department has arrived and a skilled firefighter has begun manual cervical spine stabilization. You begin your primary survey. You open the airway by using a jaw thrust. You notice no signs of any bleeding around the patient's face and mouth. She appears young and you notice that she has signs of spontaneous breathing. She appears to be breathing shallowly at a rate of 6 breaths/min. You notice her chest is rising uniformly. She has a pulse of 128 beats/min and it is thready. She is moving her arms but not her legs.

Questions

4. What are the next most appropriate actions?
5. What are concerns with this patient's presentation and vital signs?
6. Which part of the focused physical examination will be important?
7. If the patient is unconscious, what should be evaluated? If the patient is conscious, what additional information would be helpful?

If resuscitate after 10-12 mm., BG will be high since brain not using it. keep body temp low & gradually warm. keeps metabolism lower. Allows BG to ↓. Better neurological function after resus.

910 Chapter 23 Disorders of the Nervous System

ALTERED MENTAL STATUS

[OBJECTIVES 4, 5]

Description and Definition

Altered mental status is a disruption of a person's emotional and intellectual functioning and, as previously described, results from dysfunction of the reticular formation, cerebral cortex, or both. Alterations in mental status range from very subtle to comatose. The paramedic should carefully assess the patient to avoid missing subtle presentations.

Etiology

Altered mental status may or may not be caused by a condition related to the central nervous system. For example, metabolic problems, infectious diseases, trauma, and poisonings are some of the possible causes of altered mental status (Box 23-1).

The cause of altered mental status can be divided into two broad categories: toxic metabolic states and structural lesions. Toxic metabolic states exist when a toxin is in the body or when a metabolic substrate, such as oxygen or glucose, is decreased. Structural lesions are space-occupying lesions that cause altered mental status as a result of their encroachment on the reticular formation. Within these two categories are the following six general causes of altered mental status:

1. Structural causes such as intracranial bleeding, head trauma, brain tumor, or space-occupying lesions

2. Metabolic dysfunction such as anoxia, hypoglycemia, diabetic ketoacidosis, thiamine deficiency, kidney or liver failure, or postictal phase of a seizure
3. Medications and street drugs such as barbiturates, narcotics, hallucinogens, depressants, or alcohol
4. Cardiovascular dysfunction such as hypertensive encephalopathy, hypoperfusion, dysrhythmias, or stroke
5. Respiratory dysfunction such as hypercapnia, hypoxia, or toxic inhalations
6. Infectious process such as meningitis, sepsis, or septicemia

> **PEDIATRIC***Pearl*
>
> The most common causes of altered mental status in a pediatric patient are hypoxia, head trauma, seizures, infection, hypoglycemia, and drug or alcohol ingestion.

History and Physical Findings

A patient with altered mental status displays changes in personality, behavior, or responsiveness. The patient may appear agitated, combative, sleepy, withdrawn, slow to respond, or completely unresponsive.

General impression findings that indicate altered mental status include unusual agitation, irritability, confusion, reduced responsiveness, or moaning. Other general impression findings associated with altered mental status include abnormal muscle tone or body position, abnormal work of breathing, and pallor. During the primary survey, determine the patient's level of responsiveness with the AVPU scale. A GCS score should be obtained during the secondary survey.

In addition to the history of the present illness and the past medical history for a patient with an altered mental status, ask a family member or friend (if available) if the patient's behavior appears unusual. Consider the following questions:

- When did the patient's symptoms begin?
- Was the onset of symptoms gradual or sudden?
- What was the patient doing when they started or occurred?
- How rapidly have the patient's symptoms progressed?
- Any history of a similar episode?
- Any history of head trauma, seizures, poisoning, infection with fever (suggesting sepsis), meningitis, a shunt in the brain, or brain tumor?
- Any use of alcohol, sedatives, or hypnotic agents?

BOX 23-1	**Possible Causes of Altered Mental Status (AEIOU TIPPS)**

A Alcohol, Abuse

E Epilepsy, Electrolyte disorders, Encephalopathy, Endocrine

I Insulin, Intoxication

O Overdose (opiates, lead, sedatives, aspirin, carbon monoxide)

U Uremia (kidney failure) and other metabolic causes, Underdosage

T Trauma, Temperature, Tumor

I Infection (encephalitis, meningitis, Reye's syndrome, sepsis)

P Psychological (fake, hysterical, or pseudoseizures)

P Poisoning

S Shock, Sickle cell disease, Subarachnoid hemorrhage, Space-occupying lesion, Shunt-related problems

- Any history of exposure to extremes of temperature (hot or cold)?
- What medication is the patient currently taking? What are the dosages? Does the patient take the medication as prescribed?
- Any history of diabetes or anorexia (potential causes of hypoglycemia)? If the patient is a diabetic, does he or she take insulin injections or oral diabetic medication? When did the patient last eat? Any unusual exercise or recent illness?

The physical examination can provide important clues regarding the cause of the patient's altered mental status. Note the presence of any odors that may help determine the cause of the patient's altered mental status. For example, a fruity odor on the breath may indicate diabetic ketoacidosis, and an odor of almonds can indicate cyanide exposure. Patients with an altered mental status may breathe shallowly, even when skin color and respiratory rate appear normal. Close observation is necessary to ensure adequate ventilation. Examine the patient's skin for bruises (which may suggest trauma or abuse) or rashes (may suggest sepsis or meningitis). Abnormal heart rates and rhythms indicate a cardiac cause, which may be correctable in the prehospital setting. Variations in vital signs can indicate increasing intracranial pressure or the presence of metabolic acidosis. An increased temperature may be associated with an infectious process, whereas a decreased temperature may be associated with dehydration and certain overdoses. Evaluate the head for signs of trauma, pupil responses, and bite marks to the tongue. Constricted pupils may be associated with narcotic overdoses, whereas fixed and dilated pupils are associated with cerebral hypoxia and some overdoses. Examine the extremities for asymmetrical strength and movement, which may indicate a stroke.

Toxic metabolic states and structural lesions create different presentations in the patient with an altered mental status. Although the exact cause of the altered mental state may not be evident in the prehospital setting, the history and physical findings should help the paramedic determine which of these categories is the most likely cause.

Toxic metabolic states often are slow in onset, have symmetric neurologic findings, and cause pupil responses (normal or abnormal) to be equal bilaterally (preserved pupillary responses).

The altered mental status associated with structural lesions often is sudden in onset and presents with asymmetric neurologic findings, unresponsive or asymmetric pupils, and a progressive pattern of deterioration caused by the focal pressure on the brain. These patients also may have signs of increasing intracranial pressure such as an increased blood pressure, decreased pulse, and altered respirations. The findings of increased intracranial pressure are discussed in more detail later in this chapter and in Chapter 47.

PARAMEDIC Pearl

The airway of a patient with an altered mental status is at risk of airway obstruction because of decreased muscle tone and depressed gag and cough reflexes. This may lead to airway obstruction, resulting in hypoxemia and respiratory failure or respiratory arrest. Repeat the initial assessment often throughout your care of these patients and revise your treatment plan based on the patient's response to your interventions.

Therapeutic Interventions

Regardless of the cause of the patient's altered mental status, the priorities of care remain the same—airway, breathing, and circulation. Treatment is directed at the underlying cause of the patient's altered mental status only after these issues are addressed. If cervical spine injury is suspected (by examination, history, or mechanism of injury), manually stabilize the head and neck in a neutral, in-line position or maintain spinal stabilization if already completed.

Difficulty with secretions, vomiting, and inadequate tidal volume are common and significant problems in the patient with an altered mental status. Use positioning or airway adjuncts as necessary to maintain an open airway. Suction as needed. Avoid the use of an oral airway unless the patient is unresponsive. Use of an oral airway in a semiresponsive patient may cause vomiting if a gag reflex is present. Begin positive-pressure ventilation as needed. Intubation may be necessary to ensure an open airway and adequate ventilation if the condition is not easily reversed, such as in hypoglycemia or a narcotic overdose (Box 23-2).

PARAMEDIC Pearl

Pulse oximetry, capnography, and continuous cardiac monitoring should be routinely performed for any patient who has an altered mental status.

Initiate intravenous access, draw blood, and check the patient's blood glucose level. If the blood glucose level is low, treat with dextrose or glucagon. If malnutrition or chronic alcohol abuse is suspected, administer thiamine before glucose to avoid the possibility of Wernicke-Korsakoff syndrome. Administer naloxone if the patient has an altered mental status and signs suggestive of an opioid overdose, such as pinpoint pupils and respiratory depression. Recall, however, that not all opioids result in pupil constriction. Provide specific treatment for any other conditions found during the physical examination.

PARAMEDIC Pearl

Always check the blood glucose level of any patient with altered mental status.

Patient and Family Education

A patient who has chronic altered mental status may need assistance with daily activities such as bathing, eating, dressing, and toileting. A physician will discuss the patient's decision making capacity with the patient's family. Arrangements may need to be made to identify an individual who can make decisions on the patient's behalf. This decision may need to be modified if the patient's decision-making capacity improves after treating the cause of the patient's altered mental status.

WERNICKE'S ENCEPHALOPATHY
Reversible   *Alcoholics*

Description and Definition

First described in 1881 by Carl Wernicke, Wernicke's encephalopathy is caused by a deficiency of vitamin B$_1$ (thiamine). Classic presentation of this condition includes confusion, ataxia, and oculomotor disturbances such as nystagmus.

Etiology

Thiamine is a crucial component in the metabolism of carbohydrates, including the breakdown of glucose in the Kreb's cycle. When the brain, with its high metabolic demands, is unable to derive energy from the metabolism of glucose, damage to the neurons results. Thiamine also plays a role in the maintenance of the myelin sheath of the nervous system. In the absence of thiamine the myelin sheath begins to break down, slowing nervous impulse transmission. This results in dysfunction of the nervous system. Further effects of decreased thiamine are a decrease in the electrical stimulation of neurons.

Thiamine must be taken in through the diet, and in its absence stores in the body will be depleted in 1 month. However, signs and symptoms of thiamine deficiency develop within 1 week in the thiamine-deprived patient. The most common cause of thiamine deficiency is chronic alcoholism. These patients generally have a decreased intake of thiamine as well as an impaired ability to store thiamine. Chronic malnutrition is another common cause of thiamine deficiency because of decreased dietary intake.

Epidemiology and Demographics

The incidence and prevalence of Wernicke's encephalopathy are difficult to determine because the condition often goes unrecognized in patients. The incidence is believed to be between 0.8% and 2.8% of the general population; it can be as high as 12.5% of chronic alcoholics (Salen, 2006). Wernicke's encephalopathy also occurs in other situations in which nutrition is compromised, such as patients with AIDS or cancer, with or without chemotherapy. Wernicke's encephalopathy is a medical emergency, with a mortality rate approaching 20%. A male predominance exists, most likely because a greater number of men abuse alcohol compared with women.

History and Physical Findings

As described above, the classic presentation of Wernicke's encephalopathy includes confusion, ataxia, and oculomotor disturbances, but this presentation only occurs in 12% of patients. Newer diagnostic criteria include any two of the following: malnutrition, altered mental status, ataxia, and oculomotor disturbances. This process should be a strong consideration when faced with a chronic alcoholic with these signs. Additional findings may include disinterest or inattention, agitation, speech disturbances, paresthesia, depressed reflexes, stupor, signs of cerebellar dysfunction, hypothermia, dysfunction of extraocular movements, and coma (rarely).

Closely associated with Wernicke's encephalopathy is Korsakoff's psychosis. This results from the same mechanism as Wernicke's but is manifested by memory impairments, the inability to learn new information, the inability to remember information that was learned at an earlier time, and apathy. These patients also often exhibit confabulation. This is the process by which they fill in memory gaps with information spontaneously created. They are unable to recall this information once they have said it. The paramedic who suspects confabulation should repeat a question previously asked to ascertain if the patient provides the same information. Although confabulation is common, it is not required for the diagnosis of Korsakoff's psychosis. It remains unknown if this is a conscious effort to conceal memory loss or a subconscious mechanism. Wernicke's encephalopathy is a reversible disorder but Korsakoff's psychosis is not. These two conditions can exist together as Wernicke-Korsakoff syndrome.

Korsakoff's—long term alcoholism not reversible

Differential Diagnosis

Differential diagnoses include the following:

- Psychotic illness
- Hypoxia

- Hypercarbia
- Cerebellar infarction
- Head injury
- Amnesia
- Hydrocephalus
- Complex partial seizure
- Postictal phase of a seizure
- Stroke
- Hepatic encephalopathy

Therapeutic Interventions

Address and correct any life threats found during the primary survey. This may include airway management, oxygenation, or assisted ventilations as a result of an altered mental status. Administer fluids as necessary to support the blood pressure and warm the patient if hypothermia is present.

The primary treatment for these conditions is the administration of thiamine. The speed of response to thiamine varies and depends on the patient and the amount of neuronal damage present. Altered mentation, ataxia, and oculomotor disturbances may respond quickly or take days to months. Many patients may not show any response to treatment. If the patient has Korsakoff's psychosis, the amnesia, recall, and inability to learn new things will not be reversed.

The administration of glucose to thiamine-deficient patients can result in the depletion of their thiamine stores and lead to the development of these conditions. Therefore thiamine must be administered before glucose in any patient in whom thiamine deficiency is suspected.

National Standard

Patient and Family Education

Educate the patient and family of the importance of maintaining a healthy diet to ensure the intake of adequate amounts of thiamine. In addition, explain the effects of chronic alcohol abuse on the ability to store thiamine.

DELIRIUM VERSUS DEMENTIA

Description and Definition

10-12% of people w/OSS dic during 1st episode

[OBJECTIVES 4, 5]

You have no doubt often heard a patient called delirious or have been told a patient has dementia. These two terms are different, and recognizing the correct meaning of each is important. **Delirium** is short-term and temporary mental confusion and fluctuating level of consciousness. **Dementia** is a long-term decline in mental faculties such as memory, concentration, and judgment.

Can't be reversed

Etiology

Delirium is the result of a widespread dysfunction in brain tissue. It often is caused by a condition outside the central nervous system. For example, heart failure, heart attack, cardiac dysrhythmias, pneumonia, chronic respiratory problems, urinary tract infections, and strokes are common causes. In the elderly, cardiovascular conditions, infections, and medications are the most common causes of delirium. Medications that can cause profound delirium are listed in Box 23-3.

Dementia often is seen in the elderly, especially those with degenerative neurologic disorders. Although Alzheimer's disease is the most common cause of dementia, it also has many other causes.

BOX 23-3	Medications That Can Cause Delirium

- Digitalis
- Steroids
- Antihypertensives
- Salicylates
- Oral hypoglycemics
- Tricyclic antidepressants
- Benzodiazepines

PARAMEDIC*Pearl*

The general causes of delirium can be remembered by the mnemonic MADCAP:

- **M**edication reactions and **m**etabolic derangements (e.g., hypoglycemia)
- **A**lcohol and **a**nticholinergics
- **D**ementia
- **C**ardiac disorders and **c**erebrovascular accident
- **A**lterations in hemodynamic or respiratory status
- **P**neumonia and associated sepsis, or any sepsis

Reprinted from Bosker, G., Weins, D., & Sequeira, M. *The 60-second EMT: Rapid BLS/ALS assessment, diagnosis, and triage* (2nd ed.). St. Louis: Mosby.

PARAMEDIC*Pearl*

Because the brain requires so much of the body's resources (e.g., cardiac output, glucose), it often is the first organ to be affected when homeostasis is disrupted. Therefore altered mental status always is considered a serious sign and should be assessed and treated accordingly.

Epidemiology and Demographics

Despite its prevalence in the elderly, dementia is *not* part of the normal aging process. It is estimated that 6.8 million people in the United States are currently affected with dementia and that 1.8 million of those show severe symptoms (National Institute of Neurological Disorders and Stroke, 2004).

History and Physical Findings

Delirium is one of the most common presenting symptoms of a physical illness in the elderly and is more common than fever, tachycardia, and pain (Drake, 1996). Assume that every patient you encounter is completely alert and oriented with a GCS of 15 until proven otherwise by the history given by someone who knows the patient well. Remember, even in patients with a baseline altered mental status, changes can occur. Any deviation from baseline mental status should be taken seriously.

Especially in its end stages, dementia can cause patients to exhibit bizarre, irrational, and even violent behavior. You may have to reassure family and friends that the patient's behavior is a result of a medical condition and that the patient is not aware of his or her actions.

Differential Diagnosis

Differential diagnoses include the following:

- Brain abscess
- Brain neoplasm
- Diabetic ketoacidosis
- Encephalitis
- Epidural and subdural infections
- HIV infection and AIDS
- Heat illness
- Herpes simplex
- Hepatic encephalopathy
- Hypercalcemia
- Hypernatremia
- Hypertensive emergencies
- Hypoglycemia
- Hypothyroidism
- Panic disorders
- Schizophrenia
- Subarachnoid hemorrhage
- Subdural hematoma
- Wernicke's encephalopathy
- Withdrawal syndromes

Therapeutic Interventions

Treatment for delirium is focused on finding and correcting its cause. Care for the patient with dementia primarily is supportive. When providing care, maintain eye contact. Speak to the patient in a calm manner. Ask only one question at a time and allow the patient time to answer. Calmly reorient the patient as necessary. Sedation is sometimes needed for severe agitation.

Patient and Family Education

A patient with dementia usually requires continuous supervision. The family should identify a primary caregiver and other potential caregivers. The caregiver should establish a regular, structured daily routine and encourage the patient's participation. Tasks should be broken down into several simple steps. The caregiver and family should be realistic about what the patient can and cannot do. Caregivers should be taught about the signs and symptoms of potentially complicating medical problems such as urinary tract infection and incontinence. Encourage caregivers to attend caregiver support groups.

SEIZURES

Description and Definition

[OBJECTIVES 4, 5]

A **seizure** is a temporary alteration in behavior or consciousness caused by abnormal electrical activity of one or more groups of neurons in the brain.

Etiology

Just as myocardial cells in the heart can become irritated and begin firing, causing ectopy and dysrhythmias, nerve cells in the brain can also randomly fire, causing sudden changes in behavior. During a seizure, neurons in the brain may fire up to 500 times per second, far above the normal rate of approximately 80 times per second (Weiderholt, 2000).

Irritation to the brain cells can result from a variety of causes. Hypoxia, whether systemic or localized, can cause profound changes in brain function and can lead to seizures. Hypoglycemia can cause seizures because the cells of the brain do not have the energy needed for normal function. Hypoxia and hypoglycemia are the two most common organic causes of seizures; fortunately they are both easily treated in the prehospital setting. Anything that applies pressure to or moves brain tissue can cause seizures. This includes bleeding in the cranial cavity, brain tumor, brain abscess, and head trauma. Metabolic imbalances such as hypoglycemia, hypocalcemia, low magnesium levels, and sodium imbalances can also trigger a seizure. A rapid rise in body temperature can cause a **febrile seizure;** however, this normally is seen in children younger than 2 years. Lastly, exposure to or withdrawal from alcohol, certain medications, and street drugs can cause seizure activity as well. A specific cause is found only in approximately half of all seizure cases (Weiderholt, 2000). Possible causes of seizures are listed in Box 23-4.

Epidemiology and Demographics

Approximately 2.5 million Americans will have a seizure in their lifetimes. Each year in the United States more than 181,000 people are diagnosed with **epilepsy,** a disease of recurrent seizures, often of unknown cause (Cross, 2004). Approximately 20% of patients with epilepsy cannot control their seizures, even with medication (Weiderholt, 2000). The most common organic causes of seizures have been mentioned; however, the paramedic must realize that the most common cause of seizures in general is the failure of patients to take their anticonvul-

BOX 23-4 Possible Causes of Seizures

- Idiopathic (unknown cause)
- Metabolic (hypoxia, hypoglycemia, thyrotoxicosis, hypocalcemia, low magnesium levels, sodium imbalance)
- Eclampsia
- Bleeding in the cranial cavity
- Brain tumor or abscess
- Head trauma
- Fever
- Infection
- Vascular disorders
- Cardiac dysrhythmias
- Genetic and hereditary factors
- Drug intoxication or withdrawal
- Cerebral degenerative diseases
- Failure to take anticonvulsant medication

BOX 23-5 Simple Partial Seizures

- Average seizure lasts 10 to 20 seconds
- Patient remains conscious
- May verbalize during the seizure
- No postictal event after the seizure
- Characterized by motor or sensory symptoms without impairment of consciousness
- Motor: forceful turning of the head and eyes to one side, clonic movements beginning on one side of the face or extremities
- Sensory: paresthesias or pain localized to a specific area

BOX 23-6 Complex Partial Seizures

- Most common type of seizure in children and adults.
- Consciousness is always impaired.
- May begin as a simple partial seizure and progress or may begin as a complex seizure.
- Average duration is 1 to 2 minutes.
- Often preceded by a sensory aura (visual, auditory, or olfactory).
- Often includes automatisms (purposeless repetitive movements such as picking at clothes, lip smacking, chewing, eye blinking, rubbing or caressing objects, walking or running in a nondirective, repetitive fashion). Automatisms are not remembered by the patient.
- Postictal confusion or sleep may follow the seizure.

sant medications. Always inquire about compliance of all medications, especially anticonvulsants.

Types of Seizures

The two categories of seizures are partial and generalized. Partial seizures can evolve into generalized seizures, particularly in patients who are not taking their anticonvulsant medications.

Partial Seizures

Partial seizures affect only part of a cerebral hemisphere. The area involved is called the *focus*. Partial seizures may be simple or complex. **Simple partial seizures** do not alter consciousness, whereas **complex partial seizures** do alter consciousness or awareness. *"space out" - kids*

Simple Partial Seizures. Simple partial seizures also are known as *focal motor* or *focal sensory seizures* because the excess electrical activity is only at one focus (location) in the brain. Patients with simple partial seizures may have visual, auditory, or olfactory hallucinations. Involuntary twitching or other rhythmic muscle contractions centralized in one part of the body, or unusual sensations such as gastrointestinal discomfort, may also be seen in these patients (Box 23-5). *"petit mal" - old terminology resolve by adulthood*

Complex Partial Seizures. Complex partial seizures are also called *temporal lobe seizures* because they are associated with focal lesions of the temporal lobe. A complex partial seizure may manifest as a blank stare accompanied by lip smacking, chewing, or twitching movements of the mouth and face. Patients having a complex partial seizure may have blocked communication. They often mumble and may understand spoken words but are unable to respond. These patients may appear dazed and unaware of their surroundings. They may display clumsy, undirected actions and disorientation and wandering. They are frequently oblivious to obstacles that may be in their path (Box 23-6). Reports have been made of some patients

"marching" seizure - progresses to other areas

psychomotor seizure - conscious but unaware of anything (old terminology)

becoming extremely violent during a complex partial seizure (formerly called a *psychomotor seizure*); therefore the paramedic should always be alert for scene safety issues in these situations.

Sometimes a partial seizure may spread from one part of the brain to the entire brain. This is known as a *partial seizure with secondary generalization* and is the cause of an **aura**—a sensory hallucination that precedes a generalized seizure. Patients who experience auras may report an unpleasant taste, smelling an odd or noxious smell, or seeing halos of light around objects. These are examples of partial seizures occurring in an area of the brain responsible for the senses and then spreading to the entire brain. A thorough description of the aura must be obtained for comparison to prior seizures. If the aura is abnormal, it may indicate a different pathologic cause of the seizure. If the seizure is a first seizure for the patient, the description of the aura can help the neurologist determine the likely focus of the seizure.

Generalized Seizures

Frontal lobe - generalized

Generalized seizures are caused by excessive electrical activity in both hemispheres of the brain at the same time. All generalized seizures have an abrupt onset and involve an alteration of consciousness. The presentation of a generalized seizure can vary widely, from subtle eye fluttering to the more commonly recognized rhythmic stiffening and jerking of the body. An unconscious patient showing any repetitive movements should be considered as having a generalized seizure until proven otherwise.

Absence Seizures. An **absence seizure** (also called a *petit mal seizure*) is a transient loss of awareness of surroundings without a loss of motor tone. The patient stares vacantly into space. An absence seizure may manifest with eye fluttering and rarely lasts longer than 30 seconds. A patient may have hundreds of absence seizures per hour and often is misdiagnosed as daydreaming. The patient may have automatisms. They are not associated with an aura and the patient does not enter a postictal state. Absence seizures are uncommon before the age of 5 years and are more prevalent in girls. Many of these patients develop tonic-clonic seizures by the time they reach adolescence (Weiderholt, 2000).

Tonic-Clonic Seizures. Tonic-clonic seizures (also called *generalized motor seizures* or *grand mal seizures*) are the most dramatic of seizures. Beginning suddenly and without warning, the tonic-clonic seizure shows four characteristic phases: aura (in some patients), tonic phase, clonic phase, and postictal period.

An aura is a peculiar sensation that precedes a seizure. Auras include an unusual taste, a dreamy feeling, a visual disturbance (such as a flashing light or floating light), an unpleasant odor, or a rising or sinking feeling in the stomach. The most common auras experienced by a child are epigastric discomfort or pain and a feeling of fear.

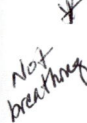

During the tonic phase, the patient suddenly becomes unconscious and experiences widespread muscle contraction, becoming stiff and rigid. The patient may cry out as the respiratory muscles contract and force exhalation. The tonic phase usually lasts 15 to 20 seconds.

The clonic phase is characterized by rhythmic jerking of all the muscles, alternating with relaxation. This is the longest phase of the seizure, lasting approximately 90 seconds to 2 minutes. Sphincter control is lost, particularly the bladder (urinary incontinence). The diaphragm tenses and jerks like other muscles during the tonic-clonic seizure. Therefore the patient is not able to breathe effectively. Blood oxygen saturation dramatically drops, especially if the seizure is prolonged. The clonic phase slows toward the end of the seizure. The patient often sighs as the seizure comes to an abrupt stop. Most tonic-clonic seizures cause no lasting damage or neurologic problems.

After the tonic and clonic phases, the patient enters the **postictal** (literally "after the seizure") **phase.** This phase, also known as the *quiet phase,* is a period of gradual awakening after a seizure characterized by confusion, disorientation, and fatigue. This phase ends with the patient returning to a level of normal behavior. The muscle contractions of a tonic-clonic seizure are extremely tiring. The patient's blood glucose level may have dropped from the excess demands of the muscles and brain tissue. Any or all of the following may last minutes to hours:

- Change from unresponsive to drowsy, confused, or combative
- Deep respirations
- Salivation, tachycardia, headache, partial paralysis (Todd's paralysis); usually transient
- Amnesia for the seizure

As the patient awakens, he or she may be combative and resist being touched. The patient often appears anxious and fearful. Keep in mind that the patient's brain has to, in effect, "reboot" after a seizure. The patient probably has little conscious idea or control over his or her actions. The patient may report an intense headache, general fatigue, and muscular pain. Vomiting is common in the postictal phase. For most patients, this phase usually lasts 15 to 30 minutes. However, some patients have much longer postictal periods.

A good history of the seizure episode from bystanders is essential. If this is the first time the patient has had a seizure, assume an underlying cause such as trauma, overdose, or brain injury and aggressively treat the patient. Questions to consider include the following:

- What was the patient doing at the time of the seizure?
- Did the patient cry out or attract your attention in any way?
- What did the seizure look like? A tonic-clonic seizure is often described as "jerking," "shaking," or "flopping like a fish out of water."
- Did the seizure begin in one area of the body and progress to others?
- When did the seizure start? How long did the seizure last? (Be aware that this information is often inaccurate.)
- Does the patient have a history of seizures or epilepsy? If so, is the patient taking antiseizure medications as prescribed? Has the dosage recently been changed?
- Did the patient lose bowel or bladder control?
- When the patient awoke, did he or she show any change in speech or ability to move the extremities?
- Did the patient hit his or her head or fall?
- Has the patient recently had a fever or headache or complained of a stiff neck?
- Has the patient experienced any recent trauma or falls?

PARAMEDIC*Pearl*

Alcohol use decreases the effectiveness of seizure medications and often is the cause of seizure activity, despite medication compliance.

Febrile Seizures. A febrile seizure is a generalized seizure that occurs with fever in childhood. It occurs in 2% to 3% of children, with a greater risk in those who have a first-degree relative who had febrile seizures.

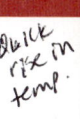

Recurrent febrile seizures occur in 30% to 50% of cases. Criteria for a febrile seizure include the following:

- Age 3 months to 5 years (most occur between ages 6 and 18 months)
- Fever greater than 38.8°C (101.8°F)
- No central nervous system infection

Most febrile seizures are simple febrile seizures. A simple febrile seizure is usually associated with a core body temperature that increases rapidly to 38.8°C (101.8°F) or greater. The seizure is usually tonic-clonic and lasts a few seconds to 15 minutes. It is followed by a brief postical period of drowsiness. A complicated (also known as *atypical* or *complex*) febrile seizure lasts longer than 15 minutes or is associated with a postictal phase. The child may have repeated seizures within the same day. Febrile seizures lasting longer than 30 minutes are called febrile status epilepticus. The risk of epilepsy after febrile seizures is low.

Pseudoseizures. Pseudoseizures also are called *fake, hysterical,* or *psychological seizures*. Pseudoseizures typically occur between 10 and 18 years of age and are more frequent among girls. They occur in many patients with a history of epilepsy and in some with ongoing true seizures. A pseudoseizure may appear realistic but frequently is bizarre, with unusual postures, verbalizations, and uncharacteristic tonic or clonic movements. A physician will diagnose a pseudoseizure only after a thorough history and physical examination and exclusion of true seizures.

Differentiating between a pseudoseizure and a true seizure is sometimes difficult. Distinguishing features of a pseudoseizure may include the following:

- Lack of cyanosis
- Normal reaction of the pupils to light
- No loss of sphincter control
- Uncoordinated movement (versus rhythmic tonic-clonic movement)
- No physical injury (absence of tongue biting during the seizure)
- Moaning or crying
- The ability to have a seizure on request

Therapeutic Interventions

For patients who have a history of epilepsy, treatment for a generalized seizure is generally supportive. If the patient is seizing on your arrival, do not attempt to restrain him or her or place anything in the mouth. This can cause damage to the patient's teeth and can cause injury to you. Move any nearby objects and furniture out of the patient's way so that the patient does not injure himself or herself. Administering 100% oxygen by nonrebreather mask is beneficial, and if the patient becomes cyanotic or the seizure is prolonged, assist ventilation with a bag-mask device. If airway management is needed, place a nasal airway because the patient may have clenched teeth, prohibiting insertion of an oral airway and intubation. Administration of a benzodiazepine is indicated to stop

seizure activity. A child having a febrile seizure should be cooled to reduce fever. Removal of thick clothing and blankets usually is all that is necessary to lower the patient's body temperature. More intense cooling methods should be attempted cautiously and only after consulting medical direction because they can rapidly cause hypothermia.

If the patient is in the postical phase, monitor him or her closely, including pulse oximetry and the electrocardiogram (ECG). The postictal phase is one of the most dangerous times for airway compromise because the tongue is flaccid and can occlude the pharynx. Therefore the patient should be placed in the lateral recumbent position unless trauma is suspected. The patient should remain on oxygen, and a blood glucose level should be obtained. Give dextrose if the blood glucose level is less than 60 mg/dL. Obtain intravenous access to prepare for the possibility of another seizure. Assess the patient for potential causes of the seizure and for any injuries that may have been sustained during the seizure. Because some dysrhythmias can cause seizure-like behavior, apply a cardiac monitor. Consider spinal stabilization if the possibility of head or neck trauma exists (Box 23-7).

Patient and Family Education

Family members of a patient with seizures likely have witnessed a seizure before, but reassuring them is helpful. Although dramatic, seizure activity often does not cause long-term neurologic damage. When the patient is in the postical phase, explain to the family that the bizarre behavior they may witness is a normal part of the postictal phase.

Status Epilepticus

[OBJECTIVES 4, 5]

Seizures are not usually life threatening. In some cases, seizure activity is prolonged and can cause permanent brain damage or death. **Status epilepticus** is a single

---

BOX 23-7 | **Patient Management: Seizures (Adult)—Prolonged, Repetitive, or Status Epilepticus**

- ABCs; establish an airway, apply SpO$_2$ monitor, give oxygen, and ventilate the patient as needed.
- Administer a benzodiazepine to stop the seizure activity
- Establish IV (if not already done) and check blood glucose level. If hypoglycemic, give dextrose IV. If unable to establish IV, give glucagon IM. Give thiamine IV or IM if possible alcoholism or patient appears malnourished.
- If blood glucose level is within normal range, give benzodiazepine in small increments per local protocol.
- When seizure resolves, obtain vital signs and apply cardiac monitor.
- Contact medical direction for further instructions.

ABCs, Airway, breathing, and circulation; *IV,* intravenous; *IM,* intramuscular.

seizure lasting longer than 30 minutes or repeated seizures without full recovery of responsiveness between seizures and lasting longer than 30 minutes. Any seizure may evolve into status epilepticus. *2 seizures w/out lucid interval*

Etiology

Status epilepticus is a medical emergency and must be treated as such. Prolonged seizure activity is extremely taxing on brain cells. The high rate of firing is believed to cause the neurons to generate toxic byproducts, thereby causing cell death. As the seizure continues, the patient's hypoxia worsens. This lack of oxygen causes cells throughout the body, which are already under high metabolic stress, to undergo anaerobic metabolism and generate more toxic waste products. This can create systemic metabolic acidosis. Generally, this acidosis resolves itself when the seizure ends (Jans et al., 1998).

lactic acid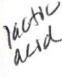

History and Physical Findings

In some patients, seizure activity and status epilepticus may continue after tonic and clonic movements stop. This is sometimes called *silent status epilepticus*. Because of the high levels of activity, the motor neurons that carry signals from the brain to the muscles have become exhausted, causing the patient to become limp while seizure activity continues in the brain. Assume that any patient who appears to be in a postictal state without an improving level of consciousness is still seizing, particularly if the patient was in status epilepticus before. If you are unsure, discuss the patient's condition and treatment with medical direction (Jans et al., 1998).

Therapeutic Interventions

Status epilepticus requires immediate treatment. The goal of treatment is rapid termination of the seizure activity. The patient likely will not be able to protect the airway or breathe effectively during prolonged seizure activity. Remove any tight clothing that could compromise the airway, such as a necktie. Place a nasopharyngeal airway, consider nasal intubation, and assist the patient's ventilations with a bag-mask device attached to 100% oxygen. Unfortunately, because the body's metabolic demands are so high during seizure activity, even the best ventilation and oxygenation are unable to keep pace, and cell injury and death will still occur. Therefore quickly stopping seizure activity is essential and can prevent permanent brain damage.

Prehospital treatment of status epilepticus usually relies on benzodiazepines to stop seizure activity. The two most commonly used are diazepam (Valium) and lorazepam (Ativan). Because these drugs can cause respiratory depression, be prepared to assist ventilations aggressively. Both drugs can be given intravenously (IV), intramuscularly (IM), or rectally. The IV route is preferred because IM and rectal absorption can be slow, unpredictable, and ineffective. Rectal administration is often effective in pediatric patients (Weiderholt, 2000). Lorazepam is often used in emergency departments because it has a longer duration of action. Treatment and transport should be performed rapidly to ensure the best possible patient outcome.

SYNCOPE

[OBJECTIVES 4, 5]

Description and Definition

Blood not getting to brain

Syncope is a transient loss of consciousness and inability to maintain postural tone, typically resulting in a ground-level fall. Syncope is commonly known as *fainting, passing out, blacking out,* or *falling out.*

In near syncope (i.e., presyncope), signs and symptoms of imminent syncope occur, including dizziness with or without blackout (called a *gray-out*), anxiety, pallor, diaphoresis, thready pulse, and low blood pressure. Near syncope may be accompanied by partial or complete loss of vision or hearing but no loss of consciousness.

The progression to syncope is marked by loss of consciousness, atony, and falling. The loss of consciousness typically occurs within a few seconds of the onset of symptoms and is associated with complete recovery shortly after the patient assumes a supine position. Syncope causes no residual neurologic problems.

Etiology

Syncope has many causes, many of which have no neurologic pathology. Non–life-threatening causes include the following:

- Increased vagal tone
- Psychogenic reactions
- Prolonged standing, fatigue, dehydration

Potentially life-threatening causes include the following:

- Dysrhythmias including supraventricular tachycardia, bradycardia, prolonged QT syndrome
- Cardiac abnormalities that decrease blood flow to the heart, lungs, brain, and body
- Myocardial ischemia
- Certain drug intoxications
- Hypoglycemia, anemia, hypoxia, head trauma

Types of Syncope

Cardiac Syncope. Cardiac syncope may be caused by structural heart disease (such as aortic stenosis or pulmonary stenosis) or may be the result of dysrhythmias. Extremely fast or slow heart rates can result in insufficient cardiac output, shock, and increased cardiac workload. Consider a cardiac cause of syncope when the following occur:

- Syncope occurs in a recumbent position.
- Syncope is provoked by exercise.
- Chest pain is associated with syncope.
- A family history of fainting or sudden death exists.
- No warning signs occurred before the event.

BOX 23-8 Causes of Vasovagal Syncope

- Anxiety
- Fright
- Pain
- Needlestick, blood drawing
- Sight of blood
- Fasting
- Witnessing violence
- Hot and humid conditions
- Crowded places
- Prolonged and motionless standing
- Bearing down during urination or bowel movements

↓ HR, pale, cool, diaphoretic   can sit up when HR ↑

Noncardiac Syncope. Vasovagal syncope is the most common cause of fainting. Vasovagal syncope also is called vasodepressor, neurocardiogenic, or common syncope. Warning signs and symptoms last a few seconds to a minute and consist of dizziness, lightheadedness, pallor, palpitations, nausea, and diaphoresis, followed by a loss of consciousness and muscle tone. Unconsciousness does not last more than a minute and the patient gradually awakens. Causes of vasovagal syncope are listed in Box 23-8.

Some people are prone to episodes of syncope in particular situations. Examples of situational syncope include the following:

- Cough syncope (also called *tussive syncope*) occurs in people with lung disease when coughing forcefully. This type of syncope may be seen in asthmatic children. It occurs shortly after the onset of sleep. A coughing spasm abruptly awakens the child. The child sweats, becomes agitated, and is frightened. A loss of consciousness is associated with a generalized loss of muscle tone, upward gaze, and clonic muscle contractions lasting for several seconds. Urinary incontinence is frequent. Recovery begins within seconds, and consciousness is usually restored a few minutes later. The child has no recollection of the episode except for the events surrounding the coughing spasm.
- Swallow syncope occurs during swallowing in some people who have throat or esophageal disease.
- Postprandial syncope can occur in people (particularly older adults) when their blood pressure falls approximately 1 hour after eating.
- Carotid sinus hypersensitivity occurs in some people with minimal stimulation of the carotid sinus in the neck. For example, turning the neck, shaving with an electric razor, or wearing a tight collar may cause fainting in susceptible individuals.
- Micturition syncope occurs in some individuals when they empty an overfilled bladder.

Postural syncope (orthostatic hypotension) may be precipitated by prolonged bed rest, prolonged standing, and conditions that decrease the circulating blood volume (e.g., bleeding, dehydration). Normal vasoconstriction of the arterioles and veins in the upright position is absent or inadequate, resulting in hypotension without a reflex increase in heart rate. Syncope may be the first sign of unrecognized bleeding caused by conditions such as gastrointestinal bleeding, leaking aortic aneurysm, or ruptured ectopic pregnancy. Drugs that interfere with vasoconstriction (e.g., calcium channel blockers, antihypertensive drugs, vasodilators, phenothiazines) and diuretics may worsen orthostatic hypotension.

Hypoglycemia may cause syncope. Syncope may be preceded by confusion, headache, altered mental status, weakness, and nausea. Neurologic syncope may be caused by a stroke, transient ischemic attack (discussed later in this chapter), migraine headaches, and other neurologic conditions.

Psychogenic syncope often is associated with experiencing or anticipating an unpleasant situation. Examples include feeling afraid, seeing blood, feeling pain, and witnessing violence or other disturbing experiences. In psychogenic syncope, an initial temporary sympathetic response is followed by a reflex vagal reaction.

Epidemiology and Demographics

Facts about syncope include the following:

- Syncope and near syncope are common reasons for EMS response.
- Syncope represents 3% of all emergency department admissions and 6% of all inpatient hospital admissions yearly (Morag, 2004).
- Syncope is uncommon before age 10 to 12 years but is quite common in adolescent girls.
- Minor injuries are common (25%); serious injuries occur in 1% to 2% of patients.
- If syncope is recurrent, it may have a major effect on lifestyle and/or quality of life.
- The family history is positive for similar episodes in 90% of patients.

History and Physical Findings

Assessment of syncope can be tricky because the patient is likely conscious when you arrive. Because many people confuse syncope with other conditions such as seizures or psychiatric episodes, find out from bystanders if the patient actually became unconscious and unarousable. Try to find out the length of the episode and the events leading to the episode and afterwards. Tremulousness often is reported before syncope. Be sure to differentiate between this event and a seizure. Did the patient immediately become alert and oriented, or did a period in which the patient was awake but with altered mental status follow?

The history of the present illness is the best way to find out the underlying cause of a syncopal episode. Watch for several red flags when assessing a patient with syncope. They are divided into three categories: before the episode, during the episode, and after the episode (Box 23-9).

BOX 23-9 Red Flags When Assessing Syncopal Patients

- Before syncope, stay on the SCENT:
  - **S**upine posture at onset
  - **C**ardiac symptoms before syncope (chest pain, dyspnea, palpitations)
  - **E**lderly patients
  - **N**o warning of syncope; implies a cardiac or neurologic cause
  - **T**rauma associated with syncope, either as a cause or result
- During the syncopal episode, watch for TIPS:
  - **T**ongue biting; may indicate a seizure
  - **I**ncontinence, particularly of stool
  - **P**rolonged duration, longer than 1 minute
  - **S**eizure activity
- After the syncopal episode, be like Jackie CHAN:
  - **C**onfusion
  - **H**eadaches
  - **A**bnormal vital signs
  - **N**eurologic dysfunction, particularly focal deficits

- Hyponatremia
- Hypovolemia
- Internal cardiac defibrillator malfunction
- Mitral stenosis
- Myocardial infarction
- Pacemaker malfunction
- Pulmonary embolism
- Valvular heart disease
- Restrictive cardiomyopathy
- Subarachnoid hemorrhage
- Tetralogy of Fallot

PARAMEDIC*Pearl*

Syncope can usually be differentiated from a seizure because of its short duration, associated symptoms of nausea and sweating, and complete orientation after the event.

Differential Diagnosis

Differential diagnoses include the following:

- Adrenal insufficiency or crisis
- Aortic aneurysm or dissection
- Aortic stenosis
- Cardiac dysrhythmias
- Dehydration
- Drug toxicity
- Ectopic pregnancy
- Hypoglycemia

Therapeutic Interventions

Management of syncope is focused on identifying and treating the underlying cause. As always, problems found in the primary survey should be managed first. However, in a true case of syncope, the patient is usually conscious on your arrival. Initiate pulse oximetry and cardiac monitoring. Obtain IV access and give a fluid challenge of normal saline or Ringer's lactate if the patient is hypotensive. Infuse fluids at a rate appropriate to the patient's condition, such as preexisting dehydration. All patients with a history of syncopal episode should have their blood glucose monitored and a 12-lead ECG.

Patients with a syncopal episode may want to refuse transport because their symptoms have often resolved before EMS arrival. Nonetheless, always attempt to transport these patients. Determining the true cause of a syncopal episode often is difficult in the emergency department and almost impossible in the field.

Patient and Family Education

Teach the family how to care for a person who has fainted or who has frequent episodes of fainting. Tell them to help the patient to the ground, bed, or couch to reduce the risk of injury. Teach them to loosen any tight clothing and call 9-1-1 right away if the patient does not respond to his or her name after lying down.

Case Scenario CONCLUSION

You have supplied supplemental oxygen. You have placed the patient on a backboard and secured the cervical spine with the appropriate head blocks and fasteners. En route to the hospital, you have started two large-bore IV lines, given a fluid challenge of normal saline, and performed a head-to-toe physical examination during transport. The patient initially moves her upper extremities in flexion with painful stimulus. She does not move her lower extremities. She opens her eyes to pain only. Her speech is incomprehensible. You notice no open wounds but an obviously deformed femur. The patient's vital signs reveal a blood pressure of 90/40 mm Hg, pulse of 128 beats/min, and respirations spontaneous at 12 breaths/min, slightly labored.

Questions

8. *What is this patient's current GCS score?*
9. *What do the vital signs indicate?*
10. *What is the appropriate verbal and written documentation for this patient?*

HEADACHE

[OBJECTIVES 4, 5]

Description and Definition

A headache, or pain felt in or around the head, is a common complaint that almost everyone has experienced at some time or another. Headaches usually resolve without treatment, but they can be extremely debilitating and may be a symptom of other underlying problems.

Etiology

Headaches are generally placed in two categories: vascular and nonvascular.

Vascular Headaches

Vascular headaches involve changes in the diameter or size and chemistry of blood vessels that supply the brain. This causes a throbbing pain that is not easily relieved. A **migraine headache** is a recurrent headache with symptom-free intervals and at least three of the following characteristics: *Find in dark room*

- Accompanying abdominal pain, nausea, or vomiting
- Throbbing or pulsatile character of the pain
- Located on one side of the head (but bilateral in 40% of patients)
- Associated aura (visual, sensory, motor)
- Relief after rest or sleep
- Positive family history

The exact cause of migraine headaches is not clearly understood. Some researchers believe that migraines may be caused by changes in the trigeminal nerve pathway in the nervous system. Others believe that migraines are caused by a combination of the expansion of blood vessels in the brain and imbalances in brain chemicals, such as dopamine and serotonin. Migraine headache triggers are listed in Box 23-10.

BOX 23-10	**Migraine Headache Triggers**

- Minor head injuries
- Sleep deprivation
- Strong or unusual smells
- Emotional stress or depression
- Changes in hormone levels
- Bright lights, flashing lights, flickering lights, television
- Noise
- Irregular eating patterns
- Substance abuse or withdrawal
- Specific foods and chemicals (monosodium glutamate, nuts, chocolate, cola drinks, hot dogs, or spicy meats)
- Often no trigger can be identified

The pain of a migraine headache usually lasts from 1 to 3 hours but may last as long as 72 hours. Migraines may be accompanied by intense nausea and vomiting and may be preceded for hours or days by pallor, decreased or increased appetite, mood changes, dizziness, or ringing in the ears (tinnitus). They usually are described as throbbing pain with accompanying nausea and vomiting, sweats, and pain when exposed to bright lights (photosensitivity).

Cluster headaches are attacks of severe stabbing pain, primarily localized behind or around the eye, temple, forehead, or cheek region. They tend to occur on one side of the head and are accompanied by nasal congestion and a watery eye on the affected side. Cluster headaches usually last 20 to 60 minutes. Patients typically hold the eye, rock back and forth or pace, and rub the head. The exact mechanism of cluster headaches remains uncertain. Men and women can be affected by either type of vascular headache (Weiderholt, 2000). However, cluster headaches are more common in males. The typical patient is the young to middle-aged male smoker, with a peak incidence in the late 20s.

Nonvascular Headaches

Nonvascular headaches have many different causes. These include headaches caused by hypertension, stroke, subarachnoid hemorrhage, brain tumors, abscesses, and other diseases of the eyes and nervous system. A tension headache is a benign headache also known as a *muscle contraction headache* or *stress headache*. This type of headache affects more than 75% of the population. Women are more commonly affected than men, and the prevalence peaks during middle age. The pain associated with a tension headache often is describes as constant and dull or as a tight band encircling the head. The muscles of the neck may tighten as well.

Some disease processes can bring on headaches. Sinus infections, meningitis, and encephalitis are notorious for causing headaches. Infectious headaches often are accompanied by fever and, depending on the pathogen, also may be seen with a rash, neck stiffness (nuchal rigidity), confusion, altered mental status, nausea, and vomiting.

Epidemiology and Demographics

An estimated 60% to 80% of Americans report having had a headache at one time or another (Sahai-Srivastava, 2005).

History and Physical Findings

When interviewing the patient with a headache, keep in mind the possible causes of the headache. Determining when the headache started and what the patient was doing at the time of onset is important. Has the patient taken any medications for the headache, either over the counter or prescription? If so, have they helped? A complete neurologic assessment should be performed to look for any signs of a serious neurologic problem, such as a stroke.

Therapeutic Interventions   *Sleep!*

As for most other neurologic conditions, prehospital management of a headache is mostly supportive. If an infectious disease is suspected as the cause, proper standard precautions, including respiratory protection, should be taken. Supplemental oxygen given by nonrebreather mask or nasal cannula can be helpful in reducing pain from a headache and should always be considered. Use common sense to help ease a patient's headache pain. During transport, turn down the lights in the back of the ambulance and avoid sirens, horns, and loud noises as much as possible. Consider IV access, analgesics such as ibuprofen or acetaminophen, and antiemetics for vomiting.

Patient and Family Education

The patient should be taught to call 9-1-1 if a headache is preceded or accompanied by visual disturbances, weakness on one side or part of the body, or difficulty speaking. Teach the patient to follow up with a physician for any severe headache (particularly if it is unusual for the patient), headache accompanied by stiff neck or high fever, or headache that occurs after a head injury.

BRAIN TUMOR

[OBJECTIVES 4, 5, 6]

Description and Definition

A brain tumor (**neoplasm**) is especially dangerous because of the confined space of the cranium. A primary brain tumor starts in the brain. A secondary brain tumor results from cancer that began in another part of the body and has spread to the brain.

Etiology

Just as any other tumor, a brain tumor can be benign (noncancerous) and stay in one place or malignant and spread cancer (metastasizing) to other parts of the body. A benign brain tumor usually grows more slowly and is less likely to return after removal than a malignant brain tumor. Either type can have severe and wide-ranging neurologic symptoms. Possible risk factors for brain cancer include radiation to the head, HIV infection, various environmental toxins, cigarette smoking, and some inherited conditions.

Epidemiology and Demographics

Brain tumors are most common in persons older than 65 years. Brain tumors are the leading cause of cancer death in patients younger than 50 years and are almost always fatal.

History and Physical Findings

The signs and symptoms of a brain tumor are often caused by increased intracranial pressure and depend on the location of the tumor, its size, and how quickly it grows. The most common symptom in the setting of a brain tumor is a headache. Signs and symptoms of a brain tumor are shown in Box 23-11. These signs and symptoms often present off and on over the course of days and weeks, especially if the tumor fluctuates in size.

Differential Diagnosis

Differential diagnoses include the following:

- Arteriovenous malformation
- Metastatic disease to the brain

Therapeutic Interventions

Diagnosing a brain tumor in the field is impossible and should not be attempted. Many times when EMS is contacted for a patient with a brain tumor, the patient already has a diagnosis and is under hospice care at home. In these cases, determine what has changed to make the patient or family call EMS.

As always, correcting life-threatening problems found in the primary survey comes first in the management of a patient with a brain tumor. If the patient already has a diagnosis of a brain tumor, ask about the presence of a do not resuscitate order. Regardless of the patient's status, give supportive care including oxygen, electrocardiographic monitoring, and additional care per medical direction instructions. Pharmacologic interventions may include analgesics, anticonvulsants in the case of seizures, and antiemetics.

Patient and Family Education

Teach the patient to call 9-1-1 or see a physician if he or she develops any of the following symptoms:

- Unexplained, persistent vomiting

BOX 23-11	Brain Tumor: Signs and Symptoms

- Recurrent and severe headaches
- Nausea and vomiting
- Gradual loss of sensation or movement in an extremity
- Lack of coordination
- Dizziness
- Changes in personality or behavior
- Double vision, blurred vision, loss of peripheral vision
- Nosebleed
- Difficulty speaking
- Hearing problems
- Seizures without a prior history

- Double vision or blurring of vision, particularly on only one side
- Increased sleepiness
- Seizures
- Headaches of a different type or pattern than usual

If the patient has a known brain tumor, tell him or her to call 9-1-1 if symptoms suddenly change or rapidly worsen.

BRAIN ABSCESS

[OBJECTIVES 4, 5]

Description and Definition

An **abscess** is a collection of pus within the body. A brain abscess can be dangerous because no space for swelling is available in the cranial cavity. As a result, pressure is put on the brain tissue, causing neurologic dysfunction.

Etiology

A brain abscess may occur after a penetrating head injury or neurosurgery. It can also result from an infection of nearby structures. For example, an ear or sinus infection can spread to the brain. Frontal lobe abscesses may occur after dental procedures. The organism causing the infection may be bacterial, viral, parasitic, or fungal. In some cases the source of the infection is never found.

Epidemiology and Demographics

This condition is estimated to be the cause of 1 of every 10,000 hospital admissions, equaling approximately 1500 to 2500 cases annually (Brook, 2005).

History and Physical Findings

Signs and symptoms of a brain abscess include headache, altered mental status, focal neurologic deficits, fever, seizures, nausea and vomiting, and neck stiffness.

Differential Diagnosis

Differential diagnoses include the following:

- Meningitis
- Encephalitis
- Stroke
- Brain tumor

Therapeutic Interventions

Most patients who have a large brain abscess require surgery to drain the abscess. A small brain abscess may be treated with drugs targeted to destroy the responsible organism. Prehospital management of a patient with a brain abscess is primarily supportive.

Patient and Family Education

Patients who have been prescribed antibiotics for an ear or sinus infection should be taught to take the medication as instructed. Because a dental infection is a potential source of brain infection, maintaining good dental hygiene is important.

CEREBROVASCULAR ACCIDENT (STROKE)

[OBJECTIVES 4, 5]

Stroke Center - has to have CT

Description and Definition

Time = brain

A **cerebrovascular accident** (commonly called a *stroke* or *brain attack*) is a sudden change in neurologic function caused by an alteration in cerebral blood flow. The brain requires a constant, abundant blood flow to function normally. When the brain's blood supply is disrupted, the patient may undergo significant changes in mental status; consciousness; and even vital life functions such as heart rate, respiratory rate, and blood pressure. If this disruption continues for longer than 10 to 20 minutes, the cells of the brain become injured and begin to die (Weiderholt, 2000).

Cerebral Blood Flow

carotids
circle of Willis
vertebral
foramen magnum

To meet its metabolic demands, the brain requires an extremely high amount of oxygen. In fact, the brain consumes 20% of the oxygen in the body and requires 20% of the total cardiac output to obtain the oxygen it needs. Blood reaches the brain by way of the anterior and posterior circulation. Eighty percent of cerebral perfusion is from the anterior circulation, which originates in the carotid system and is provided by the internal carotid arteries, which supply the frontal lobe, anterior parietal lobes, and the anterior temporal lobes, among other structures. The remaining 20% of cerebral perfusion is from the posterior circulation, which originates in the vertebral arteries. The posterior circulation is crucial to survival because it supplies the brainstem, cerebellum, posterior parts of the cerebrum, and other structures.

To ensure a constant supply of blood to the brain, even in the event of blockage of the anterior or posterior circulation, a system of redundancy exists is the cerebral circulation. The two internal carotids end by forming the anterior cerebral arteries and the middle cerebral arteries, which then supply the aforementioned areas of the brain. The two vertebral arteries end by forming the basilar artery, which then forms the posterior cerebral arteries. All these vessels are interconnected by communicating arteries forming the circle of Willis. In this manner a complete circle is formed that allows perfusion to continue if either the anterior or posterior circulation is blocked. After the circle of Willis, however, collateral circulation is limited to vessels in the dura mater and arachnoid membrane. Therefore redundant circulation is limited beyond the circle.

Once levels of the brain beyond the dura mater and arachnoid membrane are reached there is no collateral circulation. Blockages occurring in these areas must be alleviated to avoid death of brain tissue.

Etiology

Two main types of stroke are diagnosed: ischemic stroke and hemorrhagic stroke. An **ischemic stroke** occurs when blood flow in one of the arteries in the brain is blocked. Ischemic strokes account for 80% of all strokes. Blockage is most commonly caused by a blood clot. If the blood clot develops at the blockage site, it is called a *thrombus;* if it develops elsewhere in the body and then travels to the site of blockage, it is called an *embolus.* When blood flow to a part of the brain is stopped, that area ceases to function, causing a deficit in the body region controlled by that area of brain tissue. This pathology is similar to that of a heart attack or pulmonary embolus.

The majority of ischemic strokes are the result of a cerebral thrombus created by the presence of atherosclerotic plaques that form in the cerebral vasculature. These patients often have a long history of cardiovascular disease and risk factors for the formation of arterial plaques. These often occur in areas of turbulent blood flow, such as the bifurcation of arteries. This location is especially dangerous because both branches at the bifurcation can be blocked, causing widespread cerebral ischemia. A specific type of thrombotic stroke is known as a lacunar stroke. These occur in small vessels beyond any point of collateral circulation and can be devastating. Patients with a history of hypertension or diabetes are at particular risk for this type of stroke. Lacunar strokes often are localized and generally do not result in cognitive impairment or the inability to speak. Common presentations include the following:

- *Pure motor hemiparesis:* Unilateral paralysis.
- *Pure sensory dysfunction:* Unilateral numbness, tingling, or loss of sensation.
- *Ataxic hemiparesis:* Unilateral weakness and loss of coordination. This generally affects the lower extremities more than the upper extremities.

Embolic strokes generally have an identifiable cause, such as atrial fibrillation. In this situation a clot called a *mural thrombus* forms on the walls of the atria. When a piece of the thrombus breaks off and floats freely in the vascular system, it becomes an embolus. If this occurs in the left atrium the embolus can easily travel to the cerebral circulation, where it will lodge in a vessel and cause the cessation of blood flow and the onset of a stroke. Other kinds of emboli include air, fat, amniotic fluid, foreign bodies, tumors, bacteria, and fungus.

Sometimes a blood vessel in the brain can rupture, causing bleeding. This is called a **hemorrhagic stroke.** These account for 20% of all strokes. If the bleeding occurs within the brain tissue, it is classified as an **intracerebral hemorrhage.** If the bleeding is beneath the arachnoid membrane, it is classified as a **subarachnoid hemorrhage.** Intracerebral hemorrhages account for the majority of hemorrhagic strokes and often occur in patients with a history of hypertension, arteriovenous malformations, or existing aneurysms. Subarachnoid hemorrhages are generally caused by the rupture of a saccular (or berry) aneurysm in the subarachnoid space. Hemorrhagic strokes can occur in patients of any age. When they occur in young patients they generally are caused by the rupture of an aneurysm or an arteriovenous malformation. Rarely do these patients have a history of hypertension. Both intracranial and subarachnoid hemorrhages can occur as a result of trauma as well. This also is more common in younger patients than in older patients and is discussed in more detail in Chapter 47.

Regardless of the cause of the stroke, the outcome is the same. The part of the brain deprived of blood flow is termed the *area of primary injury.* All electrical activity in this area stops because of the lack of oxygen and glucose, resulting in a neurologic deficit. These cells initially are salvageable and the cell membranes remain intact; however, if the ischemia continues the cell membranes lose their integrity, causing increased permeability to electrolytes and eventual death. Surrounding the primary injury is an area called the *ischemic penumbra.* The cells in this area remain salvageable because of collateral circulation. However, if ischemia continues, the area of primary injury and the ischemic penumbra increase, resulting in the involvement of a greater area of the brain and greater neurologic dysfunction.

Time is crucial in the neurologic survival of the patient having a stroke. If the ischemic areas of the brain can be reperfused before permanent cell damage occurs, the patient can often recover with minimal neurologic deficits. This has led to the concept of the "window of treatment" for patients having a stroke. If reperfusion is accomplished with fibrinolytics, treatment must be complete within 3 hours of the onset of symptoms. Intraarterial therapy available at some stroke centers has extended this window to 6 hours after the onset of symptoms. The paramedic therefore must accurately identify the time of onset of symptoms whenever possible. An unknown or estimated time of onset makes patients ineligible for reperfusion therapy because the risks outweigh the benefits if the time limit has been exceeded. In addition, the paramedic must transport the patient to an appropriate facility. If available, a stroke center is the destination of choice when the patient is within the window of treatment. Much like bypassing community hospitals with a trauma patient to reach a trauma center, bypassing such facilities to reach a stroke center generally provides the best possible outcome for a stroke patient.

Epidemiology and Demographics

[OBJECTIVE 6]

- Stroke is the third leading cause of death in the United States, behind cardiovascular disease and cancer.

- Stroke affects more than 700,000 patients per year.
- Current costs of stroke-associated care is greater than $53 billion annually.
- Most strokes occur in persons older than age 65 years.
- Stroke is the most common cause of acquired disability in adults.
- Ischemic strokes are the most common type of stroke, representing 80% of all strokes (Bogousslausky, 2003).
- Hemorrhagic strokes have a much higher mortality rate than ischemic strokes, approaching 80%.
- Ten percent of patients die during the stroke and another 20% to 40% die within a few months. Forty percent have a mild, persistent neurologic deficit, and 10% require permanent institutional care (Weiderholt, 2000).
- African Americans have a much higher rate of stroke than other races.
- Stroke risk factors are listed in Box 23-12.

The Centers for Disease Control and Prevention have identified a "Stroke Belt" in the United States composed of states that have a higher incidence of stroke and a 10% or higher mortality rate from stroke than the national average. Most of these are in the south, including Alabama, Arkansas, Georgia, Indiana, Kentucky, Louisiana, Mississippi, North Carolina, South Carolina, Tennessee, Virginia, Oregon, and Washington.

History and Physical Findings

The history and symptoms of a patient with an ischemic stroke can vary widely depending on whether the blockage is a thrombus or an embolus. As a thrombus forms in a cerebral vessel over time, the patient may report symptoms such as **hemiparesis** or **hemiplegia.** These symptoms usually come and go or slowly worsen with time. Depending on the location of the stroke they may progress in a period of minutes to 3 days. The paramedic must not rule out the possibility of a stroke because of a perceived slow progression of signs and symptoms. An embolic stroke, on the other hand, usually occurs

suddenly, with the maximal severity of the symptoms at onset without worsening or improving. Thrombotic strokes may occur while a patient is asleep. This results in the patient awakening in the morning with neurologic impairments. In these situations determining if the stroke is thrombotic or embolic is difficult because whether it developed slowly or suddenly during sleep cannot be determined.

The symptoms of hemorrhagic stroke tend to occur with a higher severity and progress more rapidly than those of ischemic stroke. Patients often report a sudden onset "thunderclap" headache, or the "worst headache of my life." The headache is made worse by lying down and by movement. Signs and symptoms may quickly progress to forceful vomiting (often without nausea), neurologic deficits, visual disturbances such as blurry or double vision, unconsciousness, and seizures. The patient also may show signs and symptoms of rising **intracranial pressure (ICP),** unilateral pupil dilation, nausea, vomiting, and vital sign changes.

Under normal circumstances, very little extra room exists in the cranial cavity. The brain and its blood vessels sit inside the skull, cushioned on all sides by CSF. When a blood vessel ruptures, blood begins to fill the cranial cavity. This causes a rise in pressure within the cavity, and something must be moved out of the skull to make room. The blood filling the cerebral arteries is first to go. As the vessels are collapsed by the rising ICP, cerebral perfusion pressure markedly decreases. **Cerebral perfusion pressure (CPP)** is the pressure of the blood filling the arteries of the brain. CPP can be calculated as:

$$CPP = MAP - ICP$$

where *MAP* is mean arterial pressure, calculated as the diastolic blood pressure plus one third of the pulse pressure (PP):

$$MAP = DBP + \frac{1}{3}PP$$

ICP is usually less than 15 mm Hg and the normal range of CPP is approximately 70 to 150 mm Hg. If a patient has a blood pressure of 120/80 mm Hg, then the MAP is approximately 93 mm Hg. Therefore if this patient has an ICP of 13 mm Hg, then CPP is approximately 80 mm Hg, a normal level. However, if this patient's ICP increases to 50 mm Hg because of cerebral hemorrhage, then CPP will drop to 43 mm Hg. If the patient's ICP rises enough to equal MAP, then the patient will begin to undergo brain cell death because CPP will be zero and the brain will receive no oxygen or nutrients (Moraine et al., 2000).

To offset the rise in ICP, the body increases systemic blood pressure to try to perfuse the brain. However, this situation carries the risk of the increased systolic pressure increasing the ICP further, making the situation worse. If ICP continues to rise, CSF will be pushed out of the cavity. Finally, as the pressure increases further, the brain also will be pushed out **(herniate)** of the cranium through the foramen magnum. This twofold process causes severe damage and death to brain tissue and the characteristic pattern of **Cushing's triad:** hypertension (often with a widening pulse pressure), bradycardia, and abnormal respirations. An increase in body temperature often is seen; however, this is not considered part of Cushing's triad. This pattern continues for only a short time before the patient's blood pressure and heart rate drop and the patient dies. Compensatory mechanisms for increased intracranial pressure are explained in greater detail in Chapter 47.

Obtain a history of the event, including the time of onset; prior strokes or neurologic events; the progression of the stroke; recent or preceding factors, signs, or symptoms; and a past medical history including risk factors for strokes.

An effective tool to use with patients suspected of having a stroke is the Cincinnati Prehospital Stroke Scale. This scale assesses three major signs of stroke: facial droop, speech, and arm drift (Box 23-13). The outcome of the Cincinnati Prehospital Stroke Scale is reported as normal or abnormal; it does not have a numeric scale. If any single element is abnormal, a 72% chance exists that the patient is having a stroke.

Another tool used to assess for the presence of a stroke is the Los Angeles Prehospital Stroke Screen (LAPSS) (Figure 23-20). In addition to assessing for motor dysfunction and facial droop, this tool incorporates other information obtained as part of the normal assessment of the patient. This includes the patient's age, the time of onset, the presence of a history of seizures, blood glucose level, and the patient's baseline mobility status. With the addition of these elements the LAPSS has a sensitivity (ability to detect) of 93% and a specificity (accuracy) of 97% in the setting of a stroke.

The signs and symptoms often associated with a stroke are listed in Box 23-14. However, a few findings warrant further discussion. Recall from Chapter 7 the presence of Broca's area and Wernicke's area and their relation with the formation of speech and understanding of the spoken word. Strokes that affect either of these areas can result in aphasia, also called dysphasia.

Expressive aphasia occurs when the stroke affects Broca's area and often is called *Broca's aphasia*. In this situation the patient is able to understand and comprehend language but is unable to communicate verbally. Although the patient is able to articulate words clearly, communication is ineffective because sentence structure is poor and disjointed and often is limited to a few broken words. Receptive aphasia occurs when the stroke affects Wernicke's area and often is called *Wernicke's aphasia*. In this situation the patient cannot comprehend the spoken word. As a result, the patient has clear and articulate speech but it is not appropriate for the situation or questions being asked. Sentences also may be long and contain unnecessary or made-up words.

Aphasia, or dysphasia, should not be confused with dysarthria. Dysarthria is the inability to form words as a

---

BOX 23-13 Cincinnati Prehospital Stroke Scale

Facial droop/weakness: Ask patient to "Show me your teeth" or "Smile for me."
- Normal: Both sides of face move equally well.
- Abnormal: One side of face does not move at all.

Motor weakness (arm drift): With eyes closed, ask patient to extend arms out in front 90 degrees (if sitting) or 45 degrees (if supine). Drift is scored if the arm falls before 10 seconds.
- Normal: Both arms move the same *or* both arms do not move at all.
- Abnormal: One arm either does not move *or* one arm drifts down compared with the other.

Aphasia (speech): Ask the patient to say "A rolling stone gathers no moss," "You can't teach an old dog new tricks," "The sky is blue in Cincinnati," or a similar phase.
- Normal: Phrase is repeated clearly and correctly.
- Abnormal: Patient uses inappropriate words, words are slurred, or the patient is unable to talk.

Reprinted from Kothari, R.U., Pancioli, A., Liu, T., Brott, T., & Broderick, J. (1999). Cincinnati Prehospital Stroke Scale: Reproducibility and validity. *Annals of Emergency Medicine, 33*(4), 373-378.

BOX 23-14 Signs and Symptoms Associated with a Stroke

- Dysarthria
- Dysphagia
- Inability speak
- Inappropriate emotions
- Ataxia
- Hemiparesis
- Hemiplegia
- Paresthesia
- Aphasia
- Dysphasia
- Diplopia
- Hemianopsia
- Monocular blindness
- Deviated gaze
- Nystagmus
- Incontinence
- Convulsions
- Headache
- Altered mental status
- Confusion
- Coma
- Nausea and vomiting
- Vertigo
- Dizziness
- Facial droop
- Cerebellar dysfunction

■ **Los Angeles Prehospital Stroke Scale**

Criteria	Yes	Unknown	No
1. Age >45	☐	☐	☐
2. No history of seizures	☐	☐	☐
3. Symptoms <24 hrs	☐	☐	☐
4. Not wheelchair-bound or bedridden at baseline	☐	☐	☐
5. Glucose 60–400	☐	☐	☐

Assess symmetry in facial movement, hand grip, or arm strength

	Normal	Right	Left
Facial smile/grimace	☐	☐ Droop	☐ Droop
Grip	☐	☐ Weak	☐ Weak
		☐ None	☐ None
Arm strength	☐	☐ Drifts down	☐ Drifts down
		☐ Falls rapidly	☐ Falls rapidly

	Yes	No
6. Based on exam, patient has only unilateral weakness	☐	☐

Items 1-6 all Yes or Unknown, then LAPSS criteria are met. If LAPSS criteria are met, then call the receiving hospital with a "code stroke"; if not, then return to the appropriate treatment protocol. (NOTE: The patient may still be experiencing a stroke even if the LAPSS criteria are not met.)

Figure 23-20 Los Angeles Prehospital Stroke Scale.

result of the loss of control of the muscles required for speech. With dysarthria the patient understands and responds appropriately because Broca's and Wernicke's areas are not affected. However, because of the inability to control the muscles of speech, the words often are slurred and may be difficult to understand.

These terms also can be confused with dysphagia, which refers to difficulty in swallowing.

Differential Diagnosis

Differential diagnoses include the following:

- Trauma (such as subdural hematoma)
- Transient ischemic attack
- Meningitis or encephalitis
- Hypertensive encephalopathy
- Intracranial mass
- Spinal cord or peripheral nerve disease
- Brain abscess
- Seizures or Todd's paralysis
- Infections
- Complex migraines
- Bell's palsy
- Guillain-Barré syndrome
- Hypoglycemia
- Drug or alcohol intoxication

Therapeutic Interventions

If the patient's signs and symptoms suggest an acute stroke, begin transport and notify the receiving facility. Perform a focused or detailed physical examination en route to definitive care as dictated by the patient's condition.

As with any patient, your immediate concerns lie with the problems found in the primary survey. Level of consciousness is rarely decreased in patients having a stroke. Unconsciousness should point to another cause, such as seizures or hypoglycemia (Bogousslausky, 2003). However, do not rule out stroke as a possibility in the unconscious patient because hemorrhagic strokes and ischemic strokes involving the posterior circulation can render the patient unconsciousness. Make sure the patient's airway remains open. Patients with an acute stroke may lose the ability to swallow if the cranial nerves are affected. They may not be able to breathe effectively if the brainstem is involved. Apply a pulse oximeter and cardiac monitor. Give oxygen as needed and per medical direction instructions. Monitor the patient's breathing effort and be prepared to assist ventilations. If inadequate breathing is present, consider intubation, particularly if the patient's GCS score is less than 8. Consider the use of pharmacologically assisted intubation if necessary and approved by medical direction. Lidocaine is usually given IV approximately 90 seconds before intubation to prevent a further increase in ICP.

> **PARAMEDIC Pearl**
>
> Keep a close watch on a stroke patient's airway, breathing, and circulation; they may worsen quickly.

Establish IV access with a saline lock or an IV line containing normal saline or Ringer's lactate and run at a keep-open rate (30 mL/hr). Avoid giving large volumes of fluids unless hypotension is present. Obtain a 12-lead ECG. Do not delay transport to definitive care to perform these procedures.

Check the patient's blood glucose level. Hypoglycemia often mimics the signs and symptoms of a stroke. If the patient's blood glucose level is below 60 mg/dL, give dextrose. Otherwise, avoid giving dextrose-containing solutions because the hypertonic molecules may worsen brain swelling (Adams et al., 2003).

Use a prehospital stroke alert checklist to screen patients for stroke signs and symptoms, time of onset, and contraindications to fibrinolytic therapy or other therapies that may become available. Obtaining this information should not delay patient transport. However, do not allow urgency to leave the scene cause important information, such as the time of onset, to be missed. Any information obtained should be relayed to the receiving facility.

Be familiar with the categorization and designation of hospitals in your area. As previously discussed, patients showing signs and symptoms of an acute stroke should be transported to a designated stroke center if delivery to the center within the window of treatment is possible. Notify the center of your impending arrival. If transport to a stroke center is not possible or practical, consult medical direction to determine the appropriate receiving facility based on local and available resources.

Seizures are most likely to occur within 24 hours of stroke. Persistent seizures should be treated with benzodiazepines.

PARAMEDIC*Pearl*

While caring for a stroke patient, keep in mind that even though the patient may not be able to communicate, he or she may be fully aware of the surroundings. Assume the patient can hear you and talk to him or her as you provide care.

Patient and Family Education

The patient's family should be taught the following signs and symptoms of a stroke:

- Sudden numbness or weakness of the face, arm, or leg, especially on one side of the body
- Sudden severe headache with no known cause
- Sudden dimness or loss of vision, particularly in one eye
- Sudden confusion, difficulty speaking, or trouble understanding speech
- Unexplained dizziness, unsteadiness, or sudden falls, especially with any of the other signs

Stroke victims and their families must be taught to activate the EMS system immediately on recognition of signs and symptoms. Psychological support is essential for these patients and their families.

PARAMEDIC*Pearl*

The three *R*'s of stroke are *r*educe risk, *r*ecognize symptoms, and *r*espond by calling 9-1-1.

TRANSIENT ISCHEMIC ATTACK

[OBJECTIVES 4, 5]

Description and Definition

A **transient ischemic attack (TIA)** is a reversible episode of localized neurologic dysfunction that typically lasts a few minutes to a few hours, resolving within 24 hours.

Etiology

The etiology of a TIA is similar to an ischemic stroke. Blood flow is decreased in cerebral arteries that may have a partial blockage or undergo vasospasm. This decreased flow prevents oxygen and nutrients from reaching brain tissue.

Epidemiology and Demographics

More than 50,000 Americans sustain a TIA each year. TIAs subside with no long-term impairment but are often an indicator of things to come. Studies show that 20% to 30% of major strokes are preceded by a TIA or minor stroke.

History and Physical Findings

[handwritten: 30% have CVA within 3 months if don't change anything]

A TIA shows the same signs and symptoms as a stroke and often are called *mini-strokes*. The difference is that the symptoms of a TIA resolve within 24 hours from onset, usually within 10 to 20 minutes (Weiderholt, 2000). Differentiating between a stroke and a TIA in the field is impossible and the worst should always be suspected.

The symptoms of a TIA may be subtle and more noticeable to the patient's family than to the patient. If the symptoms have resolved on your arrival, obtain and document a detailed description of the symptoms and determine if they are now completely resolved. Ask about a history of cardiac dysrhythmias, particularly atrial fibrillation. Atrial fibrillation can cause blood pooling and clotting. Ask about the use of stimulants such as cocaine. Cocaine can cause vasospasm.

Differential Diagnosis

Differential diagnoses include the following:

- Bell's palsy
- Brain tumor
- Hemorrhagic stroke
- Hypoglycemia

- Ischemic stroke
- Migraine headache
- Subarachnoid hemorrhage

Therapeutic Interventions

Treatment for a TIA is the same as for stroke. A patient who has had a TIA that has resolved must be evaluated by a physician.

Patient and Family Education

Teach the patient and family the signs and symptoms of stroke. Explain that a TIA often is a predictor of a stroke. The patient or a family member should call 9-1-1 if any of the signs and symptoms of a stroke are observed. Although clot-busting drugs are not used to treat a TIA, patient evaluation by a physician may help decrease the risk of an impending stroke.

INFECTIOUS NERVOUS SYSTEM DISORDERS

Meningitis

[OBJECTIVES 7, 8]

Description and Definition

Meningitis is a potentially deadly infection of the layers of connective tissue covering the brain and spinal cord. The blood supply of the meninges lies next to the venous system of the nasopharynx, mastoid process, and middle ear. The organism that causes meningitis penetrates vulnerable sites of the blood-brain barrier and spreads throughout the subarachnoid space. Because the meninges are continuous around the central nervous system and CSF flows in the arachnoid space, infection quickly spreads through the coverings of the brain. The inflammatory response causes the brain to become swollen and covered with a layer of pus (Figure 23-21).

Meningitis can be caused by viruses, bacteria, and fungi. Viral (aseptic) meningitis is the most common type of meningitis. Bacterial meningitis usually is caused by *Streptococcus pneumoniae*, *Neisseria meningitidis*, or *Haemophilus influenzae* type b (Hib).

Etiology

Following are common causes of meningitis:

- Approximately 90% of cases of viral meningitis are caused by enteroviruses. Herpes viruses and the mumps virus also can cause viral meningitis.
- In older infants and children, the infection that causes meningitis usually is secondary to another bacterial infection, such as an upper respiratory, ear, or sinus infection or pneumonia.
- Bacterial meningitis also may occur from direct entry of bacteria into the central nervous system.

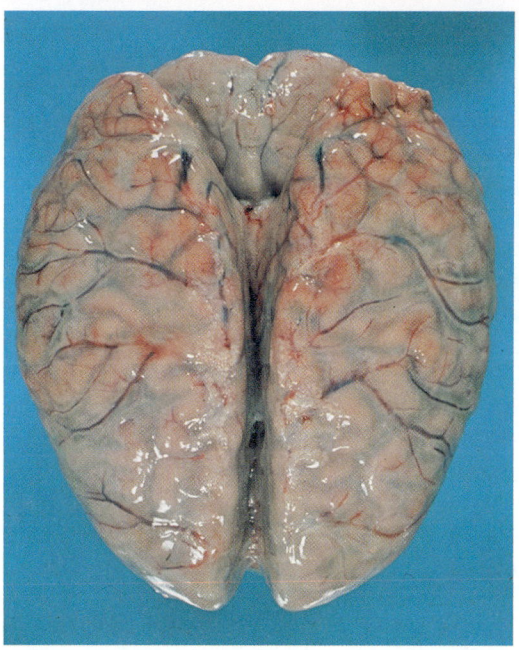

Figure 23-21 Brain with pus covering the cerebral hemispheres in meningitis.

For example, bacteria may enter the central nervous system through a penetrating injury of the skull or skull fracture (CSF leak).

Epidemiology and Demographics

Facts about meningitis include the following:

- Vaccines now given to all children as part of their routine immunizations (beginning at approximately 2 months of age) have reduced the occurrence of Hib meningitis. *S. pneumoniae* and *N. meningitidis* are now the leading causes of bacterial meningitis.
- Although bacterial meningitis can occur at any time of the year, the incidence increases in late winter and early spring. The incidence of viral meningitis increases during the summer months.
- Meningitis caused by *S. pneumoniae* (also called *pneumococcal meningitis*) has the following characteristics:
  - Most commonly occurs in infants younger than 8 months and after head injury
  - Has a higher incidence in African Americans than in whites
  - Has an increasing incidence of antibiotic resistance
- Meningitis caused by *N. meningitidis* (also called *meningococcal meningitis*) has the following characteristics:
  - From 2% to 15% of healthy individuals (particularly adults) are asymptomatic carriers of the organism in their nasopharynx.
  - It most often occurs in children younger than 5 years; peak attack is at 6 to 12 months of age, and another peak attack occurs in adolescence.

History and Physical Findings

Signs and symptoms of meningitis vary depending on the organism responsible for the infection. Viral meningitis often is mistaken for the flu.

High fever, headache, and stiff neck are common symptoms of meningitis in patients older than 2 years. Additional findings include signs of meningeal irritation, headache, photophobia, lethargy, altered mental status, chills, vomiting, and seizures. In patients younger than 2 years, signs and symptoms are more subtle and may be limited to increased irritability and decreased feeding. Symptoms can develop over several hours, or they may take 1 to 2 days. In newborns and infants younger than 2 to 3 months, fever, headache, and neck stiffness may be absent or difficult to detect. The patient may have a nonblanching rash; when pressure is applied to the area of the rash, the rash does not blanch white, as is normally seen.

Differential Diagnosis

Differential diagnoses include the following:

- Brain abscess
- Encephalitis
- Migraine headache

Therapeutic Interventions

Prehospital care of any patient suspected of having meningitis warrants standard precautions, including gloves and mask protection. Care for viral meningitis is primarily supportive. Care usually includes pain management and monitoring for seizures.

Bacterial meningitis is a life-threatening medical emergency with a mortality rate of 25% to 50%. Death can occur within 30 to 60 minutes; therefore recognition is key to survival. Prehospital care for bacterial meningitis starts with establishing and maintaining a patent airway. Suction as necessary. Give oxygen and place the patient on a cardiac monitor and pulse oximeter. Establish IV access. If signs of shock or dehydration are present, give normal saline or Ringer's lactate as instructed by medical direction and then reassess. Do not overhydrate. Check the patient's blood glucose level and give dextrose if hypoglycemic. Assess mental status, neurologic signs, and vital signs every 5 minutes. Be prepared to treat seizures.

On arrival at the receiving facility, be sure to inform the physician of your suspicions so that the patient's family members and others with whom the patient may have been in close contact can be tested for meningitis.

Patient and Family Education

Persons in the same household or daycare center or anyone in direct contact with the oral secretions of a patient infected with meningococcal meningitis are at increased risk of acquiring the infection. Close contacts should see their physicians and receive antibiotic prophylaxis.

Encephalitis

[OBJECTIVES 7, 8]

Description and Definition

Encephalitis is an infection of the brain tissue.

Etiology

Encephalitis is most often caused by a viral infection, but it can be bacterial or parasitic. The same organisms responsible for viral meningitis may also be associated with encephalitis. However, encephalitis is much less common. In rare cases encephalitis may be caused by brain injury or adverse reactions to medications or poisons.

West Nile virus is a type of encephalitis. First isolated in the West Nile region of Uganda in 1937, West Nile virus first appeared in the United States in 1999. Since then, cases of human infection have appeared in every state in the continental United States.

Epidemiology and Demographics

Like most cases of encephalitis, West Nile virus rarely is fatal but can be dangerous to pediatric patients, the elderly, and those with compromised immune systems.

History and Physical Findings

Signs or symptoms of mild to moderate encephalitis are flulike and include fever, fatigue, sore throat, headache, nausea and vomiting, drowsiness, and photophobia. Altered mental status occurs in virtually all patients. As the disease progresses, signs of serious nervous system dysfunction may develop, such as muscle weakness or paralysis, memory loss, impaired judgment, a decreased level of consciousness, and seizures.

Differential Diagnosis

Differential diagnoses include the following:

- Brain abscess
- Brain tumor
- Hypoglycemia
- Meningitis
- Psychiatric disorder
- Status epilepticus
- Subarachnoid hemorrhage

Therapeutic Interventions

Prehospital treatment primarily consists of supportive care. If the patient is alert and has stable vital signs, give oxygen, apply a pulse oximeter, and transport to the closest appropriate facility. If the patient has an altered mental status, closely monitor the patient's airway. Give oxygen and apply a pulse oximeter and cardiac monitor. Because seizures may occur with encephalitis, establish IV access and treat seizures with benzodiazepines per local protocol. If signs of shock are present, give normal saline or Ringer's lactate as instructed by medical direction. Transport to the closest appropriate facility.

Patient and Family Education

Vaccination is available against Japanese encephalitis virus. Vaccination is recommended for people who perform extensive outdoor activities.

Shingles

[OBJECTIVES 7, 8]

Description and Definition

Shingles is an extremely painful infection of a spinal nerve by the varicella-zoster virus, the same virus responsible for chickenpox.

Etiology

Shingles can develop in patients in two ways. Patients historically were only able to develop shingles after being exposed to the varicella-zoster virus, which results in chickenpox. After the case of chickenpox subsides the virus travels to a sensory nerve deep within the body and lies dormant, usually for decades. Later, usually when the patient is much older, the virus is reactivated for unknown reasons and infects and irritates a sensory nerve, usually a spinal nerve. However, because of the advent of the varicella virus vaccine, shingles can now develop in patients who never had chickenpox. This is because the vaccine contains a live virus, meaning a subinfectious dose of the virus is injected into the patient. This causes an immune response that develops immunity to chickenpox. However, the virus undergoes the same process as a natural exposure, in which it travels to a sensory nerve and remains dormant until reactivation.

Epidemiology and Demographics

An estimated 50,000 cases of shingles occur in the United States per year. Because of vaccination against chickenpox, however, the rate of infection may change in the future (Moon, 2005). Shingles is most common among people older than 50 years but can develop at any age. In fact, the number of shingles cases in the pediatric population has increased since the introduction of the varicella-zoster virus vaccine.

History and Physical Findings

The infection has three phases, each with distinct symptoms. First, in most patients extreme sensitivity and pain develop along a unilateral dermatome. After 1 to 3 days, this progresses to a reddened rash with raised bumps and blisters along the same area (Figure 23-22). These bumps and blisters fill with pus and scab over within 10 to 12 days. The scabs then fall off and the rash disappears within 2 to 3 weeks. Scarring of the area may result. The pain associated with shingles usually lasts from 3 to 5 weeks.

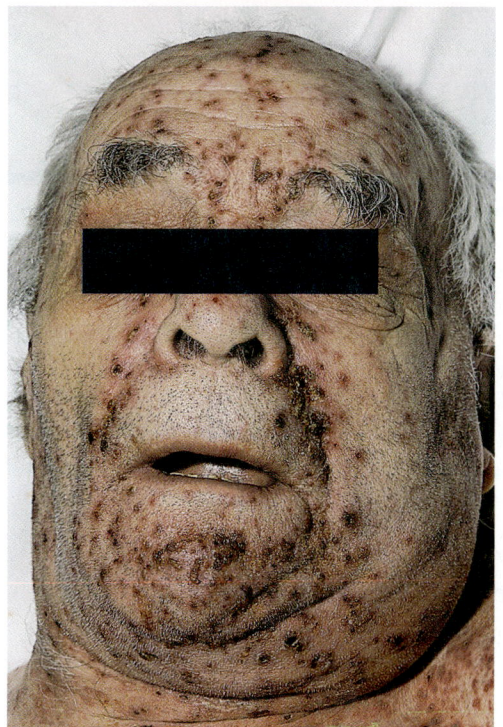

Figure 23-22 Shingles in the cervical dermatomes.

Differential Diagnosis

Differential diagnoses include the following:

- Acute appendicitis
- Bell's palsy
- Cholecystitis
- Conjunctivitis
- Herpes simplex
- Herpes zoster
- Kidney stone
- Trigeminal neuralgia

Therapeutic Interventions

Take appropriate standard precautions. Varicella-zoster is not contagious except to immunocompromised patients. Examples of immunocompromised patients include those with HIV infection or who receive cancer treatments or organ transplants. Varicella-zoster does not cause any threats to the airway or respirations, but the pain can be severe. Give supportive care and consider analgesics as dictated by local protocols.

Patient and Family Education

A patient who has shingles may find that applying a baking soda paste or calamine lotion or taking baths helps relieve itching. The patient should call 9-1-1 or seek medical help if the rash spreads near the eyes because eye damage, including loss of vision, can occur.

Poliomyelitis

[OBJECTIVES 7, 8]

Description and Definition

Poliomyelitis, commonly called *polio,* is a highly infectious viral disease.

Etiology

Poliovirus is usually transmitted by direct fecal-oral contact, indirect contact with saliva or feces, or contaminated water. The virus enters the body through the mouth, multiplies in the intestine, and then spreads to lymph nodes and the blood. Once multiplied, the virus tends to attack the motor neurons of the spinal cord and brainstem. This can cause total paralysis in a matter of hours.

Epidemiology and Demographics

Facts about poliomyelitis include the following:

- Children are more susceptible to infection, but the risk of paralysis is higher in adults. Polio mainly affects children younger than 5 years.
- The incubation period of poliomyelitis is approximately 7 to 14 days.
- No cure is available, but the disease can effectively be prevented with a multiple-dose vaccination program. Worldwide, cases of polio have decreased 99% since 1988 because of a strong vaccination initiative.

History and Physical Findings

Most patients (95%) infected with poliovirus are asymptomatic. Initial symptoms in some patients include fever, nausea, vomiting, fatigue, headache, neck stiffness, and pain in the extremities. Paralysis occurs in less than 10% of patients and usually peaks within 48 hours. One in 200 cases leads to irreversible paralysis, usually of the legs. Among these patients, 5% to 10% die when the paralysis spreads to the phrenic nerve, which is responsible for contraction of the diaphragm and therefore breathing.

From 10% to 20% of patients with paralytic polio have postpolio syndrome develop 20 to 30 years after the initial infection. This syndrome consists of excessive fatigue and progressive weakness of formerly paralyzed muscles. The etiology of this condition is unknown.

Differential Diagnosis

Differential diagnoses include the following:

- Encephalitis
- Guillain-Barré syndrome
- Meningitis

Therapeutic Interventions

Prehospital care for the patient who has poliomyelitis is mainly supportive. Maintain an open airway. Watch for difficulty swallowing and signs of inadequate breathing. Positive-pressure ventilation is usually needed in patients who are paralyzed. Analgesics may be needed for back pain and leg spasms. In general, narcotics should be avoided because of the risk of additional respiratory depression.

Patient and Family Education

The patient and family should be taught to wash their hands thoroughly after contact with the patient and his or her secretions to reduce the spread of infection. Parents should be encouraged to have their children vaccinated against polio.

DEGENERATIVE NERVOUS SYSTEM DISORDERS

Alzheimer's Disease

[OBJECTIVES 9, 10]

Description and Definition

First described by Alois Alzheimer in 1907, **Alzheimer's disease** is a devastating degenerative nervous system disorder causing a dementia marked by slowly declining function in thinking, reasoning, and especially memory.

Etiology

On the cellular level, abnormal proteins called *clumps* (senile plaques) and *bundles* (neurofibrillary tangles) are believed to form and grow onto and between neurons. These choke neurons, which leads to widespread cell death over time. Eventually, as more and more neurons die, the brain becomes atrophied and wasted in appearance. This process usually begins in the hippocampus, the brain's memory switchboard. As the disease progresses, the clumps and bundles spread to the frontal and temporal lobes of the cerebrum, affecting personality, causing hallucinations, and affecting motor function. Eventually this spreads to most of the brain, though the occipital lobe often remains unaffected.

Epidemiology and Demographics

Alzheimer's disease is the most common cause of senile dementia, affecting an estimated 5 million people in the United States and 30 million people worldwide. This equals approximately 10% of the elderly population in the United States. The disease is present in 40% to 50% of those older than 84 years (Weiderholt, 2000). The number of persons affected by Alzheimer's disease is estimated to triple by the year 2050 (Kuljis, 2005).

History and Physical Findings

Signs and symptoms of Alzheimer's disease vary widely as the condition progresses. In its early stages, patients may have slight lapses in memory and cognition, such as trouble recognizing familiar family and friends or remembering recent events and activities. The patient may seem to have problems finding a particular word to describe something or may show difficulty performing familiar tasks. These signs often go unnoticed or are simply credited to age by the patient's friends and family.

This decrease in mental function continues as the patient becomes unable to think clearly or solve problems and develops communication issues (problems with reading, speaking, and writing). At this stage, patients begin to lose the ability to perform simply daily functions such as bathing, grooming, dressing, preparing meals, and remembering to take scheduled medications. Even in familiar surroundings, the patient becomes increasingly confused and disoriented and has a greater risk of falls and accidents. A common phenomenon of increasing restless, anxiety, and a tendency to wander away from home is referred to as *sundowner syndrome,* because it often happens around dusk.

In its most advanced stages, victims of Alzheimer's disease sustain a complete loss of both short-term and long-term memory and may be unable to recognize even close family and friends. These patients often undergo drastic changes in personality, perhaps becoming hostile, anxious, or angry. Severely disoriented, they become dependent on others for all their daily needs and usually are under almost full-time nursing care. The patient's motor function eventually declines to a point at which the patient has a complete loss of mobility, becoming bedridden. The patient also may be unable to swallow and eat normally, likely requiring placement of a feeding tube.

Alzheimer's patients likely are very poor historians and may even be outright combative and hostile. These patients can be very difficult to interact with. Always remember that this is not intentional. The patient is not aware of his or her actions and words. Prescription medications now on the market have been shown to slow the progression of Alzheimer's disease, particularly when taken in the earliest stages. No cure is available, however, and the disease is chronic and devastating. Patients usually do not die of Alzheimer's disease itself, but instead succumb to complications of the condition, including trauma from falls, aspiration of food and liquid into the lungs, and sepsis from infections caused by the inability to care for oneself.

Differential Diagnosis

Differential diagnoses include Parkinson's disease and stroke.

Therapeutic Interventions

Prehospital treatment for this condition includes supportive care.

Patient and Family Education

Provide emotional support to the patient and family. Encourage the family to create a routine for the patient.

As the disease progresses, the patient may need assistance with activities of daily living, including eating, bathing, dressing, and toileting. A physician will discuss the patient's decision-making capacity with the patient's family. Arrangements may need to be made to identify an individual who can make decisions on the patient's behalf.

Parkinson's Disease

[OBJECTIVES 9, 10]

Description and Definition

Parkinson's disease (also called *shaking palsy*) is a degenerative disorder of the brain.

Etiology

Parkinson's disease affects the extrapyramidal system, which is responsible for fine motor coordination and posture. It is believed to occur from a deficiency of dopamine in the cerebellum.

Epidemiology and Demographics

Parkinson's disease is one of the more common degenerative nervous system disorders, affecting 1% of the population older than 60 years. It is more common in men than in women. Approximately 1 million people are currently affected, with roughly 50,000 new cases diagnosed each year (Hauser, 2004). Parkinson's disease has an average age of onset of 60 years, but as the disease has become better recognized younger diagnosis is becoming more common, but rarely before age 40 years.

History and Physical Findings

The four key signs of Parkinson's are a resting tremor, rigidity, bradykinesia, and postural instability. A resting tremor is usually asymmetrical and initially appears as a "pill rolling" tremor, as if the patient were moving a round pill back and forth between the thumb and index finger. This tremor may progress to the entire limb and often is aggravated by stress. The rigidity of Parkinson's disease is a stiffness of the muscles and leads to jerky, irregular motions when an extremity is moved. Bradykinesia, or slowed movements, describes a gradual muscle weakness and decrease in muscle function. Signs such as poor or small handwriting, soft speech, a decreased blink rate and lack of facial expression are examples. In the later stages of the illness, postural instability develops, which is an imbalance of the body caused by the loss of the normal reflexes used to keep the body upright. These tremors and movement problems may complicate assessment and often are the cause of falls and related injuries in patients with Parkinson's disease.

Differential Diagnosis

Differential diagnoses include Alzheimer's disease and stroke.

Die from respiratory failure

Therapeutic Interventions

Prehospital treatment for this condition includes supportive care. Patients who have Parkinson's disease are at risk of choking and aspiration. Closely monitor the patient's airway and breathing. Use positioning or airway adjuncts as necessary to maintain an open airway. Suction as needed. These patients often take levodopa, which is a precursor to dopamine, in an attempt to increase dopamine levels.

Patient and Family Education

Provide emotional support to the patient and family. Talk to them about the benefits of installing or using handrails in halls and stairs. Throw rugs should be removed from floors to decrease the likelihood of falls and be replaced with nonskid mats where needed. As the disease progresses, the patient often finds dressing easier if clothing is fitted with hook-and-loop closures rather than zippers or buttons. Slip-on shoes that fit well should be used instead of shoes that must be tied.

Amyotrophic Lateral Sclerosis

[OBJECTIVES 9, 10]

Description and Definition

More commonly known as *Lou Gehrig's disease,* **amyotrophic lateral sclerosis (ALS)** is a degenerative disease of the motor spinal nerves. At the onset, only upper or lower motor neurons are involved; however, the disease progresses to involve both. The site of onset is random and the progression is asymmetric.

Etiology

The exact cause of ALS is unknown. Motor spinal nerves begin to break down because of an unknown process and the patient starts to lose voluntary muscle control. As this happens, the muscles controlled by these dying nerves become weak and shrink from lack of activity. The muscles also twitch (fasciculate). The patient's sensation and mental abilities remain unaffected, as are the anal and bladder sphincter muscles and the muscles that move the eye. The disease usually progresses until the phrenic nerve that controls the diaphragm (originating from C3, C4, and C5) dies and the patient is unable to breathe. Early respiratory paralysis is possible, which often leads to death before advanced stages of the disease set in.

Epidemiology and Demographics

ALS strikes approximately five out of every 100,000 people, most between the ages of 40 and 70 years. Currently no cure is available.

History and Physical Findings

Symptoms often begin as clumsiness or weakness in one hand, such as being unable to button a shirt or having difficulty swallowing. The weakness then spreads up to the arm and shoulder, then quickly throughout the body. Most patients with ALS die within 5 years of diagnosis (Dangond, 2004). Even in late stages sensory, bowel, and bladder function are intact. Dementia is not a component of ALS and cognitive function remains intact. Additional signs and symptoms are shown in Box 23-15.

Differential Diagnosis

Differential diagnoses include the following:

- Brain tumor
- Dementia
- Diabetic neuropathy
- Myasthenia gravis

Therapeutic Interventions

Patients with ALS have home mechanical ventilators and often are under nursing care. EMS is commonly called for an equipment malfunction; catheter infection; and conditions associated with chronic illness, including pneumonia, respiratory failure, and aspiration. Use positioning or airway adjuncts as necessary to maintain an open airway. Suction as needed. Many patients with ALS have a do not resuscitate order.

Patient and Family Education

Provide emotional support to the patient and family. Promote safety in the home. Discuss the use of nonskid mats instead of throw rugs. Explain the benefits of installing and using handrails in tub, shower, and toilet areas as well as in halls and stairs. A home health care agency should be contacted to assist the family in caring for the patient. The patient and family should be referred to a local ALS support group.

PARAMEDIC*Pearl*

When caring for a patient with ALS, remember that although the patient's body may be losing muscle function, his or her mind, personality, intelligence, and memory remain intact. Although the patient may have difficulty communicating with you, he or she can still see, smell, taste, hear, and recognize touch. As with all patients, explain what you are doing and why as you provide care. Be compassionate and respectful.

Multiple Sclerosis

Difficult to diagnose

[OBJECTIVES 9, 10]

Description and Definition

Multiple sclerosis (MS), an autoimmune disorder in which the body's immune system attacks the nervous system, is a puzzling disease.

Etiology

Peripheral nerves in the body are wrapped in a myelin sheath, which in effect insulates a neuron much like rubber insulation on a wire. In MS the myelin sheath

BOX 23-15	Signs and Symptoms of ALS

Lower Motor Neuron Disease

- Asymmetric weakness that generally begins distally in one limb
- Recent development of cramping
- Progressive wasting and atrophy of muscles
- Spontaneous twitching
- Difficulty in chewing, swallowing, or moving the face

Upper Motor Neuron Disease

- Hyperactivity of reflexes (tendon jerks)
- Spastic resistance to movement of affected limbs
- Muscle stiffness out of proportion to weakness
- Exaggeration of motor expressions of emotion

ALS, Amyotrophic lateral sclerosis.

comes under attack, causing dysfunction of the peripheral nervous system. This affects both sensory function and motor control.

Epidemiology and Demographics

An estimated 123,000 patients with MS live in the United States, and approximately 10,000 new cases are diagnosed each year. Women are affected at twice the rate of men, and the average age at onset is 33 years (Weiderholt, 2000). Scientists have shown MS to have a genetic link, though the extent of this link is unclear.

History and Physical Findings

The symptoms of MS depend on the part of the nervous system affected. Dysfunction in the occipital lobe causes a painful vision loss, and trouble in the cerebellum causes a loss of fine motor control. If the peripheral nerves are affected, the patient has weakness and pain in the extremities; problems with the cranial nerves can cause facial pain and paralysis, hearing loss, and vertigo. Symptoms of MS follow an unpredictable course, coming and going at random times. The severity of MS also is mysterious; some patients live most of their lives symptom free, whereas others are confined to bed because of the disease. Often the cause of EMS intervention is a fall. Through investigation the paramedic is able to learn of increased or intermittent muscle weakness and suspicion of this disease becomes evident.

Differential Diagnosis

Differential diagnoses include brain tumor.

Therapeutic Interventions

Prehospital treatment for this condition includes supportive care. Use positioning or airway adjuncts as necessary to maintain an open airway. Suction as needed.

Patient and Family Education

Provide emotional support for the patient and family. Patients who have MS are prone to falls. Discuss the need for keeping pathways and stairs free of clutter. Discuss installing and using handrails and the importance of adequate lighting.

Guillain-Barré Syndrome

[OBJECTIVES 9, 10]

Description and Definition

Guillain-Barré syndrome is an autoimmune disorder that attacks the peripheral nervous system.

Etiology

Guillain-Barré syndrome usually occurs after some insult to the immune system, such as a surgery or medication therapy.

Epidemiology and Demographics

Guillain-Barré syndrome is exceedingly rare (National Institute of Neurological Disorders and Stroke, 2005).

History and Physical Findings

The patient typically reports weakness initially, a tingling or a "pins and needles" sensation in the legs. In many patients this spreads up the legs and to the rest of the body. As the immune system attacks more and more peripheral nerves, the patient's muscle strength in the extremities becomes weaker and weaker, and the patient often loses deep tendon reflexes. Eventually the patient may become paralyzed. Weakness usually peaks approximately 3 weeks after the onset of symptoms and then usually slowly goes away. Some patients may have to be placed on a mechanical ventilator in the meantime because the nerves that control respiration may be impaired. The recovery period may be a little as a few weeks but may last as long as a few years. A small percentage of patients may relapse into further episodes of weakness. *usually self resolves*

Differential Diagnosis

Differential diagnoses include the following:

- Encephalitis
- Heavy metal poisoning (lead, thallium, arsenic)
- Hyperkalemia
- Hypermagnesemia
- Hypokalemia
- Meningitis
- Myasthenia gravis
- Organophosphate poisoning
- Poliomyelitis
- Snake envenomation
- Spinal cord infection or injury

Therapeutic Interventions

A patient who has Guillain-Barré syndrome is at risk of airway and breathing problems. Use positioning or airway adjuncts as necessary to maintain an open airway. Suction as needed. Apply a pulse oximeter and cardiac monitor. Give oxygen and begin positive-pressure ventilation as needed. Tracheal intubation may be needed in cases of respiratory failure. Monitor for cardiac dysrhythmias. Changes in heart rate ranging from bradycardia to tachycardia are common. Tachycardia rarely requires treatment. Atropine is typically used for symptomatic bradycardia. Because hypotension or hypertension is common, establish IV access. Hypotension usually responds to IV fluids and supine positioning. Transport to the closest appropriate facility for physician evaluation.

Patient and Family Education

Depression is common in patients with this condition. Provide emotional support for the patient and family.

Myasthenia Gravis

[OBJECTIVES 9, 10]

Description and Definition

Myasthenia gravis, literally meaning *grave muscle weakness,* is another autoimmune neurologic disorder that causes muscle weakness and fatigue.

Etiology

Myasthenia gravis is caused by the lymphocytes attacking the acetylcholine receptors found on the voluntary skeletal muscle side of neuroeffector junctions. Fewer receptors are available to be stimulated, and the antibodies of the immune system often attach to the receptors, blocking them from being stimulated. When the presynaptic neuron releases acetylcholine, instead of stimulating a muscle contraction as normal, the neurotransmitter is blocked. This condition is usually an acquired immunologic disorder, but it can be caused by inherited problems of the neuroeffector junction. The cause of this disorder is believed to be related to the thymus, an endocrine gland important in the body's immunity.

Epidemiology and Demographics

Approximately 36,000 cases of myasthenia gravis have been estimated to exist in the United States, but given that many patients are undiagnosed or misdiagnosed, that number probably is much higher (Howard, 1997). Women younger than 40 years and men older than 60 years are most commonly affected.

History and Physical Findings

Myasthenia gravis can affect any voluntary muscle, but the muscles that control eye and eyelid movement, facial expression, and swallowing are most often affected. Ptosis, or a drooping of the eyelid, often results. The onset of the condition may be sudden, and the disorder often is misdiagnosed. The severity of muscle weakness fluctuates. In many patients it is better in the morning and worsens as the day goes on, particularly in muscles that are extensively used. Myasthenia gravis usually becomes worse over time. The symptoms often go away for periods, only to return. After 15 to 20 years, the condition becomes the most severe, and the muscles that are affected most atrophy and shrink. A myasthenic crisis occurs when the muscles of respiration become involved. In this case the respiratory rate and tidal volume slow until the patient enters respiratory arrest. This often occurs without any findings other than a history of myasthenia gravis.

Differential Diagnosis

Differential diagnoses include the following:

- Acute respiratory distress syndrome
- ALS
- Aspiration pneumonia
- Brain tumor
- Brown-Séquard syndrome
- Chronic obstructive pulmonary disease
- Guillain-Barré syndrome
- Heart failure
- Hypercalcemia
- Hypermagnesemia
- Hypokalemia
- Hypothyroidism
- Ischemic stroke
- Spinal cord injury

Therapeutic Interventions

Generalized muscle weakness is a potential cause of respiratory failure. Use positioning or airway adjuncts as necessary to maintain an open airway. Suction as needed. Apply a pulse oximeter and cardiac monitor. Give oxygen and begin positive-pressure ventilation as needed. Tracheal intubation may be needed in cases of respiratory failure. Monitor for cardiac dysrhythmias. Establish IV access. Transport to the closest appropriate facility for physician evaluation.

Patient and Family Education

Teach the patient and family that frequent rest periods should be taken throughout the day. Stress, strenuous exercise, and excessive exposure to the sun or cold weather can worsen symptoms and should be avoided.

Huntington's Disease

[OBJECTIVES 9, 10]

Description and Definition

Huntington's disease (also known as *Huntington's chorea*) is a devastating, degenerative neurologic condition.

Etiology

Huntington's disease is a hereditary illness in which certain neurons within the brain undergo genetically programmed cell death. As more neurons die, the brain becomes shrunken in appearance and the patient undergoes radical personality changes, loses intellectual function, and becomes physically debilitated.

Epidemiology and Demographics

Huntington's disease is rare. An estimated four to eight people in 100,000 currently have the disease. It usually strikes middle-age adults (ages 35 to 44 years), but can occur at any age. Huntington's disease is always fatal. Patients who have this disease usually die 10 to 15 years after onset, usually from heart failure or pneumonia (Revilla, 2004).

History and Physical Findings

Huntington's disease usually begins with behavioral symptoms, such as irritability, moodiness, and depression. The patient also starts to experience a decline in cognitive function as a progressive dementia sets in. At the same time, the patient develops movement disorders, beginning with involuntary, purposeless movements, such as shuffling the feet or flexing fingers. As the disease continues, the symptoms worsen and the patient may develop psychotic symptoms such as hallucinations and delusions, a sharp decline in mental functions with an increasing dementia, and worsening movement problems, such as tremors and slowed movements similar to Parkinson's disease.

Differential Diagnosis

Differential diagnoses include the following:

- Alcoholism
- Alzheimer's disease
- Bipolar disorder
- Parkinson's disease

Therapeutic Interventions

Prehospital treatment for this condition includes supportive care.

Patient and Family Education

Because Huntington's disease is hereditary, each child of a parent who has this disease has a 50% chance of inheriting it. Everyone who carries the gene will develop the disease. Family members should be encouraged to seek genetic counseling. A home healthcare agency should be contacted to assist the family in caring for the patient. The patient and family should be referred to a local support group.

SPINAL CORD DISORDERS

Spinal Cord Compression

[OBJECTIVE 11]

The spinal cord is well protected inside the vertebrae of the spine. However, the protection afforded by the small space of the vertebral canal also can worsen spinal cord injuries. Usually caused by trauma, compression and penetration of the spinal cord can have drastic consequences to the rest of the body. The cord may be compressed directly by vertebrae that are out of line, bone fragments, torn ligaments, swelling from a tumor or other disease process, penetrating objects, or vertebral discs that are out of place. Compression of the spinal cord can quickly lead to neuronal death. Neurologic dysfunction below the site of injury soon results. Damage to blood vessels causes ischemia of the cord, and the spinal cord immediately begins to swell inside the canal, further limiting blood supply. The cell bodies of neurons may rupture and die. Spinal cord injury or compression can lead to spinal shock because the brain cannot regulate blood pressure below the site of injury. If the lesion is high enough on the cervical spine, respirations can be compromised.

Several specific spinal cord syndromes can cause characteristic symptoms. Anterior cord syndrome, in which the front portion of the spinal cord is injured but not the rear portion, presents with paralysis and loss of pain and temperature sensation below the site of injury, but the patient retains touch, vibration, and position sense. Brown-Séquard syndrome occurs when a lateral half of the spinal cord has been injured, leaving the other side unaffected. This presents with paralysis and loss of vibration and position sense on the same side as the injury and loss of pain and temperature sensation on the opposite side (Gondim & Thomas, 2005).

Any patient with a potential spinal cord injury or who has been victim of trauma with a significant mechanism of injury warrants a full neurologic examination and spinal immobilization. In cases of high spinal cord injury, respiratory assistance may be necessary with a bag-mask device. In cases of spinal shock, IV fluids may be needed.

Autonomic Dysreflexia

[OBJECTIVE 12]

Autonomic dysreflexia is a life-threatening potential complication of spinal injury. Recall that the sympathetic nervous system originates in the mid-thoracic region of the spinal cord (T1 to L2). In fact, most of the sympathetic system is centered around T5 or T6. Injuries to the spinal cord above this level leave the brain unable to communicate with the sympathetic nervous system. Autonomic dysreflexia occurs when a stimulus below the site of injury travels through the intact spinal nerve and up the spinal cord until it is blocked by the injury. On the way, this stimulus causes an increase in sympathetic tone and the release of neurotransmitters such as norepinephrine and dopamine. This quickly results in arterial vasoconstriction and a sharp increase in blood pressure. The brain senses this hypertension and activates the parasympathetic nervous system, which is found at the brainstem, causing bradycardia and parasympathetic stimulation above the site of injury. Any painful, irritating, or strong stimuli can cause this sympathetic stimulation. Examples include urinary tract infections, hemorrhoids, menstruation, and insect bites. However, this most often is caused by either a distended bladder or a distended rectum impacted with feces. An estimated 50% to 90% of patients with a spinal cord injury at T6 or above develop autonomic dysreflexia (Campagnolo, 2005).

The typical patient with autonomic dysreflexia has had a spinal cord injury at T6 or above and is paraplegic, perhaps even quadriplegic. The normal systolic blood pressure for a patient with a spinal cord injury is approximately 90 to 100 mm Hg. A systolic blood pressure 20 to 40 mm Hg above this may signify autonomic dysreflexia. Patients may have systolic blood pressures that approach 300 mm Hg. This hypertension typically is associated with bradycardia. The patient may appear flushed and diaphoretic above the site of injury and pale and dry below.

Autonomic dysreflexia is a life-threatening emergency because severe hypertension can cause rupture of blood vessels in the brain and subsequent hemorrhage. You must act quickly. First, if possible, try to move the patient to an upright position to lower the blood pressure. This will only slightly lower the patient's blood pressure, if at all. Fortunately, reversing autonomic dysreflexia is as easy as removing the stimulus causing it. As noted previously, this most often is caused by a distended bladder or impacted bowel. First check the patient's indwelling urinary catheter if the patient has one. Look for twisting or kinking or a bag that is too full and correct these problems. Flush the catheter to clear any blockages that may be present that cannot be seen outside the body. If the patient does not have a urinary catheter, insert one if so trained. Next, manually remove any impacted feces from the rectum with a gloved hand. If the patient's blood pressure remains high, quickly transport the patient to the emergency department and monitor closely (Tomassoni, 2003). Educate patients with a spinal cord injury about the importance of closely monitoring for blockage of indwelling catheters and fecal impactions.

Hydrocephalus

[OBJECTIVE 13]

Hydrocephalus describes a condition of an excessive amount of CSF. It can be caused by too much CSF being created, a blockage in flow, or a problem with the absorp-

tion of CSF into the bloodstream. Hydrocephalus also may be congenital, affecting three per 1000 live births, or may occur from injuries and illnesses of the central nervous system. The rate of acquired hydrocephalus is not known. If the amount of CSF rises, then ICP also will rise and the patient may develop related symptoms, as previously explained. Often the pressure rises to the point at which a shunt must be surgically replaced to remove CSF from the central nervous system and deposit it into the abdominal cavity, where it can be reabsorbed into the body. Seventy-five percent of patients treated for hydrocephalus become dependent on these shunts. As with any tubing, these shunts may clog or kink and hydrocephalus may recur (Hord, 2004).

Spina Bifida

[OBJECTIVE 14]

Normally the meninges and spine develop around the brain and spinal cord in the womb, and when a baby is born his or her central nervous system is completely covered and protected. Sometimes, however, this does not occur and the meninges may herniate through the spine or even outside the skin, causing the spinal cord to develop incorrectly. This set of malformations of the meninges and spinal cord is collectively known as **spina bifida** and leads to a wide variety of neurologic impairments and usually means physical disability. This condition affects approximately one to two per 1000 live births annually (Foster, 2004).

Spina bifida is categorized according to the level of exposure of the meninges and the spinal cord. In spina bifida occulta these structures are not exposed; only a hole exists in the spinal column. Often a small dimple and tuft of hair in the midline lower lumbar region are the only external signs of this defect. In spina bifida meningocele, the spinal cord remains in the spinal column but a bulging of the meninges occurs. This creates a pouch, or sac, filled with CSF and is evident on the exterior lower lumbar spine. A myelomeningocele is the most severe form of spina bifida. As with the meningocele an exterior pouch originates in the hole in the lumbar spine. However, in this case the spinal cord also protrudes from the spine. Hydrocephalus, epilepsy, cerebral palsy, and developmental delays are commonly associated with this condition. The paramedic should use caution with latex-containing products around these patients because latex allergies also are common.

The spinal cord and meninges often are surgically re-placed into the vertebral canal, sometimes in utero. No matter how early surgical correction is performed, however, the patient almost always has some sort of disability. Spina bifida that does not involve herniation of the contents of the spinal canal rarely requires treatment.

OTHER DISORDERS

Muscular Dystrophy

[OBJECTIVE 15]

Although not technically neurologic in nature, **muscular dystrophy (MD)** describes a group of hereditary conditions that causes progressive muscle degeneration and increasing weakness that spreads over the entire body. Duchenne MD is the most common type of MD and is attributed to a sex-linked gene. Therefore only males can be affected by this form of MD. First described in the nineteenth century, it is caused by a defective gene that encodes for dystrophin, a protein normally found in muscle tissue and the brain. Without dystrophin, muscles develop incorrectly and are weak.

All types of MD have progressive muscle weakness as the defining symptom, which usually begins proximally and moves distally. Typically, this is noticed between the ages of 3 and 6 years when the patient demonstrates difficulty standing from a sitting position. Instead, the patient rolls onto the stomach and pushes himself or herself up (Grower's sign). The affected child often develops spinal and skeletal abnormalities such as lordosis, or swayback, and tends to walk on the toes for compensation (toe walking). Because dystrophin is also found in the brain, some degree of mental retardation often is seen. By puberty, many patients with MD are unable to walk and become wheelchair bound. This immobility causes the skeletal muscles and other soft tissues to become contracted and further shrink. Living past age 30 years is extremely rare because most die from cardiopulmonary complications of malformed cardiac muscle (Do, 2002). You may be required to make special accommodations, such as transporting a patient's wheelchair.

Dystonic Reactions

[OBJECTIVE 15]

Dystonia literally means "abnormal muscle tone." This usually involves involuntary muscle contractions and spasms, most often in the head, neck, and tongue. Although this can occur from many different causes, it is often an adverse side effect of certain antipsychotic drugs, such as chlorpromazine (Thorazine), prochlorperazine (Compazine), and haloperidol, and is termed a *dystonic reaction*. Cogentin - can take w/ Haldol to prevent rxn

A typical presentation of a dystonic reaction is a twisting of the head and neck to one side from muscle spasm, a swelling and protrusion of the tongue, and possibly the twisting and contortion of an arm. This can be dramatic in appearance and onset can be quite fast. Even though a patient may have been taking a certain medication for years, a dystonic reaction can still occur without warning or apparent cause. Fortunately this reaction does not involve the mental functions of the brain, usually does not cause airway or breathing problems, and almost always presents with a set of normal vital signs. Reversal of a dystonic reaction can be done by administering 25 to 50 mg diphenhydramine IV or IM. In most cases this causes the reaction to subside in minutes. Reassure the patient that this condition is temporary and reversible.

Trigeminal Neuralgia

[OBJECTIVE 15]

Widely considered to be one of the most painful afflictions in medicine, **trigeminal neuralgia** is a condition causing sharp, violent pain in the face. Trigeminal neuralgia stems from irritation of the trigeminal nerve. This condition is most often caused by a problem with the cranial nerve itself but also may be related to a lesion in the pons, where the trigeminal nerve connects to the brain. Most often the exact cause is unknown. It is a relatively uncommon illness and affects women more than men at a 3:2 ratio.

Sometimes known as *tic douloureux*, trigeminal neuralgia causes pain along the areas innervated by the trigeminal nerve (CN V), often at the upper and lower jaw. This pain is often described as stabbing or like a shock and is brief in duration, typically lasting from a few seconds to 1 to 2 minutes. These episodes may occur dozens of times a day and often are triggered by shaving, face washing, chewing, or touching the face in a certain way. Antiepileptic medications have been found to ease the symptoms of trigeminal neuralgia and often are used in its treatment (Huff, 2005).

Bell's Palsy

[OBJECTIVE 15]

Imagine waking up one morning and looking in the mirror to find that half of your face is paralyzed. This is exactly what happens in **Bell's palsy,** a paralysis of the facial nerve (CN VII) that affects approximately 23 in 100,000 persons. Most patients suspect that they have had a stroke, but no other neurologic abnormalities exist. Patients also report pain behind the ears, altered senses of sight and hearing, drooling, and tearing of the eyes. The exact cause of Bell's palsy is unknown, but a popular theory is the inflammation and swelling of the facial nerve causes it to be compressed against the skull where it exits the temporal bone. The herpes simplex virus is suspected to be the most common cause of inflammation of the facial nerve. Bell's palsy has no cure, but treatment may involve steroids to reduce inflammation, antiviral agents, and physical therapy if necessary. This condition usually resolves within 3 months, but some cases may require up to 1 year to resolve. Some patients are left with residual effects, such as nasal dryness, excessive tearing of the eyes, and inadequate eyelid closure. No prehospital interventions exist for Bell's palsy except for a thorough neurologic assessment to discount the possibility of stroke.

Case Scenario SUMMARY

1. *What is critical in the assessment of this scene?* With a scene of this magnitude a number of initial parts of the assessment are critical. Scene safety should not be overlooked. Ensure your safety as well as that of other EMS providers. If it is dark or a possibility of electrical wires or other hazards exists, lights are important. Triage may be needed based on the help available and the number of EMS personnel that have arrived.

2. *What should be the initial actions?* The patient should receive a primary survey. As you approach the patient, look for obvious signs of deformity or bleeding. No doubt exists that significant trauma has occurred. Open the airway by using a jaw thrust maneuver with cervical spine precautions. View the patient's airway for foreign bodies, blood, or possible obstructions. Assess breathing. If breathing is spontaneous, assess it for adequacy. If no breathing is present and the airway has been opened, provide positive-pressure ventilation until the airway can be secured with an endotracheal tube. Then assess circulation.

3. *What is the mechanism of injury and how does this affect the assessment?* This patient was thrown from a vehicle. The mechanism of a rollover with damage to three sides of the vehicle is significant enough to assume a severe injury. Be sure to consider that injury could occur to the head, brain, neck, spinal cord, chest, abdomen, pelvis, and extremities.

4. *What are the next most appropriate actions?* The patient demonstrates inadequate breathing and should receive supplemental oxygen. Her respirations should be supplemented with a bag-mask device and 100% oxygen. This patient also is showing significant signs of injury, so arrangement for rapid treatment and transport also would be appropriate.

5. *What are concerns with this patient's presentation and vital signs? What is appropriate initial therapy?* The patient has a thready pulse, which can indicate shock. The mechanism of injury is significant and can indicate bleeding, spinal cord injury, or significant head trauma. The respirations are not adequate, which can indicate a central brain injury or a chest injury. This patient is unstable, and rapid treatment and transport to a trauma center are essential. The patient should receive positive-pressure ventilation and IV access. The rate of fluid administration for a patient with a possible head injury and hypovolemic shock should be guided by your trauma protocols and/or consultation with medical direction. Note any obvious significant external bleeding and address immediately.

6. *Which part of the focused physical examination will be important?* The patient should receive a thorough physical examination during transport or while waiting for transport. After initial stabilization, the following should be assessed. The patient should have a thorough examination of the head and scalp. Note obvious skull deformities, bleeding, Battle's sign, or blood from the ears. Assess the neck and stabilize the cervical spine with a well-fitting cervical collar. Check the eyes for reactivity of the pupils. Check the nose for CSF or bleeding. Recheck the airway. Auscultate the lungs for breath sounds. Evaluate the chest wall for adequate rise and fall as well as symmetry. Gently palpate to evaluate for crepitus. Evaluate the abdomen for distention, rigidity, open injury, and bruising. Assess the integrity of the pelvis. Evaluate the extremities for deformity, bruising, and obvious bleeding. Address all significant injuries with the appropriate therapy and treatment.

7. *If the patient is unconscious, what should be evaluated? If the patient is conscious, what additional information would be helpful?* If the patient is unconscious, still evaluate for responsiveness. The AVPU mnemonic can be used. Is the patient alert? Is the patient alert when you speak to her? Is she alert to painful stimulus? Is she unresponsive? The GCS can be used to evaluate mental status. For adults, the GCS evaluates eye opening, verbal response, and motor response. If the patient is conscious, the GCS can be used. Ask the patient subjective questions regarding pain, numbness, tingling, and ability to move extremities.

8. *What is this patient's current GCS score?* The patient's GCS score is 7. The patient receives a 2 for eye opening to pain, a 2 for incomprehensible sounds for verbal response, and a 3 for flexion to painful stimuli. This is a score of 7 and an objective measurement of the patient's neurologic status that can be followed through the course of treatment. In general, a patient with a GCS score lower than 8 should be intubated.

9. *What do the vital signs indicate?* The patient has hypotension, which can be consistent with spinal injury or her femur fracture. The patient is tachycardic, possibly because of multiple injuries. Her respirations are improving. Because knowing whether an intracranial bleed or contusion is present is impossible, remember that a significant head injury is possible. This patient is still in very serious condition and requires rapid transport for definitive medical care.

10. *What is the appropriate verbal and written documentation for this patient?* The appropriate prehospital care report will include a brief description of the mechanism of injury as well as the initial patient position. This should be followed by the primary survey findings, secondary survey findings (including vital signs), and interventions. In this case be sure to relay the change in the patient's heart rate and the findings with the blood pressure. The written care report also should have this documented.

Chapter Summary

- The most basic portion of the nervous system is the neuron, or nerve cell.
- Each neuron has three parts: the dendrites, cell body, and axon.
- Neurons send impulses to other cells by neurotransmitters, chemicals that cross the synapse.
- The central nervous system is composed of the brain and spinal cord.
- The central nervous system is covered by three layers of connective tissue called the *meninges*.
- The meninges contain CSF, which circulates throughout the central nervous system.
- All nervous tissue not in the brain or spinal cord comprises the peripheral nervous system.
- The peripheral nervous system has two parts: the somatic, which controls voluntary muscle movements and sensation from the skin, and the visceral, which comprises the ANS.
- The spinal nerves branch off of the spinal cord and are named for the vertebra level where they exit.
- The ANS has two divisions that work against each other: the sympathetic, or fight-or-flight response, and the parasympathetic, or rest-and-digest response.
- Twelve cranial nerves branch off the brain and spinal cord.
- Perform a complete neurologic assessment if your patient has or has had altered mental status, a loss of consciousness, an alteration in strength or sensation, or a loss of function of an extremity.
- One of the primary goals of the neurologic assessment is to find focal deficits—absent or altered functions of sensations of a body part caused by damage to a portion of the nervous system.
- All patients with altered mental status should have their blood glucose levels monitored.
- Dementia is a slow, progressive decline in mental functions. Delirium is an acute, temporary state of mental confusion and/or fluctuating level of consciousness.
- Disruption of blood flow to an area of brain tissue is known as a cerebrovascular accident or stroke.
- A seizure is massive, excessive neuronal firing in the brain that alters behavior.
- Seizures are divided into partial seizures, which only affect part of the brain, and generalized seizures, which affect the entire brain.
- After a generalized seizure, the patient goes through a postictal period in which he or she may be combative, confused, and fearful.
- Status epilepticus is a single seizure lasting longer than 30 minutes or repeated seizures without full recovery of responsiveness between seizures and lasting longer than 30 minutes. It is a life-threatening condition requiring aggressive care.
- Syncope is a transient loss of consciousness, often resulting in a ground-level fall.
- Headaches are either vascular (caused by dilation of blood vessels within the head) or nonvascular (caused by something else).
- A brain neoplasm is a tumor within the brain that may be benign or malignant.
- A brain abscess is a collection of pus within the brain.
- An ischemic stroke is caused by a blocked blood vessel in the brain.
- A hemorrhagic stroke is caused by a ruptured, bleeding blood vessel in the brain.
- Hypertension, bradycardia, and abnormal respirations are the hallmarks of Cushing's triad, signifying rising ICP.
- A TIA shows the same signs and symptoms as a stroke but resolves within 24 hours.
- Alzheimer's disease is a degenerative, progressive decline in memory, reasoning, and cognition. It is the most common cause of senile dementia in the elderly.
- Parkinson's disease is a degenerative nervous disorder affecting fine motor control and the extrapyramidal system.
- Any injury to the spinal cord affects sensation and movement below the site of injury.

REFERENCES

Adams, H. P., Jr., Adams, R. J., Brott, T., del Zoppo, G. J., Furlan, A., Goldstein, L. B., et al. (2003). Guidelines for the early management of patients with ischemic stroke: A scientific statement from the Stroke Council of the American Stroke Association. *Stroke, 34*(4), 1056-1083.

Anderson, K. N., & Anderson, L. E. (1994). *Mosby's pocket dictionary of medicine, nursing and allied health* (2nd ed.). St. Louis: Mosby.

Bogousslausky, J. (2003). *Stroke prevention by the practitioner* (2nd ed.). New York: Karger.

Bosker, G., Weins, D., & Sequeira, M. (1996). *The 60-second EMT: Rapid BLS/ALS assessment, diagnosis, and triage* (2nd ed). St. Louis: Mosby.

Brook, I. (2005). *Brain abscess.* Retrieved February 3, 2005, from http://www.emedicine.com.

Campagnolo, D. I. (2005). *Autonomic dysreflexia in spinal cord injury.* Retrieved September 9, 2005, from http://www.emedicine.com.

Dangond, F. (2004). *Amyotrophic lateral sclerosis.* Retrieved September 9, 2005, from http://www.emedicine.com.

Do, T. (2002). *Muscular dystrophy.* Retrieved September 9, 2005, from http://www.emedicine.com.

Foster, M. (2004). *Spina bifida.* Retrieved September 9, 2005, from http://www.emedicine.com.

Frosh, M. P., Anthony, D. C., & Girolami, U. D. (2005). The central nervous system. In V. Kumar, A. K. Abbas, & N. Fausto (Eds.). *Robbins and Cotran pathologic basis of disease* (7th ed.). Philadelphia: Elsevier.

Gondim, F. A. A. G., & Thomas, F. P. (2005). *Spinal cord trauma and related diseases.* Retrieved May 29, 2008, from http://www.emedicine.com.

Hauser, R. A. (2004). *Parkinson disease.* Retrieved May 29, 2008, from http://www.emedicine.com.

Howard, J. F., Jr. (1997). *Myasthenia gravis—A summary.* Retrieved September 9, 2005, from http://www.myasthenia.org.

Hord, E. D. (2004). *Hydrocephalus.* Retrieved September 9, 2005, from http://www.emedicine.com.

Huff, J. S. (2005). *Trigeminal neuralgia.* Retrieved September 9, 2005, from http://www.emedicine.com.

Jans, M. K., Jundt, C. M., & McNeil, M. A. (1998). *When seizures are medical emergencies: Pre-hospital management of status epilepticus.* St. Paul, MN: Epilepsy Foundation of Minnesota.

Kuljis, R. O. (2005). *Alzheimer's disease.* Retrieved September 9, 2005, from http://www.emedicine.com.

Moon, J. (2005). *Herpes zoster.* Retrieved September 9, 2005, from http://www.emedicine.com.

Morag, R. (2004). *Syncope.* Retrieved September 9, 2005, from http://www.emedicine.com.

Moraine, J., Berre, C., & Melot, J. (2000). Is cerebral perfusion pressure a major determinant of cerebral blood flow during head elevation in comatose patients with severe intracranial lesions? *Journal of Neurosurgery, 92,* 606-614.

National Institute of Neurological Disorders and Stroke. (2004). *Dementias: Hope through research.* Retrieved September 9, 2005, from http://www.ninds.nih.gov.

National Institute of Neurological Disorders and Stroke. (2005). *Guillain-Barré syndrome fact sheet.* Retrieved September 9, 2005, from http://www.ninds.nih.gov.

Ramachandran, V. S. (1998). *Phantoms in the brain: Probing the mysteries of the human mind.* New York: HarperCollins.

Revilla, F. J. (2004). *Huntington disease.* Retrieved September 9, 2005, from http://www.emedicine.com.

Sahai-Srivastava, S. (2005). *Pathophysiology and treatment of migraine and related headache.* Retrieved September 9, 2005, from http://www.emedicine.com.

Salen, P.N. (2006). *Wernicke encephalopathy.* Retrieved May 29, 2008, from http://www.emedicine.com.

Tomassoni, P. J., & Campagnolo, D. I. (2003). Autonomic dysreflexia: One more way EMS can positively affect patient survival. *Journal of Emergency Medical Services, 28*(12), 46-50.

Weiderholt, W. C. (2000). *Neurology for non-neurologists* (4th ed.). Philadelphia: W. B. Saunders.

SUGGESTED RESOURCES

An interactive online guide to the neurological examination. http://www.neuroexam.com.

The brain atlas from the Lundbeck Institute. http://www.brainexplorer.org.

LeDoux, J. (2002). *The synaptic self: How our brains become who we are.* New York: Viking Adult.

National Institute of Neurological Disorders and Stroke. http://www.ninds.nih.gov.

Ratey, J. J. (2001). *A user's guide to the brain: Perception, attention and the four theaters of the brain.* New York: Pantheon.

Chapter Quiz

1. The central nervous system is composed of _____.
  a. the brain and spinal cord
  b. all nervous tissue within the body
  c. the brain, spinal cord, and spinal nerves
  d. the brain

2. The parts of a neuron are _____.
  a. the nucleus, axon, and nervous branches
  b. the cell body, axon, and dendrites
  c. the neural projections, cytoplasm, and organelles
  d. the synaptic membrane, nucleus, and axon

3. The frontal lobe of the brain is responsible for _____.
  a. the sense of hearing
  b. the sense of sight
  c. fine tuning of motor functions
  d. speech, abstract thinking, and personality

4. The visceral nervous system innervates which of the following?
  a. Skin
  b. Muscles
  c. Organs
  d. Muscles of the face and eyes

5. The somatic nervous system innervates which of the following?
  a. Skin
  b. Tongue
  c. Organs
  d. Muscles of the face and eyes

6. Which of the following is a component of the GCS?
  a. Skin response
  b. Flexion response
  c. Eye opening
  d. Pupillary response

7. The layers of the meninges, in order from the outside of the body inward, are _____.
  a. dura mater, pia mater, arachnoid membrane
  b. subarachnoid space, dura mater, pia mater
  c. dura mater, arachnoid membrane, pia mater
  d. pia mater, arachnoid membrane, dura mater

8. A 24-year-old man has ingested four hits of LSD and is telling you he sees parakeets flying inside the ambulance and hears voices telling him to catch the birds and eat them. This is an example of a(n) _____.
  a. delusion
  b. hallucination
  c. affect
  d. nervous dissociation

9. The patient's condition in question 8 is an example of _____.
  a. dementia
  b. affect
  c. senility
  d. delirium

10. You respond to a local community college for a 32-year-old man reporting "the worst headache of my life" that came on suddenly a few minutes ago. On your arrival, that patient is vomiting forcefully. As you assessing him, your patient suddenly begins to seize. His vital signs are heart rate, 52 beats/min; blood pressure, 190/140 mm hg; respirations, 32 breaths/min and irregular; and GCS, 4 (E = 1, V = 1, M = 2). This patient most likely is having a(n) _____.
    a. ischemic stroke
    b. TIA
    c. hemorrhagic stroke
    d. absence seizure

11. Management of the patient in question 10 would most likely include which of the following?
    a. Oxygen, glucose monitoring, fluid bolus of an isotonic solution, and rapid transport
    b. Oxygen, glucose monitoring, placement of IV (to keep vein open), benzodiazepines, and rapid transport
    c. Oxygen, glucose monitoring, placement of IV (to keep vein open), morphine sulfate, and rapid transport
    d. Oxygen, fluid bolus of an isotonic solution, benzodiazepines, and rapid transport

12. You respond to a local laundromat for a 65-year-old woman reporting right-sided hemiparesis and headache. Bystanders state that 5 minutes ago she was standing in front of a dryer when she collapsed on the floor and became unable to speak. Vital signs are heart rate, 100 beats/min; blood pressure, 160/100 mm Hg; respirations, 20 breaths/min and regular; and GCS, 9 (E = 4, V = 1, M = 4). This patient most likely has or is having a(n) _____.
    a. ischemic stroke
    b. ALS
    c. hemorrhagic stroke
    d. absence seizure

13. Status epilepticus is defined as which of the following?
    a. Any seizure
    b. Seizures lasting longer than 30 minutes
    c. Seizures lasting longer than 5 minutes
    d. Any seizure caused by epilepsy

14. You respond to a large church for a patient who has "passed out." Bystanders report that your patient stood up rapidly during a sermon, stated she felt dizzy, and then fell to the ground unconscious. After approximately 30 seconds the patient awoke and is now completely alert and oriented. She denies any current pain or discomfort. Which of the following best describes this condition?
    a. Absence seizure
    b. Tonic-clonic seizure
    c. Syncope
    d. TIA

15. You respond to a residence for a 45-year-old woman reporting a headache. You find her lying in bed with the shades drawn and also complaining of nausea and sweating. She states her headache is "throbbing" and began late last night and woke her from sleep. She has taken 800 mg ibuprofen with no relief. This patient most likely has or is having a _____.
    a. TIA
    b. cluster headache
    c. simple partial seizure
    d. migraine headache

16. You respond to a local college dormitory for a 20-year-old woman with "altered mental status." On arrival, your patient is lying in bed and is responsive to verbal stimuli. Her roommate reports that the patient has been reporting a headache, nausea, and fever for 3 days. When you ask the patient to tuck her chin to her chest, she cries out in pain. This patient most likely has _____.
    a. encephalitis
    b. meningitis
    c. myasthenia gravis
    d. MS

17. An infectious disorder of the nervous system that causes painful rashes to develop along unilateral dermatomes is _____.
    a. myasthenia gravis
    b. MS
    c. shingles
    d. Guillain-Barré syndrome

18. You respond to a residence for a 68-year-old woman who is "not acting right." You arrive to find the patient's daughter, who tells you that her mother's mental function has "been going downhill" for some time, but now her mother has locked herself in the bedroom and is talking about people who are not there. This presentation is most consistent with which of the following?
    a. MS
    b. ALS
    c. Parkinson's disease
    d. Alzheimer's disease

19. The two most common causes of autonomic dysreflexia are
    a. additional injury below the site of spinal injury and cold stimulus.
    b. fecal impaction and urinary bladder distention.
    c. pressure sores and infection below the site of spinal injury.
    d. reactions to medications and allergic reactions.

20. The term *hydrocephalus* describes a condition of _____.
    a. too much CSF
    b. an infection in the CSF
    c. blood in the CSF
    d. not enough CSF

Chapter Quiz—continued

21. You are called to the home of a 36-year-old man who woke this morning with complete paralysis of the right side of his face. He also reports a headache centered around his right ear. He has no other neurologic deficits. You think this condition probably is Bell's palsy, an inflammation of _____.
    a. CN VII, the trigeminal nerve
    b. CN X, the vagus nerve
    c. CN VII, the facial nerve
    d. CN VIII, the acoustic nerve

22. You are transporting a 28-year-old woman who has been having a tonic-clonic seizure for almost 10 minutes and has not responded to repeated doses of diazepam. This patient's condition is best described as _____.
    a. status epilepticus
    b. petit mal seizure
    c. absence seizure
    d. complex partial seizure

Terminology

Abscess A collection of pus.

Absence seizure A generalized seizure characterized by a blank stare and an alteration of consciousness.

Affect Description of the patient's visible emotional state.

Altered mental status Disruption of a person's emotional and intellectual functioning.

Alzheimer's disease Progressive dementia, seen mostly in the elderly and marked by decline of memory and cognitive function.

Amyotrophic lateral sclerosis (ALS) Autoimmune disorder affecting the motor roots of the spinal nerves, causing progressive muscle weakness and eventually paralysis.

Anesthesia Absence of normal sensation, particularly pain.

Arachnoid membrane Weblike middle layer of the meninges.

Aura Sensory disturbances caused by a partial seizure; may precede a generalized seizure.

Autonomic dysreflexia Massive sympathetic stimulation unbalanced by the parasympathetic nervous system because of spinal cord injury, usually at or above T6.

Autonomic nervous system (ANS) Branch of the peripheral nervous system that provides control of the automatic functions of the body, such as heart rate, blood pressure, and digestive and excretory functions.

Axon Branching extensions of the neuron where impulses exit the cell.

Bell's palsy Paralysis of the facial nerve (CN VII), often caused by infection by the Herpes simplex virus.

Blood-brain barrier Dense network of blood vessels that only allow a select group of molecules into the brain from the systemic circulation.

Brainstem Lowest portion of the brain; composed of the diencephalon, midbrain, pons, and the medulla oblongata; center for control of basic life functions, such as heart rate and respirations.

Cell body Portion of the neuron containing the organelles, where essential cellular functions are performed.

Cerebellum Structure approximately the size and shape of two walnuts at the rear and bottom of the brain that coordinates fine motor control.

Cerebral perfusion pressure (CPP) Pressure inside the cerebral arteries and an indicator of brain perfusion; CPP = MAP − ICP.

Cerebrospinal fluid (CSF) Clear, watery fluid that circulates beneath the arachnoid membrane and bathes the brain and spinal cord.

Cerebrovascular accident (CVA) Blockage or hemorrhage of the blood vessels in the brain, usually causing focal neurologic deficits; also known as a *stroke*.

Cerebrum Outermost and most superior portion of the brain.

Cluster headaches One-sided vascular headaches usually accompanied by nasal congestion and a watery eye on the affected side.

Complex partial seizure A seizure affecting only one part of the brain that does alter consciousness.

Cranial nerves Twelve pairs of nerves that exit the brain and innervate the head and face; some also are part of the visceral portion of the peripheral nervous system.

Cranium The vaultlike portion of the skull, behind and above the face.

Cushing's triad Characteristic pattern of vital signs during rising ICP, presenting as rising hypertension, bradycardia, and abnormal respirations.

Delirium Short-term and temporary mental confusion and fluctuating level of consciousness, often caused by intoxication from various substances, hypoglycemia, or acute psychiatric episodes.

Delusion A false idea about a situation.

Dementia Long-term decline in mental faculties such as memory, concentration, and judgment; often seen with degenerative neurologic disorders such as Alzheimer's disease.

Dendrite Branchlike projections from a neuron that receive impulses or sensory information.

Dermatomes Areas of the body innervated by specific sensory spinal nerves.

Diencephalon Highest part of the brainstem; location of the thalamus, hypothalamus, and the limbic system.

Dura mater Outermost layer of the meninges.

Dystonia Impairment of muscle tone, particularly involuntary muscle contractions of the face, neck, and tongue; often caused by a reaction to certain antipsychotic medications.

Encephalitis Inflammation and usually infection of brain tissue.

Epilepsy Group of neurologic disorders characterized by recurrent seizures, often of unknown cause.

Extension posturing (decerebrate) Occurs as a result of an injury to the brainstem; presents as the patient's arms at the side with wrists turned outward.

Febrile seizure Seizure caused by too rapid of a rise in body temperature; rarely seen after age 2 years.

Flexion posturing (decorticate) Occurs from an injury to the cerebrum; presents as a bending of the arms at the elbow, the patient's arms pulled upwards to the chest, and the hands turned downward at the wrists.

Focal deficit Alteration or lack of strength or sensation in the body caused by a neurologic problem.

Foramen magnum Opening in the floor of the cranium where the spinal cord exits the skull.

Form of thought Ability to compose thoughts in a logical manner.

Frontal lobe Part of the cerebrum beneath the frontal bone; responsible for high-level functions such as speech, abstract thinking, and personality.

Generalized seizure Excessive electrical activity in both hemispheres of the brain at the same time.

Glasgow Coma Scale (GCS) Neurologic assessment of a patient's best verbal response, eye opening, and motor function.

Guillain-Barré syndrome Autoimmune neurologic disorder marked by weakness and paresthesia that usually travel up the legs.

Hallucination A false sensory perception originating inside the brain, such as hearing the voices of people who are not present.

Hemiparesis Muscle weakness affecting half of the body.

Hemiplegia Paralysis of one side of the body.

Hemorrhagic stroke Rupture of a blood vessel in the brain causing decreased perfusion and potentially leading to rising ICP.

Herniation Protrusion of the brain through an abnormal opening, often the foramen magnum.

Huntington's disease Programmed cell death of certain neurons in the brain, leading to behavioral abnormalities, movement disorders, and a decline in cognitive function.

Hydrocephalus An excessive amount of CSF.

Hypothalamus Interface between the brain and the endocrine system; provides control for many autonomic functions.

Intracerebral hemorrhage Bleeding within the brain tissue, often from smaller blood vessels.

Intracranial pressure (ICP) Pressure inside the brain cavity; should be very low, usually less than 15 mm Hg.

Ischemic stroke Lack of perfusion to an area of brain tissue caused by a thrombus or embolus.

Medulla oblongata Lowest portion of brain tissue and the interface between the brain and the spinal cord; responsible for maintenance of basic life functions such as heart rate and respirations.

Meninges Layers of connective tissue that wrap and protect the central nervous system.

Meningitis Irritation of the connective tissue covering the central nervous system, often from infection or hemorrhage.

Midbrain Lies below the diencephalon and above the pons; works with the pons to route information from higher within the brain to the spinal cord and vice versa.

Migraine headaches Recurrent headaches usually described as throbbing pain with accompanying nausea and vomiting, sweating, and photosensitivity.

Motor cortex Area of brain tissue on the frontal lobe that controls voluntary movements.

Multiple sclerosis (MS) Autoimmune disorder in which the immune system attacks the myelin sheath surrounding neurons, causing widespread motor problems and pain.

Muscular dystrophy (MD) Hereditary condition causing malformation of muscle tissue and leading to malformation of the musculoskeletal system and physical disability.

Myasthenia gravis Autoimmune disorder affecting acetylcholine receptors throughout the body, causing widespread muscle weakness.

Myotomes Areas of the body controlled by specific motor spinal nerves.

Neoplasm Cancerous growth; a tumor that may be malignant or benign.

Nerve Neurons and blood vessels wrapped together with connective tissue; the body's information highways.

Neuroeffector junction Interface between a neuron and its target tissue.

Neuron Basic nerve cell.

Neurotransmitters Chemicals that cross the synapse to stimulate a target tissue.

Terminology—continued

Occipital lobe Most rearward portion of the cerebrum; mainly responsible for processing the sense of sight.

Parasympathetic division of the ANS Opposes the sympathetic division of the ANS; when stimulated causes a rest-and-digest response, causing decreased heart rate, pupil constriction, and shunting of blood to the digestive and reproductive organs.

Paresthesia Abnormal sensation described as numbness, tingling, or pins and needles.

Parietal lobe Portion of the cerebrum that assists with language processing and body position sense; found beneath the parietal bone of the skull.

Parkinson's disease Progressive movement disorder caused by dysfunction in the cerebellum; rigidity, tremor, bradykinesia, and postural instability are characteristic.

Peripheral nervous system Composed of all nervous tissue in the body outside the brain and spinal cord.

Pia mater Thin, innermost layer of the meninges.

Poliomyelitis Viral infection that tends to attack the motor roots of the spinal nerves, often leading to physical disability and even paralysis of the diaphragm.

Pons Brain structure below the midbrain and above the medulla oblongata, which works with the midbrain to route information from higher within the brain to the spinal cord and vice versa.

Postictal State that begins at the termination of seizure activity in the brain and ends with the patient returning to a level of normal behavior.

Preoccupation A topic or theme that consistently recurs in a person's thought process and conversations.

Reticular formation A cloud of neurons in the brainstem and midbrain responsible for maintaining consciousness.

Reuptake Absorption of neurotransmitters from the synapse into the presynaptic neuron to be reused or destroyed.

Seizure A temporary alteration in behavior or consciousness caused by abnormal electrical activity of one or more groups of neurons in the brain.

Sensory cortex Area of brain tissue on the frontal lobe responsible for receiving sensory information from different parts of the body.

Shingles Infection of a nerve, often by the herpes zoster virus, causing severe pain and a rash along a unilateral dermatome.

Simple partial seizure A seizure affecting only one part of the brain without an alteration in consciousness.

Somatic Portion of the peripheral nervous system that carries impulses to and from the skin and

musculature; responsible for voluntary muscle control.

Spina bifida Malformation of the meninges and spinal cord in utero, often leading to permanent physical disabilities.

Spinal cord Long stalk of nerve tissue that is the interface between the brain and the body; extends from the foramen magnum to the lumbar spine.

Spinal nerves Paired nerves that originate from the spinal cord and exit the spine on either side between vertebrae; each has a sensory root and a motor root.

Status epilepticus A single seizure lasting longer than 30 minutes or repeated seizures without full recovery of responsiveness between seizures and lasting longer than 30 minutes.

Subarachnoid hemorrhage Bleeding from the arteries between the arachnoid membrane and the pia mater that occurs suddenly and is often fatal.

Sympathetic division of the ANS When stimulated, provides a fight-or-flight response, including increased heart rate, pupil dilation, bronchodilation, and the shunting of blood to the muscles.

Synapse Microscopic space at the neuroeffector junction that neurotransmitters cross to stimulate target tissues.

Syncope A transient loss of consciousness and inability to maintain postural tone, typically resulting in a ground-level fall; also known as *passing out* or *fainting*.

Temporal lobe Cerebrum beneath the temporal bone; area where processing of hearing and language occurs.

Thalamus The sensory switchboard; area through which almost all sensory information passes.

Thought content The dominant themes and ideas of a patient; may include delusions, hallucinations, and preoccupations.

Tonic-clonic seizure Form of generalized seizure with a tonic phase (muscle rigidity) and a clonic phase (muscle tremors).

Transient ischemic attack (TIA) Neurologic dysfunction caused by a temporary blockage in blood flow; by definition the symptoms resolve within 24 hours but usually within 1 or 2 hours.

Trigeminal neuralgia Irritation of the seventh cranial nerve (trigeminal nerve), causing episodes of severe, stabbing pain in the face.

Vascular headaches Headaches that involve changes in the diameter or size and chemistry of blood vessels that supply the brain.

Visceral Portion of the peripheral nervous system that processes motor and sensory information from the internal organs, includes the ANS.

Endocrine Emergencies and Nutritional Disorders

Objectives *After completing this chapter, you will be able to:*

1. Describe the incidence, morbidity, and mortality rates of endocrine emergencies, including the need for rapid assessment and intervention.
2. Discuss the anatomy and physiology of the organs and structures involved in endocrinologic diseases.
3. Describe normal glucose metabolism.
4. Describe the pathophysiology of type 1 and type 2 diabetes.
5. Discuss the pathophysiology of diabetic metabolism.
6. Describe the assessment findings of the hypoglycemic patient.
7. Develop a treatment plan based on the assessment findings of the hypoglycemic patient.
8. Describe the assessment findings of the hyperglycemic patient.
9. Develop a treatment plan based on the assessment findings of the hyperglycemic patient.
10. Describe the assessment findings of the patient with diabetic ketoacidosis.
11. Develop a treatment plan based on the assessment findings of the patient with diabetic ketoacidosis.
12. Describe the assessment findings of the patient with hyperosmolar hyperglycemic nonketotic coma.
13. Develop a treatment plan based on the assessment findings of the patient with hyperosmolar hyperglycemic nonketotic coma.
14. Discuss the pathophysiology of pituitary gland disorders.
15. Describe the assessment findings of patients with pituitary gland disorders.
16. Develop a treatment plan based on the assessment findings of the patient with a pituitary gland disorder.
17. Discuss the pathophysiology of thyroid gland disorders.
18. Describe the assessment findings of patients with thyroid gland disorders.
19. Develop a treatment plan based on the assessment findings of the patient with a thyroid gland disorder.
20. Discuss the pathophysiology of parathyroid gland disorders.
21. Describe the assessment findings of patients with parathyroid gland disorders.
22. Develop a treatment plan based on the assessment findings of the patient with a parathyroid gland disorder.
23. Discuss the pathophysiology of adrenal gland disorders.
24. Describe the assessment findings of patients with adrenal gland disorders.
25. Develop a treatment plan based on the assessment findings of the patient with an adrenal gland disorder.
26. Discuss the etiology of nutritional disorders.
27. Discuss the pathophysiology of nutritional disorders.
28. Describe the assessment findings of patients with nutritional disorders.
29. Develop a treatment plan based on the assessment findings of the patient with a nutritional disorder.

Chapter Outline

Anatomy and Physiology
Endocrine Disorders

Nutritional Disorders

Case Scenario

You are called to the scene of a 34-year-old woman who is having chest pain, palpitations, and fatigue. You find her sitting still, sweating, and uncomfortable. She states she has been losing weight and has noticed that she has been getting steadily worse. She has been taking birth control pills but is otherwise not taking any other medications. She has no past medical history except two normal vaginal deliveries. Her pulse is 144 beats/min, blood pressure is 148/98 mm Hg, respirations are 28 breaths/min and labored, pulse oximetry is 98% on room air, and her skin is hot and moist. Her husband states that she has been having periods of confusion.

Questions

1. *What is your impression of this patient?*
2. *What are some key factors that should be investigated during the physical examination?*
3. *What are the most appropriate initial interventions?*
4. *What is the significance of the confusion?*

[handwritten: Exocrine - through a duct]

[handwritten: Hormones — Protein - attaches to receptor on cell wall - affects inside. Steroid - fat soluble - go through cell wall & attach inside - is 1° messenger]

[OBJECTIVE 1]

The endocrine system consists of eight glands: the hypothalamus, pituitary, thyroid, parathyroid, thymus, pancreas, adrenal, and the gonads. These glands send chemical messengers called **hormones** throughout the body to maintain **homeostasis.** The endocrine glands secrete these hormones directly into the bloodstream without the use of ducts. Glands with ducts (such as the sweat glands) are called exocrine glands and are not part of the endocrine system.

Specialized cells in the various endocrine glands throughout the body release hormones. This is known as **endocrine communication** (Table 24-1). These hormones are deposited into the bloodstream. From the bloodstream, they are distributed evenly to all body tissues. Different body systems have target cells that are activated by the specific hormones floating in the bloodstream. Once these cells have been activated, they have preprogrammed responses that regulate important body functions. Most hormones have antagonizing hormones that act to balance, or buffer, each other. Two competing hormones, insulin and glucagon, provide a good example; through complex mechanisms insulin acts to lower blood glucose levels, whereas glucagon acts to raise blood glucose levels. In this manner the body is better able to achieve homeostasis.

As an EMS professional, you most often will see endocrine emergencies related to diabetes mellitus. According to the National Institute of Health (NIH), in 2005, 20.8 million people (7% of the population) had diabetes in the United States (National Diabetes Information Clearinghouse, 2005). Of those, 14.6 million were diagnosed and 6.2 million were undiagnosed. In addition to diabetic patients, you will see patients with other endocrine disorders that you may have to identify and treat. Some of these disorders include thyrotoxic crisis, myxedema, nonketotic hyperosmolar coma, and hyperadrenalism. These disorders are all examples of episodes of when the human body has lost homeostasis. Some of these conditions may be fatal if they are not rapidly detected and properly treated. Others can lead to a progression of syndromes that may ultimately lead to the patient's death unless they are diagnosed and treated.

The human body is a complex organism composed of multiple interconnected systems. To function effectively, these body systems must be regulated and coordinated down to the cellular level. To achieve this level of coordination, cells from within a body system and between body systems must be able to interact. In a few special situations, cells with the same function may communicate with each other through a process known as **direct communication.** For direct communication to occur, the cells must share extensive physical contact. This communication occurs through the exchange of ions and molecules directly from one cell to the other. Another form of intercellular communication is known as **para-**

TABLE 24-1	Intercellular Communication	
Type of Communication	**Route of Communication**	**Messenger**
Endocrine	Bloodstream (slow)	Hormone
Neural	Synaptic (rapid)	Neurotransmitter
Paracrine	Extracellular fluid	Paracrine factors or cytokines
Direct	Contact with contiguous cell	Ions and molecules

[handwritten: Exocrine - tear ducts]

crine communication. A cell uses paracrine communication to communicate with other cells within the same tissue set but not in direct contact with that cell. Chemical messengers called *paracrine factors,* or *cytokines,* are released into the extracellular tissue and migrate to the surrounding tissue. Cells with appropriate receptor sites are then activated by these paracrine factors. Because the paracrine factors are released into the extracellular fluid, they generally only affect the tissue surrounding the cells that released them. In contrast, hormones are released into the bloodstream and affect target sites throughout the body.

The nervous system also relies on chemical messengers to communicate between cells. This process is called **synaptic communication.** In the case of the nervous system, these chemical messengers are called *neurotransmitters.* These neurotransmitters are released into the synapse between nerve cells and rapidly trigger receptors on the next neuron. Neurotransmitters are rapidly broken down and reabsorbed for future use. Because the nervous system is located throughout the entire body, this form of intercellular communication is capable of transmitting messages over long distances. Moreover, it is a rapid form of communication.

ANATOMY AND PHYSIOLOGY

Overview of the Endocrine System

[OBJECTIVE 2]

As previously stated, the endocrine system consists of eight major glands (Figure 24-1). The pineal gland is also a part of the endocrine system. The effects of the hormone it releases, melatonin, remain somewhat vague. Melatonin has been suggested to play a part in inhibiting reproductive functions, protecting against free radicals, and setting circadian rhythms (Martin, 2002). Also suggested is the theory that many other body tissues play a part in endocrine function, including tissues found in the placenta, heart, kidneys, and digestive tract.

The glands of the endocrine system are ductless and vascular. Exocrine glands contain ducts and release their chemical products through those ducts directly to the site where they are to be used. For example, the lacrimal glands produce lacrimal secretions and are exocrine glands. These secretions are deposited directly onto the eye by the lacrimal ducts to bathe the eye with nutrients and protect it. In contrast, the endocrine glands deposit hormones into the bloodstream to be distributed to the entire body. Some hormones may only affect tissues in one body system; other hormones may have target tissues in many body systems.

Hypothalamus

The human body regulates itself by communicating at the cellular level through the nervous and endocrine systems. As a result, a link must exist between the two

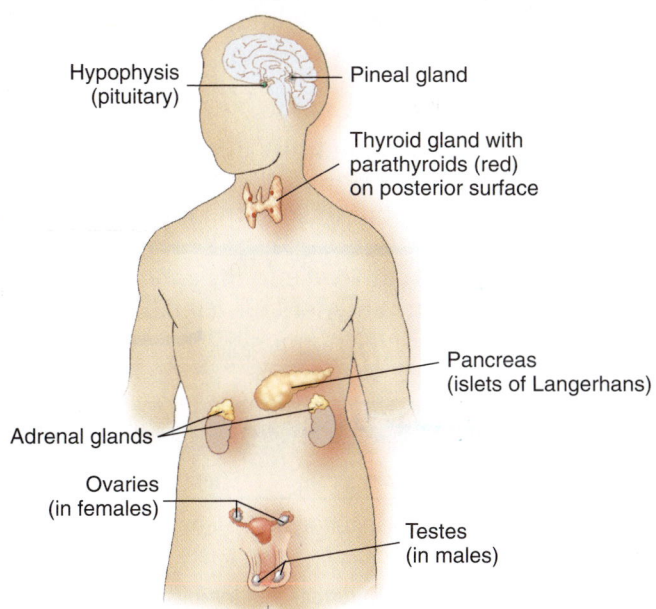

Figure 24-1 Endocrine glands.

systems, such as a command and control center. The hypothalamus serves this function. The hypothalamus is located deep in the cerebrum of the brain. It contains cells that function both as nerve cells and as glandular cells. The neuron functions of these cells receive input from the autonomic nervous system. This input includes feedback from the body's self-monitoring system. Information processed by the hypothalamus includes, among other things, reports on blood pressure, heart rate, body temperature, and blood glucose levels. Some hypothalamic neural cells pass this information on to the central nervous system, some neural cells conduct impulses to the posterior pituitary gland, and some glandular cells produce and release hormones that trigger target tissue in the anterior and posterior lobes of the pituitary gland. These hormones, sometimes called regulatory hormones, regulate the release of hormones by the pituitary gland.

The regulatory hormones released by the hypothalamus into the bloodstream that target tissues in the pituitary gland include the following (Table 24-2):

- Growth hormone–releasing hormone (GHRH)
- Growth hormone–inhibiting hormone (GHIH)
- Corticotropin-releasing hormone (CRH)
- Thyrotropin-releasing hormone (TRH)
- Gonadotropin-releasing hormone (GnRH)
- Prolactin-releasing hormone (PRH)
- Prolactin-inhibiting hormone (PIH)

The primary effect of these regulatory hormones is to direct the pituitary gland to increase or decrease production of hormones that coordinate body systems. In addition to the regulatory hormones listed, the hypothalamus manufactures and transports antidiuretic hormone (ADH) and oxytocin directly into the pituitary gland for release into the bloodstream from that point.

Pituitary Gland #2

The pituitary gland is found just inferior to the hypothalamus inside a depression in the sphenoid bone and rests just above the roof of the mouth. The pituitary acts as a sort of thermostat for most of the body's hormone-producing glands. It is divided into the anterior lobe and the posterior lobe. The anterior lobe contains endocrine cells that produce several hormones. Some of the hormones released by the anterior lobe of the pituitary gland do not directly affect body systems. Instead, they stimulate other glands to release hormones that regulate body functions. The anterior lobe of the pituitary gland is regulated by hormones produced by the hypothalamus and deposited into the bloodstream. The hormones released by the anterior lobe of the pituitary gland include the following (Table 24-3):

- Growth hormone (GH)
- Adrenocorticotropic hormone (ACTH)
- Thyroid-stimulating hormone (TSH)
- Follicle-stimulating hormone (FSH)
- Luteinizing hormone (LH)
- Prolactin

The posterior lobe of the pituitary gland contains the distal ends of some hypothalamic neurons. These hypothalamic neurons produce hormones but do not release them directly into the bloodstream. Instead, the axons that originated in the hypothalamus extend directly into the posterior lobe of the pituitary gland, where they are stored in secretory vesicles. These hormones are then secreted into the bloodstream when stimulated by nerve impulses from the hypothalamus. This form of transportation is called axoplasmic transport. The hormones released in the posterior lobe of the pituitary gland include ADH and oxytocin. ADH, also called *arginine vasopressin*, increases the reabsorption of water into the bloodstream. In the absence of ADH, an individual may develop diabetes insipidus, in which the kidneys pass copious amounts of water because they are not told to retain it. Arginine vasopressin also acts as a peripheral vasoconstrictor and is used in the management of patients in cardiac arrest. Oxytocin stimulates milk release and smooth muscle contractions in the uterine wall, prompting fetal delivery.

TABLE 24-2	Hypothalamus Hormones	
Hormone	Target Site	Effect
GHRH	Anterior pituitary	Stimulates release of GH
GHIH	Anterior pituitary	Inhibits release of GH
CRH	Anterior pituitary	Stimulates release of ACTH
TRH	Anterior pituitary	Stimulates release of TSH
GnRH	Anterior pituitary	Stimulates release of LH and FSH
PRH	Anterior pituitary	Stimulates release of prolactin
PIH	Anterior pituitary	Inhibits release of prolactin

GHRH, Growth hormone–releasing hormone; *GH*, growth hormone; *GHIH*, growth hormone–inhibiting hormone; *CRH*, corticotropin-releasing hormone; *ACTH*, adrenocorticotropic hormone; *TRH*, thyroid-releasing hormone; *TSH*, thyroid-stimulating hormone; *GnRH*, gonadotropin-releasing hormone; *LH*, luteinizing hormone; *FSH*, follicle-stimulating hormone; *PRH*, prolactin-releasing hormone; *PIH*, prolactin-inhibiting hormone.

TABLE 24-3	Pituitary Hormones	
Hormone	Target Site	Effect
Pituitary Gland, Anterior		
GH	All cells, especially growth cells	Stimulates cell growth and replication, especially in skeletal muscles and cartilage
ACTH	Adrenal cortex	Stimulates release of steroidal hormones by the adrenal cortex
TSH	Thyroid	Stimulates release of thyroid hormones
FSH	Ovaries or testes	Stimulates development of ovum or sperm
LH	Ovaries or testes	Stimulates release of hormones by the ovaries or testes
Prolactin	Mammary glands	Stimulates production and release of milk
Pituitary Gland, Posterior		
ADH	Kidneys	Stimulates increased reabsorption of water into bloodstream
Oxytocin	Uterus and breasts of women	Stimulates uterine contractions and milk release

GH, Growth hormone; *ACTH*, adrenocorticotropic hormone; *TSH*, thyroid-stimulating hormone; *FSH*, follicle-stimulating hormone; *LH*, luteinizing hormone; *ADH*, antidiuretic hormone.

Thyroid Gland #3

The thyroid is located on the anterior neck over the trachea, just below the cricoid cartilage. The gland consists of two lobes connected by an isthmus in the middle and extends laterally and caudally on either side of the midline. The thyroid affects almost every organ in the body, including the nervous, cardiovascular, and gastrointestinal systems; reproductive organs; and even the skin, hair, and nails. It is critical for normal metabolism.

The thyroid gland contains a large number of hollow spheres called thyroid follicles. These spheres are filled with a viscous colloid that contains large quantities of suspended proteins. The thyroid gland's two main hormones, thyroxine (T_4) and triiodothyronine (T_3), are produced in the thyroid follicles by using iodine absorbed through the digestive tract (Table 24-4). TSH, which is released by the pituitary gland, or environmental factors such as cold, cause the thyroid gland to release T_4 and T_3. This release in turn increases the body's rate of cellular metabolism.

The thyroid gland also produces calcitonin in the perifollicular, or C (clear) cells. Calcitonin regulates concentrations of calcium (Ca^{++}) in body fluids. When calcitonin levels in the body increase, body fluid calcium levels decrease. This effect is caused by an increased reuptake of calcium by the bones and a decrease in the breakdown of bone tissue.

Parathyroid Glands #4

Four parathyroid glands are embedded in the thyroid gland (Figure 24-2). They are located on the posterior aspect of the thyroid gland, with one in the superior and one in the inferior aspect of each of the two lobes. The parathyroid glands are quite small and weigh approximately 1.6 g. The C cells of the thyroid gland act to decrease fluid calcium levels, whereas the chief cells of the parathyroid glands act to increase fluid calcium levels (Table 24-5). This is accomplished by releasing parathyroid hormone (PTH). This hormone causes the bones to release calcium into the blood and the kidneys to reab-

sorb calcium. Homeostasis is maintained through the antagonistic effects of PTH and calcitonin balancing the levels of calcium in the body.

Thymus #5

The thymus is located in the mediastinum, just behind the sternum. During childhood an individual's thymus is quite large. It diminishes in size as the person reaches adulthood. The thymus, which is often associated with the lymphatic system, releases several hormones that are together called *thymosin* (Table 24-6). Thymosin promotes the maturation of T lymphocytes, the white blood cells primarily responsible for immunity.

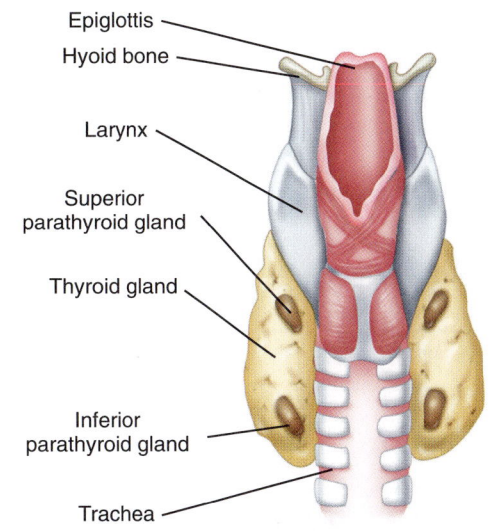

Labels: Epiglottis, Hyoid bone, Larynx, Superior parathyroid gland, Thyroid gland, Inferior parathyroid gland, Trachea

Figure 24-2 Thyroid and parathyroid glands.

TABLE 24-4	Thyroid Hormones	
Hormone	**Target Site**	**Effect**
T_4	All cells	Stimulates cellular metabolism
T_3	All cells	Stimulates cellular metabolism
Calcitonin	Bone	Stimulates calcium uptake by bones and decreases blood calcium levels; less important in healthy, nonpregnant adults

T_4, Thyroxine; T_3, triiodothyronine.

TABLE 24-5	PTH Hormones	
Hormone	**Target Site**	**Effect**
PTH	Bones, intestines, kidneys	Stimulates calcium release from bones, calcium uptake from intestinal tract, and calcium reabsorption in kidneys, with a net increase in blood calcium levels

PTH, Parathyroid hormone.

TABLE 24-6	Thymus Hormones	
Hormone	**Target Site**	**Effect**
Thymosin	White blood cells	Promotes the development and maturation of lymphocytes

1 Islet produces 0.6u insulin/day

Pancreas   #6   *Exocrine & endocrine*

[OBJECTIVE 3]

The pancreas is located partially in the retroperitoneal space behind the stomach (see Figure 24-1). It is a slender, pale organ with both endocrine and exocrine functions (Table 24-7). Approximately 99% of the pancreatic volume consists of exocrine gland cells called *pancreatic acini*. These cells connect to ducts that deposit an alkaline, enzyme-rich fluid directly into the digestive tract.

17. The remainder of the pancreas is composed of clustered endocrine cells forming islets. These pancreatic islets are also known as the **islets of Langerhans.** Four types of cells are found in the islets of Langerhans (Figure 24-3). Alpha cells, which produce glucagon, comprise approximately 25% of the cells found in the islets. Beta cells, which produce insulin, comprise approximately 60% of the islets of Langerhans. Delta cells, which produce somatostatin, comprise 10% of the islets. Somatostatin is

TABLE 24-7	Pancreatic Hormones	
Hormone	**Target Site**	**Effect**
Glucagon	All cells, primarily in liver, muscle, and fat	Stimulates glycogenolysis and gluconeogenesis in the liver, thus increasing serum glucose levels
Insulin	All cells, primarily in liver, muscle, and fat	Stimulates cellular uptake of glucose; increases rate of synthesis of glycogen, proteins, and fats, thus decreasing blood glucose levels
Somatostatin (identical to GHIH)	Alpha and beta cells in the pancreas	Inhibits secretion of glucagon and insulin within pancreas acting as a buffer
Pancreatic polypeptide	Gallbladder, pancreatic exocrine glands	Inhibits gallbladder contraction, regulates some pancreatic enzymes

GHIH, Growth hormone–inhibiting hormone.

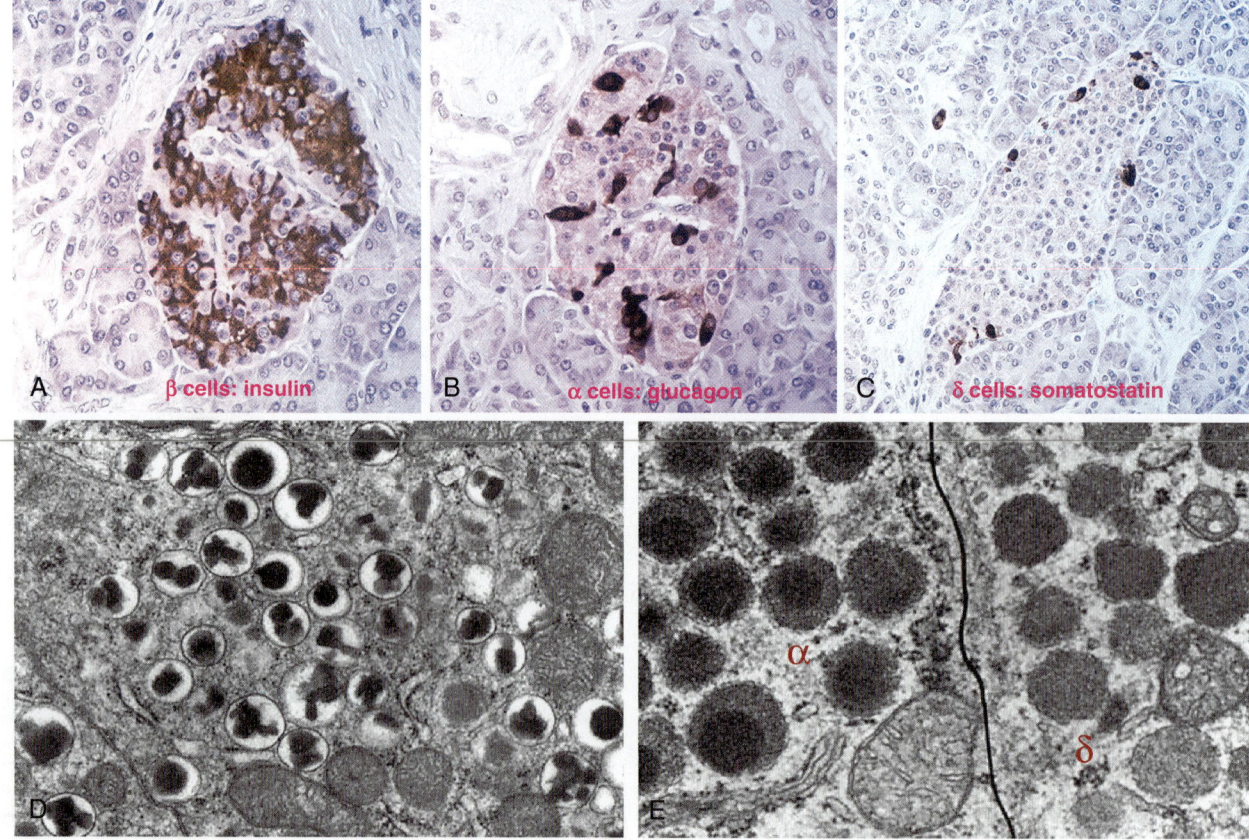

Figure 24-3 Islets of Langerhans. **A,** Beta cells. **B,** Alpha cells. **C,** Delta cells. **D,** F cells. **E,** Portions of an alpha cell *(left)* and a delta cell *(right)* also exhibit granules.

identical to GHIH released by the hypothalamus. The remaining cells in the islets of Langerhans are F cells, which produce pancreatic polypeptide.

Insulin and glucagon play an important role in maintaining a proper blood glucose balance between 60 and 120 mg/dL. As the body senses a rise in blood glucose levels, insulin is released into the bloodstream. Insulin decreases blood glucose levels by aiding the movement of glucose from the bloodstream into cells. (Note that brain cells do not depend on insulin to help move glucose from the bloodstream into the cells.) Insulin also prompts the liver to convert circulating glucose into glycogen. Glycogen is used by the body when blood glucose levels may not be high. Glycogen is also stored in skeletal muscle cells in a lesser amount that is not readily available for systemic use. Insulin also increases amino acid absorption, protein synthesis, and triglyceride synthesis and inhibits the release of glucagon.

When the blood glucose levels begin to drop glucagon is released into the bloodstream, which inhibits the release of insulin. Glucagon causes the liver and skeletal muscles to convert glycogen back into glucose. This process is known as **glycogenolysis.** In addition, glucagon causes an increase in the breakdown of fats into fatty acids and body proteins into amino acids for conversion by the liver into glucose. This formation of glucose synthesis in the liver is called **gluconeogenesis.**

Somatostatin, produced by the delta cells in the islets of Langerhans, antagonizes both insulin and glucagon

production. By inhibiting the release of both of these hormones, the body is able to avert wide swings in blood glucose levels as insulin and glucagon compete.

Adrenal Glands

The adrenal glands are located on each side of the body on the superior aspect of each kidney. Each adrenal gland is a yellow, pyramid-shaped gland divided into two distinct sections, the adrenal cortex and the adrenal medulla (Table 24-8). The adrenal cortex completely surrounds the inner adrenal medulla.

Like the hypothalamus, the adrenal medulla contains cells that function both as neural cells and as endocrine cells. The medulla interacts closely with the sympathetic component of the autonomic nervous system. When stimulated by the neurons of the sympathetic division of the autonomic nervous system, the medullar cells release epinephrine (adrenalin) and norepinephrine into the bloodstream. These catecholamines cause an increase in cardiac activity, vasoconstriction, and glycogenolysis, which are all key components in the sympathetic nervous system fight-or-flight response.

The adrenal cortex releases three steroidal hormones sometimes called **adrenocortical steroids,** but are more simply known as **corticosteroids.** These corticosteroids are essential to life. Without external replacement of these corticosteroids, the person will die. Between them, these corticosteroids assist in the regulation of

TABLE 24-8 Adrenal Hormones

Hormone	Target Site	Effect
Adrenal Gland, Cortex		
Glucocorticoid: cortisol	Most cells	Stimulates release of amino acids from skeletal muscles, lipids from adipose tissue, and glucose and glycogen from liver (mimics effects of glucagon); antiinflammatory effects
Mineralocorticoids; aldosterone	Kidneys, blood	Increases renal reabsorption of sodium and water (more so in the presence of ADH) and increases urinary loss of potassium; net increase in blood volume
Estrogen	Most cells	Stimulates development of secondary sexual characteristics
Progesterone	Uterus	Stimulates uterine changes in preparation for gestation
Testosterone	Most cells	Stimulates development of secondary sexual characteristics
Adrenal Gland, Medulla		
Epinephrine	Muscle, liver, cardiovascular system	Stimulates cardiac activity, increases vasoconstriction, stimulates glycogenolysis, raises blood glucose levels
Norepinephrine	Muscle, liver, cardiovascular system	Stimulates vasoconstriction

ADH, Antidiuretic hormone.

TABLE 24-9	Gonad Hormones	
Hormone	**Target Site**	**Effect**
Estrogen	Most cells, primarily those in the female reproductive system	Stimulates development of secondary sexual characteristics
Progesterone	Uterus	Stimulates uterine changes in preparation for gestation
Testosterone	Most cells, primarily those in the male reproductive system	Stimulates development of secondary sexual characteristics

blood glucose levels, promote the peripheral use of lipids, stimulate the kidneys to reabsorb sodium, and have anti-inflammatory effects.

Gonads

In both males and females the primary functions of the gonads are to promote sexual maturation to puberty and fulfill any subsequent reproductive needs (Table 24-9). In the male the gonads (testes) are located directly below and behind the penis, inside the scrotum. The interstitial cells of the testes produce male hormones known as *androgens*. The most prominent of these hormones is testosterone. Testosterone promotes healthy sperm production, determines secondary male sex characteristics such as hair production, and stimulates growth. Testosterone has also been shown to affect muscle production and aggressive behavioral responses.

In females the gonads (ovaries) are located inside the pelvic cavity on either side of the uterus. The anterior pituitary gland directs the actions of the ovaries through FSH and LH. The ovaries produce estrogen, progesterone, and a small amount of testosterone. Estrogen promotes follicular maturation (egg development) before ovulation, secondary sex characteristics, and associated behaviors. Progesterone prepares the uterus for implantation of the fertilized egg. During pregnancy, progesterone ensures that the uterine wall maintains functionality and prepares the mammary glands for activity.

ENDOCRINE DISORDERS

Disorders of the Pituitary Gland

Diabetes Insipidus

Description
[OBJECTIVE 14]

Diabetes insipidus (DI) is defined literally as the passing of water. The disorder has an effect on the concentration of sodium in the blood and therefore on blood concentration. The posterior pituitary secretes ADH in response to high sodium content or elevated serum osmolality. Its action on the collecting tubules of the kidneys results in increased reabsorption of water from

the urine, helping increase blood volume and lower abnormally elevated serum sodium levels. Posterior pituitary deficiencies can present as DI (lack of ADH). Central DI is caused by a lack of ADH production. This can result from surgery, edema, trauma, or infiltration by tumor. A deficit of ADH results in poor ability to reabsorb free water properly. With increasing losses of free water in the urine and poor absorption into the bloodstream, the urine and serum osmolality are low, serum sodium is elevated, and urine sodium is low. If untreated, symptoms progress and may result in death. Central DI usually occurs in the extremes of age and is seen in less than 1% of all hospitalized patients.

A patient typically knows he or she has central DI. Moreover, it often is a long-term result of a cerebrovascular accident (stroke) pituitary tumor, and/or surgery. A patient's current symptoms of dehydration, muscle spasms, confusion, or hyperreflexia may be a result of central DI. However, because of the rarity of DI and the broad range of differentials, it is not often considered by the paramedic in the field.

In renal, or nephrogenic, DI, patients have sufficient levels of ADH but the kidneys do not respond normally to ADH. Nephrogenic DI can be inherited in some cases, but it more often is a result of the side effects of some medications, polycystic kidney disease, sickle cell disease, or electrolyte disturbances. Nephrogenic DI may be a short-term or chronic syndrome.

History and Physical Findings
[OBJECTIVES 15, 16]

Patients with DI present with polydipsia and polyuria, muscle spasms, hyperreflexia, coma, altered mentation, and other similar signs and symptoms of hypernatremia and dehydration.

The signs and symptoms of DI are vague and resemble the general signs and symptoms of hypernatremia. Many of these signs and symptoms also are present with other more common central nervous system and metabolic disorders; therefore you should consider those first.

Therapeutic Interventions. Treatment of the patient with DI includes intravenous fluid replacement with isotonic saline or Ringer's lactate if possible. These fluids are used because the sodium content in them is still hypotonic compared with the serum sodium levels seen in DI. Hormone replacement can begin once the patient is stabilized. Treatment often results in significant improvement in serum sodium levels with appropriate fluids alone. ADH is rapidly metabolized by the body and has a half-life of 5 minutes. Desmopressin is a preparation that is not metabolized as quickly and can be given as a pill, subcutaneous injection, or intranasal spray. In patients with nephrogenic DI, desmopressin therapy is not effective and alternate treatment modalities must be used. These alternate modalities include identifying treatable underlying disorders and increasing fluid intake to match urine output. In both central and nephrogenic DI, serum sodium and urine volume should be closely monitored with treatment.

General Hypopituitarism Not emergency

Hypopituitarism is a deficiency of one, some, or all of the pituitary hormones previously described. The cause may be injury to the pituitary from tumor, surgery, or trauma or certain genetic causes that reveal themselves over time. The abnormal regulation of TSH results in hypothyroidism. Patients have poor growth, cold intolerance, dry skin, and constipation. The treatment involves oral thyroid replacement.

GH deficiency is increasingly common. Patients may have mild forms that go undiagnosed or severe GH deficiency. The severe deficiency results in short stature as well as hypoglycemia. GH is an important hormone responsible for blood sugar regulation, helping to raise the blood sugar level during hypoglycemia. Patients with GH deficiency may have a history of hypoglycemia during infancy. The treatment is hormone replacement with recombinant human GH given as subcutaneous injections once nightly. Adults with GH deficiency, either from childhood or acquired as adults from trauma or surgery, may benefit from treatment with hormone replacement. GH treatment provides benefits in both body composition and cardiovascular health in those who are deficient. Excessive GH secretion usually is caused by a pituitary tumor. It may result in gigantism, called acromegaly.

LH and FSH deficiency is rare unless associated with other pituitary hormone deficiencies. Patients with these gonadotropin deficiencies have delayed puberty. In addition, they are at risk for osteoporosis from low levels of estrogen production during the important years when bone density increases. Women may have a lack of ovulation and late or absent menses (beyond age 16 years). Men might present with small testes compared with the expected size for age. Treatment, if needed, includes replacement hormone therapy—estrogen and progesterone in women and testosterone in men. Excessive LH and FSH or premature pulsing leads to early puberty, called central precocious puberty. This may result from a tumor, the effects of radiation, or unknown causes.

Pituitary adrenal insufficiency results from a lack of ACTH secretion, which is necessary to stimulate the adrenal production of steroids. A reduction in the secretion of ADH is a critical signal, especially during stressors such as trauma, surgery, and even fever or illness. Patients may have ACTH deficiency as the result of trauma, surgery to the pituitary, hemorrhage, or idiopathic causes. Typically the signs of underfunction may not be evident except in times of extreme stress or illness. These patients have ample production of cortisol because their adrenals are healthy, but the signal to the adrenals is absent. This prevents the appropriate rise in cortisol during important times.

Disorders of the Thyroid Gland

Hyperthyroidism (Thyrotoxicosis)
Description
[OBJECTIVES 17, 18]

Hyperthyroidism is an overactive thyroid. It can be caused by an accidental overdose of thyroid hormone (rare but important to consider) or an autoimmune process that produces antibodies that stimulate the gland rather than inhibit it, as in Hashimoto's thyroiditis.

History and Physical Findings. Patients with hyperthyroidism have tachycardia, rapid respirations, heat intolerance, diarrhea, weight loss despite polyphagia, sweating, and irritability. In a child, hyperthyroidism often is misdiagnosed as attention deficit–hyperactivity disorder as the child's school performance becomes affected. Graves disease is a commonly described form of autoimmune thyroid disease that results in hyperthyroidism. It affects the ocular muscles, leading to protrusion of the eyes or exophthalmia.

The excessive blood levels of thyroid hormone (regardless of origin) result in a state known as **thyrotoxicosis.** The causes of thyrotoxicosis can come from the gland itself or from stimulation of the thyroid gland by antibodies that stimulate excessive thyroid hormone production. The classic example of this is Graves disease. Patients with thyrotoxicosis may present with an enlarged thyroid gland or goiter. Moreover, involvement of the eyes often results in protrusion of the globe (exophthalmos) and impairment of normal ocular and eyelid movements.

A **thyroid storm** refers to thyrotoxicosis in its most extreme form. Patients with this degree of thyrotoxicosis are a true medical emergency. The presenting signs and symptoms are the result of an extreme hypermetabolic state. Those that should be of concern include inadequate ventilation because of extreme tachypnea, tachycardia, and often sinus tachycardia or atrial fibrillation, resulting in decreased cardiac output, shock, hyperthermia, delirium, and cardiovascular collapse. Additional signs and symptoms include bounding pulses, a wide pulse pressure, systolic murmurs, heat intolerance, irritability, hyperactivity, fatigue, palpitations, weight loss despite an increased appetite, tremor, warm and moist skin, diarrhea, and polyuria.

Therapeutic Interventions
[OBJECTIVE 19]

Prehospital care of the patient with thyroid storm is symptomatic. It includes airway support, shock management, dysrhythmia management, and possibly the administration of beta-blockers, calcium channel blockers, and steroids (Box 24-1).

Hypothyroidism (Myxedema)

Description. A thyroid deficiency is not life threatening. However, patients with low levels are significantly affected. Poorly controlled hypothyroidism results in an elevated TSH level, which can lead to the development of pituitary enlargement from hypertrophy of these TSH-producing cells.

Hypothyroidism can result from iodine deficiency, an important element used by the thyroid gland to make thyroid hormone. In the United States iodine deficiency is rare. However, in some developing countries it is still encountered. These patients may have low thyroid function and an enlarged thyroid gland or goiter. The body's response to low thyroid hormone is to increase the TSH production to stimulate the gland further. Much like a thermostat, the thyroid hormone level is regulated by the feedback to the pituitary, and TSH responds appropriately. Congenital hypothyroidism can result from abnormal formation of the thyroid gland itself. In addition, the neonatal thyroid gland may not form thyroid hormone correctly because of an enzyme defect. Regardless of the cause, congenital hypothyroidism requires treatment. It is relatively common and most states have adopted mandatory newborn thyroid screening.

History and Physical Findings
[OBJECTIVES 18, 19]

Thyroid hormone is critical in brain growth, which occurs in the first 2 to 3 years of life. Inadequate thyroid hormone levels in the bloodstream can lead to mental retardation and poor development overall. The classic example of untreated congenital hypothyroidism is cretinism. These infants present with short stature, protruding tongues, and poor tone with delayed development. Hypothyroidism also can result from an autoimmune process in which the body makes antibodies that attack the thyroid gland or its enzymes, making the gland inactive. Hashimoto's thyroiditis is an example of this and is especially common in adolescent girls. The treatment of hypothyroidism involves replacement hormone (levothyroxine) taken as a pill or suspension.

In its most severe state, hypothyroidism is commonly called **myxedema.** This term is sometimes used generally to describe all levels of hypothyroidism, but it most often represents the most severe state. The signs and symptoms of myxedema are shown in Box 24-2. Patients with myxedema have exacerbated effects when subjected to stress, trauma, cold, drugs and alcohol, hypoglycemia, and hypothermia. The hallmarks of myxedema include hypothermia in the absence of accidental cold exposure, hypoglycemia in the absence of insulin replacement therapy, and coma. Hypotension and respiratory depression also may accompany coma, and you should assess patients for hypercarbia and hypoxia.

Therapeutic Interventions. The prehospital treatment of these patients is supportive. Care should include close attention to airway management, temperature regulation, and shock prevention. Although myxedema and myxedema coma are serious and possibly life-threatening conditions, they occur in less than 0.1% of all patients with hypothyroidism. In addition, consider that most, if not all, of the signs and symptoms are indicative of other, more common pathologic conditions. Therefore in the

---

BOX 24-1	Signs, Symptoms, and Treatment of Thyroid Storm

Signs and Symptoms
- High fever
- Irritability
- Tachycardia
- Hypotension
- Vomiting
- Diarrhea
- Delirium
- Coma

Treatment
- ABCs
- Oxygenation
- Ventilatory support
- Fluid resuscitation
- Cardiac monitoring
- Beta-blockers, per local protocol
- Steroids, per local protocol

ABCs, Airway, breathing, and circulation.

BOX 24-2	Myxedema: Signs and Symptoms

- Edematous face
- Periorbital edema
- Masklike effect
- Impaired memory
- Slowed speech
- Decreased initiative
- Somnolence
- Cold intolerance
- Hypothermia
- Dry, coarse skin —"doughy"
- Muscle weakness and swelling
- Constipation
- Weight gain
- Hair loss
- Hoarseness

absence of a thyroidectomy scar or a solid history of hypothyroidism, myxedema should be a remote consideration. Treatment is directed toward presenting signs and symptoms such as problems with airway, breathing, and circulation.

Disorders of the Parathyroid Gland

Hyperparathyroidism

Description. Hyperparathyroidism is defined as an oversecretion of PTH. Most cases of hyperparathyroidism are caused by a tumor of one of the four parathyroid glands.

History and Physical Findings. The signs and symptoms of hyperparathyroidism are often attributable to excess calcium and can include muscle weakness, fatigue, nausea, vomiting, and volume depletion.

Therapeutic Interventions. Prehospital care of the patient with hyperparathyroidism is supportive. Hospital treatment is typically directed at lowering calcium levels. Ultimately, if hyperparathyroidism is caused by a tumor, surgical intervention may be warranted.

Hypoparathyroidism

Description

[OBJECTIVES 20, 21, 22]

Poor function of the parathyroid gland may result from autoimmune disease. It also can be the result of lack of formation or surgical removal, as in a complete thyroidectomy.

History and Physical Findings. Because PTH works with vitamin D to regulate total body calcium, the signs and symptoms of hypoparathyroidism are usually the same as those of hypocalcemia: altered mental status, paresthesia of the extremities, muscle cramping and spasms, twitching, tremors, and seizures.

Therapeutic Interventions. Prehospital care for the patient with hypoparathyroidism is supportive. Hospital treatment includes calcium and vitamin D replacement.

Disorders of the Pancreas

Brain doesn't require insulin to work

[OBJECTIVE 4]

Diabetes has become a growing epidemic in the United States and other countries. It is responsible for many health complications that have increased rates of mortality and morbidity. The categories of diabetes have changed from year to year as new forms of diabetes have been recognized. For the sake of simplicity, this text addresses type 1 diabetes and type 2 diabetes and the common endocrine emergencies that develop from these disease processes.

The beta cells of the islets of Langerhans produce an important hormone called *insulin*. Insulin is responsible for decreasing blood sugar. It promotes the uptake of glucose into cells as well as fatty acids and amino acids. Insulin works opposite from glucagon and stimulates

enzymes that are responsible for storing glucose and generating glycogen in the liver.

The delta cells secrete somatostatin, the regulating hormone for the other endocrine hormones of the pancreas. Somatostatin inhibits the secretion of insulin as well as glucagon and centrally inhibits GH.

Type 1 diabetes, formerly called insulin-dependent diabetes mellitus or juvenile diabetes, results in a lack of insulin production from autoimmune destruction of the islet cells of the pancreas, in particular the beta cells that make insulin. Type 2 diabetes, formerly known as non-insulin-dependent diabetes mellitus or adult-onset diabetes, results from a resistance to insulin at the cells on which it acts or a decrease in insulin production. With the increased duration of the disease, patients with poorly controlled type 2 diabetes eventually develop a lack of insulin production as well.

usually young but it can be older it autoimmune or post chemo

obesity ↑ sugar consumption oral meds

usually older pt. but can be young

As a paramedic, you will commonly encounter diabetic emergencies. These problems include complications from a blood sugar level that is too low (hypoglycemia), resulting in seizure or coma, or a blood sugar level that is too high (hyperglycemia), resulting in diabetic ketoacidosis or hyperosmolar hyperglycemic nonketotic coma.

Hypoglycemia

Region XI - below 60 treat

Description

[OBJECTIVE 5]

Hypoglycemia is a common problem experienced by both patients with type 1 and patients with type 2 diabetes. The diabetic patient must intensively control his or her diabetes to prevent long-term complications. The Diabetes Control and Complications Trial (1997) emphasized intensive control of diabetes in the prevention of long-term complications. Approximately 1500 patients with diabetes participated in this study. After more than 10 years, the patients receiving intensive diabetes control had a significant reduction in nephropathy, neuropathy, and retinopathy. However, those without intensive diabetes control had a threefold increase in the incidence of moderate to severe hypoglycemia compared with those with conventional diabetes control. Therefore, as the medical community strives to prevent long-term complications, patients with diabetes should be counseled on the risks and prevention of hypoglycemia.

Mild to moderate hypoglycemia is common and, although not completely preventable, it is easily treated. It can be detected with close blood glucose monitoring. Moreover, it rarely results in complications to the patient. Serious hypoglycemia requires intervention and treatment. As an EMS professional, you will most commonly see serious hypoglycemia. You will need to promptly provide treatment to these patients. If untreated or not detected, serious hypoglycemia can lead to coma or death.

Counterregulation is the body's natural defensive ability to maintain blood sugar. An understanding of this concept is critical. It will help you treat and hopefully prevent severe hypoglycemia. The body's first line of defense against low blood sugar is to reduce insulin production by the pancreas and increase glucagon production by the alpha cells. The body's second line of defense is the secretion of catecholamines by the adrenal gland. These include epinephrine and norepinephrine production. The effects of this catecholamine release can be seen in the hypoglycemic patient as tachycardia and diaphoresis. This second line of defense also includes cortisol. The term *cortisol* comes from the word *cortex*, which is where the adrenocorticosteroids are produced in the adrenal gland. Cortisol is another important counterregulatory hormone. It allows an increase in blood sugar and counteracts insulin action. Other hormones produced by the intestine and GH from the pituitary increase blood sugar as well. Lastly, be sure to note the contribution of the autonomic nervous system. Stimulation of the nervous system contributes to signals that allow counterregulatory hormone increase. This stimulation also triggers symptoms that tell the body that sugar is low. This should lead a person to consume a source of sugar. In response to the action of these hormones, the body mobilizes fatty acids and amino acids from adipose and muscle, respectively. The liver uses these products to make new sugar for the body; this process is called gluconeogenesis.

Patients with type 1 diabetes do not make insulin on their own. As a result, the body's first line of defense from hypoglycemia is lost and a decrease of insulin levels is not possible. Often a low blood sugar in diabetes is caused by elevated exogenous insulin from inaccurate dosing, intentional overdose, or perhaps a mismatch with carbohydrate intake and exogenous insulin intake. In addition, increased use of glucose, as in exercise, causes the blood sugar to drop sharply, resulting in hypoglycemia.

Patients with type 2 diabetes are able to make insulin from their pancreas and can suppress insulin production from their own bodies. However, their bodies may be resistant, or over time they may not make enough insulin to lower the blood glucose adequately. Medications given to treat type 2 diabetes act by either stimulating the body's ability to secrete insulin or by improving insulin action. These medications also have a tendency to contribute to hypoglycemia, especially in certain groups of patients—the elderly and those who are not metabolizing these medications properly because of liver or kidney disease. Often if the hypoglycemia is caused by excessive insulin dosing by the patient or the prolonged or exaggerated effect of oral diabetes medication, the low blood sugar effect will be prolonged and a more long-term treatment may be needed.

Some patients who have had type 1 diabetes for many years, and to a lesser degree patients who have had type 2 diabetes for many years, have been shown to have a lack of glucagon release from the pancreas in response to hypoglycemia (Gerich et al., 1973). Lack of glucagon response makes the body more dependent on epinephrine to overcome the effects of hypoglycemia, yet there may be some lack of responsiveness to epinephrine in diabetes as well (Guy et al., 2004; Guy et al., 2005). Prolonged disease can also decrease a patient's ability to recognize a low blood sugar, preventing him or her from taking the necessary measures of self-treatment. This is called *hypoglycemic unawareness*.

History and Physical Findings
[OBJECTIVE 6]

Hypoglycemia is defined as a blood glucose level of 60 mg/dL or less. Significant signs and symptoms often are seen near 50 mg/dL. In the field, a standard practice for advanced life support providers is the determination of blood glucose. Whenever possible, determine a patient's blood glucose level to confirm that the clinical findings are consistent with hypoglycemia. Box 24-3 demonstrates a generic approach to blood glucose determination with a standard glucometer. Many glucometers are available on the market. Familiarize yourself with the model you will be using and follow all manufacturer recommendations for maintenance and calibration.

The clinical presentation of hypoglycemia can take many forms. All eventually lead to unconsciousness and death in the diabetic patient if not treated. Note that although most of the body's cells can withstand a drop in blood glucose level, the brain is dependent on and sensitive to glucose levels. That explains why many of the signs and symptoms of hypoglycemia reflect neurologic changes and deficiencies. Some of the most common signs and symptoms are the following:

- Hunger
- Agitation or combative behavior that cannot be explained
- Altered mentation
- Nausea /Vomiting
- Weakness
- Confusion
- Tachycardia (poor cardiac output)
- Cool, clammy skin
- Seizures

Therapeutic Interventions
[OBJECTIVE 7]

Treatment of the patient with hypoglycemia always involves increasing the blood glucose level (Box 24-4). Three basic methods are used to accomplish this. The least invasive and most available method is to have the patient ingest glucose in the form of a glucose paste applied buccally or tablets that dissolve in the mouth. Food sources, such as orange juice or hard candy, can be used if other sources are unavailable. However, these food sources often are not glucose (i.e., orange juice is fructose) and therefore do not work as well or as fast. In addition, they may pose an airway risk if the patient loses consciousness. In any case, if a source of glucose is to be administered in the mouth, the patient must be able to manage his or her own airway (swallow and gag). More-

BOX 24-3　Blood Glucose Sampling

1. Take appropriate infection control precautions.
2. Verify patient condition warrants use of device.
3. Verify that device has been calibrated and is within normal testing limits.
4. Select a finger that will result in proper sampling.
5. Turn on unit and follow the manufacturer's instructions.
6. Clean fingertip with alcohol pad and allow to dry.
7. Use sterile lancet or lancet pen on the side of selected finger.
8. Penetrate skin to obtain a hanging drop of blood.
9. Apply blood to pad according to the manufacturer's instructions.
10. Properly position testing strip into device according to the manufacturer's instructions.
11. Properly dispose of lancet.
12. Correctly read and interpret findings.
13. Properly dispose of testing strip.
14. Place sterile dressing on penetrated finger as necessary.
15. Record blood glucose test result.

BOX 24-4　Signs, Symptoms, and Treatment of Hypoglycemia

Signs and Symptoms

Hunger
Nausea
Weakness
Weak, rapid pulse
Pale, cool, clammy skin
Seizures
Altered mental status

- Agitated
- Confused
- Combative
- Lethargic
- Unresponsive

Treatment

ABCs
Oxygenation
Ventilatory support
Oral glucose; 15-30 g

- Ensure the patient can manage his or her own airway

IV D50: 12.5-25 g based on blood glucose initial value, reassessment, and/or resolutions of signs and symptoms.

- Ensure IV site is patent

IV or IM glucagon: 0.5-1.0 mg

ABCs, Airway, breathing, and circulation; *IV,* intravenous; *IM,* intramuscular.

over, you must monitor the patient's level of consciousness at all times.

If the patient cannot manage his or her own airway or if the level of consciousness might change, intravenous (IV) dextrose is the treatment of choice. IV dextrose works almost immediately in increasing the patient's blood glucose level. Moreover, it can be administered regardless of the patient's airway or level of consciousness. Ensure the IV line is patent because dextrose 50% is hypertonic and can cause tissue necrosis if extravasation occurs.

If the patient is not a candidate for oral glucose and patent vascular access is not possible, glucagon is the last option. As previously mentioned, glucagon increases blood glucose levels by a different mechanism than glucose. Glucagon initiates the breakdown of glycogen from stores in the liver (glycogenolysis). Patients who have inadequate glycogen stores in the liver cannot benefit from glycogenolysis; you cannot release what you do not have in the first place. The most common reasons that a patient would not have adequate glycogen liver stores are chronic alcoholism or malnutrition, young age, illness, history of seizure, or some kind of trauma.

In all cases, when the patient's blood glucose level is increased, an immediate decrease or disappearance of signs and symptoms should occur. Soon after, the patient should ingest a more complex source of carbohydrates, such as peanut butter and crackers. This will ensure that his or her blood glucose levels remain above 80 mg/dL. All patients need monitoring after treatment because the longevity of treatment is directly related to the level of imbalance of insulin in the patient's system, and a return of hypoglycemia is common. Additionally, take care to determine the cause of the hypoglycemic episode. Simply correcting the signs and symptoms is not enough. In regard to hypoglycemic episodes in the diabetic patient, you must take steps to educate the patient and his or her family members about its cause. Also instruct them about the steps that should be taken in the future to prevent reoccurrence.

Hyperglycemia
[OBJECTIVES 8, 9]

Hyperglycemia is almost always a result of diabetes mellitus. By itself, and at a level lower than approximately 250 mg/dL, it represents no immediate life threat. In fact, these patients may go several years without diagnosis of type 2 diabetes. It does, however, cause several physiologic changes that have detrimental long-term effects. Largely because of the increased hyperosmolarity it causes, hyperglycemia puts undue strain on the cardiovascular system, kidneys, and other end organs that are sensitive to increased serum viscosity and subsequent pressures. The result over time is seen as increased incidence of disorders such as renal failure, congestive heart failure, retinopathy, coronary artery disease, and neuropathy. The signs and symptoms of simple hyperglycemia are usually mild, if present at all. They can include blurred vision, polyuria, polydipsia, polyphagia, orthostatic syncope, frequent infections, and skin ulcerations. If you encounter a patient with simple hyperglycemia who has not progressed to the more serious syndromes covered in the following paragraphs, treatment should include supportive care and transport.

When serum glucose levels rise above tolerable levels, other physiologic changes occur. These changes represent actual pathologic conditions called diabetic ketoacidosis (blood glucose above 350 mg/dL, approximately, and usually in type 1 diabetics) and hyperosmolar hyperglycemic nonketotic coma (blood glucose levels greater than 600 mg/dL, approximately, and usually in type 2 diabetics).

[margin: 3-Sluns Diabetic coma; Slower onset]

Diabetic Ketoacidosis

[margin note: On insulin, a cetone breath occurs over 3-5d]

Description. **Diabetic ketoacidosis (DKA)** is a life-threatening emergency that results from persistent hyperglycemia caused by a complete lack of—or too little—insulin in the body. It can occur in patients who are newly diagnosed with type 1 diabetes, diabetics who have an increased release of glycogen in response to stress or illness and do not adjust their insulin intake accordingly, as well as those with poorly controlled diabetes. This results in elevated blood sugar level, excessive breakdown of the body's energy stores, and the resulting accumulation of acids in the body that cause dehydration, electrolyte abnormalities, and metabolic acidosis.

DKA is a complex metabolic problem that arises from the combination of several adaptive mechanisms in the body resulting from too little insulin action. A lack of insulin leads to an inability of the body to manage glucose. As a result, a rise in blood glucose ensues. The other hormones that affect blood sugar in the body now become unopposed. This then leads to an imbalance in glucose metabolism. These other hormones include glucagons, epinephrine, and cortisol. Hyperglycemia with very little glucose entering into the cells leads to a catabolic state or breakdown of the body's stores. The body tries to mobilize glucose stores in an effort to provide glucose to the cells. Counterregulatory hormones such as glucagon, epinephrine, and cortisol make the situation worse by mobilizing glycogen stores from the liver. This, in turn, leads to an elevated blood glucose level as well. The low insulin levels result in an increase in serum free fatty acids becoming mobilized from adipose tissue because of lipolysis. Fatty acids are then broken down primarily by the mitochondria in liver cells. As part of this process, ketone bodies are released into the bloodstream. Ketone bodies consist of acetoacetate, beta-hydroxybutyrate, and acetone. Large quantities of ketone bodies in the bloodstream cause a decrease in the blood's pH and a resultant acidosis. This acidosis results in the body's attempt to buffer the acidity with HCO_3, and the blood pH lowers because of an inability to keep up with the ongoing acidity. In addition to fat tissue breaking down its stores, muscle is also mobilizing its stores in an effort to create more sugar for the body. This creates

amino acids that may be used by the liver to make glucose (gluconeogenesis). Lactate increases in the bloodstream as well and contributes to lowering the body's pH.

History and Physical Findings
[OBJECTIVE 10] *[margin: Warm, dry skin]*

The load of glucose to the kidneys results in the spilling of glucose in the urine, causing the body to become hyperosmotic. This leads to the mobilization of water toward the bloodstream and ultimately dehydration. In addition to the spilling of glucose in the urine because of osmotic diuresis, the kidneys also help clear ketone bodies. Because of the significant amount of water loss from diuresis, patients also lose excessive amounts of sodium, potassium, and phosphates in the urine. This combination of effects leads to both dehydration and metabolic acidosis with associated electrolyte imbalances. Signs and symptoms manifest themselves through these factors. Patients have symptoms of dry mucous membranes, orthostatic hypotension, supine hypotension, fatigue, increased thirst (polydipsia), increased urination (polyuria), increased hunger (polyphagia), tachycardia, abdominal pain, vomiting from the acidosis, altered mental status and, with time, weight loss from the hypermetabolic state. The patient's respiratory rate is usually elevated and the tidal volume is increased (Kussmaul's respirations) because of **ketonemia**, acidosis, and the body's attempt to relieve itself of CO_2. This results in hypocapnia, which is recognized by lower than normal end-tidal CO_2 levels. A fruity odor to the patient's breath is consistent with ketones as well. Patients usually appear thin or dehydrated and have warm, dry skin.

In patients with type 2 diabetes, DKA is rare because insulin is still present, at least early on in the disease, and despite elevated blood sugar the level of insulin is enough to prevent uncontrolled breakdown of glycogen, adipose tissue, and muscle. In all patients with type 2 diabetes, regardless of the duration of the disease, ketones can be found in the urine with hyperglycemia. With increased duration of type 2 diabetes, a loss of pancreatic insulin production may occur. In fact, patients may develop elevated serum ketones, reduced blood pH, and DKA similar to those patients with type 1 diabetes.

Therapeutic Interventions *[margin: RMC]*
[OBJECTIVE 11]

Treatment of DKA includes fluids and insulin (Box 24-5). However, the replacement of losses must be slow. The majority of patients with DKA became ill and dehydrated over a prolonged period—days and up to weeks. The replacement of fluids also should be gradual to prevent complications of overaggressive treatment. Therefore carefully consider bolus administration with fluids based on the patient's cardiovascular status. If a patient is stable, often the administration of fluids is best given as a continuous infusion of 1.5 to 2 times the maintenance rate for the patient. If the patient is hypotensive, rapidly

Insulin: Different peaks / onset of action
R - fast acting.
L - slower acting

http://evolve.elsevier.com/Aehlert/paramedic   **961**

BOX 24-5 — Signs, Symptoms, and Treatment of Diabetic Ketoacidosis

Signs and Symptoms

- Polyuria
- Polydipsia
- Polyphagia
- Warm, dry skin
- Dry mucus membranes
- Tachycardia
- Postural hypotension
- Kussmaul respirations
- Sweet, fruity breath (acetone odor)
- Decreased level of consciousness
- Coma in late stages

Treatment

- ABCs
- Oxygenation
- Ventilatory support
- Fluid resuscitation

ABCs, Airway, breathing, and circulation.

Hypomagnesemia is commonly associated with DKA as a result of the loss of magnesium through the urine. This can worsen vomiting and cause alterations in mental status, as well as induce other electrolyte abnormalities, and lead to potentially fatal cardiac dysrhythmias. Magnesium deficiency from DKA is generally not addressed in the prehospital setting; however, if the paramedic suspects severe deficiency he or she can, in consultation with medical control, consider mixing 0.35 mEq/kg of magnesium in the initial fluid boluses.

The associated increase of relative serum potassium levels emphasizes the need to monitor the patient's electrocardiogram. The monitoring of potassium can be assisted by evaluation of T waves, P waves, and width of the QRS complex on the electrocardiographic pattern. Children are less likely than adults to have cardiovascular complications as potassium rises. However, this does not preclude the need for monitoring the cardiovascular status of all patients with DKA closely.

PARAMEDIC*Pearl*

Aggressive hydration, particularly with hypotonic fluids, has been shown to contribute to complications of therapy, such as cerebral edema. Conservative fluid management is key.

administer isotonic fluids until the systolic pressure is 80 mm Hg, then slow the infusion. As with any patient in whom fluid boluses are being administered, closely monitor the patient for the development of pulmonary edema. The elevated osmolality of the serum from hyperglycemia results in a prolonged and progressive shrinking (crenation) of the body's cells as water moves out into the hypertonic intravascular compartment. The rapid administration of intravascular fluids promotes the rapid movement of fluid into the cells of the body and increases the risk for edema. Of particular concern is cerebral edema, which can lead to changes in mental status, coma, and death. This is particularly true in the pediatric patient. In pediatric patients IV fluid boluses should be limited to 10 mL/kg at a time with fluids such as normal saline or Ringer's lactate solution. These IV fluid boluses should not be repeated unless significant conditions exist. In adults, 1 to 1.5 L is typically given over the first hour. Also monitor neurologic status.

The use of NaHCO$_3$ (sodium bicarbonate) to treat the metabolic acidosis of DKA is controversial and generally not considered unless the pH is less than 7.0. It should not be used outside a hospital setting and must be deemed necessary by the medical team. Arbitrary administration of sodium bicarbonate can cause a paradoxic acidosis in the cerebrospinal fluid as well as several other complications that worsen the patient's condition and outcome. The patient's vital signs should be closely monitored for blood pressure, heart rate, respiratory rate, and assessment of neurologic status (Umpierrez & Kitabchi, 2003).

You do not need to administer insulin immediately; often simple IV fluid management and transport to the hospital are enough to establish significant improvement of the hyperglycemia as well as help correct the metabolic acidosis. Insulin ideally is given as a drip. Large boluses before drip therapy are discouraged, especially in pediatric patients. Excessive bolus administration of insulin rapidly decreases the serum glucose and serum potassium levels along with the fluid administration. It promotes rapid movement of potassium and hydrogen ions and water into cells. Patients may develop hypoglycemia or hypokalemia from overly aggressive insulin administration. A significant decrease in morbidity is noted with continuous low-dose therapy. IV insulin is significantly more effective than intramuscular (IM) or subcutaneous administration, at least in the initial treatment. Also consider in a patient with poor perfusion that subcutaneous insulin may not absorb appropriately. This can lead to a slowing of onset of action.

Regular insulin 1st bolus then slow IV infusion

Hyperosmolar Hyperglycemic Nonketotic Coma

older pts. comorbid conditions - HTN, TY

Description. **Hyperosmolar hyperglycemic nonketotic coma (HHNC)** is the result of elevated glucose from poor or little insulin action (Kitabchi et al., 2004). It is typically described in a patient with type 2 diabetes; however, it has been reported in children with type 1 diabetes. Similar to DKA, secretion of hormones is exaggerated. This results in an increase of the blood glucose level because of mobilization of glucose stores. However, patients with hyperosmolar hyperglycemia have some

Not on insulin, occurs over days - weeks

insulin action remaining compared with those with DKA. Therefore the breakdown of fatty acids and excessive formation of ketone bodies is less dramatic. These patients have smaller amounts of ketones present in the urine and serum than do patients with DKA, but they have higher blood sugar levels (often much higher) because of excessive hormone action and insulin resistance. Glucose is present in the urine and dehydration occurs because of elevated serum osmolality and free water losses in an effort to rid the body of sugar. HHNC generally occurs in elderly patients, who may have decreased renal function and a decrease in the ability to eliminate glucose. This, along with the insulin resistance, leads to the extremely elevated glucose levels (more than 600 mg/dL) associated with the condition. Because of the insulin resistance associated with HHNC, insulin therapy often is not effective, leading to a mortality rate approaching 70%.

History and Physical Findings
[OBJECTIVE 12]

The clinical presentation of these patients is similar to the dehydration component of DKA. The acidotic signs and symptoms, such as fruity breath and Kussmaul's respirations, are absent. The time of onset between HHNC and DKA also is different. DKA may occur in a matter of hours to days, whereas HHNC has a more insidious onset and can take days to weeks. Signs and symptoms manifest themselves through severe volume depletion and the central nervous system. These include warm, dry skin, dry mucous membranes, poor skin turgor, tachycardia, weakness, polyuria, polydipsia, polyphagia, orthostatic hypotension, supine hypotension, altered mental status, lethargy, coma, and possibly seizures.

Therapeutic Interventions
[OBJECTIVE 3]

The treatment is as described for DKA. It includes fluid therapy and insulin, with close monitoring of vital signs and cardiovascular status (Box 24-6).

Gestational Diabetes

Description. Patients who are pregnant have the chance of developing gestational diabetes. This form of diabetes does not have a pancreatic component, but rather results from impaired glucose tolerance. During the first trimester the presence of increased levels of progesterone and estrogen causes an increased sensitivity to insulin. This, along with the glucose demands of the placenta and fetus, can lead to episodes of hypoglycemia, especially in the patient with preexisting diabetes. During the second trimester resistance to insulin occurs and peaks in the third trimester. This can lead to significant elevations in blood glucose levels, or gestational diabetes. If untreated the risk of fetal death significantly increases; however, if discovered early and appropriate treatment is initiated, the impact is minimal. The diabetes may resolve at the end of the pregnancy or continue for life. However, even

BOX 24-6	Signs, Symptoms, and Treatment of HHNC

Signs and Symptoms
- Polyuria
- Polydipsia
- Polyphagia
- Warm, dry skin
- Dry mucus membranes
- Tachycardia
- Postural hypotension
- Decreased level of consciousness
- Coma in late stages

Treatment
- ABCs
- Oxygenation
- Ventilatory support
- Fluid resuscitation

HHNC, Hyperosmolar hyperglycemic nonketotic coma; *ABCs,* airway, breathing, and circulation.

if the diabetes resolves, the woman has a significant chance of developing diabetes within the next 10 years.

History and Physical Findings. Patients at risk for gestational diabetes include patients who are older than 25 years, are obese, have a history of impaired insulin secretion, had a prior delivery of a child greater than 9 pounds, have a first-degree relative with a history of diabetes, have recurrent infections, had complications or poor outcome in a prior pregnancy, and who are of African or Hispanic ancestry. Signs and symptoms are the same as for hyperglycemia as previously described.

Therapeutic Interventions. Treatment is similar to any patient with hyperglycemia. Long-term treatment includes dietary modification and insulin therapy if needed. Historically, oral hypoglycemics have been avoided because of possible effects on the fetus; however, glyburide has been determined to be safe and effective.

Complications of Diabetes

Diabetes is a systemwide disease process and is not limited to the pancreas. These complications often lead to significant morbidity and mortality. For example, impairment of the immune system places these patients at higher risk of complicated infections. Complications can be divided into vascular and nonvascular, with vascular complications further divided into microvascular and macrovascular. The primary complications of concern to the paramedic are the vascular complications.

Microvascular Complications. Diabetic retinopathy is the leading cause of adult blindness in the United States. This condition can cause a variety of deficiencies in vision, which can lead to an increase in falls and other traumatic injuries. Diabetic nephropathy can lead to renal dysfunction and resulting hypertension. Preexisting hypertension can accelerate the damage to the kidneys, further exacerbating hypertension and hypertensive emergencies. Neuropathy results from poor perfusion to the nerves and subsequent dysfucntion. It is particularly evident in the distal peripheral nerves and results in either pain, hypersensitivity to pain, or the absence of pain sensation. This often leads to the "stump hands and feet" experienced by patients with diabetes. Foot complications such as ulcers are common in these patients because of a loss of sensation in the feet. Constant pressure can lead to necrosis of the affected area and potentially life-threatening infections. Autonomic neuropathy can develop and manifests through the autonomic system affected. This can result in delayed gastric emptying, constipation, nocturnal diarrhea, bladder dysfunction, hypotension, tacycardia at rest, syncope, and even sudden cardiac arrest.

Macrovascular Complications. Peripheral vascular disease, cerebovascular disease, and coronary artery disease are all complications of diabetes. In fact, the American Heart Association has classified diabetes in the same category of risk factors for cardiovascular disease as smoking, hypertension, and high cholesterol. This is because an increase in arthrosclerosis and platelet activity causes the formation of thrombi and thromboemboli. Reduced circulation to the extremities exacerbates distal neuropathies, accounting for the disproportionately high number of amputations in diabetic patients. Decreased blood flow to the brain and increased thrombus formation make cerebrovascular accidents (strokes) common in this population. Coronary artery disease is also common in diabetic patients for the same reason. This, combined with a decrease in pain sensation, makes diabetic patients especially susceptible to atypical myocardial infarctions. Often these present simply as weakness, fatigue, or general malaise. This presentation often is termed a "silent" myocardial infarction because of the lack of chest pain or other typical signs and symptoms of a heart attack. The paramedic must carefully evaluate for the presence of a myocardial infarction in the diabetic patient with vague complaints. The same principles should be applied to any elderly patient with vague complaints because neuropathies can be part of the aging process.

Disorders of the Adrenal Glands

Adrenal Insufficiency

Description
[OBJECTIVE 23]

Acute adrenal insufficiency is a life-threatening emergency. Treatment of these patients cannot be delayed. These patients show a rapid deterioration of cardiovascular and metabolic status. Primary adrenal insufficiency, or Addison's disease, is the inability of the adrenal cortex to produce aldosterone, cortisol, or both. This results from the destruction of 90% or more of the adrenal

glands. Addison's disease can result from an autoimmune process, an infectious disease such as tuberculosis or HIV and associated opportunistic infections, or a genetic disorder such as congenital adrenal hyperplasia Tumors, trauma, and chemotherapeutic agents also are related to adrenal injury that results in insufficiency of cortisol production (Arlt & Allolio, 2003). Secondary adrenal insufficiency is the result of pituitary disorders, as previously described, or hypothalamic disorders. In these situations ACTH production is decreased, which results in the inability of the body to produce adequate amounts of cortisol during times of stress, when it is most needed. In these patients, however, adequate amounts of aldosterone are present because of stimulation by the rennin-angiotensin response. Finally, adrenal insufficiency can occur in patients who have been on long-term steroid therapy such as prednisone. In these patients the adrenal cortex reduces its production of cortisol and aldosterone as a result of the ingestion of oral steroid medications. If the patient suddenly stops taking these medications, a life-threatening adrenal insufficiency can occur. More often than not adrenal insufficiency is secondary to a chronic condition with the acute presentation of signs and symptoms rather than the acute cessation of the production of cortisol and aldosterone.

History and Physical Findings
[OBJECTIVE 24]

The signs and symptoms of adrenal insufficiency include weakness, fatigue, darkening of skin pigmentation (Addison's disease only), anorexia, hypoglycemia, weight loss, early morning nausea, vomiting, abdominal pain, salt craving, diarrhea, fainting, and dizziness. The presentation is not specific, but patients generally demonstrate hypotension (often refractory to fluid therapy) and tachycardia with signs of dehydration, hyperkalemia, and hyponatremia. The electrocardiogram may show characteristics of hyperkalemia (peaked T waves, flattened P waves, and widening of the QRS complex) and/or low voltage in all leads.

Therapeutic Interventions
[OBJECTIVE 25]

Treatment of these patients is immediately directed toward airway, breathing, and circulation. IV access is critical. The best first treatment is the correction of electrolyte abnormalities such as hypoglycemia or hyponatremia with appropriate IV fluids. Fluid replacement may include a fluid bolus of 10 to 20 mL/kg depending on hemodynamic status.

Cushing Syndrome

Description
[OBJECTIVES 24, 25]

Cushing syndrome, more often found in women than in men, is a disorder of overproduction or above-average levels of corticosteroids. The cause of this increase of circulating corticosteroids is most often a tumor on the adrenal gland. However, it also can be caused by tumors of the pituitary gland, long-term corticosteroid use as treatment for other disorders (asthma), or enlargement of the adrenal glands from a congenital or unknown etiology.

History and Physical Findings. Patients with Cushing syndrome have physical manifestations of the disorder that include a "moon face" and fat accumulation above the clavicles and on the upper back (buffalo hump). Other signs and symptoms of this condition are shown in Box 24-7.

Therapeutic Interventions. Cushing syndrome is rarely a prehospital emergency. Treatment of this patient should be focused on symptom management.

BOX 24-7 Cushing Syndrome: Signs and Symptoms

- Thin skin
- Acne
- Moon face
- Hump on upper back (buffalo hump) *C7*
- Supraclavicular fat pad
- Thin extremities *— muscle loss 2° to excess cortisol*
  mobilizes amino acids
- Ecchymosis
- Slow healing
- Mood swings
- Pendulous abdomen
- Purplish abdominal striae
- Weight gain
- Increased facial hair
- Weakness

Hyperglycemia — excess cortisol
mobilizes fatty acids w/amino acids
liver makes more sugar — gluconeogenesis

Case Scenario—continued

Further history reveals that the patient is normally healthy. She has no surgical history. She does not drink, smoke, or take any illicit drugs. She has been getting more ill over the past few days, with unintentional weight loss occurring over the last month. You place the patient on supplemental oxygen and the cardiac monitor. The cardiac monitor reveals a sinus tachycardia. You establish IV access and infuse normal saline at a rate of 150 mL/hr. The patient starts acting confused. She is moving all extremities and not making any sense. You begin a thorough physical examination and note that she has very prominent eyes. Her mucous membranes appear dry. You note a large nodule near her throat, but her trachea is midline. Auscultation of lung sounds reveals bilateral crackles. Heart sounds are normal. Her abdomen is soft with normal bowel sounds. Her extremities are moist and warm.

Questions

5. *What are possible diagnoses for this patient?*
6. *What are the most important treatment considerations for this patient?*
7. *What additional interventions should be done?*

NUTRITIONAL DISORDERS

Malnutrition

[OBJECTIVE 26]

Malnutrition is still a prevailing medical problem worldwide. It results from the body receiving inadequate energy to meet its metabolic needs. It can result from poor intake of calories, vitamins, or certain portions of the body's required nutrients, such as protein.

In mild nutritional disorders the symptoms may not be evident. As malnutrition progresses, as in starvation, the symptoms may include dizziness, fainting, weight loss, and neurologic changes. Eating disorders such as anorexia nervosa and bulimia are psychologically influenced forms of malnutrition. Rarely will you be called to treat a patient with a nutritional disorder. More frequently these patients seek care from primary care practitioners as their signs and symptoms worsen. When you are called for emergent signs and symptoms, you should relate the patient's symptomatology to an underlying nutritional disorder. At times, your observations in the field may be the clues that ultimately lead to a diagnosis of a nutritional disorder. Prehospital management of the patient with a nutritional disorder deals more with the treatment of the patient's symptoms than reversing the disorder.

Case Scenario CONCLUSION

The patient becomes more confused. She is sweating profusely. Her heart rate is still 144 beats/min. You begin to prepare for urgent transport.

Looking Back

8. What comfort measures can be done for this patient?

9. What documentation should be done for this patient both in the written and oral report?

Inadequate Caloric Intake

[OBJECTIVE 27]

Marasmus is malnutrition from an overall lack of calories. It may be from poor intake or a complication of other diseases possibly related to poor absorption. These patients have poor weight gain usually followed by weight loss. Subcutaneous fat is lost, particularly at the buttocks and thigh area. Treatment is supportive and based on laboratory findings and physical deterioration (e.g., dehydration, hyponatremia). The prevention of marasmus may be increased through public assistance and education programs that target at-risk populations.

Kwashiorkor is a form of malnutrition caused by the body receiving inadequate protein calories compared with the total calorie intake, which may be enough to maintain weight. Although rare in the United States compared with developing countries, kwashiorkor is seen more commonly in elderly patients in nursing home settings. The symptoms include lethargy, fatigue, irritability, and most importantly edema, which may be generalized. Patients usually have a distended abdomen. Blood tests reveal low serum albumin. The treatment is supportive, with close observation and rapid treatment of shock if it develops. The patient's blood pressure is low because of low blood volume from hypoalbuminemia. The refeeding of these patients should be done slowly, or poor absorption and further loss of calories from the gastrointestinal tract may result. Most patients recover if treatment is provided early; however, permanent disability and possibly death may result if treatment is delayed. Kwashiorkor may be avoided in the elderly population through nutritional education.

Alcohol can cause myriad nutritional disorders, including the ability to store and use electrolytes and minerals. This is because of poor intake, vomiting, diarrhea, or impaired function. Patients may be hypokalemic, hyponatremic, or hypocalcemic. Long-term alcohol abuse is the most common cause of hypomagnesemia. Hypoglycemia, although rare, can result from alcohol abuse. When found it is more likely to be in the patient who chronically abuses alcohol. It is often caused by poor intake, the depletion of glycogen, decreased cortisol, and impaired glucogenesis.

Alcoholic ketoacidosis (AKA) is a condition that can easily be confused with DKA. This condition commonly occurs 1 to 3 days after an episode of binge drinking with minimal intake of food. Because of malnutrition resulting from abdominal pain, nausea, vomiting, or resistance to eating, the body will resort to alternative sources of energy, such as in DKA. However, in AKA the blood glucose level is generally normal or low rather than elevated. As fats are broken down for energy, fatty acids are formed and acidosis ensues. Further complications of acidosis can occur as a result of vomiting and hyperventilation, which can result in mixed acid-base disorders. Signs and symptoms include tachypnea (often Kussmaul's respirations), hypocapnia, evidence of dehydration, and a fruity odor to the breath. Treatment includes managing any disorder associated with the airway, breathing, or circulation. Fluid boluses are indicated as appropriate to correct the patient's hemodynamic status. Because these patients often are thiamine deficient (discussed in the following section), consider the administration of thiamine. If hypoglycemia exists administer IV dextrose, but only after the administration of thiamine. As previously mentioned, patients who abuse alcohol likely have hypomagnesemia. The addition of 1 to 2 g magnesium sulfate to the first liter of fluid administered is reasonable to correct this condition. As with DKA, sodium bicarbonate should not be administered in an attempt to correct metabolic acidosis. Finally, be sure to consider other causes of abdominal pain in the chronic alcohol abuser. Acute pancreatitis and gastrointestinal bleeding are common in these patients and can present along with AKA.

Inadequate Vitamin Intake

[OBJECTIVE 27]

Vitamins are a vital part of nutrition. They help the body function in many ways. Essential vitamins are divided into fat soluble (vitamins A, D, E, and K) and water soluble (vitamins B complex and C) (Table 24-10). Fat-soluble vitamins are stored in the body in the liver. They are not required on a daily basis. Water-soluble vitamins are not stored in the body and therefore must be replaced daily in the diet. The B-complex vitamins come from whole grains, meats, eggs, fish, poultry, milk products, and fresh vegetables.

The B-complex vitamins include thiamine (vitamin B_1), riboflavin (vitamin B_2), niacin, vitamin B_6, folate, vitamin B_{12}, biotin, and pantothenic acid. These vitamins help the body optimize the production of energy from food. Thiamine deficiency leads to beriberi disease.

TABLE 24-10 Vitamins and Their Sources	
Vitamin	**Source**
Fat Soluble	
Vitamin A (retinol)	Eggs, meat, milk, cheese, cream, liver, kidney, codfish oil, carrots, pumpkins, sweet potatoes, winter squashes, cantaloupe, pink grapefruit, apricots, broccoli, spinach, and most dark green, leafy vegetables
Vitamin D	Produced in the skin on exposure to ultraviolet rays; cod, halibut, salmon, and fortified milk products
Vitamin E (alpha tocopherol)	Nuts, whole grains, seed oils, spinach
Vitamin K	Wide variety of meats and vegetables
Water Soluble	
Vitamin B_1 (thiamine)	Whole grains
Vitamin B_2 (riboflavin)	Lean meats, legumes, nuts, leafy green vegetables, dairy products
Vitamin B_3 (niacin)	Lean meats, dairy products, poultry, fish, nuts, eggs
Vitamin B_6 (pyridoxine)	Poultry, fish, liver, eggs, broccoli, cabbage
Vitamin B_{12} (cyanocobalamin)	Only present in animal-derived products

Fat-Soluble Vitamins

Vitamin A

[OBJECTIVES 28, 29]

Vitamin A (also known as *retinol*) is an important fat-soluble vitamin that plays essential roles in vision, growth, and development; the development and maintenance of healthy skin, hair, and mucous membranes; immune functions; and reproduction. Its precursor is known as *beta-carotene*. Beta-carotene is an important antioxidant that helps the body fight toxins and prevents cell damage and possibly prevents cancer. Animal sources of vitamin A include eggs, meat, milk, cheese, cream, liver, kidney, and cod and halibut fish oil. Plant sources of beta-carotene include carrots, pumpkin, sweet potatoes, winter squashes, cantaloupe, pink grapefruit, apricots, broccoli, spinach, and most dark green, leafy vegetables. The plant sources are fat-free sources of vitamin A. Most milk products in the United States have been fortified with vitamin A.

Vitamin A deficiency is common in developing countries and is a leading cause of blindness (Institute of Medicine, 2001). However, in the United States diet restrictions and alcoholism contribute to vitamin A deficiency (U.S. Department of Health and Human Services, 2004). Zinc deficiency can also contribute to vitamin A deficiency because it is required to process vitamin A from the body's stores.

Symptoms of vitamin A deficiency can include poor growth and increased incidence of respiratory and gastrointestinal diseases in mild deficiency. In more moderate deficiency states, patients may present with night blindness and immune deficiency.

A deficiency can occur when intake of fat is inadequate or losses of fat are increased, as in pancreatic disease or cystic fibrosis. In addition, patients with chronic gastrointestinal disease do not absorb vitamin A appropriately, which can lead to deficiency. Vitamin A is stored in the liver, and patients with alcoholism may use up stores excessively. Treatment with vitamin A must be approached with care because, as a fat-soluble vitamin, it can be toxic in high levels. In patients with alcoholism and liver disease, this threshold of toxicity may be lower because of poor liver function.

Hypervitaminosis A refers to high storage levels of vitamin A in the body that can lead to toxic symptoms. It can lead to liver damage, poor bone mineralization, and resulting osteoporosis. Vitamin A can contribute to birth defects if it is taken in excessive amounts by pregnant mothers. Toxic symptoms include constipation, nausea and vomiting, headache, dizziness, blurred vision, and poor muscle tone. In addition, patients may develop hydrocephalus. Skin and hair become brittle, and the patient may experience hair loss.

Certain drugs contain derivatives of vitamin A, such as retinoic acid, which is used to treat acne and other skin conditions. Excessive use of these agents also may result in similar toxicity. Prehospital treatment of the patient with vitamin A toxicity includes supportive care along with discontinuation of the drug or vitamin supplement.

Vitamin D

[OBJECTIVES 28, 29]

Vitamin D is a fat-soluble vitamin. It is often called a hormone because it sends messages in the body that affect absorption of calcium and phosphorus. Vitamin D is taken in the diet and also is produced in the skin on exposure to ultraviolet rays from the sun. On conversion in the skin, vitamin D is then activated by enzyme pathways present in the liver and the kidney to form its active form, called calciferol, or 1,25-OH vitamin D (vitamin D_3). PTH increases the activity of the converting enzyme present in the liver, stimulating the activation of vitamin D and contributing to its ability to raise blood calcium levels.

Vitamin D is naturally present in fatty fish such as cod, halibut, and salmon and in fortified food and milk products. Vitamin D was added to milk products in the 1930s because of a growing epidemic of rickets (deficiency of vitamin D) in the United States (Institute of Medicine, 1999). The active form of vitamin D is produced in the kidney and stimulates calcium and phosphorus absorption from the gut.

Rickets can develop as a result of poor exposure to sunlight or poor ability to absorb ultraviolet rays, such as in dark-skinned individuals. In addition, breast-fed babies who do not receive vitamin D supplementation can be at risk for vitamin D deficiency, especially if the mother is also deficient and provided low stores to the baby during pregnancy. Poor absorption or the inability to convert vitamin D can result in rickets, as seen in those with gastrointestinal or hepatic or renal disorders.

Symptoms of hypovitaminosis D are consistent with those symptoms of hypocalcemia. Long-term sequelae can lead to poor bone density and osteoporosis, predisposing individuals to fractures, as seen in elderly patients. Osteoporosis is being seen at earlier ages, and the vitamin D intake in diet is becoming more and more emphasized as a contributor (Reid, 1996).

Acute treatment of rickets should focus on recognizing and treating cardiac dysrhythmias caused by hypocalcemia followed by supportive care. The long-term treatment of vitamin D deficiency includes vitamin D as well as calcium. Osteoporosis may require treatment with medications that prevent bone resorption and increase bone density.

Toxicity of vitamin D also can be a concern. Symptoms include nausea, vomiting, constipation, weakness, and weight loss. Symptoms are usually related to hypercalcemia resulting from the elevated effect of vitamin D. Excessive exposure to the sun and high consumption of vitamin D–containing foods are likely causes of vitamin D toxicity. Toxicity typically results from the excessive intake of supplements. Nausea, constipation, bone pain, and cardiac dysrhythmias may be present. Treatment of these patients is supportive and calls for monitoring for cardiac dysrhythmias resulting from hypercalcemia.

Vitamin E
[OBJECTIVES 28, 29]
Vitamin E (alpha tocopherol) is a fat-soluble vitamin found in nuts, whole grains, seed oils, and spinach. It functions as an antioxidant and stimulates the immune system. In addition, it influences platelet activity and prevents excessive clotting in the body. In some studies antioxidants have been shown to slow the effects of atherosclerosis. Moreover, the use of antioxidants, vitamin E in particular, has been recommended as an adjunctive treatment in those with cardiac risk factors. Other studies have shown that the routine use of vitamin E by people with low cardiac risk factors has little benefit (Ueda & Yasunari, 2006). Deficiency can be caused by poor absorption, as in fat-losing states from malabsorption, or dietary deficiency. Symptoms can include poor reflexes and muscle tone with an effect on the eye muscles, resulting in poor upward gaze. Neurologic symptoms include poor balance and coordination.

Treatment is based on etiology. If the patient has poor absorption, IM vitamin E replacement may be required. Assessing clotting factors in the blood is critical. Toxicity is rare, and treatment should be supportive if suspected until confirmed.

Vitamin K
[OBJECTIVES 28, 29]
Vitamin K is an important vitamin that assists clotting. Vitamin K controls the formation of blood clotting factors II (prothrombin), VII, IX, and X. Its deficiency causes an increased risk of bleeding. Babies are not able to manufacture prothrombin well in their liver, and vitamin K is not transferred in breast milk. This puts them at risk for vitamin K deficiency and clotting problems at birth, called *hemorrhagic disease of the newborn*. In the United States vitamin K is routinely given as an IM injection to infants at birth to prevent hemorrhagic disease of the newborn. If unprotected, babies may develop bleeding early or later in the newborn period, which may lead to intracranial hemorrhage if severe. Certain drugs such as phenytoin (Dilantin) or warfarin (Coumadin) may interfere with the ability to produce vitamin K, and infants born to mothers taking such medications are at risk for this disorder as well.

Vitamin K deficiency is rare in adults because it is present in a wide variety of vegetable and meat products. Deficiency usually develops in the face of poor absorption, as in a patient who has had intestinal surgery or disease or in those with liver disease. In addition, certain medications such as cephalosporin antibiotics, anticonvulsants, salicylates, and excessive vitamin A and E intake can affect vitamin K levels. Bleeding is the main manifestation of deficiency of vitamin K. Blood tests reveal a prolonged prothrombin time and normal platelets, fibrinogen, and bleeding time.

Treatment is preventative in newborns, as previously stated. Often a test dose of vitamin K is given and the prothrombin time before and after treatment is compared and evaluated to confirm diagnosis. Toxicity is rare, depending on the type of vitamin K. Effects may include jaundice in newborns, hemolytic anemia, and hyperbilirubinemia. Toxicity also blocks the effects of oral anticoagulants. A precursor to vitamin K (menadione) can be toxic and can cause hemolytic anemia, hyperbilirubine-mia, and kernicterus in infants. This is typically associated with formula-fed infants or those receiving synthetic vitamin K_3 (menadione) injections. Because of its toxicity, menadione is no longer used for treatment of vitamin K deficiency. However, vitamin K_1 (phylloquinone) is considered nontoxic even at levels as high as 500 times the recommended daily allowance.

Water-Soluble Vitamins
Vitamin B_1 (Thiamine)
[OBJECTIVES 28, 29]

Vitamin B_1 is a water-soluble vitamin that is important in carbohydrate metabolism. It is present in whole grains. Thiamine deficiency (beriberi) results from poor intake, impaired absorption, or increased requirement such as in patients with fever or hyperthyroidism or those who are pregnant or lactating. Patients with liver disease or alcoholism are known to be particularly at risk for B_1 deficiency. Symptoms of early deficiency include fatigue, memory and sleep disturbances, decreased appetite, nausea, and constipation.

Dry beriberi refers to the complex presentation of neurologic symptoms that include burning and tingling of the feet and lower extremities. Symptoms usually involve both sides of the body. Patients may have loss of the ankle jerk reflex and poor strength in their upper legs, causing difficulty rising from a seated position. With the progression of the disease, impairment of nerve function may spread to the lower extremities, resulting in foot drop. The upper extremities are typically affected later.

Wet beriberi results from the effect of thiamine deficiency on the cardiovascular system. Cardiac output increases, with vasodilation and warm extremities. Symptoms of tachycardia, wide pulse pressure, sweating, warm skin, and lactic acidosis develop. Eventually heart failure occurs and patients develop shock.

Wernicke-Korsakoff syndrome is a neurologic disorder most often associated with patients who are chronic alcoholics. Chronic alcoholism often interferes with the intake, absorption, and utilization of thiamine. Although Wernicke's encephalopathy and Korsakoff's psychosis are separate disorders, they usually occur together in the chronic alcoholic. Symptoms for Wernicke syndrome include ataxia, nystagmus, eye muscle weakness, and mental derangement caused by an acute but reversible encephalopathy. Korsakoff psychosis is of greater concern because once it is established it is usually irreversible. This syndrome is characterized by amnesia, disorientation, delirium, and hallucinations. Chronic alcoholics with hypoglycemia are at some risk for developing Wernicke-Korsakoff syndrome if administered IV D50 without also being administered thiamine. Follow local protocols for consideration of administering 100 mg of thiamine IV or IM in these situations. Thiamine toxicity is rare. The symptoms are usually nonspecific but may

include tachycardia, headache, weakness, vasodilation, hypotension, cardiac dysrhythmias, and convulsions. Wernicke's encephalopathy, Korsakoff's psychosis, and Wernicke-Korsakoff syndrome are discussed in greater depth in Chapter 23.

Vitamin B_2 (Riboflavin)
[OBJECTIVES 28, 29]

Vitamin B_2 is a water-soluble vitamin important for body growth and red blood cell production. It is found in lean meat, eggs, legumes, nuts, green leafy vegetables, and dairy products. Vitamin B_2 deficiency is rare in the United States because breads and cereals are often fortified with riboflavin. Riboflavin is broken down by direct sunlight, so products rich in vitamin B_2 should not be stored in glass containers in direct sunlight. Symptoms of deficiency include sore throat, swollen mucosal membranes, sores in the mouth and lips, skin disorders, and anemia. Prehospital treatment of these patients includes supportive care until replacement therapy can be initiated.

Vitamin B_3 (Niacin)
[OBJECTIVES 28, 29]

Vitamin B_3 is a water-soluble vitamin important in many aspects of health, growth, and reproduction. It may be obtained by consuming lean meats, dairy products, poultry, fish, nuts, and eggs. When not enough niacin is consumed, a disease called pellagra may occur. Pellagra is characterized by an increased sensitivity to light, aggression, dermatitis, insomnia, weakness, confusion, diarrhea, and dementia in later stages. Patients who overdose on niacin may expect peptic ulcers, skin rashes, or liver damage. Prehospital treatment of patients having either too much or too little vitamin B_3 should be supportive in nature.

Vitamin B_6 (Pyridoxine)
[OBJECTIVES 28, 29]

Vitamin B_6 is a water-soluble vitamin important in neurologic function. It helps in protein metabolism in the body and is present in poultry, fish, liver, and eggs as well as in beans, broccoli, and cabbage. A deficiency is rare because vitamin B_6 is added to many food products, even vegetarian foods. Typically poor absorption or the effects of medications are the main causes for B_6 deficiency. Common medications known for this effect include isoniazid (used to treat tuberculosis), hydralazine, and penicillamine (used to treat lead toxicity). B_6 is converted to its active form by the intestine. Therefore gastrointestinal disorders also can contribute to low levels in the serum. Symptoms of deficiency are nonspecific and can include muscle weakness and fissures at the corners of the mouth. In infants failure to thrive, irritability, and seizures may develop. The treatment of this deficiency involves food or dietary supplements. Toxicity is rare, and treatment is supportive.

Vitamin B₁₂ (Cyanocobalamin)

[OBJECTIVES 28, 29]

Vitamin B_{12} is a water-soluble vitamin important in nerve cell and red blood cell production. It is only available in animal-derived products. Causes of deficiency include a vegetarian diet that excludes all meats, eggs, and dairy products. In addition, patients with inflammatory bowel disease, chronic alcoholism, or pernicious anemia can develop B_{12} deficiency. Vitamin B_{12} is absorbed from the intestine with the help of a substance known as intrinsic factor. B_{12} deficiency resulting from a lack of intrinsic factor is called pernicious anemia. Low B_{12} levels lead to an abnormal production of red blood cells that are large (macrocytic) and easily broken down (hemolytic). Symptoms of B_{12} deficiency include anorexia, diarrhea, shortness of breath, fatigue, and weakness. Neurologic symptoms also are present, including tingling of the hands and feet. Treatment involves replacement either orally when appropriate or IM if malabsorption or pernicious anemia is the cause. Neurologic sequelae from chronic deficiency may be irreversible. Take special care with the administration of the IM injection because the pigment of the preparation can cause tattooing of the skin if given superficially to the muscle tissue. Interestingly, vitamin B_{12} is also used as a treatment option for cyanide poisoning. B_{12} toxicity is rare, and treatment is supportive.

Inadequate Mineral Intake

[OBJECTIVES 28, 29]

Iron is a mineral essential for body function. Its deficiency is the most common nutritional deficiency. Iron is present in red meats, egg yolks, liver, raisins, spinach, and broccoli. Its deficiency is caused by either poor dietary intake or excessive loss from bleeding. Iron deficiency results in anemia. Hemoglobin contains iron; therefore the oxygen-carrying ability of the red blood cells depends on the iron level of the body. In addition, iron is a component of myoglobin, an energy provider for muscles. Symptoms of iron deficiency include dizziness, irritability, decreased appetite, muscle weakness, tiredness, and pallor. In children, iron deficiency can be caused by lead poisoning. The treatment of the underlying cause is essential. Adults in particular should be evaluated for sources of gastrointestinal blood loss. Replacement therapy can be either oral or IM. Vitamin C is necessary for absorption, and oral supplementation is best absorbed when taken with a food source high in vitamin C, such as fruit or juice.

Symptoms of iron toxicity include vomiting and diarrhea. Toxicity can result from excessive intake, repeated blood transfusions, or chronic alcoholism. Hemochromatosis is an inherited disorder in which patients absorb excessive iron. Treatment of iron toxicity is directed at binding the iron.

Potassium, magnesium, and calcium are additional minerals that are integral to the function of the human body. An in-depth look at these minerals can be found in Chapters 7 and 8.

Case Scenario SUMMARY

1. *What is your impression of this patient?* This patient has vital signs that are very concerning. She is tachycardic, tachypneic, and diaphoretic. The key is to try to figure out what is causing these vital signs and treat accordingly. Obtain a detailed history, including information about the patient's medical history, surgical history, allergies, medications, and all events leading up to this point.

2. *What are some key factors that should be investigated during the physical examination?* The patient should have a thorough head-to-toe physical examination. Attention to the head for signs of trauma could possibly explain the confusion. Signs of infection such as neck stiffness (meningitis), crackles (pneumonia or heart failure), pharyngitis, or abdominal pain should be investigated. The interesting part of this case is that this patient's symptoms could have many possible causes.

3. *What are the most appropriate initial interventions?* Place the patient on a cardiac monitor and establish IV access. Immediately perform a blood glucose measure-

ment. The patient also should be placed on supplemental oxygen. Nitroglycerin and aspirin should be considered because of the report of chest pressure. Pharmacologic interventions to reduce fever should be considered if protocol allows.

4. *What is the significance of the confusion?* Any confusion is important. This patient is having episodes of periodic confusion. This could be from fever, infection, or a possible stroke and should prompt careful investigation and rapid transport. Details regarding the patient's confusion also are helpful. If the patient is having one-sided weakness, speech abnormalities, or visual changes, this may indicate stroke. Generalized confusion can indicate delirium from infection, fever, or an endocrine emergency.

5. *What are possible diagnoses for this patient?* This patient may have any of the following:
   - *Infection:* Fever, meningitis, pneumonia, urinary tract infection, sepsis

Continued

Case Scenario SUMMARY—continued

- *Stroke:* The patient may be having paroxysmal atrial fibrillation with symptoms of transient ishemic attack or even stroke
- *Cardiac:* Atrial fibrillation, atrial flutter, acute myocardial infarction, cardiomyopathy, congestive heart failure
- *Endocrine:* New-onset diabetes, dehydration, electrolyte abnormalities, thyroid disorder

6. *What are the most important treatment considerations for this patient?* This patient should receive IV fluids. Dehydration may cause the heart rate increase, and certainly with the possibility of fever fluids would be helpful. Careful reassessment of heart tones would be helpful. The patient has exophthalmos, which can be seen in hyperthyroidism. Considering the patient's other symptoms, the patient most likely has thyroid storm. Contact medical direction for further orders. Propranolol is often a first-line agent for this condition. Prehospital care of the patient with thyroid storm is symptomatic and includes airway support, shock management, dysrhythmia management, and possibly the administration of beta-blockers, calcium channel blockers, and steroids.

7. *What additional interventions should be done?* Make the patient as comfortable as possible. Contact medical direction. This patient could at any point go into an unstable cardiac rhythm or go into respiratory arrest. The patient must be continually monitored and rapid transport arranged.

8. *What comfort measures can be done for this patient?* This patient should be placed in a position of comfort for transport. The patient should receive fluids and supplemental oxygen. If the patient is having continued pain, it should be addressed. Morphine sulfate may be used based on blood pressure and the patient's condition.

9. *What documentation should be done for this patient both in the written and oral report?* The oral report should be done promptly. The receiving facility should be notified that this patient will be transported and an estimated time of arrival should be provided. The receiving facility should be given a detailed history, physical examination findings, electrocardiographic findings, and interventions. Be sure to relay the finding of the proptotic eyes. The written report also should contain the above information. Any changes in the patient's condition should be documented with an accurate time. Repeat vital signs should also be documented.

Chapter Summary

- The endocrine system, along with the neurologic system, is responsible for helping the body maintain homeostasis. Although the neurologic system is able to respond more rapidly to changes and the endocrine system takes longer to respond, those changes may remain in effect longer. The endocrine system communicates with tissues throughout the body through the release of hormones by eight main endocrine glands: the hypothalamus, pituitary, thyroid, parathyroid, thymus, pancreas, adrenal, and gonads. Hormones interact with target tissues in all parts of the body to effect changes to balance body systems and maintain homeostasis.
- The most prominent endocrine disorders you will encounter will be related to diabetes mellitus. In the patient with type 1 diabetes, the beta cells, found in the islets of Langerhans located in the pancreas, have ceased producing insulin. Insulin is responsible for aiding the movement of glucose across the cell wall and into the cell for metabolizing. It also prompts the liver to convert circulating glucose into glycogen for later use. In type 2 diabetes, either insulin production has diminished to the point where it can no longer meet metabolic demands, or cellular receptor sites have decreased sensitivity and no longer respond effectively to current insulin levels. Glucagon is released by the alpha cells in the pancreas. Glucagon acts on the liver to convert glycogen back to glucose, a process called glycogenolysis.
- Although rare, some endocrine disorders besides diabetes may prove rapidly fatal to the patient. Thyrotoxicosis, or thyroid storm, is caused by overactivity of the thyroid gland. Signs and symptoms of a thyroid storm include tachypnea, tachycardia, shock, hyperthermia, and delirium. Treatment includes dysrhythmia management, shock management, airway support, beta-blockers, and steroids. The other rare but lethal endocrine disorder you may encounter is myxedema. Myxedema is an underactivity of the thyroid gland. Signs and symptoms include unexplained hypothermia, unexplained hypoglycemia, hypotension, respiratory depression, and coma. Prehospital treatment includes supportive care, airway management, temperature regulation, and treatment for shock.

- Other than diabetes, most metabolic and nutritional disorders are not life threatening. They build over a period and are diagnosed by the patient's family physician. You usually become aware of these conditions during the history component of the patient assessment. Be aware of the pathophysiology of these disorders, how they interact with other disease processes, and what modifications you may need to make to current protocols to accommodate these interactions.

REFERENCES

Arlt, W., & Allolio, B. (2003). Adrenal insufficiency. *Lancet, 361*(9372), 1881-1893.

The Diabetes Control and Complications Trial Research Group. (1997). Hypoglycemia in the Diabetes Control and Complications Trial. *Diabetes, 46,* 271-286.

Gerich, J. E., Langlois, M., Noacco, C., Karam, J., & Forsham, P. H. (1973). Lack of a glucagon response to hypoglycemia in diabetes: Evidence for an intrinsic pancreatic alpha-cell defect. *Science, 182,* 171-173.

Guy, A. D., Sandoval, D., Richardson, M. A., Tate, D., & Davis, S. N. (2004). Effects of glycemic control on target organ responses to epinephrine in type 1 diabetes. *American Journal of Physiology, Endocrinology, and Metabolism, 289*(2):E258-E265.

Guy, D. A., Sandoval, D., Richardson, M. A., Tate, D., Flakoll, P. J., & Davis, S. N. (2005). Differing physiological effects of epinephrine in type 1 diabetes and nondiabetic humans. *American Journal of Physiology, Endocrinology, and Metabolism, 288*(1), E178-E186.

Institute of Medicine. (1999). *Dietary reference intakes: Calcium, phosphorus, magnesium, vitamin D and fluoride,* Washington, DC: National Academy Press.

Institute of Medicine. (2001). *Dietary reference intakes for vitamin A, vitamin K, arsenic, boron, chromium, copper, iodine, iron, manganese, molybdenum, nickel, silicon, vanadium, and zinc,* Washington, DC: National Academy Press.

Kitabchi, A. E., Umpierrez, G. E., Murphy, M. B., Barrett, E. J., Kreisberg, R. A., Malone, J. I., & Wall, B. M. (2004). Hyperglycemic crises in diabetes. *Diabetes Care, 27*(suppl 1), S94-102.

Martin, F. H. (2002). *Fundamentals of anatomy and physiology (6th ed.),* Upper Saddle River, NJ: Prentice Hall.

National Diabetes Information Clearinghouse. (2005). *National diabetes statistics.* Retrieved September 9, 2006, from http://diabetes.niddk.nih.gov.

Reid, I. R. (1996). Therapy of osteoporosis: Calcium, vitamin D, and exercise. *American Journal of Medical Science, 312,* 278-286.

Ueda, S., & Yasunari K. (2006). What we learnt from randomized clinical trials and cohort studies of antioxidant vitamin? Focus on vitamin E and cardiovascular disease. *Current Pharmaceutical Biotechnology, 7*(2), 69-72.

Umpierrez, G. E., & Kitabchi, A. E. (2003). Diabetic ketoacidosis: Risk factors and management strategies. *Treatments in Endocrinology, 2*(2), 95-108.

U.S. Department of Health and Human Services. (2004). *Advance Data from Vital and Health Statistics. Dietary intake of selected vitamins for the United States Population: 1999-2000, number 339,* Washington, DC: National Center for Health Statistics.

SUGGESTED RESOURCES

Kronenberg, H. M., Melmed, S., Polonsky, K. S., & Larson, P. R. (2008). *Williams textbook of endocrinology* (10th ed.). Philadelphia: Elsevier Saunders.

Sperling, M. A. (2002). *Pediatric endocrinology* (2nd ed.). Philadelphia: Saunders.

Food and Nutrition Board. (1989). *Recommended dietary allowances* (10th ed.). Washington, DC: National Academy Press.

U.S. Department of Agriculture. (2000). Nutrition and your health: Dietary guidelines for Americans (5th ed.). *Home and garden bulletin no. 232,* Washington, DC: U.S. Government Printing Office.

Chapter Quiz

1. Which gland functions primarily to regulate other glands to maintain homeostasis?

_____
_____
_____
_____

2. Which gland releases TSH, and what is that hormone's primary function?

_____
_____
_____
_____

3. What are the three main types of cells located in the islets of Langerhans that assist the body in regulating blood glucose levels, and what hormones do they release?

_____
_____
_____

4. What disorder is caused by a lack of ADH from the posterior pituitary gland, and what are its signs and symptoms?

_____
_____
_____
_____

Chapter Quiz—continued

5. What term is used to describe thyrotoxicosis in its most extreme form, and what are its signs and symptoms?

_____

_____

_____

_____

6. When a patient has myxedema, what gland is malfunctioning? Is the malfunction from overactivity or underactivity of the gland, and what signs and symptoms might you expect?

_____

_____

_____

_____

7. Describe the pathophysiology behind why a patient with DKA has ketonemia, whereas a patient with HHNC does not.

_____

_____

_____

_____

8. Describe the signs, symptoms, and treatment for a patient having a hypoglycemic episode.

_____

_____

_____

_____

9. What nutritional disorder is caused by the body receiving inadequate protein caloric uptake, and in what population is this disorder most commonly seen?

_____

_____

_____

_____

10. What disorder is caused by an insufficiency of vitamin B_1 and may be encountered in the chronic alcoholic? In what scenario might you inadvertently cause this condition?

_____

_____

_____

_____

Terminology

Adrenocortical steroids Hormones released by the adrenal cortex essential for life; assist in the regulation of blood glucose levels, promote peripheral use of lipids, stimulate the kidneys to reabsorb sodium, and have antiinflammatory effects.

Alcoholic ketoacidosis (AKA) Condition found in patients who chronically abuse alcohol accompanied by vomiting, a build-up of ketones in the blood, and little or no food intake.

Beriberi Disease caused by a deficiency of thiamine and characterized by neurologic symptoms, cardiovascular abnormalities, and edema.

Corticosteroids See *Adrenocortical steroids.*

Cushing syndrome Disorder caused by the overproduction of corticosteroids; characterized by a "moon face," obesity, fat accumulation on the upper back, increased facial hair, acne, diabetes, and hypertension.

Diabetes insipidus (DI) Disorder caused by insufficient production of ADH in the posterior pituitary gland, causing a larger than normal increase in the secretion of free water in the urine and poor absorption of water into the bloodstream.

Diabetic ketoacidosis (DKA) Condition found in diabetic patients caused by the lack or absence of insulin, leading to an increase of ketone bodies and acidosis in the blood.

Direct communication Method of intercellular communication in which one cell communicates with the cell adjacent to it by using minerals and ions.

Endocrine communication Method of intercellular communication in which one cell communicates with target cells throughout the body by using hormones.

Gluconeogenesis Creation of new glucose in the body by using noncarbohydrate sources such as fats and proteins.

Glycogenolysis Creation of glucose in the body through the breakdown of glycogen.

Homeostasis A state of equilibrium in the body regarding functions and composition of fluids and tissues.

Hormones Chemicals within the body that reach every cell through the circulatory system.

Hyperosmolar hyperglycemic nonketotic coma (HHNC) Condition caused by a relative insulin insufficiency that leads to extremely high blood sugar levels while still allowing for normal glucose metabolism and an absence of ketone bodies.

Islets of Langerhans Groups of cells located in the pancreas that produce insulin, glucagon, somatostatin, and pancreatic polypeptide.

Ketonemia The presence of ketones in the blood.

Kwashiorkor A form of malnutrition caused by inadequate protein intake compared with the total needed or required calorie intake.

Marasmus A form of nutritional deficiency from an overall lack of calories that results in wasting.

Myxedema Severe form of hypothyroidism characterized by hypothermia and unresponsiveness.

Paracrine communication Method of intercellular communication in which cells communicate with cells in close proximity through the release of paracrine factors, or cytokines.

Synaptic communication Method of intercellular communication in which neural cells communicate to adjacent neural cells by using neurotransmitters.

Thyroid storm Severe form of hyperthyroidism characterized by tachypnea, tachycardia, shock, hyperthermia, and delirium.

Thyrotoxicosis Excessive blood levels of thyroid hormone.

Wernicke-Korsakoff syndrome Neurologic disorder caused by a thiamine deficiency; most often seen in chronic alcoholics; characterized by ataxia, nystagmus, weakness, and mental derangement in the early stages. In later stages, the condition is much more likely to become permanent and is characterized by amnesia, disorientation, delirium, and hallucinations.

Immune System Disorders

Objectives *After completing this chapter, you will be able to:*

1. Review the specific anatomy and physiology of the immune system and pathophysiology pertinent to immune system disorders.
2. Describe characteristics of the immune system, including the categories of white blood cells, the reticuloendothelial system, and the complement system.
3. Describe the processes of the immune system defenses, including humoral and cell-mediated immunity.
4. Define *natural* and *acquired immunity*.
5. Define *antigens* and *antibodies*.
6. Discuss the formation of antibodies in the body.
7. Define specific terminology identified with immune system disorders.
8. Discuss the following relative to the human immunodeficiency virus: causative agent, body systems affected and potential secondary complications, modes of transmission, the seroconversion rate after direct significant exposure, susceptibility and resistance, signs and symptoms, specific patient management and personal protective measures, treatments, and research exploring possible immunization.
9. Discuss the following autoimmune disorders: systemic lupus erythematosus, insulin-dependent diabetes mellitus, rheumatoid arthritis, celiac disease, chronic active hepatitis, and multiple sclerosis.
10. Define *allergic reaction*.
11. Define *anaphylaxis*.

12. Describe the incidence, morbidity, and mortality rates of anaphylaxis.
13. Identify the risk factors most predisposing to anaphylaxis.
14. Discuss the anatomy and physiology of the organs and structures related to anaphylaxis.
15. Describe the prevention of anaphylaxis and appropriate patient education.
16. Discuss the pathophysiology of allergy and anaphylaxis.
17. Describe the common methods of entry of substances into the body.
18. List common antigens most frequently associated with anaphylaxis.
19. Describe physical manifestations and pathophysiologic principles of anaphylaxis.
20. Differentiate manifestations of an allergic reaction from anaphylaxis.
21. Recognize the signs and symptoms related to anaphylaxis.
22. Differentiate the various treatment and pharmacologic interventions used in the management of anaphylaxis.
23. Describe the clinical significance of abnormal findings in the patient with anaphylaxis.
24. Develop a treatment plan for the patient with allergic reaction and anaphylaxis.
25. Discuss the principles of and disorders related to transplantation surgery.
26. Discuss public health principles relevant to immune system disorders.

Chapter Outline

Immune System Physiology (Defense against Infection)
Immune System Pathophysiology and Treatment

Field Management of Immune System Disorders
Public Health and Immunity
Chapter Summary

Case Scenario

You and your partner are called to the airport to meet an arriving commercial flight. When you arrive at the gate (before arrival of the flight) you learn that a 39-year-old male passenger had become acutely short of breath during a 4-hour flight. After arrival of the flight, the patient is removed from the plane by airline personnel. He is sitting upright and is alert and oriented with two- to three-word dyspnea. He is pale on 6 L of oxygen by nasal cannula and has a rapid, strong radial pulse. He is tachypneic and appears to be extremely short of breath. He informs you that he is HIV positive and was diagnosed with hepatitis B 10 years ago.

Questions

1. What is your general impression of this patient?
2. What are some possible causes of this patient's respiratory distress, pallor, and tachypnea?
3. Are these symptoms related to the patient's history of HIV and hepatitis? How should you protect yourself?
4. What intervention should you initiate at this time?

The immune system forms the body's defense against infection and infestation. Every day the body is exposed to millions of agents that could injure or infect it. The immune system constantly works to prevent or limit such problems. This chapter explores the types of infectious organisms that can cause illness, the mechanisms the immune system uses to stop them, and the ways in which EMS professionals can assist the body in its effort to protect itself.

In some cases the immune system itself can attack the body or react to other agents in ways that cause more harm than good. This chapter explores ways in which this occurs, the diseases or injuries that can result, and how EMS professionals can intervene to prevent further damage.

IMMUNE SYSTEM PHYSIOLOGY (DEFENSE AGAINST INFECTION)

[OBJECTIVE 1]

Pathogenic Agents

The environment is filled with organisms that threaten to infect or invade the human body. Most of these organisms fall into one of five groups: prions, viruses, bacteria, parasites, or fungi.

Prions are infectious agents composed of only proteins. Known prion diseases affect the structure of the brain or other nervous tissue in animals and human beings. Prion diseases also are known as *transmissible spongiform encephalopathies*. These diseases include bovine spongiform encephalopathy ("mad cow" disease) in cattle, Creutzfeldt-Jakob disease in human beings, scrapie in sheep, and chronic wasting disease in deer and elk. At this time, much about these diseases remains unknown. Because of their protein-only composition, they are impossible to cure. The only way to do so is to denature the protein through heat, chemical, or other methods that also would kill the organism.

Viruses differ from the other organisms because they are not composed of cells, the basic building block of most living things. Instead they consist of genetic material (RNA or DNA) that must use the machinery of other organisms to reproduce. Viruses cannot migrate on their own and need some outside mechanism to move from one host to another. Medications that limit viruses are called **antivirals.**

Bacteria (singular, *bacterium*) do not have a true nucleus. Instead, they contain a less-sophisticated nucleoid. Cells with a nucleoid are prokaryotes, and cells with a nucleus are eukaryotes. Eukaryotes and prokaryotes also differ in the cell membranes and the contents of the cells; prokaryotes do not have the more-sophisticated organelles contained in eukaryotes. Some bacteria have flagella (e.g., a whiplike tail) that make them motile (able to move on their own), but most are nonmotile. Medications that kill or limit bacteria are called **antibacterials.** The term **antibiotic** technically refers to a medication that kills any living thing, but usually it refers to bacteria.

PARAMEDIC *Pearl*

Antibiotics only kill bacteria and generally are not effective in stopping other organisms. This fact is frequently misunderstood; many patients request an antibiotic thinking it will kill or stop an infection by a virus.

Bacteria are often classified by their shape: cocci (spheres), bacilli (rods), and spirochetes (coils). Further terminology marks their arrangement, such as diplococci (balls in pairs), streptococci (balls in chains), and staphylococci (balls in clusters). Another categorizing system uses their response to a laboratory test called a *Gram stain*. Gram-negative bacteria turn red with this test and gram-positive bacteria turn blue. This is a quick and useful way to help identify bacteria and determine which antibiotic to choose in treating it. For instance, gram-positive bacteria are killed much more easily by the antibiotic penicillin G than are gram-negative bacteria.

Parasites are organisms that live in or on another organism (the host) and use it to survive without contributing to the host's survival. In infectious disease terms, parasites refer to worms and protozoa. Worms are multicellular organisms categorized in the animal kingdom. They include parasites such as tapeworms and hookworms. Protozoa are much smaller organisms and are categorized in the kingdom Protista. They include parasites such as *Trichomonas vaginalis,* which causes the sexually transmitted disease trichomoniasis.

Fungi (singular, *fungus*) also are protists and are plant-like organisms; unlike plants, however, they do not contain chlorophyll. Fungi are categorized as **yeasts** or **molds.** Yeasts are single cells that reproduce by budding, whereas molds are multicellular organisms that grow long filaments known as hyphae. Medications that kill fungi or control a fungal infection are known as **antifungals.**

External Defenses

The body has a number of defense mechanisms to prevent infection by prions, viruses, bacteria, parasites, or fungi (Figure 25-1).

Externally, the skin serves as a mechanical barrier between internal tissue and infective agents.

Because the gastrointestinal (GI) tract, upper respiratory tract, and genitourinary (GU) tract communicate with the outside world, they are considered external barriers. Each of these body systems prevents pathogenic agents from reaching internal tissues by serving as a mechanical barrier. They also have unique features that further prevent infection.

The GI and GU tracts normally have extensive bacteria living in them, known as *normal flora* or *resident flora,* that help the GI system perform its functions (Figure 25-2). They also prevent colonization by pathogenic bacteria. One important complication of antibiotics is secondary infection of the GI or GU system by bacteria that are not killed by the antibiotic but can proliferate, because the normal florae were killed by the antibiotic. Normal flora also can become pathogenic if they grow in areas where they should not be found. For example, *Escherichia coli* is a common normal flora in the GI tract but also a common cause of urinary tract infection if it is allowed to enter the GU tract.

In addition, the GI tract also contains acids in the stomach that kill potential pathogens. Pathogens can be removed from the body in feces passed out of the GI tract. The GU tract also removes potential pathogens from the body by urine. Elements in the urine itself, as well as prostatic fluid in men, can help slow or stop the growth of bacteria.

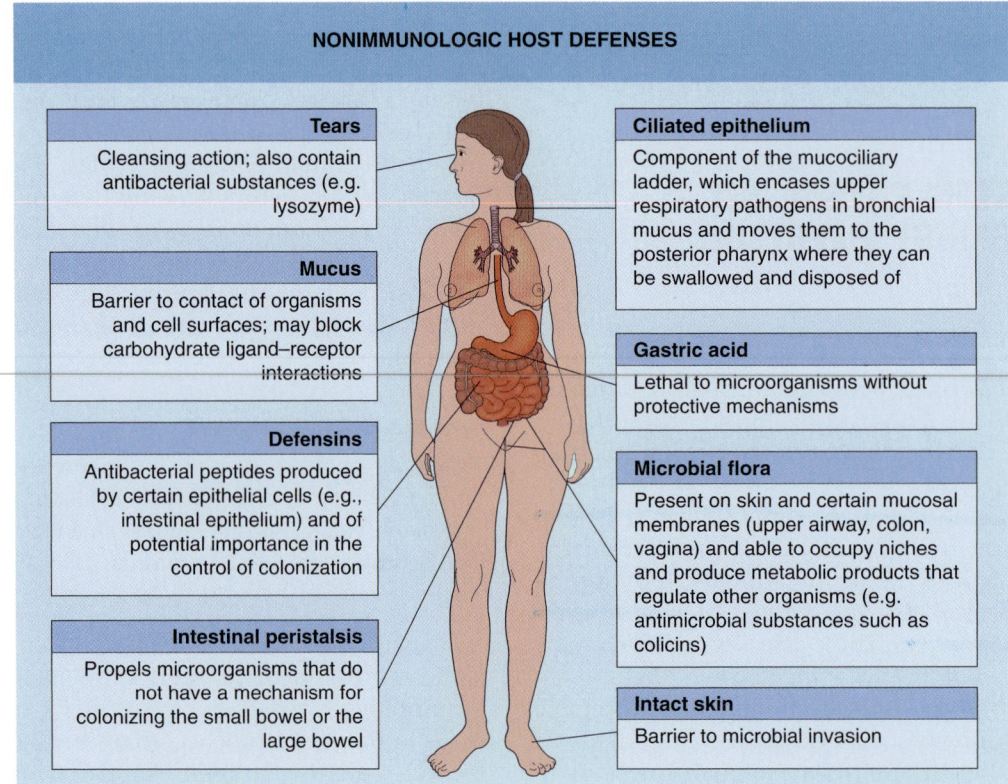

NONIMMUNOLOGIC HOST DEFENSES

Tears
Cleansing action; also contain antibacterial substances (e.g. lysozyme)

Mucus
Barrier to contact of organisms and cell surfaces; may block carbohydrate ligand–receptor interactions

Defensins
Antibacterial peptides produced by certain epithelial cells (e.g., intestinal epithelium) and of potential importance in the control of colonization

Intestinal peristalsis
Propels microorganisms that do not have a mechanism for colonizing the small bowel or the large bowel

Ciliated epithelium
Component of the mucociliary ladder, which encases upper respiratory pathogens in bronchial mucus and moves them to the posterior pharynx where they can be swallowed and disposed of

Gastric acid
Lethal to microorganisms without protective mechanisms

Microbial flora
Present on skin and certain mucosal membranes (upper airway, colon, vagina) and able to occupy niches and produce metabolic products that regulate other organisms (e.g. antimicrobial substances such as colicins)

Intact skin
Barrier to microbial invasion

Figure 25-1 The body has a number of defense mechanisms to prevent infection.

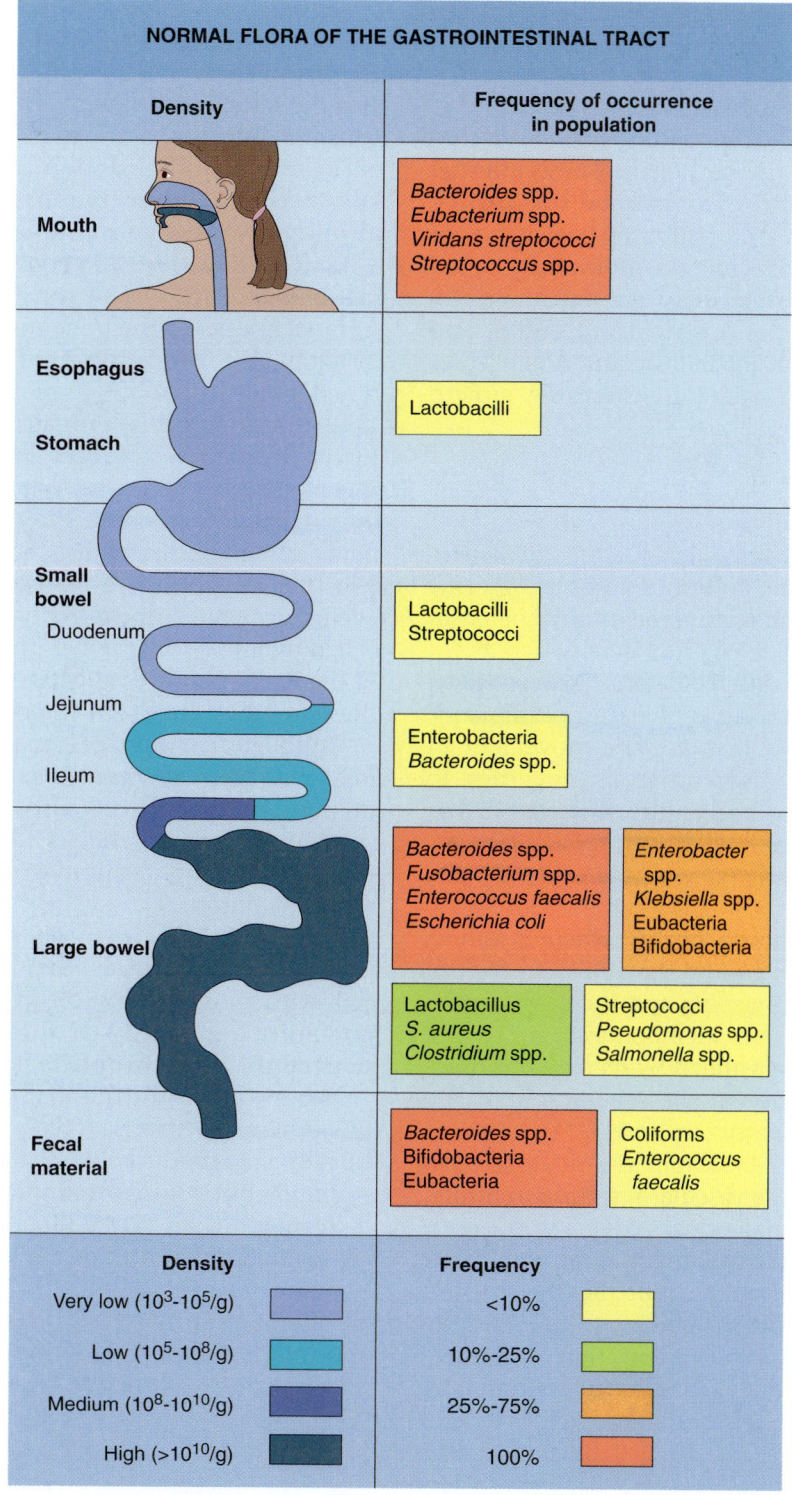

NORMAL FLORA OF THE GASTROINTESTINAL TRACT

Density	Frequency of occurrence in population

Mouth

Bacteroides spp.
Eubacterium spp.
Viridans streptococci
Streptococcus spp.

Esophagus

Stomach

Lactobacilli

Small bowel
Duodenum

Lactobacilli
Streptococci

Jejunum

Ileum

Enterobacteria
Bacteroides spp.

Large bowel

Bacteroides spp.
Fusobacterium spp.
Enterococcus faecalis
Escherichia coli

Enterobacter spp.
Klebsiella spp.
Eubacteria
Bifidobacteria

Lactobacillus
S. aureus
Clostridium spp.

Streptococci
Pseudomonas spp.
Salmonella spp.

Fecal material

Bacteroides spp.
Bifidobacteria
Eubacteria

Coliforms
Enterococcus faecalis

Density		Frequency	
Very low (10^3-10^5/g)		<10%	
Low (10^5-10^8/g)		10%-25%	
Medium (10^8-10^{10}/g)		25%-75%	
High (>10^{10}/g)		100%	

Figure 25-2 The gastrointestinal (GI) and genitourinary (GU) tracts normally have extensive bacteria (normal flora) living in them that help these body systems perform their functions and prevent infection.

The upper respiratory tract helps remove pathogens through coughing and sneezing. Nasal hairs and cilia in the tract collect pathogens and prevent them from further movement into the body. The tonsils are part of the lymphatic system, which fights infection and helps kill potential pathogens found in the oropharynx.

Internal Defenses

[OBJECTIVES 2, 3]

If organisms penetrate the body's external defense system and are able to enter internal tissues, further mechanisms act to slow or kill the pathogen. These internal immune defenses are categorized as **natural immunity** or **acquired immunity.** The effects of both types of immunity are regulated by protein hormones called **cytokines.** Cytokines that mediate natural immunity include tumor necrosis factor, interleukin 1 and 6, and chemokines. Cytokines that mediate acquired immunity include interleukin 2 and 4 and transforming growth factor.

Natural Immunity

[OBJECTIVE 4]

Natural immunity is sometimes called *nonspecific immunity* because its mechanisms do not identify the specific invading organism. It provides universal internal defenses against pathogens that evade external defenses.

Inflammatory Response and Mediators. Inflammation is one of the most familiar forms of natural immunity. The inflammatory response involves the movement of agents to an area, or changes in an area's properties, to help fight infection and/or heal injury. Triggers for the inflammatory response can be infection, such as a bacterial invasion, or injury, such as a chemical burn or a sprained joint.

The inflammatory response begins when a cell is injured. Injured cells begin to lose the ability to control their metabolism, causing swelling and increasing cellular acidity. Eventually the cell's membranes begin to leak and the cell begins to be consumed by its own enzymes. This swelling and destruction at the cellular level is the beginning of the inflammatory response.

Next arterioles, venules, and capillaries dilate to rush blood to the area. This is the vascular response to injury. This change in permeability produces edema in the area, which is the beginning of the swelling that can eventually be grossly visible in an infected or injured body part.

The initial cell injury and changes in vascular permeability trigger various agents and systems that fight infection and clear destroyed tissue. The reticuloendothelial system consists of cells in many different body systems that reabsorb fluids and clear debris by a process known as **pinocytosis.** Pinocytosis, or reabsorption, differentiates the reticuloendothelial system from cells that act to consume invading pathogens (Abbas, 1994). The process of ingestion and digestion of invading pathogens is known as **phagocytosis** and is performed by cells known as **phagocytes** (Figure 25-3).

Phagocytosis is performed by the mononuclear phagocyte system. This system consists of mobile cells formed from stem cells in the bone marrow. In the marrow they develop into **monoblasts** and are released into the blood. Once in the blood, monoblasts are called **monocytes.** Monocytes eventually settle into tissues and mature into **macrophages.** Macrophages absorb foreign materials, kill foreign microbes (by enzymes and other materials), and slow the spread of infection. They have many other specific names. Some are simply synonyms (e.g., histiocyte); others refer to the tissue in which they eventually reside: in the central nervous system they are called microglia, in the liver they are called Kupffer cells, in the lungs they are called alveolar macrophages, and in the bone they are called osteoclasts.

Although macrophages are general defensive cells that fight any agent recognized as foreign or debris (natural immunity), their effects also can be amplified when a specific foreign material is identified (acquired immunity). This amplification is described further under Acquired Immunity.

Other cells also perform phagocytosis in a similar fashion as macrophages. **Granulocytes** are white blood cells with an important role in inflammation and natural immunity and consist of three different types of cells: **neutrophils, eosinophils,** and **basophils.**

Neutrophils form the major cell population in acute inflammatory response. Like macrophages, they nonspecifically consume foreign agents and debris but can be amplified by acquired immunity processes.

Eosinophils are white blood cells that respond generally to inflammation but are thought to be most active against certain classes of pathogens. They are particularly effective at destroying parasites, and a high level of eosinophils in a patient's blood sometimes indicates infection with a parasite, particularly helminths (worms).

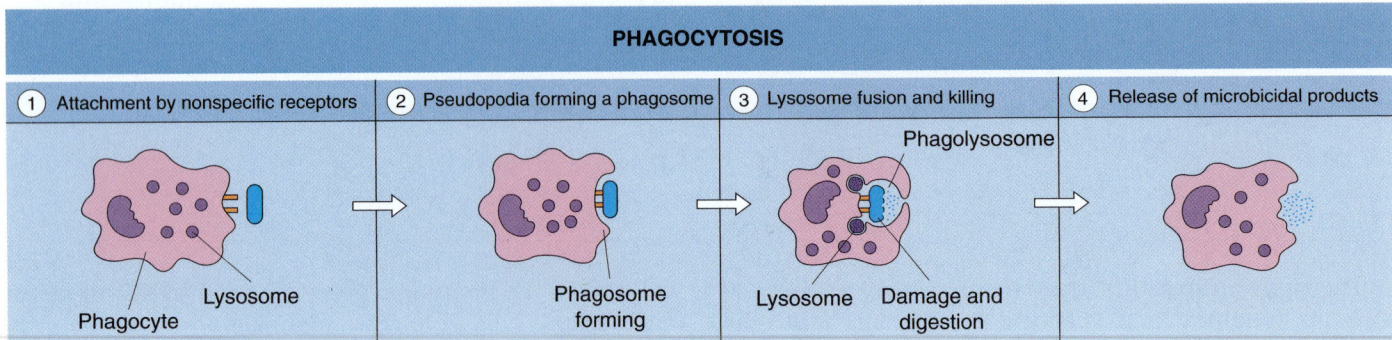

PHAGOCYTOSIS

| 1 Attachment by nonspecific receptors | 2 Pseudopodia forming a phagosome | 3 Lysosome fusion and killing | 4 Release of microbicidal products |

Phagocyte — Lysosome

Phagosome forming

Phagolysosome — Lysosome — Damage and digestion

Figure 25-3 Phagocytosis.

Basophils also are white blood cells, with some structural and functional differences, that enter inflammatory sites and mediate responses to foreign agents or materials. Their actions are most similar to mast cells, described below.

The Lymphatic System. The lymphatic system includes the tonsils, spleen, and thymus gland, which help clear infective agents and provide additional natural immunity protection. It also contains a circulatory liquid, known as **lymph,** that flows away from body tissue and toward the heart, removing debris and pathogens from the tissue. Lymph is clear and colorless except the lymph draining from the small intestine, which is opaque and milky-colored from material drained from the intestine (called chyle). Lymph passes through **lymph nodes,** which filter out foreign materials and collect infection-fighting cells that kill pathogens, on its way to the heart.

The structure of the lymphatic system generally mirrors the venous and arterial circulation. Lymph capillaries begin in the tissues and gradually merge to form larger vessels, called *ducts.* Lymph capillaries are spread throughout most of the body; the only tissues without lymphatic drainage are the central nervous system (CNS), bone marrow, and tissues that also do not have blood supply. The lymphatic drainage eventually feeds into the right lymphatic duct (which drains the right thorax, right upper limb, and right side of the head and neck) or the thoracic duct (which drains the left thorax, left upper extremity, and left side of head and neck). These ducts feed back into the central veins entering the heart.

Although the structure is similar to blood circulation, the action of lymph is different in a number of ways. Lymph carries debris and dangerous materials away from tissue, whereas blood carries nutrients and gases to and from tissue. Lymph does not circulate back and forth between heart and tissue as with blood, but instead follows a one-way path from tissue to the heart. To facilitate this one-way movement, lymph capillaries contain one-way valves that prevent movement of debris and infective agents back into the tissues—another structural difference from the venous system, which has no such valves. As previously mentioned, lymph vessels also contain unique filtration structures, known as *lymph nodes,* that filter out debris and foreign agents from the lymph as it passes through them. Lymph nodes contain concentrations of lymphocytes and macrophages, which destroy pathogens. Major groups of lymph nodes are located in the inguinal nodes (groin), axillary nodes (armpit), and cervical nodes (neck) (Figure 25-4). When an infection is present, these nodes often fill with foreign material, resulting in lymph node enlargement, or **lymphadenopathy.** Finally, lymph contains unique cells known as **lymphocytes.** Most lymphocytes are a key part of the acquired immunity system. However, one type of lymphocyte, called **natural killer cells,** is perhaps the best example of natural immunity cells in the body. They destroy many (but not all) pathogens and

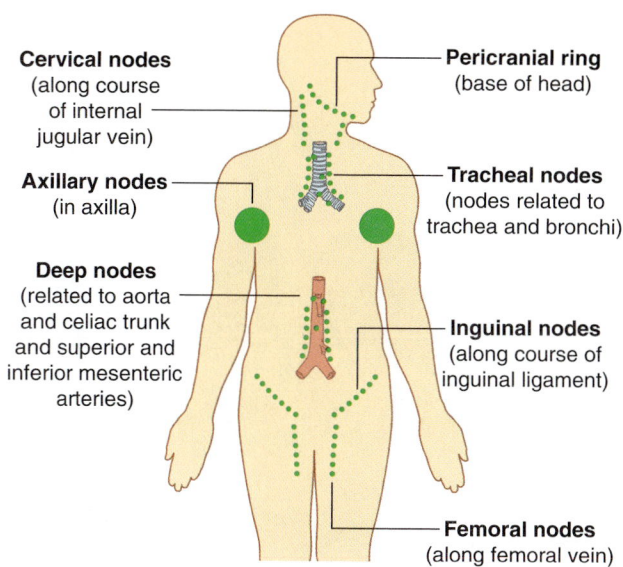

Figure 25-4 Regions associated with clusters or a particular abundance of lymph nodes.

are not specifically configured for certain targets and so are nonspecific (natural) killers. However, they do not destroy normal tissue, so their action is not random but part of an intentional immune response.

Figure 25-5 demonstrates a schematic representation of lymphatic system action.

Acquired Immunity

[OBJECTIVES 4, 5, 6]

Physiology of Antigens and the Immune Response. Acquired immunity is the process by which the body recognizes foreign substances and mounts a specific defense against them. Foreign substances that trigger specific immune responses are called **antigens.** Acquired immunity can be thought of as an enhancement to the inflammatory response. Functionally, acquired immunity offers two more specialized features beyond the basic inflammatory response.

First, acquired immunity builds memory for certain antigens so that encounters with the same antigen in the future prompt increasingly powerful and effective defense responses. Second, acquired immunity amplifies the effect of natural immunity, acting on cells such as macrophages, neutrophils, and basophils to make them more effective against certain recognized targets.

Acquired immunity accomplishes these functions through the actions of lymphocytes, known as B lymphocytes and T lymphocytes, which identify specific antigens and then respond in one of two ways. A detailed description of the inflammatory response and immune system, as well as their interactions, is presented in Chapter 8.

Humoral Immunity. B lymphocytes respond to antigens by producing **antibodies,** which destroy bacteria.

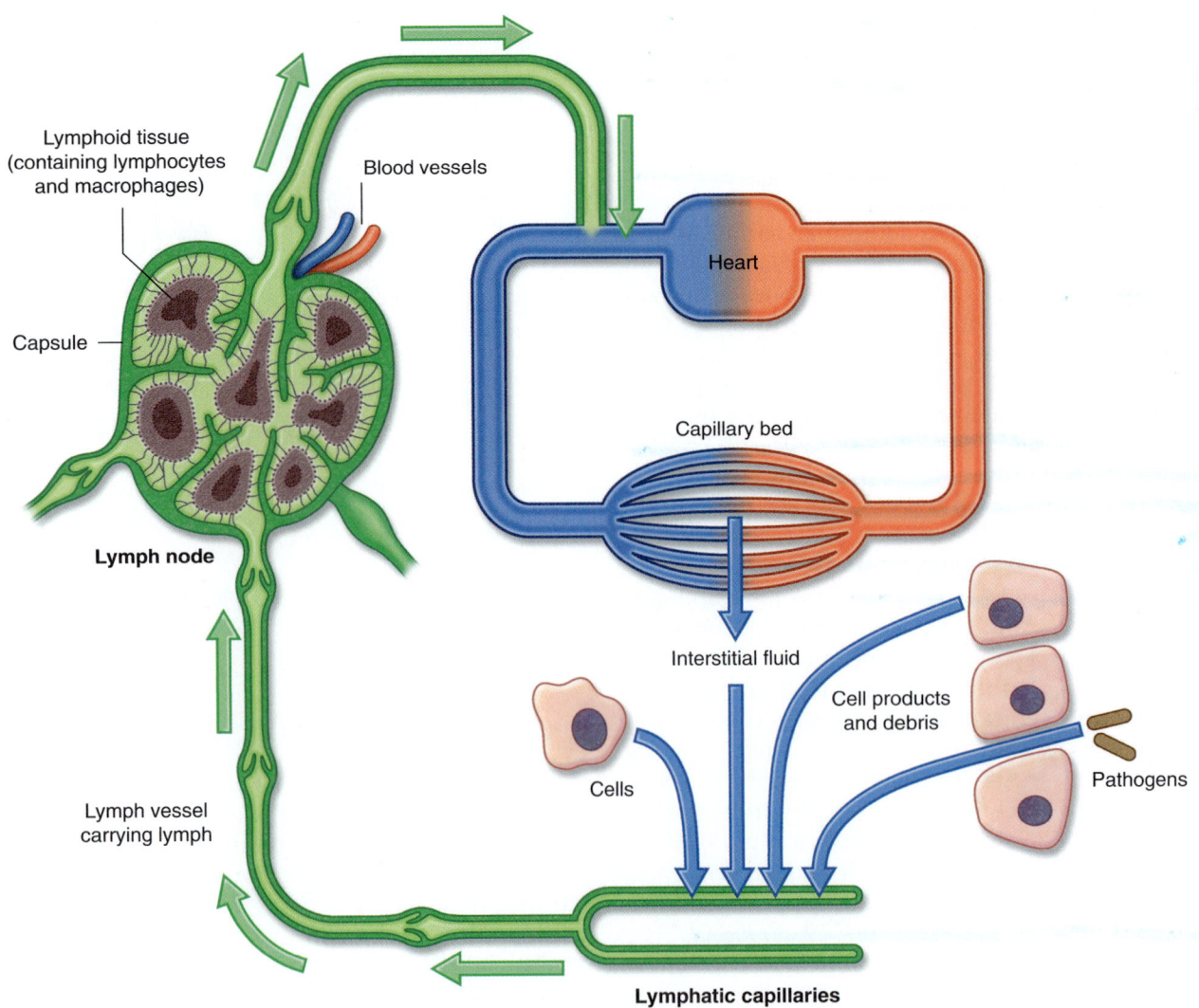

Figure 25-5 Lymphatic vessels and blood vessels carry lymph through the body.

This activity is known as **humoral immunity.** Humoral immunity is used primarily to kill bacteria that are freely moving throughout the body's tissues and fluids ("humors") and can thus be found and killed by mobile antibodies (Figure 25-6). Humoral immunity also triggers mast cells and the complement cascade. Mast cells act like basophils, but whereas basophils circulate, mast cells are found inside tissues and come from different origins. The complement cascade is a series of proteins that interact with each other in a highly structured manner to destroy pathogens.

Cell-Mediated Immunity. T lymphocytes act through **cell-mediated immunity.** In this response, pathogens found within body cells or trapped within the body's macrophages are killed by the action of T lymphocytes. In the case of macrophage-trapped pathogens, the T lymphocyte further activates the macrophage, allowing it to kill the pathogen. In the case of intracellular infection (particularly viruses), T lymphocytes directly **lyse** (destroy) the body cell to kill the indwelling pathogen.

Humoral and cell-mediated immunity are powerful mechanisms for fighting infection and play a role in nearly all physiologic and pathophysiologic actions of the immune system. The process by which they are activated is known as the phases of immune response.

Phases of Immune Response. To mount an effective cell-mediated immune response, the body must first recognize that a foreign antigen is present. This is known as the **cognitive phase.** In this phase antigens bind to specific receptors on lymphocytes that are unique to that antigen. When this particular receptor is bound, the lymphocyte knows that the particular antigen it represents is present in the body.

The process by which that lymphocyte activates other lymphocytes is known as the **activation phase.** During this phase the lymphocytes specific to the identified antigen create copies of themselves, leading to vastly increased numbers of clones of the lymphocyte specific to that antigen. This process is known as *amplification.* The lymphocytes themselves also change during this phase, converting from antigen-recognizing cells to

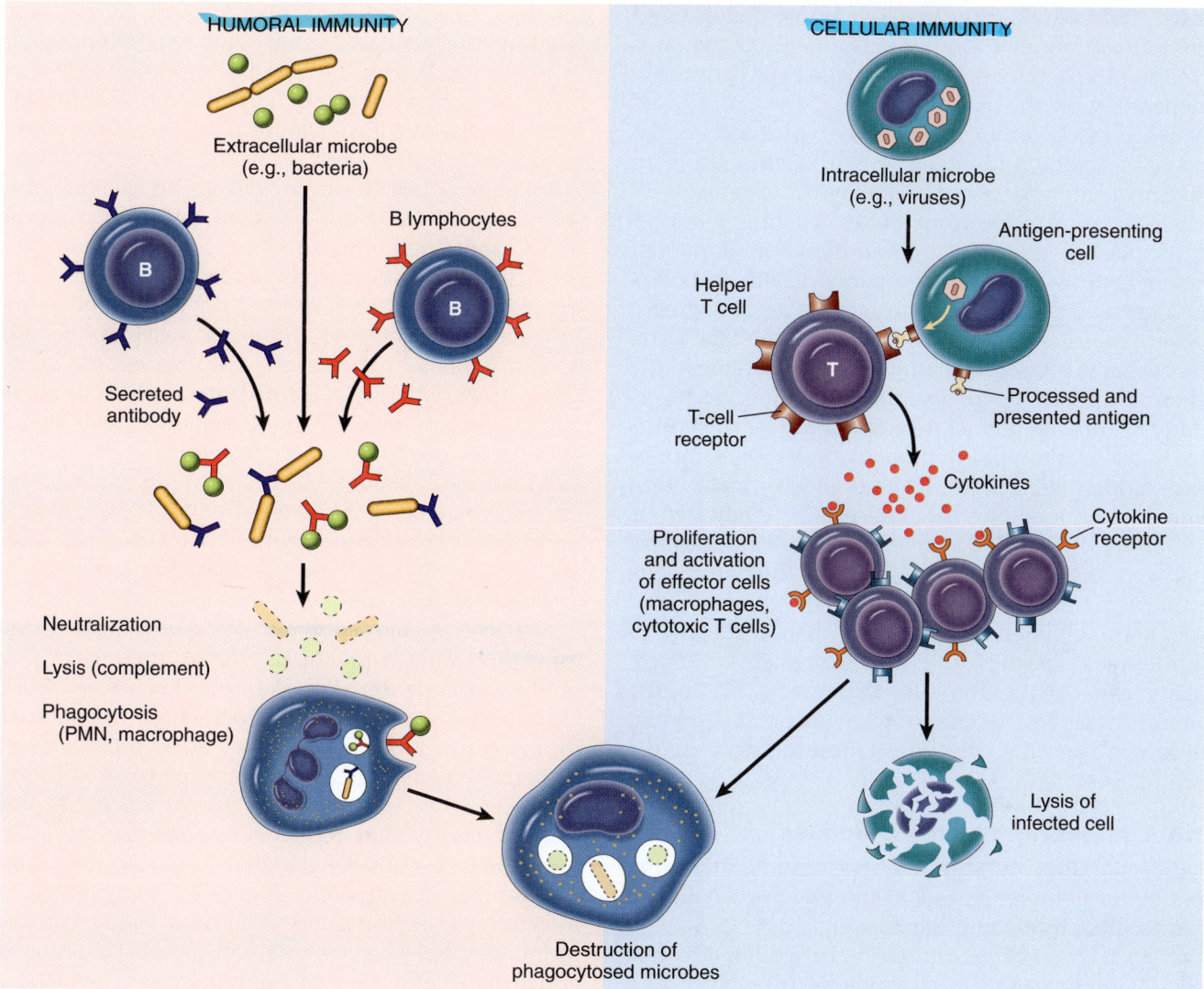

Figure 25-6 Humoral and cell-mediated immunity. *PMN,* Polymorphonuclear neutrophil.

antibody-secreting cells. To use a military analogy, the same cells convert from intelligence-gathering surveillance units to soldier units once they have identified the antigen they are programmed to detect and destroy. These cells then migrate to the sites where antigen or inflammatory responses are found. This is known as *lymphocyte migration*. Through amplification and lymphocyte migration, the body needs to maintain only a small number of passive surveillance cells attuned to a particular antigen; but if that antigen is discovered, they can quickly form an entire army of combat cells dedicated to the complex task of eradicating the infection.

The process of infection eradication is known as the **effector phase.** Cells that operate during the effector phase are called effector cells and include activated lymphocytes and inflammatory components of natural immunity such as complement, cytokines, basophils, mast cells, and macrophages. This highlights a key point to understand in immune response: although activated T cells are the cells acquired immunity adds to the effector phase, one of their principal purposes is to trigger a more enhanced and focused response in the many cells involved in natural immunity. In the absence of B- and T-lymphocyte activation, all these agents also can be active, but to a much less focused and powerful degree. Effector cells control an infection and kill or contain the pathogen causing it.

Factors Affecting the Immune System

Many factors can improve or detract from the healthy functioning of the immune system.

Factors Affecting External Defenses

The external defenses of the human body can be amplified by other means. The skin is an outstanding natural barrier to infection, but personal protective equipment is even better at preventing pathogenic exposure. This equipment supplements the skin in places where it may not be intact, prevents pathogenic invasion by agents that can erode or bypass the skin, and can cover the body in places where the skin is not present (such as the mouth). This is why healthcare providers wear gloves and are sometimes required to wear personal protective suits and masks or respirators of varying degrees of permeability, depending on the pathogen.

In other cases, rather than prevent pathogen entry, exposure of healthy individuals to pathogens exiting an already-invaded host must be prevented. Examples of this can range in scale from individual interventions, such as placing a paper surgical mask on a patient with tuberculosis, to large-scale public health interventions, such as quarantining a hospital or neighborhood. However, an intervention anywhere on this spectrum shares the same purpose as natural external defenses—the prevention of body tissue invasion by pathogens.

Many factors can detract from the ability of the body's external defenses to operate properly. Skin can be torn or burned. Cough reflexes can be blunted with medication or unconsciousness. Normal flora can be eradicated as a side effect of antibiotics given for other indications. Ulcers and diverticuli (cryptlike extrusions from the intestines) can impair the lining of the stomach and bowel. Many different sources can change the pH of the urine and stomach. Tonsils can be surgically removed. Smoking can destroy the cilia that are useful in the respiratory tract for trapping foreign material. Diet and medications can slow the transit time of stool in the bowel.

Factors Affecting Internal Defenses

An understanding of acquired and natural immunity allows better comprehension of interventions designed to add to this physiologic response.

Just as a B lymphocyte can secrete antibodies designed to kill a certain pathogen, antibodies can be given to a patient as a medication. These antibodies are called **immunoglobulins.** Examples include rabies immunoglobulin, tetanus immunoglobulin, and hepatitis B immunoglobulin. The administration of immunoglobulin confers **passive immunity,** which means that the patient is immune as long as the antibodies are active and present in sufficient numbers. However, in this model the body itself is not involved in the additional immune response. Examples of this include giving tetanus or rabies antibodies to patients already known or suspected to be infected with these agents.

Active immunity can also be induced. In this model patients are exposed to a synthetic, dead, or modified pathogen in subinfectious amounts. In this manner the pathogen cannot hurt them, but it induces the same immune response as the true pathogen. Through the mechanisms of acquired immunity the patient then has the apparatus needed to fight off the pathogen if ever exposed to the true antigen.

The best example of this type of induced active immunity is **vaccination.** Vaccinations are familiar to paramedics, all of whom should be vaccinated against hepatitis B. Other vaccinations currently required or recommended in the U.S. general population include those against pertussis, diphtheria, *Staphylococcus pneumoniae*, measles,

mumps, chickenpox, and rubella. These are all administered in childhood, although some require boosters.

Vaccinations can be vitally important for certain higher risk populations, such as children and the elderly. Both populations have significantly decreased mortality rates from infections now prevented by vaccination.

Influenza vaccinations are developed each fall to fight the strains of influenza expected to be most prevalent that season. The Centers for Disease Control and Prevention (CDC) publishes recommendations each year regarding influenza vaccination based on supply and demand. In general, inactivated influenza vaccinations during certain periods of the season are reserved for high-risk populations, whereas **attenuated vaccinations** can be given to any nonallergic, nonpregnant patient aged 5 to 49 years at any time (CDC, 2005) (Box 25-1). Because vaccinations depend on adequate immune response, the response may be variable in patients with unpredictable response, such as those with HIV (Melvin & Mohan, 2003). Live vaccinations are contraindicated in HIV-infected patients.

A high-risk population is a group at increased risk for infection. Some individuals are at high risk because of their occupation. For example, healthcare workers, even healthy ones, are considered a high-risk population for many infections because they are frequently exposed to pathogens. Others are similarly considered high risk simply by living in areas where the pathogens are present in an unusually high frequency (**pandemic** areas). Some individuals are considered high risk because their immune systems are impaired in some way; examples include infection of the immune system itself (e.g., HIV), absent immune system components (e.g., removal of the spleen), and reduced efficiency of the immune system (the very young and very old). Identifying and protecting individuals who may be at high risk is an important public health mission and boosts the body's own defense mechanisms.

BOX 25-1   Vaccination Controversies

Vaccinations are associated with a certain amount of controversy. The safety of vaccinations is continually monitored. Some vaccinations have been discontinued because they were found to be ineffective or caused more harm than good. An example of a vaccination causing unexpected side effects was the formulation for rotavirus. It was discontinued when it was found to be associated with very high rates of an intestinal condition known as *intussusception*. Another concern that has been raised about vaccinations relates to the use of mercury derivatives (such as thimerosol) as a preservative, which are thought to possibly cause a form of mercury poisoning resembling autism. Although no definitive scientific evidence links vaccinations with these conditions, many vaccinations are now preservative and thimerosal free.

IMMUNE SYSTEM PATHOPHYSIOLOGY AND TREATMENT

[OBJECTIVE 7]

The immune system sometimes malfunctions or becomes infected itself. This can lead to increased infection risk as well as illness and injury. Immune systems that are inadequate in some way are referred to as immunodeficient. **Immunodeficiencies** can be acquired or congenital (present at birth). Congenital, or primary, immunodeficiencies include severe combined immunodeficiency disease (the lack of production of B cells and T cells), agammaglobulinemia and hypogammaglobulinemia (the absence or low levels of immunoglobulins), and DiGeorge syndrome (the lack of T cells). Secondary immunodeficiencies result from an outside agent affecting a previously functioning immune system. These outside agents include cancer, chemotherapy, some disease processes such as diabetes, malnutrition, loss of immunoglobulins, loss of protective barriers such as in burns, and infectious diseases such as HIV. The immune system can also malfunction by misrecognizing and attacking its own body's tissues (autoimmune disorders) or producing a massive, disproportionate, and harmful response to an antigenic stimulus (**hypersensitivity disorders**). Finally, advances in transplantation surgery have allowed foreign organs to be transplanted into patients. This requires bypassing the normal functioning of the immune system because **rejection** occurs when the immune system attacks the transplanted organ or when the transplanted organ triggers a hypersensitivity disorder.

Acquired Immunodeficiency

Acquired immunodeficiency disorders are not present at birth, but are acquired by infection or malfunction of the immune system.

HIV and AIDS

[OBJECTIVE 8]

The prototype of acquired immunodeficiency is the **human immunodeficiency virus (HIV)** and the syndrome it causes: **acquired immunodeficiency syndrome (AIDS).**

AIDS is a syndrome reflecting a defect in cell-mediated immunity, causing increased susceptibility to infection. The first cases of AIDS were seen in 1981 when increased rates of normally rare infections were found in previously healthy homosexual men. In 1983 researchers discovered that HIV was the causative pathogen in AIDS.

HIV is a ribonucleic acid (RNA) virus that infects the immune system. It specifically targets T lymphocytes with a surface marker known as CD4. In 1985 the first test was developed to identify HIV in a patient's body, allowing researchers to track the progression of the virus around the world. If AIDS develops, clinicians directly count the number of CD4 T lymphocytes to track the progression of the syndrome.

It is critical to understand the fact that AIDS is always caused by infection with HIV, but infection with HIV does not always cause the specific syndrome of AIDS. With the introduction of highly active antiretroviral therapy and early treatment, many patients currently live asymptomatically with HIV infection without signs of AIDS. However, AIDS continues to be a massive public health threat worldwide. An estimated 40.3 million people worldwide were infected with HIV by the end of 2005, with 3 million AIDS-related deaths in that year alone. Of these deaths, more than half a million were children (Joint United Nations Programme on AIDS, 2005). More alarmingly, in 2005 alone approximately 5 million new cases of HIV-infected patients were identified (Joint United Nations Programme on AIDS, 2005). Overall, 25 million people have died of AIDS worldwide since its appearance in the 1980s—one of the most destructive epidemics in recorded history (Joint United Nations Programme on AIDS, 2005).

In North America approximately 1 million people live with HIV or AIDS (Joint United Nations Programme on AIDS, 2005). In the United States approximately 80% of cases occur in adult men, 18% in adult women, and 1% in children. Almost 50% of these cases occur before the patient is 30 years old, and most die long before they are 45 years old. HIV and AIDS are seen disproportionately in minority groups; in 2001 more than 70% of AIDS cases appeared in minority racial or ethnic groups, with almost half being African American (Rothman et al. 2006).

HIV infection is now established by testing with enzyme-linked immunosorbent assay (ELISA) and Western blot assay technology. Overall sensitivity and specificity of this testing is greater than 99.9% (Rothman et al., 2006). False-negative results, when they occur, usually are attributable to testing during the period when a patient has been infected with HIV but no antibodies demonstrating it have yet appeared in the blood. This window is present for the first several months of infection. False-negative rates can be as high as 0.3% in areas of high HIV prevalence but are less than 0.001% in low-prevalence areas (Rothman et al., 2006). False-positive tests are extraordinarily rare, on the order of less than 0.0004% (Rothman et al., 2006).

HIV infection can be asymptomatic, cause symptoms of its own, and develop into full-blown AIDS. To clarify where patients fall on this spectrum, the CDC has developed an HIV classification system that applies to all patients older than 13 years (Castro, 1992). This classification system uses numbers (categories 1, 2, and 3) to categorize CD4 T-lymphocyte count and an alphabetical system to categorize clinical symptoms.

In regard to CD4 count, category 1 is defined as more than 500 cells/mcL, category 2 is defined as 200 to 499 cells/mcL, and category 3 is defined as fewer than 200 cells/mcL. Categorizing patients with regard to CD4 count is clinically important. Antiretroviral therapy is considered at counts of less than 500/mcL; prophylaxis against *Pneumocystis carinii* pneumonia, the most common serious infection of AIDS, is recommended for all persons with CD4+ T-lymphocyte counts of less than 200/mcL.

In regard to clinical categorization, category A represents asymptomatic HIV infection. These patients are HIV positive and may have persistent generalized lymphadenopathy and some viral symptoms, but they do not have any conditions listed in categories B or C.

Patients in category B have symptomatic infections believed by a clinician to be caused by the HIV infection or represent an immunodeficiency defect. Examples include fever or diarrhea for longer than 1 month, shingles, pelvic inflammatory disease, and peripheral neuropathy. Category C denotes infection with AIDS.

Once HIV infection is documented, clinicians must vigilantly monitor for the development of AIDS. The most recent definition of AIDS was established by the CDC in 1993. It is currently defined as present when the patient either demonstrates an AIDS-defining illness (Box 25-2) or has fewer than $200/mm^3$ of CD4 cells (Rothman et al., 2006).

[OBJECTIVES 8, 9]

Risk Factors. HIV is present in the blood, semen, vaginal, and cervical secretions of infected individuals. It can be directly transmitted through vaginal or anal intercourse, the fetal placenta, or open mucous membranes or wounds making contact with body fluids containing HIV.

BOX 25-2 AIDS-Defining Illnesses

- Candidiasis, esophageal or pulmonary
- Cervical cancer
- Coccidioidomycosis, extrapulmonary
- Cryptococcosis, extrapulmonary
- Cryptosporidiosis (with diarrhea for more than 1 month)
- Cytomegalovirus infection (of any organ system other than the liver, spleen, or lymph nodes)
- Herpes simplex virus (mucocutaneous ulcer for more than 1 month, pneumonitis, or esophagitis)
- HIV-associated dementia (with functional impairment)
- HIV wasting syndrome
- Histoplasmosis, extrapulmonary
- Isosporiasis (with diarrhea for less than 1 month)
- Kaposi's sarcoma
- Lymphoma
- Mycobacterium tuberculosis (pulmonary or disseminated)
- *Pneumocystis carinii* pneumonia
- Progressive multifocal leukoencephalopathy
- Bacterial pneumonia (recurrent)
- Progressive multifocal leukoencephalopenia
- *Salmonella septicemia*, recurrent
- Toxoplasmosis (of internal organ)

Reprinted from Rothman, R. E., Marco, C. A., Yang, S., & Kelen, G. D. (2006). AIDS and HIV. In J. Marx, R. S. Hockerberger, & R. M. Walls (Eds.). *Rosen's emergency medicine: Concepts and clinical practice* (pp. 2072-2073, 2087, 2091). Philadelphia: Elsevier.

The following are defined as primary risk factors for acquiring HIV infection:

- Intravenous (IV) drug abuse
- Heterosexual sexual activity with a partner at risk
- Homosexual or bisexual sexual activity
- Blood transfusion before 1985
- Prenatal, perinatal, and postnatal maternal-neonatal transmission

Each of these factors carries independent risk, and overall risk of infection increases along with the number of risk factors present (CDC, 1996). From 1985 to 2001, the greatest relative increase of AIDS cases was seen in patients contracting HIV through heterosexual exposure, and the greatest relative decrease was seen in homosexual patients. However, exposure through male homosexual activity remained the highest proportion of AIDS cases as of 2001 (Rothman et al., 2006).

The overall risk that a healthcare worker may have some type of body fluid exposure is not small. However, the performance of your duties as a paramedic is not considered a primary risk factor, and the overall risk of contracting HIV is small. As of June 2000, 57 cases of HIV infection have been documented in healthcare workers that appeared at the same time as an occupational exposure, with another 138 cases considered possibly caused by exposure (Gerberding, 2003).

Healthcare worker exposure risk can be significantly reduced by following CDC guidelines for standard precautions, which recommend the use of protective equipment (including gloves, gown, mask, and eye protection) for any situation with a potential exposure.

If an exposure does occur, healthcare pofessionals should follow their agency's exposure plan, consulting with their personal physicians as necessary. The CDC postexposure prophylaxis guidelines currently advise case-by-case evaluation of risk in consultation with a physician (Panlilio et al., 2005). Risk evaluation includes determination of the type of exposure and HIV status (or risk factors for HIV infection if unknown status) of the source. Higher risk exposures include deep injuries, visible blood on a device, and injuries sustained when placing a catheter into a vessel; lower risk exposures include superficial injuries and solid needles (Rothman et al., 2006). Most protocols call for rapid testing of the source, with negative findings considered adequate to withhold prophylactic treatment (Rothman et al., 2006). If exposure to a known HIV-positive source occurs, postexposure prophylaxis should be strongly considered.

If an exposed individual, in consultation with his or her physician, elects to start prophylactic treatment the CDC guidelines (Panlilio et al., 2005) include tables that recommend the number and type of medications to use based on source and exposure risk factors.

Research is ongoing to optimize treatment options with antiviral medications. The incidence of death from AIDS declined rapidly through 1998 after the introduction of highly active antiretroviral therapy in 1996 (Rothman et al., 2006). Living asymptomatically with HIV-positive status is now possible if viral loads are kept low and AIDS does not develop. In addition, researchers continue to attempt to develop a vaccination against HIV. The HIV Vaccine Trials Network, supported by the U.S. National Institutes of Health and National Institute of Allergy and Infectious Diseases, currently has clinical trial programs worldwide (HIV Vaccine Trials Network, 2008). Promising research also is being pursued in other countries. As of May 2008, however, no vaccine is available.

Field Evaluation and Treatment

[OBJECTIVE 8]

Because HIV and AIDS are usually detected secondary to another illness, infection should be considered in your differential diagnosis whenever numerous, rare, or AIDS-defining illnesses are present, especially in patients in whom HIV/AIDS risk factors are present.

When taking a history for patients with known HIV infection, ask whether AIDS has developed. Directed questions looking for symptoms of the AIDS-defining illnesses (such as fever, diarrhea, weight loss, or mental status changes) are indicated.

The physical examination of patients with HIV/AIDS should be directed toward identifying signs of increased immunosuppression or AIDS-defining illnesses. This includes a careful oropharyngeal examination looking for thrush or unusual lesions; a careful mental status examination looking for signs of dementia or encephalopathy; and complete vital signs, including temperature. No specific field treatment for HIV/AIDS is available, although symptomatic treatment often is necessary.

Patient and Family Education. Patient and family education may be necessary to explain the difference between HIV and AIDS, to discuss ways it can and cannot be transmitted, and to discuss risks of transmission. Expanded-scope EMS systems can include prevention programs that could be of great assistance in reducing HIV transmission rates. At this time many myths and misunderstandings prevail about HIV and AIDS. An empathetic and well-educated paramedic can be helpful in educating the public about this dangerous but often-misunderstood condition.

PARAMEDIC Pearl

When taking a history for patients suspected of HIV or AIDS, evaluate risk factors. Great sensitivity is needed when exploring these topics because some risk factors (such as drug abuse and homosexuality) are culturally stigmatized. You must be empathetic and realize that, like cancer, AIDS is a diagnosis that is greatly feared by many individuals. Suggestions that he or she may have this syndrome could be alarming to the patient.

Case Scenario—Continued

You transfer the patient to your oxygen supply and increase flow to 15 L by nonrebreather mask as you continue your assessment. The patient reports that he became acutely short of breath approximately 3 hours into the flight. He states that he has been in good health until 3 to 4 days ago (during a business trip), when he developed a productive cough and intermittent stabbing pain in the left side of the chest. He had made an appointment to visit his physician today on returning home. The patient has retractions and shows use of accessory muscles of respiration. Chest wall movement is symmetric. Breath sounds reveal coarse rhonchi and are very diminished in the right upper lobes and moderately diminished at the left apex. Vital signs are blood pressure, 124/82 mm Hg; pulse, 132 beats/min; respirations, 40 breaths/min; and SpO$_2$, 84%.

Questions

5. Is this patient high priority? Why or why not?
6. What conditions are consistent with a productive cough, diminished breath sounds, stabbing chest pain, and hypoxia?
7. How does the history of HIV and hepatitis fit into the picture?
8. What treatment will you initiate at this time?

Lymphoma

Lymphoma represents another type of acquired immunodeficiency, in this case a cancerous type. It afflicts B lymphocytes, T lymphocytes, or stem cells and manifests itself in the lymph nodes. The etiology of most lymphomas is unknown, although some are associated with viral sources. In addition, the risk of developing lymphoma is increased with the presence of other acquired and congenital immunodeficiency disorders (Rubin, 1994). Symptoms and demographics vary with the type of lymphoma. Taken together, lymphoma accounts for 5% of all cancers; it is found more often and is more often lethal in white populations, in whom incidence is higher than 20 cases per 100,000 (National Cancer Institute, 2006).

Leukemia

Leukemia is a cancer disorder of blood cells. Many of the forms of leukemia, such as chronic myelogenous forms, principally involve immunity cells such as granulocytes. However, clinical manifestations of leukemia are usually less significant in terms of immune system function and more consistent with other generalized cancer presentations.

Autoimmune Disorders

[OBJECTIVE 9]

Autoimmune disorders, in which the immune system inappropriately attacks its own host tissue, are numerous and frequently devastating.

Systemic lupus erythematosus (SLE) is an autoimmune disease that attacks multiple body systems. It occurs at a rate of 17 to 48 cases per 100,000 people in North America and northern Europe and is seen most commonly in black women of childbearing age (1 case per 250) (Sercombe, 2006). The pathophysiologic failure is the production of a line of B cells that produce abnormal **autoantibodies** (antibodies that attack the body). In other cases the antibodies can bind with tissue, causing hypersensitivity reactions. According to the American College of Rheumatology definitions, patients must have four of 11 conditions associated with SLE to be diagnosed with the condition (Tan et al., 1982). The classic presentation is fever, joint pain, and rash in a female of childbearing years, but much more serious manifestations can be present, including life-threatening failure of the kidneys and neurologic system. Cardiac presentations of SLE include pericarditis, endocarditis, and myocarditis. Acetaminophen and nonsteroidal antiinflammatory drugs (NSAIDs) are useful for pain control, although NSAIDs should be withheld if SLE nephritis is present. Physicians may prescribe corticosteroids for additional inflammatory control. SLE is a complex condition and families and patients may need to be educated regarding the wide range of symptoms that can be caused by the disease and about the autoimmune source of the condition.

Type 1 (insulin-dependent) diabetes mellitus occurs when the islet cells of the pancreas stop making sufficient quantities of insulin, which must then be administered as a medication. Autoantibodies against the pancreatic islet cells are the usual cause of this type of diabetes, making it an autoimmune disorder. Diabetes, as well as its complications and treatment, is more extensively discussed in Chapter 24.

Rheumatoid arthritis most commonly develops in women between the ages of 30 and 50 years. Granulocytes are inappropriately stimulated to secrete enzymes destructive to joint tissue. Ultimately the joint can be destroyed by granulation tissue. Hypersensitivity reactions, such as complexes of antigen and antibody that deposit directly into the joint, also can cause extensive damage. Rheumatoid factor, an antibody, is positive in approximately 85% of patients with rheumatoid arthritis (Anderson, 1997). An important factor to the prehospital management of patients with rheumatoid arthritis is the knowledge that chronic rheumatoid arthritis can degrade the ligament that binds the C2 dens to C1 in the cervical spine. Because of this, great care must be taken when intubating patients with a longstanding history of rheumatoid arthritis. Many different types of medications are used to control this condition. Prehospital care centers on pain relief. Unlike other sources of arthritis, patients with this condition may need to be educated about the autoimmune source of their problem.

Progressive systemic sclerosis, the newer and more preferred term for *scleroderma,* is an autoimmune disease that appears as a severe and progressive disease of the skin, often associated with organ complications (Figure 25-7).

The earliest symptom of progressive systemic sclerosis is *Raynaud phenomenon,* which is characterized by episodes of poor color, pain, and paresthesias of the fingers consistent with poor blood flow (Figure 25-8). This is followed by edema and thickening of the skin, including tightening of the facial skin that can result in a "stone face" (Figure 25-9). This progression is caused by excessive deposition of collagen in the skin. Collagen deposition can spread to internal organs, causing pulmonary,

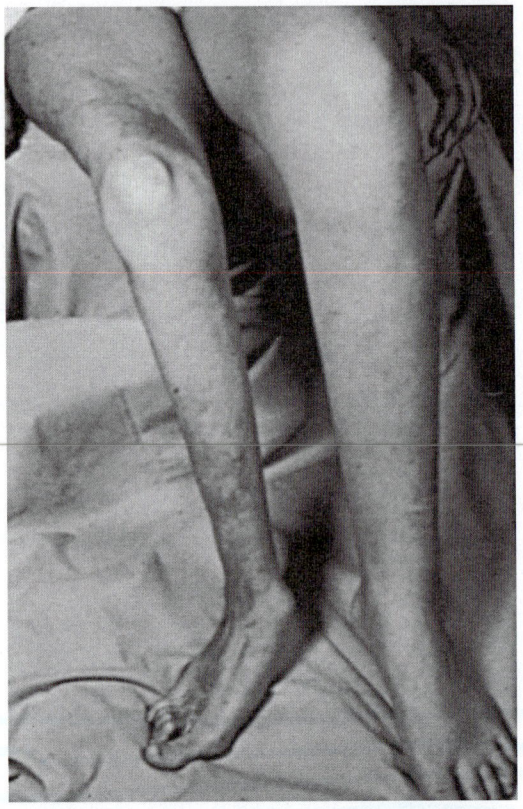

Figure 25-7 Progressive systemic sclerosis of the right leg of a 14-year-old girl. The condition began at the age of 6 years and resulted in severe muscle wasting and shortening of the extremity.

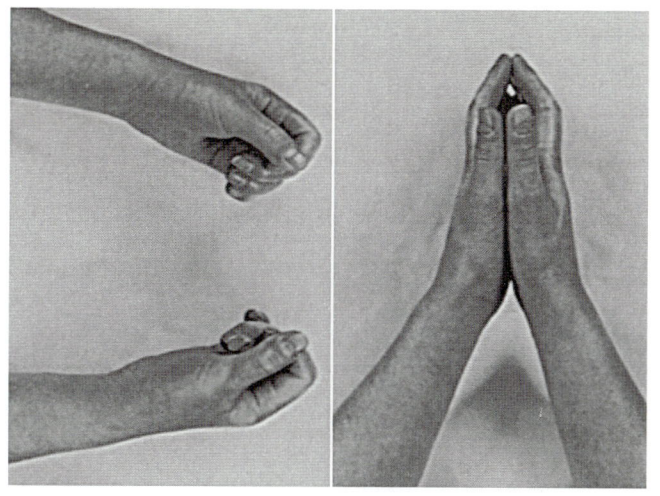

Figure 25-8 The hands of a young woman with rapidly progressing systemic sclerosis. The skin of her hands is taut, limiting fist closure and finger extension.

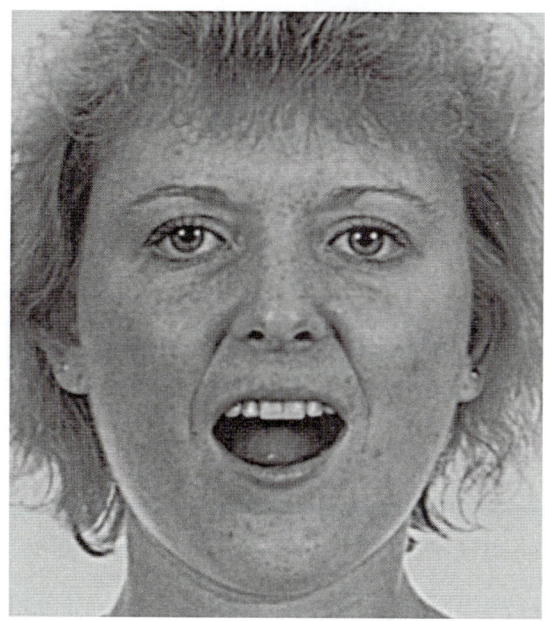

Figure 25-9 A young woman with rapidly progressing systemic sclerosis. The skin of her face is taut, limiting mouth opening.

renal, cardiac, vascular, and GI complications. The pulmonary system is of particular importance to the paramedic because it is implicated in two thirds of patients with progressive systemic sclerosis and is the leading cause of death in this group. Common pulmonary symptoms include dyspnea with exertion, nonproductive cough, and rales (crackles). Cardiac abnormalities, including dysrhythmias, various degrees of conduction blocks, pericarditis, and heart failure, are common in patients with progressive systemic sclerosis.

Estimates for the number of people in the United States with progressive systemic sclerosis range from 40,000 to 165,000 (National Institutes of Health, 2001). Raynaud phenomenon also can be seen without progressive systemic sclerosis and can be quite uncomfortable for patients. However, connective tissue disorders such as progressive systemic sclerosis, SLE, and rheumatoid arthritis are the most common causes of Raynaud phenomenon. The term *overlap syndrome* or *mixed connective tissue disease* is used to describe patients who have signs and symptoms of multiple connective tissue diseases. Smoking tobacco greatly exacerbates these symptoms. Patients and families who smoke should be advised to stop smoking and avoid any exposure to tobacco smoke if they have these conditions. Patients also should be educated about the importance of preventive measures recommended by their physician; for example, influenza and pneumonia vaccinations become particularly important in patients with pulmonary manifestations of progressive systemic sclerosis. Because so many organ systems can be involved, patients with this condition often have many specialists involved in their care and thus may have many treatments. Calcium channel blockers may be used to reduce Raynaud phenomenon. Various cardiac medications may be used if the heart activity is restricted, which can cause myocarditis, cardiomyopathy, or dysrhythmias. Various lotions and creams can be used to treat taut skin. A comprehensive physical examination is required to identify any new manifestations of the disease. When taking a history, carefully review the medications the patient is taking for clues regarding the manifestations already being treated. Prehospital treatment is symptomatic.

Celiac disease (also known as *gluten-sensitive enteropathy* or *nontropical sprue*) is characterized by generalized difficulty absorbing foods, which resolves when gluten-containing foods are withdrawn from the diet. Gluten is a water-insoluble portion of wheat. Celiac disease is believed to be caused at least in part by the inappropriate action of B and T cells stimulated by gluten and gliadin (an alcoholic extract with similar effect as gluten), although the exact pathophysiology of the disease and the autoantibodies' role in it is not fully understood. Celiac sprue occurs in approximately 1 in every 3000 persons in the United States. The highest prevalence is in Western Europeans, where rates can be as high as 1 in 250 to 300 persons. The disease is rare in Africans and Asians (Klapproth & Yang, 2005). When taking the patient's medical history, ask about recent dietary changes, bowel function, and weight changes, with specific questions regarding the presence of diarrhea, flatulence, weight loss, abdominal bloating, or cramping. Patients may describe (or physical examination may reveal) extraintestinal symptoms such as bleeding, osteopenia with consequent fractures, hypocalcemia causing neurologic symptoms (ataxia, motor weakness, seizures, sensory loss), itchy vesicular or ecchymotic skin disorders, peripheral edema, and hormonal disorders (including amenorrhea, delayed periods, and infertility in women and impotence or infertility in men) (Klapproth

& Yang, 2005). Prehospital treatment is symptomatic. Patients and families may need to be educated about the source of their dietary difficulties, with specific attention to the immune system's role and the importance of avoiding gluten products.

Chronic active hepatitis and *chronic persistent hepatitis* often are categorized as autoimmune conditions. Hepatitis is more completely discussed in Chapter 31.

Multiple sclerosis (MS) is an inflammatory disorder affecting the CNS. It is believed to be an autoimmune disorder. MS is present in 0.1% of the U.S. population, with the most common age of onset being 25 to 30 years. It is almost twice as common in women compared with men (Stettler & Pancioli, 2006). Although the exact autoimmune mechanisms are not known, a leading theory suggests that genetic predisposition interacts with an environmental trigger or an infection to produce T cells oriented to attack the CNS, causing areas of scarring called *lesions* or *plaques* that result from destruction of the myelin sheath, a process known as *demyelination*. After demyelination ceases, the process of healing progresses over several weeks to months, forming areas of scarring. Later, another stressor trigger activates these T cells, which produces a pathologic inflammatory response, resulting in another exacerbation (Stettler & Pancioli, 2006).

The neurologic effects of MS can either be positive or negative. Positive effects are the result of the formation of ectopic neurologic impulses or inappropriate communication between neurons—much like a short circuit. Other effects result from conduction blocks, or conduction delays of the nervous impulses. The presence of blocks and delays can vary, which explains why the severity of symptoms can change from day to day and even hour to hour. Symptoms can be so subtle the patient may not seek treatment for years. Symptoms of MS are listed in Box 25-3 and can be divided into the following major classifications according to the part of the brain affected:

- Changes in mental status and impaired thinking
- Cranial nerve abnormalities
- Difficulties with motor function and sensory function
- Sexual, bowel, and bladder dysfunction

To be diagnosed with this condition, a patient must have at least two clinical episodes of different neurologic symptoms that occurred at different times. Field diagnosis is impossible. However, it is a condition to be suspected in young, otherwise healthy patients (especially female) who have recurrent neurologic impairments (with visual changes often being the first described). History taking must be comprehensive to connect the many different symptoms occurring at different times, which at first may not seem to be related. Physical examination should be equally comprehensive because many organ systems are involved. Prehospital treatment involves control of symptoms or supportive care. MS

BOX 25-3	Signs and Symptoms of Multiple Sclerosis

- Weakness
- Fatigue
- Facial weakness
- Coordination difficulties
- Cerebellar dysfunction
- Loss of dexterity
- Hyperreflexia
- Ataxia
- Increased falls
- Sensory loss
- Paresthesia
- Visual disturbances
- Nystagmus
- Vertigo
- Memory disorders
- Attention difficulties
- Difficulty solving problems
- Impaired judgment
- Urinary urgency
- Urinary hesitancy
- Urinary incontinence
- Constipation
- Impotence

represents a classic case emphasizing the importance of empathetic and sensitive paramedical care even in apparently frustrating cases. Patients with MS can be inappropriately "written off" as psychiatric patients, malingerers, or drug seekers by many providers because of their many vague, migratory, and intermittent neurologic symptoms before the correct diagnosis is made.

Crohn's disease is a chronic inflammatory bowel disease that is discussed in Chapter 26. The exact cause of this condition is unknown, but environmental, inflammatory, immunologic, and genetic factors are thought to be involved. Whether this disease has an autoimmune component is a subject of great debate and remains unknown. Contemporary thought is that the disorder occurs as a result of an overreaction of the immune system to an environmental, infectious, or dietary agent rather than an autoimmune disorder.

Hypersensitivity Disorders

Hypersensitivity represents a pathologic immune response in which a body is reexposed to an antigen. The response is pathologic because, instead of functioning to harm a foreign material, the body either attacks its own cells or mounts such an inappropriately large response to foreign antigens that it causes harm. Hypersensitivity disorders are divided into four types: immediate hypersensitivity, cytotoxic hypersensitivity, immune complex–mediated hypersensitivity, and T cell–mediated hypersensitivity.

Type I: Immediate Hypersensitivity

[OBJECTIVES 10 TO 24]

Immediate hypersensitivity is the most familiar of these disorders. The mildest form is the **allergic** (or atopic) **reaction.** Some patients have a predisposition toward allergic responses and are known as *atopic.* Allergy occurs when the body is exposed to an antigen (in this situation called **allergens**) to which it has already developed antibodies, and these antibodies overreact to the exposure. In immediate hypersensitivity reactions, the antibodies involved are known as *immunoglobulin E* (IgE) *antibodies.* They are produced during the initial exposure to an antigen and are stored bound to basophils and mast cells. When the antigen appears again, IgE antibodies recognize it and trigger massive release of **histamines.** Histamines dilate capillaries and cause vessels to become more permeable, causing flushing and edema and potentially the loss of intravascular volume as fluid leaks out into tissue. Hypotension and cardiac failure eventually can result. Histamines also cause the itchiness seen in allergic reactions. *Leukotrienes* are also released and cause bronchoconstriction, resulting in coughing, sneezing, wheezing, and potentially respiratory collapse. The cascade begun by activation of the basophils and mast cells also can cause nausea, vomiting, diarrhea, and abdominal pain and cramping. Secondary effects from primary hypoxia and/or shock can be seen in many other systems, such as the nervous system, including confusion, weakness, headache, syncope, seizures, and ultimately possible coma. Findings associated with allergic reactions are listed in Box 25-4.

In its mildest forms, an allergic reaction manifests as itchiness and whelplike or plaquelike rashes (known as **urticaria** or *hives*) caused by release of histamine. The patient also may complain of flushing, warmth, and tingling. Prehospital treatment of an allergic reaction usually consists of the intravascular or intramuscular administration of **antihistamines** such as diphenhydramine. Local measures at the site of exposure, if external, include dependent positioning of an extremity and application of ice if not otherwise contraindicated.

Moderate allergic reactions can have respiratory involvement such as mild wheezing and mild complaints of difficulty breathing. Perfusion is not affected in moderate reactions. These findings are not life threatening and patients generally respond well to the administration of diphenhydramine. However, the patient should be closely monitored for any increase in difficulty breathing, bronchoconstriction, or respiratory distress.

Anaphylaxis represents the most serious manifestation of immediate hypersensitivity, causing up to 1500 deaths each year (Tran, 2006). It is characterized by respiratory distress and failure, hypotension, cardiovascular collapse, and multisystem involvement and appears within seconds to minutes of exposure to the allergen.

BOX 25-4 Signs and Symptoms of Allergic Reaction

Skin
- Flushing
- Pruritus (itching)
- Urticaria (hives)
- Edema
- Tingling
- Warmth

Cardiovascular System
- Vasodilatation
- Vascular permeability
- Tachycardia
- Hypotension
- Lightheadedness

Airway
- Angioedema
- Laryngeal edema
- Rhinitis
- Cough
- Sneezing
- Hoarseness
- Throat tightness

Gastrointestinal System
- Nausea
- Vomiting
- Cramping
- Diarrhea

Respiratory System
- Bronchospasm
- Wheezing
- Pulmonary edema
- Retrosternal tightness
- Dyspnea

Nervous System
- Dizziness
- Headache
- Convulsions
- Confusion
- Syncope
- Coma

The hallmark of anaphylaxis is cardiovascular collapse, which can occur without preceding respiratory symptoms. Untreated, death from hypoxia (caused by airway edema and bronchospasm) or cardiovascular failure can be rapid. Any patient with an atopic history should be considered at risk for an anaphylactic reaction at some time.

At the first sign of anaphylaxis (respiratory distress or cardiovascular compromise), administer epinephrine. If

[handwritten notes at top of page:]

IV Epi 1:10,000 = cardiac arrest (10ml = 1mg)
anaphylaxis (1ml = 0.1mg)

25-50mg Benadryl IV or IM
IM Epi 1:1000 0.3mg (0.3ml)

the patient is hemodynamically stable, administration of subcutaneous 1:1000 epinephrine is indicated. If the patient is hemodynamically unstable (evidenced by hypotension or cardiovascular collapse), administration of IV 1:10,000 epinephrine may be ordered. The benefit of epinephrine in allergic reactions is threefold. Unlike diphenhydramine, which only blocks H1 receptors, epinephrine reduces the release of vasoactive amines from mast cells and basophils. In addition, the alpha effects cause vasoconstriction and the beta effects cause bronchodilation. Therefore the release of vasoactive amines is decreased and the effects of those already circulating are reversed. Administer diphenhydramine IV or IM. As always, airway, breathing, and circulation take priority in assessment and treatment. Airway management is critical. Anaphylaxis represents an airway emergency in an otherwise healthy, nontraumatized patient. Consider any complaint of tightness of the throat or shortness of breath as potential impending respiratory failure. Administer high-concentration oxygen and monitor pulse oximetry and capnography. Obtain IV access and administer fluids as appropriate according to the patient's hemodynamic status. Patients who have cardiovascular collapse as a result of vasodilation may need large amounts of isotonic fluids to correct hypotension. The paramedic should closely monitor for the development of pulmonary edema because the vessels surrounding the alveoli dilate and become "leaky" along with the rest of the vascular system. Pressor agents such as dopamine may be considered in the setting of pulmonary edema or hypotension refractory to the administration of fluids and epinephrine.

Once cardiopulmonary stability has been assured, all interventions for less severe allergic reactions should also be used for anaphylaxis. Aerosolized epinephrine may be given if available and if the patient has respiratory symptoms. Any antigenic material still in contact with the patient should be removed. If an insect stinger remains, do not squeeze it. Squeezing the stinger can result in the release of more venom. Glucagon may be ordered by medical direction if the patient is taking a beta-blocker. Beta-agonists such as albuterol can be helpful for bronchospasm refractory to epinephrine. Steroid medications, such as methylprednisolone sodium succinate (Solu-Medrol), are available to paramedics in some EMS systems. These medications do not immediately relieve the signs and symptoms associated with an allergic reaction or anaphylaxis, but they do reduce the inflammatory effects associated with these reactions. Because steroid medications exert their effects through their antiinflammatory actions, their onset is slow and they should be administered after medications with a more rapid onset. However, their benefit in long-term patient outcome should not be discounted and they should not be ignored simply because they do not have an immediate action. Some patients may have already self-administered epinephrine by a prescribed EpiPen. This should be considered if further epinephrine is being

given. However, at least one study has demonstrated that more than 35% of anaphylactic cases required more than one dose of epinephrine, so self-administration of epinephrine should not be considered definitive treatment (Davis, 2005).

PARAMEDIC *Pearl*

The generic names of beta-blockers typically end in "olol"—for example, propranolol, timolol, esmolol, atenolol, metoprolol.

A careful history can sometimes indicate the trigger for the patient's reaction. Known patient allergies are especially important to obtain in cases of suspected anaphylaxis. Common allergens include latex (Box 25-5), drugs, foods (nuts and crustacean seafood being the most common sources), and insect stings (most often from the Hymenoptera order). Food is the most common source among these; 4% of Americans are afflicted with food allergies, which cause approximately 30,000 anaphylactic reactions and 150 to 200 deaths each year (Glauser, 2005). Penicillin is the most common drug allergy, occurring at a rate of one to five reactions per 10,000 treatments, with one death per 50,000 to 100,000 treatments (Tran, 2006). Taking great care to avoid contact with allergens triggering allergic responses is the best prevention of this condition. Major public health efforts have been mounted to help consumers avoid exposure to common allergens. Many airlines no longer routinely serve products containing nuts, and many food items now have stamped on their packaging whether they are produced in factories or shops that also process nut products.

Angioedema represents a particular dermatologic manifestation of immediate hypersensitivity. It can occur in conjunction with a generalized allergic reaction or may appear as the sole manifestation of a hypersensitivity reaction. It is similar to urticaria, and both usually are considered similar processes on an allergic spectrum, but angioedema involves deeper dermal tissue and usually is not as itchy. In addition, it is usually confined to the face, mouth, lips, and tongue. It sometimes appears in the extremities and, in men, the genitalia. Angioedema also

BOX 25-5 | Latex Allergies

Latex is a natural rubber harvested from the rubber tree *(Hevea brasiliensis)* found in the southern Amazon river basin. From 0.1% to 1% of the population is allergic to latex or the chemical products contained in latex materials. Healthcare workers are at increased risk, with rates from 5% to 12% (Tran, 2006). Because of this high rate of allergy and the corresponding importance of personal protective equipment, all healthcare workers should have access to nonlatex equipment if necessary to avoid an allergic reaction.

can occur from the use of angiotensin-converting enzyme inhibitors. It is managed in the prehospital arena in the same way as other type I hypersensitivity reactions. In some cases other mechanisms may cause angioedema, the most well known being a hereditary source. Hereditary angioedema is known for its poor response to typical allergic and anaphylactic medications, and although they are still indicated, proactive and vigilant airway management is the most critical intervention in these cases. Incidence in the United States may be as high as 15%, with a predominance in females (Dodds & Sinert, 2005).

Anaphylactoid reactions mimic anaphylaxis (including the release of mediators from mast cells and basophils) clinically but are not mediated by IgE antibodies. Therefore prior sensitization is not required. These types of reaction cannot be differentiated in the field and doing so would not be helpful. Treatment is the same as that for a true anaphylactic reaction.

Type II: Cytotoxic Hypersensitivity

Cytotoxic hypersensitivity occurs when a particular cell membrane triggers IgG or IgM antibodies directed against it. The complement cascade is then initiated, a membrane-attack complex is generated, and the cell membrane is damaged or destroyed. Complement initiation also attracts phagocytes that release enzymes, further damaging the cell membrane.

Type III: Immune Complex Hypersensitivity

Immune complex hypersensitivity appears when antigen-antibody complexes are not promptly removed by the reticuloendothelial system. If they are not appropriately removed, they deposit in tissues and cause an inflammatory response. Wherever they are deposited the complement cascade is activated, with results similar to cytotoxic hypersensitivity.

Serum sickness is the classic historic type III hypersensitivity disorder. This condition was seen when foreign serum was injected and, if it cleared slowly, bound with antibodies to form immune complexes. This is more often seen now with certain drugs, such as penicillin. Foreign serum is rarely used in modern medicine.

Type IV: Delayed Hypersensitivity

Unlike the other hypersensitivity disorders, delayed hypersensitivity is not caused by antibodies, but rather CD4 lymphocytes such as those targeted by HIV. It is delayed because the time frame for lymphocytic response is hours to days after contact with the antigen. Many examples of contact dermatitis are caused by delayed hypersensitivity; it is the mechanism, for example, of allergic responses to poison ivy, chemical skin allergies such as nickel allergy, and skin allergies to some cosmetics and soaps. Delayed hypersensitivity also is the mechanism used by the tuberculin skin test. Purified protein derivative, or tuberculin, is injected intradermally, with no initial reaction. Gradually some local reaction may occur, with the degree of reaction indicating whether a patient has been infected in the past (a greater reaction indicates prior sensitization).

Transplantation Disorders

[OBJECTIVE 25]

The ability to treat organ failure by transplantation of a foreign organ into a patient is one of the most significant medical advances of the modern era. Successfully transplanted solid organs currently include the heart, liver, lung, kidney, bowel, and pancreas. Many other tissues also have been successfully transplanted, including hands, corneas, skin, pancreatic islet cells, bone and bone marrow, blood and blood vessels, and heart valves. This has given rise to an entirely new field of medicine. You should be familiar with the many terms used in describing transplants and associated procedures. **Cadaveric transplantation** is transplantation of organs from an already deceased person to a living person. **Crossmatch** is the process by which blood compatibility is determined (by mixing blood samples from the donor and recipient). A positive crossmatch means the donor and recipient are not compatible. **Human leukocyte antigens** (also referred to as the *major histocompatibility complex*) are antigens that transplant surgeons attempt to match to prevent incompatibility, which is insufficient similarity between donor and recipient characteristics, particularly blood types and organ types. **Allografting** is transplanting organs or tissues from genetically nonidentical members of the same species. Most medical transplants are allografts. If the transplanted tissue is from a genetically identical person (i.e., identical twin), the process is termed **isografting.** If the transplanted tissue is from a member of a different species, the process is termed **xenografting** (e.g., porcine heart valves, which are harvested from pigs). **Autografting** is transplanting organs or tissues within the same person. This is used when skin or veins are moved from one site to another.

Despite the successes of transplantation surgery, the process can cause significant immune system complications. The immune system, as it is designed to do, recognizes the organ as foreign and attempts to eradicate it from the body through the mechanisms previously discussed. To prevent this, transplant recipients must be immunosuppressed (normal immune function must be hindered) for the remainder of their lives to prevent the native immune system from rejecting the transplanted organ. One exception to this are transplants between identical twins. Unsuccessful immunosuppression can lead to rejection of the transplanted organ. Rejection types are classified as hyperacute, acute, and chronic.

Physicians track histocompatibility antigens, such as ABO blood types and human leukocyte antigens, and try to match them between donor and recipient before transplantation to prevent rejection. However, if preformed antibodies exist in the host, a hyperacute rejection can occur. Preformed antibodies can form through prior exposure to the histocompatability antigen such as from prior transplant, blood transfusions, or pregnancy. These antibodies usually are directed at the vascular endothelium of the transplanted organ, trigger the complement cascade, and are usually IgG or IgM. This is another example of type II (cytotoxic) hypersensitivity, although some researchers also believe components of type IV (delayed) hypersensitivity may be present in hyperacute rejection as well. Effects of hyperacute rejection usually are seen during the operation or in the immediate postoperative period.

Acute rejection occurs within the first months after transplantation. Acute rejection also can occur at any time if immunosuppressive drugs are stopped. Acute rejection represents type IV (delayed) hypersensitivity.

Chronic rejection is characterized by fibrosis and loss of organ function. It occurs over a span of years and represents combined elements of humoral and cell-mediated immunities (type II and type IV hypersensitivities)—precise pathophysiologic processes that are not completely understood.

In all transplant recipients, direct the prehospital history and physical examination at careful evaluation of the function of the transplanted organ. Ask patients about any history of pain, fever, or weight loss in addition to specific questions regarding transplant function. Field treatment is symptomatic. Many transplant recipients require care at a specialty center (usually a tertiary care center) providing posttransplant care and often require transport to these facilities, even for conditions

that might otherwise be cared for at a community facility. Patients and families always should be advised of the importance of rapid medical evaluation for any illness in a transplant recipient. Patients may need to be reminded of the absolute need, given the financial and medical resources dedicated to their transplantation, to avoid lifestyle choices that might endanger the transplanted organ (e.g., tobacco abuse in lung transplants, alcohol abuse in liver transplants).

PARAMEDIC*Pearl*

Rejection rates after transplantation surgery have significantly improved. Kidney transplant rejection currently affects 10% to 15% of patients, with 1-year organ survival of 95% (Benfield, 2002). In heart transplant recipients (in whom infection is a more common cause of death), 1-year survival rate is 85%. Patients average one to two rejection episodes per year (Lyn et al., 2004). The International Society for Heart & Lung Transplantation reports 1-year lung transplant survival rates of 71%. Only 5% of deaths are caused by rejection; more common causes of death include heart failure and graft failure, with the most common cause (35%) being infection (Sharma & Unruh, 2004). Liver transplant recipient survival at 1 year is 86%. As many as 40% of patients have at least one episode of acute rejection during the first 3 months after transplantation (Manzarbeitia, 2005).

Case Scenario **CONCLUSION**

Your partner starts an IV as you complete your assessment and prepare to transport. En route to the hospital you apply the cardiac monitor, which reveals a sinus tachycardia without ectopy. After consultation with medical direction, you administer albuterol by small-volume nebulizer. Little impact is made on the patient's symptoms. The patient's condition is largely unchanged on arrival at the emergency department. After a brief evaluation in the emergency department, the patient is sent to radiography, where he is found to have bilateral pneumonia with a 90% pneumothorax on the left and a 35% pneumothorax on the right. After insertion of bilateral chest tubes (with a tremendous reduction in his dyspnea) the patient is admitted to the intensive care unit with a diagnosis of *Pneumocystis carinii* pneumonia.

Looking Back

9. *Is the pneumothorax related to the patient's pneumonia or his HIV/hepatitis history? How?*
10. *Given the patient's final disposition, was your treatment appropriate? Why or why not?*

FIELD MANAGEMENT OF IMMUNE SYSTEM DISORDERS

Patient Assessment

Patient assessment in immune system disorders, as in all emergency care, is driven by attention to life-threatening conditions. Assess the airway and assist ventilations or intubate the patient as indicated. Give supplemental oxygen and establish an IV line per local protocol. Assess circulation. A complete secondary survey is crucial

because many immune system disorders manifest in the areas not adequately evaluated during the primary survey, such as in the integumentary and GU systems. A complete history is helpful to you, as the paramedic, and the hospital provider who receives your report to assess the patient's current condition adequately. Patient assessment is more completely discussed in Chapter 17.

Patients with immune system disorders require the same meticulous attention to standard precautions and personal protective equipment on your part as all other patients. However, in patients with communicable diseases this becomes even more important for your safety. Some EMS systems recommend double-gloving when caring for patients with blood-borne communicable diseases when invasive procedures are being performed. In every case, sensitivity must be maintained for the patient's situation. The empathetic provider recognizes that many communicable and immune system diseases carry social and medical stigmas, and strict patient confidentiality and professionalism should be maintained at all times.

Treatment Summary

Few specific treatments are available for immune system disorders, with the exception of allergic reactions, which are managed with antihistamines. Further interventions that may be needed for allergic reactions (depending on patient condition) include IV hydration, beta agonists, epinephrine, glucagon, steroids, vasopressors, and oxygen.

PUBLIC HEALTH AND IMMUNITY

Immunization Summary

Immunizations represent a key public health measure to prevent acquired immune system disorders. Immunizations use the immune system to prevent disease; some immunizations also are being developed to prevent immune system disorders. The range of immunizations available, as well as a further discussion of their indications and possible complications, is presented in Chapter 31.

Immunizations Recommended for EMS Providers

EMS professionals are required to have more immunizations than the general public because of their increased exposure to communicable diseases. In addition to the standard childhood vaccinations (such measles, mumps, rubella, and polio), EMS employment also generally requires immunization against hepatitis B. Annual influenza vaccinations are usually recommended, as is maintenance of tetanus toxoid vaccination. Weaponized infectious diseases have become more of a concern after the September 11 terrorist attacks in the United States, and for a brief period smallpox immunization was considered for select EMS providers. Initial interest in widespread smallpox vaccination has waned because of the small but measurable immunization mortality rate, even in selected populations, and cases of immunization-rated deaths in the military when smallpox immunization programs were implemented after the terrorist attacks. EMS professionals involved in specialized response may require additional immunizations. Members of federal disaster medical assistance teams are generally required to maintain hepatitis A immunity, and individuals vaccinated against polio with an oral vehicle are required to obtain injected polio virus. Vaccinations against other potentially weaponized diseases are available, such as anthrax (HBO vaccine, Emergent Biosolutions, Rockport, Md.); these may become more widely used for select EMS providers (e.g., military, disaster, or terrorism response) if bioterrorism activities continue to increase globally.

HIV and Public Health

[OBJECTIVE 26]

HIV is an immune system disorder considered a global public health threat, particularly in developing and impoverished countries. Numerous international, governmental, and nongovernmental agencies are involved in three major efforts to control the spread of this disease: developing mechanisms to reduce transmission, developing treatments to control viral load if the disease is contracted, and developing a vaccine to prevent transmission and ultimately eradicate the disease. Despite this attention HIV infection continues to be epidemic and even pandemic in some parts of the world. The fact that high mortality rates occur in the most productive years of life also has tremendous economic and public health implications for the most heavily affected countries and regions.

Case Scenario SUMMARY

1. *What is your general impression of this patient?* He is a high-priority patient. His two- to three-word dyspnea, coupled with the onset of symptoms during flight, suggest that rapid evaluation and transportation to the emergency department are warranted.

2. *What are some possible causes of this patient's respiratory distress, pallor, and tachypnea?* Several possibilities exist for the patient's sudden onset of respiratory distress, including pulmonary embolus (a relatively high risk related to prolonged flight), spontaneous pneumo-

thorax, allergic reaction or mild anaphylaxis, exacerbation of preexisting respiratory condition (such as asthma), or even anxiety.

3. *Are these symptoms related to the patient's history of HIV and hepatitis? How should you protect yourself?* It is too early to tell. The patient's HIV status places him at risk for almost any infectious disease, some of which result in respiratory compromise and/or distress. HIV is transmitted by blood and body fluids. Adequate protection includes wearing gloves when starting IV lines or

Continued

Case Scenario SUMMARY—continued

coming in contact with body fluids. If the patient is coughing, or you anticipate performing suction or intubation, you also should wear goggles.

4. *What intervention should you initiate at this time?* Initial interventions should include continuation of oxygen therapy, starting an IV, applying a pulse oximeter and cardiac monitor, and performing additional assessment.

5. *Is this patient high priority? Why or why not?* Yes. His two- to three-word dyspnea, retractions, use of accessory muscles, tachycardia, and low SpO$_2$ level all signal significant respiratory distress with hypoxia.

6. *What conditions are consistent with a productive cough, diminished breath sounds, stabbing chest pain, and hypoxia?* Pneumonia is the most likely possibility. Chest pain, cough, and hypoxia also may be caused by pulmonary embolus, but a pulmonary embolus typically does not result in sputum production or breath sound changes. The decreased breath sounds may be the result of consolidation related to pneumonia or may signal the presence of a pneumothorax.

7. *How does the history of HIV and hepatitis fit into the picture?* As previously noted, HIV increases susceptibility to infectious disease. Patients with HIV frequently develop pneumonia. The history of hepatitis B probably is not related.

8. *What treatment will you initiate at this time?* If the patient does have pneumonia (or even a severe upper respiratory tract infection), administering an inhaled bronchodilator may be beneficial, as would increasing oxygen administration. The patient's history and presentation also are consistent with dehydration, so infusion of isotonic fluid is appropriate. The patient's condition should be carefully monitored and, if he develops altered mental status or worsening SpO$_2$, intubation may be considered.

9. *Is the pneumothorax related to the patient's pneumonia or his HIV/hepatitis history? How?* Both. The patient likely began to develop pneumonia 2 to 3 days before his flight. Susceptibility was increased because of his HIV status. His significant respiratory distress and coughing may have caused small tears in his pleura, resulting in development of the pneumothorax. His respiratory distress was likely to increase, as was the size of each pneumothorax, related to the commercial airliner's pressurized environment.

10. *Given the patient's final disposition, was your treatment appropriate? Why or why not?* Yes. Treatment of pneumonia, regardless of the patient's immune status, should include bronchodilation, oxygen administration, and IV fluid infusion.

Chapter Summary

- The immune system includes both internal and external defenses to protect against pathogens.
- Pathogens include prions, viruses, bacteria, parasites, and fungi.
- Internal defenses are divided into natural and acquired immunity. Natural immunity is nonspecific and defends against all potential pathogens in a similar way (e.g., inflammatory response). Acquired immunity is specific to a particular pathogen (e.g., vaccination).
- The immune system can fail, causing immunodeficiencies, which may be acquired or congenital. Congenital immunodeficiencies, such as severe combined immunodeficiency syndrome, are present at birth and often are genetic. Acquired immunodeficiencies, such as HIV, must be transmitted to a patient and usually are infectious.
- Autoimmune diseases are present when the immune system response attacks its own tissue (e.g., MS and SLE).
- Hypersensitivity disorders manifest themselves as excessive responses to an antigen that are uncomfortable or dangerous for the patient. They are divided

into four types: type I (immediate), type II (cytotoxic), type III (immune complex–mediated), and type IV (delayed).

- Anaphylaxis is a good example of type I hypersensitivity. Drug reactions are an example of type II. Poststreptococcal glomerulonephritis is an example of type III, and tuberculosis skin testing is a good example of type IV hypersensitivity.
- Transplant recipients can have two different types of problems involving the immune system. Their immune system can function too well and reject the transplanted organ. On the other hand, when the immune system is suppressed to avoid rejection, other opportunistic infections can develop because of the lack of normal immune response.
- Meticulous attention to personal protective equipment and standard precautions are important when treating all patients, especially those with communicable immune system disorders. This also includes complying with vaccination requirements for health providers and specific missions and encouraging the public to comply with universal vaccination recommendations.

REFERENCES

Abbas, A. K., Lichtman, A. H., & Pober, J. S. (1994). *Cellular and molecular immunology* (2nd ed.) (pp. 5, 21, 23). Philadelphia: W.B. Saunders.

Anderson, R. J. (1997). Rheumatoid arthritis: Clinical and laboratory features. In J. H. Klippel (Ed.). *Primer on the rheumatic diseases* (11th ed.). Atlanta, GA: Arthritis Foundation.

Benfield, M. (2002). Repeated transplant rejection. *aakpRENALIFE, 18,* 2.

Castro, K. G. (1992). Revised classification system for HIV infection and expanded surveillance case definition for AIDS among adolescents and adults. *Morbidity and Mortality Weekly Report, 41,* RR-17.

Centers for Disease Control and Prevention. (1996). Update: Trends in AIDS incidence, death, and prevalence—United States. *Morbidity and Mortality Weekly Report, 46,* 165.

Centers for Disease Control and Prevention. (2005).Update: influenza vaccine supply and recommendations for prioritization during the 2005-06 influenza season. *Morbidity and Mortality Weekly Report, 54*(34), 850.

Davis, J. E. (2005). Allergies and anaphylaxis: Analyzing the spectrum of clinical manifestations. *Emergency Medicine Practice, 7*(10), 19.

Dodds, N., & Sinert, R. (2005). *Angioedema.* Retrieved March 7, 2006, from http://www.emedicine.com.

Gerberding, J. L. (2003). Occupational exposure to HIV in health care settings. *New England Journal of Medicine, 343,* 826.

Glauser, J. (2005). Food allergy. *Emergency Medicine Reports, 26*(5), 1.

HIV Vaccine Trials Network. (2008). *HIV Vaccine Trials Network.* Retrieved June 1, 2008, from http://www.hvtn.org.

Joint United Nations Programme on HIV AIDS/World Health Organization. (2005). *Global summary of the AIDS epidemic.* Retrieved February 14, 2006, from http://www.unaids.org.

Klapproth, J. M., & Yang, V. W. (2005). *Celiac sprue.* Retrieved March 7, 2006, from http://www.emedicine.com.

Klippel, J. H. (Ed.). (1997). *Primer on the rheumatic diseases* (11th ed.). Atlanta, GA: Arthritis Foundation.

Lyn, E. T., Perkins, A. M., & Conrad, S. A. (2004). *Heart transplants.* Retrieved March 7, 2006, from http://www.emedicine.com.

Manzarbeitia, C. (2005). *Liver transplantation.* Retrieved March 7, 2006, from http://www.emedicine.com.

Melvin, A. J., & Mohan, A. M. (2003). Response to immunization with measles, tetanus, and *H. influenza type b* vaccines in children who have human immunodeficiency virus type 1 infection and are treated with highly active antiretroviral therapy. *Pediatrics, 111,* e641.

National Cancer Institute. (2006). *A snapshot of lymphoma.* Retrieved March 7, 2006, from http://planning.cancer.gov.

National Institutes of Health. (2001). *Handout on health: Scleroderma.* Washington, DC: National Institutes of Health.

Panlilio, A. L., Cardo, D. M., Grohskopf, L. A., Heneine W., & Ross, C. S. (2005). Updated U.S. Public Health Service Guidelines for the Management of Occupational Exposures to HIV and Recommendations for Postexposure Prophylaxis. *Morbidity and Mortality Weekly Report, 54*(RR09), 1-17.

Rothman, R. E., Marco, C. A., Yang, S., & Kelen, G. D. (2006). AIDS and HIV. In J. Marx, R. S. Hockberger, & R. M. Walls (Eds.). *Rosen's emergency medicine: Concepts and clinical practice* (pp. 2072-2073, 2087, 2091). Philadelphia: Mosby Elsevier.

Rubin, E. (1994). *Pathology* (pp. 138, 1074). Philadelphia: J.B. Lippincott.

Sercombe, C. T. (2006). Systemic lupus erythematosus and the vasculitides. In J. Marx, R. S. Hockberger, & R. M. Walls (Eds.). *Rosen's emergency medicine: Concepts and clinical practice* (p. 1805). Philadelphia: Mosby Elsevier.

Sharma, S., & Unruh, H. (2004). *Lung transplantation.* Retrieved March 7, 2006, from http://www.emedicine.com.

Stettler, B., & Pancioli, A. M. (2006). Brain and cranial nerve disorders. In J. Marx, R. S. Hockberger, & R. M. Walls (Eds.). *Rosen's emergency medicine: Concepts and clinical practice* (p. 1671). Philadelphia: Mosby Elsevier.

Tan, E. M., Cohen, A. S., Fries, J. F., Masi, A. T., McShane, D. J., Rothfield, N. F., et al. (1982). The 1982 revised criteria for the classification of systemic lupus erythematosus (SLE). *Arthritis and Rheumatism, 25,* 1271.

Tran, T. P. (2006). Allergy, hypersensitivity, and anaphylaxis. In J. Marx, R. S. Hockberger, & R. M. Walls (Eds.). *Rosen's emergency medicine: Concepts and clinical practice* (p. 1819). Philadelphia: Mosby Elsevier.

SUGGESTED RESOURCES

Cydulka, R., & Hancock, M. (2006). Dermatologic presentations. In J. Marx, R. S. Hockberger, & R. M. Walls (Eds.). *Rosen's emergency medicine: Concepts and clinical practice* (p. 1857). Philadelphia: Mosby Elsevier.

Fischer, A. (2000). Severe combined immunodeficiencies (SCID). *Clinical and Experimental Immunology, 122,* 143-149.

Chapter Quiz

1. Antibiotics, as the term is generally used in medicine, are most commonly given to kill _____.

a. bacteria
b. fungi
c. parasites
d. viruses

2. Viruses _____.

a. are motile
b. have a cell wall
c. need to invade other cells to survive and replicate
d. are usually killed by antibiotics

3. Anaphylaxis is an example of which type of hypersensitivity disorder?

a. I
b. II
c. III
d. IV

4. A young adult who already has been exposed to a bacteria is again exposed to the same bacteria. Describe the steps his body takes to prevent a bacterial infection from occurring, from the initial exposure to the elimination of the bacteria. Include the following terms: antigen, antibody, cognitive phase, activation phase, effector phase, lymphocyte, phagocytosis.

Chapter Quiz—continued

5. Which of the following immunizations is currently recommended or required for all EMS providers?
   a. HBO vaccine
   b. Hepatitis B
   c. Smallpox
   d. Varicella

6. Which of the following is considered a possible field treatment for anaphylaxis?
   a. Antibiotic
   b. Antihistamine
   c. Antiviral
   d. Penicillin

7. True or False: If standard antirejection measures are taken after transplant surgery, little attention needs to be paid to typing an organ and its new host before transplantation.

8. Every year anaphylaxis is responsible for _____ of deaths in the United States.
   a. dozens
   b. hundreds
   c. millions
   d. thousands

9. MS is an example of a(n) _____.
   a. acquired immunodeficiency disorder
   b. autoimmune disorder
   c. congenital immunodeficiency disorder
   d. hypersensitivity disorder

10. The GI tract is a part of the body's _____.
    a. external defenses
    b. internal defenses

11. The phase of immune response in which a pathogen is killed is the

    _____.
    a. activation phase
    b. cognitive phase
    c. effector phase
    d. lytic phase

Terminology

Acquired immunity Specific immunity directed at a particular pathogen that develops after the body has been exposed to it once (e.g., immunity to chickenpox after first exposure).

Acquired immunodeficiency syndrome (AIDS) An acquired immunodeficiency disease that can develop after infection with HIV.

Activation phase In phases of immunity, the stage at which a single lymphocyte activates many other lymphocytes and significantly expands the scope of immune response in a process known as amplification.

Active immunity Induced immunity in which the body can continue to mount specific immune response when exposed to the agent (e.g., vaccination).

Allergen A substance that can provoke an allergic reaction.

Allergic reaction An abnormal immune response, mediated by IgE antibodies, to an allergen that should not cause such a response and to which the patient has already been exposed; usually involves excessive release of immune agents, especially histamines.

Allografting Transplanting organs or tissues from genetically nonidentical members of the same species.

Anaphylactoid reaction Reaction that clinically mimics an allergic reaction but is not mediated by IgE antibodies, so not a true allergic reaction.

Anaphylaxis Life-threatening allergic reaction.

Antibacterial Medication that kills or limits bacteria.

Antibiotic In common medical terms, a drug that kills bacteria.

Antibody Agents produced by B lymphocytes that bind to antigens, thus killing or controlling them and slowing or stopping an infection; also called immunoglobulin.

Antifungal Agent that kills fungi.

Antigen A marker on a cell that identifies the cell as "self" or "not self"; antigens are used by antibodies to identify cells that should be attacked as not self.

Antihistamine Medication that reduces the effects of histamine.

Antiviral Medication that kills or impedes a virus.

Attenuated vaccine A vaccine prepared from a live virus or bacteria that has been physically or chemically weakened to produce an immune response without causing the severe effects of the disease.

Autoantibodies Antibodies produced by B cells that mistakenly attack and destroy "self" cells belonging to the patient; autoantibodies are the pathophysiologic agent of most autoimmune disorders.

Autografting Transplanting organs or tissues within the same person.

Bacteria Prokaryotic microorganisms capable of infecting and injuring patients; however, some bacteria, as part of the normal flora, assist in the processes of the human body.

Basophils Type of granulocyte (white blood cell or leukocyte) that releases histamine.

B lymphocytes Cells present in the lymphatic system that mediate humoral immunity (also known as B cells).

Cadaveric transplantation Transplantation of organs from an already deceased person to a living person.

Cell-mediated immunity Form of acquired immunity; results from activation of T lymphocytes that were previously sensitized to a specific antigen.

Cognitive phase In the phases of immune response, the stage at which a foreign antigen is recognized to be present.

Crossmatch The process by which blood compatibility is determined by mixing blood samples from the donor and recipient.

Cytokines Agents produced by many types of cells that control inflammation (e.g., monokines, lymphokines, interleukins, some interferons, and tumor necrosis factor).

Effector phase In phases of immunity, the stage at which the infection is eradicated.

Eosinophils Type of granulocyte (white blood cell or leukocyte) involved in immune response to parasites as well as in allergic responses.

Fungi Plantlike organisms that do not contain chlorophyll; the two classes of fungi are yeasts and molds.

Granulocyte A form of leukocyte that attacks foreign material in the wound.

Histamine A substance released by mast cells that promotes inflammation.

Human immunodeficiency virus (HIV) The virus that can cause AIDS.

Human leukocyte antigen Leukocyte antigen that transplant surgeons attempt to match to prevent incompatibility.

Humoral immunity Immunity from antibodies in the blood.

Hypersensitivity disorder A disorder in which the immune system responds inappropriately and excessively to an antigen (in this response, known as allergens).

Immunodeficiency Deficit in the immune system and its response to infection or injury.

Immunoglobulin See *Antibody*.

Isografting Transplanting tissue from a genetically identical person (i.e., identical twin).

Lymph Fluid that flows through lymphatic ducts and aids in immune response and debris removal.

Lymph nodes Fluid within the lymphatic system.

Lymphadenopathy Swelling of lymph nodes.

Lymphocyte A form of leukocyte.

Lyse To destroy a cell.

Macrophages A monocyte that has matured and localized in one particular type of tissue; active in the immune system by activating agents that kill pathogens, absorbing foreign materials, and slowing infections and infectious agents.

Mold A multicellular type of fungus that grows hyphae.

Monoblasts Immature monocytes.

Monocytes Type of white blood cell (leukocyte) designed to consume foreign material and fight pathogens; generally become macrophages within a few days after release into the bloodstream.

Natural immunity Nonspecific immunity that mounts a generalized response to any foreign material or pathogen (e.g., inflammation).

Natural killer cells Lymphocytes that kill most foreign agents they encounter without specifically identifying them; a classic example of a cell involved in natural immunity response.

Neutrophils A form of granulocyte that is short lived but often first to arrive at the site of injury; capable of phagocytosis.

Pandemic A disease that affects the majority of the population of a single region or that is epidemic at the same time in many different regions.

Parasites An organism that lives within or on another organism (the host) but does not contribute to the host's survival.

Passive immunity Induced immunity that only lasts as long as the injected immune agents are alive and active (e.g., immunoglobulin injection).

Phagocytes A cell that has the ability to ingest and destroy foreign substances.

Phagocytosis Ingestion and digestion of foreign materials by phagocytes (cells, such as macrophages, designed to perform this function).

Pinocytosis Absorption or ingestion of nutrients, debris, and fluids by a cell.

Prions Infectious agents composed of only proteins.

Rejection In terms of organ transplantation, the process by which the body uses its immune system to identify a transplanted organ and kill it; the medical management of posttransplant patients is largely directed at preventing rejection.

T lymphocytes Cells present in the lymphatic system that mediate cell-mediated immunity (also known as T cells).

Urticaria A vascular skin reaction that may appear as part of an allergic response; characterized by wheals and itchiness.

Virus Microorganism that invades cells and uses their machinery to live and replicate; cannot survive without a host, does not have a cell wall of its own, and consists of a strand of DNA or RNA surrounded by a capsid.

Xenografting Transplanting tissue from a member of a different species (e.g., porcine heart valves harvested from pigs).

Yeast A unicellular type of fungus that reproduces by budding.

Gastrointestinal Disorders

Objectives *After completing this chapter, you will be able to:*

1. Describe the incidence, morbidity, and mortality rates of gastrointestinal emergencies.
2. Identify the risk factors most predisposing to gastrointestinal emergencies.
3. Discuss the anatomy and physiology of the organs and structures related to gastrointestinal diseases.
4. Discuss the pathophysiology of inflammation and its relation to acute abdominal pain.
5. Define *somatic pain* as it relates to gastroenterology.
6. Define *visceral pain* as it relates to gastroenterology.
7. Define *referred pain* as it relates to gastroenterology.
8. Differentiate hemorrhagic from nonhemorrhagic abdominal pain.
9. Discuss the signs and symptoms of local inflammation relative to acute abdominal pain.
10. Discuss the signs and symptoms of peritoneal inflammation relative to acute abdominal pain.
11. List the signs and symptoms of general inflammation relative to acute abdominal pain.
12. Based on assessment findings, differentiate local, peritoneal, and general inflammation as they relate to acute abdominal pain.
13. Describe the questioning technique and specific questions the paramedic should ask when gathering a focused history in a patient with abdominal pain.
14. Describe the technique for performing a comprehensive physical examination on a patient with abdominal pain.
15. Define *abdominal wall hernia*.
16. Define *incarcerated hernia*.
17. Define the etiology of an incarcerated hernia.
18. Describe signs and symptoms of an incarcerated hernia.
19. Describe the treatment for an incarcerated hernia.
20. Define *esophagitis*.
21. List the common causes of esophagitis.
22. Describe the signs and symptoms of esophagitis.
23. Describe the treatment of esophagitis.
24. Define *candidiasis of the esophagus*.
25. Describes the etiology of candidiasis esophagitis.
26. Describe the signs and symptoms of candidiasis esophagitis.
27. Describe the treatment for candidiasis esophagitis.
28. Describe gastroesophageal reflux.
29. Define the cause of gastroesophageal reflux.
30. Describe the symptoms of reflux and how they differ from other forms of esophagitis.
31. Describe the treatment for gastroesophageal reflux.
32. Define *caustic substances*.
33. Provide examples of caustic substances.
34. Define the type of necrosis that occurs with acidic and alkali substances.
35. Describe the importance of obtaining a history in caustic ingestion.
36. Describe the pertinent parts of the physical examination in caustic ingestion.
37. Define treatment for caustic ingestion.
38. Define *Boerhaave syndrome*.
39. Describe the signs and symptoms of Boerhaave syndrome.
40. Describe the treatment of Boerhaave syndrome.
41. Define *esophageal foreign body*.
42. Describe the signs and symptoms of esophageal foreign body.
43. Describe the appropriate treatment for esophageal foreign body.
44. Define *hiatal hernia*.
45. Describe the signs and symptoms of a hiatal hernia.
46. Define *Mallory-Weiss syndrome*.
47. Describe the signs and symptoms of Mallory-Weiss syndrome.
48. Describe the appropriate treatment for Mallory-Weiss syndrome.
49. Define *esophageal stricture* and *stenosis*.
50. Describe the signs and symptoms of esophageal stricture and stenosis.
51. Describe the appropriate treatment for esophageal stricture and stenosis.
52. Define *tracheoesophageal fistula*.
53. Describe the signs and symptoms of a tracheoesophageal fistula.
54. Describe the appropriate treatment for tracheoesophageal fistula.
55. Define *esophageal varices*.
56. Discuss the pathophysiology of esophageal varices.
57. Describe the signs and symptoms related to esophageal varices.
58. Describe the appropriate management for esophageal varices.
59. Integrate pathophysiologic principles and assessment findings to formulate a field impression and implement a treatment plan for the patient with esophageal varices.
60. Define *cirrhosis*.
61. Describe the pathophysiology of cirrhosis.
62. Describe the signs and symptoms of cirrhosis.
63. Describe the appropriate treatment of cirrhosis.
64. Define *hepatorenal failure*.
65. Describe the signs and symptoms of hepatorenal failure.

Objectives—continued

66. Describe the appropriate treatment of hepatorenal failure.

67. Define *acute hepatitis*.

68. Discuss the pathophysiology of acute hepatitis.

69. Recognize the signs and symptoms related to acute hepatitis.

70. Describe the management of acute hepatitis.

71. Integrate pathophysiologic principles and assessment findings to formulate a field impression and implement a treatment plan for the patient with acute hepatitis.

72. Define *hepatic tumors*.

73. Describe the signs and symptoms of hepatic tumors.

74. Describe the appropriate treatment of hepatic tumors.

75. Define *cholecystitis, cholelithiasis, cholangitis,* and *choledocholithiasis*.

76. Discuss the pathophysiology of cholecystitis.

77. Recognize the signs and symptoms related to cholecystitis.

78. Describe the management of cholecystitis.

79. Integrate pathophysiologic principles and assessment findings to formulate a field impression and implement a treatment plan for the patient with cholecystitis.

80. Define *pancreatitis*.

81. Discuss the pathophysiology of pancreatitis.

82. Recognize the signs and symptoms related to pancreatitis.

83. Describe the management of pancreatitis.

84. Integrate pathophysiologic principles and assessment findings to formulate a field impression and implement a treatment plan for the patient with pancreatitis.

85. Define *pancreatic tumors*.

86. Define *adenocarcinoma, cyst adenoma,* and *neuroendocrine tumors*.

87. Describe the signs and symptoms of pancreatic tumors.

88. Describe the appropriate treatment of pancreatic tumors.

89. Define *peritonitis*.

90. Describe the signs and symptoms of peritonitis.

91. Describe the appropriate treatment for peritonitis.

92. Define *gastritis*.

93. Describe signs and symptoms of gastritis.

94. Describe the appropriate treatment for gastritis.

95. Define *peptic ulcer disease*.

96. Discuss the pathophysiology of peptic ulcer disease.

97. Recognize the signs and symptoms related to peptic ulcer disease.

98. Describe the management of peptic ulcer disease.

99. Integrate pathophysiologic principles and assessment findings to formulate a field impression and implement a treatment plan for the patient with peptic ulcer disease.

100. Define *upper gastrointestinal bleeding*.

101. Discuss the pathophysiology of upper gastrointestinal bleeding.

102. Recognize the signs and symptoms related to upper gastrointestinal bleeding.

103. Describe the management of upper gastrointestinal bleeding.

104. Integrate pathophysiologic principles and assessment findings to formulate a field impression and implement a treatment plan for the patient with upper gastrointestinal bleeding.

105. Define *lower gastrointestinal bleeding*.

106. Discuss the pathophysiology of lower gastrointestinal bleeding.

107. Recognize the signs and symptoms related to lower gastrointestinal bleeding.

108. Describe the management of lower gastrointestinal bleeding.

109. Integrate pathophysiologic principles and assessment findings to formulate a field impression and implement a treatment plan for the patient with lower gastrointestinal bleeding.

110. Define *acute gastroenteritis*.

111. Discuss the pathophysiology of acute gastroenteritis.

112. Recognize the signs and symptoms related to acute gastroenteritis.

113. Describe the management of acute gastroenteritis.

114. Integrate pathophysiologic principles and assessment findings to formulate a field impression and implement a treatment plan for the patient with acute gastroenteritis.

115. Define *bowel obstruction*.

116. Discuss the pathophysiology of bowel obstruction.

117. Recognize the signs and symptoms related to bowel obstruction.

118. Describe the management of bowel obstruction.

119. Integrate pathophysiologic principles and assessment findings to formulate a field impression and implement a treatment plan for the patient with bowel obstruction.

120. Define *appendicitis*.

121. Discuss the pathophysiology of appendicitis.

122. Recognize the signs and symptoms related to appendicitis.

123. Describe the management of appendicitis.

124. Integrate pathophysiologic principles and assessment findings to formulate a field impression and implement a treatment plan for the patient with appendicitis.

125. Define *colitis*.

126. Discuss the pathophysiology of colitis.

127. Recognize the signs and symptoms related to colitis.

128. Describe the management of colitis.

129. Integrate pathophysiologic principles and assessment findings to formulate a field impression and implement a treatment plan for the patient with colitis.

130. Define *Crohn's disease*.

131. Discuss the pathophysiology of Crohn's disease.

132. Recognize the signs and symptoms related to Crohn's disease.

133. Describe the management of Crohn's disease.

134. Integrate pathophysiologic principles and assessment findings to formulate a field impression and implement a treatment plan for the patient with Crohn's disease.

135. Define *diverticulitis*.

136. Discuss the pathophysiology of diverticulitis.

137. Recognize the signs and symptoms related to diverticulitis.

138. Describe the management of diverticulitis.

139. Integrate pathophysiologic principles and assessment findings to formulate a field impression and implement a treatment plan for the patient with diverticulitis.

140. Define *hemorrhoids.*
141. Discuss the pathophysiology of hemorrhoids.
142. Recognize the signs and symptoms related to hemorrhoids.
143. Describe the management of hemorrhoids.
144. Integrate pathophysiologic principles and assessment findings to formulate a field impression and implement a treatment plan for the patient with hemorrhoids.

145. Integrate pathophysiologic principles of the patient with a gastrointestinal emergency.
146. Differentiate gastrointestinal emergencies on the basis of assessment findings.
147. Correlate abnormal findings in the assessment with the clinical significance in the patient with abdominal pain.
148. Develop a patient management plan based on field impression in the patient with abdominal pain.

Chapter Outline

Anatomy and Physiology
Assessment
Management
Abdominal Wall Hernias
Esophageal Disorders
Hepatic Disorders

Biliary Disorders
Pancreatic Disorders
Stomach Disorders
Bowel Disorders
Gastrointestinal Illness
Chapter Summary

Case Scenario

You and your partner are called to a private residence around 10:00 PM on a midsummer night. On arriving at the residence, you are greeted by a concerned man who states that he thinks his wife is having a heart attack. He leads you into the master bedroom, where you find a 42-year-old Hispanic woman complaining of epigastric pain radiating to her back and chest. She states, "It's really bad and I can hardly catch my breath." A brief assessment reveals a middle-aged, slightly overweight woman sitting on her bed, propped up by several pillows. She appears to be in acute distress. Her skin is warm and dry. A quick assessment of her radial pulse reveals a strong pulse with no irregularity.

Questions

1. *What is your initial impression?*
2. *What do you think could be causing the woman's chest pain?*
3. *What additional information do you need to complete your assessment?*

RMC d Transport !

[OBJECTIVES 1, 2]

Abdominal pain often is the first sign of a gastrointestinal (GI) disorder. It also may be the only sign. Abdominal pain is among the most common reasons why patients seek emergency care, accounting for up to 10% of emergency department visits (Marx et al., 2006). Approximately 7% of all patients who have abdominal pain may have a life-threatening condition. Older adults and immunocompromised patients are at increased risk for serious morbidity and mortality (Marx et al., 2006). The etiology of GI disease varies with age and individual risk factors. However, abdominal pain and disorders of the GI tract can affect almost anyone at almost any time. Therefore you should be well acquainted with the anatomy, physiologic features, and pathologic conditions of the GI system.

ANATOMY AND PHYSIOLOGY

[OBJECTIVES 3 TO 12]

The GI tract includes all structures involved in eating and processing food, including the degradation of food, absorption of nutrients, and elimination of waste. Starting from the pharynx, the esophagus proceeds distally through the chest cavity, passes through the diaphragm, and terminates at the stomach (Figure 26-1). The esophagus is a hollow muscular organ that contracts as swallowed food moves downward from the mouth to the stomach. It lies posterior to the trachea and is a compressible structure. It begins to the right of the aorta and then passes anterior to the aorta as it traverses inferiorly.

The stomach lies just inferior to the diaphragm in the left upper quadrant of the abdomen. It is partially covered

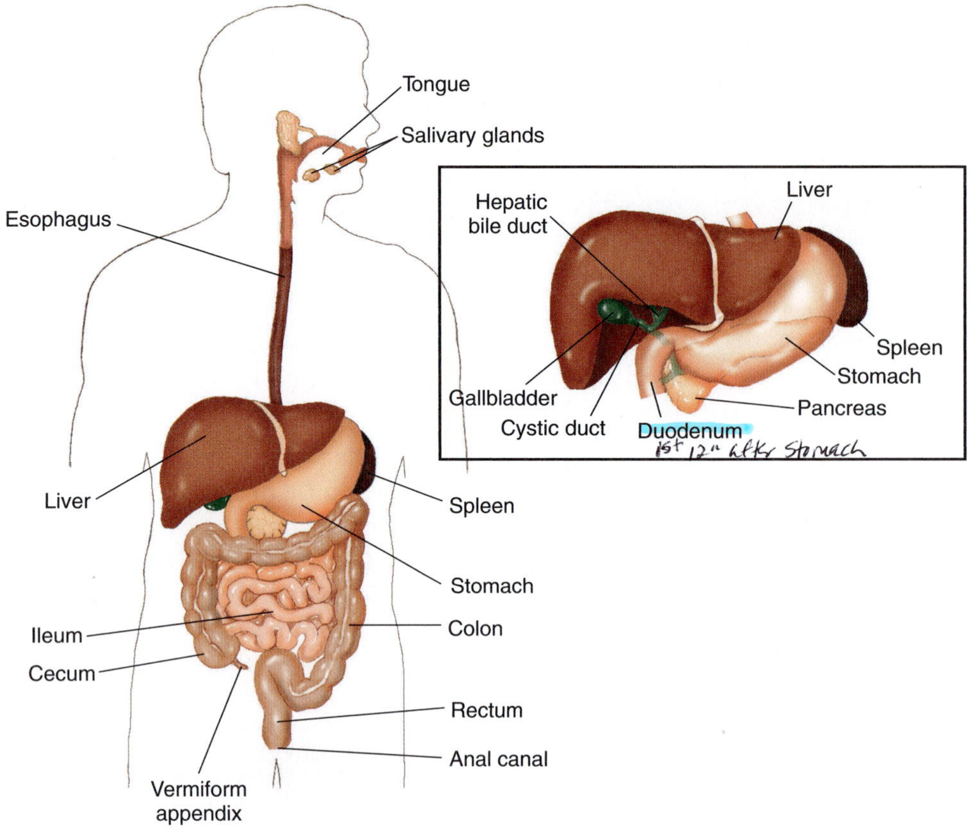

Tongue

Salivary glands

Esophagus

Hepatic bile duct

Liver

Spleen

Stomach

Pancreas

Gallbladder

Cystic duct

Duodenum
1st 12" after stomach

Liver

Spleen

Stomach

Colon

Ileum

Cecum

Rectum

Anal canal

Vermiform appendix

Figure 26-1 Anatomy of the gastrointestinal tract.

21 ft. of small intestine
5 ft. of large intestine

by the left lobe of the liver and protected by the ribcage. As food passes from the stomach, it enters the duodenum through the pyloric sphincter. The duodenum is the first part of the small intestine. Here nutrients are absorbed as food moves through the small intestine by muscular contractions called **peristalsis.** The food then progresses from the duodenum through the jejunum and ileum. The ligament of Treitz is located at the junction of the duodenum and jejunum. The appendix is a small appendage that arises from the initial part of the colon. This portion of the bowel can become inflamed and infected.

rhythmic

Next, food enters the large intestine or colon, where water is absorbed and bacteria break down ingested food into nutrients (Figure 26-2). The small intestine is a long structure, 6 to 7 m, curled back and forth within the abdominal cavity. The colon, by comparison, is relatively short, at approximately 1.5 m long. The large intestine is further subdivided into the ascending, transverse, and descending colon (Figures 26-3 to 26-5).

The remaining byproducts of ingested food are considered waste products. The term **feces** is used for the undigested food particles that travel through the descending colon. The feces then progress to the sigmoid colon and then through the rectum to exit the body by the anus.

Also considered part of the GI system are the various other organs involved in the digestion of food and elimination of waste, such as the liver, gallbladder, and pan-

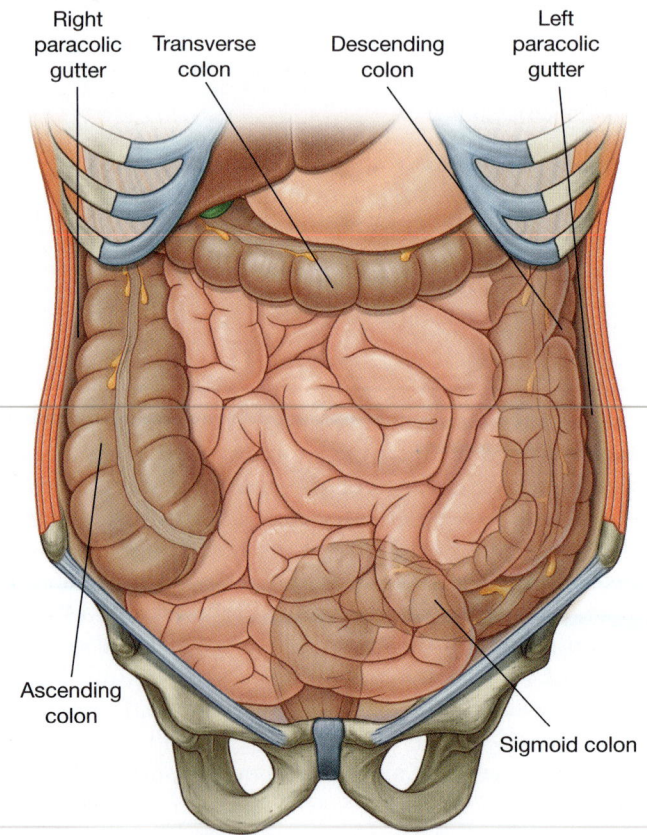

Right paracolic gutter

Transverse colon

Descending colon

Left paracolic gutter

Ascending colon

Sigmoid colon

Figure 26-2 The small and large colon.

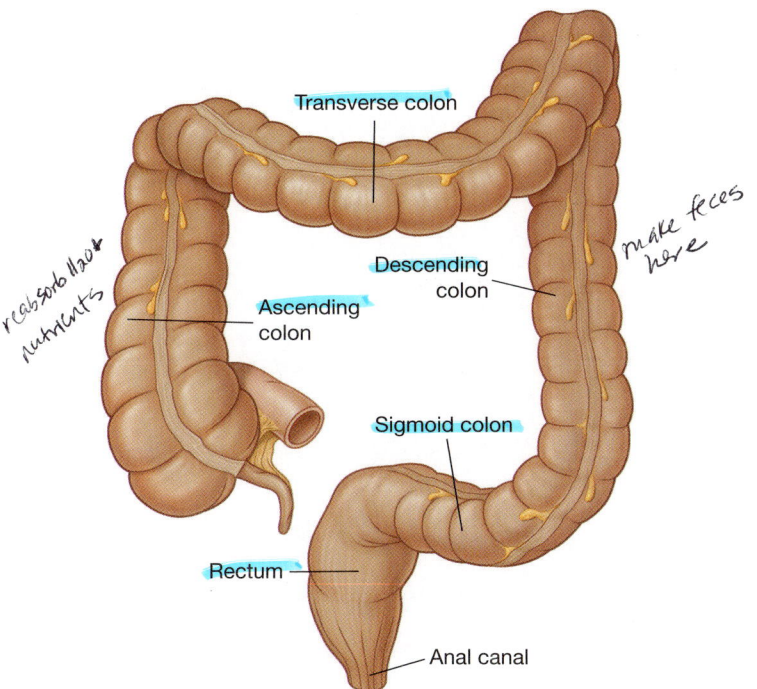

reabsorb H2O nutrients (handwritten)
make feces here (handwritten)

Figure 26-3 The colon.

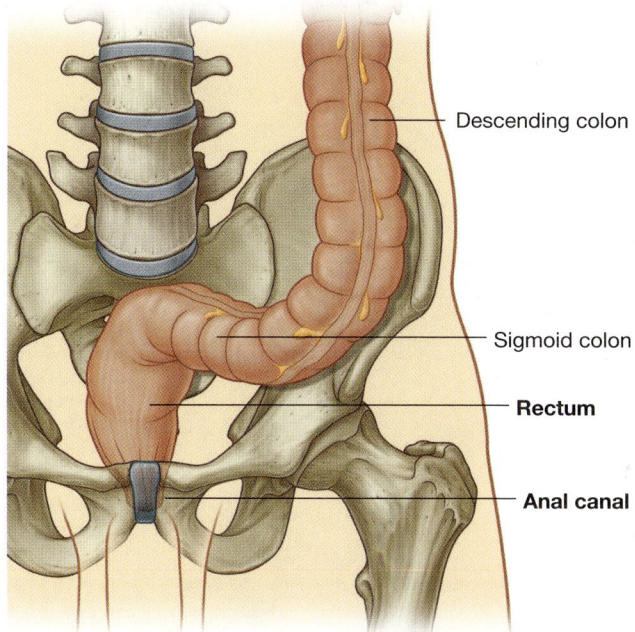

Figure 26-5 Descending colon, rectum, and anal canal.

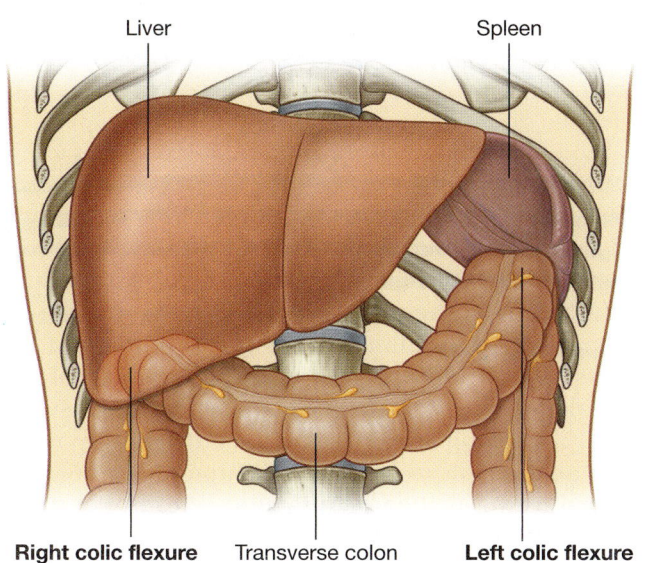

Figure 26-4 Transverse colon.

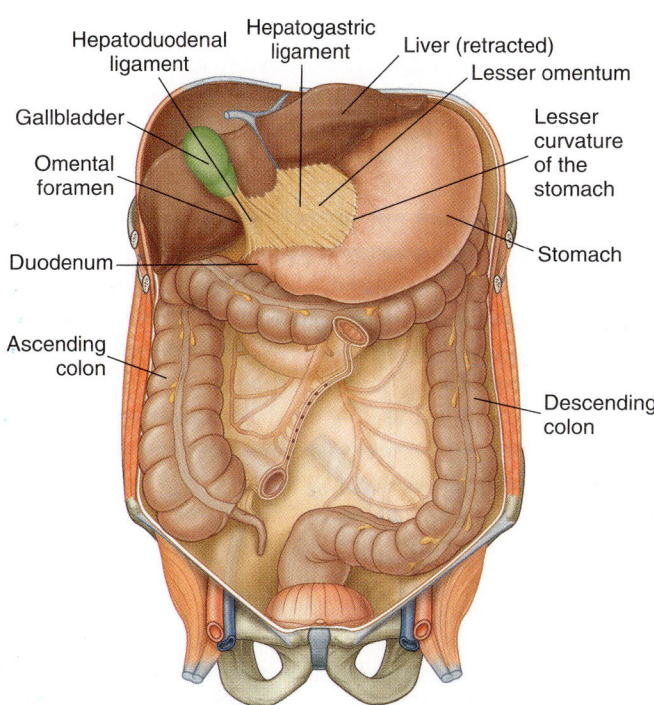

Figure 26-6 Liver, gallbladder, and stomach.

creas (Figures 26-6 and 26-7). The liver is a complex organ with many functions. It is responsible for the maintenance of blood glucose. It also is responsible for detoxification of drugs, hormones, and other foreign substances. The liver produces plasma proteins that aid in blood clotting. Bile salts are produced in this organ that help with the digestion of ingested food. The gallbladder is a small pouch located near the liver that stores bile. Bile is produced in the liver and is necessary to digest fats in ingested food. Bile is expelled through the common bile duct into the duodenum. The sphincter of Odi is located at the end of the common bile duct and regulates the movement of

bile into the duodenum. The pancreas is located in the mid-epigastric region. The pancreas is unique in that it performs both endocrine and exocrine functions. Through its endocrine functions it is responsible for the synthesis of glucagon, insulin, and somatostatin. Glucagon and insulin are critical in the maintenance of blood glucose. Its exocrine functions include the production of pancreatic digestive juices (pancreatic amylase, trypsin, chymotrypsin, and carboxypeptidase), which aid in the digestion

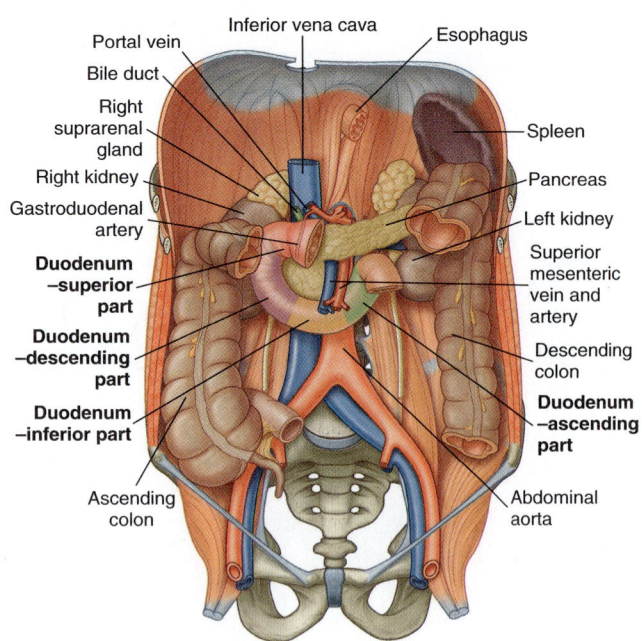

Figure 26-7 Abdominal contents.

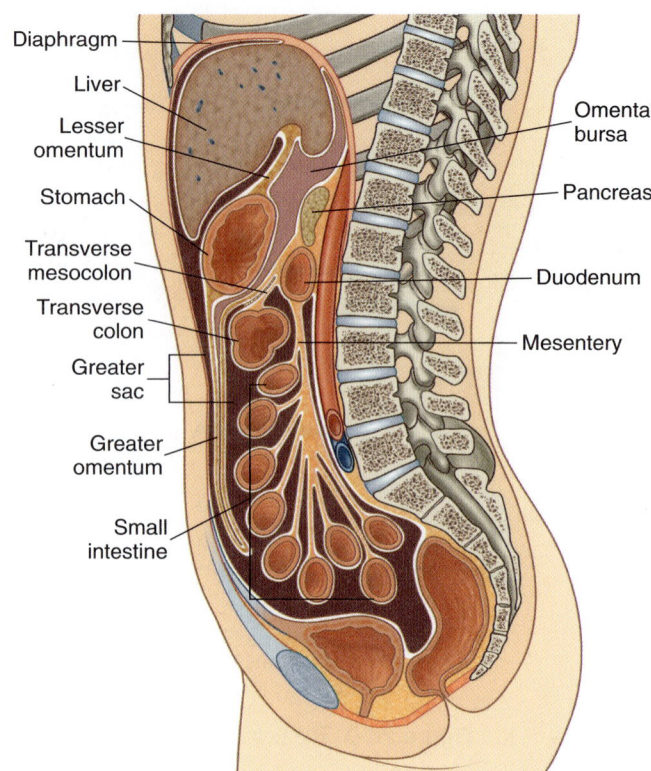

Figure 26-8 Omentum.

of carbohydrates, fats, proteins, and nucleic acids. The pancreatic duct expels these substances at its junction with the duodenum that is adjacent to the opening of the common bile duct. Indicators of pancreatic failure include foul-smelling stool that contains undigested material.

Most of the intraabdominal structures are covered by a thin layer of tissue called the **peritoneum.** The peritoneum is composed of two parts: the parietal peritoneum, which lines the walls of the abdominal cavity, and the visceral peritoneum, which covers the organs within the abdominal cavity. The potential space between these two layers is the peritoneal cavity. The abdominal organs are suspended within the abdominal cavity by folds of peritoneum called **mesentery** (Figure 26-8). The mesentery contains the nerves, arteries, veins, and lymph vessels that supply the intestines and other intraabdominal structures.

Abdominal pain may be classified as one of three categories: visceral pain, somatic pain, and referred pain. **Visceral pain** is deep pain caused by activation of pain receptors in internal areas of the body that are enclosed within a cavity, such as the chest, abdomen, or pelvis. Visceral sensory nerve fibers travel with autonomic nerves to communicate with the central nervous system (Figure 26-9). The pain is usually dull and poorly localized in the midline—epigastrium, periumbilical region, or lower mid-abdomen—because abdominal organs transmit sensory nerve signals to both sides of the spinal cord (Figure 26-10) (Feldman, 2006). Visceral pain is generally described as cramping, burning, or gnawing and often is accompanied by sweating, restlessness, nausea, vomiting, perspiration, and pallor. The patient may move about in an effort to relieve the discomfort.

Somatic pain is caused by the activation of pain receptors in the cutaneous tissues of the body's surface or deep tissues of the body, such as musculoskeletal tissue or parietal peritoneum. In contrast to visceral pain, somatic pain is generally more intense and more precisely localized (Feldman, 2006). The discomfort that accompanies acute appendicitis is an example of both visceral and somatic pain associated with the GI system. In early acute appendicitis, the patient typically reports vague abdominal pain in the area around the umbilicus (visceral pain). As the inflammation spreads, the patient is able to localize the pain in the right lower quadrant of the abdomen (somatic pain).

Referred pain is pain perceived as occurring in one part of the body other than its true source (Figure 26-11). This occurs frequently with GI disorders. For example, pain from gallbladder disease often is described as, or accompanied by, pain in the right shoulder.

Disorders of the GI tract commonly encountered in the prehospital setting are hemorrhage and **inflammation.** Hemorrhage can occur from trauma and may result in rupture of a solid or hollow organ. Solid organs such as the liver or spleen are covered with a tough, fibrous capsule. This capsule can become distended from bleeding, causing considerable pain. Hollow organs also can bleed. This can occur from a bleeding ulcer or from rupture. Blood can be irritating to the abdominal

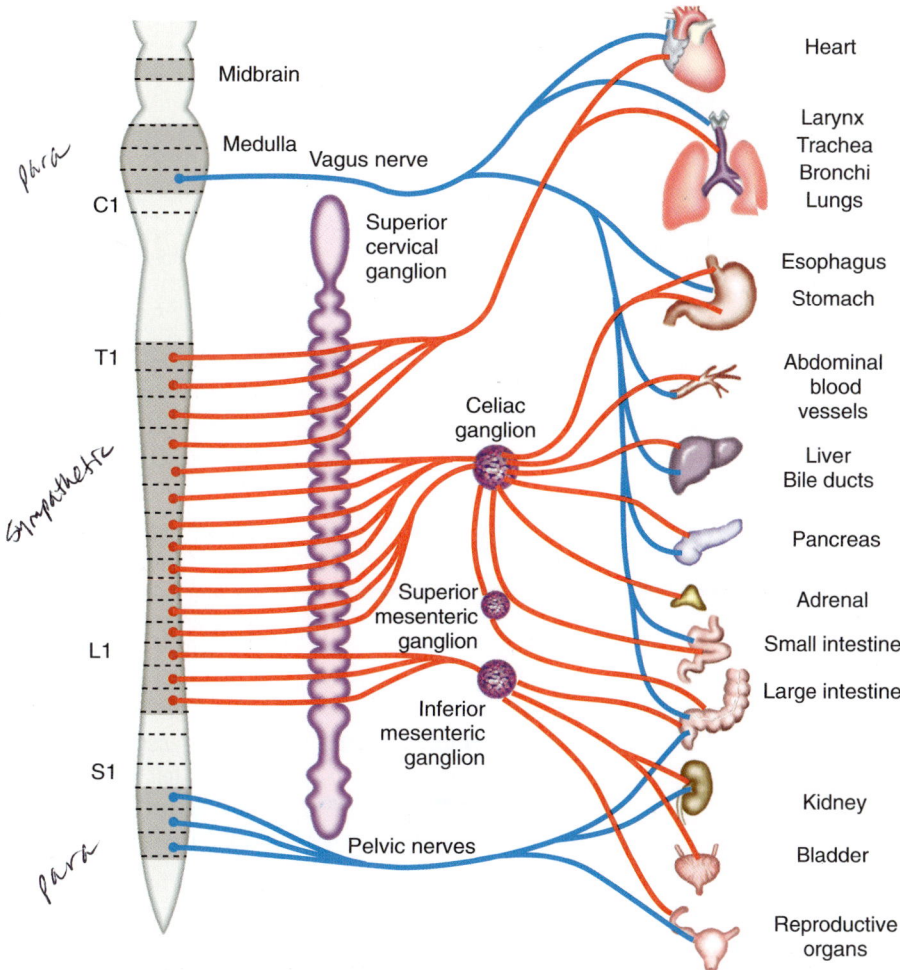

Figure 26-9 Pathways of visceral sensory nerve innervation. Visceral nerve fibers mediating pain travel with autonomic nerves to communicate with the central nervous system. In the abdomen, these include both vagal and pelvic parasympathetic nerves and thoracolumbar sympathetic nerves. Sympathetic fibers are shown as *red lines;* parasympathetic fibers are shown as *blue lines.*

lining and the organs. Patients may have bleeding or pain.

Inflammation is another common cause of pain in GI disorders. It is caused by the body's reaction to injury. Common causes of inflammation include infection, chemical irritation, toxins, and autoimmune conditions. The source and location of inflammation can be important in determining the cause of the disorder. Signs and symptoms are helpful in the treatment of GI disorders. Local inflammation may be poorly localized and described by the patient as a vague, dull ache. It is usually described as originating from deep within the abdomen. Reproducing the pain may be difficult during palpation or percussion of the abdomen. Diffuse inflammation occurs when the surrounding peritoneum has been affected. Palpation or percussion of the abdominal wall irritates the parietal peritoneum and causes increased abdominal pain.

ASSESSMENT

[OBJECTIVES 12, 13, 14]

When assessing a patient with abdominal symptoms, first obtain an adequate history and a thorough physical examination. The importance of an adequate history cannot be emphasized enough. In the patient with abdominal symptoms, the history is as valuable, if not more so, than the physical examination. Because pain is the most common GI complaint, a complete description of the patient's pain is appropriate. At a minimum, the paramedic must determine the time of onset, the speed of onset, activity at onset, the location and character of the pain, the progression of the pain, and any radiation of the pain. This can be described by the OPQRST mnemonic discussed in Chapter 17 and provided in Box 26-1. Determining whether the pain is constant or intermittent can provide valuable information. Constant pain is often

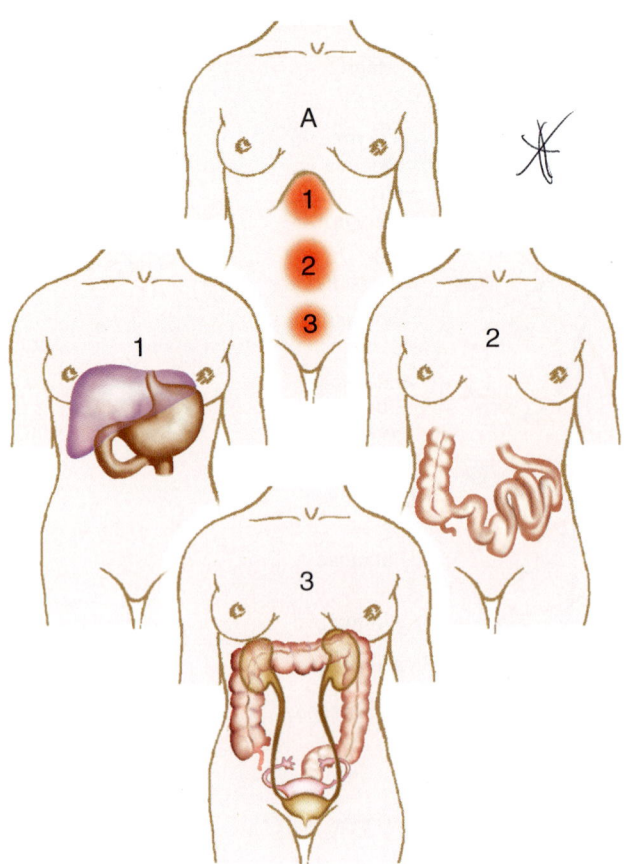

Figure 26-10 Localization of visceral pain. Pain arising from organ areas shown in *1, 2,* and *3* is felt in the epigastrium, mid-abdomen, and hypogastrium (the middle portion of the most inferior region of the abdomen), respectively, as shown at *A.*

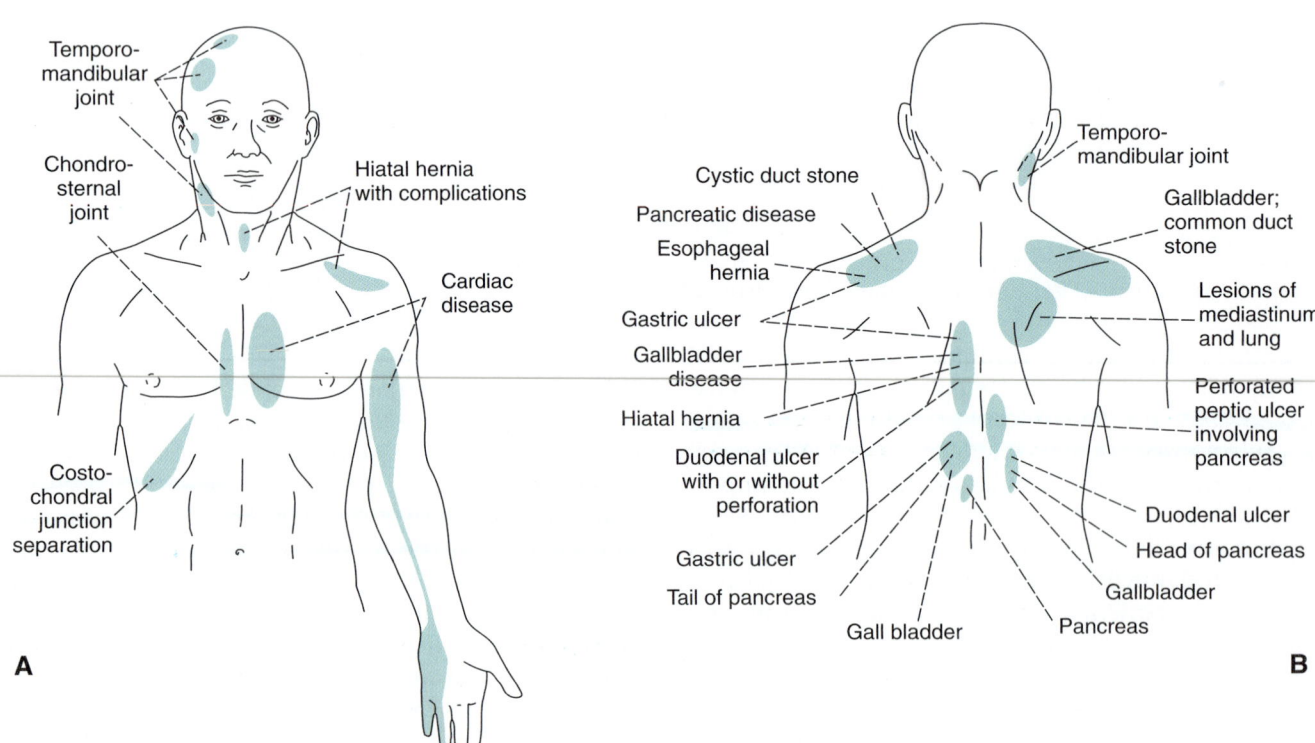

Figure 26-11 Patterns of referred pain from visceral and somatic structures. **A,** Anterior distribution. **B,** Posterior distribution.

| **BOX 26-1** | **OPQRST Mnemonic** |

Onset
Provocation, **p**alliation, **p**osition
Quality
Radiation, **r**adiation
Severity
Timing (duration)

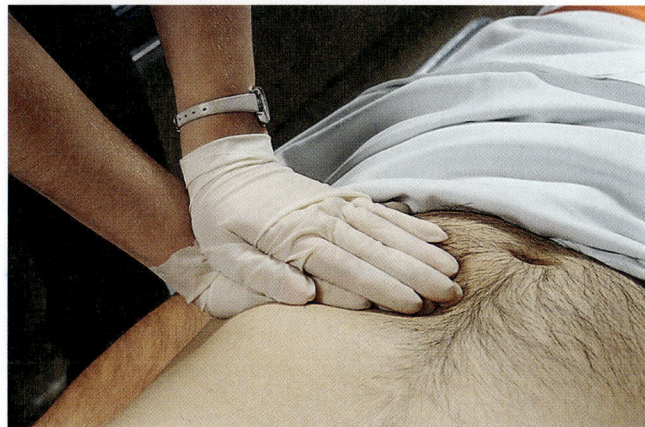

Figure 26-12 Palpation of the abdominal quadrants.

associated with inflammation of a solid organ, ischemia, or peritonitis, whereas intermittent pain often is associated with an obstructed hollow organ. Pain from peritoneal irritation is associated with rigidity of the abdominal wall and intensifies when the patient coughs or moves. The patient's activity, or lack thereof, can also provide important clues. The patient with peritonitis typically lies still, but the patient with ischemia of the bowel often moves about, trying to find a comfortable position.

Additional information should be elicited, such as the presence or absence of associated symptoms that often accompany GI disorders: nausea, vomiting, diarrhea, constipation, or bleeding. Inquire about family history, past medical problems, social history, and the use of medications and drugs. Questions should be open ended. That is, the patient should be encouraged to describe the symptoms in his or her own words. For example, a patient with vomiting should be asked an open-ended question such as, "What does the vomitus look like?" instead of a closed-ended question such as, "Is there any blood in your vomitus?" Questioning also is usually more informative and meaningful if it progresses from the general to the specific.

Physical assessment of the patient with GI symptoms follows the same basic sequence as outlined in Chapter 17. The examination should begin with inspection, followed by auscultation, palpation, and percussion. Alternatively, this may be described as the look, listen, and feel approach. The patient's airway, breathing, and circulation (ABCs) and any other immediately life- or limb-threatening conditions must be addressed before obtaining a complete history and physical examination for any medical problem.

Inspection involves looking at the abdomen and pelvis. These body areas should be evaluated for distention, bruising, swelling, scars, pulsations, or discoloration. Next auscultate the abdomen. Gently place the stethoscope on the abdominal wall. This step should be performed once in each of the four abdominal quadrants. As peristalsis moves food through the intestines, the resulting displacement of solids, fluid, and air can be heard as a gurgling sound when the stethoscope is applied to the anterior abdominal wall. With some practice, the pitch and timbre of normal bowel sounds can be learned. A partial bowel obstruction may force the intestinal contents through a smaller than usual luminal opening, resulting in bowel sounds of a higher than normal pitch.

Conversely, a complete bowel obstruction may result in absent bowel sounds because no contents are moving through the occluded lumen. Some conditions, such as hemorrhage, lead to an increased rate of peristalsis and hyperactive bowel sounds, whereas others, such as **ileus,** lead to decreased peristalsis and hypoactive bowel sounds.

If such abnormalities of auscultation are understood, they provide valuable clues regarding the etiology of the patient's problem. However, two conditions may limit the usefulness of prehospital auscultation. First, in the noisy and uncontrolled prehospital environment hearing bowel sounds clearly may be difficult. Second, abnormal bowel sounds are a late finding in many GI disorders, and the patient can have significant disease and still have normal bowel sounds. Despite these two caveats, prehospital auscultation is a valuable skill and should be part of the assessment for all patients with abdominal symptoms.

Palpation is probably the mainstay of the assessment of the patient with abdominal pain or other GI symptoms (Figure 26-12). As previously mentioned, tenderness can be either localized or diffuse depending on the etiology and location of the disorder. However, the presence or absence of tenderness is not the only valuable information to be obtained from palpation of the abdomen. The presence of guarding, masses, organomegaly, or rebound tenderness also should be evaluated at this stage of the physical examination.

Guarding is the conscious or unconscious tensing of the abdominal wall muscles. This often occurs when a patient believes pain will occur with the act of palpation. Its presence often indicates a significant pathologic condition under the involved area. Abdominal rigidity is much more serious than involuntary guarding. **Rebound tenderness** (or often simply *rebound*) denotes the finding that an irritated peritoneum often hurts more when the abdominal wall relaxes back to its original position than it did when it was first compressed. This can be elicited by asking the patient, "Which hurts more, when I press or when I let go?" while palpating the abdomen. Alter-

Bowel sounds 2-37 x/min
usually don't auscult in field

natively, tenderness on percussion of the abdomen also indicates peritoneal irritation.

In addition, the presence of any abnormal mass or enlargement of any organ on the abdominal examination is an important physical finding and may provide direction to isolating the cause of the patient's symptoms. Palpation of the abdomen also can yield valuable clues to other, non-GI-related diseases as well, such as the presence of a pulsatile abdominal mass associated with an abdominal aortic aneurysm.

Finally, percuss the abdomen. **Percussion** is not always taught to prehospital professionals, but it is simple to learn and provides valuable information. The technique is described in Chapter 17. Similar to auscultation, a little practice will teach the provider to appreciate the sound of a normal percussion note. If the intestines are filled with more air than usual, then a **hyperresonant** or tympanitic percussion note may be heard. Excess fluid in the abdominal cavity may result in dullness to percussion.

On the basis of the findings of the physical examination, assess for any disease-specific findings as appropriate for your differential diagnoses. This may include Murphy's sign, rebound tenderness, Rovsing's sign, psoas sign, obturator sign, cutaneous hyperesthesia, Cullen's sign, Grey Turner's sign, and Kehr's sign (Table 26-1).

MANAGEMENT

Although the GI system is complex, the prehospital management is straightforward. GI problems can be severe, but few (with the exception of active bleeding) are immediately life-threatening. Your goal is to determine the presence of an acute abdominal emergency with the assessment tools described above. Although these tools may provide valuable clues regarding the etiology of the patient's symptoms, rarely is an exact diagnosis possible or even desirable in the field. Instead, your job is to recognize the existence of any serious GI or abdominal problem. Treatment should begin with

TABLE 26-1	Specific Abdominal Signs	
Sign	**Indication**	**Procedure**
Murphy's sign	Cholecystitis	Place the fingers under the right costal margin as the patient exhales. As the patient inhales, a positive finding is an abrupt cessation in inhalation caused by pain.
Rebound tenderness	Peritoneal irritation	Depress the abdomen. A positive finding is an increase in pain on release of the abdominal wall.
Rovsing's sign	Appendicitis	Apply pressure to the left lower quadrant. A positive finding is the presence of pain in the right lower quadrant.
Psoas sign	Appendicitis	With the patient supine place your hand above the right knee and have the patient raise the leg. Increased abdominal pain is a positive finding.
Obturator sign	Appendicitis	With the patient supine, have the patient flex the right leg at the hip and knee. Apply lateral pressure to the knee and rotate the lower leg laterally. This causes internal rotation of the femur. An increase in abdominal pain is a positive finding.
Cutaneous hyperesthesia	Appendicitis	Lift folds of skin on the abdomen without pinching. A painful response in the right lower quadrant is a positive finding.
Cullen's sign	Periumbilical hemorrhage	Check for bluish discoloration of the umbilicus.
Grey-Turner's sign	Hemorrhagic pancreatitis	Check for bruising over the flanks.
Kehr's sign	Splenic hemorrhage	Referred pain in the left shoulder. (Pain may refer to the right shoulder as a result of hemorrhage of the liver, but this finding does not have a specific name)
Fothergill's sign	Differentiation of intraabdominal pain and masses versus pain and masses located in the abdominal wall	Have the patient tense the abdominal muscles while you palpate the abdomen. A decrease in pain or a disappearing mass indicates intraabdominal origin. An increase in pain or a mass that is still palpable indicates an origin in the abdominal wall.

a primary survey. Immediately address the ABCs and treat any life-threatening conditions, such as shock. Next address comfort measures, including pharmacologic treatment (per local protocol) of pain and nausea. The patient should be transported safely and comfortably to the nearest appropriate receiving facility.

Case Scenario—continued

The patient states that she has no medical history or allergies, and she is not taking any medication except birth control pills. She tells you that she was taking a shower when the pain started. She initially felt the pain just above her stomach and points to the area of her xyphoid process. She further states that the pain moved up to her chest and taking a breath became difficult. When asked, the patient rates her discomfort as an 8 on a 10-point scale. She tells you that nothing she does helps ease the pain. Her vital signs are as follows: pulse, 96 beats/min and regular; respirations, 22 breaths/min and shallow; and blood pressure, 118/88 mm Hg. Breath sounds are equal bilaterally. Your partner has placed the patient on supplemental oxygen, applied the cardiac monitor, and obtained a 12-lead ECG. You observe an ECG that appears normal in all 12 leads. The monitor shows a sinus rhythm with no ectopy or evidence of ST-segment changes. On the basis of the patient's report of chest pain, you administer aspirin and sublingual nitroglycerin. The patient's condition does not change, although she tells you that she now has a headache.

Questions

4. Has your initial impression changed?
5. What other conditions may mimic an acute myocardial infarction or give the impression that one has occurred?
6. What are your treatment options for this patient?

ABDOMINAL WALL HERNIAS

[OBJECTIVES 15, 16, 17, 18, 19]

An abdominal (or ventral) **hernia** occurs when the intraabdominal contents, usually the small intestines, protrude through a weakness or defect in the muscles of the abdominal wall. These defects can be either congenital or acquired. Common causes of acquired weakness in the abdominal wall include age, obesity, and prior abdominal surgery. Although often large, occasionally painful, and of great concern to patients, abdominal wall hernias are seldom dangerous. They only present a problem if they become **incarcerated.** This occurs when the abdominal contents will not return through the defect into the abdominal cavity. These cases require rapid evaluation and treatment because they can lead to **strangulation,** a condition in which the blood supply to the involved area is stopped, putting the bowel at risk for ischemia and infarction. This is a true emergency and requires prompt surgical evaluation.

The hernia itself is usually easy to diagnose because it is visible. Incarceration is recognized by the patient's history; he or she will describe a hernia that will not "go back in." As the incarcerated bowel swells and the blood supply decreases, the patient may become systemically ill with abdominal pain, fever, nausea, vomiting, and other signs of obstruction, such as the absence of bowel movements or flatus. The signs and symptoms of an incarcerated hernia are similar to those of small bowel obstruction, appendicitis, colitis, and peritonitis.

Do not attempt to reduce a possible incarcerated hernia. Supportive care, intravenous (IV) fluids, and rapid transport to an appropriate receiving facility are the proper treatments for a possible incarcerated or strangulated abdominal hernia. Reducible ventral hernias require no specific prehospital treatment.

ESOPHAGEAL DISORDERS

[OBJECTIVES 20, 21, 22, 23]

Esophagitis

Esophagitis refers to any inflammation or infection of the esophagus (Figure 26-13). Common causes include candidiasis, infection, caustic ingestions, esophageal reflux, and esophageal rupture. Pill esophagitis is estimated to occur in 10,000 people each year (Marx et al., 2006). This occurs when a patient swallows a pill but it becomes lodged in the esophagus. As the pill erodes, it can cause inflammation of the esophagus. The occurrence of esophagitis is increased in patients with diabetes, HIV, alcoholism, or cancer; patients who are pregnant; and patients who take corticosteroids. Esophagitis is associated with burning in the center of the thorax. This pain gets worse with swallowing, which may become difficult. Although uncomfortable, most forms of esophagitis (caustic ingestions being one important exception) are not dangerous.

Taking a thorough history is important. The patient may provide information on medical problems related to

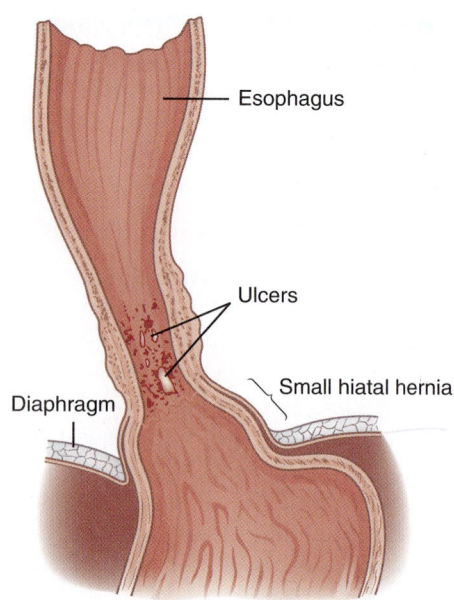

Figure 26-13 Esophagitis with esophageal ulcerations.

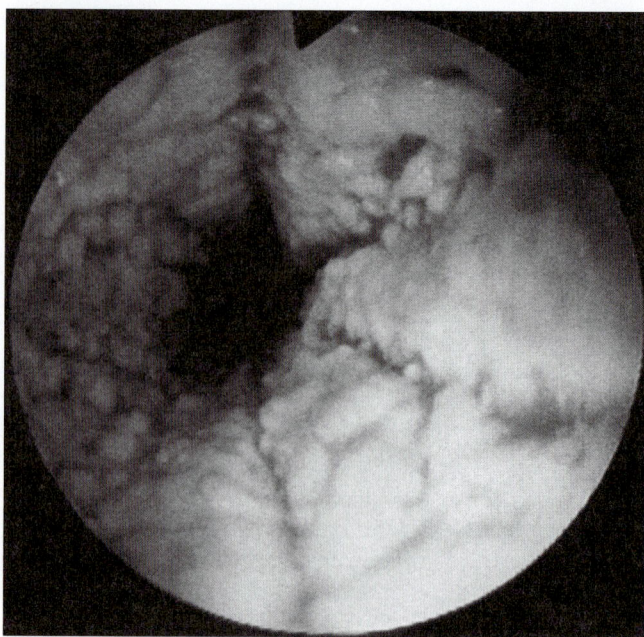

Figure 26-14 Endoscopic view of severe candida esophagitis. The opening of the esophagus is obscured by thick, white-yellow plaques.

the GI system. The patient should also provide a history if similar events have occurred in the past. If pain is present, a thorough investigation with the OPQRST mnemonic should be used as a guide. Remember that GI symptoms may be the only presenting complaint of true anginal (heart) pain. Physical examination should include a focused examination of the neck, chest, and abdomen.

Most forms of esophagitis have no specific treatment. IV fluids may be helpful in severe cases accompanied by dehydration. Pain medication also may have a role in the management of esophagitis.

Esophageal Candidiasis

[OBJECTIVES 24, 25, 26, 27]
Yeast species, especially *Candida albicans,* commonly colonize the human body. Thrush is a common yeast infection of the oropharynx, particularly in infants. Many women develop vaginal yeast infections at some time in their lives. These types of yeast infections are common, even in otherwise healthy patients, and are easy to treat with prescription and over-the-counter medications.

However, more serious yeast infections also occur, especially in patients with weakened immune systems. Infections can occur in patients with cancer or those infected with HIV. In such patients, *Candida* species may grow in the oropharynx and down into the esophagus as well (Figure 26-14). Patients with these conditions typically provide this information in their history. They often are quite knowledgeable regarding their disease and its complications. Symptoms include a burning pain in the esophagus and pain on swallowing. The pain may be so severe that the patient may be clinically dehydrated because of a decrease in oral intake.

No prehospital treatment is available for esophageal candidiasis alone, but if the patient is weak or dehydrated, IV fluids are appropriate. Hospital treatment includes antifungal medications.

Educate family members on handwashing. Candidiasis does not usually affect healthy people in their GI tracts. However, immunocompromised patients are at risk for a number of diseases, and handwashing is effective in preventing their spread.

Esophageal candidiasis is part of a larger classification—infectious esophagitis. In addition to *Candida* species infections, infectious esophagitis can be caused by a variety of bacteria and viruses, including herpes simplex virus (both type 1 and type 2), varicella-zoster virus, and cytomegalovirus. Signs and symptoms of these infections can include hemorrhage, nausea, vomiting, fever, chills, necrosis of the esophagus, chest pain, and difficult and/or painful swallowing. As with esophageal candidiasis, treatment is supportive and should include airway management, oxygen, and IV fluids as the patient's condition determines. If chest pain is present, a cardiac evaluation should be performed.

Gastroesophageal Reflux Disease

[OBJECTIVES 28, 29, 30, 31]
Another specific form of esophagitis is gastroesophageal reflux disease (GERD). This common disorder affects people from infancy to adulthood. Statistics show that 7% of adults have heartburn or reflux daily in the United States (Marx et al., 2006). GERD occurs when the lower esophageal sphincter, which normally separates the

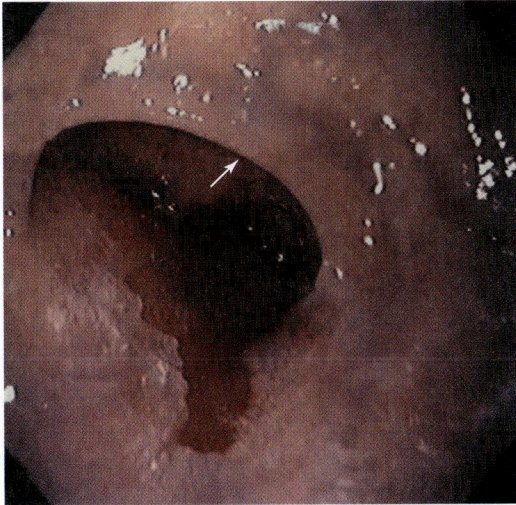

Figure 26-15 Endoscopic view of the distal esophagus from a patient with gastroesophageal reflex disease.

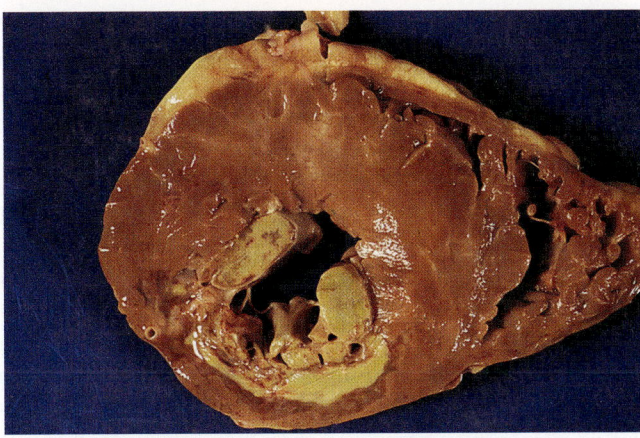

Figure 26-16 Coagulative necrosis.

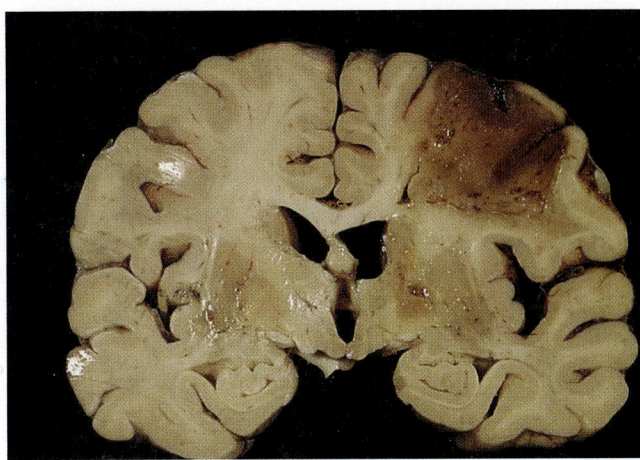

Figure 26-17 Liquefaction necrosis.

esophagus from the stomach, is weakened (Figure 26-15). This allows the stomach contents to move backward up into the esophagus, causing burning and irritation. Obesity, smoking, and alcohol use weaken the lower esophageal sphincter and predispose to GERD. In addition, heavy meals, spicy foods, and supine posture shortly after eating increase the symptoms of GERD.

Symptoms are similar to those of other forms of esophagitis and include a burning pain in the center of the thorax. Patients often refer to this as heartburn. Unlike some forms of esophagitis, the pain from GERD often occurs shortly after meals rather than with the act of swallowing. Patients with more significant GERD often describe a hot, acidic liquid (acid brash) traveling all the way back up into their mouths.

In addition to over-the-counter medicines, a variety of prescription medicines also are available to treat GERD. Patients are usually advised to stop smoking, limit alcohol intake, and control their weight. In addition, they should avoid large meals and foods that worsen their symptoms. Patients are also advised not to eat before going to bed in the evening. They should also elevate the head of their bed. This may decrease the occurrence of reflux symptoms by using gravity to help fight the backward flow of stomach contents. Acute reflux is not immediately dangerous. Chronic reflux may cause further weakening of the sphincter and may predispose the esophageal cells to **dysplasia.** No prehospital treatment is indicated for acute reflux. However, in the setting of chest pain, a cardiac etiology should be considered and an appropriate evaluation performed.

Caustic Ingestions

[OBJECTIVES 32, 33, 34, 35, 36, 37]

Caustic ingestions can occur from intentional or accidental ingestion. Caustic substances include both acidic and

alkali substances. These injuries mostly occur in patients younger than 2 years who swallow such substances accidentally and in older patients who swallow them during suicide attempts. Caustic acid ingestions include toilet bowl cleaners, fertilizers, and photography chemicals. Caustic alkali or basic ingestions include drain cleaners, oven cleaners, bleach, and batteries. Acids cause **coagulation necrosis,** which limits their penetration through tissues (Figure 26-16). Alkali ingestions cause **liquefaction necrosis,** which can lead to full-thickness esophageal burns (Figure 26-17).

The history of a caustic ingestion is usually clear. Either the patient admits to the ingestion or, in the case of small children, the parents usually find the substance near the child or even find the child with the substance in the hand or mouth. Your role is usually to record an accurate history and relay it to the receiving facility personnel. Identify the substance and transport the container if safe and possible.

When obtaining a history, ask questions regarding the time of the ingestion, the amount, and any self-treatment. Patients may complain of pain but are often asymptomatic immediately after a caustic ingestion. Acid

kids w/ button batteries, magnets

ingestions may be associated with hematemesis, melena, and gastric perforation with resultant peritonitis. Most acids are foul tasting and the amount ingested is usually small. Alkali ingestions are usually tasteless, and the amount ingested is therefore often greater. Alkali ingestions may present with orofacial burns, drooling, vomiting, and pain on swallowing. If the larynx and epiglottis are involved the patient may have hoarseness or stridor. Patients may report chest pain if the esophagus has perforated and mediastinitis has developed.

The major problem with caustic ingestions is late complications, such as tissue sloughing 2 to 3 days after injury and long-term sequelae such as scarring, esophageal stricture formation, or gastric outlet obstruction. If perforation has not immediately occurred, it may occur 5 to 14 days later. These are serious injuries, even in patients who initially are asymptomatic. All such patients should be transported to a hospital for further evaluation.

Before or during transport little specific prehospital treatment is possible. If the patient is drooling, he or she should be transported in a way that protects the airway. The patient may be kept in a sitting position or a position of comfort. Intubation may be necessary if stridor or significant drooling is present. Cricothyrotomy may even be necessary if upper airway edema is extensive. Shock may occur and should be treated with IV fluids. Vomiting may occur, and again the patient's airway should be protected to decrease the risk of aspiration. Under no circumstances should emesis be induced. Do not place a nasogastric tube without specific orders from medical direction. Finally, do not attempt to neutralize the substance with any other chemical unless specifically instructed to do so by medical direction.

Patient education can include instructions on the storage of cleaning and caustic chemicals. Instruction on safety proofing a house with small children also may be helpful.

Boerhaave Syndrome

[OBJECTIVES 38, 39, 40]

Boerhaave syndrome is perforation of the esophagus after forceful vomiting. The mortality rate can be as high as 50% if surgery is not performed within 24 hours (Marx et al., 2006). Patients usually give a history of diffuse pain in the chest that radiates to the neck, back, and abdomen. The pain often is severe and distracting. The patient also may complain of difficulty breathing or swallowing and may vomit blood. In severe cases the patient may be cyanotic, and in late cases (if the esophageal contents have entered the **mediastinum,** pleura, or peritoneum) infection can result, leading to shock and death.

Physical examination findings depend on the severity of the perforation and the time since it occurred. **Subcutaneous emphysema** is common if the perforation is in the neck, but perforation into the mediastinum, pleural space, or peritoneum may not be apparent on initial physical examination. Tachycardia and tachypnea are common. A rigid abdomen, fever, and hypotension also may be seen.

The treatment for Boerhaave syndrome is early surgical intervention, so rapid transport to an appropriate receiving facility should be a priority. Airway compromise, hypoxia, and shock should be treated aggressively while en route.

Esophageal Foreign Bodies

[OBJECTIVES 41, 42, 43]

As with caustic ingestions, swallowed foreign bodies are most common in young children, with a peak age of incidence of 18 to 48 months. Patients with mental disorders or those with dentures are also prone to esophageal foreign bodies. Almost anything may be swallowed if it is small enough to fit into the mouth of a toddler or a motivated adult. Depending on the shape of the object, some foreign bodies may easily pass through the GI tract without incident. Esophageal foreign bodies can create problems. If the object is too large to pass easily through the esophagus and into the stomach, it may become lodged. This will inhibit food, liquid, and saliva from passing through the esophagus. If the object is large, it may possibly cause pressure on the trachea, which lies anteriorly to the esophagus. This can cause an airway emergency. The esophagus narrows in four places: the cricopharyngeal muscle, the aortic arch, the left mainstem bronchus, and the diaphragmatic hiatus. The narrowest spot, and therefore the site of most esophageal foreign bodies, is at the level of the cricopharyngeal muscle (Figure 26-18). A few esophageal foreign bodies themselves are hazardous and some may even cause esophageal erosion. For example, button batteries are essentially a caustic alkali ingestion and should be treated as such.

When taking a history be sure to obtain as much information as possible regarding the object that has been ingested. Signs and symptoms of esophageal foreign body include an acute onset of difficulty swallowing, inability to swallow, pain with swallowing, foreign body sensation, and pooling of oral secretions. Physical examination should include a thorough assessment of airway and breathing. Pooling and inability to swallow oral secretions also should raise suspicion of esophageal obstruction.

Anything swallowed by the patient, even a button battery, is unlikely to cause a problem once it has entered the stomach. However, you cannot reliably determine the object's location, so all such patients should be transported for further evaluation. Most cases require radiographs and continual reassessment. Treatment is generally limited to airway management and transport. If the object is in the oropharynx and easily visualized, removal may be considered. However, this is rarely the case; most objects lodge in the esophagus beyond the paramedic's view.

If the patient's complaints indicate the obstruction is in the lower esophagus, glucagon may be ordered because of its relaxation effect on esophageal smooth muscle. However, glucagon has no effect on the upper third of the esophagus and minimal effects on the middle third of the esophagus. Therefore its use should be limited to situations in which lower esophageal obstruction is strongly suggested. Glucagon has no effect on peristalsis. The use of glucagon should not be considered if the patient may have ingested a sharp object. Glucagon is not recommended for this use in children because most obstructions occur in the upper third of the esophagus. Rapid administration has been associated with vomiting, which could cause esophageal rupture or airway compromise. The onset of action is approximately 45 seconds, with a duration of 25 minutes. Approximately 1 minute after administration the patient should be given water because drinking stimulates normal peristalsis to move the obstruction through the relaxed esophagus.

The use of meat tenderizer has been discussed in the past for esophageal obstructions from the ingestion of inadequately chewed meat. This should not be considered because the meat tenderizer can cause damage to the esophagus itself.

Prevention education for the family should involve information on the proper storage of small objects. Keeping all small objects away from curious toddlers often is difficult for families with children of various ages. Tips on placing objects on tables or in childproof cabinets may be helpful.

Hiatal Hernia

[OBJECTIVES 44, 45, 46]

The esophagus enters the stomach through a hole in the diaphragm known as the **hiatus.** On occasion the stomach extends proximally, upward through a weakness in the diaphragm. This is known as a hiatal hernia, a form of internal **hernia.** Two main types of hiatal hernias occur: sliding and paraesophageal (Figure 26-19). Hiatal hernias may be asymptomatic but often patients report symptoms similar to those of GERD or esophagitis. Heartburn is usually the predominant symptom, and patients often state that they have burning in the chest or with swallowing. A thorough history often prompts the patient to discuss a previous diagnosis of hiatal hernia. He or she may also describe chronic heartburn symptoms. Physical

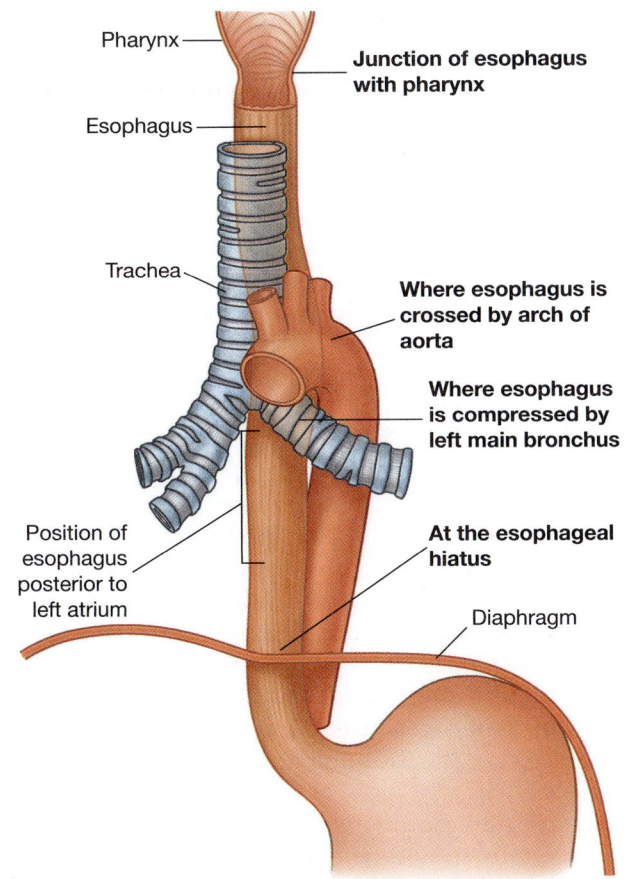

Figure 26-18 Sites of normal esophageal constriction and foreign body obstruction.

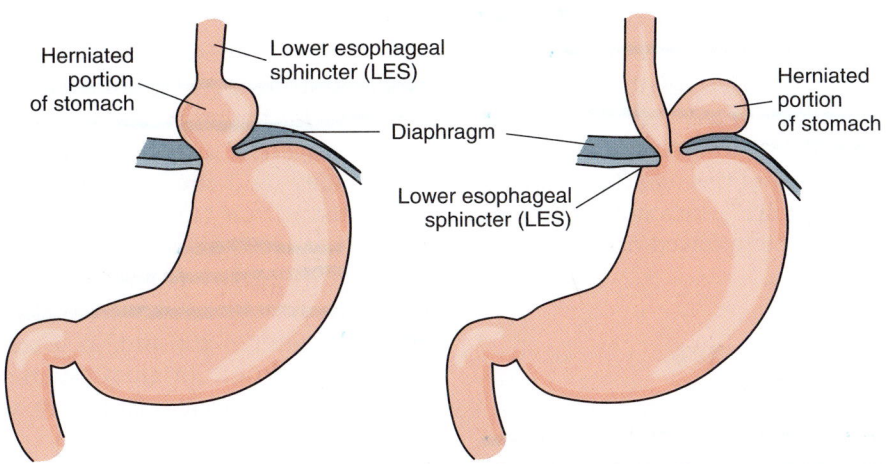

Figure 26-19 Hiatal hernias.

examination should include an assessment of the ABCs. Observe for signs and symptoms of esophageal rupture. No specific prehospital treatment exists for a hiatal hernia.

The pain of an acute myocardial infarction may present in the epigastrium. Therefore any patient complaining of abdominal pain should receive an appropriate cardiac examination to ensure the cause of the pain is not cardiac. Patients with a history of a hiatal hernia may want to blame their pain on that mechanism rather than consider a cardiac source. Patients should be educated on immediately following up with any type of abdominal or chest pain.

Mallory-Weiss Syndrome

[OBJECTIVES 46, 47, 48]

Protracted vomiting, or occasionally short bouts of intense vomiting, can lead to longitudinal tears in the distal esophagus or proximal stomach. Most of these tears occur at the level of the stomach (75%), with the remainder near the gastroesophageal junction (Marx et al., 2006). These tears are called *Mallory-Weiss tears* or the *Mallory-Weiss syndrome* and often involve arterial bleeding into the esophagus and stomach. The swallowed blood is irritating to the GI tract, which can lead to more vomiting.

Hematemesis, or blood-tinged emesis, after a period of nonbloody vomiting is the usual presentation of Mallory-Weiss syndrome. However, patients may not give a clear history of antecedent vomiting, instead only reporting the current symptom of GI bleeding.

When obtaining a history, ask questions regarding vomiting, including the frequency of vomiting, the color of the emesis, and whether any blood was present. Digested blood often looks like coffee grounds (i.e., "coffee ground" emesis).

En route to the hospital, transport patients in a position of comfort that minimizes further vomiting and swallowing of blood. If the patient continues to vomit, antiemetics may be useful. IV fluids may be used to replace the fluids lost through vomiting and to treat hemorrhagic or hypovolemic shock, if present. Mallory-Weiss syndrome is not usually diagnosed in the field. All GI bleeding should be treated seriously with appropriate transport. In reality, Mallory-Weiss tears are usually self-limiting, with only 3% being fatal (Marx et al., 2006).

Bleeding that occurs with vomiting can be alarming for patients. They should receive education indicating that all bloody emesis should be followed up for further diagnosis and treatment.

Esophageal Stenosis and Stricture

[OBJECTIVES 49, 50, 51]

Stenosis describes any abnormal narrowing in any part of the body. A **stricture** is a specific form of narrowing, usually from scar tissue formation. Both strictures and

stenosis may occur in the esophagus, usually because of prior injury. As previously discussed, caustic ingestion may lead to stenosis or stricture formation.

Most patients with stenosis or stricture are already aware of their diagnosis at the time of EMS contact. A standard history should elicit appropriate information. Symptoms are related to the abnormal narrowing: pain on swallowing or a sensation that swallowed food is stuck in the esophagus. In more advanced cases, food may indeed become lodged in the esophagus; in severe cases, the patient may not even be able to swallow liquids or handle his or her own secretions. Physical examination should focus on the ABCs and the management of oral secretions.

Although uncomfortable, the symptoms of stenosis and stricture are seldom life threatening unless they progress to an inability to handle secretions. These cases should be handled as you would any patient at risk of airway compromise. Otherwise, no specific prehospital treatment is available. If the patient's oral intake has been markedly decreased for a lengthy period, IV fluids may be warranted. The patient should be transported in a position of comfort.

Endoscopy or surgery is often needed to remove impacted food or repair esophageal stenosis or strictures. A number of pharmacologic interventions are sometimes used to aid the passage of impacted food boluses. Glucagon may be considered as previously described; however, in the setting of a stenosis or stricture, it is unlikely to be effective. All patients who believe they have a food bolus stuck in their throat or who cannot tolerate swallowed liquids or their own secretions, with or without a prior history of esophageal stenosis or stricture, should be transported to the hospital for further evaluation or treatment.

Patients who are unable to swallow food, liquids, or oral secretions should be encouraged to be transported. Education regarding the risk of aspiration and serious illness or death should be given if the patient refuses transport.

Tracheoesophageal Fistula

[OBJECTIVES 52. 53, 54]

A tracheoesophageal fistula (TEF) is a communication between the trachea and the esophagus. This condition can be congenital or acquired. The majority are congenital in etiology and are present since birth. Commonly associated with a TEF is another congenital abnormality called *esophageal atresia*. In this condition the esophagus is not continuous from the mouth to the stomach. The portion originating in the mouth ends in a blind pouch (Figure 26-20) and, as a result, is not connected with the portion originating in the stomach. These conditions are usually associated with other congenital abnormalities such as cardiac, digestive, and renal malformations and/or chromosomal disorders such as trisomy 13, 18, or 21.

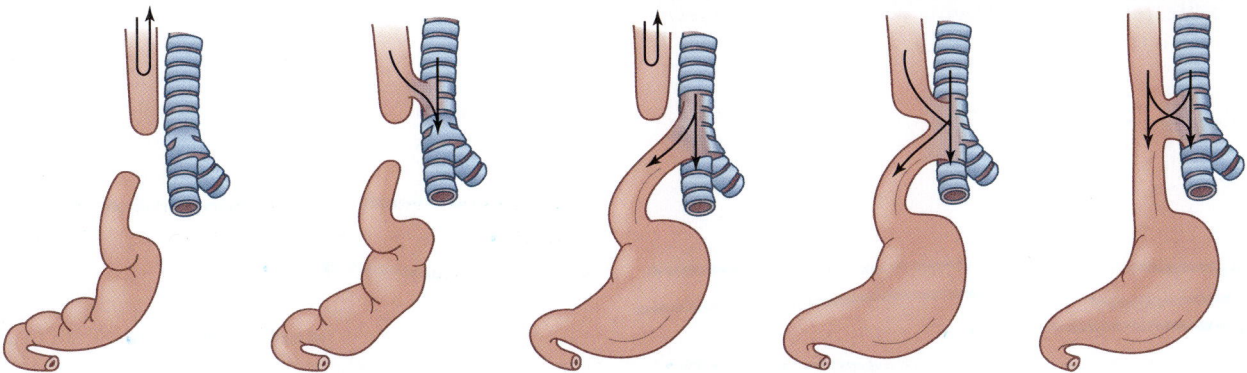

Figure 26-20 Five types of esophageal atresia and tracheoesophageal fistula.

TEFs usually appear with severe and potentially fatal respiratory complications immediately after birth or in early infancy. Most patients with a congenital TEF have a diagnosis before you encounter them.

Acquired TEFs usually occur after a malignancy, infection, or trauma. Intubation and prolonged mechanical ventilatory support also may rarely lead to a TEF. Acquired tracheoesophageal fistulas, however, are rare.

An undiagnosed TEF in an infant appears as copious frothy white bubbles in the mouth and nose that recur despite suctioning. The infant also may develop a rattling cough or even have choking and cyanosis. Symptoms worsen during feeding.

Acquired TEF in an adult may result from malignancy or infection. Patients may have cough, fever, chills, and respiratory distress. This may progress to pulmonary infections and death despite aggressive treatment. Acquired TEFs from trauma or prolonged intubation may have a somewhat better prognosis. However, the overall morbidity and mortality rates of this condition remain high.

Surgical repair is required for all confirmed TEFs, so these patients must be evaluated at the hospital. During transport reduce the risk of aspiration with suctioning and elevation of the patient's head. IV hydration may be indicated. If acute respiratory failure develops, perform endotracheal intubation.

The patient's family typically is already educated on the disease process. If they do have any questions, have them contact their pediatrician or GI specialist.

Esophageal Varices

[OBJECTIVES 55 TO 59]

A varix (plural, **varices**) is a dilated vein that has become enlarged from increased pressure. It is associated with damage to the valves normally found within the vein. In the case of esophageal varices, obstruction of blood flow through the portal vein causes a rise in the venous pressure. Because the portal venous system lacks valves, this increased pressure results in retrograde flow of blood and transmission of the elevated pressure back through gastroesophageal collaterals. As the collateral veins become enlarged, they are known as esophageal varices.

Esophageal varices are usually asymptomatic unless they bleed. Although bleeding is rare, when it does occur it can be quite serious. It is the most common clinical manifestation of **portal hypertension** (McCance & Huether, 2006). Cirrhosis, either alcoholic or viral, is the most common cause of esophageal varices in the United States (University of Michigan Health System, 2005). Therefore a history of heavy alcohol use and/or other symptoms of liver disease such as anorexia, nausea, vomiting, weight loss, and jaundice may be associated with esophageal varices. However, the patient may have sudden and massive hematemesis and even shock. A detailed history is important in these patients. Information regarding frequent bleeding, bruising, nonsteroidal antiinflammatory drug use, or recent vomiting may make severe bleeding more likely.

On physical examination, frank hematemesis may be evident. Signs and symptoms are directly related to the amount of blood loss and may range from mild tachycardia to profound shock. Patients at risk for varices are also at risk for other GI hemorrhage. Therefore internal bleeding also may occur. Patients with internal bleeding may exhibit signs of pallor and unexplained shock. In addition, patients may be cyanotic, dyspneic, and tachypneic. Jaundice may be observed in the sclera or under the tongue. Other signs of liver disease, such as gynecomastia, palmar erythema, and ascites, also may be noted. If a patient has upper GI bleeding and a history of ascites, esophageal varices should be suspected.

Ruptured esophageal varices are a life-threatening emergency. Although many textual and verbal descriptions of the bleeding associated with this condition have been put forward, none is able to provide justice to the amount of hemorrhage that can be associated with this condition. Prehospital management is directed toward problems associated with the ABCs. Airway management may be necessary in situations of copious hemorrhage, which may include intubation. Hypoxia should be corrected or avoided through the administration of oxygen. Treatment for hemorrhagic shock with IV crystalloid often is indicated, and for patients with significant bleeding, two large-bore IV lines are necessary.

HEPATIC DISORDERS

Cirrhosis

[OBJECTIVES 60 TO 63]

Cirrhosis is a consequence of chronic liver disease and has many etiologies. It is characterized by replacement of liver tissue by fibrotic scar tissue (Figure 26-21). This leads to progressive loss of liver function. In the United States alcoholic liver disease is the most common cause of cirrhosis. Viral hepatitis, especially hepatitis C, also is a frequent cause of cirrhosis.

Patients usually call 9-1-1 because of symptoms and complications, not the disease itself. The symptoms range from mild to life-threatening and vary significantly from individual to individual. They may include fatigue,

weakness, muscular atrophy, weight loss, and easy bruising. Additional findings are listed in Box 26-2 (Figure 26-22).

In general, the symptoms of cirrhosis are varied because the liver fulfills a variety of important functions in the body. The liver produces clotting factors. When cirrhosis damages the liver, the production of clotting factors is decreased. If the level falls enough, the patient may have severe bruising and bleeding from a variety of sites. In addition, the deposition of bile products in the skin can cause intense **pruritus** (itching). These bile products are metabolized by a normally functioning liver. The fluid that collects in the peritoneum can become infected (**spontaneous bacterial peritonitis**) and may appear as severe sepsis. Cirrhosis and liver failure have wide-ranging effects throughout the body, including the immune system, coagulation cascade, kidneys, central nervous system, sexual organs, and bone formation.

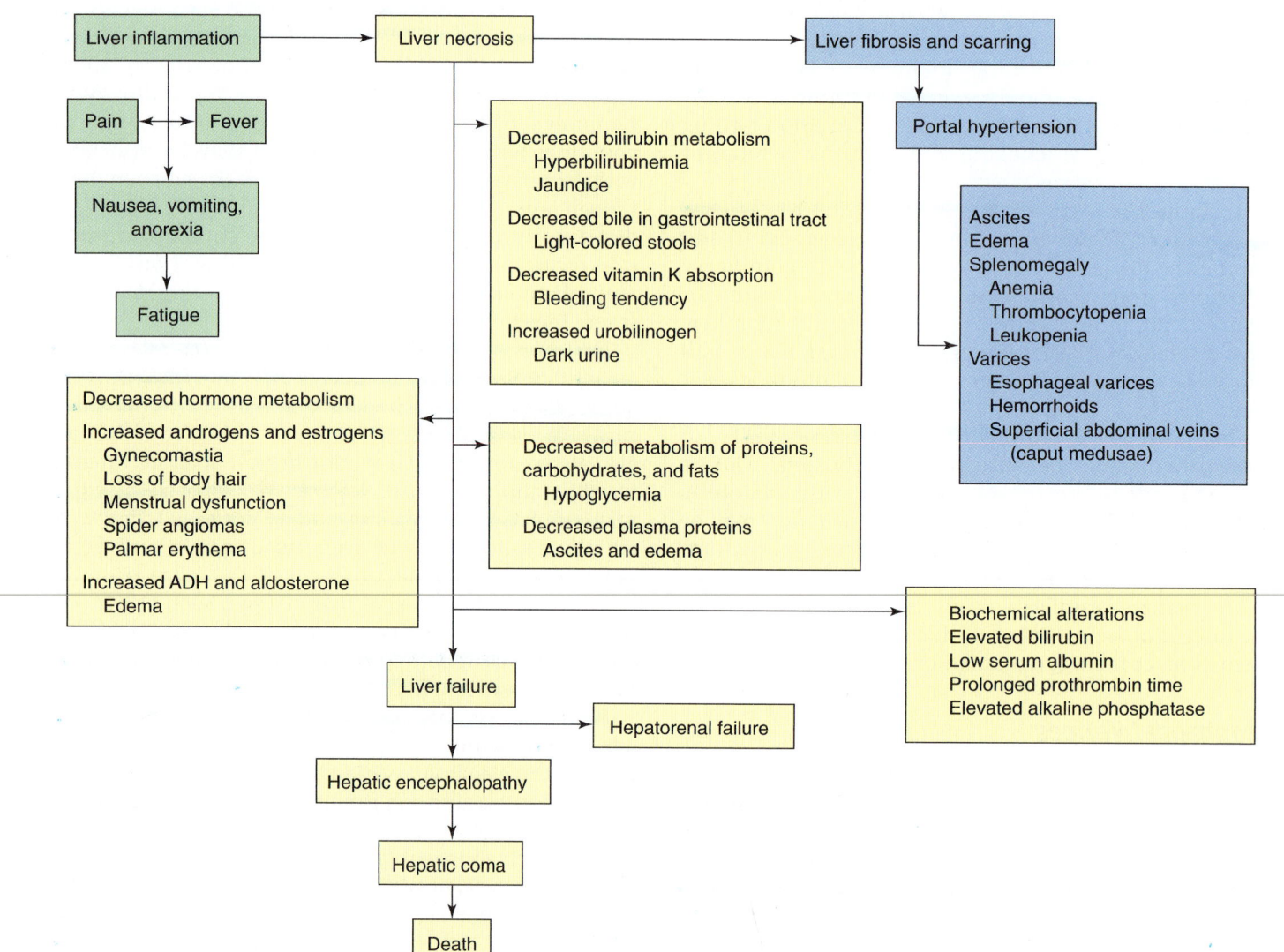

Figure 26-21 Common signs and symptoms of cirrhosis. *ADH,* Antidiuretic hormone.

BOX 26-2 Common Signs and Symptoms of Cirrhosis

Spider angiomata: vascular lesions caused by altered sex hormone metabolism

Palmar erythema: mottled, reddened palms from altered sex hormone metabolism

Dupuytren's contracture: flexion deformities of the fingers caused by disordered collagen deposition

Gynecomastia: benign breast enlargement in men caused by altered sex hormone metabolism

Testicular atrophy: atrophy caused by altered sex hormone function

Ascites: accumulation of fluid in the peritoneal cavity; may be noted on physical examination by dullness to percussion that moves as the level of the fluid changes with body position (shifting dullness) (see Figure 26-22)

Caput medusa: distention of the veins (varices) of the abdominal wall from portal hypertension

Fetor hepaticus: pungent breath odor caused by portal-systemic shunting and failure of the liver to break down waste products

Jaundice: yellowing of the skin and especially sclera and mucous membranes caused by the inability of the liver to break down bilirubin; also may be found in dark urine

Asterixis: flapping of the outstretched, dorsiflexed hands associated with hepatic failure, renal failure, or encephalopathy

Encephalopathy: altered mental status caused by a buildup of toxins usually metabolized by the liver

Esophageal varices: dilated veins from increased venous pressure

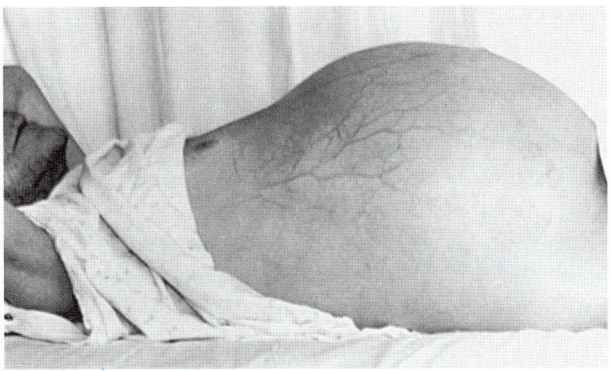

Figure 26-22 Ascites.

While taking a history, obtain as much information as possible about the patient's condition. Information on past signs and symptoms and the onset of new symptoms is helpful. The physical examination should include a head-to-toe examination. Examination of the abdomen for signs of ascites, distention, and abdominal pain will provide significant information regarding the progression of the patient's disease. Observation of the skin and sclera for **icterus** (jaundice) also provides information. Physical examination findings indicate the stage of the disease, not necessarily the duration of time that the disease has been present. Early on, the liver may be enlarged and tender, but as cirrhosis progresses the size may return to normal; in late-stage cirrhosis the liver shrinks to less than normal size.

Little prehospital therapy is available for most of the complications of cirrhosis. Patients with hepatic encephalopathy may need airway support, including intubation. Those in shock from infection or hemorrhage may require IV fluids. If local protocol allows, symptomatic treatment for itching and nausea may be helpful as well.

Although cirrhosis may not manifest immediately, patients who have severe alcohol abuse problems are at risk. Education is essential for these patients. Avoid confrontation with patients who are currently intoxicated, however.

Hepatorenal Failure

[OBJECTIVES 64, 65, 66]

Hepatorenal failure, or the hepatorenal syndrome (HRS), is the onset of kidney dysfunction in patients with acute or chronic liver disease in the absence of any other identifiable reason for renal pathology. The exact pathophysiology of HRS is unknown; however, decreased renal blood flow is believed to play a major role. The reason for this decreased flow to the kidneys is unclear but may involve the effects of the diseased liver itself, compression of the venae cavae by ascites, and a complex interplay between local and systemic factors that influence renal hemodynamics.

The history of a patient with HRS includes signs and symptoms of liver failure or a previous diagnosis of liver failure. Patients may state they have decreased urine output, increased swelling of their legs, and dyspnea. These symptoms indicate that the body is not eliminating excess fluid. Patients who have spontaneous bacterial peritonitis are at increased risk of developing HRS. In addition, patients with a history of GI bleeding also are at increased risk of developing HRS.

Physical examination likewise should focus on the primary survey. Assess and support airway and breathing as necessary. Observe the patient's mental status for signs of possible **encephalopathy.** Ascites may be noted on physical examination but also may be found in patients who do not have HRS.

No prehospital treatment is available for renal failure or HRS. Care for these patients should be as described for the patient with cirrhosis or liver failure.

Acute Hepatitis

[OBJECTIVES 67 TO 71]

Hepatitis refers to any inflammation of the liver. Damage to the liver cells from inflammation and loss of normal liver function can occur, resulting from a variety of

---

BOX 26-3 | **Some Causes of Hepatitis**

- Viral
  - Hepatitis A
  - Hepatitis B
  - Hepatitis C
  - Mumps
  - Cytomegalovirus
  - Epstein-Barr virus
- Toxic
  - Alcohol
  - Drug induced
- Metabolic
- Obstructive
- Autoimmune
- Miscellaneous
  - Alpha$_1$ antitrypsin deficiency
  - Nonalcoholic steatohepatitis

---

causes (Box 26-3), although the viral forms are most commonly encountered and of most interest to EMS providers. Fortunately the number of viral hepatitis cases has been declining over recent years. This is likely because of the availability of vaccinations, increased public awareness, and modern blood bank screening procedures.

In general, hepatitis is associated with a history of malaise, joint aches, abdominal pain, anorexia, fever, vomiting, dark urine, and jaundice. When taking a history, the patient may provide information on viral exposure, alcohol consumption, recent illness, autoimmune disease, drug overdose, or congenital anomaly. You may need to ask specific questions to elicit important information from the patient. Patients may complain of abdominal pain, nausea, vomiting, fatigue, headache, and photophobia. On physical examination the patient may have abdominal tenderness, especially in the right upper quadrant. The patient's liver may also be enlarged on palpation. Dullness may be heard on abdominal percussion in the right upper quadrant. Prehospital treatment options for hepatitis are limited and generally symptomatic. IV access, appropriate fluid therapy, and antiemetics if necessary are the mainstay of treatment for cirrhosis.

The signs, symptoms, and treatment of hepatitis in the prehospital setting are generally the same regardless of etiology. However, some specific features of the various types of hepatitis are worth mentioning.

Hepatitis A, or infectious jaundice, is a virus transmitted by the fecal-oral route; that is, it is transmitted by direct person-to-person contact or contaminated food and water. The avoidance of raw and unpeeled foods—and, importantly for EMS providers, strict personal hygiene and good handwashing—can help prevent the spread of hepatitis A infection. Symptoms associated with hepatitis A infection are often mild. Patients are frequently misdiagnosed as having gastroenteritis or the flu. They may not seek medical care, and their diagnosis is only made retrospectively. Once recovered from a bout of hepatitis A, the patient has lifelong immunity. However, symptoms may relapse for 6 months to a year after initial diagnosis before complete recovery is made. A vaccine is available that confers similar immunity. Hepatitis A does not usually have a chronic phase, and long-term sequelae are rare. If this condition is suspected in the prehospital environment, IV fluid administration would be appropriate.

The hepatitis B virus, however, can cause both acute and chronic hepatitis. This virus is transmitted by contact with infected blood or body fluids. Common routes of transmission include tattoos, sexual contact, and infected needles; an infected mother can also pass the virus to her unborn child. Importantly, in approximately 50% of cases the source of infection is unknown. Most patients develop antibodies against the hepatitis B virus and are immune from further infection. However, 5% to 15% of patients develop chronic hepatitis B. Although treatment for chronic hepatitis B infection is available, it is expensive and effective in less than half of cases. Complications of chronic hepatitis B infection include chronic hepatitis, cirrhosis, liver failure, and hepatocellular carcinoma. Fortunately a vaccine against hepatitis B infection is available. All healthcare workers and others at risk for blood or body fluid exposure are strongly encouraged to receive this vaccine. The goal of prehospital treatment is to treat the symptoms.

Hepatitis C also is transmitted through infected blood or body fluids and can lead to chronic hepatitis and cirrhosis. In contrast to hepatitis B, no vaccine is available. In addition, patients infected with hepatitis C may remain asymptomatic for up to 20 years. Therefore EMS providers and other healthcare workers must rigorously apply standard precautions in every patient contact to prevent infection with this serious virus. The goal of prehospital treatment is to treat the symptoms and any life-threatening conditions.

Alcoholic hepatitis is another form of the disease commonly encountered by prehospital providers. Alcoholic hepatitis usually occurs after a period of increased alcohol consumption. Acute inflammation of the liver is caused by the toxic effect of ethanol on the liver cells. Most cases are mild and only determined on the basis of liver function tests performed at the hospital. However, alcoholic hepatitis can lead to jaundice and liver failure. Mortality rate in these cases is high. Alcoholic hepatitis does not necessarily lead to cirrhosis, but long-term alcohol use is a common cause of cirrhosis.

A variety of other drugs and toxins can cause hepatitis as well. Common examples include halothane (an anesthetic agent), INH (a tuberculosis-specific antibiotic), phenytoin, zidovudine (an anti-HIV drug), ketoconazole (an antifungal), nonsteroidal antiinflammatory drugs, some herbs and nutritional supplements, *Amanita* spp. mushrooms, and acetaminophen (Tylenol and others). Hepatitis is more common in overdoses in which the detoxification methods of the liver are overwhelmed. Hepatitis also can occur from other viruses, other diseases, inborn errors of metabolism, and even from obesity alone (nonalcoholic steatohepatitis). The clinical features of these various forms of hepatitis vary greatly with the etiology and physiology of the particular patient. Fortunately, however, you do not need to determine the etiology of the hepatitis to treat the patient properly. Remember to perform a primary survey and treat all life-threatening conditions.

Providers, patients, and patients' families should be encouraged to follow strict handwashing guidelines. This is particularly helpful with hepatitis A. For hepatitis B and C, stress safe body fluid behavior. This may be difficult to discuss; however, if the opportunity presents itself, good hygiene and the avoidance of unsafe sexual practices and IV drug use are critical.

PARAMEDIC*Pearl*

Exercise caution when establishing IVs in patients with hepatitis. Although we frequently worry about HIV transmission, the transmissibility of hepatitis is much higher than HIV.

Hepatic Tumors

[OBJECTIVES 72, 73, 74]

The liver is prone to develop cancerous tumors after infection with the hepatitis B virus. The liver is also a common site for both primary and **metastatic** cancers as well as benign tumors from a variety of other causes.

The signs and symptoms of liver tumors depend on the nature and stage of the disease. Many liver nodules, masses, and tumors are asymptomatic and are noted only at the time of evaluation for another disease or only at autopsy. Other such lesions may be associated with mild elevations in liver function tests or may mimic mild cases of hepatitis. Still other lesions, such as those associated with larger or more aggressive benign or malignant tumors, may cause pain, abdominal distention, and signs and symptoms of cirrhosis or liver failure. Patients may also have general signs and symptoms of cancer and no findings specifically relating to the liver. Such patients may have fever, chills, night sweats, weight loss, abdominal distention, and pain. Patients already diagnosed with cancer and who are undergoing therapy may have complications of that therapy such as nausea, vomiting, and signs of systemic infection related to the immunocompromise associated with chemotherapy or radiation therapy.

Treatment for hepatic tumors involves attention to any life-threatening conditions. Supportive care also may be necessary. Patients with any form of cancer may have severe dehydration, nausea, vomiting, diarrhea, and pain. Treating these conditions per protocol is appropriate.

BILIARY DISORDERS

Cholecystitis, Cholelithiasis, and Choledocholithiasis

[OBJECTIVES 75, 76, 77, 78, 79]

The gallbladder is prone to a spectrum of diseases ranging from asymptomatic gallstones at one end to **cholangitis** (a bacterial infection superimposed on gallbladder obstruction, usually from stones) at the other. Along this spectrum, the problems of **cholecystitis, cholelithiasis,** and **choledocholithiasis** are most important for the prehospital provider.

Bile is secreted by the gallbladder and aids in the digestion of food, especially fatty foods. Bile may form a semisolid sludge or solidify as gallstones. These stones are primarily formed of cholesterol (80%), but stones composed mostly of bile pigments also occur (20%) (Figure 26-23). The presence of these stones alone is known as *cholelithiasis* and is common, with an incidence of 10% to 20% (McCance & Huether, 2006). However, these stones often are diagnosed only as part of the evaluation for another medical problem or at autopsy.

Gallstones become symptomatic when they obstruct the cystic duct through which bile normally flows into the intestine. The cystic duct occasionally becomes obstructed not from actual stones, but from gallbladder sludge or inflammation alone (**acalculous cholecystitis**). The symptoms associated with obstruction of the cystic duct are known as *gallbladder* or *biliary colic*.

If this obstruction persists, the gallbladder itself becomes inflamed and distended. This can lead to gallbladder wall edema, ischemia, and necrosis. This stage of an inflamed gallbladder is known as *cholecystitis*. Early in the process the bile is sterile and cholecystitis is primarily an inflammatory process. However, if left untreated bacterial infection follows in up to 75% of cases. Infection that spreads to the remainder of the biliary tree is known as *cholangitis*. This is a life-threatening illness but is relatively rare.

Stones also may become stuck in or form in the common bile duct. This is known as *choledocholithiasis*. Again, the symptoms of any stage or variety of gallbladder disease are essentially the same, although the severity of symptoms often parallels the severity of disease.

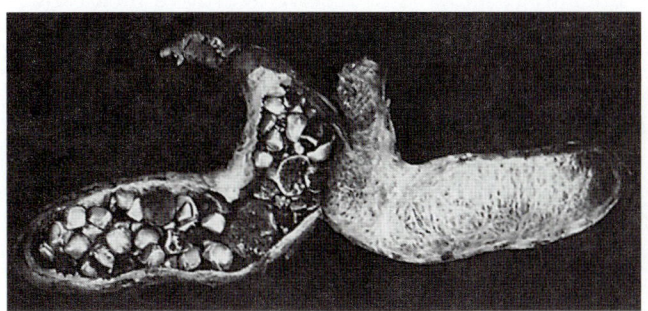

Figure 26-23 Gallstones.

The risk of developing gallstones is strongly associated with racial and ethnic factors. The major risk factors are sometimes referred to as the five *F*'s: *f*air, *f*at, *f*ertile, *f*emale, and *f*orty. Hispanics also have an increased incidence of gallstones. Although women have more gallstones overall, men with gallstones are more likely to develop cholecystitis than are women.

In most patients gallstones are asymptomatic. When obtaining a history, be sure to discuss the type and location of pain. When biliary colic develops it is usually described as a constant pain in the epigastric region or right upper quadrant. The pain may radiate to the right upper back, right shoulder, or scapula. Other symptoms associated with gallbladder disease include nausea, vomiting, and fever. Indigestion, belching, bloating, and fatty food intolerance are frequently believed to represent typical symptoms of gallbladder disease. However, these symptoms also are common in people without gallstones. On physical examination, patients are often tender in the right upper quadrant or epigastric areas. They also may exhibit guarding and a positive **Murphy's sign**—an inspiratory pause when the right upper quadrant is palpated—because of pain.

Patients with cholecystitis may appear more ill than those with simple symptomatic gallstones. They are more likely to be febrile and occasionally even be hypotensive or tachycardic. Patients with cholecystitis quite frequently have a history of similar symptoms that have spontaneously resolved. This may represent a prior history of symptomatic cholelithiasis without inflammation that has now become acute cholecystitis. However, overall the symptoms of cholelithiasis, cholecystitis, and choledocholithiasis are much the same.

The prehospital treatment for all these entities, as well as for the far less common acalculous cholecystitis and cholangitis, is also much the same. In other words, you do not need to be concerned with whether the patient's symptoms are from cholelithiasis, cholecystitis, or choledocholithiasis because all biliary tract disorders are treated with IV fluids, pain medications, and antiemetics. Some sources recommend against the use of morphine in biliary pain. The belief is that this drug can theoretically increase the tone of the sphincter, which controls the release of bile, and thereby increase the patient's symptoms. However, in practice this seldom presents a problem. Therefore some prehospital protocols may recommend an alternative analgesic.

Encourage patients to receive definitive medical care. If they refuse, patients should be encouraged to receive help in the near future. Although cholelithiasis may not be life threatening, it has the potential to develop into a serious medical condition with infection and sepsis.

PANCREATIC DISORDERS

Pancreatitis

[OBJECTIVES 80 TO 84]

Pancreatitis is an inflammation of the pancreatic gland. A hallmark of this disease is that the pancreatic enzymes

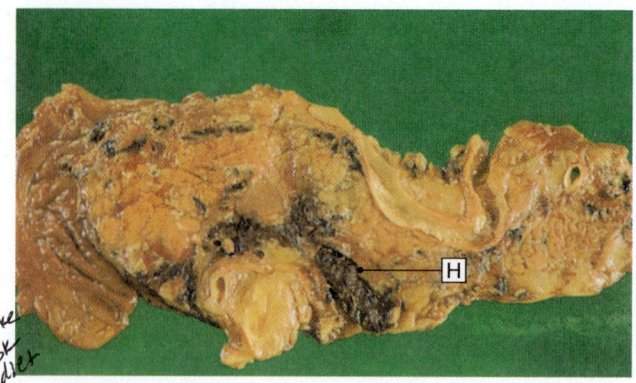

Figure 26-24 Acute pancreatitis. The pancreas appears edematous and is commonly hemorrhagic *(H)*.

that normally aid in digestion of food autodigest the pancreatic tissue itself, leading to inflammation. This can occur as an acute process or as intermittent attacks of chronic pancreatitis (Figure 26-24). Irritation of surrounding tissues is common in pancreatitis, as is movement of fluid into the interstitial space. This can result in associated edema of the bowel wall and a decrease in peristalsis. The incidence of acute pancreatitis is 100 cases per 100,000 people in the United States. The mortality rate has been decreasing steadily over the last 20 years and is currently 4% to 7%. The incidence of chronic pancreatitis is four cases per 100,000 people in the United States.

In the United States, the major causes of pancreatitis are excess alcohol consumption and gallbladder disease. In 70% to 80% of cases chronic alcohol use is the underlying factor. In contrast, 45% of cases of acute pancreatitis are caused by gallstones and 35% of cases of acute pancreatitis are caused by alcoholism. The paramedic should obtain an adequate history of all possible causes rather than assume alcohol is the underlying factor. Alcohol consumption directly damages the pancreas and allows digestive enzymes to leak out and further damage pancreatic tissue. Gallstones that obstruct the pancreatic duct can cause digestive enzymes to leak back into the pancreatic parenchyma. Although these are by far the most common causes of pancreatitis, a variety of medications, viral diseases, and trauma can also cause the condition.

Patients may report constant, severe mid-epigastric pain that radiates directly to the back. However, the severity of the pain does not correlate with the severity of the disease. The pain also may travel to the right or left upper quadrant of the abdomen. In severe cases the pain may be diffuse. A history should focus on the OPQRST format for pain. Patients may provide a history of a drinking binge, but generally no relation to the onset of pain and eating exists. However, be sure to ask questions regarding trauma, medication ingestion, and any other illness. Fever, nausea, and vomiting are common symptoms.

Once the digestive enzymes begin to destroy the pancreatic tissue, a variety of inflammatory and vasoactive substances are released from the pancreas. Therefore pancreatitis is more than a local disease and is associated with a variety of systemic manifestations, especially on physical examination. Patients are often in distress and appear systemically ill. They frequently are restless and have tachycardia and tachypnea. They may be febrile and hypotensive. Jaundice may be present, although it is usually mild. On abdominal examination the epigastrium or right upper quadrant may be tender and breath sounds may be diminished or even absent. Distention, guarding, and rigidity of the abdomen may develop. Peritoneal findings often are absent because the pancreas is primarily a retroperitoneal organ.

Prehospital treatment for pancreatitis consists of symptomatic treatment. Based on history and physical examination, pancreatitis and gallbladder disease may present quite similarly. The treatment for each condition is similar. Complete the primary survey and address life-threatening conditions. If the patient is hypotensive, dehydrated, or appears in shock, provide IV crystalloids. A nasogastric tube often is helpful in the vomiting patient, as are antiemetics. Because these patients often are in severe pain, analgesia is imperative. Early pain management with narcotic analgesics is indicated, as is continual monitoring for the return of pain and readministration of narcotics as needed.

Pancreatic Tumors

[OBJECTIVES 85, 86, 87, 88]
As in most organs in the body, tumors in the pancreas can be either **malignant** or benign. In addition, tumors in the pancreas are further divided according to the type of cells involved. Pancreatic exocrine cells form the ducts and other tissues but are not hormonally active. Approximately 95% of all pancreatic cancers are adenocarcinomas derived from exocrine cells. Benign tumors also can arise from pancreatic exocrine cells and are known as cyst adenomas.

Endocrine cells of the pancreas also can develop tumors. These tumors are known as *neuroendocrine tumors* or *islet cell tumors*. Endocrine cell tumors that are not hormonally active are called *nonfunctioning islet tumors*.

Pancreatic cancer is one of the most serious and deadly of all malignancies. It usually occurs in middle-age or older patients who often have a history of chronic alcohol use. The first symptom is typically a dull pain in the upper abdomen that radiates to the back, similar to pancreatitis. However, symptoms of pancreatic cancer frequently do not develop until late in the life of the disease. In addition, although pain is common, the classic symptom of pancreatic cancer is painless jaundice that develops as the tumor obstructs the bile duct.

The symptoms of endocrine tumors may be similar to the hormone produced. For example, one of the most common islet cell tumors is one that secretes insulin. Patients may be weak, dizzy, and hypoglycemic.

Prehospital treatment for pancreatic tumors is supportive care. The patient should receive a primary survey and all life-threatening emergencies should be treated.

Per protocol, treat pain, nausea, and vomiting. Transport should be to the appropriate medical facility.

Peritonitis

[OBJECTIVES 89, 90, 91, 92]
Peritonitis is an inflammation of the peritoneal membrane, usually caused by infection. It can be associated with a number of other diseases as well as be a primary problem itself (spontaneous bacterial peritonitis).

Peritonitis can occur from multiple causes, including infection, trauma, and bowel rupture. It is discussed in detail in the relevant sections elsewhere in this text. In general, peritonitis regardless of cause has a similar presentation. The initial signs and symptoms may be those referable to the original disease, such as abdominal pain and fever, nausea, vomiting, and anorexia in appendicitis. As inflammation spreads, often because of organ perforation with resultant contamination of the peritoneal cavity, rebound tenderness can develop. Patients may appear to be frankly septic with fever, hypothermia, chills, and hypotension. On physical examination, bowel sounds frequently are decreased or absent.

Spontaneous bacterial peritonitis (SBP); however, often manifests differently. This disease usually occurs in the setting of liver cirrhosis and often is asymptomatic, especially early in its course. It occurs because the portal hypertension associated with cirrhosis causes the bowel wall and mucosa to swell and become porous, allowing bacteria to enter the peritoneal cavity and potentially the bloodstream as well.

Although patients may not report specific symptoms with SBP, it is a common cause of worsening hepatic or renal function in patients with underlying liver disease. It also is a common reason for ascites or hepatic encephalopathy to develop or worsen. However, when SBP does cause symptoms, they are similar to the signs and symptoms of peritonitis.

Prehospital treatment for peritonitis includes careful attention to the ABCs. Patients may have significant airway and breathing difficulties as complications of peritonitis and infection. Septic shock is also a reality and may suddenly develop. IV fluids for tachycardia or shock are an appropriate prehospital intervention. Pain and nausea medications also may be indicated in these patients.

STOMACH DISORDERS
Gastritis

[OBJECTIVES 92, 93, 94]
Gastritis refers to inflammation of the gastric mucosa from a wide variety of causes. Gastritis can be acute or chronic (Figure 26-25). Chronic gastritis may be caused by *Helicobacter pylori*, the same bacteria responsible for peptic ulcer disease. Acute gastritis is usually the result of some local injury to the gastric mucosa. This may occur from viral infection or ingestion of a substance that irri-

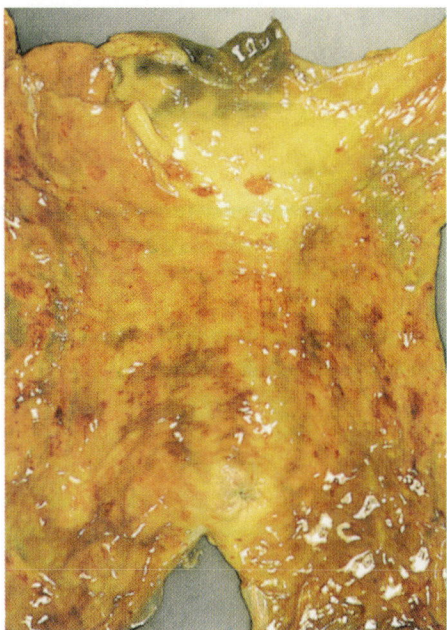

Figure 26-25 Acute gastritis.

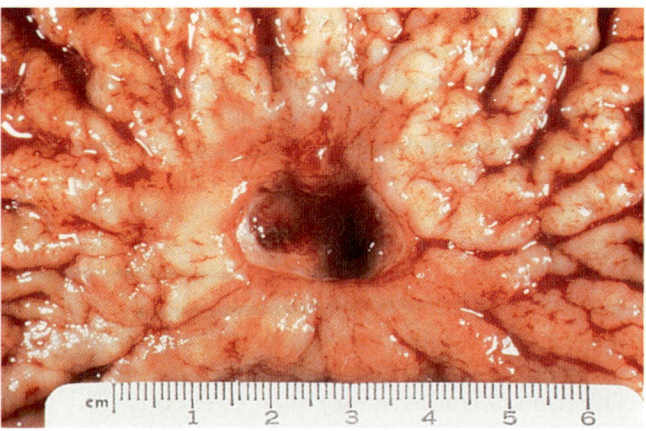

Figure 26-26 Chronic peptic ulcer.

Proton pump inhibitors (H2blockers)
Prilosec

Peptic Ulcer Disease

[OBJECTIVES 95 TO 99]

Peptic ulcers are defects in the gastric mucosa of the stomach and small intestine. These ulcers can bleed, causing pain, morbidity, and death. Approximately 5 million people in the United States have peptic ulcer disease (Figure 26-26), and the annual estimated healthcare costs for the condition are more than $15 billion.

The interior of the stomach is a harsh environment because of the secretion of hydrochloric acid and pepsinogen by the gastric mucosa in response to gastrin and H_2 receptor stimulus. Although pepsinogen itself has no digestive capacity, as soon as it is exposed to hydrochloric acid or previously formed pepsin, it is transformed into pepsin, which is highly acidic. Hydrochloric acid and pepsin are crucial for proper digestion of proteins in the stomach. The stomach is protected from these chemicals by a heavy coating of mucus produced by mucous cells in the stomach. The duodenum is protected by pancreatic secretions, which contain large amounts of sodium bicarbonate. Recall the location of the pancreatic duct; its placement effectively neutralizes the contents of the stomach as they enter the duodenum. When acid enters the duodenum, gastric emptying is delayed and the production of pancreatic juices is increased. This provides further protection against an acidic environment in the duodenum. Peptic ulcers are formed when production of hydrochloric acid and pepsin by the gastric mucosa is increased, causing a decrease in the protective ability of the mucous coating, or when the ability to neutralize these substances is lost.

As previously mentioned, *H. pylori* has a close association with chronic gastritis and peptic ulcer disease. Other common causes of peptic ulcer disease include aspirin and other nonsteroidal antiinflammatory drugs, cigarette smoking, and heavy or prolonged alcohol consumption. In general, all peptic ulcers are caused by an imbalance between the production of stomach acids (hydrochloric

tates the gastric mucosa. The use of alcohol or a variety of prescription and over-the-counter medications are some of the most common causes of gastritis. Medications implicated in the development of gastritis include aspirin, steroids, nonsteroidal antiinflammatory drugs, and narcotic pain medications, such as acetaminophen with codeine. Regardless of the cause, up to 50% of the population has evidence of gastritis by the age of 50 years.

Signs and symptoms of gastritis include **dyspepsia**, bloating, indigestion, heartburn, and belching. Nausea and vomiting may occur. If vomiting is severe or prolonged, tachycardia, dehydration, and electrolyte disturbances may develop. If hemorrhagic gastritis develops, as often occurs with alcohol-induced gastritis, hematemesis, melena, and even hemorrhagic shock may develop.

A thorough history, including a discussion on current pain, medical history, medications, and social history, is helpful. Physical examination should begin with the primary survey. Treat any life-threatening conditions. If hemorrhagic shock is suspected, do not delay treatment with IV crystalloids and rapid transport. Perform a thorough abdominal examination during the secondary survey.

Prehospital treatment is limited. Place the patient in a position of comfort for transport. Manage pain and nausea and perform continual reassessment. Support the ABCs if the patient's condition deteriorates or the patient demonstrates the signs of shock.

Gastritis may be a benign condition. However, other serious conditions present similarly to gastritis. Therefore all patients with abdominal pain should be encouraged to receive a thorough medical evaluation.

acid and pepsin) and the ability of the gastric mucosa to prevent damage from these acids. *H. pylori,* for example, increases gastric acid production and decreases mucosal integrity.

Approximately 1% of peptic ulcers are caused by Zollinger-Ellison syndrome. Patients with this syndrome have gastrin-secreting tumors. Gastrin is an endogenous hormone that regulates the production of stomach acids; unregulated gastrin release by these tumors causes an increase in the production of stomach acids. In addition, the gastric epithelial cells responsible for producing stomach acids undergo hypertrophy, which further increases the amount of acid produced. This can lead to peptic ulcer disease, erosive esophagitis, and diarrhea. Diarrhea is present in 73% of patients with Zollinger-Ellison syndrome, whereas it is not commonly associated with other causes of peptic ulcer disease.

Ulcers can occur either in the stomach (gastric ulcers) or in the first parts of the duodenum (duodenal ulcers). In either case they are referred to as *peptic ulcers.* Symptoms can help determine the location of the ulcer to some extent. However, a large amount of overlap occurs in these symptoms. The pain of duodenal ulcers classically occurs 90 minutes to 3 hours after a meal, often awakening the patient at night several hours after eating dinner. The classic presentation is the patient who awakes at 3:00 AM; in most of the population gastric acid production is highest at 2:00 AM. This pain is often relieved by the morning, when gastric acid production is lowest. The pain from gastric ulcers, on the other hand, often is described as being made worse with eating; in fact, nausea and anorexia may limit the patient's food intake with a gastric ulcer. In either case, the pain is usually described as burning or gnawing in nature and located in the epigastric region. However, the pain can be located in other areas of the abdomen, chest, or back. Some patients may complain of a vague or cramping pain. The pain of peptic ulcers is relieved by antacids 90% of the time. Colicky pain, nausea and vomiting, or constant pain lasting weeks to months is rarely caused by peptic ulcers and should initiate a search for another cause of the patient's signs and symptoms.

The major area of concern for the prehospital provider is the complications that may accompany peptic ulcer disease. Ulcers may perforate, producing peritoneal signs such as a rigid, boardlike abdomen and generalized rebound tenderness. This looks and is treated much like peritonitis from any cause. Alternatively, an ulcer may cause sufficient local inflammation and swelling to create an acute obstruction. The most worrisome and most common complication of peptic ulcer disease, however, is hemorrhage. This may manifest as either hematemesis and/or **melena.** The bleeding from a peptic ulcer may be mild. Significant bleeding accompanied by pallor, tachycardia, hypotension, and frank hemorrhagic shock is not unusual.

History should focus on the symptoms, the type of pain, the relation of pain with food, and previous diagnosis. Physical examination should begin with the primary survey. Treat any patient with frank hematemesis, melena, or shock with fluid resuscitation and rapid transport. If the patient appears stable, perform a complete abdominal examination. No specific prehospital treatment is available for uncomplicated peptic ulcer disease; however, the administration of antacids or H_2 blockers, such as cimetidine, may reduce the patient's pain. The measures described above for gastritis may be useful here as well.

Patients may believe that their peptic ulcer disease is a chronic condition and does not warrant any further investigation. Educate patients and their families on signs of possible erosion and perforation of the peptic ulcer. If the patient has severe pain, hematemesis, or signs of shock, he or she must be transported immediately because this can indicate a perforation of the bowel.

Upper and Lower Gastrointestinal Bleeding

[OBJECTIVES 100 TO 109]

Bleeding from the GI tract is described as either upper or lower GI bleeding depending on the location. If it is above the ligament of Treitz, it is considered upper GI bleeding. If is distal to the ligament of Treitz it is considered lower GI bleeding. Upper GI bleeding affects 50 to 150 people per 100,000 annually, accounting for 90% of GI bleeds, with a mortality rate of approximately 10%. Lower GI bleeding accounts for approximately 10% of GI bleeds annually. These conditions can occur at any age, but they peak between 40 and 70 years of age with most deaths occurring in those older than 60 years. A male predominance is found in upper GI bleeding and a female predominance in lower GI bleeding.

Common causes of upper GI bleeding include entities previously discussed, such as caustic ingestions, Mallory-Weiss tears, esophageal varices, and gastritis and peptic ulcer disease. Of these, peptic ulcer disease is the most common cause and is responsible for 50% of upper GI bleeds. The most common causes of lower GI bleeding are discussed in the following section according to their anatomic location in the bowel. These include diverticular disease, tumors, polyps, hemorrhoids, autoimmune disease, and anal fissures.

The signs and symptoms of upper and lower GI bleeding can be similar, and distinguishing between the two on clinical factors alone can be difficult. However, some important differences exist between these two types of bleeding. Upper GI bleeding is more commonly associated with abdominal pain, usually described as sharp or burning pain located in the epigastric region. It may be described as radiating to the back. Hematemesis and coffee ground emesis also are more commonly associated with upper GI bleeding. Lower GI bleeding is often painless and is typically not associated with hematemesis. Melena may occur in either condition; however, the prognostic implications of this clinical feature vary depending on the source of bleeding. Melena from upper GI bleeding is a relatively common occurrence because blood must remain in the GI tract for 8 to 14 hours before taking on this characteristic. Although melena is possible with lower GI bleeds, it is uncommon because the blood rarely remains in the GI tract that long unless an underlying decrease in GI motility is present. Because bismuth-containing solutions such as Pepto-Bismol can turn stools black, be sure to ask about use of this medication when obtaining the history. Bright red blood in the stool **(hematochezia)** is most often associated with lower GI bleeds. However, this finding can occur from an upper GI source and, when present, implies a larger and more rapid loss of blood. When the history suggests hematochezia the paramedic should be sure to rule out other possible sources of hemorrhage. Small amounts of blood from hemorrhoids can produce blood-streaked stools, evidence of blood on toilet paper, and bright-red water in the toilet bowl.

In either upper or lower GI bleeding the degree of hemorrhage and therefore symptoms may vary from occult (noted only by the presence of heme-positive stools or a new anemia) to massive. In occult cases, the patient may report symptoms such as fatigue and weakness and may appear pale, especially at the nail beds and conjunctiva. Occult GI bleeding is more common with lower bleeding than with upper bleeding. When symptomatic the patient usually reports the passage of bright-red blood from the rectum or blood in the toilet bowl. Black stools and melena may occur with either upper or lower GI bleeding. Milder cases may exhibit only the history of abdominal pain and hematemesis. Major cases may exhibit the signs and symptoms of hypovolemic shock, such as tachypnea; tachycardia; restlessness and anxiety; pale, cool, and moist skin; and decreases in blood pressure. Only later is the history of prior abdominal pain and bleeding elicited. Cases between these two extremes may exhibit a history of abdominal pain and bleeding as well as the signs of moderate blood loss, such as orthostatic hypotension, lightheadedness, and tachycardia.

A good history can provide important information. Patients often provide a medical history of bleeding and are able to tell you what caused their bleeding. Information on social history, such as smoking and alcohol consumption, also is helpful. Questions regarding fatigue, weakness, shortness of breath, and vomiting provide information regarding the extent of symptoms. Also ask the patient about the presence of hematemesis, blood in the stool, or black and tarry stool. Begin the physical examination with the primary survey. Immediately treat severe symptoms. Rapid transport is essential. Milder cases should have a thorough history and physical examination.

Treatment of the patient with upper and lower GI bleeding depends on the severity of the bleeding and the symptoms. Mild cases are treated with supportive care. Massive cases are treated as hypovolemic shock, with special attention given to protecting the patient's airway. This may include early intubation. Massive bleeding and hematemesis can rapidly lead to aspiration and respiratory failure. After protecting the airway, administer oxygen and monitor oxygen saturation, capnography, and cardiac function. IV access is appropriate for all patients with GI bleeding. If the bleeding is severe, two large-bore IVs are appropriate. Transport the patient with continual reassessment. Perform a secondary survey en route to the receiving facility if possible. Perform other potential treatments, such as nasogastric intubation and medication administration, according to local protocol.

Case Scenario CONCLUSION

In questioning the woman, she tells you that she ate dinner approximately 1 hour before her symptoms began. You ask what she had for dinner, and she tells you that she ate a breakfast meal consisting of fried eggs, hash brown potatoes, toast, and orange juice. A focused physical examination reveals tenderness in the epigastrium and right upper abdominal quadrant. While palpating the right upper quadrant and applying pressure to the area, the patient exhibits a pause in her breathing (Murphy's sign). The patient's breath sounds are bilaterally equal and no indication of hypoxia is present. Pulse oximetry reveals an SpO$_2$ of 98% on room air. Her blood glucose level is 104 mg/dL. The patient repeatedly belches while you perform the focused assessment and reassess her vital signs. She expresses slight relief after each belch.

Looking Back

7. *What is your final impression of the patient's condition?*
8. *What did the meal contribute to the patient's chief complaint?*
9. *What are contributing factors that help determine the cause of the woman's chest pain?*

BOWEL DISORDERS

Gastroenteritis

[OBJECTIVES 110, 111, 112, 113, 114]

Acute **gastroenteritis** is inflammation of the lining of the stomach and intestines that causes disruption in the normal mucosal lining functioning, such as water and nutrient absorption. Typical symptoms include cramping, abdominal pain, nausea, vomiting, fever, anorexia (loss of appetite), malaise, headache, and watery diarrhea. Depending on the infectious agent responsible for the condition, the diarrhea may be discolored (green or bloody) and contain mucus and undigested food. This condition may come on suddenly with significant vomiting and diarrhea, which can cause loss of electrolytes and dehydration. Many different causes of gastroenteritis exist. Viruses and bacteria commonly cause gastroenteritis. Viruses are typically passed from person to person (fecal-oral route) or by eating contaminated food. Good handwashing is essential.

One of the most common viruses is the Norwalk virus. This virus commonly occurs in small children and often is transmitted at day care and school. In recent history outbreaks of this virus have occurred on cruise ships. Other common viruses that can cause acute gastroenteritis include norovirus, adenovirus, astrovirus, and rotavirus. *Norovirus* was recently approved as the official genus name for the group of viruses provisionally described as Norwalk-like viruses. Bacterial infection can be caused by *Salmonella* spp., *Escherichia coli*, *Campylobacter* spp., and *Staphylococcus* spp. Transmission occurs by the fecal-oral route and from poorly cooked meat, poorly refrigerated food, and contaminated food. Parasites, such as *Giardia* spp., have also been known to cause gastroenteritis. Other causes include wheat intolerance, lactose intolerance, allergies, autoimmune conditions, medications, radiation therapy, and chemical toxins.

Chronic gastroenteritis occurs from long-term changes to the mucosal lining of the stomach and the intestines. The causes of chronic gastritis include infection, medication use, inflammatory conditions, and toxins. The symptoms typically last longer with a more insidious onset.

When obtaining a history, questions regarding time of onset, symptoms, and pain are important. Duration of symptoms also is helpful. Questions regarding exposure to chemicals, possible food poisoning, camping or hiking activity, foreign travel, swimming in potentially infected water, and previous medical conditions are quite helpful. Physical examination should include a primary survey. Address and treat all serious medical conditions. The physical examination also should include a detailed abdominal examination. Increased bowel sounds are commonly heard on auscultation. On palpation the patient may have mild tenderness in all four quadrants. Check the patient's skin for tenting as a sign of dehydration. The patient also may exhibit signs of muscle spasm as a result of electrolyte imbalances.

Treatment should include IV access and fluid administration as dictated by the patient's presentation. Medications for nausea and abdominal cramping should be considered. All other care is symptomatic and supportive.

Obstruction

[OBJECTIVES 115, 116, 117, 118, 119]

Obstruction occurs when the lumen of the small or large bowel is blocked. Large-bowel obstructions are much less common than small-bowel obstructions and generally are caused by a malignant disease. Normal bowel contents cannot flow forward, which disrupts the normal function of the digestive system. An ileus occurs when the bowel loses its normal peristaltic movement. This can occur from illness, abdominal injury, recent surgery, or medication. Ileus can mimic a bowel obstruction and often cannot be distinguished in the prehospital environment. A true obstruction usually results from a complete mechanical blockage of the intestine, which can be caused by adhesions, a hernia, polyps, tumors (inside and outside the lumen), foreign body, impacted stool, intussusception, and volvulus. **Intussusception** typically occurs in children. This occurs when a part of the bowel telescopes into another portion of the bowel. In the adult patient, 80% of intussusceptions occur in the small bowel and 90% of the time have a pathologic lesion as the cause. **Volvulus** is twisting of the bowel (Figure 26-27). If the bowel twists on itself, obstruction can occur. In the adult patient, a volvulus of the small bowel is rare. In the large bowel, most volvuli occur in the colon in patients between the ages of 60 and 70 years. Approximately three cases per 100,000 people are reported annually, accounting for up to 7% of large-bowel obstructions.

Signs and symptoms of a bowel obstruction include nausea, vomiting, abdominal pain, lack of bowel movements (complete obstruction), diarrhea (partial obstruction), inability to pass bowel gas, and abdominal distention. The pain associated with obstructions is typically described as crampy or colicky as it increases and decreases (although may never totally subside) with waves of peristalsis. The timing of increases and decreases in pain varies according to the location of the obstruction. In small-bowel obstructions, proximal obstructions are abrupt in onset and have a more frequent pain cycle, whereas a distal obstruction typically presents with a slower pain cycle that has progressed over a period of 1 to 2 days. Distal obstructions and large-bowel obstructions are more commonly associated with abdominal distension. Pain that becomes constant indicates bowel ischemia.

A good history should focus on past medical history. Previous bowel obstructions, abdominal surgery, cancer, radiation therapy, chemotherapy, hernia, and abdominal illness predispose a person to bowel obstruction. Specific questions on nausea, vomiting, and bowel habits provide

Stomach   Pylorus   Duodenum

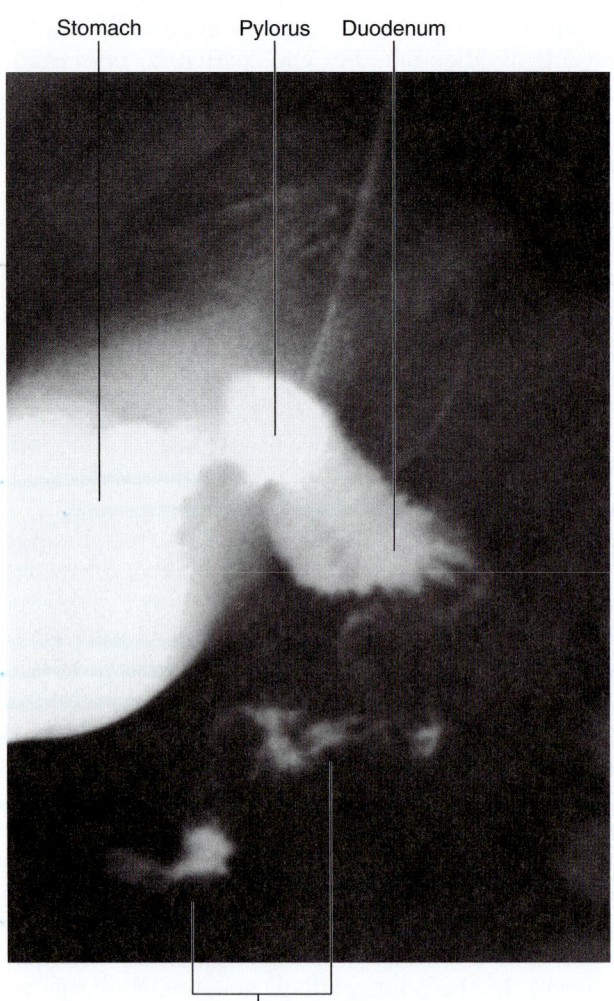

Ribbon-twisted duodenum and proximal jejunum

Figure 26-27 Volvulus.

Thickened wall

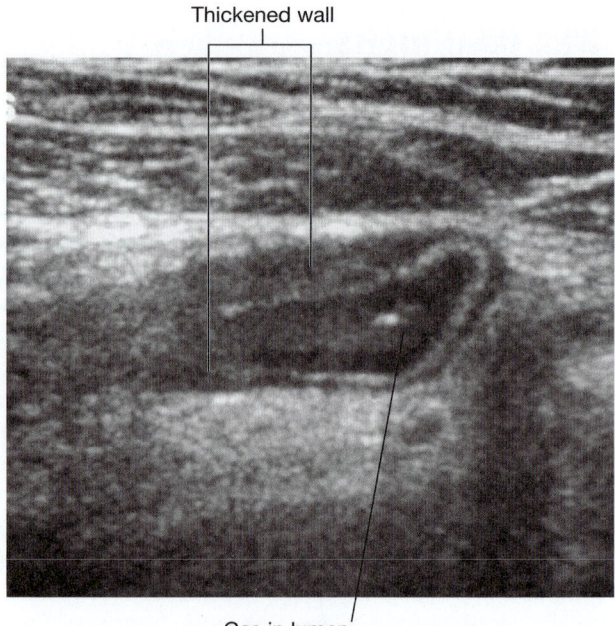

Gas in lumen

Figure 26-28 Inflamed appendix.

valuable information. Begin the physical examination with the primary survey. A thorough abdominal examination with special consideration on abdominal auscultation, palpation, and percussion is essential and provides significant information. Auscultation may reveal either absent or high-pitched bowel sounds. This occurs when bowel contents that attempt to move forward slam into the obstruction and are pushed backward. Percussion may elicit hollow or high-pitched notes as the bowel lumen is filled with air that cannot pass the obstruction. Palpation may reveal a firm, painful, distended abdomen because normal bowel contents, including digested food and air, cannot pass the obstruction.

Although diagnosis of a bowel obstruction is not always evident in the prehospital environment, it does have some unique symptoms, recognition of which is key. If bowel obstruction is suspected, place the patient in a position of comfort. Obtain IV access with appropriate fluid administration. If the patient appears dehydrated, provide fluids; otherwise maintenance fluids are indicated. The patient should avoid taking any food or water by mouth. A nasogastric tube may be placed to

remove the normal fluids produced by the stomach by gentle suction. Medication administration may be appropriate for pain and nausea control. Bowel obstructions can be a surgical emergency; therefore patients should be transported to a facility with immediate surgical capability when possible.

Bowel obstructions may spontaneously resolve. Educate the patient on the significant risks of bowel instruction, including the risk of bowel perforation and severe systemic infection.

Appendicitis

[OBJECTIVES 120, 121, 122, 123, 124]

Appendicitis is inflammation of a small tubular structure that arises off the colon near the cecum. Appendicitis usually results from infection or obstruction, commonly a **fecalith.** The obstruction causes the appendix to become distended, the normal drainage is decreased, and blood flow is altered. The appendix may become highly distended, inflamed, and gangrenous. This is considered a surgical emergency. If the appendix ruptures, bowel contents may spill into the abdomen and cause peritonitis (Figure 26-28).

Appendicitis is a common condition and occurs in the young and old, with a peak incidence between 20 and 40 years of age. Approximately 7% of people develop this condition. Predicting who will have appendicitis is not possible. Patients typically have a fever, nausea, and abdominal pain. The initial symptom may be poorly localized, dull pain in the periumbilical area. This occurs from the visceral pain common with bowel disorders and typically lasts 4 to 6 hours. As the appendix becomes more inflamed, the patient may find that the pain localizes to the right lower quadrant or to the right lower back, becoming steady and severe. However, this classic presentation of appendicitis does not occur in many patients and depends on the anatomic location and orientation of the appendix.

When obtaining a history, be sure to discuss surgical history. If the patient has already had the appendix removed, the pain obviously has another etiology. Information on appetite, pain location, onset of pain, and fever is helpful. On physical examination, focus on the abdominal examination. Perform auscultation. Absent, normal, or hyperactive bowel sounds may be heard. Because of the inflammation, the peristaltic activity of the bowel typically ceases and causes decreased bowel sounds and an ileus. Palpation may reveal pain in the periumbilical area. In addition, the patient may have pain with movement of the pelvis or hips. Palpation in the left lower quadrant may illicit pain in the right lower quadrant. This is called **Rovsing's sign.** A positive obturator sign, psoas sign, and cutaneous hyperesthesia also may be present; however, these are often late findings (see Table 26-1). Anatomically, the appendix may vary in location from person to person. Some patients have a retrocecal appendix, which means the appendix is tucked behind the cecum. This situation may produce low back pain (Figure 26-29). The most common location for the appendix is at McBurney's point, which is halfway between the umbilicus and the right anterior superior iliac spine. The patient may have point tenderness and pain in this area. However, because of this location variability, the patient may have localized pain and tenderness in other areas of the abdomen. If the appendix

ruptures peritonitis can result, causing signs of peritoneal irritation such as rebound tenderness and involuntary guarding.

Begin treatment by obtaining IV access. Provide fluids; food and beverages should be avoided. Administer pain and nausea medication as dictated by the patient's condition. Transport the patient in a position of comfort to a facility with immediate surgical capability.

Appendicitis is a difficult diagnosis to make. Encourage patients to receive a complete workup with any abdominal pain that has signs and symptoms of appendicitis.

Ulcerative Colitis

[OBJECTIVES 125 TO 129]

Ulcerative colitis is an inflammatory condition of the large bowel in which ulcerations form on the mucosal surface of the intestine. It is often simply referred to as *colitis*. Colitis predominantly affects the rectum but may affect any part of the colon (Figure 26-30). The exact cause is unknown, but speculation is that the immune system may overreact to a viral or bacterial insult, causing this exaggerated inflammatory response. Patients may complain of diarrhea, abdominal cramping, bloody stools, and purulent stools. They also may have fatigue, weakness, weight loss, and loss of appetite.

History is important. Many patients may already have a diagnosis of ulcerative colitis, which is helpful. Other patients may provide a history of recurrent problems with fatigue, diarrhea, and abdominal discomfort. Physical examination should include a thorough abdominal

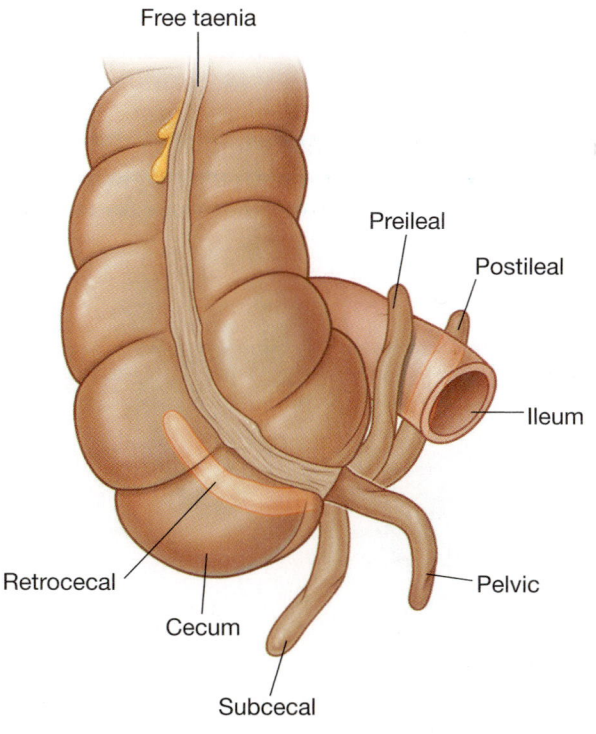

Figure 26-29 Positions of the appendix.

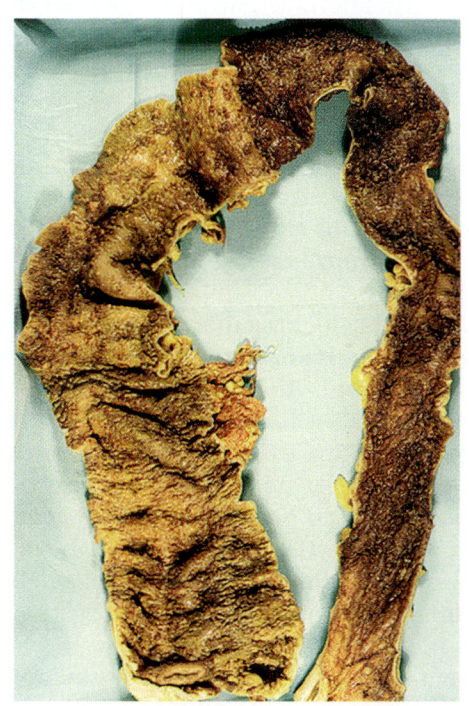

Figure 26-30 Acute ulcerative colitis.

examination. Remember that even people with a diagnosis of ulcerative colitis may have appendicitis, obstruction, or even gastroenteritis.

Treatment should be supportive. IV fluids may be helpful for dehydration because of volume loss with diarrhea. Provide medications for pain, nausea, and vomiting. Transport with the patient placed in a position of comfort.

Crohn's Disease

[OBJECTIVES 130, 131, 132, 133, 134]

Crohn's disease is an inflammatory bowel condition that affects both the small and large intestine. Historically, it has been believed to be an autoimmune-related condition. However, this belief is increasingly being questioned. The disease has definite genetic tendencies and tends to run in families. The inflammation in Crohn's disease causes significant swelling, ulcerations, scar tissue, and obstruction. The difference between Crohn's disease and ulcerative colitis is that in Crohn's disease the ulcerations may go through all layers of the bowel. In ulcerative colitis, the ulcerations tend to remain in the mucosa or most superficial layer. The location of these two inflammatory conditions also is slightly different. Crohn's disease affects all areas of the bowel and ulcerative colitis tends to affect only the colon or lower bowel.

Signs and symptoms of Crohn's disease are similar to other inflammatory conditions. In fact, Crohn's disease and ulcerative colitis are collectively referred to as *inflammatory bowel disease*. Patients may report nausea, vomiting, severe diarrhea, abdominal pain, abdominal cramping, weight loss, and loss of appetite. Crohn's disease also can involve other organ systems. Patients may have skin conditions, arthritis, gallbladder disease, inflammatory eye conditions, ulcerations of the nose and mouth, and kidney stones.

Obtaining a history is important. The patient may be aware of his or her diagnosis. If not, asking questions regarding other findings may allude to Crohn's disease. If the patient has diarrhea, abdominal cramping, right upper quadrant pain, kidney stones, and arthritis, he or she may have Crohn's disease. The ulcerations can perforate through the bowel wall. Patients also may have problems in the bladder, vaginal area, or skin. The patient may report pus or stool leaking from an ulcer in their skin. This can occur if the ulceration of the bowel erodes through the bowel wall and creates a **fistula** (tunnel) through the skin. Physical examination should include a complete head-to-toe examination because this condition can obviously cause multiple organ system ailments. Be sure to perform a thorough abdominal examination. Peritonitis may develop from a ruptured bowel. Abdominal distention, rebound tenderness, fever, and severe sepsis can occur.

Treatment should include rapid assessment and treatment of life-threatening conditions. IV access is important, and fluid hydration should be appropriately managed. Administer pain medication according to the patient's condition. These patients require rapid transport.

Diverticulosis and Diverticulitis

[OBJECTIVES 135, 136, 137, 138, 139]

The normal lumen of the bowel is smooth. Small sacs or outpouches called *diverticula* can form along the bowel wall. Diverticula can develop as people age and have been attributed to fiber-deficient diets. **Diverticulosis** is the medical condition of a bowel wall that has multiple diverticula. Diverticula develop from stretching of the bowel wall. As stool is moved by peristaltic contraction of the bowel, stretching of the bowel wall occurs. This stretching causes weakness in the bowel wall, forming these pouches or diverticula (Figure 26-31). **Diverticulitis** is a condition in which the diverticula get inflamed and infection may develop. Digested food matter may become trapped in these pouches, causing infection. Patients with diverticulosis may be asymptomatic. If they have symptoms, they may have irregular bowel movements. They also may have painless bloody stools. Patients with diverticulitis typically have signs of illness, including fever, shaking chills, nausea, vomiting, abdominal pain, and diarrhea.

While taking a history, a patient may provide a medical history of diverticulosis or even diverticulitis. Questions regarding nausea, vomiting, fever, chills, and pain are helpful. Asking the patient to relate this experience to previous abdominal complaints also may provide information. The physical examination should include a comprehensive examination with attention to the abdomen and pelvis. Treatment is mainly supportive. IV access is appropriate, and fluid replacement should be instituted if the patient appears dehydrated or has been vomiting. Finally, provide medications for pain and nausea as needed.

Patients with diverticulosis should follow a strict diet rich in fiber. Patients also should not eat any small seeds that can get trapped in the diverticular outpouches. Refer

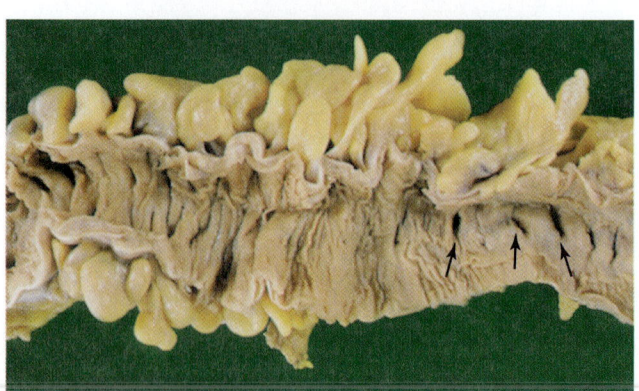

Figure 26-31 Diverticular disease.

Lips flat from dehydration
Hypokalemic, hypocalcemic
Cardiac dysrhythmias

the patient to his or her physician for more information on avoiding diverticulitis or the inflammation of diverticulosis.

Hemorrhoids

[OBJECTIVES 140, 141, 142, 143, 144]

Hemorrhoids are swollen venous tissue that originates from the anal area. They may be internal (not visualized) or external (around the external anal opening). Hemorrhoids commonly occur from increased pressure or straining while defecating. Signs and symptoms of hemorrhoids include itching, pain, burning, and bleeding. Patients typically do not call for prehospital care if they know they have hemorrhoids. However, the initial presenting symptoms may be rectal bleeding, which may prompt the call.

When obtaining a history, ask about bowel habits and the presence of hemorrhoids. If the patient states he or she has rectal bleeding, ask the patient to explain in more detail. Bleeding that drips into the toilet after a bowel movement or stains the tissue pink is consistent with a hemorrhoid. Large bloody stools should be treated as a GI bleed. Physical examination should include a thorough examination of the abdomen. This is important if the presenting symptom is rectal bleeding. Hemorrhoids should be a diagnosis of exclusion. Most bleeding from hemorrhoids is self-limiting, and pain typically resolves with topical creams. Treatment is supportive.

GASTROINTESTINAL ILLNESS

[OBJECTIVES 145, 146, 147, 148]

In summary, when addressing a GI complaint an accurate history is important. Many GI disorders are not true emergencies, but others can be life-threatening. Distinguishing the difference and treating accordingly are important. A thorough history and physical examination are critical to effective treatment and transport for GI emergencies. When obtaining information, apply this information to the pathophysiologic causes of the various GI diseases. Critical thinking skills can be used to form a differential diagnosis. When taking a history, ask basic questions. Open-ended questions and asking the patient to explain the symptoms yield the most information. Use the OPQRST mnemonic to elicit specific information regarding pain. Ask the patient questions regarding nausea, vomiting, diarrhea, stool consistency/color, and any bleeding. Treatment should immediately address any life-threatening conditions. Patients who appear to be in shock or who are losing large quantities of blood should be assessed quickly and transported. Start IV fluids en route. Remember that a correct diagnosis for the GI complaint is not necessary, but all emergent conditions should be treated rapidly. Through a combination of past medical history, the chief complaint, history of present illness, and physical examination, you should be able to formulate a basic assessment and treatment plan for the patient.

Case Scenario SUMMARY

1. *What is your initial impression?* A primary consideration is chest pain from an acute myocardial infarction.

2. *What do you think could be causing the woman's chest pain?* The woman's chest pain may have a number of causes, including acute myocardial infarction, pulmonary embolism, spontaneous pneumothorax, and referred pain from an abdominal disorder.

3. *What additional information do you need to complete your assessment?* Additional information includes a SAMPLE history and evaluation of OPQRST regarding the current condition.

4. *Has your initial impression changed?* A normal ECG does not completely rule out a cardiac etiology of the chest discomfort.

5. *What other conditions may mimic an acute myocardial infarction or give the impression that one has occurred?* Patients with epigastric distress and chest pain need a thorough assessment. Other possible causes of the patient's symptoms include indigestion, hiatal hernia, and pulmonary embolism.

6. *What are your treatment options for this patient?* Supplemental oxygen is appropriate for any patient with chest discomfort. The MONA protocol (*m*orphine, *o*xygen, *n*itroglycerin, and *a*spirin) also may be appropriate. In the event that the chest pain is caused by something other than a cardiac etiology, the protocol does not pose any significant problem. The patient in this case study has chest pain that originates in the epigastrium and is caused by cholecystitis. Analgesics are indicated in such cases.

7. *What is your final impression of the patient's condition?* Based on the patient's clinical picture, she is exhibiting signs and symptoms characteristic of biliary pain or cholecystitis.

8. *What did the meal contribute to the patient's chief complaint?* Patients with gallstones typically have intolerance for fatty foods such as eggs and acidic beverages such as orange juice.

9. *What are contributing factors that help determine the cause of the woman's chest pain?* The patient who typically suffers from gallstones has the five *F*'s of cholelithiasis: *f*air, *f*at, *f*ertile, *f*emale, and *f*orty. In addition to her clinical presentation, this patient exhibited all five *F*'s.

Chapter Summary

- Abdominal pain is one of the most common reasons why patients seek emergency care.
- Etiology of abdominal pain varies with the patient's age and risk factors.
- The GI system includes all organs responsible for the ingestion and digestion of food.
- Pain that is well localized is called *somatic pain*.
- Pain that is poorly localized is called *visceral pain*.
- Pain that is felt at a distant location is called *referred pain*.
- Pain assessment should follow the OPQRST mnemonic.
- The assessment should contain open-ended questions.
- Management of GI symptoms should include a primary survey, a secondary survey, pain and nausea management, and fluid replacement.
- Local protocols should be followed for appropriate treatment and management.
- Hernias that become strangulated or incarcerated can pose a serious medical condition.
- Esophagitis is inflammation of the esophagus and has many causes.
- GERD is a common disorder that leads to esophagitis.
- Caustic ingestions can cause trauma to the esophagus.
- Historical facts such as time of ingestion, chemical ingestion, and amount ingested are important.
- Airway control is important in caustic ingestions.
- Esophageal obstruction can occur with caustic ingestions.
- Most foreign objects will pass through the GI tract if they enter the stomach.
- Vomiting may lead to longitudinal tears in the esophagus called Mallory-Weiss tears.
- Hematemesis (frank bloody emesis) may occur with a Mallory-Weiss tear.
- Esophageal stenosis can occur from esophagitis.
- Tracheoesophageal fistula and esophageal atresia are congenital conditions.
- Tracheoesophageal fistula can lead to aspiration of food and liquids into the lungs.
- Esophageal varices can be caused by portal hypertension.
- Hematemesis may occur with varices and may be serious.
- Cirrhosis can lead to liver failure.
- Cirrhosis is caused by damage to the liver cells.
- Cirrhosis can lead to ascites or fluid in the abdominal cavity.
- Ascites can become infected and lead to sepsis (SBP).
- Cirrhosis often can cause encephalopathy or altered consciousness or coma.
- Renal failure may follow liver failure.
- Hepatitis is an inflammatory condition of the liver.
- Hepatitis may be self-limiting or progress to liver failure.
- Hepatitis A is transmitted by the fecal-oral route.
- Hepatitis B is transmitted by sexual contact, body fluid, tattoos, and blood transfusions.
- Hepatitis C is transmitted by infected blood or body fluids.
- Cholelithiasis is the presence of stones in the gallbladder.
- Cholelithiasis has an incidence of 10% to 20% of the population in developed countries.
- Pancreatitis is inflammation of the pancreas.
- Pancreatitis can present with severe abdominal pain, nausea, and vomiting.
- Peritonitis occurs when the lining of the abdominal cavity is inflamed.
- Rebound tenderness may be present with peritonitis.
- Gastritis is inflammation of the gastric mucosa.
- Gastritis can present with significant abdominal pain.
- Peptic ulcers can cause significant GI bleeding.
- GI bleeding has many causes.
- Treatment begins with a primary survey for GI bleeding.
- Appendicitis usually begins with periumbilical pain.
- Appendicitis can lead to sepsis if the luminal cavity ruptures.
- Ulcerative colitis typically affects the rectum. Ulcerative colitis is an inflammatory condition that involves the mucosal lining of the GI tract.
- Crohn's disease can affect the small and large intestines. It can cause erosion through all layers of the bowel, leading to fistula formation.
- Patients who have Crohn's disease may have arthritis, skin conditions, and inflammatory conditions of the eye in addition to bowel symptoms.
- Diverticular disease is caused by stretching of the bowel during straining and low-fiber diets. Diverticulosis is the disease of colonic diverticula (small outpouchings of the colon). Diverticulitis is inflammation of one or more of the outpouchings.
- Hemorrhoids are distended veins either internal or external to the anal opening.

REFERENCES

Feldman, M., Friedman, L., & Brandt, L. J. (2006). *Sleisenger & Fortran's gastrointestinal and liver disease: Vol. 2. Pathophysiology, diagnosis, management* (8th ed.). Philadelphia: Saunders.

Marx, J. A., Hockberger, R. S., & Walls, R. M. (Eds.). *Rosen's emergency medicine: Concepts and clinical practice* (6th ed.). Philadelphia: Elsevier.

McCance, K. L., & Huether, S. E. (2006). *Pathophysiology: The biologic basis for disease in adults and children* (5th ed.). St. Louis: Mosby.

University of Michigan Health System. (2005). *Esophageal varices.* Retrieved June 1, 2008, from http://www.med.umich.edu.

SUGGESTED RESOURCE

Drake, R. L., Vogl, W., & Mitchel, A. W. M. (2005). *Gray's anatomy for students.* Philadelphia: Churchill-Livingstone.

Chapter Quiz

1. You arrive on scene to find a 27-year-old man who states that he is having severe nausea, vomiting, diarrhea, bloody stools, and pus coming out of a small skin ulcer near his rectum. Which of the following diseases does this patient most likely have?
   a. Crohn's disease
   b. Gastritis
   c. Gastroenteritis
   d. Hemorrhoids

2. You arrive on scene to find a 55-year-old man who states he feels weak. The weakness has been getting worse over the last few days. Which of the following questions would be the most helpful in determining if the patient has GI bleeding?
   a. Are you experiencing any vomiting?
   b. Are you nauseated?
   c. Are your stools dark and tarry?
   d. Do you have abdominal pain or cramping?

3. You arrive on scene to find a 43-year-old woman who has hematemesis. She has a heart rate of 144 beats/min and a blood pressure of 72/40 mm Hg. Her skin is pale, cool, and diaphoretic. Which of the following is the most important appropriate initial treatment?
   a. Abdominal examination
   b. Assessment of airway and breathing
   c. IV fluid administration
   d. Supplemental oxygen

4. A patient has nausea, abdominal cramping, and diarrhea. The symptoms started approximately 2 hours ago. He has no significant past medical history. He does not drink alcohol or use any recreational drugs. Physical examination reveals a patient who has hyperactive bowel sounds, soft abdomen, and normal percussion sounds. Which of the following is the most likely cause of his symptoms?
   a. Cirrhosis
   b. Gastritis
   c. Gastroenteritis
   d. Small bowel obstruction

5. You arrive on scene to find a 54-year-old man who states he went on a drinking binge. He is reporting pain in the middle of his abdomen that radiates to his back. He denies any previous history of liver problems. He states he is nauseated and cannot keep any food down. On physical examination, you notice the patient has tenderness in the epigastric area. Which of the following is a likely cause of his pain?
   a. Crohn's disease
   b. Hemorrhoids
   c. Pancreatitis
   d. Ulcerative colitis

6. A patient has abdominal pain. His symptoms include vomiting of green liquid, loss of appetite, and abdominal pain. He states he has had multiple bowel surgeries and this feels like a previous bowel obstruction. His vitals are respirations, 14 breaths/min and nonlabored; blood pressure, 128/86 mm Hg; oxygen saturation, 100% on room air; and pulse, 98 beats/min. Which of the following would be appropriate treatment?
   a. A large glass of water for rehydration
   b. Insertion of a nasal airway
   c. IV access with a normal saline bolus
   d. Placing the patient in the shock position

7. You arrive on scene to find a 17-year-old male patient who is reporting right lower abdominal pain. He states he has fever, nausea, vomiting, and no appetite. When you palpate the left side of his abdomen, the patient states he feels pain in the right lower quadrant. Which of the following disease processes does this describe?
   a. Appendicitis
   b. Gastritis
   c. Hepatitis
   d. Pancreatitis

8. A patient calls 9-1-1 for rectal bleeding. He states he has had bright red blood filling the toilet. He denies pain and states he is feeling fine. He has not had this happen before. Which of the following is the most likely cause of his bleeding?
   a. Diverticulitis
   b. Diverticulosis
   c. Gastritis
   d. Hemorrhoids

9. You are examining a patient with abdominal pain. He cannot describe to you the exact location. Which of the following best describes this patient's pain?
   a. Rebound
   b. Referral
   c. Somatic
   d. Visceral

10. You arrive on the scene of a 43-year-old woman who has pain in the right upper quadrant of her abdomen. She complains that it is a sharp pain that is worse after eating. You palpate her right upper quadrant and she has guarding and reproducible pain. Which of the following is the most likely cause of her pain?
    a. Cholecystitis
    b. Crohn's disease
    c. Gastroenteritis
    d. Pancreatitis

11. You arrive on the scene of a patient with abdominal pain. He has pain that he rates at a 10 of 10. He states he is having nausea, vomiting, diarrhea, and he feels very ill. Which of the following is an appropriate treatment plan?
    a. Oral fluids administration
    b. Orogastric tube
    c. Pain and nausea management
    d. Supine transport

Terminology

Acalculous cholecystitis Inflammation of the gallbladder in the absence of gallstones.

Appendicitis Inflammation of the appendix, a tubular process that extends from the colon.

Cholangitis Inflammation of the bile duct.

Cholecystitis Inflammation of the gallbladder.

Choledocholithiasis The presence of gallstones in the common bile duct.

Cholelithiasis The presence of stones in the gallbladder.

Cirrhosis A chronic degenerative disease of the liver.

Coagulation necrosis Dead or dying tissue that forms a scar or eschar.

Diverticulitis Inflammation of a diverticulum, especially of the small pockets in the wall of the colon that fill with stagnant fecal material and become inflamed.

Diverticulosis A condition of the colon in which outpouches develop.

Dyspepsia Epigastric discomfort often occurring after meals.

Dysplasia Abnormal cell growth; cells take on an abnormal size, shape, and organization as a result of ongoing irritation or inflammation.

Encephalopathy A condition of disturbances of consciousness and possible progression to coma.

Esophagitis Inflammation of the esophagus.

Fecalith A hard impacted mass of feces in the colon.

Feces Undigested food material that has been processed in the colon.

Fistula An abnormal tunnel that has formed from within the body to the skin.

Gastritis Inflammation of the stomach.

Gastroenteritis Inflammation of the stomach and the intestines.

Guarding The contraction of abdominal muscles in the anticipation of a painful stimulus.

Hematemesis Vomiting of bright red blood.

Hematochezia Bright-red blood in the stool.

Hemorrhoids Swollen, distended veins in the anorectal area.

Hepatitis Inflammation of the liver.

Hernia Protrusion of any organ through an abdominal opening in the muscle wall of the cavity that surrounds it.

Hiatus A gap or a cleft.

Hyperresonant A high-pitched sound.

Icterus Jaundice.

Ileus Decreased peristaltic movement of the colon.

Incarcerated hernia Hernia of intestine that cannot be returned or reduced by manipulation; it may or may not become strangulated.

Inflammation A tissue reaction in an injury, infection, or insult.

Intussusception Invagination of a part of the colon into another part of the colon; also referred to as *telescoping*.

Liquefaction necrosis Dead or dying tissue in which the necrotic material becomes softened and liquefied.

Malignant Very dangerous or virulent; often used to describe a deadly form of cancer or a spreading of cancer.

Mediastinum Located in the middle of the thoracic cavity between the two plural sacs; contains the heart, great vessels, trachea, and esophagus among other structures; extends from the sternum to the vertebral column.

Melena Foul-smelling, dark, tarry stools stained with blood pigments or with digested blood, often indicating GI bleeding.

Mesentery Layers of connective tissue found in the peritoneal cavity.

Metastatic Spread of cancerous cells to a distant site.

Murphy's sign An inspiratory pause when the right upper quadrant is palpated.

Pancreatitis Inflammation of the pancreas.

Percussion A diagnostic technique that uses tapping on the body to differentiate air, solids, and fluids.

Peristalsis The wavelike contraction of the smooth muscle of the GI tract.

Peritoneum Serous membrane that lines the peritoneal cavity.

Peritonitis Inflammation of the peritoneum, typically caused by infection or in response to contact with blood or digestive fluids.

Portal hypertension Increased venous pressure in the portal circulation.

Pruritus Itching of the skin.

Rebound tenderness Discomfort experienced by the patient that occurs when the pressure from palpation is released.

Referred pain Pain felt at a site distant to the organ of origin.

Rovsing's sign Pain in the right lower quadrant elicited by palpation of the abdomen in the left lower quadrant.

Somatic pain Pain that arises from either the cutaneous tissues of the body's surface or deep tissues of the body, such as musculoskeletal tissue or the parietal peritoneum.

Spontaneous bacterial peritonitis (SBP) Infection of cirrhotic fluid in the abdominal cavity.

Stenosis Abnormal constriction or narrowing of a structure.

Strangulation Compression of the vessels that carry blood, leading to ischemia.

Stricture A specific form of narrowing, usually from scar tissue formation.

Subcutaneous emphysema Air entrapped beneath the skin, typically caused by rupture of a structure containing air; feels like crackling when palpated.

Varices Distended veins.

Visceral pain Deep pain that arises from internal areas of the body that are enclosed within a cavity.

Volvulus Intestinal obstruction caused by a knotting and twisting of the bowel.

Renal and Urogenital Disorders

Objectives   *After completing this chapter, you will be able to:*

1. Discuss the anatomy and physiology of the urogenital organs and structures.
2. Describe the questioning technique and specific questions the paramedic should use when gathering a focused history in a patient with abdominal pain.
3. Describe the techniques used in performing a comprehensive physical examination of a patient reporting abdominal pain associated with the urologic system.
4. Describe the incidence, morbidity, and mortality rates and risk factors predisposing to urologic emergencies.
5. Describe the etiology, history, and physical findings of acute renal failure.
6. With the patient history and physical examination findings, develop a treatment plan for a patient in acute renal failure.
7. Describe the etiology, history, and physical findings of chronic renal failure.
8. With the patient history and physical examination findings, develop a treatment plan for a patient in chronic renal failure.
9. Define *renal dialysis*.
10. Discuss the common complication of renal dialysis.
11. Describe the etiology, history, and physical findings of renal calculi.
12. With the patient history and physical examination findings, develop a treatment plan for a patient with renal calculi.
13. Describe the etiology, history, and physical findings of urinary retention.
14. With the patient history and physical examination findings, develop a treatment plan for a patient with urinary retention.
15. Describe the etiology, history, and physical findings of a urinary tract infection.
16. With the patient history and physical examination findings, develop a treatment plan for a patient with a urinary tract infection.
17. Describe the internal and external male anatomy.
18. Describe the incidence and signs and symptoms associated with genital lesions, including genital herpes, syphilis, chancroid lesions, granuloma inguinale, lymphadenoma, genital warts, and *Molluscum contagiosum.*
19. Discuss the signs and symptoms associated with blunt genital trauma in the male patient.
20. Describe the prehospital care for blunt genital trauma in the male patient.
21. Discuss male genitourinary infections, including epididymitis, orchitis, Fournier's gangrene, prostatitis, and urethritis.
22. Describe the signs and symptoms of male genitourinary infections, including epididymitis, orchitis, and Fournier's gangrene.
23. Describe the etiology, history, and physical findings of phimosis and paraphimosis.
24. With the patient history and physical examination findings, develop a treatment plan for a patient with paraphimosis.
25. Describe the etiology, history, and physical findings of priapism.
26. With the patient history and physical examination findings, develop a treatment plan for a patient with priapism.
27. Discuss the epidemiology of benign prostate hypertrophy.
28. Discuss the effects of an enlarged prostate gland, including urinary retention, increased risk of urinary tract infections, and renal failure.
29. Discuss the etiology of testicular masses.
30. Describe the etiology, history, and physical findings of testicular torsion.
31. With the patient history and physical examination findings, develop a treatment plan for a patient with testicular torsion.

Chapter Outline

Urinary System Anatomy
Functions of the Urinary System
General Assessment Considerations

Kidney Diseases
Urinary System Conditions
Chapter Summary

Case Scenario

At 9:15 AM you receive a call to a private residence involving difficulty breathing. You arrive within minutes of receiving the call and are greeted by a distraught older woman who tells you that her husband is "gurgling when he breathes." She escorts you into the master bedroom, where you find a 70-year-old man unresponsive in his bed. The sounds of pulmonary edema are obvious from several feet away. You ask about his current condition and the woman states, "He was like this when I woke up this morning." She has not been able to arouse her husband. A quick head-to-toe assessment reveals cool skin coated with crystals. A distinct odor of urine permeates the air. When palpating the patient's arms, you note a large, pulsating bulge in the right forearm and a nonpulsatile bulge in the left forearm.

Questions

1. What is your initial impression of this patient?
2. What additional information do you need?
3. What may be causing the patient's pulmonary edema?

A patient reporting abdominal pain can have one of many problems, including conditions involving the urinary system. Thus the paramedic should gain an understanding of the urinary system to perform a complete assessment and determine the nature of the patient's chief complaint.

URINARY SYSTEM ANATOMY

[OBJECTIVE 1]

The urinary system is composed of organs that serve many functions, including the elimination of dissolved organic waste products from the vascular system and body (Figure 27-1). Structures of the urinary system include the following:

- Kidneys, which produce urine
- Ureters, which drain urine from each kidney into the urinary bladder
- Urinary bladder, which stores urine before elimination from the body
- Urethra, which transports urine out of the body

Structure of the Kidneys

The kidneys are located on either side of the spine between the twelfth thoracic vertebra and the third lumbar vertebra. The right kidney is positioned lower than the left to make room for the liver. Both kidneys are located between the back muscles and the peritoneum. The kidneys are located in the retroperitoneal space, which is behind and outside the peritoneal cavity.

As shown in Figure 27-1, B, each kidney is shaped like a bean. Each kidney has a medial indentation (known as the **hilus**) through which the renal artery, vein, lymphatic vessels, and nerves enter and leave the kidney. Each kidney has three main regions: the renal cortex, the renal medulla, and the renal pelvis. The outer layer of the kidney is the renal cortex. The renal medulla, found deeper within the kidney, forms cone-shaped areas called renal pyramids. Renal columns, which are extensions of the renal cortex, separate the renal pyramids. The renal pyramids point toward the renal pelvis, which collects urine and forms the upper portion of the ureter. The edges of the renal pelvis are called calyces, which collect urine. Urine production begins in the renal pyramids and renal cortex.

Nephrons

Nephrons are the functional (urine-producing) units of the kidney. Nephrons filter the blood; collect excreted water and waste products; and reabsorb water, nutrients, and electrolytes (Figure 27-2). Each normal adult kidney contains more than 1 million nephrons. Blood flow to the kidneys is supplied by the renal arteries, which divide into arterioles and capillaries.

A nephron contains a **glomerulus,** which is a clump of interconnected capillaries. The glomerulus projects into a cup-shaped capsule, called *Bowman's capsule.* The space inside Bowman's capsule is called *Bowman's space.* The glomerulus and Bowman's capsule compose the renal corpuscle. Blood enters the glomerulus by an afferent arteriole and leaves by an efferent arteriole. Pores in the walls of the capillaries in the glomerulus allow the blood to be filtered. Filtered water and wastes (known as filtrate) flow from Bowman's capsule through renal tubules (Figure 27-3). These tubules are divided into sections, each having several functions (Table 27-1).

Nephrons reabsorb all useful organic materials as well as more than 90% of the water from the filtrate. Approximately 6 m² of filtration space is found in the kidneys. Nephrons are typically able to produce about 125 mL/min of filtrate. However, nearly 99% of the filtrate is reabsorbed, and only 1 mL/min of filtrate reaches the collecting tubules that empty into the urinary bladder. One measure of kidney function is assessing the

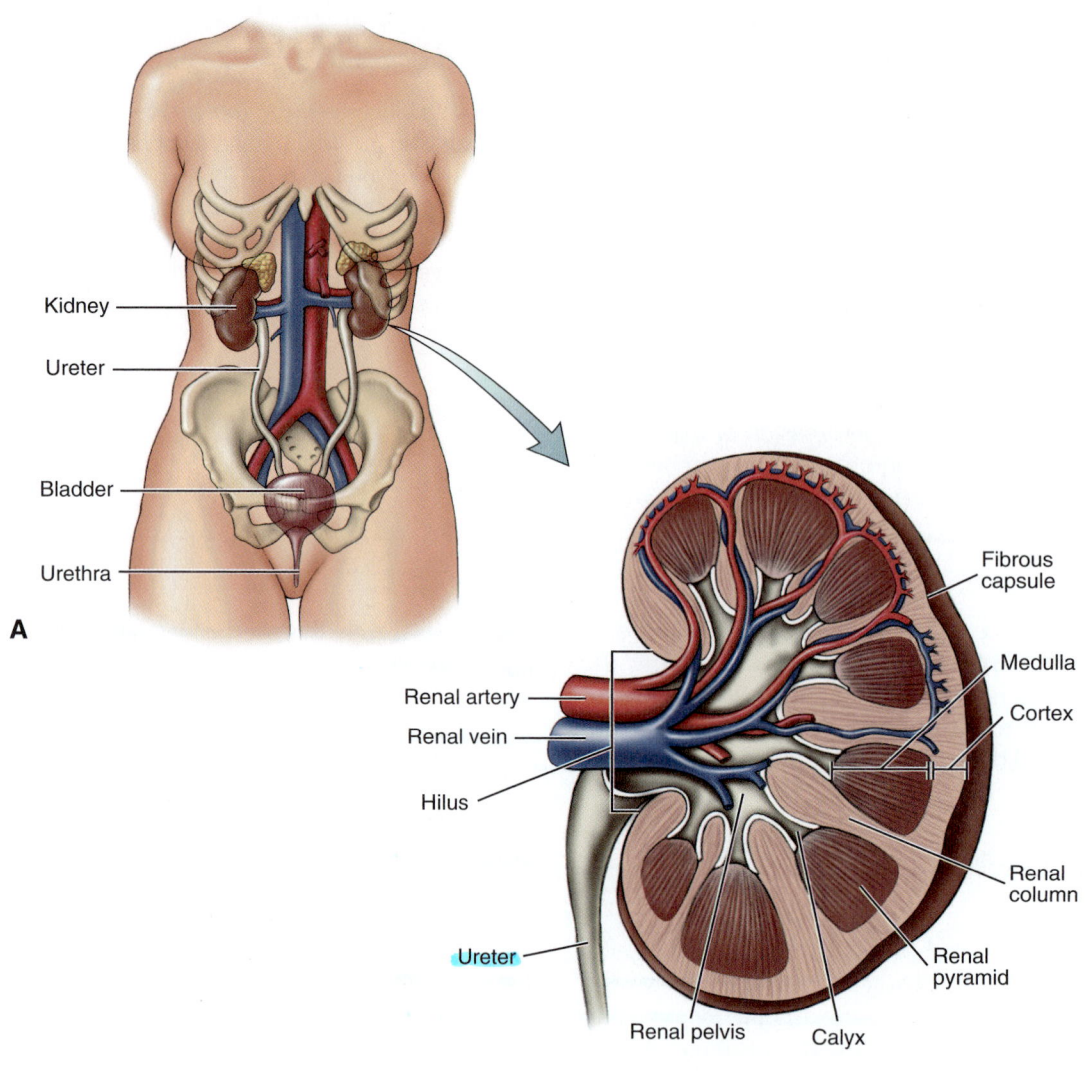

Figure 27-1 A, Organs of the urinary system. **B,** Diagram of the kidney.

TABLE 27-1	Functions of the Renal Tubules
Renal Tubule	**Function**
Proximal convoluted tubule	Reabsorbs water, ions, and organic nutrients
Loop of Henle	Reabsorbs water, sodium, and chloride ions
Distal convoluted tubule	Secretes ions, acids, drugs, and toxins
Collecting tubule	Reabsorbs water; secrets sodium, potassium, hydrogen, and bicarbonate ions

amount of urine produced per hour. In a catheterized patient, urine production of 30 mL/hr or more is considered adequate. *up to 60-120 ml/hr is normal*

Many factors influence urine production, including state of hydration, renal blood flow, medications, and levels of hormones such as antidiuretic hormone (ADH) and aldosterone. Of particular note is the effect of diuretics on filtration, reabsorption of water and electrolytes, and urine formation. For example, osmotic diuretics such as mannitol inhibit water and sodium reabsorption in the proximal tubules. Loop diuretics such as furosemide reduce sodium, potassium, and chloride reabsorption in the loop of Henle. Thiazide diuretics inhibit sodium and chloride reabsorption in the distal tubules. *HCTZ*

Ureters and Urinary Bladder

Urine is drained from each kidney through thin-walled muscular tubes called **ureters.** These tubes are approximately 30 cm (12 inches) in length. Urine is moved out of the kidney by peristaltic contractions that begin inside the kidney and minor and major calyces. These contractions continue in the renal pelvis and move the urine along the ureters toward the urinary bladder.

The **urinary bladder** is a muscular sac responsible for storing urine before it is eliminated from the body

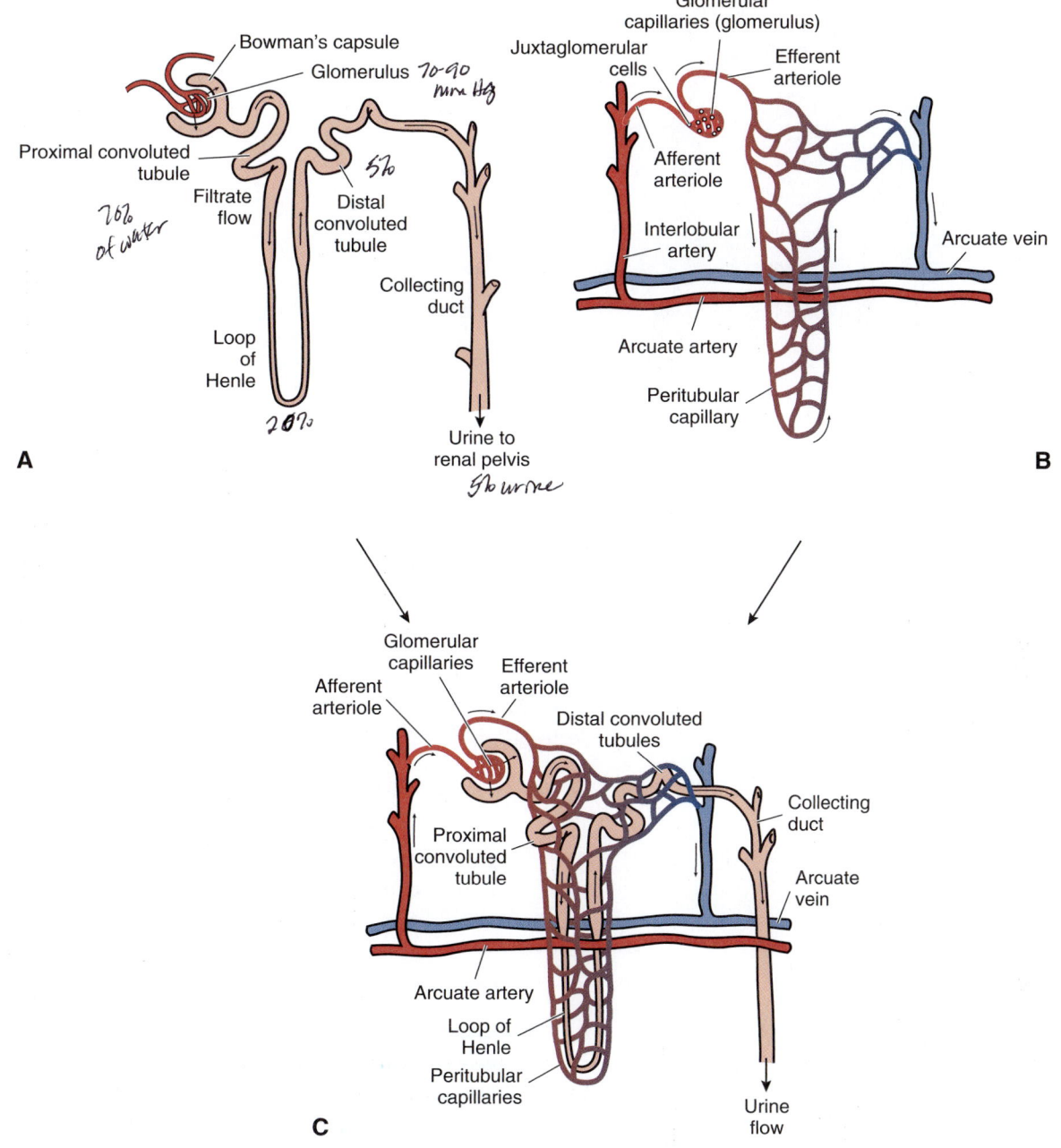

Figure 27-2 The tubular and vascular structures of the nephron. **A,** Glomerulus and tubules. **B,** Blood supply to the nephron. **C,** Complete nephron.

(Figure 27-4). In males, the urinary bladder is located between the rectum and the pubic bone (pubic symphysis). In females, the urinary bladder is below the uterus and in front of the vagina. Because it can expand to accommodate an increasing amount of urine, the size of the bladder varies. At capacity, the adult urinary bladder can hold up to 1 L of urine.

Urethra

The **urethra** is a short tube that transports urine from the urinary bladder outside the body. In both sexes the urethra passes through a band of skeletal muscle known

as the external urethral sphincter, which helps control the flow of urine.

FUNCTIONS OF THE URINARY SYSTEM

The urinary system has several functions, as described in Chapter 7. A brief review of these functions is provided here. The most obvious function is water and waste removal. However, this important system carries out many other functions, including:

• Regulating water and electrolytes
• Regulating acid base balance

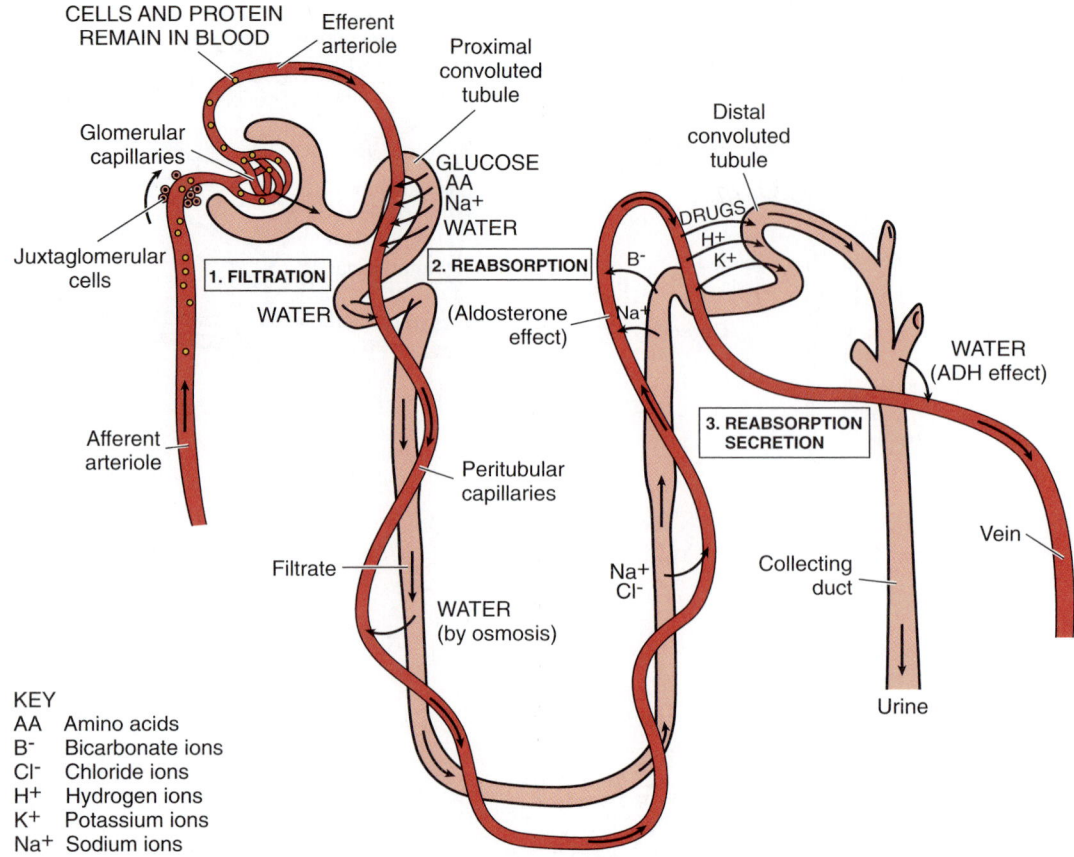

Figure 27-3 The process of urine formation. *ADH*, Antidiuretic hormone.

- Excreting waste products and foreign chemicals
- Regulating arterial blood pressure
- Secreting hormones
- Producing red blood cells (erythrocytes)
- Producing new sugar (glucose)

Water and Electrolyte Regulation

Water and electrolyte excretion must be matched to water and electrolyte intake to achieve homeostasis. The kidneys alter their filtration and excretion rates to match the body's intake of water and electrolytes.

Acid-Base Balance   *Na Bicarb*

Along with the lungs and other body buffer systems, the kidneys help regulate acid-base balance by excreting acids and regulating the body's stores of buffers. For example, the kidneys are the only way that the body can eliminate sulfuric and phosphoric acids created by the metabolism of proteins.

Excreting Waste Products and Foreign Chemicals

The kidneys are the primary means of eliminating waste products generated by metabolism, including urea, creatinine, uric acid, and bilirubin (from breakdown of hemoglobin). They also eliminate other foreign chemicals ingested or produced by the body such as toxins, food additives, and medications.

Hormone Secretion

Erythropoietin (EPO) and calcitriol are hormones secreted by the kidneys. EPO acts on the bone marrow to increase the production of red blood cells. Calcitriol is the active form of vitamin D. It promotes the absorption of calcium from food and mobilizes calcium from bones to the blood.

Renin is a hormone formed in the kidney that initiates the eventual formation of angiotensin II, which is discussed in more detail in the following section.

Arterial Blood Pressure Regulation

The kidneys primarily regulate blood pressure by excreting large amounts of sodium and water. However, over a short period the kidneys exert control over arterial blood pressure by the renin-angiotensin-aldosterone mechanism (Figure 27-5). This mechanism consists of secreting renin, which leads to the formation of angiotensin II, a powerful vasoconstrictor. This is an important concept, especially when considering a patient in shock. When a patient goes into shock, the kidneys respond by producing renin. Renin combines

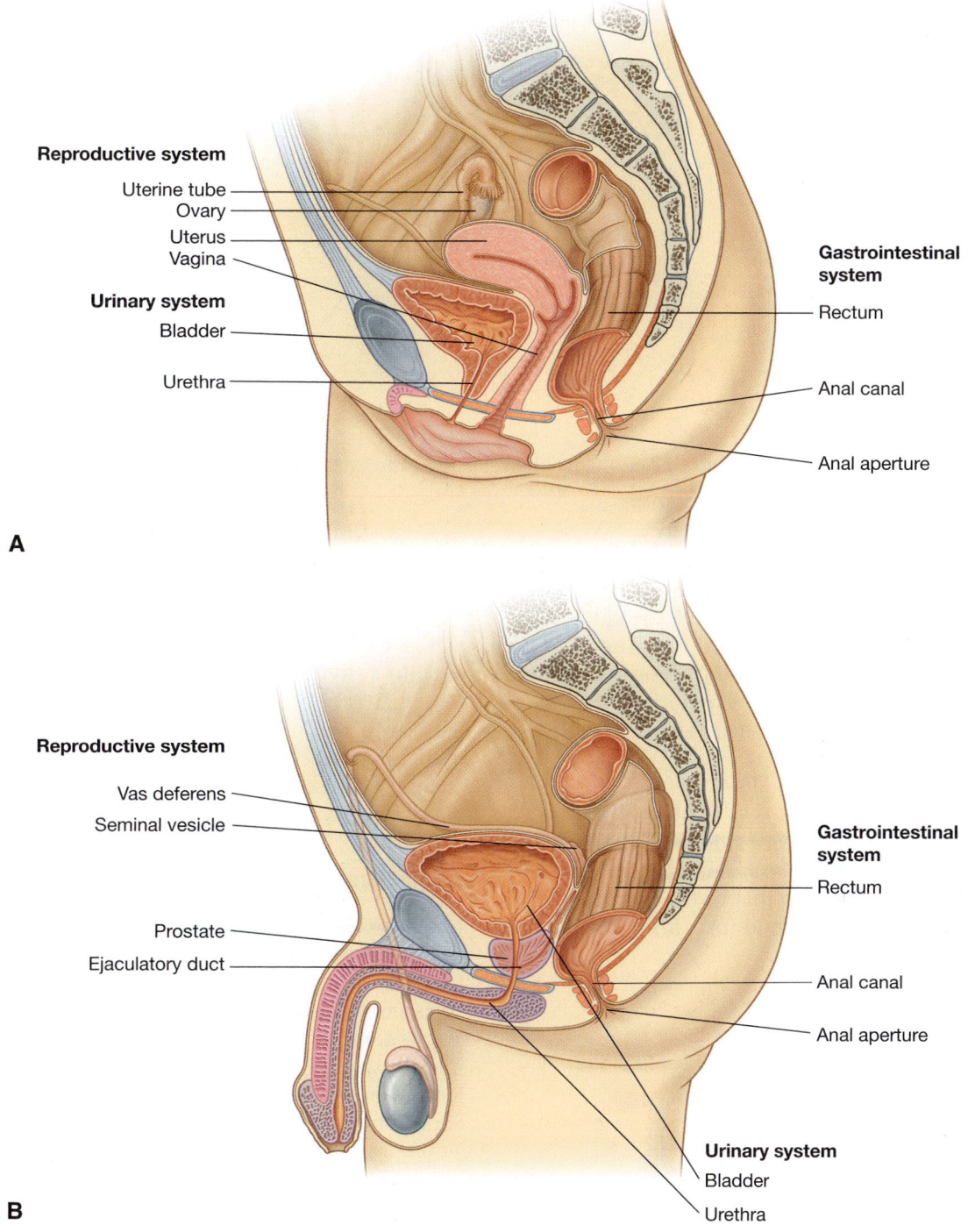

Reproductive system
Uterine tube
Ovary
Uterus
Vagina

Urinary system
Bladder
Urethra

Gastrointestinal system
Rectum

Anal canal

Anal aperture

A

Reproductive system
Vas deferens
Seminal vesicle

Prostate
Ejaculatory duct

Gastrointestinal system
Rectum

Anal canal

Anal aperture

Urinary system
Bladder
Urethra

B

Figure 27-4 Location of the urinary bladder. **A,** Female. **B,** Male.

with angiotensinogen to produce angiotensin I. In the lungs angiotensin-converting enzyme converts angiotensin I to angiotensin II, which constricts the peripheral arteries as a compensatory mechanism to maintain the patient's blood pressure. In addition, angiotensin II stimulates the production of aldosterone. Kidney function is regulated by several hormones produced in other areas of the body. Aldosterone, produced by the adrenal glands, exerts an effect on the kidneys by increasing the reabsorption of sodium into the circulatory system. As sodium is reabsorbed, so is water and the circulating fluid volume is maintained. ADH is produced by the hypothalamus and released by the posterior pituitary. Increases in ADH cause decreased elimination of water, whereas decreases in ADH cause increased elimination of water. Atrial naturietic peptide (ANP) is produced by the atria when they are distended by increased blood volume. ANP inhibits the absorption of water and sodium in the renal tubules, thereby increasing the elimination of water.

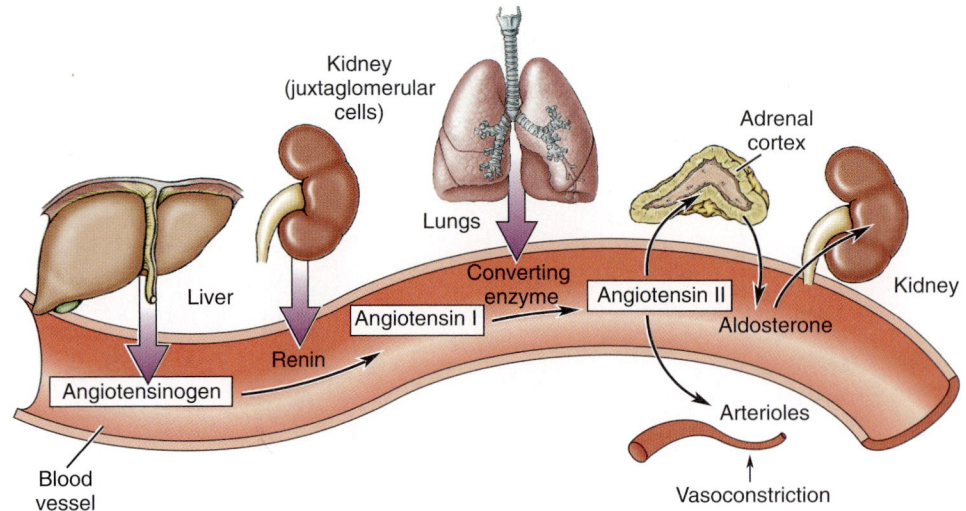

Figure 27-5 The renin-angiotensin-aldosterone system.

Erythrocyte Production

The kidneys secrete an EPO to stimulate the production of red blood cells. In healthy individuals, the kidneys are responsible for nearly all EPO production in the body. In patients with renal failure or other kidney disease or those who have had their kidneys removed, the reduction in EPO typically results in severe anemia.

Gluconeogenesis

During prolonged fasting, the kidneys produce new glucose from amino acids and other chemicals. This gluconeogenesis is comparable to that of the liver when the individual has gone without food for a long time.

> **PARAMEDIC*Pearl***
>
> The kidneys have multiple functions and are major regulatory organs affecting water, blood pressure, red blood cells, acid-base balance, and blood sugar.

GENERAL ASSESSMENT CONSIDERATIONS

[OBJECTIVES 2, 3]

Patients with acute abdominal pain need a careful evaluation to discover the nature of their discomfort. The astute paramedic should conduct a focused examination that includes the following:

- Detailed recent medical history
- History of the present complaint
- Any changes in bladder or bowel habits?
- Any increased or decreased frequency in urination?
- Any pain or burning sensation when urinating?
- Any unusual color or odor to the urine?
- Any blood in the urine?

- Any unusual discharge?
- Any unusual lumps or recent swelling?
- Thoroughly evaluating the presenting pain, including the OPQRST method
- Determining whether the pain is visceral, such as in a ureter or the bladder, or somatic in nature

Perform a complete and focused physical examination including inspection, auscultation, palpation, and percussion of the abdomen to help identify the cause of the patient's discomfort.

Inspection

Uncover the patient's abdomen and thoroughly examine it, noting size and whether it is flat, concave, or round. Look for any scars or wounds and, if present, ask about their relevance to the patient's current condition. Note any abdominal movement, such as pulsation. Such movements are more likely to be noticeable in a thin person. Finally, note the presence of edema, asymmetry, or other appearance that may be abnormal.

Auscultation

With the diaphragm of the stethoscope, listen to the patient's abdomen in various quadrants. Bowel sounds are gurgling or clicking sounds that appear from five to 35 times per minute. Hypoactive bowel sounds are heard less than five times per minute. In contrast, hyperactive bowel sounds are heard more than 35 times per minute. The paramedic also should note the absence of bowel sounds.

> **PARAMEDIC*Pearl***
>
> The value of listening to bowel sounds in the prehospital setting is questionable. Prehospital care for patients with a genitourinary complaint is primarily supportive. Although listening to bowel sounds can be informative, the information obtained is unlikely to alter the paramedic's treatment plan.

Palpation

After listening to the patient's abdomen, palpate it. Note the temperature and moisture of the abdominal skin as well as the presence of any tenderness, swelling, or pulsations. Place the pads of your fingers on the abdomen and, using the fingers of your other hand, press firmly and indent the patient's abdomen by a few inches. Note the presence of any tenderness.

PARAMEDIC*Pearl*

When palpating the abdomen, always begin in the quadrant farthest from the site of the pain indicated by the patient.

Percussion

Place the palm and fingers of your flattened hand over each quadrant of the abdomen. With two fingers of the other hand, tap on the index and middle fingers of the hand on the abdomen. This action creates a shock wave transmitted into the abdominal cavity. The paramedic should observe two things: sounds created by the percussion and any pain that may be caused by the technique. The sounds created by tapping on the abdomen vary depending on the nature of the tissue, as follows:

- Muscle tissue produces a flat sound
- Solid organs produce a dull, thudding sound
- Hollow organs produce tympanic sounds (drumlike) because they contain air and fluid

Percussion over the kidney is slightly different from percussion of the abdomen. With the patient sitting or lying on one side, place the palm and open fingers of one hand directly over the kidney. With the other hand formed in a fist, firmly strike your flattened hand. The patient should feel a thud, but no pain. The presence of pain could indicate a pathologic condition of the kidney or associated structures.

In the event the patient has an acute urologic emergency, the paramedic should consider treatment alternatives that may include the following:

- Airway, ventilatory, and circulatory support as needed
- Initiating intravenous (IV) therapy
- Pain medication, depending on the nature of the problem
- Prompt transportation while monitoring level of consciousness and vital signs

KIDNEY DISEASES

[OBJECTIVE 4]

A number of different kidney diseases afflict millions of people throughout the United States. These illnesses are associated with high rates of morbidity and mortality along with significant costs to provide ongoing care. According to the National Kidney and Urologic Diseases

Information Clearinghouse, approximately 4.5% of adults older than 20 years have evidence of chronic kidney disease (National Institutes of Health [NIH], 2004).

Renal insufficiency is a decrease in renal function to approximately 25% of normal. When renal function is significantly lost, renal failure is present.

Acute Renal Failure

[OBJECTIVES 5, 6]

Etiology and Epidemiology

Acute renal failure (ARF) is seen when the kidneys suddenly stop functioning either partially or completely but eventually recover full or nearly full functioning over time. ARF can result from problems in the following three areas:

1. Decreased blood supply to the kidneys (prerenal)
2. Abnormalities within the kidneys (intrarenal)
3. Blockage in the urine collecting system (postrenal)

ARF typically results from a major insult to the body. Once the insult has been identified and promptly corrected, ARF reverses. Failure to correct the problem can lead to chronic renal failure.

Prerenal Acute Renal Failure. Prerenal ARF is caused by a reduction in blood supply to the kidneys. The name *prerenal* stems from the problem occurring before the kidney. Prerenal failure is the most common cause of ARF. Causes of prerenal ARF include the following:

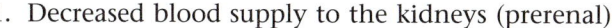

- Hypovolemia from blood loss (trauma, surgery, diarrhea, vomiting, burns)
- Cardiac problems such as acute myocardial infarction or damage to cardiac valves
- Abnormalities in kidney hemodynamics such as stenosis, embolism, or thrombosis in the renal artery as well as blockage of prostaglandin synthesis caused by excessive aspirin intake
- Hypotension caused by peripheral vasodilation, including neurogenic or anaphylactic shock or septicemia

Patients with prerenal ARF can regain kidney function as long as blood flow to the kidney remains at least 20% of normal and the cause of the decreased blood flow is corrected before the cells of the kidney are damaged.

Intrarenal Acute Renal Failure. When the disease develops within the kidneys, the patient is said to have intrarenal ARF. Causes of this condition include the following:

- Injury to the small blood vessels and/or glomerulus from inflammation of the blood vessels, emboli from cholesterol, malignant hypertension, and acute glomerulonephritis
- Injury to the structures of the tubules, such as necrosis from ischemia or toxins such as heavy metals, ethylene glycol, insecticides, or poisonous mushrooms

BOX 27-1	Substances That May Cause Acute Renal Failure

- Heavy metals, such as mercury, arsenic, and lead
- Solvents such as methanol and ethylene glycol
- Antibiotics such as sulfonamides, aminoglycosides, penicillins, cephalosporins, and acyclovir
- Angiotensin-converting enzyme inhibitors
- Antidepressants and anticonvulsants such as citalopram hydrobromide (Celexa), phenytoin, and carbamazepine
- Analgesics and nonsteroidal antiinflammatory drugs, including acetaminophen and aspirin
- Anticancer drugs
- Pesticides and herbicides
- Drugs that can form methemoglobin, such as nitrates, nitrites, potassium chloride, and benzocaine

- Interstitial injury of the kidneys caused by acute pyelonephritis

To identify intrarenal causes of ARF, carefully assess the patient, paying attention to the following:

- **Hematuria** (blood in the urine), edema, and hypertension, which indicate a glomerular etiology
- A recent history of hypotension after hemorrhage, drug overdose or abuse, sepsis, surgery, or cardiac arrest, all of which can lead to tubular intrarenal ARF
- Any exposure to toxins, including new medications that could damage the kidneys or cause rhabdomyolysis
- Recent blood transfusion

Of particular note is the exposure to toxins. Ingestion, inhalation, injection, or absorption of many chemicals can be **nephrotoxic.** Substances that can be poisonous to the kidneys are shown in Box 27-1.

PARAMEDIC*Pearl*

Nonsteroidal antiinflammatory drugs can be dangerous, especially in patients at risk of hypovolemia (Ulinksi, 2004). When obtaining a patient's history, question the patient about the use of nonsteroidal antiinflammatory drugs, including the quantity taken, period over which they are taken, and the reason they are taken.

Postrenal Acute Renal Failure. Any condition that can block the flow of urine can lead to postrenal ARF. Causes of postrenal ARF include the following:

- Blockage of the renal pelvis or ureters by large kidney stones (**renal calculi**) or blood clots
- Obstruction of the urinary bladder
- Urethral obstruction

When only one kidney is affected, the composition of body fluids typically changes little because the other kidney assumes an increase in urinary output. However, if both kidneys are affected or if the patient has only one kidney, ARF quickly develops. When the condition involves both kidneys, it must be resolved with a few hours before permanent kidney damage.

History and Physical Examination Findings

As previously mentioned, the three general types of ARF are prerenal, intrarenal, and postrenal. Regardless of the cause the end result is a buildup of nitrogen-containing waste products, such as urea, in the blood. This buildup of nitrogenous waste products is called **azotemia.** This condition has negative effects on nearly every system in the body and causes disorders such as metabolic acidosis and hyperkalemia. Although determining the specific cause of the condition may be difficult, a careful patient evaluation may provide clues to the cause of the illness. Signs and symptoms of ARF common to all types include the following:

- Reduced urine output (oliguria)
- No urinary output (anuria)
- Excessive urination at night
- Swelling of feet, ankles, and legs
- Neuropathies of hands and feet
- Anorexia
- Altered mental status, including agitation, lethargy, delirium, coma, alternating moods, hallucinations
- Metallic taste in mouth
- Hand tremors
- Seizures
- Easy bruising and prolonged bleeding
- Flank pain
- **Tinnitus**
- Hypertension

When evaluating the patient for possible ARF from postrenal causes, ask the patient about a medical history of the following:

- Kidney stones
- Prostate enlargement
- Gout
- Use of medications that can cause crystal formation, such as sulfonamides, acyclovir, and methotrexate

Therapeutic Interventions

Prehospital care for patients in ARF includes airway and ventilatory support, establishing IV access, monitoring the patient's vitals signs and ECG, prompt treatment for shock (hypovolemic and other types), maintenance of an adequate blood pressure after a cardiac event, proper treatment for ingested toxins, and prompt transport to the emergency department.

The keys to managing ARF are prevention and correcting the pathology that can lead to the condition. Prevention is aimed at reversing hypovolemia and treating toxic exposures that put the kidneys at risk. Be alert for signs and symptoms related to hypovolemia, such as thirst, decreased urine output, orthostatic hypotension, and severe dehydration. These conditions, if treated promptly with fluid resuscitation, can reverse ARF. In patients with severe cardiac disease, orthopnea and paroxysmal nocturnal dyspnea can indicate a predisposition for ARF. In the elderly, be aware that insensible fluid loss such as normal fluid loss during breathing can reduce circulating volume in patients who are unable to provide hydration for themselves. This is particularly true during prolonged heat waves during the summer.

PARAMEDIC Pearl

The National Kidney Foundation and other resources publish information on coping with kidney failure for patients and their families. Key tips include the following:

- Evaluating all treatment options, such as dialysis and transplantation
- Paying attention to a proper diet that includes increased calories, but reduced protein intake
- Monitoring water intake to avoid overhydration

Brochures are available for download from the National Kidney Foundation (http://www.kidney.org).

Chronic Renal Failure

[OBJECTIVES 7, 8]

Etiology and Epidemiology

By definition, **chronic renal failure** is a structural or functional abnormality of the kidneys that is present for more than 3 months. Chronic renal failure is caused by an irreversible loss of a large number of nephrons. The loss can be rapid or gradual depending on the underlying cause. The patient's clinical picture usually appears reasonably normal until 70% or more of the nephrons have ceased functioning.

Two of every 1000 people currently have chronic renal failure and its terminal counterpart, **end-stage renal disease (ESRD).** Similar to ARF, chronic renal failure can have prerenal, intrarenal, and postrenal causes (Box 27-2). <10-20 ml/hr

Patients with chronic renal failure are at risk for progression to ESRD and cardiovascular disease. This is accounted for in part by the fact that many risk factors are common to both progression of kidney disease and cardiovascular complications, such as diabetes, hypertension, and high cholesterol (Toto, 2004). Diabetes mellitus and hypertension are among the strongest risk factors for chronic renal failure. African Americans, Mexican Americans, Native Americans, Asians, and Pacific Islanders have a markedly higher risk for chronic renal failure than the general population (Toto, 2004). Other important risk factors include autoimmune disease, chronic systemic

---

BOX 27-2 Causes of Chronic Renal Failure

- Glomerulonephritis
- Polyarteritis nodosa
- Lupus erythematosus
- Diabetes mellitus
- Hypertension
- Atherosclerosis
- Toxins
- Renal calculi
- Prostate enlargement
- Constriction of the urethra
- Polycystic disease (congenital)

BOX 27-3 Signs and Symptoms of Chronic Renal Failure

- Headache
- Weakness
- Mental status changes
- Loss of appetite (anorexia)
- Nausea, vomiting
- Diarrhea
- Weight loss
- Increased urination (the kidneys cannot conserve water)
- Rusty or brown-colored urine
- Increased thirst (loss of water leads to dehydration)
- Hypertension
- Puffiness around the eyes
- Uremic frost
- Itching (pruritus)

---

infection, urinary tract infection, obstruction of the urinary tract, cancer, family history of chronic kidney disease, reduced renal mass, low birth weight, drug exposure, and recovery after ARF (Toto, 2004).

Many vital processes within the body are affected as kidney function declines. For example, increased amounts of sodium, water, and potassium are retained, upsetting the balance among blood volume and water, electrolytes, and pH. Disruption of the renin-angiotensin system results in hypertension. The ability to retain glucose and excrete urea is disrupted, resulting in a buildup of urea in the blood and a loss of glucose. Red blood cell development is disrupted, resulting in the development of chronic anemia.

History and Physical Examination Findings

Uremia is a term used to describe the signs and symptoms that accompany chronic renal failure. Typical signs and symptoms of chronic renal failure are shown in Box 27-3. As kidney function declines, signs and symptoms typically worsen as toxins accumulate in the bloodstream (Figure 27-6). Signs and symptoms of chronic renal failure by body system are shown in Table 27-2.

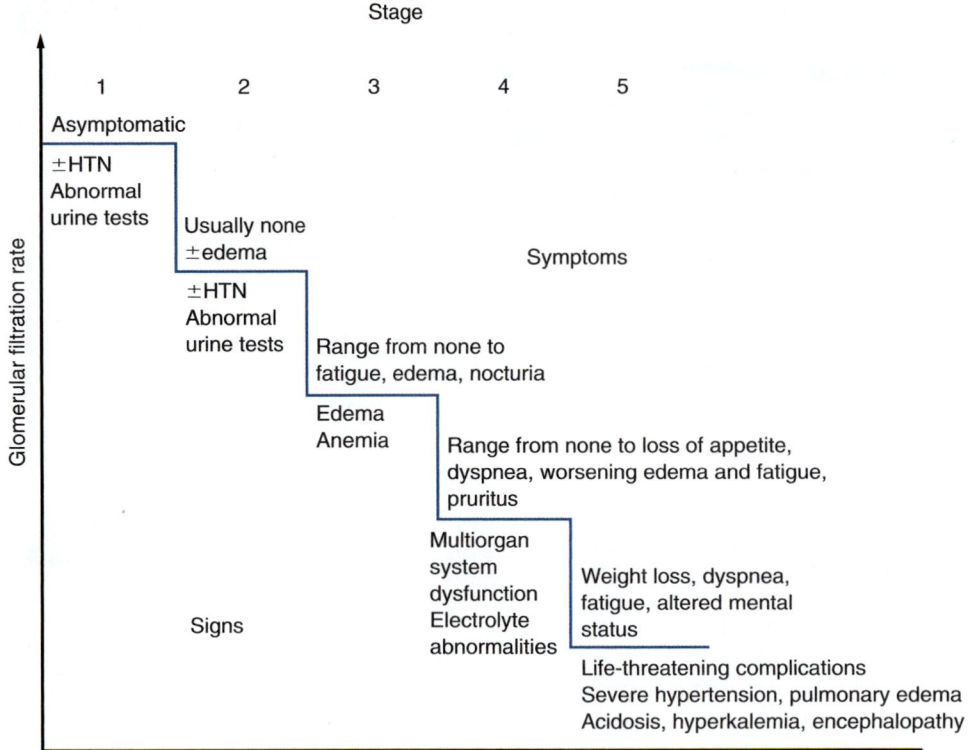

Figure 27-6 Signs and symptoms in chronic kidney disease according to stage. *HTN,* Hypertension.

PARAMEDIC*Pearl*

Kundhal and Lok (2005) found that a significant number of patients with chronic renal failure also have underlying cardiovascular pathology. The authors found that the rate of cardiovascular disease in chronic renal failure patients is three to four time higher that in control subjects matched for age.

Therapeutic Interventions

Prehospital care for the patient with chronic renal failure includes airway and ventilatory support, establishment of IV access, monitoring of the patient's vitals signs and ECG, and transport to an appropriate facility for further care.

Patients with chronic renal failure are advised to consider all treatment options, including hemodialysis, home hemodialysis, peritoneal dialysis, and transplantation. Of special importance is monitoring the diet. Patients should do the following:

- Eat diets that have balanced amounts of protein-rich foods, including beef, poultry, and fish
- Avoid fruits and vegetables that are high in potassium, such as bananas and tomatoes, as well as chocolate and nuts
- Restrict fluid intake
- Avoid or restrict salt
- Restrict foods and beverages containing phosphorous, such as cheese and nuts

Acidosis

End-Stage Renal Disease

Etiology and Epidemiology

Over time, chronic renal failure may progress to the total loss of functioning nephrons and, ultimately, to ESRD. ESRD has been described as a federal government term indicating the long-term need for dialysis or transplantation. Unlike chronic renal failure, in which some renal function is left, ESRD presents with minimal, if any, kidney function—usually less than 10% of baseline. ESRD cannot be reversed. The patient must be treated with dialysis or undergo transplantation. In the United States more than 300,000 patients diagnosed with ESRD receive dialysis and more than 20,000 have a functioning kidney they received by transplantation (U.S. Renal Data System, 2005).

Many causes of ESRD are possible. According to the National Kidney and Urologic Diseases Information Clearinghouse (NIH, 2004), the primary causes of ESRD include the following:

- Diabetes mellitus (35.3%)
- Hypertension (23.3%)
- Glomerulonephritis (15.5%)
- Polycystic kidney disease (4.4%)
- All other conditions (21.4%)

History and Physical Examination Findings

Signs and symptoms of ESRD are relatively mild until kidney function is 15% or less of normal, as shown in

TABLE 27-2	Systemic Effects of Uremia		
System	**Manifestations**	**Mechanisms**	**Treatment**
Skeletal	Osteitis fibrosa (bone inflammation with fibrous degeneration); bone demineralization (principally subperiosteal loss of cortical bone in the fibers, lateral ends of the clavicles, and lamina dura of the teeth); spontaneous fractures, bone pain; osteomalacia (rickets) with ESRD	Bone resorption associated with hyperparathyroidism, vitamin D deficiency, and demineralization; lowered calcium and raised phosphate levels	Control of hyperphosphatemia to reduce hyperparathyroidism; administration of calcium and aluminum hydroxide antacids, which bind phosphate in the gut, together with a phosphate-restricted diet; vitamin D replacement; avoidance of magnesium antacids because of impaired magnesium excretion
Cardiopulmonary	Pulmonary edema, Kussmaul respirations	Fluid overload associated with pulmonary edema and acidosis leading to Kussmaul respirations	Angiotensin-converting enzyme inhibitors; combination of propranolol, hydralazine, and minoxidil for those with high levels of renin; bilateral nephrectomy with dialysis or transplantation
Cardiovascular	Hypertension, pericarditis with fever, chest pain, and pericardial friction rub	Extracellular volume expansion; hypersecretion of renin also associated with hypertension; anemia increases cardiac workload	Volume reduction with diuretics that are not potassium sparing (to avoid hyperkalemia)
Neurologic	Encephalopathy (fatigue, loss of attention, difficulty with problem solving); peripheral neuropathy (pain and burning in the legs and feet, loss of vibration sense and deep tendon reflexes); loss of motor coordination, twitching, fasciculations, stupor, and coma with advanced uremia	Uremic toxins associated with ESRD	Dialysis or successful transplantation
Hematologic	Anemia, usually normochromic normocytic; platelet disorders with prolonged bleeding times	Reduces EPO secretion associated with loss of renal mass, leading to reduced red cell production in the bone marrow; uremic toxins associated with shortened red cell survival	Dialysis; recombinant human EPO and iron supplementation; conjugated estrogens; DDAVP (1-desamino–8-D–arginine vasopressin); transfusion
Gastrointestinal	Anorexia, nausea, vomiting; mouth ulcers, stomatitis, urinous breath (uremic factor), hiccups, peptic ulcers, gastrointestinal bleeding, and pancreatitis associated with ESRD	Retention of metabolic acids and other metabolic waste products	Protein-restricted diet for relief of nausea and vomiting

ESRD, End-stage renal disease; *EPO,* erythropoietin.

TABLE 27-2 **Systemic Effects of Uremia**—continued

System	Manifestations	Mechanisms	Treatment
Integumentary	Abnormal pigmentation and pruritus	Retention of urochromes, contributing to sallow, yellow color; high plasma calcium levels and neuropathy associated with pruritus	Dialysis with control of serum calcium levels
Immunologic	Increased risk of infection that can cause death; increased risk of carcinoma	Suppression of cell-mediated immunity; reduction in number and function of lymphocytes; diminished phagocytosis	Routine dialysis
Reproductive	Sexual dysfunction; menorrhagia, amenorrhea, infertility, and decreased libido in women; decreased testosterone levels, infertility, and decreased libido in men	Probably related to dysfunction of ovaries and testes	No specific treatment

Modified from Keane, W. F. (2000). *Kidney International Supplement, 75,* S27-S31; and Uribarri, J. (2000). Acidosis in chronic renal insufficiency. *Seminars in Dialysis, 13*(4), 232-234.

BOX 27-4 **Signs and Symptoms of End-Stage Renal Disease**

- Confusion
- Decreased levels of consciousness
- Dyspnea
- Peripheral edema
- Chest pain
- Bone pain
- Itching skin
- Nausea and vomiting
- Diarrhea
- Anemia
- Easy bruising
- Muscle twitching
- Anxiety
- Decreased mental acuity
- Delirium
- Hallucinations
- Seizures

Box 27-4. Differential diagnoses of ARF, chronic renal failure, and ESRD are shown in Table 27-3.

Similar to chronic renal failure, patients and their families are urged to review all treatment options as well as modify their diet. Additionally, patients and families are urged to seek support groups in their areas to help cope with the life-altering nature of the illness.

Therapeutic Interventions

[OBJECTIVE 9]

Dialysis is the process of diffusing blood across a semipermeable membrane to remove substances that the kidney would normally eliminate. Patients with ESRD receive dialysis treatments until a transplant can be arranged or until the patient succumbs to the illness. For the older adult, a transplant may not be a viable option because of advancing age, concurrent medical conditions, or cost. In such cases, dialysis is a life-long treatment. Over time, the survival rate of patients on dialysis significantly decreases (NIH, 2004) as shown by the following:

- 1 year—77.8% survival (data from 2000 to 2001)
- 2 years—62.9% survival (data from 1999 to 2001)
- 5 years—31.9% survival (data from 1996 to 2001)
- 10 years—9.0% survival (data from 1991 to 2001)

Immediate survival depends on dialysis. Two types of dialysis treatments are available: hemodialysis and peritoneal dialysis (Figure 27-7). Most hemodialysis is typically performed at a clinic, but home machines are available. Peritoneal dialysis often is performed in the home.

Hemodialysis cleans and filters the blood by removing waste products and fluids. To accomplish this, the blood is slowly filtered through a machine called a dialyzer. Once filtered, the blood is returned to the patient. The hemodialysis process usually takes from 2 to 5 hours to complete. Most patients must undergo dialysis three times per week to remain healthy.

The patient's blood is accessed by a shunt, graft, or fistula. A **shunt** is typically used while awaiting other access routes to be created and allowed to heal. With a shunt, catheters are inserted into an artery and a vein from outside the body. Most shunts are located on the forearm. When not in use during dialysis, the catheters are connected to each other with clear tubing, allowing the continuous flow of blood from artery to vein. The

TABLE 27-3 Differential Diagnosis of ARF, Chronic Renal Failure, and ESRD

System	ARF	Chronic Renal Failure	ESRD
Central nervous	Altered mental status, agitation, lethargy, delirium, coma, alternating moods, hallucinations; neuropathies of hands and feet; hand tremors, seizures, tinnitus	Headache, weakness, lethargy	Confusion, decreased levels of consciousness, anxiety, decreased mental acuity, delirium, hallucinations, seizures
Respiratory			Dyspnea
Circulatory	Swelling of feet, ankles, and legs; easy bruising, prolonged bleeding; hypertension	Hypertension, pericarditis	Peripheral edema, chest pain, anemia, easy bruising
Gastrointestinal	Metallic taste in mouth, anorexia	Loss of appetite, vomiting, increased thirst	Nausea and vomiting, diarrhea
Genitourinary	Excessive urination at night, oliguria, anuria	Polyuria, rusty or brown-colored urine	Minimal if any urine output
Musculoskeletal	Flank pain		Bone pain, muscle twitching
Skin		Puffiness around eyes, itching, yellow-brown color, uremic frost	Itching, uremic frost

ARF, Acute renal failure; *ESRD*, end-stage renal disease.

catheters are covered with self-adhering roller gauze for protection.

The two other access routes, a graft and a fistula, require surgery to create. With a **graft,** a surgeon connects a piece of the patient's saphenous vein to an artery and vein. In lieu of using the patient's own blood vessel, a cow's artery or a synthetic graft may be used. In creating a **fistula,** an artery and vein in the arm or leg are surgically connected to each other under the skin. After healing, the graft or the fistula can be used to withdraw blood from and return it to the patient.

Peritoneal dialysis is performed at home. The treatment consists of using the peritoneum in the abdomen to filter and cleanse the blood. The procedure uses a catheter that has been surgically implanted into the abdomen. Once the catheter is ready to use, it is attached to a bag of solution called *dialysate* that is infused into the abdomen.

In one form of peritoneal dialysis called *continuous ambulatory peritoneal dialysis,* the catheter is sealed and covered after the solution has been administered, and the patient keeps the dialysate in the abdomen for several hours. After a specified time, usually 4 to 6 hours later, the dialysate, which has cleansed and filtered the blood, is drained. The process is then repeated. This method of peritoneal dialysis is performed daily and repeated four to five times per day.

Another form of peritoneal dialysis performed at home is continuous cycle peritoneal dialysis. The procedure is essentially the same as the one described above; however, the patient's catheter connects to a machine that automatically fills and drains the dialysate four to five times. This procedure is generally done at night while the patient is sleeping or resting, taking from 10 to 12 hours to complete.

A paramedic should remember a few things when caring for a patient who receives dialysis treatments. These tips apply regardless of whether the call for assistance is related to the dialysis or another medical emergency. The following guidelines will prevent inadvertent clotting of the graft or fistula:

- Do not take the patient's blood pressure on the extremity with the access device. Some patients may have more than one graft or fistula because one of the access sites has failed. Ask which site is being used. If the patient is unable to answer or is uncertain, gently touch the access site. The presence of a "thrill" or vibration to the touch indicates a patent site that should be avoided.
- Do not apply firm, direct pressure on the arm with the site, even if bleeding is present. Gentle pressure usually suffices.
- Loosen tight or restrictive clothing on the extremity of the access site.
- Do not use the access device to give drugs and/or fluids unless it is the only access site available and establishing vascular access by other means is not possible. Use of the access device for this purpose should be an absolute last resort.
- If the tubing of the external shunt becomes disconnected, the patient will bleed profusely. Direct pressure will not control the hemorrhage. Reconnect the shunt or use hemostats to temporarily stop the flow of blood until the tubing can be reconnected.

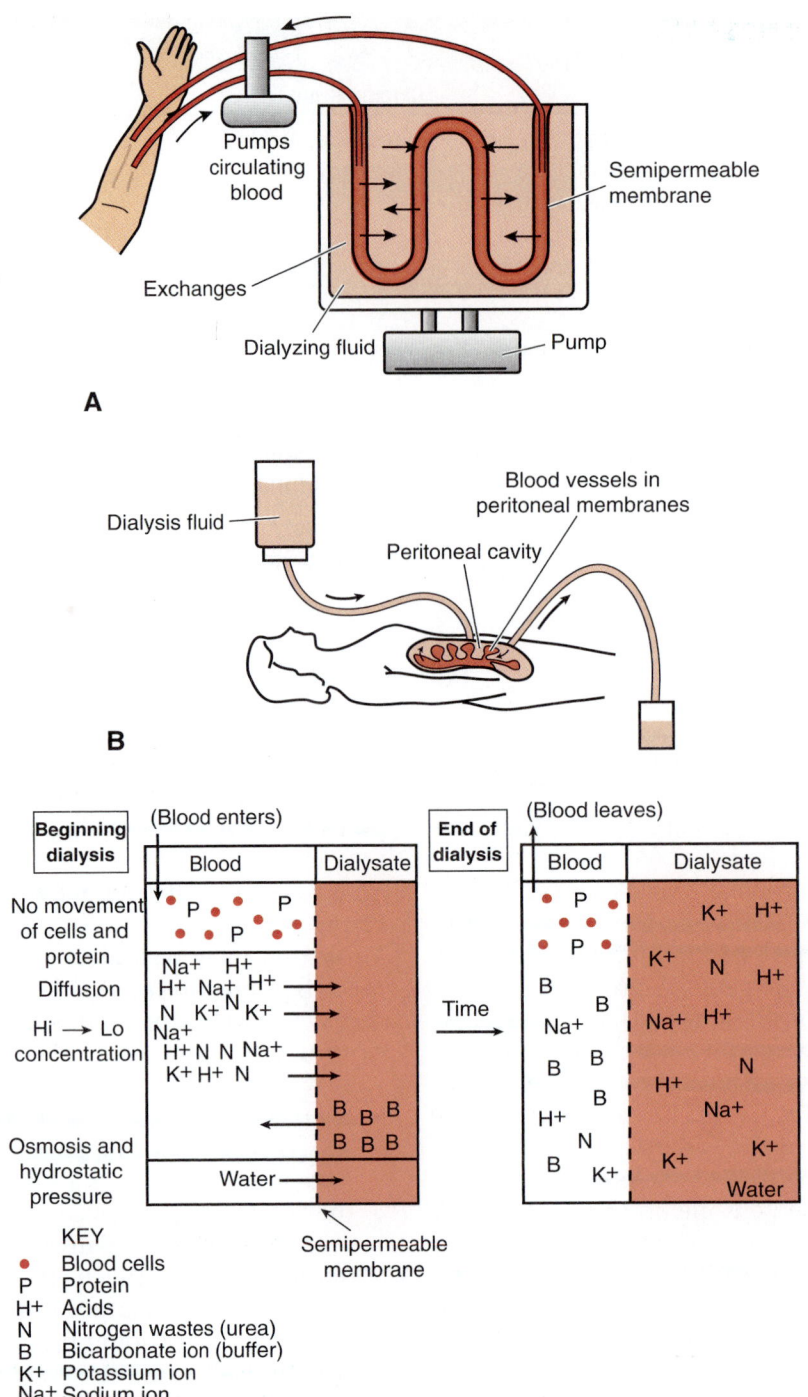

Figure 27-7 A, Hemodialysis. **B,** Peritoneal dialysis. **C,** Principles of dialysis.

Complications of Dialysis

[OBJECTIVE 10]

Paramedics may be called to assist a dialysis patient who has posttreatment complications. The adverse effects of dialysis are shown in Box 27-5.

These complications usually occur at the dialysis center where medical treatment is provided by the center's staff. EMS may be called to transport the patient to the emergency department. If the patient becomes hypotensive

BOX 27-5 Adverse Effects of Dialysis

- Hypotension from the sudden loss of circulating fluid volume.
- Muscle cramps caused by sudden change in electrolytes.
- Nausea and vomiting.
- Disequilibrium syndrome caused by a change in osmolality between intracellular and extracellular fluids. Patients may report headache, restlessness, nausea, and fatigue. Severe conditions may present with confusion, seizures, and coma.
- Hemorrhage from the use of anticoagulants; dialysis patients are at risk for bleeding that may be difficult to control.
- Air embolism from malfunctioning of the dialyzer.
- Chest pain from myocardial ischemia, which can be caused by hypotension and hypoxia brought on by the dialysis treatment. In addition, cardiac dysrhythmias may develop and must be treated according to current resuscitation guidelines. If dysrhythmias develop during dialysis, the treatment should be stopped.

after leaving the dialysis treatment center or while being treated at home, paramedics begin emergency care by treating for shock, including giving oxygen and elevating the patient's legs. IV therapy may or may not be indicated. Some hypotensive patients respond to a 200- to 300-mL fluid challenge. The best procedure is to consult medical direction regarding the management of these patients.

Occasionally after a dialysis treatment, some bleeding may occur at the catheter insertion site. Apply gentle, direct pressure to the area, cover it with a sterile dressing, and transport the patient to the emergency department.

For patients on peritoneal dialysis, infection at the catheter site could lead to peritonitis or sepsis. If peritonitis is suspected, prompt transport to the emergency department is essential while providing other emergency care as needed.

Occasionally a patient is unable to complete dialysis because of complications before or during therapy. These patients usually return home until the next scheduled treatment. Patients are advised to monitor diet and fluid intake closely to avoid serious and potentially life-threatening problems associated with fluid overload, waste accumulation, and electrolyte imbalance. Signs and symptoms of fluid overload associated with incomplete dialysis include the following:

- Acute pulmonary edema
- Hypertensive crisis
- Elevated blood potassium level (hyperkalemia)
- Uremic frost

High potassium levels can quickly become life-threatening; the patient may develop asystole without warning.

Physical signs and symptoms of hyperkalemia include the following:

- Slow, irregular pulse
- Muscular weakness
- Tingling of the hands, feet, and tongue
- ECG changes such as depressed P waves, widened QRS complex, and peaked T waves; with severe hyperkalemia the QRS complex can widen to the point that it resembles a sine wave
- **Uremic frost,** created when the body tries to rid excess urea through sweating; when the water dries, it leaves a crystal residue on the skin that resembles a frost and smells like urine

When called to assist a patient in acute distress from fluid overload, the paramedic is faced with a dilemma. Taking a blood pressure may not be recommended depending on the location of the access site. Starting an IV is usually not indicated because the patient has too much fluid volume, and diuretics do not work because the patient's kidneys are not functioning properly. The most effective treatment is to monitor the airway and give high-flow supplemental oxygen, prepare to intubate the patient and assist ventilation, and monitor the patient's ECG. Be prepared to begin cardiopulmonary resuscitation in the event of cardiac arrest. Transport the patient to the closest appropriate facility. In most cases the most appropriate facility will be one that has dialysis capability. The decision to transport to a closer facility for immediate patient stabilization versus a facility with dialysis capabilities should be made in consultation with medical direction.

PARAMEDIC Pearl

Beware the dialysis patient in fluid overload with uremic frost. The potassium levels may be extremely high and the patient could lapse into cardiac arrest at any time.

If hyperkalemia is suspected, immediate treatment must be provided to avoid potential cardiac arrest. If the patient is in cardiac arrest, hyperkalemia must be suspected as a cause and treated. The goals in treatment of this condition include antagonizing the effects of the hyperkalemia and promoting movement of potassium into the intracellular space, both of which are done pharmacologically. Calcium chloride (or gluconate) antagonizes the cardiotoxic effect of hyperkalemia by restoring the cardiac resting membrane potential. The metabolic alkalosis caused by sodium bicarbonate has a twofold effect in these patients. In addition to treating metabolic acidosis, the induced alkalosis causes a shift of potassium into the cells in exchange for hydrogen ions. Glucose and insulin also promote the movement of potassium into the cells. The administration of glucose in the absence of insulin administration has been debated; however, its use alone is recommended. Finally, if the patient is not in cardiac arrest, albuterol promotes the movement of potassium into the intracellular space.

URINARY SYSTEM CONDITIONS

The paramedic may be called to care for patients with acute urinary system problems that are not currently causing renal failure and perhaps will not in the future. Some of these conditions include the following:

- Renal calculi
- Urinary retention
- Urinary system infection such as cystitis and pyelonephritis

In addition, males may experience unique urinary system problems that need to be evaluated by the paramedic. Urinary system problems unique to male patients include the following:

- Genital lesions
- Blunt trauma
- Infection such as epididymitis, orchitis, Fournier's gangrene, prostatitis, and urethritis
- Structural emergencies such as phimosis or paraphimosis, priapism, benign prostate hypertrophy, and testicular masses

Some of these conditions may present with emergent symptoms requiring prompt paramedic intervention and transport to the emergency department.

Renal Calculi

[OBJECTIVES 11, 12]

Etiology and Epidemiology

Kidney stones (nephrolithiasis), or renal calculi, occur in a certain number of patients. Of the total U.S. population, 5.2% had kidney stones during 2001. Men (6.3%) have a higher incidence of renal calculi than do women (4.2%). Kidney stones have resulted in 2.2 million physician visits along with nearly 180,000 hospital discharges.

Renal calculi develop when the urine becomes highly concentrated with substances such as calcium salts, uric acid, and cystine. These substances create crystals that lead to stones inside the kidney. The presence of renal calculi causes significant alteration in renal blood flow, resulting in a reduction of glomerular filtration. Renal infection is also commonly associated with renal calculi, which can lead to complications such as pyelonephritis, abscesses, and sepsis. Small stones or pieces of larger stones can break off and pass into the ureter, where they may result in blockage of the ureter (ureterolithiasis). The ability of the stone to pass through the ureter is a function of its size. Stones less than 5 mm generally pass spontaneously within 4 weeks, whereas stones larger than 8 mm require surgery or lithotripsy. Stones between 5 and 8 mm may pass spontaneously but often require surgery or lithotripsy.

History and Physical Examination Findings

The patient's history often includes risk factors for the development of renal calculi. Patients often have a family history of renal calculi, and the most common patient is the middle-age professional white male with a sedentary lifestyle. Other factors can also promote the formation of renal calculi, including Crohn's disease, hyperparathyroidism, recurrent urinary tract infections, living in a hot and dry climate, and a history of prior calculi formation.

As the stone passes through the ureter, the signs and symptoms of renal calculi develop, including the following:

- Severe flank or back pain, often described as extreme, colicky, or spasmlike, with the patient unable to remain still
- Abdominal pain
- Pain radiating to the pelvis, groin, or genitals
- Nausea and vomiting

- Increased urinary urgency
- Painful urination
- Hematuria
- Fever and chills

Because the overt symptom of renal calculi is flank pain, the paramedic should carefully assess the patient to rule out kidney infection, shingles, arthritis of the spine, muscle spasm, or disease or injury of an intervertebral disc.

Therapeutic Interventions

Prehospital treatment is aimed at care and comfort. Transport the patient to the emergency department in a position of comfort (may be difficult to obtain). Narcotic analgesics or IV nonsteroidal antiinflammatory drugs such as ketorolac (Toradol) often are needed to reduce the pain. Antiemetics may be necessary to control nausea and vomiting. Patients who are prone to renal calculi often are advised to monitor their fluid intake that can lead to stones. Some medications, including over-the-counter drugs such as vitamin C, may increase uric acid levels. Patients are urged to talk with their physicians about continuing these medications.

Urinary Retention

[OBJECTIVES 13, 14]

Etiology and Epidemiology

Urinary retention is the inability to empty the bladder or completely empty the bladder when urinating. Acute urinary retention is a relatively infrequent condition; however, advancing age, moderate or severe lower urinary tract symptoms, benign prostatic hypertrophy, and specific drug therapies may increase the occurrence (Meigs et al., 1999). Urinary retention is more common in men than in women.

Urinary retention can be new and short term or it can be chronic. It can be caused by failure of the urinary bladder muscle, damage to the nerves, or blockage of the urethra, possibly from an enlarged prostate gland.

History and Physical Examination Findings

Signs and symptoms of urinary retention include the following:

- Sudden inability to urinate
- Distention of the urinary bladder
- Acute lower abdominal pain
- Delirium in the elderly patient

Therapeutic Interventions

Prehospital care for urinary retention is primarily supportive. The patient must be transported to the hospital so that the excess urine can be drained, typically through the insertion of a urinary catheter. Transport the patient in a position of comfort. Once at the hospital the physician will alleviate the excessive distention of the urinary bladder and treat the underlying cause.

GERIATRIC *Considerations*

Urinary retention in the older adult may lead to delirium. Carefully question the recent urinary history and bladder habits for any older adult who has a sudden onset of delirium.

Urinary System Infections

[OBJECTIVES 15, 16]

Etiology and Epidemiology

Infections of the urinary system can include cystitis (urinary bladder infection) and pyelonephritis (kidney infection). Thirty-four percent of the population older than 20 years has reported at least one episode of urinary tract infection (UTI). More women (53.5%) than men (13.9%) have UTIs. The most common bacterium involved in UTIs is *Escherichia coli;* however, other causes of UTI include gonorrhea and *Chlamydia* spp. (NIH, 2004).

History and Physical Examination Findings

If left untreated, a simple bladder infection can result in cystitis. Signs and symptoms of cystitis include the following:

- Burning sensation or pain during urination
- Sense of increased urgency of urination
- More frequent urination
- Cloudy urine
- Rust-colored urine
- Foul-smelling urine
- Low-grade fever

Children may have fewer specific symptoms, and older women may have no symptoms other than weakness, falls, or confusion.

If the infection is untreated, it can spread to the kidneys. Signs and symptoms of pyelonephritis include all the above signs and symptoms plus the following:

- Flank or back pain
- Abdominal pain (occasionally)
- Persistent fever with body temperature above 102° F
- Chills accompanied by shaking
- Flushed skin
- Diaphoresis
- Headache
- Urinary frequency
- Dysuria
- Hematuria

Differential diagnoses of urinary tract infection and renal calculi are shown in Table 27-4.

Therapeutic Interventions

Prehospital care includes prompt transportation to the emergency department, where the patient can undergo tests to determine the nature of infection and proper

TABLE 27-4 **Differential Diagnosis of UTI and Renal Calculi**

System	UTI	Renal Calculi
Central nervous	Weakness, confusion (older adult)	NA
Respiratory	NA	NA
Circulatory	NA	NA
Gastrointestinal	NA	NA
Genitourinary	Polyuria, urinary urgency, burning sensation, cloudy urine, foul-smelling urine, hematuria	Hematuria, urinary urgency, painful urination, hematuria
Musculoskeletal	Flank pain if kidneys involved, back pain, chills and shaking	Severe flank pain; inability to remain still; back pain; abdominal pain; may radiate to pelvis, groin, genitals; chills if fever present
Skin	Low-grade fever, may increase to 102° F; flushed skin, diaphoresis	Normal body temperature, may develop fever

UTI, Urinary tract infection; *NA,* not applicable.

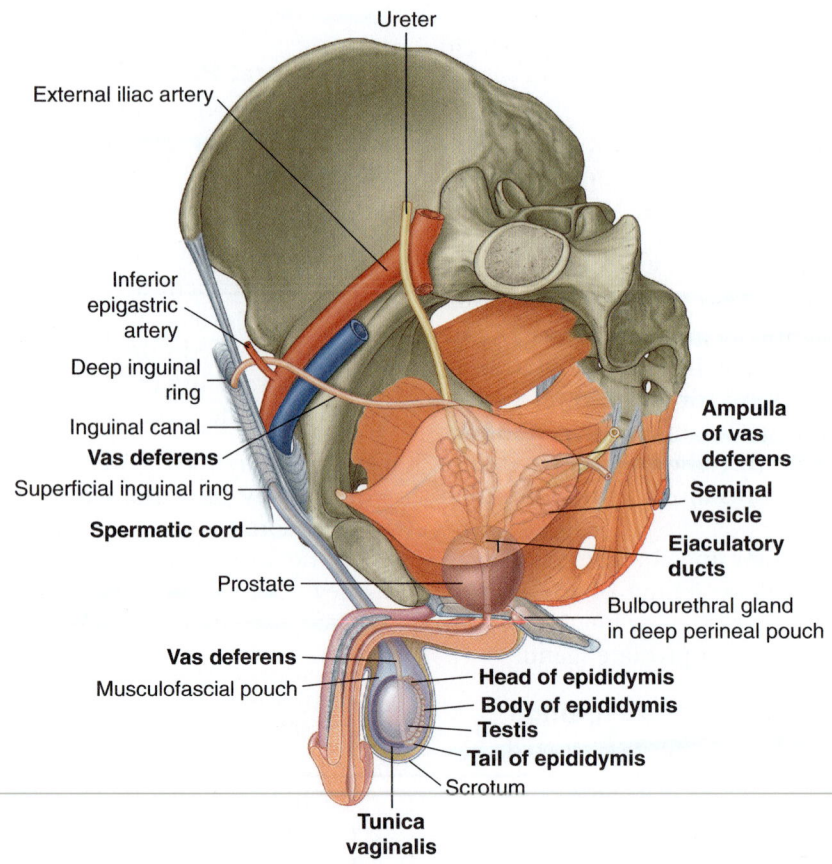

Figure 27-8 Anatomy of the male reproductive system.

course of antibiotics. If septicemia develops, prehospital care for septic shock may be needed.

Urinary System Conditions Limited to Males

Male Genitourinary Structures

[OBJECTIVE 17]

The penis is a tube-shaped organ consisting of a root, body, and extremity known as the *glans penis* or *head* (Figure 27-8). The root of the penis is connected to the pelvis by strong ligaments. The body of the penis consists of three cylinders containing tissue that can become erect.

Two of the internal chambers lying side by side are called the *corpus cavernosa* (cavernous body). These cylinders, when filled with blood, cause the penis to enlarge and become erect. The third chamber called the *corpus spongiosum* (spongy body) surrounds the urethra. It allows the urethra to elongate during an erection.

The scrotum, a pouch located beneath the penis, is the other visible component of the male reproductive system and contains the testes. When allowed to hang free, the left side of the scrotum is larger than the right because the spermatic cord on the left is longer. The skin of the scrotum has a large number of blood vessels that, when injured, can bleed heavily.

Another layer of the scrotum located under the skin is also highly vascular and has a strong ability to contract. Because the testes need to be cooler than the rest of the body to produce sperm, the ability of the tissue to contract and expand is important. For example, when the scrotum is exposed to cold, this layer contracts, bringing the testes closer to the body for warmth. In contrast, when the temperature is warm, this layer relaxes and the testes are allowed to hang away from the body.

Inside the scrotum, the testes are suspended by the spermatic cords. These oval-shaped organs are responsible for producing sperm and the male hormone testosterone. Each testis contains a large number of blood vessels and nerve endings. Injury to the testes can cause bleeding and a tremendous amount of pain.

Sperm are produced in tiny, coiled tubes and are transported to a flattened area called the epididymis that runs along the back edge of each testis. The epididymis consists of 18 to 20 feet of convoluted tubes that temporarily store the sperm (Figure 27-9).

From the epididymis, sperm are transported to a tube called the *vas deferens,* eventually arriving at the seminal vesicles next to the urinary bladder, where the sperm are stored before ejaculation.

Several problems related to the penis can prompt a call to 9-1-1. Although most of these conditions are not life threatening, paramedics should understand a few to provide appropriate patient care.

Genital Lesions

[OBJECTIVES 18]

Genital lesions can be found in either gender but are more common in males. Common causes of genital lesions include the following:

- Genital herpes, which inflicts more than 45 million people in the United States (Centers for Disease Control and Prevention [CDC], 2005a)
- Primary and secondary syphilis (2.7 cases per 1 million population [CDC, 2005b])
- Chancroid lesions (243 cases in 1997 [Crowe & Hall, 2005])
- Granuloma inguinale—rare bacterial and sexually transmitted disease causing a red lump in the genital or anal areas that easily bleeds and spreads while destroying genital tissues (100 cases per year in the United States [Medline Plus, 2005])
- Lymphadenoma—rare malignancy of lymph nodes
- Genital warts (1 million cases in the United States [CDC, 2005c])
- *Molluscum contagiosum*—viral disease considered a sexually transmitted disease causing papules, typically in the genital region; most often found in patients with HIV
- Allergic reactions

Rarely are these lesions life-threatening, but they can be disconcerting to the patient. The signs and symptoms of these lesions are highlighted in Table 27-5.

Patients with genital lesions should be referred to the emergency department physician for thorough assessment, diagnosis, and treatment. Because most of these lesions are sexually transmitted diseases, patients should learn about preventing transmission of the illness to sexual partners.

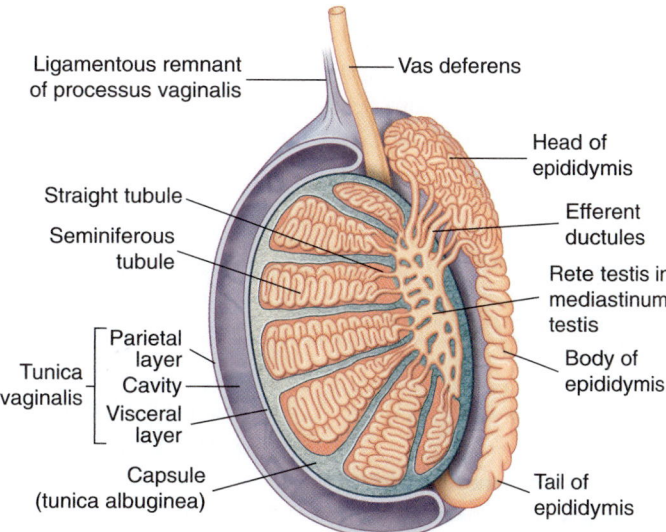

Figure 27-9 Anatomy of a testis and surrounding structures.

TABLE 27-5 Genital Lesions

Lesion	Signs and Symptoms	General Treatment
Genital herpes	Initially, tingling and tenderness; painful red bumps; fever; headache; muscle aches; painful or difficult urination; swollen glands in groin	No prehospital treatment; antiviral medications; acyclovir, famciclovir, valacyclovir
Syphilis	First degree: Painless chancre at site of infection, disappears over time Second degree: Brown rash over skin, fever, headache, sore throat, swollen lymph glands	Early diagnosis and treatment with antibiotics; without treatment, progresses to tertiary syphilis with central nervous system and other organ system damage
Chancroid lesions	Tender, reddened papule; becomes pustule; develops painful ulcer; swollen glands in groin	Prehospital: cover ulcer; antibiotic therapy; azithromycin, ceftriaxone, ciprofloxacin
Granuloma inguinale	Painless red lump on genitals; forms red nodule; will bleed easily if injured; spreads and destroys genital tissue	Prehospital: control bleeding and cover injured tissues; antibiotic therapy; tetracycline, doxycycline, ciprofloxacin
Lymphadenoma	Swollen lymph node; lesion may be squamous or sebaceous cell carcinoma; may be other form of cancer	Prehospital: none; refer to physician
Genital warts	Flesh-colored or white lesions; cauliflower in appearance; increased moisture around lesions; itching may be present	Prehospital: none; prescription medication; cauterization, laser therapy, surgical removal
Molluscum contagiosum	Virus of family Poxviridae; painless; small lesion with dimple; initially firm, dome shaped; becomes soft, gray; may drain; core of white, waxy material	Prehospital: none; spontaneously heal in people with normal immune systems; compromised immune systems may need scraping, freezing, or electrosurgery

Case Scenario CONCLUSION

You opt to transport the patient to a facility with emergency dialysis capabilities. After administering high-flow oxygen by nonrebreather mask, you assess the patient's SpO$_2$. It reads 88 mg/dL. You opt to intubate the patient before transporting him. Once the patient's airway has been secured, you notify the receiving facility and begin transporting the patient. You decide to forego IV access because of the possibility of worsening his fluid overload and potentially interfering with the dialysis site. As you proceed to the facility, you note the man's ECG indicates asystole. You verify pulselessness and begin cardiopulmonary resuscitation. Within a few moments the patient's ECG returns to a sinus rhythm with pulses. A few minutes later, you arrive at the emergency department and turn over care to the hospital staff. After cleaning your vehicle, you check on the patient. He is responding well to emergency dialysis. The emergency department physician tells you the patient was hyperkalemic.

Looking Back

7. Can you use venous access ports such as the dialysis fistula or graft to initiate IV access?
8. What did the hyperkalemia contribute to the patient's condition?

Blunt Trauma

[OBJECTIVES 19, 20]

Because of the vascular nature of the male urinary tract and genitals, blunt trauma causes significant bleeding in the genital region (Figure 27-10). Signs and symptoms of blunt trauma include the following:

- Scrotum may fill with blood and become swollen
- Severe pain
- Peritonitis if the urinary bladder has ruptured
- Pelvic fracture depending on mechanism of injury
- Spinal injury depending on mechanism of injury

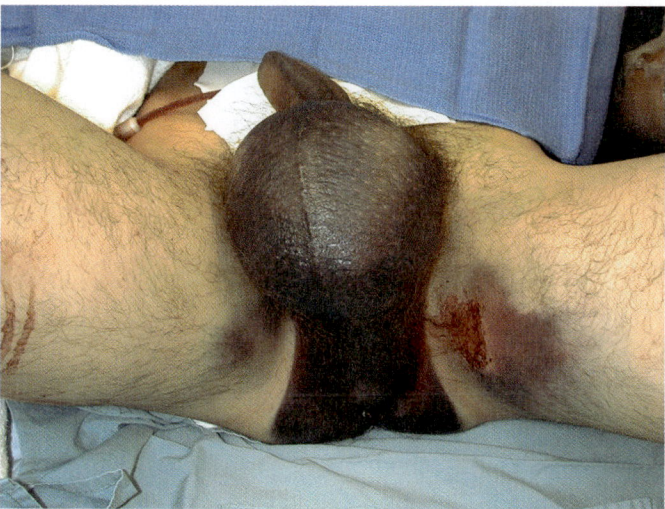

Figure 27-10 Straddle injury.

Patients complaining of pain, swelling, and discoloration of the scrotum may be bleeding into the abdomen. The peritoneum lines the abdominal cavity and also extends into the scrotum. Bleeding in the lower abdomen may present with blood in the scrotum. A careful examination of the patient is required to rule out intraabdominal injury.

> **PARAMEDIC***Pearl*
>
> Blood from an abdominal injury may drain into the scrotum. Carefully assess the abdomen of any patient with swelling and discoloration of the scrotum.

Prehospital treatment for blunt trauma of the genitourinary system is similar to the treatment of blunt trauma to other areas of the body. If appropriate and the injury is localized to the genitalia, cold compresses can be used to reduce pain and swelling. Treat for shock with high-flow oxygen and IV fluids. Depending on the mechanism of injury, the paramedic may need to treat for a pelvic fracture or take spinal precautions and place the patient on a long spine board.

Genitourinary Infection
[OBJECTIVES 21, 22]
Other than UTIs, males can experience several other infectious processes of the genitourinary system, including the following:

- *Epididymitis:* inflammation of the epididymis
- *Orchitis:* inflammation of one or both testes
- *Fournier's gangrene:* bacterial infection of the genitals
- *Prostatitis:* inflammation of the prostate
- *Urethritis:* inflammation of the urethra

Epididymitis and Orchitis. Epididymitis and orchitis are conditions that can be extremely painful. The signs and symptoms include the following:

- Swelling and pain of the scrotum
- Enlarged testes
- Swollen testicle on the affected side
- Swollen groin on the affected side
- Testicular pain that worsens during a bowel movement
- Fever
- Urethral discharge

Because this is an infectious process, the patient needs transportation to the emergency department. Care and comfort is the aim of prehospital care. Occasionally analgesics may be needed to reduce pain and discomfort.

Fournier's Gangrene. Fournier's gangrene is an infection caused by bacteria, typically in combination with yeast. The infection invades the skin of the genitals and perineum and spreads rapidly. Men, especially those with a predisposing condition such as alcoholism, Crohn's disease, diabetes mellitus, obesity, and immune system disorders (e.g., HIV), are more prone to the infection than are women. Signs and symptoms of Fournier's gangrene include the following:

- Crepitus of the skin
- Gray-black discolored tissues
- Pus draining from the tissues
- Fever
- Genital pain and redness
- Odor
- Severe genital pain along with swelling of the penis and scrotum

This condition is emergent because, without treatment, the infection will spread and can result in septicemia, heart failure, and death. Prompt transport to the emergency department is required. Patients at risk for Fournier's gangrene include those with diabetes mellitus or alcoholism, of advanced age, with poor nutrition, or on steroids. Prehospital care should include treatment for shock while ensuring proper hydration and adequate ventilation.

Structural Conditions

Structural conditions of the genitourinary system may be the precipitating call to 9-1-1. Although the majority of structural problems are not urgent, the paramedic must be able to recognize the conditions for which prompt transportation is required.

Phimosis and Paraphimosis
[OBJECTIVES 23, 24]
Two of the more urgent structural conditions are phimosis and paraphimosis. These conditions are described as the inability to retract the foreskin over the glans of the penis (Figure 27-11). Because of this, the patient may develop an infection under the foreskin and report a discharge. **Paraphimosis** is the more serious of the two

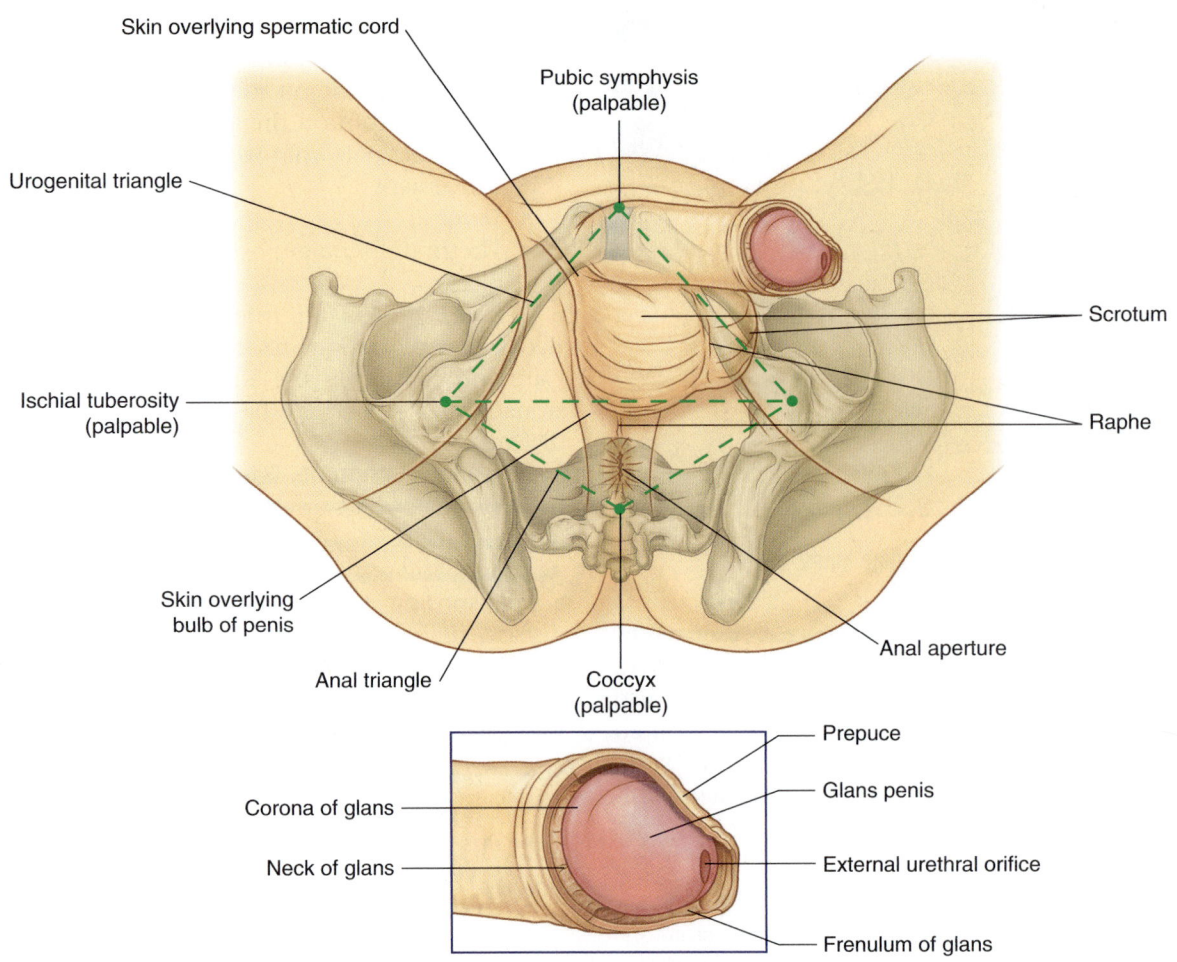

Figure 27-11 Glans and foreskin.

conditions and occurs when the foreskin cannot be replaced over the glans after it has been retracted. The result is a tight ring around the glans that acts as a tourniquet, leading to swelling of the glans. These conditions are found in 1% of the adult male population and are more common in men who are hospitalized or in skilled nursing facilities.

Treatment for paraphimosis includes squeezing the glans firmly for 10 minutes or longer to reduce swelling. If approved by medical direction, wrap the glans in gauze, then apply an elastic wrap from the distal end of the penis onto the shaft to produce constant and gentle compression. An alternative treatment is to wrap the penis in plastic, then apply cold packs to reduce the swelling. Transport the patient to the emergency department when the compression dressing can be removed and the foreskin replaced over the glans. If this fails, the emergency department physician may need to incise the foreskin to alleviate the constriction. Any underlying infection must also be treated.

Priapism
[OBJECTIVES 25, 26]

Priapism is a prolonged and painful erection. Before the marketing of medications for erectile dysfunction such as sildenafil (Viagra), tadalafil (Cialis), and vardenafil (Levitra), the term *priapism* was not often heard or discussed. The incidence of priapism is rare; however, it has been known to occur in 40% of patients with sickle cell disease. Although the specific cause of priapism is debated, several possible causes include the following:

- Disorders of the blood, such as sickle cell anemia, myeloma, and leukemia
- Accidental or surgical trauma
- Nervous system damage caused by multiple sclerosis or diabetes mellitus
- Erectile dysfunction drugs
- Drugs injected to enhance sexual performance
- Certain psychotropic medications such as trazodone and chlorpromazine
- Spinal trauma

An erection that lasts more than 4 hours is a medical emergency that needs treatment. Prehospital treatment includes supportive care, which may include the use of analgesics in consultation with medical direction.

Priapism may spontaneously resolve, or it may need intervention with oral or injected medications. Blood occasionally may need to be drained from the penis to reduce the erection and allow normal flow of blood out

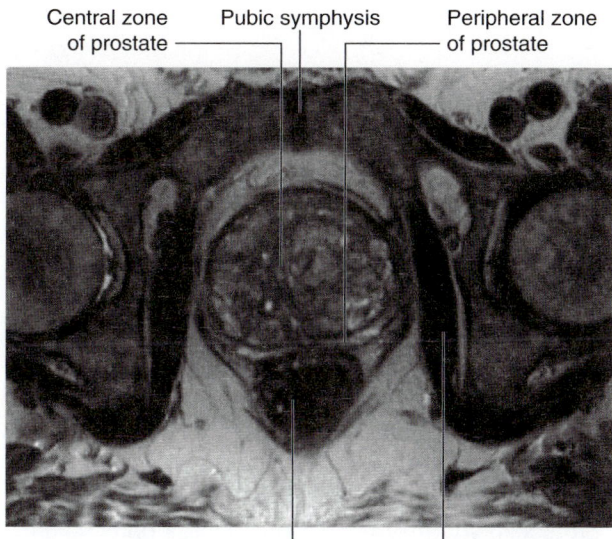

Figure 27-12 Benign prostatic hypertrophy.

of the corpus cavernosa. In rare cases untreated priapism may lead to structural damage inside the penis that could interfere with erections and sexual performance.

Benign Prostatic Hypertrophy
[OBJECTIVES 27, 28]

Benign prostatic hypertrophy also is known as *benign prostatic hyperplasia* (Figure 27-12). Simply stated, the condition is a noncancerous enlargement of the prostate gland. According to the American Urological Association, approximately 50% of men will have some degree of prostate enlargement by the time they reach 60 years of age. The incidence increases to 90% by 90 years of age (American Urological Association, 2005).

Because of its location, an enlarged prostate can put pressure on the urethra and restrict the flow of urine out of the urinary bladder. Complications of benign prostatic hypertrophy include urinary retention and an increased risk of urinary tract infections, renal calculi, and renal failure from obstruction. Benign prostatic hypertrophy does not cause cancer; however, both can be found together in the same patient.

Paramedics probably will not be called to assess a patient with benign prostatic hypertrophy. Rather, the paramedic may be called to attend the patient because of urinary retention or ARF. Remember that the causes of these conditions could be structural and attributed to an enlarged prostate gland. A complete routine physical examination of the patient by an emergency department physician is in order. Prehospital treatment for this condition is primarily supportive.

GERIATRIC *Considerations*
Older men at risk of an enlarged prostate are also at risk of urinary retention that can, in turn, lead to delirium because of either infection or renal failure.

Testicular Masses
[OBJECTIVE 29]

Patients with a testicular mass generally do not call 9-1-1. However, in assessing a male patient with a specific or vague complaint, the paramedic may be informed of an unusual mass on a testis. Testicular cancer is of concern to all men. Between 6000 and 8000 men are diagnosed with cancer of the testes annually.

The patient may report a painless lump on a testicle or pain in the scrotum. The pain, if present, can be described as a dull ache that gets worse with exercise or pain that is severe. The pain may be localized to the scrotum or may radiate along the spermatic cord into the lower abdomen.

Because an exact assessment of a testicular mass is difficult without a comprehensive examination, the patient should see a physician as soon as possible. A testicular mass can be something emergent such as testicular torsion, strangulated hernia, or malignancy. Benign causes of testicular masses include **hydrocele, varicocele,** or **spermatocele,** which can be cared for under a nonemergent or routine basis. Men are strongly advised to perform self-examinations to detect lumps or masses in the scrotum.

Testicular Torsion
[OBJECTIVES 30, 31]

Testicular torsion is a medical emergency caused by the twisting of the spermatic cord inside the scrotum. Although it typically occurs in infants younger than 1 year, it can occur in older boys and men, especially after trauma when swelling of the scrotum occurs. The incidence of testicular torsion in men younger than 25 years is one case in 4000. Occasionally no cause is known.

When the spermatic cord twists, it cuts off the blood supply to the testis. Without blood, the affected testicle can atrophy and may need to be surgically removed. Signs and symptoms of testicular torsion include the following:

- Sudden onset of severe pain in one testis
- Possible predisposing event such as blunt trauma
- Swelling on one side of the scrotum
- Lump on testis
- Blood in semen
- Nausea and/or vomiting
- Lightheadedness

Treatment involves prompt surgery. In the prehospital setting, treatment should include care and comfort along with prompt transportation to the emergency department and possibly analgesics to reduce severe pain. The salvage rate for patients undergoing surgery less than 6 to 8 hours after onset ranges from 80% to 100%. Those waiting more than 12 hours have a minimal if any salvage rate. Without surgery, the affected testicle can become necrotic, atrophy, and cause infection.

Case Scenario SUMMARY

1. *What is your initial impression of this patient?* The patient is unresponsive with obvious pulmonary edema. The exact nature of the problem is not completely evident on the initial approach to the patient.

2. *What additional information do you need?* A SAMPLE history and physical evaluation are key. In addition, assess the OPQRST of the present condition. A head-to-toe evaluation is in order. All this information may identify the cause of the problem and explain why an odor of urine is in the room.

3. *What may be causing the patient's pulmonary edema?* Pulmonary edema can have a number of causes, including congestive heart failure, toxic inhalation, medication overdose, and fluid overload. You need to identify the cause and treat the underlying etiology if possible. The smell of urine, coupled with the bulges in the patient's arms, should begin to highlight the nature of the problem.

4. *Has your initial impression changed?* Based on the additional information, the etiology of the pulmonary edema is becoming clear—fluid overload from ESRD, incomplete dialysis, and excessive fluid intake. The ECG changes indicate the possibility of hyperkalemia.

5. *What treatment options are available?* Treatment options are limited in this case. Supporting the airway and supplemental oxygen are indicated. But do you initiate IV access and administer medications? Establishing IV access may worsen fluid overload and medications may be ineffective or, perhaps, toxic. Intubation and airway management with positive-pressure ventilation are indicated, especially in light of a low SpO_2.

6. *The nearest emergency department is 2 miles away, but the nearest facility with dialysis capability is 10 miles away. What is your best transport option?* Transportation should consider the nearest *most appropriate* facility. In this case, a facility with emergency dialysis capabilities is the most appropriate destination.

7. *Can you use venous access ports such as the dialysis fistula or graft to initiate IV access?* Depending on local protocols, you may use venous access ports, shunts, and fistulas in the event emergency access is critically needed. In this case, the patient has one access site that is functioning (it is pulsing) and one that is nonfunctional (not pulsing). If you opt to establish IV access in the functioning dialysis access site, you may cause the loss of that site for emergency dialysis.

8. *What did the hyperkalemia contribute to the patient's condition?* The patient's hyperkalemia contributed to the sudden onset of asystole. Because of prompt intervention, the patient had a quick return of spontaneous circulation. Prompt arrival at the emergency department and access to dialysis were able to resolve the hyperkalemia and pulmonary edema.

Chapter Summary

- Patients complaining of abdominal pain or discomfort pose a challenge to paramedics. One source of the patient's chief complaint is the urinary system.
- Functions of the urinary system include water and electrolyte regulation, acid-base balance, excretion of waste products and foreign chemicals, hormone excretion, arterial blood pressure regulation, erythrocyte production, and gluconeogenesis.

- Conditions including renal failure (acute or chronic plus ESRD), renal calculi, urinary retention, urinary system infections, and male genitourinary problems (including structural problems) can contribute to acute abdominal discomfort.
- A thorough assessment coupled with an understanding of the urinary system help identify the nature of the patient's condition and lead to the best course of treatment.

REFERENCES

American Urological Association. (2005). *Diagnosis of BPH*. Retrieved October 30, 2006, from http://www.urologyhealth.org.

Centers for Disease Control and Prevention. (2005a). *Sexually transmitted diseases: Genital herpes.* Retrieved October 30, 2006, from http://www.cdc.gov.

Centers for Disease Control and Prevention. (2005b). *Sexually transmitted diseases: Syphilis.* Retrieved October 30, 2006, from http://www.cdc.gov.

Centers for Disease Control and Prevention. (2005c). *Sexually transmitted diseases: Human papillomavirus (HPV) infection.* Retrieved October 30, 2006, from http://www.cdc.gov.

Crowe, M., & Hall, M. A. (2005). *Chancroid.* Retrieved February 5, 2008, from http://www.emedicine.com.

Kundhal, K., & Lok, C. E. (2005). Clinical epidemiology of cardiovascular disease in chronic kidney disease. *Nephron Clinical Practice, 101,* c47-c52.

Medline Plus. (2005). *Medical encyclopedia: Granuloma inguinale*. Retrieved October 30, 2006, from http://www.nlm.nih.gov.

Meigs, J. B., Barry, M. J., Giovannucci, E., Rimm, E. B., Stampfer, M. J., & Kawachi I. (1999). Incidence rates and risk factors for acute urinary retention: The health professionals follow-up study. *Journal of Urology, 162*(2), 376-382.

National Institutes of Health. (2004). *Kidney and urologic diseases statistics for the United States*. Retrieved October 30, 2006, from http://kidney.niddk.nih.gov.

Toto, R. D. (2004). Approach to the patient with kidney disease. In Brenner, B. M. (Ed.), *Brenner & Rector's the kidney* (7th ed.). Philadelphia: Saunders.

United States Renal Data System. (2005). *Annual data report*. Retrieved October 30, 2006, from http://www.usrds.org.

SUGGESTED RESOURCES

Guyton, A. C., & Hall, J. E. (2006). *Textbook of medical physiology* (11th ed.). Philadelphia: W. B. Saunders.

Kahsai, D. (2001). Geriatric urologic emergencies. *Topics in Emergency Medicine, 23*(3), 61-67.

Kent, T. H., & Hart, M. N. (1998). *Introduction to human disease* (4th ed.). Stamford, CT: Appleton and Lange.

Litwin, M. S., & Saigal, C. S. (2004) *Urologic diseases in America*. Washington, DC: U.S. Government Publishing Office, NIH Publication No. 04-5512.

National Kidney Foundation: *NKF brochures in PDF formation*. Retrieved April 30, 2008, from http://www.kidney.org.

Thomas, K., Chow, K., & Kirby, R. S. (2004). Acute urinary retention: A review of the etiology and management. In *Prostate cancer and prostatic diseases* (7th ed.). Nature Publishing Group.

Chapter Quiz

1. What are two major risk factors that can lead to chronic renal failure?

_____

_____

2. How is ARF best defined?

_____

_____

3. How does the use of nonsteroidal antiinflammatory drugs contribute to ARF?

_____

_____

4. A common cause of urinary retention in men is benign prostatic hypertrophy. Why does this condition result in urinary retention?

_____

_____

5. What are the treatment options for a patient with ESRD?

_____

_____

6. A patient had a severe episode of dehydration and hypotension several days earlier. Now the patient is reporting a metallic taste in the mouth and tremors in the hands. What is (1) the most likely cause of the patient's condition and (2) the best prehospital treatment for this patient?

_____

_____

7. A young woman is reporting severe burning when she urinates along with cramping pain over the lower abdomen. She tells you her urine is cloudy, has a brown color, and has a bad odor. What condition does the paramedic suspect?

_____

_____

8. An elderly dialysis patient is found at home midway between dialysis treatments. He is unresponsive to verbal or physical stimuli and appears to have a large quantity of dried crystals on the skin. What condition does the patient have and what is the cause?

_____

_____

9. A 22-year-old man complains of penile pain that started after showering. He states that it feels like there is a tourniquet around his penis. Inspection reveals a swollen glans with what appears to be a constricting band of foreskin immediately behind the head of the penis. The shaft of the penis is soft. What is the patient's condition and how should it be treated in the prehospital setting?

_____

_____

Terminology

Acute renal failure (ARF) When the kidneys suddenly stop functioning, either partially or completely, but eventually recover full or nearly full functioning over time.

Azotemia The increase in nitrogen-containing waste products in the blood as a result of renal failure.

Chronic renal failure The gradual, long-term deterioration of kidney function.

Dialysis The process of diffusing blood across a semipermeable membrane to remove substances that the kidney would normally eliminate.

End-stage renal disease (ESRD) When the kidneys function at 10% to 15% of normal and dialysis or transplantation is the only option for the patient's survival.

Fistula Surgical connection of an artery and vein in the arm or leg to each other under the skin.

Glomerulus A clump of interconnected capillaries within a nephron.

Graft Connection by a surgeon of a piece of the patient's saphenous vein to an artery and vein; in lieu of using the patient's own blood vessel, a cow's artery or a synthetic graft may be used.

Hematuria Blood in the urine.

Hilus Indentation through which the renal artery, vein, lymphatic vessels, and nerves enter and leave the kidney.

Hydrocele Collection of fluid in the scrotum or along the spermatic cord.

Nephron The functional unit of the kidney.

Nephrotoxic Chemicals, medications, or other substances that can be toxic to the kidneys.

Paraphimosis Tight, constricting band caused by the foreskin when it is retracted behind the glans penis.

Priapism A prolonged and painful erection.

Renal calculi Kidney stones formed by substances such as calcium, uric acid, or cystine.

Renal insufficiency A decrease in renal function to approximately 25% of normal.

Shunt Insertion of catheters into an artery and a vein from outside the body. Most shunts are located on the forearm. When not in use to provide dialysis to a patient, the catheters are connected to each other with clear tubing, allowing the continuous flow of blood from artery to vein, and are covered with self-adhering roller gauze for protection.

Spermatocele Benign accumulation of sperm at the epididymis presenting as a firm mass.

Tinnitus Ringing or buzzing in the ears.

Testicular torsion Twisting of the spermatic cord inside the scrotum that cuts off the blood supply to the testis.

Uremia A term used to describe the signs and symptoms that accompany chronic renal failure.

Uremic frost Dried crystals of urea excreted through the skin that appear to be a frosting on the patient's body.

Ureters A thin-walled pair of tubes that drain urine from each kidney to the bladder.

Urethra A short tube that transports urine from the urinary bladder outside the body.

Urinary bladder A muscular sac responsible for storing urine before it is eliminated from the body.

Urinary retention The inability to empty the bladder or completely empty the bladder when urinating.

Varicocele Dilation of the venous plexus and internal spermatic vein, presenting as a lump in the scrotum.

Musculoskeletal Disorders

Objectives *After completing this chapter, you will be able to:*

1. Discuss and describe the basic anatomy and function of the musculoskeletal system.
2. Discuss the general assessment, physical examination findings, and treatment of patients with musculoskeletal conditions.
3. Discuss the causes, identification, and prehospital management of acute and chronic low back pain.
4. Discuss the causes, identification, and prehospital management of acute and chronic neck pain.
5. Discuss the causes, identification, and prehospital management of overuse injuries.
6. Discuss the causes, identification, and prehospital management of generalized muscle disorders.
7. Discuss the causes, identification, and prehospital management of generalized joint disorders.
8. Discuss the causes, identification, and prehospital management of infectious diseases of the musculoskeletal system.
9. Discuss the causes, identification, and prehospital management of neoplastic disorders of the musculoskeletal system.
10. Discuss the causes, identification, and prehospital management of a child with a limp not associated with trauma.

Chapter Outline

Anatomy and Physiology
General Assessment and Treatment of Patients with Musculoskeletal Disorders
Acute and Chronic Back Pain
Acute and Chronic Neck Pain
Injuries and Overuse Syndromes

Generalized Muscle Disorders
Generalized Joint Disorders
Infectious Diseases of the Musculoskeletal System
Neoplastic Disorders of the Musculoskeletal System
Special Circumstances: The Child with a Limp
Chapter Summary

Case Scenario

You are called to the scene of a 35-year-old man whose leg is trapped under a car. He was changing a flat tire when the jack broke. He rates his pain as 10 out of 10 and states he cannot feel his lower leg. His vital signs are pulse, 112 beats/min; blood pressure, 128/86 mm Hg; respirations, 16 breaths/min and non-labored. His skin is moist. You cannot see the leg that is trapped under the car.

Questions
1. What is your impression of this patient?
2. What possible conditions should be anticipated that are associated with this mechanism of injury?
3. What comfort measures would be appropriate for this patient?

When thinking of the musculoskeletal system, traumatic injuries (particularly fractures) often come to mind. However, EMS professionals must be able to identify and treat many other disorders of the musculoskeletal system. In general, these diseases and injuries are immobilizing and painful and routinely faced in the prehospital setting. This chapter describes the basic anatomy and functions of various components of the musculoskeletal system and discusses various conditions, including neck and back pain, complications of traumatic injuries, overuse injuries, infectious diseases, and neoplastic processes. Finally, some special situations are discussed, such as the child with a limp.

ANATOMY AND PHYSIOLOGY

[OBJECTIVE 1]

The musculoskeletal system is the supporting and movement structure for the body. It also protects the vital organs of the head, chest, and abdomen. Like other organ systems, the musculoskeletal system has blood vessels, nerves, and lymph vessels. It has nutrient and metabolic requirements and can become diseased.

The adult skeleton is composed of 205 bones (Moore, 1992). It consists of two parts, the **axial skeleton,** which is the skull, vertebral column, sternum, and ribs, and the **appendicular skeleton,** consisting of the bones of the shoulders, pelvis, and limbs.

Bones also can be classified by shape. **Long bones** are found in limbs. They have a body (called a *shaft*) and two ends that permit movement at joints. These bones have attachment points for muscles, which allow the mechanical basis of movement. The humerus, ulna, radius, femur, tibia, and fibula are good examples of long bones. The individual bones of the fingers and toes (phalanges) are examples of long bones even though they are relatively small.

Short bones are cuboidal (square) in shape and are found only in the feet and wrists. They assist with fine movements in several anatomic planes and are compact and strong. **Flat bones** usually protect and encase vital organs and often are curved to help form walls of cavities. The ribs and bones of the skull are examples of flat bones. **Sesamoid bones,** such as the patella (kneecap), develop in certain tendons to protect the tendons from excessive wear where they cross major joints. **Irregular bones** have unique shapes and functions and are mostly found in the face and vertebral column (Moore, 1992).

Bones have five main functions: (1) protection of vital structures; (2) support for the body; (3) a mechanical basis for movement; (4) production of blood cells; and (5) storage and supply of salts, such as calcium, phosphorus, and magnesium (Moore, 1992).

Each bone is covered with a fibrous connective tissue called the **periosteum.** Blood vessels enter the periosteum and supply the bone with vital nutrients. A bone stripped of its periosteum will ultimately die, just as the heart muscle dies when the arteries supplying the muscle become blocked. The periosteum is richly supplied with nerves (innervated), and when the periosteum is disrupted (such as with a fracture), pain results.

Joints are where bones and ligaments meet to allow movement or form a connection. **Ligaments** are bands of fibrous connective tissue that connect bone to bone. The most common joint is the synovial joint, a type of joint lined with cartilage and containing **synovial fluid,** which allows easy joint motion (Figure 28-1). Joints can be subjected to traumatic injuries (e.g., a shoulder dislocation) and nontraumatic conditions (e.g., gout), which are discussed later. Joints have rich vascular and nerve supplies, just as bones do. Excessive stretching or twisting of the joint can be quite painful. Another impor-

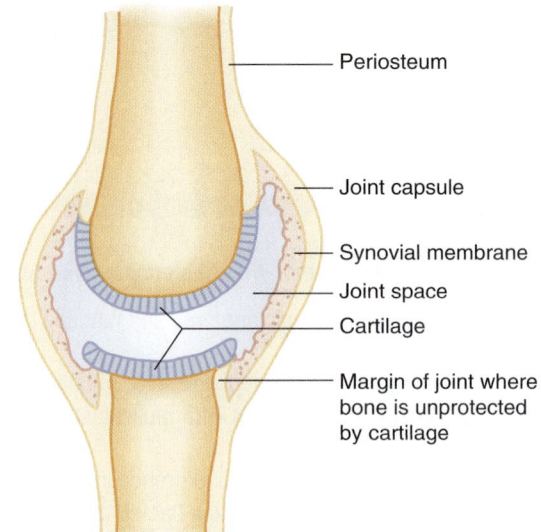

Figure 28-1 Anatomy of a synovial joint.

tant function of joints is to allow **proprioception,** the perception of motion and position of a body part.

Skeletal muscles, or voluntary muscles, are responsible for movements of the skeleton. The human body is composed of more than 600 muscles, which constitute approximately 40% of our body weight (Moore, 1992). The structural unit of a muscle is a muscle cell or fiber. Skeletal muscles have at least two attachments, described as an origin and an insertion, and produce movement by contracting, resulting in a pulling motion (never a pushing motion). Muscles may taper into dense, collagenous fibers where they attach to a bone. This connective, fibrous tissue is a **tendon.** Muscles, like all other parts of the musculoskeletal system, are supplied by a rich collection of blood vessels and nerves. Loss of proper blood supply or innervation results in muscle wasting, called **atrophy.** In patients with permanent nerve injuries (e.g., spinal cord injuries) or poor distal circulation, muscle atrophy often is observed and may be a clue regarding an underlying disease process.

GENERAL ASSESSMENT AND TREATMENT OF PATIENTS WITH MUSCULOSKELETAL DISORDERS

[OBJECTIVE 2]

As with all initial patient assessments, life-threatening conditions must be first and foremost identified and treated. The ABCDE mnemonic (see Chapter 17) is the preferred approach for the primary survey. Fortunately, most nontraumatic musculoskeletal conditions are not life-threatening and, as such, treatment can be aimed toward alleviating pain and providing comfort.

Assuming that no immediate life threat is identified, musculoskeletal symptoms often are addressed in a focal manner, meaning obtaining an adequate history and performing a physical examination that focuses on the affected body area.

Important Elements of the History

Following are important elements of the history for the focused musculoskeletal symptom (Seidel et al., 1995):

- How long has the pain been present? Was the onset sudden or gradual? Sudden pain often is associated with an acute injury, such as a sprain. Slowly developing and worsening pain may be associated with a gradual process, such as arthritis or a bone tumor.
- What is the quality and severity of the pain? Sudden, sharp, tearing, or throbbing pain can be associated with an acute injury, whereas a dull, aching, constant pain may be more indicative of an inflammatory or infectious process.
- Does the pain radiate to another area? Pain that originates in the neck or back and radiates to the arms or legs may suggest a central cause, such as a herniated disc.
- Is the pain isolated to one limb or joint, or are multiple limbs and/or joints involved? Many acute injuries involve just one area, but multiple affected areas mays suggest a diffuse inflammatory process.
- Is the pain associated with activity and, if so, what kind? Running, twisting, lifting, repetitive motions (such as painting), direct contact, or trauma?
- Is the pain better, worse, or unchanged with movement or rest? Many sprain and strain injuries improve with rest and worsen with movement, whereas morning stiffness and pain that improve with light movement may suggest rheumatoid arthritis.
- What physical signs has the patient noticed? Are erythema, joint swelling, edema of the affected limb, ecchymosis, deformity, or open wounds present? Joint swelling may be the result of bleeding into the joint, an acute injury, or an inflammatory disease such as gout.
- What associated symptoms are present? Does the patient report fever, general weakness, or any other generalized symptoms? Fever and a swollen, tender joint always suggest septic arthritis.
- What has the patient done for the pain, and did it help? For example, has the patient been taking over-the-counter medications (such as ibuprofen or acetaminophen), trying ice or heat packs, or using a brace or a splint?

The Focused Musculoskeletal Examination

Once the pertinent history is obtained, the focused musculoskeletal examination is performed, looking at the following key factors (Seidel et al., 1995).

Symmetry

How does the affected area compare with the opposite side? Is it swollen in comparison, or is atrophy present? Is one limb shorter than the other? Is one limb rotated when compared with the opposite side? Although perfect symmetry is not absolute, gross differences should not exist from joint to joint or limb to limb.

Deformity

Does the affected area show gross deviation? Is the affected joint tense, or swollen? Is a prior surgical scar visible?

Skin Findings

Is the overlying skin erythematous or warm to the touch? Is a rash present, which may indicate an infectious etiology? Is an open wound visible and, if so, is bleeding present? This may suggest an open fracture or dislocation. Is this skin tense or firm? This finding in the right context could indicate compartment syndrome.

Palpation of Affected Muscles and Bony Points

Feel for any tenderness, heat, laxity, or swelling.

Strength of Affected Muscles

Again, comparison of the affected side with the unaffected side is important. Weakness of the muscle may be from pain, fatigue, overstretching, or atrophy.

Range of Motion

Testing range of motion should be done in accordance with agency policy and medical director approval. Test **passive range of motion,** which is the movement of the joint while the patient is relaxed and the examiner moves the affected area. Then test **active range of motion,** which is movement of the joint as done by the patient using his or her own muscles. Discrepancies between passive and active range of motion may indicate true muscle weakness or joint disorder. Movements at the joint should be smooth, without pain or crepitus. Pain, limitation of movement, joint instability, or spastic movement may indicate a problem with the joint, related muscle group, or nerve supply.

Assessment of Sensation and Circulation

A sensory stimulus, such as a light touch with a cotton swab, should feel equal from side to side. Is sensory perception unequal at the affected area? Is blood flow to the affected area adequate, or is it cold, pale, and poorly perfused? Are distal pulses equal when comparing one side with the other?

General Treatment Principles

Once the history and physical examination are done, the condition must be stabilized and treated. Of course, follow local protocols. But in general, the following concepts may apply:

- Immobilization is a good technique for painful joints. The affected joint should be splinted in a position of comfort and in an anatomically correct position if possible, immobilizing the bones above and below.
- Cervical and spinal stabilization should be considered for patients with traumatic injuries and acute neck and/or back pain in conjunction with local protocols.
- The application of an ice pack to a painful joint or limb may be beneficial in an acute condition, such as a sprain.
- Elevation of the affected extremity may help reduce swelling, which in turn can lead to pain relief.
- Pain medications can be considered in conjunction with pain control protocols. The choice of pain medications will depend on local rules and the availability of oral versus intravenous or intramuscular medications.

Some specific conditions, discussed in the following setions, may require additional advanced life support measures.

ACUTE AND CHRONIC BACK PAIN

[OBJECTIVE 3]

Low back pain is a common chief complaint as well as a symptom complex. Indeed, low back pain is a significant and costly problem in society, as shown by some of the following statistics (Lehrich et al., 2006):

- Approximately 80% of individuals in the general population will have at least one episode of low back pain during their lifetimes.
- Low back pain occurs in roughly 25% of the working population each year and to a disabling degree in 2% to 8%.
- Back pain lasting at least 2 weeks affects approximately 14% of adults each year, and approximately 1% to 2% have sciatica.

Low back pain is a common symptom of persons frequently involved in repetitive bending and lifting activities. The presentation may be acute, such as in a situation of a motor vehicle crash or industrial lifting accident (the classic lumbosacral strain), or chronic, as in a person with degenerative joint disease of the spine or a spinal bony tumor. Although exact definitions may vary, chronic back pain often is thought of as pain lasting more than 4 weeks (Lehrich & Sheon, 2006).

The best approach to patients with acute or chronic back pain is to obtain an adequate history from the patient. In addition to the general concepts presented earlier, the following key risk factors, if present, may suggest a more serious cause of back pain (Tintinalli, 2004):

- Pain more than 6 weeks in duration, age greater than 50 years, history of cancer, weight loss, night pain, unremitting pain even when supine, motor weakness, sensory loss, or bowel or bladder incontinence may suggest a tumor.
- Fever, chills, history of intravenous drug abuse, history of an immune system disorder, or unremitting pain may suggest an infectious process.
- Abdominal pain, passage of blood with bowel movements or urination, pulsatile masses in the abdomen, or vomiting may be associated with an acute intraabdominal process such as an abdominal aortic aneurysm.
- Sharp, unilateral pain that originates in the low back and radiates to the flank and groin, associated with hematuria, may be related to a kidney stone.
- Mid-back pain may be a presentation of a serious or even life-threatening condition such as cardiac ischemia, pancreatitis, pneumonia, or aortic dissection.

The most common cause of back pain is strain of soft tissue elements in the back, with more serious causes of back pain such as infections or malignancies being less common (Lehrich et al., 2006). A **strain** is a stretching injury of a muscle or its associated tendon, sometimes resulting in a partial or complete tear of the tendon. Back strain tends to be acute, or sudden, and often is a result of a mechanical process such as lifting or bending. The pain may be achy or dull in nature and may radiate to one or both buttocks. Pain usually improves with rest and worsens with movement. Pain that radiates down the legs is less common, and limping or leg weakness is typically not associated with a back strain. Findings include localized tenderness and possibly firm, tense muscles that might be in spasm.

Sciatica is a specific cause of low back pain. The vertebral column is composed of 33 bones. Beginning at the space between the second and third vertebral bodies, and continuing down to the end of the spine, plates of fibrocartilage called *intervertebral discs* are found. Discs play a role in weight bearing and movement. Sometimes a portion of the disc can weaken and protrude out of position, compressing the adjacent nerve roots. This condition is known as a **herniated disc** (Figure 28-2). If the affected nerve root is the sciatic nerve, the term **sciatica** can also be used. The pain of a herniated disc often is described as sharp, electric, or shooting and radiates down the posterior aspect of one leg. The affected leg also can feel numb.

Many patients know they have disc problems, so history taking is important. Herniated discs are rare in patients younger than 20 years. In those with new back pain, particularly in the prehospital setting, discerning disc pain from low back strain is not important. Rather, get the patient to a facility where the diagnostic

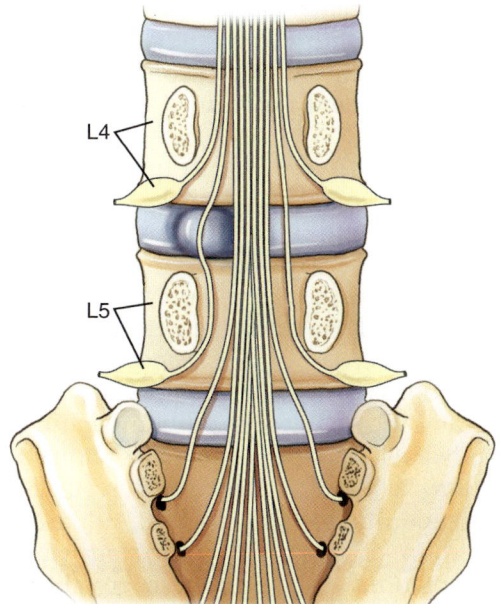

Figure 28-2 Lateral lumbar disc herniation involving the L4-L5 disc and compressing the L5 nerve root.

process can be started and provide pain control en route. Typically disc pain has some degree of radiation along a dermatome and is aggravated by a specific motion. Dermatomes correspond to specific spinal nerves (see Chapter 23). Approximately 80% of patients with a herniated disc ultimately improve without surgery to repair the displaced disc (Tintinalli, 2004). Most do quite well with physical therapy and pain control measures.

Cauda equina syndrome is a group of symptoms associated with the compression of the peripheral nerves still within the spinal canal below the level of the first lumbar vertebra. From 85% to 90% of cauda equina syndrome cases are caused by a mass or tumor from malignant cancer (Schiff, 2003). Because peripheral nerves are involved, both weakness and decreased sensation are present and the symptoms are bilateral. The distribution is typically the posterior thighs and gluteal muscles, with associated bowel and bladder dysfunction. Compare this with sciatic nerve pain with unilateral symptoms but normal bowel and bladder function. Findings suggestive of cauda equina syndrome include localized back pain in the presence of motor weakness of the legs, loss of the ability to walk, paralysis, sensory defects, and loss of bowel or bladder continence.

Acute and chronic low back pain have many other causes, some of which are presented later in this chapter. However, making an exact diagnosis in the field is generally not feasible or necessary, and the exact cause of the pain may not even be found in the emergency department. As previously noted, the best course of action is to be aware of risk factors signifying more serious causes of back pain and provide appropriate analgesia while transporting the patient in a position of maximal comfort. If

a traumatic injury has occurred, follow local protocols for spinal immobilization.

ACUTE AND CHRONIC NECK PAIN

[OBJECTIVE 4]

Neck pain is a fairly common condition. Approximately 10% of the adult population will have neck pain at least once, but less than 1% develop any neurologic deficits (Isaac & Anderson, 2006). In the prehospital setting many, if not most, of the patients with neck pain have had a traumatic injury (e.g., from a motor vehicle crash, sports injury, or fall). However, you should be cognizant of other causes of neck pain.

The general history and examination principles presented earlier are a good reference for the evaluation of patients with neck pain You also should observe the position in which the patient is holding the neck at rest. In addition, assess the bilateral shoulders and arms to evaluate for weakness or numbness, which may suggest cervical nerve root involvement.

As with back pain, one the most common causes of neck pain is cervical strain. Cervical strain is a non-specific diagnosis often used to describe an injury and spasm of the cervical and upper back muscles (Isaac & Anderson, 2006). The presumption of cervical strain is reasonable in patients with acute neck and trapezius pain with no neurologic symptoms. Cervical strain can have many causes, including traumatic injuries, the carrying of heavy items, and even physical stresses of everyday life, including poor posture and sleeping habits (Isaac & Anderson, 2006). Symptoms are experienced as pain, stiffness, and tightness in the upper back or shoulder and last for up to 6 weeks (Isaac & Anderson, 2006). Localized muscle warmth and spasm may be palpable.

Cervical spondylosis is a progressive, degenerative condition that can cause neck pain and loss of flexibility (Tintinalli, 2004). This condition tends to occur in older adults, and the soft tissues of the spinal column, the cervical discs, or the intervertebral joints can be affected. Symptoms can include cervical stiffness, pain with movement, and limitations of range of motion.

Cervical disc herniations can also result in neck pain. The most frequently affected discs are those between the fifth and sixth, and sixth and seventh, cervical vertebrae. Symptoms include neck pain, headache, pain that radiates to the shoulder or arm, and sensory deficits in the shoulder or arm (Tintinalli, 2004).

As with patients with back pain, provide the patient with neck pain appropriate analgesia and transport in a position of comfort. Cervical spine immobilization should be done for patients with neck pain and a history of trauma.

INJURIES AND OVERUSE SYNDROMES

[OBJECTIVE 5]

The two most common musculoskeletal injuries you may encounter are sprains and strains.

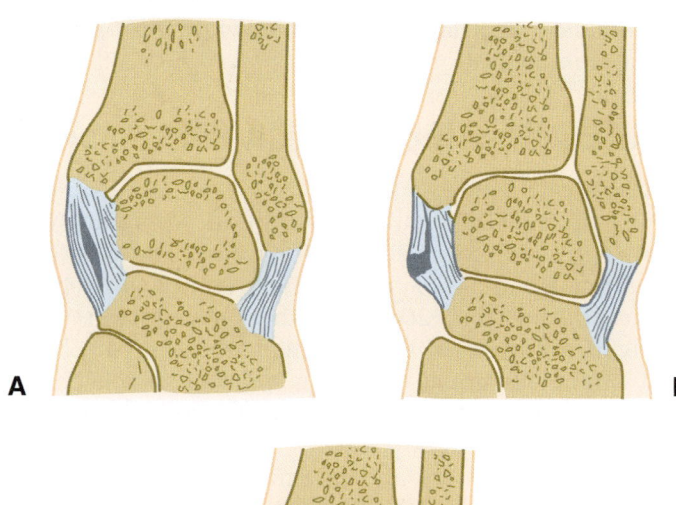

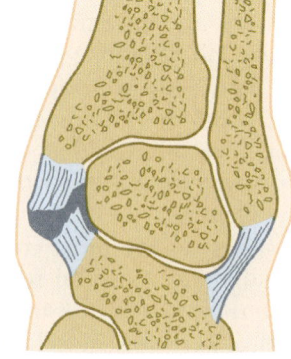

Figure 28-3 Types of ankle sprains. **A,** Mild (first degree). **B,** Moderate (second degree). **C,** Severe (third degree).

Sprains and Strains

A **sprain** is an injury to a *ligament* that results when it is overstretched, leading to a tear or complete disruption of the ligament (Figure 28-3). Sprains occur when a joint is forced into an unnatural position. The classic sprain is an inversion injury to the ankle, resulting in an overstretching of the lateral ankle ligaments (including the anterior talofibular, the posterior talofibular, and the calcaneofibular ligaments).

A strain is an injury to a *muscle* that results when it is overstretched, leading to tearing of the individual muscle fibers. This injury is commonly referred to as a *pulled muscle.* Lumbar back strains (previously discussed) and hamstring strains in the thigh are common.

Findings common to both of these injuries include sudden pain, often associated with some activity such as running, jumping, lifting, or twisting; a report of a popping sound; and localized swelling, ecchymosis, erythema, warmth, and pain on palpation of the affected area. Examine the joints immediately above and below the injury to assess for other injuries. If the injury resulted in a fall, assess the neck and back.

In the prehospital setting distinguishing between a sprain and a strain is not necessary. The treatment principles are the same: immobilization, compression of the affected joint with an elastic wrap, elevation of the affected part, application of an ice pack, and appropriate

analgesia. These patients must receive a thorough evaluation for compartment syndrome because compressive elastic wraps and elevation are contraindicated in the setting of compartment syndrome.

Tendonitis

Tendonitis is simply inflammation of a tendon, often as a result of overuse. This condition can affect virtually any tendon, but the most common areas are the rotator cuff tendons of the shoulder, the wrist flexor and extensor tendons that insert at the elbow, the patellar and popliteal tendons at the knee, the posterior tibial tendon in the leg, and the Achilles tendon at the posterior ankle (Steele & Norvell, 2006). Middle-age adults are most susceptible to tendonitis (Steele & Norvell, 2006). The causes of tendonitis include repeated, intense, and sustained exertion of the tendon; awkward or sustained postures; vibration; insufficient recovery time between activities; cold temperatures; and monotonous or repetitive motions (Steele & Norvell, 2006).

The diagnosis of tendonitis is made after a careful history is obtained, with physical examination findings confirming pain at the attachment points of the affected tendon, pain on active range-of-motion testing, and sometimes **crepitus** (a grating, crackling, or popping sensation heard or palpated at the affected tendon). Prehospital treatment is the same as for sprains and strains.

Carpal Tunnel Syndrome

Carpal tunnel syndrome (CTS) is a condition characterized by wrist pain caused by compression of the medial nerve in the wrist. CTS is the most frequently encountered peripheral compressive neuropathy. The estimated lifetime risk of acquiring CTS is 10%, the annual incidence is 0.1% among adults, and overall prevalence of CTS is 2.7% (Norvell & Steele, 2006). The median nerve passes through a tunnel bounded by the carpal bones of the wrist and the ligaments bridging the arch of the carpal bones. Frequent use of the wrist, particularly with repeated flexion and/or constant pressure on the volar wrist joint, can cause thickening of this ligament. Repetitive movements are thought to be a factor, such as using computer keyboards or playing certain musical instruments. As the ligament thickens, it causes pressure on the median nerve. The presentation is normally numbness (paresthesia) in the first three fingers of the hand with associated weakness (Figure 28-4). Pain can radiate to the elbow or even the neck. Findings can include weakness of thumb abduction, pain in the distribution of the medial nerve with hyperflexion of the wrist for 60 seconds, and paresthesia in the medial nerve distribution while tapping the volar wrist over the medial nerve. Prehospital treatment involves appropriate analgesia and immobilization of the wrist.

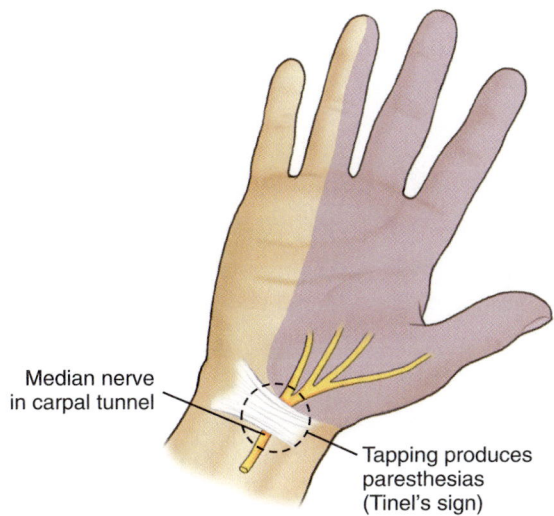

Median nerve in carpal tunnel

Tapping produces paresthesias (Tinel's sign)

Figure 28-4 Distribution of pain and/or paresthesias *(shaded area)* when the median nerve is compressed by swelling in the wrist (carpal tunnel).

GENERALIZED MUSCLE DISORDERS

[OBJECTIVE 6]

Myositis

Myositis is a rare muscle disease in which the body's immune system is activated, resulting in inflammation and pain of muscle tissue. Prevalence rates are estimated at approximately one per 100,000 in the general population. The female/male predominance is approximately 2:1 and, in adults, the peak incidence occurs in the fifth decade, although all age groups may be affected (Miller, 2006). Myositis can be associated with any of the inflammatory diseases (rheumatoid variants), infectious illnesses (particularly viral diseases), alcohol, drugs (including certain prescription drugs or even illicit drugs such as cocaine), or trauma. Findings include muscle pain and weakness, especially the proximal muscles of the limbs. No sensory loss should occur in the affected limbs (Tintinalli, 2004). If the neck or chest muscles are involved, trouble swallowing or breathing could be present. Some cases of myositis also can result in a skin rash. The diagnosis is made by muscle biopsy, although it is inferred through the use of an elevated creatine phosphokinase level in blood serum analysis. Supportive care yields the best results.

Rhabdomyolysis

Rhabdomyolysis is a clinical syndrome in which skeletal muscle is injured, resulting in muscle tissue necrosis and subsequent release of intracellular contents. It has a variety of causes, including direct muscle injury (e.g., crush injuries, electrical injuries, or lightning injuries), drugs of abuse, infections, medications, temperature disorders (hyperthermia, hypothermia), toxins (e.g.,

brown recluse spider bites), and metabolic disorders (Tintinalli, 2004). It can occur in bedridden patients who are not being turned or not having pressure points addressed. Also consider the patient who fell and was unable to get up or get assistance for several hours or days.

As the muscle tissue is injured, muscle cells break down and release creatine phosphokinase, myoglobin, potassium, and other substances into the interstitial spaces and vascular system. These substances can then result in "clogging" of the filtration system of the kidneys' glomeruli. Renal failure ensues if aggressive measures are not taken; rhabdomyolysis accounts for an estimated 8% to 15% of all cases of sudden renal failure (Craig, 2004). Signs and symptoms include myalgia, stiffness, weakness, malaise, and possibly dark-brown urine. Nausea, vomiting, abdominal pain, and tachycardia can occur in severe cases. Remember that rhabdomyolysis can still be present in patients without any signs or symptoms (Tintinalli, 2004).

Prehospital care typically should include brisk, adequate hydration in the form of intravenous fluids. Normal saline solution initially is the preferred fluid and should be infused at 500 mL/hr to maintain urine output at 200 to 300 mL/hr (Craig, 2004). Definitive treatment includes alkalinization of the urine (by adding sodium bicarbonate to intravenous fluids), which prevents precipitation of the myoglobin. This is typically done in the hospital setting once laboratory testing confirms the suspicion of rhabdomyolysis.

Compartment Syndrome

Compartment syndrome (CS) is a condition in which increased pressure within a fixed anatomic compartment results in compromised blood flow and subsequent nerve injury and tissue death. Technically CS does not solely affect the muscles, but discussion of this syndrome fits well with general muscle disorders. CS can occur in any limb: the upper arm, the forearm, the hand, the gluteal compartments, the thigh, or the leg. The classic and most common CS results when a tibia fracture causes bleeding and soft tissue swelling in the compartments of the leg (Paula, 2006). Besides fractures, other causes of CS include soft tissue injuries, thermal injuries, constrictive casts and dressings, arterial spasm or thrombosis, venous disease, snakebites, bleeding disorders, and even intravenous infiltration. An estimated 30% of limbs develop CS after vascular injury (Paula, 2006).

CS should be suspected in patients with limb pain and a history of a precipitating event (such as a fracture or snakebite). Findings can include severe resting pain, pain on palpation of the affected area, a tense or firm extremity, and particularly pain on passive or active flexion of the involved muscles.

CS is considered an orthopedic emergency, and once its presence is confirmed in the emergency department (usually by measuring the pressure inside the affected limb), a surgical procedure may be performed to relieve the dangerously high pressure. Therefore prehospital treatment should be aimed at rapid transport to the hospital while providing adequate pain control. If CS is suspected, do not elevate the limb, which could worsen CS.

Case Scenario—continued

The fire department arrives and begins to move the vehicle off the patient's leg. You have already notified the receiving hospital of the patient's condition, mechanism of injury, and an estimated time of arrival.

Questions

4. *What should be done before extrication?*
5. *What changes may occur in the patient's condition?*
6. *After the primary survey, what assessments should be performed next?*

GENERALIZED JOINT DISORDERS

[OBJECTIVE 7]

Many diseases are specific to joints and their related structures, the most common of which are discussed here.

Arthritis

Arthritis is a nonspecific term referring to any inflammatory condition of a joint. Several types of arthritis can occur. **Osteoarthritis,** or **degenerative joint disease,** is a disorder in which the cartilaginous covering of the joint surface starts to wear away (Figure 28-5). This disease typically strikes adults older than 40 years, and age is the strongest risk factor (Kalunian et al., 2005). Many other factors contribute to the development of degenerative joint disease, including local inflammation, mechanical forces, genetics, and joint integrity or history of joint trauma (Kalunian et al., 2005). Typically the synovial fluid is or becomes thickened. The joints start to swell as the body attempts to decrease the pain associated with the cartilage rubbing against cartilage. With increased and thickened synovial fluid, the joints become stiff and painful. Eventually, as a result of the inflammation, calcium deposits can occur in the cartilage or the supporting ligaments, further increasing the pain and decreasing the range of motion. Physical findings include pain on palpation of the joint, crepitus, joint effusions, bony enlargement, malalignment, decreased range of motion, and generalized signs of inflammation, including warmth and erythema (Kalunian et al., 2005).

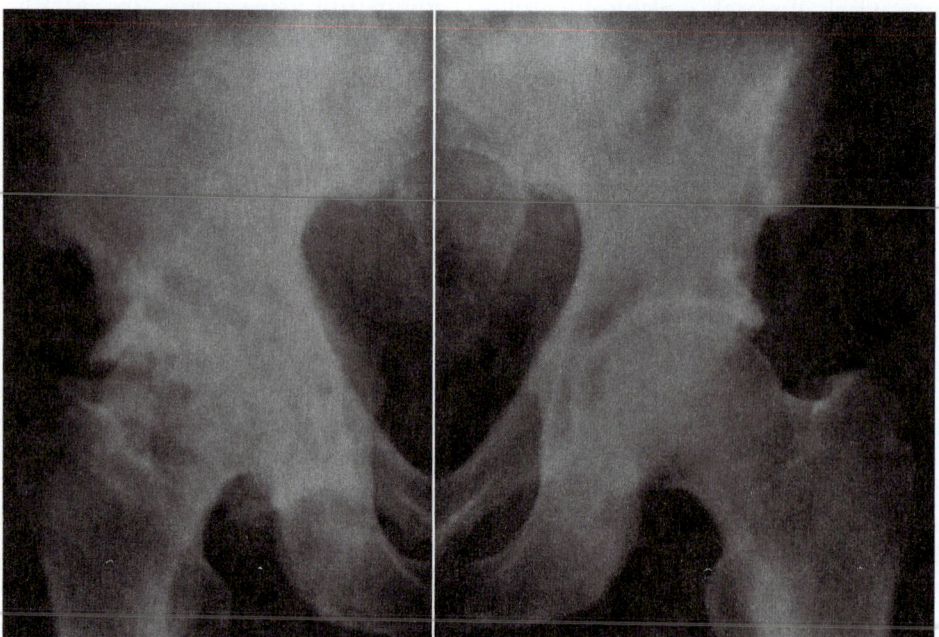

A

B

Figure 28-5 Severe osteoarthritis of hip **(A)** compared with normal hip **(B).**

Rheumatoid Arthritis

In contrast, **rheumatoid arthritis (RA)** is an inflammatory process mediated through an immune complex disease. This disease tends to affect women up to three times more than men and has an estimated incidence of 30 per 100,000 people (Venables & Maini, 2006). Joint complaints tend to be similar, but at the cellular level the inflammation starts when byproducts of an autoimmune system response cause joint swelling and pain. Some form of vascular involvement is typical. The following specific criteria are required to diagnose RA (Venables & Maini, 2006):

- Morning stiffness for at least 1 hour and present for at least 6 weeks
- Swelling of three or more joints for at least 6 weeks
- Swelling of wrist, metacarpophalangeal, or proximal interphalangeal joints for at least 6 weeks
- Symmetric joint swelling
- The presence of specific radiographic changes typical of RA and positive blood tests for rheumatoid factor

Up to one third of patients with RA also have systemic symptoms, including weight loss, fatigue, low-grade fevers, and depression.

Gout

Gout is a metabolic disease typically affecting the large joints of the body, classically the foot's first metatarsophalangeal joint (the great toe). It is usually unilateral and not associated with trauma. The etiology is the deposition of uric acid crystals in the joint space. The crystals mechanically irritate the joint lining by sticking into the **synovium.** This is a fairly common disease, affecting up to 0.8% of the U.S. population (Becker, 2006). Gout is most common in men between the age of 30 to 45 years and in women between ages 55 and 70 years (Becker, 2006).

Known risk factors for developing gout include obesity, trauma to a joint, consuming excessive amounts of alcoholic beverages (particularly beer, whiskey, gin, vodka, and rum) on a regular basis, overeating, ingestion of large quantities of meat and seafood, and medications that affect blood levels of urate (especially diuretics) (Becker, 2006).

Signs and symptoms of gout include the usual manifestations of an inflamed joint, such as severe pain, warmth, swelling, and erythema (Figure 28-6). Patients commonly awaken from sleep with the pain. The pain from an acute flare-up of gout is usually much more intense than pain from degenerative joint disease or RA. Even light touch is perceived as being quite painful, such as a blanket draped over the affected toe.

In all cases of joint disorders the prehospital treatment is the same. Adequate analgesia can be given while transporting the patient in a position of comfort. If any sus-

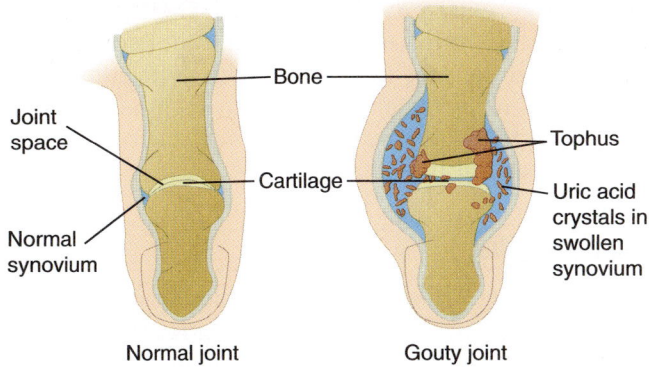

Figure 28-6 Comparison of a normal joint and a gouty joint.

picion of a possible traumatic injury to the joint exists, immobilization, ice packs, and elevation can be used to help alleviate pain.

INFECTIOUS DISEASES OF THE MUSCULOSKELETAL SYSTEM

[OBJECTIVE 8]

Septic Arthritis

Septic arthritis is the invasion of microorganisms, such as bacteria, into the joint space. This condition is rare, affecting an estimated 20,000 people per year in the United States (Brusch, 2005). It can affect any age group, including children and infants. One source reports that 45% of cases are found in adults older than 65 years (Brusch, 2005). Any joint can be infected, but the knee is the most common (Tintinalli, 2004). Risk factors for septic arthritis include a history of prior joint trauma, artificial (prosthetic) joints, a history of intravenous drug abuse, sexually transmitted diseases, or a history of immunosuppression.

A joint can become infected by one of three primary mechanisms: (1) direct inoculation (such as introducing a needle into a joint), (2) spread from an adjacent osteomyelitis (see following section), or (3) hematogenous spread (microorganisms are carried by the blood from a remote part of the body). Of these three, the hematogenous route is the most common (Tintinalli, 2004).

Once present in the joint space, bacteria (or other organisms) trigger the host's immune system. As a result, the joint space becomes a battleground where the host's defenses and the microorganisms' products of metabolism both result in local tissue, cartilage, and bone destruction. This tends to be a gradual process, sometimes over several days to several weeks, which is one clue when asking about the nature of the joint pain.

Physical examination findings of an infected joint can include localized pain and swelling, erythema, warmth, and limitations of passive and active range of motion. The patient may walk with a limp, particularly children, if the lower extremity is involved. The examination should not be limited to the affected joint because other systemic findings may be present, such as fever or a rash. Also important to remember is that more than one joint can be affected at the same time, such as from disseminated gonococcal infections.

Osteomyelitis

Osteomyelitis, the invasion of microorganisms into bone, shares many similarities with septic arthritis. Bone infections also occur by direct inoculation (such as an open fracture allowing bacteria to invade the bone), direct extension of an adjacent skin wound, or hematogenous spread from other sites. All age groups, including children and infants, are susceptible. The risk factors for osteomyelitis are also similar to those of septic arthritis. Additional risk factors include a history of sickle cell disease, recent orthopedic surgery, vascular disease, and long-term steroid use (Bo-Eisa & Al-Omran, 2005). The incidence of chronic osteomyelitis is estimated to be one case per 5000 people. The tibia is the most commonly affected bone (50%), followed by the femur (30%) and the fibula (12%) (Bo-Eisa & Al-Omran, 2005). Any bone can potentially be subject to osteomyelitis, including the vertebral bodies, so this condition should be included in the differential diagnosis for patients with back or neck pain.

Elements of the history of illness and physical examination findings also are similar to septic arthritis. Osteomyelitis could be suspected in a patient with appropriate risk factors, a history of gradually worsening pain, pain with weight bearing or use of the affected limb, fever, chills, and findings of erythema, swelling, and pain with movement of the limb.

In all cases of infectious diseases of the musculoskeletal system, the definitive diagnosis is made in the hospital setting, and treatment is directed toward providing the optimal antibiotics in conjunction with possible surgical drainage of the infection, debridement of the infected bone, or removal of the prosthetic joint. In the prehospital setting you can provide appropriate analgesia while transporting to the hospital. If the patient exhibits signs of sepsis (hypotension, tachycardia, fever or hypothermia, altered mental status), initiate fluid resuscitation and oxygen therapy in conjunction with local protocols while carefully monitoring the patient's hemodynamic status during transport.

NEOPLASTIC DISORDERS OF THE MUSCULOSKELETAL SYSTEM

[OBJECTIVE 9]

Tumors

Tumors that affect the bone and soft tissues of the musculoskeletal system can be divided into primary tumors and secondary tumors. Primary tumors originate in the bone directly, whereas secondary tumors originate from areas beyond the bone and metastasize (spread) to the bone.

Primary Tumors

Primary tumors of the bone are exceedingly rare, with fewer than 3000 cases expected to be diagnosed per year (Rosenthal & Hornicek, 2006). Multiple types of primary bone tumors are ultimately diagnosed after radiographs, biopsies, and other studies are performed.

Secondary Tumors

Secondary tumors are much more prevalent. The most common cancers to spread to bone include breast, prostate, thyroid, lung, kidney, and pancreas, which together account for approximately 80% of all secondary bone tumors (Rosenthal & Hornicek, 2006). Cancers typically spread by the hematogenous route, but direct invasion from adjacent tumors also can occur.

Pain is the most frequent symptom. It usually develops gradually over weeks, is localized, and is more severe at night (Patel & Benjamin, 2005). Bone metastases exert a major adverse effect on quality of life in patients with cancer.

If the bone tumor is in the spine, the presence of neurologic signs or symptoms, such as weakness, numbness, or loss of sensation, are worrisome. This may indicate compression of spinal nerve roots or the spinal cord itself.

Pathologic Fractures

Pathologic fractures occur as a result of an underlying disease process that weakens the mechanical properties of the bone. Bone tumors are common causes of pathologic fractures, but other metabolic diseases, such as osteoporosis, can cause these fractures as well. Pathologic fractures may be the first presentation of a primary bone tumor in up to 10% of cases (Levine & Aboulafia, 2003). The tumor or metabolic process results in a destruction of the bone, which can give way with even minor trauma or something as benign as a sneeze that results in a rib fracture. Patients with a suspected fracture without a history of significant trauma should be asked about any prior history of known cancer or chronic pain in the affected area before the fracture occurred. The findings of a pathologic fracture are the same as for other fractures: pain, deformity, swelling, loss of function. Prehospital treatment is also the same: analgesia with adequate immobilization of the affected area.

SPECIAL CIRCUMSTANCES: THE CHILD WITH A LIMP

[OBJECTIVE 10]

You may, on occasion, encounter a child with a limp, which can be alarming for both the child and the parents. In one study, the estimated incidence of children with an acute limp without a known history of trauma was 1.8 per 1000, with a median age of just over 4 years old (Clark, 2005a).

The number of possibilities for the limping child is extensive but can be broken down into the following broad categories:

- Infections (e.g., septic arthritis, osteomyelitis)
- Inflammatory disorders, such as transient synovitis (a benign inflammation of the synovial fluid and synovium)
- Trauma, both accidental and nonaccidental
- Bony deformities, both congenital and acquired
- Neoplastic diseases: bony tumors, both benign and malignant
- Neuromuscular causes (e.g., muscular dystrophy)
- Vascular disease: diseases that affect the blood supply of the affected joint, leading to localized tissue and bony ischemia and necrosis

Important elements of the history include when the limp started, gradual or sudden onset, any history of trauma, any recent illnesses or fever, whether the limp improves or worsens with activity, and any history of illnesses. One important fact to consider is that the location of pain may not reflect the actual site of the problem; for example, problems in the hip can cause pain in the knee or thigh.

Physical examination principles are generally the same as presented earlier. In children, complete the general examination first, focusing on areas of least concern before the area of most concern (Clark, 2005a).

Transient Synovitis

A few special causes of limp in children merit extra discussion. **Transient synovitis,** a nonspecific inflammation of the synovium and synovial fluid, is the most common cause of nontraumatic hip pain in children (Clark, 2005b). The exact cause is not known, although it is thought to be related to recent minor trauma, recent illness, or a result of a medication reaction in children with allergic tendencies (Whitelaw & Schikler, 2006). It typically affects children between the ages of 3 and 8 years, with a higher risk in boys than girls (Clark, 2005b). Children have usually had symptoms less than 1 week, which include pain and limitation of movement at the joint. Children generally appear well and do not have a fever (or merely a low-grade fever).

Slipped Capital Femoral Epiphysis

Slipped capital femoral epiphysis is a disease in which a displacement of the growth plate of the femur (the epiphysis) occurs posteriorly (Figure 28-7). This condition typically affects overweight preteen and early teenaged boys, although girls can be affected as well. It is usually a gradual process, with children reporting pain for weeks or months before the diagnosis is made. Sometimes the history reveals a slowly progressing pain that became suddenly worse after a minor trauma, such as jumping off of a relatively low height. Children may only report knee or thigh pain with this condition even though the hip is the site of the problem. Findings can reveal a hip rotated slightly outward. Joint effusion is usually not present. Radiographs confirm the diagnosis.

As is the case with many musculoskeletal diseases, the exact cause of a limp in a child may not be found in the prehospital setting, nor is it necessary. After obtaining a careful history and performing a good physical examination, treatment principles are the same.

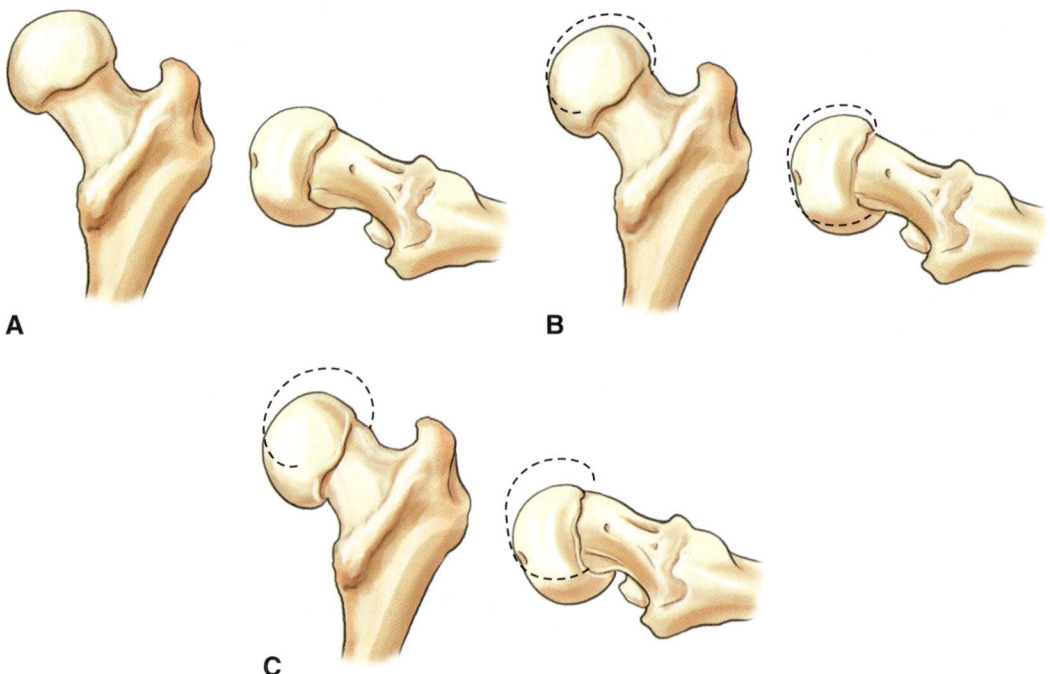

Figure 28-7 Slipped capital femoral epiphysis. **A,** Mild. **B,** Moderate. **C,** Severe.

Case Scenario SUMMARY

1. *What is your impression of this patient?* This patient has a crush injury, which could be life-threatening. Because visualizing the leg is impossible, assessing the damage is difficult. The patient could be losing significant blood. He also has significant pain. The patient requires advanced life support care and rapid transport to a receiving facility that can handle a possible amputation.

2. *What possible conditions should be anticipated that are associated with this mechanism of injury?* The patient has a crush injury. Anticipate hemorrhagic shock. The crush injury can lead to rhabdomyolysis and CS, which can have serious ramifications. CS can lead to loss of function or amputation of the limb.

3. *What are comfort measures that would be appropriate for this patient?* Comfort care should include analgesia with a narcotic such as morphine if vital signs are stable. Other comfort care to be considered in this patient (once extricated) would be splinting the leg.

4. *What should be done before extrication?* Prehospital care in this situation typically would include administering supplemental oxygen, applying a pulse oximeter and cardiac monitor, and administering brisk, adequate IV hydration. Normal saline solution initially is the preferred IV fluid and should be infused at 500 mL/hr to maintain urine outputs at 200 to 300 mL/hr (Craig, 2004). Provide pain medication per protocol. Other considerations before extrication include anticipating the

need for a leg splint, pressure dressings, and a backboard to facilitate patient movement once freed from the vehicle.

5. *What changes may occur in the patient's condition?* The patient may have increased pain during or immediately after extrication. Careful attention to comfort measures should be performed. This may include pain medication and careful patient movement. The crush injury causes destruction of the muscle cells, which can lead to the release of potassium; a hyperkalemic state therefore may ensue. This can cause significant cardiac dysrhythmias and even death. In anticipation of this, placing a cardiac monitor would be appropriate. Monitor the patient for any sudden electrocardiographic changes, such as peaked T waves or widening of the QRS duration. If these changes occur, contact medical direction for further orders for the treatment of possible hyperkalemia. Other changes to anticipate before extrication include hypotension as a result of blood loss.

6. *After the primary survey, what assessments should be performed next?* After the primary survey, do a brief secondary survey looking for other potential injuries (chest, abdomen, back, pelvis). Then focus on the leg: pulses, color, sensation, and movement.

7. *What is the significance in the change in the vital signs?* The patient has had a significant drop in blood pressure. The heart rate also has increased, which indicates that

the patient is in hemorrhagic shock. The patient should be rapidly treated, stabilized, and transported.

8. *What is the appropriate treatment?* Because of the patient's hypotension, further pain medications should now be withheld. Intravenous normal saline should be now running wide open (or at a rate infused per local protocol), with a systolic blood pressure goal of at least 100 mm Hg. Monitor blood pressure frequently, preferably at least every 5 minutes. Gentle attempts at repositioning the leg in its normal anatomic position may improve blood flow to the distal extremity. Place pressure dressings over any areas of bleeding. Splint the leg in a position that affords the greatest patient comfort while keeping bleeding to a minimum. Splinting the leg also may provide some additional pain relief. The patient should be treated and stabilized as rapidly and efficiently as possible; consider transport to the closest appropriate trauma center.

9. *What should be monitored during transport?* The patient should receive continual cardiac and vital sign monitoring. Monitor the patient's mental status. Document any changes in skin color, vital signs, and the affected limb. Give the receiving facility frequent updates regarding the patient's condition.

Chapter Summary

- In addition to fractures, the musculoskeletal system is subject to many other injuries and disease processes.
- In the prehospital setting, making the exact diagnosis for most musculoskeletal disorders is usually not possible, or necessary, because treatment principles are generally the same.
- A careful history and physical examination may provide clues to a more serious condition, such as an infectious or neoplastic disease.

- The majority of musculoskeletal diseases and injuries are not life-threatening, and prehospital treatment can be directed toward appropriate analgesia and comfort measures such as splinting, ice packs, elevation, and transportation in a position of comfort.
- When evaluating the patient with back pain, be sure to consider nonmusculoskeletal causes of pain, including cardiac, pulmonary, and abdominal conditions.

REFERENCES

Becker, M. (2006). *Gout.* Retrieved October 2006, from http://www.utdol.com.

Bo-Eisa, A., & Al-Omran, S. (2005). *Osteomyelitis.* Retrieved October 2006, from http://www.emedicine.com.

Brusch, J. (2005). *Septic arthritis.* Retrieved October 2006, from http://www.emedicine.com.

Clark, M. (2005a). *Approach to the child with a limp.* Retrieved October 2006, from http://www.utdol.com.

Clark, M. (2005b). *Overview of the causes of limp in children.* Retrieved October 2006, from http://www.utdol.com.

Craig, S. (2004). *Rhabdomyolysis.* Retrieved October 2006, from http://www.emedicine.com.

Isaac, Z., & Anderson, B. (2006). *Evaluation of the patient with neck pain and cervical spine disorders.* Retrieved October 2006, from http://www.utdol.com.

Kalunian, K., Brion, P., & Wollaston, S. (2005). *Clinical manifestations of osteoarthritis.* Retrieved October 2006, from http://www.utdol.com.

Lehrich, J., Katz, J., & Sheon, R. (2006). *Approach to the diagnosis and evaluation of low back pain in adults.* Retrieved October 2006, from http://www.utdol.com.

Lehrich, J., & Sheon, R. (2006b). *Treatment of chronic low back pain.* Retrieved October 2006, from http://www.utdol.com.

Levine, A., & Aboulafia, A. (2003). Pathologic fractures. In B. D. Browner (Ed.). *Skeletal trauma: Basic science, management, and reconstruction* (3rd ed.). Philadelphia: Saunders.

Miller, M. (2006). *Clinical manifestations and diagnosis of adult dermatomyositis and polymyositis.* Retrieved October 2006, from http://www.utdol.com.

Moore, K. (1992). *Clinically oriented anatomy* (3rd ed.). Baltimore: Williams & Wilkins.

Norvell, J., & Steele, M. (2006). *Carpal tunnel syndrome.* Retrieved October 2006, from http://www.emedicine.com.

Patel, S., & Benjamin, R. (2005). Soft tissue and bone sarcomas and bone metastases. In D. Kasper (Ed.). *Harrison's principles of internal medicine* (16th ed.). New York: McGraw-Hill.

Paula, R. (2006). *Compartment syndrome, extremity.* Retrieved October 2006, from http://www.emedicine.com.

Rosenthal, D., & Hornicek, F. (2006). *Bone tumors: diagnosis and biopsy techniques.* Retrieved October 2006, from http://www.utdol.com.

Schiff, D. (2003). *Clinical features and diagnosis of epidural spinal cord compression, including cauda equina syndrome.* Retrieved October 2006, from http://www.utdol.com.

Seidel, H., Ball, J., Dains, J., & Benedict, G. (1995). *Mosby's guide to physical examination* (3rd ed.). St. Louis: Mosby–Year Book.

Steele, M., & Norvell, J. (2006). *Tendonitis.* Retrieved October 2006, from http://www.emedicine.com.

Tintinalli, J. E. (Ed.) (2004). *Emergency medicine: A comprehensive study guide* (6th ed.). New York: McGraw-Hill.

Venables, P., & Maini, R. (2006). *Clinical features of rheumatoid arthritis.* Retrieved October 2006, from http://www.utdol.com.

Whitelaw, C., & Schikler, K. (2006). *Transient synovitis.* Retrieved October 2006, from http://www.emedicine.com.

SUGGESTED RESOURCES

Delee, J., & Drez, D. (2003). *Delee and Drez's orthopaedic sports medicine* (2nd ed.). Philadelphia: Saunders.

Kasper, D. L., Braunwald, E., Fauci, A., Hauser, S., Longo, D., & Jameson, L. J. (2005). *Harrison's principles of internal medicine* (16th ed.). New York: McGraw-Hill.

Chapter Quiz

1. Which bone is considered a part of the appendicular skeleton?
   a. Mandible
   b. Radius
   c. Ribs
   d. Vertebral column

2. Which of the following findings is of concern as a potentially serious cause of low back pain?
   a. Associated with hypotension and abdominal pain
   b. Improves with rest
   c. Sudden onset after lifting a heavy box
   d. Worsens with movement

3. Which of the following is typically associated with sciatica?
   a. A tumor
   b. Back pain that radiates down the posterior aspect of one leg
   c. Inflammation of a tendon
   d. Loss of bowel or bladder continence

4. Which of the following is true concerning sprains and strains?
   a. A "pop" heard or felt at the time of injury always suggests a fracture.
   b. Both injuries are treated in the same manner.
   c. Distinguishing between the two in the prehospital setting is important and necessary.
   d. Local soft tissue swelling is uncommon.

5. CTS affects the _____.
   a. ankle
   b. elbow
   c. knee
   d. wrist

6. Which of the following is true concerning rhabdomyolysis?
   a. Bright yellow urine may be one sign of rhabdomyolysis.
   b. One serious complication of rhabdomyolysis is low blood sugar.
   c. Prehospital treatment includes withholding intravenous fluids to prevent volume overload.
   d. This condition may be associated with nausea, vomiting, abdominal pain, and tachycardia.

7. One key finding that may help differentiate gout from other joint diseases such as osteoarthritis is _____.
   a. pain on movement of the joint
   b. pain with even light touch of the affected area
   c. the presence of local warmth and erythema
   d. the presence of local swelling

8. Which of the following are three risk factors for septic arthritis or osteomyelitis?
   a. A history of immunosuppression, local swelling, and dark-brown urine
   b. A history of prior joint or bone trauma or surgery, history of immunosuppression, and intravenous drug abuse
   c. Intravenous drug abuse, hypotension, and pain associated with a tumor
   d. Pain with even the lightest touch, hypotension, and a history of immunosuppression

9. Which of the following is true regarding neoplastic diseases of the musculoskeletal system?
   a. Bone pain associated with tumors often is sudden and worse during the daytime.
   b. In the prehospital setting, pathologic fractures cannot be treated the same as traumatic fractures.
   c. Secondary tumors are less common than primary tumors.
   d. Tumors may result in pathologic fractures of bone.

10. Which of the following is true regarding the child with a limp?
    a. A careful history and examination will not elicit any clues to the cause of a limp.
    b. Slipped capital femoral epiphysis typically affects girls aged 3 to 6 years.
    c. The most common cause of nontraumatic hip pain in children is transient synovitis.
    d. Limping in children has only one cause.

Terminology

Active range of motion The degree of movement at a joint as determined by the patient's own voluntary movements.

Appendicular skeleton Part of the skeleton that consists of all the bones not within the axial skeleton: upper and lower extremities, the girdles, and their attachments.

Atrophy Wasting away of a part of the body, such as a muscle, often as a result of disrupted nerve or blood supply.

Axial skeleton Part of the skeleton composed of the skull, hyoid bone, vertebral column, and thoracic cage.

Carpal tunnel syndrome (CTS) A medical condition in which the median nerve is compressed at the wrist (within the carpal tunnel), resulting in pain and numbness of the hand.

Cauda equina syndrome A group of symptoms associated with the compression of the peripheral nerves still within the spinal canal below the level of the first lumbar vertebra, characterized by lumbar back pain, motor and sensory deficits, and bowel or bladder incontinence.

Cervical spondylosis Degeneration of two or more cervical vertebrae, usually resulting in a narrowing of the space between the vertebrae.

Compartment syndrome (CS) A condition in which compartment pressures increase in an injured extremity to the point that capillary circulation is stopped; often only correctable through surgical opening of the compartment.

Crepitus Grating, crackling, or popping sounds and sensations heard and felt under skin and joints.

Degenerative joint disease See *Osteoarthritis.*

Flat bones Specialized bones that protect vital anatomic structures (e.g., ribs and bones of the skull).

Gout A metabolic disease in which uric acid crystals are deposited on the cartilaginous surfaces of a joint, resulting in pain, swelling, and inflammation.

Herniated disc A condition in which an intervertebral disc weakens and protrudes out of position, often affecting adjacent nerve roots.

Irregular bones Unique bones with specialized functions not easily classified into the other types of bone (e.g., vertebrae).

Joints Point where two or more bones make contact to allow movement and provide mechanical support.

Ligaments Fibrous connective tissue that connects bones to bones, forming joint capsules.

Long bones Bones that are longer than they are wide, have attachments for muscles to allow movement, and are found in limbs (e.g., the femur).

Myositis A rare muscle disease in which the body's immune system is activated, resulting in inflammation and pain of muscle tissue.

Osteoarthritis A disorder in which the cartilaginous covering of the joint surface starts to wear away, resulting in pain and inflammation of a joint; also known as *degenerative joint disease.*

Osteomyelitis An infection of bone.

Passive range of motion Degree of movement at a joint determined when the examiner moves the joint with the patient at rest.

Pathologic fracture Fractures that occur as a result of an underlying disease process that weakens the mechanical properties of the bone.

Periosteum Fibrous connective tissue rich in nerve endings that envelops bone.

Proprioception Sense of position and location of a limb relative to the body.

Rhabdomyolysis Complex series of events that occur in patients with severe muscle injury (e.g., crush injuries); destruction of the muscle tissues results in a release of cellular material and acidosis that can lead to acute renal failure.

Rheumatoid arthritis (RA) A painful, disabling disease in which the body's immune system attacks the joints.

Sciatica Pain in the lumbar back and leg caused by irritation and impingement of the sciatic nerve, usually from a herniated disc.

Septic arthritis Invasion of microorganisms into a joint space, causing infection of the joint.

Sesamoid bones Specialized bones found within tendons where they cross a joint; designed to protect the joint (e.g., the patella [kneecap]).

Short bones Specialized bones of the skeleton designed for compactness and strength, often with limited movement (e.g., bones of the wrist [carpals]).

Skeletal muscles Muscles that affect movement of the skeleton, usually by voluntary contractions.

Slipped capital femoral epiphysis A disease in which a posterior displacement of the growth plate of the femur (the epiphysis) occurs.

Sprain An injury to a ligament that results when the ligament is overstretched, leading to tearing or complete disruption of the ligament.

Strain An injury to a muscle that results when the muscle is overstretched, leading to tearing of the individual muscle fibers.

Synovial fluid Fluid located within the joint capsules of synovial joints; provides lubrication and cushioning during manipulation of the joint.

Synovium Soft tissue that lines the noncartilaginous surfaces of a joint.

Tendonitis Inflammation of a tendon, often caused by overuse.

Tendons Tough, fibrous bands of connective tissue that connect muscle to muscle and muscle to bones.

Transient synovitis A nonspecific inflammation of a joint, usually the hip, that affects the synovium and synovial fluid in children.

Cutaneous Disorders

Objectives *After completing this chapter, you will be able to:*

1. Describe the three layers of the skin, their composition, and their functions.
2. Describe the morphology of primary skin lesions.
3. Describe the morphology of secondary skin lesions.
4. Describe the recognition and treatment of skin cancer.
5. Describe malignant melanoma and how it is best recognized.
6. Recognize and treat decubitus ulcers.
7. Recognize and treat atopic dermatitis.
8. Recognize and treat contact dermatitis.
9. Recognize and treat psoriasis.
10. Recognize and treat impetigo.
11. Recognize and treat folliculitis.
12. Recognize and treat furuncles and carbuncles.
13. Recognize and treat cellulitis.
14. Recognize and treat fungal infections.
15. Recognize and treat *Candida* species infections.
16. Recognize and treat pediculosis.
17. Recognize and treat scabies.
18. Recognize and treat common warts.
19. Recognize and treat *Varicella* species infections.
20. Recognize and treat herpes simplex.
21. Recognize and treat herpes zoster.
22. Recognize and treat urticaria.
23. Recognize and treat erythema multiforme.

Chapter Outline

Anatomy and Physiology of the Skin
Primary Skin Lesions
Secondary Skin Lesions
Cancers of the Skin
Decubitus Ulcers
Atopic Dermatitis (Eczema)
Contact Dermatitis

Psoriasis
Bacterial Skin Infections
Fungal Skin Infections
Parasitic Infestations
Viral Skin Infections
Specialized Erythema
Chapter Summary

Case Scenario

At 11:20 PM on a warm summer night your crew is called to a private residence, where you are greeted by a concerned man who states that his wife is acting "funny." As you walk into the home, the man tells you that his wife woke up screaming, "I am going nuts! This itching is driving me crazy!" As you approach the patient, you see an approximately 30 year-old woman wringing and scratching her hands. She is in tears and appears distraught. Just before reaching the woman's side, the husband whispers, "She's been under a lot of stress at the nursing home where she works. I think she's having trouble there."

Questions

1. What is your initial impression of the patient?
2. What additional information do you need to complete your assessment?
3. What may be causing the woman's distress?

The skin is considered the largest organ of the body and has many different functions. Because of its size and availability for inspection, examination of the skin can provide many answers to external and internal pathologic questions. The challenge for any clinician in examining cutaneous disorders lies in distinguishing normal from abnormal. The next challenge is to distinguish significant findings from nonsignificant findings and then integrate pertinent signs and symptoms into an appropriate differential diagnosis. Because some cutaneous conditions are transmissible, remember to use appropriate standard precautions when providing emergency care.

This chapter prepares you to recognize, diagnose, and initially manage common cutaneous diseases. Selected eruptive diseases are discussed and illustrated to show their characteristics and common variations.

ANATOMY AND PHYSIOLOGY OF THE SKIN

[OBJECTIVE 1]

The skin is the body's largest organ. It covers the external surface of the body and weighs approximately 6 lb. The skin serves as a protective barrier against the environment (e.g., heat, light, injury, infection); regulates body temperature; and stores water, fat, and vitamin D. The skin also can sense painful and pleasant stimulation.

The skin is composed of three layers—the epidermis, dermis, and subcutaneous layer—with each layer performing specific protective functions.

The **epidermis** is the top layer and is primarily composed of epidermal cells, called **keratinocytes.** The epidermis is the barrier that protects the skin from environmental conditions. It also helps prevent desiccation (dryness) and provides immune surveillance.

The next layer, called the **dermis,** is primarily composed of collagen. The dermis also houses hair follicles, sebaceous glands, eccrine glands, and apocrine glands. The third layer of skin is the subcutaneous layer; it houses nerves, larger blood vessels, and adipose tissue. The anatomy of the skin is discussed in greater detail in Chapter 7.

The language of cutaneous disorders is always descriptive. You should learn the skill of describing various primary, secondary, and special skin lesions. When describing skin lesions, always use the terms noted in the template shown in Box 29-1.

PRIMARY SKIN LESIONS

[OBJECTIVE 2]

A **primary skin lesion** is best described as a lesion that has not been altered by scratching, rubbing, scrubbing, or other types of trauma. You should be comfortable in describing the following 10 primary lesions:

1. A **macule** is a flat, circumscribed (well-defined) discolored lesion that is less than 1 cm in diameter (Figure 29-1). One example is a freckle.
2. A **papule** is an elevated solid lesion usually less than 0.5 cm in diameter (Figure 29-2). Papules may arise from the epidermis, dermis, or both. Examples include verruca (warts) and elevated nevi (moles).
3. A **plaque** is an elevated, solid lesion usually greater than 0.5 cm in diameter that lacks any deep component (Figure 29-3). A plaque is often formed by coalescence of papules. Actinic keratosis is an example.
4. A **patch** is a flat, circumscribed, discolored lesion greater than 1 cm. It also can be described as a large macule. An example is a Mongolian spot (Figure 29-4).
5. A **nodule** is an elevated solid lesion in the deep skin or subcutaneous tissues. Nodules are usually larger and deeper than papules and are greater than 0.5 cm in diameter. Nodules also can be described as larger and deeper papules (Figure 29-5).
6. A **wheal** is a firm, rounded, flat-topped elevation of skin that is evanescent (has a short duration) and pruritic (itches). It also is known as a *hive* (Figure 29-6).

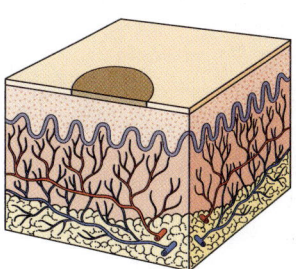

Figure 29-1 Macule.

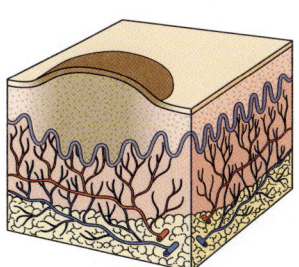

Figure 29-2 Papule.

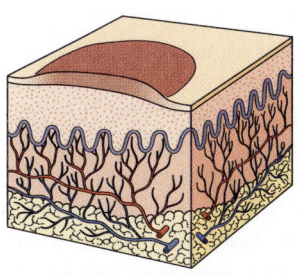

Figure 29-3 Plaque.

BOX 29-1	**Template for Describing Skin Lesions**

- **Size:** in millimeters
- **Color:** pigmentation
- **Type:** primary, secondary, special
- **Arrangement:** grouped lesions
- **Distribution:** generalized, truncal
- **Shape:** round, irregular
- **Moisture:** moist, dry
- **Elevation:** flat, elevated

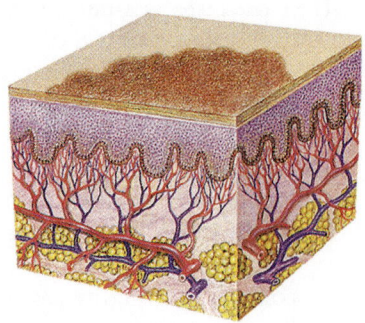
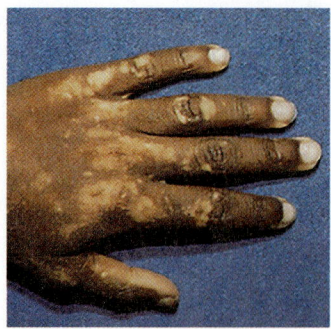

Figure 29-4 Patch.

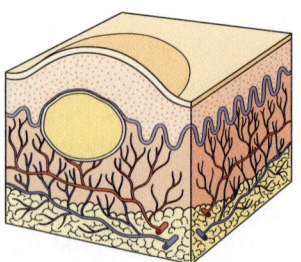

Figure 29-5 Nodule.

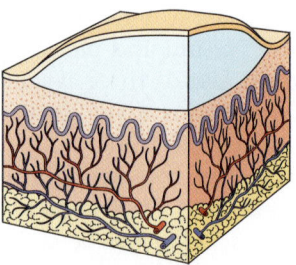

Figure 29-8 Bulla.

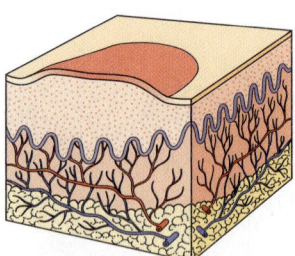

Figure 29-6 Wheal.

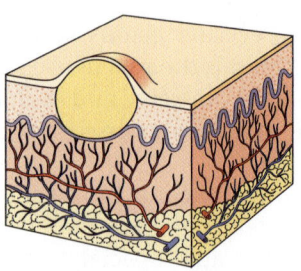

Figure 29-9 Pustule.

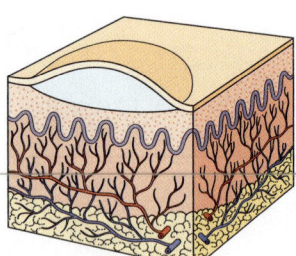

Figure 29-7 Vesicle.

7. A **vesicle** is an elevated lesion that contains clear fluid and is less than 0.5 cm. It sometimes is called a *water blister* (Figure 29-7). The vesicles associated with chickenpox are an example.
8. A **bulla** is a localized, fluid-filled lesion usually greater than 0.5 cm (Figure 29-8). Blisters are an example.
9. A **pustule** is a lesion that contains purulent material (Figure 29-9). Acne is an example.

10. A **cyst** is described as an elevated and circumscribed, walled cavity that contains fluid or purulent material (Figure 29-10).

SECONDARY SKIN LESIONS

[OBJECTIVE 3]

A **secondary skin lesion** is best described as a primary lesion that has been altered by scratching, scrubbing, or other types of trauma or caused by a type of injury or insult. You should be comfortable describing the following seven secondary lesions:

1. A **crust** is a collection of cellular debris or dried blood. It often is called a *scab* (Figure 29-11).
2. An **erosion** is a partial focal loss of epidermis. This lesion is depressed, moist, and does not bleed. Rupture of a vesicle or bulla is an example. It usually heals without scarring (Figure 29-12).

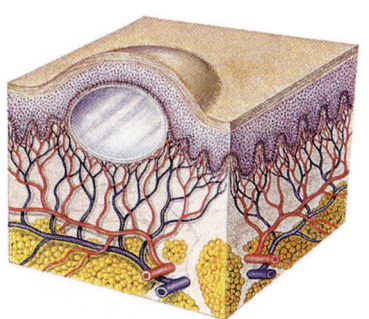
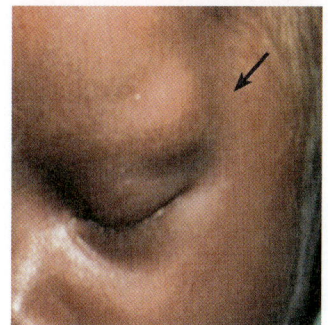

Figure 29-10 Cyst.

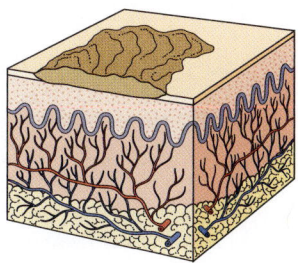

Figure 29-11 Crust.

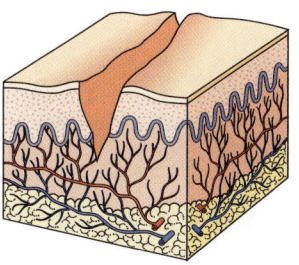

Figure 29-14 Fissure.

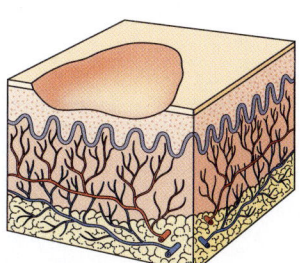

Figure 29-12 Erosion.

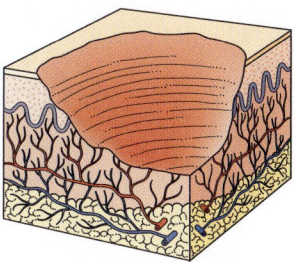

Figure 29-13 Ulcer.

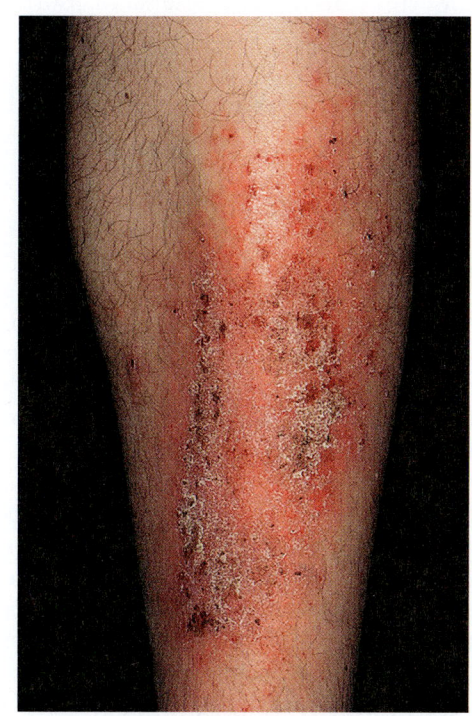

Figure 29-15 Excoriation.

3. An **ulcer** is a full-thickness crater that involves the dermis and epidermis, with loss of the surface epithelium. This lesion is depressed and may bleed. It usually heals with scarring (Figure 29-13).

4. A **fissure** is a vertical loss of epidermis and dermis with sharply defined walls. It is sometimes called a *crack* (Figure 29-14).

5. An **excoriation** is a linear erosion created by scratching. It is a hollowed-out area that is sometimes crusted (Figure 29-15).

6. A **scar** is a collection of new connective tissue. It may be hypertrophic or atrophic and implies dermoepidermal damage (Figure 29-16).

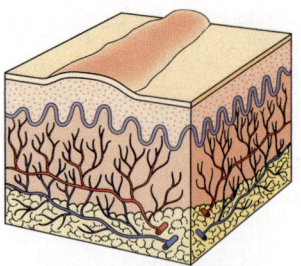

Figure 29-16 Scar.

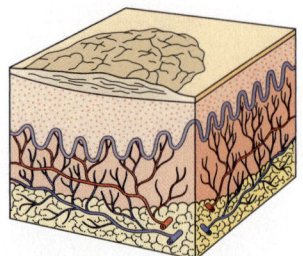

Figure 29-17 Scale.

7. A **scale** is thick stratum corneum that results from hyperproliferation or increased cohesion of keratinocytes (can include eczema or psoriasis) (Figure 29-17).

CANCERS OF THE SKIN

[OBJECTIVE 4]

Description, Definition, Etiology

Cancer of the skin is the most common human malignancy. It begins when cells grow out of control and take over healthy cells. Two common categories of skin cancer are named after the type of skin cell affected: **nonmelanoma** skin cancer, which refers to either basal cell carcinoma (Figure 29-18) or squamous cell carcinoma, and **malignant melanoma** (Figure 29-19). Malignant melanoma is the most dangerous. The overwhelming majority of cancerous skin lesions are caused by exposure to ultraviolet sunlight; hence they occur on portions of the skin chronically exposed to the sun. A history of severe sunburn may be associated with the development of melanoma (Rivers, 1996).

Epidemiology and Demographics

Figures from the American Cancer Society (2006) suggest more than 1 million cases of nonmelanoma skin cancer in 2006. The most common of the skin cancers is basal cell carcinoma, with an incidence ranging from approximately 800,000 to 900,000 cases per year in the United States. Squamous cell cancers occur less often, with an incidence of approximately 200,000 to 300,000 cases per year (American Cancer Society, 2006). Melanoma is the sixth most common cancer in the United States.

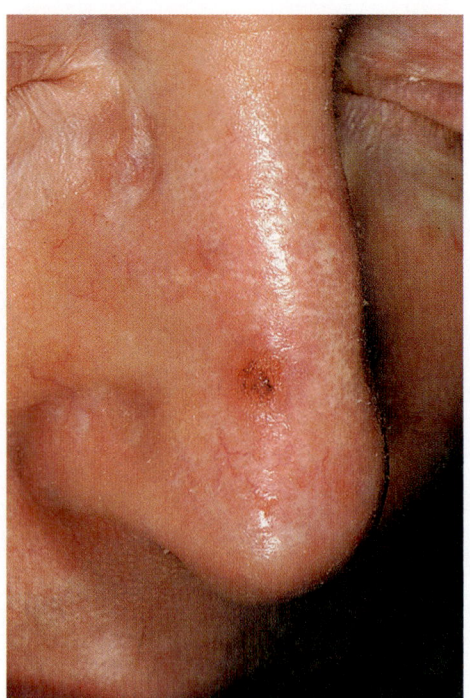

Figure 29-18 Basal cell carcinoma.

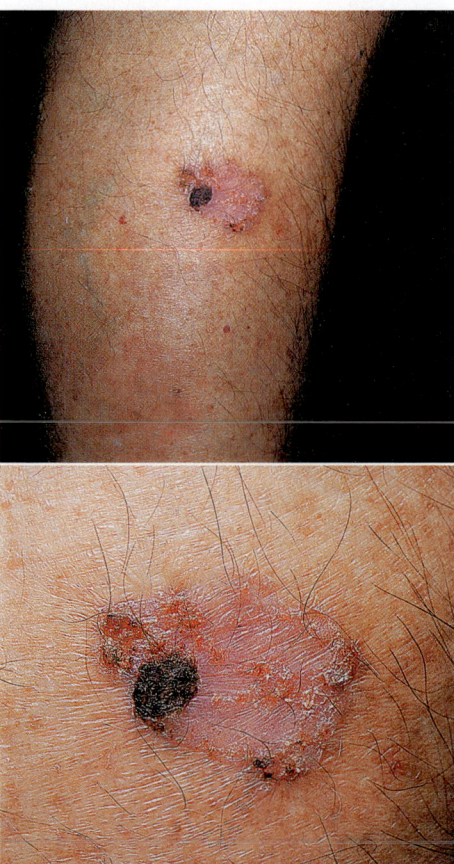

Figure 29-19 Malignant melanoma.

Incidence rates are increasing faster than any other form of cancer (Jernal et al., 2006).

History and Physical Findings

As in most areas of healthcare, a careful history and full examination of the patient are essential. The duration and evolution of the lesion, its color, morphology, and distribution often provide more information than most investigations. For instance, approximately 60% of all basal cell carcinomas occur on the nose; it also is the most common malignant tumor in persons with pale skin. Squamous cell carcinoma is found more prominently on the backs of hands, face, lips, and ears. Squamous cell carcinoma is the most common malignant tumor of the oral mucosa.

Differential Diagnosis

Determining whether a skin lesion is malignant is the primary motive for evaluation, but this determination is not an EMS priority.

Therapeutic Interventions

The diagnosis of nonmelanoma skin cancer is by inspection, but histologic confirmation is usually indicated. The most common treatment is excision; however, superficial lesions may respond to radiation therapy, electrosurgery, photodynamic therapy, or topical treatments. Melanoma, on the other hand, requires early staging and complete surgical removal. Moles that constantly change shape, are discolored (brown with shades of blue, purple, red, black, white, and gray), or are elevated are of particular concern.

Patient and Family Education

[OBJECTIVE 5]

Avoiding sun exposure is the best approach to preventing skin cancer. Parents should protect young children and teach older children about sun protection with sunscreen (with at least a sun protection factor of 15), appropriate clothing, and hats as well as avoidance of midday sun exposure. Early detection of melanoma can be life saving. Self-examination may be a more valuable early detection method than physician examination (Howell, 1997). Melanoma recognition is enhanced through careful evaluation (Box 29-2). Early aggressive treatment decreases the mortality rate related to melanomas.

DECUBITUS ULCERS

Description, Definition, Etiology

[OBJECTIVE 6]

Decubitus ulcers, also known as *pressure ulcers,* are localized areas of tissue damage that develop when soft tissue is compressed between a bony prominence and a firm

BOX 29-2	Melanoma Recognition

- **A**symmetry
- **B**order irregularities
- **C**olor variegation (different colors within the same region)
- **D**iameter greater than 6 mm
- **E**nlargement

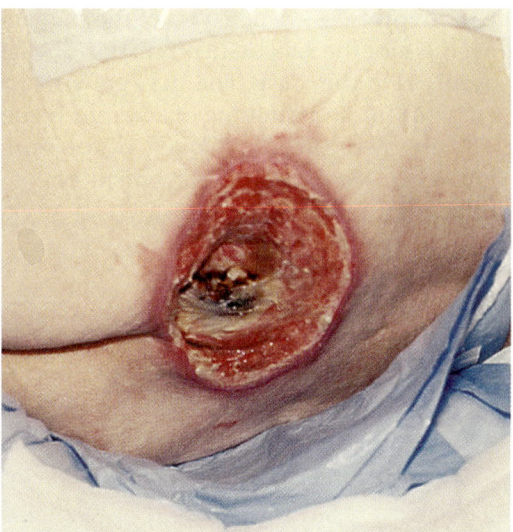

Figure 29-20 Decubitus ulcer.

external surface for a prolonged period (Garibaldi et al., 1981) (Figure 29-20). The factors that contribute to pressure ulcers include breaks in the integrity of the skin and pressure-induced changes such as ischemia. This causes decreased blood flow and contamination, often leading to bacterial infection at the site.

Epidemiology

Decubitus ulcers may be the chief complaint in approximately 5% of patients (Lookingbill & Marks, 2000). The frequency depends on the different types of skin ulcers according to the location and circumstances of the patient population.

History and Physical Findings

Physical findings include the presence of a lesion, from nonblanching skin to a full-thickness wound, over a bony prominence. The sacrum and heels are the most common locations of pressure ulcers. Lesions often present with localized signs of soft tissue involvement, such as warmth, erythema, tenderness, purulent discharge, and a foul odor (Livesley & Chow, 2002). Note that a visual break in the skin may not adequately represent the amount of underlying damage. Decubitus ulcers progress through the following four stages during their development:

1. Stage I presents with intact skin and findings such as warm, tender, inflamed, thickened, red skin that blanches under pressure. These findings indicate that an ulcer is likely to form. If the pressure is allowed to continue, redness that does not blanch with pressure may occur, which is the first sign of tissue destruction. Finally, the skin may turn white as ischemia develops.
2. Stage II involves loss of the epidermis and possibly the dermis. This may present as an abrasion, blister, or superficial ulceration.
3. Stage III involves loss of all layers of the skin and involvement of the subcutaneous tissue. The fascia is not involved in this stage. This may present as a crater with or without undermining of adjacent tissue.
4. Stage IV involves loss of all layers of the skin and subcutaneous tissue with involvement of underlying structures such as muscle, bone, tendon, and joint capsules.

Differential Diagnosis

The diagnosis of decubitus ulcer is by physical examination, history, and location of lesion. Rarely are laboratory tests valuable except for determining the cause of infected lesions.

Therapeutic Interventions

Management of pressure ulcers consists of local wound care including debridement of necrotic tissue, application of an appropriate wound dressing, nutritional support, and pressure relief. Relief of pressure is the most important treatment measure because without the relief of pressure, the wound cannot heal.

Patient and Family Education

The most important component for caretakers of a patient with decubitus ulcers (or the risk of) is to understand what causes them and make every effort to prevent them. Prevention of pressure ulcers is one of the most important aspects of care of the immobile patient. Efforts to minimize skin pressure and stress are pivotal in the prevention of pressure ulcers. This includes avoiding pressure of greater than 2 hours to any single area of the body and keeping areas susceptible to decubitus ulcers clean and dry. Patients who are immobile or confined to bed should have clothing and bed linens changed frequently.

ATOPIC DERMATITIS (ECZEMA)

Description, Definition, Etiology

[OBJECTIVE 7]

Dermatitis literally means "inflammation of the skin," but it almost always refers to a specific group of inflammatory diseases. Atopic dermatitis and eczema often are used interchangeably, but atopic dermatitis is a chronic inflammatory skin disease considered familial with allergic features. It often coincides with asthma and allergic rhinitis.

The exact pathogenesis of atopic dermatitis is not completely understood. Patients appear to have a genetic disposition that is exacerbated by a number of factors.

Epidemiology and Demographics

Atopic dermatitis affects 8% to 25% of the population worldwide and is predominantly a disease of childhood. It may occur in any race or geographic location. A higher incidence appears to be found in urban areas in developed countries (Trepka et al., 1996). Almost 50% of patients with atopic dermatitis report a family history of allergy problems. Most patients have manifestations of atopic dermatitis by age 5 to 7 years, although it may improve with time.

History and Physical Findings

Sometimes called "the itch that rashes," no primary lesion has ever been established in atopic dermatitis. Beltrani (1999) states that "Atopic dermatitis is an itch which when scratched erupts." Three of four clinical features must be present to make the diagnosis: (1) pruritus; (2) typical morphology and distribution; (3) chronic or relapsing course; and (4) personal or family history of asthma, allergic rhinitis, or atopic dermatitis (McGovern, 2001). Acute skin lesions in children appear as intensely pruritic patches with papules and some scaling on the face, scalp, extremities, or trunk. In adults the flexural areas such as the neck, antecubital fossae, and popliteal fossae are most commonly involved (Figure 29-21).

Differential Diagnosis

The differential diagnosis of atopic dermatitis includes other eczematous disorders such as contact dermatitis, seborrheic dermatitis, psoriasis, and drug reactions. A

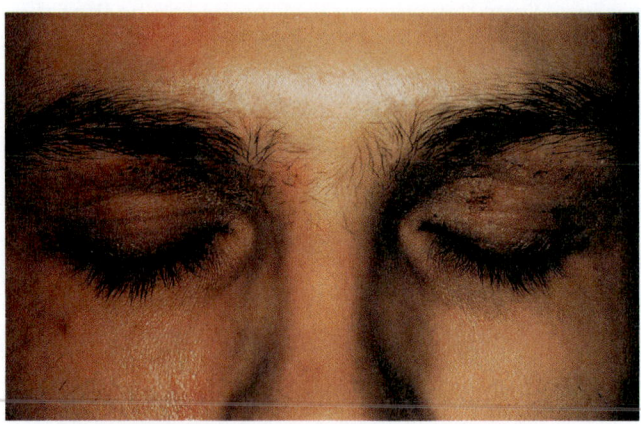

Figure 29-21 Atopic dermatitis of the upper eyelids.

good history and physical examination will help determine the cause and treatment of the dermatitis.

Therapeutic Interventions

Standard modalities in the treatment of atopic dermatitis include potent topical antiinflammatory preparations and lubrication of the skin (Charman, 1999).

CONTACT DERMATITIS
Description, Definition, Etiology

[OBJECTIVE 8]

Contact dermatitis refers to any dermatitis arising from direct skin exposure to a substance. The cause may either be allergic or irritant induced, the latter being the more common. Contact dermatitis is caused by exposure to an allergen or by direct irritation of the skin (such as by metals, cosmetics, soaps, tape, plants, and detergents). Sensitization occurs on the first exposure, and on subsequent exposures a pruritic rash develops at the site. The rash is erythematous and edematous, often covered with small vesicles.

Epidemiology, Demographics

In a prospective study reported in the *American Journal of Contact Dermatitis,* contact dermatitis represented a relatively large proportion of visits for dermatitis. Irritant dermatitis represented 2.3% of all first visits and 1.6% of all total visits. Allergic contact dermatitis accounted for 3.1% of all first and 2.4% of all total visits. Other types of dermatitis were found in 12.5% of all first and 11.1% of all total visits. Contact dermatitis ranked first among types of dermatitis, being seen in 30.0% of first visits for dermatitis and in 27.0% of total visits for dermatitis (Shenefelt, 1996). Both allergic and irritant reactions are twice as common in females as in males. For the healthcare worker, exposure to latex from wearing protective gloves has become a common problem and is related to a hypersensitivity reaction.

History and Physical Findings

Contact dermatitis usually appears with an intensely pruritic rash. In some cases an exposure of up to 2 weeks before the onset of the rash can be identified. In chronic cases the dermatitis may have been present for years (Figure 29-22).

Differential Diagnosis

Contact dermatitis is identical to many other eczematous-type rashes. No standard laboratory test assists in the diagnosis. Patch testing may help identify the allergen. The history and physical examination help determine the most likely diagnosis.

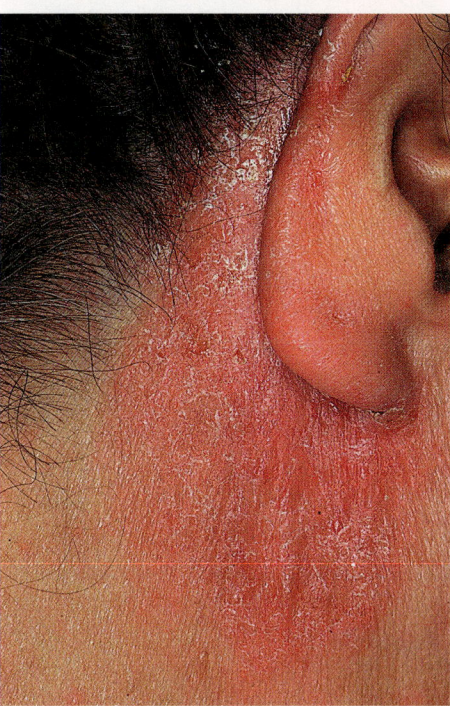

Figure 29-22 Contact dermatitis.

Therapeutic Interventions

Prevention of contact dermatitis is the best therapeutic intervention. This is often difficult because avoiding particular irritants or allergens requires a change in lifestyle and sometimes a change in occupation. Severe contact dermatitis may be treated with a short course of tapered systemic steroids followed by topical steroids and astringent dressings.

PSORIASIS
Description, Definition, Etiology

[OBJECTIVE 9]

Psoriasis is a common chronic skin disorder characterized by erythematous papules and plaques with a silver scale. Most evidence suggests that psoriasis has a genetic predisposition, although environmental and behavioral factors may play a role (Naldi, 2004). Approximately 40% of patients with psoriasis have a family history of the disorder (Gladman et al., 1986).

Epidemiology and Demographics

Worldwide psoriasis prevalence rates range from 0.6% to 4.8% (Naldi, 2004).

History and Physical Findings

Typical psoriasis is recognized with ease because of red, discrete, flat-topped persistent plaques and papules with

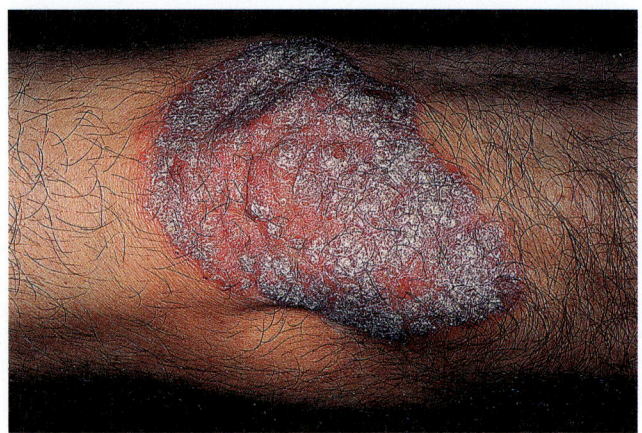

Figure 29-23 Psoriasis.

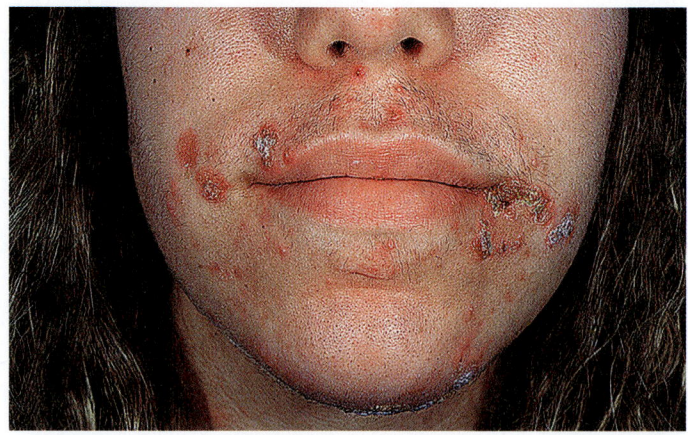

Figure 29-24 Impetigo.

thick silvery scales. Because of this presentation, the diagnosis is made by physical examination (and in some cases biopsy). No laboratory tests confirm or exclude the condition (Figure 29-23).

Differential Diagnosis

The diagnosis of psoriasis is usually not difficult because of the characteristics of the lesions. If the typical silvery scale is not present, lesions may be mistaken for fungal infections.

Therapeutic Interventions

The goal of therapeutic intervention in psoriasis is to decrease the proliferation of the epidermal and dermal inflammation. Numerous topical and systemic therapies are available to treat psoriasis. Treatment is based on severity, patient preference, and response.

BACTERIAL SKIN INFECTIONS
Description, Definition, Etiology

[OBJECTIVE 10]

The majority of bacterial infections of the skin are caused by *Staphylococcus aureus* or group A beta-hemolytic streptococci.

S. aureus has the potential of colonizing the skin and gains entry through damaged skin or a hair follicle (Lookingbill & Marks, 2000). Skin colonization of *S. aureus* causes impetigo. Entry through a hair follicle results in folliculitis or a furuncle (also known as a boil). Note that group A beta-hemolytic streptococci do not colonize skin, rather the bacteria gain entry through damaged skin.

Impetigo

Impetigo is a superficial vesicopustular skin infection that primarily occurs on exposed areas of the face and extremities from scratching infected lesions. Impetigo is readily passed by skin-to-skin contact, especially among children.

Epidemiology

Impetigo usually is caused by *S. aureus*. It rarely requires hospitalization and responds well to local treatment. Impetigo is most common in children but can be found in adults, particularly if they have children in the household who also have impetigo. This skin infection usually occurs in warm, humid conditions. It is easily spread with close contact (as in crowding) and poor personal hygiene. The infection typically arises at sites of minor skin trauma.

History and Physical Findings

Impetigo usually begins at a traumatized region of skin, where a combination of vesicles and pustules develop. The pustules then rupture and crust. This leaves a characteristic thick, golden or honey-like appearance. These are most often seen on exposed facial surfaces, particularly around the nose and mouth (Figure 29-24). Burning and pruritus are often associated with this condition.

Differential Diagnosis

Impetigo may be mistaken for contact dermatitis or other forms of dermatitis. Many lesions present with a crusted surface. The depth of the lesion assists in the diagnosis because impetigo has superficial crusts.

Therapeutic Interventions

Stevens et al. (2005) recommend topical antibiotic treatment for patients with minimal numbers of lesions and oral antibiotic therapy for more severe cases.

Patient and Family Education

Inform patients and family members to withhold children from daycare settings for the first 24 hours after treatment. Frequent handwashing with soap, avoiding sharing personal items, and avoiding contaminated linen are important measures to reduce the incidence of impetigo among children.

Folliculitis

Epidemiology and Etiology
[OBJECTIVE 11]

Folliculitis is localized to hair follicles and is more common in immunocompromised patients. Folliculitis is generally caused by *S. aureus* or *Pseudomonas aeruginosa*, the latter through exposure to swimming pools, whirlpools, and hot tubs with inadequate chlorination. It also is acquired by inadequately cleaned spa pedicure chairs.

History and Physical Findings

The lesions of folliculitis are usually multiple and measure 5 mm or less in diameter. The lesions are erythematous, pruritic, and frequently have a central pustule on top of a raised lesion, often with a central hair. These lesions usually come in clusters and may drain; they usually resolve without scarring (Figure 29-25).

Differential Diagnosis

The distribution of the pustules determines the diagnosis in folliculitis and should be differentiated from acne.

Therapeutic Interventions

Warm salt water compresses and topical antibiotic ointments or creams usually resolve the problem. Sometimes the pustule may need to be drained. Systemic antibiotics do not seem to be effective.

Furuncles and Carbuncles

Description, Definition, Etiology
[OBJECTIVE 12]

Furuncles (boils) are inflammatory nodules that involve the hair follicle (and many times follow an episode of folliculitis), whereas a **carbuncle** is a series of abscesses in the subcutaneous tissues that drain through hair follicles.

S. aureus is the most common cause of both furuncles and carbuncles. These lesions appear when areas of skin containing hair follicles are exposed to friction and perspiration. This usually occurs on the face, neck, buttocks, and underarms.

Epidemiology

According to Lookingbill and Marks (2000), abscesses and furuncles account for 2% of all patient visits to the emergency department. Recurrent furuncles usually are treated by a dermatologist.

History and Physical Findings

Furuncles are painful and usually drain pus. Carbuncles are essentially interconnected furuncles that drain through openings in the skin (Figures 29-26 and 29-27).

Differential Diagnosis

Furuncles and carbuncles should be differentiated from other types of skin abscesses, although their characteristics are rarely confused with other conditions.

Therapeutic Interventions

The main treatments for furuncles and carbuncles are warm compresses, incision, and drainage when needed. Antibiotics are considered when indications of systemic infection are present.

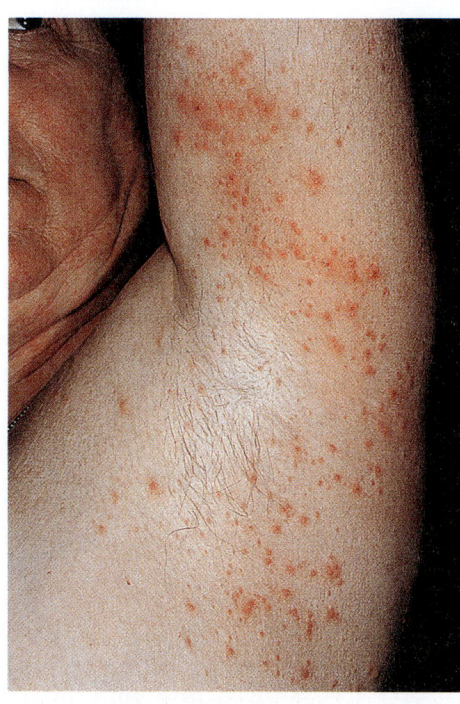

Figure 29-25 Folliculitis.

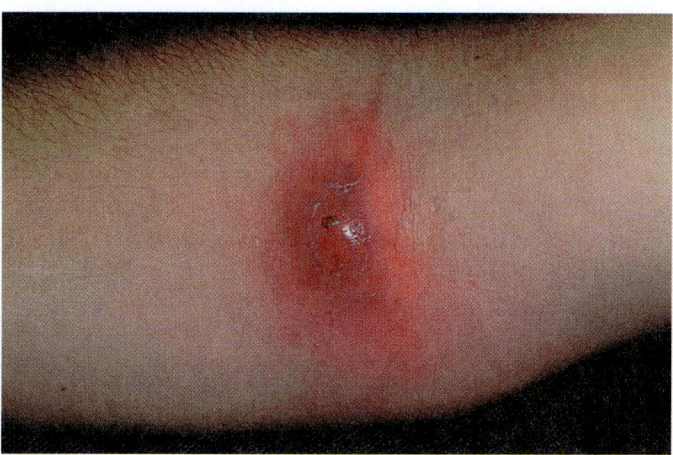

Figure 29-26 Furuncle.

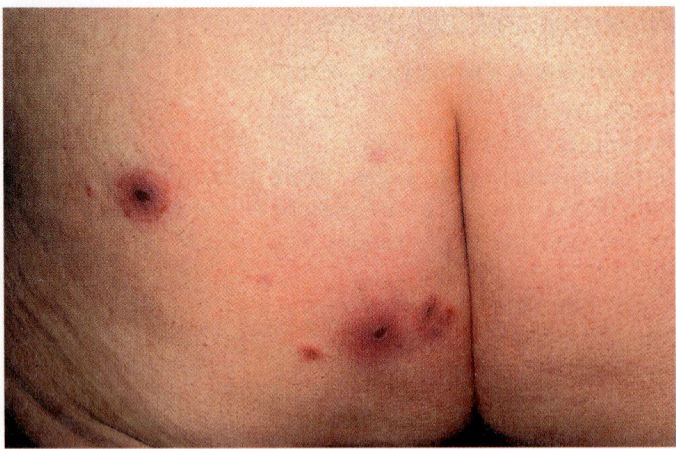

Figure 29-27 Carbuncle.

Cellulitis

Description, Definition, Etiology

[OBJECTIVE 13]

Cellulitis infections of the skin have many different names to describe the various types of infection, although they often have a similar pathology.

Epidemiology and Demographics

According to Auwaerter (2006), skin and soft tissue infections account for 7% to 10% of hospitalizations in North America.

History and Physical Findings

Cellulitis may appear as a swollen, red area of skin that feels hot and tender and may spread rapidly. The skin on the face or lower legs is most commonly affected by this infection, though cellulitis can occur on any part of the body. Cellulitis initially may be superficial, affecting only the epidermis, but it also may affect the subcutaneous tissue and can spread to the lymph nodes and bloodstream.

If untreated, the spreading bacterial infection can rapidly turn into a life-threatening condition. You must be able to recognize the signs and symptoms of cellulitis. Most importantly, look for red, swollen, warm, and tender areas of skin (Figure 29-28).

Differential Diagnosis

Because any crack or break of the skin may lead to an infection, a physician needs to determine the type of infection as rapidly as possible before it progresses. The appearance of the skin helps make a proper diagnosis. Cellulitis in the lower leg is characterized by signs and symptoms that may be similar to those of a clot occurring deep in the veins (e.g., warmth, pain, swelling). Blood tests, a wound culture, or other tests help rule out a blood clot.

Therapeutic Interventions

With bacterial cellulitis an oral antibiotic must be given as soon as possible. If a fever is present or the extent of

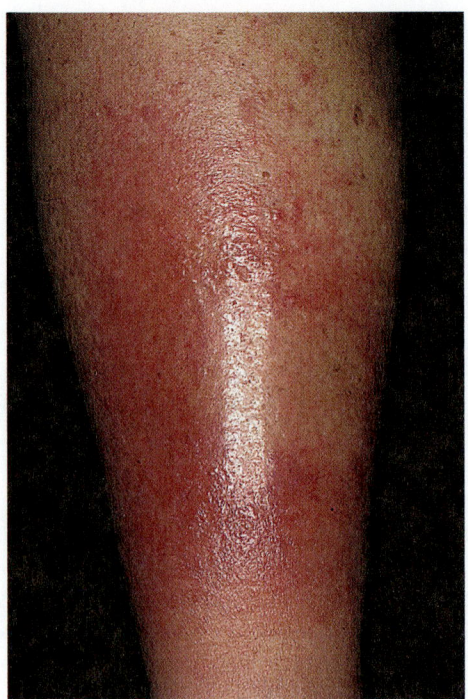

Figure 29-28 Cellulitis.

the cellulitis is large, the patient may be hospitalized and receive intravenous antibiotics.

FUNGAL SKIN INFECTIONS

Dermatophyte Infections

Description, Definition, Etiology

[OBJECTIVE 14]

Fungal infections of the skin are common and usually superficial. They most commonly result from a group of fungal infections called *dermatophytes*. Most fungal infections are superficial and are identified by the word *tinea* and then followed with a term that denotes the location of the lesion. Table 29-1 lists the most common tinea infections and their locations. These are also shown in Figures 29-29 to 29-33.

Epidemiology and Demographics

Dermatophyte infections are quite common and represent approximately 2.5% of new patients (Lookingbill & Marks, 2000). The incidence is much higher in warm, humid climates.

History and Physical Findings

The history and physical findings vary with the types of tinea. In most cases the patient has a scaly rash and associated itching.

Differential Diagnosis

The differential diagnosis varies with the type of tinea (see Table 29-1). Other types of dermatitis may mimic tinea. The best way to diagnose tinea is through a test

TABLE 29-1	Tinea Infection Sites	
Name	**Location**	**Appearance**
Tinea capitis	Head, scalp	Round, scaly area where no hair is growing; diffuse scaling (Figure 29-29)
Tinea corporis	Body	Annular; ringworm
Tinea cruris	Groin, genitalia	Sharply demarcated area with elevated scaling, geographic borders (Figure 29-30)
Tinea pedis	Feet	Maceration between the toes, scaling on soles or sides of the foot, sometimes vesicles and/or pustules (Figure 29-31)
Tinea manuum	Hands	Dry, diffuse scaling, usually on palm (Figure 29-32)
Tinea unguium	On or under fingernails or toenails	Dark debris under nails
Tinea versicolor	Trunk	Pink, tan, or white patches with fine, desquamating scale (Figure 29-33)

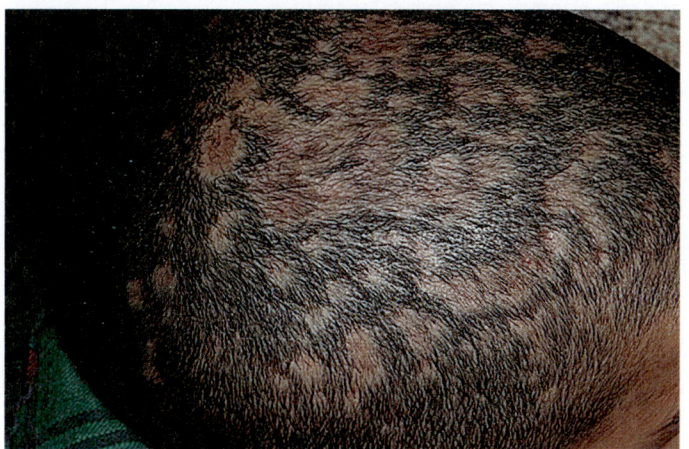

Figure 29-29 Tinea capitus.

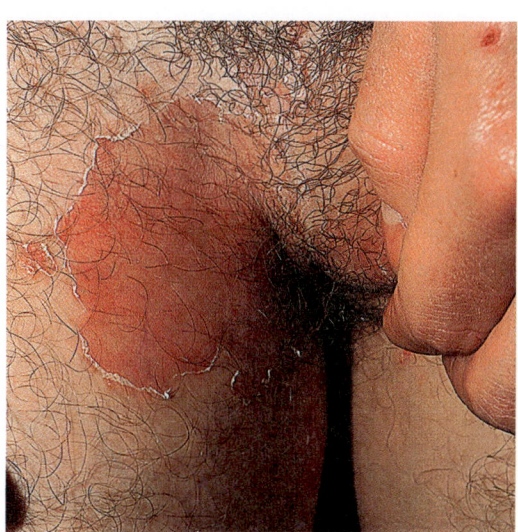

Figure 29-30 Tinea cruris.

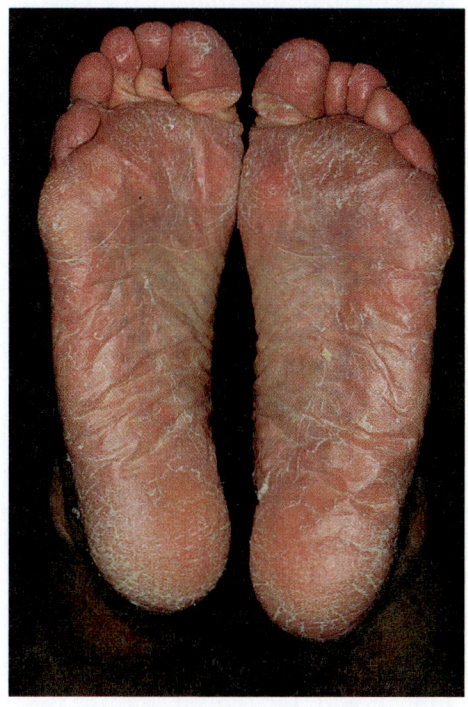

Figure 29-31 Tinea pedis.

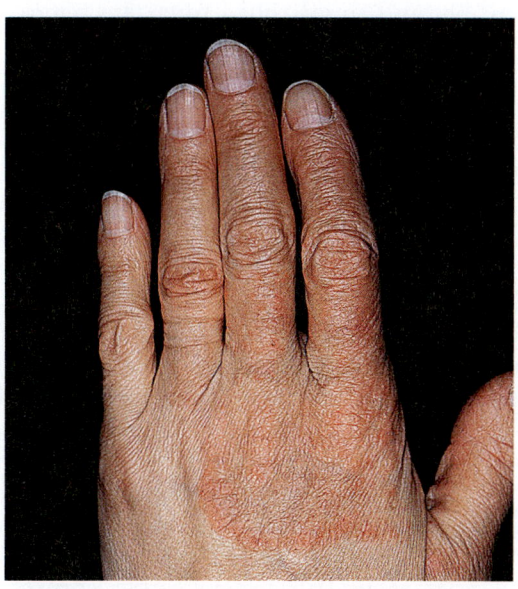

Figure 29-32 Tinea manus.

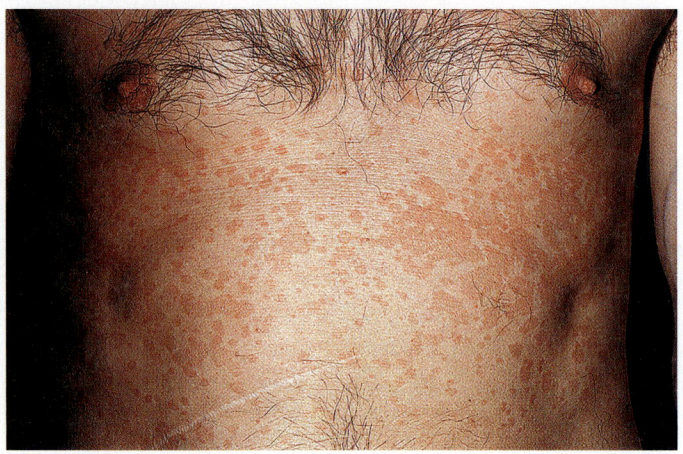

Figure 29-33 Tinea versicolor.

called a *KOH preparation,* which differentiates a dermatophyte from a candidal infection. Rarely is skin biopsy indicated.

Therapeutic Interventions

Because most dermatophyte infections involve limited areas, they respond well to topical antifungal agents. Complications are rare.

Candida Infections

Description, Definition, Etiology

[OBJECTIVE 15]

Candida species infections are inflammatory reactions in the epidermis from infection with the fungus *Candida albicans. Candida* species infections may also occur in the bloodstream in immunocompromised patients. *Candida* species infections in the oral cavity are called *thrush.* These infections are commonly referred to as *yeast infections,* because single-celled fungi are referred to as *yeast.*

Epidemiology

Candidiasis affects patients of all ages. Only approximately 0.3% are new patients (Lookingbill & Marks, 2000). The disease is much more common in infants and hospitalized patients.

History and Physical Findings

The most common symptom of candidiasis is itching and burning of the skin. Candidiasis is more common in moist environments and more often seen on the hands, between fingers, in the perineal area, and under the breasts. The common characteristics are bright-red erythema of the affected skin surrounded by satellite pustules and papules (see Figures 29-2 and 29-9). The patient's history may include recent use of antibiotics. Normal bacterial flora keeps this fungus under control; when the bacteria are eradicated, such as when taking an antibiotic, a fungal overgrowth results in a *Candida* species infection.

Differential Diagnosis

The differential diagnosis depends on the location of the lesions but can easily be mistaken for other forms of dermatitis. Usually the clinical findings are enough to make the diagnosis and skin biopsies are rarely needed.

Therapeutic Interventions

Topical antifungal preparations (e.g., nystatin) are the mainstay of treatment. Widespread infection may require systemic therapy. Fluconazole (Diflucan) is an oral antifungal used for systemic infections or infections not cleared with topical medications.

PARASITIC INFESTATIONS

Pediculosis

Description, Definition, Etiology

[OBJECTIVE 16]

Human infestation with lice is referred to as **pediculosis.** Lice are ectoparasites that live on the body. Three types of lice can infect human beings: the body louse *(Pediculus humanus corporis),* the head louse *(Pediculus humanus capitis),* and the pubic louse *(Pthirus pubis).*

Lice are spread from person to person by close physical contact or contact with items such as combs, clothing, hats, blankets, or linens. Overcrowding (such as in daycare centers) encourages the spread of lice.

Epidemiology and Demographics

Lice have claws on their legs that are used for feeding and clinging to hair or clothing. The pubic louse is distinct, with pincerlike claws resembling those of sea crabs (hence the term *crabs*). Lice stay close to the skin for moisture, food, and warmth. They move freely and quickly, which explains their ease of transmission. A fertilized female louse lays approximately 10 eggs per day for up to 1 month until it dies. The eggs (called *nits*) are attached to the hair shaft, close to the skin surface, where the temperature is optimal for incubation. The eggs hatch in approximately 6 to 10 days. Nits are cemented to the hair shaft and are difficult to remove. Nits can survive for up to 10 days away from the human host.

Pubic lice may be found on the short hairs of the body—areolar hair, axillary hair, beard, scalp margins, eyebrows, and eyelashes—in addition to pubic hair.

Pediculosis affects 6 to 12 million people annually. *P. capitis* is common among school children. Head lice are rare among African Americans; this may be attributable to the twisted nature of the hair shaft and the use of hair pomades (Rubeiz & Kibbi, 2006).

Body lice and their eggs are predominantly found on clothing and should be looked for in the seams of clothes.

History and Physical Findings

Lice infestations are usually asymptomatic, although itching may occur as an allergic reaction to the saliva of the lice injected during feeding (Maunder, 1993) (Figure 29-34). The diagnosis is made through identification of the louse or the residual nits. Lice or nits are best found with a fine-toothed comb. Nits also can be found at the base of the scalp.

Differential Diagnosis

Identification of the lice or nits makes the diagnosis. When they are not found, other conditions that cause scalp itching must be explored, such as dandruff.

Therapeutic Interventions

Lice and nits are best removed with a fine-toothed comb. Soaking the hair in a solution of equal parts water and white vinegar and then wrapping in a wet towel for at least 15 to 20 minutes may facilitate the removal of lice and nits. Solutions or shampoos that kill lice are the mainstays of therapy. Common treatments are permethrin 5% (Elimite) or Nix Lotion 1% and are available over the counter.

Patient and Family Education

All household members should be examined and treated at the same time. With appropriate treatment the condition has a more than 90% cure rate. No treatment is 100% effective, and most treatments must be repeated. Tell parents to wash all bedding, towels and clothing in hot water and soap to kill the lice and their nits. If more than one child is in the house, all children should be treated. Pubic lice in children may be an indication of sexual abuse.

Scabies

Description, Definition, Etiology

[OBJECTIVE 17]

Scabies is a contagious skin disease of the epidermis marked by itching and small, raised, red spots caused by the itch mite. The cause of this condition is the mite *Sarcoptes scabiei,* which burrows into the skin, causing an itchy eruption.

Epidemiology

Scabies is common although the incidence varies. Transmission is usually from person to person through direct contact, although the condition has been known to occur through contact with recent contaminated clothing or bedding of an infested person. Infection is more common in the fall and winter months in developed countries.

History and Physical Findings

The most outstanding feature of scabies is pruritus. It is often severe and at its worst at night. The skin lesion is usually small and red, with nondescript papules that often are excoriated with blood. Although the mite can be seen by the naked eye, the diagnosis is traditionally made by identification of the S-shaped burrows noted on the skin (Figure 29-35). A small papule or vesicle may appear at the end of the burrow. The areas most likely to attract mites are between the fingers, sides of the hands, wrists, elbows, axillae, groin, breasts, and feet. The head is usually spared in adults but may be affected in children.

Differential Diagnosis

Because the mite is rarely seen and is not needed to make the diagnosis, when only excoriations are seen in the face

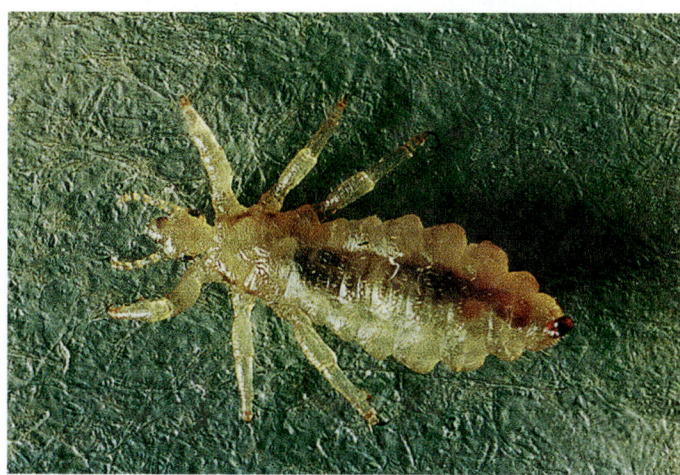

Figure 29-34 Body louse.

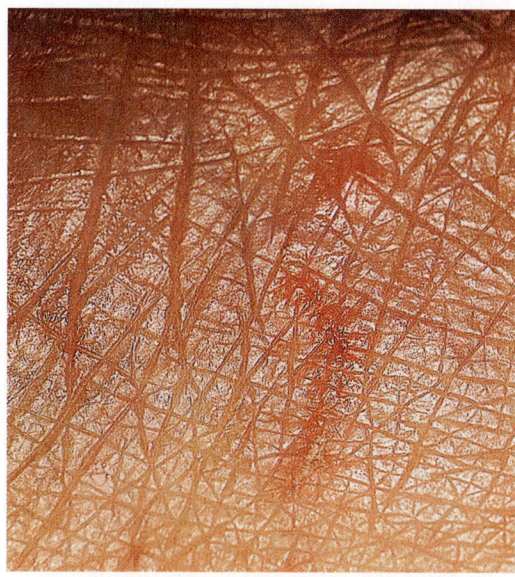

Figure 29-35 Scabies burrow lesion.

of intense itching this condition may be misdiagnosed as atopic dermatitis.

Therapeutic Interventions

The treatment for scabies is generally a topical application of medications that kill the mite. When done properly, the cure rate is close to 100%. Common treatments includes benzoate, crotamiton, lindane, and permethrin. Most of these products are available by prescription. Benadryl may also be used to help alleviate the itching.

Patient and Family Education

All members of the family of the infested person should be treated at the same time to avoid a rebound effect. Some possibility exists that infested clothing or bedding could result in the spread of scabies. Appropriate washing in hot water or even drying in a hot dryer may destroy the mites. As with lice, all items the infected person has been in contact with must be cleaned in hot, soapy water. If one child in a family is infected, all children should be examined for signs of infestation and treated if necessary.

Case Scenario—continued

The primary survey reveals no significant abnormalities and no indication of trauma. The woman states that her hands have been itching the past 2 days, but it seems to get worse at night when she is trying to rest. The itching does not seem to persist during the day. The woman also tells you that the skilled nursing facility where she works recently received several older adults from a retirement home that was forced to close because of substandard conditions. The staff at the skilled nursing facility has been nearly overwhelmed. As you continue your assessment, you note that the woman's hands are inflamed, with small raised papules particularly noted in the webs of her fingers. Both hands are affected. You ask about the lesions, and the patient tells you that some of the new admissions have red rashes on their body; the staff members have been treating the rashes with hydrocortisone. The woman denies using any new soaps or detergents at work or home.

Questions

4. Has your first impression changed?
5. What conditions might cause red papules between the fingers?
6. What additional assessment and treatment options for the woman should be considered?

VIRAL SKIN INFECTIONS

Viruses are common causes of skin infections. The three types of viruses usually causing skin infections are noted in Table 29-2.

Description, Definition, Etiology

[OBJECTIVE 18]
Skin viruses usually establish infection through direct inoculation into the epidermal cells of the skin.

Warts and Papillomavirus

History and Physical Findings

Warts are benign lesions caused by the papillomavirus. The common wart (known as *Verruca vulgaris*) is a flesh-colored, firm nodule that interrupts normal skin lines. A single wart or clusters of warts may be present. These warts are commonly found on hands and around fingernails (Figure 29-36). Plantar warts (named for their location) are found, usually as a single painful lesion, on the bottom of the foot. Venereal warts (known as *Condylomata acuminatum*) are found on or around the rectum,

TABLE 29-2	Common Viral Skin Infections	
Type	**Introduced**	**Examples**
Papova	Direct inoculation into skin	Warts, human papillomavirus
Pox	Direct inoculation into skin	*Molluscum contagiosum* virus
Herpes	Direct inoculation into skin (except for varicella-zoster virus, which is acquired through the respiratory route)	Herpes simplex virus, varicella-zoster virus

perineal area, inguinal folds, or external genitalia. They have a cauliflower-like appearance. These may be caused by the human papillomavirus (Figure 29-37).

Differential Diagnosis

Although common warts are fairly easy to recognize, they may be confused with a callus. Nonetheless, the location

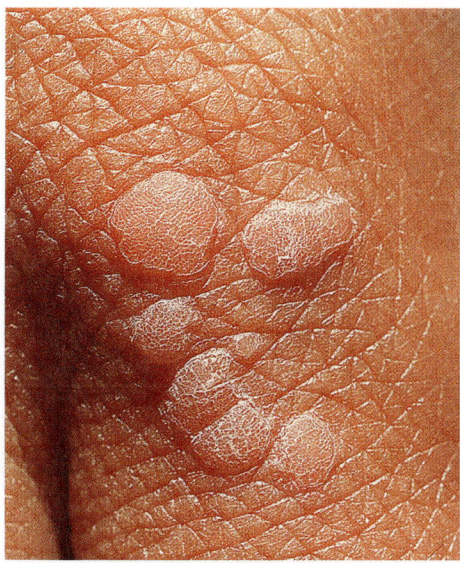

Figure 29-36 Warts.

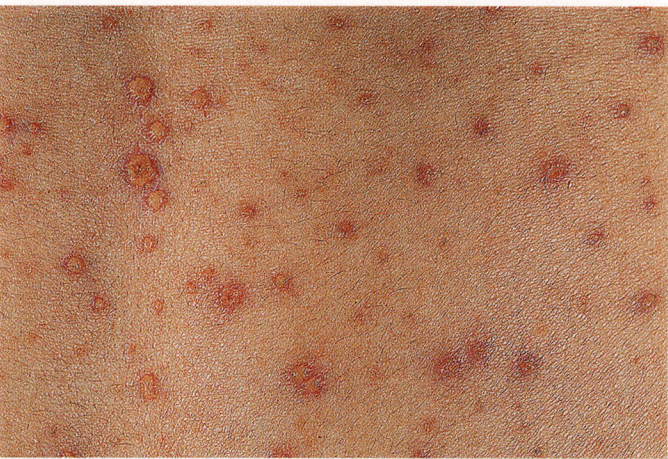

Figure 29-38 Chickenpox.

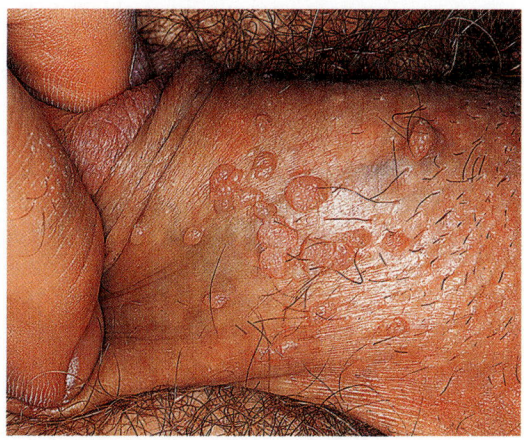

Figure 29-37 Human papillomavirus.

of the lesion helps in the diagnosis. Warts are rarely biopsied unless carcinoma is suspected. Human papillomavirus is the major cause of cervical cancer in women.

Therapeutic Interventions

Treatment of warts is usually based on location and for cosmetic reasons. Removal is by destruction and is usually painful. Common modalities are cryotherapy with liquid nitrogen, electrodessication and curettage, and surgical excision or laser therapy.

Varicella (Chickenpox) and Variola (Smallpox)

Description, Definition, Etiology

[OBJECTIVE 19]

Varicella (chickenpox) is an acute contagious vesicular skin eruption caused by the varicella-zoster virus. Varicella is usually a childhood disease, with most cases occurring before the age of 10 years (Lookingbill & Marks,

2000). However, varicella can occur in adults and is generally more serious in this population. Adults who did not contract varicella during childhood should be vaccinated against the disease.

Epidemiology and Demographics

An estimated 3.5 to 4.0 million cases of chickenpox occur each year in the United States. The disease occurs during all months of the year but peaks between March and May. Varicella is spread through airborne droplets from one person to another by coughing, sneezing, and so forth.

History and Physical Findings

The hallmark of varicella is a generalized pruritic vesicular rash that is mostly found on the trunk but also may be found on the head and mucous membranes (Figure 29-38). It is characterized by an onset of macules, which progress into papules and vesicles, and concludes with crusting lesions. All three of these characteristics may be present at the same time.

Differential Diagnosis

Diagnosing varicella is usually not difficult, although some conditions, such as herpes simplex, may mimic it. Cultures of the lesions can make the diagnosis.

Variola (smallpox) outbreaks have occurred from time to time for thousands of years, but the disease is now eradicated after a successful worldwide vaccination program. The last case of smallpox in the United States was in 1949. The last naturally occurring case in the world was in Somalia in 1977. After the disease was eliminated, routine vaccination against smallpox among the general public was stopped because it was no longer necessary for prevention (Centers for Disease Control and Prevention, 2007).

NOTE: Smallpox occurs on the palms of the hands and soles of the feet. Chickenpox does not. All smallpox vesicles are at the same stage of eruption at the same time (chickenpox lesions may be in all three stages of erup-

TABLE 29-3	Differences between Smallpox and Chickenpox	
	Smallpox	**Chickenpox**
Incubation period	Exposure to the virus is followed by an incubation period during which infected individuals do not have any symptoms and may feel fine. This incubation period averages 12 to 14 days but can range from 7 to 17 days. During this time the patient is not contagious.	The incubation period of chickenpox is between 10 and 20 days. During this time the patient is contagious.
Initial symptoms (prodrome)	The first symptoms of smallpox include fever, malaise, head and body aches, and sometimes vomiting. The fever usually is high, in the range of 101° to 104° F (38° to 40° C). At this time, infected individuals are usually too sick to carry on their normal activities. This prodrome phase may last for 2 to 4 days.	The first symptoms may be fever, abdominal pain or loss of appetite, mild headache, general feeling of unease and discomfort (malaise) or irritability, mild cough and runny nose the first 2 days of illness before the rash appears.
Symptoms	By the end of the second week the lesions have scabbed over. When the scabs fall off the patient is no longer contagious.	The best-known sign of chickenpox is a red, itchy rash that breaks out on the face, scalp, chest, and back, but it can spread across the entire body, even into the throat, eyes, and vagina. The chickenpox rash usually appears less than 2 weeks after exposure to the virus and begins as superficial spots. These spots quickly turn into small, liquid-filled blisters that break open and crust over. New spots continue to appear for several days and may number in the hundreds. Itching may range from mild to intense.
Transmission	Direct transmission requiring fairly prolonged face-to-face contact through infected body fluids or contaminated objects. Rarely carried by air. Human beings are the only natural hosts.	The virus is transmitted through the air, by direct contact with someone with chickenpox, and by breathing infected droplets.

tion). These are the differentiating characteristics (Table 29-3).

Therapeutic Interventions

Because the diagnosis is fairly obvious, rarely are diagnostic tests ordered. The treatment of varicella is mostly symptomatic and aimed at relieving the symptoms. Antihistamines and topical lotions or creams may be used to reduce the itching. Antiviral drugs such as acyclovir, valacyclovir, and famciclovir also may be used to shorten the course of the infection.

Patient and Family Education

Active vaccination against varicella is safe and indicated to avoid this disease. However, a person may have an outbreak of varicella more than one time in his or her life. A common misconception is that people can be infected by chickenpox only once.

NOTE: In the event of a smallpox outbreak, vaccination will be indicated. The smallpox vaccine carries numerous risks, so benefits versus risks should be weighed before administration of the vaccine.

Case Scenario CONCLUSION

You continue your assessment and note nothing significant. The patient's vital signs are normal and her skin is warm and dry. She is begging you to give her something to relieve the itching. Because her condition does not appear to be an allergy, you contact medical direction, which instructs you to give 25 mg of diphenhydramine intramuscularly. You give the medication and convince the woman to seek medical attention at the emergency department.

You and your partner ready the patient for transport. En route to the hospital, she is more relaxed. The transport continues without incident and you transfer care to the emergency department staff.

Looking Back

7. What is your final impression of the patient?
8. What treatment options are available for this patient?
9. What precautions should you and your partner take after transporting the patient?

Herpes Simplex

Description, Definition, Etiology

[OBJECTIVE 20]

Herpes simplex is a skin eruption caused by the herpes simplex virus and is divided into two types; HSV-1 causes oral infection and HSV-2 causes genital infection. Patients with either of these types frequently have recurrent episodes.

Epidemiology and Demographics

According to Lookingbill and Marks (2000), more than 100 million episodes of HSV-1 are estimated to occur yearly in the United States. HSV-2 infection has increased in the past 20 years.

History and Physical Findings

The lesions usually begin with painful, indurated erythema, which is followed by grouped vesicles (Figure 29-39). The vesicles rapidly become pustules, which then rupture and drain. The affected skin sometimes becomes necrotic.

Differential Diagnosis

Herpes simplex may be confused with impetigo, contact or atopic dermatitis, or fungal infections. The correct diagnosis is mostly made by history and physical examination, although a culture of the vesicle will confirm the diagnosis of herpes simplex.

Therapeutic Interventions

A number of medications are used to treat herpes simplex (e.g., acyclovir, valacyclovir, famciclovir). They work well and may be administered in topical or oral forms. However, these medications reduce the incidence of outbreaks, but they do not cure the disease. Even when using the medication, spreading the virus to others is possible when an outbreak occurs.

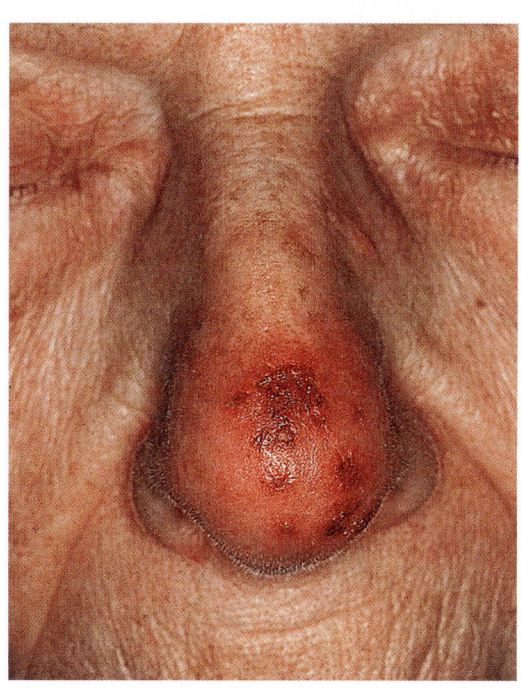

Figure 29-39 Herpes simplex.

Patient and Family Education

Herpes simplex is spread by direct contact with infected individuals who may be asymptomatic but shedding the virus.

Herpes Zoster (Shingles)

Description, Definition, Etiology

[OBJECTIVE 21]

Herpes zoster, also known as *shingles,* is a skin eruption that follows a particular nerve distribution (dermatome). This disease is caused by the varicella-zoster virus in persons who have had varicella sometime in his or her life. As described in Chapter 23, after an initial infection with the varicella-zoster virus it travels to the dorsal root ganglia, where it becomes dormant, often for decades. Later in life, for reasons unknown, the virus reactivates and causes irritation to a spinal sensory nerve. This often occurs during times of stress and/or when the immune system is weakened or compromised and unable to keep the virus under control.

Epidemiology

Herpes zoster occurs in all age groups but is mostly found in older individuals, with 30% being older than 55 years (Donahue et al., 1995). The incidence seems to increase with age. However, the number of cases of pediatric herpes zoster has increased in recent years. This is likely attributable to vaccination with a live virus.

History and Physical Findings

The usual manifestations of herpes zoster start with fever; malaise; a feeling of numbness, pruritus, or burning in the affected area; and headache (called a *prodrome*) followed by scattered vesicles that appear to follow a pattern or direction associated with the dermatome of the affected spinal nerve (Figure 29-40). This occurs more often on the trunk but has been known to occur on the head and face. Rarely is it seen on extremities or on both sides of the body.

Differential Diagnosis

The distribution of herpes zoster makes the diagnosis, but other skin disorders may mimic this condition, such as herpes simplex.

Therapeutic Interventions

Rarely are laboratory tests needed except to rule out other conditions. Because of the frequent pain of this condition, analgesics are used in concert with astringent compresses. Acyclovir and other antiviral medications are commonly prescribed, and steroids are occasionally used in severe cases.

Patient and Family Education

Herpes zoster that occurs on or near the eye may be a serious condition, and the patient should be seen by an ophthalmologist.

SPECIALIZED ERYTHEMA

Two specialized erythema conditions (Urticaria and erythema multiforme) are presented because of their distinctive characteristics.

Urticaria (Hives)

Description, Definition, Etiology
[OBJECTIVE 22]

Urticaria, also known as *hives,* is a skin condition in which a wheal on the skin forms from edema. This condition is often caused by a reaction to a drug or through contact with substances (skin contact or even inhaled) causing hypersensitivity in the patient. For urticaria that lasts longer than 6 weeks, a cause is usually not found.

Epidemiology

Urticaria is common and is more often found in young adults. A reported 20% of the population has had urticaria at some point in life (Lookingbill & Marks, 2000).

History and Physical Findings

A careful history of drug use (both prescription and illicit) is essential in determining the cause of this condition. Determining potential exposures to allergens, chemicals, or foods also is important. Urticarial lesions are easily recognized as edematous plaques, which may have pale centers and reddish borders (Figure 29-41). They are often described as geographic in shape and may be scattered or clustered. Pruritus is a common symptom.

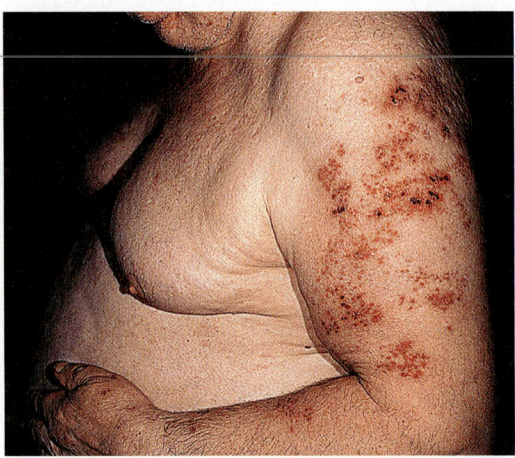

Figure 29-40 Herpes zoster.

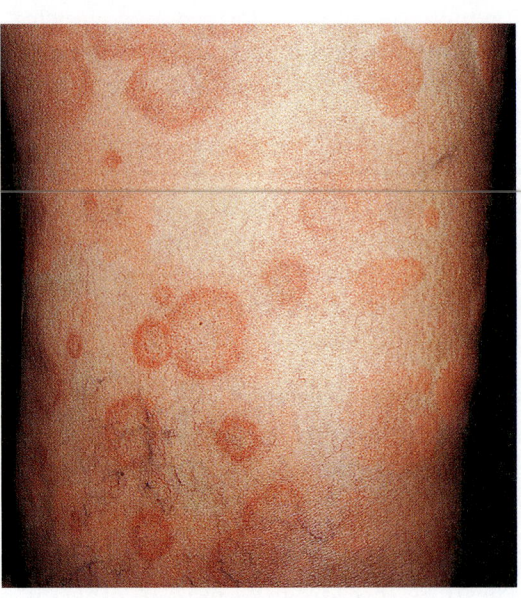

Figure 29-41 Urticaria.

Differential Diagnosis

Urticaria may be mistaken for erythema multiforme or other skin conditions. Urticarial lesions rarely last longer than 24 hours, whereas other conditions may last a great deal longer. The patient also may have a respiratory reaction from inhaling the offending substance.

Therapeutic Interventions

Laboratory testing is rarely helpful in determining the etiology, although it may be appropriate in ruling out other systemic conditions that may be part of the cause. Obviously any suspicious medication (such as aspirin or penicillin) should be discontinued. Suspicious exposures also should be avoided (e.g., shrimp, latex). Relief is usually achieved with antihistamines.

Patient and Family Education

Urticaria may reoccur and should be closely monitored.

Erythema Multiforme

Description, Definition, Etiology

[OBJECTIVE 23]

Erythema multiforme is an internal (immunologic) reaction in the skin characterized by a variety of lesions.

Epidemiology

This condition is uncommon, affecting less than 1% of the population (Lookingbill & Marks, 2000). It affects older children and young adults.

History and Physical Findings

As in urticaria, a complete history of drug use should be taken because this is the most common source implicated—particularly penicillins, barbiturates, hydantoins, and sulfonamides. This condition is known for its "target" lesions with three zones of color, which makes the diagnosis (Figure 29-42). The epidermis may be normal or

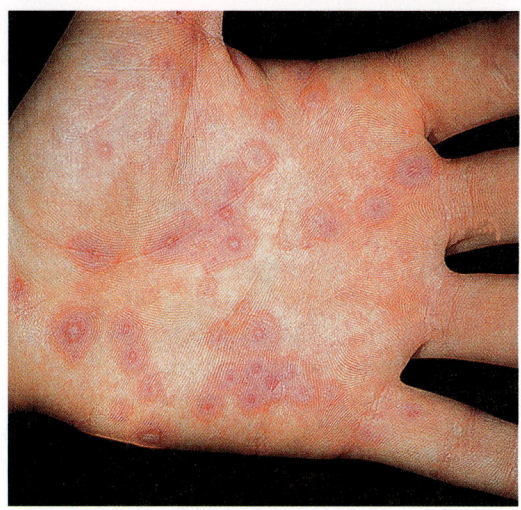

Figure 29-42 Purpura.

blistered. The dermis may be erythematous, and the epidermis may be normal or necrotic.

Differential Diagnosis

This condition may be mistaken for urticaria or viral or bacterial skin conditions.

Therapeutic Interventions

This disease is so distinctive because of the target lesions that a biopsy is rarely required. Treatment of the precipitating cause, whether infection or drug reaction, is the critical component.

Patient and Family Education

This is a serious condition and should not be taken lightly. It may last 2 to 3 weeks, with more severe involvement up to 6 weeks.

Case Scenario SUMMARY

1. *What is your initial impression of the patient?* Your initial impression may include a psychiatric disorder caused by stress. It also may include an allergic reaction or contact dermatitis from contact with some allergen either at home or at work.

2. *What additional information do you need to complete your assessment?* Additional information needed includes a head-to-toe evaluation and a SAMPLE history. You should ask whether the patient has changed laundry detergents or started to use a new type of soap to wash her hands at work or home.

3. *What may be causing the woman's distress?* The patient's distress could be caused by a number of things, including stress. It also could be caused by the severe, unrelenting itching caused by the skin condition on her hands.

4. *Has your first impression changed?* The initial impression may be changed by the additional information. A recent influx of patients from a retirement home can be distressing. However, the presence of a rash on these new patients is cause for concern. The rash may be caused by contact dermatitis or a burrowing mite (scabies) that is easily transmitted from one person to another.

5. *What conditions might cause red papules between the fingers?* The red papules indicate the likely presence of

Continued

scabies, a burrowing mite that tends to cause severe itching, especially at night.

6. *What additional assessment and treatment options for the woman should be considered?* Additional information should include vital signs and assessing for additional evidence of mite infestation. You also may want to ask the husband if he has noticed any itching on his hands or other body surfaces. Prehospital treatment may include antiinflammatory and antiitching medications, including diphenhydramine. Depending on local protocol, you may need to request permission from medical direction to administer diphenhydramine in this situation.

7. *What is your final impression of the patient?* A final impression of this patient is the presence of scabies, perhaps contracted from one of the recent admissions to the skilled nursing facility.

8. *What treatment options are available for this patient?* Prehospital care consists of care and comfort. Diphen-

hydramine is used to reduce the itching and allow the patient to rest. However, the patient needs something to eliminate the scabies mite. Prescribed treatments, including benzoate and crotamiton, have a cure rate of nearly 100% when the directions are closely followed. The couple will need to follow additional procedures to eliminate the mite from their home, including their bedding.

9. *What precautions should you and your partner take after transporting the patient?* You and your partner will need to thoroughly disinfect the ambulance. Use any acceptable disinfecting agent and thoroughly clean all surfaces. You also may need to launder your uniforms in very hot water and dry in high heat to ensure the mites and their eggs have been destroyed. If you note any itching, especially at night, seek medical attention to determine the cause.

Chapter Summary

- As with any type of exposure, Personal protective equipment is extremely important and acts as a barrier between infectious materials and the skin, mouth, nose, and eyes (mucous membranes).
- A primary skin lesion is best described as a lesion that has not been altered by scratching, rubbing, scrubbing, or other types of trauma.
- A secondary skin lesion is best described as any lesion that has been altered by scratching, scrubbing, or other types of trauma.
- Describing skin lesions by using the names of primary and secondary lesions enables the clearest communication between paramedic and the medical director and makes documentation of skin lesions the most accurate.
- Learn the ABCDE rule to distinguish melanoma from less-harmful lesions.
- Decubitus ulcers, also known as *pressure ulcers,* are localized areas of tissue damage that develop when soft tissue is compressed between a bony prominence and a firm external surface for a prolonged period.
- Atopic dermatitis is a chronic inflammatory skin disease that is considered familial with allergic features. Atopic dermatitis and eczema are often incorrectly used interchangeably.
- Contact dermatitis refers to any dermatitis arising from direct skin exposure to a substance; the cause may be allergic or irritant induced, with the latter being more common.

- Psoriasis is a common chronic skin disorder characterized by erythematous papules and plaques with a silvery scale.
- Impetigo is a superficial vesicopustular skin infection that primarily occurs on exposed areas of the face and extremities from scratching infected lesions.
- Folliculitis is localized to hair follicles and is more common in immunocompromised patients.
- Furuncles (boils) are inflammatory nodules that involve the hair follicle (and many times follow an episode of folliculitis), whereas a carbuncle is a series of abscesses in the subcutaneous tissues that drain through hair follicles.
- Cellulitis may appear as a swollen, red area of skin that feels hot and tender and may spread rapidly. If untreated, the spreading bacterial infection can rapidly turn into a life-threatening condition.
- Most fungal infections are superficial and are identified by the word *tinea* and then followed with a term that denotes the location of the lesion. The most common result from a group of fungal infections called dermatophytes.
- The most common symptom of candidiasis is itching and burning of the skin. *Candida* infections in the oral cavity are called thrush.
- Lice are ectoparasites that live on the body. Human infestation with lice is referred to as pediculosis.
- Scabies is a contagious skin disease of the epidermis marked by itching and small, raised, red spots caused by the itch mite.

- Warts are benign lesions caused by the papillomavirus.
- Varicella (chickenpox) is an acute contagious vesicular skin eruption caused by the varicella-zoster virus. It can be distinguished from smallpox by its clinical presentation.
- Herpes simplex is a skin eruption caused by the herpes simplex virus and is divided into two types; HSV-1 causes oral infections and HSV-2 causes genital infections.

- Herpes zoster, also known as *shingles,* is a skin eruption that follows a particular nerve distribution called a *dermatome.*
- Urticaria, also known as *hives,* is a condition of a wheal on the skin resulting from edema.
- Erythema multiforme is known for its "target" lesions with three zones of color, which makes the diagnosis. The epidermis may be normal or blistered and the dermis may be erythematous.

REFERENCES

American Cancer Society. (2006). *How many people get basal and squamous cell skin cancers?* Retrieved September 4, 2006, from http://www.cancer.org.

Auwaerter, P. G. (2006). Cellulitis, skin abscesses, and community-acquired methicillin-resistant *Staphylococcus aureus. Advanced Studies in Medicine, 6,* 62-70.

Beltrani, V. S. (1999). Atopic dermatitis: The spectrum of disease, *Journal of Cutaneous Medical Surgery, 3*(suppl 2), 8-15.

Centers for Disease Control and Prevention. (2007). *Smallpox disease overview.* Retrieved March 3, 2007, from http://www.bt.cdc.gov.

Charman, C. (1999). Clinical evidence: Atopic eczema. *British Medical Journal, 318,* 1600.

Donahue, J. G., Choo, P. W., Manson, J. E., & Platt, R. (1995). The incidence of herpes zoster. *Archives of Internal Medicine, 155,* 1605.

Garibaldi, R. A., Brodine, S., & Matsumiya, S. (1981). Infections among patients in nursing homes: Policies, prevalence, and problems. *New England Journal of Medicine, 305,* 731.

Gladman, D. D., Anthorn, K. A., Schachter, R. K., & Mervart, H. (1986). HLA antigens in psoriatic arthritis. *Journal of Rheumatology, 13,* 586.

Howell, J. B. (1997). Skin self-examination for melanoma: Another golden rule. *Seminars in Cutaneous Medical Surgery, 16,* 174.

Jernal, A., Siegel, R., Ward, E., et al. (2006). Cancer statistics, 2006. *CA Cancer Journal Clinics, 56,* 106.

Lookingbill, D. P., & Marks, J. G. (2000). *Principles of dermatology* (3rd ed.). Philadelphia: W. B. Saunders.

Livesley, N. J., & Chow, A. W. (2002). Infected pressure ulcers in elderly individuals. *Clinics in Infectious Disease, 35,* 1390.

Maunder, J. W. (1993). An update on head lice. *Health Visitor, 66,* 317.

McGovern, T. W. (2001). Dermatitis (eczema). In J. E. Fitzpatrick, & J. L. Aeling (Eds.). *Dermatology secrets in color* (2nd ed.). Philadelphia: Hanley & Belfus.

Naldi, L. (2004). Epidemiology of psoriasis. *Current Drug Targets. Inflammation and Allergy, 3,* 121.

Rivers, J. K. (1996). Melanoma. *The Lancet, 347,* 803.

Rubeiz, N., & Kibbi, A. G. (2006). *Pediculosis.* Retrieved October 10, 2006, from http://www.emedicine.com.

Shenefelt, P. D. (1996). Descriptive epidemiology of contact dermatitis in a university student population. *American Journal of Contact Dermatitis, 7,* 88-93.

Stevens, D. L., Bisno, A. L., & Chambers, H. F. (2005). Practice guidelines for the diagnosis and management of skin and soft tissue infections. *Clinics in Infectious Disease, 41,* 1373.

Trepka, M. J., Heinrich, J., & Wichmann, H. E. (1996). The epidemiology of atopic diseases in Germany: An east-west comparison. *Reviews in Environmental Health, 11,* 119.

SUGGESTED RESOURCES

Fitzpatrick, J. E., Aeling, J. L. (2001). *Dermatology secrets in color* (2nd ed.). Philadelphia: Hanley & Belfus.

Lookingbill, D. P., & Marks, J. G. (2000). *Principles of dermatology* (3rd ed.). Philadelphia: W. B. Saunders.

Chapter Quiz

1. The skin serves as a protective barrier against the environment. It also regulates body temperature and stores water, fat, and _____.

2. The three layers of the skin are the epidermis, the _____, and subcutaneous fat.

3. Match the following primary skin lesions with their definitions.

   ____ Bulla

   ____ Cyst

   ____ Macule

   ____ Nodule

   ____ Papule

   ____ Patch

   ____ Plaque

   ____ Pustule

   ____ Vesicle

   ____ Wheal

   a. A firm, rounded, flat-topped elevation of skin that is evanescent and pruritic

   b. A flat, circumscribed, discolored lesion (e.g., freckle)

   c. A flat, circumscribed, discolored lesion

   d. A lesion that contains purulent material

   e. A localized, fluid-filled lesion usually greater than 0.5 cm

   f. A walled cavity that contains fluid or purulent material

   g. An elevated lesion that contains clear fluid; sometimes called a *water blister*

   h. An elevated, solid lesion in the deep skin or subcutaneous tissues

   i. An elevated, solid lesion usually greater than 0.5 cm that lacks any deep component

   j. An elevated, solid lesion usually less than 0.5 cm

Chapter Quiz—continued

4. Match the following secondary skin lesions with their definitions.

____ Crust   **a.** A collection of cellular debris or dried blood; sometimes called a *scab*

____ Erosion   **b.** A collection of new connective tissue

____ Excoriation   **c.** A full-thickness crater that involves the dermis and epidermis with loss of the surface epithelium

____ Fissure   **d.** A linear erosion created by scratching

____ Ulcer   **e.** A partial focal loss of epidermis that usually heals without scarring

____ Scar   **f.** A thick stratum corneum that results from hyperproliferation or increased cohesion of keratinocytes

____ Scale   **g.** A vertical loss of epidermis and dermis with sharply defined walls; sometimes called a crack in the skin

5. The best approach to prevent cancer of the skin is _____.
   a. always wearing a hat
   b. avoiding the sun
   c. seeing a clinician at least once a year
   d. using sunscreen with a sun protection factor of 10

6. Melanoma recognition is enhanced by _____.
   a. looking for asymmetry and border irregularities of any lesions
   b. nothing; early detection is not important
   c. watching for same colors of lesions within the different regions
   d. watching for small lesions that are less than 6 mm

7. True or False: The most important component in caring for a patient with decubitus ulcers is to understand what causes them and make every effort to prevent them.

8. True or False: *Dermatitis* literally means "inflammation of the skin."

9. True or False: Contact dermatitis is caused by exposure to an allergen or by direct irritation of the skin.

10. Match the following skin conditions with their descriptions.
    ____ Carbuncles   **a.** A red, swollen area of skin that feels hot and tender

____ Cellulitis   **b.** A combination of pustules and vesicles that, when they rupture, leave a characteristic thick, golden or honey-like appearance

____ Impetigo   **c.** Erythematous clustered lesions with a central pustule on top of a raised lesion

____ Folliculitis   **d.** Interconnected erythematous nodular lesions that drain through openings in the skin

____ Furuncles   **e.** Painful nodular lesions

____ Psoriasis   **f.** Red, discrete, flat-topped, persistent plaques and papules with thick silvery scales

11. Match the following skin conditions with their descriptions.

____ Tinea capitis   **a.** Annular lesions; sometimes called *ringworm*

____ Tinea corporis   **b.** Dark debris under fingernails or toenails

____ Tinea cruris   **c.** Dry, diffuse scaling usually seen on the palms

____ Tinea manuum   **d.** Maceration between the toes or scaling on the soles or sides of the foot

____ Tinea pedis   **e.** Pink, tan, or white patches with fine desquamating scales

____ Tinea unguium   **f.** Round, scaly area on the scalp where no hair is growing

____ Tinea versicolor   **g.** Sharply demarcated area with elevated scaling and geographic borders

12. Match the following skin conditions with their descriptions.

____ Herpes simplex   **a.** Benign lesions caused by papillomavirus

____ Pediculosis   **b.** Chickenpox

____ Scabies   **c.** HSV-1 or HSV-2

____ Warts   **d.** Lice

____ Varicella   **e.** Mites

13. Match the following skin conditions with their descriptions.

____ Erythema multiforme   **a.** Multiple presentations usually related to a drug reaction

____ Herpes zoster   **b.** Single or multiple wheals, sometimes geographic in appearance

____ Urticaria   **c.** Vesicular eruptions that follow a dermatome

Terminology

Bulla A localized, fluid-filled lesion usually greater than 0.5 cm.

Carbuncle A series of abscesses in the subcutaneous tissues that drain through hair follicles.

Cellulitis An inflammation of the skin.

Crust A collection of cellular debris or dried blood; often called a *scab*.

Cyst A walled cavity that contains fluid or purulent material.

Dermis Second layer of skin, primarily composed of collagen.

Epidermis Top layer of skin, primarily composed of epidermal cells.

Erosion A partial focal loss of epidermis. This lesion is depressed, moist, and does not bleed; usually heals without scarring.

Erythema multiforme An internal (immunologic) reaction in the skin characterized by a variety of lesions.

Excoriation A linear erosion created by scratching; a hollowed-out area that is sometimes crusted.

Fissure A vertical loss of epidermis and dermis with sharply defined walls (sometimes called a *crack*).

Folliculitis Inflammation of the follicle; localized to hair follicles and more common in immunocompromised patients; usually are multiple and measure 5 mm or less in diameter; erythematous, pruritic, and frequently have a central pustule on top of a raised lesion, often with a central hair.

Furuncles Inflammatory nodules that involve the hair follicle (e.g., boils).

Herpes simplex A skin eruption caused by the herpes simplex virus and divided into two types; HSV-1 causes oral infections and HSV-2 causes genital infections.

Herpes zoster A skin eruption that follows a particular nerve distribution (dermatome); caused by the varicella-zoster virus in persons who have had varicella sometime in their lives; also called *shingles*.

Impetigo A superficial vesicopustular skin infection that primarily occurs on exposed areas of the face and extremities from scratching infected lesions; usually begins at a traumatized region of skin, where a combination of vesicles and pustules develops; the pustules rupture and crust, leaving a characteristic thick, golden or honey-like appearance.

Keratinocytes Epidermal cells.

Macule A flat, circumscribed, discolored lesion (e.g., freckle) measuring less than 1 cm.

Nodule An elevated, solid lesion in the deep skin or subcutaneous tissues.

Papule An elevated, solid lesion usually less than 0.5 cm in diameter; may arise from the epidermis, dermis, or both.

Patch A flat, circumscribed, discolored lesion measuring greather than 1 cm.

Pediculosis Human infestation with lice.

Plaque An elevated, solid lesion usually greater than 0.5 cm in diameter that lacks any deep component.

Primary skin lesion A lesion that has not been altered by scratching, rubbing, scrubbing, or other type of trauma.

Psoriasis A common chronic skin disorder characterized by erythematous papules and plaques with a silver scale.

Pustule A lesion that contains purulent material.

Secondary skin lesion Any lesion that has been altered by scratching, scrubbing, or other type of trauma.

Scabies A contagious skin disease of the epidermis marked by itching and small, raised, red spots caused by the itch mite (*Sarcoptes scabiei*).

Scale Thick stratum corneum that results from hyperproliferation or increased cohesion of keratinocytes (can include eczema or psoriasis).

Scar A collection of new connective tissue; may be hypertrophic or atrophic and implies dermoepidermal damage.

Tinea capitis Located on the head and scalp; appears as a round, scaly area where no hair is growing; diffuse scaling is present.

Tinea corporis Located on the body; appears annular (e.g., ringworm).

Tinea cruris Located on the groin and genitalia; appears as a sharply demarcated area with elevated scaling and geographic borders.

Tinea pedis Located on the feet; appears as maceration between the toes, scaling on soles or sides of the foot, and sometimes vesicles and/or pustules.

Tinea manuum Located on the hands; appears as dry, diffuse scaling, usually on the palm.

Tinea unguium Located on or under fingernails or toenails; appears as dark debris under the nails.

Tinea versicolor Located on the trunk; appears as pink, tan, or white patches with fine, desquamating scale.

Ulcer A full-thickness crater that involves the dermis and epidermis with loss of the surface epithelium; this lesion is depressed and may bleed; usually heals with scarring.

Urticaria Also known as *hives;* a skin condition in which a wheal on the skin forms from edema; often caused by a reaction to a drug or through contact with substances (skin contact or even inhaled), causing hypersensitivity in the patient.

Varicella An acute contagious vesicular skin eruption caused by the *Varicella zoster* virus (chickenpox).

Vesicle An elevated lesion that contains clear fluid; sometimes called a *water blister*.

Warts Benign lesions caused by the papillomavirus.

Wheal A firm, rounded, flat-topped elevation of skin that is evanescent and pruritic (itches); also known as a *hive*.

Toxicology

Objectives *After completing this chapter, you will be able to:*

1. Describe the extent of injury and death associated with toxicologic emergencies.
2. Define *poison, toxicology,* and *toxicologic emergency.*
3. Describe the role of the poison control center in the treatment of toxicologic emergencies.
4. List the four routes of entry of poisons into the body and how they affect managed care of the poisoned patient.
5. Understand the need for an accurate scene size-up to ensure responder safety at toxicologic emergencies.
6. List and use available reference materials for poisonings involving household and industrial chemicals.
7. Describe the general toxidromes that can be used to classify and treat the poisoned patient.
8. Understand the importance of decontaminating patients.
9. Identify the difference between internal and external decontamination.
10. Describe the appropriate uses of activated charcoal for internal decontamination.
11. Identify the available antidotes to poisons and how they are used to treat patients.
12. Identify medications commonly involved in toxicologic emergencies and be able to list common signs and symptoms and treatment procedures that will benefit the patient.
13. Identify chemicals commonly involved in toxicologic emergencies and be able to list common signs and symptoms and treatment procedures that will benefit the patient.
14. Identify wildlife commonly involved in toxicologic emergencies and be able to list common signs and symptoms and treatment procedures that will benefit the patient.
15. Identify plants and mushrooms commonly involved in toxicologic emergencies and be able to list common signs and symptoms and treatment procedures that will benefit the patient.
16. Identify illegal drugs commonly involved in toxicologic emergencies and be able to list common signs and symptoms and treatment procedures that will benefit the patient.
17. Understand the toxicologic effects of alcohol and alcohol abuse and how to treat the signs and symptoms of alcohol poisoning.

Chapter Outline

Toxicology
Recognition and Identification of
 Poisoning Incidents

General Treatment Principles
Poisonings
Chapter Summary

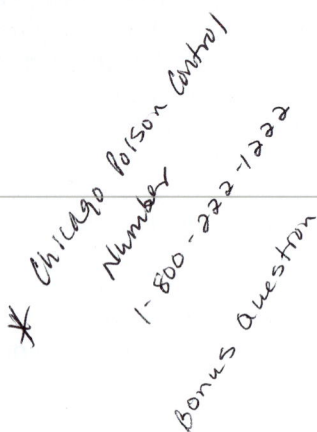

✳ Chicago Poison Control Number 1-800-222-1222

Bonus Question

Case Scenario

At 7:15 PM on a warm fall evening your crew is called to a private residence at the request of law enforcement personnel. As you walk up to the residence, an officer tells you that a group of young adults were having a dinner party when two of them reportedly started to have trouble breathing and then collapsed. As you walk into the house you see 10 or more young men and women standing around two people lying on the living room carpet. You notice a strong odor of marijuana. You also notice several empty beer cans, a tapped keg of beer, a few lines of cocaine, and a well-stocked bar. Some of the guests, although concerned about the people who are ill, have a euphoric look and others appear agitated. On reaching the patients, you find two women in their mid-20s lying on their sides in varying degrees of distress.

Questions

1. What is your initial impression of the patients?
2. What additional information do you need to complete your assessment?
3. What may be causing the women's distress?

[OBJECTIVE 1]

Poisonings present wide-ranging challenges to emergency medical personnel. For example, they can involve ensuring scene security in a suicidal overdose or locating the agent that caused a pediatric poisoning. Your prehospital treatment of these patients typically consists of providing supportive care and focusing on airway, breathing, and circulation (ABCs). Occasionally you may administer **antidotes.** Antidotes may reverse the signs and symptoms of toxic exposure. This chapter examines safe and effective responses to a wide range of poisonings, from pharmaceutical drug overdoses to illegal drug overdoses to occupational toxic industrial chemical and environmental poisonings.

According to the 2006 Annual Report of the American Association of Poison Control Centers (AAPCC) National Poison Data System, approximately 93% of poisonings occur in the home, approximately 83% of poisonings are accidental, and approximately 77% occur through the route of ingestion. More than half of the poisonings occur in children younger than 6 years. Fortunately, however, children aged 6 years and younger comprise only 3% of the fatalities. Thus statistically, as a paramedic, you most often will encounter the accidental poisoning in the home, likely involving a child. Interestingly, the most common exposure in children younger than 6 years is to cosmetics and personal care products. You must, however, be prepared for other incidents, such as the 2% of poisonings that occur in the workplace, the 8% of poisonings that involve suicide attempts, or the young child who ingested a toxic dose of medication (Bronstein et al., 2007).

TOXICOLOGY

[OBJECTIVE 2]

To perform effectively at an incident, you must understand what you are dealing with. **Toxicology** is the study of **toxins,** or **poisons.** These are substances that can harm the human body. The words *poison* and *toxin* are used interchangeably. The subject matter of toxicology ranges from the properties of the poison itself to the effect the poison has on the body. Toxicologists regularly study occupational exposure to chemicals involved in the manufacturing process. Epidemiologic studies often are carried out on exposed workers. Thus toxicology involves combining knowledge of chemistry, biochemistry, and epidemiology to understand why poisonings occur, how they affect the human body, how victims should be treated, and how to prevent further injuries. Some of the toxicologic emergencies you may encounter are listed in Box 30-1.

Poison Control Center

[OBJECTIVE 3]

The AAPCC designates poison control centers by regions. These centers are responsible for maintaining the national poison control system, elements of which include public education and research and data collection. The system

---

BOX 30-1   Toxicologic Emergencies the Paramedic May Encounter

- Therapeutic errors — *calculated wrong, elderly get confused*
- Idiosyncratic reactions
- Environmental exposures
- Occupational exposures
- Neglect and abuse
- Intentional drug and alcohol poisoning
- Suicide
- Assault
- Homicide
- Terrorism

works to improve and enhance the current system as well as provide immediate assistance to the public and EMS providers in the field. In addition, the centers advise hospitals on poisoning treatment.

These centers are an excellent resource during toxicologic emergencies. They are staffed 24 hours a day, 7 days a week by trained medical personnel. They have access to an impressive computer database of more than 350,000 drugs, chemicals, consumer products, and biologic toxins. They can advise on the most current treatment regimen and antidote treatment protocols available. The information they provide can be tailored to your initial findings, such as the suspected agent, dose, time administered, and patient weight and physical condition. Hospitals also use these centers to obtain treatment and care information.

Routes of Entry

[OBJECTIVE 4]

The *route of entry* is how a poison enters the body. The routes of entry are divided into four categories: inhalation, ingestion, absorption, and injection. All routes of entry are not created equal. The lungs and the gastrointestinal tract function as absorption and exchange membranes, whereas the skin functions as a barrier. Thus inhalation and ingestion typically are more effective routes of entry than skin absorption. Breathing is an involuntary response, whereas eating and drinking are voluntary responses. Thus inhalation poses the greatest threat to you as the emergency responder, whereas inhalation and ingestion both pose grave threats to the patient. However, do not discount absorption by the skin or eyes. Many chemicals are effectively absorbed through the skin, especially hydrocarbons and their derivatives.

Inhalation

Inhalation is the entry of a toxin into the body through the act of breathing. Inhalation is one of the most effective routes of entry because the lungs are designed to absorb oxygen from the atmosphere. Unfortunately, the lungs cannot discriminate between life-giving oxygen and toxic gases such as carbon monoxide or cyanide. Toxic gases pose a grave threat because they rapidly enter the bloodstream at the alveoli in the lungs. The bioavailability of inhaled gases is very high because they are delivered directly to the bloodstream.

Ingestion

Ingestion is the entry of a toxin into the body by eating or drinking. Ingestion is the most common route of entry for poisons. Entry by ingestion also is quite effective because the gastrointestinal (GI) system is designed to break down and absorb food. As with the lungs, the GI tract is an equal opportunity absorber. In other words, it will absorb the substance whether it is nourishment or poison. Different poisons are absorbed in different parts of the GI tract. Acids often are better absorbed in the

stomach. Bases are usually absorbed better in the small intestines because of the solubility effects of compartment pH. Most poisons are more efficiently absorbed in the small intestines because of the enormous available surface area. However, poisons must be in solution (dissolved) to be absorbed. Some pills are designed to dissolve slowly over time; thus they release the medication over a prolonged period.

Absorption

Absorption is the entry of a toxin into the body through the skin or the eyes. The skin is a highly effective barrier. Its design keeps water and nutrients inside the body and most poisons out of the body. However, many toxins effectively penetrate the skin, such as hydrocarbon solvents and fuels. The eyes also absorb many toxins quite effectively. They are the Achilles heel of the protective envelope the skin forms.

Injection

Injection is the entry of a toxin into the body by penetration. This can occur either accidentally through a puncture or intentionally by a needle injection or **envenomation.** You will most commonly encounter this route of entry in accidental and intentional overdoses from drug abuse. When a drug or toxin is directly injected into the bloodstream, this route of entry is extremely efficient. You also may encounter injection poisonings when contaminated substances accidentally enter the body. This can occur with a spray paint injection injury, for example. Another example is an occupational injury involving an impaled object. These injuries typically do not involve poisons, but sometimes these substances are contaminated with chemicals.

RECOGNITION AND IDENTIFICATION OF POISONING INCIDENTS

Your safety and the quality of patient care hinge on how rapidly and accurately you identify poisoning cases. If the causative agent is still near the patient, you may unwittingly become contaminated and poisoned if you do not promptly recognize the threat. First the toxin must be identified. Then this information must be relayed to the hospital. Antidote treatments may be available. Antidotes typically need to be rapidly administered for the patient to recover effectively. Toxicologic emergencies also can be intentionally caused. Furthermore, the side effects of a toxin can lead to violent behavior in a patient. In such cases, law enforcement must be summoned early.

Scene Size-up and Responder Safety

[OBJECTIVE 5]

Performing a good scene size-up should help minimize the risk of cross-contamination. While responding to an incident, pay close attention to the dispatch information, especially the location and chief complaint. Consider whether the location is a manufacturing facility. Determine if the chief complaint seems inconsistent with other dispatch information. The best way to protect yourself and your partner is to recognize the poisoning early, whether it is accidental or intentional. Also consider calling specialists early, such as the poison control center, hazardous materials team, and law enforcement.

Crime Scenes: Suicidal Patients and Drug Overdoses

Don't pick up foil wrappers - will explode

Law enforcement officers should secure potential crime scenes before your entry. If you find yourself in a potentially dangerous situation, leave and request backup. Suicidal patients may have weapons or be aggressive and confrontational, even if the dispatch information indicates that the call is for a poisoning. Drug overdoses pose similar problems. Several illegal drugs, such as methamphetamine, have aggressive stages in the abuse cycle. Law enforcement must immediately secure the scene, remain present during treatment, and possibly accompany the ambulance and crew to the hospital.

Chemical Release or Spill

Hazardous materials incidents pose a huge risk to paramedics. You must quickly recognize the signs of a chemical release before you become exposed or contaminated. You may be the first emergency responder at the scene. Protect yourself and others by practicing the hazardous materials awareness response mnemonic RAIN, which stands for *r*ecognize a hazardous materials incident early, *a*void the release area, *i*solate the release area, and *n*otify the properly trained agencies (hazardous materials teams). This means you may not be able to enter safely and treat the patient without proper advanced hazardous materials training and personal protective equipment.

Reference Materials

[OBJECTIVE 6]

Reference materials can be especially helpful for chemical exposures. Chemicals can be volatile. Moreover, they can pose secondary exposure hazards to paramedics. These reference materials can be kept in the response vehicle. Your partner can access them en route to the emergency if the dispatch information includes the name of the hazardous material. If the agent proves to be an inhalation hazard or skin contact hazard, you must wear the appropriate personal protective equipment. If effective respiratory protection is not available, wait for the appropriately equipped personnel, typically hazardous materials trained personnel.

NIOSH Guide

The National Institute of Occupational Safety and Health (NIOSH) has published a pocket guide to hazardous materials (2005). It contains information on the chemical and physical properties of agents, respiratory protection guidelines, and the health effect and immediate treatment regimens. The chemicals are listed alphabetically, with a synonym and trade name index in the back. You also can look up the chemicals by their **United Nations (UN) number** (the 4-digit number assigned to chemicals during transit by the U.S. Department of Transportation) or **chemical abstracts services (CAS) number** (the unique identification number of chemicals, much like a person's Social Security number) in the respective indexes in the back. This is an excellent source of information during the size-up of the incident. It provides critical information that can keep you from becoming a victim of the poison as well. You can obtain a free copy of this guide (both hardcover and CD-ROM) online at http://www.cdc.gov/niosh.

WISER Chemical Database

The Wireless Information System for Emergency Responders (WISER) is an electronic database developed by the National Library of Medicine. The database is especially useful to paramedics because of its detailed medical information. The database contains chemical and physical properties, decontamination advice, treatment guidelines (including antidote therapy), and a search engine by signs and symptoms and/or chemical and physical properties of the material. Currently 407 chemicals are in the database, and it is actively maintained. The program is free and can be downloaded to personal digital assistants, laptop computers, and tablet computers, or it can be accessed independently online. More information and download and access instructions can be found at http://www.wiser.nlm.nih.gov.

Agency for Toxic Substances and Disease Registry

The National Institutes of Health publish the currently accepted treatment guidelines for chemical exposures in volume III of the three-part series *Agency for Toxic Substances and Disease Registry*. The first two parts deal with EMS and hospital responses to hazardous materials poisonings and emergencies. Approximately 30 chemicals are covered with in-depth medical information. The medical information ranges from the medical first responder to the physician level and includes the paramedic level of care. You can obtain a free electronic copy online at http://www.atsdr.cdc.gov.

PARAMEDIC*Pearl*

In a toxicologic emergency, obtaining accurate information is critical. The poison must be identified and the time of intoxication determined to provide definitive treatment for the patient.

Patient Assessment and History

If the initial scene size-up did not raise any red flags, your next opportunity to catch a toxicologic emergency is during the initial assessment and patient history. If the patient is responsive, determine the chief complaint and the substance to which the patient was exposed, the route of entry, the amount of the substance, and how long ago the exposure occurred. Assess the ABCs quickly and thoroughly in poisoning victims. Common signs and symptoms of poisoning include altered mental status, airway and respiratory difficulty, cardiac dysrhythmias, and emesis. When obtaining the patient history, be alert to psychological illness. Accidental poisonings can occur when new medications are started or medications are switched, especially in the elderly. If the patient is unresponsive, try to obtain a history from family, friends, or bystanders. Ask if any treatment has been started or if medication dosages have been recently changed. Determine whether bystanders have given emetics (syrup of ipecac) or activated charcoal. This could affect your treatment protocol. Also be alert to unusual containers and medications. Check the prescription fill date and dosage and compare this to the contents. The presence of significantly fewer pills in the bottle than you would expect may indicate an overdose. If the patient vomits, especially in chemical poisonings, be extremely cautious of the emesis. Many chemicals are volatile, and the vomitus may emit dangerous levels of the poison into the atmosphere. If possible, contain the emesis in a sealed bag or bottle.

Toxidromes

[OBJECTIVE 7]

To treat poisoning victims effectively, you must be able to recognize quickly the signs and symptoms different toxic agents induce. These signs and symptoms are called toxidromes. Because of the complexity of toxicologic emergencies in terms of signs and symptoms and causative agents, a series of toxic syndromes has been developed (Table 30-1). This classification system is designed to associate a set of signs and symptoms with a class of causative agent and provide a treatment regimen and possibly a specific antidote. Remember, however, most poisonings require only supportive care in the field because most toxins do not have a readily available antidote. Definitive treatment by gastric lavage and any available antidotes is usually administered at the hospital emergency department.

> **PARAMEDIC Pearl**
>
> The prehospital treatment for poisonings varies widely. Be sure to check your local protocols and consult your regional Poison Control Center or medical direction when caring for patients with a toxicologic emergency.

Cholinergic Syndrome

The patient with cholinergic syndrome appears as the classic "wet" patient. The SLUDGE mnemonic applies (salivation, lacrimation, urination, defecation, gastrointestinal upset, and emesis). Fluids will come out of every orifice. In addition to the classic SLUDGE symptoms, diaphoresis (profuse sweating) and pinpoint pupils, or miosis, also will be present. Thus the acronym can be extended to SLUDGEM. Additional symptoms include bradycardia, bronchoconstriction, central nervous system (CNS) depression, confusion, convulsions, seizures, and coma.

The most common causative agents are organophosphate and carbamate pesticides; however, military nerve agents and some mushrooms also have these effects. The diagnosis is based on wet patient presentation with pinpoint pupils. The treatment includes administering the cholinergic antagonist atropine, which dries up the patient's secretions.

Anticholinergic Syndrome

As the name implies, the anticholinergic syndrome has the opposite effect of the cholinergic syndrome. This patient appears as the classic "dry" patient. The hallmarks of this syndrome are dry, flushed skin, delirium, and dilated pupils. In severe cases seizures and dysrhythmias are present. The diagnosis is based on a dry patient presentation with dilated pupils. Common causative agents include alkaloids, prescription anticholinergic medications, and incidental anticholinergic medications (such as antihistamines and tricyclic antidepressants).

Hallucinogen Syndrome

The patient with hallucinogen syndrome is one of the most dangerous and sometimes bizarre encounters. The patient has altered mental status, including possible behavioral disturbances such as aggressiveness, delusional behavior such as paranoia, and visual illusions (hallucinations). CNS effects can include stimulation or depression depending on the causative agent, the dose, and the timeline of poisoning. Other effects can include hypertension, tachycardia, chest pain, seizures, and respiratory and cardiac arrest. The diagnosis is based on behavioral abnormalities and hallucinations. The causative agents are commonly illegal drugs, such as lysergic acid diethylamide (LSD), phencyclidine (PCP), peyote, mescaline, and mushrooms.

Narcotic/Opiate Syndrome

The patient with narcotic or opiate syndrome has CNS depression (euphoria may be present with some agents), pinpoint pupils, and respiratory depression. Severe intoxication can include respiratory arrest, seizures, and coma. The diagnosis is based on euphoria, pinpoint pupils, and hypotension. Causative agents include the illegal drug heroin, which has had increased incidence over the last several years, and the prescription drugs morphine,

TABLE 30-1 Toxidromes

Syndrome (Causative Agents)	Signs and Symptoms	Treatment
Cholinergic (carbamates, nerve agents, organophosphates, some mushrooms)	Wet patient presentation: diaphoresis, SLUDGE Pinpoint pupils (miosis) CNS depression Confusion, weakness Nausea, vomiting, cramps Bronchoconstriction, wheezing Cardiac dysrhythmias Convulsions, seizures Coma	ABCs Activated charcoal *– not region XI* Atropine *– 1st – starts anticholinergic response* (*1 mg*) Pralidoxime (2-PAM) *– 2nd – releases* (*300 mg*) *acetlcholinesterase* Diazepam (Valium)
Anticholinergic (alkaloids, antihistamines, atropine, tricyclic antidepressants, antipsychotics, muscle relaxants, some plants)	Dry patient presentation: dry skin, flushed skin, thirst Delirium, lethargy, dysphagia Dilated pupils Hyperthermia Tachycardia Cardiac dysrhythmias Seizures	ABCs Activated charcoal *– not region XI but yes for national* Diazepam (Valium)
Hallucinogen (some amphetamines, LSD, marijuana, mescaline, some mushrooms, PCP)	Visual illusions Strange behavior, delusions Respiratory depression CNS depression	ABCs Calming measures (quiet, dark room) Diazepam (Valium) Restraint
Narcotic/opioid (codeine, fentanyl, heroin, meperidine, methadone, morphine, opium, oxycodone)	Euphoria, high Pinpoint pupils (miosis) Nausea, vomiting Hypotension CNS depression Respiratory depression Seizures Coma	ABCs Naloxone (Narcan)
Sympathomimetic (amphetamines, caffeine, cocaine, ephedrine, epinephrine, methamphetamine, methylphenidate [Ritalin], pseudoephedrine)	Paranoia, delusions Diaphoresis Hypertension CNS excitation, tachycardia *Severe:* Cardiac dysrhythmias Hypotension Seizures	ABCs Calming measures (quiet, dark room) Diazepam (Valium)

ABCs, Airway, breathing, and circulation; *SLUDGE,* salivation, lacrimation, urination, defecation, gastrointestinal upset, and emesis; *CNS,* central nervous system; *LSD,* lysergic acid diethylamide; *PCP,* phencyclidine.

meperidine (Demerol), and codeine. Antidote treatment includes the administration of naloxone (Narcan), an opioid antagonist. The administration of naloxone may induce withdrawal symptoms, including potentially violent behavior.

Sympathomimetic Syndrome   *Acts like epinephrine*

The patient with sympathomimetic syndrome can create one of the most dangerous situations. This is especially true when you are confronted with a "tweaking" meth-amphetamine user (explained later in this chapter). The patient will have CNS excitation, possible delusions and paranoia, hypertension, dysrhythmias, and diaphoresis. In severe cases the patient may have hypotension, dysrhythmias, and seizures. The diagnosis is based on behavioral abnormalities, diaphoresis, and hypertension. Causative agents include the illegal drugs cocaine, methamphetamine (the use of which is surging), amphetamines, and over-the-counter decongestant medications.

GENERAL TREATMENT PRINCIPLES

Unfortunately, treatment of toxicologic emergencies is usually limited to providing supportive care because of the lack of an antidote or medical control procedures. However, several poisonings do have specific antidote treatments that are extremely effective, especially when administered early. These are examined in detail in the next sections.

The first step in caring for the patient is discovering the causative agent. Accidental poisonings and overdoses are relatively easy to detect, especially in adults. Accidental poisonings in children as well as overdoses with illegal drugs or suicide attempts can be more difficult. Adult patients often are evasive about illegal drug use, children may fear disciplinary action, and young children may not be able to verbalize what they ingested. You must be persistent during your history. Use family, friends, and bystanders as much as possible. Also be alert to clues in the immediate environment, such as open or partially empty containers, the medicine cabinet, chemical residues, and drug paraphernalia.

ABCs and Supportive Care

The treatment of any **intoxication** begins with providing supportive care and maintaining the ABCs. Airway control must be maintained because many chemicals induce emesis or an emetic may have been administered before your arrival on the scene. Low-**viscosity** solvents are prone to aspiration. You may need to provide breathing assistance in cases of respiratory depression and/or arrest. Start an intravenous line (IV) for the maintenance of hemodynamic fluid balance, the administration of supportive care medications, and the administration of the antidote, if available and appropriate.

Decontamination

[OBJECTIVES 8, 9]

Decontamination is the removal of contaminants (the poisonous substance) from people or equipment. In this case, you are primarily concerned about patient decontamination. The patient may be externally contaminated, internally contaminated, or both. If the contamination is not quickly removed, the poison will continue to be absorbed or continue to damage the tissue with which it is in contact, causing further harm to the patient.

Surface contamination often occurs in industrial accidents. You must quickly and safely remove the surface contamination to prevent skin or eye absorption, inhalation of volatile vapors that off-gas, and accidental ingestion of the substance. In contrast, internal contamination may be found in the lungs, GI tract, or puncture wounds or be absorbed through the skin. Puncture wounds, aspirated chemicals in the lungs, and chemicals absorbed into the skin are extremely difficult to decontaminate.

This is usually done in the advanced care setting, if at all possible. However, in the field you can readily decontaminate the GI tract by administration of activated charcoal and, in rare cases, gastric lavage.

External Decontamination

shower for 15-20 min.

If the patient is contaminated, you must ensure that he or she is decontaminated before transport. This is a major safety consideration. Many poisons are volatile and will readily off-gas, especially in a heated ambulance or helicopter. Patients who have ingested volatile poisons should never be transported by air. You need to know which agencies in your jurisdiction can perform decontamination. Call them if you encounter a contaminated patient or if you become contaminated. The universal decontamination solution is soap and water.

Gastrointestinal (Internal) Decontamination

Consider GI decontamination in poisonings by ingestion when you arrive within 1 hour of intake. After 1 hour, the stomach contents have moved into the small intestines. At that point, most methods of internal decontamination become ineffective. Little need for internal decontamination exists when poisons with minimal toxicity are involved.

Syrup of Ipecac. The induction of vomiting with syrup of ipecac or other emetics is almost universally discouraged. In fact, this practice has steadily declined over the years. In 1985 ipecac was administered in 15% of toxic ingestions reported to poison control centers, whereas in 2006 it was administered in only 0.1% of toxic exposures. There have been several reasons for this decline in use. Studies show that emetics only reduce absorption by 30%. Although this percentage may sound impressive, outcome studies have shown no benefit in patients who received ipecac compared with those who did not. Furthermore, the drawbacks, including gastric rupture and Mallory-Weiss syndrome, generally outweigh the benefits. In a policy statement issued in 2003 the American Academy of Pediatrics recommended ipecac not be stored in the home or used in the home treatment of toxic ingestions. This negates the 1980 recommendation that ipecac be kept in all homes and used in the event of a toxic ingestion. The American Academy of Clinical Toxicology and the European Association of Poison Centers and Clinical Toxicologists recommended against the use of ipecac in the treatment of toxic ingestions in a 1997 joint position paper. This stand was reaffirmed and updated in 2004. Finally, although ipecac remains an over-the-counter medication, in 2003 a subcommittee of the Food and Drug Administration, the Nonprescription Drugs Advisory Committee, voted 6 to 4 to remove the over-the-counter approval of ipecac.

Emetics pose an increased risk of aspiration, especially if mental status unexpectedly decreases. Moreover, aspiration can possibly cause respiratory difficulty or aspiration pneumonitis. Emetics also interfere with other more effective treatments, such as activated charcoal and oral antidotes. Contraindications include altered level of consciousness, loss of gag reflex, pregnancy, ingestion of corrosives, low-viscosity hydrocarbons, and CNS depressants or irritants. Complications can include aspiration (especially with low-viscosity materials) as well as gastric and esophageal injuries (especially with corrosives). Inducing vomiting is generally considered a high-risk, low-benefit treatment. The exception to this rule may be plant poisonings.

Activated Charcoal

[OBJECTIVE 10]

The internal decontamination treatment of choice for most poisonings, especially in the field, is **activated charcoal.** The risks are low and the benefits are high. Activated charcoal has been shown to be as effective as gastric lavage. This substance is made from charred wood and comes as a finely divided black powder. The charcoal is quite effective at adsorbing (making the toxin unavailable) most chemicals because of the large surface area (1000 to 3000 m^2/g) of the finely divided material. Charcoal should be administered within 1 hour of the ingestion. **Cathartics,** such as sorbitol, are often added to the activated charcoal to increase the elimination rate. Cathartics decrease the time a poison spends in the GI tract by increasing bowel motility. This combination of adsorption and catharsis greatly reduces the absorption and internalization of the poison. Cathartics should not be used in the pediatric patient because they can cause significant electrolyte derangements. Furthermore, activated charcoal is not effective on mineral acids, ethanol, or methanol or metals such as lead, arsenic, and iron. It also is contraindicated for hydrocarbon or caustic agent ingestions, if airway reflexes are absent, or in the setting of a bowel obstruction. Therefore bowel sounds must be assessed as present before its administration. The side effects include emesis, which occurs in approximately 15% of patients.

Gastric Lavage. Gastric lavage, or pumping the stomach, is an effective method of decontamination only if performed within 1 hour of ingestion. As with ipecac, however, its use in routine treatment of toxic ingestions has been questioned; it has been shown to have no impact on outcome in non–life-threatening ingestions. As with the position change regarding ipecac, The American Academy of Clinical Toxicology and the European Association of Poison Centers and Clinical Toxicologists recommended against the use of gastric lavage in 1997 for the routine treatment of toxic ingestions. Gastric lavage only decontaminates the stomach. It is not effective once the toxin enters the small intestine. However, gastric lavage is an excellent treatment in the case of poisons that do not bind to activated charcoal and highly

toxic agents that do not have an antidote therapy. The contraindications include altered levels of consciousness (unless an endotracheal tube is in place) and the ingestion of low-viscosity hydrocarbons and corrosives. Complications of gastric lavage include possible tracheal intubation, aspiration pneumonitis, and esophageal perforation.

Whole-Bowel Irrigation. Whole-bowel irrigation (WBI) is a much more effective method of internal decontamination than gastric lavage. It is useful in poisonings that form concretions, such as salicylates and iron supplements. It also is useful for substances not readily absorbed by activated charcoal. It involves continuously administering a polyethylene glycol electrolyte solution into the stomach with a gastric tube. Typically 1 to 2 L/hr are administered until the rectal effluent is clear. The contents of the entire GI tract are cleared, which reduces toxin absorption in the intestines (especially the small intestine).

WBI has fewer complications than gastric lavage. A drawback to this technique is the lengthy time for fluid administration (2 to 6 hours); therefore it is generally not performed in the field.

Antidote Administration

[OBJECTIVE 11]

Antidotes are specific medications that counteract the effects of a poison. Antidotes are highly effective, especially when given quickly after intoxication. They can act in a number of different ways. Some antidotes increase the rate of elimination of the toxin, and other antidotes reactivate enzymes that have been damaged by the poison. Many of these mechanisms are covered in the following section. Management of the ABCs, general treatments identified in this section, and supportive care are not reiterated for each case. However, do not forget the basics.

PARAMEDIC*Pearl*

Toxicologic emergencies are unique. The nature of each emergency depends on the toxic agent, dose, route of entry, time of administration, and patient characteristics. In general, you should consult medical control and the Poison Control Center before administering specific antidotes.

POISONINGS

The various classes of poisonings are examined here in the approximate order of their occurrence (most common to least common), not necessarily in the order of those causing the most deaths. As you read through the categories, form a mental picture of how you would respond to these various toxicologic emergencies.

Medications

[OBJECTIVE 12]

The leading cause of poisoning in the United States is prescription **drug overdose,** both intentional and accidental. In 2006, sedatives, hypnotics, and antipsychotics (as a group) were listed by the AAPCC as the cause of most deaths attributed to toxic ingestion (382 deaths). When combined as a group, analgesics were responsible for the most deaths in 2006 (307 from opioids, 214 from medications containing acetaminophen, 138 from acetaminophen alone, 61 from aspirin alone, and 1 from medications containing aspirin). Acetaminophen, alone or in combination with other medications, was involved in the majority of deaths from analgesics (Bronstein et al., 2007). Approximately 80% of poisoning fatalities are attributable to intentional ingestions, although the patient may not necessarily have been suicidal. In 2006, 50% of fatalities were successful suicide attempts. When responding to and treating suicidal patients, do not forget to conduct a proper scene size-up. In addition, ensure that law enforcement accounts for scene security. Accidental poisonings can be caused by an inadvertent **overdose,** such as taking medication twice. Such poisonings also can be caused by therapeutic errors in the medical setting. Accidental poisonings are more likely to occur with medications that have a low **therapeutic index,** or a narrow effective dosage window. Small decreases in medication levels render the drug ineffective, and small increases in medication levels lead to adverse, sometimes life-threatening side effects.

The family and patient education you provide should focus on prevention. Advise patients to read the instruction sheet that comes with the medication carefully. If the pharmacist did not include one, advise the patient to ask for one. In addition, all contraindications (e.g., "do not eat within 1 hour of taking medication") and directions (e.g., "take with food") are not always listed on the bottle. Moreover, few regulations exist regarding the instructional labeling of refill medication bottles. Advise families with children to store medications in a safe place. They should be stored in locked cabinets or up high to keep them out of reach of children. Patients who take medications on a regular basis should consider using dosed and dated pillboxes to organize their medications on a weekly basis. This can help avoid accidental overdoses. These pillboxes are especially useful for geriatric patients. Advise family members to monitor medications as closely as possible (including refill status and number of pills left in the bottle). This information is helpful in the event of an overdose.

Following is a review of poisons according to their chemical properties, not the route of entry. Poisonings can have multiple routes of entry. For example, an ingestion of kerosene can be aspirated into the lungs during vomiting; therefore it has aspects of ingestion and inhalation. Treatment of patients always starts with the basics: ensuring the ABCs and providing other supportive care.

These treatments generally do not vary greatly by specific agent. However, the antidote therapy differs according to the chemical and biochemical actions of the toxin on the human body. The following text focuses on the definitive treatment of these poisoning cases.

Pain Relievers

Pain relievers have an ever-present existence in people's lives. They are available over the counter and are one of the most commonly used drugs. Unfortunately, this makes them readily available to curious children as well as individuals with depression and suicidal tendencies. Unsurprisingly, pain relievers were involved in 11.9% of all poisonings in 2006, the highest percentage of all medications (Table 30-2). To break this down further, they were the leading cause of toxic ingestions in patients older than 19 years (15.1%), and the third leading cause of toxic ingestions in patients younger than 6 years (8.4%).

Acetaminophen. Statistically acetaminophen is the medication you are most likely to encounter in a toxicologic emergency. It is an active ingredient in hundreds of over-the-counter and prescription medications. It is used to treat pain (analgesic) and fever (antipyretic). Therefore it is a preferred ingredient of cold medications. At normal doses acetaminophen is a safe and effective drug with few side effects. However, at higher doses (150 mg/kg) it can cause severe liver damage.

In the liver, acetaminophen is metabolized to a substance that causes liver toxicity. Typically, the liver can cope with therapeutic doses of acetaminophen. However, the liver's enzymes eventually cannot cope and toxic metabolites build up. The antidote for acetaminophen is N-acetylcysteine (NAC), also known as *mucomyst.* Acetaminophen toxicity is generally reversible if NAC is given within 8 hours of poisoning. Therefore NAC is generally given in the hospital setting after laboratory analysis of blood concentrations.

Salicylates. Salicylates, such as aspirin, are also common over-the-counter analgesics and are involved in many toxicologic emergencies. However, their toxicity threshold (300 mg/kg) is twice as high as acetaminophen. In addition, many nonaspirin salicylates such as methyl salicylate and bismuth salicylate are found in many products. In the pediatric patient low doses of these substances can be fatal.

Salicylates inhibit prostaglandin synthesis. This affects the acid-base balance in the body and can lead to metabolic acidosis. Salicylate poisoning has no antidote. The most effective treatment is giving activated charcoal within the first hour of ingestion. IV fluids are essential. If metabolic acidosis develops, it must be aggressively treated with sodium bicarbonate. However, determining the onset of metabolic acidosis in the field is difficult without laboratory blood work. The more important indication of sodium bicarbonate in the prehospital setting is to enhance the elimination of salicylate. By alkalinizing the urine the salicylate is trapped through an

TABLE 30-2 Pharmaceutical Poisonings: Analgesics (Pain Relievers)

Toxin	Signs and Symptoms	Treatment
Acetaminophen (APAP, Tylenol, Panadol) Combination formulas (Excedrin, Sinutab, Darvocet-N)	*Stage 1:* 0-24 hours Weakness and fatigue Nausea and vomiting Diaphoresis Pallor *Stage 2:* 24-48 hours Abdominal tenderness or pain (right quadrant; liver) Decreased urine output Elevated liver enzymes *Stage 3:* 72-96 hours Liver toxicity, jaundice Dysrhythmias Hypoglycemia Lethargy Vomiting *Stage 4:* 4-14 days Liver dysfunction resolves or patient succumbs to liver failure	ABCs Detailed patient history, especially time of ingestion Activated charcoal (within 1 hour) *Antidote:* N-acetylcysteine
Salicylates (acetylsalicylic acid, aspirin, salicylic acid)	Rapid respirations — *metabolic acidosis blow off CO2* Confusion and lethargy Abdominal pain — *GI bleed* Vomiting Hyperthermia Dysrhythmias — *SVT* Cardiac failure Coma	ABCs Detailed patient history, especially time of ingestion Activated charcoal (within 1 hour) IV fluids
NSAIDs (ibuprofen, naproxen sodium, indomethacin, ketorolac [Toradol])	Headache Tinnitus Nausea and vomiting Drowsiness Edema in extremities Rash or itchiness Dyspnea and wheezing Pulmonary edema Renal failure	ABCs Detailed patient history, especially time of ingestion Activated charcoal (within 1 hour) Monitor for hypotension and dysrhythmias

ABCs, Airway, breathing, and circulation; *IV,* intravenous; *NSAIDs,* nonsteroidal antiinflammatory drugs.

ion-trapping mechanism and eliminated from the body, thereby reducing the amount of circulating salicylate. Early symptoms of acute poisoning include gastric irritation, nausea, vomiting, diaphoresis, and tinnitus. Later signs and symptoms include hyperventilation, noncardiogenic pulmonary edema, cerebral edema, seizures, coma, and apnea.

Long-term poisoning can occur with aspirin because it is an extremely effective analgesic and is often prescribed in low doses as a preventative measure for heart trouble. Long-term poisoning symptoms can be similar to the early acute poisoning symptoms (gastric irritation and pain).

Nonsteroidal Antiinflammatory Drugs. Nonsteroidal antiinflammatory drugs (NSAIDs) are a popular variety of analgesic. They were developed in large part to reduce the stomach-related side effects of aspirin. Indeed, they live up to this intention. Ibuprofen and naproxen sodium are two common varieties of NSAIDs. NSAID poisoning has no antidote; however, activated charcoal given within the first hour of ingestion is usually effective.

Antidepressants

Antidepressants have historically been a leading cause of poisoning deaths because of their narrow therapeutic index as well as the demographic taking the medications

(Table 30-3). Traditional medications such as the cyclic antidepressants, including amitriptyline, are commonly used to treat depression. However, newer, safer medications are beginning to be prescribed more often. In 2006 antidepressants were the ninth most commonly ingested substance in all patients and the fifth leading cause of death. Serotonergic agents, which affect serotonin balance, are commonly prescribed antidepressants.

Advise family members to monitor these medications whenever possible. Keeping tabs on the refill status and how much medication is left at any given time is helpful in the event of an overdose.

TABLE 30-3	Pharmaceutical Poisonings: Antidepressants	
Toxin	**Signs and Symptoms**	**Treatment**
Tricyclic antidepressants (amitriptyline, amoxapine, clomipramine, desipramine, doxepin, imipramine, maprotiline, nortriptyline, protriptyline, trimipramine)	*Early:* Anticholinergic signs and symptoms Blurred vision *Late:* Confusion Hallucinations Respiratory depression Cardiac dysrhythmias Hypotension Seizures Death	ABCs Detailed patient history, especially time of ingestion Activated charcoal (within 2 hours) Cardiac monitoring Alkalinization with sodium bicarbonate NOTE: Do *not* use flumazenil because of seizure induction
Lithium	Thirst, dry mouth Nausea, vomiting, diarrhea Blurred vision Slurred speech Confusion, stupor Tremor, fasciculations Dysrhythmias, bradycardia Apnea, seizure, coma Renal failure	ABCs Detailed patient history IV fluid replacement therapy Alkalinization of urine with sodium bicarbonate (enhanced elimination) Activated charcoal is ineffective but may be useful in coingestions
Monoamine oxidase inhibitors (isocarboxazid [Marplan], phenelzine [Nardil], tranylcypromine [Parnate])	Headache Agitation, restlessness "Ping pong" gaze Palpitations Diaphoresis Hypertension Hyperthermia Tachycardia *Severe:* bradycardia, hypotension, coma, death	ABCs Detailed patient history, especially time of ingestion Reverse hyperthermia Cardiac monitoring Activated charcoal (within 1 hour) Seizures and hyperthermia: benzodiazepines Hypotension: norepinephrine Antagonist: cyproheptadine
Selective serotonin uptake inhibitors (citalopram, fluoxetine [Prozac], fluvoxamine, paroxetine [Paxil], sertraline [Zoloft], trazodone)	*Serotonin syndrome:* Agitation, anxiety, confusion Headache, drowsiness Diaphoresis Nausea, vomiting Salivation, diarrhea Flushed skin, cutaneous piloerection, shivering Tremors, myoclonic jerks Hyperthermia Sinus tachycardia Rigidity, incoordination Hyperactive bowel sounds	ABCs Detailed patient history, especially time of ingestion Reverse hyperthermia Activated charcoal (within 1 hour) Cardiac monitoring *Antidote:* Serotonin receptor antagonists (such as cyproheptadine and chlorpromazine)

ABCs, Airway, breathing, and circulation; *IV,* intravenous.

Tricyclic Antidepressants. Tricyclic antidepressants have historically been a leading cause of toxicologic emergencies, especially intentional overdoses. These medications have a narrow therapeutic index, which means that a fine line exists between an ineffectually low dose and an overdose. Ironically, giving too low of a dose may lead to an intentional overdose (suicide attempt), and too high of a dose could lead to an accidental overdose. As previously mentioned, the use of tricyclic antidepressants has recently declined as newer, safer alternatives have been developed. For example, in 2001 tricyclic antidepressants were the second most common cause of death from toxic ingestion. However, in 2006, tricyclic antidepressants were a component in 75 deaths, and only 13 deaths involved tricyclic antidepressants as the only agent ingested. This is a significant decrease because these medications have been responsible for large numbers of fatalities in past years.

Tricyclic antidepressants act therapeutically by increasing the amount of norepinephrine and serotonin available in the CNS by blocking the reuptake of these neurotransmitters, extending the duration of their action. This has the effect of blocking cellular ion channels and alpha-adrenergic, muscarinic, and histaminergic receptors.

Toxicity results from sodium channel inhibition in the myocardium and potassium efflux inhibition. The early signs and symptoms include classic anticholinergic toxidrome effects of dry mouth, urinary retention, constipation, and blurred vision. Late signs and symptoms include respiratory depression, confusion, hallucinations, hyperthermia, cardiac dysrhythmias from atrioventricular block (such as torsades de pointes and wide QRS), and seizures. Cardiac monitoring is critical because cardiac complications are the primary cause of death. Sudden cardiac arrest may occur days after the overdose. Tricyclic antidepressant poisoning has no antidote; however, activated charcoal given within the first hour of ingestion may be effective. Sodium bicarbonate also may be necessary to counteract the sodium channel blockade. It will help reverse the metabolic acidosis that underlies cardiac toxicity.

Lithium. Lithium is used to treat bipolar disorder (manic depression). It is a small cation (positively charged ion) that is similar to sodium. Exactly how lithium exerts its medicinal effects is unknown. Lithium is believed, however, to have some effect on the neuronal cell membrane and the cellular sodium balance. Although lithium is an effective treatment for bipolar disorder, it has a narrow therapeutic index, which increases the likelihood of accidental and intentional poisonings. To avoid accidental, therapeutic poisoning, frequent blood tests are necessary to fine tune the dosage.

Monoamine Oxidase Inhibitors. Monoamine oxidase inhibitors (MAOIs) are serotonergic agents that also have been used to treat depression. However, they are not popular because of their wide range of adverse effects and drug interactions. In fact, they also have been used as antihypertensive drugs. They have a narrow therapeutic index, multiple drug interactions, and food interactions. The enzyme monoamine oxidase breaks down monoamines into inactive metabolites. Foods containing the monoamine tyramine, such as soy sauce, shrimp paste, overripe avocados, cheese, and red wine, can bring on a hypertensive crisis. Tyramine increases the release of norepinephrine, a potent vasopressor. The use of MAOIs can increase the tyramine load in the body, making a hypertensive crisis more likely.

A new generation of MAOIs is reversible, has fewer food interactions, and is generally less toxic. Fortunately, overdoses with MAOIs have seen a steep decline over recent years. The initial signs and symptoms include headache, agitation, hypertension, hyperthermia, and tachycardia. The effects of severe poisoning may include hypotension, bradycardia, and coma. The treatment is mainly supportive, including administering activated charcoal within 1 hour of ingestion. Treat seizures and hyperthermia with benzodiazepines and late-stage hypotension with norepinephrine.

Selective Serotonin Reuptake Inhibitors. Selective serotonin reuptake inhibitors (SSRIs) have become the antidepressants and antianxiety medications of choice because they have far fewer side effects. The therapeutic index of these medications is quite wide. These antidepressants specifically limit serotonin reuptake in the brain, increasing the amount available for brain function. They have far fewer effects on the norepinephrine system, limiting many of the side effects. However, the ingestion of SSRIs with MAOIs, another serotonergic agent, can be fatal. The signs and symptoms are relatively benign. Furthermore, the treatment consists of supportive care. The antidote is generally not available in the field and is used only in severe cases of serotonin toxicity.

Sedatives, Hypnotics, and Antipsychotics

Sedatives and hypnotics also are known as *downers*. They include such common medications as benzodiazepines and barbiturates (Table 30-4). These drugs are used to calm patients and treat symptoms of anxiety, insomnia, and stress. These traits make this class of pharmaceuticals likely to be abused. In fact, an enormous black market of illegal, and often adulterated, medication exists. The effects of these drugs are accentuated with the intake of ethanol or other CNS depressants such as opioids. Indeed, many of the fatal overdoses, both from accidental abuse and intentional overdose, occur in combination with other pharmaceuticals. Barbiturates are highly addictive CNS depressants. They generally have been replaced by benzodiazepines in the medical community.

Benzodiazepines bind to the gamma-aminobutyric acid (GABA) receptor, shifting it into a high-affinity state and thereby changing chloride channel activity. GABA is an inhibitory neurotransmitter. The signs and symptoms

TABLE 30-4	Pharmaceutical Poisonings: Sedatives, Hypnotics, Antipsychotics	
Toxin	**Signs and Symptoms**	**Treatment**
Benzodiazepines (alprazolam [Xanax], chlordiazepoxide, clonazepam, diazepam [Valium], Librium, Halcion, Restoril, Dalmane, Centrax, Ativan, Serax) POTENTIAL FOR ABUSE	Drowsiness, staggering gait, slurred speech Respiratory depression Hypotension Hypothermia Dysrhythmias (bradycardia) Coma (unusual)	ABCs Respiratory support Oxygen IV fluids Detailed patient history, especially time of ingestion Activated charcoal (within 1 hour of ingestion) *Antidote:* (severe poisonings) Flumazenil (Romazicon) *(can induce seizure activity)*
Barbiturates (amobarbital, phenobarbital, secobarbital) POTENTIAL FOR ABUSE	Lethargy, drowsiness, staggering gait, slurred speech Emotional volatility Respiratory depression Fixed and dilated pupils Hypotension Fever Shock, coma	ABCs Respiratory support Oxygen IV fluids Detailed patient history, especially time of ingestion Activated charcoal (within 1 hour) Diuretics Alkalization of urine
Antipsychotics (neuroleptics) (chlorpromazine, clozapine, haloperidol [Haldol], thioridazine)	Sedation Miosis Dysrhythmias (more severe in cases of concurrent tricyclic antidepressant poisoning) Hypotension Tachycardia Seizures	ABCs Detailed patient history, especially time of ingestion Activated charcoal (within 1 hour)

ABCs, Airway, breathing, and circulation; *IV,* intravenous.

of these medications are primarily related to CNS depression, including respiratory depression with respiratory arrest. The treatment is mainly supportive. However, the benzodiazepines have the antidote flumazenil. Flumazenil has been known to induce seizures and cardiac arrest in patients taking proconvulsant or prodysrhythmic drugs. For example, a long-term diazepam (Valium) user may have a seizure if given flumazenil. Distinguishing between an overdose and withdrawal symptoms is important. Initial withdrawal symptoms from CNS depressants include anxiety, dizziness, insomnia, nausea and vomiting, tremors, mild tachycardia, and mild hypertension. More severe symptoms include confusion, hallucinations, paranoia, weakness, diaphoresis, myoclonic jerking, and seizures. These signs and symptoms can vary widely among patients and the drug involved.

Cardiovascular Drugs

Heart attack is a leading cause of death in the United States. As a result, cardiac medications are a rapidly growing sector of the pharmaceutical market. The elderly often take these drugs. Because of the arthritic conditions of these patients, the drugs may not always be stored in childproof containers, which increases the risk of accidental poisoning when, for example, grandchildren visit. Several different classes of medications each work on different components of the cardiovascular system. The majority of fatalities occur with calcium channel blockers, beta-blockers, and cardiac glycosides (Table 30-5).

Calcium Channel Blockers. Calcium channel blockers reduce blood pressure by inhibiting the contractility of vascular smooth muscle and coronary vessels, which reduces vascular resistance. They also cause negative chronotropy, negative dromotropy, and negative inotropy in the heart itself. This is accomplished by preventing voltage-gated calcium channels (L-type calcium channels) from opening. The effects on the peripheral vasculature and the heart depend on the type of calcium channel blocker ingested. Phenylalkylamines such as verapamil exhibit all these effects. On the other hand, benzothiaprines such as diltiazem primarily affect the heart, and dihydropyridines such as nifedipine primarily affect the peripheral vasculature. The signs and symptoms of overdose are hypotension, CNS and respiratory

TABLE 30-5 Pharmaceutical Poisonings: Cardiovascular Drugs

Toxin	Signs and Symptoms	Treatment
Calcium channel blockers (verapamil, amlodipine, bepridil, diltiazem, felodipine, isradipine, nicardipine, nifedipine, nimodipine) *[handwritten: Slow down HR ↑ contraction time]*	Sedation Confusion, slurred speech Nausea, vomiting Hypotension Respiratory depression Pulmonary edema Mild hyperglycemia, hyperkalemia Lactic acidosis Cardiac dysrhythmias Atrioventricular dissociation Sinus arrest, bradycardia Coma	ABCs Oxygen Detailed patient history, especially time of ingestion Activated charcoal (within 1 hour) IV fluids Cardiac monitoring Antidysrhythmics and vasopressors may be indicated *Antidote:* calcium chloride, calcium gluconate, atropine, pacing, glucagon, dopamine *[handwritten: 5mg-15mg (not done in field)]*
Beta-blockers (acebutolol, atenolol, betaxolol, esmolol, labetalol, metoprolol, nadolol, pindolol, propranolol, timolol)	Bradycardia Hypotension Respiratory depression Seizures Unconsciousness, coma	ABCs Oxygen Detailed patient history, especially time of ingestion Activated charcoal (within 1 hour of ingestion) IV access Cardiac monitoring *Antidote:* glucagons, calcium chloride, calcium gluconate, atropine, pacing, dopamine
Cardiac glycosides, digitalis glycosides, digoxin, and digitoxin (Lanoxin, Lanoxicaps, Crystodigin, Digicor, Digitaline)	Fatigue Visual disturbances *[handwritten: yellow aura]* Nausea and vomiting GI disturbances, anorexia Dysrhythmias (atrial fibrillation, atrial tachycardia, atrioventricular block, sinus bradycardia, ventricular fibrillation, tachycardia) Hyperkalemia	ABCs Oxygen Detailed patient history, especially time of ingestion Activated charcoal (within 2 hours of ingestion) IV access Cardiac monitoring *Antidote:* digoxin-specific Fab (Digibind, DigiFab)

ABCs, Airway, breathing, and circulation; *IV,* intravenous.

depression, hyperglycemia, syncope, seizures, mental status changes, and cardiac dysrhythmias (except those of ventricular conduction). The treatment includes supportive care, support of blood pressure, activated charcoal administration within 1 hour of intake, vasopressors, antidysrhythmics such as atropine (this may not be effective until after the administration of calcium), pacing, and the antidote calcium. Seizures generally respond to calcium administration; however, if they do not, benzodiazepines can be administered. Glucagon may be considered because it causes unblocked calcium channels to open and promotes calcium release from the sarcoplasmic reticulum. Unlike the standard dose for hypoglycemia, the dose for calcium channel blocker overdose (and beta-blocker overdose as described below) is 5 to 15 mg IV in adults and in 50 mcg/kg in children.

Beta-Blockers. Beta-blockers such as propranolol (Inderal) decrease cardiac output and renin secretion

from the kidneys. This, in turn, leads to lower blood pressure. Thus they are used to treat myocardial infarction (heart attack), unstable angina, and hypertension. Beta-blockers vary greatly in their specificity. Beta$_1$-receptor blocking agents are cardioselective, whereas beta$_1$- and beta$_2$-receptor blocking agents are noncardioselective.

Beta-blockers are rapidly absorbed after ingestion. Therefore rapid administration of activated charcoal is critical. The signs and symptoms vary by drug property. Common effects include hypotension, bradycardia, and cardiac dysrhythmias. Related symptoms include fatigue, dizziness, and shortness of breath. The treatment is similar to that of a calcium channel blocker overdose, including administration of activated charcoal within 1 hour of ingestion, correction of hypotension, vasopressors, antiarrhythmic administration, pacing, calcium administration, and glucagon administration. The dosing of glucagon is the same as previously mentioned for calcium channel blockers; this tends to be more effective in a beta-blocker overdose because the calcium channels are not blocked, allowing for a greater influx of calcium into the cells.

Cardiac Glycosides. Cardiac glycosides are metabolized in the body into a sugar and the active metabolite. These medications typically exert their effect on ion pumps in the cardiac cell membrane. Their primary use is to increase cardiac output; thus they are often used to treat congestive heart failure. The effects of some plant poisonings, such as foxglove leaves, can be attributable to cardiac glycosides.

Digoxin is one of the primary cardiac glycosides used. It has a narrow therapeutic index. In fact, a majority of deaths in 2006 from this medication were therapeutic errors. Digoxin increases intracellular calcium levels and inhibits the sodium-potassium activated adenosine triphosphatase. Together these actions strengthen heart contractions. These effects are seen throughout the heart, including the sinoatrial and atrioventricular nodes and Purkinje fibers. Therefore overdoses can produce almost any cardiac dysrhythmia. The core prehospital treatments include providing supportive measures, including administering activated charcoal within the first hour of intake, monitoring cardiac function, monitoring for signs and symptoms of hyperkalemia, and treating dysrhythmias. Definitive care at the emergency department includes the antidote digoxin-specific FAB (Digibind or DigiFab).

Anticonvulsants

Anticonvulsant drugs are used to treat epilepsy and seizure activity (Table 30-6). The number of such medications available has increased dramatically, as has the number of related poisonings and deaths. Anticonvulsants act in a wide variety of ways. Carbamazepine inhibits sodium channels and glutamate release as well as several CNS receptors. Phenytoin and fosphenytoin inhibit sodium and calcium channels and the sodium-potassium adenosine triphosphatase pump. How valproic acid exerts its effects is still unclear, although it may increase the concentration of the neurotransmitter GABA. Several other anticonvulsants are structurally related to GABA and likely exert their effect on the GABAergic system. The signs and symptoms of poisoning with these medications vary widely. However, CNS depression and respiratory depression are often seen. The treatment is supportive, concentrating on the ABCs. The efficacy of activated charcoal has not been sufficiently explored, but nothing indicates it is ineffective.

Antihistamines

Antihistamines are primarily used to treat cold and allergy symptoms related to runny noses (Table 30-7). They are also potent CNS depressants when taken at higher

TABLE 30-6 Pharmaceutical Poisonings: Anticonvulsants		
Toxin	**Signs and Symptoms**	**Treatment**
Carbamazepine (Tegretol)	Anticholinergic effects Movement disorders Cardiac dysrhythmias (rare) Respiratory depression Hypotension Coma	ABCs Detailed patient history, especially time of ingestion Activated charcoal (within 1 hour) Cardiac monitoring
Phenytoin-hydantoin derivatives (fosphenytoin, phenytoin [Dilantin, Epanutin]) *see a lot here*	Nystagmus Headache Ataxia (fall-related injuries) CNS depression Respiratory depression Coma	ABCs Detailed patient history, especially time of ingestion Activated charcoal (within 1 hour) IV fluids
Valproic acid (Depacon)	Drowsiness CNS depression Respiratory depression Hypotension Hypoglycemia Hypocalcemia Hypernatremia Metabolic acidosis Cerebral edema Coma	ABCs Detailed patient history, especially time of ingestion IV access Activated charcoal (within 1 hour)

ABCs, Airway, breathing, and circulation; *CNS*, central nervous system; *IV*, intravenous.

TABLE 30-7　Pharmaceutical Poisonings: Antihistamines and Asthma Medications

Toxin	Signs and Symptoms	Treatment
Diphenhydramine, hydroxyzine	Sedation Respiratory depression Anticholinergic effects Nausea, vomiting Dry patient (no sweating, dry mouth, flushing) Dilated pupils Hyperthermia Hypotension Cardiac dysrhythmias Seizures	ABCs Detailed patient history, especially time of ingestion Reverse hyperthermia IV fluids Cardiac monitoring Activated charcoal (within 1 hour)
Theophylline (aminophylline, bamifylline [Trentadil], theophylline, oxybutynin)	Agitation, tremors Nausea, vomiting, emesis Diarrhea Hypotension Hypercalcemia Hyperglycemia Clonic posturing Cardiac dysrhythmias (tachycardia) Intracranial hemorrhage Seizures	ABCs Oxygen Detailed patient history, especially time of ingestion IV access Cardiac monitoring Activated charcoal (multiple doses may be beneficial) Seizure precautions Antiemetics

ABCs, Airway, breathing, and circulation; *IV,* intravenous.

dosages. The patient often has anticholinergic signs and symptoms, including dry mouth, lack of sweating, and dilated pupils. Common signs and symptoms include respiratory depression, hyperthermia, hypotension, and cardiac dysrhythmias. The treatment is mainly supportive, focusing on the ABCs.

Asthma Therapies

Theophylline and epinephrine are used to treat breathing difficulty associated with asthma. Theophylline belongs to the xanthine family. It has a narrow therapeutic index and high toxicity. It is one of the few drugs in which therapeutic errors cause a significant percentage of deaths annually. Theophylline is a moderate bronchodilator and has mild antiinflammatory effects. It is a smooth muscle relaxant. Multiple doses of activated charcoal may be beneficial in cases of theophylline poisoning.

Household Products and Industrial Chemicals

[OBJECTIVE 13]

Household products, including cleaning agents and cosmetics, are the leading cause of toxicologic emergencies for adults and children. Fortunately, however, they cause only a small percentage of the total deaths (Table 30-8). In children, household products account for almost 25% of all exposures because of their availability around the house. Advise patients and family members to store household chemicals in locked cabinets to prevent child access. Children should also be educated about the dangers of household chemicals. Old chemicals or ones that are not used often should be disposed of properly, such as dropping them off at a hazardous materials collection center.

PARAMEDIC Pearl

In the event of a poisoning, patients and family members should immediately call 9-1-1 and *then* the Poison Control Center while waiting for the arrival of EMS.

Corrosives

Corrosives are the broad category of chemicals that corrode metal or destroy tissue on contact. Several agencies, such as the U.S. Department of Transportation (DOT) and the Environmental Protection Agency (EPA), define precise parameters for corrosive solutions. The corrosivity of a solution is measured by its pH. The standard pH scale runs from an acidic low of 0 to an alkaline high of 14. Acids have low pH. The DOT defines a strong acid as a solution with a pH less than 2. **Bases** have high pH. The DOT defines a strong base as a solution with a pH greater than 12.5. These pH values are approximate. A solution with a pH of 4 can be extremely damaging to the eyes if it is not immediately removed.

TABLE 30-8 Chemical Poisonings: Household Products and Industrial Chemicals

Toxin	Signs and Symptoms	Treatment
Acids (toilet bowl cleaners, rust removers, drain cleaners, hydrochloric acid, hydrogen chloride, sulfuric acid, phosphoric acid, acetic acid) NOTE: See below for hydrofluoric acid or hydrogen fluoride	Chemical burns Pain at the site of contact Drooling or trouble swallowing (ingestion) Respiratory difficulty (inhalation or aspiration) Shock from bleeding or vomiting	Scene size-up and safety (including rescuer PPE) ABCs External decontamination Internal decontamination (dilution with water if appropriate)
Bases (alkalis, caustics) (drain cleaners, household bleach, ammonia, hypochlorite, lye, sodium hydroxide, potassium hydroxide)	Chemical burns (liquefaction necrosis) Pain at the site of contact Drooling or trouble swallowing (ingestion) Respiratory difficulty (inhalation or aspiration) Shock from bleeding or vomiting	Scene size-up and safety (including rescuer PPE) ABCs External decontamination Internal decontamination (dilution with water if appropriate)
Carbamates (pesticides [e.g., Sevin])	Headache, dizziness Weakness Nausea, vomiting Wet patient (SLUDGE) Miosis Cardiac dysrhythmias Respiratory difficulty	Scene size-up and safety (including rescuer PPE) ABCs Detailed patient history, especially time of ingestion Activated charcoal (within 1 hour) IV fluids Diazepam for seizures *Antidote:* atropine
Carbon monoxide (incomplete combustion byproduct)	Flulike symptoms Headache, confusion Nausea, vomiting Tachypnea Loss of consciousness Coma Death	Scene size-up and safety (including rescuer PPE) ABCs Detailed patient history, especially environmental factors High-flow oxygen IV access Cardiac monitoring Rapid transport Hyperbaric oxygen
Chlorine (gas produced when ammonia reacts with bleach; water treatment plants)	Lacrimation Rhinitis Cough, wheeze Respiratory irritation Shortness of breath Pulmonary edema Respiratory arrest	Scene size-up and safety (including rescuer PPE) ABCs, high-flow oxygen Detailed patient history, especially time of ingestion IV access Nebulized sodium bicarbonate
Cyanide (rodenticide, chrome plating facilities)	Burning sensation in mouth and throat Pulmonary edema Headache, confusion, combativeness Hypertension (followed by shock-associated hypotension) Seizures, coma, death	Scene size-up and safety (including rescuer PPE) Remove patient from area ABCs Rapid administration of antidote *Antidotes:* (1) amyl nitrite and/or sodium nitrite (2) sodium thiosulfate

PPE, Personal protective equipment; *ABCs,* airway, breathing, and circulation; *SLUDGE,* salivation, lacrimation, urination, defecation, gastrointestinal upset, and emesis; *IV,* intravenous.

TABLE 30-8 **Chemical Poisonings: Household Products and Industrial Chemicals**—continued

Toxin	Signs and Symptoms	Treatment
Ethylene glycol (radiator fluid)	*Stage 1:* (1-12 hours after ingestion) CNS effects (slurred speech, ataxia, sleepiness, nausea and vomiting, convulsions, hallucinations, stupor, coma) *Stage 2:* (12-36 hours after ingestion) Cardiopulmonary effects (tachypnea, cyanosis, pulmonary edema, cardiac arrest) *Stage 3:* (24-72 hours after ingestion) Renal system effects (flank pain, oliguria, crystalluria, proteinuria, anuria, hematuria, uremia)	ABCs Detailed patient history, especially time of ingestion Activated charcoal (within 1 hour) IV fluids (volume expanding) Sodium bicarbonate for metabolic acidosis Thiamine and calcium therapy may be necessary Diazepam for seizures *Antidote:* ethanol (30 to 60 mL of 80-proof) or fomepizole Rapid transport for hemodialysis
Hydrocarbons (gasoline, diesel fuel, fuel oil, kerosene, butane, pentane, hexane, industrial solvents, dimethyl sulfoxide [DMSO], halogenated hydrocarbons, tetrahydrofuran, turpentine)	Cough indicates pulmonary injury from aspiration (alveolar instability) CNS depression Altered mental status Respiratory distress Cyanosis Nausea, vomiting Seizures Cardiac dysrhythmias	Scene size-up and safety (including rescuer PPE) ABCs External decontamination Internal decontamination (dilution with water or milk if appropriate) Intubation may be indicated Cardiac monitoring Rapid transport
Hydrofluoric acid (wheel rim cleaner, rust remover; supply for making stained glass windows)	Chemical burns Pain at the site of contact Drooling or trouble swallowing (ingestion) Respiratory difficulty (inhalation or aspiration) Shock from bleeding or vomiting	Scene size-up and safety (including rescuer PPE) ABCs External decontamination Internal decontamination (dilution with water or milk if appropriate) *Antidote:* calcium gluconate and/or calcium chloride
Iron	Hematemesis Bloody diarrhea GI hemorrhage Cardiovascular collapse	ABCs IV access Rapid transport
Isopropanol *Rubbing alcohol*	CNS depression Respiratory depression Abdominal pain, gastritis Hematemesis Hypovolemia Acetonemia, ketonuria	ABCs IV fluids Rapid transport for hemodialysis
Methanol (windshield washer fluid, gasoline additives, glass cleaner)	CNS depression Lethargy, confusion, coma, seizures Nausea and vomiting Abdominal pain Visual problems (photophobia, blurred vision, visual obstructions, slowly reacting pupils, blindness) Metabolic acidosis	ABCs Detailed patient history, especially time of ingestion Activated charcoal and/or gastric lavage (within 1 hour; controversial) IV fluids Bicarbonate for metabolic acidosis *Antidote:* ethanol (30 to 60 mL of 80-proof) or fomepizole Rapid transport for hemodialysis

Continued

TABLE 30-8	Chemical Poisonings: Household Products and Industrial Chemicals—continued	
Toxin	**Signs and Symptoms**	**Treatment**
Methylene chloride (industrial solvent)	Chemical is converted to carbon monoxide in the body	Same as for carbon monoxide
Nitrates and nitrites (hemoglobin oxidizers) (ammonium nitrate fertilizer, nitrous oxide, hydrazine fuels, isoamyl poppers)	Hypotension Methemoglobinemia Cyanosis Respiratory difficulty	*Antidote:* methylene blue
Organophosphates (pesticides)	Headache, dizziness Weakness Nausea, vomiting Wet patient (SLUDGE) Miosis Cardiac dysrhythmias Respiratory difficulty	Scene size-up and safety (including rescuer PPE) ABCs Detailed patient history, especially time of ingestion IV fluids Diazepam for seizures *Antidotes:* atropine and pralidoxime chloride

ABCs, Airway, breathing, and circulation; *CNS*, central nervous system; *IV*, intravenous; *PPE*, personal protective equipment; *GI*, Gastrointestinal; *SLUDGE*, salivation, lacrimation, urination, defecation, gastrointestinal upset, and emesis.

Acids and bases are incompatible, meaning they typically react violently when concentrated solutions come in contact. Heat is usually generated, but toxic gases also form. For example, mixing household bleach (hypochlorite) with an ammonia cleaner generates chlorine gas as well as several other noxious, and potentially fatal, gases. People mix these cleaners more often than you might imagine.

Acids. Acids are everywhere. At home, people use them as cleaning solutions, toilet bowl cleaners, drain openers, metal polishes and cleaners, wheel rim cleaners, and swimming pool treatments, among other uses. They also are found in foods. Vinegar is approximately 5% to 10% acetic acid, and many soft drinks contain phosphoric acid. In industry, acids are used as reagents in chemical plants, catalysts, industrial cleaning agents, and **neutralizing agents.** Sulfuric acid is used in such great quantities that some countries set their gross domestic product by the quantity of sulfuric acid produced and used.

Acids create a chemical burn and coagulative necrosis at the site of contact. The longer the acid remains in contact with the skin, eyes, or GI tract, the more severe the burn will be. External decontamination is quite effective in removing acids. Although acids are considered water reactive, water or soap and water are the most effective decontaminating agents. This is considered a safe practice because a relatively small quantity of acid is being washed away by a large quantity of water. This minimizes the heat generated because the cool water can easily absorb all the heat generated. In fact, you should be aware of inducing hypothermia when decontaminat-

ing patients for an extended period (more than a few minutes). Irrigate the eyes for 15 minutes with water or normal saline. Flush the skin for at least 5 minutes with water. Internal decontamination is more controversial. Emetics should never be used with corrosive ingestions. The emesis would be corrosive and burn the esophagus and mouth on the way up. In addition, the risk of aspirating the corrosive fluid into the lungs is significant. Medical control may advise you to dilute the acid with milk or water.

If decontamination is not rapidly completed, the acid will produce intense pain at the site of contact. The site of contact becomes a necrotic sore, and *eschar* may or may not form depending on the nature of the exposure. Eye exposures produce immediate and severe pain. The thin layer of cells on the cornea is rapidly destroyed, and the acid begins denaturing the **proteins** in the cornea. This may lead to visual impairment. GI damage may include mouth, esophagus, and stomach burns. The severity of the burn depends on the contact time. The stomach is usually most severely affected. The injuries include local burns up to and including ulceration and possible perforation of the stomach or esophagus. The abdominal pain is severe. The acid may be absorbed into the vasculature and cause acidosis.

Hydrofluoric acid, or hydrogen fluoride (HF), is an extremely dangerous acid. It has corrosive properties and causes acute and systemic toxicity. The burns penetrate much deeper than most acids. The fluoride ion has a strong attraction to calcium and magnesium in the body. Dermal burns may show a white or yellow-white precipitate underneath the skin. This is the calcium fluoride salt that forms. Severe HF acid exposure can cause systemic hypocalcemia and hypomagnesemia. Most deaths from HF poisoning are directly caused by cardiac dysrhythmias from hypocalcemia in the cardiac tissue. The antidote for HF poisoning is topical calcium gluconate for skin burns, IV calcium gluconate or calcium chloride for systemic burns (indicated by cardiac dysrhythmias), and eye irrigation with calcium gluconate in normal saline for eye exposure. With approval from medical direction, you should apply calcium gluconate to the burn site repeatedly and continuously (Box 30-2), even after the initial decontamination and treatment, because of the penetrating nature of HF burns. Even patients with minor or suspected HF burns should be transported and evaluated at an appropriate medical facility.

PARAMEDIC*Pearl*

In hydrofluoric acid exposures, avoid giving pain medications. The resolution of pain is the end point of burn treatment with calcium.

Bases. Alkaline materials, also known as **caustics** and **bases**, are as ever present as acids. At home they can be found in toilet bowl cleaners, drain openers, household bleach, and ammonia-based cleaning solutions. In industry they are used as reagents, neutralizing agents, and cleaning solutions.

Like acids, **alkalis** are also corrosive materials. However, the type of burn differs substantially from acid burns. Alkaline burns produce tissue **liquefaction necrosis.** This injury involves the breakdown and dissolution of cell membranes, in essence forming soap. A hallmark of caustic exposure is a slick or slimy feeling to the exposed skin. If the type of corrosive is unknown, this hallmark may indicate which type of burn it is. Pain

often is delayed in these types of exposures. Because bases dissolve the membranes of cells, liquids and solids typically are longer acting and the burns penetrate deeper than acid burns of equal strength. The external decontamination of the exposure site must be rapid and thorough.

Alkaline burns to the stomach are usually more severe than acid burns because the caustic dissolves the protective mucous layer that lines the stomach, increasing the risk of ulceration and perforation.

Ammonia is a widely used and available corrosive and flammable chemical. Farm uses include fertilization; industrial uses include refrigerants (as a liquefied gas) and reagents in chemical processes. In addition to these legitimate uses, ammonia is a chief ingredient in methamphetamine production. An increasing number of injuries occur each year from the illicit possession and use of ammonia. If you respond to an ammonia injury under suspicious circumstances, use the utmost caution. Examples of such calls may include chemical-related injury in the middle of the night in a rural area or a chemical-related injury in a primarily residential area. Law enforcement should secure the scene and the presence of other chemical hazards should be ruled out.

Hydrocarbons

Hydrocarbons are a broad class of combustible or flammable liquids typically derived from oil. These liquids are not water soluble and generally float on water. Hydrocarbons are found in small quantities around the home and in large quantities in industry. At home, people typically have small quantities of gasoline, mineral spirits, paints, and other solvents in their garages or sheds. Industry uses large quantities of hydrocarbons as fuels, solvents, and reagents for chemical processes (especially in the plastics industry).

The toxicity of hydrocarbons varies greatly. In general, hydrocarbons affect the CNS. They are readily absorbed through the skin. They are thought to change the properties (such as fluidity) of cell membranes in CNS neurons as they dissolve in the membrane. Some hydrocarbons cause cancer, whereas others are **protoxins,** which have toxic metabolites. **Volatility,** measured by **vapor pressure,** indicates the degree of risk to the respiratory system. The higher the vapor pressure, the greater the concentration of chemical in the air. This also increases the risk of flammability. You must perform a good scene size-up to determine the level of risk associated with a particular exposure. Many hydrocarbons require specialized personal protective equipment to approach the victim. Use the NIOSH guide to determine the degree of danger a particular hydrocarbon poses to both you and the victim.

The viscosity of the hydrocarbon affects the likelihood of aspiration. Thinner, less-viscous hydrocarbons are more likely to be aspirated than thicker hydrocarbons. For example, gasoline is much more likely to cause pulmonary damage than motor oil. Some hydrocarbon derivatives possess anesthetic properties, like phenol.

BOX 30-2 **Mixing and Using Calcium Jelly in the Field**

1. Request an order from medical direction for this procedure.
2. Carefully decontaminate the burn site with copious amounts of water.
3. Place approximately 3.5 g of calcium gluconate in a small container (avoid using calcium chloride because it may contribute to skin irritation).
4. Add approximately 5 oz of water-soluble jelly (e.g., K-Y Jelly, Johnson & Johnson, New Brunswick, N.J.) to the powder.
5. Mix thoroughly with a tongue depressor.
6. Liberally apply to burn area. Make sure to spread the calcium jelly beyond the visibly burned area because fluoride burns penetrate rapidly.

Phenol burns may therefore go unnoticed for longer periods; this can result in more severe burns with possible systemic effects.

A phenomenon of chemical abuse is known as *huffing.* Abusers intentionally inhale various halogenated or aromatic hydrocarbons for the "high" or euphoria. The onset of these effects is rapid and can induce severe CNS depression and respiratory depression. "Sudden sniffing death syndrome" can occur in intoxicated inhalant abusers when a sudden catecholamine release induces ventricular fibrillation. Common chemicals used by solvent abusers are chlorinated hydrocarbons, fluorocarbons, toluene, acetone, propane, and butane (Anderson & Loomis, 2003).

The signs and symptoms vary greatly depending on the specific properties of the hydrocarbon, the route of entry, and the amount of the chemical (Box 30-3). Fortunately most hydrocarbon poisonings are not serious. In fact, less than 1% require medical intervention. However, several extremely dangerous and deadly hydrocarbons and hydrocarbon derivatives exist. You must observe the patient and determine the identity of the hydrocarbon and the amount ingested. In general the most pronounced effects are on the CNS. Activated charcoal does not effectively bind all hydrocarbons. However, studies have shown it effectively binds kerosene and turpentine. Gastric lavage may be indicated in patients who have ingested camphor, halogenated hydrocarbons, aromatic hydrocarbons, heavy metals containing hydrocarbons, or pesticides containing hydrocarbons (the CHAMP mnemonic). Avoid the use of sympathomimetic drugs, such as epinephrine, in patients with hydrocarbon intoxication. These drugs may induce ventricular fibrillation in the catecholamine-sensitized heart.

Pesticides and Nerve Agents

Organophosphates and **carbamates** are two classes of widely used pesticides. They are found in insect sprays as a liquid and in rose-dusting formulations as a solid and can be applied as a mist over larger areas. The dangers these agents pose vary widely depending on the chemical structure of the pesticide and the carrier in which the pesticide is dissolved. Most of these pesticides are not water soluble and are dissolved in a hydrocarbon solvent that acts as a carrier. These two characteristics make most of them highly absorbent by the skin. The household formulations are typically more dilute, and the chemical agents in them often are not as potent. Commercially available pesticides, however, can be highly concentrated and deadly. Organophosphates and carbamates are well absorbed by ingestion, absorption, and inhalation depending on the volatility of the pesticide. However, most of the organophosphate pesticides are designed to be toxic by ingestion or contact, rather than poisonous by inhalation, to reduce the risk to the applicator.

Organophosphates were produced during World War II in Germany as nerve agents for chemical warfare. They were originally used in agriculture as pesticides. Nerve agents and organophosphate pesticides are quite similar. Nerve agents have been optimized for human toxicity, whereas pesticides have been optimized for the target pest toxicity (e.g., wasps, aphids). Nerve agents also vary in their designed battlefield use. For example, the G agents developed in Germany were comparatively volatile. If the wind conditions were not the best, they had a tendency to drift back toward the direction from which they came, injuring and possibly killing the user. To avoid this result, in the 1950s the British developed VX, which has a much lower volatility. VX is a contact poison (absorption), whereas most of the G agents are inhalation poisons.

Organophosphates, nerve agents, and carbamates all act on the acetylcholine nerve signaling system (cholinergic system). The nerve signal travels along the neuron through an electrochemical mechanism. This system stops at synapses, the junctions between neurons. At the synapse, a chemical neurotransmitter, in this case acetylcholine, must be released from the neuron and travel across the junction. At the target, acetylcholine binds to the cholinergic receptor and the electrochemical pulse continues in the next neuron or contraction starts in the muscle. Once the signal has been transmitted, the neurotransmitter must be removed. **Enzymes** are proteins that carry out vital metabolic processes and can be considered the workhorses of the cell. Acetylcholinesterase is the enzyme that breaks down the neurotransmitter acetylcholine into acetate and choline after the impulse has been transmitted. Organophosphates inhibit the enzyme acetylcholinesterase.

The signs and symptoms of organophosphate and carbamate poisoning are the same. Primarily, you will notice the "wet" patient presenting with SLUDGEM symptoms, as previously described. This is one of the stronger differential diagnoses. Other symptoms include nonspecific flulike symptoms early. In addition to the SLUDGEM symptoms, sweating and muscle fasciculations (twitching) are common. Severe poisoning can lead to respira-

---

| BOX 30-3 | Recognition of Inhalant Abuse (Huffing) |

Solvent abuse typically does not present with unique clinical findings. To uncover solvent abuse, you must maintain a high index of suspicion in the presence of the following:

- Solvent stains on skin (especially fingers, nose, and mouth) and clothing
- Irritation or sores around the mouth
- Solvent odor on the breath (such as a toluene or gasoline-like smell)
- Altered level of consciousness (dazed, disoriented, or clumsy appearance)
- Red eyes
- Runny nose
- Difficulty sleeping and/or memory loss (chronic abuse)

tory arrest. You must consider airway management a priority because of the increased bronchial secretions and muscle paralysis associated with the cholinergic effects.

However, the organophosphates and carbamates inhibit acetylcholinesterase in slightly different ways. The organophosphates and nerve agents contain an organic phosphate group but the carbamates do not. The phosphate portion of the pesticide binds to the acetylcholinesterase, and when the enzyme tries to break the organophosphate in half, it cannot. The phosphate portion gets stuck and the acetylcholinesterase is out of commission. How quickly the enzyme cuts the organophosphate and forms what is known as a *covalent complex* is the aging time of the agent. The shorter the aging time, the faster the antidote (particularly pralidoxime [2-PAM]), must be administered.

The antidotes for organophosphate poisoning are atropine and 2-PAM. The atropine treats the wet symptoms and the 2-PAM reactivates acetylcholinesterase. To be most effective, you should administer 2-PAM before the aging process occurs. In contrast, carbamates, such as the pesticide Sevin (Bayer CropScience, Research Triangle Park, N.C.), do not contain an organophosphate group but can still bind to the acetylcholinesterase enzyme. Because carbamates do not have an organophosphate group, they do not require 2-PAM as an antidote, only atropine to dry out the patient.

Carbon Monoxide

Carbon monoxide poisoning usually occurs in the home when heating or cooking appliances, such as the furnace, fireplace, outdoor grill, or gas-fueled oven, malfunction or are used improperly. Although pure carbon monoxide is a colorless and odorless gas, when it is the product of incomplete combustion odors of other substances may be noticeable. Advise patients and family members to make sure that heating and cooking appliances are properly maintained and in good working condition. Industrial carbon monoxide poisonings also can occur but are rarer. Carbon monoxide is used in suicide attempts as well. Symptoms of carbon monoxide poisoning mimic flulike symptoms in the early stages. The symptoms then progress to hypoxia and red, flushed skin.

Carbon monoxide has a high affinity for hemoglobin. Hemoglobin binds carbon monoxide 200 times stronger than oxygen, which is difficult to displace from hemoglobin. Poisoning typically requires treatment with 100% oxygen in a hyperbaric chamber. The treatment in the field is high-flow oxygen, supportive care, and rapid transport to the hospital.

Methemoglobinemia

Compounds such as nitrites and nitrates, which can oxidize the iron in hemoglobin, cause the condition known as **methemoglobinemia.** These types of poisonings can be caused by a number of different chemicals. The overuse of some medications, such as nitroglycerin, nitroprusside, and benzocaine sprays, can cause methemoglobinemia. In rural areas, biologic processes (fermentation) can create nitrites after silos are filled with grain. Peak toxicity occurs approximately 1 week after being filled. Agricultural groundwater contamination with fertilizers such as ammonium nitrate can cause methemoglobinemia in infants, called *"blue baby" syndrome.*

The effects of nitrate and nitrite poisoning include hypotension, dizziness, headache, nausea and vomiting, confusion, cerebral ischemia, cyanosis from methemoglobin production, cardiovascular collapse, and asphyxiation. The symptoms of methemoglobinemia include a slate-gray cyanosis, respiratory distress, and altered levels of consciousness, including anxiety, confusion, and stupor.

The antidote to methemoglobinemia is methylene blue, a thiazide dye. It can reduce the methemoglobin to hemoglobin by helping a second enzyme, diaphorase II, accomplish its job. Paradoxically, at higher concentrations methylene blue can act as an oxidizing agent because it must first be converted to its bioactive form (leukomethylene blue) in the body, and at higher dosages the body cannot keep up with the conversion process. Methylene blue could be called a *pro-antidote.* One contraindication of methylene blue is glucose-6-phosphate dehydrogenase (G6PD) deficiency. G6PD supplies a vital cofactor (nicotinamide adenine dinucleotide) to the enzyme involved in the activation process (diaphorase II).

Methylene blue as an antidote was discovered by Dr. Cawein in the Appalachian mountains of Kentucky in the early 1960s. The "Kentucky blue people," as they were known, have a mutation in the enzyme known as diaphorase I, which converts ferric methemoglobin back to ferrous hemoglobin. Oxygen and other oxidizers naturally convert a small percentage of hemoglobin to methemoglobin on an ongoing basis. Diaphorase enzymes have evolved to deal with this constant threat, and people with active enzymes do not succumb to even mild methemoglobinemia. Affected individuals of this population have a blue hue to their skin, similar to cyanosis. The bluish skin color was not from cyanosis associated with oxygen deprivation, but was imparted by the methemoglobin, which is a dark bluish-brown color.

Cyanides

Cyanides are prevalent in industrialized society. In the home they are found in silver polish, seeds of fruits (e.g., apples, peaches, cherries), and rodenticides. They are used in industry as reagents in processes such as electroplating and plastics manufacturing. They are found as solids, liquids, and gases. Acrylonitrile, which is converted to cyanide in the body, is a precursor to nitrile polymers, which are used in medical gloves you may currently use. Because of the large amount of plastics in homes, combustion gases from residential fires contain an increasing amount of cyanide gas. Studies show that a significant number of smoke inhalation victims have cyanide poisoning. Furthermore, studies suggest that a new investigational cyanide antidote (hydroxocobalamin) may be useful in smoke inhalation victims (Alcorta, 2004). Cyanide poisoning also can occur in patients on long-term nitroprusside therapy. Cyanide is a frequently used chemical for suicide attempts. Because of the fast-acting nature of the toxin, intentional cyanide poisoning often is fatal.

Inhalation of cyanide gas or powdered cyanide salt produces corrosive hydrocyanic acid on contact with moisture in the respiratory tract. This produces irritation and burning at the site of contact. Significant inhalation also produces pulmonary edema. Cyanide is a systemic chemical asphyxiant. Ingestion, absorption, or inhalation affect all tissues in the body.

The cyanide ion is a potent toxin at the cellular level. It binds to two proteins in the body, cytochrome oxidase and hemoglobin. Both proteins are involved in the respiratory cycle. As you know, hemoglobin transports oxygen to the cell and returns carbon dioxide to the lungs. Cytochrome oxidase is critical to the process of using oxygen to produce energy, called *oxidative phosphorylation*. Both hemoglobin and cytochrome oxidase contain iron atoms. Each protein contains a different type of iron. Hemoglobin normally contains the ferrous form of iron, which binds oxygen well. The iron of cytochrome oxidase is in the ferric state. Cyanide preferentially binds to the ferric form of iron. Few cytochrome oxidase proteins are present in each cell compared with the amount of hemoglobin circulating in the blood. This forms the basis of the two-part antidote treatment. The first part, amyl nitrite and sodium nitrite, is aimed at converting ferrous hemoglobin into ferric methemoglobin, which has a much higher affinity for cyanide. This induces a mild case of methemoglobinemia. In essence, plentiful hemoglobin is sacrificed for the scarce cytochrome oxidase. The second part of the antidote, sodium thiosulfate, complexes the cyanide into the nontoxic thiocyanate ion, which is easily eliminated.

Sulfides

Sulfides, such as hydrogen sulfide, are deadly liquids and gases. Hydrogen sulfide is involved in a large number of deaths that result from improper confined space entries and industrial accidents that involve chemical incompatibilities and the transport and use of sulfides. Several fatalities have occurred when two incompatible chemicals have been mixed and deadly hydrogen sulfide gas is generated. Below-grade confined space fatalities also occur when the entrants are overcome by hydrogen sulfide and cannot evacuate. The tragedy is magnified when would-be rescuers climb in after them and succumb as well. You must be aware of your surroundings and do a proper scene size-up when responding to possible hydrogen sulfide exposures. You should never retrieve a patient from a potentially contaminated area without chemical protective clothing, including respiratory protection. Hydrogen sulfide has a rotten egg–like odor.

However, **olfactory fatigue** sets in quickly, lulling the victim and would-be rescuer into a false sense of security. Olfactory fatigue is the loss of the sense of smell on exposure to a chemical.

Sulfides bind and inactivate various proteins vital to cell function, especially proteins containing ferric-heme, such as cytochrome oxidase. Therefore, biochemically, sulfide toxicity is quite similar to cyanide toxicity. Hydrogen sulfide is an even more powerful cellular asphyxiant than hydrogen cyanide. The signs and symptoms of sulfide poisoning are similar to cyanide poisoning and include dizziness, loss of consciousness, nausea and vomiting, respiratory tract irritation, pulmonary edema, CNS depression, respiratory distress, and seizures. Anaerobic metabolism then leads to metabolic acidosis in severe exposures.

The treatment for sulfide poisoning is primarily supportive, especially high-flow oxygen. However, sulfides, like cyanides, have an increased affinity for oxidized ferric methemoglobin over ferrous hemoglobin. The sulfur can then bind to the methemoglobin, forming sulfhemoglobin. Therefore amyl and/or sodium nitrite is an antidote to sulfide poisoning. Thiosulfate is not indicated because no comparable nontoxic metabolite to the thiocyanate ion exists. The difficulty with hydrogen sulfide toxicity is how rapidly it finds its way to the cytochrome oxidase. In practice, the administration of the antidote often is too late.

Alcohols

Alcohols are ever present in most people's lives. Ethanol, ethylene glycol, methanol, and isopropanol are the most common alcohols involved in toxicologic emergencies. They are reviewed in the approximate order of exposures and/or fatalities. Ethylene glycol and methanol are **protoxins** that are processed by the body to form toxins. Both are primarily processed by the same liver enzyme that disposes of ethanol, alcohol dehydrogenase. Unlike ethanol, which is processed into a usable fuel (hence the weight gain associated with the consumption of alcoholic beverages), ethylene glycol and methanol are processed into toxic compounds.

Ethanol. Among the alcohols, ethanol causes the most toxicologic emergencies because of its availability and classification as a food. More than 44,000 ethanol exposures were reported in 2006, with 10 fatalities caused by alcohol poisoning. Ethanol-containing substances, excluding alcoholic beverages, accounted for another 28,000 reported exposures with no fatalities. Most ethanol exposures are classified as intentional because they involve alcoholic beverages. Chronic alcohol abuse is examined later in this chapter. Ethanol is not a particularly toxic chemical, as demonstrated by its licensed use in alcoholic beverages such as beer, wine, and distilled spirits.

The signs and symptoms of toxic ingestion include euphoria, inebriation, confusion, lethargy, CNS depression, ataxia (and associated injuries from falls), stupor, respiratory depression, hypothermia, hypotension, coma, cardiovascular collapse, and death. The treatment is mainly supportive and includes maintaining the ABCs and IV access.

Ethylene Glycol.

Ethylene glycol is most commonly encountered in automotive antifreeze. It has a sweet taste and is therefore more likely to be ingested in larger quantities by children and pets. However, 70% of ethylene glycol–induced poisonings occur in adults and are mostly accidental. A total of 5343 ethylene glycol exposures were reported in 2006, with 17 fatalities. The primary route of ethylene glycol exposure is ingestion. It has a low vapor pressure and is not readily absorbed through the skin.

Ethylene glycol is metabolized into glycolic and oxalic acids, which cause most of the significant toxicity. The oxalic acid sequesters and binds calcium in the body to form calcium oxalate, which precipitates out and forms crystals. This has two detrimental effects. First, it causes hypocalcemia, with the possibility of cardiac dysrhythmias. Second, it causes severe joint pain at the sites of crystal deposition. The liver and kidneys can receive significant damage from the oxalic acid.

Toxicity occurs in three stages (see Table 30-8). The signs and symptoms include intoxication, headache, CNS depression, respiratory difficulty, metabolic acidosis, cardiovascular collapse, renal failure, seizures, and coma. The treatment consists of maintaining the ABCs and administering either ethanol or fomepizole as an antidote. Ethanol and fomepizole are both competitive inhibitors of alcohol dehydrogenase. You may use cofactor therapy consisting of pyridoxine and thiamine to assist the metabolism of ethylene glycol.

Methanol.

Methanol (wood alcohol) is a common household solvent. It is a component of windshield washer fluid, gasoline treatments, paints, and canned tabletop fuels (e.g., Sterno). Methanol is extensively used in industry as a solvent and reagent. More than 2000 methanol exposures were reported in 2006, with eight fatalities. Methanol is absorbed through the skin, but not very well. Methanol is readily inhaled because of its high volatility. Moreover, it has been ingested as an ethanol substitute.

Methanol is metabolized into formaldehyde, which is a short-lived intermediate toxin, by the enzyme alcohol dehydrogenase. Formaldehyde is then converted into formic acid, which causes most of the significant toxicity. The formic acid can cause metabolic acidosis and blindness. The signs and symptoms include sedation, ataxia, headache, vertigo, nausea and vomiting, abdominal pain, respiratory difficulty, blurred vision, seizures, and coma. The onset of symptoms can be rapid (30 minutes) or delayed up to 72 hours depending on the dose and route of entry. The treatment consists of maintaining the ABCs and administering either ethanol or fomepizole as an antidote. Ethanol and fomepizole are both competitive inhibitors of alcohol dehydrogenase. You can use cofactor therapy consisting of tetrahydrofolate to assist in the elimination of formic acid.

Isopropanol.

Isopropanol (rubbing alcohol) also is a common household and industrial solvent. It is involved in many exposures. Approximately 8000 isopropanol exposures were reported in 2006, with four fatalities.

Isopropanol is metabolized into acetone, which is not very toxic. Isopropyl alcohol toxicity is similar to ethanol toxicity in scope. Large ingestions can cause acetonemia (acetone buildup in the blood) and ketonuria (ketone buildup in the urine). The signs and symptoms include confusion, lethargy, CNS depression, respiratory depression, ketonemia, mild hypothermia, hypotension, and coma. You may notice that the patient has a fruity breath odor, similar to that of a diabetic, because of acetone production. Field treatment is mainly supportive, including maintaining ABCs and IV access. Significant exposures may need to be treated with hemodialysis in the hospital.

Metals and Heavy Metals

Overdose with heavy metals is uncommon and rarely fatal. The difficulties with metal and heavy metal poisoning are the varied effects on the body and the differing signs and symptoms. Some metals bind certain proteins preferentially, whereas others bind a wide range of proteins. This leads to both target organ–specific effects as well as systemic effects. Some heavy metals have acute effects and others have latent effects. Unfortunately, most metal poisonings have the most pronounced effects on developing infants and children.

Iron.

Iron overdose occurs more often because it is a mineral used in supplements and vitamin formulations. A total of 3953 toxicologic exposures to iron were reported in 2006, with no fatalities. Most iron exposures occur in children younger than 6 years. Symptoms of iron toxicity occur when more than 20 mg/kg are ingested. Determining the amount of iron intake in overdoses is important.

Iron is an essential mineral and vital component of several proteins, including hemoglobin. A person absorbs roughly 10% of the available iron in the small intestine. Iron can be toxic to the stomach lining in high doses. Supplements that contain iron tend to form concretions, or bezoars, in the GI tract, which may cause hemorrhaging, bloody vomitus (hematemesis), and bloody diarrhea. Significant ingestion can cause cardiovascular collapse and death within 12 to 48 hours.

Lead and Mercury.

Lead and mercury, although heavily regulated in recent years, are still present in the environment. Lead paint was used for many years until it was banned in 1978. In older buildings lead paint is still present, often under several coats of lead-free paint. Infants and children tend to put anything they can get a hold of in their mouths, and paint chips typically are small enough to swallow. Therefore long-term lead poisoning is most common in children. Advise patients and family members that lead-based paint in older houses should be well maintained. Any paint chips should be removed by scraping (not sanding), and lead-based paint should be covered with a fresh coat of nontoxic paint.

Mercury is found in many consumer products, from fluorescent bulbs and mercury thermometers to mercury switches in thermostats, electronics, and automobiles. Mercury poisoning is more common among adults because it is not as readily available to children.

Symptoms of long-term exposure include neurologic deficit. The symptoms of acute exposure vary. The treatment for heavy metal poisonings is mainly supportive. Definitive treatment consists of administering chelating agents. **Chelating agents** bind single-atom ions. These agents are generally not specific and tend to remove essential electrolytes such as potassium, sodium, calcium, and magnesium at the same time. Therefore chelation therapy must be accompanied by rigorous blood analysis and electrolyte therapy. As the paramedic, your primary role is to recognize the signs and symptoms of metal exposure and encourage follow-up evaluation at a medical facility. Early recognition of lead or mercury poisoning in children is vital to normal development and growth.

Arsenic. Arsenic has three oxidation states that lead to a variety of toxicologic effects. Arsenic can be found naturally in ground water. It also can be leached from manmade sources, such as treated lumber decks. Treated lumber contains chromated copper arsenate (CCA). Advise patients that working with CCA-treated wood, especially cutting and sanding, can create significant exposure hazards. The proper personal protective equipment must be worn and sawdust should be disposed of properly. Arsine gas is a hemolytic agent found in industry, especially the semiconductor industry. It is a potent inhalation hazard.

Arsenic manifests its toxicity by binding to various proteins vital to cell functions, such as glycolysis and the Krebs cycle. Arsine hemolysis is caused by an unknown mechanism. The signs and symptoms of acute arsenic exposure are acute GI illness, nausea and vomiting, diarrhea, lethargy, weakness, dehydration, severe anemia (arsine exposure), and renal failure. Long-term arsenic poisoning may manifest itself through skin lesions, malaise, weakness, metallic taste, headache, confusion, and neuropathy. Field treatment of these patients is mainly supportive, focusing on the ABCs. Activated charcoal is ineffective. Chelating agents such as dimercaprol are the definitive treatment in the hospital setting.

Wildlife

[OBJECTIVE 14]
Wildlife accounted for 82,133 toxicologic emergencies in 2006, yet only seven people died. The mortality rate is therefore extremely low. The **venoms** associated with wildlife vary greatly. The toxic effects can be local or systemic, immediate or delayed. Often they are a mixture of effects because of the delivery of a mixture of venoms into the injection site. The following paragraphs describe four categories of envenomations: insects, spiders, snakes, and marine animals (Table 30-9).

Insects (Hymenoptera)

Insects have a wide variety of venoms, including polypeptides, proteins, and small molecules such as histamines, serotonin, acetylcholine, and dopamine. Most severe insect envenomations result from either allergic reaction that leads to anaphylactic shock or from multiple bites or stings. Bees, wasps, and hornets accounted for 9333 reported exposures in 2006. Most insects can sting multiple times and do so until removed from contact. Honeybees are the only insects that sting only once because they leave the stinger behind. Fatalities usually occur in children or small individuals from multiple stings. Deaths have been reported from yellow jackets, fire ants, and the Africanized honeybee, which has moved into the southwest United States from South America. Fire ant venom is an alkaloid that produces necrosis at the site of contact. Multiple bites can produce systemic effects.

Symptoms of insect envenomation include localized pain, redness, swelling, and wheals at the site of injection. The treatment is mainly supportive, although the honeybee stinger should be promptly removed to stop further envenomation. Remove it by scraping the stinger away. Do not try to remove the stinger by pinching or squeezing it with forceps; this will only empty the venom sac into the wound. Wash the area and apply a cold pack to the injection site. Observe the patient for signs of anaphylactic shock, a life-threatening complication. Some patients carry epinephrine in the form of an EpiPen. When treating anaphylactic shock, try to determine whether any epinephrine has already been given before your arrival.

Spiders, Scorpions, and Ticks (Arachnida)

Spiders and scorpions are eight-legged creatures (Figure 30-1). Most spiders are harmless to human beings, but three poisonous varieties exist in the United States. Most spider bites occur from April to October.

Black Widow Spider. The black widow spider lives in all parts of the continental United States and accounted for 2522 reported exposures and no deaths in 2006. They are usually found outdoors under cover in wood piles, brush, sheds, and garages. These spiders may hitchhike into the home on outdoor storage items such as firewood or Christmas trees. The female black widow can be recognized by the bulbous, black, shiny abdomen with a red hourglass marking on the ventral side of the abdomen. It is usually an inch or less in length (see Figure 30-1, *A*). The venom is a potent neurotoxin. The male black widow is brown, approximately half the size, and nonvenomous.

The signs and symptoms include immediate and severe localized pain, redness, and swelling (papule formation) at the site of envenomation. The patient may describe the bite as a bee sting–like sensation. You may observe

TABLE 30-9 **Poisonings: Wildlife**

Toxin	Signs and Symptoms	Treatment
Honeybee (European bee and Africanized honeybee [killer bee])	Local pain, itching Swelling, edema Anaphylactic shock Headache, weakness Nausea, vomiting Respiratory distress Respiratory failure Renal failure	ABCs Rapid removal of stinger Ice pack to bite site Detailed patient history, including allergies Analgesics *Anaphylactic shock:* IV access Epinephrine (EpiPen) Rapid transport
Wasps, yellow jackets, fire ants	Local pain, itching Swelling, edema Anaphylactic shock Headache, weakness Nausea, vomiting Respiratory distress Respiratory failure Renal failure	ABCs Ice pack to bite site Detailed patient history, including allergies Analgesics
Black widow spider	Severe pain at bite site Swelling at bite site Piloerection Diaphoresis Tachycardia Hypertension Fever, hyperthermia Muscle spasms Abdominal pain	ABCs Detailed patient history, including identification Ice pack to bite site IV access Cardiac monitoring *Antidote:* antivenin
Brown recluse spider	*Local:* itchiness at bite site Erythema, edema Papule formation Necrotic lesion Bull's-eye rash *Systemic:* fever, chills Malaise, weakness Nausea, vomiting Rash Seizures Hypotension Disseminated intravascular coagulation	ABCs Detailed patient history, including identification IV fluids
Bark (sculptured) scorpion	*Mild:* local pain *Severe:* pulmonary edema Neuromotor hyperactivity Respiratory distress	ABCs Oxygen Ice pack to bite site Detailed patient history, including identification IV access Rapid transport *Antidote:* antivenin

Continued

TABLE 30-9 Poisonings: Wildlife—continued		
Toxin	**Signs and Symptoms**	**Treatment**
Pit vipers (Western rattlesnake, pigmy rattlesnake, Massasauga rattlesnake, water moccasin [cottonmouth], copperhead)	Fang marks Localized swelling, pain Weakness Diaphoresis Nausea, vomiting Paresthesia Edema (severe) Ecchymosis (severe) Shock	Scene safety ABCs Detailed patient history, including identification Cardiac monitoring Clean wound Immobilize extremity Rapid transport *Antidote:* antivenin
Coral snake	Slurred speech Dilated pupils Dysphagia Flaccid paralysis Respiratory failure	Scene safety ABCs Detailed patient history, including identification Cardiac monitoring Clean wound Immobilize extremity Rapid transport
Marine animals	Intense local pain Redness and swelling Lacerations (especially with stingrays) Nausea and vomiting Weakness Dyspnea Tachycardia Hypotension	ABCs Detailed patient history, including identification Remove stinging cells or spines Apply 110°-113° F heat to the site Cardiac monitoring

ABCs, Airway, breathing, and circulation; *IV,* intravenous.

two small fang marks 1 mm apart. The immediate effects progress to muscle spasms, abdominal rigidity in the absence of tenderness, and severe pain. The systemic effects include nausea and vomiting, diaphoresis (sweating), decreased levels of consciousness, seizures, and paralysis. The prehospital treatment is mainly supportive. Muscle spasms can be treated with muscle relaxants such as diazepam or calcium gluconate. Monitor and aggressively treat hypertension because hypertensive crisis is possible. **Antivenin** is available, so identification of the spider and rapid transport of the patient are important.

Brown Recluse Spider. The brown recluse spider lives in warmer climates, including the southern, Midwestern, and southwestern United States and Hawaii. Most envenomations occur in the south central region of the United States; this spider accounted for 1900 reported exposures and no deaths in 2006. The brown recluse lives in dark and dry locations, including houses. It is a tan to brown color. The body can be up to three quarters of an inch in length, with a characteristic violin-shaped marking on the back (it also is known as the *violin* or *fiddle-back spider*). Another identifying feature is six eyes (three pairs) arranged in a semicircle instead of the normal eight eyes of most spiders (see Figure 30-1, *B*). The venom is a cock-

tail of at least 11 peptides that possess a variety of cytotoxic properties.

Brown recluse venom is necrotic and produces a classic bull's-eye appearance around the injection site (see Figure 30-1, *F*). The bite is usually painless, and many envenomations occur at night while the victim is sleeping. The bite initially begins as a small blister (papule), possibly surrounded by a white halo. Over the next 24 hours localized pain, redness, and swelling develop. Over the next few days to weeks tissue necrosis develops at the site, and redness and swelling begin to spread. Because of the necrosis, the wound often is slow to heal and may be visible months after the bite. Systemic symptoms include malaise, chills, fever, nausea and vomiting, and joint pain. Life-threatening symptoms can include bleeding disorders such as disseminated intravascular coagulation and hemolytic anemia. The treatment is supportive because no approved antivenin is available. Clean and dress the wound, apply a cold compress, and transport the patient for medical evaluation.

Scorpions. More than 16,000 reported scorpion stings occurred in 2006, with no fatalities. More than 600 species of scorpion live in the United States. However, only the bark, or sculptured, scorpion of the southwestern states is dangerous to human beings. Scorpions are

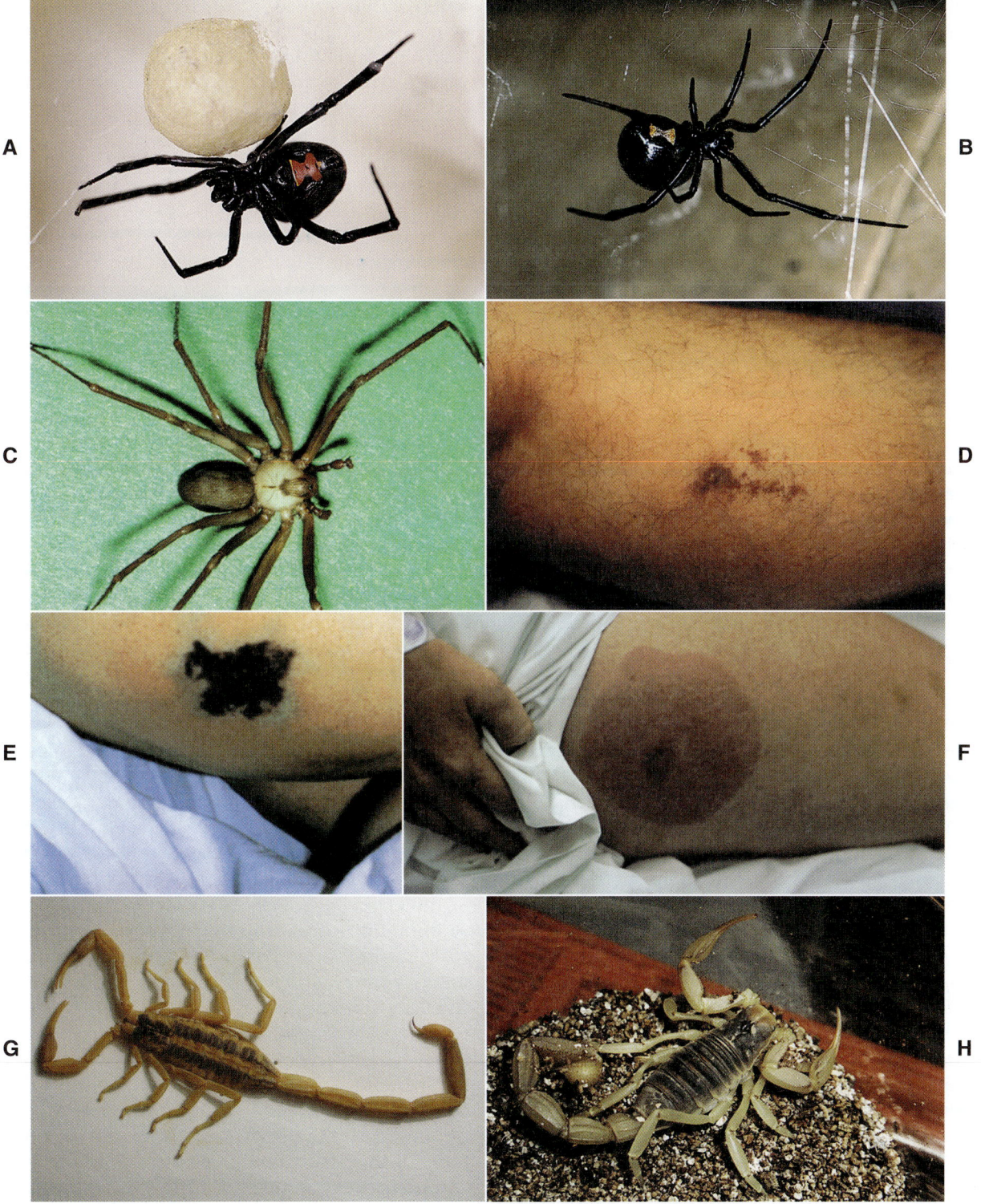

Figure 30-1 Common poisonous Arachnida found in North America. **A** and **B,** Black widow spider. Note the red hourglass marking on the ventral side of the abdomen. **C,** Brown recluse spider. Note the violin-shaped marking on the top of the head (cephalothorax). **D,** The bite of a brown recluse spider after 6 hours, 24 hours **(E),** and 48 hours **(F). G,** Striped scorpion found in the Southwest and central United States. **H,** The giant hairy scorpion found in the Southwest United States.

nocturnal and hide underneath objects and buildings during the day. Scorpions may wander into dwellings, especially at night. They are yellowish-brown, may be striped, and are approximately 1 to 3 inches long (see Figure 30-1, *G* and *H*). The sculptured scorpion is active from April to August and hibernates during the winter. They inject venom located in a bulb at the base of a stinger located on the end of the tail. They generally inject only a small amount of poison.

The bark scorpion venom is a neurotoxin. It initially produces a burning or tingling sensation followed by numbness. The toxin is a mixture of proteins and polypeptides that affect voltage-dependent ion channels, especially sodium channels, in nerve signaling. Specifically, it acts to release acetylcholine at the presynaptic terminal of neuromuscular junctions, depolarizing the junction. A secondary effect of the cocktail is CNS stimulation through sympathetic neurons. The systemic effects can include slurred speech, restlessness, salivation, abdominal cramping, nausea and vomiting, muscle fasciculations (twitching), and seizures. The symptoms typically reach their peak within 5 hours of injection. If redness and swelling are present at the injection site, the perpetrator was most likely not a bark scorpion because its venom does not induce localized inflammation.

Treatment of the patient begins with managing the ABCs and calming the patient. Supportive care should be provided for respiratory depression. Clean the wound, apply a cold compress, and immobilize the appendage, including the fingers and toes. You may place a constricting band over the site of envenomation to restrict lymphatic flow only if transport times are long. This technique is controversial and should not be confused with a tourniquet. The band should be at least 2 inches wide and should not be tighter than a watchband. It should be similar in pressure to an elastic bandage used for a sprained ankle. Avoid administration of analgesics because they may exacerbate respiratory symptoms. Provide rapid transport to the hospital because antivenin may be available, especially in Arizona.

Ticks. Ticks disseminate diseases such as Rocky Mountain spotted fever and Lyme disease. A prolonged bite by the female wood tick can lead to a rare condition known as *tick paralysis*. This is caused by a slow-acting neurotoxin secreted from the salivary glands of the tick. The symptoms usually begin within 6 days after the tick attaches to the patient. The symptoms include restlessness and itching (paresthesia) of the hands and feet. A flaccid, symmetric paralysis, which starts in the feet and progresses up the body, can develop over the next few days. Respiratory paralysis may ensue. A tick bite is important to diagnose. This helps distinguish this toxicologic emergency from other medical emergencies. The differential diagnosis also hinges on the symmetrical paralysis (rather than asymmetrical) and a progression from the feet upwards. The treatment consists of removing the tick and treating the neurologic symptoms.

Remove the tick with forceps, as close to the skin surface as possible and with steady pressure. Avoid crushing the tick, which may cause infection of the wound. Clean the wound with soap and water and dress it. Undiagnosed tick paralysis can be fatal.

Snakes

Poisonous snakes can be found in the continental United States and Alaska (Figure 30-2). Two poisonous families are native: (1) the Crotalidae (pit vipers), which include rattlesnakes (including the pigmy and Massasauga varieties), cottonmouths (water moccasins), and copperheads, and (2) the Elapidae (coral snakes). Within these two classifications were slightly more than 3000 reported venom exposures and four fatalities in 2006. An additional 1739 bites were reported from nonpoisonous domestic snakes, nonpoisonous exotic snakes, and poisonous exotic snakes, with no fatalities. Many more nonpoisonous bites were likely not reported. The snake venom toxicity and mode of action vary by family.

Pit Vipers. Pit vipers are named after a distinctive pit located on each side of the snake's head in the maxillary bone. They have triangular heads, vertical elliptical pupils, and large fangs (see Figure 30-2, *A*, *B*, and *C*). Pit vipers mainly use their venom to disable and paralyze small prey, not as a defensive weapon. Approximately 25% of pit viper bites are dry, meaning they contain little or no venom. The more severe the symptoms, the more venom was injected.

Pit viper venom contains a hydrolytic cocktail. This cocktail produces tissue necrosis at the site of envenomation and can produce systemic effects such as red blood cell destruction. These effects can lead to hemolysis, clotting defects, intravascular coagulation, and renal failure. Severe bites can kill within 30 minutes, primarily because of the effects of shock. The venom is used by the snake to immobilize and digest small prey.

The signs and symptoms include distinctive fang marks with swelling, redness, and pain at the injection site. The systemic effects include thirst, sweating, chills, weakness, dizziness, tachycardia, nausea and vomiting, diarrhea, and hypotension. Clotting defects can lead to hypovolemic shock. Remember, pit viper venom is designed to paralyze prey. Thus respiratory distress and numbness and tingling around the head are classic symptoms of their envenomation.

Treatment consists of ensuring the ABCs and slowing the absorption of the venom. Keep the bitten extremity below the heart and the patient quiet and immobile. Immobilize the limb with a splint, but do not suction, incise, or apply cold packs to the wound. Antivenin is available, so rapid transport to an appropriate medical facility is critical.

Coral Snakes. Coral snakes are much smaller than pit vipers. They are found in the Southeast (Eastern variety) and the Southwest (Arizona variety). These snakes have round pupils, a narrow head, small and fixed fangs, and

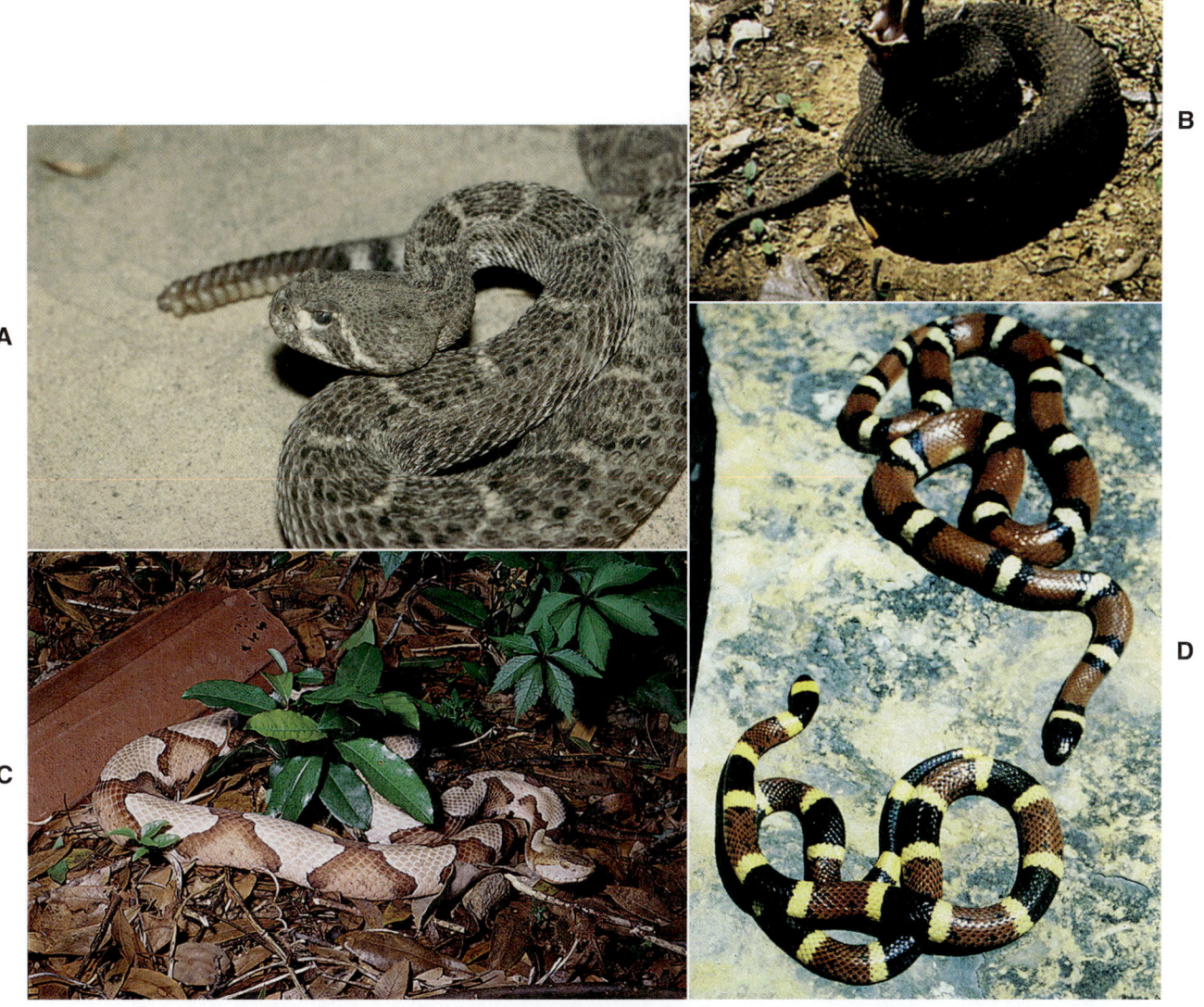

Figure 30-2 Common poisonous snakes of North America. **A,** Rattlesnake. **B,** Water moccasin. **C,** Copperhead. **D,** Coral snake.

no pits on the head. They can be recognized by a distinctive color band pattern along the length of the body. The banding pattern is black, yellow, red, yellow, black. Some nonpoisonous snakes (such as the king snake) mimic this color pattern, but imperfectly (see Figure 30-2, *D*). The old saying, "Red on yellow, kill a fellow; red on black, venom lacks," can be helpful in distinguishing the coral snake from imposters. However, the rhyme only applies to coral snakes native to the United States.

Coral snake venom contains a mixture of hydrolytic toxins and neurotoxins. The neurotoxin has a blocking effect on acetylcholine receptor sites. Severe envenomations result in respiratory and skeletal muscle paralysis. The symptoms may be delayed for 12 to 24 hours. The signs and symptoms include fang marks with swell-ing, redness, and localized numbness at the injection site. The systemic effects include weakness, drowsiness, slurred speech, ataxia, salivation, paralysis of the tongue and larynx, drooping eyelids, dilated pupils, abdominal pain, nausea and vomiting, seizures, respiratory distress, and hypotension. The neurologic effects of coral snake venom are much more pronounced than those of pit viper venom.

The treatment consists of ensuring the ABCs and slowing the absorption of the venom. Decontaminate the wound with water or normal saline. Keep the bitten extremity below the heart and the patient quiet and immobile. Immobilize the limb with a splint, apply a loose-fitting constricting band (as previously mentioned, not a tourniquet), and start an IV with a volume-expanding crystalloid fluid. Do not incise the wound or apply cold packs to the wound. Antivenin is available, so rapid transport to an appropriate medical facility is critical.

Marine Creatures

Marine creatures that can produce intense pain at the site of envenomation include jellyfish, the Portuguese man-of-war, stingrays, lionfish, sea urchins, sea anemones, fire coral, cone snails, and the blue-ringed octopus (Figure 30-3). Some of these organisms have stinging cells called **nematocysts** that inject toxin at the site of contact (jellyfish, fire coral, and sea anemones). Other organisms have spines that can inject the venom deeper into the tissue and cause secondary trauma (sea urchins and stingrays). All these toxins are heat labile and are composed of large proteins. The signs and symptoms consist of intense localized pain, redness, and swelling in combination with systemic symptoms such as respiratory difficulty and possibly cardiac dysrhythmias. The main

treatment for these injuries is supportive by washing the area in fresh, warm water (110° to 113° F). Remove any stingers or shallow spines at the wound site. Treat the lacerations from the spines. Trauma from spines, especially from stingrays, can be significant; they have caused death in divers.

Foods, Plants, and Mushrooms

Food Poisoning

Any number of different chemicals, biologic agents, or biologic toxins can cause food poisoning. The bacterium *Salmonella* sp. is often associated with food-borne illness. Other biologic agents produce toxins that can be concentrated in foods or the body during infection. Botulinum toxin is produced by the anaerobic bacterium *Clostridium botulinum*. This toxin may contaminate improperly preserved or canned foods because its spores are somewhat resistant to heat. The toxin also has been isolated and used as a biologic weapon. The signs and

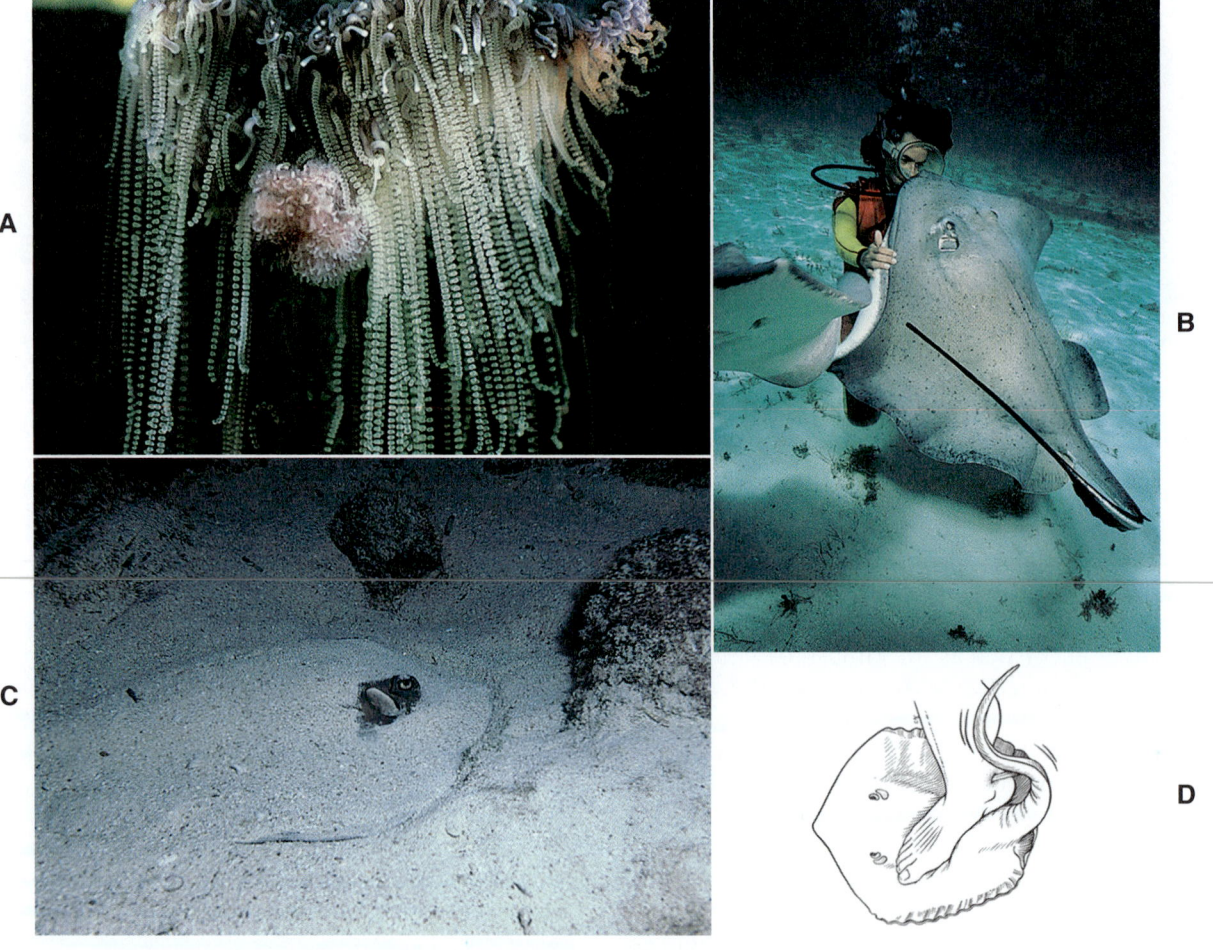

Figure 30-3 Common venomous marine creatures found in North America. **A,** Portuguese man-of-war. **B,** Stingray with a diver. **C,** Stingray nestled in the sand. **D,** The stingray lashes its tail upward and generates a deep puncture wound.

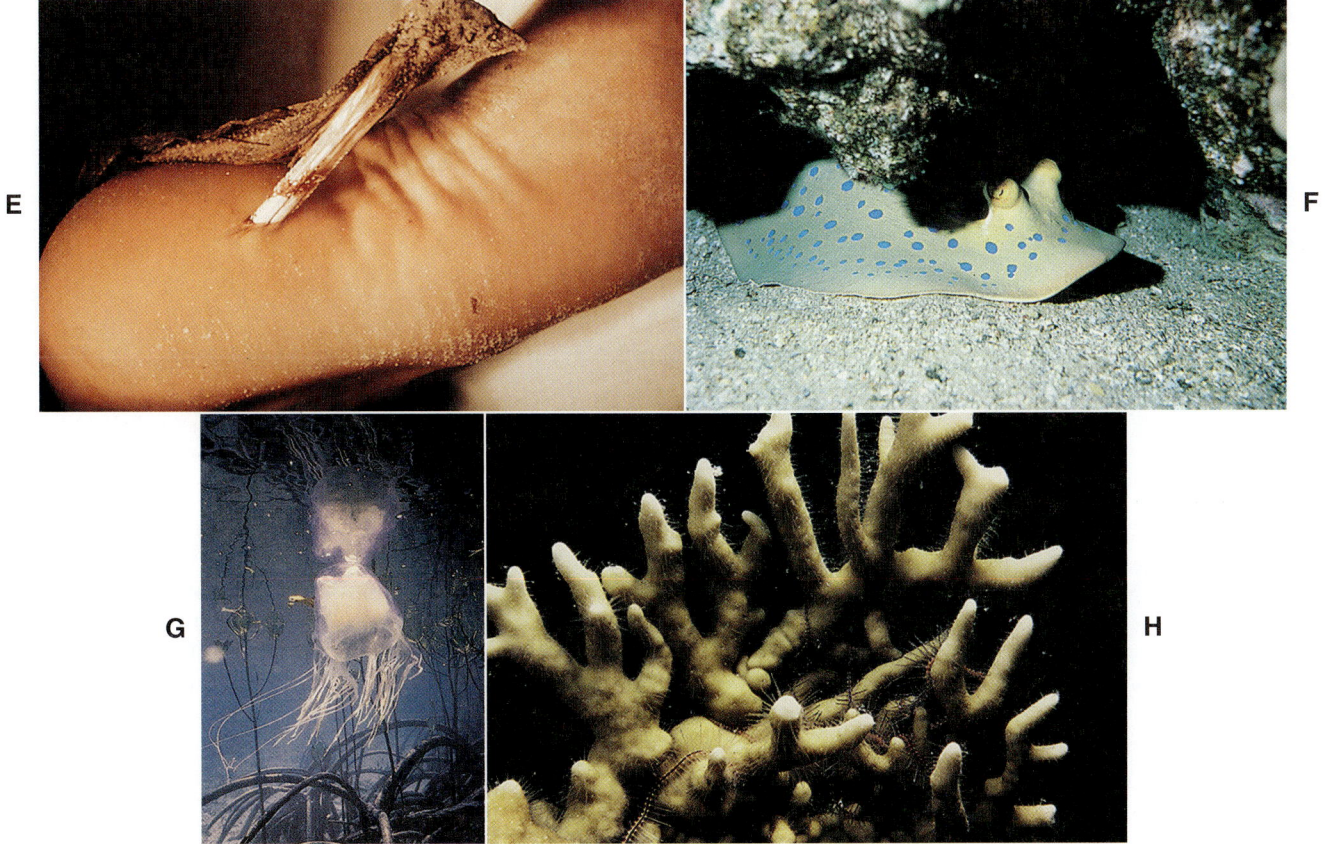

Figure 30-3, cont'd E, Stingray spine tip broken off the heel of a victim. **F,** Blue-spotted stingray. **G,** Jellyfish. **H,** Fire coral.

symptoms of botulinum toxin are severe CNS effects, including a progressive head-to-toe paralysis that can lead to respiratory arrest and quadriplegia. The early symptoms start with headache, facial droop, and blurred or double vision. In patients who go untreated, the mortality rate from respiratory failure is approximately 70%. The treatment is mainly supportive and especially involves assisting with artificial respirations as paralysis progresses. Botulinum antitoxin is available. However, most emergency departments do not routinely keep it in stock.

Plants and Mushrooms

[OBJECTIVE 15]

Most plants and mushrooms are nontoxic or slightly toxic. However, some can be highly toxic. Just over 75,000 exposures were reported in 2006. However, fatalities from plants and mushrooms are rare (four deaths in 2004). Most plant poisonings are accidental and involve household plants or ornamentals ingested by children. The primary exposure categories of plant poisonings are GI irritants, dermatitis inducers, and oxalate-containing substances. Other specific toxins are also prevalent, such as cyanogenic glycosides, cardiac glycosides, and solanine.

Mushroom poisonings occur both accidentally and intentionally. The cyclopeptide group of mushrooms, which includes the *Amanita* and *Galerina* genera, account for the bulk of lethal exposures. The cyclopeptide toxins are potent hepatotoxins (liver toxins).

Familiarity with all the different poisonous plants and mushrooms in North America is beyond the scope of a paramedic. Signs and symptoms of ingestion can vary greatly. Many plants and mushrooms contain irritating chemicals. These chemicals produce redness or irritation at the site of contact. Examine the patient's oropharynx for redness, irritation, swelling, or blistering. Excessive salivation, lacrimation, and diaphoresis also may be present. Abdominal effects may include nausea and vomiting, cramps, and diarrhea. Severe exposures may include reduced levels of consciousness and coma. The treatment for these types of poisonings is mainly supportive. It should include gathering a good patient history with a sample of the ingested material for identification or laboratory analysis.

Case Scenario—continued

A SAMPLE history reveals an altered mental status in both women. A head-to-toe survey produces similar findings of pallor, diaphoresis, weakness, and a limited ability to follow your commands. Several of the concerned guests suggest that the women were smoking pot but not using any cocaine. The party host tells you that the two girls prepared a spaghetti dinner for everyone earlier with mushrooms that they picked from outside the apartment.

Questions

4. *Has your first impression changed?*

5. *What additional assessment and treatment options for the women should be considered?*

Alcohol Abuse and Illegal Drugs

[OBJECTIVE 16, 17]

Substance abuse is a serious problem in the United States. Both illegal and prescription drugs are abused (Table 30-10). Law enforcement should be present at all overdoses, especially those with illegal drugs, for your safety as well as for legal ramifications.

Alcohol Abuse

Alcoholism is a disease of dependence on the intoxicating effects of ethanol (ethyl alcohol). It is a major problem in the United States. It leads to many deaths from accidents and drunken driving (40% of motor vehicle fatalities), injuries and deaths from violence (more than half of all assaults and murders), morbidity and mortality associated with chronic health effects, and economic losses from lost productivity (more than $100 billion annually). Many of the calls to which you will respond will be directly related to the effects of alcohol on the patient or the perpetrator.

Alcohol Dependence. Alcohol is a popular social drug because at low doses it has a stimulatory effect and lowers inhibitions. However, ethanol is a potent CNS depressant. Severe alcohol poisoning can even lead to coma and death. Accidental deaths are common from ethanol overdose, especially in the younger, inexperienced demographic such as college students. Chronic use may lead to the disease of alcoholism. Alcoholism has been shown to have a genetic component as well as an environmental component.

An alcoholic may appear as an unkempt, dysfunctional street person or, in contrast, an apparently normal, functioning next-door neighbor. Alcoholism has a wide spectrum of effects on people. Functioning alcoholics can lead productive lives, whereas other alcoholics are almost completely incapacitated. The common denominator in alcoholics is their dependence on ethanol. Some common signs of alcoholism are drinking almost every day, early in the day, and usually throughout the day. This may lead to an odor of alcohol at inappropriate times (such as during work) and a flushed appearance (especially in the face and hands). Drinking often occurs secretly to avoid detection. Some alcoholics binge drink for several days at a time, which can lead to memory loss or blackouts. Alcohol-related accidents such as bruises, lacerations, and falls may be common. Long-term ethanol ingestion can lead to GI problems (such as bleeding) and liver disease. The liver is the site of ethanol detoxification.

> **PARAMEDIC*Pearl***
>
> Do not assume a patient is intoxicated on the basis of altered mental status alone. Many conditions that affect the CNS can produce such effects, such as head injuries. Also, patients with diabetes may have an unusual smell that can be confused with ethanol. Diabetic ketoacidosis produces large amounts of acetone that can be smelled on the breath, and associated altered mental status is not uncommon. Remember to treat all patients with respect and do not jump to conclusions.

Alcohol is rapidly absorbed in the stomach, and activated charcoal has not been shown to absorb ethanol significantly. Alcohol easily passes the blood-brain barrier, and ethanol concentrations in the brain quickly approach blood levels. Alcohol is a strong vasodilator and may induce hypothermia. Dehydration may occur from the diuretic effects of ethanol. Ethanol inhibits vasopressin, a hormone responsible for fluid retention. Chronic alcoholics may combine or replace ethanol with methanol, isopropanol, or ethylene glycol. Methanol and ethylene glycol, as previously discussed, are potent toxins. A good patient history and scene survey may help you discover cases of coingestion.

Withdrawal Syndrome. Ethanol is one of the few abused drugs that can have potentially lethal withdrawal symptoms. This can occur after acute or chronic ingestion (alcoholism). The symptoms may start several hours after abstinence and can last up to a week. Seizures ("rum

TABLE 30-10   Pharmaceutical Poisonings: Street Drugs

Toxin	Signs and Symptoms	Treatment
Amphetamines (Benzedrine, Dexedrine, Ritalin, speed, uppers)	Exhilaration, hyperactivity Dilated pupils Hypertension Psychosis Tremors, seizures	ABCs Oxygen Cardiac monitor IV fluids Cardiac treatment as necessary Seizure treatment as necessary Rapid transport
Cocaine (crack, rock)	Euphoria Hyperactivity Dilated pupils Psychosis Anxiety, twitching Hypertension Hyperthermia Dysrhythmias, tachycardia Chest pain, heart attack Seizures	ABCs Respiratory support Oxygen Cardiac monitor IV fluids Cardiac treatment as necessary Seizure treatment as necessary Rapid transport
Hallucinogens (LSD, PCP, mescaline, psilocybin, ketamine)	Psychosis, suggestibility Hallucinations, distorted sensory perceptions Rambling speech Headache, dizziness Dilated pupils Nausea Seizures	Scene safety ABCs Reassure and calm patient (keep environment calm, dark, and quiet) Seizure treatment as necessary
Marijuana (grass, weed, hashish)	Euphoria, altered sensation Dilated pupils Dry mouth	ABCs Cardiac monitor
Methamphetamines (meth, speed, crank, ice, crystal, water)	Euphoria Muscle tremors Insomnia Depression Hypertension Chest pain Stroke Anxiety Hallucinations Psychosis Anorexia	Scene safety ABCs Oxygen Cardiac monitor IV fluids Cardiac treatment as necessary Seizure treatment as necessary Rapid transport
MDMA (ecstasy)	Euphoria Confusion Agitation, tremor Hyperthermia Diarrhea	ABCs Respiratory support Oxygen Cardiac monitor IV fluids Cardiac treatment as necessary Rapid transport
Narcotics (codeine, Darvocet, Darvon, heroin, hydromorphone, meperidine, methadone, morphine, oxycodone, pentazocine, propoxyphene, China white)	Euphoria CNS depression Respiratory depression Constricted pupils (miosis) Hypotension Bradycardia Pulmonary edema Coma	ABCs Respiratory support Oxygen Cardiac monitor IV fluids Cardiac treatment as necessary *Antidote:* naloxone (Narcan) IV or endotracheally until improvement Rapid transport

ABCs, Airway, breathing, and circulation; *IV,* intravenous; *LSD,* lysergic acid diethylamide; *PCP,* phencyclidine; *MDMA,* methylenedioxymethamphetamine; *CNS,* central nervous system.

fits"), which occur 24 to 36 hours after abstinence, progress into delirium tremens. Delirium tremens includes a decreased level of consciousness accompanied by hallucinations. This combination can lead to respiratory arrest and accidents from ataxia and is associated with a significant mortality rate. The signs and symptoms include anxiety, irritability, tremors, nausea and vomiting, weakness, diaphoresis, hallucinations, tachycardia, hypertension with possible orthostatic hypotension, and poor sleep. The treatment includes supportive care, especially emphasizing the ABCs. Gather a thorough patient history and determine if other drugs could be involved. The use of diazepam may be necessary to control seizures. Check for hypoglycemia and establish IV access. Have law enforcement provide scene security if possible. Transport the patient to a medical facility for evaluation and further treatment if indicated.

Amphetamines

Amphetamines were once widely used to improve task performance and prevent sleepiness. In World War II they were used to keep pilots awake for long missions, among other uses. Because of their potential for abuse, adverse effects, and addictive properties, they are rarely used medicinally. Adverse effects include hypertension, tachycardia, tachypnea, tremors, and disorganized behavior. High doses may produce seizures, hallucinations, paranoia, and psychoses. The withdrawal symptoms may include lethargy, depression, suicidal tendencies, and coma.

Cocaine

Cocaine strongly stimulates the CNS system, causing major sympathetic discharge and resulting in increased catecholamine release. The lethal dose is estimated to be approximately 1200 mg in the average adult. Most fatalities occur from cardiac dysrhythmias. These lethal effects can occur at much lower doses in susceptible individuals.

Two forms of cocaine are in common use today—the powdered form and the freebase form. Cocaine powder is a fine, white crystalline powder in its pure form. The powdered form is typically inhaled through the nose (snorting). Freebase cocaine (or crack cocaine) appears as clumps or crystals of a white or off-white solid. The freebase form of cocaine is much more potent than the powdered form. The freebase form is typically smoked. Crystals, or rocks, of the drug are heated and inhaled in a similar fashion to smoking a cigarette.

Opioids: Heroin

Opioids are CNS depressants. This factor increases the risks of respiratory failure in overdoses. Heroin is a bitter-tasting, white or off-white powder. However, it is usually adulterated, or cut, with various substances, including sugars, baking soda, starch, or any number of other substances. Opioids may be administered orally, intranasally (snorting), intradermally (skin popping), or intravenously (mainlining) or they may be smoked. You often can see tracks on abusers who mainline. However, do not dismiss a heroin or opioid overdose because of a lack of injection sites. A *speedball* is an IV injection of a mixture of heroin and cocaine. The signs and symptoms of opioid overdose include euphoria, CNS depression, respiratory depression, miosis, hypotension, bradycardia, pulmonary edema, and coma.

Naloxone (Narcan) is an opioid antagonist. It is useful for almost all opioid and opioidlike chemicals. Naloxone reverses respiratory depression, coma, and miosis (constricted pupils). The drug is typically given in small doses. The aim is to relieve respiratory depression yet leave the patient in a responsive but lethargic state. Drug abusers may become agitated and violent when their high wears off unexpectedly and they are faced with people in uniform. Naloxone should be given only in cases of respiratory depression because seizure activity is a possible side effect.

Naloxone also may induce opioid withdrawal symptoms. These signs and symptoms include irritability, diaphoresis, abdominal cramps, nausea and vomiting, hyperthermia, tremors, and tachycardia. These symptoms can generally be treated with supportive care.

Methamphetamines

Clandestine methamphetamine (meth) labs have become an epidemic in the United States. Among these are so-called mom and pop labs that can be located almost anywhere. They have been found in residences, trailers, hotels and motels, storage units, and sheds in rural, suburban, and urban areas. These labs contain many dangerous chemicals, usually stored and used improperly. Anhydrous ammonia, typically stolen from farming operations, is a primary ingredient in the "Nazi" method. The Nazi method has become the method of choice because of the tighter regulation of starting materials used in other methods, such as phenyl-2-propanone. The chemical byproducts of meth "cooking," such as phosphine gas, can pose a lethal risk to responding paramedics.

Methamphetamine is a potent CNS stimulant. The drug can be taken by all common routes (smoking, snorting, orally, and IV). Chronic meth users go through several stages during the abuse cycle. A "tweaker" is a meth abuser who typically has not slept in 3 to 10 days and is irritable and unpredictable. This stage of meth abuse can be extremely dangerous for EMS personnel. Scene security is a primary consideration. The first stage lasts approximately 10 days. It is characterized by euphoria and sleeplessness. Users have a feeling of invincibility, keen senses, and keen intelligence. Chloroephedrine is a common contaminant of illicit methamphetamine. It may be responsible for much of the tachycardia.

The signs and symptoms include anxiety, restlessness, paranoia, delirium, hallucinations, chest pain, palpitations, difficulty breathing, pulmonary hypertension, hyperthermia, hypertension, strokes, and seizures. Chronic users may be malnourished and anorexic. Scene safety is crucial because of the psychiatric effects of methamphetamines. The meth lab itself poses serious risks (e.g., booby traps, risk of explosion). The treatment consists of providing supportive care, especially the ABCs. IV access and cardiac monitoring are indicated. Seizures may be treated with diazepam. Rapid transport is usually indicated.

Drugs Used in Sexual Abuse Crimes

Methylenedioxymethamphetamine (MDMA), or ecstasy, is a modified form of methamphetamine. It is also a CNS stimulant. The signs, symptoms, and treatment are the same as for amphetamines. Although ecstasy is a derivative of methamphetamine, the potentially violent stage is not seen with MDMA abuse. This drug has been popular in the teenage and college student demographic.

Rohypnol (flunitrazepam) also is known as the "date rape" drug. It is a potent CNS depressant in the benzodiazepine class. Because of the strong sedative and amnesia effects these drugs possess, they have been used covertly in social settings such as parties and nightclubs. The signs, symptoms, and treatment are the same as for any of the benzodiazepines. However, you must treat the consequences of sexual abuse or rape as well. Law enforcement should be involved in these poisonings because a crime likely has been committed (food tampering, sexual abuse, and/or rape).

Hallucinogens: Phencyclidine

The most common hallucinogen is PCP. It was originally used as a veterinary tranquilizer. After its abuse potential was discovered, it was replaced with other, safer alternatives in this setting. PCP has CNS stimulatory and depressant properties.

At low doses (10 mg or less) phencyclidine produces a mixture of psychoactive effects, including euphoria, disorientation and confusion, and sudden mood shifts (e.g., rage). The signs of PCP use include flushing, diaphoresis, hypersalivation, and vomiting. In general the pupils remain reactive. Facial grimacing and nystagmus, or involuntary movement of the eyes, are identifiable effects of low-dose PCP use. PCP users are much less sensitive to pain. As a result, this may lead to the appearance of superhuman strength from overexertion. At low doses, death is associated with self-destructive behaviors related to the analgesic and CNS depressant effects of PCP. Remember, patients under the influence of hallucinogens pose a risk to themselves and others, including the paramedics on scene.

High doses (greater than 10 mg) may produce extreme CNS depression, including coma. Respiratory depression, hypertension, and tachycardia are not uncommon effects. The hypertension may cause cardiac difficulties, encephalopathy, intracerebral hemorrhage, and seizures. High-dose overdoses may require you to manage respiratory arrest, cardiac arrest, and status epilepticus. Rapidly transport these patients to the hospital.

The acute onset of PCP psychosis may result after even low doses. This is a true psychiatric emergency and may last for days to weeks after the exposure. Patients' behavior ranges from unresponsiveness (catatonic state) to violent behavior and rage. These patients can be extremely dangerous. As a result, law enforcement should accompany you to the appropriate medical facility.

Other common hallucinogens include LSD, mescaline, psilocybin mushrooms, and marijuana.

Case Scenario CONCLUSION

As you continue your assessment you learn that, because of recent rains and damp conditions, the group had been harvesting an abundance of mushrooms from a local field. Both patients' vital signs reveal hypotension, tachycardia, and dilated pupils. While comparing assessment findings with your partner, one of the girls begins to seize. The seizure terminates with the administration of diazepam.

You and your partner ready the patients for transport, including IV access and supplemental oxygen at 15 L/min by nonrebreather mask. The transport continues without incident and you transfer care to the emergency department staff.

Looking Back

6. *What is your final impression of the patients?*
7. *What treatment options are available for these women?*

Case Scenario SUMMARY

1. *What is your initial impression of the patients?* Your initial impression may include acute intoxication of alcohol or drugs.
2. *What additional information do you need to complete your assessment?* Additional information needed includes a head-to-toe assessment and a SAMPLE history. You should ask what substances or beverages both women ingested to identify a potential common intoxicant. Ask the bystanders for any relevant information pertaining to recent events leading to the women's current condition.
3. *What may be causing the women's distress?* The women's condition could be caused by a number of things, including acute alcohol overdose, the use of any illicit drug alone or in combination with other drugs, or food poisoning.
4. *Has your first impression changed?* The initial impression may be changed by the additional information.

Learning that the women fell ill after ingesting spaghetti and sauce may suggest food poisoning. However, food poisoning does not typically present with such an immediate onset.

5. *What additional assessment and treatment options for the women should be considered?* Additional information needed includes vital signs. You also may want to ask about the ingredients of the spaghetti sauce and if the women ingested anything other than the meal. Treatment options are somewhat limited and include supplemental oxygen and IV access.
6. *What is your final impression of the patients?* A final impression of these patients is mushroom poisoning from self-harvested mushrooms.
7. *What treatment options are available for these women?* Prehospital care consists of ventilatory support, supplemental oxygen, and IV access.

Chapter Summary

- Toxicologic emergencies can cover a wide range of signs and symptoms depending on the toxin.
- Toxins can affect any organ system in the body.
- In an unknown medical emergency, you must quickly assess the signs and symptoms and determine the nature of the emergency.
- If an underlying medical condition seems implausible, a good patient history or examination of the area may reveal the source of illness as poisoning.

- Poisons can be found almost anywhere—in the home, in the workplace, and in nature.
- Poisonings may be accidental or intentional.
- You must always be cautious when responding to a toxicologic emergency.

REFERENCES

Alcorta, R. (2004). Smoke inhalation and acute cyanide poisoning. *JEMS Communications, Summer,* 6-17.
Anderson, C. E., & Loomis, G. A. (2003). Recognition and prevention of inhalant abuse. *American Family Physician, 68,* 869-874.
Bronstein, A. C., Spyker, D. A., Cantilena, L. R. Jr., Green, J., Rumack, B. H., & Heard, S. E. (2007). 2006 Annual report of the American Association of Poison Control Centers' National Poison Data System (NPDS). *Clinical Toxicology, 45*(8), 815-917.
National Institute of Occupational Safety and Health. (2005). *Publication No. 2005-149: NIOSH pocket guide to chemical hazards.* Retrieved February 1, 2006, from http://www.cdc.gov.

SUGGESTED RESOURCES

Agency for Toxic Substances and Disease Registry: http://www.atsdr.cdc.gov.
Auerbach, P. S. (2007). *Wilderness medicine* (5th ed.). Philadelphia: Elsevier.
Bronstein, A. C., & Currance, P. (1999). *Emergency care for hazardous materials exposure* (2nd ed.). St. Louis: Mosby.
Currance, P., & Bronstein, A. C. (1999). *Hazardous materials for EMS: Practices and procedures.* St. Louis: Mosby.
Dart, R. C. (2004). *Medical toxicology* (3rd ed.). Philadelphia: Lippincott Williams & Wilkins.
Department of Health and Human Services. (2000). *Managing hazardous materials incidents: A planning guide for the management of contaminated patients.* Washington, DC: U.S. Government Printing Office.
National Institute of Occupational Safety and Health: http://www.cdc.gov.
Wireless Information System for Emergency Responders: http://www.sis.nlm.nih.gov.

Chapter Quiz

1. True or False: The scene size-up is one of the most important steps in responding safely to a toxicologic emergency.

2. Identify the four routes of entry.

   _____

   _____

   _____

   _____

3. Good reference materials available for a hazardous materials incident do not include which of the following?
   a. NIOSH guide
   b. *Physicians' Desk Reference*
   c. 2008 Emergency Response Guidebook

4. True or False: The Poison Control Center can generally give you specific advice regarding the agent involved in a toxicologic emergency.

5. List four common toxidromes and describe the signs and symptoms you would find.

   _____

   _____

   _____

   _____

6. The preferred method of GI decontamination is _____.

7. The medication most often involved in toxicologic emergencies is
   _____.
   a. acetaminophen
   b. epinephrine
   c. tricyclic antidepressants.

8. *Therapeutic index* refers to _____.
   a. the card catalog system used by the Food and Drug Administration to keep track of drugs
   b. the degree of dependence the drug induces in users
   c. the effective dosage window of the medication

9. True or False: Bases are chemicals that have a pH less than 7.

10. True or False: Hydrocarbons with a high viscosity are more likely to be aspirated.

11. Organophosphates, carbamates, and nerve agents inhibit which enzyme?
    a. Acetylcholinesterase
    b. Alcohol dehydrogenase
    c. Cytochrome C

12. True or False: Methemoglobinemia causes SLUDGEM symptoms.

13. Cyanides inhibit which enzyme?
    a. Acetylcholinesterase
    b. Alcohol dehydrogenase
    c. Cytochrome C

14. The antidote for methanol poisoning is _____.
    a. atropine and pralidoxime
    b. ethanol
    c. methylene blue

15. True or False: Chelating agents can be used to eliminate heavy metals from the body.

Terminology

Activated charcoal An adsorbent made from charred wood that effectively binds many poisons in the stomach; most effective when administered within 1 hour of intake.

Alkali A substance with a pH greater than 7; also known as a *base* or *caustic*.

Antidote A substance that can reverse the adverse effects of a poison.

Antivenin A substance that can reverse the adverse effects of a venom by binding to it and inactivating it.

Base A substance with a pH greater than 7; also known as an *alkali* or *caustic*.

Carbamate A pesticide that inhibits acetylcholinesterase.

Cathartics Substances that decrease the time a poison spends in the GI tract by increasing bowel motility.

Caustic A substance with a pH greater than 7; also known as a *base* or *alkali*.

Chelating agent A substance that can bind metals; used as an antidote to many heavy metal poisonings.

Chemical Abstracts Services (CAS) number Unique identification number of chemicals, much like a person's Social Security number.

Corrosive A substance able to corrode tissue or metal (e.g., acids and bases).

Decontamination The process of removing dangerous substances from the patient; may involve removing substances from the skin (external decontamination)

Terminology—continued

and/or removing substances from the GI tract (internal decontamination).

Drug overdose Internalization of more than the safe amount of a medication or drug; often associated with illegal drugs when a user administers too great an amount of substance; may be used to commit suicide.

Envenomation The process of injecting venom into a wound; venomous animals include snakes, insects, and marine creatures.

Enzyme A large molecule (protein) that performs a biochemical reaction in the cell.

Gastric lavage A method of internal decontamination that involves emptying the stomach contents through an orogastric or nasogastric tube.

Hydrocarbon A member of a large class of chemicals belonging to the petroleum derivative family; they have a variety of uses, such as solvents, oils, reagents, and fuels.

Intoxication Being under the effect of a toxin or drug; common terminology (nonmedical) refers to intoxication as being under the effect of alcohol or illegal drugs.

Liquefaction necrosis The injury seen when skin and cells are dissolved and die; bases (alkalis) commonly cause this injury.

Methemoglobinemia The oxidation of hemoglobin from the ferrous iron to the ferric iron state.

Nematocyst The stinging cells many marine creatures use to envenomate and immobilize prey.

Neutralizing agent A substance that counteracts the effects of acids or bases; brings the pH of a solution back to 7.

Olfactory fatigue Desensitization of the sense of smell.

Organophosphate A pesticide that inhibits acetylcholinesterase.

Overdose The accidental or intentional ingestion of an excess of a substance with the potential for toxicity.

Poison Any substance that can harm the human body; also known as a *toxin*.

Protein Any one of a number of large molecules composed of amino acids that form the structural components of cells or carry out biochemical functions.

Protoxin A substance converted to a toxin through a biochemical process in the body; would be harmless if not converted (e.g., methanol and ethylene glycol).

Therapeutic index The ratio of the amount of drug to produce a therapeutic dose compared with the amount of drug that produces a lethal dose; a narrow therapeutic window is dangerous because of the greater possibility of undermedicating and the greater possibility of overdosing.

Toxicology The study of poisons.

Toxidrome A classification system of toxic syndromes by signs and symptoms.

Toxin Any substance that can harm the human body; also known as a *poison*.

United Nations (UN) number The 4-digit number assigned to chemicals during transit by the U.S. DOT; the 2008 Emergency Response Guidebook lists useful information about these chemicals.

Vapor pressure The pressure exerted by a vapor against the sides of a closed container; a measure of volatility—high vapor pressure means it is a volatile substance.

Venom The poison injected by venomous animals such as snakes, insects, and marine creatures.

Viscosity The thickness of a liquid; a high-viscosity liquid does not flow easily (e.g., oils and tar); a low-viscosity liquid flows easily (e.g., gasoline) and poses a greater risk for aspiration and consequent pulmonary damage.

Volatility A measure of how quickly a material passes into the vapor or gas state; the greater the volatility, the greater its rate of evaporation.

Infectious and Communicable Diseases

Objectives *After completing this chapter, you will be able to:*

1. Review the specific anatomy and physiology pertinent to infectious and communicable diseases.
2. Define specific terminology identified with infectious and communicable diseases.*
3. Discuss public health principles relevant to infectious and communicable diseases.
4. Identify public health agencies involved in the prevention and management of disease outbreaks.
5. For specific diseases, identify and discuss the issues of personal protection.
6. Describe and discuss the rationale for the various types of personal protective equipment.
7. Discuss what constitutes a significant exposure to an infectious agent.
8. List and describe the steps of an infectious process.
9. List and describe the stages of infectious diseases.
10. List and describe infectious agents, including bacteria, viruses, fungi, protozoans, helminths (worms), and prions.
11. Describe host defense mechanisms against infection.
12. Describe the processes of the immune system defenses, including humoral and cell-mediated immunity.
13. Describe characteristics of the immune system, including the categories of white blood cells, the mononuclear phagocyte system, and the complement system.
14. Describe the assessment of a patient suspected of, or identified as having, an infectious or communicable disease.
15. Discuss the proper disposal of contaminated supplies (e.g., sharps, gauze sponges, tourniquets).
16. Discuss the following relative to the human immunodeficiency virus: causative agent, body systems affected and potential secondary complications, modes of transmission, the seroconversion rate after direct significant exposure, susceptibility and resistance, signs and symptoms, specific patient management and personal protective measures.
17. Discuss hepatitis A (infectious hepatitis), including the causative agent, body systems affected and potential secondary complications, routes of transmission, susceptibility and resistance, signs and symptoms, patient management and protective measures, and immunization.
18. Discuss hepatitis B (serum hepatitis), including the causative agent, the organ affected and potential secondary complications, routes of transmission, signs and symptoms, patient management and protective measures, and immunization.
19. Discuss the susceptibility and resistance to hepatitis B.
20. Discuss hepatitis C, including the causative agent, the organ affected, routes of transmission, susceptibility and resistance, signs and symptoms, patient management and protective measures, and control measures.
21. Discuss hepatitis D (hepatitis delta virus), including the causative agent, the organ affected, routes of transmission, susceptibility and resistance, signs and symptoms, patient management and protective measures, and control measures.
22. Discuss hepatitis E, including the causative agent, the organ affected, routes of transmission, susceptibility and resistance, signs and symptoms, patient management and protective measures, and control measures.
23. Discuss tuberculosis, including the causative agent, body systems affected and secondary complications, routes of transmission, susceptibility and resistance, signs and symptoms, patient management and protective measures, and control measures.
24. Discuss meningococcal meningitis (spinal meningitis), including causative organisms, tissues affected, modes of transmission, susceptibility and resistance, signs and symptoms, patient management and protective measures, and immunization and control measures.
25. Discuss other infectious agents known to cause meningitis, including *Streptococcus pneumoniae, Haemophilus influenzae* type b, and other varieties of viruses.
26. Discuss pneumonia, including causative organisms, body systems affected, routes of transmission, susceptibility and resistance, signs and symptoms, patient management and protective measures, and immunization.
27. Discuss tetanus, including the causative organism, the body system affected, modes of transmission, susceptibility and resistance, signs and symptoms, patient management and protective measures, and immunization.
28. Discuss rabies and hantavirus as they apply to regional environmental exposures, including the causative organisms, the body systems affected, routes of transmission, susceptibility and resistance, signs and symptoms, patient management and protective measures, and control measures.
29. Identify pediatric viral diseases.
30. Discuss chickenpox, including the causative organism, the body system affected, mode of transmission, susceptibility and resistance, signs and symptoms, patient management and protective measures, and immunization and control measures.

*Objectives 1 and 2 are addressed throughout this chapter to provide a comprehensive overview of anatomy and physiology and terminology associated with communicable disease.

Objectives—continued

31. Discuss mumps, including the causative organism, the body organs and systems affected, mode of transmission, susceptibility and resistance, signs and symptoms, patient management and protective measures, and immunization.

32. Discuss rubella (German measles), including the causative agent, the body tissues and systems affected, modes of transmission, susceptibility and resistance, signs and symptoms, patient management and protective measures, and immunization.

33. Discuss measles (rubeola, hard measles), including the causative organism; the body tissues, organs, and systems affected; mode of transmission; susceptibility and resistance; signs and symptoms; patient management and protective measures; and immunization.

34. Discuss the importance of immunization and diseases, especially in the pediatric population, that warrant widespread immunization.

35. Discuss pertussis (whooping cough), including the causative organism, the body organs affected, mode of transmission, susceptibility and resistance, signs and symptoms, patient management and protective measures, and immunization.

36. Discuss influenza, including the causative organisms, the body system affected, mode of transmission, susceptibility and resistance, signs and symptoms, patient management and protective measures, and immunization.

37. Discuss mononucleosis, including the causative organisms; the body regions, organs, and systems affected; modes of transmission; susceptibility and resistance; signs and symptoms; patient management and protective measures.

38. Discuss the characteristics of and organisms associated with febrile and afebrile respiratory disease, including bronchiolitis, bronchitis, laryngitis, croup, epiglottitis, and the common cold.

39. Discuss syphilis, including the causative organism; the body regions, organs, and systems affected; modes of transmission; susceptibility and resistance; stages of signs and symptoms; patient management and protective measures.

40. Discuss gonorrhea, including the causative organism, the body organs and associated structures affected, mode of transmission, susceptibility and resistance, signs and symptoms, patient management and protective measures.

41. Discuss chlamydia, including the causative organism; the body regions, organs, and systems affected; modes of transmission; susceptibility and resistance; signs and symptoms; patient management and protective measures.

42. Discuss herpes simplex type 1, including the causative organism, the body regions and system affected, modes of transmission, susceptibility and resistance, signs and symptoms, patient management and protective measures.

43. Discuss herpes simplex 2 (genital herpes), including the causative organism; the body regions, tissues, and structures affected; mode of transmission; susceptibility and resistance; signs and symptoms; patient management and protective measures.

44. Discuss scabies, including the etiologic agent, the body organs affected, modes of transmission, susceptibility and resistance, signs and symptoms, patient management and protective measures.

45. Discuss lice, including the infesting agents, the body regions affected, modes of transmission and host factors, susceptibility and resistance, signs and symptoms, patient management and protective measures, and prevention.

46. Describe Lyme disease, including the causative organism, the body organs and systems affected, mode of transmission, susceptibility and resistance, phases of signs and symptoms, patient management and control measures.

47. Discuss gastroenteritis, including the causative organisms, the body system affected, modes of transmission, susceptibility and resistance, signs and symptoms, patient management and protective measures.

48. Discuss the local protocol for reporting and documenting an infectious or communicable disease exposure.

Chapter Outline

Infectious Diseases and Public Health
Process of Infection
Approach to Patients with a Possible Infectious
  Disease
Infectious Diseases

Exposures to Infectious and Communicable
  Diseases
Preventing Disease Transmission
Chapter Summary

Case Scenario

On a cool spring evening you are dispatched to a private residence in an affluent section of town. The call reference is shortness of breath. You arrive at a single-family home and are greeted by a woman who states that her husband is having trouble breathing. According to the woman, he has been feeling ill for the past month and recently developed a fever and congestion. She adds that his condition seems to have gotten worse in the last few days. Tonight, she continues, he cannot sit still, is coughing a lot, and has trouble catching his breath. As you approach the bedroom to find the patient, you can hear a very wet cough.

Questions

1. What is your initial impression?
2. What additional information do you need?
3. What common personal protective equipment would you use or consider using at this point?

[OBJECTIVES 1, 2]

This chapter discusses numerous communicable diseases that you will encounter in the prehospital setting. At the conclusion of this chapter you should be knowledgeable and able to identify multiple diseases and infections, describe their signs and symptoms, and know the prehospital and definitive treatment. This chapter discusses the local and federal response to local infections and outbreaks as well as widespread outbreaks and these agencies' roles in the process of identification, treatment, and confinement of such infections. It covers protection against these infections, including the importance of personal protective equipment and why it should be emphasized in training.

INFECTIOUS DISEASES AND PUBLIC HEALTH

[OBJECTIVE 3]

Many public health principles affect daily care of the population. When protecting the public, the paramedic must understand the demographic characteristic of the local community because infectious diseases affect entire populations. The study and treatment of infectious diseases is, by its nature, regional. Populations display varying **susceptibilities** to infection and, conversely, have varying degrees of disease. When dealing with infectious diseases, the paramedic must understand the needs of the patient, the consequences to public health, and the risk of person-to-person contact with family members and friends.

Agencies Involved in Prevention and Management of Infectious Diseases

[OBJECTIVE 4]

Each large municipality has public health agencies involved in the prevention and management of disease outbreaks. The local health agencies are the first line of defense in disease surveillance and outbreaks. State agencies are frequently involved in regulation and enforcement of federal guidelines. At the private sector level they are responsible for influence of local protocols and guidelines for dealing with disease surveillance and response to outbreaks. At the federal level, Congress plays an integral role in national health policy by enacting public laws and by drafting the federal budget for agencies such as Occupational Safety and Health Administration and the U.S. Department of Public Health and Human Services, which in turn is in charge of the Centers for Disease Control and Prevention (CDC), National Institute of Occupational Safety and Health, and the Federal Emergency Management Association.

Exposure Plans for Health Agencies

[OBJECTIVES 5, 6, 7]

Your agency has a responsibility to protect the public from disease. Components of the healthcare agency's exposure plan are health maintenance and surveillance of its employees, a designated officer to serve as a liaison between the agency and community health agencies involved in monitoring response to communicable diseases, identification of job classifications, and a schedule of when and how the provisions of blood-borne pathogen standards will be implemented. The service should ensure that its blood-borne pathogen standard includes engineering and work practice controls, personal protective equipment (PPE), baseline employee evaluations, immunizations, and follow-up training. The employees also have a responsibility to themselves and the public to use PPE. Gloves, gowns, face shields, masks, protective eyewear, and aprons should be used any time that the paramedic's eyes, mucous membranes, broken skin, or work clothes may come in contact with blood or other potentially infectious bodily fluids.

Other responsibilities of the agency include procedures involving exposure and postexposure counseling, which includes the employee's right to know of any exposure to a communicable disease. Your employer is also responsible for interfacing with and notifying local health authorities and state and federal agencies as well as maintaining personal, vehicular, and building disinfection and storage. Hazardous materials education should be provided for employees regarding disinfection agents, after-action reports of agency response, correct disposal of needles into containers, and the correct handling of body fluid–tinged linens and supplies used in patient care.

Paramedic Responsibilities ~yourself~

You also have a responsibility to adopt an attitude relative to infection control. This attitude includes maintenance of personal hygiene; attention to wounds and maintenance of the skin; effective handwashing after every patient contact; removal, disposal, and cleaning of work garments that have been infected; maintenance of physiologic and psychological health to prevent distress; and correct handling and disposal of needle and body fluid–tinged supplies. You should become aware of and avoid tendencies to wipe your face and rub your mucous membranes with gloved hands.

Cleaning surfaces: 1 part bleach : 10 parts water

> **PARAMEDIC***Pearl*
>
> **Latex Allergy**
>
> As an EMS professional, you are at risk for developing latex allergy. Equipment that may contain latex includes blood pressure cuffs, stethoscopes, disposable gloves, oral and nasal airways, endotracheal tubes, and syringes. Some proteins in latex can cause a range of mild to severe allergic reactions. If you develop symptoms after latex exposure such as nasal, eye, or sinus irritation; hives; shortness of breath; coughing; wheezing; or unexplained shock, seek medical attention for your immediate symptoms, then follow up with a physician experienced in treating latex allergy.

PROCESS OF INFECTION

[OBJECTIVE 8]

The infectious process has several steps. It starts with the infectious reservoir (human being, animal, or environment). The environmental factors dictate the presence of endemic species outside the host and climatic conditions. Successful transmission of a disease requires a number of conditions be met. The conditions for transmission depend on the **virulence** (strength of the organism) of the disease or its dose, the immune status of the host, and the correct mode of entry. All three factors are required to create a risk of exposure and subsequent infection. The life cycle of an infectious agent also depends on the demographics of the host, such as the population's ability to move, age distributions, socioeconomic considerations, and population migration dictated by religion.

Stages of Infectious Disease

[OBJECTIVE 9]

If an infection occurs, the infectious disease progresses through stages. Those stages are the incubation, window, communicable, latent, and disease periods. The **incubation period** is the interval between exposure to an agent and the first appearance of symptoms. The **window phase** is the period after infection in which the antigen is present but no antibody is detectable. The **communicable period** is a period after an infection when the infectious disease can be transmitted to another host, with significant manifestations appearing at this point. The **latent period** is the opposite of communicable period; at this point the infectious agent cannot be transmitted. The **disease period** is the interval between the first appearance of symptoms associated with the infection and resolution of the same or death. Always remember that the resolution of symptoms does not mean the infectious disease agent is destroyed.

Types of Infectious Agents

[OBJECTIVE 10]

As discussed in previous chapters, infectious agents include bacteria, viruses, fungi, protozoa, helminths, and prions.

Bacteria can be prokaryotic, which means the nuclear material is not contained in a distinct envelope. They also can be self-reproducing without a host cell. Bacteria create localized or systemic infections. Signs and symptoms of bacteriologic infection depend on the cells and tissues infected.

A virus must invade a host's cell to reproduce. A virus also must be eukaryotic, which means the nuclear material must be contained within a distinct envelope.

Fungi have protective capsules to surround the cell and protect it from the host's phagocytes. Protozoans are single-cell organisms that can move and feed on organic compounds. Helminths (worms) are not necessarily microorganisms, as the previous examples are. Lastly, prions are infectious proteins that do not contain a nucleic acid, trigger no immune response, and are not destroyed by heat or cold.

Host Defense Mechanisms

[OBJECTIVES 11, 12, 13]

As described in Chapter 8, the body has specific defense mechanisms to protect itself from infectious agents. The first lines of defense are anatomic barriers and associated nonspecific defenses. In addition to the skin, the respiratory system has turbinates to create turbulent air flow and nasal hairs to trap foreign material. Mucus has the ability to trap foreign material and expel the material as sputum or phlegm.

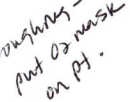

Another nonspecific defense mechanism is the normal bacterial flora. In the gastrointestinal and genitourinary systems, competition between colonies of microorganisms for nutrients and space helps prevent the spread of pathogenic organisms. In the same systems normal flora create environmental conditions that are not conducive to pathogens, and stomach acids may destroy some microorganisms or deactivate their toxic products. These systems also facilitate the elimination of pathogens by feces.

If the infectious agent bypasses the first lines of defense the body displays an inflammatory response caused by local cellular injury. The injury may be physical, thermal, or chemical or, as covered in this chapter, an invasion by microorganisms. The inflammatory response constitutes the second line of defense against infectious diseases and includes responses by neutrophils, macrophages, eosinophils, basophils, and natural killer cells.

If the first two lines of defense fail, the third line of defense, the immune system, must stop the agent. The lymphocyte is the backbone of the immune response. The immune system has two different components to help the body fight foreign agents: humoral **immunity** and cell-mediated immunity. The humoral immunity component is a time-consuming response in which B lymphocytes produce daughter cells. The daughter cells then produce plasma cells that eventually produce antibodies. Cell-mediated immunity also is a time-consuming response in which T lymphocytes coordinate the activity of other components of the immune system to deal with foreign materials. The different T cells are helper T cells, suppressor T cells, killer T cells, and inflammatory T cells. The complement system complements, or enhances, the immune response. This is a system of approximately 20 proteins that, once activated, result in a cascade occurring on the crystallizable fragment (Fc) of antibodies. This process enhances many of the functions of the immune system, including lysis of the organism, agglutination of the organism, or neutralizing viruses. It also enhances properties of the inflammatory response, including an increased ability for phagocytosis of the organism and an increase in chemotactic factors, which attract additional neutrophils and macrophages to the area.

A compartment of the immune response is the reticuloendothelial system (RES). This system consists of fighter cells in the spleen, lymph nodes, liver, bone marrow, lungs, and intestines. The RES works in conjunction with the lymphatic system to help rid the body of cellular debris that the immune system has created from fighting infection. The RES structures also assist in communication between the intracellular environment, extracellular environment, and lymphatic system as well as serve as storage sites for mature B and T cells until the immune system needs them to fight intruders.

APPROACH TO PATIENTS WITH A POSSIBLE INFECTIOUS DISEASE

[OBJECTIVES 14, 15]

The responsibilities of public health systems and individual paramedics require a detailed approach to patient care in the presence of suspected infectious or communicable diseases. Always suspect infectious diseases in a patient, respect visceral and intuitive suspicions that the dispatched call may involve infectious diseases, and wear gloves and glasses on all calls as well as gowns when needed. You should become knowledgeable and proficient in patient assessment techniques and interviewing. The focused history and physical examination should include history of present illness, including details such as the illness onset (gradual or sudden), any fever, antipyretic use, neck pain or rigidity, rashes, difficulty swallowing or secretions, and changes in signs and symptoms over time. Assessment of the patient's past medical history should include chronic infections, use of steroids or antibiotics, organ transplantation, diabetes or other endocrine disorders, and chronic obstructive disease or respiratory complications. The detailed history and physical examination, once the present medical history has been established, should be comprehensive and include skin temperature, hydration, and color. Assess the sclera for icterus, the patient's reaction to neck flexion, the patient's breath sounds, any abdominal tenderness, and extremity or digit lesions. Complete the call by properly disposing of supplies once transfer of the patient has been completed.

INFECTIOUS DISEASES

Human Immunodeficiency Virus

[OBJECTIVE 16]

The human immunodeficiency virus (HIV) is thought to have originated in western Africa, with reported cases as early as the 1950s. In the United States, HIV is an evolving disease transmitted through fluids between human beings during sex or by percutaneous routes. Two strands of HIV (1 and 2) have been identified, with the major difference being that HIV2 develops more slowly into acquired immunodeficiency syndrome (AIDS). The diagnosis for HIV is made by documenting the decrease of infection-fighting cells called CD4 or T helper cells.

In 2003 an estimated 1,039,000 to 1,185,000 persons in the United States were living with HIV or AIDS, and in 2005 37,331 new cases of HIV or AIDS were diagnosed. The CDC estimates that approximately 40,000 persons in the United States become infected with HIV each year (CDC, 2007a).

HIV is spread through vaginal and anal intercourse. HIV is also spread through intravenous drug use when needles are shared and plunger aspiration spreads fluids from one user to another in an attempt to get most of the drug being injected. The infected person may not know of infection for years until opportunistic diseases lead to the diagnosis, thus allowing transmission to occur without the host's knowledge. The infected host will usually notice **malaise** and swelling of the lymph nodes, with an increase in diarrhea, unintended weight loss, evening fevers, and episodes of sweating. Physical signs include purplish lesions called *Kaposi sarcoma* (Figure 31-1). These symptoms in an already immune-suppressed person could become debilitating. HIV can take weeks to years before it progresses to AIDS. The diagnosis of AIDS is made when the CD4 cells or T-cell count falls below 250 mm³. At this point the patient is highly susceptible to opportunistic infections such as *Pneumocystis carinii*, which is a cause of pneumonia and the most common life-threatening opportunistic infection in patients with AIDS.

Once a person receives a diagnosis of HIV, he or she usually becomes despondent and goes through a period of depression related to the fear of loss of life, family, and friends. When the diagnosis is made, the patient is usually advised to talk to a psychiatrist as a part of treatment. To date no definitive cure for HIV or AIDS exists other than supportive care that allows the body to maintain its T-cell count and the administration of vitamins A, B, and C in response to the sometimes excessive diarrhea.

Healthcare providers will encounter patients with HIV or AIDS in the field and not know it. The only protection for the provider is to follow standard precautions at all times when the risk of contact with infectious materials is present, during patient contact, and during any biohazard cleanup after the run is completed. Healthcare providers who may have been exposed to HIV through an errant needlestick typically show a seroconversion rate of 0.2% to 0.3%. Protection advice for the public is to follow safe sex practices and, if available in the area, use of a needle exchange program for intravenous drug abusers.

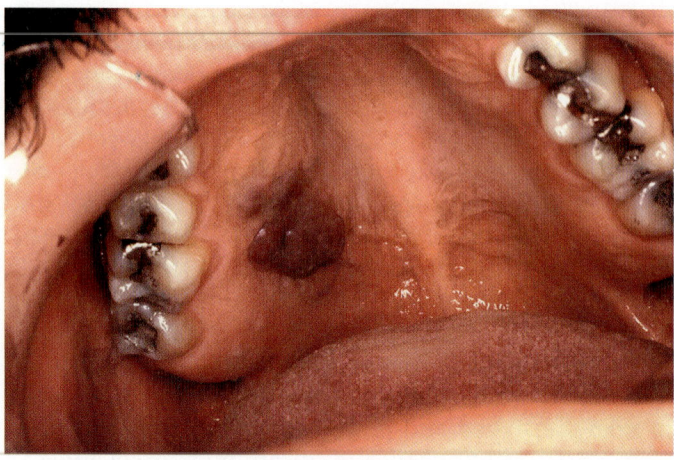

Figure 31-1 An HIV-infected patient with Kaposi sarcoma.

Hepatitis

[OBJECTIVE 17]

The history of viral hepatitis dates to around 1885, when approximately 200 German shipyard workers became jaundiced after being inoculated for smallpox from a vaccination created with human lymph nodes. At least six different strains of hepatitis have been identified (A, B, C, D, E, and G), with different effects seen in different socioeconomic groups and in underdeveloped countries, where drainage is still a problem.

Hepatitis A (HAV) and B (HBV) were initially discovered during World War II and became a major problem for military forces. Around 1989 a specific test for both HAV and HBV was found. Apparently posttransfusion infections were not HAV or HBV, but a third form of hepatitis called hepatitis C. Since then, other cases of hepatitis have found to not be A, B, or C. A water-borne form has been found and is called hepatitis E. Fortunately, cases of hepatitis A, B, and C have declined over the past several years. This decline is believed to be the result of effective vaccination programs, modern blood bank screening techniques, and public education leading to a decrease in activities that carry a high risk of infection. Hepatitis E is most commonly found in Asia, Africa, and the countries of the former Soviet Union, but is uncommon in the United States.

Hepatitis A Virus

HAV (formerly known as *infectious hepatitis*) is spread by the oral-fecal route, either directly by person-to-person contact or through contaminated water or food. Infection can spread quickly under conditions of poor sanitation and overcrowding. Persons at risk for HAV infection include staff and residents of institutions for the mentally handicapped, children and workers at day care centers, sexually active male homosexuals, intravenous drug abusers, sewage workers, military personnel, and certain low socioeconomic groups in defined community settings (Zuckerman & Zuckerman, 2004).

HAV enters the body by ingestion and then spreads to the liver. The incubation period for HAV is approximately 30 days, with a range of 15 to 45 days. Less than 14% of children infected with HAV have symptoms. In contrast, adults are more likely to have signs and symptoms of the disease. In most cases involving adults, jaundiced coloring is the predominant symptom, with abrupt onset of fever, weakness, anorexia, abdominal discomfort, nausea, and darkening of the urine, with liver failure being rare with treatment. Prognosis in most cases of HAV is good.

HAV can be prevented by good personal hygiene and proper sanitary disposal of human waste. Vaccines also are available for long-term prevention of HAV infection in persons 12 months of age and older. Immune globulin is available for short-term prevention of HAV infection. For example, immune globulin may be given to individuals who have close contact with a person who has HAV, to those exposed to contaminated food, or to persons traveling to areas in which HAV infection is common. Immune globulin can be given before and within 2 weeks after coming in contact with HAV.

Prehospital treatment for HAV is usually supportive. Hospitalization for HAV infection is usually unnecessary unless secondary problems arise, such as encephalopathy, coagulopathy, or intractable nausea and vomiting with abdominal pain. In most cases HAV infection is self-limiting. Prolonged illness and symptoms have been known to occur in some patients; however, chronic HAV infection does not occur.

Hepatitis B Virus

B & C are blood borne

[OBJECTIVES 18, 19]

People with HBV infection may have many of the same symptoms as HAV infection. After exposure, asymptomatic seroconversion is common, with age being the determining factor in the development of symptoms. Of note, acute HBV infections cannot be clinically distinguished from other hepatitis infections without laboratory testing.

HBV is transmitted through blood and other bodily fluids, including saliva, tears, semen, and vaginal secretions. Blood contains the highest concentrations of virus and saliva contains the lowest. HBV is commonly transmitted through sexual activity, drug use with nonsterile syringes, and percutaneous and mucosal exposure to infected secretions.

The patient's age at the time of infection is the largest factor in whether the patient will develop chronic HBV infection (Figure 31-2). In otherwise healthy patients, up

to 90% of exposed infants develop chronic infection; 25% to 50% of children ages 1 to 5 years become chronically infected after exposure. Only 6% to 10% of adolescents and adults develop chronic HBV infection after exposure (CDC, 2006a).

No specific treatment is available for HBV infection, though effective vaccinations exist. People who have not been vaccinated against HBV infection are the most susceptible. Those who have not been vaccinated against HBV should become so unless a medical reason not to exists.

Passive immunizations are recommended with a dose of immune globulin to help prevent hepatitis if exposed and reduce some symptoms in an infected person. Preventive measures such as meticulous hygiene and vigorous handwashing when in contact with contaminated materials also are recommended. After handwashing, the most important thing the healthcare worker can do to prevent infection with HBV or any infectious disease is to practice good sharps handling techniques. One of the most common routes of exposure to HBV in healthcare workers is through inadvertent needlesticks. Always immediately place needles in an appropriate sharps container and never recap a needle.

Hepatitis C

[OBJECTIVE 20]

blood borne

The hepatitis C virus (HCV) is a blood-borne virus most commonly transmitted by contaminated needles. Ten percent of patients with the disease have a history of a prior blood transfusion, 4% to 8% of cases are in healthcare workers who contracted it from occupational exposure, and 23% to 60% of cases are linked to intravenous drug abuse. Transmission of HCV through sexual contact is possible but uncommon. Before 1992, HCV was most commonly associated with contaminated blood products received during transfusion.

Because HCV can be spread easily through contaminated needles, it is a cause of great concern for healthcare workers who find themselves the victim of an errant needlestick. Up to 85% of healthcare workers who become infected with HCV become chronic carriers of the disease.

The disease is also seen for unknown reasons in persons with alcoholic liver disease. Alcoholics with cirrhosis and HCV sometimes lose liver function at a greater rate than do patients with either disease alone.

HCV infection has an average incubation period of 7 to 9 weeks, although the accepted clinical incubation period ranges from 2 to 25 weeks.

When transmission of HCV occurs, the signs and symptoms are similar to other types of hepatitis infections, including jaundice, malaise, fever, and change in stool and urine color. Many people infected with HCV appear completely asymptomatic.

Prehospital patient management for patients infected with HCV is primarily supportive. EMS and all other healthcare personnel should always use standard

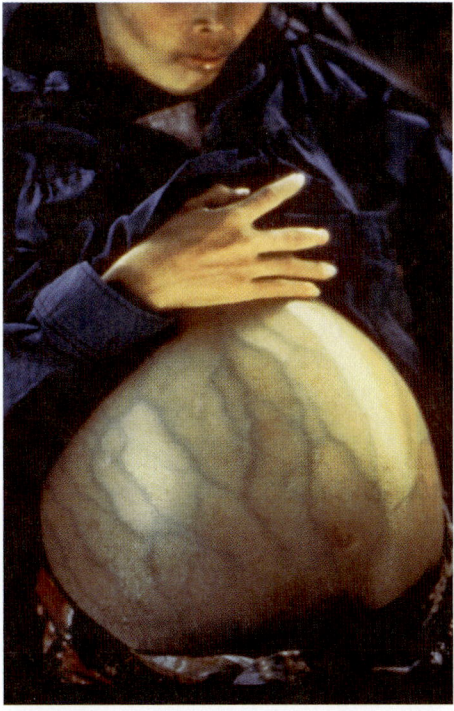

Figure 31-2 A female patient with a distended abdomen caused by a liver tumor resulting from chronic hepatitis B infection.

precautions and practice proper handwashing (American Academy of Pediatrics, 2003; Hoeprich et al., 1994).

Hepatitis D, E, and G

more common in other countries – probably fecal-oral

[OBJECTIVES 21, 22]

Further testing and treatment have detected hepatitis viruses in addition to A, B, and C. Hepatitis D is a delta virus, which means that it is not a complete virus but does infect the cell with other than the A, B, or C virus. When infected with HBV, hepatitis D becomes pathogenic. Hepatitis E is spread like HAV, and hepatitis G is a newly identified hepatitis virus. All treatment is the same and is usually supportive, involving intravenous fluids to lessen the chance of shock.

Tuberculosis

can get into other organs besides lungs

[OBJECTIVE 23]

In 2006 a total of 13,779 cases of tuberculosis (TB) were reported, resulting in 657 deaths in the United States. This is an all-time low in TB cases since national reporting began in 1953. However, the rate of decline was slower compared with 2005. The incidence of TB in patients born in other countries was 9.5 times higher compared with patients born in the United States (CDC, 2007g).

TB, although primarily a lung disorder, can affect all organs with acute, latent, or chronic problems. The causative agent for TB is *Mycobacterium tuberculosis,* which is primarily transmitted person to person through aerosolized nuclei or prolonged exposure to a person with active TB. Contamination usually comes from droplet nuclei expelled during a cough, sneeze, or prolonged talking. The infection is active in the air, but once it hits the ground it becomes inactive. Specific high-risk populations include nursing homes, healthcare facilities, prisons, medically underserved low-income populations, alcoholics, intravenous drug users, and the homeless. Paper and cloth masks provide no protection. Healthcare providers should use disposable particulate respirators.

TB is difficult to diagnose and cure because the patient cannot usually pinpoint when symptoms began; some asymptomatic diagnoses result from radiographic examination. Symptoms start gradually, usually with fever, malaise, and weight loss. The fever is usually noticed more at night, with the trademark night sweats, and the cough that is nonproductive early in the disease later becomes productive and associated with hemoptysis. Some blood streaking may occur as a result of the necrotic walls of cavities that the disease has created and from massive bleeding from ruptured vessel walls inside the lung. Pleuritic chest pain results from infection of the parietal pleural surface, and effusions are usually present. Dyspnea occurs if damage to the lung is extensive, and respiratory failure may follow as the disease progresses. On physical examination, crackles or rales may be detected over areas of consolidation, and a hollow sound resembling the sound made by blowing across the mouth of a bottle (amphoric breath sounds) may be heard over

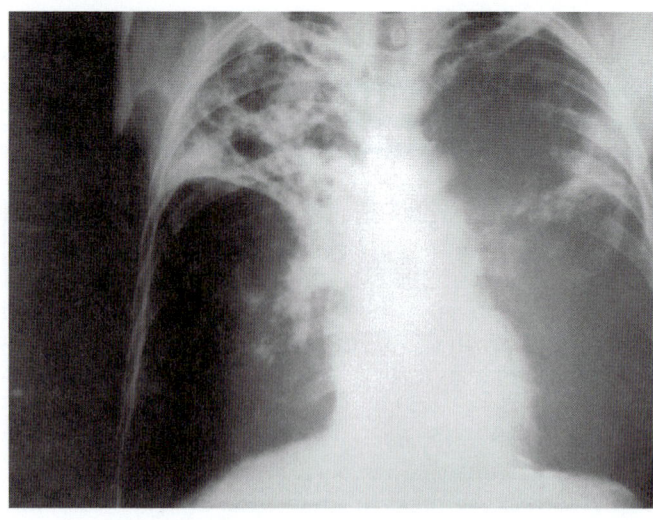

Figure 31-3 A radiograph of a patient with bilateral tuberculosis.

supposed to take TB drugs for 1 year – often don't so drug resistant strains

cavities (Figure 31-3). The differential diagnosis of TB symptoms includes asthma, pneumonia, pleural effusion, meningitis, septic shock, and both adult and pediatric respiratory distress syndrome.

Treatment for TB has been possible for more than four decades, with five drugs as the first line of treatment. Some drug resistance occurs, requiring second-line drugs. The first-line drug isoniazid, which was developed in 1952, remains the drug of choice. Rifampin, ethambutol, pyrazinamide, and streptomycin are the next choices in order of decreasing toxicity. Drug-resistant TB has increased in the United States for several reasons. The first is the closing of TB sanatoria, which terminated the direct supervision of treatment by physicians. The second reason is the pandemic infection rate of HIV-infected immigrants from countries with a high incidence of drug-resistant strains. Prehospital treatment is aimed at respiratory supportive care.

In 1989 the CDC published a plan to eradicate TB by 2010 (CDC, 1989). The plan focused on three groups of people: those with active, contagious pulmonary TB; infected persons without disease; and the uninfected. The paramount objectives are for the physician to identify the disease in a patient, work to keep transmission from occurring again, and then ensure that treatment is adhered to by encouraging family members to protect themselves from infection, ensuring treatment is mandated (Hoeprich et al., 1994; Li & Brainard, 2006).

Meningitis

[OBJECTIVES 24, 25]

Meningitis is an inflammatory disease of the central nervous system caused by the growth of a virus, bacteria, or fungus in and adjacent to the leptomeninges. Viral meningitis often is referred to as *aseptic meningitis.* This condition is often associated with an existing viral illness and is self-limited with complete recovery.

Bacterial meningitis is the more severe and potentially life-threatening form of meningitis. The most common cause is *Streptococcus pneumoniae* because most healthy people harbor this bacteria in the nasopharynx. However, it also can be caused by *Neisseria meningitides,* and *Listeria monocytogenes*. It also is caused to a lesser extent by *Haemophilus influenzae* type b because of the introduction of the *H. influenzae* vaccine in 1988; in fact, meningitis caused by this bacteria is almost nonexistent in the United States. The spread of meningitis is usually from direct or prolonged exposure to an infected person; to the prehospital provider, spread is usually during intubation and cardiopulmonary resuscitation. The causes of meningitis vary with age and the clinical setting in which the bacteriologic infection occurred. The bacteria initially colonize in the nasopharynx, where they proliferate; they then reach the subarachnoid space by crossing the blood-brain barrier. Although the mechanism by which this happens is not completely understood, patients often have decreased defense mechanisms, including the complement system, opsonization, and immunoglobulins. Inflammation of the meninges occurs as a result of the influx of leukocytes to the area to combat the infection along with the associated cytokine production, bacterial lysis, and other mediators of inflammation (see Chapter 8). This results in an increase in vascular permeability, edema and, ultimately, intracranial pressure. Males are more susceptible to the bacteria than are females when the infection is caused by gram-negative bacteria such as *Neisseria meningitides;* however, females are more commonly affected by *L. monocytogenes*. Because children have little protection without prior inoculation, meningitis is primarily a childhood disease. Meningitis is usually a metastatic infection typically associated with infections such as pneumonia, otitis media, and endocarditis. The actual causative agent is largely unknown (Lazloff, 2005) (Figure 31-4).

The affected person can have a variety of symptoms depending on the type of infection and, more importantly, his or her age. The usual presentation of fever, stiff neck, a petechial rash, an altered level of consciousness, diffuse neurologic deficits, vomiting, Kernig sign, Brudzinski sign, and increased intracranial pressure are not present in neonates and young infants. In these patients the initial signs and symptoms are quite subtle and may include refusal to eat, unexplained irritability, and lethargy. As the disease progresses fever, bulging fontanelles, and seizures can occur. Elderly patients may have only fever and delirium. The differential diagnosis of meningitis includes subarachnoid hemorrhage, herpes simplex encephalitis, and delirium tremens.

The primary function of the paramedic is to recognize the presence of meningitis and treat the signs and symptoms such as seizures. Without rapid treatment outcome can be poor, including death. Treatment for meningitis centers around several different antibiotics chosen for the specific bacteria that caused the infection. The primary choices are chloramphenicol, ampicillin and

Kids & college students

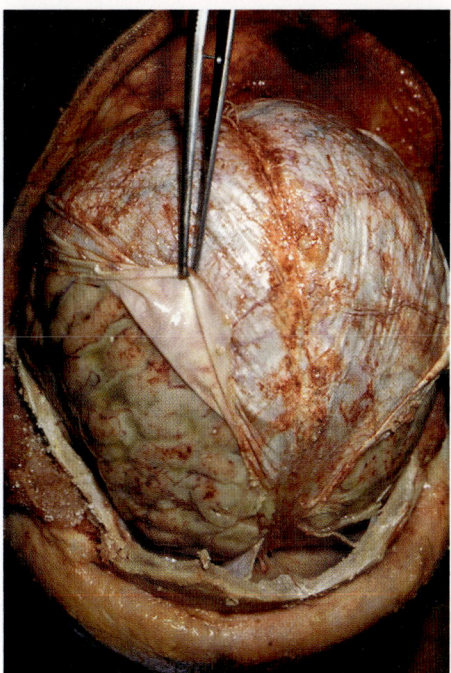

Recognized w/in 24 hrs. or may die.

Figure 31-4 Pneumococcal meningitis.

other penicillins, and cephalosporins. Supportive therapy in and out of the hospital is still recommended to protect against dehydration from vomiting and decreased intake.

Prevention of meningitis uses early inoculation from purified polysaccharide vaccines with minimal and infrequent side effects. Take precaution and adhere to hand and respiratory protection whenever possible. Any exposure to meningitis should be covered in the exposure control plan of that service. Patients' families also should be educated on the importance of proper exposure procedures, including the use of standard precautions and prophylaxis with rifampin (Berkow, 1999; Hoeprich et al., 1994).

Pneumonia

[OBJECTIVE 26]

As described in Chapter 21, pneumonia is an inflammatory respiratory infection that affects the alveoli and surrounding tissues. Pneumonia is most common in the winter months; upwards of 3 million cases causing approximately 500,000 hospital admissions are seen in the United States annually. This disease is particularly deadly in the elderly population. The disease may be caused by a host of bacterial, fungal, and viral organisms that attack the respiratory and central nervous systems. Agents commonly known to cause pneumonia include *S. pneumoniae, Staphylococcus aureus, Mycoplasma pneumoniae, H. influenzae, Legionella* spp., and other viral and fungus causative agents. Treatment regimens depend on a number of factors, including the health of the host and

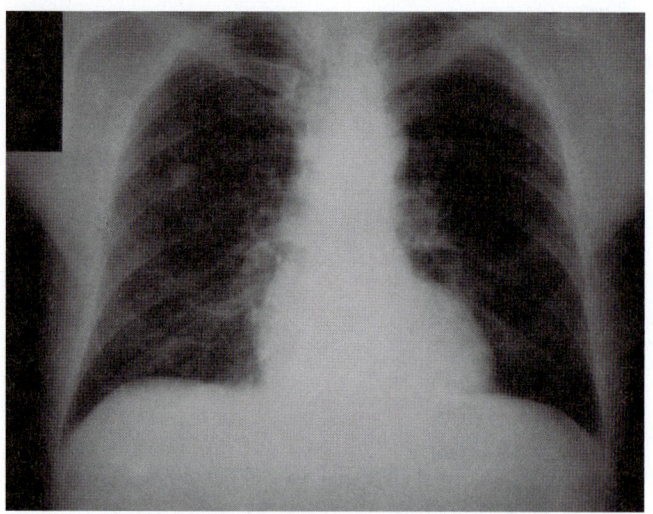

Figure 31-5 A patient with pneumonia in the upper right lobe.

whether pneumonia is the primary infection or developed secondary to another illness (Figure 31-5).

Pneumonia often is classified as community acquired or hospital acquired. Although the latter form specifies "hospital," it can be acquired in any healthcare facility. In general, community-acquired pneumonia is managed in the outpatient setting and has a low mortality rate. However, its incidence is increasing. Infections acquired in a healthcare setting have a higher mortality rate because they tend to be more virulent strains of infectious organisms and may be resistant to medications.

The transmission of pneumonia is usually by droplet or direct contact with the host or through linens contaminated by respiratory secretions. The susceptibility of the host is directly proportionate to the status of the respiratory tissues (e.g., pulmonary edema, influenza, chronic lung disease) and aspiration in any form (e.g., alcohol intoxication, aspirated gastric contents). The groups of most concern regarding susceptibility are those with sickle cell disease, cardiac disease, diabetes mellitus, chronic renal failure, HIV, organ transplantation, and different forms of lymphoma. Pneumonia has accounted for approximately 15% of all hospital-associated infections and 27% and 24% of all infections acquired in the intensive care unit and critical care unit, respectively (CDC, 2004).

Physical findings and associated symptoms of pneumonia are directly related to the causative organism. The onset of typical pneumonia may be sudden, with chills, fever, chest discomfort with respiration, and difficulty breathing. Physical examination of the patient may reveal varying degrees of respiratory distress, fever, tachycardia, tachypnea, and potentially low oxygen saturation. Crackles may be present over affected lobes (with other lobes normal) in lobar pneumonia, scattered crackles in bronchopneumonia, and scattered crackles and wheezes in interstitial pneumonia.

Certain agents cause atypical pneumonia. In these cases the patient may have a gradual onset of the disease, a nonproductive cough, a low-grade fever or the absence of fever, chills, headache, nausea and vomiting, a sore throat, and extrapulmonary symptoms. Although the determination of typical or atypical pneumonia is unnecessary in the prehospital setting, the paramedic must be aware of the distinction in order to not miss the diagnosis of pneumonia in the absence of a productive cough and fever.

In the elderly, pneumonia often manifests with nonspecific complaints such as acute confusion or changes in the normal ability to function. In many cases, pneumonia in these patients may be severe by the time it is recognized, and the patient may be septic without prior indicators of an infection.

In children, fever, tachypnea, and chest retractions are ominous signs. The patient may cough up yellow-green phlegm. Several effective antibiotics treat bacterial pneumonia; however, drug-resistant strains have been reported. As far as isolation is concerned, most patients do not require it unless they are in a facility with other patients who are more susceptible to drug-resistant infections. Immunizations do exist for some strains but are usually not indicated in EMS personnel.

Encourage patients with pneumonia to remain compliant with treatments as prescribed by their physicians, even if they begin to feel better before the completion of therapy. Also encourage patients to cover their mouths when coughing. Advise families of patients to observe proper handwashing techniques and seek medical attention at the first sign of infection.

Tetanus

[OBJECTIVE 27]

Tetanus is caused by a bacterial spore that attacks the musculoskeletal system exclusively. The causative agent is *Clostridium tetani*, which is commonly found in the soil and gastrointestinal tracts of animals. *C. tetani* is a spore-forming gram-positive bacteria. It also is a strict anaerobe that is highly susceptible to heat. This means that if the bacterium is exposed to a harmful environment, such as oxygen or heat, it will form a spore for survival. Unlike the bacterium itself, the spores are highly resistant to heat, antiseptics, phenol, and other chemicals, which allows them to survive in the soil and other environments. Tetanus is introduced into the body through wounds, burns, or other injuries to the skin. The infection also can be introduced when material such as soil, street dust, or feces penetrates the skin, such as in the setting of a puncture wound with a contaminated object.

Once inside the body and in the absence of oxygen, the spores germinate and the bacterium *C. tetani* is reformed. *C. tetani* releases two toxins, tetanolysin and tetanospasmin. The role of tetanolysin is unknown, but tetanospasmin is the cause of tetanus. It spreads to nearby motor nerves, where it binds to the nerves and spreads up the axons to the ventral horns of the spinal cord. There it interferes with neurons that inhibit muscular contraction. The incubation period for the disease is 3 to 21 days.

The susceptibility of tetanus is rather general, meaning anyone can contract it; this is the reason immunization is recommended for the general population. The vaccine was first introduced in 1924 and became widely used in the military during World War II. This resulted in a significant decrease in the cases of tetanus compared with World War I. The vaccination became a part of routine childhood vaccinations in the late 1940s, and booster shots are recommended every 10 years. Because of this tetanus is a rare disease in the United States. All infections reported in recent years have been in patients who were either never vaccinated or did not receive the recommended booster. Infection and cure do not result in immunity to the disease.

Signs and symptoms of tetanus are muscular **tetany** (prolonged muscular contractions) of the jaw and neck muscles. These can be strong enough to cause fractures. In children abdominal rigidity may be the first sign. For the adult, facial contortion known as **risus sardonicus** may be seen. If left untreated, tetanus can lead to respiratory failure. Management of a patient with tetanus is administration of tetanus immune globulin or tetanus antitoxin (equine origin) generally followed by active tetanus immunization with a booster. EMS workers should keep their immunizations up to date and counsel patients with breaks in the skin to receive treatment while inquiring their immunization status.

Rabies

[OBJECTIVE 28]

Rabies, a viral infection of mammals caused by a *rhabdovirus* of the genus *Lyssavirus,* is usually transmitted by the spread of infected saliva into a bite wound. More than 60 different viruses are in this genus, and the causative virus of rabies has a distinct bulletlike appearance with protruding glycoprotein spikes. Transmission is rare in the United States, with five to 10 cases annually, but is much more prominent in less-developed countries, which report 40,000 to 70,000 deaths from rabies per year. In 2006 a total of 6940 animal cases and three human cases were reported to the CDC in the United States (CDC, 2007b).

The rabies virus and at least five related viruses (Mokola virus, Duvenhage virus, two European bat viruses, and Lagos bat virus) constitute the causative agent and are classified as rhabdoviruses according to morphology, host range, tissue tropism, and susceptibility to chemical reagents. Rabies occurs nearly worldwide in wildlife, although it is absent in many insular areas such as the United Kingdom, Australia, New Zealand, Japan, and Hawaii. Rabies occurs in a cyclic, widespread migration that alternates with periods of endemicity. During 2005,

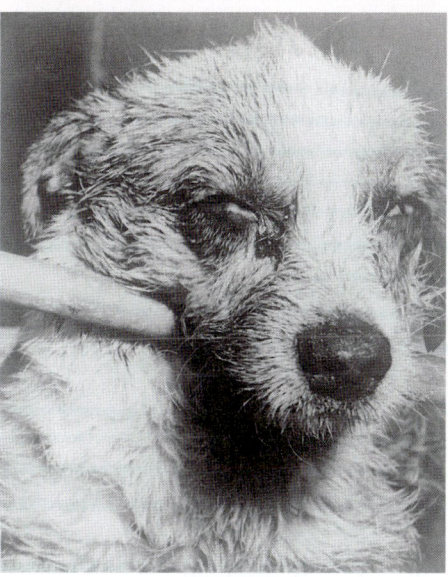

Figure 31-6 Close-up of a dog's face during late-stage "dumb" paralytic rabies.

92% of the 6417 cases of nonhuman rabies reported in the United States were in wildlife (Blanton et al., 2006). Wildlife rabies is complex, involving many species of hosts and viral strains or variants. In general, each rabies strain is well adapted for serial transmission. The domestic dog is the principal **vector** in Africa, Latin America, Asia, and Turkey (Figure 31-6). Wild animals are the principal vectors for Europe, Canada, and the United States.

Except for a relatively brief period before the appearance of signs of the disease, no infectious, clinically healthy carrier state has been shown to exist in the species infected with typical rabies. The virus is usually transmitted by a bite that implants saliva containing an infective dose of virus in a muscle. The virus then multiplies in the muscle and travels along the nerves from the point of inoculation to the central nervous system. While the infection progresses, it is largely isolated from the immune systems of the host. Viral replication in the brain is followed by migration to the eyes, heart, skin, and mouth. The cycle is complete when the virus replicates in the salivary glands and is shed into the saliva. The dense sensory concentration of nerve endings in the face, head, neck, and fingers explains the higher fatality rate when one of these sites is the point of inoculation. The rabies virus has been shown to be infective through contact with the mucous membranes. Transplacental transmission did not occur in several reliable reports of pregnant women with rabies.

The clinical phases of rabies are generally the same in terrestrial species, including human beings: **prodrome,** excitatory, and paralytic. In human beings, until advancement to the paralytic phase, mental faculties are well preserved. The incubation period is 1 to 3 months but is extremely variable, ranging from 10 days to 14 months. Cases with latency periods of up to 7 years have been confirmed. Death usually follows the appearance of rabies after 4 to 14 days, but predominately paralytic cases may last longer.

The prodromal phase usually lasts 2 to 10 days, with patients having nonspecific symptoms such as fever, malaise, headache, anorexia, nausea and vomiting, sore throat, poorly defined sensory changes, rhinitis, anxiety, agitation, and gastrointestinal symptoms. Paresthesia, pruritus, or pain at the site of the bite may be the first neurologic symptoms.

The excitatory phase is seen in approximately 80% of cases but can be absent, be quickly transitory, or may last a week. This phase usually begins gradually and may persist until death. Progressive anxiety, agitation, and apprehension are usually present, with an impending feeling of doom. Patients may become disoriented and have spasm of the neck muscles, twitching, and seizures. Weakness is present in the muscle group at the site of inoculation. Hydrophobia, the classic diagnostic manifestation of rabies, is a forceful, painful expulsion of liquids when the patient attempts to swallow.

The last phase, the paralytic phase, occurs in approximately 20% of cases and may precede death by 1 to 4 weeks. In this phase, a progressive, general flaccid paralysis develops; apathy changes into stupor, progressing to coma. Urinary incontinence is followed by peripheral vascular collapse, then death.

Diagnosis of rabies comes when a bite has occurred from a rabid animal and the bitten person shows typical signs. In many instances a history of exposure is lacking and the diagnosis of rabies is revealed in postmortem laboratory tests.

Clinical rabies is almost always fatal; no specific therapy is available for overt rabies. The only means proved useful are preventive and must be initiated as quickly as possible after exposure.

Prevention of rabies in human beings includes avoiding exposure to infected animals, cleansing wounds, and immunizing persons who have been exposed. The biggest step in the prevention of rabies is adequate surveillance.

Hantaviruses

Food storage n warehouses otherwise rare

[OBJECTIVE 28]

Hantavirus is a disease that consists of hemorrhagic fevers with renal syndromes (HFRS) in Eurasia and hantavirus pulmonary syndrome (HPS) in the Americas. The infection is primarily rodent borne and caused by a number of different hantaviruses, each with a specific rodent reservoir.

The clinical syndrome of the hantavirus was identified as early as AD 960 in China. In 1940 the Japanese first inoculated human beings and monkeys with a bacteria-free serum from patients already infected; the recipients then developed the same symptoms, proving to the scientists that the etiology is both infectious and viral.

HFRS occurs in early summer and late fall. It still continues to be a cause of considerable infections in certain countries in Asia. The disease is chronic, with lifelong secretions of the virus. Adult men who hunt rodents and laboratory workers who handle infected rodents are at the greatest risk. Human-to-human transmission has not been documented. The virus enters the human body through the respiratory mucosa.

Hantavirus renal syndrome involves fever, hemorrhage, and renal failure, with severe cases presenting with headache, abdominal and lumbar pain, and proteinuria. The patient is initially febrile, then develops hypotension and oliguria. Most patients develop diuresis, leading to prolonged convalescence. Survival usually entails complete recovery, but chronic renal insufficiency may result.

During the febrile stage the patient has blurred vision, photophobia, and retroorbital pain. The face, neck, and back are flushed, and pharyngeal and conjunctival stain is seen. Petechiae are seen in the conjunctivae, axillae, and at pressure points.

During the hypotensive phase, a rising hematocrit level corresponds with capillary leak syndrome. Massive proteinuria and oliguria are present.

The oliguric phase is associated with severe hemorrhagic phenomena. The majority of deaths are seen in this phase. Less severe cases develop fever with gastrointestinal symptoms followed by brief oliguria.

HPS displays a febrile, respiratory failure pattern with prominent capillary leak syndrome. Hypotension and hemorrhagic manifestations are frequent. Tachycardia, tachypnea, and hypotension are common and promote hypotension and pulmonary edema. If frank shock with severe hypoxemia present promptly, mortality rate is much higher.

Diagnosis can be confirmed serologically by a fourfold immunoglobulin G antibody rise. Detection of viral antigens also can be made from serum samples. Isolation of the virus is difficult and not generally available for diagnostic purposes.

Treatment of hantavirus infection is difficult. Ribavirin has been shown to work for HFRS if administered in the first 7 days but has not been shown to be of any benefit to HPS. Studies are currently underway, but supportive care is still the mainstay of treatment.

Prevention is difficult because rodents are still hunted for food, but household hygienic precautions have been shown to be useful.

Viral Diseases of Childhood

Varicella Zoster (Chickenpox)

[OBJECTIVES 29, 30]

Chickenpox is a common childhood ailment endemic in all parts of the world. It primarily affects the integumentary system with a generalized vesicular rash consisting of 250 to 500 lesions. The infection is caused by the varicella zoster virus, which is a member of the herpesvirus family. Human beings are the only source of the virus, which is primarily airborne. Although most people who have had chickenpox remain immune after the primary infection, the virus establishes latency in the dorsal root ganglia and can reactivate later in life, resulting in herpes zoster (shingles).

also airborn

The infection is spread when the virus comes in contact with the mucosa of the upper respiratory tract or the conjunctiva of a susceptible person. The virus also may be spread through contact with ruptured vesicles.

After exposure to the virus, the incubation period is between 10 and 21 days. A low-grade fever and general feeling of malaise typically precede the onset of the rash by 24 hours. After the rash appears the fever may continue for several days. Lesions may appear anywhere on the body but are more numerous on the trunk, with the legs typically becoming the last area to be involved (Figure 31-7). The rash begins as small red spots that become blisters on an erythematous base. Lesions continue to form for up to 5 days in the otherwise healthy child and typically heal over a 3-week period.

Children with chickenpox should be kept home from school and remain as isolated as possible until all lesions have dried and crusted over. **Antiviral** drugs, such as acyclovir, shorten the duration and severity of the symptoms as well as pain in older patients. Keep children's fingernails short during the duration of the illness to prevent scratching of blisters and secondary bacteriologic infections. Drugs such as acetaminophen may be used to control fevers and pain, but aspirin should be avoided to prevent Reye syndrome.

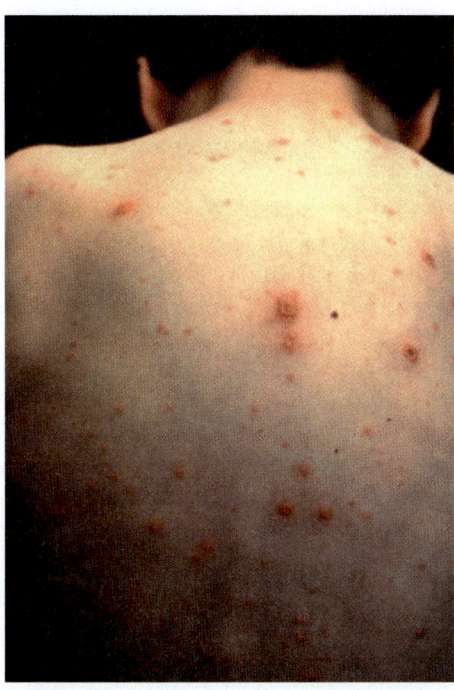

Figure 31-7 A patient with chickenpox lesions.

Observe standard precautions when in contact with patients and while handling dirty linens. Personnel who have never had chickenpox are encouraged to undergo vaccination. Of adults who receive the chickenpox vaccine, 82% show antibody production after the initial dose and 92% antibody production after two doses. Varivax, the vaccination for chickenpox, contains a weakened but live agent that prevents chickenpox in 70% to 90% of all cases. The remaining 10% to 30% of patients show a significant decrease in the severity of the disease. The vaccine should not be given to patients who have taken high doses of systemic steroids in the past month. For pregnant women with a significant exposure, the varicella-zoster immune globulin is recommended (American Academy of Pediatrics, 2003; Hoeprich et al., 1994; Newton et al., 2000).

Mumps

[OBJECTIVE 31]

Mumps is an acute viral infection caused by a member of the Paramyxovirus family that most commonly affects children and young adults. The mumps virus causes a general infection characterized by tenderness and swelling of the parotid and salivary glands. Although the prevalence of mumps has decreased with the measels, mumps, and rubella (MMR) vaccination, infections are still seen at a rate of fewer than 500 per year in the United States. Fully one third of cases may be asymptomatic. Patients with mumps are at risk for developing aseptic meningitis because the most common extraglandular site of mumps is the central nervous system. Although mumps accounts for only 1% of aseptic meningitis infections in the United States, only 40% to 50% of patients with mumps meningitis have inflammation of the parotid glands (parotitis).

Mumps is spread through droplet transmission and contact with the saliva of an infected person. Patients are most contagious for 1 to 2 days before parotid swelling and for up to 5 days after parotid swelling. The incubation period of the mumps virus can range from 12 to 25 days.

Although children are now required by law to receive vaccinations against mumps, a single vaccination does not always confer immunity. Immunity from vaccination lasts well into adulthood, as confirmed by laboratory tests. Patients who contract the infection despite vaccination or because of a lack of vaccination are typically immune from further infection.

Although one third of cases remain asymptomatic, the illness usually presents with low-grade fever, headache, malaise, anorexia, and upper and lower respiratory symptoms a few days before the onset of parotitis. Mumps is characterized by the swelling of the parotid and other salivary glands that progresses for up to 3 days and then subsides over the following 7 to 10 days (Figure 31-8). Parotitis is seen bilaterally in 75% of cases, yet one gland often will swell a few days before the others. The swelling may range from tenderness to a painful enlargement of

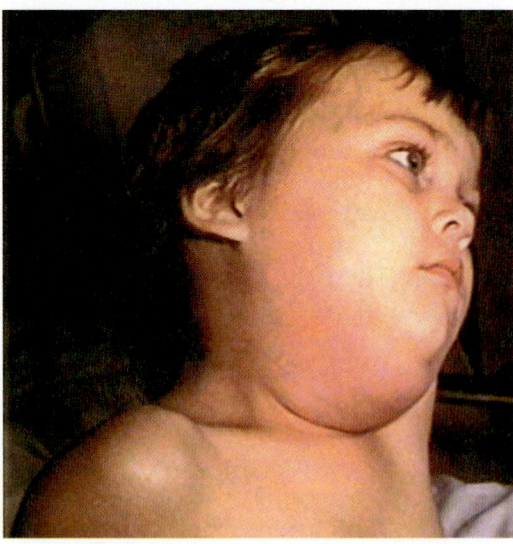

Figure 31-8 A patient with mumps.

the face and jaw, causing the angle of the jaw to disappear and asymmetry of the neck. Mumps also may cause swelling of the sublingual glands, leading to dysphagia and swelling of the tongue. Less commonly mumps also may cause hearing loss, pancreatitis, and arthritis.

Because mumps is caused by a virus, treatment for the condition is aimed at supportive care. Acetaminophen and ibuprofen can be given to relieve pain and swelling, and the patient should be encouraged to stay hydrated and fed, although patients with mumps can sometimes find eating and drinking painful.

EMS personnel should not be working without having been vaccinated by either a mumps vaccine alone or the combination MMR immunization. Use standard precautions when treating patients with mumps. Give patients a surgical mask to wear, and thoroughly wash hands and arms after patient contact. Because mumps is spread through contact with an infected patient's saliva, take special care when handling anything that has come into contact with the patient's mouth or mucous membranes (e.g., thermometers, tissues) (American Association of Pediatrics, 2003; Hoeprich et al., 1994; Newton et al., 2000).

Rubella   *Not as severe as Rubeola unless PG woman*
[OBJECTIVE 32]

Rubella often is referred to as the *German measles* or *3-day measles* and is caused by the rubella virus. Rubella affects the integumentary and musculoskeletal systems as well as the lymph nodes.

The virus is spread through the inhalation of virus from the respiratory tract of an infected person. A single, brief exposure to an infected patient is not likely to cause infection; close, prolonged contact is more consequential. Rubella also may be spread through nasopharyngeal secretions.

Rubella may be transmitted from mother to fetus with severe consequences. This is referred to as *congenital*

Rubella syndrome (CRS). Infants exposed to rubella in the first trimester have a 90% chance of being born with some degree of CRS. Infant anomalies associated with CRS include ophthalmologic (glaucoma, cataracts), cardiac, auditory (hearing impairment), and neurologic (mental retardation, behavioral disorders) abnormalities as well as retarded growth. Infants born with CRS also exhibit a large degree of viral shedding in secretions and should be considered contagious until they are at least 1 year of age.

Human beings are the only known natural carriers of the rubella virus. The incidence of rubella has decreased by 99% in the United States after the invention of the MMR vaccine (Zimmerman & Reef, 2002). Most outbreaks now occur in unvaccinated young adults at work and on college campuses. After vaccination or natural infection, active immunity is acquired and generally lasts for life.

Rubella is generally a mild disease of moderate contagiousness with a 1- to 5-day incubation period, after which a mild prodrome may occur. The prodrome, most commonly seen in adolescents and young adults rather than young children, is characterized by headache, low-grade fever, **conjunctivitis,** malaise, and respiratory symptoms. Cervical, postauricular, and occipital lymph nodes become swollen and tender. As the prodromal symptoms decrease the rash appears, starting at the face and quickly moving down the trunk and extremities, often in a matter of hours. The rash, sometimes mistaken for scarlet fever, is an erythematous maculopapular rash lasting for up to 3 days that quickly fades in the order it appeared (Figure 31-9). Although rare, acute rubella encephalitis can occur in approximately 1 in 6000 cases and is more common in children. Approximately 33% of females who contract the disease develop a self-limiting arthritis involving the fingers, wrists, and knees. The arthritis usually clears without residual effects within 2 to 30 days.

EMS personnel who encounter patients with suspected rubella infections must use standard precautions, including a mask to avoid exposure to respiratory secretions. Use effective handwashing, as with all patients. No specific treatment for rubella is available, only supportive care. All personnel should be vaccinated against rubella before working, especially women, because infections during pregnancy can lead to CRS. The MMR vaccine protects against measles, mumps, and rubella and has shown to be 98% to 99% effective. The vaccine, however, is not recommended for pregnant women because it carries a theoretical risk to the fetus (American Academy of Pediatrics, 2003; Hoeprich et al., 1994; Newton et al., 2000).

Measles (Rubeola, Hard Measles)
[OBJECTIVES 33, 34]

Measles is an acute, highly contagious disease caused by the measles virus of the Paramyxoviridae family. Measles affects the respiratory system, central nervous

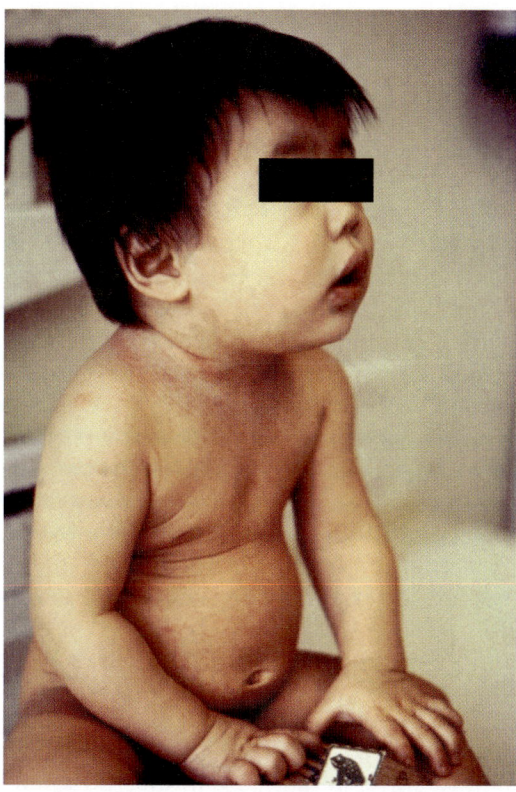

Figure 31-9 A patient with a rubella rash.

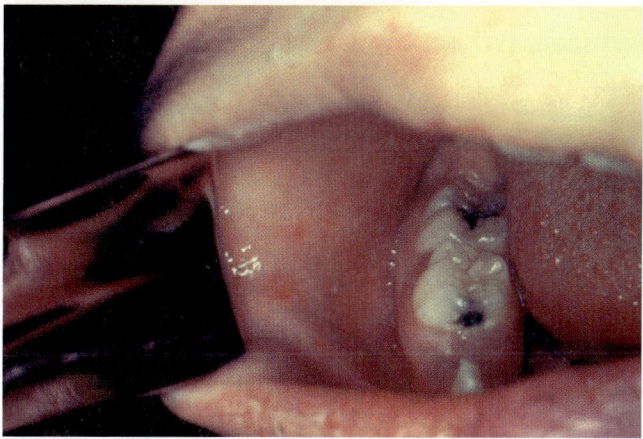

Figure 31-10 A patient with Koplik spots on the oral mucosa.

system, mouth, and pharynx, with a rash appearing on the skin. The virus is highly contagious and is spread through direct contact and droplets from the nasopharynx.

Measles is considered one of the most contagious of all infectious diseases. Patients are contagious from 1 to 2 days before the onset of any prodromal symptoms and up to 4 days after the appearance of the rash. Measles has an incubation period of between 8 and 18 days.

Incidence has been reduced 98% to 99% in the United States since vaccination efforts began in 1963. Although vaccine failure occurs in up to 5% of people who received a single dose at 1 year or older, immunity acquired after natural infection is lifelong.

Measles first appears as a series of prodromal symptoms that include a hacking cough, conjunctivitis, swelling of the eyelids, photophobia, and a body temperature of up to 105° F. During this prodromal period characteristic Koplik spots (Figure 31-10) appear on the buccal mucosa either on the inner lip or just opposite the lower molars. These spots appear as reddish bumps with tiny blue-white specks in their centers. Koplik spots are difficult to find during the early prodromal phase but quickly spread to the entire mucous membrane. These spots appear up to 2 days before the appearance of rash and tend to vanish as the rash reaches its peak.

The rash normally first appears behind the ears, on the forehead, and in the hairline as flat, reddened patches before quickly progressing to the maculopapular rash that spreads down over the trunk and abdomen, usually reaching the feet by the third day. The measles rash first appears thicker over the head and shoulders and then begins to clear, following the same pattern toward the feet. It typically lasts 6 days.

Patients with measles sometimes have secondary infections such as laryngitis, otitis media, myocarditis, and damage to the eyes. Pneumonia is frequently seen as a secondary infection, with an incidence rate between 3.5% and 50%. Pregnant women are at increased risk. The most dangerous complication from measles is the development of subacute sclerosing panencephalitis (SSPE). SSPE is seen as a complication in 1 of every 1000 cases and carries a mortality rate of 5% to 10%. The highest fatality rate is seen in children younger than 4 years. Of all patients who develop SSPE, 30% to 35% are left with mild to severe neurologic impairments.

The symptoms of SSPE usually begin between the first and seventh days of infection with a rash and first present as general drowsiness and irritability. These symptoms may progress to seizure activity and coma within hours. Vomiting and sudden rises in temperature are commonly seen as well. Coma may lighten after 1 to 3 days, with a variable period of recovery.

Because measles is caused by a virus, no cure is available; management is aimed at supportive care. As with every patient, use standard precautions, including a mask and proper handwashing. All personnel should be immunized with the MMR vaccination, which has shown to confer 99% immunogenicity.

The importance of immunization, especially in the pediatric population, cannot be overstated. Although many of the diseases of childhood generally are self-limiting, they can cause lifelong disabilities, suffering, and death. The MMR vaccination in particular has drastically decreased the number of cases of measles, mumps, and rubella seen today (American Academy of Pediatrics, 2003; Hoeprich et al., 1994; Newton et al., 2000).

Pertussis (Whooping Cough)

[OBJECTIVE 35]

Pertussis, which means *forceful cough,* is caused by the gram-negative bacillus *Bordetella pertussis* and is commonly referred to as *whooping cough.* It affects the oropharynx and is transmitted by airborne droplets from an infected host.

Many cases of pertussis in the United States go unrecognized or misdiagnosed. Nearly all people are vaccinated against pertussis, but older children and adults may still become infected, implying that immunity may decrease over time. Many of the cases in young children and previously immunized persons do not follow the classic pattern, allowing for misdiagnosis.

Pertussis has an incubation period of 6 to 20 days, after which patients exhibit signs of an upper respiratory infection. The initial phase, the catarrhal phase, of pertussis is indistinguishable from upper respiratory infection except that the symptoms worsen and the cough becomes more persistent.

The next phase, the paroxysmal phase, of the illness lasts for 2 to 4 weeks and is characterized by episodic sudden coughing, which may be so severe that the patient may not be able to eat or sleep adequately. The cough most associated with pertussis is noted for the violent inspiratory stridor forced by air hunger caused by a prolonged paroxysm of coughing. This also may be associated with cyanosis, protrusion of the tongue, diaphoresis, salivation, lacrimation and vomiting. Periods of syncope and apnea also may occur. However, many patients have a cough but do not "whoop," especially children younger than 6 months and adults. Infants may simply have periods of apnea and no other associated signs or symptoms.

Patients in the final phase, the convalescent phase, have a cough that may last for weeks to months.

Be cautious in patients with a recent history of a paroxysmal cough and always use standard precautions and mask the patient with a surgical mask. Patients are thought to be most contagious *before* the onset of the paroxysmal cough. Erythromycin has been shown to be effective at decreasing the communicability period but only if administered during the incubation period and *before* the onset of paroxysmal cough.

Vaccinations are available as the diphtheria, tetanus, and pertussis (DTP) immunization. Unlike some vaccinations, immunity wanes over time so booster doses are recommended (American Academy of Pediatrics, 2003; Hoeprich et al., 1994; Newton et al., 2000). This is particularly important for healthcare workers (CDC, 2006b).

Other Viral Diseases

Influenza

[OBJECTIVE 36]

Influenza is one of the most common infectious diseases primarily affecting the respiratory system. It accounts for a large degree of suffering, morbidity, and mortality. Of the three influenza viruses (A, B, and C) only one serologic form of influenza B exists. Influenza A, however, undergoes antigenic drift and mutates so often that variants are named by geographic location of isolation, culture number, and year of isolation. For example, the A/USSR/90/77 influenza strain is influenza A, found in the former Soviet Union, culture number 90, in 1977. Influenza A is further characterized by the types of surface glycoproteins, hemagglutinin and neuraminidase. Seven hemagglutinin types and up to nine neuraminidase glycoproteins are capable of producing any variation of influenza A virus (H1N1, H1N2, H5N1, etc.). Influenza A is the most common cause of the influenza virus, whereas influenza B causes regional or widespread epidemics every 2 to 3 years. Influenza C rarely causes epidemics, but rather small outbreaks in children; no significant variants are known. Nearly 100% of the population has developed antibodies against influenza viruses by age 15 years.

Influenza is an extremely infectious virus that can be spread through the air in crowded places and through direct contact with an infected person. The virus can live outside the body for up to several hours in settings with low humidity and low temperature.

Influenza has an incubation period of 24 to 96 hours, though viral shedding in infected patients may begin 1 day before the onset of symptoms. All persons are susceptible to influenza infection; however, the disease can be fatal in the very young and very old. The yearly influenza vaccine is not a guarantee of immunity, but rather scientists' best guess at which strain of influenza will affect the population that winter based on the South American flu season. Mutation or antigenic drift after the vaccine has been created is not uncommon. After influenza infection, patients are typically **resistant** to additional influenza infections but only to the same strain.

Influenza usually begins with a sudden onset of fever, with body temperature ranging from 102° F to 104° F, followed by headache, chills, muscle aches, diaphoresis, anorexia, joint stiffness, fatigue, malaise, and upper respiratory symptoms. The cough that accompanies influenza is not typically productive and may be accompanied by a sore throat and nasal congestion as well as nausea and vomiting.

Treatment for patients with influenza is often limited to supportive care only. If a diagnosis of influenza is made within 48 hours of infection, a patient may be given amantadine hydrochloride, rimantadine hydrochloride, oseltamivir phosphate (TamiFlu), or zanamivir (Relenza). These medicines have been shown to decrease the duration and severity of influenza infection. Persons exposed to influenza also may be given amantadine, rimantadine, or oseltamivir prophylactically.

Closely observe standard precautions and have the patient with influenza wear a a surgical mask. Also be cautious in handling any dirty linens, thermometer probes, respiratory supplies, and oxygen delivery devices that have come into contact with infected patients. EMS workers and other healthcare employees are encouraged to be immunized by mid-September each year so that immunity peaks during the U.S. flu season, which begins in November and continues through March.

Special attention has been paid to an emerging influenza threat commonly referred to as *bird flu, avian influenza,* or its subtype, *H5N1.* Currently this strain of influenza A can be passed directly from infected birds to human beings but has not been shown to be communicable from person to person, except in rare cases. The H5N1 strain of influenza causes symptoms typical of influenza, but because of the severity of the disease many people die from respiratory failure.

Currently the disease in human beings has been confined to Asia, though birds have tested positive for the virus across Europe. As of November 2006 the World Health Organization had confirmed 258 cases of human infection, with 154 cases proving fatal. Scientists do not know when or if the virus will mutate but warn that a pandemic of avian influenza could cause the deaths of millions worldwide. No vaccine can be created for H5N1 until the virus mutates to a form that is communicable from person to person (American Association of Pediatrics, 2003; CDC, 2006c; Hoeprich et al., 1994; World Health Organization, 2007).

Mononucleosis
[OBJECTIVE 37]

Infectious mononucleosis is an acute disease caused by the Epstein-Barr virus (EBV), a member of the herpes family. EBV infections affect the oropharynx, tonsils, and lymphatic system.

Infectious mononucleosis is extremely contagious and is spread by oropharyngeal secretions and saliva. In children the transmission from caregivers and other family members is common. In adults, kissing is implicated in the spread of the disease. EBV also can be spread through blood transfusions but rarely causes clinical disease.

Most EBV infections are seen in young adults between the ages of 15 and 25 years. In college settings more cases are seen in early fall and early spring, but no seasonal variance exists for the general population. Exposure to EBV does not guarantee the development of clinical disease, but infection usually provides a high degree of resistance.

Infectious mononucleosis has an incubation period of 30 to 50 days, after which the disease is characterized by varying fevers, sore throat, oropharyngeal discharges, lymphadenopathy (especially of the cervical lymph nodes), conjuctival hemorrhage (Figure 31-11), and splenomegaly. Rupture of the spleen is rare but not unprecedented and is commonly the only cause of abdominal pain in patients with the disease.

No specific treatment or vaccine is available for infectious mononucleosis. Nonsteroidal antiinflammatory

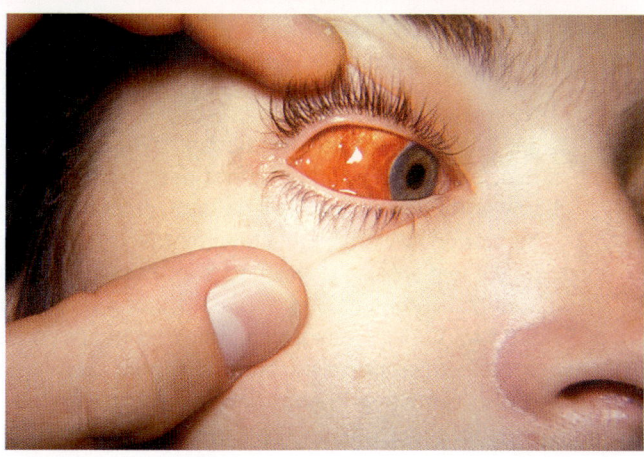

Figure 31-11 A conjunctival hemorrhage of the eye in a patient with mononucleosis.

drugs may provide some symptomatic relief. The disease is usually self-limiting and recovery occurs in a few weeks, but patients may not recover their former level of energy for months.

As always, use standard precautions in dealing with patients infected with EBV and wash hands thoroughly.

Other Viral Respiratory Diseases
[OBJECTIVE 38]

Other viruses may cause acute respiratory disease. Symptoms can be divided into two groups: acute afebrile and acute febrile.

Acute afebrile respiratory diseases may cause laryngitis, rhinitis, and pharyngitis in the upper respiratory tract or croup, bronchitis, or bronchiolitis in the lower respiratory tract. Children are most often adversely affected by these symptoms. Although infection can lead to secondary bacterial infections, antibiotics should be reserved for known bacteriologic infections. The frivolous use of antibiotics in the past has given rise to a new generation of multi–drug-resistant pathogens.

Acute febrile respiratory diseases may cause tonsillitis, croup, bronchiolitis, bronchitis, pharyngitis, and pneumonitis. The primary viruses responsible for causing these diseases are the parainfluenza viruses types 1, 2, and 3 and the respiratory syncytial virus (RSV). Parainfluenza viruses are the leading cause of bronchiolitis.

RSV is a major viral pathogen in children younger than 2 years and is usually spread from November through April. RSV immune globulin (RespiGam) may prevent the illness in children.

Place surgical masks on all patients with unknown respiratory pathogens and always practice standard precautions.

Case Scenario—continued

As you approach the patient, you see a 40-year-old man wearing pajamas and lying on a bed. Used tissues are in the wastebasket and cough syrup and a thermometer are on the nightstand. The patient states that this "cold" started after he got back from a business trip to London a month ago. He started feeling run down about 3 to 4 days later and came down with "this bug that I can't shake." He adds that 2 days ago he started having trouble breathing and the cough got worse, as did the tightness in his chest. According to the patient, he developed shortness of breath that morning and it has gotten steadily worse. Breath sounds reveal crackles. You ask about a fever and the patient indicates that he has been running a fever of 101° to 102° F. At night he states he becomes very sweaty. He denies any allergies. He admits to taking some leftover penicillin, but that did not seem to work. He states the over-the-counter cough medicine has not helped either. He has no significant past medical history. The man's wife states that he has eaten a little chicken soup, but nothing much else.

Questions

4. *Has your initial impression changed?*
5. *What do you think may be causing the man's upper respiratory infection?*
6. *What treatment options should you consider at this time?*

Sexually Transmitted Diseases

The United States has the highest incidence of sexually transmitted diseases (STDs) in the industrialized world, with more than 12 million cases diagnosed annually. The history and physical examination provide the majority of the information needed to make the diagnosis of an STD. Recognition and quick treatment of these conditions are key to preventing complications and the spread of these diseases. The paramedic must therefore be comfortable questioning patients about their sexual history when these conditions are suspected. This includes numbers of partners, gender of partners, the use of contraception and barrier devices, and menstrual history in women. Although physical examination of the genitalia is not commonly needed, the paramedic should ask questions to gain this information. STDs often are broken into two categories: those that appear with genital ulcers (sores) and those that do not. Those that do not often result in genital discharge. In this case determine the color, odor, frequency, and amount of the discharge.

Syphilis

[OBJECTIVE 39]

In 2006 more than 36,000 cases of syphilis were reported in the United States, including 9756 primary and secondary cases. Interestingly, half of all the primary and secondary cases occurred in 20 counties and 2 cities. The incidence of primary and secondary syphilis declined by nearly 90% between 1990 and 2000. However, from 2000 to 2006 cases of syphilis have risen steadily. In 2006 there was a 12% increase in cases compared with 2005. Cases of syphilis are highest in women ages 20 to 24 years and men ages 35 to 39 years (CDC, 2007f).

Syphilis is a sexually transmitted disease caused by a spirochete bacterium called *Treponema pallidum*. It starts as an ulcer, called a *chancre,* at the site of inoculation; if left untreated the disease progresses through secondary, latent, and tertiary stages.

Transmission of syphilis is usually through sexual contact. Persons with untreated syphilis during the initial and secondary stages are highly contagious when moist mucocutaneous lesions are present. These are typically genital lesions, but they can be found on other areas of the body. An estimated one third of persons having sexual contact with an infected person who has primary or secondary syphilis will acquire the disease. Absence of open lesions does not ensure lack of infectiousness because other body fluids may contain the agent. Congenital syphilis usually occurs from transplacental infection of the fetus. The greatest risk occurs during stages of heavy spirochetemia. Half of the infants born to women with primary or secondary syphilis are stillborn, premature, or die shortly after birth. Perinatal infection also may occur from contact by the neonate when in the birth canal.

The several stages of syphilis are difficult to diagnose because some patients do not have early manifestations or do not know they are infected.

The first stage, the incubation stage, averages 3 weeks but can range from 10 to 90 days. During this time the bacteria adheres to and penetrates the epithelium. As the bacteria multiply, they disseminate. Patients are asymptomatic during this stage.

The primary stage, called *primary syphilis,* is noted by a chancre at the site of inoculation. The classic chancre is a painless primary lesion with a clean base and rounded, discrete borders that have a rubbery consistency. The chancre starts as a small, red, hard papule that enlarges and subsequently breaks down, causing a crater with an encrusted surface. The majority of these lesions are genital, but they can occur in the mouth and on the lips, fingers, and rectum. The area of the lesion below the crusted surface has a high bacteria count. Untreated, this stage lasts from 2 to 6 weeks with spontaneous resolution. Because these lesions are painless and eventually resolve spontaneously without scarring, they can go unnoticed. However, resolution does not indicate cure. The bacteria have simply moved to the bloodstream, where they continue to infect and replicate. This stage is known as *primary latency* and can last from 2 to 8 weeks, during which time the patient is asymptomatic.

The secondary stage, called *secondary syphilis*, usually appears 6 to 24 weeks after initial infection, or 5 to 8 weeks after resolution of the primary chancre. Because of bacterial replication and migration during primary latency, several body systems are affected and symptoms are more profuse and widespread. The patient begins to complain of fatigue, malaise, fever, anorexia, sore throat, and weight loss. The most common finding of this stage is a rash that encompasses the entire body, including the palms of the hands and soles of the feet. Secondary syphilis can affect every organ system and has come to be known as "the great imitator." This name comes from the fact that the disease can involve diverse organ systems and mimic other clinical conditions during this stage. Among the systems most commonly involved, in addition to the skin (Figure 31-12), are the lymphatic system, gastrointestinal tract, joints, bones, liver, kidneys, eyes, and the central nervous system. As with the primary stage, this stage spontaneously resolves in 2 to 6 weeks.

Latent syphilis is noted when the lesions from secondary syphilis have disappeared. This stage is divided into early latency and late latency and can last from 6 months to 8 or more years. If left untreated the infected person will have secondary relapses at a rate of 90% in the first year and 95% within the first 2 years. The CDC uses the 1-year mark to demarcate early from late latency. During this stage patients are asymptomatic but still infected. If tested during this stage the patient shows antibodies for the bacteria, but the bacteria itself is not detectable.

Tertiary syphilis refers to one of three outbreaks that appears years to decades after infection and is separated into late benign syphilis, cardiovascular syphilis, and neurosyphilis. Damage to the organ systems is the result of the infection and the body's response to the infection. Patients may have tumors, called *gummas,* in the mucous membranes, liver, skin, bone, and cartilage. Weakening of arterial walls can lead to an aortic aneurysm or damage to the aortic valves and subsequent heart failure. Any part of the nervous system can be affected by syphilis; however, the central nervous system, cranial nerves, and dorsal roots of the spinal cord are the most common. This can result in headaches, seizures, alterations in mental status, cognitive impairment, ataxia, slurred speech, and destruction of the optic nerve. The pupils may exhibit a condition known as *Argyll Robertson pupil.* In this condition the pupil constricts to accommodation but does not constrict in response to light. Fortunately, tertiary syphilis is rare because of the widespread use of antibiotics for other conditions.

The diagnosis of syphilis is difficult because it is a pathogen that cannot be cultivated on an artificial medium. If the physician is unfamiliar with syphilis a presumptive diagnosis is acceptable to administer appropriate therapy.

Therapy for syphilis is penicillin for all stages. Some of the newer cephalosporins, most notably ceftriaxone, have excellent track records in vitro. Persons who have an allergy to penicillin or who are pregnant can be treated with tetracycline and doxycycline.

Prevention of syphilis in the post-penicillin age has been found not to be cost effective, but serologic testing of expectant mothers has been found to be useful in the first and third trimesters and at the time of delivery. Complete eradication of syphilis probably requires development of an effective vaccine. In 1999 the CDC launched the Syphilis Elimination Effort in the United States in response to the declining rates of syphilis between 1990 and 2000. Ironically, as mentioned above, syphilis rates have been increasing each year since 2000. Several speculations for the cause of this are beyond the scope of this chapter (Hutto, 2001; CDC, 2007f; CDC, 2008b).

Gonorrhea

[OBJECTIVE 40]

Gonorrhea is the second most common STD in the United States, with an estimated 700,000 new cases each year. The CDC estimates only half of annual cases are reported. In 2006 a total of 358,366 new cases were reported to the CDC. The incidence of gonorrhea dropped dramatically (74%) from 1975 to 1997 because of the implementation

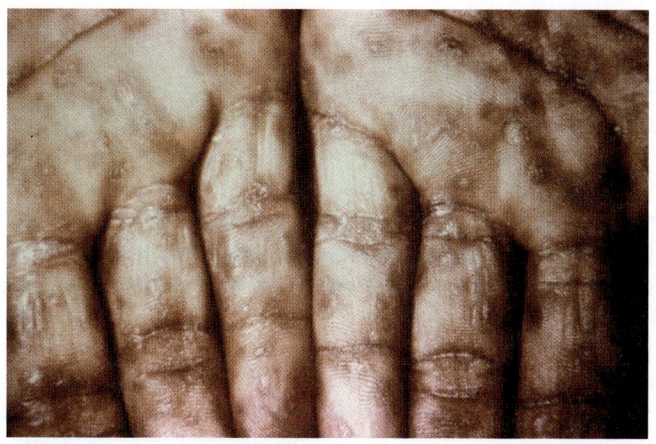

Figure 31-12 Keratotic lesions on the palms of a patient's hands caused by a secondary syphilitic infection.

of a national gonorrhea control program in the mid 1970s. However, after several years of stable rates, incidence is on the rise. The year 2006 showed the second consecutive year in which the rates of gonorrhea increased. The highest reported rates of infection are among sexually active teenagers, young adults, and African Americans (CDC, 2007e).

Gonorrhea is a sexually transmitted disease caused by the bacterium *Neisseria gonorrhoeae* that can directly affect the urethra, anal canal, pharynx, and conjunctivae. Other areas of the body can become infected and result in endometritis, salpingitis, and peritonitis. Bartholinitis can occur in the female and periurethral abscess and epididymitis can occur in the male. Systematic complications may include arthritis, dermatitis, endocarditis, and meningitis.

The spread of gonorrhea and the signs and symptoms completely depend on the site of inoculation, age of the patient, the duration of the infection, and the occurrence of local or systemic spread of the gonococci. These factors are greatly influenced by the individual's sexual practices.

The human being is the only natural host of the gonococcal infection. In heterosexual men the infection usually involves only the urethra; in homosexual men the urethra, anal canal, and pharynx can become infected. The usual incubation period is 2 to 7 days, although it can be longer. Signs and symptoms occur 2 to 14 days after exposure, although some men never experience symptoms. In women the most common site is the cervix, followed in decreasing order by the urethra, anal canal, and pharynx. Urethral, rectal, and pharyngeal infection rarely lead to local complications, but salpingitis occurs in approximately 20% of women with cervical gonorrhea, which can lead to complications such as ectopic pregnancy or infertility from damage to the fallopian tubes. Symptoms of gonorrhea in the male are a purulent urethral discharge commonly associated with dysuria, frequency, and meatal erythema. Most symptomatic men seek treatment and are able to halt the disease without progression. Men who do not show symptoms or have minimal symptoms sometimes ignore the infection, causing primary spread to women, who become at risk for local or systemic complications. In women any visible epithelium that is exposed becomes dusky red and friable. There may be purulent exudate causing vaginal discharge perceived by the patient as more copious and yellow than normal. Additional findings include abnormal vaginal bleeding, abdominal or pelvic pain, and burning or painful urination. Contiguous spread from the discharge may occur by the perineum to the anus and urethra. Gonorrhea may be spread to the eyes from self-inoculation by rubbing the eyes with infected fingers. Gonococcal conjunctivitis presents with red conjunctiva and purulent discharge. Without treatment it can lead to blindness. This condition can affect newborns who pass through the vaginal canal of infected mothers.

Treatment for gonorrhea has improved. Until 1986 penicillin G, ampicillin or amoxicillin, tetracycline, and spectinomycin were the treatments of choice, but widespread resistance has been encountered. Ceftriaxone is now the recommended choice of the CDC, with a 125-mg intramuscular dose for uncomplicated gonorrhea. All patients who have been treated for gonorrhea should be tested for syphilis and receive counseling. Hospitalization is recommended for women who have pelvic inflammatory disease to facilitate parenteral therapy with combinations of antimicrobials active against other vaginal anaerobic organisms.

Gonorrhea has no definitive cure, and outbreaks may occur. EMS workers should protect themselves with everyday personal protective equipment use.

Chlamydia

[OBJECTIVE 41]

Chlamydia infection is the most common sexually transmitted disease in most parts of the world, including the United States. In 2006 a total of 1,030,911 cases were reported to the CDC. However, underreporting is common; estimates of actual cases range from 3 to 5 million annually. This underreporting is because in 75% of women and 50% of men the infection often is asymptomatic, or silent. However, even when asymptomatic the infection can cause multiple complications, including salpingitis, damage to the uterus and fallopian tubes, increased risk of ectopic pregnancy, infertility in women, and epididymitis in men. As with other STDs, the incidence of clamydia was higher in 2006 than in 2005 (CDC, 2007d).

Clamydia is caused by the gram-negative bacteria *Chlamydia trachomatis*. The bacteria can only survive inside the host's cell by using the host's adenosine triphosphate. Chlamydia infection can affect the eyes, respiratory system, oropharynx, and the genital area and associated organs.

Chlamydia may be spread through sexual activity, the sharing of contaminated clothing or towels, and hand-to-hand transmission from infected eye secretions, making children the major reservoir. All people are susceptible to chlamydial infections, and up 25% of men have been estimated to be carriers. After infection no immunity is acquired.

The symptoms depend on the site of infection and the stage of the disease and appear 1 to 3 weeks after the initial infection. In sexually active adults and teenagers, the most common site of infection is the urethra and endocervix; in children it is the respiratory tract and conjunctiva.

In men the most common symptom associated with urethral infection of chlamydia is dysuria and discharge. In women the onset may be asymptomatic, although endocervical infection often is characterized by discharge. The similar symptoms of chlamydia and gonorrhea make

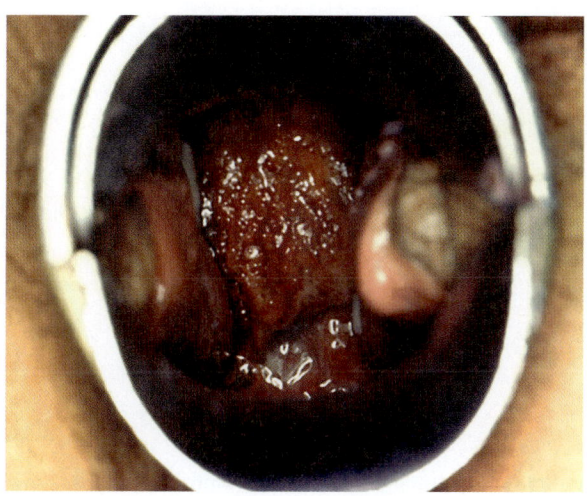

Figure 31-13 A female patient's cervix has signs of erosion and erythema from chlamydial infection.

diagnosis difficult in the absence of laboratory confirmation (Figure 31-13).

Patients also may develop conjunctivitis from infection. Chlamydia is the leading cause of preventable blindness worldwide. Pneumonia in infants may be caused by chlamydia infection after passing through the birth canal of an infected mother. The same gynecologic conditions that result from gonorrhea infection also may result from chlamydia.

As with other STDs treatment is with antibiotics, including azithromycin and doxycycline. Concomitant infections with gonorrhea are common; therefore many patients are treated for both if one is suspected. Reinfections are common unless the patient's sexual partners are not infected.

EMS personnel who come in contact with patients suspected to have chlamydia should observe standard precautions and practice proper handwashing. Chlamydia has no vaccine, but the condition may be treated with antibiotics such as doxycycline, azithromycin, tetracycline, and erythromycin.

Herpes

[OBJECTIVES 42, 43]

Herpes simplex virus (HSV) is an infection that affects human beings and causes asymptomatic infections or mild skin and mucosal diseases. HSV is subdivided into HSV-1 and HSV-2. An estimated 80% of the population is seropositive for HSV-1 infection. HSV-1 typically affects trigeminal ganglia, and outbreaks occur in the oropharyngeal area. However, genital HSV-1 infections are possible. HSV-2 typically affects the sacral ganglia, and outbreaks occur in the genital area. However, oral and anal infections are possible. After the initial infection, HSV enters a latent nonreplicative state that reactivates on occasion. Reactivation is often the result of emotional or physical stress, trauma, fever, ultraviolet light expo-

sure, or immunosuppression. The primary HSV infection may be severe, especially in the neonate, and reactivated disease can cause encephalitis as well as **keratitis** and blindness in normal hosts.

Herpes is the most common cause of ulcerative STDs in the United States. An estimated 50 million individuals have had the disease, and 200,000 to 300,000 new cases are reported each year. Genital herpes shows a female predominance of 2:1. It is estimated to affect one out of every four women and one out of every eight men (CDC, 2008a).

Although HSV may infect a wide variety of hosts, human beings are the natural reservoir. The spread of HSV is usually the result of close personal contact because of the instability of the infection and the presence of the virus in the sores it causes. The major portals of entry are broken skin and the mucous membranes. The disease can be spread in the absence of sores. The infection may spread quickly in non-Westernized cultures, lower socioeconomic populations, and patients in hospitals or wards that house children. No evidence shows that HSV is spread through aerosols or inanimate objects such as toilet seats or pools. The primary infection is spread through mucous membranes or injured and diseased skin. Newborns can be infected if the mother has active lesions during delivery. Ideally in this situation a cesarean section should be performed in the hospital as opposed to a prehospital or hospital vaginal delivery.

HSV can be a latent infection in which the primary infection is asymptomatic or unrecognized by the host, making the spread of HSV an important source for others. If the primary infection is symptomatic, it is generally more severe than recurring infections. These situations involve an incubation period of 2 to 7 days before signs and symptoms appear. Before the development of herpetic sores is a prodrome period of burning and itching to the area, typically the lips or genitals depending on the type of infection. After the prodrome, painful vesicular or ulcerative lesions appear that heal over the course of several weeks. A systemic infection can include findings of fever, malaise, headache, confusion, and fatigue.

Therapy of HSV-1 and HSV-2 is still being studied. Antiviral chemotherapy is effective in improving the severity and duration of infections caused by HSV. Effective topical agents for HSV are trifluorothymidine, acyclovir, vidarabine, and idoxuridine. Vidarabine is effective in immunosuppressed patients and neonatal patients, whereas acyclovir is the preferred agent because it is less toxic and has a greater clinical efficacy.

Prevention is most easily accomplished by avoiding contact with potentially infected secretions. Always wear personal protective equipment when in contact with oral, respiratory, or genital secretions. Avoid sexual contact with infected persons who are at high risk. Condoms should be used because of their ability to protect against infection, and spermicides should be used for their ability to prevent some viral activity (Tyring, 2002).

Scabies and Lice

[OBJECTIVE 44]

Scabies

Scabies is an infectious disease of the skin caused by a parasitic infestation of *Sarcoptes scabiei,* a mite. The female mite invades the upper layers of the skin, where a hypersensitivity reaction occurs in response to the mite's protein and feces. Norwegian scabies is the most severe variety.

Scabies is spread by person-to-person contact, including sexual contact. The mite can also be spread through contact with the dirty linens of an infected person, but only if contact is within 24 hours. The scabies mite is capable of burrowing into skin in 2.5 minutes.

All persons are susceptible to scabies infestation, though people with past exposure develop symptoms within 1 to 4 days, whereas people without a previous exposure do not develop symptoms for 2 to 6 weeks. Fewer mites are seen on additional exposures as well.

Scabies causes intense itching, especially at night. The inseminated female mites burrow into the skin, leaving S-shaped tunnels behind them where they lay eggs and feed on the epidermis. Vesicles and papules form on the patient's skin at the end of these burrows.

In men, lesions are most often seen around finger webs, thighs, external genitalia, armpits, the waist, and the anterior wrists. Females most often have lesions on the nipples, abdomen, and the lower portion of the buttocks. In infants, areas not typically seen in adults become involved, including the head, neck, palms of the hands, and soles of the feet.

Although scabies cause severe discomfort, complications are typically only seen from lesions that have been broken open by scratching and then have become infected.

EMS personnel should follow standard precautions when handling patients, clothing, and any linens. Separately bag any dirty ambulance linens. Washing and drying clothes and linens in hot water is of questionable efficacy, unlike in head lice, and is more important in Norwegian scabies infestation.

Scabies are treated with topical solutions of drugs chosen according to physician preference and patient age. Topical solutions should be used exactly as directed to avoid toxicity.

No immunization exists for scabies, and families should be educated on proper use of insecticides and environmental decontamination of clothes and linens.

Lice

[OBJECTIVE 45]

Lice can infest the head (*Pediculosis humanus capitis*), the body (*Pediculosis humanus corporis*), and the pubic region (*Pthirus pubis*). Body lice have been involved in epidemic

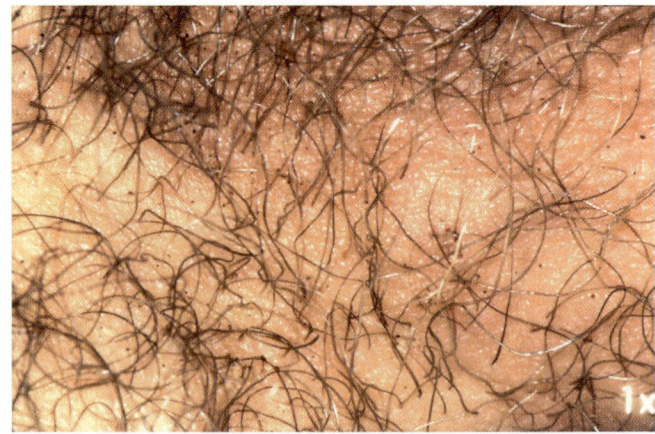

Figure 31-14 A patient with crab lice; note the reddish-brown crab feces.

spread of typhus, trench fever in World War I, and relapsing fever.

Head lice are spread through direct contact with a person or by direct contact with an item used on the affected region of the body. Body lice can be spread through direct contact and indirect contact with infested items. Pubic lice are spread through sexual contact (Figure 31-14).

Lice leave a host that has become febrile, so fevers and overcrowding favor the transmission of lice. The eggs of head lice do not hatch at temperatures less than 72° F.

Lice have a three-stage life cycle, from egg to nymph to adult. Eggs take 7 to 10 days to hatch, after which the nymph stage lasts 7 to 13 days depending on temperature. The cycle from egg to egg takes approximately 3 weeks.

All persons are susceptible to lice. The primary symptom of lice infestation is itching. Head lice infestation is seen in the hair, eyebrows, eyelashes, mustaches, and beards. Body lice infestation is seen along the seams of clothing, especially the inner seams.

Lice can be treated with topical medicines and mechanical removal of all eggs, nymphs, and adults from the body. Follow standard precautions when handling these patients and their belongings and bag all linen separately. Spray the inside of the ambulance with a commercially available insecticide known to be effective at killing lice and mites. Most commercial sprays contain carbamates, malathion, or pyrethrins and should be adequate.

Unlike fleas, lice and mites are not known to jump great distances, so cleaning the patient compartment around the stretcher as well as the head of the stretcher should prove sufficient. Rinse all areas cleaned with insecticide afterwards. Wear gloves at all times during the procedures.

Prevention of lice infestation can be accomplished by practicing good personal hygiene and washing clothing and linens in hot water to destroy nits and lice.

Case Scenario CONCLUSION

As you complete your primary survey, you apply supplemental oxygen by nonrebreather mask at 15 L/min. The patient indicates a little relief. As you prepare for transport, you ask about his trip from London. He tells you it was OK, but a woman seated behind him coughed quite a bit. According to the patient, it was annoying: "She hacked for 6 hours." He added that he thinks she was from some third-world country because she seemed to have a distinct non-British and non-American accent. As the patient tells you this latest piece of information, he begins a paroxysm of coughing and expels bloody mucus into a tissue. You ask if this has happened before. The patient states he has been coughing up blood-tinged mucus since last night.

Looking Back

7. What is your final impression?

8. What precautions should you use during and after transport?

9. What process should you use to clean the ambulance after the call?

Lyme Disease

[OBJECTIVE 46]

Lyme disease is a tick or arthropod-borne disease that infects many people in temperate regions of the world but is most common in the United States, Europe, and Russia. The disease is caused by a spirochete bacteria (*Borrelia burgdorferi*) that affects the skin, central nervous system, cardiovascular system, and the joints. Ticks are the vector of transmission and are responsible for its spread to human beings. The reservoirs and hosts of *B. burgdorferi* vary according to geographic region, as does the type of tick that acts as the vector. Described here is the classic cycle that occurs in the Northeast United States, where the disease was first identifed. In this model adult female deer ticks lay their eggs on the white-tailed deer. After hatching, the larval ticks feed on the white-footed mouse, which is the reservoir of *B. burgdorferi,* and the tick becomes infected. After releasing from the mouse, the infected tick, now a nymph, continues its maturation until adulthood, when it returns to the white-tailed deer to complete the reproduction cycle. During the nymph stage, however, the nymph is not particular regarding which animal it feeds on, as long as it is a vertebrate. Human beings are more likely to be infected at this time, as are other vertebrates such as dogs.

All persons are susceptible to the disease. Reinfection has been known to occur in patients previously treated for the disease, so no immunity is believed to occur.

Lyme disease is the most common vector-borne disease in the United States, with approximately 20,000 new cases reported each year. In 2006 a total of 19,931 cases were reported. The first known cases occured in the 1970s in Lyme and Old Lyme, Conn., although they initially were misdiagnosed as juvenile rheumatoid arthritis. Although these were the first confirmed cases, the disease is believed to have been present in North America for centuries. The incidence and prevalence of Lyme disease has been steadily increasing since it became a reportable event in 1991. This is likely attributable to an actual increase in the incidence of the disease as well as increased detection.

As with syphilis, Lyme disease occurs in stages. The first stage is a localized reaction at the site of the bite that produces a painless, warm rash called *erythema migrans* and flulike symptoms such as fever, chills, headache, malaise, a stiff neck, and myalgia.

Erythema migrans begins as a flat, round rash that spreads outwards from the site of the bite. The outside of the rash remains red, with the center turning white, blue, or sometimes black and necrosing. The incubation period from bite to the appearance of erythema migrans is between 3 and 32 days from the initial tick exposure.

The second stage of Lyme disease is the early disseminated stage, during which the pathogen invades the skin, heart, nervous system, and joints. The skin of the patient develops multiple lesions. As the bacteria invade the nervous system the patient is affected in several ways. The cranial nerves, especially the seventh cranial nerve, may be invaded, causing Bell's palsy (Figure 31-15). The disease may involve the brain, causing meningitis, and invade the motor and sensory nerves of the patient, producing peripheral neuropathy. Lyme disease also affects the heart and may cause varying atrioventricular blocks, more commonly in adults than children. Less commonly the disease may cause myocarditis and left ventricular dysfunction. Additional signs and symptoms found during stage two include musculoskeletal pain, sore throat, dry cough, fatigue, lethargy, and sensitivity to light.

The late stage of Lyme disease most often is characterized by recurrent arthritis that affects the large joints, especially the knees. Arthritis associated with Lyme disease may not be preceded by the earlier stages of the disease. Arthritis is a complication that occurs in up to 60% of untreated patients and is seen less commonly in Europe. Approximately 10% of patients develop chronic arthritis that lasts for more than a year. Patients with Lyme disease also may have an encephalopathy characterized by depression, sleep disorders, and cognitive deficits.

Educate patients regarding the proper removal of ticks. The tick should be grasped as close as possible to the

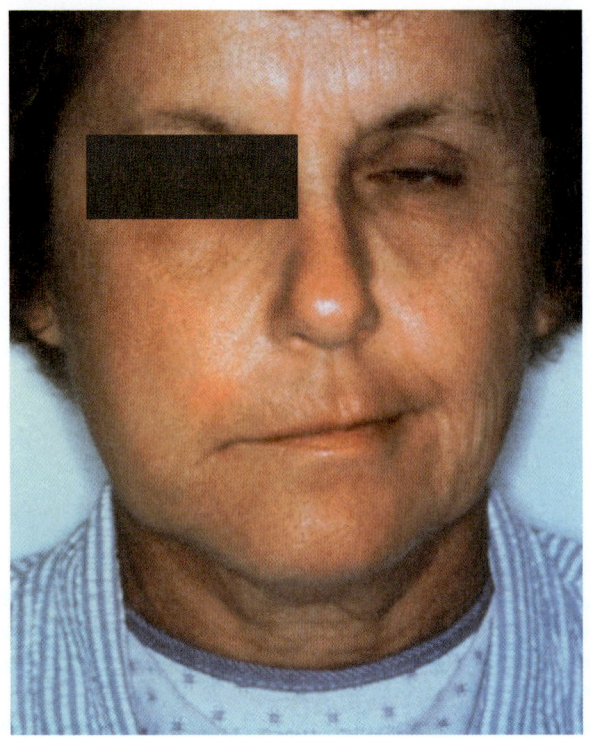

Figure 31-15 A patient with facial palsy caused by Lyme disease.

surface of the skin with tweezers or forceps and pulled out. Patients and providers should take care not to crush or squeeze the body of the tick. Avoid older methods of removing ticks, such as with the hot head of a match or nail polish, because they are ineffective and may contribute to the transmission of disease if the tick regurgitates. Wash the site with hot soap and water and dress it appropriately.

Patients and providers at risk for tick exposure should attempt to protect themselves with a commercially available tick repellent. Wearing white or light-colored clothing makes ticks easier to discover. Peak seasons are summer and early fall, when tick activity and the number of people outside are both increased.

EMS personnel who treat patients in forested or wilderness areas should inspect themselves and their patients for the presence of ticks. Treat the patient compartment of the ambulance with an insecticide effective at killing ticks.

No evidence of person-to-person communicability for Lyme disease has been found. Congenital transmission between an infected mother and her fetus also has not occurred.

Although Lyme disease may be treated with antibiotics, no vaccine is available (Edlow, 2006; CDC, 2007c).

Gastroenteritis

[OBJECTIVE 47]

Gastroenteritis refers to any infection that, as a primary symptom, causes an inflammation of the stomach lining and intestinal tract. Gastroenteritis accounts for a large number of illness and deaths worldwide, especially in developing countries.

Gastroenteritis may be caused by any number of pathogens, including viruses such as the rotovirus, the Norwalk virus, and enteric adenoviruses as well as parasitic infections caused by *Giardia lamblia, Cryptosporidium parvum,* and *Cyclospora cayetanensis.* Bacterial infections such as those caused by *Salmonella* spp. and *Shigella* spp., which are not normal intestinal flora, also may cause gastroenteritis. Overgrowth of normal intestinal flora such as *Escherichia coli, Klebsiella pneumoniae, Enterobacter* spp., *Vibrio cholerae,* and *Campylobacter jejuni* also may cause gastroenteritis.

Pathogens causing gastroenteritis are typically transmissible through contaminated food or water or by the fecal-oral route. In developing countries natives typically develop some degree of resistance to endemic pathogens, whereas travelers are much more susceptible to endemic pathogens. Personnel and victims in disaster areas (e.g., floods, tornados, combat zones) also are much more susceptible to the development of gastroenteritis.

Gastroenteritis presents with the onset of abdominal pain and cramps, diarrhea, nausea and vomiting, fever, anorexia, and frank shock. Ulcers, chronic gastritis, and heartburn are caused by *Helicobacter pylori* infection. Differentially, many of the same symptoms may be caused by *Salmonella* spp. infection, botulism, appendicitis, inflammatory bowel disease, or a bowel obstruction (large or small).

When in contact with patients with gastroenteritis, be careful to avoid any habits that may facilitate oral-fecal transmission. Always use careful handwashing and follow standard precautions. Do not report for work when ill.

Personnel working in disaster areas should pay careful attention to the procurement of potable water and sanitation. Workers should always know the source of their water supply and ensure it has been decontaminated before consumption.

Although some organisms that cause gastroenteritis are susceptible to antibiotic treatment, care is usually based on symptoms. Vaccines do not exist for most of the pathogens that cause gastroenteritis (Diskin, 2006).

EXPOSURES TO INFECTIOUS AND COMMUNICABLE DISEASES

[OBJECTIVE 48]

An exposure incident occurs when any potentially infectious material comes in contact with the eyes, nose, mouth, mucous membranes, or nonintact skin. Immediately report any potential exposure.

The importance of reporting any exposure cannot be overstated. Reporting an exposure allows for immediate medical screenings and permits identification of possible infectious agents and proper treatment. Every EMS agency should have a designated individual who documents and investigates exposures, commonly referred to as an *infection control officer.* The infection control officer may then evaluate the circumstances under which the person was exposed and make recommendations on procedural changes to avoid future exposures. Immediate reporting of an exposure also allows the source patient to be tested if permission can be obtained. Failure to report an exposure incident can result in a lack of care and follow-up regarding the incident. Always report any incident, no matter how minor it may seem. A disease may present itself years to decades after the intitial exposure.

Under the Ryan White Act, exposed employees have the right to request a patient's infection status from that patient's healthcare provider. However, neither the employee nor the agency he or she represents may force the patient to be tested. Federal law requires employers to have an exposure control plan that tells the employee the proper steps to take if an exposure occurs.

The Ryan White Act requires that employers designate a person or officer within the organization to whom exposed employees should report. On notification of an employee exposure, the officer then initiates the appropriate measures of the organization's exposure control plan based on the type of exposure and within local guidelines.

Employers are required by law to provide employees with appropriate medical care and treatment in the event of an exposure. Such care and treatment should include counseling about the risks, signs and symptoms, and the clinical probability of developing a disease as well as information on how to prevent further spread. The employee should be offered appropriate treatment based on the U.S. Public Health Service's guidelines. Exposed employees should be offered appropriate medication and given information on the medicine's side effects, interactions, and contraindications. The infection control officer or physician also should evaluate any reports of illness in the employee to determine if the condition could be related to HIV or hepatitis infection.

After an exposure the employee, upon agreement, should have his or her blood tested. The employee has the right to donate a blood sample but to refuse HIV testing at the time the sample is given. The employer must retain the employee's blood sample for 90 days in case the employee changes his or her mind regarding the blood tests or in case HIV or hepatitis-like symptoms should develop.

A healthcare provider must provide the employee with information regarding the results of the tests as well as information about prophylactic treatment and other therapeutic regimens and may implement treatment at the request of the employee.

Vaccinations should be made available to employees who may have occupational exposure to blood and other potentially infectious materials.

After an appropriate medical screening and treatment, the healthcare professional should provide a statement to the employer's designated officer. This report simply identifies whether vaccination was recommended to the exposed employee and if the employee received that vaccination. The report also must document that the employee was informed of the results of the examination and was told of any medical conditions resulting from the exposure that may require additional treatment or evaluation.

A copy of the report is provided to the designated officer and the employee. All other elements of the medical examination are confidential and are not released to the designated officer or the employer without the expressed, written permission of the employee. Records of employee exposures must be maintained for the duration of employment, plus 30 years, per Occupational Safety and Health Administration standards.

PREVENTING DISEASE TRANSMISSION

Do not report for duty if you have any of the following conditions:

- Diarrhea
- Draining wound or wet lesions
- Body temperature >100.5° F
- Positive mononucleosis status
- Jaundice
- Lice or scabies
- You have been taking antibiotics for *less* than 24 hours for strep throat

Make sure your immunizations are up to date for the following:

- MMR
- Hepatitis B and A (if appropriate)
- DTP
- Polio
- Chickenpox
- Influenza

Approach all patients with caution and an appropriate attitude. Make every effort to control the scene because an uncontrolled scene increases the chances for an exposure to bodily fluids. Always observe standard precautions by wearing gloves and, if conditions exist, goggles or a face shield, a gown, or N-95 respirator.

Patients with headache, fever, cough, stiff neck, and recent weight loss and who are taking medications that suggest an infectious process should be treated appropriately. Never treat patients differently or refuse to do something for a patient out of fear of infection. Most infections can be prevented with proper use of standard precautions, proper handwashing (including the webs of the fingers), and disinfection of used equipment.

Prehospital personnel handle few infectious processes that are true emergencies. However, always be aware of the risks to yourself, patients, and co-workers with exposure to unknown infectious agents, which occurs on a nearly daily basis. Always follow standard precautions and assume that any bodily substance or fluid is infectious.

Case Scenario SUMMARY

1. *What is your initial impression?* The initial impression should include upper respiratory infection from any number of causes, including the common cold, influenza, pneumonia, sudden acute respiratory syndrome, TB, and other conditions.

2. *What additional information do you need?* Additional information that could help determine the nature of the illness includes a SAMPLE history and OPQRST evaluation of the patient's complaint.

3. *What common personal protective equipment would you use or consider using at this point?* Gloves initially should be worn, but in the presence of protracted coughing consider using an N-95 respirator. A simple cloth or paper surgical mask is ineffective in screening bacteria such as *Mycobacterium tuberculosis.*

4. *Has your initial impression changed?* The clinical assessment begins to point toward TB as the problem.

5. *What do you think may be causing the man's upper respiratory infection?* Clinical findings such as fever, night sweats, and crackles further confirm the suspicions.

6. *What treatment options should you consider at this time?* Treatment options include administering high-flow oxygen by nonrebreather mask, placing the patient on a pulse oximeter and cardiac monitor, and establishing IV access. If the patient appears dehydrated, an increased IV flow rate of normal saline may be needed (in consultation with medical direction).

7. *What is your final impression?* A history of close exposure to someone from a third world country with a significant cough points in the direction of TB. In addition, hemoptysis or coughing up blood-tinged sputum is suggestive of TB. Transport the patient in a position of comfort.

8. *What precautions should you use during and after transport?* When you suspect TB as the presenting condition, wearing gloves and an N-95 mask is essential. A gown is appropriate, especially if the patient has a productive cough. In preparing to transport the patient, remove or cover any nonessential equipment. During transport, be sure to use the exhaust fan in the rear of the patient compartment to help remove droplets exhaled or coughed by the patient. Once at the receiving facility, follow your organization's postexposure response plan. Be sure to report the exposure and secure a follow-up TB skin test.

9. *What process should you use to clean the ambulance after the call?* Clean all surfaces of the ambulance with an approved disinfectant. Wipe down the cabinets, squad bench, stretcher, and any exposed equipment. At the receiving facility, leave the doors open to air out the vehicle while turning the patient over to the emergency department staff. During daylight hours, leave the vehicle in the sun because ultraviolet radiation from the sun helps destroy the bacteria.

Chapter Summary

- When treating patients with communicable diseases and infections, first protect your partner and yourself; then treat the patient while protecting the public from a widespread outbreak.

- Wearing personal protective equipment and staying up to date with inoculations against infections are important aspects of patient care.

- Transmission of an infectious disease depends on a number of factors, including virulence, correct mode of entry into the body, and the immune status of the host.

- The stages of an infectious disease are the incubation period, window period, communicable period, latent period, and disease period.

- A disease may be caused by a bacterium, virus, fungus, protozoan, helminth, or prion.

- The body has multiple defense mechanisms, including the skin, white blood cells, the RES, and the complement system.

- A detailed history and physical examination of the patient should alert you to clues that an infectious disease may be present.

- HIV has two strains, HIV-1 and HIV-2. Both are communicable through unprotected sexual intercourse and contact with infected secretions or blood.

- HIV is incurable and has no vaccination.

- Hepatitis affects the liver and is communicable sexually and by infected blood and secretions.

- Hepatitis has no cure, although vaccinations are available for some strains.

- TB primarily affects the lungs but can affect other organs. It is spread through respiratory secretions from an infected person and may be treated with antibiotics.

- Meningitis may be caused by many pathogens. Bacterial meningitis is caused by bacteria reaching the meninges through the blood.

- Treatment for bacterial meningitis is antibiotic therapy based on the type of bacterium responsible for infection.
- Bacterial pneumonia is a lung infection caused by bacteria and is transmissible through respiratory droplets or prolonged direct contact with an infected person.
- Bacterial pneumonia is treated with antibiotics.
- Tetanus is caused by a spore that enters the body through a wound, burn, or other injury to the skin.
- Tetanus is treated by vaccination.
- Herpes is a viral infection that may affect many organ systems.
- Herpes has no cure and no vaccination and may be spread through direct contact with infected persons.
- Gonorrhea is primarily a sexually transmitted disease that can affect different body systems depending on the site of exposure.
- Gonorrhea is treated with antibiotics.
- Syphilis is a sexually transmitted disease that begins as a chancre at the site of infection.
- Syphilis is treated with antibiotics and is spread through direct contact.
- Chickenpox is a common childhood disease that is highly communicable through contact with infected persons and is airborne. Chickenpox is usually self-limiting and currently has a vaccination, though no cure.
- Mumps is an infection that affects the parotid and salivary glands. Mumps infection is self-limiting and has a vaccination.
- Rubella is a viral infection spread through contact with infected persons. Rubella is self-limiting and has a vaccination.
- Measles is a highly contagious viral infection that has no cure, is self-limiting, and has a vaccination.
- Pertussis, meaning *forceful cough,* is a disease caused by a gram-negative bacterial infection. Pertussis is spread through infected respiratory secretions and may be treated in its early stages with antibiotics. Pertussis does have a vaccine, but its effectiveness has been shown to wane over time.
- Influenza is one of the most common and contagious infectious diseases that commonly affects the respiratory system. It has no cure, and vaccines are released yearly based on predictions of which strain will affect the general population that year.
- Avian influenza (H5N1) is an emerging strain of influenza A that has primarily been shown to be contagious from bird to human being; only limited cases of human-to-human transmission have been documented. Avian influenza in human beings has an extremely high mortality rate, and scientists warn that mutation of the virus could cause a worldwide pandemic.
- Mononucleosis is caused by a virus spread through infected secretions. Mononucleosis has no cure or vaccination, and symptoms may persist for several months.

- HSV-1 is a viral infection that affects the oropharynx, mouth, lips, skin, fingers and toes, and possibly the central nervous system. No cure or vaccination is available, and infection is lifelong.
- Acute afebrile respiratory distress can cause multiple upper and lower airway infections. Antibiotics are used only for bacterial infections with resistant strains.
- RSV is a major viral infection in children younger than 2 years. RSV is largely spread from April to November. It can be prevented in children with a medication called *RespiGam.*
- Scabies is an infectious parasitic disease caused by the infestation of a mite. Females of the species invade the upper layer of the skin, causing irritation. Scabies is spread by person-to-person contact and infected linens in a 24-hour window. Infestation occurs at any site of female burrowing where eggs have been laid. Lesions form at sites of infestation. It is treated with a topical solution taken as prescribed by the physician to avoid toxicity.
- Lice infect the head, body, and pubic region. Lice have been known to spread typhus, relapsing fever, and trench fever (during World War I). Lice can be spread through direct and indirect contact, with pubic lice spread through sexual contact. Lice leave a febrile host, so overcrowding populations favor transmission for spread of lice. Itching is the primary symptom. Topical solutions and mechanical removal of eggs are the only treatments available.
- Gastroenteritis is any infection that causes swelling to the stomach or its lining. Gastroenteritis is responsible for morbidity and mortality worldwide, especially in developing countries. Gastroenteritis is caused by multiple pathogens and is transmissable through contaminated food and water and fecal-oral contamination. Gastroenteritis manifests with abdominal pain and cramps, nausea, vomiting, diarrhea, fever, and frank shock.
- Standard precautions and handwashing should be practiced when in contact with infected persons and in disaster areas. In the latter situation, a source of potable water must be ensured.
- Chlamydia is the most commonly spread sexually transmitted disease in the world today. The bacteria can only survive in the host using the cell's adenosine triphosphate. Chlamydia affects the eyes, respiratory, sexual, and associated organs. It is spread through sexual contact, hand-to-hand contact, and contaminated towels and clothes. No acquired immunity to chlamydia is possible, and symptoms depend on the site and stage of the disease. Chlamydia is the leading cause of preventable blindness worldwide.
- EMS personnel who come in contact with infected persons should practice standard precautions and handwashing.
- Lyme disease is a bacterial infection spread by ticks and is most common in the United States, Europe, and Russia. Lyme disease often appears in stages, with the

Chapter Summary—continued

first stage presenting as a rash around the site of inoculation. The second and third stages begin the systemic infection. No vaccination against Lyme disease is available, and no immunity is acquired after infection. Lyme disease may be treated with antibiotics.

- Any exposure to potentially infectious diseases or materials should be immediately reported to the designated officer.
- Further medical testing and treatment are provided at no cost to the employee as appropriate.

REFERENCES

American Academy of Pediatrics. (2003). *Red Book: 2003 report of the committee on infectious diseases* (26th ed.). Elk Grove Village, IL: American Academy of Pediatrics.

Berkow, R. (1999). *The Merck manual of medical information, home edition.* New York: Pocket Books.

Blanton, J. D., Krebs, J. W., Hanlon, C. A., Rupprecht, C. E. (2006). Rabies surveillance in the United States during 2005. *Journal of the American Veterinary Medical Association, 229*(12), 1897-1911.

Centers for Disease Control. (1989). A strategic plan for the elimination of tuberculosis in the United States. *Morbidity and Mortality Weekly Report, 38*(suppl S-3), 1-25.

Centers for Disease Control and Prevention. (2004). *Overview of pneumonia in healthcare settings.* Retrieved February 2007 from http://www.cdc.gov.

Centers for Disease Control and Prevention. (2006a). *Hepatitis B virus.* Retrieved February 10, 2008, from http://www.cdc.gov.

Centers for Disease Control and Prevention. (2006b). Preventing tetanus, diphtheria, and pertussis among adults: Use of tetanus toxoid, reduced diphtheria toxoid and acellular pertussis vaccine. *Morbidity and Mortality Weekly Report, 55*(RR-17), 1-33.

Centers for Disease Control and Prevention. (2006c). Sexually transmitted diseases treatment guidelines, 2006. *Morbidity and Mortality Weekly Report, 55*(RR-11), 1-100.

Centers for Disease Control and Prevention. (2007a). *A glance at the HIV/AIDS epidemic.* Retrieved February 10, 2008, from http://www.cdc.gov.

Centers for Disease Control and Prevention. (2007b). *Epidemiology.* Retrieved February 10, 2008, from http://www.cdc.gov.

Centers for Disease Control and Prevention. (2007c). *Learn about Lyme disease.* Retrieved February 10, 2008, from http://www.cdc.gov.

Centers for Disease Control and Prevention. (2007d). *STD surveillance 2006: National profile—chlamydia.* Retrieved February 10, 2008, from http://www.cdc.gov.

Centers for Disease Control and Prevention. (2007e). *STD surveillance 2006: National profile—gonorrhea.* Retrieved February 10, 2008, from http://www.cdc.gov.

Centers for Disease Control and Prevention. (2007f). *STD surveillance 2006: National profile—syphilis.* Retrieved February 10, 2008, from http://www.cdc.gov.

Centers for Disease Control and Prevention. (2007g). *Trends in tuberculosis, 2006—United States.* Retrieved February 10, 2008, from http://www.cdc.gov.

Centers for Disease Control and Prevention. (2008a). *Genital herpes—CDC fact sheet.* Retrieved February 10, 2008, from http://www.cdc.gov.

Centers for Disease Control and Prevention. (2008b). *Syphilis—CDC fact sheet.* Retrieved February 10, 2008, from http://www.cdc.gov.

Diskin, A. (2006). *Gastroenteritis.* Retrieved February 28, 2007, from http://www.emedicine.com.

Edlow, J. A. (2006). *Tick-born diseases, introduction.* Retrieved February 28, 2007, from http://www.emedicine.com.

Hoeprich, P. D., Jordan, M. C., & Ronald, A. R. (1994). *Infectious diseases: A treatise of infectious processes* (5th ed.). Philadelphia: J.B. Lippincott Company.

Hutto, B. (2001). Syphilis in clinical psychiatry: a review. *Psychosomatics, 42,* 453-460.

Lazloff, M. (2005). *Meningitis.* Retrieved February 28, 2007, from http://www.emedicine.com.

Li, J., & Brainard, D. (2006). *Tuberculosis.* Retrieved February 28, 2007, from http://www.emedicine.com.

Newton, D., Olendorf, D., Jeryan, C., & Boyden, K. (2000). *Sick! Diseases and disorders, injuries and infections, vols. 1-3.* Detroit: U-X-L.

Tyring, S. K. (2002). *Mucocutaneous manifestations of viral diseases.* New York: Marcel Dekker.

World Health Organization. (2007). *Epidemic and pandemic alert and response (EPR): Avian influenza.* Retrieved February 28, 2007, from http://www.who.int.

Zimmerman, L., & Reef, S. (2002). *VPD surveillance manual* (3rd ed.). Atlanta, GA: Centers for Disease Control and Prevention.

Zuckerman, J. N., & Zuckerman, A. J. (2004). Hepatitis viruses. In *Cohen & Powderly: Infectious diseases* (2nd ed.). St. Louis: Mosby.

SUGGESTED RESOURCES

Centers for Disease Control and Prevention
1600 Clifton Road
Atlanta, GA 30333
(404) 639-3311
Public Inquiries: (404) 639-3534 or (800) 311-3435
http://www.cdc.gov

Infectious Diseases Society of America
66 Canal Center Plaza, Suite 600
Alexandria, VA 22314
http://www.idsociety.org

United States Army Medical Research Institute of Infectious Diseases
Attn: MCMR-UIZ-R
1425 Porter Street
Frederick, MD 21702-5011
http://www.usamriid.army.mil

Chapter Quiz

1. How many types of HIV have been identified?
   _____

2. List three examples of the transmission of HIV.
   _____
   _____
   _____

3. List three symptoms of HAV.
   _____
   _____
   _____

4. What is the organ infected by HCV?
   _____

5. Is meningitis contracted from direct or indirect contact?
   _____

6. Name four of the seven types of diseases that make some populations more susceptible for pneumonia.
   _____
   _____
   _____
   _____

7. What system is affected by tetanus?
   _____

8. In children, what is the most prominent sign of tetanus?
   _____

9. What is the incubation period for tetanus?
   _____

10. What is the primary body system affected by chickenpox?
    _____

11. What is the incubation period for mumps?
    _____

12. Which systems of the body are affected by Rubella?
    _____

13. What is the mode of transmission for measles?
    _____

14. When is pertussis (whooping cough) thought to be the most communicable?
    _____

15. What is the most popular mode of transmission for mononucleosis?
    _____

16. What are gummas?
    _____

17. What areas are affected by chlamydia?
    _____

18. What systems are affected by Lyme disease?
    _____

19. What cardiac abnormalities can occur with Lyme disease?
    _____

Terminology

Antiviral An agent that kills or impedes a virus.

Communicable period The period after infection during which the diease may be transmitted to another host.

Conjunctivitis Inflammation of the conjuctiva.

Disease period The interval between the first appearance of symptoms and resolution.

Immunity A body's ability to resist a particular disease.

Incubation period The time between exposure to a disease pathogen and the appearance of the first signs or symptoms.

Keratitis Inflammation and swelling of the cornea.

Latent period Period during and after infection in which the diease is no longer transmissable.

Leptomeningitis Inflammation of the inner brain coverings.

Malaise General feeling of illness without any specific symptoms.

Prodrome A symptom indicating the onset of a disease.

Resistance The ability of the body to defend itself against disease-causing microorganisms.

Risus sardonicus Distorted grinning expression caused by involuntary contraction of the facial muscles.

Terminology—continued

Susceptibility Vulnerability or weakness to a specific pathogen; the opposite of resistance.

Tetany Repeated, prolonged contraction of muscles, especially of the face and limbs.

Vector A mode of transmission of a disease, typically from an insect or animal.

Virulence A term used to refer to either the relative pathogenicity or the relative ability to do damage to the host of an infectious agent.

Window phase The period after infection during which the antigen is present but no antibody is detectable.

Psychiatric Disorders and Substance Abuse

Objectives *After completing this chapter, you will be able to:*

1. Define *behavior* and distinguish between normal and abnormal behavior.
2. Define *behavioral emergency*.
3. Discuss factors that may alter the behavior or emotional status of an ill or injured individual.
4. Discuss the pathophysiology of psychiatric disorders.
5. Describe appropriate measures to ensure the safety of the patient, paramedic, and others.
6. Correlate the abnormal findings in assessment with the clinical significance in patients using the most commonly abused drugs.
7. Define the following terms:
   - Affect
   - Anxiety
   - Fear
   - Open-ended question
   - Posture
   - Phobia
   - Dysphoria
   - Euphoria
8. Describe the circumstances when relatives, bystanders, and others should be removed from the scene.
9. Describe the techniques that facilitate the systematic gathering of information from the disturbed patient.
10. Identify techniques for physical assessment in a patient with behavioral problems.
11. Be able to recognize various psychiatric disorders on the basis of assessment and history of present illness.
12. Integrate pathophysiologic principles with the assessment of the patient with psychiatric disorders.
13. Discuss the prevalence of behavior and psychiatric disorders.
14. Describe the history and physical findings associated with psychiatric disorders.
15. Describe management strategies for various psychiatric disorders.
16. List the clinical uses, street names, pharmacologic characteristics, assessment findings, and management for patients who have taken or been exposed to the following substances:
    - Cocaine
    - Marijuana
    - Methamphetamines
    - Barbiturates

- Sedative-hypnotics
- Narcotics or opiates
- Common household substances
- Drugs abused for sexual purposes or gratification
- Alcohols
- Hydrocarbons
- Psychiatric medications
- Newer antidepressants and serotonin syndromes
- Lithium
- Monoamine oxidase inhibitors
- Club drugs
- Hallucinogens
- Dissociatives

17. List situations in which you may have to transport a patient forcibly and against his or her will.
18. List the risk factors for suicide.
19. List behaviors that indicate a patient may be at risk for suicide.
20. Describe the verbal techniques useful in managing the emotionally disturbed patient.
21. Describe methods of restraint that may be necessary in managing the emotionally disturbed patient.
22. Describe the medical and legal considerations for management of emotionally disturbed patients.
23. Describe the condition of restraint asphyxia and why you must never restrain a patient in a prone position.
24. Define the following terms:
    - Substance or drug abuse
    - Tolerance
    - Withdrawal
    - Addiction
25. List the most commonly abused drugs by chemical name and street name.
26. Discuss the incidence of drug abuse in the United States.
27. Describe the pathophysiology of commonly abused drugs.
28. Differentiate the various treatments and pharmacologic interventions in the management of the most commonly abused drugs.
29. Integrate pathophysiologic principles and the assessment findings to formulate a field impression and implement a treatment plan for patients using the most commonly abused drugs.
30. Discuss the signs and dangers of clandestine drug manufacturing laboratories.

Chapter Outline

[Handwritten margin notes:]
Neurosis: obsessed w/something but behavior OK

Psychosis: behavior becomes erratic/obsessive

Case Scenario

On a brisk autumn afternoon you receive a call to a convenience store on South Main Street. According to the dispatcher, the police department is requesting that you transport a patient with a suspected mental illness.

You arrive in the parking lot of the convenience store to find two officers standing next to a young adult male. The patient is dressed in a plaid flannel shirt and blue jeans. The situation is unusual in that the patient is barefoot and standing motionless in a small puddle of water in the middle of the asphalt parking lot. His eyes are open and he appears to be staring at the ground. One of the police officers states that the store manager found him this way approximately 20 minutes ago and that the man has not moved. The officer further states that he found the patient's wallet and the department is attempting to contact the patient's mother, with whom he lives. The officer adds that the patient is 22 years old according to his driver's license.

Questions

1. What is your initial impression?
2. What additional information do you need?
3. What sources can you use to obtain the necessary information?

Patients with behavioral emergencies present some of the most moving and challenging cases you will encounter in your career as a paramedic. You will be required to use your most refined assessment techniques to arrive at a differential field diagnosis. In addition to the complete neurologic assessment, you must be skilled in listening. This is one of the most essential skills an effective paramedic can master. To elicit the details to determine your patient's current problem, you must create an atmosphere of trust and empathy. To do that, you must truly want to help your patient.

Patients call EMS because they have a medical emergency and they need help. Patients with behavioral emergencies and mental illness are no different, and you should treat them with the same respect, attention, and compassion you would give a patient with any illness or injury. The stigma surrounding mental illness in the United States is overwhelming. Many people, even many healthcare workers, often express the belief that a patient's mental illness is "made up" or that a patient "could feel better if he wanted to." This idea not only worsens illnesses and hurts patients' recoveries, it also kills. Suicide was the eleventh most common cause of death in the United States in 2002 (Kochanek et al., 2005) and is the tragic result of too many cases of psychiatric illnesses.

This chapter also discusses substance abuse, which is shamed perhaps even more than other mental disorders. As a paramedic, your function is not to judge. Instead, your role is to assess, treat, and support. This chapter was written with these goals in mind. Emphasis is placed on the recognition and treatment of patients under the influence of intoxicating substances and those experiencing withdrawal syndromes. Most of the substances discussed are illegal under current laws, though that is not the focus of this chapter. When confronted with a patient abusing substances, many providers fall victim to the same thinking as for mental illness: "He's bringing this on himself; he can stop if he wanted to." Addiction is no less a disease than is diabetes or AIDS, and like those afflictions it is chronic but treatable. By keeping an open mind and remaining compassionate, the majority of your contacts with patients having behavioral emergencies or using substances will be smooth and easy to handle.

BEHAVIOR

[OBJECTIVES 1, 2]

Behavior is defined as a person's observable activities. No established definitions categorize "normal" behavior and "abnormal" behavior. Behavior that you may consider bizarre and abnormal may be normal and mundane to others. In general, normal behavior is measured against the norms and expectations of society. Although not necessarily tasteful, a man walking down the sidewalk without a shirt in the summertime is considered normal. That same man walking down the same sidewalk with a shirt but no pants on is considered abnormal. Religious and cultural factors should be taken into account when deciding what is normal. If a person told you that when he drank wine from a cup it turned to blood in his mouth, you might consider that abnormal and bizarre. Yet millions of Catholics worldwide believe that this phenomenon, called *transubstantiation,* occurs during communion. In the context of religious belief, many ideas and concepts that may seem abnormal to some are considered normal.

How is a mental disorder defined? Broadly, a mental disorder is present when abnormal behavior affects a person's life functions, such as eating, sleep, sexual relations, socialization, and career.

A **behavioral emergency** is loosely defined as actions or ideations by a patient that are harmful or potentially harmful to the patient or others. These include suicidal, homicidal, and aggressive behaviors and ideations. However, outside such obvious indicators, differentiating what is normal and acceptable from what is abnormal and dangerous is difficult.

Symptoms associated with the disorders covered in this chapter may vary widely from patient to patient. No two patients are alike, and no two cases of mental illness present the same way. As prehospital professionals, paramedics sometimes witness the more extreme cases of these disorders. Remember that modern psychology and medicine are effective at treating most mental disorders, and most patients with these illnesses lead normal lives.

PSYCHOPATHOLOGY

Limbic System

[OBJECTIVES 3, 4]

Beneath the cerebral cortex of the brain lies a group of structures collectively termed the **limbic system.** The limbic system is neuronal circuitry that controls motivation and emotion (Figure 32-1). The outermost portion of the limbic system is the limbic lobe—a band of neurons that encircles the inner structures of the limbic system and the innermost layer of the cerebral cortex. This position allows the limbic lobe to interact with each of the lobes of the cerebral cortex.

At the base of the limbic system are two structures approximately the size and shape of two plums. Together, these structures form the **thalamus.** This region functions as the "switchboard" of the brain, through which almost all incoming and outgoing signals travel as they are relayed to the appropriate destinations (the sense of smell is one notable exception). Enveloping the thalamus and flanking the limbic system are the **hippocampi** (singular, *hippocampus*). These chili pepper–shaped structures are the primary centers for the processing and consolidation of long-term memory. In simple terms, the hippocampi filter incoming sensory information, determining which stimuli are dangerous, beneficial, or

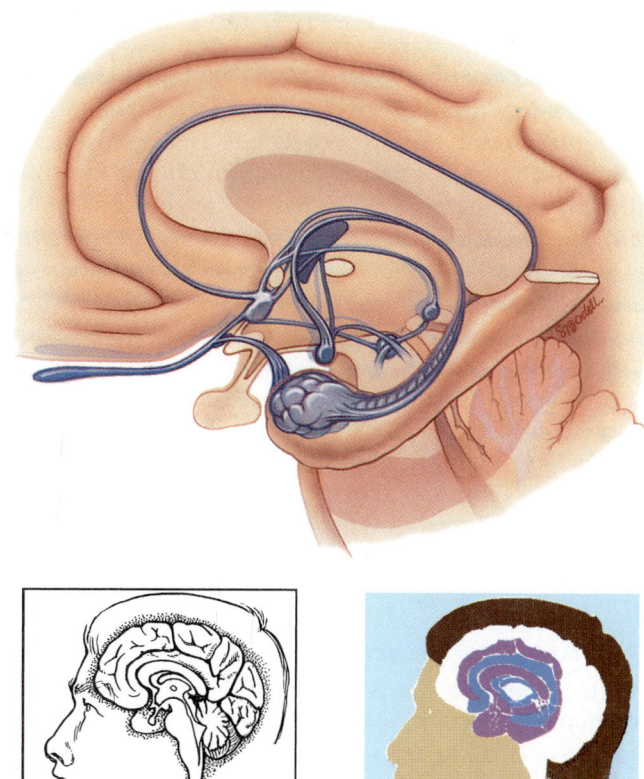

Figure 32-1 The limbic system.

generally useful. If the hippocampi determine something to be important, it is committed to memory. The hippocampi are believed to be responsible for processing information from several parts of the brain at the same time. Putting these memory puzzle pieces together provides the experience of memory as complete and whole instead of broken into fragments (Whybrow, 1997).

At the blunt end of each hippocampus lies an **amygdala** (plural, *amygdale*). Each is approximately the size and shape of a small almond. They are the emotional sentinels of the brain. Working closely with the other limbic structures, the amygdale attach emotional significance to stimuli passing through them. An impulse corresponding to the image of a tree is not likely to elicit much of a reaction from the amygdale. Conversely, the sound of a growling pack of wolves is likely to set the amygdale into alarm mode, bringing about potentially life-saving emotions of fear and anxiety. Animal studies have shown that damage to the amygdala produces a state best described as a near-total lack of emotion. Other studies have shown that the amygdale are integral in the production of the movements of the face associated with emotional expression. The amygdale have close associations with all the other limbic structures, especially the thalamus, hippocampi, and the hypothalamus (Whybrow, 1997).

In the center of the limbic system is the **hypothalamus,** a small, bulblike structure that hangs from the thalamus. The hypothalamus is connected to the thalamus on its superior aspect and the pituitary gland on its inferior aspect. This relation makes the hypothalamus the bridge between the nervous system and the endocrine system. Although it accounts for less than 1% of the brain's mass, the hypothalamus is responsible for almost all the body's housekeeping functions. By stimulating the endocrine system and other portions of the brain, the hypothalamus controls arterial blood pressure, water conservation responses, thirst, body temperature, and hunger responses. Exceptions to this are the maintenance of a steady pulse and respiratory rate, which is controlled by the medulla oblongata. In addition, the hypothalamus is the seat of the autonomic nervous system (see Chapter 23). The close association of the hypothalamus with the limbic system allows physiologic responses to emotions, such as an increase in heart rate and respirations from intense fear or blushing of the skin when embarrassed.

> ### PARAMEDIC*Pearl*
>
> Although the brain is a single organ, picturing it as several different organs (amygdala, hypothalamus, cerebral cortex, medulla oblongata, etc.) working together in harmony often is helpful. Like the members of a symphony, different areas of the brain contribute parts that, when taken together, form images, thoughts, and feelings.

Pathologic changes in body systems often can be traced to malfunctions of specific tissues. For example, myocardial infarction can be caused by a blockage of the blood flow within a coronary artery. This lack of perfusion to the myocardium causes irritation, injury, and cell death. Disorders of behavior are rarely caused by a single source or tissue pathology. Although science's understanding of the physiologic roots of mental illness and abnormal behavior has grown exponentially in the past 100 years, much is left to be learned.

Disorders of behavior arise from a complex interaction of many factors, including the layout of the brain from the genetic codes of DNA, experiences during the formative years of life, and the complex interactions of hormones. An exact definition of what has gone wrong to produce a depressive illness or schizophrenia is impossible to create. For a paramedic, the exact causes do not matter. However, discussing some general risk factors and possible causes of mental illness is helpful.

Organic Etiology

[OBJECTIVES 3, 4]

Behavioral emergencies often have very little, if any, psychological basis. Consider the case of a patient with diabetes who does not eat and yet still takes their insulin. These actions may cause a sudden drop in blood glucose levels, causing confusion and abnormal behavior. The patient may show symptoms that could be considered part of a psychiatric disorder, such as odd speech and mannerisms, hallucinations, and even delusions. In such cases, abnormal behavior stems from a biologic cause and is said to be **organic.** Examples of organic conditions that can cause abnormal behavior are shown in Box 32-1.

When assessing a patient behaving abnormally, the paramedic's primary concern is to rule out an organic cause. Effective and accurate performance on a full mental status examination (discussed later in this chapter) on all patients with abnormal behavior is crucial. Always suspect organic causes in any patient with a sudden onset of abnormal behavior and no prior medical or psychiatric history.

> **BOX 32-1** **Organic Conditions That Can Cause Abnormal Behavior**
>
> - Alzheimer's disease
> - Brain abscess
> - Brain neoplasm
> - Brain trauma
> - Hypoglycemia
> - Dehydration
> - Hypoxia
> - Hypothermia
> - Substance intoxication
> - Substance withdrawal
> - Stroke

Genetic Predisposition

[OBJECTIVES 3, 4]

Many studies have shown higher rates of certain mental illnesses within families. For example, an estimated 80% of people with bipolar disorder have a bipolar parent. A large amount of supportive data comes from twin studies, in which data from identical twins (who share all the same genes) are compared with data from fraternal twins (who only share approximately half of their genes). This has led many researchers to conclude that mental illness has a genetic basis. However, this does not mean that everyone who has bipolar disorder will have a child with bipolar disorder. Some genes may make the development of a mental illness *more likely*. Many other factors also are thought to play a role.

Biochemical Factors

[OBJECTIVES 3, 4]

In the 1930s researchers studying a new drug used to treat tuberculosis noted that patients taking the medication reported feeling happier and more optimistic than before. With further study, these researchers concluded that the medication could be used to treat depression. Hence the first antidepressant was born. Since then, the number of antidepressants in use around the world has increased as a result of the idea that mental illness is related to the biochemistry of the brain.

Recall that nerve cells do not physically touch; instead, neurons are separated by a microscopic space—the synapse. The axon of a transmitting neuron releases chemical signaling agents called *neurotransmitters* that bind to receptor sites on a gland, muscle, or dendrite of a receiving neuron. As Ramachandran (1998) states in *Phantoms in the Brain*:

A piece of your brain the size of a grain of sand would contain one hundred thousand neurons, two million axons, and one billion synapses, all "talking to" each other. Given these figures, it's been calculated that the number of possible brain states—the number of permutations and combinations of activity that are theoretically possible—exceeds the number of elementary particles in the universe. Given this complexity, how do we begin to understand the functions of the brain? Obviously, understanding the *structure* of the nervous system is vital to understanding its functions.

For the purposes of this chapter, this structure includes the specific parts of the brain discussed above as well as the chemical language of neurons—neurotransmitters. Different areas of the nervous system use different neurotransmitters. For example, the parasympathetic division of the autonomic nervous system uses acetylcholine, whereas the sympathetic division primarily uses norepinephrine. Various regions of the brain communicate within themselves with specific chemicals. These regions are called neurotransmitter pathways and often control specific functions. For example, the neurotransmitter

serotonin is theorized to have a role in cognitive functions, control of some movements, emotions (particularly panic and anxiety), appetite regulation, and the sleep-wake cycle.

One model of mental illness asserts that relative imbalances in the levels of neurotransmitters in the brain are responsible for psychiatric disorders. This view has become increasingly popular, with pharmaceutical companies advertising medications to "fix" these imbalances. Unfortunately, the roots of psychiatric disorders are not that simple, and no medical tests can be performed to diagnose or predict mental illnesses accurately. Some patients may have a major depressive episode that can be resolved entirely through psychotherapy (talk therapy) without the use of medications. Nonetheless, millions of people nationwide regularly take these medications for all varieties of mental illness.

Biochemical imbalances may be only a symptom of mental illness, not the underlying cause. The brain is a dynamic organ; it performs functions to create life experiences and is equally affected by those life experiences. Because of the large number of functions controlled by certain neurotransmitter pathways, imbalances of neurotransmitters are probably responsible for the *symptoms* of various disorders. One of the primary symptoms of major depression is a change in appetite. Some patients may experience a dramatic decrease in appetite with accompanying weight loss, whereas others overeat and gain weight. Drugs that affect the levels of serotonin in the brain, including most antidepressants, help alleviate *symptoms* of depression, such as changes in appetite. The primary neurotransmitters thought to be involved in mental illness are serotonin, dopamine, and norepinephrine. Altering the levels of these neurotransmitters is the primary mechanism of action for most psychiatric drugs in use today.

Psychosocial Factors

[OBJECTIVES 3, 4]

Events in life clearly affect a person's emotional state. For example, the death of a loved one can bring about a period of sadness and grieving, or a promotion at work can make someone feel joy and optimism. These **psychosocial factors** are life changes and events that cause or aggravate mental disorders. How a psychosocial factor will affect someone cannot be predicted because everyone is affected differently by life events. Relocating to another city may elicit feelings of excitement and hope in one person, but in another it may cause overwhelming feelings of anxiety and worry about the changes such a move will bring.

Studies have shown that psychosocial factors often are key factors in mental illness. However, psychosocial factors are only one part of the picture. People develop mental disorders even when no major psychosocial stressors exist, and not everyone who has lost a loved one or been fired from a job develops mental illness.

Developmental Factors

[OBJECTIVES 3, 4]

Some researchers point to the events of childhood as a causative factor of mental illness. Emotional crises experienced during the developmental years are believed by some to predispose some people to mental illness later in life. Indeed, studies have shown that children who experience the death of a parent, particularly before the age of 5 years, have much higher rates of depression later in life. Other developmental factors associated with mental illness include divorce of one's parents, sexual abuse, physical abuse, and parental substance abuse.

Biopsychosocial Concept

[OBJECTIVES 3, 4]

In the 1970s George Engel, a practicing physician, proposed a new way of thinking about mental illness called the *biopsychosocial model*. This concept proposed that biologic makeup (bio), behavior (psycho), and surroundings (social) all relate and interact. Biology can affect behavior, as in a case of depression resulting from thyroid dysfunction or cancer. However, behavior can affect biology, such as people who have a terminal illness and die soon after "losing the will to live." Social circumstances can affect behavior. For example, consider the development of depression and posttraumatic stress disorder after a tragic or traumatic event. A mother's depression surely affects her children—an example of a person's behavior affecting surroundings. All three of these components interact to "cause" mental illnesses.

PARAMEDIC*Pearl*

Although the causes of psychiatric illnesses have been speculated about since the dawn of medicine, modern research shows that these disorders are almost never attributable to one simple cause. Instead, they arise from a highly complex mix of factors, including those outside the realm of biology and traditional medicine, and vary widely from patient to patient.

ASSESSMENT OF THE PATIENT WITH A BEHAVIORAL EMERGENCY

PARAMEDIC*Pearl*

When a paramedic has completed initial training, he or she is adept in many skills such as airway management, obtaining IV access, and giving medications. At times, patients with behavioral emergencies will require these skills. All patients, however, require use of one essential skill—the ability to empathize and listen.

Rescuer Safety and Scene Assessment

[OBJECTIVES 5, 6]

As with any scene, the safety of you and your crew is most important. Staging for police is recommended for the majority of behavioral emergencies, including all cases of suicidal, homicidal, and assaultive ideations or actions. Just as you would scan the scene of a motor vehicle crash for downed power lines and leaking chemicals, you should study the area of *every* call. Do not be misled by dispatch information; the call for a "man down," "unknown problem," or "altered mental status" can be caused by or quickly lead to a violent situation. Heightened awareness begins as soon as you arrive on scene and exit the vehicle. In addition to being vigilant for conditions that may compromise your safety, remember personnel at the receiving facility are usually not able to view the patient's living environment. The state of someone's dwelling may yield important clues about the nature of a mental illness. The following guidelines use a house as an example, but they can be applied to almost any setting.

Look at the residence you have responded to. Does the house appear suspicious or out of place with the other residences on the block? Is it dark and closed up? Has the lawn been mowed and taken care of, or is it cluttered with trash and random objects? Entering the residence requires extra awareness. Approach the entrance from the side. Before you knock and announce your presence, stand beside the door and listen for a moment. Do you hear shouting, loud noises, or other signs of a violent situation inside? If not, then stay to the side, knock, and wait for someone to answer.

As you enter, look for signs that violence has occurred. The presence of weapons or ammunition should be a warning. What is the condition of the patient's living area? Although few people clean the house when calling EMS, a residence should appear relatively well maintained. Does the furniture appear to have been pushed around recently? Are objects from tables and shelves knocked onto the floor? These may be signs of violence or a struggle. How clean is the house? Many residences are messy, but filth and a lack of basic hygiene may indicate the patient has been incapacitated and unmotivated—possible consequences of a depressive illness. Remember, you are the patient's advocate. If a patient appears to be unable to care for himself or herself, your duty is to help by reporting the situation. With the patient's permission, look inside the refrigerator. Is food present? Is it fresh or has it decayed? Is alcohol inside? The contents of a patient's kitchen can provide valuable insight into a patient's recent state of mind.

While you are in the patient's home, look for signs of substance abuse, which is sometimes seen with mental illness. Note any bottles and cans of alcohol or drug paraphernalia such as plastic bags, razor blades, syringes, spoons that have been burned, cigarette rolling papers, and empty cigar wrappers. Also be alert for empty pill bottles, which could indicate an overdose.

Patient Contact and Interview

[OBJECTIVES 5, 7, 8, 9, 10]

Once you make patient contact, you must maintain awareness of your patient's actions and behavior no matter how calm he or she initially seems. Most patients with behavioral emergencies are not violent and sincerely want your help. Patients rarely transition from being calm and cooperative to enraged and violent without cause or warning, even in the context of mental illness. Human behavior runs along a continuum, with quiet, withdrawn behavior at one end and loud, aggressive actions at the other. As a paramedic, you must be able to recognize where on this continuum your patient is and to which end behavior is moving. Take special note of the patient's **posture,** which is a reflection of the patient's overall attitude and frame of mind. Tone and volume of voice, facial expression, body position, and tension all comprise posture. A patient may seem comfortable and calm, with a relaxed posture. On the other hand, a yelling patient with a furrowed brow, clenched fists, and reddened face displays an aggressive posture. This person may be only seconds away from violent behavior.

As with any response, assess safety throughout the incident. Monitor the posture of your patient and others on scene at all times. If you feel threatened, *leave immediately* and stage away from the scene until law enforcement can arrive and secure the patient. In the rare circumstance that you are unable to avoid a physical confrontation, use the minimal amount of force necessary to allow your escape and avoid harming the patient.

> **PARAMEDIC***Pearl*
>
> Go with your instincts—if your gut tells you that a patient will soon become violent, it is probably true.

As with any patient, your first concern lies with the initial assessment. Violent patients can injure themselves or others. A suicidal patient may be bleeding from an intentional injury or may have overdosed on medications that could compromise breathing and mental status. If life-threatening problems are found during the initial assessment, managing them takes priority over any other aspects of patient care. If the patient is awake and alert, exercise caution when first approaching. Many patients view EMS personnel as authority figures. Suddenly advancing individuals may cause fear or anxiety in some patients and send them into a defensive mode.

As you get closer to the patient, watch your positioning. Be aware of the patient's "personal space" and respect it. Getting too close can cause fear and apprehension and

may even incite violence if the patient is already agitated. In general you should remain somewhere between 18 and 48 inches away. Do not stand or sit directly in front of the patient; this can be intimidating, and if you are attacked you have less chance to dodge. Instead, stand at an angle. Start at a distance and then move closer as you feel appropriate. As with any scene be aware of exits and make sure they remain accessible at all times. Standing in front of doorways can cause patients to feel trapped and isolated, however, potentially making your interview more difficult.

To gain the most from an interview with a patient with a behavioral problem, you must maintain a quiet, nonthreatening atmosphere and give the patient a sense that you are there to help. Your attitude and body language tell the patient more about how you feel than your words do. Keep your hands in the patient's view at all times and do not make sudden moves or gesture too much with your hands. Make frequent eye contact but do not stare. This lets the patient know you are listening to and focused on him or her. Avoid threatening language or tone of voice; a feeling of trust takes time build, and only one callous sentence can break destroy relationship. Your role is that of a healthcare professional, not a police officer, parent, or judge. Maintain compassion but avoid friendliness. Attempting to become the "buddy" of a patient with paranoid delusions can quickly provoke deep feelings of mistrust and caution.

> **PARAMEDIC***Pearl*
>
> Under no circumstances should you ever lie to a patient. Telling a patient that you are not going to force him to go to the hospital immediately before you and your team restrain him may make things easier for you but will cause numerous problems later. Do not forget that you are part of a continuum of healthcare. To many patients, you are part of the same organization as nurses, doctors, and therapists. By lying, you create a deep mistrust and compromise the efforts of all the professionals who follow you.

Part of scene management includes people management. Remove the patient from any crisis or threatening situation such as angry or arguing family members. Attempt to limit the number of personnel present while maintaining a safe environment. Separate the patient from friends and family members unless absolutely necessary (e.g., the patient will not calm down without certain people present). Others may have a tendency to answer questions for the patient; their presence may prohibit the patient from giving you honest answers regarding feelings and activities. Elicit information from all sources separately and compare them later. The patient's loved ones can be invaluable for providing information about the current problem in addition to details about any previous or similar episodes and conditions. Provide emotional support for family and friends;

unusual behavior and suicide attempts often are quite distressing.

History of the Present Illness

[OBJECTIVES 7, 9, 10]

Establish the current problem—why you have been called. This is best obtained by asking the patient a simple question, such as "How can I help you today?" Some patients may be forthcoming and give detailed explanations of their current issue, and some may provide only one- or two-word responses. Avoid interrupting the patient, but keep him or her focused on what you need to know. Gently redirect the patient to the main topic when necessary. On the other hand, do not fear silence. Many patients, particularly those with depressive symptoms, are withdrawn and quiet.

Ask specific, open-ended questions about what the patient is telling you. **Open-ended questions** are questions that cannot be answered by a simple "yes" or "no." Examples include "How did that make you feel?" and "Why do you think that happened?"

Expand on the behavioral patient's chief complaint as you would with any other patient. For example, take the complaint of "feeling down." How long has the patient been feeling this way? Has anything made these feelings subside or intensify, such as problems with family or troubles at work? Is this the first time the patient has ever felt this way? If not, when was the last time the patient had these feelings? Did the patient seek treatment then? If so, what type of treatment and what was the outcome?

Many paramedics fall in to the trap of thinking that all patients with a particular disorder appear in the same way. This is not true. For example, some patients with major depression may exhibit little to no appetite, whereas others may overeat. This is discussed in more depth later in this chapter.

Check vital signs of all patients, including those exclusively with a behavioral problem. Psychiatric and substance abuse patients often demonstrate both medical and behavioral symptoms. You must investigate these symptoms as you would any other patient, with detailed questioning and a physical examination. Do not allow yourself to think that "it's just a psychiatric problem" or that "it's all in her head." Failure to investigate a complaint or withholding care is unprofessional and may constitute negligence.

Past Psychiatric History

[OBJECTIVE 9]

Ask about allergies, medications, and any past medical history your patient may have. Many patients do not view "medical history" and "psychiatric history" in the same light and therefore may not mention previous psychiatric diagnoses and treatments. Thus you must specifically ask about psychiatric disorders. If a patient reports a psychiatric history, find out more details. What kind of psychiatric disorder? Most patients will be forthcoming, particularly when asked, but some patients may shy away from these topics or even question their past diagnoses. Asking, "What did the doctor/mental health professional you were seeing say your diagnosis was?" is often helpful. Several psychiatric disorders, by their very nature, lead patients to question the opinions of their caregivers. However, as previously stated, mental illness cannot be simply tested for; diagnosis can be difficult and take years. Note both the reported diagnosis and how the patient feels about the condition. You should not determine what is correct; simply record your observations.

Also ask about psychiatric hospitalizations. For patients who have been admitted to inpatient facilities several times, detailed recording of each incident is impractical and unnecessary. Instead, find out the date and duration of the patient's most recent hospitalization and determine any consistent reasons for inpatient treatment. Asking such questions often reveals crucial information. Consider a patient with a history of schizophrenia who states he has been hospitalized three times over the past 4 years. You may be quick to assume that his hospitalizations would be for his schizophrenia, but further questioning could reveal that he had actually been admitted for alcohol detoxification. Knowing this, you can open a new line of questioning about abuse of alcohol and other substances, which currently may be affecting your patient.

Today's standard treatment for many psychiatric disorders is drug therapy, often with psychotherapy and other treatments. Many individuals who have been diagnosed with psychiatric illnesses have difficulty with medication compliance, which can lead to acute behavioral crises. Therefore you must determine what medicines the patient is prescribed and whether he or she has been taking them. Attempt to view the patient's pill containers, particularly with patients suspected of being suicidal. You do not have to open the containers and start counting pills to match the actual number with the expected number. A simple glance is usually enough to see a surplus of pills, indicating the patient may not be taking the medication as prescribed, or see that fewer pills than expected are there, possibly because the patient has overdosed. Be mindful that many people repackage their medications, so do not jump to conclusions. Be sure to ask the patient about other treatments he or she may be undergoing, such as psychotherapy. Ask about the general nature of the treatments and if the patient has recently missed any appointments.

Mental State Examination

[OBJECTIVE 10]

After learning the history of the current problem, examine the patient's mental state. This is almost exactly like the mental status component of the full neurologic examination detailed in Chapter 23. As in cases of neurologic disorders, you are studying the patient's cognitive processing and looking for abnormalities that may signify underlying problems. Remember that your goal is not to diagnose or correct specific psychiatric disorders but to note your findings and convey them to the staff of the receiving facility.

Appearance and Behavior

As you approach, observe where the patient is found and what he or she is doing. Compare what you see with what you would expect to see. Is the patient still in her bedclothes, lying in bed? This is probably normal in the middle of the night, but what about the middle of the afternoon? What if this same patient has not been out of bed for several days? This is abnormal and could be a sign of a major depressive illness. Is the patient sitting down? Standing up? Pacing around the room? Look for signs of **psychomotor agitation,** which is excessive motor activity resulting from inner tensions that is usually nonproductive and tedious. Examples include pacing, fidgeting, hand wringing, pulling at one's clothes, and generally not being able to sit still. Note anything that seems out of place and remember that safety is paramount.

Observe the patient's clothing; is it appropriate for the situation or season? A patient standing in his front yard wearing only a pair of shorts may be appropriate in the summertime, but this is probably abnormal when snow is on the ground. Look at the patient's personal hygiene, taking his or her social status and income into account. Does he seem well groomed or disheveled? Some psychi-

atric illnesses may cause a patient to neglect personal appearance and hygiene.

Speech and Form of Thought

Form of thought describes the ability of a patient to process information and create logical, flowing ideas. Speech patterns and mannerisms are a window into a patient's form of thought. No specific tests or questions let you assess speech. Instead, note this information while interviewing the patient. First assess for disorganized speech, a disorder of thought form or process. These findings generally can be divided into two categories: rate of thought and speech production and quality of associations.

Rate of speech and thought ranges from mutism at one end of the spectrum to pressured speech at the other. **Mutism** describes a condition in which the patient simply will not speak. This can have its root in several conditions, such as the negative symptoms of schizophrenia (discussed later in this chapter) or the interruptions of thought seen in mood disorders. Although somewhat more verbal than patients with mutism, those showing **poverty of speech** offer few spontaneous answers and talk very little. Poverty of speech is easily recognized; you will find yourself asking far more questions than normal (Carlat, 2005). Consider the following example:

Paramedic:	Why do you think your mother is concerned about you?
Patient:	I don't know.
Paramedic:	She feels that you may be thinking about hurting yourself. Is that true?
Patient:	Maybe, I don't know.
Paramedic:	How has school been for you lately? Have you had any trouble?
Patient:	No.

A patient exhibiting poverty of speech can be easily confused with a patient who is angry and resentful of your presence. A patient with a disorder causing poverty of speech may show other depressive, psychotic, or substance-related symptoms. A related symptom is **thought blocking,** a phenomenon in which a patient starts to say something, then stops mid-thought, completely forgetting what he or she had to say. Thought blocking is a frequently seen symptom of the thought disorder caused by schizophrenia.

Some patients have speech patterns that are more rapid than normal. **Pressured speech** is rapid, loud, and intense. This constant, often uninterruptible speech usually results from **racing thoughts,** a subjective patient complaint that one's thoughts are going so fast one cannot keep up. Racing thoughts are directly converted into pressured speech during a manic episode, part of bipolar disorder. Racing thoughts also are seen in anxiety disorders, stimulant drug intoxication, seizures, and some forms of drug withdrawal.

Put simply, **looseness of associations** describes a departure from the subject at hand. Looseness of associations runs along a continuum from circumstantiality to word salad. Patients exhibiting **circumstantial thinking** make many detours and add extra details when answering questions but eventually return to the main topic. You may become inpatient and interrupt the patient to return to the main focus. Such a speech pattern is not always abnormal; those for whom it is normal often are known as being long winded. Circumstantial thinking also is seen in anxiety states, early forms of dementia, some forms of psychosis, and substance intoxication (Carlat, 2005).

Patients exhibiting **tangential thinking** go off topic but never return, unlike patients with circumstantial thinking. These patients follow a progression of ideas that are related to each other; however, each step is farther and farther from the initial topic. For example:

Paramedic:	Have you ever felt suicidal?
Patient:	No, I could never kill myself. I had a friend who committed suicide by jumping off of the Memorial Bridge last year. That was the same month that I went on vacation to Alaska. It's truly beautiful up there in the summer. Everything's green and lush and you would never know that it's so cold and snowy a few months later. A few years ago my car got stuck in the snow and it took me hours to find someone . . .

Even more disjointed associations are known as **flight of ideas.** A patient with flight of ideas rapidly moves from topic to topic with no clear transition or reason. This can be difficult to follow and often is present in manic episodes and psychotic illnesses.

Paramedic:	Do you have any allergies?
Patient:	I don't know. I might be getting sick. There are people all around me that don't believe in what I'm doing, always telling me what to do. It's the right thing, something that must be done. My mother hasn't been there for me, but she will be. I can't go to the hospital because no one will take care of my dog.

Note that although following a patient exhibiting flight of ideas is impossible, all sentences are grammatically correct and make sense when taken individually. When a patient's form of thought becomes even more disjointed, he or she may lose the ability to form sentences and logical thoughts; this is known as **word salad.** Like flight of ideas, thoughts lack a coherent pattern. In word salad, however, even words within sentences are disjointed and confused. You may even feel that your patient is speaking a different language:

Paramedic:	Have you been hearing voices of people that are not there?
Patient:	I work in compared clocks. Sixteen books to have five people. There is a rounding of their timing. Would you like to have some?

Notice that in word salad a patient strays off topic between sentences and within sentences themselves. This is an extreme version of looseness of associations and indicates severe illness, often schizophrenia and sometimes dementia (Carlat, 2005).

Thought Content

After examining a patient's form of thought, look for abnormalities of thought content, such as psychosis. **Psychosis** is a state of highly distorted perceptions of reality, often evidenced by hallucinations and delusions. It may be a part of many psychiatric disorders as well as organic illnesses. Abnormal thought content also includes suicidal and homicidal ideations (discussed in more detail later in this chapter) and preoccupations.

A **hallucination** is false sensory information originating from within the brain without an external stimulus. The brain does not differentiate between vividly imagined and real stimuli. Therefore hallucinations are real to the person experiencing them and can be quite frightening. They can be heard (auditory) and may take the form of constantly hearing footsteps from behind, hearing gunshots, but most often hearing voices. These voices may talk to no one in particular or they may speak directly to the patient and try to influence behavior. They may even talk to each other, and patients may be observed talking to them. Patients may also have visual hallucinations. Examples include seeing people and objects that are not there as well as more subtle distortions of reality, such as slight alterations in people's faces. Objects may change shape as perception of depth and size are distorted. Hallucinations can also involve the senses of taste, touch, and smell, though these are not as common. A patient may realize that a hallucination is not real, or it may be a part of his or her reality. People can experience transient hallucinations without the presence of a psychiatric disorder, such as when very tired or under the influence of certain drugs.

Delusions are false perceptions of situations and events that a patient believes to be true no matter how convincing evidence is to the contrary. These firmly held false beliefs may be blatant and dramatic, as in the case of a patient who thinks that he is invincible and believes he may jump from a tall building without harm. Delusions often can be more subtle, however, such as a recurrent belief that one's spouse is being unfaithful or that people are not to be trusted. These often are complex and involve events and situations that have been misinterpreted and become woven into the delusion. An estimated 60% of patients who have delusions have **paranoid delusions** that involve persecution or the belief that they are being attacked, harassed, or conspired against. This paranoia often involves large organizations and institutions, such as the government, the Central Intelligence Agency, or the mafia. As an authority figure, your presence may worsen these delusions.

Inflated perceptions of one's worth, power, or knowledge are called **grandiose delusions.** Sometimes called *delusions of grandeur,* these often are seen in manic states and psychosis. A common type of grandiose delusion is one of a religious nature. A patient may believe that he or she is godlike, with special powers. An example is a patient who was found barefoot in the street, grabbing pedestrians as they passed. When asked what she was doing, she replied that she was the Messiah and was simply healing people as they walked past.

A delusion may focus on the appearance or functioning of one's body and is called a **somatic delusion.** These may be present in anorexia nervosa, in which a patient steadfastly believes she is overweight even when dangerously starved and thin, or in body dysmorphic disorder, in which a patient believes he has an ugly disfigurement when none exists. All the disorders mentioned are covered in more detail later in this chapter.

Another common type of delusion is a **delusion of reference,** sometimes known as *ideas of reference.* In this type of delusion a patient believes ordinary events have a special, and often dangerous, significance. A patient may believe that everyone she sees, from children riding bicycles down the street to people chatting at a bus stop, are discussing her. In a delusion of reference, a car honking its horn while driving past may be taken as a warning or that someone is trying to communicate with the patient. In extreme forms, the patient may believe that people on television or radio programs are speaking about and directly to her.

Preoccupations are topics and ideas that consistently and constantly return to one's mind, dominating thoughts. Preoccupations may include the obsessions seen in obsessive-compulsive disorder. For example, the feeling that serious harm will come to the patient or a loved one or that one's surroundings are contaminated or poisoned. Of course, these preoccupations have little basis in reality. The patient often realizes his preoccupations are false and silly yet is unable to rationalize them away. Preoccupations are the "theme songs" of the mind, often telling what a patient is thinking. The heightened sexuality of mania (discussed in detail later) often shows itself during conversation as sexual topics are brought up again and again.

Two specific preoccupations are depersonalization and derealization. **Depersonalization** describes feelings of detachment or estrangement from the self. **Derealization** is a feeling that the external world is strange, or not real, as though it were being watched on television or in a movie. These feelings often are seen in anxiety disorders and, needless to say, can be extremely disconcerting and frightening.

When encountering patients with delusions and hallucinations, acknowledge what the patient is experiencing without lending credence to it. For example, telling a patient that you also see the hallucination of a 6-foot rabbit standing next to him is inappropriate. Tell the patient that you believe that *he* is seeing the rabbit, but you must be honest and tell the patient that you do not see anything. Do not buy into a patient's delusions, but do not directly confront or dispute them either. Do not

tell a delusional patient that you believe he is a secret agent of the government. Trying to convince a delusional patient that he is not a secret agent, on the other hand, is pointless. Instead, acknowledge what the patient is telling you and courteously move on to other parts of your assessment.

Delirium often is referred to as *a clouding of consciousness.* This condition is characterized by the rapid onset of a state of confusion often associated with auditory or visual hallucinations, misinterpretations, and illusions. During this condition patients maintain a normal or possibly mildly decreased level of consciousness. The have difficulty concentrating or maintaining a thought process. Patients may believe they are in a different location, be confused regarding the time of day, or be unaware of the current situation.

Delirium may have intracranial or extracranial causes, including fever, head injuries, nutritional deficiencies, stress, neurologic conditions, infections, medications and drugs, and intoxication. With correct diagnosis of the cause, delirium is reversible. Unfortunately, the diagnosis of delirium can be evasive and often is missed by clinicians. Instead, the patient's presentation is attributed to dementia, mania, depression, or part of the aging process. The paramedic must realize this condition is not a part of the normal aging process, and although more common in the elderly, it can affect patients of any age. Delirium is a common condition, particularly in nursing homes. It has been found to be present in 10% to 20% of elderly patients at the time of hospital admission. An additional 20% to 30% of patients develop it during the course of hospitalization, and it is found in 40% of patients in the intensive care unit. Delirium should be suspected in the presence of an acute history of a change in cognition, behavior, or life function.

Unlike delirium, which occurs over a short period, dementia can be defined as memory loss associated with at least one cognitive deficit that occurs over time. Severe and excessive intellectual changes often are present. Dementia is not part of the normal aging process. Alzheimer's disease is the classic example of dementia; however, it has many other causes. An estimated 6.8 million people in the United States have dementia, and 3% of the population likely has it at any given time. The prevalence of dementia increases with age. An estimated 1% to 2% of individuals older than 65 years and an estimated 15% of those older than 80 years have dementia.

In addition to Alzheimer's disease, more than 70 different causes of dementia have been identified, including nutritional disorders, vascular disorders, Pick's disease, Creutzfeldt-Jacob disease, Huntington disease, other neurologic disorders, metabolic disorders, and infectious diseases. In some situations the underlying condition can be addressed, causing a resolution in the dementia. Findings may include personality and behavioral changes, anxiety, agitation, and depression, all of which may progressively deteriorate.

Emotion, Affect, and Mood

[OBJECTIVE 7]

When assessing a patient's mental state, you should get a sense of the patient's emotions. Observe and record these for every patient with a behavioral disturbance. The first way to describe a patient's emotional state is by observing the outward expression of emotion, as perceived by you, the interviewer. This is known as **affect.** Affect is generally described on three levels: stability, appropriateness, and intensity. Stability of affect ranges from a stable affect to one that rapidly and frequently changes, known as **labile.** A patient who is sullen and withdrawn might stare at the floor while talking. Although this affect might not be considered "appropriate," it is stable. A patient who is laughing hysterically one minute and sobbing the next has a labile affect. While interviewing the patient, listen to what is being said and compare it to the presenting affect. Is it what you would expect to see? A patient who is giggling while discussing his or her plans for suicide does not have an appropriate affect.

Normal, healthy persons exhibit a range of emotions. A patient who exhibits no emotion is considered to have a **flat affect,** sometimes called a *blunted affect.* Patients who show some emotion but to a lesser degree than normal are said to have a **constricted affect.** For example, when a patient smiles slightly and lets out a short, small chuckle in response to a joke that most people would find particularly funny, he or she probably has a constricted affect. Patients showing negative symptoms of schizophrenia often have a flat or blunted affect; many patients with depression show a constricted affect. Conversely, patients who are heated and passionate are said to have an **intense affect.** Bear in mind, however, that many normal, healthy people are passionate or quiet and reserved.

In common usage, the terms *affect* and *mood* are used interchangeably. Sometimes affect is used to describe what emotions the interviewer sees on the patient's face, and mood is defined as the patient's own description of his or her feelings. For the purposes of this chapter, however, **mood** is defined as the dominant and sustained emotional state of a patient. It is the lens through which a patient views and experiences the world. Unlike affect, which can be observed to change rapidly, mood is steadier and typically changes over the course of days or weeks.

The two extremes of mood are dysphoria and euphoria. **Dysphoria** is an unpleasant emotional state characterized by depression, sadness, and irritability. **Euphoria** (also known as an **elevated mood**) is an exaggerated sense of happiness or well-being in which a person feels "on top of the world," "high," or "ecstatic." A normal mood is referred to as a **euthymic mood.** You will not assess mood during your examination of mental state, but these definitions are important in the discussion of mood disorders that follows.

PARAMEDIC *Pearl*

Consider the thermostat for a furnace found in the home. Mood can be compared to the temperature at which the thermostat is set. The actual temperature fluctuates around the set point. This is analogous to emotion. A person with a depressed mood may still have emotional highs and lows, but these emotional variations are still lower than normal. Affect is synonymous with the reading of a digital thermometer at an exact point and time within the house (Whybrow, 1997). Another way to think of affect is as emotional weather that varies around an emotional climate, which is mood (American Psychiatric Association, 2000).

Orientation, Memory, and Attention

Use standard questioning to determine a person's orientation to person, place, time, and event. This often is recorded as A&O×4 ("alert and oriented times four"). Orientation to person is a simple matter of asking the patient for his or her full name and a few other basic questions to establish identity. Orientation to time, place, and event can be assessed by asking a series of questions. Questions should begin easy and then become progressively more difficult. For orientation to place, start by asking the patient what country he or she is currently in. Follow this with the state, then city, and finally the specific address. Orientation to time can be assessed in the same way, first asking the patient for the current year, then season, month, day of the week, and date. Keep in mind that many healthy people do not keep track of the date or day of the week, and in many situations a patient would not be expected to know the exact address of the current location. Orientation to event is assessed by asking the patient what events led up to his or her call for assistance.

The three divisions of memory also should be tested: hold function memory, recent memory, and remote memory. Hold function and recent memory are tested by telling the patient three specific words (such as cat, television, and truck, though the specific words are not important). The patient should then immediately repeat them back to you (testing hold function memory), then repeat them back to you again in 5 minutes (testing recent memory). Remote memory is tested by asking general knowledge questions. These questions could include the names of the past five presidents of the United States (Bush, Clinton, Bush, Reagan, Carter) or what buildings were attacked on September 11, 2001 (the World Trade Center and the Pentagon).

Assessing for Substance Abuse

[OBJECTIVE 6]

Attempt to determine whether the patient is under the influence of any substances. Start with direct questioning, such as "Have you used any alcohol or drugs within the past 48 hours?" In addition to looking for paraphernalia or empty bottles and cans, as mentioned under scene assessment, observe the patient for signs of drug and alcohol use. These signs may include needle marks on the arms or the smell of alcohol on the patient's breath. Your patient may deny use of substances even though your assessment indicates otherwise. Document these signs and your patient's responses to your questions, then avoid pressing the issue further. Questioning a patient about any history of substance abuse is appropriate, but avoid direct confrontation and argument.

SCHIZOPHRENIA

Description and Definition

[OBJECTIVE 11]

Schizophrenia describes a set of conditions marked by three types of symptoms: psychotic symptoms, thought disorder symptoms, and negative symptoms. Psychotic symptoms include bizarre and often damaging behavior, usually related to delusions and hallucinations. These abnormal perceptions often are violent and frightening. Examples may include voices shouting insults and belittling comments at the patient or hallucinations involving being attacked or raped. Symptoms that indicate thought disorder are primarily looseness of associations (including flight of ideas and word salad) and thought blocking. Taken together, psychotic symptoms and thought disorders comprise the positive symptoms of schizophrenia. The negative symptoms of schizophrenia are marked by a sharp decrease in interactions with others as patients turn the focus of their attentions inward. Examples include a lack of motivation, poverty of speech, flat affect, and **anhedonia,** the lack of enjoyment in activities that a patient used to take pleasure in.

Five classes of schizophrenia are generally used: paranoid, disorganized, catatonic, undifferentiated, and residual. For the most common type, **paranoid schizophrenia,** positive symptoms are dominant. This type is characterized by frequent hallucinations and delusions of persecution. Patients who exhibit more negative symptoms such as extreme disorders of thought and disorganized speech are considered to have **disorganized schizophrenia.** These patients typically have severe social impairment and at times may have difficulty and exhibit extremely odd behaviors. Other patients instead show disorders of movement. Individuals with **catatonic schizophrenia** show hyperactivity, excessive agitation, or excitement, or they may be extremely withdrawn or show symptoms such as mutism or **catatonia.** Patients with schizophrenic symptoms that do not fall into one of these three types are considered to have undifferentiated schizophrenia. For a person to be diagnosed with schizophrenia of any type, he or she must show a disturbance in behavior for at least 6 months, with positive symptoms occurring for at least 1 month. Finally, a patient who previously had a schizophrenic episode but does not currently show any symptoms is said to have residual schizophrenia. Patients with symptoms of schizophrenia and mood disorders (discussed later) are said to have schizoaffective disorder.

Know meds for diseases

Case Scenario—continued

As you approach the patient, he remains absolutely motionless. His eyes do not blink or change their gaze. He continually looks down, as if staring at something on the ground. You do not see anything that would attract such attention. The patient's hands are in his pockets, but you can palpate a radial pulse at 72 beats/min. His respirations are shallow, almost imperceptible, at a rate of 8 breaths/min. While attempting to assess the patient's blood pressure, he mutters to himself quietly but quickly returns to his motionless state. His blood pressure is 110/70 mm Hg. Other pertinent physical findings include cool and dry skin, normal skin color, and no indication of cyanosis or evidence of hypoxia. You do not notice any unusual odor on the patient's breath. No indication is present of trauma to the head, chest, abdomen, or extremities. No information is yet available regarding the patient's past medical history, including allergies, medications, last oral intake, or events leading up to the current situation. Your partner suggests asking the patient to lie on the stretcher and be more comfortable. He also suggests starting an IV and obtaining a glucose level.

Questions

4. *Has your initial impression changed?*
5. *What do you think may be causing the man's motionless state?*
6. *What treatment options should you consider at this time?*

Etiology

[OBJECTIVE 12]

The etiology of schizophrenia is as unclear as its definition. Some have speculated that schizophrenia is actually several disorders with several etiologies, but this is currently unclear. Schizophrenia is not well understood as an illness, and almost every case is different. The previously discussed categories are meant to be broad classifications. Schizophrenia most likely results from a combination of factors. Studies have shown a strong genetic predisposition to developing schizophrenia; however, despite this genetic predisposition, most children of schizophrenics do not develop the disease and most schizophrenic patients do not have schizophrenic relatives. Developmental factors, particularly during childhood and in the womb, have been linked to the condition. A number of studies have demonstrated a significant link between maternal infection by the influenza virus during the second trimester of pregnancy and a higher risk of the child developing schizophrenia later in life. Some hypothesize that hurtful comments and a negative family environment contribute to schizophrenia as a child and into adulthood.

Schizophrenia is linked to an excess of dopamine in certain areas of the brain (Sue et al., 2002). Support for this idea comes from the action and effects of certain antipsychotic drugs known as phenothiazines. These medications block dopamine receptors in the brain and in most patients dramatically help practically all the symptoms of schizophrenia. The evidence for the dopamine hypothesis is far from conclusive, however. Many patients with schizophrenia do not respond well or at all to antipsychotic medications. In addition, some schizophrenic patients show a resolution of symptoms without the use of antipsychotic medications.

Detailed studies of the brains of those with schizophrenia—using magnetic resonance imaging, positron emission tomography scans, and examination at autopsy—have shown several brain abnormalities. These oddities include a decrease in the amount of nervous tissue in the cerebrum and the thalamus and enlargement of the ventricles (spaces deep inside the brain where cerebrospinal fluid is stored). The rate of use of glucose by brain cells and the blood flow in certain areas of the brain are lower in schizophrenic patients than in those without the disorder. These studies are far from conclusive because neurologic abnormalities are not present in all schizophrenic patients. In fact, these changes are more prevalent in patients primarily exhibiting the negative symptoms of schizophrenia.

Epidemiology and Demographics

[OBJECTIVE 13]

Schizophrenia is one of the more common mental disorders. One out of every 100 adults around the world is schizophrenic. The illness strikes males and females in equal numbers but tends to be more severe in men than

in women. The onset of schizophrenia also is earlier in males (18 to 24 years old) than in females (25 to 44 years old). Diagnosis before puberty and in the elderly is rare.

Higher rates of schizophrenia have been linked to lower socioeconomic status, though the reasons for this are unclear. Schizophrenia is twice as common among blacks (2.1%) than the general population, whereas the rate for Hispanics is slightly lower than average (0.8%).

History and Physical Findings

[OBJECTIVES 11, 12, 14]

Symptoms of schizophrenia are typically seen in three stages. Schizophrenia starts with a slow increase in social withdrawal, poor communication, inappropriate affect, and neglect of hygiene and grooming. Patients undergo a sharp decrease in cognitive ability that takes a heavy toll on education, career, and social life. Most of this decline occurs in the first 5 to 10 years, with relative stability thereafter.

A major event or psychosocial stressor often causes patients to enter the second stage, or active phase. During this stage, a patient has all the symptoms of schizophrenia, including severe distortions of reality, little social interaction, severe disorders of thought, and flat or highly inappropriate affect. During this time patients are most likely to be hospitalized. The severity of the symptoms of schizophrenia then usually subsides, marking the third stage. Patients may have complete remission, a level of symptoms just below that of the active phase, or anywhere in between. Some schizophrenic patients may never show any symptoms again, though most will have later episodes that are equal to or worse than previous ones.

The onset of symptoms often is confusing and frightening for those with schizophrenia, leading some to seek treatment during the early phases of the disease. However, this is not always the case because many patients are even more fearful of hospitalization and being labeled as "crazy" or "insane." Given the social isolation and withdrawal that is part of the illness, schizophrenic patients in the full-blown active phase are not likely to call EMS. However, because of the bizarre behavior often exhibited during this phase, others that are close to the patient are likely to request your services.

No physical findings are associated with schizophrenia. Remember that anyone with altered mental status should receive a full assessment, including measurement of blood glucose. Carefully assess for suicidal and assaultive ideations and involve law enforcement if necessary.

Differential Diagnosis

[OBJECTIVE 11]

Differential diagnosis of schizophrenia includes the following diseases or conditions (Frankenberg, 2005):

- Addison disease
- Alcohol intoxication

- Bipolar disorder
- Brain abscess
- Brief psychotic disorder
- Cocaine intoxication
- Depression
- Encephalopathy
- Head trauma
- Huntington disease
- Hypoglycemia
- Hypokalemia
- Hypothyroidism
- Phencyclidine (PCP) intoxication
- Schizoaffective disorder
- Wernicke-Korsakoff syndrome

Therapeutic Interventions

[OBJECTIVE 15]

Acute interventions in the field are focused on assessing for and treating suicidal or homicidal ideations as well as calming violent or distressing psychotic episodes. Always attempt to transport the patient to a facility that will have records of prior psychiatric treatments and therapies.

Long-term care of schizophrenic patients is usually a twofold process—administration of antipsychotic drugs (e.g., haloperidol, risperidone, clozapine, olanzapine) to control positive symptoms combined with psychotherapy to develop coping mechanisms, good behavioral habits, and positive social skills.

Patient and Family Education

Although the literal meaning of schizophrenia is "split mind," the idea that the condition involves multiple personalities or personas is completely incorrect. Schizophrenia is quite distressing and confusing to family members. A patient's family may become the enemy when seen with the twisted worldview of schizophrenia. Comfort the loved one by explaining that hallucinations and delusions are part of the disorder and to be expected (Box 32-2).

BOX 32-2	**Schizophrenia: Main Symptoms**

Positive Symptoms

Thought disorders
- Thought blocking, loosening of associations (flight of ideas, word salad), decreased cognitive abilities

Psychotic Symptoms

Hallucinations, delusions, bizarre behavior

Negative Symptoms

Social withdrawal, isolation, anhedonia

TARDIVE DYSKINESIA

[OBJECTIVE 16]

Haldol causes it Cogentin - RX for pt. can give Benadryl in field

Description and Definition

Long-term use of antipsychotic drugs is associated with degenerative neurologic symptoms known as **tardive dyskinesia.** Patients with tardive dyskinesia exhibit involuntary and repetitive movements of the mouth and face, such as sucking, chewing, grimacing, or pouting. Patients also may rock back and forth or tap their feet. The patient is usually not aware of these movements.

Etiology

Tardive dyskinesia usually results from suppression of the dopamine pathways in the brain by antipsychotic drugs over long-term use. This pathology is similar to the lack of dopamine found in the brains of patients with Parkinson disease.

Epidemiology and Demographics

An estimated 15% to 30% of patients receiving antipsychotic medication therapy develop tardive dyskinesia. Tardive dyskinesia is most common among populations of patients who have been treated with antipsychotic medications for a long period, but the disorder also occurs in others. Older women are at higher risk for developing this condition, as are blacks. The prevalence of tardive dyskinesia is higher in cigarette smokers (Brasic, 2005).

History and Physical Findings

History is notable for long-term antipsychotic drug therapy. Primary physical findings are repetitive, involuntary motions of the facial muscles and extremities.

Differential Diagnosis

Differential diagnosis for tardive dyskinesia includes the following:

- Dystonic reaction
- Parkinson's disease
- Seizure disorders

Therapeutic Interventions

Often lowering the dose of the drug causing the symptoms of tardive dyskinesia can be helpful, but the disorder has no cure. No acute interventions are possible in the field.

Patient and Family Education

Caution caregivers regarding the risks of falls. Patients should never alter the dosage of their medications without first consulting their prescribing physician. An abrupt cessation of antipsychotic medications often causes a rapid return of severe psychotic symptoms.

MOOD DISORDERS

Human emotion runs a continuum. Dysphoria, depression, despair, and sadness lie at one end; euphoria, joy, happiness, and elation are at the other. As mentioned in the beginning of this chapter, the relations among mood, affect, and emotion are important in the patient with a behavioral condition. Recall that the emotional experiences of most people center around a midpoint on this scale, at a euthymic mood. Mood disorders are characterized by periods of time spent at the extremes of this scale (Table 32-1).

Major Depression and Dysthymia

Description and Definition

[OBJECTIVE 11]

Everyone has felt "down" at one time or another. Feelings of sadness and the blues are at their worst during a grief response, such as when someone close dies. For most, this grief response passes within a month. For others, mood sinks past sorrow into dysphoria and **melancholy.** These episodes may not be associated with a triggering event and are marked by major disruptions of homeostasis, activities, and thought. Melancholic episodes also are known as major depressive episodes and are part of major depressive disorder. In this chapter, these terms are used interchangeably to describe a period of dysphoric mood: sadness, depression, and/or irritability.

Dysthymia is chronic, constant, low-grade depression that lacks the more severe symptoms of melancholy such as suicidal ideations or delusions. Many patients with dysthymia experience a double depression, or an episode of melancholy on top of chronic dysthymia (Callaway, 2004).

Etiology

[OBJECTIVE 12]

Dysthymia and melancholy are thought to be different severities of the same disease (Callaway, 2004). The exact pathology of depression is unknown. Research has linked

TABLE 32-1	Comparison of Episodes Occurring in Mood Disorders			
	Melancholy	**Hypomania**	**Mania**	**Mixed**
Energy level	Low	Elevated	High	High
Sleep	Increased or decreased	Decreased	Dramatically decreased or absent	Dramatically decreased or absent
Psychomotor activity	Psychomotor retardation; flat or constricted affect	Hyperactive; intense affect	Psychomotor agitation; very intense, labile affect	Psychomotor agitation; very intense, labile affect
Description	"I doubt completely my ability to do anything well. It seems as though my mind has slowed down and burned out to the point of being virtually useless . . . [I am] haunt[ed] . . . with the total, the desperate hopelessness of it all. Others say, "it's only temporary, it will pass, you will get over it," but of course they haven't any idea of how I feel, although they are certain they do. If I can't feel, move, think, or care, then what on earth is the point?"	"At first when I'm high, it's tremendous. Ideas are fast . . . like shooting stars you follow until brighter ones appear. All shyness disappears, the right words and gestures are suddenly there. Sensuality is pervasive, the desire to seduce and be seduced is irresistible. Your marrow is infused with unbelievable feelings of ease, power, well-being, omnipotence, euphoria—you can do anything. But, somewhere, this changes."	"The fast ideas become too fast and there are far too many. Overwhelming confusion replaces clarity. You stop keeping up with it— memory goes. Infectious humor ceases to amuse. Your friends become frightened, everything is now against the grain. You are irritable, angry, frightened, uncontrollable, and trapped."	"You feel as if you're going to crawl out of your skin, to get up and move but no exercise satisfies. Thoughts flood your head, thoughts of death, thoughts you can't remember, frightening images . . . Suicide appears as a soothing alternative, quieting the horrible madness within."

From the National Institute of Mental Health. (2008). *Bipolar disorder.* Retrieved June 27, 2008, from http://www.nimh.nih.gov.

it to alterations of serotonin availability in the brain and an increase of activity in the limbic system, especially the amygdala.

Many developmental factors are associated with depression, including divorce and the death of a parent, particularly of the same sex, during childhood. Psychosocial events of loss, such as death, divorce, and unemployment, frequently precipitate a major depressive episode, but in many cases no trigger is clearly identified.

Epidemiology and Demographics

[OBJECTIVE 13]

Major depression is the most commonly diagnosed mental illness in the United States. Thirteen percent of the population will have at least one episode of major depression during their lifetimes. Estimates put the lifetime rate of dysthymia at approximately 6% (Callaway, 2004). Depression is twice as common in women than men. Although the average age at onset is approximately 30 years old, depression can strike at any age (Hasin et al., 2005). Before puberty, girls and boys are equally affected. Newer data suggest that the average age at onset is decreasing and the percentage of people affected is increasing (American Psychiatric Association, 2000). Studies show higher rates of depression among Native Americans and lower rates among blacks, Asians, and Hispanics. Estimates suggest that major depression disorders will cost society more than any other illness by the year 2020 (Hasin et al., 2005).

Immediate family members of someone with major depression are 1.5 to three times more likely to develop the disorder. Higher rates of alcohol and substance abuse are also noted among patients diagnosed with major depression and their families. Risk factors include advanced age, terminal illness, low socioeconomic status, childhood loss of a parent (particularly of the same sex), and other stressful life events.

The most devastating course a melancholic episode can take is suicide. One study showed that an estimated 8% of patients attempted suicide, 36% "thought a lot about suicide," and 45% "felt that they wanted to die" during a melancholic episode (Hasin et al., 2005). More than half of all suicide attempts happen in the context of melancholy. The death rate from suicide among those with mood disorders can exceed 15% (Aronson, 2005).

History and Physical Findings

[OBJECTIVES 11, 12, 14]

During a melancholic episode, nothing seems to satisfy. As anhedonia settles in, people and activities that once brought enjoyment now only disappoint. Self-worth and self-esteem are nonexistent. Thinking becomes tedious and difficult; the mind feels as though it is in a haze. For someone deep in depression, even the simplest of choices can be agonizingly difficult and crushing. Deciding whether to leave a door open or close it when entering a room can seem like an impossible task. As melancholy worsens, thoughts of death and suicide become frequent. In its most severe forms, major depression can have psychotic features, particularly delusions involving death and dying.

Depressive episodes may last for days, weeks, or even months. These bouts may resolve themselves, but patients experiencing a major depressive episode usually require treatment and many require inpatient hospitalization. Although many patients have only one episode during their entire lifetimes, approximately half of those who have had one period of major depression will have another episode within their lifetimes. Some patients have these depressive periods frequently, whereas others may go for years between episodes. The average duration of a treated melancholic episode is 20 weeks (Reus, 2000).

Patients with major depression may not initially or directly complain of a down mood or sadness and demonstrate a normal affect and a normal appearance. Many patients, particularly young men, show irritability and anger during an episode of melancholy. Those with more severe symptoms may show a lack of grooming and hygiene as well as a blunted or flat affect. Psychomotor retardation is common, but psychomotor agitation may be present.

During melancholy, the world becomes a painful place as feelings of worthlessness, hopelessness, and guilt dominate the mind. Suicidal ideations, preoccupations with death and dying, and an obsession with one's own mortality are common. Patients often report an inability to concentrate and continual short-term memory loss.

Dysfunction of the limbic system and hypothalamus during depression causes a major disruption of homeostasis. Disturbance of sleep is almost always seen, typically insomnia, but hypersomnia (dramatically increased sleep levels) is also seen. Patients often report waking up hours earlier than intended and then being unable to return to sleep. Appetite also is usually affected as part of major depression. During melancholic episodes, appetite may be dramatically increased or decreased, leading to weight gain or loss. Libido and the desire for social interaction are lost. The body becomes fatigued, tired, and unmotivated, and patients often report body aches and pains.

Patients with dysthymia exhibit many of the symptoms of depression such as poor appetite, sleep disturbances, low self-esteem, and feelings of hopelessness; however, they are less severe.

Differential Diagnosis

[OBJECTIVE 11]

The differential diagnosis for major depression includes the following:

- Alcoholism
- Anemia

- Anorexia nervosa
- Anxiety disorders
- Bipolar disorder
- Bulimia nervosa
- Chronic fatigue syndrome
- Cushing syndrome
- Dissociative disorders
- Dysthymia
- Graves disease
- Hypercalcemia
- Hyperthyroidism
- Hypochondriasis
- Hypoglycemia
- Hypothyroidism
- Insomnia
- Lyme disease
- Marijuana abuse
- Menopause
- Obsessive-compulsive disorder
- Personality disorders
- Posttraumatic stress disorder
- Schizoaffective disorder
- Schizophrenia
- Somatoform disorders
- Syphilis
- Systemic lupus erythematosus
- Wernicke-Korsakoff syndrome

Therapeutic Interventions

[OBJECTIVE 15]

Patients need definitive psychiatric care during an episode of melancholy, particularly if they experience suicidal or homicidal ideations. If a patient is potentially a threat to self or others, he or she must be transported for evaluation. Patients who are suicidal are not considered rational and may have to be transported against their will. Consult medical direction and follow local protocols. As a paramedic, you should not conduct an in-depth psychiatric interview with the patient. If the patient wishes to talk, listen attentively and document important details. This is therapeutic for the patient and may provide more detailed information about the patient's current state of mind to receiving facility staff. Over the long term, depressive disorders are mainly treated with psychotherapy and antidepressant medications.

Antidepressants

[OBJECTIVE 16]

Three main types of antidepressants are currently prescribed: monoamine oxidase inhibitors (MAOIs), tricyclic antidepressants (TCAs), and selective serotonin-reuptake inhibitors (SSRIs). All work by increasing the levels of serotonin, norepinephrine, and/or dopamine (collectively known as monoamines) in the synapses of the brain. As their name implies, MAOIs block the action of monoamine oxidase, an enzyme that breaks apart these monoamines into their amino acid building blocks to help remove them from the synapse. TCAs stop the reuptake of norepinephrine, dopamine, and serotonin into presynaptic neurons. The SSRIs block the reuptake of serotonin only and are commonly used today.

Because suicidal ideations are common in melancholy, antidepressants are often used during suicide attempts. SSRIs are targeted to only serotonin reuptake and have a large therapeutic index. During an overdose, the most common finding is lethargy, and serious complications are rare. In extremely large ingestions, seizures, nonspecific ECG changes, and central nervous system (CNS) depression can occur. When combined with another drug that increases serotonin levels in the brain, such as ecstasy (discussed later) or another type of antidepressant, SSRIs can cause a potentially lethal condition known as serotonin syndrome. The syndrome usually manifests after a change in dosage or the addition of another medication, but its onset and severity vary widely. Symptoms may range from mild confusion and tachycardia and mild tremors to unresponsiveness, life-threatening hyperthermia, and severe muscle rigidity (Williams & Keyes, 2001). Treatment of SSRI overdose consists of supportive care.

TCAs are much more toxic, and even small doses over therapeutic levels can be fatal. In large doses, TCAs cause profound anticholinergic symptoms such as tachycardia, hyperthermia, dilated pupils, altered mental status, and seizures. In addition, they block the sodium and potassium channels of the myocardium, slowing depolarization in the heart and causing a widened QRS complex, prolonged QT interval, and even ventricular tachycardia and cardiac arrest. Hypotension may also be present. Patients who have overdosed on TCA medications should be closely monitored and rapidly transported. Treat seizures with benzodiazepines and hypotension with fluid replacement. Medical control may order intravenous (IV) sodium bicarbonate to counteract the sodium channel–blocking effects of TCAs and increase the pH of the blood.

MAOI therapy can also have fatal complications. These drugs are powerful and cause a buildup of catecholamines (dopamine and norepinephrine) throughout the body. Any other medication that causes direct or indirect sympathetic stimulation, such as decongestants, steroids, and beta-agonists, can quickly cause a state of sympathetic overload. Tyramine is an amino acid that stimulates the release of norepinephrine from neurons. It is also broken down by monoamine oxidase, and patients undergoing long-term MAOI therapy have an excess of this compound in their blood. Tyramine is present in many foods, particularly aged foods such as wine, cheese, and smoked meats as well as nuts and soy products. Taking even a little more tyramine into the body through the diet can be enough to trigger a sympathetic overload in patients taking MAOIs. For these reasons they often are not used today and are generally reserved for severe episodes of melancholy. However, new research has shown MAOIs may be beneficial in cases of migraine headaches, Parkinson's disease, and anxiety disorders, among other conditions.

Patient and Family Education

A common misconception of major depression is that the person has the ability to "snap out of it" and spontaneously recover. This could not be further from the truth. Remind others that depression is a serious illness and more than a simple case of the blues. Educate family and close friends of a patient with a history of melancholic episodes about the warning signs of suicide and where to turn for help.

PARAMEDIC*Pearl*

Symptoms of a melancholic episode can be remembered by the mnemonic In SAD CAGES.

Interest level in activities (anhedonia)
Sleep disturbances (insomnia or hypersomnia)
Appetite (increased or decreased)
Depressed mood
Concentration difficulties
Activities decreased (psychomotor retardation)
Guilt or excessive, constant worrying
Energy levels decreased
Suicidal thoughts or preoccupations with death and dying

Bipolar Disorder and Cyclothymia

Description and Definition

[OBJECTIVE 11]

Some people who suffer the deep lows of depression also experience periods at the euphoric end of the mood spectrum. Although mood is a smooth continuum, two levels of elevated mood above normal are recognized: hypomania and mania. Episodes of **hypomania** are not usually thought of as bad by those experiencing them (see Table 32-1). As a patient moves from a euthymic mood to hypomania, he or she becomes filled with an overwhelming sense of well-being and confidence. Shyness disappears and the person becomes talkative and outgoing; libido is incensed as he or she starts to feel more attractive to the opposite sex. During hypomania, the mind moves quickly, seeming to come up consistently with the right line in a conversation or the correct answer to a question. Those having a hypomanic episode often show poor judgment and distractibility. As a hypomanic episode progresses, patients often smoothly move into the bizarre and dangerous irrationality that is mania.

Mania is everything that melancholy is not (see Table 32-1). Self-worth is dangerously inflated, often to the point of grandiose delusions. A patient having a manic episode has noticeably elevated mood and limitless energy, taking on project after project. Judgment becomes highly impaired and the person behaves in an irrational and risky manner. Others often see someone in an episode of hypomania as witty, charming, and funny. During mania, an unintelligible blur of thoughts comes at extreme speed; other people become fearful and intimi-

dated. Some patients do not feel the inflated self-worth and elevated mood of mania but instead experience the guilt and worthlessness of depression combined with the energy and agitation of mania. These periods are termed **mixed episodes** and can be quite dangerous because patients in the midst of these often have suicidal ideations. Mixed episodes occur in 40% of bipolar patients (Jacobson & Jacobson, 2001).

Bipolar disorder is an illness of extremes of mood. Bipolar I shifts from melancholy to full-blown mania or a mixed episode. Bipolar II also manifests with depression, but elevation of mood stops at hypomania. The frequency of manic, hypomanic, melancholic, or mixed episodes varies widely from patient to patient. At the conclusion of a hypomanic or manic episode, most patients rapidly descend into the depths of melancholy. Some may have only one manic episode in a lifetime, whereas others may have episodes yearly or, in severe cases, several times a day. If a patient has more than four episodes each year, the disorder is called *rapid cycling*. Melancholy in someone who has never had an episode of mania is sometimes called *unipolar depression*.

Cyclothymia is a less-severe form of bipolar disorder. Patients have periods of hypomania and episodes of depression that do not meet the criteria for an episode of melancholy. In patients with cyclothymia, episodes of mood disturbance are usually shorter and much more frequent than those seen in bipolar disorder.

Etiology

[OBJECTIVE 12]

Bipolar disorder is thought to have a different etiology than major depression. As with major depressive disorder, bipolar disorder is believed to result from changes in brain neurotransmitter levels and their receptors. These changes are highly complex, affecting many neurotransmitters and different parts of the brain. Bipolar disorder also is associated with significant structural changes to the limbic system, but the cause is unknown (Reus, 2000).

Manic or melancholic episodes have many causes or triggers that vary widely from person to person. For many patients sudden changes in the sleep/wake cycle can precipitate a manic or depressive episode. Other triggers include psychosocial stressors such as moving, marriage, or divorce. Hormonal changes associated with pregnancy and birth have been known to cause a manic episode in susceptible individuals.

Epidemiology and Demographics

[OBJECTIVE 13]

More than 2 million Americans are estimated to have bipolar disorder. Many with bipolar II are misdiagnosed with unipolar depression because patients only seek treatment during depressive episodes. The illness usually emerges in late adolescence and early adulthood, but for some patients episodes begin in early childhood. For others, bipolar disorder does not present until middle age or later. Five percent to 15% of those with bipolar II disorder have a manic episode within 5 years, shifting their diagnosis to bipolar I disorder (American Psychiatric Association, 2000). If untreated, bipolar disorder becomes progressively worse as episodes of both extremes of mood become more frequent and severe. Bipolar disorder has a 60% lifetime rate of associated substance abuse (Reus, 2000).

Overall, bipolar I disorder affects men and women equally, but women are more likely to have the rapid-cycling type. Bipolar II disorder is more common in women than in men. Cyclothymia also affects approximately 1% of Americans, usually starting during late puberty and early adulthood. Cyclothymia progresses to bipolar disorder in approximately 15% to 50% of cases. Both bipolar disorder and cyclothymia show strong genetic components (American Psychiatric Association, 2000).

History and Physical Findings

[OBJECTIVES 11, 12, 14]

The defining symptom of bipolar disorder is the manic episode. A decreasing need for sleep is usually one of the earliest signs; most episodes either begin with the patient going to sleep later and later each night or waking earlier and earlier each morning. As mania intensifies, patients go from healthy levels of sleep to 3 or 4 hours per night, then to little or none at all.

An elevated, elated mood must last for at least 1 week to be considered part of a manic episode. The euphoria of mania is infectious; the manic patient can often persuade family and friends to loan him or her money for impractical inventions or foolish business ideas, against better judgment. This euphoria can quickly turn to irritability and anger, particularly when the patient is crossed or confined. Labile affect is common and ranges from elated to angry (American Psychiatric Association, 2000).

During mania, individuals have an elevated self-image, often to the point of delusion. Patients typically engage in expansive, goal-oriented behavior. For example, despite having no talent or experience, a patient may attempt to write a novel or compose a symphony. Patients may explain that they are in high-level positions of power, such as those within the government. They may excessively plan or engage in goal-directed activities at work, school, or church.

Thoughts come at the mind in a torrential downpour during mania. Patients display rushed, pressured speech and feel that they cannot keep up with their own minds. Many patients compulsively write things down to remember them, generating dozens of lists and notes. However, these scribblings are typically illegible or make little sense when read by others. In conversation, patients display looseness of associations.

Mania is marked by a loss of rationality and control. Patients often have an intense desire to socialize and may call distant acquaintances late at night "to catch up," oblivious to the irritation of the other party. A manic patient may dramatically change his or her appearance and dress in a more sexually suggestive style. Clothes may seem to have been quickly and haphazardly put on or appear bright, tasteless, and out of place (Soreff, 2004). During a manic episode, persons often say and do things they normally would not, such as making unethical business deals or criticizing and lying to family and friends. An inflated sense of self-esteem typically leads to risky and dangerous behaviors, such as substance abuse, promiscuous sex, reckless driving, risky investments, or shopping sprees totaling thousands of dollars. These behaviors are unusual for the patient and continue despite painful consequences, such as motor vehicle collisions, sexually transmitted disease, and an inability to pay for purchased merchandise. Patients may exhibit assaultive or suicidal ideations, particularly when psychotic features are present.

Hypomania is a lesser form of mania without bizarre behavior and psychosis (American Psychiatric Association, 2000). In addition to becoming more talkative and social, a hypomanic person becomes increasingly involved in projects at school, work, or home but to a more manageable level. Once hypomania turns downward to depression, however, commitments that seemed effortless may now seem impossible.

Substance abuse is common among those with bipolar disorder. Individuals frequently attempt to self-medicate, using depressant drugs to bring them down from manic highs and stimulant drugs to lift up their depressive lows. Alcohol use is common during both depressive and manic episodes.

Differential Diagnosis

[OBJECTIVE 11]

Differential diagnosis of bipolar disorder includes the following (Soreff, 2004):

- Anxiety disorders
- Cushing syndrome
- Head trauma
- Hyperthyroidism
- Hypothyroidism
- Posttraumatic stress disorder
- Schizoaffective disorder
- Schizophrenia
- Cancer
- Neurosyphilis
- Epilepsy
- AIDS
- Multiple sclerosis
- Medication effects
- Attention deficit–hyperactivity disorder, especially in children and adolescents
- Multiple personality disorder
- Oppositional defiant disorder (in children)
- Alcohol abuse and withdrawal
- Stimulant abuse and withdrawal
- Hallucinogen abuse
- Opiate abuse and withdrawal

Therapeutic Interventions

[OBJECTIVES 15, 16]

During a manic episode, determine whether the patient's reckless behaviors are a danger to self or others because suicidal ideations are not uncommon. A person who has been manic for several days has probably slept and eaten or rested little during that time and may be malnourished or exhausted. For a few patients, the psychotic symptoms of severe mania may lead to delusions of persecution. To defend against perceived threats, a delusional, manic patient may turn to violence.

Manic episodes commonly require inpatient hospitalization. Most manic patients are likely to say that they feel nothing wrong and refuse transport. In these cases, a legal order for involuntary transport may be needed. For approximately three fourths of manic patients, lithium carbonate (Librium) or divalproex (Depakote) is effective but takes 10 to 14 days to take effect. For acute mania, a sedative such as a benzodiazepine may be necessary. Treatment of bipolar depression is problematic because antidepressant medications often precipitate manic episodes (Reus, 2000).

Lithium carbonate is a powerful drug that has helped many patients with bipolar disorder lessen the frequency and duration of manic episodes. However, little difference exists between a therapeutic dose of lithium and a toxic one. This narrow window of safety, combined with the suicidal ideations common during the depressive episodes of bipolar disorder, cause approximately 10,000 cases of lithium toxicity each year. Symptoms range from mild confusion, tremor, and weakness to seizures and cardiovascular collapse. Because lithium toxicity is a potentially lethal condition, focus on initial assessment findings, secure venous access, and monitor the patient's electrocardiogram during rapid transport to the hospital (Linakas, 2004).

Patient and Family Education

The behavior of a patient in a manic episode can be distressing and hurtful to family and friends. Reassure the patient's loved ones that patients lose control during a manic episode and frequently say and do things they do not mean.

PARAMEDIC*Pearl*

Affect and behavior may change rapidly during a manic episode. Always be cautious, watch where you position yourself, and avoid threatening gestures or tones.

ANXIETY DISORDERS

Description and Definition

[OBJECTIVES 7, 11]

Fear refers to the physical and emotional reaction to a real or perceived threat. **Anxiety** is a state of apprehension and worry about real or perceived *future* threats.

Differentiation between fear and anxiety is not necessary; the two often happen together and cause similar reactions. Everyone suffers from anxiety at some point in life. The tension you feel en route to a potentially "bad" call or as you await test results from your examinations are two examples of anxiety. For those who have anxiety disorders, however, worry and apprehension become an everyday occurrence, a painful fact of life. The anxiety disorders, although different in specifics and presentation, all have a common symptom—excessive worrying and anxiety that disrupts daily activities. Although most patients with anxiety disorders realize that their anxiety and fear are irrational, they cannot stop or decrease their reactions.

A **panic attack** is a sudden, paralyzing anxiety reaction. These attacks frequently are encountered in the emergency setting. An attack may have a definite trigger or no obvious cause and is characterized by an overwhelming sense of fear, apprehension, and impending doom. When someone has panic attacks often enough to cause worry in daily life about having another, the condition is termed *panic disorder*. A diagnosis of panic disorder is not required to have panic attacks, and panic attacks are common symptoms of many other anxiety disorders. Panic attacks often are self-reinforcing; patients have feelings of "going crazy" or "losing it," which intensify anxiety and fear.

A **phobia** is an intense fear of a particular object or situation. Phobias are generally classified into broad groups such as animal phobias (e.g., cats, spiders, dogs), natural environment phobias (e.g., water, heights, storms), blood injection injury phobias (e.g., the sight of blood, being injected with a needle), and situational phobias (e.g., tight and enclosed spaces, bridges, tunnels) (American Psychiatric Association, 2000).

Agoraphobia is a phobia of places and situations where escape during a panic attack would be difficult or embarrassing. Many of those who have agoraphobia become homebound because the thought of being trapped in a crowd or a public place is paralyzing and can trigger a panic attack. Excessive, intense fear of social gatherings and situations is relatively common and termed *social phobia*. Patients may worry about specific aspects of a phobia, such as being bitten by a dog or falling from a height. Others may have fears related to the effects of the intense anxiety related to the stimulus, such as fainting, losing control, or screaming. Some may have no basis or rationale for their phobias.

Instead of severe, acute reactions, some patients have a constant, excessive worry about everyday life, called **generalized anxiety disorder (GAD).** This excessive anxiety cannot be controlled and produces symptoms of prolonged stress such as muscle tension, fatigue, sleep difficulties, and irritability. The concerns and anxiety of GAD are usually related to routine activities, such as family members' health, financial responsibilities, or job pressures. The intensity, duration, and frequency of these worries are highly disproportionate to the actual likelihood or consequences of the feared event (American Psychiatric Association, 2000). Someone with GAD may focus on one particular matter or switch from worry to worry.

A stressful, traumatic event that involves threatened or actual death or serious injury can cause anxiety symptoms experienced long afterwards. This reaction is termed **posttraumatic stress disorder (PTSD)** and may also be a product of witnessing something terrible happen to someone else. Events that can cause PTSD include violent physical assault, military combat, rape, torture, severe motor vehicle crashes, and natural and manmade disasters. Molestation ahead of a child's developmental age also can cause episodes of PTSD. Exposure to this extreme trauma causes an alternating pattern of emotional numbness and reliving of the event through vivid memories and dreams.

Some patients have considerable anxiety and distress over unwanted and recurring ideas or impulses. These intrusive thoughts are called *obsessions*. These are not simply worries about everyday life. Instead they are bothersome and sometimes disturbing thoughts that most patients try to ignore, at least initially. To neutralize these obsessions, a patient may develop compulsions, or certain rituals that *must* be performed. A patient with obsessions of accidentally burning down his home may develop compulsions related to fire, such as repeatedly searching the house for flammable objects. Compulsions are usually performed in a specific, ritualistic fashion. A patient may believe that he or she has to touch each corner of the bedroom, in a certain order, exactly 24 times before going to bed each night. Another patient may feel an uncontrollable need to make sure the doors to the house are locked dozens of times before feeling secure. This cycle of obsessions and compulsions is called **obsessive-compulsive disorder (OCD)**. Do not confuse this with obsessive-compulsive personality disorder, detailed later in this chapter. Types of anxiety disorders are summarized in Box 32-3.

Etiology

[OBJECTIVE 12]

Patients with anxiety disorders often have marked hyperactivity in the region of the pons controlling sympathetic stimulation. This may explain the increased heart rate, breathing rate, and hypertension associated with anxiety states. Patients with anxiety disorders typically have heightened sensitivity to substances that increase activity in this area of the brain, such as caffeine and epinephrine. A serotonin deficiency in certain areas of the brain has been strongly linked to OCD (Greist & Jefferson, 2000).

Epidemiology and Demographics

[OBJECTIVE 13]

Approximately one fourth of Americans will have symptoms of an anxiety disorder at least once during their lives. A direct connection exists between anxiety and

| BOX 32-3 | Types of Anxiety Disorders |

- *Panic attacks:* Acute reactions of intense fear and anxiety that may or may not be related to a specific stimulus
- *Phobias:* Reactions of fear and anxiety related to a specific stimulus
- *Generalized anxiety disorder (GAD):* Constant and excessive worry about everyday occurrences and events
- *Posttraumatic stress disorder (PTSD):* Episodes of acute panic and distress regarding a traumatic event experienced or witnessed by the patient, alternating with periods of feeling numb
- *Obsessive-compulsive disorder (OCD):* Recurrent, excessive anxiety caused by obsessions; patient attempts to relieve anxiety by performing rituals, called compulsions

depression; at least three fourths of those diagnosed with depression disorders report feeling anxious, worried, and fearful (Greist & Jefferson, 2000).

Among the general population, animal phobias predominate; however, situational phobias are much more commonly seen in clinical settings. Only 12% to 30% of those with specific phobias are estimated to seek help for their disorders. The onset of specific phobias is during childhood for most patients, although those who experience situational phobias show a peak of onset in the late 20s. More than half of those with a phobia have an additional mental illness, particularly other anxiety disorders, mood disorders, or substance abuse.

PTSD affects approximately 1% of the general population over a lifetime, but this rate is much higher in populations who have experienced severe, traumatic events. In a sampling of employees at the Pentagon 2 years after the terrorist attacks of September 11, 2001, approximately 14% were found to have probable PTSD. This rate was higher in those employees who were actually at the Pentagon that day and even higher in those who had witnessed dead bodies or severe injuries (Grieger et al., 2005).

OCD is a relatively common disorder, affecting approximately 2% to 3% of Americans. Unlike the other anxiety disorders, OCD affects men and women equally. Patients usually begin to show symptoms of the disorder in their early 20s.

History and Physical Findings

[OBJECTIVES 11, 12, 14]

A patient in the middle of a panic attack may report any number of physical symptoms in addition to overwhelming and paralyzing terror. Patients commonly have chest pain and discomfort, including palpitations and a pounding heartbeat. Shortness of breath, often associated with feelings of choking or smothering, is common. Other symptoms during a panic attack often include nausea, diaphoresis, lightheadedness, and dizziness. Patients often report tremors, numbness and tingling sensations (particularly in the hands and feet), and chills or hot flashes. A person in the middle of a panic attack may express intense fears of "losing control," "going crazy," or dying. Patients often describe feelings of extreme detachment from the environment, such as derealization and depersonalization.

Exposure to a phobia-related stimulus provokes intense anxiety and avoidance reactions. A true, pathologic phobia interferes with daily activities. For example, a child may refuse to go to school for fear of encountering a dog (American Psychiatric Association, 2000). The degree of terror elicited by a phobia depends on how close the individual is to the feared object or situation. Even the thought of a phobia-inducing stimulus can cause a panic attack in some. A patient with a fear of flying may feel uneasy looking at an airplane; if he were on that plane he may become terrified and develop chest pain and dyspnea. Patients may be able to endure limited contact with their phobias, but only with extreme dread and difficulty. Children may react to phobias with crying, tantrums, and clinging.

Symptoms of PTSD may appear days after a traumatic event or may not come for 6 months or more. Vivid and frightening recollections come at inopportune times and cause much stress and disruption. These episodes often are triggered by stimuli related to the traumatic event. For example, for a victim of a major automobile accident, riding in a car afterwards may trigger a flood of intense, painful memories and anxiety (American Psychiatric Association, 2000).

Patients with OCD recognize that their obsessions and compulsions are products of their own mind and usually believe that they are silly, foolish, or senseless. Nevertheless, these individuals believe they *must* perform these rituals, usually to prevent "something terrible" from happening. The specific harm often is unnamed, and no connection may exist between a compulsion and the harm it is meant to neutralize. Patients may spend hours each day performing these ritualistic acts. Symptoms of OCD may be constant or come and go, but the disorder is typically chronic.

Differential Diagnosis

Differential diagnosis of anxiety disorders includes the following (Yates, 2005):

- Addison disease
- Alcohol intoxication or withdrawal
- Anaphylaxis
- Anorexia nervosa
- Asthma
- Marijuana intoxication or withdrawal
- Conversion disorders
- Major depression
- Diabetes mellitus
- Digitalis toxicity
- Encephalopathy
- Factitious disorder
- Fibromyalgia
- Hallucinogen intoxication or withdrawal
- Inhalant intoxication or withdrawal
- Malingering
- Meningitis
- Personality disorders
- Autism
- Pulmonary embolism
- Schizophrenia
- Somatoform disorders
- Stimulant intoxication or withdrawal
- Unstable angina
- Shock

Therapeutic Interventions

[OBJECTIVE 15]

In any patient, somatic symptoms such as chest pain and dyspnea must be investigated with a full, detailed assessment and physical examination. Try to calm and focus the thoughts of a patient having a panic attack. Remove external stimuli, such as loud or abusive bystanders, or move the patient to a quiet, calm environment such as the back of the ambulance. Coaching a patient to focus on the process of breathing can take his or her mind away from anxiety and apprehension. Position yourself at or below the patient's eye level and hold the patient's hands if allowed. While making eye contact, reassure the patient that he or she is safe and protected by using a calm, even tone.

Giving oxygen probably has limited benefit during a panic attack but should be attempted. Patients often do not tolerate a nonrebreather mask during a panic attack because it may worsen feelings of smothering or suffocation. Having a patient breathe in and out of a paper bag is not an acceptable therapy. Most panic attacks are self-limiting, peaking after approximately 10 minutes. For extreme, prolonged attacks, medical direction may authorize the administration of a benzodiazepine such as diazepam or lorazepam. Decrease anxiety associated with phobias by moving the patient away from the stimulus causing the reaction. Starting an IV in those with blood or needlestick phobias may cause a brief syncopal episode.

Long-term behavioral therapy can reduce the symptoms associated with OCD by 60% to 80% in approximately three fourths of patients. SSRI antidepressants such as fluoxetine (Prozac) have been shown to reduce the symptoms of anxiety disorders and obsessive-compulsive behaviors and feelings (Greist & Jefferson, 2000). For patients having recurrent panic attacks, SSRIs often can decrease the number of attacks or prevent them altogether.

Patient and Family Education

You may need to remind family and bystanders that patients have little control over their symptoms during a panic attack. By keeping the surroundings calm, you will help the patient become calm.

SOMATOFORM DISORDERS

Description and Definition

[OBJECTIVE 11]

Patients with **somatoform disorders** have preoccupations with their bodies. Physical complaints may suggest a medical illness but cannot be explained by clinical findings such as vital signs and laboratory tests. Some would say that the complaints of these patients "are all in their head." Although this is true to a degree, patients do experience the pain and symptoms they describe. Four main types of somatoform disorders occur: conversion disorder, hypochondriasis, somatization disorder, and body dysmorphic disorder.

Patients with conversion disorder unknowingly convert their psychological distress into pseudoneurologic symptoms. These symptoms can be motor or sensory related and may present as seizures. Conversion symptoms usually are exacerbated after a psychologically stressful event.

Hypochondriasis is a preoccupation with having a specific serious medical illness founded on misinterpretations of bodily signs and symptoms. Patients with hypochondriasis maintain they are afflicted with an illness despite medical evaluations and tests that say otherwise. These patients stop short of being delusional, however, because they can acknowledge that they may be exaggerating symptoms and not actually be sick.

Somatization disorder is characterized by multiple, recurring complaints resulting in medical treatment or the impairment of life functioning. Symptoms occur in a pattern and cannot be explained by any known medical condition. Diagnosis of the disorder is made by the following:

- Pain in at least four different sites or functions
- At least two gastrointestinal symptoms other than pain
- At least one sexual or reproductive symptom other than pain
- At least one symptom other than pain that suggests a neurologic condition

Patients preoccupied with a defect in their appearance often have body dysmorphic disorder. A flaw may be an excessive, exaggerated response to a minor abnormality or completely imagined. This "fault" causes substantial distress, and patients often describe their supposed deformity as "intensely painful," "tormenting," or "devastating." Preoccupations are difficult to control. Patients may spend hours each day thinking about their supposed

---

BOX 32-4	Somatoform Disorders

- *Conversion disorder:* Psychological stress converted into neurologic symptoms
- *Hypochondriasis:* Preoccupation about having a specific medical condition; symptoms are related to same condition
- *Somatization disorder:* Symptoms relating to many body systems and functions
- *Body dysmorphic disorder:* Preoccupation about a real or imagined physical flaw or ugliness

---

defect and become so self-conscious they avoid work, school, and other public situations (American Psychiatric Association, 2000). A summary of somatoform disorders is shown in Box 32-4.

Etiology

[OBJECTIVE 12]

Symptoms of conversion disorder are thought to be a protective mechanism used to shield the patient from emotional trauma and pain. When a disturbing event or emotion occurs, it is suppressed into the subconscious and reformed into physical symptoms. Converting this pain blocks the upsetting emotions and nets the attention and help of others.

Hypochondriasis is believed to stem from a failed attempt to cope with psychological needs or conflicts. Unable to express emotions effectively, patients focus on physical symptoms instead.

The etiology of somatization disorder is unknown. Some studies have shown a fairly strong link between childhood abuse and trauma and somatization disorder, but the reasons for this are unknown (Loewenstein et al., 2000).

Epidemiology and Demographics

[OBJECTIVE 13]

In the United States somatoform disorders are primarily seen in women, except for hypochondriasis, which seems to present equally in both sexes. Conversion disorder is present in as many as one out of every 2000 Americans, but rates among patients in hospitals and the healthcare system are much higher. Hypochondriasis is thought to be common in medical practice, through definitive numbers are lacking. Lifetime prevalence of somatization disorder is estimated at approximately 2% of women and 0.2% of men.

History and Physical Findings

[OBJECTIVES 11, 12, 14]

Symptoms of conversion disorder are usually motor and sensory nervous deficits, typically in response to a stressful event. Sensory problems may present as blindness, deafness, double vision, or a loss of touch sensation. Motor symptoms include acute paralysis or weakness, difficulty swallowing, or an inability to speak. Patients may exhibit pseudoseizures, which often resemble generalized seizures but are not caused by abnormal conduction within the brain. These symptoms may closely mimic actual medical conditions, or they may seem out of place and odd. Patients with more medical knowledge tend to display symptoms more accurately.

Defining symptoms of hypochondriasis are typically part of one particular disease or condition. For example, a woman may believe she has breast cancer and feels pain and discomfort in that breast. She also may complain of associated weakness and other related symptoms. These symptoms persist despite medical tests and proof that the condition does not exist. As with other somatoform disorders, symptoms of hypochondriasis depend on the patient's medical knowledge and experience. Patients often do extensive research on the condition they believe they have, subconsciously reaffirming their symptoms.

Patients diagnosed with somatization disorder typically have multiple complaints involving several body systems. Pain is commonly experienced at several locations, such as the head, abdomen, chest, back, and extremities. Bodily functions such as menstruation, urination, or sexual intercourse often are painful as well. Gastrointestinal symptoms such as nausea and bloating are common, as is sexual dysfunction. Finally, patients describe neurologic problems such as those seen with conversion disorder, amnesia or altered mental status, and loss of consciousness.

Because they are usually the most visible parts of the body, patients with body dysmorphic disorder typically focus on flaws located on the face and head. Examples include acne, wrinkles, scars, paleness, thinning hair, excessive facial hair, and facial asymmetry. Patients may obsess about the shape and size of facial features such as the eyes, eyebrows, ears, and mouth. The breasts, genitals, abdomen, or overall body build and size can also be the focus of patients with body dysmorphic disorder. Some patients avoid discussing specific flaws and instead only refer to their perceived overall "ugliness."

Episodes of pain and dysfunction related to somatoform disorders usually begin during adolescence and young adulthood. Some patients may have only one episode in a lifetime, but recurring episodes are more common.

Differential Diagnosis

[OBJECTIVE 11]
Differential diagnosis of somatoform disorders includes the following:

- GAD
- Major depression
- Cerebrovascular accident or transient ischemic attack
- Factitious disorder
- Substance intoxication or withdrawal
- Hundreds of medical conditions

Therapeutic Interventions

[OBJECTIVE 15]
No prehospital treatment is possible for somatoform disorders. Avoid dismissing patient complaints because these symptoms feel very real and are not intentionally produced. Assess and treat for all symptoms as you would with any patient.

Patients with somatization disorder and hypochondriasis often resist psychiatric treatment because they firmly believe they are physically ill. Psychotherapy concentrated on modifying behavior and learning coping mechanisms is the most effective treatment. Treatment of conversion disorder is centered on finding deep, underlying emotional problems causing the disorder's symptoms. This is typically done with psychotherapy and hypnotherapy.

FACTITIOUS DISORDER AND MALINGERING
Description and Definition

[OBJECTIVE 11]
Unlike the somatoform disorders, patients with **factitious disorder** intentionally produce signs and symptoms of illness in an effort to assume the sick role. The word *factitious* means "artificially produced," and severe forms of the disorder are known as *Munchausen syndrome*. Patients with this disorder often are quite knowledgeable about the disease or illness for which they feign symptoms.

Those with factitious disorder are often seen at various physicians' offices, clinics, and emergency departments. They may sit through countless, painful, and expensive medical tests, all of which usually show normal findings. Complaints often are related with dramatic flair and show. The majority of patients with factitious disorder have worked in healthcare in some capacity and are quite knowledgeable about medical testing and procedures. They may even suggest diagnostic tests, remedies, and surgeries to a physician. They characteristically abuse high-dose narcotic analgesics and directly ask for them, often by name and dose. They tend to become angry when their requests are denied (Eisendrath & Guillermo, 2000).

If admitted to the hospital, patients with factitious disorder commonly allow themselves to be discovered. This often prompts feelings of anger and resentment in medical staff after being deceived. When discovered, patients typically discharge themselves against medical advice and quickly leave the premises, only to be admitted to another hospital a few hours later. In severe cases, patients must move frequently from city to city to avoid detection (American Psychiatric Association, 2000). The majority of patients with factitious disorder only inflict minor illnesses on themselves, such as skin infections.

Another much rarer form of this disorder is factitious illness by proxy. In this form of the disease, the patient inflicts illness in another person. The patient's need for attention from medical personnel is fulfilled when he or she seeks treatment for their victim. Factitious disorder by proxy almost always takes the form of a mother intentionally making her child ill.

Malingering is the act of faking illness for a tangible gain. Examples include a child who pretends to have the flu to avoid a test at school or a patient who has been arrested feigning shortness of breath to delay incarceration. Others examples include reporting neck pain that does not exist after a motor vehicle crash or pretending to have an illness to receive food, shelter, and lodging at a hospital. Malingering is not considered a mental disorder because the patient deliberately feigns symptoms and has a clear goal in mind.

Etiology

[OBJECTIVE 12]

Patients with factitious disorder often lacked emotional care and support in early childhood, possibly because of the death of a parent or neglect. Many with this disorder were hospitalized for a period during childhood. During hospitalization, their emotional and physical needs were met by physicians and nurses. Some researchers hypothesize that patients with factitious disorder attempt to regain this comfort level in response to deep emotional and psychological trauma. Others believe factitious illness allows patients to take control of being ill and being treated in the hospital—something they were not able to do as a sick child (Eisendrath & Guillermo, 2000).

Malingering has an infinite number of motives. Common reasons include monetary gain, an excused absence from work or school, and avoidance of incarceration or prosecution.

Epidemiology and Demographics

[OBJECTIVE 13]

The nature of factitious disorder and malingering prevents accurate and thorough epidemiologic studies. Patients with severe factitious disorder may have several aliases used at different hospitals and clinics. They often discharge themselves abruptly and quickly from inpatient care, making them difficult to track (Eisendrath & Guillermo, 2000).

One study, based on the impressions of neurologists, has estimated malingering to be a factor in approximately 30% of cases involving disability or personal injury litigation and 20% of cases involving criminal prosecution (Mittenberg et al., 2002).

History and Physical Findings

[OBJECTIVES 11, 12, 14]

As with patients having somatoform disorders, those with factitious disorder report multiple symptoms, such as pain; however, they also go to extreme lengths to produce physical signs of illness. Patients might inject saliva into the layers of their skin to produce abscesses, place a thermometer in warm water to fake a fever (American Psychiatric Association, 2000), or inject insulin to cause hypoglycemia (Eisendrath & Guillermo, 2000). In extreme cases a patient may inject urine into his or her bloodstream to cause septic shock. Although less common, signs and symptoms falsified by these patients may be psychological in nature.

Complaints and symptoms of illness and pain in factitious disorder are limited only by the patient's imagination and medical knowledge. In some persons, both can be expansive. Patients usually relate their symptoms with drama and flair, often giving detailed accounts that may or may not fit a specific diagnosis. Those with factitious illness usually have extensive histories of multiple tests, treatments, and surgeries for an illness never specifically diagnosed (American Psychiatric Association, 2000).

Differential Diagnosis

[OBJECTIVE 11]

Differential diagnosis of factitious disorder and malingering includes the following:

- Medical illness
- Somatoform disorders

Therapeutic Interventions

[OBJECTIVE 15]

Refrain from confronting a patient about feigning symptoms unless you have witnessed something that contradicts the patient's history. Even then, challenging the patient is likely to result in anger and even violence toward you and your crew (Greer et al., 2005). Instead, discretely inform the receiving physician of your suspicions and document appropriately.

Patients with factitious disorder generally show a poor prognosis, and severe cases often are considered untreatable. Nonconfrontational and nonpunishing tactics are preferred to expose patients with factitious disorder, followed by psychotherapy.

PARAMEDIC*Pearl*

Determining the presence of factitious illness is not the paramedic's job. Carefully document your findings and suspicions and relay them to the receiving physician.

EATING DISORDERS

Description and Definition

[OBJECTIVE 11]

Extreme attitudes, beliefs, and practices related to eating and food are known as eating disorders. As well as causing emotional and psychological pain, eating disorders have drastic and frightening physical consequences. They are debilitating and can be lethal if untreated.

Anorexia nervosa is characterized by a distorted body image, leading to drastic, intentional weight loss and bizarre behavior and attitudes related to food. Anorexics look in a mirror and see themselves as overweight, even when dangerously emaciated and thin. Patients go to great lengths to lose weight by drastically reducing caloric intake and avoiding high-carbohydrate and high-fat foods altogether. Patients with anorexia nervosa are hyperactive, constantly running, biking, swimming, or doing any aerobic, calorie-burning exercise. Despite eating very little, persons with anorexia nervosa develop preoccupations with food and cooking. Anorexic patients typically have many food-associated rituals and bizarre eating behaviors. These activities are often done in secret, and food may be hoarded or hidden. Some patients with anorexia nervosa also may eat large amounts of food in one sitting (binging), then use vomiting or laxatives to remove food from the body (purging) to avoid gaining weight—a practice known as *bulimia*.

PARAMEDIC*Pearl*

The term *anorexia* means a lack of appetite, leading to an inability to eat. Anorexia nervosa is the name given to the eating disorder.

Bulimia nervosa is a disorder characterized by this pattern of binging and purging of food. Although patients with anorexia nervosa characteristically become drastically underweight, those with bulimia nervosa usually maintain a normal body weight or are slightly overweight. Individuals with bulimia nervosa typically have normal eating patterns until they have an episode of binge eating. The term *binge* describes secretly eating large amounts of food in one sitting—much more than would be considered a normal meal. Food eaten while binging is typically high-carbohydrate, high-calorie junk food. Binges usually last about an hour but may continue for longer. When binging, patients have no recognition of hunger or satiety and typically do not stop until they develop nausea or severe abdominal pain, fall asleep, are interrupted, or induce vomiting. Patients may force themselves to vomit by triggering the gag reflex mechanically or ingesting emetics such as syrup of ipecac (Norman, 2000). Eventually many patients with bulimia nervosa develop the ability to vomit at will. Depression, sadness, and isolation typically precede binges, which temporarily relieve these feelings. These negative emotions typically return soon after a binge is over and often are worse as the individual chastises himself or herself for losing control.

Etiology

[OBJECTIVE 12]

Research shows that eating disorders may result from abnormalities of brain chemistry and structure, much like mood disorders. Much attention has been given to the relation between eating disorders and the media pushing an image of thin, angst-ridden models to young women as the ideal shape and figure. Indeed, eating disorders are practically nonexistent in developing countries with more traditional standards of beauty.

Persons with anorexia nervosa often fiercely resent any attempts to curb their behaviors, asserting that they are fully capable of controlling their dieting. Below the surface, however, they are immobilized by fear and helplessness. These feelings may be directly related to eating and body image, or they may be connected to other factors such as family conflicts or academic performance. By controlling their eating habits and weight, patients maintain a sense of self-control and independence. The inability of those with anorexia nervosa to see themselves as anything but overweight perpetuates this loss of control and reinforces cycles of self-destruction.

The self-depreciation and low self-esteem seen in bulimia nervosa have led many researchers to theorize that the disease is related to an imbalance of neurotransmitters in the brain, much like depression or anxiety disorders. Bulimia nervosa typically responds well to antidepressant medications, lending support to this idea. In fact, bulimia may be a direct manifestation of depression or anxiety disorders in some patients. Bulimia nervosa is typically a chronic condition, and patients may have it for years before seeking treatment, if they do at all.

Mood and anxiety disorders are common in patients with eating disorders. Personality disorders (typically those from clusters B and C, discussed later in this chapter) also are commonly associated with eating disorders.

Epidemiology and Demographics

[OBJECTIVE 13]

Between 1% and 3% of high school and college-age females in the United States are estimated to have anorexia or bulimia. The number of females with an eating disorder outnumbers males by a factor of 9:1. However, research shows that more males may have eating disorders than previously thought. Eating disorders are most common in the upper and upper-middle socioeconomic classes of society (Norman, 2000). They are more prevalent (particularly bulimia) among those involved in sports and activities where thinness is valued, such as cheerleading, gymnastics, and modeling. The incidence of eating disorders is currently increasing.

History and Physical Findings

[OBJECTIVES 11, 12, 14]

Patients with anorexia nervosa go to extreme lengths to lose weight, typically appearing very thin, frail, and gaunt. Malnutrition is common. Even though anorexic individuals may appear weak, hyperactivity is common and patients feel compelled to exercise constantly. Detailed, often bizarre rituals and procedures are associated with food and eating.

As food intake decreases, the body turns on protective mechanisms to fight starvation. Young girls may have a delayed onset of menstruation, and the monthly menstrual cycle may significantly decrease or even stop. Gastrointestinal problems such as vomiting and constipation are common, and gastric emptying times are significantly increased. Other common symptoms associated with anorexia are headaches, frequent urination, and intolerance to cold. In addition to an extremely thin appearance, other physical findings include dehydration, hypotension, bradycardia, and cardiac arrhythmias. A thin coating of hair, called *lanugo*, grows all over the anorexic patient's body to help maintain warmth. Patients with eating disorders often display a flat affect and psychomotor retardation.

By contrast, patients with bulimia nervosa typically have a normal or slightly elevated body weight. The binging and purging of food that define bulimia are quite damaging to the body. Frequent vomiting irritates the throat and causes swelling of the salivary glands and abdominal pain. The acidic emesis wears down the enamel of the teeth, often causing decay. Menstrual irregularities are common. Electrolyte imbalances lead to lethargy and fatigue. In severe cases, excessive purging may lead to dehydration and electrolyte imbalances. Death from rupture of the stomach and esophagus has been reported (Norman, 2000).

Differential Diagnosis

[OBJECTIVE 11]

Differential diagnosis of anorexia or bulimia includes the following:

- Brain abscess
- Cancer
- Major depression
- Anxiety disorders
- AIDS

Therapeutic Interventions

[OBJECTIVE 15]

You may be called to treat the complications of anorexia and bulimia, such as syncopal episodes or abdominal pain. Treat complaints and abnormal findings as with any other patient. Avoid directly confronting the patient with suspicions of an eating disorder. Instead, inform the receiving physician of your suspicions and the signs you have observed.

Inpatient hospital treatment of anorexia nervosa is initially focused on halting starvation and helping the patient learn to eat normally again. Bulimia nervosa tends to respond well to antidepressant medications.

Patient and Family Education

Research points to the idea that eating disorders stem from abnormal brain function, as with major depression or schizophrenia. Long-held ideas that high expectations or cold indifference from parents contributes to eating disorders have lately come into question. Traditionally, treatment of eating disorders focused on separating the patient from her parents based on the thinking that overbearing parents often caused or worsened the disease. Newer treatment methods actively include the family, helping to restore self-esteem and control to the patient.

PERSONALITY DISORDERS

Everyone has "enduring patterns of perceiving, relating to, and thinking about the environment and oneself" that are with us "in a wide range of important social and personal contexts" (American Psychiatric Association, 2000). These patterns are known as *personality traits*. The expression of these traits often changes in different situations. How you display your personality traits around your supervisor usually differs from the way you show them around friends, but overall you still have the same traits. In some individuals these patterns are less flexible and become harmful, causing problems in relationships, on the job, and in other parts of life.

When this happens, personality traits become **personality disorders.** These are not like other psychiatric disorders that are characterized by episodes that come and go. Instead, personality disorders are typically always present. Persons with personality disorders commonly have mood and anxiety disorders as well. However, those with only anxiety or mood disorders are typically aware of their personal shortcomings and the hurt they cause others (behavior during a manic episode is a notable exception). On the other hand, those with personality disorders are blind to the hurt they cause others and unable to appreciate the impact of their actions (Marmar, 2000). Although personality disorders often cause major disturbances in life functioning, no sustained disturbances of thought usually occur, such as the hallucinations and delusions seen in schizophrenia. When psychosis is part of a personality disorder, it is usually short lived, self-limiting, and does not require medication or hospitalization. Personality disorders are divided into three categories known as clusters (Table 32-2). Personality disorders are among the most controversial of psychiatric diagnoses. To determine the presence of a

TABLE 32-2	Personality Disorders	
Cluster Type	**Personality Disorders**	**Characteristics**
A: odd and eccentric	Paranoid, schizoid, schizotypal	Self-imposed social isolation, perception of others as hostile, trusts no one, jumps to strange conclusions, odd beliefs (e.g., magic, conspiracy, psychic abilities)
B: emotional and dramatic	Histrionic, borderline, antisocial, narcissistic	Labile and excessive emotions, impulsivity, difficulty making and keeping relationships, over-the-top behavior
C: anxious and fearful	Avoidant, dependent, compulsive	Crippling anxiety and shyness, avoidance of conflict, perfectionism

personality disorder, a mental health clinician must examine data and experiences over time throughout a patient's life. Many researchers believe that personality disorders often are misdiagnosed, creating a stigma that may prevent a patient from gaining effective mental health treatment for years. You may recognize characteristics of people you know described in this section, but remember that the diagnosis of a personality disorder often is difficult for a well-trained mental health professional. It should not be attempted by paramedics.

Cluster A, Odd and Eccentric

Description and Definition

[OBJECTIVE 11]

The **cluster A personality disorders** are dubbed the odd and eccentric type. These include paranoid personality disorder, schizoid personality disorder, and schizotypal personality disorder (see Table 32-2). People with cluster A personality disorders interact with others in a distant, often bizarre manner. They may feel uncomfortable when dealing with others and have trouble picking up on affective clues during conversations, such as a sarcastic or joking tone (Marmar, 2000). These disorders have a common thread of social isolation and odd thought processes. Like other personality disorders, those with cluster A disorders typically see nothing abnormal regarding the way they live and behave.

Those with paranoid personality disorder often avoid social contact because of a deep mistrust of others. They may perceive almost everyone else as hostile with bad intentions and remain constantly on guard. They may be easily offended and harbor long-standing grudges and resentments. Relationships with others are strained; successful friendships and marriages are rare because of an extreme lack of trust. They are seen by others as cold and humorless and may form uneasy truces with acquaintances such as neighbors or co-workers.

Schizoid personality disorder is characterized by self-imposed isolation and distance from others. These individuals often have little desire for relationships with others and typically pursue solitary activities and careers. Patients with schizotypal personality disorder also are distant and detached from others and are seen by others as weird or eccentric. These patients also have odd thoughts and unusual ideas about the world around them. Schizotypal personalities often have strong beliefs in superstition or psychic abilities, such as mind reading and fortune telling (Marmar, 2000). People with schizoid and schizotypal personality disorder often daydream and may have difficulty separating reality from fantasy.

Etiology

[OBJECTIVE 12]

Some researchers speculate that cluster A personality disorders share a similar etiology with schizophrenia. In fact, these disorders are sometimes known as the *schizophrenic spectrum cluster* because they show many similarities to schizophrenia in terms of behavior and response to treatment. A genetic predisposition to cluster A personality disorders may exist because a higher occurrence is present in families with a history of schizophrenia.

Epidemiology and Demographics

[OBJECTIVE 13]

Because of their solitary nature, obtaining an accurate count of those with cluster A personality disorders is difficult. The most common is schizotypal personality disorder, estimated to affect approximately 3% of the general population. Paranoid personality disorder is less common, affecting 0.5% to 2% of the population (Moore & Jefferson, 2004). The prevalence of schizoid personality disorder is not known but is thought to be relatively rare (Marmar, 2000). Cluster A personality disorders affect men more often than women and emerge around late childhood and early puberty, though many patients are described as lifelong loners.

History and Physical Findings

[OBJECTIVES 11, 12, 14]

Patients with cluster A personality disorders avoid social contact by nature and often shy away from the healthcare system. Their beliefs and behaviors often put these patients at odds with society and interfere with social and occupational functioning. For example, someone with a cluster A disorder may live an isolated lifestyle with dozens of cats, ignoring hygiene and health codes (Giese, 2001). During a history-taking interview, patients with cluster A disorders may seem emotionless, with a blunted affect. However, some patients, particularly those with paranoid personality disorder, may become overtly hostile and angry if they have strong feelings over an issue or if they feel threatened. When under stress, those with cluster A personality disorders may have delusions or hallucinations, but these are almost always short lived (less than a day).

Differential Diagnosis

[OBJECTIVE 11]

Differential diagnosis of cluster A personality disorders includes the following:

- Schizophrenia
- Major depression
- Avoidant personality disorder
- Borderline personality disorder

Therapeutic Interventions

[OBJECTIVE 15]

Avoid directly challenging odd or abnormal beliefs of a person with a cluster A personality disorder. Explain medical diagnoses and procedures in clear, plain language. Do not expect your tone of voice or facial expressions to carry any meaning; what may be a funny joke to you may be taken as insulting by the patient (Marmar, 2000).

PARAMEDIC*Pearl*

Be clear and concise. Avoid jokes, puns, and turns of phrase.

Cluster B, Emotional and Dramatic

Description and Definition

[OBJECTIVE 11]

Persons with **cluster B personality disorders** are characterized as impulsive, unpredictable, and labile (see Table 32-2). This cluster of disorders, collectively known as the *emotional and dramatic type,* includes histrionic personality disorder, borderline personality disorder, antisocial personality disorder, and narcissistic personality disorder (American Psychiatric Association, 2000). Persons with these disorders usually display over-the-top behavior, with chaotic and excessively emotional responses to crises (Giese, 2001). Others are generally put off by these dramatic reactions. Those with cluster B personality disorders frequently have difficulty making and keeping close friends, and romantic relationships tend to be emotional, stormy, and short lived. These

patients often have extensive histories of "doctor shopping," discharges, and refusals of treatment against medical advice (Moore & Jefferson, 2004).

Histrionic personality disorder is characterized by frequent drama, with a need to be at the center of attention at all times. Patients with this disorder are drawn to drama and tragedy and are often bored with the mundane, day-to-day details of life. These persons tell melodramatic and exciting stories that usually lack detail or depth. Speech patterns are likely to be dramatic and colorful, with exaggerated mannerisms. They tend to be impressionable and suggestible and rely heavily on intuition, making important decisions from the gut instead of thinking them through. When they are not the center of attention, those with histrionic personality disorder can become upset, even throwing angry temper tantrums or pouting and crying to elicit pity. As a result, others often find patients with a histrionic personality disorder to be shallow, insincere, and overly dramatic, lacking genuine emotions.

The defining characteristic of **borderline personality disorder** is instability—of emotions, relationships, and attitudes. People with a borderline personality often have rapid shifts in mood and affect from depression to anger or joy to despair, often changing over the course of hours (contrasted with the mood swings of bipolar disorder, which typically take place over weeks or months). Feelings about themselves or others are subject to unpredictable and sometimes violent change; they are unable to form stable pictures of themselves. People with borderline personality disorder have a persistent sense of loneliness and emptiness and go to extraordinary lengths to avoid abandonment. Others are able to bring order and comfort into the lives of people with borderline disorder, but this is usually short lived. These patients view others in all-or-nothing terms—people are either all good or all bad. Someone with borderline personality disorder has difficulty understanding that a person could love someone but also be angry with them at the same time.

A person with antisocial personality disorder lacks the ability to sympathize with or understand the feelings of others. In the most pathologic state, a patient may show a complete disregard for the law or any potential consequences of his or her actions. Without inhibitions, antisocial personalities behave recklessly and dangerously, acting on whims and doing as they please. Persons with this disorder have been termed *sociopaths* in the past, and the synonym endures today. These individuals frequently commit acts of violence, including assault, destruction of property, and theft. They can be aggressive, violent, and cruel, hurting others or destroying property for the sake of doing so. Decisions are made without thinking, possibly leading to changes in jobs, relationships, and residences on the spur of the moment (American Psychiatric Association, 2000). Many antisocial personalities make up what they lack in morality with intelligence and people skills. They may appear as caring, likeable, and endearing when it suits their needs, but these feelings often are empty and hollow (Moore & Jefferson, 2004). Deceit and manipulation are tools commonly used by the person with antisocial personality disorder to get what he or she wants, such as money or sex (American Psychiatric Association, 2000). Most of these patients usually come across as slick rather than cunning and clever (Moore & Jefferson, 2004).

Persons with narcissistic personality disorder see themselves as better than everyone else no matter what their actual achievements and status may be. Accomplishments are highly exaggerated, and individuals are boastful and arrogant (American Psychiatric Association, 2000). They feel entitled to the respect and admiration of others yet have little regard for the feelings and opinions of those around them. A person with narcissistic personality disorder is envious of others who have achieved higher status and believes that he or she deserves more. These individuals usually only enter into friendships and relationships to boost their own self-esteem and do not hesitate to push others aside for their own personal gain. Like the other cluster B disorders, narcissistic personalities have difficulty sensing the feelings of others and are uncaring and oblivious to any hurt they cause. They are highly sensitive to criticism, becoming angry and even enraged. This rage may be masked by an attitude of arrogance and indifference.

Etiology

[OBJECTIVE 12]

The etiology of the cluster B disorders is largely unknown. Some evidence suggests a genetic component of histrionic and borderline personality disorders, but the exact relation is unknown. Patients with borderline personality disorder usually describe extensive histories of childhood neglect and abuse, frequently sexual (Paris, 2005a).

Epidemiology and Demographics

[OBJECTIVE 13]

Approximately 10% to 15% of persons in treatment for psychiatric disorders are estimated to have histrionic personality disorder, but the prevalence among the general population is unknown (Marmar, 2000). Borderline personality disorder is one of the most commonly diagnosed psychiatric illnesses in women. It is estimated to affect approximately 2% of the general population and up to 20% of those in inpatient psychiatric treatment centers (Marmar, 2000).

Antisocial personality disorder affects approximately 4% of males and 1% of females. The percentage of those affected with borderline and antisocial disorders is much higher among institutionalized populations. Up to half of current prison inmates are estimated to have antisocial personality disorder.

A high association exists between the cluster B disorders and substance abuse, particularly alcohol. Cluster B disorders usually begin to show symptoms during puberty and early adulthood (antisocial personality disorder is a notable exception). In boys, the disorder often begins early in childhood, sometimes appearing as gradually escalating harmful behaviors. Other times the disorder may show itself with a dramatic event such as the murder of a playmate or family member (Moore & Jefferson, 2004).

History and Physical Findings

[OBJECTIVES 11, 12, 14]

Psychosocial events prompt endless lamentation from someone with a histrionic personality to anyone who will listen. Women with histrionic personality disorder tend to dress seductively and provocatively. Men often sport a "macho" image with revealing clothing and excess jewelry. Both genders often are flirtatious. Promiscuity is common. Those with histrionic personality disorder often display symptoms similar to those seen in conversion disorder, particularly when stressed.

Patients with borderline personality disorder lack control of their emotions, particularly anger. Self-injury, discussed later in this chapter, is commonly used by borderline personalities to regulate these emotional swings. Strong suicidal impulses may be a part of borderline personality disorder for some patients. When in a low mood, suicide may seem to be a saving grace from the instability of life. When in a better mood, suicide may seem like a logical alternative. Regardless, the suicidal impulse is present most of the time in many with borderline personality disorder, and an estimated 5% to 10% of patients do commit suicide (Moore & Jefferson, 2004).

An inability to form close relationships with others leads to a lonely emptiness common in cluster B disorders. This is often masked, such as with arrogance and indifference in the person with narcissistic personality or with anger and violence in the person with antisocial personality.

Differential Diagnosis

[OBJECTIVE 11]

Differential diagnosis of cluster B personality disorders includes the following:

- Cyclothymia
- Bipolar disorder
- Atypical depression
- Substance abuse

Therapeutic Interventions

[OBJECTIVE 15]

EMS is frequently contacted for the consequences of the violent, self-destructive behavior of antisocial personality disorder, such as motor vehicle crashes, drug overdoses, and suicide attempts. Suicidal behavior and ideations are a frequent part of borderline personality disorder and may be present in the other cluster B disorders. Initial management is focused on the consequences of self-destructive behavior, such as cutting or overdose.

Cluster B personality disorders present some of the biggest challenges seen in long-term psychiatric care. Diagnosis of personality disorders is difficult and takes years. Patients often have little respect for boundaries and may attempt to become too close to their therapists, only to become angry and find another practitioner when told their behavior is inappropriate. Long-term treatment focuses on teaching patients how to regulate their emotions and choose behaviors that prove to be more adaptive in their lives.

Cluster C, Anxious and Fearful

Description and Definition

[OBJECTIVE 11]

Avoidant personality disorder, dependent personality disorder, and obsessive-compulsive personality disorder comprise the **cluster C personality disorders** (see Table 32-2). Like cluster A personality disorders, those with cluster C disorders frequently have few friends. For those with cluster C personality disorders, however, this isolation is not by choice, but instead may stem from a crippling shyness and anxiety.

Patients with avoidant personality disorder feel awkward and socially inept. Despite a desperate desire for close relationships, they remain withdrawn and shy because of an intense fear of embarrassment. Even in situations where acceptance is fairly certain, avoidant personalities stay tense and unwilling to relax, afraid of being humiliated.

Dependent personality disorder is marked by an excessive and constant need to be taken care of. Persons with this disorder are clingy, needy, and unable to make decisions. Minor choices common in everyday life, such as what color shirt to wear or where to eat for lunch, are impossible without getting opinions and reassurance from others (American Psychiatric Association, 2000). Someone with dependent personality disorder prefers others to make decisions, most often a specific individual such as a parent or spouse. This person is unable to express any disagreement with others, particularly those on whom he or she depends. Being alone, even for a short time, causes intense feelings of anxiety and depression; patients often are preoccupied with a fear of abandonment (Marmar, 2000).

Obsessive-compulsive personality disorder is characterized by extreme attention to detail and a preoccupation with lists, orders, and schedules—to a degree that the original reasons for the tasks are lost. Productivity and creativity dwindle because of an obsession with control and intense perfectionism. No matter what, those with compulsive personality disorder always believe that their performance is not good enough. These individuals often are self-admitted pack rats and keep excessive amounts of stuff around "just in case I need it." Persons with obsessive-compulsive personality disorder are uncomfortable with emotions and express them in a carefully chosen, restrained manner (American Psychiatric Association, 2000). Almost three quarters of persons with obsessive-compulsive personality disorder also have obsessive-compulsive disorder.

Etiology

[OBJECTIVE 12]

Many researchers believe that avoidant personality disorder is a social phobia with an early onset, though no proof of this exists. Some evidence shows a genetic component to dependent personality disorder, but its extent is unknown. Higher rates of dependent disorder are found among the youngest children in families. Some speculate the development of dependent disorder is related to a lack of maternal attention during key developmental stages (Marmar, 2000). Compulsive personality disorder may have a genetic component; it is most common in the oldest children of families.

> **PARAMEDIC*Pearl***
>
> Cluster C personalities often are self-barred from social interaction by preoccupations and anxiety.

Epidemiology and Demographics

[OBJECTIVE 13]

Avoidant personality disorder is estimated to affect 0.5% to 1% of the general population and strikes males and females equally. The rate of dependent personality disorder among the general population is unknown but is estimated to affect approximately 2% of those seeking psychiatric treatment. Dependent disorder is more common in women than in men. Compulsive disorder is seen approximately twice as frequently in men and is present in roughly 1% of the general population (Marmar, 2000). Depression and anxiety disorders commonly coexist with cluster C personality disorders.

History and Physical Findings

[OBJECTIVES 11, 12, 14]

Avoidant personalities are wallflowers and become tense when forced to attend social gatherings. They often may look as though they want to socialize but also seem conflicted. Those with dependent personality disorder typically appear submissive and often go out of their way to be cooperative and helpful. Medical complaints are frequently exaggerated and require excessive attention. If the complaints of a person with a dependent personality are not promptly attended to, the person may believe he or she is being treated unfairly and may erupt into angry outbursts. Patients with compulsive personality disorder become particularly upset when they experience a loss of control, such as in the face of an authority figure or during a physical illness. Their attention to detail may prompt them to ask about procedures constantly and frequently.

Differential Diagnosis

[OBJECTIVE 11]

Differential diagnosis of cluster C personality disorders includes the following:

- Anxiety disorders
- Major depression
- Obsessive-compulsive disorder

Therapeutic Interventions

[OBJECTIVE 15]

Patients with cluster C personality disorders often require reassurance and comforting. Long-term treatment is focused on recognizing and correcting poor coping mechanisms.

THE SUICIDAL PATIENT AND SELF-INJURY

[OBJECTIVES 17, 18, 19]

As a paramedic, you will almost certainly encounter a patient who has attempted suicide. **Suicide** is defined as the act of ending one's own life by any means. *Suicidal ideation* refers to thoughts, fantasies, or plans of suicide. A suicide attempt is an unsuccessful effort to end one's own life.

Approximately half of those who kill themselves have a history of intentional **self-injury** (Hawton et al., 1998), also known as *self-mutilation, parasuicidal behavior,* or *cutting*. In reality, self-injury is typically not an attempt at suicide but instead a coping mechanism, though not a healthy one. The subconscious goal of most self-injury is emotional control. Some individuals become so overwhelmed by emotional pain that they become numb; they use self-injury to bring themselves back to feeling. Others use self-injury for the opposite effect—to bring themselves down when emotional pain becomes too great or as a distraction from their anguish. Researchers point to the body's release of natural opiates in response to pain and speculate that some who practice self-injury seek this biochemical high (Kluger, 2005). Although unusual, some patients report using self-injury as a means of gaining attention or as a cry for help. However, most who practice self-injury hide their injuries under bracelets and long sleeves and keep their activities secret. Many practice self-injury in the heat of emotion, without thinking or fully realizing their actions (Nock & Prinstein, 2005).

Epidemiology and Demographics

Approximately 10% of Americans consider suicide during their lifetimes. However, only approximately 0.3% of the population attempt it, and less than one tenth of those succeed (Moore & Jefferson, 2004). Persons younger than 45 years are more likely to attempt suicide, but the elderly (older than 60 years) are more likely to be successful. The rate of attempted suicide is higher among younger people, estimated to be 3% to 10% of teenagers (Rossow et al., 2005). For all ages, females are more likely to attempt suicide, but males have much higher completion rates (Moore & Jefferson, 2004). Suicide by firearm injury is the most common method of completed suicide (Kochanek et al., 2005).

Self-injury is estimated to be practiced by approximately 4% of the adult population of the United States. The prevalence of self-injury is much higher among adolescents; studies report rates of up to 40% (Nock & Prinstein, 2005). Although long reported to be practiced almost solely among females, some estimate up to 30% of those who self-injure are male (Kluger, 2005). A higher rate of self-injury is associated with personality disorders, particularly borderline personality disorder (Paris, 2005b) and obsessive-compulsive personality disorder. Self-injury also is linked to depression and substance abuse (Hayes, 2005).

Risk Factors

[OBJECTIVE 18]

A patient who has previously attempted suicide is much more likely to do so again within 1 to 2 years (Moore & Jefferson, 2004). Patients with mood disorders are at higher risk, particularly those with mixed episodes or melancholy. Persons attempting suicide are more likely to do so while under the influence of drugs or alcohol (Rossow et al., 2005). Persons who have recently quit using alcohol and other substances also are at increased risk. Chronic, terminal illnesses are associated with a higher risk for suicide. Patients with easy access to lethal methods, particularly firearms, are at a much higher risk for completing suicide. Recent tragedy or loss, such as a recent divorce; the loss of a job; or the death of a parent (particularly by suicide), spouse, or child increases the likelihood of a suicide attempt.

Assessment

Although technically part of the thought content portion of the mental status examination, assessing for suicidal and homicidal thoughts and ideations deserves special attention. Doing so may be difficult, but you should ask all patients about suicidal and homicidal thoughts. Being direct and open is the best way to broach this subject. Examples of questions include, "Are you feeling suicidal?" "Have you thought about hurting yourself or anyone else?" "Do you feel like you would be better off dead?" and "Is there anyone you feel would be better dead?" Simply determining whether a patient is suicidal or homicidal is not enough.

PARAMEDIC *Pearl*

If a patient says that he is suicidal, ask if he has already taken any actions to hurt himself. Then ask if he has a plan to do so. Those who have specific, lethal plans are much more serious about suicide than are patients without a plan. A man who states that he has thought about taking a gun into a deserted field and shooting himself is very different from a woman who says she has considered taking a handful of sleeping pills and lying down beside her sleeping husband to die. The former is considering using a highly lethal method in a situation where rescue is not likely (Moore, 2004). Plans that involve specific locations, times, or dates also are more serious.

Trauma resulting from self-injury is typically superficial and not serious enough to be life threatening. The most common method of self-injury is superficial cutting of the skin, often on the fleshy and convenient forearms. The tool of choice is typically the most convenient, including razors, scissors, knives, and sharp glass (Petronic-Rosic, 2005). However, many reported methods of self-injury exist, such as intentionally breaking one's own bones, repeatedly banging one's head against a wall, or burning oneself with heat or acid. Whatever the method, the act is usually done several times in one session. A person may make small incisions into the skin over and over again, typically only enough to draw blood and cause pain.

Management

[OBJECTIVE 17]

For safety, consider all suicidal patients to be violent until proven otherwise. Stage away from the scene and wait for law enforcement personnel before entering. Thoroughly assessing for and discovering suicidal attempts and ideations is the most essential part of treatment. If a patient has already attempted suicide, your first priorities lie within the initial assessment, finding and treating life-threatening problems. A patient who has taken a large dose of benzodiazepines may be at risk for respiratory depression and failure. Someone who has cut herself or himself may be in danger of life-threatening hemorrhage.

PARAMEDIC *Pearl*

A suicidal patient rarely threatens anyone else, but only one incident is needed to end a rescuer's career or life. Remember scene safety throughout your assessment and treatment of a suicidal patient. Stay aware of your patient's tone of voice and body posture and be on the lookout for weapons.

After finding and correcting physical problems, turn your attention to the patient's psychological state. Most suicidal patients require no more than your respect, your ability to listen, and dignified transport. Avoid pressuring patients to talk about the details of their ideations any more than necessary. Do not expect a person to have a specific reason for wanting to harm himself or herself; suicide is not a rational, thought-out act.

Once a patient has told you that he or she is considering suicide, you have an ethical and often legal obligation to help the patient receive proper treatment. Every suicide attempt or threat, no matter how seemingly trivial, must be taken seriously. Applied to the wrong patient, a diagnosis of attention seeking or melodrama can mean death. An order for involuntary transport and treatment may be needed for a suicidal patient. Most suicidal patients want help and remain cooperative as long as you remain respectful, nonjudgmental, and interested in helping them.

When managing a patient who has self-injured, treat physical injuries while being kind and compassionate. Serious injury is uncommon, but extensive scarring may result and patients may unintentionally injure themselves more severely. Your attitude may greatly affect the patient. Providers who act horrified and shocked by self-injury may cause patients to feel they are horrible and not worthy of help. Reactions of puzzlement or disbelief may leave the impression that you are unwilling to help (Abraham & Hardi, 2005). Reacting with judgment or criticism may cause feelings of shame and distrust.

IMPULSE CONTROL DISORDERS

Impulse control disorders can be defined as the failure to resist an impulse, drive, or temptation to perform acts that are harmful to the self or others. They are often a sign of underlying personality disorders such as antisocial disorder, borderline personality disorder, bipolar disorder, substance-related disorder, or schizophrenia. To that end they can be difficult to differentiate from disorders such as obsessive-compulsive disorder, anxiety disorder, depression, and personality disorders.

The patient with an impulse control disorder generally has a feeling of increased arousal, excitement, or tension before performing the impulsive act, then feels a sense of relief or pleasure after performing the act. In addition, the patient may or may not have feelings of regret or guilt after the impulsive act. More often than not, the act itself does not drive the patient—rather, the feelings of intense excitement and relief that result from its performance do. Disorders in this category include pathologic gambling, kleptomania, trichotillomania, intermittent explosive disorder, and pyromania.

Pathologic Gambling

Definition and Description

The most common impulse control disorder is pathologic gambling. This can be defined as a persistent and recurrent preoccupation with gambling that results in great excitement and interferes with normal life functions such as work and social activities. An estimated 1% to 3% of adults and many adolescents have this disorder. However, it can be difficult to distinguish from other forms of gambling. Findings that distinguish this disorder from other forms of gambling disorders include the addictive nature of the disorder and associated excitement, not the amount of money spent. Individuals often become upset or irritable if they are forced to reduce their gambling. They are consumed with thoughts of gambling, often reliving prior winning and losing experiences, planning their next bet, and attempting to gain funds with which to gamble. Pathologic gamblers are unable to walk away from a wager and continue the behavior in response to repeated losses. They often neglect financial obligations; embezzle money from employers and family; exploit relationships to finance their gambling; and lie to family, friends, and employers about their gambling.

Etiology and Epidemiology

The causes of pathologic gambling are difficult to determine; however, individuals with this disorder show some consistent traits. They tend to have a high tolerance for stress and high energy levels. Many have a positive experience early in their gambling career that convinces them the benefits of gambling outweigh the risks. Women afflicted with this condition tend to start gambling later in life, whereas men often start as adolescents or in early adulthood.

History

Pathologic gambling tends to progress through four progressive phases: winning, losing, desperation, and hopelessness. Diagnosis often is made when five or more of the following characteristics are exhibited:

- Lies to conceal the gambling habit
- Increases frequency or funds to gamble with to increase the associated excitement
- Feels anxiety or irritability when unable to gamble
- Views gambling as an escape from life's problems
- Has been unsuccessful in repeated attempts to reduce or eliminate gambling
- Has stolen money from employers or individuals to support gambling
- Ignores other financial obligations to finance gambling
- Borrows money from others to finance gambling
- Continues gambling to recover losses
- Had jeopardized family or work relationships because of gambling

Differential Diagnosis

Diagnoses to consider include the following:

- Social gambling
- Manic episode
- Antisocial or narcissistic personality disorders

Therapeutic Interventions

The prehospital paramedic is rarely called on to treat an individual with pathologic gambling. However, the paramedic who works in a nontraditional setting may interact with these patients. Emergency treatment often is not required. The key to treatment is recognition of the problem, acceptance of the problem by the patient, and psychological counseling. Because of its prevalence, this disorder has had more focus than any other impulse control disorder.

Kleptomania

Definition and Description

Kleptomania is the recurrent and compulsive theft of items. These items are not stolen for personal gain, for monetary value, as an act of rebellion, to support a substance abuse habit, or out of need. The theft is associated purely with the tension-release sensation of performing the impulsive act. In fact, kleptomaniacs usually have enough money in their pockets to pay for the stolen item.

Etiology and Epidemiology

Kleptomania is a relatively rare condition; fewer than 5% of thefts are estimated to be associated with the disorder. The cause remains unknown, but suspicions include abnormalities in serotonin levels. Its clinical classification has been questioned by many psychologists; some consider it an obsessive-compulsive disorder. However, it may be more prevalent than historically thought and often is associated with mood and eating disorders. The disorder is more common in women than in men, although the exact prevalence is unknown.

History

Patients may have a long history of theft and possibly multiple convictions before the disorder is recognized. The primary indicator of kleptomania is a feeling of tension or arousal before the theft and a feeling of release or pleasure after the theft. Additional findings include the fact that the theft was not for financial gain or any of the reasons mentioned previously, and the reasons are not better explained by personality disorders, conduct disorders, or manic episodes.

Differential Diagnosis

Diagnoses to consider include the following:

- Manic episodes
- Antisocial personality disorder
- Conduct disorder
- Ordinary criminal acts
- Delusional acts

Therapeutic Interventions

The prehospital paramedic is rarely called on to treat an individual with kleptomania. However, the paramedic who works in a nontraditional setting may interact with these patients. Emergency treatment is usually not required. The key to treatment is recognition of the problem, acceptance of the problem by the patient, and psychological counseling. SSRIs have had some success in treating these patients.

Trichotillomania

Definition and Description

Trichotillomania is the habitual pulling out of one's hair to the point of noticeable hair loss. Although currently classified as an impulse control disorder, many psychologists and psychiatrists believe it is better classified as an obsessive-compulsive disorder.

Etiology and Epidemiology

The disorder is much more common in women than in men. Common areas of the body affected are the scalp, eyebrows, and eyelashes. The disorder is predominant in children and adolescents, as opposed to adults, and increases in life stress are believed to be the cause. As with other impulse control disorders, it is historically believed to be associated with a tension-relief sensation but, again, many believe it is an obsession rather than an impulse. To be classified as trichotillomania the hair loss cannot be associated with other medical conditions.

History

Patients with this disorder have evidence of noticeable hair loss caused by pulling. This often results in distress and impairment of normal life functions because of issues associated with their resulting appearance. The patient may feel an increase in tension and excitement before removing the hair, with resulting pleasure or tension relief after its removal. Hair loss cannot be explained by medical conditions such as alopecia or other psychiatric disorders.

Differential Diagnosis

Diagnoses to consider include the following:

- Alopecia
- Obsessive-compulsive disorder
- Munchausen syndrome

Therapeutic Interventions

The prehospital paramedic is rarely called on to treat an individual with trichotillomania. However, the paramedic who works in a nontraditional setting may interact with these patients. Emergency treatment is usually not required. Behavior modification and habit reversal are the mainstays of treatment. Patients often are taught to recognize events that lead to hair pulling and to perform another act, such as flexing and extending their fingers, in response to the event rather than pulling their hair.

Intermittent Explosive Disorder

Intermittent explosive disorder (IED) is of particular concern to the paramedic because of the scene safety issues it can cause. It is defined as recurring episodes of violent and aggressive outbursts that are grossly out of proportion to the initiating stimulus. To be classified as IED, these outbursts must result in either physical assaults on other individuals or animals or the destruction of property. In addition, they cannot be attributable to another psychological disorder, a medical condition such as head trauma, or an intoxicated state, and the violence cannot be premeditated or preplanned.

Etiology and Epidemiology

Aggression can be defined as behavior directed at another person or object in which either verbal or physical force is used to injure, coerce, or express anger. Disproportionate impulsive aggression and loss of control are the hallmarks of IED. The condition is much more common in males than females, and the patient often does not accept responsibility for his or her actions. This denial is believed to be a subconscious mechanism to avoid guilt associated with their actions. They commonly blame the victim, outside circumstances, or statements by third parties. This is of particular concern to the paramedic. As an "outsider" to the situation, you may be the target of the aggression because of seemingly innocuous comments made during interaction at the scene.

The causes of IED are suspected to include experiencing aggression as a child, witnessing aggression as a child, and experiencing a dysfunctional parental relationship. Fortunately it is a rare disorder, but it may be more common than historically thought.

History

Patients with this disorder generally have a history that includes the following:

- Physical or verbal aggression toward people, animals, or property that occurs an average of twice a week for a period of 1 month or at least three times over a 1-year period
- The intensity of the outburst is grossly disproportionate to the initiating stimulus
- The intent of the aggression is not to obtain a tangible objective
- The behavior causes feelings of guilt or distress or affects personal or professional relationships
- The aggression cannot be explained by other causes such as psychological disorders, medical conditions, or intoxication

Differential Diagnosis

Diagnoses to consider include the following:

- Head trauma
- Dementia

- Personality disorders
- Conduct disorders
- Psychotic disorders

Treatment

First and foremost, the paramedic should ensure the safety of the crew on scene. Treatment often is for traumatic injuries sustained by the individual with IED or someone who is injured during the outburst. Standard trauma guidelines should be followed. Treatment for IED itself includes psychiatric counseling and antidepressant medications and mood stabilizers. If able to be done safely, the paramedic should attempt to determine if the patient with a known history of IED is compliant with his or her medications. This can help determine whether an outburst is likely to occur.

Pyromania

Description and Definition

Pyromania is the repeated and intentional setting of fires for the pleasure associated with the tension-release cycle. Fires are not set for monetary gain, insurance claims, covering of a crime, an expression of anger, or any other reason beyond the inability to resist the impulse.

Etiology and Epidemiology

This rare condition is much more common in male children than in female children or adults and tends to be episodic rather than a consistent behavior. To receive the diagnosis, the individual must have set two or more destructive fires that cannot be attributed to another psychiatric illness or any issue identified in the preceding section. Diagnosis is often difficult because it requires the differentiation of the disorder of impulse from other psychiatric disorders or childhood curiosity with fire. Most children are intrigued by fire at some point and may occasionally set them as a result of this fascination. However, this is a normal stage of development attributed to curiosity and not an impulse control disorder. The majority of childhood fires are set for reasons other than pyromania.

Pyromania is poorly understood and its causes are unknown. Associations with individual personality, poor social skills, and dysfunctional relationships with parents have been found. In addition, these patients often have poor learning skills and emotional difficulties. Research of this condition has been difficult because of the low incidence of cases and the difficulty of distinguishing it from arson and other causes of fire setting.

History

The pyromaniac may have a history of the following:

- The intentional setting of fires on two or more occasions
- A feeling of tension or excitement before the event followed by a feeling of pleasure, relief, or gratification after the event

- An obsession or preoccupation with fire
- Fires not set for monetary gain, personal profit, vengeance or anger, or curiosity or to hide a crime; they also are not the result of impaired judgment, another psychiatric illness, or other explainable cause
- Poor relationships with parents
- Poor social skills
- Poor learning ability
- Emotional difficulties and disorders

Differential Diagnosis

Diagnoses to consider include the following:

- Childhood curiosity
- Arson
- Malicious intent
- Personality disorders
- Conduct disorders
- Manic episodes

Therapeutic Interventions

The prehospital paramedic is rarely called on to treat an individual with pyromania. More likely interactions are to treat resulting burns. In this case normal burn therapy should be performed. Paramedics who work in a nontraditional setting may interact with these patients. Emergency treatment is typically not required. The key to treatment is recognition of the problem, which, as described above, can be difficult. Treatment primarily includes behavior modification that directs interest away from setting fires into more socially acceptable methods of addressing the tension-release cycle.

GENERAL PRINCIPLES FOR MANAGEMENT OF PATIENTS WITH BEHAVIORAL EMERGENCIES
Patient Rights and Expectations

[OBJECTIVES 15, 20]

To assess and manage patients with behavioral emergencies, you must move out of a mindset characterized by invasive procedures and drugs to one of observation, evaluation, and emotional support (Loyola Emergency Medical Services System, 2005). As with any other patient, those with mental illness deserve respect and attention. Even a psychotic patient can sense a provider's annoyance through body language and tone. Your actions during the first few seconds of patient contact set the tone for its duration. Behavioral patients have a right to their dignity and privacy. You would not ask a patient with abdominal pain to provide a detailed and potentially embarrassing medical history in front of bystanders, family, or friends. Therefore you should not expect a behavioral patient to discuss his or her psychiatric history and private feelings in the presence of others. Ensure that enough personnel are present to maintain your safety, but try to limit the number of people present as much as possible. Consider asking the patient to consent to a pat-down search by law enforcement for your safety if you suspect the patient to be violent or harboring a weapon.

Verbal Restraint

[OBJECTIVES 15, 20, 21]

The best way to stop a violent situation is to prevent it from happening. Spotting a knife or a gun is easy. Interpreting the subtle signs of a patient's increasing anger and agitation can be more difficult. Patients rarely go from quiet and reserved to combative and violent without reason. In fact, they often are provoked. Your tone of voice and response to the patient's concerns and questions determine how the patient will react to you. Providers who are standoffish and dismissive can anger patients to the point at which they will react, possibly causing harm to themselves, you, or your crew. After a violent confrontation with a patient, hearing someone involved say "I saw that coming" is common.

When a patient becomes irritated and angry, your reactions usually determine where the situation will lead. Do not take insults personally; psychotic patients or those under the influence of substances often are not completely aware of their actions. Confrontational and argumentative patients may try to goad you into a fight. Never raise your voice toward a patient. Direct confrontation and threats only intensify the patient's emotions toward you and may provoke him or her further. Even if you say things the patient wants to hear, shouting causes your message to be lost. Keep your tone businesslike and courteous. Many paramedics defuse loud situations by using an increasingly softer tone as the patient's tone becomes louder. This forces the patient to stop and listen to what you are saying. If a patient shows increasing hostility toward you, have another paramedic talk to the patient to help calm him or her. Never agree to a patient's demands to the effect of, "if you leave the room, I'll talk to your partner but not you." The safety of your partner is just as important as your own.

Involuntary Transport and Patient Restraint

[OBJECTIVES 15, 17, 20, 21, 22] *Document !*

Sometimes conditions necessitate the restraint and involuntary transport of a patient. Three forms of patient restraint are used: verbal, physical, and chemical. Verbal restraint, detailed above, always comes first. After verbal attempts have failed, physical and/or chemical restraints may be required. Physical and chemical restraints are always last resorts and should be applied *only to prevent the patient from harming himself or others*. Restraints should never be used out of anger or as punishment. A competent patient has a right to refuse any or all treatments. Restraining someone who is capable of making informed, rational decisions is never permissible, even to provide life-saving medical care (Annas, 1999). Those under the influence of alcohol or drugs and suicidal patients are not considered rational.

Law enforcement personnel should be present when restraining someone, but a patient being transported in an ambulance should be restrained by EMS providers. Every agency should have a protocol dictating when and how to use physical and chemical restraints. However, most agencies in the United States have weak standards or no such plan in place (Tintinalli, 1993). Restraint may be needed in situations outside behavioral emergencies, such as in the case of a nasally intubated patient attempting to extubate himself.

The first step in restraining a patient is to have a plan. Five personnel should be present: a provider for each extremity and one to manage the head and help others as needed. Before anyone touches the patient, designate a team leader and be sure everyone involved knows exactly what his or her role is. Careful coordination will prevent injury to your crew and the patient. Do not forget standard precautions. Restraining a patient can expose you and your team to blood, saliva, urine, and feces. Ensure everyone is wearing the proper personal protective equipment (Kupas & Wydro, 2002).

Have the proper equipment on hand. Your goal is almost always to restrain the patient for transport to a facility. This is best accomplished by using the stretcher and a long backboard. You must restrain the patient to the backboard at four points—both wrists and both ankles. Use soft restraints such as cravats, gauze, or commercial devices secured with hook-and-loop closure material. Avoid any hard or possibly cutting objects, such as leather straps, rope, cord, cables, or tape. These objects can cause injury and occlude circulation easier than soft restraints. Do not use police handcuffs. To be effective, handcuffs should be in place with the arms behind the back. Not only is this painful for a supine patient, but it also prohibits you from accessing the patient's arms to take a blood pressure reading or start an IV. If the patient's condition suddenly deteriorates or you are involved in a vehicle crash, you may need to access the patient's torso and arms quickly; handcuffs prevent this (Figure 32-2). Ideally, any patient you are to transport who is handcuffed on your arrival should be restrained with soft restraints by you. If a law enforcement officer refuses to remove handcuffs from a patient for transport, that officer *must ride with you in the ambulance* to the hospital in case of an emergency.

After you have assembled your team and equipment, carefully approach the patient. Explain again why the patient must be transported to the hospital against his or her will. Offer one more opportunity to be voluntarily transported. If the patient refuses, each team member should perform his or her role and begin the process of physical restraint. Place a long spinal immobilization board on top of a stretcher. Position the patient on top of the backboard in a supine position, as you would if you were immobilizing the patient for spinal protection. With soft restraints, secure the patient's wrists and ankles

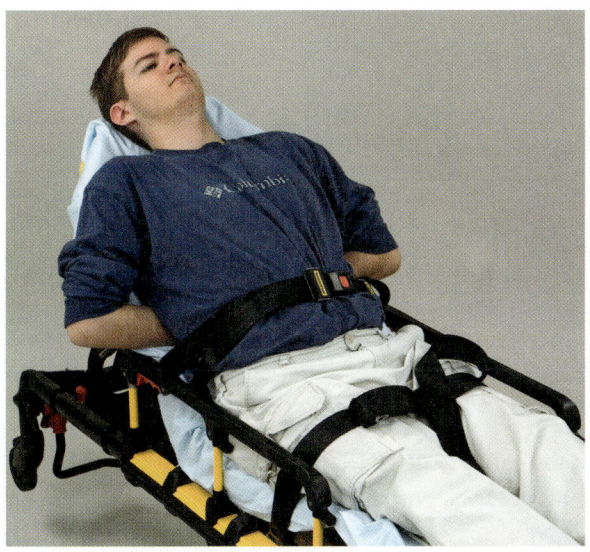

Figure 32-2 Restraining a patient on a stretcher with handcuffs prevents easy access to the patient's arms and hands and should be avoided.

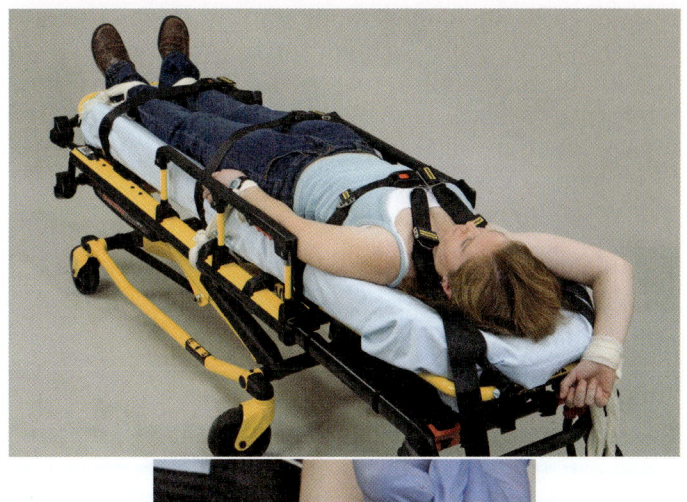

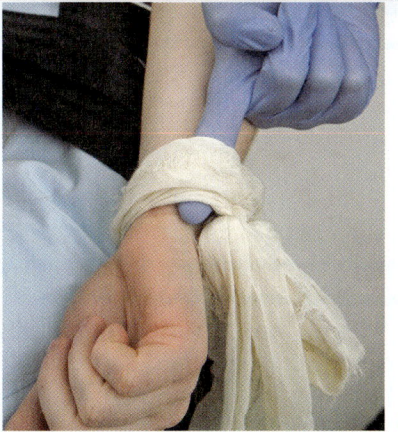

Figure 32-3 Proper restraint techniques. **A,** Patient is restrained to a long backboard for ease of transferring the patient at the destination; note placement of patient's arms to prevent them from working together. **B,** You should be able to slip one finger easily underneath any restraint.

to the backboard, not the stretcher. Prevent the patient's muscle groups from working together by restraining one wrist in a raised position next to the head and the other by the hips (Figure 32-3, *A*). Securing the legs with a seat belt across the thighs just above the knees prevents kicking better than ankle restraints do (Kupas & Wydro, 2002). A nonrebreather mask connected to oxygen or a loosely applied surgical mask can prevent spitting (Kupas & Wydro, 2002). By using a long backboard, you will not have to release the restraints to move the patient to a hospital bed. You should be able to slip one finger underneath any restraint with ease (Figure 32-3, *B*). If not, that restraint is tied too tightly and must be retied. Check distal pulse, movement, and sensation in each hand and foot immediately before and after restraint as well as every few minutes thereafter.

After a patient is physically restrained, he or she likely will continue to struggle and fight. Use calming and verbal restraint techniques. Never antagonize or tease a patient in restraints or allow others to do so. Continued struggling against restraints has been associated with a syndrome known as *excited delirium* (detailed later in this chapter). To prevent this lethal condition, patients who are physically restrained should also be chemically restrained.

Chemical restraint is the use of medications to decrease agitation and increase patient cooperation (Kupas & Wydro, 2002). The goal is to calm the patient's behavior without altering the patient's level of consciousness or causing amnesia. In emergency settings, a benzodiazepine, a butyrophenone, or both are typically used for chemical restraint. The two most common benzodiazepines used are lorazepam (Ativan) and midazolam (Versed). The most dangerous side effects of benzodiazepines are respiratory depression and hypotension (Kupas

& Wydro, 2002). Droperidol (Inapsine) and haloperidol (Haldol) are the most commonly used butyrophenones. Both have a rapid onset of action, but droperidol often is preferred in the prehospital setting for its shorter duration (Richards et al., 1998; Kupas & Wydro, 2002). Butyrophenones commonly cause extrapyramidal symptoms and orthostatic hypotension and have been known to cause a prolonged QT interval and torsades des pointes. All four of these medications are given IV or intramuscularly (Kupas & Wydro, 2002). Carefully monitor the patient's respiratory rate, pulse oximetry, mental status, and ECG when using any of these agents.

The use of neuromuscular-blocking agents to restrain a patient chemically is never acceptable. In cases of hypoxia, head injury, and other situations for which rapid-sequence induction is indicated, it may be used as restraint. Rapid-sequence induction is an acceptable method only when the complete protocol is followed; no drugs may be omitted or added for the purposes of restraint. These situations are rare, and less-restrictive methods should be used in most cases (Kupas & Wydro, 2002).

The decision to restrain a patient should never be taken lightly. Use of physical restraints can have lethal consequences, including restraint asphyxia (discussed in the next section) and excited delirium (discussed later in this chapter). Restraint that is not indicated or done improperly may be considered assault, battery, or false imprisonment (Kupas & Wydro, 2002). As a rule of thumb, plan on encountering legal issues with any patient you restrain.

Restraint Asphyxia

[OBJECTIVES 22, 23]

Description and Definition

Restraint asphyxia results from an inability to expand the chest cavity and create a negative pressure inside the lungs for inspiration in relation to immobilization or restraint. Restraint asphyxia is controversial and often is seen in situations in which excited delirium is present. No proven link exists between the two (Stratton et al., 2001).

Etiology

Restraint asphyxia may result from improper positioning and is sometimes called *positional asphyxia*. It has a high association with restraint in the prone position, particularly in overweight individuals. Especially dangerous is the "hog tying" method of restraint, in which the subject's wrists and ankles are handcuffed or bound and the ankles and wrists are bound to each other. This position elevates the shoulders and hips, placing all the patient's weight squarely on the abdomen (Figure 32-4). This can prevent movement of the abdominal organs and therefore the "pulling down" of the diaphragm required for inspiration.

Restraint asphyxia may also result from devices applied too tightly or incorrectly. A patient may be strangled while attempting escape from an improperly applied restraint device. Belts or other restraints secured too tightly across the chest, abdomen, or neck also seriously impair ventilation.

Mechanical complications of restraint may combine with the increased metabolic requirements of a body that has been involved in a struggle to cause asphyxia. A patient usually requires restraint because of violent and combative behavior. An exhausted patient whose bloodstream has high circulating levels of epinephrine and norepinephrine after a chase or struggle requires large amounts of oxygen. In these situations patients can develop asphyxia faster when placed in a position that decreases oxygen intake.

Epidemiology and Demographics

A 1998 study found 142 restraint-related deaths nationwide over the previous decade, but the actual number was probably much higher (Annas, 1999).

History and Physical Findings

In cases of restraint asphyxia, patients often shift from normal breathing and circulation to asystole and apnea within a matter of minutes. Cases have involved a period of slowed, irregular respirations before cardiac arrest. During this period the patient ceases struggling and becomes quiet. For patients who are restrained or are at other risk for excited delirium, this should raise a red flag (Stratton et al., 2001). Despite respiratory arrest often being witnessed by qualified personnel who immediately take action, resuscitation efforts are usually unsuccessful (Stratton et al., 1995).

Differential Diagnosis

Differential diagnosis for restraint asphyxia includes the following:

- Suicide attempt
- Excited delirium
- Complications from an unknown medical condition
- Overdose or adverse effects of drugs and alcohol

Therapeutic Interventions

The best treatment for restraint asphyxia is prevention. Proper use of restraint devices is essential. Never place any restraint where it could potentially constrict the chest or abdomen or crush the neck. Observe a restrained patient at all times. If the patient attempts to escape, prevent him or her from becoming entangled or injured.

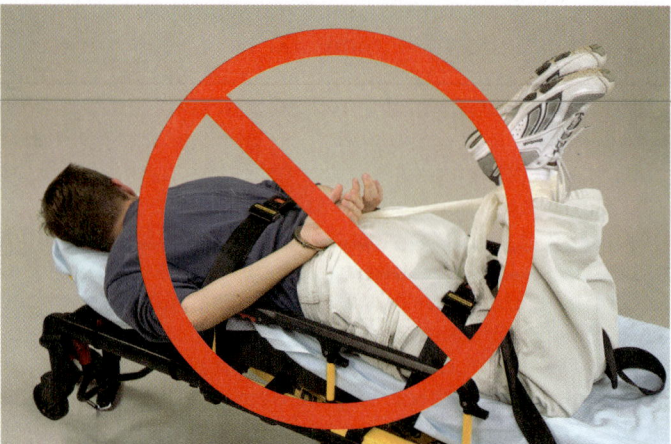

Figure 32-4 In the hog-tied position, the shoulders and hips are elevated. The patient's weight rests squarely on the abdomen, potentially leading to restraint asphyxia.

PARAMEDIC*Pearl*

If your agency uses commercial restraint devices, you must be familiar with their use. While attempting to restrain a patient is not the time to learn how your agency's restraint devices work.

If still fighting in restraints, give Versed. Can prevent asystole from continued fighting

http://evolve.elsevier.com/Aehlert/paramedic **1209**

Contrary to the National Standard Curriculum for paramedics issued by the National Highway and Traffic Safety Administration in 1994, it is *never* appropriate to restrain a patient in the prone position. This includes "sandwiching" a patient between two long spine boards. You may hold a patient in a prone position for a brief period while gaining control during a violent episode. While in this position, a patient's range of motion and visual field are limited, helping you and your team gain the upper hand (Kupas & Wydro, 2002). Avoid placing any weight (such as a hand or knee) on the patient's back, which can further compress the abdomen and chest (Stratton et al., 2001). Move a restrained patient to a lateral or supine position as soon as possible and maintain proper positioning throughout transport.

Remember that you are the advocate for the patient's health and best interests. In most studied cases of death related to hobble restraint, law enforcement initially placed the patient in a harmful position (Stratton et al., 2001). You are responsible for ensuring that no other personnel use restraining techniques that may be harmful. You must step forward and order the patient to be placed in a better position—your patient's life may depend on it.

> **PARAMEDIC** *Pearl*
>
> Imagine yourself in the place of a restrained patient and show him the same respect you would want. Visualize potentially dangerous positions the patient could move into.

SUBSTANCE ABUSE

Use, Abuse, and Addiction

[OBJECTIVE 24]

When a person uses a substance for something other than its accepted purpose or in greater amounts than prescribed, the action is called **abuse.** For the purposes of this chapter, abuse has nothing to do with the law. Some commonly abused substances, such as marijuana and heroin, are illegal in the United States. Others are legal but tightly regulated, such as cocaine and amphetamines. Still others are legal and loosely regulated or not regulated at all, such as alcohol and inhalants. Table 32-3 lists characteristics, names, effects, and illustrations of the substances discussed in this chapter.

For many, substance use and abuse is a pastime—something to be enjoyed once in a while on the weekends or when out with friends. For others, however, achieving the high from drugs of abuse becomes an all-consuming compulsion. These individuals may abuse substances to influence their emotional state—for example, using cocaine to get "pumped" for a night of drinking and dancing or smoking marijuana after work each day to "relax." Others may drink alcohol to overcome shyness or use inhalants to avoid boredom. Many soon discover they are controlled by a continuing need to use that substance—a state known as **addiction** or dependence.

Loss of control shows itself in many ways. Those addicted may set limits for themselves on substance use—"just a drink or two" or "only one cigarette after dinner"—only to break them. People who are addicted may become aware of their consistent cravings and strongly desire to curb their use, only to find that they are slaves to the drug. Persons addicted to a substance often have a history of several attempts to quit, with each one failing. More and more time is spent obtaining, using, and recovering from the drug. Individuals begin to experience problems related to their addiction at school, work, or within the family, such as repeated absences and tardiness or child neglect. Another sign of addiction may be the abuse of a substance early in the morning, soon after waking up. Those who are addicted frequently use substances despite having important things to do, such as going to work.

Addicted people may put themselves in harm's way to obtain a substance. For example, they may engage in prostitution or theft to raise money for their habit. Use of the drug can have harmful effects as well, such as driving while intoxicated or being arrested for substance-related offenses. Malnutrition becomes common in cases of addiction; even the essential act of eating is eclipsed by an ever more powerful psychological and often physical need for a drug. Despite all negative effects, those who are addicted continue to use because they have to.

Most patients who abuse substances have a drug of choice that they use regularly and often. However, most people who abuse substances use many drugs—sometimes together, sometimes not (Clark et al., 2000). Many people who are dependent on the effects of a certain drug that is unavailable will use a similar drug instead. Abusers often combine drugs to intensify or offset each drug's effects. For example, a user might snort cocaine to be able to drink more alcohol without feeling drowsy.

Tolerance and Withdrawal

[OBJECTIVE 24]

A metaphor for an abused drug's effects on body homeostasis is a seesaw. Without the presence of the drug, the seesaw is balanced and the body is at homeostasis. When an abuser takes a drug, the seesaw tilts in one direction, causing noticeable effects such as tachycardia, hypertension, or subjective feelings such as euphoria. These effects are typically quite powerful the first time a drug is used. Over time and repeated use, receptors stimulated by a particular substance become less sensitive. Users may report that the same amount of drug that once had a powerful effect now does nothing. Therefore higher doses of the drug are needed to cause the same effects. This is known as **tolerance** to a drug. Some opioid abusers have been known to require upwards of 10 times the normal dosage for pain control, amounts that would be fatal to many first-time users.

TABLE 32-3 Comparison of Commonly Abused Drugs

Category and Name	Examples of *Commercial* and Street Names	DEA Schedule*/How Administered†
Cannabinoids		
Hashish	Chronic, gangster, hash, hash oil, hemp	I/Swallowed, smoked
Marijuana	Blunt, dope, ganja, grass, herb, joints, Mary Jane, pot, reefer, skunk, weed	I/Swallowed, smoked
Depressants		
Barbiturates	*Amytal, Nembutal, Seconal, Phenobarbital;* barbs, reds, red birds, phennies, tooies, yellows, yellow jackets	II, III, V/Injected, swallowed
Benzodiazepines (other than flunitrazepam)	*Ativan, Halcion, Librium, Valium, Xanax;* candy, downers, sleeping pills, tranks	IV/Swallowed, injected
Flunitrazepam‡	*Rohypnol;* forget-me pill, Mexican Valium, R2, roche, roofies, roofinol, rope, rophies	IV/Swallowed, snorted
GHB‡	*Gamma-hydroxybutyrate;* G, Georgia home boy, grievous bodily harm, liquid ecstasy	I/Swallowed
Dissociatives		
Ketamine	*Ketalar SV;* cat Valium, K, special K, vitamin K	III/Injected, snorted, smoked
PCP and analogs	*Phencyclidine;* angel dust, boat, hog, love boat, peace pill	I, II/Injected, swallowed, smoked
Dextromethorphan	*Robitussin-DM, Coricidin Cough and Cold;* DXM, robo, robo-trippin', dodo	Not scheduled/Swallowed
Hallucinogens		
LSD	*Lysergic acid diethylamide;* acid, blotter, boomers, cubes, microdot, yellow sunshines	I/Swallowed, absorbed through mouth tissues
Mescaline	Buttons, cactus, mesc, peyote	I/Swallowed, smoked
Psilocybin	Magic mushroom, purple passion, shrooms	I/Swallowed
Opioids and Morphine Derivatives		
Codeine	*Empirin with Codeine, Fiorinal with Codeine, Robitussin A-C, Tylenol with Codeine;* Captain Cody, Cody, schoolboy; (with glutethimide) doors & fours, loads, pancakes and syrup	II, III, IV/Injected, swallowed
Fentanyl and fentanyl analogs	*Actiq, Duragesic, Sublimaze;* Apache, China girl, China white, dance fever, friend, goodfella, jackpot, murder 8, TNT, tango and cash	I, II/Injected, smoked, snorted
Heroin	*Diacetylmorphine;* brown sugar, dope, H, horse, junk, skag, skunk, smack, white horse	I/Injected, smoked, snorted
Morphine	*Roxanol, Duramorph;* M, Miss Emma, monkey, white stuff	II, III/Injected, swallowed, smoked
Opium	*Laudanum, paregoric;* big O, black stuff, block, gum, hop	II, III, V/Swallowed, smoked
Oxycodone HCL	*Oxycontin;* Oxy, OC, killer	II/Swallowed, snorted, injected
Hydrocodone bitartrate, acetaminophen	*Vicodin;* vike, Watson 387	II/Swallowed

*Schedule I and II drugs have a high potential for abuse. They require greater storage security and have a quota on manufacturing, among other restrictions. Schedule I drugs are available for research only and have no approved medical use; Schedule II drugs are available only be prescription (unrefillable) and require a form for ordering. Schedule III and IV drugs are available by prescription, may have five refills in 6 months, and may be ordered orally. Most Schedule V drugs are available over the counter.

†Taking drugs by injection can increase the risk of infection through needle contamination with staphylococci, HIV, hepatitis, and other organisms.

‡Associated with sexual assaults.

Intoxication Effects	Potential Health Consequences
Euphoria; slowed thinking and reaction time, confusion; impaired balance and coordination	Cough, frequent respiratory infections; impaired memory and learning; increased heart rate, anxiety; panic attacks; tolerance, addiction
Reduced anxiety; feeling of well-being; lowered inhibitions; slowed pulse and breathing; lowered blood pressure; poor concentration Also for barbiturates: sedation, drowsiness Also for benzodiazepines: sedation, drowsiness	Fatigue; confusion; impaired coordination, memory, judgment; addiction; respiratory depression and arrest, death Also for barbiturates: depression; unusual excitement; fever; irritability; poor judgment; slurred speech; dizziness; life-threatening withdrawal Also for benzodiazepines: dizziness Also for flunitrazepam: visual and gastrointestinal disturbances; urinary retention; memory loss for the time under the drug's effects Also for GHB: drowsiness; nausea and vomiting; headache; loss of consciousness; loss of reflexes; seizures; coma, death
Increased heart rate and blood pressure; impaired motor function Also for ketamine: at high doses, delirium, depression, respiratory depression, and arrest For PCP and analogs: possible decrease in blood pressure and heart rate, panic, aggression, violence	Memory loss; numbness; nausea and vomiting for PCP and analogs: loss of appetite, depression
Altered states of perception and feeling; nausea Also for LSD and mescaline: increased body temperature, heart rate, blood pressure; loss of appetite; sleeplessness, numbness, weakness, tremors Also for LSD: persistent mental disorders Also for psilocybin: nervousness, paranoia	Persisting perception disorder (flashbacks)
Pain relief; euphoria; drowsiness Also for codeine: less analgesia, sedation, and respiratory depression than morphine Also for heroin: staggering gait	Nausea, constipation; confusion, sedation; respiratory depression and arrest; tolerance, addiction; unconsciousness, coma, death

Continued

TABLE 32-3	Comparison of Commonly Abused Drugs—continued	
Category and Name	**Examples of *Commercial* and Street Names**	**DEA Schedule*/How Administered†**
Stimulants		
Amphetamine	*Biphetamine, Dexedrine;* bennies, black beauties, crosses, hearts, LA turnaround, speed, truck drivers, uppers	II/Injected, swallowed, smoked, snorted
Cocaine	*Cocaine hydrochloride;* blow, bump, C, candy, Charlie, coke, crack, flake, rock, snow, toot	II/Injected, smoked, snorted
MDMA	Adam, clarity, ecstasy, Eve, lover's speed, peace, STP, X, XTC	I/Swallowed
Methamphetamine	*Desoxyn;* chalk, crank, crystal, fire, glass, go fast, ice, meth, speed	II/Injected, swallowed, smoked, snorted
Inhalants	Solvents (paint thinners, gasoline, glues), gases (butane, propane, aerosol propellants, nitrous oxide), nitrites (isoamyl, isobutyl, cyclohexyl); laughing gas, poppers, snappers, whippets	Not scheduled/Inhaled through nose or mouth
ETOH	*Far t oo many to name;* booze, hooch, sauce, suds	Not scheduled/Swallowed

Modified from National Institute of Drug Abuse. (2006). *Commonly abused drugs.* Retrieved March 28, 2008, from http://www.drugabuse.gov/DrugPages/DrugsofAbuse.html.
MDMA, 3,4-Methylenedioxymethamphetamine (ecstasy); *ETOH*, ethanol; *CNS*, central nervous system.

As long-term substance abuse continues, the body changes its chemistry to compensate for a drug's effects. The seesaw becomes even again as the body's tolerance grows and homeostasis is maintained. Abruptly stopping the regular use of a drug tilts the seesaw in the other direction as the body's compensatory mechanisms become unchecked. This imbalance causes a specific set of signs and symptoms called **withdrawal.** Withdrawal symptoms usually begin as blood plasma levels of the drug begin to drop. The withdrawal symptoms of a drug are usually the opposite of its effects. For example, use of stimulant drugs such as cocaine causes an increase in energy level and a suppression of appetite. Withdrawal from cocaine is marked by lethargy and hunger. Withdrawal symptoms can be relieved by small doses of the substance. Presence of tolerance or withdrawal symptoms is a strong indicator of addiction.

Case Scenario CONCLUSION

As you complete your assessment, one of the police officers approaches and informs you that he spoke with the man's mother, who agrees to meet the patient at the psychiatric facility. She indicated that her son has been diagnosed with paranoid schizophrenia with catatonic tendencies. He can become violent if forcefully aroused from a catatonic state. The officer has implemented the necessary process for involuntary commission for psychiatric evaluation.

Questions
7. What is your final impression?
8. What treatment options should be considered for this patient?
9. How should you prepare the man for transport?

Intoxication Effects	Potential Health Consequences
Increased heart rate, blood pressure, metabolism; feelings of exhilaration, energy, increased mental alertness Also for amphetamine: rapid breathing Also for cocaine: increased temperature Also for MDMA: mild hallucinogenic effects; increased tactile sensitivity; empathic feelings Also for methamphetamine: aggression, violence, psychotic behavior	Rapid or irregular heartbeat; reduced appetite, weight loss; heart failure; nervousness; insomnia Also for amphetamine: tremor, loss of coordination; irritability, anxiousness, restlessness; delirium, panic, paranoia, impulsive behavior, aggressiveness; tolerance, addiction; psychosis Also for cocaine: chest pain; respiratory failure; nausea; abdominal pain; stroke, seizure; headaches; malnutrition; panic attacks Also for MDMA: impaired memory and learning; hyperthermia; cardiac toxicity, renal failure, liver toxicity Also for methamphetamine: memory loss, cardiac and neurologic damage; impaired memory and learning; tolerance, addiction
Stimulation, loss of inhibition; headache; nausea or vomiting; slurred speech, loss of motor coordination; wheezing	Unconsciousness; cramps; weight loss; muscle weakness; depression; memory impairment; damage to cardiovascular and nervous systems; sudden death
Increased energy, suppressed inhibitions, intense affect (at low doses); profound CNS depression, combativeness, aggression (at high doses)	Hypotension; dehydration; dysrhythmias; loss of airway control; aspiration; alcoholism; liver damage; neurologic damage; Wernicke-Korsakoff syndrome

[handwritten: 0.08 legal limit]
[handwritten: ★ Healthy liver – 1 drink/hour]

ETHANOL

[OBJECTIVES 16, 25]

Description and Form

Ethanol (ETOH) is the intoxicating ingredient in liquor, beer, and wine. A colorless, odorless liquid, it is also found in mouthwash, cologne, perfume, deodorant, aftershave, and some over-the-counter medications. ETOH is commonly referred to as *alcohol,* which is misleading because many other alcohols have different toxic syndromes.

Beer and wine are made from the products of fermented grains and grapes, whereas liquors are distilled from fermented fruits and vegetables. The concentration of ETOH in alcoholic beverages is measured by volume and is expressed as a proof. An alcoholic beverage that is 100 proof contains 50% ETOH by volume; one that is 50 proof is 25% ETOH. The remainder of this volume is composed of water and congeners—substances other than ETOH and water present in alcoholic beverages that are responsible for their wide variety of flavors.

The price of alcohol varies widely. Some brands of malt liquor may cost less than $2, whereas bottles of expensive vintage wine may cost hundreds or even thousands of dollars. ETOH is almost always ingested and is present in hundreds of brands of alcoholic drinks available at convenience stores, grocery stores, liquor stores, bars, and restaurants throughout the United States.

Epidemiology and Demographics

[OBJECTIVE 26]

ETOH is the most commonly used and abused drug in the world. Consumption of alcoholic beverages crosses social and economic lines and is ingrained in many cultures as a part of celebrations and leisure activities. An estimated 22 million Americans regularly abuse alcohol (Substance Abuse and Mental Health Services Administration, 2004). Five percent to 15% of them have **alcoholism,** which is addiction and dependence on ETOH. More than 200,000 Americans die of alcoholism each year, more than all other illicit drugs combined (Yip, 2002).

ETOH's effect of erasing inhibitions, coupled with its popularity, ensures that many prehospital calls—particularly trauma-related incidents—feature a patient under the influence of ETOH. Among 15- to 45-year-olds, ETOH is associated with half of all traffic fatalities, half of deaths by fire, two thirds of drownings and homicides, and 35% of suicides. Overall, ETOH is involved in an estimated 38% of all traffic fatalities. Alcoholism is the leading cause of death and disability in the United States. Twenty percent of the money spent on hospital care in the United

States is for treatment of ETOH-related illness and injury (Nelson, 2002).

Routes and Pathophysiology

[OBJECTIVE 27]

ETOH is absorbed into the bloodstream through the digestive tract—approximately 20% by the stomach and the remainder by the small intestine. Absorption of ETOH is enhanced by increased gastric emptying, consumption of ETOH on an empty stomach, and carbonation. Under ideal conditions, 80% to 90% of ingested ETOH is absorbed within 60 minutes, but absorption may be delayed up to 2 or 3 hours (Nelson, 2002).

One drink is defined as a 1-oz shot of 100-proof liquor, one 4-oz glass of wine (12% ETOH), or a 10-oz bottle of beer for a person weighing 70 kg (154 lb). In the bloodstream ETOH concentration is measured as **blood alcohol content (BAC).** This is equivalent to milligrams of ETOH per deciliter of blood (mg/dL) divided by 100. One drink contains approximately 15 g ETOH, but most of this is metabolized by the liver before entering the bloodstream. Therefore one drink raises the BAC of a 70-kg person by 0.036 on average (3.6 mg/dL). Although BAC is most definitively measured by blood testing, breathalyzers are used to obtain an accurate BAC reading quickly when venipuncture is impractical.

ETOH easily passes across most membranes in the body, including the blood-brain barrier. The exact mechanisms of action of ETOH are unknown. It is believed to interact with several neurotransmitters, particularly enhancing the effects of gamma-aminobutyric acid (GABA, the inhibitory neurotransmitter) in the brain. ETOH has both CNS depressant and stimulant properties at low doses and is a complete CNS depressant at higher doses.

Approximately 5% of ingested ETOH is directly excreted through the urine, and approximately 5% is exhaled through the lungs. The remainder is metabolized by the liver and excreted in the urine. On average, an adult can metabolize one drink of ETOH per hour. Heavy drinkers may metabolize more per hour (up to three drinks), whereas persons with liver disease may metabolize alcohol much more slowly.

Paraphernalia

[OBJECTIVE 6]

Alcoholic beverages are primarily packaged in bottles, cans, and kegs. Alcoholic drinks, particularly liquors, are mixed with a host of fruit juices, sodas, and other alcoholic and nonalcoholic beverages to make them more palatable.

Alcohol has a high rate of consumption in combination with illicit drugs, such as cocaine and marijuana. In 2004, 32% of heavy drinkers were also current illicit drug users, and 61% smoked cigarettes (Substance Abuse and Mental Health Services Administration, 2004).

TABLE 32-4	Effects of ETOH Related to BAC
BAC (%)	**Effects**
0.02	Few obvious effects, slight intensification of mood
0.05	Loss of emotional restraint, feeling of warmth, flushing of skin, mild impairment of judgment
0.10	Slight slurring of speech, loss of fine motor control, unstable emotions, inappropriate laughter
0.12	Coordination and balance difficult, distinct impairment of mentation and judgment
0.20	Responsive to verbal stimuli, very slurred speech, staggering gait, diplopia (double vision), difficulty standing upright, memory loss
0.30	Briefly aroused by painful stimuli, deep snoring respirations
0.40	Unresponsiveness, incontinence, hypotension, irregular respirations
0.50	Death possible from apnea, hypotension, or aspiration of vomitus

ETOH, Ethanol; *BAC,* blood alcohol concentration.

Subjective Effects and Physical Findings

[OBJECTIVE 6]

Symptoms of ETOH intoxication are directly related to BAC levels (Table 32-4). Because BAC depends on weight and other factors, the effects of ETOH vary widely from person to person. At low doses alcohol often causes people to become energetic and intensifies mood. Persons become talkative and inhibitions lessen. People may demonstrate more emotional and even flirtatious behavior than they normally would. Patients lose the ability to make insightful decisions and often engage in risky behaviors. At higher doses patients can be emotionally unstable, dramatic, and confrontational. As the dose of ETOH increases and an intoxicated patient moves toward unresponsiveness, behavior may become bizarre, unpredictable, and dangerous.

The most easily recognized symptoms of ETOH intoxication are neurologic. These findings include impaired coordination and slurred speech in the early stages of intoxication, progressing to an inability to maintain balance when standing upright (Wilson & Saukkonen, 2004). Visual changes such as blurry or double vision also are common as the pupils dilate and the occipital lobe of the cerebrum is affected. The patient's level of consciousness steadily decreases. At high levels patients are unresponsive to even deep, painful stimuli. Incontinence of the bladder or even bowels may be present. Snoring respirations develop as the patient loses the ability to control his or her airway, making the patient vulnerable to vomiting and aspiration (Wilson & Saukkonen, 2004). Seizures can result from ETOH ingestion, particularly in children who also are hypoglycemic. Just as with any case of altered mental status, decreased level of consciousness from ETOH abuse is a medical emergency.

ETOH use causes tachycardia and vasodilatation. Widespread vasodilation may cause hypothermia, particularly if the patient is malnourished and environmental conditions are favorable. ETOH may decrease cardiac output in patients with preexisting cardiac conditions and may contribute to dysrhythmias such as atrial fibrillation, runs of ventricular tachycardia, and atrioventricular blocks. The odor of alcohol on the breath is not a reliable indicator of a patient's intoxication level.

Tolerance and Withdrawal

[OBJECTIVE 6]

A hangover the day after heavy drinking is the most common form of ETOH withdrawal. Characterized by headache, lethargy, inability to focus, nausea, and vomiting, it appears within 6 to 12 hours after drinking stops. This is a mild withdrawal syndrome, and symptoms are relieved by the ingestion of more ETOH (Jain, 2004). More severe ETOH tolerance and withdrawal usually develop in patients who abuse ETOH daily for at least 3 months or have consumed large quantities for at least 1 week. At first patients show ETOH craving and mild anxiety. After a day or so sympathetic stimulation occurs, causing tachycardia, hypertension, hyperventilation, diaphoresis, fever, anxiety, tremor, and insomnia.

Approximately 5% of alcoholics experience the most serious form of ETOH withdrawal, **delirium tremens (DT).** DT is characterized by psychosis and confusion (delirium) and generalized seizures (tremens). The condition typically develops 2 or 3 days after stopping drinking and often begins with a sudden seizure. Profound sympathetic stimulation causes intense diaphoresis, hyperthermia, and hyperventilation, which may lead to dehydration. If untreated, DT is fatal for 35% of patients (Gossman, 2005).

Long-Term Effects

[OBJECTIVE 6]

Abuse of ETOH over many years causes a host of problems. The drug is especially toxic to the liver and may cause a fatty liver, hepatitis, and cirrhosis. Blood backing up from a diseased liver is known as *portal hypertension* and can cause esophageal varices. High rates of pancreatitis and malnutrition are associated with chronic ETOH abuse.

Alcoholism

Alcoholism is a chronic, progressive illness with biologic, psychologic, and social symptoms (see Table 32-4). The onset of alcoholism is slow. A person may be a heavy drinker for decades before becoming an alcoholic. Persons with an ETOH problem often continue drinking despite negative consequences. Alcoholics are unable to control their ETOH intake and often consume more drinks than intended. They may go on binges that last days at a time, neglecting work, school, and family. As with any addiction, those with alcoholism spend a substantial portion of their time drinking ETOH and recovering from binges. Many mask their illness, remaining functional on the surface. An alcoholic may hold down a job but might be frequently absent while recovering from binges. The families of alcoholics also suffer. In addition to neglect, alcoholism has a high association with domestic and child abuse. As with any addiction, alcoholics experience withdrawal when without alcoholic beverages and may consume other ETOH-containing products. In desperate situations, they may drink more dangerous alcohols such as methanol or isopropyl, leading to toxicity.

Wernicke-Korsakoff Syndrome

ETOH interferes with the digestive system's ability to absorb thiamine, also known as vitamin B_1. Thiamine is required by the neurons of the brain to use glucose effectively. Long-term deficiency causes a disorder called *Wernicke-Korsakoff syndrome*. During the first phase of this illness, sometimes called *Wernicke encephalitis,* the patient demonstrates confusion, odd movements, paralysis of the muscles controlling the eye, and an abnormal gait. Hypothermia and hypotension may result. These symptoms are usually temporary and can be reversed by thiamine administration.

In approximately 80% of patients this syndrome progresses to a second irreversible stage, sometimes known as *Korsakoff psychosis.* This phase is characterized by all the symptoms seen in the first stage, plus amnesia, an inability to learn new information, and permanent psychosis (Salen, 2001).

Differential Diagnosis

Differential diagnosis for ETOH intoxication includes the following (Egland, 2005):

- Hyperosmolar hyperglycemic nonketotic coma
- Pancreatitis
- Diabetic ketoacidosis
- Hypoglycemia
- Meningitis and encephalitis
- Status epilepticus
- Subarachnoid hemorrhage
- Ethylene glycol poisoning
- Lithium toxicity

Therapeutic Interventions

[OBJECTIVES 28, 29]

As with any patient presenting with altered mental status, focus on protecting the airway. During mild intoxication, this may be as simple as waking the patient so that he or she can control his or her own breathing. In severe cases, endotracheal intubation may be required. The use of bag-mask ventilation with supplemental oxygen in conjunction with a nasopharyngeal airway often is the best initial airway management for an unresponsive patient. Be vigilant for vomiting and act quickly to prevent aspiration.

Assess for other causes of altered mental status, particularly opiate overdose and hypoglycemia. Give naloxone or dextrose as needed. Consider giving IV thiamine, which is often depleted after heavy alcohol use. Thiamine should be given before 50% dextrose if both are available and indicated (Yip, 2002).

For patients with DT, treat the symptoms of sympathetic overload. Give oxygen and start an IV of normal saline. Consider a fluid bolus if the patient appears dehydrated. Give thiamine if available and 50% dextrose if the patient's blood glucose level is below 60 mg/dL. Seizures associated with DT are usually short and self-limiting, but status epilepticus develops in a small percentage of patients, warranting the administration of benzodiazepines.

Patient and Family Education

A patient with altered mental status must be transported and is considered to give implied consent, no matter how much friends and family may ask you to let the patient "sleep it off" or assure that they will "keep him rolled on his side." You may need to explain to friends and family the potential consequences of high blood alcohol levels such as aspiration, hypotension, and death.

> **PARAMEDIC*Pearl***
>
> Alcohol intoxication and withdrawal are potentially deadly and should always be taken seriously.

STIMULANT DRUGS

Cocaine

[OBJECTIVE 16]

Description and Form

[OBJECTIVE 25]

Derived from the leaves of the coca plant (*Erythroxylon coca*), cocaine is a powerful, highly addictive CNS stimulant. The drug is typically found in two forms: **cocaine hydrochloride,** a fine white powder that can be purified and processed into **crack cocaine,** a solid, brownish-white crystal. The term *crack* comes from the crackling and popping sounds the drug makes when heated. Powdered cocaine (referred to in this text as *cocaine*) is known as *blow, coke, snow,* or *yayo.* Crack cocaine (referred to in this text as *crack*) is frequently called *rock* or simply *crack.*

Cocaine is known to have been used during the religious ceremonies of the inhabitants of Peru in the sixth century and the Incas in the eleventh century. In 1884 cocaine was first used as a local anesthetic, and by the early twentieth century its use was widespread. The drug

was an ingredient in many medications and health products, including Coca-Cola (Hollander & Hoffman, 2002). Today cocaine is classified as a schedule II medication by the federal Drug Enforcement Agency and is used as a topical or intranasal anesthetic.

Epidemiology and Demographics

[OBJECTIVE 26]

In 1999, 3.7 million Americans were reported to use cocaine, and 1.5 million were estimated to use the drug monthly. Cocaine is the most frequent cause of drug-related visits to the emergency department (Hollander & Hoffman, 2002). It is used by all races, socioeconomic levels, and both genders. Geographic patterns of use typically vary from year to year.

Routes and Pathophysiology

[OBJECTIVE 27]

Cocaine can be smoked (called *freebasing*), melted and then injected, or taken orally, but it is most often taken intranasally (snorted). A user may inhale tiny amounts of cocaine, called *bumps,* from a small spoon or may divide the cocaine into narrow bands called *lines* or *rails* and then use a hollow tube to inhale them intranasally. A 1-inch line typically contains 25 to 100 mg of cocaine, and a user may snort many over several hours. Crack is always smoked. A typical dose is a crystal weighing approximately one eighth of a gram.

When smoked, snorted, or injected, both forms of cocaine act on the CNS within 30 seconds. The duration of the effects varies widely from person to person. A cocaine high usually lasts 15 to 20 minutes. Crack is highly purified (85% to 90% cocaine) and has a very high rate of absorption. Its effects are more intense but disappear within 5 to 7 minutes. Users may smoke repeated doses for 12 to 24 hours if more crack is available and the user does not become exhausted and fall asleep.

Both forms block the reuptake of dopamine by neurons in the brain, causing massive CNS stimulation and heavy activation of the brain's reward system. This artificial reward is primarily responsible for the drug's highly addictive qualities. Patients may alternate doses of heroin and cocaine, a process known as *speedballing.* The user experiences intense, pleasurable stimulation from the cocaine and is then brought down to a dreamy, relaxed state with heroin. Although speedballing greatly increases the effects of the two drugs, it also makes users more likely to overdose and causes an extremely powerful addiction to both.

Paraphernalia

[OBJECTIVE 6]

Mirrors and razor blades are used to separate powdered cocaine into lines. Small, hollow tubes, such as shortened straws or rolled-up paper currency, are used for snorting. Crack is smoked out of a crack pipe, a glass tube approximately 4 to 6 inches long that is either slightly tapered or has steel wool at one end to hold the burning crystal.

Subjective Effects and Physical Findings

[OBJECTIVE 6]

Users of cocaine and crack report feelings of euphoria and intense energy, often appearing talkative and mentally alert. Massive release of dopamine in the brain can cause seizures. Some patients may have tactile hallucinations known as *cocaine bugs,* a crawling sensation underneath the skin. Users with this disturbance often scratch themselves very deeply, leading to ulceration and bleeding. Users have been known to exhibit bizarre, erratic, and even violent behavior, particularly after using large doses.

Sympathetic stimulation causes dilated and sluggish pupils, tachycardia, and widespread vasoconstriction leading to hypertension. Use of cocaine and crack has a high association with sudden death. Tachycardia from sympathetic stimulation can lead to potentially lethal tachydysrhythmias that often are refractory to adenosine or cardioversion. Vasospasm of the coronary or cerebral arteries can lead to a heart attack or stroke. Extreme hypertension may rupture a cerebral artery, causing a subarachnoid hemorrhage and rapid death. The risk of stroke is seven times higher when a person is intoxicated by cocaine (Hollander & Hoffman, 2002).

A twenty-fourfold increase in the risk of a heart attack exists within 1 hour of cocaine use. Cocaine-related myocardial infarction typically appears differently from other heart attacks. Patients often describe an atypical character to the chest pain. These feelings may be delayed for hours or days after last use of the drug. A 12-lead electrocardiogram may show nonspecific ST-segment changes, ST-segment elevation, or inverted T waves. Because cocaine causes vasoconstriction in all coronary arteries at once, several areas of the heart may be affected (Hollander & Hoffman, 2002).

Cocaine increases motor activity and heat production and decreases heat loss by systemic vasoconstriction. The drug also is thought to affect the temperature-regulating centers in the hypothalamus, but this has not been proven. Hyperthermia is one of the most serious complications of cocaine toxicity, and proper management has been shown to have positive effects of patient outcome (Hollander & Hoffman, 2002).

Long-Term Effects

[OBJECTIVE 6]

The most serious consequence of long-term use of cocaine and crack is dependence and addiction. When an addicted person is not using, even minor mentions of cocaine use or exposure to people or things related to use can trigger intense and powerful cravings (National Institute on Drug Abuse, 2004). Long-term use has been linked to many types of heart disease, including coronary artery disease and dilated cardiomyopathy. Over time cocaine also causes a narrowing of the cerebral arteries, decreasing blood flow to the brain and impairing cognition. Regularly snorting cocaine can lead to a loss of the sense of smell, chronic nosebleeds, an inflamed and constantly runny nose, and even destruction of the septum of the nose. Because cocaine is an appetite suppressant, many users experience significant weight loss and malnutrition (National Institute on Drug Abuse, 2004).

Tolerance and Withdrawal

[OBJECTIVE 6]

Users of cocaine and crack experience a withdrawal syndrome characterized by lethargy, severe depression, anxiety, anhedonia, and intense cravings for the drug almost immediately after stimulant effects subside. Tolerance often develops over time, and physical and psychological addiction is common.

Differential Diagnosis

Differential diagnosis of cocaine intoxication includes the following:

- Alcohol intoxication
- Encephalitis
- Hypoglycemia
- Hyponatremia
- Panic attack
- Ischemic stroke
- Subarachnoid hemorrhage
- Anticholinergic toxicity
- Antidepressant toxicity
- Benzodiazepine intoxication
- Methamphetamine intoxication
- Hallucinogenic mushroom intoxication
- PCP intoxication

Therapeutic Interventions

[OBJECTIVES 28, 29]

When dealing with a patient under the influence of crack or cocaine, the safety of you and your crew comes first. Users have been known to become violent quickly, sometimes without warning or provocation, so carefully monitor the patient's behavior and body language. Avoid being confrontational or making sudden, unexpected movements. Evacuate the scene and call for law enforcement as needed. Treatment of uncomplicated intoxication is merely supportive care. Administer 100% oxygen by nonrebreather mask, obtain and monitor a 12-lead ECG, and obtain IV access with an isotonic crystalloid. Avoid giving large amounts of fluid and transport quietly to a facility of the patient's choosing.

Patients with cocaine-related chest pain, dysrhythmias, or ischemic ECG changes require more aggressive care. Oxygen administration and constant ECG monitoring are required. Look for ischemic ST-segment changes and changes in QRS complexes on a 12-lead ECG. Because the cardiac-related effects of cocaine and crack are primarily caused by CNS stimulation, the brain must be calmed to treat them effectively. Start an IV and give doses of benzodiazepines as ordered by medical direction. Follow advanced cardiac life support protocols to treat chest pain and dysrhythmias after or concurrent with benzodiazepine administration. Transport to a facility capable of cardiac catheterization and advanced cardiac care.

Ecstasy

[OBJECTIVES 16, 25]

Description and Form

Tablets of the powerful stimulant drug **3,4-methylenedioxymethamphetamine (MDMA)** are called **ecstasy.** A clear liquid in its pure form, MDMA is structurally similar to methamphetamine and the hallucinogen mescaline. Originally synthesized by a German pharmaceutical company in 1914, the drug has been designated schedule I by the Drug Enforcement Agency.

MDMA is a synthetic designer drug made in clandestine laboratories. It is formed into tablets, usually with a logo, design, or cartoon character imprinted on the pill's face. An ecstasy pill's color and design is limited only by the producer's imagination and has no relation to the amount of MDMA present. To increase profits, producers of ecstasy may cut or mix it with other compounds to maximize the number of pills produced. These substances are most often other stimulants such as caffeine, cocaine, or pseudoephedrine. Other examples include dextromethorphan, vitamins, and heroin. Known as *E, X, XTC,* or *Adam,* one tablet of ecstasy usually costs $20 to $40 and contains approximately 50 to 200 mg MDMA.

Epidemiology and Demographics

[OBJECTIVE 26]

Use of ecstasy is on the rise. The Drug Abuse Warning Network found an 800% increase in patients with MDMA-related symptoms seen at major metropolitan emergency departments in the United States from 1995 to 2002. Its use is most prevalent among adolescents and young adults (Yew, 2005).

Routes and Pathophysiology

[OBJECTIVE 27]

MDMA is effective at doses of 1 to 2 mg/kg. It is almost always sold on the streets as tablets but may be seen in its liquid form. Ecstasy is typically ingested, and initial effects begin within 20 to 40 minutes. Intoxication peaks within 90 minutes; effects may last for more than 10 hours but usually subside after 6 hours. Like all amphetamines, MDMA causes the release of dopamine and norepinephrine. The drug also prevents serotonin from moving back into the presynaptic neurons in certain areas of the brain. MDMA blocks these reuptake molecules on the presynaptic neuron and causes them to pull serotonin *out* of the presynaptic neuron. This floods the synapses of the brain with serotonin (Chiang, 2002).

Some users intensify the effects of MDMA by stacking, or ingesting multiple doses of ecstasy spaced over several hours.

Ecstasy is sometimes taken with other hallucinogens and dissociatives such as LSD, dextromethorphan, or ketamine. This is known as *candy flipping.* Either greatly increases the likelihood of dangerous side effects and overdose.

Paraphernalia

[OBJECTIVE 6]

Although no paraphernalia is needed to ingest ecstasy, users may play with soft stuffed animals that feel exceptional because of heightened tactile sensation. Glow sticks, twirled while dancing, produce trails of light that are amplified by a user's dilated pupils and MDMA's hallucinogenic properties. A menthol rub or spray may be applied to the skin and eyes because the intense odor and tingling, cooling sensation are especially pleasurable. Many users characteristically keep a lollipop or pacifier in their mouths to prevent grinding their teeth.

Subjective Effects and Physical Findings

[OBJECTIVE 6] *Hyperthermia & Dehydration*

Users report dramatically increased energy, a strong sense of euphoria and well-being, heightened sexuality, and expanded consciousness. Heightened senses (particularly touch) and mild hallucinations such as light trails (bright streaks following moving light sources) are common. Sympathomimetic effects are evident, including tachycardia, hypertension, hyperthermia and dilated, sluggish pupils. Powerful CNS stimulation causes a clenched jaw; users often unconsciously grind their teeth (Chiang, 2002). Cases have been reported of chronic users grinding away all the enamel from their teeth.

High energy and CNS stimulation cause many users of ecstasy to frequent dance clubs playing electronic "techno" music with rapid, bounding beats. The loud music and dark atmosphere in these clubs, known as *raves,* are conducive to heightening a user's experience while minimizing detection. For more about raves, see the section on club drugs and drugs used for sexual purposes at the end of this chapter.

During MDMA abuse a number of factors can come together to produce a potentially lethal condition. Doses of 4 to 5 mg/kg can cause a sharp spike in body temperature. Combined with frenzied dancing, low fluid intake, and possibly alcohol ingestion, this hyperthermia can cause rapid and severe dehydration. Raves are crowded, dimly lit, and play very loud music for hours. Reports have been made of ecstasy users becoming unresponsive from heat exhaustion and dehydration only to be left lying on the floor or in a corner for hours. Prolonged hyperthermia such as this leads to brain damage and death. Dehydration can lead to acute renal failure and cardiac dysrhythmias. Circumstances similar to these cause most MDMA-related deaths.

Tolerance and Withdrawal

[OBJECTIVE 6]

MDMA causes short-term effects that persist even after the drug is eliminated from the body. As mentioned,

MDMA causes a massive release of serotonin and dopamine into the synapses of brain cells. Neurons increase production of these neurotransmitters to keep up, but eventually the supply of serotonin becomes exhausted. After MDMA leaves the body, much less serotonin is present in brain cells than normal. This causes "E depression," a dysphoric mood with feelings of anxiety and fear lasting for 24 to 48 hours after the MDMA high is over.

Tolerance to the psychoactive properties of MDMA develops rapidly, and an increase in adverse effects is reported after frequent use. Repeated doses can result in sympathomimetic toxicity.

Long-Term Effects

[OBJECTIVE 6]

Effects of long-term MDMA use are not well defined. Monkeys given high, repeated doses of MDMA (two doses a day for 4 days) show damage to serotonin-producing neurons in their brains up to 7 years later. Other studies have shown a link between ecstasy use, decreased memory, and cognitive impairment.

Differential Diagnosis

Differential diagnosis of MDMA intoxication includes the following:

- Alcohol intoxication
- Encephalitis
- Hypoglycemia
- Hyponatremia
- Panic disorder
- Ischemic stroke
- Subarachnoid hemorrhage
- Anticholinergic toxicity
- Antidepressant toxicity
- Benzodiazepine intoxication
- Cocaine intoxication
- Methamphetamine intoxication
- Hallucinogenic mushroom intoxication
- PCP intoxication

Therapeutic Interventions

[OBJECTIVES 28, 29]

Treatment of a patient under the influence of MDMA consists of close monitoring of mental status and vital signs. Give 100% oxygen. Patients may rapidly become hyperthermic. When indicated, use cooling measures to make sure that the patient's body temperature does not rise too high or too quickly. Start an IV with an isotonic crystalloid and a large-bore catheter for rapid administration of fluid as needed. Monitor the patient's ECG rhythm and treat dysrhythmias according to advanced cardiac life support protocols. Patiently and calmly explain what you are doing as you do it, taking into account your patient's altered sensations and perceptions. Transport the patient for physician evaluation.

Patient and Family Education

A common misconception is that MDMA is a "safe" drug of abuse. Explain the potential consequences of MDMA use, including hyperthermia, and stress the importance of fluid intake and avoidance of ETOH. Point out that the contents of an MDMA pill are unknown and that pills are made in illegal laboratories without any regulation or safety tests.

Methamphetamine

[OBJECTIVES 16, 25]   *Cheap*

Description and Form

Methamphetamine is another powerful CNS stimulant made in clandestine laboratories. Methamphetamine comes in a white, powdered form and as a clear crystal, known as *crystal meth*. The powdered form, known as *speed*, can be snorted, injected, or smoked; crystal meth is smoked in the same manner as crack cocaine. Crystal meth is typically more pure than powdered methamphetamine because it is clear and impurities are easily spotted. For an infrequent user, a dose may be 10 to 50 mg. This is commonly repeated every 3 to 8 hours to stay awake or every half hour to 4 hours to maintain euphoria and the rush.

Epidemiology and Demographics

[OBJECTIVE 26]

In 2004, 1.4 million (0.6%) persons aged 12 years and over were estimated to have used methamphetamine within the past year (Substance Abuse and Mental Health Services Administration, 2004). The rate of use in 2004 was highest for young adults aged 18 to 25 years. Males use methamphetamine more often than do females. The highest rates of methamphetamine use were found among Native Hawaiians and Pacific Islanders (2.2%) and American Indians (1.7%), whereas the lowest rates were seen in blacks (0.1%) and Asians (0.2%). Western states show the highest rates of methamphetamine use (Substance Abuse and Mental Health Services Administration, 2004).

Routes and Pathophysiology

[OBJECTIVE 27]

Though chemically related to MDMA and prescription amphetamines, such as those used in the treatment of attention deficit disorder or narcolepsy, methamphetamine is more powerful. Crystal meth is smoked, whereas powdered methamphetamine can be smoked, ingested, injected, or snorted. Both have an onset of action of approximately 30 seconds or less, and effects may last up to 24 hours. Like other stimulant drugs, methamphetamine causes the release of massive amounts of dopamine in the brain.

Paraphernalia

[OBJECTIVE 6]

A pipe is used to smoke crystal meth, much like crack cocaine. Powdered methamphetamine use may be associated with syringes or short straws and rolled-up paper currency if injected or snorted. Methamphetamine also may be smoked in its powdered form. Users often remove the metal end and filaments from an ordinary glass light bulb and place the powder inside. The outside is heated with a lighter and the user inhales the smoke that exits the globe.

Subjective Effects and Physical Findings

[OBJECTIVE 6]

Methamphetamine users often follow an up-and-down pattern of binging and craving. When moderate to heavy levels of the drug first reach the brain, users experience a rush of intense euphoria, high energy, feelings of increased physical strength, and sexual stimulation lasting approximately 5 minutes. Signs of sympathomimetic stimulation are obvious and include tachycardia, hypertension, tachypnea, hyperthermia, palpitations, premature ventricular contractions, dry mouth, abdominal cramps, suppressed appetite, twitching, pallor, and dilated pupils. Within about an hour, this initial rush fades away.

Over the next few days a patient uses more and more methamphetamine in an attempt to regain the initial euphoria and pleasure of the rush phase. A strong tolerance builds, and taking the drug begins to have little or no effect. A user starts "tweaking," or experiencing a period of intense craving for methamphetamine. Behavior during this time often mimics that of paranoid schizophrenia. Tweaking patients may demonstrate dysphoric mood, disorganized thoughts, paranoia, anxiety, and irritability. Hallucinations (auditory and tactile) and delusions are common. Pupils appear normal during this stage, which lasts from 4 to 24 hours. Finally the user crashes, beginning a period of intense fatigue, uncontrollable sleepiness, and even worse drug cravings. These symptoms continue for up to 3 days. The user gradually returns to a state of normalcy over the next 2 to 7 days. After that, he or she is able to go on another meth binge.

Tolerance and Withdrawal

[OBJECTIVE 6]

In addition to the short-term tolerance described above, long-term tolerance can develop. A withdrawal syndrome of depression, anxiety, fatigue, paranoia, aggression, and intense craving for the drug is associated with stopping methamphetamine use (National Institute on Drug Abuse, 2002).

Long-Term Effects

[OBJECTIVE 6]

Methamphetamine causes severe, permanent damage to the body. Overuse of dopamine and norepinephrine neurons in the brain burns them out. A long-term decline of cognitive function becomes evident as more and more brain tissue is lost. Frequent users of methamphetamine age prematurely and typically appear years older than they are.

Differential Diagnosis

Differential diagnosis of methamphetamine intoxication includes the following:

- ETOH intoxication
- Encephalitis
- Hypoglycemia
- Hyponatremia
- Panic disorders
- Ischemic stroke
- Subarachnoid hemorrhage
- Anticholinergic toxicity
- Antidepressant toxicity
- Benzodiazepine intoxication
- Cocaine intoxication
- Hallucinogen intoxication
- PCP intoxication

Therapeutic Interventions

[OBJECTIVES 28, 29]   *RMC + benzo*

Management of methamphetamine toxicity is the same as for cocaine toxicity. Users under the influence of methamphetamine tend to be more violent and unpredictable, however. Stay on guard. Physical restraint may be required for safety. If so, chemical restraint is necessary to prevent excited delirium (described below).

> **PARAMEDIC*Pearl***
>
> The behavior of patients under the influence of methamphetamines can be erratic and dangerous. Be careful.

EXCITED DELIRIUM

[OBJECTIVES 6, 22]

Description and Definition

Excited delirium is a form of abnormal behavior characterized by paranoia, aggression, hyperthermia, dramatically increased strength, and insensitivity to pain. Although it is a controversial diagnosis, you should be aware of the condition because it often ends in sudden death (Mets, 1996), particularly after patient restraint and when the patient is under the influence of stimulant drugs.

Etiology

The causes of excited delirium are even more controversial. Some speculate that death from excited delirium is related to long-term stimulant abuse and related heart disease. Stimulant use can easily result in delirium, tachycardia, and hyperthermia, particularly when the patient is provoked. Other researchers believe excited delirium is related to a genetic fault that prevents the brain from adjusting the number of drug receptors in the limbic system. The brain becomes unable to remove the large amount of excess neurotransmitters present from stimulant drug abuse. A sharp increase in these chemicals in the amygdala can bring on severe delirium, paranoia, and aggression (Paquette, 2003). Elevated levels of catecholamines (dopamine, norepinephrine, epinephrine) also have been shown to increase the toxicity of cocaine in the body (Mets, 1996).

Excited delirium probably develops from several factors occurring together. Risk factors highly associated with excited delirium and sudden death include patient restraint (particularly in the prone position), long-term stimulant drug use, underlying heart disease, and struggling during and after physical restraint (Stratton et al., 2001).

Epidemiology and Demographics

Excited delirium is typically seen in men aged 20 to 40 years, but cases have been reported in women. Patients often have a long history of stimulant drug abuse, usually cocaine or methamphetamine. Tolerance to stimulant drugs increases with long-term use, and so does the likelihood of excited delirium. Reports exist of excited delirium deaths related to psychotic episodes, but most cases are associated with stimulant drug abuse.

History and Physical Findings

A typical case of excited delirium might involve a 32-year-old man with a long history of cocaine abuse. After snorting a usual amount of cocaine one night, he suddenly becomes paranoid and aggressive. He forces his way into the home next door and verbally and physically assaults the family living there, accusing them of stealing and conspiring against him. When the police arrive, they are surprised by the man's extreme physical strength and call for backup to subdue him. Eight police officers are finally able to restrain the man and place him under arrest. The neighbors later tell police they had seen the man before but had never spoken to him. Concerned about his bizarre behavior and minor injuries from the scuffle, the police request an EMS response to evaluate the man.

The paramedic who evaluates the patient finds that he is tachycardic, hypertensive, and hyperthermic. He is still combative and agitated, so the paramedics and police officers forcefully restrain him to a long backboard with proper technique. While en route, the attendant in charge notices that the patient has become quiet and compliant and seems to have fallen asleep. Although dramatically different from his earlier agitated state, the paramedic assumes that the patient has given up struggling. Within a few minutes, the patient's respiratory rate becomes slow and irregular. After placing him on an ECG monitor, the paramedic finds that the patient is now in asystole. Despite early recognition and rapid treatment, including intubation and advanced cardiac life support protocols, the man remains in cardiac arrest and is pronounced dead at the hospital.

The details of specific episodes of excited delirium may differ, but several symptoms from this example often are seen. An abnormal episode of agitation and violence begins suddenly, usually requiring the patient be restrained. The patient often displays far greater strength than would be expected for a person of a certain size and build, making restraint difficult. Finally, in cases of sudden death related to excited delirium, the patient becomes calm and quiet for a short period (5 minutes or less) immediately before going into respiratory and cardiac arrest (Stratton et al., 2001).

Differential Diagnosis

Differential diagnosis for excited delirium includes the following:

- Restraint asphyxia
- Cocaine toxicity
- Methamphetamine toxicity

Therapeutic Interventions

[OBJECTIVE 28]

As with restraint asphyxia, the best treatment for excited delirium is prevention. Chemical restraints should be given as soon as possible after the physical restraint of patients with risk factors for excited delirium. This will end the struggle and hopefully prevent the possible peak of delirium that leads to sudden death. Administer 100% oxygen and continually and carefully monitor the patient's respirations and ECG rhythm. Be aware of hyperthermia and initiate rapid cooling measures as needed.

> **PARAMEDIC Pearl**
> Sudden calm and quiet after intense struggling in a restrained patient is an ominous sign and could indicate impending respiratory and cardiac arrest.

DEPRESSANT DRUGS

Sedative-Hypnotics

[OBJECTIVES 16, 25]

Description and Form

Certain prescription depressant drugs can cause powerful relaxation and euphoria. These medications are typically known as **sedative-hypnotics,** drugs that calm, relax, and/or induce sleep. These drugs are used for sedation and relief of anxiety, treatment of insomnia, and control and treatment of seizures. The two most commonly abused sedative-hypnotics are barbiturates and benzodiazepines. Other sedative-hypnotics include buspirone (BuSpar), zolpidem (Ambien), chloral hydrate, meprobamate (Equanil), and carisoprodol (Soma) (Cooper, 2005). Gamma-hydroxybutyrate is a sedative-hypnotic discussed later in this chapter.

Barbiturates were first used in medicine around the beginning of the twentieth century. Examples of barbiturates still in use include methohexital (Brevital), thiopental (Pentothal), amobarbital (Amytal), pentobarbital (Nembutal), butalbital (Fiorinal), butabarbital (Butisol), and phenobarbital. Because their use may cause drastic side effects and addiction, barbiturates are prescribed less often today in favor of the relatively safer benzodiazepines. Commonly prescribed short-acting benzodiazepines are estazolam (ProSom), flurazepam (Dalmane), temazepam (Restoril), triazolam (Halcion), and midazolam (Versed). Long-acting benzodiazepines include alprazolam (Xanax), chlordiazepoxide (Librium), diazepam (Valium), and lorazepam (Ativan). Most abused prescription drugs are either illegitimately prescribed or stolen from pharmacies and clinics (Joseph, 2005).

Epidemiology and Demographics
[OBJECTIVE 26]

In 2002 approximately 1.5 million Americans abused CNS depressants, and more than 100,000 cases of persons seeking emergency medical treatment related to benzodiazepines were reported (National Institute on Drug Abuse, 2005c). Women are more likely than men to be prescribed these medications.

Routes and Pathophysiology
[OBJECTIVE 27]

Benzodiazepines and barbiturates are usually ingested when prescribed or abused but may be injected IV or intramuscularly. Both types of drugs affect the concentrations and actions of the neurotransmitter GABA within the brain, producing a CNS depressant effect.

Subjective Effects and Physical Findings
[OBJECTIVE 6]

Benzodiazepine and barbiturate intoxication causes a sleepy, sedated feeling and reduces anxiety and worry. Use of CNS depressants and alcohol can lead to bradycardia, slowed respiratory rate, and death (National Institute on Drug Abuse, 2005c). Most cases of severe sedative-hypnotic toxicity are from suicide attempts.

Tolerance and Withdrawal
[OBJECTIVE 6]

Tolerance to barbiturates and benzodiazepines develops quickly with repeated use. Withdrawal from these medications is similar to that for ETOH. Suddenly stopping use can cause a surge of activity in the brain and lead to seizures (National Institute on Drug Abuse, 2005c).

Long-Term Effects
[OBJECTIVE 6]

Prolonged use of CNS depressant drugs leads to addiction and tolerance. Other symptoms associated with long-term abuse of CNS depressant drugs are amnesia, irritability, and anger.

Differential Diagnosis

Differential diagnosis of sedative-hypnotic intoxication includes the following (Cooper, 2005):

- ETOH abuse
- Brain abscess
- ETOH withdrawal
- DT
- Diabetic ketoacidosis
- Epidural hematoma
- Hyperosmolar hyperglycemic nonketotic coma
- Hypertensive emergencies
- Hypoglycemia
- Metabolic acidosis
- Brain tumor

Therapeutic Interventions
[OBJECTIVES 28, 29]

A major side effect of sedative-hypnotic overdose is respiratory depression. Securing a patent airway and ensuring adequate ventilation and oxygenation are essential. Obtain IV access to keep a vein open. In cases of CNS depressant withdrawal, be prepared to manage seizures with diazepam or lorazepam.

Patient and Family Education

Many believe that simply because a drug is a prescription medication it is safe to use and abuse. This is not true; many prescription drugs are addicting and have severe side effects.

PARAMEDIC*Pearl*

The generic names of barbiturates typically end in "-tal," and generic names of benzodiazepines usually end in "-pam."

Gamma-Hydroxybutyrate

[OBJECTIVES 16, 25]

Description and Form

Gamma-hydroxybutyrate (GHB) is a white powder usually dissolved in water and sold at $5 to $10 per dose. GHB also is known as *liquid ecstasy, scoop, easy lay, Georgia home boy, grievous bodily harm, liquid X,* and *goop* (Britt & McCance-Katz, 2005). It is sold in the United States under the name Xyrem, a Schedule III medication used to treat narcolepsy, but abuse of this form is rare.

GHB is easily manufactured from industrial chemicals purchased over the Internet. Detailed instructions for GHB production also are available online, and some amateurs may attempt to synthesize the drug. If done incorrectly highly toxic chemicals are left mixed with the product, potentially leading to serious adverse effects. Improper manufacturing techniques also lead to wide variations in the strength of homemade GHB.

Epidemiology and Demographics
[OBJECTIVE 26]

The number of medical emergencies related to GHB has greatly increased over the past 15 years. Sixty deaths were reported from GHB overdose in 2000 (Gahlinger, 2004).

Routes and Pathophysiology

[OBJECTIVE 27]

GHB is ingested, often with ETOH, which increases its effects. One dose ranges from 2 to 30 g. GHB is structurally similar to the inhibitory neurotransmitter GABA, which probably is the reason for its potent CNS depressant effects.

Subjective Effects and Physical Findings

[OBJECTIVE 6]

Effects of GHB are similar to ETOH but much more intense. GHB has been described as "a case of beer in a capful of liquid." The drug initially produces euphoria and at higher doses rapidly causes unresponsiveness. Other effects include nausea, vomiting, tremors, agitation (in lower doses), confusion, hallucinations, and bradycardia (Britt & McCance-Katz, 2005). Overdoses may cause Cheyne-Stokes respirations, seizures, and death (Gahlinger, 2004).

Tolerance and Withdrawal

[OBJECTIVE 6]

Within 12 hours of a final dose of GHB a chronic user may develop mild withdrawal symptoms such as tachycardia, insomnia, hypertension, tremor, confusion, nausea, and vomiting. Two or 3 days after the last dose, withdrawal symptoms may become severe and patients may experience hallucinations, paranoia, anxiety, and disorientation. The entire syndrome may last 3 to 15 days. Withdrawal from GHB is rare and is almost exclusively seen in users who have used large amounts of the drug over long periods.

Long-Term Effects

[OBJECTIVE 6]

The long-term effects of GHB abuse are unknown.

Differential Diagnosis

Differential diagnosis of GHB intoxication includes the following:

- Opioid intoxication
- ETOH intoxication
- Suicide attempt
- Neurologic illness or injury
- Date rape

Therapeutic Interventions

[OBJECTIVES 28, 29]

Protect the airway and ensure adequate ventilation with 100% supplemental oxygen. Reports have been made of seemingly unresponsive patients under the influence of GHB suddenly becoming violent and combative, particularly when the pharynx is stimulated during airway management and intubation attempts. Consider the use of nasopharyngeal airways. Bradycardia associated with GHB toxicity responds well to standard doses of atropine (0.5 mg IV).

PARAMEDIC*Pearl*

GHB is frequently abused with ETOH, which intensifies its effects. One or both may be used to facilitate sexual assault.

Opioids

[OBJECTIVE 16]

Description and Form

[OBJECTIVE 25]

Opioids are drugs with extensive analgesic properties. This class includes tightly regulated prescription drugs such as morphine, codeine, and oxycodone as well as the illegal drugs heroin and opium. Some of these drugs are produced by processing the extracted seed pods of the poppy plant and are called *opiates*. The term *narcotic* was originally coined to describe opiates but has been used by the public and law enforcement to mean any illegal psychoactive substance. The term *opioids* includes the naturally derived opiates and drugs that are synthesized in the laboratory and cause similar effects (Nelson, 2002).

Prescription opioids come in pills, tablets, and syrups taken orally; in suspensions that can be injected; and in transdermal patches that deliver medication through the skin. Opium is a milky sap obtained from poppy seed pods and typically contains approximately 10% morphine (Nelson, 2000). Morphine can be extracted from opium, but today it is more commonly synthesized in the laboratory. **Heroin (diacetylmorphine)** is derived from morphine and is sold on the streets as a white or brownish powder. It is sometimes seen in the form of a black, sticky substance known as *black tar heroin.* To maximize profits, heroin sold on the street often is cut with other substances such as sugar, starch, and powdered milk. Users are at severe risk for overdose and death because the actual content of heroin in a dose sold on the street can vary widely (National Institute on Drug Abuse, 2005a).

Epidemiology and Demographics

[OBJECTIVE 26]

An estimated 2.5 million Americans used prescription opioids for nonmedical purposes in 2002 (National Institute on Drug Abuse, 2005c). Almost 4 million people in the United States have used heroin at some point in their lives, and an estimated 281,000 have received treatment for heroin abuse (National Institute on Drug Abuse, 2005a).

Routes and Pathophysiology

[OBJECTIVE 27]

Opioids can be taken through a variety of routes, including ingestion, injection, intranasal inhalation, and smoking. IV injection provides the most potent effect and an onset of action within 10 seconds. The onset of opioids injected intramuscularly is slower, approximately 5 to 8 minutes. Heroin causes effects within 10 to 15 minutes when snorted or smoked (National Institute on Drug Abuse, 2005a).

Once an opioid reaches the brain, it binds to a variety of opiate receptors. Some decrease the sensation of pain within the brain itself. Other opiate receptors produce feelings of euphoria. A powerful feeling of euphoria after extensive, exhausting exercise, known as a *runner's high,* is an example of natural opiate receptor stimulation (Nelson, 2002).

Paraphernalia

[OBJECTIVE 6]

To administer heroin IV, users melt powdered heroin with a flame and a spoon (a "cooker"). The liquid heroin is drawn into a syringe through a cotton ball to filter it, then injected.

Subjective Effects and Physical Findings

[OBJECTIVE 6]

As opioids flood the brain, users typically describe a rush of euphoria. The intensity of this surge of pleasure depends on the particular opioid used and the route of administration. IV injected heroin produces the strongest response. Less-powerful orally ingested opioids, such as codeine, have less-dramatic effects. This rush is accompanied by a warm, flushed feeling in the skin; heaviness in the extremities; dry mouth; and sometimes nausea, vomiting, and severe itching (National Institute on Drug Abuse, 2005a). Users become drowsy and thought processes are slowed and clouded for several hours.

After a potent dose of stronger opioids such as heroin or morphine, the CNS is profoundly depressed. Depressed brain activity leads to a decrease in heart rate, breathing rate, and tidal volume, potentially leading to hypoxia and death. Heroin purchased on the street is particularly dangerous because the exact dose is never known (National Institute on Drug Abuse, 2005a). Orthostatic blood pressure changes may be seen. A patient's pupils typically become extremely constricted and pinpoint, but this is not seen in all cases of opioid toxicity. Patients who have been without oxygen and sustained brain injury may present with dilated, fixed pupils. Whenever this slowed state is reversed, either naturally or with the assistance of medications, the patient is at risk for opioid-induced pulmonary edema (Nelson, 2002).

Tolerance and Withdrawal

[OBJECTIVE 6]

To avoid withdrawal symptoms, a person addicted to heroin may use the drug approximately four times each day. Opioid withdrawal typically occurs within a few hours of the last dose. Worsening drug cravings, yawning, and a runny nose give way to nausea, vomiting, diarrhea, sweating, muscle pain, bone pain, anxiety, and tachycardia. Although quite painful, opiate withdrawal is rarely

life threatening as long as dehydration and electrolyte imbalances are avoided (Hamilton, 2002). Symptoms typically peak 1 to 2 days after last use and subside after a week or so. Relapse, abusing after a period of quitting, is common in cases of opioid addiction.

Long-Term Effects

[OBJECTIVE 6]

Long-term injection of opioids causes scarred and collapsed veins and infections of the blood and heart valves. Subcutaneous and intramuscular injection with nonsterile needles causes skin abscesses and other infections. Many substances used to cut heroin do not readily dissolve in the blood and can clog the vessels of the heart, lungs, kidneys, and brain, causing a variety of ischemic conditions. Because heroin users typically have limited resources, syringes, needles, cookers, and cotton often are shared, leading to a much higher risk of contracting HIV, hepatitis, and other infectious diseases. Paraphernalia sharing is common among users of any injected drug of abuse, and so are these blood-borne diseases.

Differential Diagnosis

Differential diagnosis of opioid intoxication includes the following:

- Cardiac arrest
- ETOH intoxication
- GHB intoxication
- Dissociative intoxication

Therapeutic Interventions

[OBJECTIVES 28, 29]

For a patient who has overdosed on opioids, ensure an open airway and adequate ventilation with a nasal airway and a bag-mask. Because the patient may soon be revived with naloxone, avoid oral airways and endotracheal intubation at first. After the patient's lungs are adequately ventilated with supplemental oxygen, give naloxone IV or intramuscularly. Patients who have been revived on scene with naloxone must be transported to a facility for observation. The effects of naloxone usually do not last as long as the opioids it has reversed, potentially leading to a recurrent episode of unresponsiveness, decreased respirations, and hypoxia.

Patient and Family Education

Many users believe smoking or snorting heroin is less addictive and less dangerous than injecting it. This is not true.

PARAMEDIC*Pearl*

A common stereotype of a heroin abuser is a junkie covered in track marks from extensive IV injections. In reality, most heroin users ingest or snort the drug to avoid telltale signs and deadly hazards associated with needle use.

MARIJUANA

[OBJECTIVES 16, 25]

Description and Form

Marijuana is the dried mixture of shredded leaves, stems, and seeds of the Indian hemp plant *Cannabis sativa*. Delta-9-tetrahydrocannabinol (THC) is the primary psychoactive substance found within the plant, but approximately 60 other chemicals called *cannabinoids* are found within the plant. Some of these compounds have minor psychoactive effects. *C. sativa* grows throughout the world and was one of the earliest plants cultivated by human beings—to make clothing and rope as well as to use for its intoxicating effects. The plant's flowers can be processed into a concentrated resin, hashish, and even further into hashish oil, both of which contain higher concentrations of THC. The THC content of marijuana today is approximately 20 times higher on average than 25 years ago because of advanced cultivation practices. The concentration of THC varies widely depending on the variety of the plant and its growing and harvesting conditions. Marijuana also is known as *reefer, weed, pot, herb, ganja, Mary Jane, grass,* and *trees.* A typical marijuana joint contains approximately 20 mg of THC. Approximately 80 joints can be produced from 1 oz of marijuana, which costs approximately $280. Marijuana is typically sold in smaller quantities, such as one eighth of an ounce for $30 to $40.

Marijuana is a Schedule I drug, meaning it has no accepted medical use, but this is controversial among researchers. Studies have shown marijuana has medicinal effects such as reducing nausea and easing pain in chronic diseases such as AIDS, cancer, and multiple sclerosis. Dronabinol (Marinol), a Schedule III medication, is a synthetic form of THC available for regulated prescription use. Dronabinol has been shown to have the antinausea properties of marijuana but is much less psychoactive and less effective for pain control. Because of this, dronabinol is not typically abused.

Epidemiology and Demographics

[OBJECTIVE 26]

Marijuana is by far the most widely used illegal drug in the United States. Forty percent (94 million) of Americans older than age 12 years have tried marijuana at least once. People of all ages use marijuana, but use is more widespread among adolescents and young adults (National Institute on Drug Abuse, 2005b). Overall, abuse has been steadily increasing over the past 30 years (Otten, 2000). Hashish is much less commonly seen in the United States but may be common abroad.

Routes and Pathophysiology

[OBJECTIVE 27]

When smoked, THC and other compounds from marijuana are absorbed into the blood from the alveoli, reach-ing the brain within 15 seconds. Marijuana's effects peak within 10 to 30 minutes and last for 1 to 4 hours (Otten, 2000). The drug has a longer duration when eaten (4 to 6 hours) but also a longer onset of action (20 to 30 minutes). Because of erratic absorption from the acidic stomach and first-pass metabolism, much higher concentrations of THC enter the bloodstream from smoking marijuana (National Institute on Drug Abuse, 2005b). Marijuana may still affect the body hours or even days after use because THC is stored in fatty tissues and slowly released into the bloodstream. Marijuana often is used with other drugs, such as heroin, ketamine, crack, PCP, and opium. It also is commonly used with ETOH; the two drugs greatly enhance each other's effects, producing a more intoxicated state (Otten, 2000).

Paraphernalia

[OBJECTIVE 6]

Marijuana is usually smoked in cigarettes (joints), cigars (blunts), or pipes (bowls or bongs) but can also be ingested. Hashish and hashish oil are usually sprinkled on tobacco and smoked. When burned, marijuana has a strong, characteristic odor.

Subjective Effects and Physical Findings

[OBJECTIVE 6]

Psychological effects of marijuana include changes in sensation, perception, thinking, and coordination. Users report a relaxed euphoria with a slowed sense of time and more intense perception of colors and sounds. Typically this relaxation gradually turns into sleepiness. For some users, particularly those with little experience with the drug, marijuana can cause paranoia, anxiety, panic, derealization, and depersonalization. These feelings are frightening but pass within a few minutes. A person solely under the influence of marijuana is completely alert and oriented, even in cases of acute panic (Marx, 2002). In rare cases high doses of marijuana can cause temporary psychosis (National Institute on Drug Abuse, 2005b).

Overdosing on marijuana is nearly impossible. Even frequent smoking over several hours is unlikely to cause any major adverse effects. Within a few minutes of use, marijuana causes mild tachycardia and bronchodilation (Marx, 2002). Its effects on blood pressure and pupil reactions are usually negligible. Blood vessels in the eyes become engorged with blood, causing the reddened conjunctiva seen with intoxication. The strong relaxation associated with use may cause the user to have a slouching posture. Muscle tremors and weakness may occur. Users frequently report increased appetite, dry mouth, and urinary retention.

Some individuals develop dyspnea or chest pain after smoking marijuana, but these symptoms usually pass and are rarely life-threatening (Otten, 2000). However, the risk of angina and myocardial infarction is greatly increased within the first few hours of using marijuana. Many users underestimate the decreased reaction time and impaired perceptions associated with marijuana intoxication. These effects can be particularly hazardous when driving. Short-term memory is impaired, reducing the ability to perform complex tasks. Effects on cognition and memory may persist for days after use. Although drivers under the influence of marijuana typically drive slower than the posted speed limit, the drug's effects are dramatically enhanced by other drugs, particularly ETOH.

Adult users smoking or ingesting even highly potent marijuana may gradually become more and more sedated but do not exhibit a decreased level of consciousness, even after hours of heavy use. However, oral ingestion of potent marijuana can cause rapid-onset drowsiness, limp muscles, and lethargy and carries the potential of a more severe coma and airway obstruction (Marx, 2002).

Tolerance and Withdrawal

[OBJECTIVE 6]

After repeated, successive uses of marijuana over a few hours, a user soon develops tolerance to its effects, but that tolerance typically goes away within one to two days. Marijuana abuse can lead to dependence and addiction, particularly of a psychological nature. Withdrawal has been seen with long-term marijuana use and is characterized by irritability, insomnia, nausea, decreased appetite, and restlessness. Symptoms can be reduced with small doses of THC (Otten, 2000) and are reported to peak approximately 1 week after stopping use (National Institute on Drug Abuse, 2005b).

Long-Term Effects

[OBJECTIVE 6]

Long-term marijuana smoking is damaging to the throat and pulmonary tree, probably even more so than tobacco. Marijuana smoke contains approximately three times as much tar as filtered cigarette smoke and five times more carbon monoxide (Otten, 2000). Marijuana smoke contains 50% to 70% more carcinogenic compounds than tobacco smoke. Regular marijuana users typically develop the same pulmonary symptoms as tobacco users, such as increased phlegm production, chronic cough, sore throat, and a higher risk of pulmonary infections (National Institute on Drug Abuse, 2005b). Marijuana users typically inhale more deeply and forcefully than tobacco users, increasing exposure to toxic smoke and increasing their risk of a spontaneous pneumothorax or pneumomediastinum.

 Heavy marijuana use disrupts the hippocampus, affecting the user's ability to form and recall memories. Long-term use is associated with decreased intellectual and emotional development, particularly around the crucial period of adolescence and puberty, when marijuana use is most common. Depression, anxiety, and personality disturbances are associated with long-term use. Long-term users overwhelmingly report that the drug has adversely affected their social lives, physical and mental health, careers, and cognitive abilities (National Institute on Drug Abuse, 2005b).

Differential Diagnosis

Differential diagnosis of marijuana intoxication includes the following (Daly, 2004):

- Alcoholism
- Anxiety disorders
- Bipolar disorder
- Depressive disorders
- Hallucinogen abuse
- Inhalant abuse
- Opioid abuse
- Panic attack
- Schizophrenia
- Cocaine abuse
- Dissociative drug abuse

Therapeutic Interventions

[OBJECTIVES 28, 29]

Episodes of panic are transient and managed by calming and coaching the patient. In the rare event that a patient under the influence of marijuana is extremely panicked and agitated, a low dose of a benzodiazepine may be ordered to reduce anxiety and calm the patient. Assess and treat reports of dyspnea and chest pain as with any other patient by administering oxygen, obtaining a 12-lead ECG, and obtaining IV access.

Patient and Family Education

Despite a low potential for acute adverse effects, marijuana is not a "safe" drug. Its long-term consequences can be harmful.

PARAMEDIC*Pearl*

Effects of marijuana are usually benign, and emergency treatment is not needed. Patients with serious signs and symptoms probably are under the influence of one or more other drugs.

INHALANTS

[OBJECTIVES 16, 25]

Description and Form

Inhalants are volatile substances (producing fumes at room temperature) that are deliberately inhaled to induce a mind-altering high. The most commonly abused inhalants are glue, shoe polish, and gasoline, but the abuse of almost any product containing **hydrocarbons** can produce these effects. Hydrocarbons are large molecules commonly found in toluene (an additive in metallic paints), rubber cement, lacquer, dry cleaning fluids, butane fuel, and cooking sprays (Wilson & Saukkonen, 2004). Virtually all aerosol products contain hydrocarbons and can be abused (American Academy of Pediatrics, 1996).

Abusing nitrous oxide (N_2O), an odorless, colorless gas used as an anesthetic, also is common. Some EMS agencies use Nitronox, N_2O mixed with oxygen, as a pain reliever for patients with isolated trauma. Commonly known as *laughing gas,* N_2O also is used in the manufacture of whipped cream.

Epidemiology and Demographics

[OBJECTIVE 26]

Inhalant abuse is almost wholly seen in teenagers and young adults. After marijuana, inhalants are the most commonly abused substances among eighth and tenth graders. In one survey of adolescents aged 12 to 17 years, almost one in 10 reported inhalant abuse at some point in life, equal to approximately 2 million teenagers nationally. Eighty percent of inhalant abusers report their first use before age 15 years, with some as early as 6 to 8 years old. The rate of abuse peaks at age 15 years. A sharp decline occurs after age 18 years, though some users continue into adulthood. Use has always been reported as higher among young males, but newer data show that boys and girls equally abuse inhalants. Inhalant abuse is widespread throughout the world, particularly in poor communities and developing countries. Inhalants are particularly attractive to young people from suburban, rural, and lower socioeconomic backgrounds because they are cheap and easily obtained. However, children and teenagers from all income groups are known to abuse inhalants (Wu, et al., 2004). A strong association has been reported between inhalant use and antisocial personality disorder.

Routes and Pathophysiology

[OBJECTIVE 27]

Fumes from hydrocarbon-containing substances are breathed into the lungs and easily absorbed into the bloodstream through the alveoli (Wilson & Saukkonen, 2004). Only a few deep inspirations are usually needed to produce effects depending on the specific chemical. Inhalants are quickly transported throughout the body, and most pass freely through the blood-brain barrier. In the brain, effects of inhalants are twofold. Inhaled hydrocarbons and other chemicals likely affect the actions of GABA within the brain, much like ETOH and benzodiazepines. Hypoxia and hypercarbia result from use, which intensify the effects of inhalants. Oxygen saturation of hemoglobin is even worse inhaling from a closed plastic bag (Anderson & Loomis, 2003).

Paraphernalia

[OBJECTIVE 6]

The biggest draws of younger users to inhalants are availability and ease of use. Most of those who regularly abuse inhalants use several different chemicals. Users may breathe in fumes directly from a container (sniffing), from a chemical-soaked rag (huffing), or from liquid poured into a plastic or paper bag (bagging).

N_2O can be inhaled from canisters of whipped cream available at any grocery store. In some states selling small, metal canisters of N_2O used to make whipped cream is legal. These canisters are known as *whippets* and may be sold with a cracker, a device designed to puncture the metal tube containing the gas and deliver it into a balloon, from which it can be inhaled.

Subjective Effects and Physical Findings

[OBJECTIVE 6]

Within seconds of breathing an inhalant, the user is stimulated by a rush of euphoria. As the brain is starved of oxygen, speech becomes slurred and the user develops a staggering gait. Hallucinations are common. This high lasts only a few seconds to a minute, so users commonly continue to inhale the chemical, sometimes for hours. Cycles of inhaling soon give way to drowsiness and sleep, usually before a user can inhale enough to become unresponsive (American Academy of Pediatrics, 1996).

Inhalants cause an individual to become uninhibited and impulsive, often resulting in trauma. Dangerous behaviors lead to drowning, jumping from a height, hypothermia, and falls (American Academy of Pediatrics, 1996). A large number of chemicals abused as inhalants are flammable. Thoughtlessness and impaired judgment may lead to extensive burns and property damage. Many inhalants are compressed gases that could become cold enough to cause frostbite when expanding (Wu et al., 2004). Suffocation becomes a danger if a user loses consciousness and the airway becomes occluded by a plastic bag (American Academy of Pediatrics, 1996).

An estimated half of inhalant-related deaths result from sudden sniffing death syndrome (Anderson & Loomis, 2003). Chemicals in some inhalants cause the myocardium to become highly sensitized to epinephrine. When a sensitive user is suddenly startled, such as by an authority figure or a vivid hallucination, a surge of epinephrine rushes to the heart, resulting in fatal arrhythmias and death. More than one fifth of those who die suddenly from inhalant use have never used inhalants before (American Academy of Pediatrics, 1996).

Inhalant use is most easily recognized by a strong chemical odor that lingers on the breath for hours. Clothing may be stained with paint or chemicals. Flecks of paint may be found on the patient's face, lips, and hands. Over time, harsh fumes dry the skin surrounding the mouth, causing small cracks that form a pus-filled rash (American Academy of Pediatrics, 1996).

Tolerance and Withdrawal

[OBJECTIVE 6]

Tolerance has been reported in some cases of inhalant abuse but is easily avoided by using another chemical. Cases of inhalant dependence have been documented, but many progress to abusing other substances as they get older. Some point to a cycle of inhalant abuse that results in damage to the frontal lobe of the brain. This neurologic damage lowers intelligence, impairs decision-making skills, and leads to further abuse (Yip et al., 2005). A withdrawal syndrome is rare. Symptoms are similar to ETOH withdrawal and include insomnia, irritability, jitteriness, nausea, vomiting, and tachycardia. Withdrawal may last a month or longer (Anderson & Loomis, 2003).

Long-Term Effects

[OBJECTIVE 6]

In a study of delinquent youths, those using inhalants reported more personal and family dysfunction than their nonusing counterparts, such as suicidal ideations and abuse of other substances (Wu et al., 2004). Youths using inhalants commonly have difficulty in school and social settings. Inhalant abuse causes severe damage to the heart, lungs, liver, kidneys, and brain within only a few years of regular abuse. Congestive heart failure, renal failure, and inhibition of the immune system are linked to inhalant abuse (Anderson & Loomis, 2003). Long-term use causes permanent damage to the brain, resulting in atrophy, dementia, decreased intelligence, and a loss of coordination. Heavy inhalant abusers often show weight loss from a decreased appetite and poor hygiene and grooming (American Academy of Pediatrics, 1996).

Differential Diagnosis

Differential diagnosis of inhalant intoxication includes the following:

- ETOH intoxication
- Stimulant intoxication
- Dissociative intoxication
- Hallucinogen intoxication
- Traumatic brain injury

Therapeutic Interventions

[OBJECTIVES 28, 29]

Be alert to scene safety in cases of inhalant abuse. Open containers of volatile liquids can fill an entire room with poisonous, flammable fumes in a few minutes. Multiple unconscious patients and strong chemical odors are ominous signs of a rescuer safety risk. Request personnel specialized in hazardous materials if needed. Remove contaminated clothing before loading a patient into a closed ambulance. Establish airway control and effective ventilations. Apply 100% high-flow oxygen by nonre-breather mask or bag-mask. Monitor ECG for dysrhythmias and treat according to advanced cardiac life support protocols. Some recommend that epinephrine be avoided in cases of sudden sniffing death syndrome (Anderson & Loomis, 2003). Follow local protocols. Attempt to identify the specific substance by its container and contact the local Poison Control Center for further information.

Prevention and education are the most effective methods of combating inhalant abuse. Treatment of long-term inhalant abuse is difficult, expensive, and not very effective. The federal government requires special labeling of any substances that could potentially be used for inhalant abuse, but critics say that this only shows young people which chemicals to abuse. Many states and the federal government have made potentially abused products illegal to sell to minors, but these laws are difficult to enforce.

Patient and Family Education

Many parents stop worrying about the chemicals under the sink after their child is a toddler. Parents should consider either disposing of or locking away chemicals that could be inhaled and abused.

> **PARAMEDIC*Pearl***
>
> Look for chemicals, rashes, and/or discolorations around the mouth and hands.

HALLUCINOGENS

[OBJECTIVES 16, 25]

Description and Form

As the name suggests, **hallucinogens** are substances that cause hallucinations and distort perceptions of reality. Some of them have been used during religious and social ceremonies throughout the world since prehistoric times (Marx, 2002).

Various species of mushrooms have hallucinogenic properties because they contain a compound called *psilocybin*. These mushrooms grow wild throughout the world, including the United States. One variety is commonly found growing in cow dung and is concentrated in parts of the southern United States. Another is found in the Pacific Northwest growing on lawns (Marx, 2002). Hallucinogenic mushrooms, also known as *psychedelic mushrooms, shrooms,* or *caps,* are picked and dried, then sold for $20 to $40 per dose.

Certain varieties of cactus found in the American Southwest and Mexico also have hallucinogenic properties. The fleshy tops of these cacti, called *peyote buttons,* are removed and eaten whole or processed into a hallucinogenic liquid called *mescaline.* People avoid eating peyote itself because it has an extremely bitter taste and frequently causes nausea and vomiting (Marx, 2002). Mescaline also can be produced synthetically.

In 1938 Albert Hofmann, a Swiss chemist, created a new hallucinogenic drug in his laboratory from ergot, a fungus that grows on rye grass. After accidentally ingesting a small amount of this synthesized compound, known as **LSD** (an abbreviation for the German words for lysergic acid diethylamide), Hofmann discovered its intense hallucinogenic effects (National Institute on Drug Abuse, 2001). A similar hallucinogenic compound also is found in very small amounts in the seeds of the morning glory plant. LSD is classified as a Schedule I drug and is made in clandestine laboratories. Also known as *acid*, LSD is a clear or white crystal that easily dissolves in water. Liquid or crystal LSD may be ingested directly, but it is usually soaked into sugar cubes or encased in thin squares of gelatin called *window panes*. The most common form of LSD is blotter acid, sheets of paper soaked in the drug and then cut into quarter-inch squares called *tabs*. Each square is one dose (National Institute on Drug Abuse, 2001). These sheets of paper are typically colorfully printed with cartoon characters or intricate geometric designs (Marx, 2002). One tab of LSD costs approximately $5, but users frequently take two to four at a time.

Epidemiology and Demographics

[OBJECTIVE 26]

For thousands of years the use of hallucinogens was limited to where mushrooms and peyote were found or could be grown. With the discovery of LSD, which can be synthesized anywhere, hallucinogen use spread throughout the world, exploding in the 1960s. The number of people using hallucinogens dropped during the 1970s and 1980s but increased during the 1990s, particularly among adolescents and young adults.

Although 10% to 20% of Americans occasionally use hallucinogens, only approximately 0.5% regularly abuse these drugs (Moore & Jefferson, 2004). An estimated 8% of Americans will try hallucinogens at least once during their lifetimes. They are the third most commonly abused substances among high school students after ETOH and marijuana. Use is most common among white men aged 18 to 25 years (Cameron, 2004).

Routes and Pathophysiology

[OBJECTIVE 27]

Hallucinogens are almost always ingested, but LSD can be absorbed through the skin. The exact mechanisms of hallucinogens are unknown, but they are believed to alter concentrations of serotonin and norepinephrine significantly within the brain, particularly at the cerebral cortex. Most have an onset of action within 30 to 90 minutes, and effects may last up to 12 hours. LSD can produce hallucinations after approximately 20 mg are ingested, but typical street doses range from 50 to 300 mg.

Paraphernalia

[OBJECTIVE 6]

Little paraphernalia is associated with hallucinogen use because squares of LSD, hallucinogenic mushrooms, and peyote are eaten whole. The colorful blotter paper impregnated with LSD is rarely seen whole because it is cut up for distribution.

Subjective Effects and Physical Findings

[OBJECTIVE 6]

The effects of hallucinogens are collectively called *trips*. The defining symptoms of use are visual hallucinations and distortions of spatial perception. Emotions often are labile, changing widely and frequently, although anger is uncommon. Most trips contain pleasant and unpleasant aspects, but the drug's effects are unpredictable. A person's mood, expectations, and surroundings can dramatically alter the drug's effects. Patients remain fully alert and oriented. Trivial, everyday objects may suddenly be intensely fascinating and filled with meaning. In fact, the user has an overall sense that his or her thoughts are profound and may feel a sense of cosmic unity. Visual hallucinations, such as geometric forms with rippling, flowing colors, are common. At times hallucinations may take the form of complex images of people and things that are not there. Patients recognize that these visual disturbances are not real yet they are amazed by them. Memories while under the influence of hallucinogens also seem extremely vivid and altered. Sounds and smells are intensified, but auditory hallucinations are rare and less complex (Moore & Jefferson, 2004). Sometimes a user may experience a blending of senses called synesthesia—"hearing colors" or "seeing sounds" (National Institute on Drug Abuse, 2001).

Other altered perceptions include feelings that time is moving very slowly or that one's body is changing shape. Most users have mentally stimulating and emotionally satisfying trips. Some, however, may have bad trips that include nightmarish imagery and terrifying feelings of anxiety and despair. Because a trip is so lengthy, fears often center around thoughts that these effects are not going to stop or that the user is going insane. Physiologic effects of hallucinogens include hypertension, tachycardia, dizziness, dry mouth, sweating, tremors, and loss of appetite.

Tolerance and Withdrawal

[OBJECTIVE 6]

A tolerance to the euphoria of hallucinogens develops quickly, within a few days. However, users do not develop tolerance to the physiologic effects. Despite rapidly developing tolerance, withdrawal syndromes from hallucinogens are rare (Moore & Jefferson, 2004).

Long-Term Effects

[OBJECTIVE 6]

For a few days after a trip some users may experience moods that resemble those seen in episodes of melancholy and, less commonly, mania. When they occur, these changes only last a few days. A psychosis may result shortly after a trip in a small minority of users. These patients have hallucinations similar to those experienced during a trip, only now the patient believes they are real. This, too, usually lasts only a few days, although cases of longer duration have been reported.

When not using hallucinogens, up to a quarter of people who use these drugs have flashbacks—brief hallucinations similar to those seen during a trip. Many flashbacks last only a few seconds and may be as simple as a burst of color or shapes. Although some users may have chronic flashbacks over many years, most do not experience flashbacks more than a few weeks after use.

Differential Diagnosis

Differential diagnosis of hallucinogen intoxication includes the following:

- Dissociative intoxication
- ETOH intoxication
- MDMA intoxication
- ETOH withdrawal
- Excited delirium

Therapeutic Interventions

[OBJECTIVES 28, 29]

The most likely reason that someone using a hallucinogen may seek emergency medical attention is for a bad trip marked by fears of "going crazy." A bad trip generally can be managed by calming and comforting the patient. Reassure the patient that what is being experienced is caused by the hallucinogen and that the effects will go away. Trauma resulting from the impaired perception of hallucinogens is the other reason EMS is likely to be called and should be managed as usual.

PARAMEDIC Pearl

Permanent symptoms resulting from hallucinogen abuse are rare.

DISSOCIATIVES

[OBJECTIVE 16]

Description and Form

[OBJECTIVE 25]

Like hallucinogens, **dissociatives** distort perceptions of sight and sound, but they also cause feelings of detachment (dissociation) from the surroundings as well as the self. Phencyclidine (PCP) and ketamine are two often-abused dissociative drugs originally used as anesthetics (drugs that decrease or block sensation) (National Institute on Drug Abuse, 2001). PCP was developed in the 1950s as an IV anesthetic and was used in veterinary medicine. It was never approved for use in human beings because patients given it during clinical trials became combative and violent when waking up. In the 1970s a powdered form of PCP appeared on the streets known as *ozone, hog, rocket fuel, angel dust,* and *embalming fluid* (National Institute on Drug Abuse, 2001). In its purest form, PCP is a white powder. Most PCP sold on the streets today comes from clandestine laboratories and may be gummy and tan or brown from contaminants. Powdered PCP is sprinkled on tobacco, parsley, or marijuana and smoked (Joseph, 2005).

Ketamine was developed as an anesthetic to replace PCP in the early 1960s, but its use also was discontinued after similar reports of hallucinations. Children show much milder side effects when given ketamine, and it is sometimes used as an anesthetic agent during brief but painful procedures (Britt & McCance-Katz, 2005). Today ketamine is primarily used in veterinary medicine as an anesthetic for smaller animals such as cats and dogs. In fact, most ketamine sold on the street has been stolen from veterinary clinics and offices. When the fluid of the injectable solution is evaporated, a white powder remains. This is the form of ketamine usually seen on the streets and it is known as *K, special K, vitamin K, bump, cat Valium,* or *jet.* Ketamine is odorless, colorless, and easily mixed with alcoholic beverages; because it also has effects of sedation and amnesia, ketamine often is used to facilitate rape.

Dextromethorphan (d-3-methoxy-*N*-methylmorphine) is a cough suppressant with a similar molecular structure to the opiate codeine. It is found in many over-the-counter cough and cold preparations. Two common brands are Robitussin and Coricidin Cough and Cold, giving dextromethorphan the nicknames *robo, robotrippin, CCC,* or *triple C.* Dextromethorphan also is known as *DXM* (Haroz & Greenburg, 2005). In higher doses it causes dissociative effects similar to ketamine and PCP.

Epidemiology and Demographics

[OBJECTIVE 26]

Because the effects of PCP are highly unpredictable and often bizarre, its use has significantly declined after peaking in the 1970s and 1980s. Approximately 3% of the population (mostly male) of the United States has used PCP at least once. Between 1993 and 2003 the percentage of white PCP users decreased by half while the percentage of black PCP users doubled—to 54% (Drug and Alcohol Services Information System, 2005). Exact rates of ketamine and dextromethorphan abuse are difficult to find.

Routes and Pathophysiology

[OBJECTIVE 27]

PCP and ketamine can be injected IV, taken orally, snorted intranasally, or smoked with tobacco and marijuana. Ketamine is typically snorted and PCP smoked. Dextromethorphan is ingested orally in the form of cough medicine. Dissociative drugs act by affecting glutamate, a neurotransmitter in the brain involved in perception of pain, memory, and responses to the external environment (National Institute on Drug Abuse, 2001).

The effects of ketamine and PCP are felt within seconds to minutes depending on the route of administration. PCP is long acting, lasting for several hours (National Institute on Drug Abuse, 2001); the effects of ketamine have a much shorter duration, usually 30 to 45 minutes (Gahlinger, 2004). Because it is taken orally, dextromethorphan has a slower onset of action of 30 to 45 minutes, and its effects may last from 2 to 6 hours (Haroz & Greenburg, 2005).

Paraphernalia

[OBJECTIVE 6]

Abusers of ketamine may use a plastic intranasal inhaler known as a *bullet*. Indeed, this device is shaped like a bullet, with a vial in the base and a hole at the rounded end to deliver the drug. Between is a valvelike device that only allows a single dose, or bump, of ketamine to be inhaled at once.

Subjective Effects and Physical Findings

[OBJECTIVE 6]

In low doses PCP causes euphoria, agitation, violence, rage, and unpredictable behavior. As the dose increases, the user becomes unresponsive and may develop extension posturing or other muscle rigidity. PCP causes tachycardia and hypertension, which may increase to critical levels in patients who have taken high doses. Hyperthermia is common and body temperature may reach 108° F (Williams & Keyes, 2001). Effects of PCP are highly unpredictable and change each time a user takes it. One time an individual may have mild experiences of detachment and relaxation. The next time the person takes PCP, he or she may develop a psychosis characterized by insensitivity to pain and belief that he or she has superhuman strength and abilities. In this state PCP users are at extremely high risk for trauma and confrontations with others and law enforcement. Those under the influence of PCP may exhibit slurred speech, loss of coordination, a blank stare, or rapid and random eye movements (Joseph, 2005).

Low doses of ketamine produce a feeling of warmth and relaxation, sometimes called *K-land*. Higher doses of ketamine cause the user to enter a dreamlike state in which he or she may experience vivid hallucinations and visual distortions. Increasing amounts produce a power-ful dissociation, described by many to be like sitting at the bottom of a dark well, looking up and seeing a circle of light that is the rest of the world. This effect is known as a *K-hole* and often is described as a "near-death experience" (Britt & McCance-Katz, 2005). At extremely high doses ketamine produces unresponsiveness and amnesia. Ketamine also can decrease sensitivity to pain, so unintentional trauma is an issue. These effects are not nearly as strong as those seen with PCP. In addition, psychosis and rage are absent (Gahlinger, 2004). Unlike most anesthetics, PCP does not cause respiratory depression and actually excites the cardiovascular system (Joseph, 2005).

Most cough syrups contain approximately 3 mg of dextromethorphan per 1 mL; one 12-oz bottle of Robitussin contains 710 mg. At doses of 15 to 30 mg, up to three to four times daily, dextromethorphan acts on the brain to inhibit the coughing reflex. Dextromethorphan is abused at doses that range from 100 mg to 1500 mg. Effects increase with dose and include euphoria, altered perception of time, hallucinations (auditory and visual), and paranoia. At extremely high doses dextromethorphan causes tachycardia, diaphoresis, lethargy, muscle rigidity, and tremors. A person abusing dextromethorphan typically demonstrates slurred, garbled speech and a stiff, robotic walk (Haroz & Greenburg, 2005). Approximately 10% to 15% of whites metabolize dextromethorphan differently and experience only sedation and dysphoria with use.

The primary complication of dextromethorphan abuse comes from the consumption of large amounts of cold and cough preparations. These medications usually contain other ingredients, such as acetaminophen, diphenhydramine, and pseudoephedrine, which can cause significant problems. High doses of acetaminophen cause severe liver damage, diphenhydramine is associated with anticholinergic symptoms, and pseudoephedrine causes sympathomimetic effects. These other toxicities may dramatically increase the effects of dextromethorphan (Haroz & Greenburg, 2005).

Tolerance and Withdrawal

[OBJECTIVE 6]

Tolerance to and withdrawal from dissociatives is highly uncommon (Moore & Jefferson, 2004). Addiction and severe withdrawal symptoms have been reported in long-term ketamine users (Gahlinger, 2004). Dextromethorphan has a withdrawal syndrome characterized by craving, dysphoria, and sleep disturbances (Horaz, 2005).

Long-Term Effects

[OBJECTIVE 6]

Long-term use of dissociative drugs is associated with decreased memory, attention, and cognition (Britt & McCance-Katz, 2005). Users of ketamine may experience flashbacks similar to those seen with hallucinogen abuse (Gahlinger, 2004).

Differential Diagnosis

Differential diagnosis of dissociative intoxication includes the following:

- Hallucinogen abuse
- ETOH abuse
- MDMA abuse
- Psychosis
- Schizophrenia
- ETOH withdrawal

Therapeutic Interventions

[OBJECTIVES 28, 29]

Users of PCP can be extremely violent, irrational, and combative. They also may exhibit superhuman strength, and attempts to confront or restrain them can be quite dangerous. Excited delirium is a possibility in these patients and should be prevented. As opposed to patients intoxicated with hallucinogens, patients under the influence of PCP often cannot be talked down. In fact, these tactics can make violent and combative patients worse. Instead, PCP-related psychosis should be treated with physical and chemical restraint (Moore & Jefferson, 2004).

Users of dissociatives (including PCP) usually appear in a withdrawn, quiet state or as unresponsive. Ensure a patent airway and adequate ventilation with supplemental oxygen. Tachycardia and hypertension should resolve with calming of agitation, which can usually be talked down. In more extreme cases, benzodiazepines can be given as needed (Britt & McCance-Katz, 2005). Symptoms associated with ketamine usually resolve within 1 hour.

Patient and Family Education

The concentration and quality of PCP is frequently unknown and varies from sample to sample. PCP often is sold as or mixed with other drugs, including MDMA, ketamine, marijuana, and cocaine.

> **PARAMEDIC***Pearl*
>
> Dissociatives produce detachment (dissociation) between a user's mind, body, and environment.

CLANDESTINE LABORATORIES

[OBJECTIVE 30]

Many drugs, such as MDMA and methamphetamine, are synthesized in clandestine laboratories commonly known as *meth labs.* Methamphetamine is made from many common, legally purchased ingredients. Although the procedure is fairly lengthy, methamphetamines can be manufactured in many locations. In fact, the space inside a car trunk is large enough to accommodate a meth lab. Strong odors during synthesis make isolated locations preferred. Making methamphetamine is not easy, however. In addition to being caught, those operating labs run the risk of toxicity from the strong vapors produced. Many of these chemicals are highly flammable and burn for long periods at high temperatures. A meth lab is an extremely dangerous place and must be disassembled and decontaminated by personnel with hazardous materials training and equipment.

Most clandestine laboratories are located in inconspicuous places far away from other people. However, they have been found in car trunks, basements, sheds, and garages. Windows, if present, are painted over or covered with paper or foil. All labs contain large amounts of various chemicals, including camping fuel, solvents, rock salt, denatured or rubbing alcohol, iodine, muriatic acid, packages of over-the-counter drugs containing pseudoephedrine, and many others. Labels are usually covered or removed and chemicals often are transferred to different containers. Common equipment found in a clandestine lab includes heat-resistant cookware, canning jars, funnels, plastic soda bottles, plastic hoses, gasoline cans, and fans for ventilation. The most obvious sign of a meth lab is the strong chemical odors of acetone, ether, or ammonia. Meth labs often are said to have a strong smell of cat urine.

You are not likely to be dispatched to known clandestine labs, which are dangerous places associated with illness and injury. If you find yourself in a meth lab, you must quickly evacuate. Leave along the exact route you used to enter and do not touch anything inside; operators often booby trap their facilities. Do not attempt to stop any chemical reactions present by turning off heat sources or pouring out chemicals. Immediately move a safe distance away and request law enforcement and hazardous materials teams.

CLUB DRUGS AND DRUGS ABUSED FOR SEXUAL PURPOSES

[OBJECTIVE 16]

Club drugs is a term given to drugs that facilitate social interactions. MDMA (ecstasy) creates powerful feelings of empathy and love toward others. At lower doses ketamine and dextromethorphan cause stimulant effects and make users feel sociable. These drugs are frequently used in dance clubs, called *raves.* Raves often are single-concert events held in large, empty spaces such as warehouses or open fields. They are elaborate productions; the venue is typically garishly decorated and partygoers dress in colorful, coordinated outfits. The popularity of raves peaked around the beginning of the current decade. Law enforcement has become much more aware of their presence, dramatically decreasing the number of raves nationwide.

Drugs can be abused for sexual purposes in two ways: to increase the duration or pleasure of sex or to facilitate sexual assault. The heightened tactile stimulation associated with MDMA abuse highly increases sexual pleasure, but it may cause impotence. For this reason it often is combined with medications used to treat erectile dysfunction, such as sildenafil (Viagra), vardenafil (Levitra), and tadalafil (Cialis), to increase sexual stamina and erection duration. Methamphetamine's sexual effects (hypersexuality and decreased inhibitions) and its emotional effects (increased self-esteem and confidence) often are used to enhance erotic experiences. Its stimulant properties prolong and intensify sex. The drug is particularly popular among gay and bisexual men. Its use is associated with a higher rate of unprotected sex and higher risk of HIV infection (Halkitis et al., 2005). Nitrites, specific types of nonhydrocarbon inhalant drugs, can be taken at the point of sexual climax to heighten the pleasure of orgasm. The drugs also are known as *poppers* because they are typically packaged in small vials that are popped open when used. Nitrites are illegal in the United States but are common in Great Britain and Europe.

Agents used to facilitate sexual assault are typically CNS depressants that cause amnesia or profound unresponsiveness, such as ETOH, sedative-hypnotic drugs, and GHB. ETOH is most commonly associated with sexual assault, either by itself or in combination with other drugs. Drinking ETOH lowers inhibitions, leads to poor decision making, and can cause amnesia. The strong

taste of liquor drinks is often used to mask the taste of other agents. GHB has an unpleasant salty or soapy taste that is easily masked by alcoholic beverages. It is inexpensive and fairly available, and its effects are amplified by ETOH. Flunitrazepam (Rohypnol), also known as *roofies, rophie, roche,* and *forget-me,* is a benzodiazepine not currently sold in the United States but can be obtained from pharmacies across the Mexican border or by mail order. It is odorless and tasteless, making it particularly well suited for date rape. Other sedative-hypnotics, such as diazepam and midazolam, have been reported as being used for purposes of rape. Despite media focus on flunitrazepam, it is less commonly seen in the United States. However, "roofies" has become a generic term among the public for any pharmacologic agent used to facilitate rape.

A typical scenario of drug-facilitated sexual assault begins with the victim ingesting an altered alcoholic beverage that is bought by an unknown individual. Victims may awaken many hours later in unfamiliar surroundings, sometimes in a state of undress or partial dress. Memories of events that occurred during these hours often are spotty or not present at all (Scott-Ham & Burton, 2005). In cases of sexual assault, provide emotional support and attempt to preserve evidence but also assess and treat for potential adverse effects of these drugs.

Case Scenario SUMMARY

1. *What is your initial impression?* Your initial impression can include a variety of assessments, including psychiatric disorders and drug intoxication or overdose. Head or other trauma cannot be ruled out on initial arrival at the scene.

2. *What additional information do you need?* Additional information needed includes a SAMPLE history as well as a detailed evaluation of the patient's current condition.

3. *What sources can you use to obtain the necessary information?* Because the patient is uncommunicative, his medical history must be obtained from another source, including friends, family, or available medical records. Asking the police officer for information about the patient would help. The officer can contact relatives if available for appropriate medical history and current medication use.

4. *Has your initial impression changed?* The patient has no indication of accidental injury and his vital signs are within normal limits; thus his current condition is most likely medical or psychiatric in nature. A more thorough assessment is warranted.

5. *What do you think may be causing the man's motionless state?* The man's motionless state is typical of catatonia.

6. *What treatment options should you consider at this time?* Treatment options might include IV access and obtaining a glucose level to rule out a diabetic emergency as a possible cause of the patient's symptoms. However, you must consider these options carefully because you do not want to arouse the patient forcefully from his catatonic state.

7. *What is your final impression?* Based on the history obtained by the police officer and your assessment findings, your final impression is that the patient is in a catatonic state related to his psychiatric condition.

8. *What treatment options should be considered for this patient?* Treatment options based on the final assessment include quiet transportation to a receiving psychiatric facility.

9. *How should you prepare the man for transport?* In preparation to transport this patient, you should consider a calm, subdued approach. Be constantly alert for the potential of the patient's violently coming out of the

Continued

Case Scenario SUMMARY—continued

catatonic state. Depending on local laws and protocols, you may seriously consider placing the patient in physical restraints as a precaution. If the patient awakens and becomes violent, you, your partner, and the patient are at substantial risk for injury. With police assistance, place a backboard behind the patient and secure his arms and legs to the board with commercial cloth restraints, cravats, or roller gauze. Gently lean the backboard to a reclining position while the patient is in a supine position. Place the patient onto the stretcher and secure him with straps across his chest, hips, and thighs. Transport without emergency lights and siren unless the patient's condition worsens and such equipment is necessary.

Chapter Summary

- The most essential skill for dealing with behavioral emergencies is listening.
- "Normal" behavior is usually measured against the standards and expectations of society.
- A behavioral emergency results when a patient's ideas or actions are harmful or potentially harmful to himself or others.
- The majority of human emotional experience originates in the limbic system of the brain.
- Organic behavioral emergencies have biologic causes (e.g., stroke, hypoglycemia).
- Alterations in the concentrations or actions of neurotransmitters in the brain are linked to many psychiatric and substance abuse disorders.
- Psychosocial factors are life changes and events that may worsen psychiatric problems.
- Events during childhood help cause mental illness and are called *developmental factors*.
- The biopsychosocial concept of mental illness proposes that mental illnesses result from a complex interaction among biologic makeup, behavior, and a person's environment.
- For the majority of behavioral emergencies, such as a violent or suicidal patient, you should stage away from the scene and wait for law enforcement before entering.
- Careful study of a patient's residence and surroundings can yield important clues about his or her state of mind and illness.
- When interviewing a patient with a behavioral emergency, maintain a quiet, nonthreatening environment with equal, open access to exits for you and the patient.
- Do not be afraid to request bystanders, family, or friends to leave the scene or move the patient to your ambulance to create a private, quiet setting.
- Open-ended questions about how the patient has been feeling and acting yield the best results.
- Assess and treat all reports of pain or discomfort per local protocols; do not dismiss somatic complaints of patients with behavioral emergencies.
- Always suspect organic illness in patients with a sudden-onset behavioral emergency and no prior history.
- Perform a neurologic examination as well as a detailed interview in all patients with behavioral emergencies.
- Speech patterns and mannerisms can be assessed to learn more about a patient's form of thought, specifically rate of speech and looseness of associations.
- Psychosis is a state of highly distorted perceptions of reality with hallucinations and delusions.
- A hallucination is false sensory information that originates within the brain; a delusion is a false perception or interpretation of events and situations.
- Preoccupations are ideas that consistently and constantly return to a patient's mind.
- Affect is the outward expression of a patient's emotions as observed and described by the interviewer.
- Mood is the dominant, sustained emotional state of a patient and is the lens through which he or she sees the world.
- Affect can be thought of as emotional weather that fluctuates around mood, the emotional climate.
- Dysphoria is an extremely depressed, low mood; euphoria is an exaggerated feeling of joy and happiness.
- Schizophrenia is a neurologic illness marked by psychotic symptoms, disorders of thought, and a decrease of social interactions.
- Anhedonia is defined as the lack of enjoyment of activities and people a patient used to find pleasurable.
- Long-term use of antipsychotic medications often leads to tardive dyskinesia, a neurologic disorder characterized by involuntary movements of the mouth and face.
- Mood runs a continuum from melancholy at the low end and mania at the high end.
- Dysthymia is a chronic, constant, low-grade depression.
- Patients who have melancholic episodes only are said to have unipolar depression, whereas patients whose melancholic episodes alternate with hypomania, mania, or mixed episodes have bipolar disorder.

- Cyclothymia is a lesser form of bipolar disorder.
- Fear is the physical and emotional reaction to a real or perceived threat; anxiety is apprehension and worry about a future event.
- Panic attacks are sudden, severe, paralyzing anxiety reactions.
- Phobias are intense fears of specific objects or situations.
- Excessive, persistent worrying about everyday events is termed *generalized anxiety disorder.*
- Episodes of vivid, disturbing memories and dreams alternating with periods of emotional numbness after a traumatic event define posttraumatic stress disorder.
- Obsessive-compulsive disorder consists of unwanted, intrusive ideas (obsessions) and specific, repetitive rituals that the patient feels he or she must perform (compulsions).
- Somatoform disorders are characterized by abnormal preoccupations with the body and physical symptoms.
- Patients with factitious disorder intentionally produce signs and symptoms of an illness to assume the sick role.
- Faking an illness for a tangible gain is called *malingering.*
- Patients with anorexia nervosa consistently see themselves as overweight, take drastic measures to become thin, and have strange behaviors and rituals associated with food and eating.
- Eating large amounts of food in one setting (binging) and then forcing oneself to vomit or use laxatives (purging) to avoid gaining weight is characteristic of bulimia.
- Personality disorders are abnormal and damaging ways of thinking about and interacting with the world that are always present.
- Three groupings of personality disorders exist: odd and eccentric disorders (cluster A), emotional and dramatic disorders (cluster B), and anxious and fearful disorders (cluster C).
- Suicide is the act of ending one's own life. Thoughts of suicide are called *suicidal ideations,* and unsuccessful tries to end one's own life are known as *suicide attempts.*
- Cutting, burning, or hurting oneself is known as self-injury and is an unhealthy coping mechanism for overwhelming and troubling emotions.
- To care for behavioral patients, you must move out of a mindset characterized by invasive procedures and drugs and into one of observation, evaluation, and emotional support.
- Stop violent situations by preventing them.
- Physical and chemical restraints are last resorts used only to prevent the patient from harming himself or others.
- Patient restraint carries medical, legal, and ethical risks.
- Patients should never be restrained in the prone position and should never be transported while handcuffed.
- Chemical restraint should be used after physical restraint to prevent continued struggling and the development of excited delirium.
- Restraint asphyxia results from an inability to expand the chest cavity and create a negative pressure for inspiration.
- Using a substance for any reason other than its approved, accepted purpose is known as *abuse.*
- Addiction, or dependence, is an uncontrollable need to use a substance despite negative consequences.
- Long-term use of a drug makes its receptors in the brain less sensitive, forcing users to take more of the substance to achieve the same effects, known as *tolerance.*
- Withdrawal symptoms result when a patient abruptly stops using a drug after his or her body has adapted to its constant presence.
- Those who abuse drugs rarely only choose one; poly-substance abuse and overdose are common, making assessment and treatment difficult.
- The intoxicating agent in alcoholic beverages such as wine, beer, and liquor is called ETOH.
- Stimulant drugs such as cocaine, methamphetamine, and MDMA are highly addictive and carry high risks of side effects and withdrawal syndromes.
- Excited delirium can produce wildly abnormal behavior characterized by aggression, paranoia, hyperthermia, superhuman strength, and insensitivity to pain.
- Excited delirium is related to the use of stimulant drugs and often ends in sudden death.
- Drugs that relax, relieve anxiety, and/or induce sleep are called *sedative-hypnotics.*
- Opioids are powerful pain-killing drugs with a high potential for abuse and addiction.
- Sedative-hypnotics, GHB, ketamine, and ETOH are used separately or together to facilitate sexual assault.
- Marijuana is the dried and shredded leaves, stems, and seeds of the hemp plant, which is smoked or eaten to cause euphoria and relaxation.
- Abuse of inhalants causes a rush of euphoria of short duration and is most common among older children and teenagers.
- Hallucinogens, such as LSD, psilocybin mushrooms, peyote, and mescaline, cause hallucinations and distort perceptions of reality.
- Dissociatives, such as ketamine, PCP, and dextromethorphan, create a feeling of detachment (dissociation) of the mind, body, and the user's surroundings.

REFERENCES

Abraham, G., & Hardi, D. (2005). Self-mutilation: Inward pain turned inside out. *School Nurse News, 22*(2), 28-31.

American Academy of Pediatrics. (1996). Inhalant abuse. *Pediatrics, 97*(3), 420-423.

American Psychiatric Association. (2000). *Diagnostic and statistical manual of mental disorders* (4th ed.). Washington, DC: American Psychiatric Association.

Anderson, C. E., & Loomis, G. A. (2003). Recognition and prevention of inhalant abuse. *American Family Physician, 68*(5), 869-874.

Annas, G. J. (1999). The use of physical restraints during emergencies. *The New England Journal of Medicine, 241*(18), 1408-1412.

Aronson, S. C. (2005). *Depression.* Retrieved November 12, 2005, from http://www.emedicine.com.

Brasic, J. R. (2005). *Tardive dyskinesia.* Retrieved October 16, 2005, from http://www.emedicine.com.

Britt, G. C., & McCance-Katz, E. F. (2005). A brief overview of the clinical pharmacology of "club drugs." *Substance Use and Misuse, 40,* 1189-1201.

Callaway, E. (2004). *Dysthymic disorder.* Retrieved November 12, 2005, from http://www.emedicine.com.

Cameron, S. (2004). *Hallucinogens.* Retrieved December 21, 2005, http://www.emedicine.com.

Carlat, D. J. (2005). *The Psychiatric Interview* (2nd ed.). Philadelphia: Lippincott Williams and Wilkins.

Chiang, W. K. (2002). Amphetamines. In L. R. Goldfrank et al. (Eds.). *Goldfrank's toxicologic emergencies* (7th ed.). New York: McGraw-Hill.

Clark, H. W., McClanahan, T., Kanas, N., Smith, D., & Landry, M. J. (2000). Substance-related disorders: Alcohol and drugs. In H. H. Goldman (Ed.). *Review of general psychiatry* (5th ed.). New York: McGraw-Hill.

Cooper, J. S. (2005). *Toxicity, sedative-hypnotics.* Retrieved January 6, 2006, from http://www.emedicine.com.

Daly, R. C. (2004). *Cannabis compound abuse.* Retrieved December 21, 2005, from http://www.emedicine.com.

Drug and Alcohol Services Information System. (2005). *Trends in admissions for PCP: 1993-2003.* Arlington, VA: Substance Abuse and Mental Health Services Administration.

Egland, A. G. (2005). *Toxicity, ethanol.* Retrieved November 11, 2005, from http://www.emedicine.com.

Eisendrath, S. J., & Guillermo, G. G. (2000). Factitious disorders. In H. H. Goldman (Ed.). *Review of general psychiatry* (5th ed.). New York: McGraw-Hill.

Frankenberg, F. R. (2005). *Schizophrenia.* Retrieved December 17, 2005, from http://www.emedicine.com.

Gahlinger, P. M. (2004). Club drugs: MDMA, gamma-hydroxybutyrate (GHB), rohypnol and ketamine. *American Family Physician, 69*(11), 2619-2626.

Giese, A. A. (2001). Personality disorders. In J. L. Jacobson, A. M. Jacobson (Eds.). *Psychiatric secrets* (2nd ed.). Philadelphia: Hanley & Belfus.

Gossman, W. (2005). *Delirium tremens.* Retrieved November 11, 2005, from http://www.emedicine.com.

Greer, S., Chambliss, L., & Mackler, L. (2005). What physical exam techniques are useful to detect malingering? *Journal of Family Practice, 54*(8), 719-722.

Greist, J. H., & Jefferson, J. W. (2000). Anxiety disorders. In H. H. Goldman (Ed.). *Review of general psychiatry* (5th ed.). New York: McGraw-Hill.

Grieger, T. A., Waldrep, D. A., Lovasz, M. M., & Ursano, R. J. (2005). Follow-up of Pentagon employees two years after the terrorist attack of September 11, 2001. *Psychiatry Services, 56*(11), 1374-1378.

Halkitis, P. N., Fischgrund, B. N., & Parsons, J. T. (2005). Explanations for methamphetamine use among gay and bisexual men in New York City. *Substance Use and Misuse, 40,* 1331-1345.

Hamilton, R. J. (2002). Substance withdrawal. In R. Goldfrank et al. (Eds.). *Goldfrank's toxicologic emergencies* (7th ed.). New York: McGraw-Hill.

Haroz, R., & Greenberg, M. I. (2005). Emerging drugs of abuse. *Medical Clinics of America, 89*(6), 1259-1276.

Hasin, D. S., Goodwin, R. D., Stinson, F. S., & Grant, B. F. (2005). Epidemiology of major depressive disorder. *Archives of General Psychiatry, 62,* 1097-1106.

Hawton, K., Arensman, E., Townsend, E., Bremner, S., Feldman, E., Goldney, R., et al. (1998). Deliberate self harm: Systematic review of efficacy of psychosocial and pharmacological treatments in preventing repetition. *British Medical Journal, 317*(7156), 441-447.

Hayes, V. M. (2005). Self-inflicted harm is not an indication of suicidal behavior. *American Family Physician, 72*(7), 1172.

Hollander, J. E., & Hoffman, R. S. (2002). Cocaine. In R. Goldfrank et al. (Eds.). *Goldfrank's toxicologic emergencies* (7th ed.). New York: McGraw-Hill.

Jacobson, J. L., & Jacobson, A. M. (2001). *Psychiatric secrets* (2nd ed.). Philadelphia: Hanley & Belfus.

Jain, A. (2004). *Withdrawal syndromes.* Retrieved November 11, 2005, from http://www.emedicine.com.

Joseph, D. E. (2005). *Drugs of abuse.* Washington, DC: U.S. Department of Justice.

Kluger, J. (2005). The cruelest cut: Often it's the one teens inflict on themselves. *Time, 165*(20), 48.

Kochanek, K. D., Murphy, S. L., Anderson, R. N., & Scott, C. (2005). Deaths: Final data for 2002. *National Vital Statistics Reports, 53*(5), 2, 10.

Kupas, D. F., & Wydro, G. C. (2002). Patient restraint in emergency medical services systems. *Prehospital Emergency Care, 6*(3), 340-345.

Linakas, J. (2004). *Toxicity, lithium.* Retrieved December 5, 2005, from http://www.emedicine.com.

Loewenstein, R. J., McKay, S., & Purcell, S. D. (2000). Somatoform and dissociative disorders. In H. H. Goldman (Ed.). *Review of general psychiatry* (5th ed.). New York: McGraw-Hill.

Loyola Emergency Medical Services System. (2005). *An EMS approach to behavioral emergencies.* Retrieved February 26, 2006, from http://www.loyolaems.com.

Marmar, C. R. (2000). Personality disorders. In H. H. Goldman (Ed.). *Review of general psychiatry* (5th ed.). New York: McGraw-Hill.

Marx, J. A. (Ed.). (2002). *Rosen's emergency medicine: Concepts and clinical practice* (5th ed.). St. Louis: Mosby.

Mets, B., Jamdar, S., & Landry, D. (1996). The role of catecholamines in cocaine toxicity: A model for cocaine "sudden death." *Life Sciences, 59*(24), 2021-2031.

Mittenberg, W., Patton, C., Canyock, F. M., & Condit, D. C. (2002). Base rates of malingering and symptom exaggeration. *Journal of Clinical Experimental Neuropsychology, 24*(8), 1094-1102.

Moore, D. P., & Jefferson, J. W. (2004). *Handbook of medical psychiatry* (2nd ed.). Philadelphia: Mosby Elsevier.

Nock, M. K., & Prinstein, M. J. (2005). Contextual features and behavioral functions of self-mutilation among adolescents. *Journal of Abnormal Psychology, 114*(1), 140-146.

National Institute on Drug Abuse. (2001). *Hallucinogens and dissociative drugs.* Washington, DC: National Institutes of Health.

National Institute on Drug Abuse. (2002). *Methamphetamine abuse and addiction.* Washington, DC: National Institutes of Health.

National Institute on Drug Abuse. (2004). *Cocaine abuse and addiction.* Washington, DC: National Institutes of Health.

National Institute on Drug Abuse. (2005a). *Heroin abuse and addiction.* Washington, DC: National Institutes of Health.

National Institute on Drug Abuse. (2005b). *Marijuana abuse.* Washington, DC: National Institutes of Health.

National Institute on Drug Abuse. (2005c). *Prescription drugs: Abuse and addiction.* Washington, DC: National Institutes of Health.

Nelson, L. S. (2000). Opioids. In R. Goldfrank et al. (Eds.). *Goldfrank's toxicologic emergencies* (7th ed.). New York: McGraw-Hill.

Norman, K. (2000). Eating disorders. In H. H. Goldman (Ed.). *Review of general psychiatry* (5th ed.). New York: McGraw-Hill.

Otten, E. J. (2000). Marijuana. In R. Goldfrank et al. (Eds.). *Goldfrank's toxicologic emergencies* (7th ed.). New York: McGraw-Hill.

Paquette, M. (2003). Excited delirium: Does it exist? *Perspectives in Psychiatric Care, 39*(3), 93-94.

Paris, J. (2005a). Borderline personality disorder. *Canadian Medical Association Journal, 172*(12), 1579-1583.

Paris, J. (2005b). Understanding self-mutilation in borderline personality disorder. *Harvard Review of Psychiatry, 13,* 179-185.

Petronic-Rosic, V. (2005). Self-mutilation: An addictive, contagious, and easily spotted cry for help. *SKINmed, 4*(3), 136-137.

Ramachandran, V. S. (1998). *Phantoms in the brain: Probing the mysteries of the human mind.* New York: HarperCollins.

Reus, V. (2000). Mood disorders. In H. H. Goldman (Ed.). *Review of general psychiatry* (5th ed.). New York: McGraw-Hill.

Richards, J. R., Derlet, R. W., & Duncan, D. R. (1998). Chemical restraint for the agitated patient in the emergency department: Lorazepam versus droperidol. *The Journal of Emergency Medicine, 16*(4), 567-573.

Rossow, I., Groholt, B., & Wichstrem, L. (2005). Intoxicants and suicidal behavior among adolescents: Changes in levels and associations from 1992 to 2002. *Addiction, 100,* 79-88.

Salen, P. (2001). *Wernicke encephalopathy.* Retrieved November 11, 2005, from http://www.emedicine.com.

Scott-Ham, M., & Burton, F. C. (2005). Toxicological findings in cases of alleged drug-facilitated sexual assault in the United Kingdom over a 3-year period. *Journal of Clinical Forensic Medicine, 12*(4), 175-186.

Soreff, S. (2004). *Bipolar affective disorder.* Retrieved December 4, 2005, from http://www.emedicine.com.

Stratton, S. J., Rogers, C., Brickett, K., & Gruzinski, G. (2001). Factors associated with sudden death of individuals requiring restraint for excited delirium. *American Journal of Emergency Medicine, 19*(3), 187-191.

Stratton, S. J., Rogers, C., & Green, K. (1995). Sudden death in individuals in hobble restraints during paramedic transport. *Annals of Emergency Medicine, 25*(5), 710-712.

Substance Abuse and Mental Health Services Administration. (2004). *The national survey on drug use and health.* Rockville, MD: U.S. Department of Health and Human Services.

Sue, D., Sue, D. W., & Sue, S. (2002). *Understanding abnormal behavior.* Boston: Houghton-Mifflin.

Tintinalli, J. E. (1993). Violent patients and the prehospital provider. *Annals of Emergency Medicine, 22,* 1276-1279.

Whybrow, P. (1997). *A mood apart: The thinker's guide to mood and its disorders.* New York: Harper-Collins.

Williams, L. C., & Keyes, C. (2001). Psychoactive drugs. In M. D. Ford, et al. (Eds.). *Clinical toxicology.* St. Louis, Saunders.

Wilson, K. C., & Saukkonen, J. J. (2004). Acute respiratory failure from abused substances. *Journal of Intensive Care Medicine, 19*(4), 183-193.

Wu, L. T., Pilowsky, D. J., & Schlenger, W. E. (2004). Inhalant abuse and dependence among adolescents in the United States. *Journal of the American Academy of Child and Adolescent Psychiatry, 43*(10), 1206-1214.

Yates, W. R. (2005). *Anxiety disorders.* Retrieved December 12, 2005, from http://www.emedicine.com.

Yew, D. (2005). *Toxicity, MDMA.* Retrieved October 16, 2005, from http://www.emedicine.com.

Yip, L. (2002). Alcohols and drugs of abuse. In R. Goldfrank et al. (Eds.). *Goldfrank's toxicologic emergencies* (7th ed.). New York: McGraw-Hill.

Yip, L., Mashhood, A., & Naudé, S. (2005). Low IQ and gasoline huffing: The perpetuation cycle. *American Journal of Psychiatry, 162*(5), 1020-1021.

SUGGESTED RESOURCES

Erowid: http://www.erowid.org
The Good Drugs Guide: http://www.thegooddrugsguide.com
Miller, C. D.: http://www.charlydmiller.com/index.html
Jamison, K. R. (1997). *An unquiet mind: A memoir of moods and madness.* New York: Vintage.
Jamison, K. R. (2000). *Night falls fast: Understanding suicide.* New York: Vintage.
National Institute on Drug Abuse: http://www.drugabuse.gov

Psych Central: http://www.psychcentral.com
The Virtual Psychology Classroom at AllPsych Online: http://www.allpsych.com.
Walton, S. C. (2001). *Get the dope on dope: First response guide to street drugs* (vol. 1, 2nd ed.) Calgary, AB: Burnand Holding Co. Ltd.
Whybrow, P. (1998). *A mood apart: The thinker's guide to mood and its disorders.* New York: Harper-Collins.

Chapter Quiz

1. Which of these parts of the brain is not part of the limbic system?
  a. Amygdala
  b. Cerebellum
  c. Hippocampus
  d. Thalamus

2. Which of the following is an example of an organic etiology?
  a. Amnesia caused by a stroke
  b. Development of borderline personality disorder as a result of childhood abuse
  c. Onset of an episode of melancholy after the recent loss of a job
  d. Pressured speech from a manic episode

3. You respond to the home of a 28-year-old woman who is reported to be "not acting right." On your arrival, you hear shouting inside the door and sounds of a struggle. The best action is to _____.
  a. call for law enforcement and wait in the yard
  b. knock loudly, shouting "EMS, open up!"
  c. leave the scene immediately and wait for law enforcement to clear the scene before reentering
  d. quickly open the door and surprise the occupants, giving you the advantage to control the situation

4. Tardive dyskinesia is a condition resulting from long-term _____.
  a. antidepressant medication therapy
  b. antipsychotic medication therapy
  c. electroshock therapy
  d. schizophrenia

5. The opposite of melancholy is _____.
  a. cyclothymia
  b. dysthymia
  c. hypomania
  d. mania

6. A patient who was raped 6 months ago reports that she has been having terrible nightmares and periods of reliving the experience. In between these episodes, she says that she feels emotionally "numb." This patient is most likely suffering from _____.
  a. agoraphobia
  b. bipolar disorder
  c. delusions
  d. PTSD

Chapter Quiz—continued

7. A 19-year-old patient in police custody is reporting shortness of breath. After evaluation and transport by you and your crew and a lengthy evaluation at the emergency department, she admits that she never actually felt short of breath but only wanted to avoid going to jail. This is an example of _____.
 a. conversion disorder
 b. factitious disorder
 c. malingering
 d. somatization disorder

8. A 16-year-old male patient complains of abdominal pain. He appears frail and thin yet seems to have substantial energy. His mother states that he has not been eating very much for weeks and has been exercising constantly. This presentation is most likely related to which of the following?
 a. Anorexia nervosa
 b. Body dysmorphic disorder
 c. Bulimia nervosa
 d. Marijuana use

9. You respond to the home of a 47-year-old man who is "out of his head." On your arrival he is pacing back and forth, mumbling incoherently. When you try to talk to him, he becomes very agitated and yells for you to leave him alone. You are unable to obtain any information from him, but you think he may be violent. Medical control orders you to transport the patient involuntarily to the hospital for psychiatric evaluation. Which of the following steps is appropriate?
 a. Ensure you have at least three team members: one for the head, one for the arms, and one for the legs.
 b. Have your partner attempt to distract the patient while you sneak up behind him and inject intramuscular haloperidol to calm him down.
 c. Restrain the patient to a long backboard for ease of transfer and transportation.
 d. Tie the patient's hands behind his back and his feet to the stretcher and transport rapidly.

10. Which of the following is inappropriate to use for chemical restraint?
 a. Succinylcholine (Anectine)
 b. Droperidol (Inapsine)
 c. Haloperidol (Haldol)
 d. Midazolam (Versed)

11. All the following are potential long-term consequences of alcohol abuse except _____.
 a. alcoholism
 b. DT
 c. dystonic reaction
 d. Wernicke-Korsakoff syndrome

12. Most MDMA-related deaths result from _____.
 a. an overdose, leading to myocardial rupture
 b. cerebral atrophy
 c. contaminated pills
 d. hyperthermia and dehydration

13. The most effective prevention of death from excited delirium is probably _____.
 a. administering 100 mg thiamine IV
 b. chemically restraining patients who are physically restrained yet continue to struggle
 c. fanning and pouring water over the patient to prevent overheating
 d. limiting communication with the patient and ignoring complaints until he calms down

14. What is a dissociative?
 a. A drug that causes hallucinations
 b. A drug that decreases the connection between mind and body
 c. A drug that is illegal and not approved for use
 d. A drug that may cause toxicity in very small quantities

15. You respond to the home of a 30-year-old woman reporting substernal chest pain after snorting cocaine 3 hours ago. A 12-lead ECG shows nonspecific ST changes throughout all leads. The most appropriate treatment order for this patient is _____.
 a. oxygen, aspirin, and fluid bolus of 10 mL/kg of an isotonic crystalloid
 b. oxygen, diazepam, aspirin, nitroglycerin, and morphine
 c. oxygen, fluid bolus of 20 mL/kg of an isotonic crystalloid, and diazepam
 d. oxygen, nitroglycerin, diazepam, and morphine

16. You are trying to comfort a 15-year-old boy who ingested LSD 5 hours ago and is having a bad trip. The patient tells you that he feels like the floor he is sitting on is swallowing him whole and that he thinks he is going crazy. The best course of actions is to ___.
 a. blindfold the patient so that he cannot see anything to fear
 b. reassure him that what he is experiencing is caused by the drug and eventually will pass
 c. remind him that LSD can cause bizarre hallucinations and that what he is experiencing is his fault
 d. tell him to move to the ceramic tile flooring because it is hard and will not let him sink

17. You are dispatched for a "man down" inside a residence. On your arrival you find an approximately 20-year-old woman lying supine on the floor with a respiratory rate of approximately 6 breaths/min. She is unresponsive to painful stimuli and her pupils are pinpoint and nonreactive. Of the following, the most likely cause of this patient's condition is _____.
 a. cocaine toxicity
 b. ETOH toxicity
 c. GHB toxicity
 d. heroin toxicity

18. Of the following, which is the most appropriate treatment for the patient in question 17?
    a. Insert nasopharyngeal airway, ventilate the lungs with 100% oxygen, and administer 1 mg atropine IV or intramuscularly.
    b. Insert nasopharyngeal airway, ventilate the lungs with 100% oxygen, and administer 1 mg naloxone IV or intramuscularly.
    c. Insert oropharyngeal airway, ventilate the lungs with 100% oxygen, and prepare to intubate.
    d. Orally intubate patient and administer 1 mg naloxone by endo-tracheal tube.

19. You are treating a 24-year-old woman who became unconscious while at a dance club. The patient's friend informs you that they had just arrived at the club an hour ago and that the patient has only had three alcoholic beverages all night and that the patient does not use any illegal drugs. The patient is unresponsive, even to deep painful stimuli. Of the following, which is the most likely explanation for this patient's condition?
    a. Cocaine toxicity
    b. ETOH toxicity
    c. GHB toxicity
    d. Marijuana toxicity

20. You respond to assist a 12-year-old girl with altered mental status and no medical history. Her friends tell you that they were all watching TV when the patient "looked sleepy and then wouldn't wake up." You notice a rash around the patient's mouth and smell a strong chemical odor on her breath. The most likely cause of this patient's condition is _____.
    a. a seizure
    b. ETOH abuse
    c. inhalant abuse
    d. marijuana abuse

Terminology

Abuse Use of a substance for other than its approved, accepted purpose or in a greater amount than prescribed.

Addiction A pattern of compulsive seeking of a substance and an uncontrollable need to use that becomes more important than almost everything else in a person's life.

Affect The observable, dominant outward expression of emotion.

Agoraphobia Consistent anxiety and avoidance of places and situations where escape during a panic attack would be difficult or embarrassing.

Alcoholism Addiction and dependence on ETOH; often develops over many years.

Amygdala Almond-shaped structure at the end of each hippocampus that attaches emotional significance to incoming stimuli; has a large role in the fear response (plural, *amygdale*).

Anhedonia Lack of enjoyment in activities one used to find pleasurable.

Anorexia nervosa Eating disorder characterized by a preoccupation that one is obese; drastic, intentional weight loss; and bizarre attitudes and rituals associated with food and exercise.

Anxiety The sometimes vague feeling of apprehension, uneasiness, dread, or worry that often occurs without a specific source or identified cause; also a normal response to a perceived threat.

Behavior The conduct and activity of a person that is observable by others.

Behavioral emergency Actions or ideations by the patient that are harmful or potentially harmful to the patient or others.

Bipolar disorder An illness of extremes of mood, alternating between periods of depression and episodes of mania (type I) or hypomania (type II).

Blood alcohol content (BAC) Milligrams of ETOH per deciliter of blood divided by 100; a fairly standard measure of how intoxicated a person is.

Borderline personality disorder Cluster B disorder marked by unstable emotions, relationships, and attitudes.

Bulimia nervosa Eating disorder consisting of a pattern of eating large amounts of food in one sitting (binging) and then forcing oneself to regurgitate (purging), with associated guilt and depression.

Catalepsy Abnormal state characterized by a trancelike level of consciousness and postural rigidity; occurs in hypnosis and in certain organic and psychological disorders such as schizophrenia, epilepsy, and hysteria.

Catatonia A state of psychologically induced immobility with muscular rigidity, at times interrupted by agitation.

Catatonic schizophrenia A form of schizophrenia characterized by alternating periods of extreme withdrawal and extreme excitement. During the withdrawal stage stupor, waxy flexibility, muscular rigidity, mutism, blocking, negativism, and catalepsy

Terminology—continued

may be seen; during the period of excitement, purposeless and impulsive activity may range from mild agitation to violence. See *Catatonia*.

Circumstantial thinking Adding detours and extra details to conversations but eventually returning to the main topic.

Cluster A personality disorders Odd and eccentric type of personality disorders, including paranoid, schizoid, and schizotypal; characterized by social isolation and odd thought processes.

Cluster B personality disorders Emotional and dramatic type of personality disorders, including histrionic, borderline, antisocial, and narcissistic; characterized by impulsive, unpredictable behavior and manipulation of others.

Cluster C personality disorders Anxious and fearful type of personality disorders, including avoidant, dependent, and compulsive; marked by anxiety, shyness, and avoidance of conflict.

Cocaine hydrochloride Fine, white powdered form of cocaine, a powerful CNS stimulant; typically snorted intranasally.

Constricted affect Emotion shown in degrees less than expected.

Crack cocaine Solid, brownish-white crystal form of cocaine, a powerful CNS stimulant; typically smoked.

Cyclothymia A less-severe form of bipolar disorder marked by more frequently alternating periods of a dysphoric mood that does not meet the criteria for depression and hypomania.

Delirium tremens (DT) The most severe form of ETOH withdrawal, including hallucinations, delusions, confusion, and seizures.

Delusions False perceptions and interpretations of situations and events that a person believes to be true no matter how convincing evidence is to the contrary.

Delusions of reference A belief that ordinary events have a special, often dangerous, meaning to the self.

Depersonalization A sudden sense of the loss of one's identity.

Derealization A sudden feeling that one's surroundings are not real, as if one is watching a movie or television, not reality.

Disorganized schizophrenia A subtype of schizophrenia characterized by an earlier age of onset, usually at puberty, and a more severe disintegration of personality than occurs in other forms of the disease; symptoms include incoherence, loose associations, gross disorganization or behavior, and flat or inappropriate affect.

Dissociatives Substances that cause feelings of detachment (dissociation) from one's surroundings

and self; includes PCP, ketamine, and dextromethorphan.

Dysphoric mood (dysphoria) An unpleasant emotional state characterized by sadness, irritability, or depression.

Dysthymia A constant, chronic, low-grade form of depression.

Ecstasy (MDMA) A synthetic, hallucinogenic stimulant drug similar to both methamphetamine and mescaline.

Elevated mood (euphoria) Exaggerated sense of happiness and joy; a feeling of being on top of the world.

Ethanol (ETOH) Colorless, odorless alcohol found in alcoholic beverages such as beer, wine, and liquor.

Euthymic mood A normal, baseline emotional state.

Excited delirium Acute and sudden agitation, paranoia, aggression, hyperthermia, dramatically increased strength, and decreased sensitivity to pain related to long-term use of stimulant drugs; often ends in sudden death.

Factitious disorder Condition in which patients intentionally produce signs and symptoms of illness to assume the sick role.

Fear Physical and emotional reaction to a real or perceived threat.

Flat affect A complete or near-complete lack of emotion.

Flight of ideas Moving quickly from topic to topic during conversation but without any connection or transition.

Form of thought Ability to process information and create logical, flowing ideas.

Gamma-hydroxybutyrate (GHB) A drug structurally related to the neurotransmitter GABA, usually dissolved in liquid, that causes profound CNS depression.

Generalized anxiety disorder (GAD) Condition characterized by excessive worries about everyday life.

Grandiose delusions Dramatically inflated perceptions of one's own worth, power, or knowledge.

Hallucinations False sensory perceptions that originate within the brain.

Hallucinogens Substance that cause hallucinations and intense distortions and perceptions of reality; includes LSD, psilocybin mushrooms, peyote, and mescaline.

Heroin (diacetylmorphine) The most popular, powerful, and addictive member of the opioids.

Hippocampi Structures within the limbic system that filter incoming information, determine what stimuli is important, and commit the experiences to memory.

Hydrocarbons The psychoactive ingredient in many abused inhalants.

Hypomania An episode of a lesser form of mania that may transition into mania or alternate with depression.

Hypothalamus Small structure at the front of the limbic system that controls most of the body's housekeeping functions, such as temperature, blood pressure, thirst, and hunger; also forms the interface between the nervous system and the endocrine system.

Inhalants Substances such as aerosols, fuels, paints, and other chemicals that produce fumes at room temperature; they are breathed in, producing a high.

Intense affect Heated and passionate emotional responses.

Labile Affect that changes frequently and rapidly.

Limbic system The emotional brain; a group of structures deep within the brain that controls motivation and emotion.

Looseness of associations Going off track during conversation to varying degrees.

LSD (lysergic acid diethylamide) A powerful synthetic hallucinogen, often called acid and found on small squares of blotter paper.

Malingering Faking illness for a tangible gain (e.g., missing work, avoiding incarceration).

Mania An episode of euphoric mood characterized by very high self-esteem, seemingly limitless energy, and impaired judgment.

Marijuana Dried mixture of shredded leaves, stems, and seeds of the hemp plant that are usually smoked and contain many psychoactive compounds, most notably THC.

Melancholy An episode of dysphoric mood with disruptions of homeostasis, including alterations in appetite, activities, and sleep patterns; also called *major* or *severe depression*.

Methamphetamine A powerful, highly addictive CNS stimulant found in either a white powder form or a clear crystal form (crystal meth).

Mixed episode A period of manic-like energy and agitation coupled with the pessimism and dysphoria of severe depression.

Mood The dominant and sustained emotional state of a patient; the emotional lens through which a patient views the world.

Mutism A condition in which a person will not speak.

Obsessive-compulsive disorder (OCD) An anxiety disorder marked by frequent, intrusive, unwanted, and bothersome thoughts (obsessions) and repetitive rituals (compulsions).

Open-ended questions A form of an interview question that allows a patient to respond in narrative form to answer in his or her own way and provide details and information believed to be important.

Opioids Powerful pain-relieving drugs derived from the seed pods of the poppy plant or drugs that are similar in molecular structure.

Organic An etiology of an illness that stems from a biologic cause, such as a stroke or electrolyte imbalance.

Panic attack A sudden, paralyzing anxiety reaction characterized by an overwhelming sense of fear, anxiety, and impending doom, often with physical symptoms such as chest pain and difficulty breathing.

Paranoid delusions False perceptions of persecution and the feeling that one is being hunted or conspired against; this is the most common type of delusion.

Paranoid schizophrenia A form of schizophrenia characterized by persistent preoccupation with illogical, absurd, and changeable delusions, usually of a persecutory, grandiose, or jealous nature, accompanied by related hallucinations.

Personality disorders Patterns of interacting with others and the world that are rigid and harmful, causing social and occupational problems.

Phobia An intense fear of a particular object or situation.

Posttraumatic stress disorder (PTSD) An anxiety disorder that occurs after a traumatic, often life-threatening event.

Posture A patient's overall attitude and frame of mind.

Poverty of speech A disorder of thought form characterized by very little spontaneous, voluntary speech and short answers to questions.

Preoccupations Unwanted ideas that consistently and constantly dominate a person's thoughts.

Pressured speech Rapid, loud, and intense speech that often results from racing thoughts and is frequently seen during manic episodes.

Psychomotor agitation Excessive motor activity that is usually nonproductive and tedious, resulting from inner tensions (pacing, fidgeting, hand wringing, etc.).

Psychosis An abnormal state of widespread brain dysfunction characterized by bizarre thought content, typically delusions and hallucinations.

Psychosocial factors Life events that affect a person's emotional state, such as marriage, divorce, or death of a loved one.

Racing thoughts The subjective feeling that one's thoughts are moving so fast that one cannot keep up; often seen during manic episodes.

Restraint asphyxia Suffocation of a patient stemming from an inability to expand the chest cavity during inspiration because of restraint and immobilization.

Schizophrenia A group of disorders characterized by psychotic symptoms, thought disorder, and negative

Terminology—continued

symptoms (social isolation and withdrawal); types include paranoid, disorganized, and catatonic.

Sedative-hypnotics Prescription CNS depressant drugs that cause powerful relaxation and euphoria when abused; typically barbiturates and benzodiazepines.

Self-injury An unhealthy coping mechanism involving intentionally injuring one's own body, often through cutting or burning oneself to relieve emotional tension; also known as *self-mutilation*.

Somatic delusions False perceptions of the appearance or functioning of one's own body.

Somatoform disorders A group of disorders characterized by the manifestation of psychological problems as physical symptoms; this includes conversion disorder, hypochondriasis, somatization disorder, and body dysmorphic disorder.

Suicide The act of ending one's own life.

Tangential thinking A progression of thoughts related to each other but that become less and less related to the original topic.

Tardive dyskinesia A degenerative neurologic condition associated with long-term use of antipsychotic drugs marked by involuntary and repetitive movements of the mouth and face.

Thalamus Structure located within the limbic system that is the switchboard of the brain, through which almost all signals travel on their way in or out of the brain.

Thought blocking A symptom of thought disorder in which a patient is speaking and then stops mid-sentence, unable to remember what he or she was saying and unable to continue.

Tolerance Repeated use of a drug that leads to less of an effect from the same doses as before and/or a need for increasingly larger doses to achieve the same effects.

Withdrawal Physical and/or psychological signs and symptoms that result from discontinuing regular administration of a drug; effects are usually the opposite of the effects of the drug itself because the body has changed itself to maintain homeostasis.

Word salad The most severe form of looseness of associations in which the topic shifts so rapidly that it interrupts the flow of sentences themselves, producing a jumble of words.

Hematologic Disorders

Objectives *After completing this chapter, you will be able to:*

1. Identify the anatomy of the hematopoietic system.
2. Describe the components of blood and volume and volume control in relation to the hematopoietic system.
3. Identify and describe the blood-forming organs and how and where blood is formed.
4. Describe normal red blood cell production, function, lifespan, and destruction.
5. Explain the significance of the hematocrit regarding red blood cell size and number.
6. Explain the correlations of the red blood cell count, hematocrit, and hemoglobin values.
7. Describe normal white blood cell production, function, and destruction.
8. Identify the characteristics of the inflammatory process.
9. Identify alterations in immunologic response.
10. Describe the number, normal function, types, and lifespan of leukocytes.
11. Identify the difference between cellular and humoral immunity.
12. Describe platelets in regard to normal function, lifespan, and numbers.
13. Describe the components of the hemostatic mechanism.
14. Describe the function of coagulation factors, platelets, and blood vessels necessary for normal coagulation.
15. Describe the intrinsic and extrinsic clotting systems in regard to identification of factor deficiencies in each stage.
16. Define *fibrinolysis*.
17. Describe disseminated intravascular coagulation and its precipitating factors.
18. Identify blood groups.
19. Define *anemia*.
20. Describe the pathology and clinical manifestations and prognosis associated with:
    - Aplastic anemia
    - Hemoglobinopathy (including sickle cell disease)
    - Hemolytic anemia
    - Iron-deficiency anemia
    - Methemoglobinemia
21. Describe the pathology and clinical manifestations associated with disorders of hemostasis: platelet dysfunction, thrombocytopenia, decreased production, platelet destruction, sequestration, and hemophilia.
22. Describe the pathology and clinical manifestations associated with leukocyte disorders: leukemia, lymphoma, and multiple myeloma.
23. Identify the components of physical assessment as they relate to the hematologic system and integrate pathophysiologic principles into the assessment of a patient with a hematologic disease.

Chapter Outline

Anatomy and Physiology of the Hematopoietic
   System
Red Blood Cell Disorders
Disorders of Hemostasis

White Blood Cell Disorders
Prehospital Management
Chapter Summary

Hematology is the study of blood and its various parts and their functions. Blood acts as a means of transportation, carrying nourishment, oxygen, and waste products to and from all parts of the body. It also plays a role in regulating temperature, balancing fluid and electrolytes, regulating the pH, preventing fluid loss, and preventing disease. The various parts of the hematologic system play a key role in maintaining homeostasis, the body's physiologic balance. This chapter identifies the components of that system. In addition, it covers the disorders that commonly disturb this system.

ANATOMY AND PHYSIOLOGY OF THE HEMATOPOIETIC SYSTEM

[OBJECTIVE 1]

Two types of hematopoietic tissue are found in the body: myeloid and lymphoid. Myeloid tissue is mainly found in the bone marrow. This type of tissue produces red blood cells, white blood cells, and blood platelets. Lymphoid tissue is found in the mucosa of the digestive tract and respiratory tract. It also is found in the lymph nodes, spleen, and thymus. This type of tissue is the home to lymphocytes and other cells derived from them, such as plasma cells.

Functions and Characteristics of Blood

Blood is a connective tissue. It is composed of cells and cell fragments, which are suspended in plasma, the liquid portion of blood. In the adult body blood comprises approximately 8% of the total body weight, or approximately 5 to 6 L. Following are the primary functions of blood:

- Supply oxygen and nutrients to the cells
- Transport carbon dioxide and nitrogenous wastes from the tissues to the lungs and kidneys, where the wastes can be removed from the body
- Carry hormones from the endocrine glands to the target tissues
- Regulate body temperature
- Regulate the pH through the buffering components in the blood
- Keep fluid and electrolytes balanced through salt and plasma proteins
- Regulate the immune system through the actions of white blood cells and antibodies
- Form clots through the action of platelets

The body consists of cells that are actively involved in metabolism. These cells need a continuous supply of nutrients and oxygen. The body also consists of metabolic waste products that must be removed from the body. Blood is the chief means of transport for the nutrients, oxygen, and waste products. This vital aspect of homeostasis leads to various relations with many other organ systems, including volume regulation.

Blood Composition

[OBJECTIVE 2]
Blood is primarily composed of 55% plasma and 45% formed cellular fragments. The percentage of the blood composed of red blood cells is called the **hematocrit.** **Plasma** is the noncellular liquid portion of unclotted whole blood in which the formed elements of blood are suspended. It comprises the major portion of whole blood. Plasma is composed of 92% water, 7% protein, and 1% minerals. It contains 6.5 to 8.0 g of protein per deciliter of blood. The main proteins in plasma are albumin (60%), globulins (alpha-1, alpha-2, beta, and gamma [immunoglobulins]), and clotting proteins, especially fibrinogen. The formed elements are a mixture of red blood cells (RBCs, or erythrocytes), white blood cells (WBCs, or leukocytes), and platelets. Figure 33-1 shows the components of blood when a sample of blood has been spun in a centrifuge.

Hematopoietic Stem and Progenitor Cells

[OBJECTIVE 3]
Hematopoiesis is the formation of blood or blood cells in the body. This process starts with a common stem cell

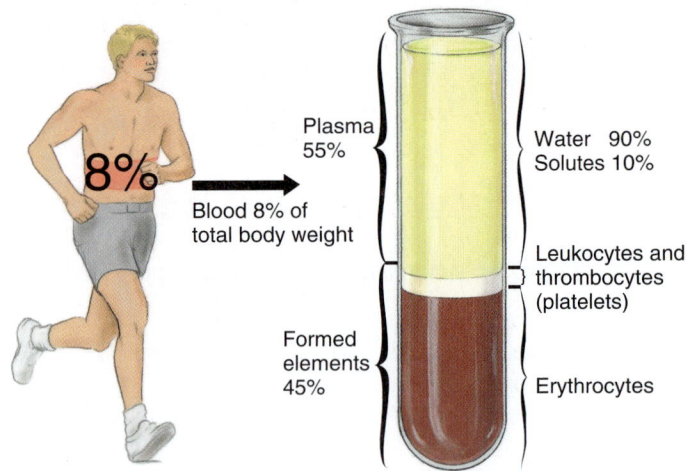

Figure 33-1 Components of a spun-down blood sample.

that has the ability to change into multiple different types of cells. The stem cell matures, or differentiates into RBCs, WBCs, and platelets (Figure 33-2). The stem cell originates in the bone marrow. The bone marrow forms a suitable environment for growth and development. The general composition of the marrow is complex. It includes **adipocytes, fibroblasts, reticular cells, endothelial cells,** and **macrophages.** Bone marrow stem cells have the ability to differentiate into a number of different cells and renew themselves. However, as stem cells become more and more differentiated, they lose the ability to self-renew. A single stem cell, after many divisions, has the ability to give rise to more than one million mature cells.

Red Blood Cells

[OBJECTIVE 4]

Normal Erythropoiesis

The body's tissues need oxygen for aerobic metabolism. This oxygen is supplied to the tissues by the circulating mass of mature RBCs, or erythrocytes. The circulating RBC population is continually being renewed by the erythroid precursor cells in the marrow. This process of renewal is under the control of both **humoral** and cellular growth factors. This cycle of normal **erythropoiesis,** or RBC production, is a carefully regulated process. Oxygen sensors within the kidney detect minute changes in the amount of oxygen available to tissue. By releasing **erythropoietin,** these sensors are able to adjust the production of RBCs to match the needs of the tissue. Thus normal erythropoiesis is best described according to (1) its major components, including the RBC structure, function, and turnover; (2) the capacity of the bone marrow to produce new RBCs; and (3) growth factor regulation.

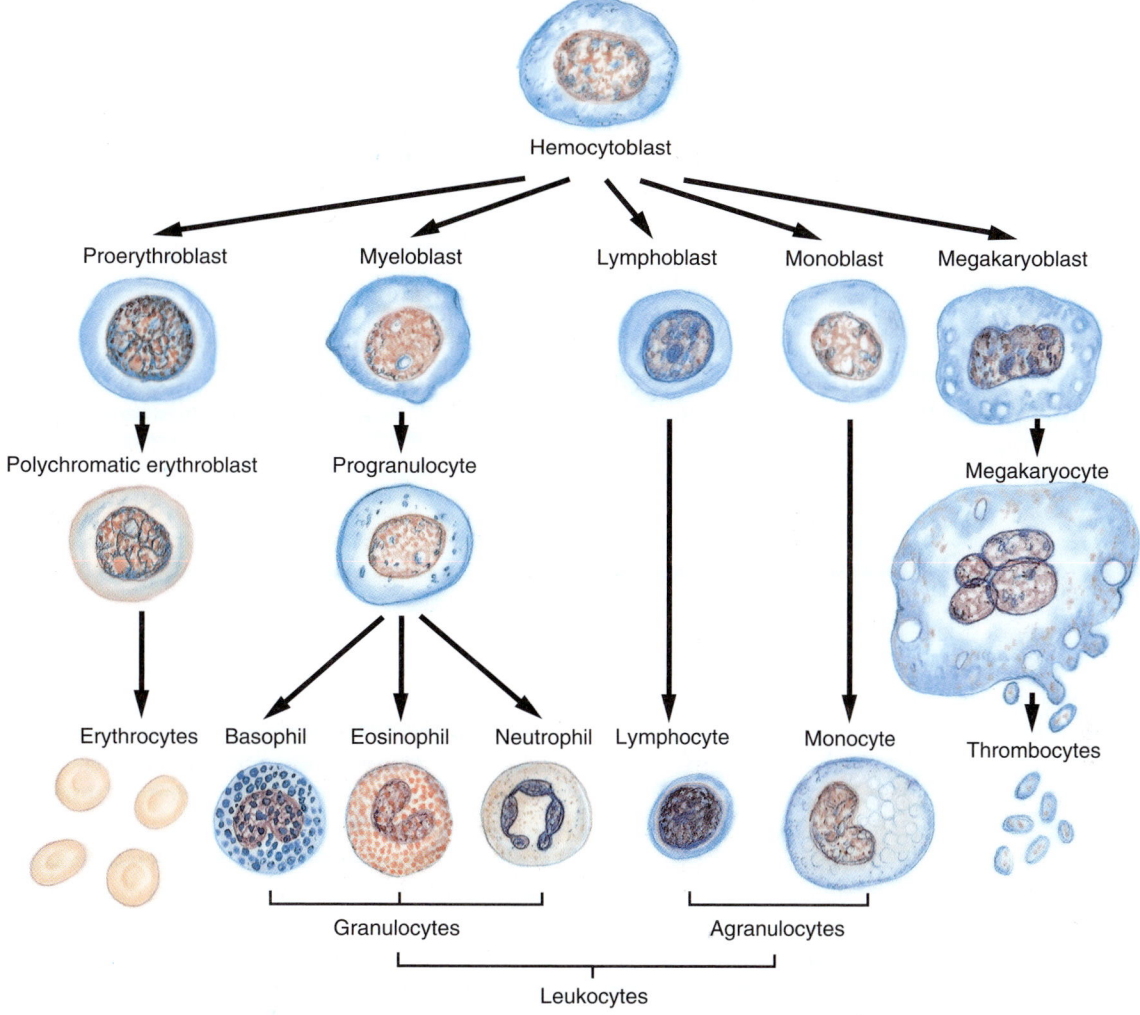

Figure 33-2 Development of the cells of the hematologic system.

Red Blood Cell Structure

The structure of the RBC is perfectly suited for its functions. Its structure allows maximal flexibility as it travels through the microvasculature. The mature red cell is a biconcave disc. It lacks a nucleus or mitochondria. Hemoglobin is the primary protein in the intracellular compartment and comprises 33% of its content. The hemoglobin molecule is a protein composed of four polypeptide chains. Each chain contains an active heme group. Each heme group can bind to an oxygen molecule and transport it to various tissues. Without a nucleus or protein metabolic pathway, the cell has a limited lifespan of 100 to 120 days. As RBCs reach the end of their lifespan, they are engulfed and destroyed by phagocytic cells of the reticuloendothelial system, primarily in the bone marrow, spleen, and liver.

Clinical and Laboratory Measures

[OBJECTIVES 5, 6]

The **hematocrit** also is called the **volume of packed red cells** or the *packed cell volume.* It measures the volume of whole blood composed of RBCs (mainly erythrocytes).

After the blood has been spun in a centrifuge, the height of the red cell column is measured and compared to the total height of the column of whole blood. The portion of the total blood volume occupied by the red cell mass is the hematocrit. Hematocrit depends mostly on the number of RBCs. However, to a much lower extent, it also is affected by the average size of the RBCs. The hematocrit typically ranges from 42% to 52% for males and 36% to 48% for females. It is usually approximately three times the hemoglobin value (assuming no marked hypochromia). The hematocrit may be affected by altitude, position of the patient, and heavy smoking by the patient in the same manner that the hemoglobin may be affected. The **RBC count** is the number of RBCs per microliter. This count gives an indirect estimate of the hemoglobin content of blood. The values typically range from 4.3 to 5.7 million cells/mcL for males and 3.8 to 4.9 million cells/mcL for females.

Hemoglobin is the molecule of the RBC that carries the oxygen. The amount of hemoglobin per 100 mL of blood can be used as an index of the capacity of the blood to carry oxygen. Total blood hemoglobin depends on the number of RBCs (the hemoglobin carriers). It also depends (to a much lower extent) on the amount of hemoglobin in each RBC. The typical values are 13.5 to 17.5 g/dL for males and 12.0 to 16.0 g/dL for females. Infants and children have very different hemoglobin values than adults.

White Blood Cells

[OBJECTIVES 7, 8, 9]

Normal Myelopoiesis

WBCs, or leukocytes, mainly work in the tissues to fight infection and aid immunity. The structure of the WBC allows movement through the capillary walls and into the tissues. The typical WBC has a nucleus. However, it lacks the hemoglobin of the RBC. The average WBC count is between 5000 and 6000 cells per cubic millimeter, and they are produced from the progenitor, or stem, cells (see Figure 33-2). Many different types of WBCs have varying functions. These jobs include phagocytosis, production of antibodies, secretion of heparin and histamine, and secretion of other chemokines. The lifespan of WBCs generally ranges from 13 to 20 days. After this time, they are destroyed in the lymphatic system.

Normal myelopoiesis produces differentiated cells. These cells go on to provide the body's host defense. This process of myelopoiesis involves the production of new myeloid cells. These cells include neutrophilic, eosinophilic, and basophilic granulocytes, monocytes, and macrophages. Myeloid cells share a common precursor cell. This precursor cell is known as the *colony-forming unit granulocyte monocyte*. This cell is able to differentiate into myeloid, megakaryocytic, and lymphoid tissue lineages. This process is driven by several growth factors, which control the rate and type of cell production. In response to an acute infection, trauma, or inflammation, WBCs release a substance called *colony-stimulating factor*. Colony-stimulating factor prompts the bone marrow to increase WBC production. In a person with bone marrow that is working properly, the numbers of WBCs can double within hours if needed. Such an increase in WBCs is referred to as **leukocytosis.**

Leukocytosis most often occurs as a result of relatively benign conditions. These conditions include infections or inflammatory processes. Much less common but more serious causes include primary bone marrow disorders. The normal reaction of bone marrow to infection or inflammation leads to an increase in the number of WBCs. These cells are mainly polymorphonuclear leukocytes and less mature cell forms (the left shift). Physical stress, as with seizures, anesthesia, overexertion, and emotional stress, also can elevate WBC counts. Certain medications, such as corticosteroids, lithium, and beta-agonists, are commonly associated with leukocytosis. Suspect primary bone marrow disorders in patients who have extremely elevated WBC counts or concurrent abnormalities in RBC or platelet counts. Also be suspicious for a marrow disorder in patients with weight loss; bleeding or bruising; liver, spleen, or lymph node enlargement; and immunosuppression. In addition, allergic reactions may result in leukocytosis.

Leukopenia, however, is an abnormal *decrease* in WBC levels. Many drugs can cause leukopenia, as can many conditions, such as bone marrow disorders. Depending on the type of WBCs involved, the terms *neutropenia* and *granulocytopenia* also may be used to describe the condition.

Types of White Blood Cells

[OBJECTIVES 10, 11]

Neutrophils. The neutrophils are the most common type of leukocyte, or WBC. They comprise approximately 70% of the total number of leukocytes. Their structure consists of a multilobed nucleus and granules spread throughout the cytoplasm. Neutrophils are the first responders to areas of tissue damage. They mainly function through phagocytosis.

Eosinophils. Eosinophils comprise approximately 2% to 4% of the total number of leukocytes. Their structure consists of a nucleus with two lobes and large granules within the cytoplasm that stain red on preparation. These cells counteract histamine and destroy parasitic infections. The percentage of these cells increases during allergic reactions.

Basophils. Basophils are the least numerous of the leukocytes. They account for less than 1% of the total leukocyte count. Their structure consists of a U-shaped nucleus with granules within the cytoplasm that stain dark blue on preparation. These cells are able to secrete histamine and heparin.

Lymphocytes. Lymphocytes also are referred to as *agranulocytes*. Their structure consists of a large nucleus and a small amount of cytoplasm. They are abundant in lymphoid tissue. Moreover, they are critical to the body's host defense. Two major types exist: T lymphocytes and B lymphocytes.

T lymphocytes mainly work to rid the body of bacteria and viruses through direct invasion. This invasion also is referred to as *cell-mediated immunity*. It involves activating macrophages and natural killer cells, producing antigen-specific cytotoxic T lymphocytes, and releasing various cytokines in response to an antigen. Cell-mediated immunity also plays a major role in the body's rejection of a transplanted organ.

B lymphocytes mainly work to rid the body of bacterial and viral organisms through the production of antibodies. This process is referred to as *humoral immunity*. It causes secreted antibodies to bind to antigens on the surfaces of invading microbes. This flags them for destruction. This highly complex process also involves the activation of many chemical mediators of the immune system and associated processes. These processes include pathogen and toxin neutralization, classical complement activation, and opsonin promotion of phagocytosis and pathogen elimination.

Platelets

[OBJECTIVES 12, 13]

Platelets are a key component of the formation of clots, or coagulation. The platelet, the vessel wall, von Willebrand factor, and fibrinogen all must work together for platelets to adhere and aggregate and a clot to form. The following steps describe how platelets normally work. First, platelets change their shape and adhere to subendothelial collagen at the wound site. Second, the platelets then aggregate to each other, a process known as *activation*. Third, multiple factors are released to stimulate further platelet activation and aggregation. This process results in the formation of fibrin. Fibrin stabilizes the platelet plug, stops the bleeding, and allows injuries to heal. The platelet count in the circulating blood is normally between 150 and 400 million per milliliter of blood.

Many factors can influence an individual's platelet count, including exercise and racial origin. The average lifespan of a platelet in the blood is 10 days.

Normal Hemostasis

[OBJECTIVES 14, 15, 16, 17]

Blood vessels are lined with the vascular endothelium. Any disruption in the vascular endothelium can activate the coagulation cascade. The cessation of bleeding after endothelial cell injury is called *hemostasis*. Hemostasis is typically achieved through vascular constriction, platelet plug formation, activation of coagulation, and clot formation. The initial reaction that reduces the flow of blood to the affected area is vascular contraction. Then the platelet formation is mediated through the connective tissue collagen in the underlying damaged endothelial cell wall. When stimulated by contact with the subendothelial tissue, the platelet undergoes an immediate shape change. This change involves the extension of pseudopods and adherence to the connective tissue surface.

The von Willebrand factor is an essential cofactor for adhesion. It binds connective tissue elements to the platelets. The **coagulation cascade** is a set of interactions of the circulating clotting factors. Figure 33-3

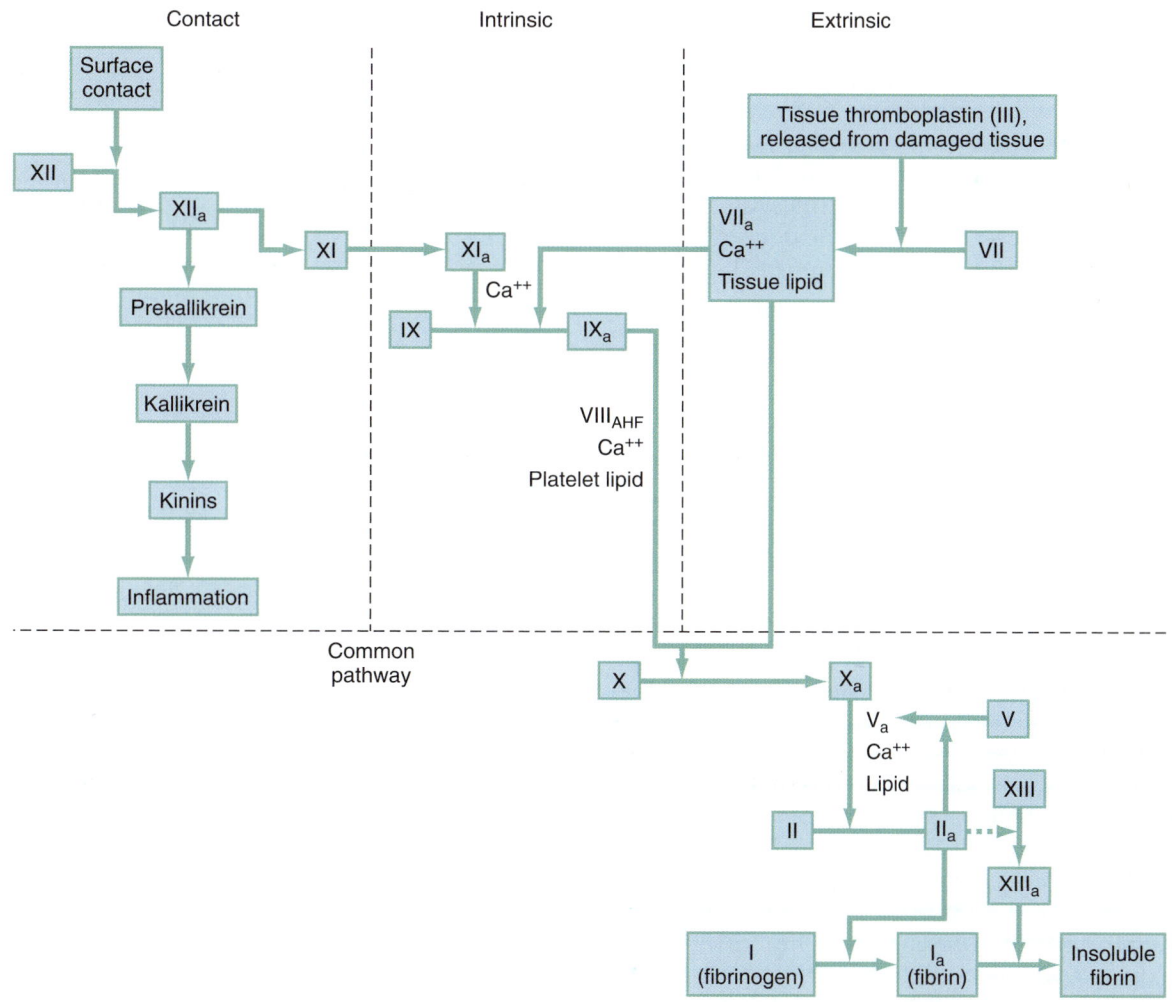

Figure 33-3 Coagulation cascade.

illustrates the complex system of events that lead to the formation of a fibrin clot. These steps are typically organized into the extrinsic and intrinsic pathways. The steps can be summarized as follows:

- Platelets and damaged tissues release chemicals. These chemicals set off a series of reactions. The reactions result in the formation of prothrombin activator.
- In the presence of calcium and prothrombin activator, prothrombin in the plasma is changed from its inactive form to active thrombin.
- Thrombin in the presence of calcium ions acts as an enzyme to convert inactive and soluble fibrinogen into active and insoluble fibrin. The fibrin threads then form a mesh that adheres to the damaged tissues. This mesh traps RBCs and platelets to form the clot.

Once the bleeding has stopped, another blood protein dissolves the clot. It does this by breaking down the fibrin into fragments. Measuring these fragments can yield information about the clot-dissolving portion of coagulation, which is called **fibrinolysis.**

Blood Typing and Transfusions: ABO and Rh Blood Groups

[OBJECTIVE 18]

Agglutinogens are specific blood type antigens found on the surface of RBCs. Antibodies to the different agglutinogens are called *agglutinins*. Many different blood types, or antigens, are on the RBC. In the clinical setting and with most uncomplicated blood transfusions, the major blood types of concern are the ABO and Rh types. The ABO blood groups are based on the presence or absence of certain agglutinogens on the erythrocyte membrane. Type A blood has A agglutinogens and B agglutinins, type B blood has B agglutinogens and A agglutinins, type AB has both A and B agglutinogens and no agglutinins, and type O has neither agglutinogen and A and B agglutinins (Figure 33-4). The Rh blood group represents another set of agglutinogens. Rh-positive blood has Rh agglutinogens, and Rh-negative blood does not have Rh agglutinogens. When transfusions are needed, the ABO and Rh types must be matched. This prevents potentially life-threatening hemolytic anemia (Figure 33-5). In general, the AB-positive blood group is referred to as the *universal recipient*. These persons can receive blood from any donor. The O-negative blood group is referred to as the *universal donor*. The blood of these persons can be donated to any recipient. Blood types of possible donors and recipients are illustrated in Table 33-1. Another situation in which the Rh blood group may present a problem is in pregnancy. If an Rh-negative mother is exposed to the Rh-positive blood of her unborn child, her immune system will develop agglutinins to the Rh agglutinogens. Although this is generally not an issue in the first pregnancy, in subsequent pregnancies if the unborn child has

Type A 40%

Agglutinogens "A" Agglutinins "anti-B"

Type B 10%

Agglutinogens "B" Agglutinins "anti-A"

Type AB 4%

Agglutinogens "A" & "B" No agglutinins

Type O 46%

No agglutinogens Agglutinins "anti-A" & "anti-B"

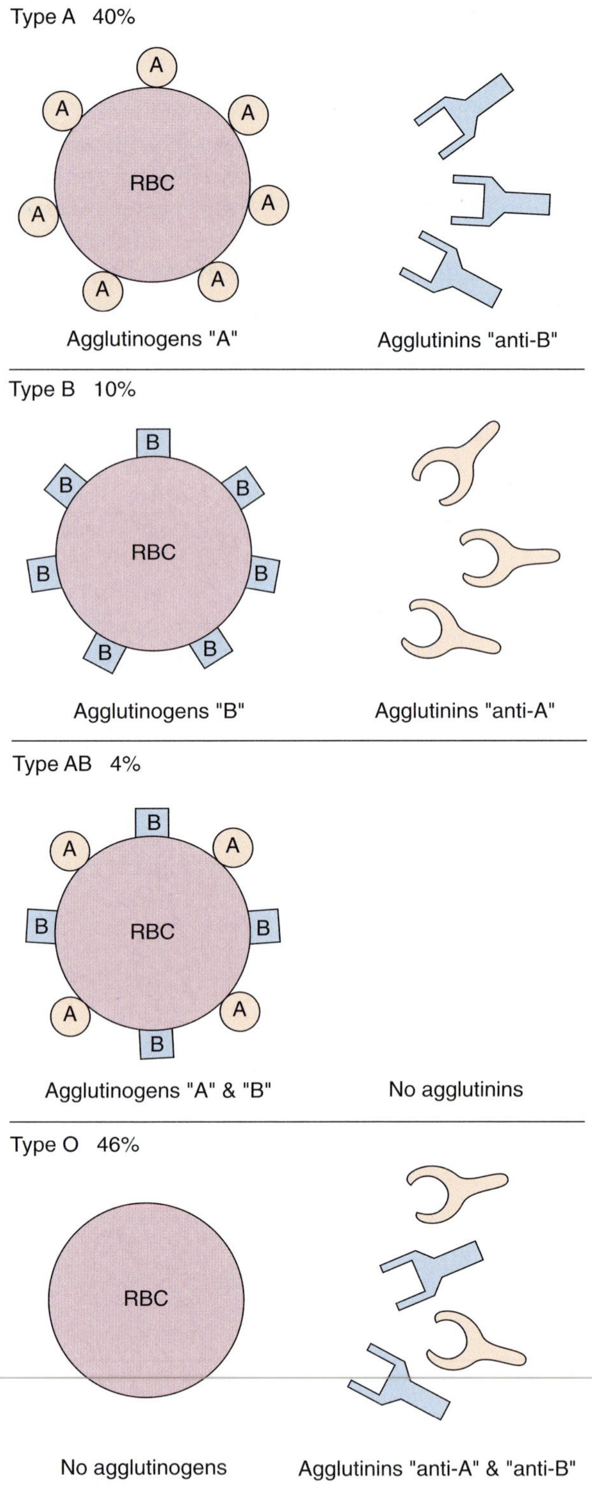

Figure 33-4 Agglutinogens and agglutinins in the ABO blood group. *RBC,* Red blood cell.

Rh-positive blood the mother's immune system will launch an attack against the RBCs of the fetus.

RED BLOOD CELL DISORDERS

[OBJECTIVES 19, 20]

In general, **anemia** is considered to be a decrease in the number of RBCs. It is reflected by a decrease in the quan-

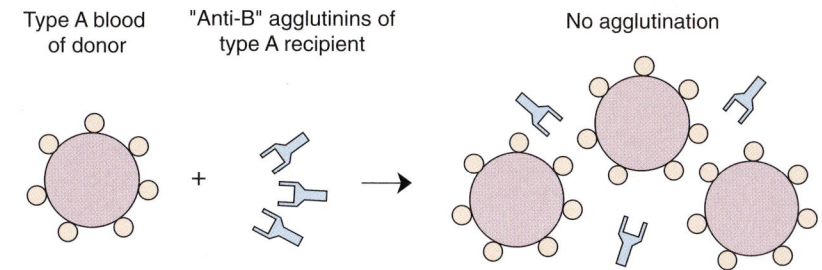

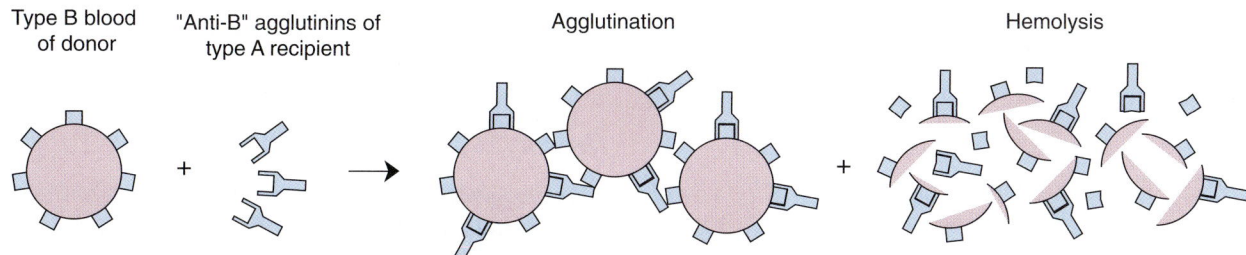

Figure 33-5 Agglutination reactions.

TABLE 33-1	ABO Rh Type and Preferred and Alternate Donor Types
Blood Type	**Donor Types**
A+	A+, A−, O+, O−
A−	A−, O−
AB+	AB+, AB−, A+, A−, B+, B−, O+, O−
AB−	AB−, A−, B−, O−
B+	B+, B−, O+, O−
B−	B−, O−

Modified from Applegate, E. J. (2006). *The anatomy and physiology learning*

tity of hemoglobin or by lowered hematocrit. This reduction in blood cell count reduces the amount of oxygen the blood can carry throughout the body. Anemia has many causes, some of which are described in the following sections.

Aplastic Anemia

Aplastic anemia is the decreased production of one or more of the major hematopoietic lineages within the bone marrow. Marrow failure can potentially occur at any number of critical points in the differentiation of the **pluripotent** stem cell. This failure is generally classified as either primary (inherited) or secondary (acquired). The term *inherited* implies that a genetic abnormality causes the bone marrow dysfunction, especially when it occurs in two or more members of the same family or is associated with congenital physical abnormalities. Some examples of acquired factors are viruses and environmental toxins.

Fanconi anemia, or congenital aplastic anemia, is the classic marrow failure disorder. It is inherited in an autosomal recessive pattern and occurs in all racial and ethnic groups. Moreover, it is often associated with growth retardation and congenital defects of the skeleton. It has a heterogenous phenotypic presentation. Patients may have typical physical defects but normal hematology, normal physical features but abnormal hematology, or physical defects and abnormal hematology.

Presentation of these patients varies. Patients with classic Fanconi anemia have both physical deformities and hematologic abnormalities. Acute presentations of either primary or secondary aplastic anemia are related to the secondary effects of the disease or the methods by which they are treated. The acute manifestations include anemia, neutropenia, or thrombocytopenia. Infections, particularly of the mouth and throat, are common. Generalized infections can be life threatening. Bruising, bleeding gums, epistaxis, and menorrhagia are the manifestations most often seen. These also are the usual presenting features of persons with symptoms of anemia.

Hemoglobinopathy

fluid + pain meds   O₂
pain in joints + abdomen

Inherited defects in globin structure are common in persons of African, Indian, Asian, and Mediterranean descent (Figure 33-6). The majority of these defects involve a single amino acid substitution in one of the globin chains. The resulting defect can be silent or produce significant anemia. The manifestations of hemoglobinopathy vary because different regions of the world are predisposed to certain genetic variants. Of the various types of hemoglobinopathy, sickle cell disease is considered the classic model with the most severe presentation. Sickle cell disease is a set of genetic abnormalities that mainly affects persons of African and Mediterranean

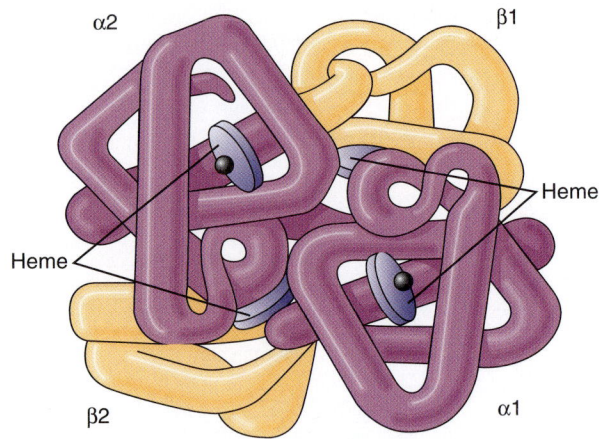

Figure 33-6 Hemoglobin is composed of two alpha-globin subunits and two beta-globin subunits.

descent. It is caused by a substitution of the amino acid valine for glutamic acid in the sixth position of the beta-globin chain (Fixler & Styles, 2002; Ingram, 1956; Serjeant, 1997; Steinberg, 1996). Several genetic variants of sickle cell disease exist. In general the most severe manifestations and disease course occur in these patients (Agarwal et al., 2002; Noguchi & Schecter, 1981). However, double heterozygotes for sickle trait and hemoglobin C or sickle trait and beta-thalassemia also manifest clinically important forms of sickle cell disease. In general, though, these typically have a more benign disease course. One benefit of sickle cell trait is that it provides some resistance against malaria. This may be why the condition is more prevalent in areas with a high incidence of malaria.

Epidemiology and Demographics

Among African Americans, the sickle cell trait occurs in 8% to 10% of newborns (Motulsky, 1972). In this population the frequency of the sickle cell (0.045%), hemoglobin C (0.015%), and beta-thalassemia (0.004%) genes (Embury, 1994) indicate that 4000 to 5000 pregnancies a year are at risk for sickle cell disease (Fleming, 1989). The burden of this disease in the United States is dwarfed by that in the rest of the world. In fact, prevalence for the sickle cell gene is as high as 25% to 30% in western Africa (Fleming, 1989); an estimated 120,000 babies are born with sickle cell disease annually on that continent. The prevalence, however, can be altered through immigration of persons from various parts of the world.

Physical Findings

The clinical manifestations of sickle cell disease largely vary between and among the major genotypes. Even within the genotype regarded as being the most severe, sickle cell anemia HbSS, some patients have no symptoms and are only incidentally detected. In contrast, other patients are disabled by recurrent pain and chronic complications. Chronic complications or severe acute crises can occur in patients who do not have recurrent pain. Patients are typically anemic but lead a relatively normal life with occasional painful episodes. Virtually every organ system in the body is subject to vaso-occlusion. This accounts for the characteristic acute and chronic multisystem failure of this disease. Important features of the disease that are less directly related to vaso-occlusion include growth retardation, psychosocial problems, and susceptibility to infection. The multiple organ systems involved are comprehensive, but they vary by each individual. They may include vaso-occlusive crisis, acute exacerbations of chronic anemia, stroke, cardiomegaly, pulmonary hypertension, repeated susceptibility to infections, right upper quadrant pain, and priapism.

Hemolytic Anemia

Hemolytic anemia results from the premature destruction of RBCs. However, the bone marrow is quite capable of making up for such losses. Thus it may increase the production of RBCs to compensate for the increased destruction. Patients may not have symptoms until the rate of destruction is less than every 30 days.

These forms of anemia are typically caused by a broad array of disorders classified as hereditary or acquired (Tabbara, 1992). Congenital, or hereditary, causes of hemolytic anemia often lead to severe problems in early childhood (e.g., beta-thalassemia major, sickle cell anemia). On the other hand, the congenital causes may remain silent until later in life, then provoke a crisis (e.g., glucose-6-phosphate dehydrogenase deficiency) (Beutler, 1994). The pathways of RBC destruction recover heme iron molecules for production in new RBCs. The process of destruction occurs either intravascularly (within the circulation) or extravascularly (by normal reticuloendothelial cell pathway). Factors in the environment or an inherent defect in the RBC structure or function can cause RBC hemolysis. Factors in the environment can affect both structurally normal and abnormal RBCs. The causes of extravascular and intravascular hemolysis are listed in Boxes 33-1 and 33-2. Although less common, patients with glucose-6-phosphate dehydrogenase (G6PD) deficiency, an enzyme that reduces nicotinamide adenine dinucleotide phosphate (NADPH, which is needed for the production of reduced glutathione and, when deficient, renders the cell susceptible to oxidant stress), are susceptible to drug-induced hemolysis.

Most forms of hemolytic anemia have few specific symptoms or signs. When the anemia is severe, however, patients may report increased fatigue or decreased exercise tolerance. They also may develop congestive heart failure. This presentation is the same for any severe anemia. In contrast, acute intravascular hemolysis may be associated with fever, chills, and severe lower back pain. This is most often seen in patients who receive incompatible or infected blood products. A patient who has had a severe hemolytic event with lysis of more than 20 to 40 mL of RBCs will have noticeable hemoglobinuria.

BOX 33-1 Causes of Extravascular Hemolysis

Autoimmune Hemolysis

- Warm-reacting (immunoglobulin G) autoimmune hemolytic anemia
- Cold-reacting (immunoglobulin M) autoimmune hemolytic anemia
- Bacterial and viral infections
- Malaria
- *Mycoplasma pneumonia*
- Infectious mononucleosis

Drug-Induced Hemolysis

- G6PD/Growth-stimulating hormone deficiency
- Autoimmune drug reactions
- Strong oxidant drugs or chemicals

Environmental Disorders

- Malignancy or DIC
- Idiopathic thrombocytopenic purpura/Henoch-Schönlein purpura
- Eclampsia or preeclampsia

Hemoglobinopathy

Membrane Structural Defect

- Hereditary spherocytosis
- Hereditary elliptocytosis
- Acanthocytosis

Modified from Hillman, R. S., & Ault, K. A. (1997). *Hematology in clinical practice: A guide to diagnosis and management.* New York: McGraw-Hill.

DIC, Disseminated intravascular coagulation.

BOX 33-2 Causes of Intravascular Hemolysis

Bacterial or Parasitic Infections

- Clostridial sepsis
- Malaria
- Bartonellosis
- *Mycoplasma pneumonia*

Blood Transfusions

- ABO mismatched transfusion
- Infected blood

Mechanical Heart Valves

Paroxysmal Hemoglobinuria

- Paroxysmal nocturnal hemoglobinuria
- Paroxysmal cold hemoglobinuria

Snake Bites

Thermal Burns

Modified from Hillman, R. S., & Ault, K. A. (1997). *Hematology in clinical practice: A guide to diagnosis and management.* New York: McGraw-Hill.

Iron-Deficiency Anemia

Iron deficiency is a leading cause of anemia in children and adults. When iron supply to the erythroid marrow is poor, RBC production is impaired. Thus the new cells released into the circulation are poorly hemoglobinated. The severity of the anemia and the degree of microcytosis (abnormally small red blood cells) and hypochromia (lack of color) generally reflect the severity and the chronic nature of the iron-deficiency state.

Iron plays an essential role in the synthesis of hemoglobin. It is relatively highly saved up within the human body. Free intracellular iron is transported to the mitochondria. There it is stored as ferritin. Iron transport pathways incorporate 80% to 90% of the iron into the creation of new RBCs. A deficiency in iron is usually a result of an imbalance between normal physiologic demands, such as rapid growth, menstrual blood loss, and dietary intake. Severe iron deficiency is usually a result of gastrointestinal tract or uterine hemorrhage, small intestinal disease, or gastric surgery. Other potential factors that could cause iron-deficiency anemia include severe malabsorption and chronic blood loss.

The clinical presentation of this anemia is relatively mild. Patients may have a profound anemia depending on the cause of the iron deficiency. The symptoms usually depend on the hemoglobin level and can range from weakness, dizziness, and shortness of breath to almost no symptoms at all. Iron-deficiency anemia is chiefly diagnosed in the laboratory.

Methemoglobinemia

The presence of methemoglobin in the blood results from the oxidation of the iron in hemoglobin from the ferrous (Fe^{2+}) to the ferric (Fe^{3+}) state. Methemoglobin composes 3% or less of the total hemoglobin in the normal human body. Under normal circumstances, these levels are maintained at 1% or less by the methemoglobin reductase enzyme system (nicotinamide adenine dinucleotide [NADH]-dehydratase, ADH-diaphorase, erythrocyte cytochrome b_3).

Methemoglobinemia can arise, however, by one of the following three distinct reasons:

- Globin chain mutations that result in increased formation of methemoglobin
- Deficiencies of methemoglobin reductase
- "Toxic" methemoglobinemia, in which normal RBCs are exposed to substances that oxidize hemoglobin iron, thus subverting or overwhelming the normal reducing mechanisms

Methemoglobin has a brownish to blue color that does not change back to red on exposure to oxygen. Thus patients with methemoglobinemia appear to be cyanotic. In contrast to truly cyanotic persons, however, these patients have PaO₂ values that are usually normal. Patients with these hemoglobins otherwise have no symptoms because methemoglobin is rarely greater than 30% to 50%, the level at which symptoms become apparent. Suspect methemoglobinemia in patients with unexplained cyanosis. A clear medical emergency exists when any patient has cyanosis and altered mental status; a normal PaO₂ should prompt you to consider methemoglobinemia. Consider the ingestion of nitrites as a suicidal act, especially in persons who are knowledgeable of chemistry, medicine, or pharmacology. Suspect methemoglobinemia from the brownish color of blood (which looks like chocolate) when it is drawn. Methylene blue is the antidote to methemoglobinemia. It can reduce the methemoglobin to hemoglobin by helping a second enzyme, diaphorase II, accomplish its job. One contraindication of methylene blue is glucose-6-phosphate dehydrogenase (G6PD) deficiency. G6PD supplies a vital cofactor(nicotinamide adenine dinucleotide) to the enzyme involved in the activation process (diaphorase II). Therefore methylene blue is ineffective in patients who have G6PD deficiency. These patients, or patients who are severely affected, may require exchange transfusion.

DISORDERS OF HEMOSTASIS

[OBJECTIVE 21]

Thrombocytopenia

Thrombocytopenia is a platelet count less than 150,000/mm³. With platelets that are working normally, thrombocytopenia is rarely the cause of bleeding unless the count is less than 50,000/mm³. When platelet levels fall to between 10,000 and 20,000, a significant increase in spontaneous bleeding occurs, especially intracranial bleeding. Thrombocytopenia can be caused by decreased platelet production, increased destruction, sequestration, or a combination of these.

Some common causes of thrombocytopenia from decreased platelet production include infections, use of certain drugs (e.g., thiazides, chemotherapeutic agents, estrogens, ethanol, alpha-interferon), radiotherapy, folate or vitamin B₁₂ deficiency, or marrow infiltration by a tumor or an infection.

A variety of immune conditions can cause platelets to be destroyed. These conditions include immune thrombocytopenic purpura; thrombotic microangiopathy; heparin-induced thrombocytopenia; diffused intravascular coagulation; and viral infections such as HIV, mumps, varicella zoster, and Epstein-Barr virus.

Moreover, a variety of conditions can cause platelet sequestration, often manifesting as hypersplenism. These conditions include liver disease or malignancy, hypothermia, and infection. Epstein-Barr virus, the agent that causes infectious mononucleosis, is well known for causing sequestration. However, other infections also may lead to splenic sequestration.

Many drugs are thought to produce thrombocytopenia. Some of the more common are heparin, sulfa-containing antibiotics, quinine and quinidine, ethanol, aspirin, indomethacin, and valproic acid.

Most platelet disorders do not present with specific symptoms or signs that clearly indicate a platelet functional defect. Von Willebrand disease is an inherited platelet disorder that may present with severe and potentially fatal bleeding. The majority of patients have mucocutaneous bleeding, gastrointestinal bleeding, or genitourinary tract bleeding.

Hemophilia

Hemophilia is a set of sex-linked genetic disorders that manifests as a blood defect characterized by delayed clotting and difficulty controlling hemorrhage (see Figure 33-3). Hemophilia A and B are the primary examples in which a defect in the production of factor VIII or IX, respectively, leads to spontaneous and excessive hemorrhage. Factor VIII or IX is reduced because of genetic mutations of a portion of the X chromosome. The disorder is relatively rare. It occurs in approximately 1 in 10,000 births for hemophilia A and 1 in 30,000 births for hemophilia B (also known as *Christmas disease*).

The severity of the hemophilia A clinical presentation varies depending on the severity of the genetic mutation and its phenotypic expression. The disorder typically manifests itself early in childhood. These patients develop frequent, spontaneous hemarthroses or hematomas and hemorrhages into joints, muscles, and vital organs, as well as intracranial hemorrhages. Intracranial hemorrhage is the major cause of death in these patients. Some patients may have relatively benign presentations. These patients may not be diagnosed until adulthood. Patients with hemophilia B have clinical characteristics similar to those with hemophilia A. In contrast, those with hemophilia B develop spontaneous hemarthroses of large joints of the upper and lower extremities. The chronic nature of hemarthroses in hemophilia B may result in the development of chronic synovitis, the destruction of cartilage and bone, and a progressive flexion contracture. Less-common manifestations of hemophilia B include hematuria, intracranial hemorrhage, and mucous membrane bleeding.

Disseminated Intravascular Coagulation

In **disseminated intravascular coagulation (DIC)** the coagulation cascade is triggered in an abnormal way. DIC is a complex systemic thrombohemorrhagic disorder that involves the production of intravascular fibrin and the consumption of procoagulants and platelets. A large amount of tissue damage—such as a burn, major trauma, a dead fetus, placental abruption, placenta previa, cancer, sepsis, or a transfusion reaction—can initiate the chain of biochemical events that lead to blood clots. The initiation of the coagulation cascade first leads to excessive clotting. This is followed by excessive bleeding as the cascade becomes overwhelmed. For a patient with trauma, the presence of DIC approximately doubles the mortality rate. DIC may be acute or chronic.

WHITE BLOOD CELL DISORDERS

[OBJECTIVE 22]

Acute Leukemia

Acute leukemia can be considered the proliferation of an immature hematopoietic progenitor that rapidly multiplies and displaces normal elements within the marrow and peripheral blood. Acute leukemia is rapidly fatal if not successfully treated. It is most often fatal as a result of infections related to granulocytopenia or bleeding related to thrombocytopenia.

Patients with acute leukemia have high levels of spontaneous cell turnover, which increases after the start of therapy. The sudden transfer of the intracellular contents and cellular breakdown products to the extravascular space can cause life-threatening elevations of uric acid, potassium, and phosphate in the so-called tumor lysis syndrome.

Hodgkin Lymphoma

Hodgkin disease probably represents a more diverse group of disorders than previously recognized. The malignant cell type is known as a *Reed-Sternberg cell*. Without the presence of this cell type diagnosis of Hodgkin disease is difficult to impossible. Hodgkin disease has a bimodal age distribution; it peaks in the second and third decades of life and then again in the sixth and seventh decades. Patients often also may have symptoms of fever, night sweats, weight loss, or pruritus. The disease is diagnosed by characteristic lymph node histology.

Long-term disease-free survival rates appear to be improving for advanced and limited-stage Hodgkin disease with the more universal application of chemotherapy. Bone marrow transplantation may be useful in the treatment of relapsed disease.

Non-Hodgkin Lymphoma

Non-Hodgkin lymphoma is chiefly derived from B cells. A patient typically has adenopathy or an abdominal mass. Non-Hodgkin lymphoma is classified on the basis of morphology, immunophenotype, genetic features, and clinical characteristics. Approximately 20% of lymphomas are B-cell follicular lymphomas, which comprise the bulk of the category previously referred to as *indolent lymphomas*. These lymphomas typically present in older patients. Diffuse, large B-cell lymphoma comprises 30% of non-Hodgkin lymphoma. Left untreated, the progression of this aggressive subtype is more rapid. It can result in death within a short period. However, a significant number of patients can be cured with chemotherapy. Lymphoblastic lymphoma, a T-cell disorder, and the B cell–derived Burkitt lymphoma are acute leukemia–like disorders. They both have onsets that tend to be explosive. These disorders frequently involve the central nervous system or other "sanctuary" sites. Both

disorders rapidly progress to death unless successfully treated.

Multiple Myeloma

Multiple myeloma is part of a spectrum of diseases labeled *plasma-cell dyscrasia*. When B cells (lymphocytes) mature in response to an infection, they develop into plasma cells. These plasma cells then are responsible for forming antibodies against bacteria and foreign proteins. For reasons that are unclear, these cells lose their ability to respond to signals from a hierarchy of immune cells. Plasma cells then divide and form abnormal proteins. This results in damage to the bone, the bone marrow, and/or other organs of the body. The rapid and repeated production of plasma cells may interfere with the normal production of blood cells. This results in leukopenia, anemia, and thrombocytopenia and leads to impaired humoral immunity.

The plasma cells may cause lytic lesions in the skeleton or in soft tissue masses. The complications include a high instance of infection, hypercalcemia, bone pain, and spinal cord compression. In addition, the overproduction of antibodies may lead to hyperviscosity, amyloidosis, and renal failure. No cure is available; however, recent advances in therapy have helped decrease the occurrence of debilitating complications.

PREHOSPITAL MANAGEMENT

The patients you see with a disorder of the hematologic system will vary in presentation. Assessing the nature of the disorder through the physical examination and the patient's presenting symptoms would be difficult. In-hospital specialized laboratory diagnostic equipment often is needed for final diagnosis. You will need to gather vital information, including the history of the acute episode and the patient's past medical history. In general, these patients may have circulatory collapse as a result of profound anemia, acute internal blood loss, febrile syndromes of WBC disorders, or multisystem organ failure. The majority of adults have acute exacerbations of chronic disorders. Pediatric patients are more challenging because their acute episode also may be the first sign of the underlying disorder.

History and Physical Examination

[OBJECTIVE 23]

Your approach to all prehospital management should begin with an assessment of the patient's *a*irway, *b*reathing, and *c*irculation. The secondary survey should be a more focused assessment and include the following:

- Assess the patient's chief complaint.
- Inquire about any pertinent review of systems (fever, bleeding, bruising, fatigue, confusion, syncope, etc.).
- Inquire about any past medical history.

- Inquire about any medications, including any recent changes or use of nonprescribed medications.
- Inquire about illicit drug use.
- Inquire about allergies.
- Inquire about any pertinent family history, especially in pediatric patients.

If the patient's history suggests a potential hematologic disorder, conduct a focused physical examination. Pertinent physical examination findings include neurologic deficits (e.g., transient ischemic attack, cerebrovascular accident), integument changes (e.g., jaundice, petechiae, ecchymosis, purpura), gastrointestinal findings (e.g., epistaxis, gum bleeding, abdominal pain with splenomegaly or hepatomegaly), and musculoskeletal findings (e.g., flexion contractures, hemarthrosis, arthritis).

Management

Management of these patients is challenging. Initially focus on stabilizing the patient's hemodynamics. Definitive therapy will be provided by in-hospital personnel (Table 33-2). Your first goal in the field is to secure the airway and breathing, bag-mask, supplemental oxygen, high-flow oxygen and, when appropriate, endotracheal intubation. The next goal in your management should

TABLE 33-2 In-Hospital Disease-Specific Treatments

Disease Entity	Current Definitive Treatment Options
Aplastic anemia	Human stem cell transplantation, androgens, antilymphocyte (thymocyte) globulin, cyclosporine
Sickle cell disease	Opiate administration, intravenous fluids, hydroxyurea, iron chelators, long- and short-term blood transfusions
Hemolytic anemia	Short-term blood transfusion
Iron-deficiency anemia	Short-term blood transfusion, dietary supplementation
Leukemia	Chemotherapy, human stem cell transplant
Hodgkin lymphoma	Chemotherapy, radiation therapy
Non-Hodgkin lymphoma	Chemotherapy, radiation therapy
Methemoglobinemia	Methylene blue
Hemophilia A and B	Recombinant factor VIII and factor IX

be to address circulation through volume replacement for hypotensive patients. In instances of significant shock and suspected blood loss, attempt to place large-bore intravenous lines. If the patient is in pain, such as in a sickle cell crisis, administer appropriate medications to provide comfort. Rapid transport of the patient to the appropriate hospital is critical.

Epidemiology

Hematologic disorders vary in nature and are either acquired or genetic. Therefore disease prevalence and incidence are difficult to assess. The prevalence varies with most of the disorders of RBCs, WBCs, and platelets. In the field, assessment of the patient's presentation will be limited without advanced diagnostic aids. The three broad symptoms a patient may demonstrate include hypoxia, infection, and anemia. The clinical presentations are provided with each disorder. The differential diagnosis for these disorders is broad. Unfortunately, unless the patient has a known diagnosis, determining the cause of the patient's symptoms is impossible without sophisticated laboratory testing and, in some cases, bone marrow biopsy.

Therapeutic Interventions

You may take some general precautions and steps. If a patient has a known or suspected bleeding disorder evident from overt bleeding, joint swelling (hemarthrosis), mental status changes, neurologic deficit, and pallor, first and foremost address the ABCs and ensure intravenous access and appropriate fluid administration. These measures will help maintain hemodynamic stability. Although many of these patients are at high risk for mental status changes as a result of intracranial hemorrhage or stroke, always evaluate for the basic, immediately reversible causes of altered mental status, including hypoglycemia, hypoxemia, possible opiate overdose, and Wernicke encephalopathy. Control of the bleeding may be difficult depending on the underlying cause. Apply the standard measures of direct pressure and elevation to sources of external bleeding. For patients with sickle cell disease who are in a painful crisis, you may typically use analgesics and isotonic intravenous fluids judiciously.

Patient and Family Education

Hematologic disorders vary in nature and are difficult to diagnose definitively in the field. Therefore provide reassurance and comfort to the family. Caution patients with known bleeding disorders about being especially careful to avoid any trauma to the head. These patients are at increased risk for intracranial hemorrhage. Alert family members to remain vigilant and maintain suspicion for intracranial hemorrhage any time they observe altered mental status. If they do, they should seek immediate medical attention.

Chapter Summary

- Blood is a connective tissue that consists of cells and cell fragments. It composes approximately 8% of the total body weight (5 to 6 L).
- Blood is composed of 55% plasma and 45% formed cellular fragments.
- RBCs are developed through a carefully regulated process known as *erythropoiesis.*
- WBCs are the body's normal host defense. They include neutrophils, eosinophils, basophils, monocytes, and macrophages.
- Platelet function requires cohesion among the platelet, the vessel wall, von Willebrand factor, and fibrinogen.

- Agglutinogens are specific blood type antigens on the surface of the RBC membrane; antibodies are made to the agglutinogens (i.e., antigens). The A, B, O, and Rh agglutinogens must be matched before transfusion.
- Diagnosis of the specific cause of the patient's hematologic symptoms in the field is impossible. However, most patients with a hematologic disorder show symptoms of hypoxia, infection, and anemia.
- Each clinical disorder can present with acute, life-threatening manifestations. As a result of limited information in the field, you must manage the ABCs and be prepared for aggressive resuscitation.

REFERENCES

Agarwal, G., Wang, J. C., Kwong, S., Cohen, S. M., Ferrone, F. A., Josephs, R., et al. (2002). Sickle hemoglobin fibers: Mechanisms of depolymerization. *Journal of Molecular Biology, 322*(2), 395-412.

Beutler, E. (1994). G6PD deficiency. *Blood, 84,* 3613-3636.

Embury, S. H. (1994). Prenatal diagnosis. In S. H. Embury, R. P. Hebbel, N. Mohandas, & M. H. Steinberg (Eds.). *Sickle cell disease: Basic principles and clinical practice* (p. 485), New York: Raven Press.

Fixler, J., & Styles, L. (2002). Sickle cell disease. *Pediatric Clinics of North America, 49*(6), 1193-1210.

Fleming, A. F. (1989). The presentation, management and prevention of crisis in sickle cell disease in Africa. *Blood Review, 1,* 18.

Ingram, V. M. (1956). A specific chemical difference between the globins of normal human and sickle-cell anaemia haemoglobin. *Nature, 178*(4537), 792-794.

Motulsky, A. G. (1972). Frequency of sickling disorders in U.S. blacks. *New England Journal of Medicine, 288,* 31.

Noguchi, C. T., & Schecter, A. N. (1981). The intracellular polymerization of sickle hemoglobin and its relevance to sickle cell disease. *Blood, 58*(6), 1057-1068.

Serjeant, G. R. (1997). Sickle-cell disease. *The Lancet, 350*(9079), 725-730.

Steinberg, M. H. (1996). Sickle cell disease: Present and future treatment. *American Journal of Medical Science, 312*(4), 166-174.

Tabbara, I. A. (1992). Hemolytic anemias: Diagnosis and management. *Medical Clinics of North America, 76,* 649-668.

SUGGESTED RESOURCES

Health on the Net Foundation, hematologic diseases: http://www.hon.ch.

Hematologic disorders: http://www.nursingplanet.com.

Hoffbrand, A. V., Pettit, J. E., & Moss, P. A. H. (2001). *Essential hematology* (4th ed.). Hong Kong: Blackwell Science.

Hoffman, R., Benz, E., Shattil, S., Furie, B., Cohen, H., Silberstein, L., et al. (2005). *Hematology: Basic principles and practice* (4th ed.). New York: Churchill Livingstone.

Noble, J. (2001). *Textbook of primary care medicine* (3rd ed.). St. Louis: Mosby.

Chapter Quiz

1. List eight normal homeostatic functions of the hematopoietic system.

_____
_____
_____
_____
_____
_____
_____

2. From what cell type do RBCs, WBCs, and platelets originate?

_____
_____

3. The average lifespan of a normal RBC is how many days?

_____
_____

4. The average lifespan of a platelet is how many days?

_____
_____

5. What are the normal ranges of hematocrit for adult males and females?

_____

_____

6. What blood type is considered the universal donor?

_____

_____

7. True or False: The etiology of most blood disorders can be determined in the field without laboratory testing.

_____

_____

8. In acute leukemia, life-threatening illness can occur from what syndrome?

_____

_____

Terminology

Adipocyte A fat cell; a connective tissue cell that has differentiated and become specialized in the synthesis (manufacture) and storage of fat.

Anemia Deficiency in RBCs or hemoglobin; most common form is iron-deficiency anemia.

Coagulation cascade A set of interactions of the circulating clotting factors.

Disseminated intravascular coagulation (DIC) A complex, systemic, thrombohemorrhagic disorder involving the generation of intravascular fibrin and the consumption of procoagulants and platelets.

Endothelial cells A thin layer of flat epithelial cells that lines serous cavities, lymph vessels, and blood vessels.

Erythropoiesis The development and differentiation of RBCs; typically occurs in the bone marrow.

Erythropoietin A hormone that stimulates peripheral stem cells in the bone marrow to produce RBCs.

Fibrinolysis The clot-dissolving portion of coagulation.

Fibroblasts A cell that gives rise to connective tissue.

Hematocrit A measure of the relative percentage of blood cells (mainly erythrocytes) in a given volume of whole blood; also called *volume of packed red cells* or *packed cell volume*.

Humoral Pertaining to elements in the blood or other body fluids.

Leukocytosis An increase in the number of WBCs in the blood; typically results from infection, hemorrhage, fever, inflammation, or other factors.

Leukopenia A decrease in the total number of WBCs in the blood.

Macrophages Large WBCs that ingest foreign substances and display on their surfaces antigens produced from the foreign substances to be recognized by other cells of the immune system.

Plasma The noncellular liquid component of unclotted whole blood.

Pluripotent Cell line that has the ability to differentiate into multiple different cell lines based on the right physiologic stimulus.

RBC count The number of RBCs per liter of blood.

Reticular cells The cells forming the reticular fibers of connective tissue; those forming the framework of lymph nodes, bone marrow, and spleen are part of the reticuloendothelial system and under appropriate stimulation may differentiate into macrophages.

Thrombocytopenia A lower than normal number of platelets circulating in the blood.

Volume of packed red cells A measure of the relative percentage of blood cells (mainly erythrocytes) in a given volume of whole blood; also called *hematocrit* or *packed cell volume.*

DIVISION 6

SHOCK

Shock and Resuscitation

Objectives
After completing this chapter, you will be able to:

1. Discuss the anatomy and physiology of the cardiovascular system.
2. Discuss the stages and types of shock, including aerobic and anaerobic metabolism, and the ischemic, stagnant, and washout phases of shock.
3. Describe the etiology, history, and physical findings of hypovolemic shock.
4. Using the patient history and physical examination findings, develop a treatment plan for a patient in hypovolemic shock.
5. Describe the etiology, epidemiology, history, and physical findings of cardiogenic shock.
6. Using the patient history and physical examination findings, develop a treatment plan for a patient in cardiogenic shock.
7. Describe the etiology, epidemiology, history, and physical findings of distributive shock.
8. Using the patient history and physical examination findings, develop a treatment plan for a patient in distributive shock.
9. Describe the etiology, epidemiology, history, and physical findings of obstructive shock.
10. Using the patient history and physical examination findings, develop a treatment plan for a patient in obstructive shock.
11. Discuss dissociative shock.

Chapter Outline

Cardiovascular System Review
Shock
Categories and Types of Shock

Special Considerations
Chapter Summary

Case Scenario

You and your partner respond to a small motel complex for an "unknown medical problem." As you arrive at the scene, a police officer motions you into room 12. As your eyes adjust from the bright sunlight to the dark, dingy motel room, you see a young man in his mid-20s sitting on the floor leaning against the couch. Empty beer cans litter the floor, and you see a pan of what appears to be coffee-ground emesis sitting next to the patient. He looks pale and seems to have difficulty focusing on you and your partner as you approach. His chest is rising and falling without distress, and he is able to speak without difficulty.

Questions

1. What is your general impression of this patient?
2. What additional assessment will be important in the evaluation of this patient?
3. What intervention should you initiate at this time?

Perfusion is the circulation of blood through an organ structure. Perfusion is the delivery of oxygen and other nutrients to the cells of all organ systems. **Shock** is defined as inadequate tissue perfusion. It results from the failure of the cardiovascular system to deliver enough oxygen and nutrients to keep vital organs functioning. The underlying cause of shock must be recognized and treated promptly. Otherwise, the patient's cells and organs may begin to malfunction and the patient could die.

CARDIOVASCULAR SYSTEM REVIEW

[OBJECTIVE 1]

For the body's tissues to be perfused adequately, the cardiovascular system must be intact. This includes an adequate fluid volume (the blood), a container to regulate the distribution of the fluid (the blood vessels), and a pump (the heart) with enough force to move the fluid throughout the container. A malfunction of or deficiency in any of these parts can affect perfusion.

Blood

The blood carries oxygen from the lungs to the body's tissues. It also carries carbon dioxide from the tissues to the lungs. Blood is composed of fluid and formed elements. The formed elements consist of red blood cells (RBCs), white blood cells (WBCs), and platelets.

Plasma

The formed elements are suspended in plasma, the liquid portion of the blood. Plasma carries many important substances, including nutrients, electrolytes, gases, wastes, and proteins such as albumin, clotting factors, antibodies, and hormones. A small amount of oxygen is dissolved in the plasma.

Red Blood Cells

RBCs account for 90% of all formed elements. In a healthy adult, RBCs compose 40% to 45% of the circulating blood volume. RBCs contain hemoglobin, an iron-containing protein that is able to bind with oxygen. When hemoglobin binds with oxygen, the blood assumes a bright red color. When oxygen is released from hemoglobin, the blood appears dark red.

The **Fick principle** describes the components needed for the oxygenation of the body's cells. It states that the oxygenation of the body's cells depends on both oxygen supply and oxygen demand. The supply of oxygen to the body's tissues depends on having an adequate number of RBCs to carry the oxygen, adequate blood flow to the tissues (perfusion), and efficient offloading of oxygen at the tissue level. The amount of oxygen used by the tissues is called the *oxygen consumption.* The amount of oxygen available to the tissues depends on the amount of oxygen taken into the body (concentration of inspired oxygen) and movement of oxygen across the alveolar/capillary membrane into the bloodstream. The tissue's demands for oxygen are met by having an adequate supply of blood and oxygen. When the tissues need more oxygen and/or cardiac output decreases, the body's tissues must extract more oxygen from the blood to meet their oxygen needs.

PARAMEDIC Pearl

All types of shock have an important feature in common; they all involve a critical reduction in the supply of oxygenated blood to the body's tissues. Without oxygen, the body's cells shift from aerobic to anaerobic metabolism.

Anemia. A person who has a decreased RBC count has a decreased oxygen-carrying ability. This condition is known as **anemia.** Anemia results in decreased tissue oxygenation, which may be caused by the loss, underproduction, or destruction of RBCs. When hemorrhage is the cause of anemia, the condition is known as **hemorrhagic anemia.** The decreased production of RBCs is seen in conditions such as leukemia and sickle cell disease. Anemia that results from the destruction of RBCs is called **hemolytic anemia.**

White Blood Cells

WBCs consume infectious organisms and produce antibodies. When an infection is present in the body, the number of WBCs increases to fight off the infecting organism. The role of WBCs is covered in more detail in Chapter 33.

Platelets

In healthy individuals, the body attempts to balance its tendency toward clotting and bleeding. Platelets take part in blood clotting. When a blood vessel is injured, platelets rush to the site to plug the leak. Because the surface of a platelet is sticky, platelets quickly clump (agglutinate) together. With the help of fibrinogen (a protein), the platelets form a clot. A scab is an example of an external blood clot. Blood clots also can form within the body. Some internal blood clots are useful. For example, a bruise is evidence of clotted blood, usually from injury to small blood vessels. In some situations an internal blood clot can cause serious problems if it cuts off the supply of oxygen and nutrients to an organ. For instance, a clot in a blood vessel of the brain can cause a stroke. A clot in a blood vessel of the heart can cause a myocardial infarction. Clot-busting drugs (fibrinolytics) are sometimes used to destroy the clot and restore blood flow to the affected area.

The body's blood-clotting ability can be affected by diseases and medications. Examples of drugs that affect blood clotting are shown in Box 34-1. Herbal products such as garlic, ginseng, and gingko also can affect blood clotting. When the number of platelets in the blood falls below its normal range, a person may bleed uncontrollably.

Blood Vessels

Arteries are conductance vessels. The main function of the large arteries is to carry blood from the heart to the arterioles (Figure 34-1). All arteries, except the pulmonary

---

BOX 34-1 Drugs That Affect Blood Clotting

- Abciximab (ReoPro)
- Aspirin
- Clopidogrel (Plavix)
- Dipyridamole (Persantine)
- Enoxaparin (Lovenox)
- Eptifibatide (Integrilin)
- Ticlopidine (Ticlid)
- Tirofiban (Aggrastat)
- Warfarin (Coumadin)

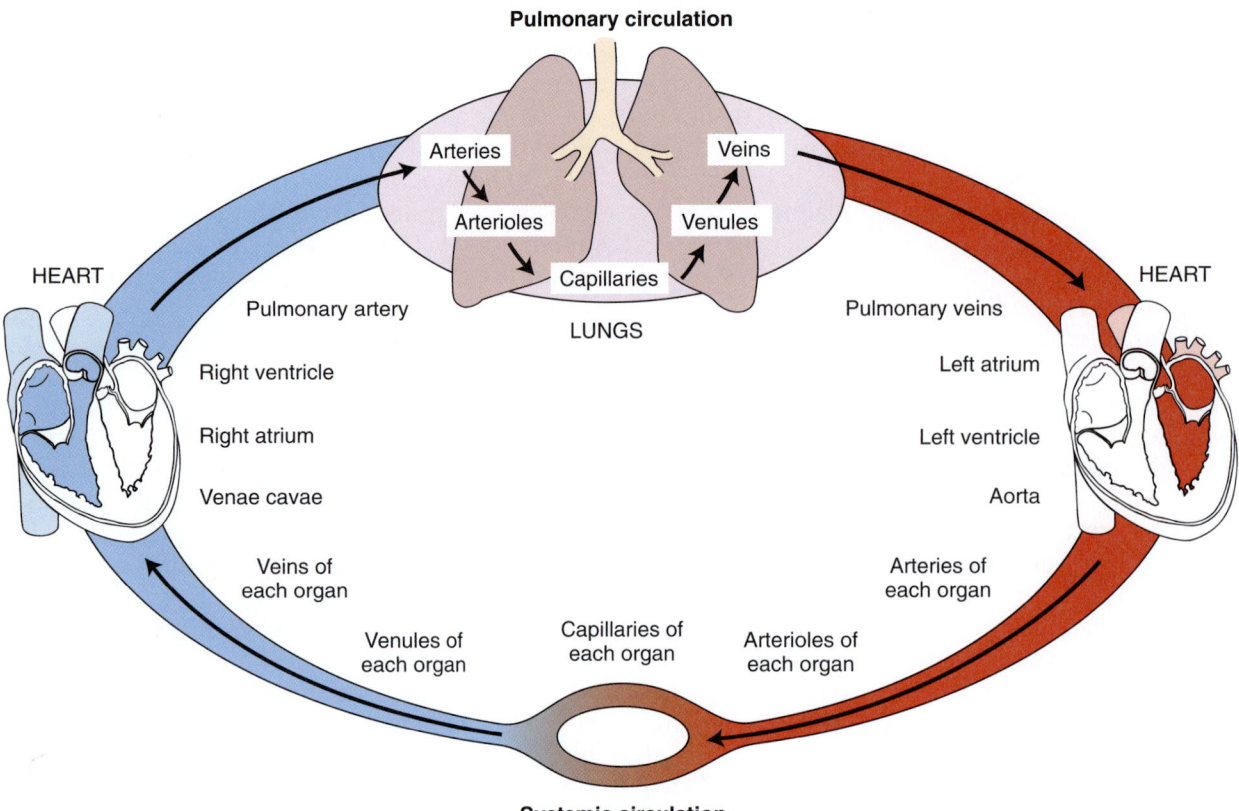

Figure 34-1 Systemic and pulmonary circulation.

arteries, carry oxygen-rich blood. Arteries are designed to carry blood under high pressure.

Arterioles are the smallest branches of the arteries. They connect arteries and capillaries. Precapillary sphincters are present where the arterioles and capillaries meet. These sphincters contract and relax to control blood flow throughout the capillaries. Precapillary sphincters respond to the needs of local tissue, opening as more blood is needed. Arterioles are composed almost entirely of smooth muscle. The presence of smooth muscle in the vessel walls allows the vessel to adjust its diameter, thereby controlling the amount of blood flow to specific tissues. Because changing the diameter of the arterioles also affects the resistance to the flow of blood, arterioles are called *resistance vessels*. A dilated (widened) vessel offers less resistance to blood flow. A constricted (narrowed) vessel offers more resistance to blood flow.

PEDIATRIC *Pearl*

Infants and children are capable of more effective vasoconstriction than are adults. As a result, a previously healthy infant or child is able to maintain a normal blood pressure and organ perfusion for a longer time in the presence of shock.

Capillaries are the smallest and most numerous of the blood vessels. They connect arterioles and venules and function as exchange vessels. The capillary wall consists of a single layer of cells (endothelium) with holes (pores) through which fluid, oxygen, carbon dioxide, electrolytes, glucose and other nutrients, and wastes are exchanged between the blood and tissues.

Venules are the smallest branches of veins. They connect capillaries and veins. Postcapillary sphincters are present where the venules and capillaries meet. They contract and relax to control blood flow from body tissues. For example, postcapillary sphincters open when blood needs to be emptied into the venous system. Venules are designed to carry blood under low pressure. The wall of a venule is slightly thicker than the wall of a capillary. The thickness of the wall increases as the venules join to form larger veins.

Veins carry deoxygenated (oxygen-poor) blood from the body to the right side of the heart. All veins, except the pulmonary veins, carry deoxygenated blood. The walls of veins are thinner than the walls of arteries. Because most (approximately 70%) of the body's blood is located in them at any one time, veins are called *capacitance* (storage) *vessels*. Venous blood flow depends on skeletal muscle action, respiratory movements, and gravity. The valves in the larger veins of the extremities and neck are arranged to allow blood flow in one direction, toward the heart.

Heart

The heart is a four-chambered muscle that pumps the blood through the blood vessels. Two thin-walled atria sit atop two thicker walled ventricles. Blood returns to the heart from the body by way of the inferior and superior venae cavae. Oxygen-depleted blood enters the right atrium and then the right ventricle. The right ventricle pumps the blood to the lungs through the pulmonary artery, where it receives oxygen. From the lungs, oxygen-rich blood returns to the left atrium by way of the pulmonary veins. The blood passes from the left atrium to the left ventricle, where it is pumped to the body by the aorta. As blood enters the two atria, 70% of the blood flows passively from the atrial chambers into the ventricles. When the atria contract, they push the last 30% of the blood into the ventricles. This final push of blood from the atria is known as **atrial kick.** Atrial kick is important to help maintain cardiac preload. **Preload** is the amount of blood in the ventricles before contraction (Figure 34-2). Preload must be maintained to maintain stroke volume. **Stroke volume** is the amount of blood pushed out of the left ventricle with each contraction. **Cardiac output** can be defined as heart rate multiplied by stroke volume. If a person's heart rate is too high or too low, or if stroke volume decreases, cardiac output decreases. When veins constrict, the amount of blood returning to the heart increases. This increases preload, which increases cardiac output. When veins dilate, less blood is returned to the heart. As a result, preload is decreased.

Constriction and dilation of arteries affect afterload. **Afterload** is the pressure in the aorta against which the left ventricle must pump to eject blood. When arteries constrict, the pressure within them increases, which increases afterload. When arteries dilate, afterload decreases, resulting in decreased perfusion pressure.

SHOCK

Adequate perfusion depends on cardiac output (CO), systemic vascular resistance (SVR), and the transport of oxygen. Remember that cardiac output is equal to stroke volume (SV) multiplied by heart rate (HR) (CO = SV × HR). Blood pressure (BP) is equal to cardiac output multiplied by systemic vascular resistance (BP = CO × SVR). Shock can result from the following conditions:

- Failure of the pump (heart), resulting in inadequate CO
- Failure of the pipes (blood vessels); significant changes in SVR (vasoconstriction causes excessive resistance and vasodilation decreases resistance)

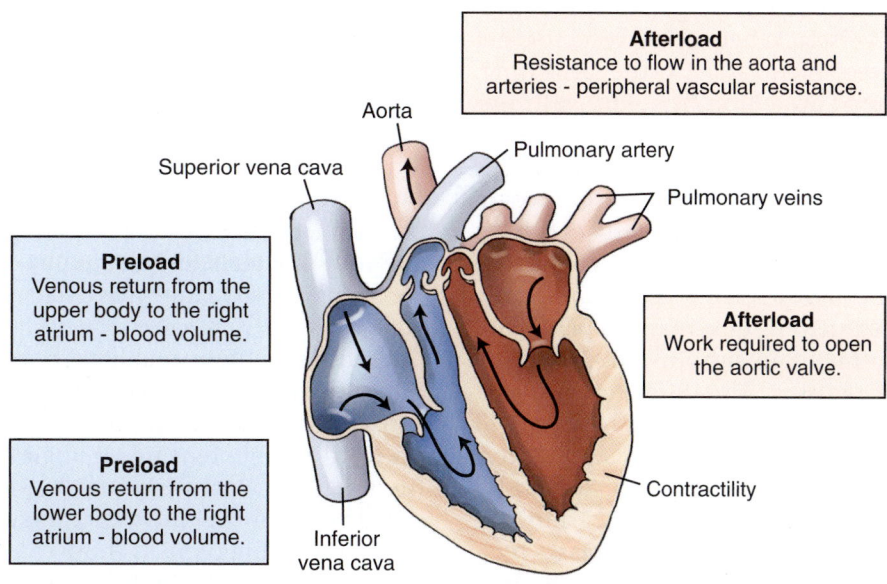

Figure 34-2 Stroke volume is determined by preload, afterload, and contractility.

- Inadequate fluid in the pipes (blood volume)
- Inability of RBCs to deliver oxygen to tissues

Stages of Shock

[OBJECTIVE 2]

When a condition sends the body into shock, the body attempts to compensate. The goal of compensation is to maintain perfusion of vital organs. If the cause of shock is not identified and halted, the body's compensation efforts begin to fail. Eventually the body reaches an irreversible point and death becomes imminent. The different stages of shock are early (compensated) shock, late (progressive or decompensated) shock, and irreversible shock.

Early (Compensated) Shock

Compensated shock is described as inadequate tissue perfusion without hypotension. Stated another way, early shock is shock with a "normal" blood pressure. Compensated shock also is called *reversible shock* because, at this stage, the shock syndrome is reversible with prompt recognition and appropriate emergency care.

When an event occurs that results in decreased perfusion (such as blood loss, a heart attack, tension pneumothorax, or a loss of vasomotor tone), the body's compensatory mechanisms attempt to preserve the vital organs. The body responds to shock in a number of ways.

Autonomic Nervous System. Chemoreceptors are stimulated by a decrease in the partial pressure of oxygen (PaO_2) and an increase in the partial pressure of carbon dioxide ($PaCO_2$). In response, ventilation increases in rate and depth. Baroreceptors are special pressure sensors found in the carotid arteries and aortic arch. When these receptors sense a decrease in cardiac output, they quickly send a message to the adrenal glands (Figure 34-3). The adrenal glands respond by releasing epinephrine and norepinephrine.

Epinephrine and norepinephrine stimulate $alpha_1$ receptors in the blood vessels. When $alpha_1$ receptors are stimulated, the blood vessels constrict. At the same time, blood flow is redistributed away from the skin, gastrointestinal (GI) tract, kidneys, fat, and muscle to vital organs such as the heart and brain. Venous constriction pushes more blood into the right ventricle, increasing preload. Increasing preload will increase SV and cardiac output. Arterial constriction increases afterload. This increases the pressure in the arteries. By increasing arterial pressure, blood pressure increases, helping ensure tissue perfusion. The overall effect is to maintain systolic blood pressure by increasing diastolic pressure. The difference between the systolic and diastolic pressures (pulse pressure) will decrease (narrow). Additionally, in a healthy adult, a correlation exists between an increase in heart rate and a decrease in systolic blood pressure. For each 1-mm Hg drop in systolic blood pressure, heart rate increases by 1 beat/min. This is not typically true for older adults, because of chronic illness and medications.

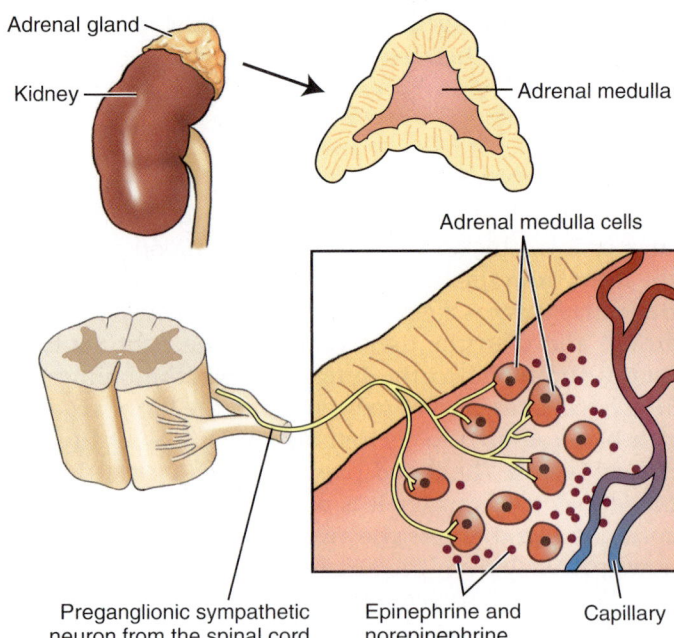

Figure 34-3 The adrenal glands release epinephrine and norepinephrine.

> **PARAMEDIC*Pearl***
> Increased afterload can be compared to placing your thumb over the end of a running garden hose. The same amount of water leaves the hose but with greater force and traveling further.

Epinephrine also stimulates $beta_1$ receptors. When these receptor sites are stimulated, the heart rate (chronotropy), the heart's force of contraction (inotropy), and the speed of impulse conduction through the heart (dromotropy) all increase. These effects work to increase cardiac output. Increased cardiac output helps maintain perfusion. Epinephrine also stimulates $beta_2$ receptors, resulting in bronchodilation and dilation of the smooth muscles of the GI tract. Through these mechanisms the body contracts the size of the container. By increasing the force of contraction, heart rate, and dilation of the lungs, perfusion through the brain and lungs is improved. This mechanism maintains the patient's systolic blood pressure and thus tissue perfusion.

Renin-Angiotensin-Aldosterone Mechanism. When blood flow to the kidneys is decreased, the juxtaglomerular complex (JGC) in the kidneys is stimulated, activating the renin-angiotensin-aldosterone system (Figure 34-4). When the JGC is stimulated by a decrease in blood flow, it releases renin. Renin converts angiotensinogen (from the liver) to angiotensin I. As angiotensin I passes through the lungs, it is converted to angiotensin II by enzymes called angiotensin-converting enzymes (ACE).

Although angiotensin II only lasts in the body a short time, it is one of the body's most powerful vasoconstricting agents. This vasoconstriction further increases preload

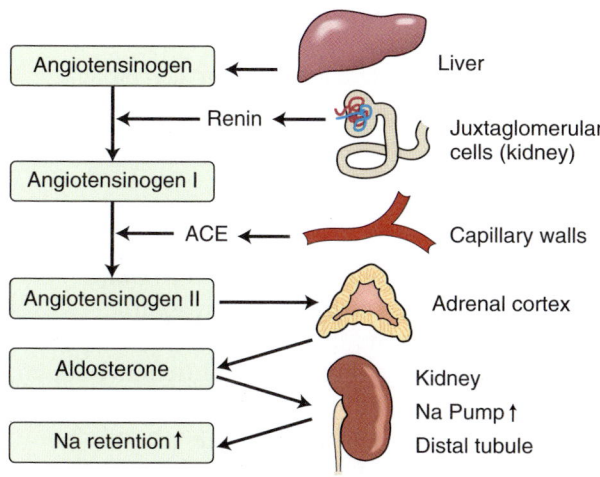

Figure 34-4 Renin-angiotensin-aldosterone mechanism.

by forcing blood in the venous system into the right side of the heart. Afterload is increased when the arteries constrict, increasing the pressure against which the heart is pushing. The more distal the blood vessel is from the heart, the greater the constriction during shock. At the most distal capillaries, the precapillary sphincter constricts, stopping blood flow *into* the capillaries. The postcapillary sphincter constricts, stopping the flow of blood *out* of the capillaries. This is known as the **ischemic phase** of shock. The goal of the body with these processes is to maintain perfusion to its vital organs. This process is known as *selective perfusion*. The distal tissues have a decreased blood supply, and the heart, brain, liver, and lungs have their perfusion maintained.

Angiotensin II stimulates the production of aldosterone. Aldosterone is released from the adrenal cortex, causing the kidneys to reabsorb sodium in the renal tubules. Water follows sodium, so more water returns to the body and less is lost as urine. Although urine output is decreased, more fluid remains within the blood vessels. Increased volume within the blood vessels increases the volume of blood returning to the right side of the heart (preload), increasing blood pressure and cardiac output.

Release of Antidiuretic Hormone. Antidiuretic hormone (ADH) (vasopressin) is secreted from the pituitary gland. ADH has vasoconstrictive properties and causes the kidneys to reabsorb water in the renal collecting ducts. These actions decrease urine output and move more volume into the venous system. Increased volume within the blood vessels increases the volume of blood returning to the right side of the heart, increasing blood pressure and cardiac output.

Intracellular Fluid Shift. The human body is approximately 60% water. Most of the body's fluid is in its cells and tissues. As the body begins to go into shock, it slowly moves fluid from the cells and tissues into the blood vessels. This helps increase blood volume and the volume of blood returning to the right side of the heart, thereby increasing blood pressure and cardiac output. If a patient

progresses into shock slowly, you may see signs of this fluid shift. The patient's skin will be dry with poor **turgor** (elasticity). When you pinch the patient's skin and then release it, the skin will stay tented. The patient's mucous membranes will be dry, and he or she may report thirst (because of cellular dehydration).

You can recognize the presence of compensated shock by taking the following actions:

- Assessing heart rate
- Assessing the presence and volume (strength) of peripheral pulses
- Assessing the adequacy of end-organ perfusion
  - Brain: assess mental status
  - Skin: assess skin temperature and capillary refill (in infants and children younger than 6 years)
  - Kidneys: assess urine output

Compensated shock is usually reversible if the cause is promptly identified and corrected. If uncorrected, shock progresses to the next stage.

PEDIATRIC Pearl

The initial signs of shock may be subtle in an infant or child. The effectiveness of compensatory mechanisms depends largely on the child's previous cardiac and pulmonary health. The pediatric patient can progress from compensated to decompensated shock suddenly and rapidly. When decompensation occurs, cardiopulmonary arrest may be imminent.

Late (Decompensated) Shock

Decompensated shock begins when the compensatory mechanisms start to fail. Decompensated shock also is called *progressive shock*. At this stage, the classic signs and symptoms of shock are evident.

During this stage of shock the protective mechanisms carried out during compensated shock now create additional complications for the body. Blood vessels respond to epinephrine and norepinephrine release with maximal constriction. The liver and spleen release stored supplies of RBCs and plasma. When precapillary sphincters dilate, blood rushes into the capillary beds. But the ongoing constriction of the postcapillary sphincters causes the blood to stand still and clot in the capillary beds. This is known as the **stagnant phase** of shock.

The capillaries become swollen and blocked with clumps of RBCs. Cells distal to the blockage become ischemic and shift to anaerobic metabolism to survive. Anaerobic metabolism is ineffective. It produces only a small amount of energy. However, it produces a large amount of lactic and pyruvic acid. The presence of excess acid causes the cell walls to break down. This cellular breakdown allows potassium to leak from the cells. Plasma also leaks from the capillaries. This results in an increase in interstitial fluid. The distance from the capillary to the cell increases. The oxygen-carrying capacity of the blood is reduced because of the increased capillary-cell distance.

As the blood pools in the capillary beds, platelets begin to stick together, forming miniclots (microemboli). This increases the thickness (viscosity) of the blood and creates blood clots throughout the body. Clotting factors are quickly exhausted. As a result, clotting does not take place where needed and bleeding occurs from multiple sites in the body. This condition is known as **disseminated intravascular coagulation (DIC).**

Pooling of blood in the capillaries causes a decrease in blood volume. Decreased blood volume causes decreased cardiac output. Decreased cardiac output causes continued hypoperfusion. Continued hypoperfusion causes increased anaerobic metabolism. Increased anaerobic metabolism results in increased acid production. Increased acid production causes decreased cardiac output and cellular damage. Shock breeds shock. Cardiac output falls and hypotension occurs (Figure 34-5). Decompensated shock is difficult to treat but is reversible if you begin appropriate aggressive care.

> **PARAMEDIC***Pearl*
>
> The presence of hypotension distinguishes compensated shock from decompensated shock.

> **PEDIATRIC***Pearl*
>
> Hypotension is a late sign of cardiovascular compromise in an infant or a child.

Irreversible Shock

In irreversible shock the body's compensatory mechanisms fail. Irreversible shock also is called *terminal shock.* In this stage of shock the continued anaerobic metabolism from hypoperfusion results in metabolic acidosis. Metabolic acidosis causes the postcapillary sphincters to open. This allows stagnated and coagulated blood that has pooled in the capillaries to be flushed through the system. This is known as the **washout phase** of shock. The excess potassium and acid, now being pushed into the body's vascular system, cause cardiac dysrhythmias that further decrease cardiac output. Clotted blood moves to the lungs, causing pulmonary emboli. This increases **hypoxemia.** As the intestines become ischemic, the flora living within them die. As the flora die, they release endotoxins as a byproduct of their death. These endotoxins are absorbed into the vascular space and circulated through the body.

In irreversible shock, cellular damage occurs throughout the body. As cells are damaged, tissue becomes damaged. As tissue is damaged, organs fail. When organs

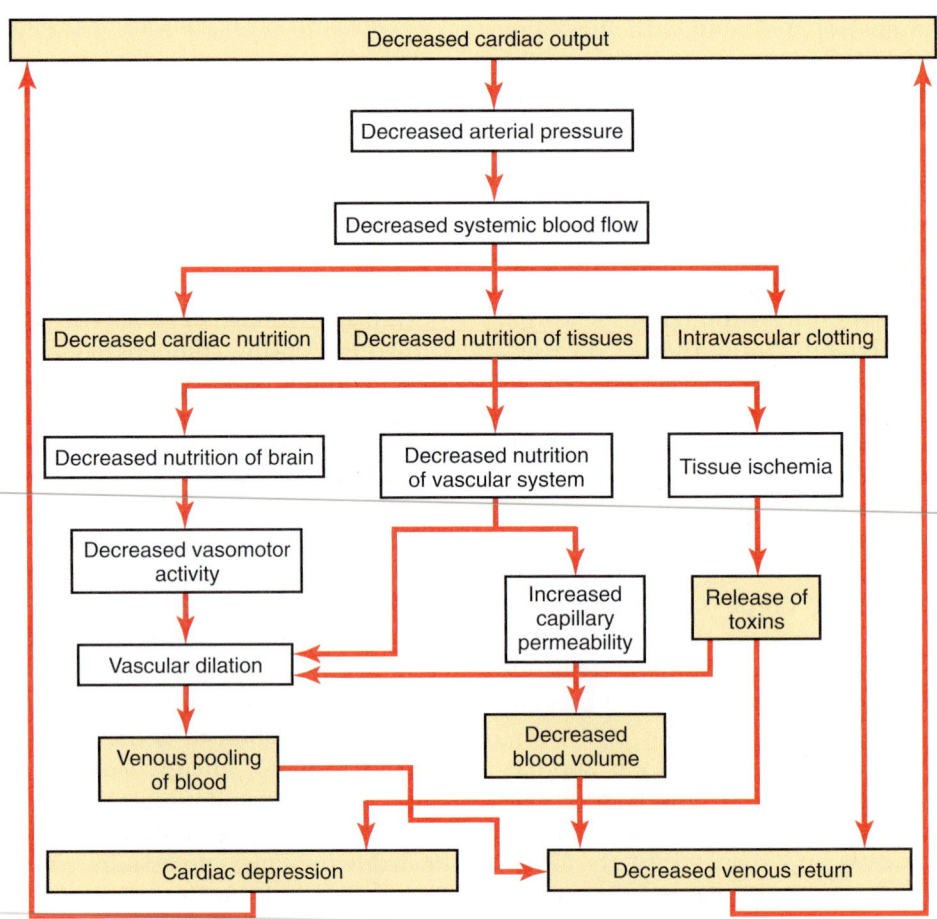

Figure 34-5 The vicious cycle of decompensated shock.

fail, body systems fail. When body systems fail, the organism (the body) dies. This is known as **multiple organ dysfunction syndrome.**

People in irreversible shock will usually die. They may survive from the field to the emergency department and perhaps into the intensive care unit, but they will develop renal failure, liver failure, **adult respiratory distress syndrome,** sepsis, or another complication that will result in death. Your goal as a paramedic is to recognize patients in danger of progressing into irreversible shock. They need rapid treatment and transport to appropriate definitive care.

Case Scenario—continued

The patient's skin is pale and dry, with poor turgor. He is alert and oriented and complains of abdominal pain, vomiting for the past 3 to 4 hours, and dizziness when he stands. He states that he has consumed four six-packs of beer in the last 18 hours and has not eaten. His medical history includes type 1 diabetes and "bleeding ulcers" for the past year. He has taken his insulin as usual throughout the episode. Vital signs are pulse, 124 beats/min; blood pressure, 84/60 mm Hg; respirations, 16 breaths/min. Blood glucose is 155 mg/dL. The remainder of the examination findings are normal.

Questions

4. Is this patient high priority? Why or why not?
5. What stage of shock is this patient in? Should you infuse intravenous (IV) fluids? If so, how much?
6. What additional treatment should be initiated?
7. What destination is most appropriate for this patient?

CATEGORIES AND TYPES OF SHOCK

Shock, by itself, is not a diagnosis. Shock is *always* attributable to some other cause. Shock is an assessment finding that should lead you to search aggressively for and find the cause of the shock (Box 34-2). After you identify the cause of the shock, you must focus patient care on stopping the cause of the shock. Some causes of shock can be halted in the field and some cannot. For example, you can stop an external arterial bleed or convert a patient out of ventricular tachycardia. Other causes of shock, such as internal hemorrhage or sepsis, cannot be stopped in the field. You must be able to recognize shock and rapidly transport the patient to definitive care.

Hypovolemic Shock

Description and Definition

Hypovolemic shock is inadequate tissue perfusion caused by inadequate vascular volume (Figure 34-6).

PARAMEDIC *Pearl*

Hypovolemic shock = ↓ intravascular volume → ↓ venous return → ↓ preload → ↓ stroke volume → ↓ cardiac output → inadequate tissue perfusion

Etiology

[OBJECTIVE 3]

Hemorrhagic shock (a type of hypovolemic shock) is caused by severe internal or external bleeding. Causes of major blood loss are shown in Box 34-3. Hypovolemic shock also may be caused by fluid loss not related to bleeding. For example, external fluid loss may occur because of dehydration, vomiting, or diarrhea. The redistribution of interstitial fluid ("third spacing") may occur in diabetes mellitus or diabetes insipidus. Plasma loss may occur because of thermal injury.

The severity of hypovolemic shock is associated with the patient's normal state of health, amount of fluid lost, and the rate at which fluid is lost. In a healthy patient, a loss of 10% to 15% of the circulating blood volume is usually well tolerated and easily compensated (Table 34-1). The circulating blood volume is proportionately larger in infants and children than it is in adults; however, their *total* blood volume is less than in adults. As a result, a small volume loss can result in serious signs and symptoms. To understand this important point, consider a 2-year-old child. By the pediatric weight formula, 8 + (2 × age in years), the child's weight is approximately 12 kg. With a value of 70 mL/kg as the normal circulating blood volume for a child this age, his or her estimated

---

BOX 34-2 | Five Primary Categories of Shock

- Hypovolemic
- Cardiogenic
- Distributive
- Obstructive/mechanical
- Dissociative

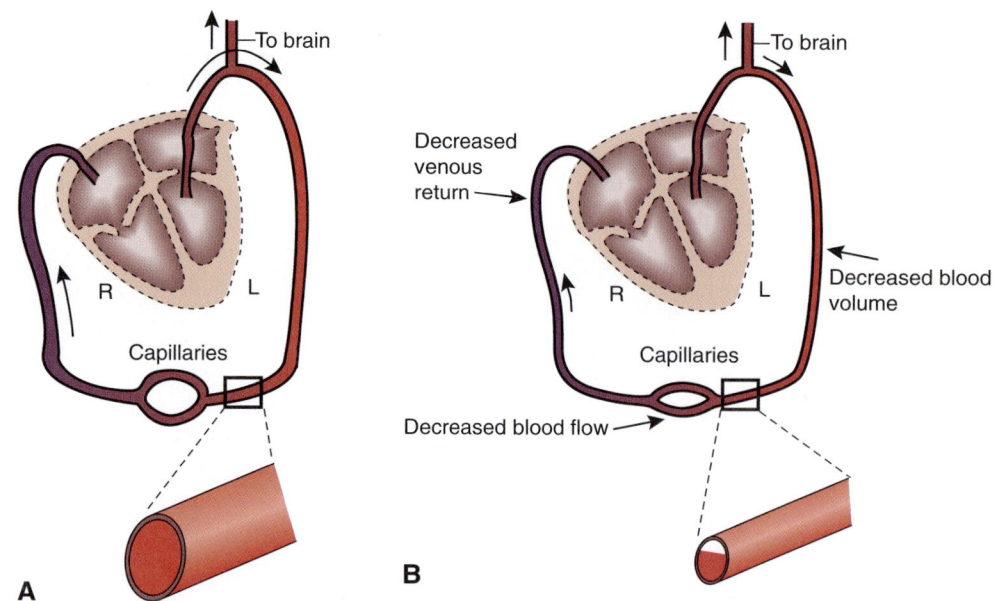

Figure 34-6 A, Normal circulation. **B,** Hypovolemic shock.

BOX 34-3 | Causes of Major Blood Loss

- Solid organ injury
- Abdominal aortic aneurysm rupture
- Vascular injury
- Penetrating trauma
- Severe gastrointestinal bleeding
- Ruptured liver or spleen
- Hemothorax
- Ruptured ectopic pregnancy
- Arteriovenous malformation
- Bleeding esophageal varices
- Pelvic fracture
- Femur fracture
- Bleeding peptic ulcer
- Placenta previa
- Abruptio placenta
- Scalp lacerations (infants/young children)
- Intracranial hemorrhage (newborn or infant)

---

blood volume is 840 mL. A volume loss of only 250 mL (approximately 30% of the blood volume) is significant and likely to produce signs and symptoms of decompensated shock in this child.

History

The amount and type of information you will be able to gather will vary depending on the patient's condition. However, obtain a history as soon as possible to help identify the type of shock present, the patient's previous health, and the onset and duration of symptoms. If the patient is too ill to answer your questions, look to other sources such as family members, friends, or law enforce-

ment personnel at the scene to provide the information you need.

> **PARAMEDIC*Pearl***
> Significant amounts of blood loss can occur with blunt trauma to the chest, abdomen, or pelvis.

Physical Findings

Begin your assessment of the patient with hypovolemic shock as you arrive on the scene. If the scene involves trauma, look at the mechanism of injury and visually assess potential injuries. As you approach the patient, form a general impression. You must identify life threats surrounding airway, breathing, and circulation in your initial assessment and treat them before proceeding.

After your initial assessment and treatment of life threats, perform a detailed physical examination. The examination should be systematic and complete. Assess the patient for external bleeding and signs of internal bleeding. Any unexplained signs of shock should be assumed to be attributable to internal hemorrhage until proven otherwise. Patients in compensated hypovolemic shock have subtle signs and symptoms. They may be anxious and confused about recent events. Their heart rate will be faster than normal for their age. Their skin may be cool and diaphoretic. Repeated blood pressure measurements will reveal a narrowing **pulse pressure** caused by blood vessel constriction in an attempt to maintain perfusion. The patient's systolic blood pressure will remain the same, but arterial constriction will increase afterload and increase the diastolic value. This will narrow the pulse pressure. A pulse pressure less than 30 mm Hg is considered narrow and suggests that significant vasoconstriction is present.

TABLE 34-1   Response to Fluid and Blood Loss

	Class I	Class II	Class III	Class IV
Stage of shock		Early (compensated)	Late (decompensated)	Irreversible
% Blood volume loss	Up to 15%	15%-30%	30%-45%	>45%
Mental status	Slightly anxious	Mildly anxious, restless	Altered, lethargic, apathetic, decreased pain response	Extremely lethargic, unresponsive
Muscle tone	Normal	Normal	Normal to decreased	Limp
Respiratory rate/effort	Normal	Mild tachypnea	Moderate tachypnea	Severe tachypnea to agonal breathing
Skin color (extremities)	Pink	Pale, mottled	Pale, mottled, mild peripheral cyanosis	Pale, mottled, central and peripheral cyanosis
Skin turgor	Normal	Poor; sunken eyes and fontanelles in infant and young child	Poor; sunken eyes and fontanelles in infant and young child	Tenting
Skin temperature	Cool	Cool	Cool to cold	Cold
Capillary refill (children <6 years)	Normal	Poor (>2 seconds)	Delayed (>3 seconds)	Prolonged (>5 seconds)
Heart rate	Typically normal if gradual volume loss, increased if sudden loss of volume	Mild tachycardia	Significant tachycardia; possible dysrhythmias; peripheral pulse weak, thready, or may be absent	Marked tachycardia to bradycardia
Blood pressure	Normal	Lower range of normal	Decreased	Severe hypotension
Pulse pressure	Normal or increased	Narrowed	Decreased	Decreased

Patients with compensated hypovolemic shock reap the most benefit from your treatment. You must be careful not to miss the signs of compensated shock or attribute the signs to other causes (Box 34-4). For example, if a patient is scared or anxious, he or she may have the same physical findings as a person in compensated shock. You must repeat vital signs and evaluate for trends. If a person is scared or anxious, his or her vital signs should return to normal as he or she relaxes. A patient in shock continues to have a faster than normal heart rate and changes in mental status, pulse pressures continue to narrow, and blood pressure eventually drops. Evaluate the mechanism of injury and maintain a high index of suspicion to avoid missing the signs of a patient progressing into shock.

Decompensated hypovolemic shock is more easily recognized. The patient's heart rate will be faster than normal for his or her age. The patient's pulse will be weak and thready. He or she will have an increased respiratory rate and systolic blood pressure will begin to drop. The patient's mental status will continue to decrease. This patient is in danger of progressing further into shock and dying. You must be able to recognize the signs of decompensated shock, aggressively treat the patient, and rapidly transport to the closest and most appropriate facility.

PARAMEDIC Pearl

Shock is a dynamic process. You must continuously reassess the patient and monitor for changes in his or her presentation and vital signs. To note changes and trends in vital signs, you must obtain more than one set.

Signs and Symptoms of Compensated Shock

- Reports of thirst, weakness
- Normal or minimally impaired mental status, peripheral vasoconstriction, skin mottling, cool extremities, mild tachycardia, normal blood pressure, and narrowed pulse pressure

Signs and Symptoms of Decompensated Shock

- Altered mental status, decreased response to pain
- Dry mucous membranes, hypotension, significant tachycardia, weak central pulses, pale, mottled skin with mild peripheral cyanosis

Signs and Symptoms of Irreversible Shock

- Extreme lethargy, may be unresponsive; limp muscle tone; severe tachypnea that decreases to occasional, gasping breaths; cold, pale, mottled skin with central and peripheral cyanosis; marked tachycardia that deteriorates to bradycardia; severe hypotension

PARAMEDIC*Pearl*

Trauma, Tachycardia, and Hypotension

Tachycardia does not always accompany hemorrhagic shock. Relative bradycardia may exist in some patients. Relative bradycardia is defined as a heart rate less than 90 beats/min and a systolic blood pressure less than 90 mm Hg. The absence of a tachycardic response to hypotension may be a protective reflex that improves stroke volume and preserves cardiac output by allowing more time for the ventricles to fill during diastole. In some severely injured patients, relative bradycardia has been associated with improved outcomes.

Do not allow the absence of tachycardia in a trauma patient to give you a false sense of security that the patient has a normal blood volume. According to one source, heart rate is not a good predictor of hypotension caused by hemorrhage. It is unreliable in the trauma patient when determining the severity of volume loss and/or degree of shock (Victorino et al., 2003).

Differential Diagnosis

Assume shock from hypovolemia until proven otherwise. Cardiogenic shock is distinguished from hypovolemic shock by the presence of one or more of the following:

- Chief complaint (chest discomfort, dyspnea, or tachycardia)
- Heart rate (bradycardia or excessive tachycardia)
- Signs of heart failure (jugular vein distention, crackles)
- Dysrhythmias

Distributive shock is distinguished from hypovolemic shock by the presence of one or more of the following:

- Mechanism that suggests vasodilation, such as spinal cord injury, drug overdose, sepsis, or anaphylaxis
- Warm, flushed skin, especially in dependent areas
- Lack of tachycardia (not always reliable because some hypovolemic patients never become tachycardic)

Obstructive shock is distinguished from hypovolemic shock by the presence of signs and symptoms suggestive of cardiac tamponade (muffled heart tones, distended neck veins) or tension pneumothorax (tracheal deviation, absent or decreased breath sounds on one side).

Therapeutic Interventions

[OBJECTIVE 4]

If trauma is the source of the patient's signs and symptoms, stabilize the cervical spine as needed. Make sure the patient's airway is open. Keep in mind that as a patient progresses further into shock, his or her level of consciousness decreases. The patient may have a respiratory drive but may lose the ability to protect his or her airway. Therefore you must be prepared to manage the airway of a patient in shock. Give high-concentration oxygen. Ensure ventilation and oxygenation are effective. Apply a pulse oximeter and use capnography, if available. Maintain oxygen saturation at greater than 95%. Suction as needed. Perform needle decompression of the chest if signs and symptoms of a tension pneumothorax are present. Control life-threatening bleeding. Apply the cardiac monitor. Avoid performing additional procedures on the scene that will delay transport to the hospital (Box 34-5).

PARAMEDIC*Pearl*

Use pulse oximetry with caution in a patient in hemorrhagic shock. The reading may not truly represent the patient's oxygenation status. Pulse oximetry measures saturated hemoglobin. Patients who hemorrhage lose hemoglobin. The hemoglobin left in the bloodstream during hemorrhagic shock therefore may be bound with oxygen, revealing a high pulse oximetry reading, but not enough hemoglobin may be present. This is known as *hemorrhagic anemia*. If in doubt, always provide high-flow oxygen to the patient in hemorrhagic shock.

To help maintain perfusion, place the patient in the supine position. Establish IV access en route to definitive care. When shock is present, the most readily available vascular access site is preferred. Attempt IV access with two large peripheral IV lines. Venous access may be difficult to obtain in a patient in shock. If immediate vascular access is needed and you cannot rapidly achieve reliable venous access, establish intraosseous (IO) access. If decompensated shock is present, immediate IO access is appropriate.

Give IV fluids per local protocol or medical direction instructions. If breath sounds are clear, an IV fluid chal-

BOX 34-5   Patient Management: Hypovolemic Shock

- ABCs, oxygen (endotracheal intubation if needed), IV, monitor
- Vital signs, pulse oximetry, capnography (if available)
- Place patient supine
- If breath sounds are clear, an IV fluid challenge of normal saline or lactated Ringer's solution is usually given
- Check patient's response; assess mental status, heart rate, respiratory effort, breath sounds, and blood pressure
- If no improvement, give additional fluids as instructed by medical direction; consider vasopressors if poor perfusion persists despite adequate ventilation, oxygenation, and volume expansion
- Recheck patient's response

ABCs, Airway, breathing, and circulation; *IV,* intravenous.

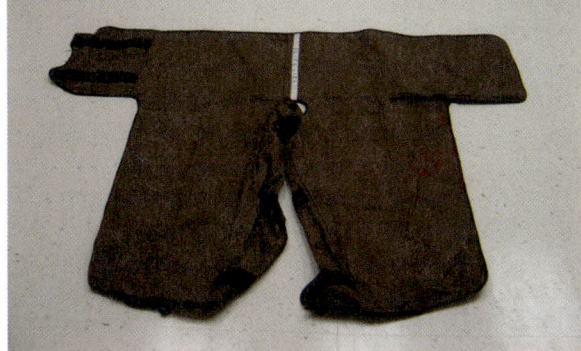

Figure 34-7 The pneumatic antishock garment (PASG).

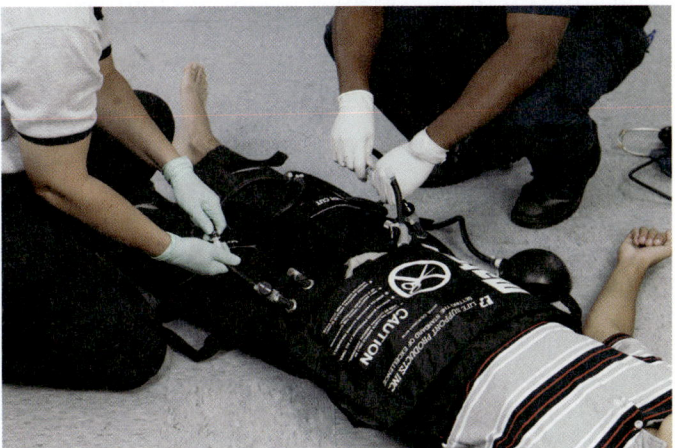

Figure 34-8 Applying the pneumatic antishock garment (PASG).

lenge of isotonic crystalloid solution is often given to maintain circulating blood volume. Crystalloid solutions do not carry oxygen and they do not clot. Therefore too much IV fluid can dilute the oxygen-carrying ability of the blood, causing further tissue hypoxia and acidosis. Too much IV fluid also can dilute the clotting ability of the blood, resulting in increased hemorrhage. Synthetic IV solutions that can carry oxygen are currently being researched. These solutions do not help with clotting but may help with tissue oxygenation. In general, IV fluids are given at a rate and volume necessary to improve perfusion but not so much as to worsen bleeding. Follow local protocol. Check the patient's response by assessing his or her mental status, heart rate, respiratory effort, breath sounds, and blood pressure. If no improvement occurs, give additional fluids as instructed by medical direction. Consider vasopressors if poor perfusion persists despite adequate ventilation, oxygenation, and volume expansion.

In some EMS systems the pneumatic antishock garment (PASG) is used to maintain blood pressure in a patient in hemorrhagic shock (Figure 34-7). The PASG may be beneficial in cases of suspected pelvic fractures with hypotension, suspected intraperitoneal hemorrhage with hypotension, suspected retroperitoneal hemorrhage with hypotension, and profound hypotension (systolic blood pressure less than 50 to 60 mm Hg). Place the PASG on the ground in an open position. Then place the patient on the PASG. The patient must be undressed. Next wrap the garment snuggly around the patient's legs and abdomen (Figure 34-8). As the patient's blood pressure drops, one leg compartment should be inflated to no more than 104 mm Hg or until the hook-and-eye closure material makes a crackling sound. Then reassess the patient's blood pressure. If the patient remains hypotensive, repeat the same procedure on the other leg. Again reassess the blood pressure. If the patient's blood pressure does not improve, inflate the abdominal compartment to no more than 110 mm Hg or until the closure material

makes a crackling sound. (Do not inflate the abdominal compartment if the patient is pregnant.) If the patient's blood pressure increases with the inflation of one of the leg compartments, do not inflate the others.

A fair amount of controversy surrounds the use of the PASG in the prehospital setting. Many argue that the PASG is ineffective in increasing blood pressure and improving perfusion. Do not delay transport to definitive care to apply this device. Do not inflate the abdominal compartment of a PASG if penetrating thoracic or abdominal injuries are present. Continuously monitor the patient's respiratory status as you apply the PASG because respiratory compromise can occur. The PASG is contraindicated in the following situations:

- Absolute contraindications
  - Congestive heart failure
  - Pulmonary edema
  - Penetrating thoracic injuries
  - Traumatic cardiopulmonary arrest
- Relative contraindications
  - Pregnancy*
  - Impaled objects in the abdomen*
  - Evisceration of abdominal organs*

*Do not inflate the abdominal compartment in these situations.

- Lower extremity compartment syndrome
- Circumferential lower extremity burns
- Lumbar spine injury
- Advanced age (Roberts & Hedges, 2004)

Removing the PASG in the prehospital setting is rarely, if ever, indicated. However, removal in the emergency department may be necessary. In these situations the paramedic may be called on by emergency department personnel who are unfamiliar with the device. Rapid deflation can be catastrophic and often is associated with a rapid drop in perfusion and blood pressure. Before deflation, assess the patient's hemodynamic status. Begin by slowly releasing a small amount of air from the abdominal compartment. If the systolic blood pressure falls by 5 mm Hg or more, stop deflation and administer IV fluids until blood pressure returns to baseline. Continue this process until the abdominal compartment is deflated; repeat the procedure for each leg compartment.

Check with medical direction and local EMS protocols about the use of the PASG in your area.

Check the patient's blood glucose level and treat if it is less than 60 mg/dL. Maintain normal body temperature. Rapidly transport a patient who has signs and symptoms of shock to the closest appropriate facility.

Patient and Family Education

In many cases hypovolemic shock is the result of a sudden illness or accident and cannot be prevented. Consequently you should provide emotional support to the patient and his or her family.

PARAMEDIC*Pearl*

Be sure to check the patient's vital signs before and after fluid resuscitation, invasive procedures, or with any sudden change in the patient's condition.

Case Scenario CONCLUSION

You and your partner place the patient on oxygen by nonrebreather mask (SpO_2 = 99%), establish two large-bore IVs, and administer normal saline (a total of 700 mL administered before arrival at the emergency department). On arrival at the hospital, the patient's mentation and color are improved. Vital signs are pulse, 104 beats/min; blood pressure, 120/88 mm Hg; respirations, 12 breaths/min. The patient receives a diagnosis of upper GI bleeding and is admitted to the hospital for further therapy and substance abuse counseling.

Looking Back

8. *Given the patient's final disposition, was your treatment appropriate? Why or why not?*

Cardiogenic Shock

Description and Definition

Cardiogenic shock is a condition in which the function of the heart muscle is severely impaired, leading to decreased cardiac output and inadequate tissue perfusion.

Etiology

[OBJECTIVE 5]

Cardiogenic shock may occur as a complication of shock from any cause. The most common cause of cardiogenic shock is a myocardial infarction (Figure 34-9). Cardiogenic shock also can occur if myocardial contractility is decreased from prolonged cardiac surgery, ventricular aneurysm, cardiac arrest, or rupture of the ventricular wall. Although rare, ventricular rupture usually occurs 4 to 7 days after a myocardial infarction. When the ventricular wall ruptures, blood leaks into the pericardial space and quickly leads to cardiac tamponade and cardiovascular collapse. Possible causes of cardiogenic shock are listed in Box 34-6.

Epidemiology and Demographics

Cardiogenic shock occurs in approximately 7% to 10% of patients with an acute myocardial infarction.

BOX 34-6 | **Possible Causes of Cardiogenic Shock**

- Myocardial infarction
- Prolonged cardiac surgery
- Ventricular aneurysm
- Ventricular wall rupture
- Cardiac dysrhythmias
- Rupture of the ventricular septum
- Myocarditis
- Cardiomyopathy
- Myocardial trauma
- Heart failure
- Hypothermia
- Severe electrolyte or acid-base imbalance
- Severe congenital heart disease

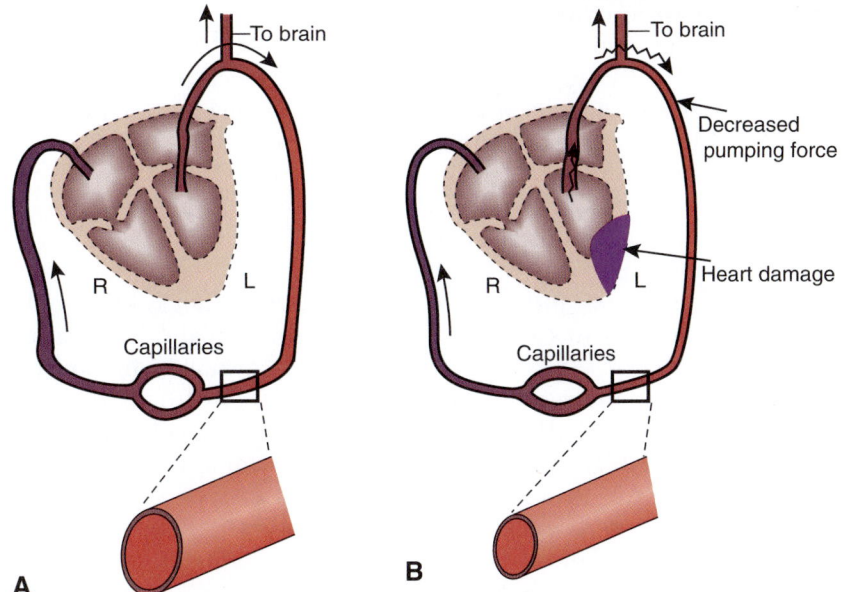

Figure 34-9 A, Normal circulation. **B,** Cardiogenic shock.

History

A patient in cardiogenic shock may be too ill to provide a medical history. If family members are present, they may be able to tell you if the patient has a history of heart disease. They may also be able to describe the patient's signs and symptoms that prompted a call to 9-1-1.

Mechanical problems from a recent MI often occur several days to a week after the infarction. If a dysrhythmia is associated with the patient's symptoms, the patient may describe recent episodes of palpitations, fainting, or lightheadedness.

Physical Findings

In compensated cardiogenic shock, the patient's mental status initially may be normal. As perfusion to the brain decreases, the patient becomes restless, agitated, and confused. In most patients, breath sounds reveal crackles. However, patients with right ventricular infarction or those who are hypovolemic may have less evidence of pulmonary congestion. Jugular venous distention (JVD), indicating right ventricular failure, may be present. If the patient is hypovolemic, JVD will be absent. Peripheral pulses often are weak and rapid. The patient's skin is usually pale or mottled. The extremities often feel cool and moist. The patient's systolic blood pressure initially may be normal, but pulse pressure is usually narrowed. If cardiogenic shock is associated with cardiac tamponade, the patient's heart sounds may be muffled.

In decompensated cardiogenic shock, the patient usually has an altered mental status or may be unresponsive. The patient's breathing is often rapid and shallow. Breath sounds usually reveal increasing pulmonary congestion and crackles. Peripheral pulses may be absent. Central pulses often are weak and rapid. The patient's

TABLE 34-2	Differential Diagnosis: Cardiogenic Shock	
Cardiovascular Causes	**Respiratory Causes**	**Other Causes**
Acute coronary syndromes	Pulmonary embolism	Hypovolemic shock
Aortic dissection		Sepsis, septic shock
Myocardial rupture		
Myocarditis		

skin is usually pale, mottled, or cyanotic. The extremities feel cold and sweaty. As ventricular function worsens and cardiac output falls, the systolic blood pressure progressively decreases.

Differential Diagnosis

Possible causes of cardiogenic shock are listed in Table 34-2.

Therapeutic Interventions

[OBJECTIVE 6]

The treatment of cardiogenic shock is generally based on increasing contractility without significantly increasing heart rate, altering preload and afterload, and controlling dysrhythmias if they are present and contributing to shock.

Administer high-concentration oxygen. Make sure oxygenation and ventilation are effective. Apply a pulse oximeter and use capnography. Maintain the patient's oxygen saturation at greater than 95%. Place the patient in a position of comfort. If pulmonary congestion is present and the patient's blood pressure will tolerate it, place him or her in a sitting position with the feet dangling. Be sure to limit the patient's physical activity while he or she is in your care. This includes ensuring the patient does not walk up or down stairs or to the stretcher.

Place the patient on a cardiac monitor and establish IV access. Obtain a 12-lead ECG (see Chapter 22). Maintain normal body temperature. Give IV fluids and medications per local protocol or medical direction instructions (Box 34-7).

Rapidly transport a patient with signs and symptoms of shock to the closest appropriate facility. Although cardiogenic shock is associated with a high mortality rate, patients who are candidates for reperfusion therapy and receive prompt treatment may have an increased chance of survival. Additional information about the treatment for cardiogenic shock is covered in Chapter 22.

BOX 34-7 | Patient Management: Cardiogenic Shock

- ABCs, oxygen (endotracheal intubation if needed), IV, monitor
- Vital signs, pulse oximetry, capnography (if available)
- Treat dysrhythmias if they are present and contribute to shock
- Check patient's response; assess mental status, heart rate, respiratory effort, breath sounds, and blood pressure

ABCs, Airway, breathing, and circulation; *IV,* intravenous.

Patient and Family Education

In many cases cardiogenic shock cannot be prevented. Be sure to provide emotional support to the patient and his or her family.

Distributive Shock

[OBJECTIVE 7]

In distributive shock, relative hypovolemia occurs when blood vessels dilate, increasing the size of the vascular space. The available blood volume must fill a greater space (Figure 34-10). This results in an altered distribution of the blood volume (relative hypovolemia) instead of actual volume loss (absolute hypovolemia). Distributive shock may be caused by a severe infection (septic shock), severe allergic reaction (anaphylactic shock), spinal cord injury (neurogenic shock), or certain overdoses, such as sedatives or narcotics.

PARAMEDIC*Pearl*

Signs and symptoms of distributive shock that are unusual in the presence of hypovolemic shock include warm, flushed skin (especially in dependent areas) and, in neurogenic shock, a normal or slow pulse rate (relative bradycardia).

Septic Shock

Description and Definition. Bacteremia is the presence of viable bacteria in the blood. **Systemic inflammatory response syndrome** is a response to infection with a change in two or more of the following: temperature, heart rate, respiratory rate, and WBC count. **Sepsis**

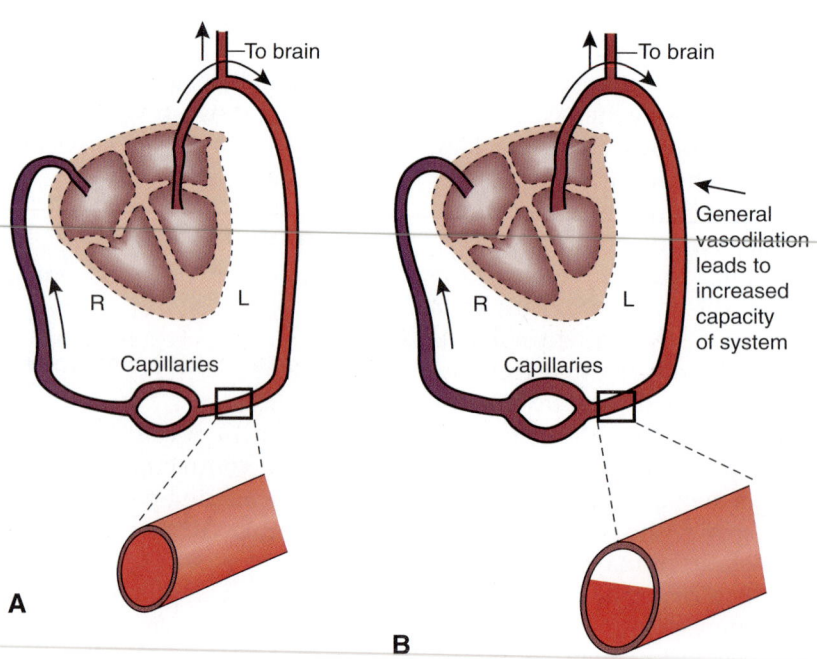

Figure 34-10 A, Normal circulation. **B,** Distributive shock.

is the systemic response to an infection. **Septicemia** refers to the multiplication of bacteria in the bloodstream, resulting in an overwhelming infection. **Severe sepsis** is associated with organ dysfunction, shock, or hypotension. Shock and perfusion abnormalities may include lactic acidosis, decreased urine output, or a sudden change in mental status.

Septic shock is sepsis with hypotension despite adequate fluid resuscitation, along with the presence of perfusion abnormalities that may include lactic acidosis, decreased urine output, or a sudden change in mental status.

Etiology. Most cases of septic shock (approximately 70%) are caused by bacteria. Common sites of bacterial infection include the kidneys (upper urinary tract infection), liver or gallbladder, bowel (usually seen with peritonitis), skin (cellulitis), and the lungs (bacterial pneumonia). Septicemia may exist for some time before septic shock develops.

Epidemiology and Demographics. Sepsis is the tenth leading cause of death in the United States. Sepsis is more likely to occur in men than in women. African Americans and other nonwhite groups are at higher risk than white patients are, and African American men are at highest risk (Martin et al., 2003).

Risk factors for sepsis include extremes of age (very young people and older adults), a compromised immune system, malnourishment, and long-term antibiotic or steroid use. Most cases of severe sepsis and septic shock occur in patients who are hospitalized for other illnesses.

The reported incidence of sepsis syndromes has dramatically increased in the past 20 years. This increase is believed to be the result of the aging of the population; growing number of patients living longer with chronic diseases; increasing use of invasive procedures; and the growing number of patients in whom sepsis develops as a result of chemotherapy, immunosuppression, or human immunodeficiency virus (HIV).

Approximately 20% to 35% of patients with severe sepsis and 40% to 60% of patients with septic shock die within 30 days. Others die within the following 6 months from poorly controlled infection, complications of intensive care, multiple organ failure, or underlying disease (Munford, 2005).

History. A patient in septic shock may be too ill to provide a medical history. If family members are present, they may be able to describe the patient's signs and symptoms that prompted a call to 9-1-1. Find out whether the patient has a history of an organ transplant or chronic illness such as AIDS or cancer. Patients with these conditions often are taking strong medications that weaken the immune system. Find out whether the patient has a history of recent invasive tests, treatments, surgery, or trauma.

Physical Findings. Septic shock occurs in two stages. The early (hyperdynamic) phase is characterized by peripheral vasodilation (warm shock) from endotoxins that prevent vasoconstriction. The patient's skin is warm, dry, and flushed. A heart rate above the normal limits for the patient's age is usually present. The patient's breathing often is rapid. His or her blood pressure may be normal or pulse pressure may be widened. The patient often has bounding peripheral pulses.

The late (hypodynamic or decompensated) phase is characterized by mottled, cool extremities (cold shock) and resembles hypovolemic shock. Peripheral pulses are diminished or absent. The patient will have an altered mental status and rapid heart rate. Patients who take medications to increase contractility (**inotropic** agents) or constrict blood vessels (vasopressor agents) may not be hypotensive. Hypotension is not a necessary finding for septic shock to be clinically diagnosed.

Fever, tachycardia, and vasodilation are common in patients with benign infections. You should suspect septic shock when these signs are present in a patient who has a change in mental status. For example, if the patient is a child, he or she may be inconsolable, not interact with parents or caregiver, or be impossible to arouse.

PARAMEDIC*Pearl*

Late septic shock is usually impossible to differentiate from other types of shock.

Differential Diagnosis. Potential causes of septic shock are listed in Table 34-3.

TABLE 34-3 Differential Diagnosis: Septic Shock

Cardiovascular Causes	Respiratory Causes	Endocrine Causes	Other Causes
Cardiogenic shock	Pulmonary embolism	Diabetic ketoacidosis	Acute renal failure
Hemorrhagic shock		Hyperthyroidism	Adrenal crisis
Myocardial infarction			Anaphylaxis
Myocardial rupture			Aspirin toxicity DIC Heatstroke

DIC, Disseminated intravascular coagulation.

Therapeutic Interventions

[OBJECTIVE 8]

Give high-concentration oxygen and ensure effective ventilation and oxygenation. Apply a pulse oximeter and use capnography. Maintain oxygen saturation at greater than 95%. Place the patient on a cardiac monitor. Establish IV access. Patients in septic shock usually require aggressive IV fluid initially because hypovolemia is an important contributor to shock. Give IV fluids and medications per local protocol or medical direction instructions (Box 34-8). A 20-mL/kg IV fluid challenge is typical. Check the patient's response to the fluids you have given by assessing mental status, heart rate, respiratory effort, breath sounds, and blood pressure. If improvement does not occur, provide the patient with additional emergency care as instructed by medical direction. Typical treatment includes repeated fluid boluses, repeating the initial assessment after *each* fluid bolus. Closely monitor the patient for increased work of breathing and the development of crackles. Check the patient's glucose level. If the serum glucose level is less than 60 mg/dL, give dextrose IV. Rapidly transport a patient who has signs and symptoms of shock to the closest appropriate facility.

PARAMEDIC*Pearl*

To manage septic shock, you must aggressively administer IV fluids. The patient in decompensated septic shock may require significant quantities of fluid. For example, some patients have required 100 to 200 mL/kg in the first few hours of resuscitation. Carefully monitor the patient for rales (crackles) and increased work of breathing during rapid fluid administration.

Patient and Family Education. Provide emotional support to the patient and his or her family. Teach patients the signs and symptoms that might signal impending serious illness; instruct those who are diabetic, being treated with chemotherapy or radiation, have had an organ transplant, or have HIV to seek medical attention if they develop a fever, chills, or rash.

BOX 34-8 | Patient Management: Septic Shock

- ABCs, oxygen, IV, monitor
- Vital signs, pulse oximetry, capnography (if available)
- Place patient supine
- If breath sounds are clear, an IV fluid challenge of 20 mL/kg normal saline or lactated Ringer's solution is usually rapidly given over a 20-minute period
- Check patient's response; assess mental status, heart rate, respiratory effort, breath sounds, and blood pressure
- If no improvement, give additional fluids as instructed by medical direction

ABCs, Airway, breathing, and circulation; *IV,* intravenous.

Anaphylactic Shock

Description and Definition. Anaphylaxis, or anaphylactic shock, occurs when the body is exposed to a substance that produces a severe allergic reaction. The reaction usually occurs within minutes of the exposure.

Etiology. Common causes of anaphylaxis are shown in Box 34-9. Type I hypersensitivity occurs when an individual is exposed to a specific allergen and develops immunoglobulin E antibodies (Figures 34-11 and 34-12). These antibodies attach to mast cells in specific body locations, creating sensitized mast cells. On reexposure to the same allergen, histamine and other chemical mediators are released. These substances cause widespread arterial and venous vasodilation and increase capillary permeability. Intravascular fluid leaks into the interstitial space, resulting in a decrease in intravascular volume (relative hypovolemia). Increased blood vessel permeability causes swelling that is noticeable in the mucous membranes of the larynx (stridor), trachea, and bronchial tree. This increases the potential for complete airway obstruction from severe swelling. The decrease in intravascular volume results in decreased preload and worsens hypotension.

PARAMEDIC*Pearl*

Patients with a latex allergy also may have a reaction to certain foods. Foods that most often result in reactions are the avocado, kiwi, banana, and chestnut (Chiu, 2005).

Epidemiology and Demographics. Anaphylaxis appears to occur more often in women as reactions to latex, aspirin, and muscle relaxants. Insect sting anaphylaxis has been reported to occur more frequently in men, probably because of more frequent exposure (Lieberman, 2003).

BOX 34-9 | Common Causes of Anaphylaxis

- Dust mites, mold, pollen extracts (ragweed, grass, trees)
- Dander from cats, dogs, horses, laboratory animals
- Foods such as milk, eggs, peanuts, tree nuts, grains, beans, shellfish, fish
- Latex rubber products
- Blood transfusion incompatibilities
- Insect venom such as that from yellow jackets, yellow and bald-faced hornets, paper wasps, honeybees, imported fire ants
- Antibiotics such as penicillins, cephalosporins, amphotericin B
- Local anesthetics such as procaine, lidocaine
- Vitamins such as thiamine, folic acid
- Nonsteroidal antiinflammatory drugs
- Radiocontrast media
- Aspirin

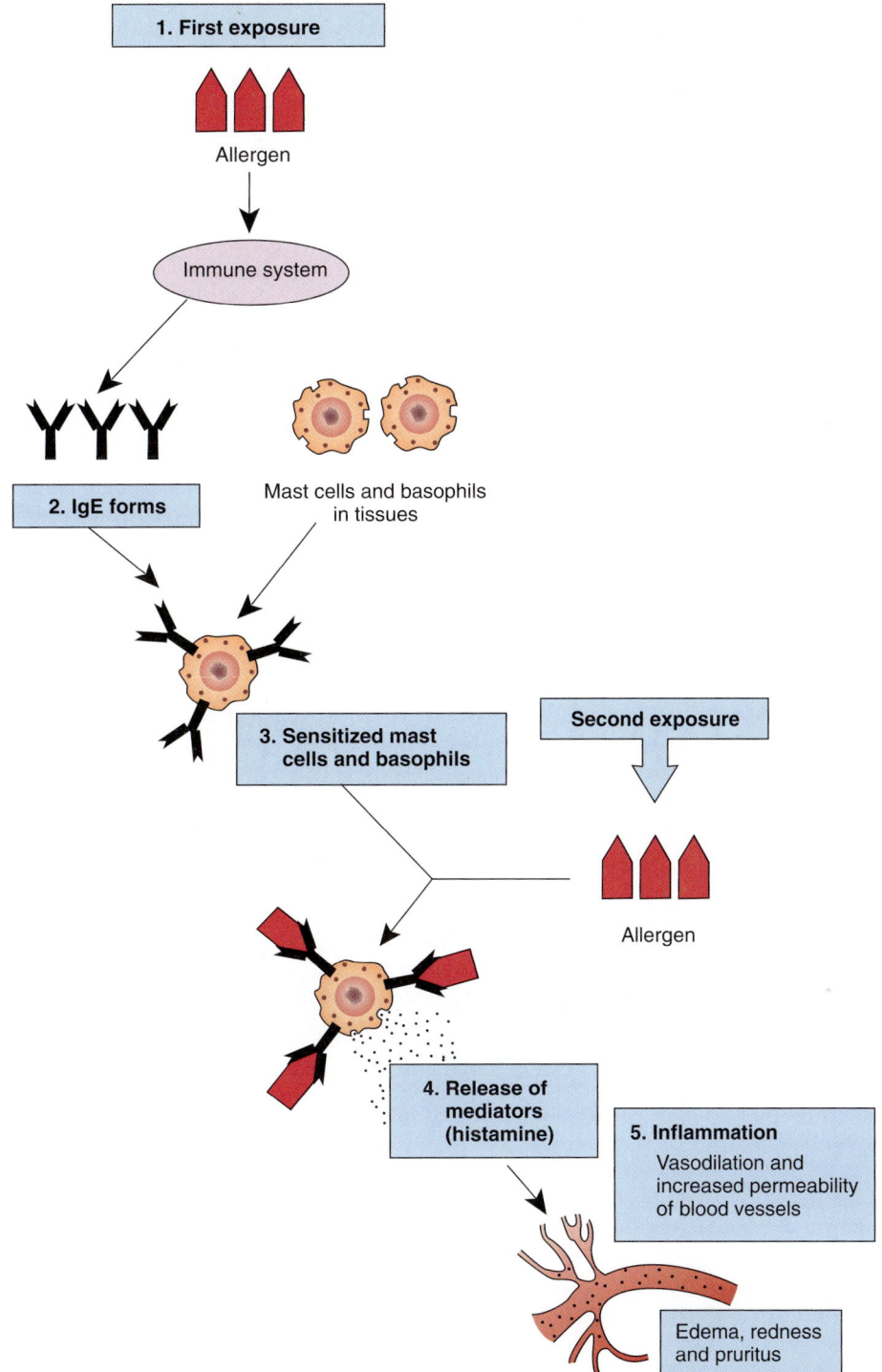

Figure 34-11 The effects of an allergic reaction (type I hypersensitivity reaction). *IgE,* Immunoglobulin E.

In the United States, most allergy deaths involving foods each year are related to peanuts and tree nuts (Chiu & Kelly, 2005). The incidence of anaphylaxis from medications increases with age (Alves & Sheikh, 2001). This may be because of the higher likelihood of multiple drug use. Most fatal reactions occur when drugs are given by the intramuscular or IV route.

History. The patient, a family member, or a bystander often will describe the patient's exposure to an allergen. Try to find out what the patient was exposed to, when the patient was exposed to it, when the patient's symptoms began, and what symptoms prompted the call to 9-1-1. Ask whether the patient has previously been exposed to the allergen. If he or she has,

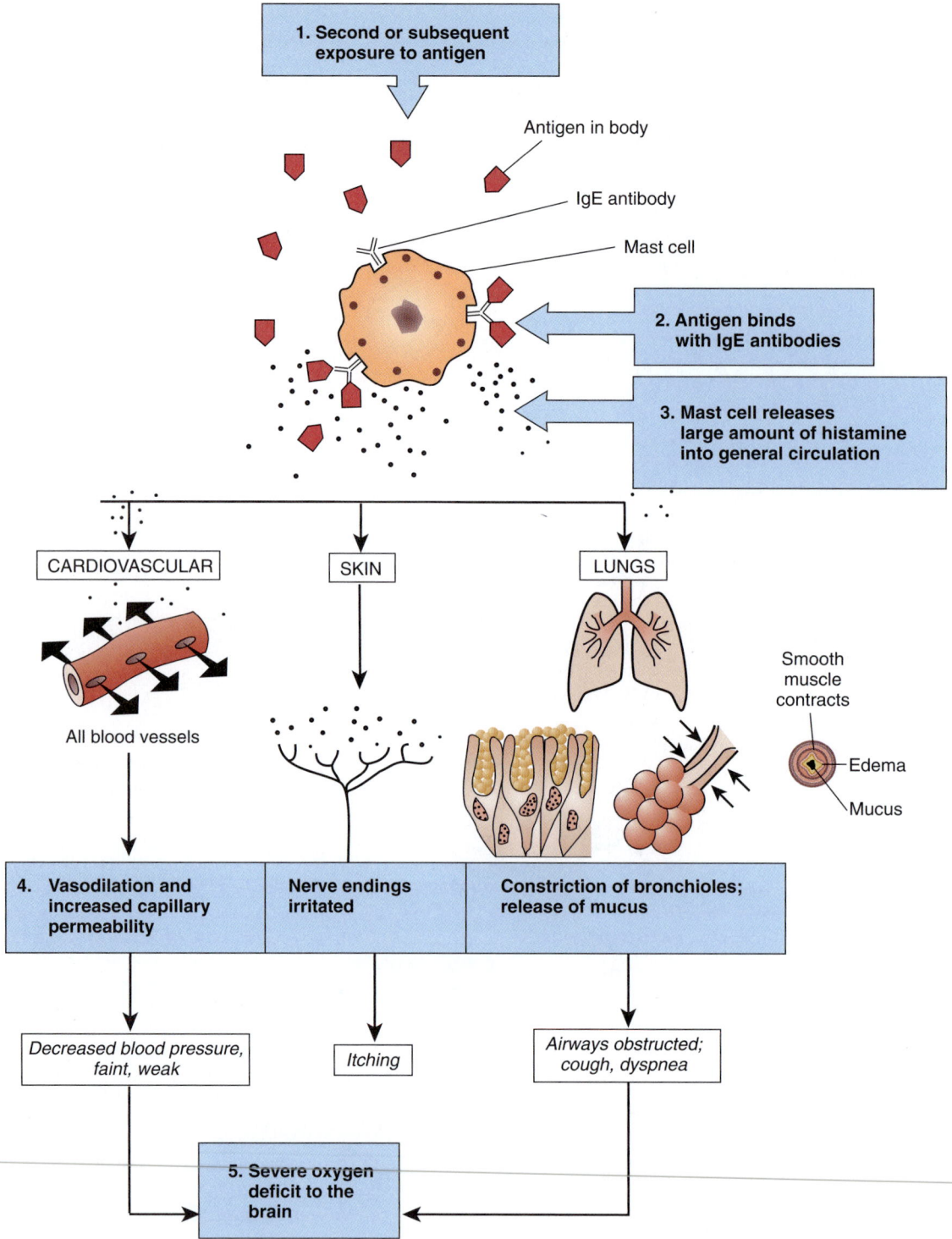

Figure 34-12 The effects of anaphylaxis (type I hypersensitivity reaction). *IgE,* Immunoglobulin E.

ask the patient what happened during that episode, if possible.

Physical Findings. The signs and symptoms typically include some or all of those shown in Table 34-4. Mild signs and symptoms may be limited to only the skin. However, up to 10% of individuals with anaphylaxis have no obvious skin signs (Sicherer & Simons, 2005).

Differential Diagnosis. Potential causes of anaphylactic shock are listed in Table 34-5.

Therapeutic Interventions. In general, the sooner the signs and symptoms start after the patient's exposure to the agent causing the reaction, the more severe the allergic reaction or anaphylaxis. You must move quickly. Establish an airway. Quickly remove the agent causing the reaction if it is still present. Administer high-concentration oxygen. Make sure oxygenation and ventilation are effective. Watch the patient's airway closely. The onset of stridor and hoarseness may indicate the need for endotracheal intubation. Apply a pulse oximeter and use capnography. Maintain oxygen saturation at greater than 95%. Establish IV access. Do not delay emergency care while establishing an IV. Place the patient on a cardiac monitor.

Give IV fluids and medications per local protocol and medical direction instructions. If the patient is having an allergic reaction, you may be asked to give diphenhydramine (Benadryl) followed by methylprednisolone (Solu-Medrol) or a similar steroid to help stop the inflammatory reaction. If the patient is experiencing anaphylaxis, the drug of choice is epinephrine. If the patient is responsive, epinephrine is typically given by the intramuscular route as a 1:1000 concentration. If the patient is unresponsive or signs of shock are present, IV epinephrine may be ordered. An IV fluid challenge may be ordered if the patient is hypotensive or tachycardic. Diphenhydramine often is given after epinephrine in cases of anaphylaxis. Additional medications that may be ordered include steroids and albuterol (Proventil). If the patient's condition does not improve after epinephrine, glucagon may be ordered. Vasopressors may be needed if the patient does not respond to IV fluids and epinephrine (Box 34-10).

Patient and Family Education. Instruct patients to call 9-1-1 if they or someone around them has serious signs and symptoms after exposure to a medication, food, insect sting, or other allergen. Give the patient examples of serious signs and symptoms, such as a rash; wheezing;

TABLE 34-4 Physical Findings: Anaphylactic Shock

Body System	Signs/Symptoms
Neurologic	Anxiety, restlessness, feeling of impending doom, fright, altered mental status, loss of responsiveness
Respiratory	Unable to speak, laryngeal edema, bronchospasm, chest or throat tightness, "lump" in the throat, stridor, wheezing, dyspnea, coughing, hoarseness, intercostal and suprasternal retractions, accessory muscle use, prolonged expiration, diminished breath sounds
Cardiovascular	Tachycardia, hypotension, dysrhythmias
Skin	Diaphoresis; urticaria (hives); flushing; pruritus (itching), especially of the palms and feet; angioedema; pallor; cyanosis
Gastrointestinal and genitourinary	Nausea, vomiting, diarrhea, abdominal pain, cramping, incontinence

BOX 34-10 Patient Management: Anaphylactic Shock

- ABCs, oxygen (endotracheal intubation as needed), IV, monitor
- Vital signs, pulse oximetry, capnography (if available)
- Do not delay treatment to establish IV access
- If IV established and breath sounds are clear, an IV fluid challenge of normal saline or Ringer's lactate is usually given if the patient is hypotensive or tachycardic
- Epinephrine is usually given IV if the patient is unresponsive or signs of shock are present or intramuscularly if the patient is responsive or if no IV access is possible
- Diphenhydramine is usually given
- A corticosteroid is usually given to help stop the inflammatory process
- Albuterol is usually given if bronchospasm is present
- Glucagon may be ordered if there is no response to epinephrine
- Vasopressors may be ordered for hypotension unresponsive to IV fluids and epinephrine
- Check patient's response after each medication/fluid challenge; assess mental status, heart rate, respiratory effort, breath sounds, and blood pressure
- If no improvement, give additional fluids as instructed by medical direction

ABCs, Airway, breathing, and circulation; *IV,* intravenous.

TABLE 34-5 Differential Diagnosis: Anaphylactic Shock

Cardiovascular Causes	Respiratory Causes	Endocrine Causes	Other Causes
Acute coronary syndromes	Foreign body aspiration	Insulin reaction	Panic attack
Aortic dissection	Pulmonary embolism		Vasovagal reaction
Cardiogenic shock	Reactive airway disease		
Dysrhythmias	Tension pneumothorax		
Hemorrhagic shock			

chest tightness; difficulty breathing; or swelling of the lips, tongue, or throat.

Patients who have had anaphylaxis should obtain a prescription from their physician for self-injectable epinephrine. The patient should be taught how to inject the medication promptly if acute anaphylaxis is suspected. The patient also should be taught to wear a medical identification emblem stating his or her allergy.

Neurogenic Shock

Description and Definition. Neurogenic shock involves a disruption in the ability of the sympathetic nervous system to control vessel dilation and constriction.

Etiology. Neurogenic shock is generalized vasodilation from a loss of sympathetic vascular tone. It may be caused by general anesthesia, spinal anesthesia, ingestion of barbiturates or phenothiazines, or a severe injury to the head or spinal cord, such as brainstem injuries or complete transection of the spinal cord (usually above T6). The injury results in a loss of sympathetic vascular tone below the level of the spinal cord injury. Examples of traumatic mechanisms of injury in which spinal cord injury may occur include the following:

- Pedestrian impact with a high-speed motor vehicle
- Motor vehicle crash involving an unrestrained or improperly restrained passenger
- Shooting or blast injury to the torso
- Fall from an extreme height
- Gymnastics injury
- Skiing accident
- Hang-gliding accident
- Horseback riding injury
- Diving accident
- Stabbing or impalement near the spinal column
- Blunt trauma to the back of the head

Epidemiology and Demographics. In a study of hypotensive patients with a spinal cord injury caused by penetrating trauma, the hypotension was not from neurogenic shock. Instead, blood loss was found to be the cause of the hypotension in 74% of patients. Only 7% had the classic findings of neurogenic shock (Zipnick et al., 1993).

Neurogenic shock usually lasts less than 24 hours, but it has been reported occasionally to last days to weeks (Shewmon, 1999; Atkinson & Atkinson, 1996).

History. In the prehospital setting, spinal cord injury is the most common cause of neurogenic shock you will encounter. Find out when the patient's injury occurred and how it occurred. Find out whether the patient was unresponsive at any time and, if so, for how long. If the patient is responsive, determine the chief complaint. Find out whether he or she has any pain, numbness, tingling, or paralysis and if any of these symptoms have changed since the time the injury occurred. Also determine whether the patient moved himself or herself or has been moved since the injury occurred. Determine whether the patient has a history of any medical illnesses and whether he or she has recently used any drugs or alcohol.

Physical Findings. In neurogenic shock, the loss of peripheral vascular tone results in widespread vasodilation below the level of the injury. This causes decreased venous return, decreased stroke volume, decreased cardiac output, and decreased tissue perfusion. The total blood volume remains the same, but blood vessel capacity is increased (relative hypovolemia). The patient's blood pressure usually reflects hypotension, with a systolic blood pressure often between 80 and 100 mm Hg. A wide pulse pressure is usually present. A decrease in blood pressure is normally accompanied by a compensatory increase in heart rate. In neurogenic shock the patient does not become tachycardic because sympathetic activity is disrupted. The patient's heart rate is usually within normal limits or is bradycardic.

The patient's respiratory rate and effort and breathing pattern may be affected depending on the location of the injury. You may see abdominal breathing if a high spinal cord injury disrupts the intercostal nerves that control rib movement. If the phrenic nerve is affected, the patient's breathing may be shallow, labored, and (possibly) irregular.

The patient's skin is usually warm and dry. Immediately after the injury, the skin appears flushed from vasodilation. Blood eventually pools, leaving the uppermost skin surfaces pale. Because widespread vasodilation may result in a loss of body heat, be aware of possible hypothermia. If neurogenic shock occurs with hypovolemia, the patient's extremities often become cool. Sweating does not occur below the level of the injury.

Motor and sensory deficits indicative of a spinal cord injury are usually present. When assessing the patient, keep in mind that an injury to the spinal cord often is associated with injury to other body areas. If the patient sustained a head injury, identifying motor and sensory deficits during the initial assessment may be difficult if he or she has an altered mental status.

PARAMEDIC*Pearl*

If a trauma patient is hypotensive but bleeding is not obvious, consider neurogenic shock.

Differential Diagnosis. Differential diagnosis includes hypovolemic shock and multisystem trauma.

Therapeutic Interventions. Because the neurogenic shock you will see in the prehospital setting is usually caused by trauma, maintain cervical spine stabilization as you assess the patient. Open the airway with a jaw thrust without head tilt maneuver if necessary. Administer high-concentration oxygen. Ensure oxygenation and ventilation are effective. You may need to assist the patient's breathing with positive-pressure ventilation. Apply a pulse oximeter and use capnography. Maintain oxygen saturation at greater than 95%. Place the patient on a cardiac monitor. Establish an IV and administer fluids and medications per local protocol or medical direction instructions. An IV fluid challenge of normal saline or lactated Ringer's solution is usually given. Monitor the patient closely for increased work of breathing and the development of crackles. Because the hypotension of neurogenic shock is not caused by actual volume loss, the administration of large volumes of IV fluids is generally not indicated. However, the careful administration of small IV fluid challenges can be beneficial. Repeat the initial assessment after each fluid challenge. Vasopressors may be ordered if the patient does not respond to IV fluids. Check the patient's glucose level; if it is less than 60 mg/dL, give dextrose IV.

Before transport, immobilize the patient's spine. If motor and sensory deficits are present, avoid further patient injury by being careful not to exert pressure on the patient's skin. The patient will not be able to tell you if something is too tight or to reposition a body area below the injury on his or her own. The patient in neurogenic shock is at risk for hypothermia. Take measures to maintain normal body temperature (Box 34-11).

Rapidly transport a patient with signs and symptoms of shock to the closest appropriate facility.

Patient and Family Education. In most cases neurogenic shock is the result of trauma. The patient who has sustained a spinal cord injury is likely to be anxious and fearful about the future. Provide emotional support to the patient and his or her family.

Obstructive Shock

Description and Definition

Shock that develops from cardiac tamponade, tension pneumothorax, or a massive pulmonary embolism is called obstructive shock because the common pathophysiologic finding in these conditions is obstruction to blood flow from the heart.

Etiology

[OBJECTIVE 9]

A tension pneumothorax can result from blunt or penetrating chest trauma, barotrauma from positive-pressure ventilation (especially when using high amounts of positive end-expiratory pressure), or a complication of central venous catheter placement (usually subclavian or internal jugular). In a tension pneumothorax, air enters on inspiration but cannot escape. Intrathoracic pressure increases, the lung collapses, and air under pressure shifts the mediastinum away from the midline toward the unaffected side. As intrathoracic pressure increases, the vena cava becomes kinked, decreasing venous return and altering cardiac output (Figure 34-13).

BOX 34-11	Patient Management: Neurogenic Shock

- ABCs, oxygen, IV, monitor
- Vital signs, pulse oximetry, capnography (if available)
- Place patient supine
- If breath sounds are clear, an IV fluid challenge of normal saline or lactated Ringer's solution is usually given
- Check patient's response; assess mental status, heart rate, respiratory effort, breath sounds, and blood pressure
- If no improvement, give additional fluids or medications as instructed by medical direction

ABCs, Airway, breathing, and circulation; *IV*, intravenous.

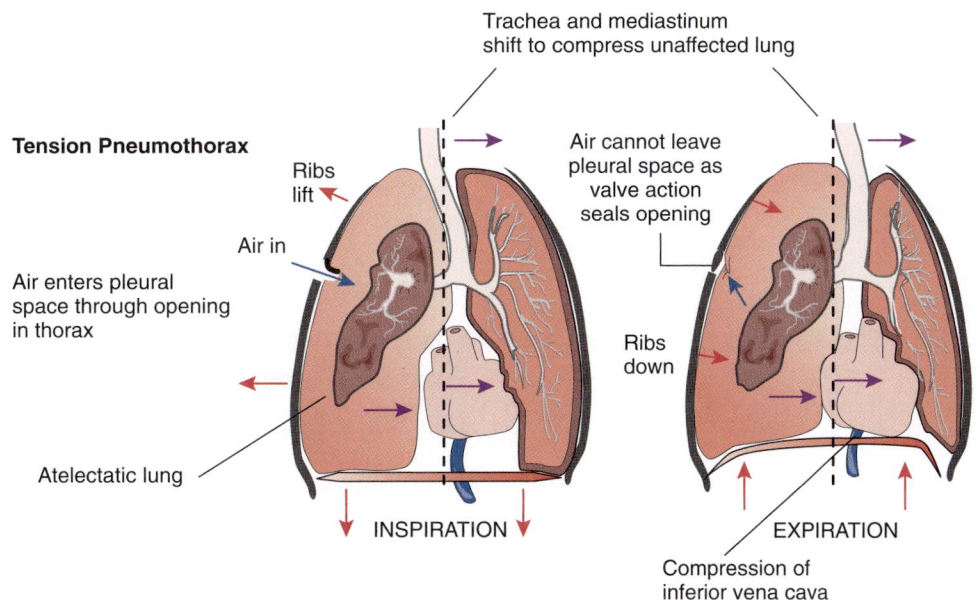

Figure 34-13 Tension pneumothorax.

Cardiac tamponade is the result of a buildup of blood or fluid in the pericardial space. The buildup of excess blood or fluid compresses the heart. This can affect the heart's ability to relax and fill with blood between contractions. If the heart cannot adequately fill with blood, the amount of blood the ventricles can pump out to the body (cardiac output) will be decreased. As a result, the amount of blood returning to the heart also is decreased. The buildup of excess blood or fluid may occur from pericarditis, after cardiac surgery, trauma, connective tissue diseases, radiation therapy, or as a complication of central venous catheters. Cardiac tamponade is covered in more detail later in this chapter.

Epidemiology and Demographics

If the left ventricle ruptures as a complication of an acute myocardial infarction (MI), cardiac tamponade and shock may develop, resulting in sudden death. This complication occurs in less than 1% of acute MIs and most often within the first week after an MI. It is most common in older women, those with a history of hypertension, and patients treated in the early period after the infarction with steroids or nonsteroidal antiinflammatory drugs (Lilly, 2001).

History

Patients with a tension pneumothorax or cardiac tamponade often are too ill to answer questions about their medical history. If a family member or a caregiver is present, attempt to learn what preceded the call to 9-1-1. If the patient has a tension pneumothorax and is able to talk, he or she will likely report shortness of breath and sudden chest pain that may radiate to the shoulder. The patient is likely to be anxious and may describe a feeling of impending doom.

The patient with cardiac tamponade is likely to be restless and report shortness of breath, chest tightness, and dizziness. If the tamponade is not caused by trauma, he or she may relay a history of a medical illness such as pericarditis or end-stage renal disease.

> **PARAMEDIC*Pearl***
>
> Consider the possibility of a tension pneumothorax if you are ventilating a patient with positive pressure, such as with a bag-mask device, and the patient's lungs become increasingly difficult to ventilate or if the condition of a patient who is on a home ventilator suddenly deteriorates. Quickly assess the patient to determine if other signs of a tension pneumothorax are present.

Physical Findings

The signs and symptoms of a tension pneumothorax reflect asphyxia and decreased cardiac output. Early signs include dyspnea, anxiety, rapid breathing, tachycardia (often more than 120 beats/min), hyperresonance of the chest wall on the affected side, and diminished or absent breath sounds on the affected side. Late signs include a decreased level of responsiveness, hypotension, and cyanosis (a very late sign). JVD may be present but difficult to detect. It may not be present if the patient is hypovolemic or in cases of severe hypotension. Tracheal deviation (displacement) toward the unaffected side often is described as a classic sign of a tension pneumothorax. However, this is an uncommon and late finding.

Classic signs of cardiac tamponade include JVD, hypotension, and muffled heart sounds **(Beck's triad).** Although these signs may be present, they appear late in the course of the buildup of pericardial fluid, occur in only 10% to 40% of patients, and are usually a preterminal event (Debehnke, 1994). Other signs include cold, pale, mottled, or cyanotic skin; tachycardia; weak or absent peripheral pulses; narrowing pulse pressure; and pulsus paradoxus. Pulsus paradoxus is a late sign and may be absent if the patient has severe hypotension.

> **PARAMEDIC*Pearl***
>
> Cardiac tamponade and tension pneumothorax present with clear lung sounds; however, lung sounds are unequal in a tension pneumothorax.

Differential Diagnosis

Possible causes of obstructive shock are listed in Table 34-6.

Therapeutic Interventions

[OBJECTIVE 10]

Management of obstructive shock depends on the cause. Tension pneumothorax and cardiac tamponade are medical emergencies. You will need to move quickly and reassess the patient's condition often while he or she is in your care.

If trauma is the source of the patient's signs and symptoms, stabilize the cervical spine as needed. Make sure the patient's airway is open. Give high-concentration oxygen. Make sure ventilation and oxygenation are effective. Apply a pulse oximeter and use capnography. Maintain oxygen saturation at greater than 95%. Suction as needed.

If signs and symptoms of a tension pneumothorax are present and the patient has a chest wound that has been

TABLE 34-6	Differential Diagnosis: Obstructive Shock
Cardiovascular Causes	**Respiratory Causes**
Acute coronary syndromes	Foreign body airway obstruction
Aortic dissection	Hemothorax
	Pulmonary embolism
	Reactive airway disease

bandaged, lift one side of the dressing to allow the release of air. Check the patient's response by assessing his or her mental status, heart rate, respiratory effort, breath sounds, and blood pressure. If signs of a tension pneumothorax are still present, perform needle decompression on the affected side of the chest. Control life-threatening bleeding. Apply the cardiac monitor. Avoid performing additional procedures on the scene that will delay transport to the hospital. Maintain normal body temperature.

Establish IV access en route to definitive care. Give IV fluids and medications per local protocol or medical direction instructions. If breath sounds are clear, an IV fluid challenge of normal saline or Ringer's lactate solution is usually given to maintain circulating blood volume. Check the patient's response by assessing his or her mental status, heart rate, respiratory effort, breath sounds, and blood pressure. Medications to increase contractility, such as dopamine or dobutamine, may be ordered if poor perfusion persists.

The definitive treatment for cardiac tamponade is pericardiocentesis. IV fluids and inotropic medications are temporizing measures. These measures should not delay transport of the patient for definitive care.

Rapidly transport a patient with signs and symptoms of shock to the closest appropriate facility.

Patient and Family Education

Explain all procedures to the patient. Provide emotional support to the patient and his or her family.

Dissociative Shock

[OBJECTIVE 11]
In dissociative shock, the heart is functioning appropriately, the vessels are intact and functioning, and an appropriate amount of blood is present in the circulatory system. In this type of shock, however, something is not allowing oxygen to reach the cells. One example is carbon monoxide (CO) poisoning. When a patient has been poisoned by CO, the CO will bind with the hemoglobin in the RBCs with a greater affinity than does oxygen. In other words, the CO will kick the oxygen off the RBCs and the oxygen will have no way to get to the tissues. This results in decreased tissue oxygenation. Other causes of dissociative shock include cyanide poisoning and anemia.

Treatment for a patient with dissociative shock is to ensure the airway is open and give oxygen. Rapidly transport the patient to a location where the cause of this shock can be stopped. For example, a patient with severe CO poisoning must be treated in a hyperbaric oxygen chamber.

SPECIAL CONSIDERATIONS

A few special considerations are worthy of covering because they can affect how the body compensates for shock.

Hydration

If a patient is dehydrated, he or she has a decreased fluid reserve. When the body attempts to pull water from the cells and tissues into the vascular space, not enough fluid is available to pull. Thus compensation is limited.

The type of tissue also affects the attempted fluid shift with shock. Muscle tissue holds more water than does lipid tissue. A patient with a greater muscle/lipid ratio may compensate for hemorrhagic shock better than the patient with a higher lipid/muscle ratio.

Age

Pediatric patients have a smaller blood volume and less fluid reserve than do adults. They can progress into hemorrhagic shock quickly. Pediatric patients can compensate for shock with increased cardiac function and vasoconstriction. However, as quickly as pediatric patients compensate, they can deteriorate. Pediatric patients tend to compensate and then move to irreversible shock with no stage in between. You must maintain a high suspicion any time a mechanism is substantial enough to cause a pediatric patient to progress to hemorrhagic shock. The signs of shock are subtle. Watch for changes in mental status and responsiveness. As a pediatric patient progresses to shock, vasoconstriction will cause the patient's extremities to become pale while the core remains pink. Treatment for these young patients must be aggressive.

As with pediatric patients, geriatric patients have a decreased fluid reserve. Unlike pediatric patients, however, older adults cannot quickly compensate for hemorrhagic shock. Older hearts cannot effectively increase rate and force of contractility. As patients age, their arteries develop arteriosclerosis. This buildup inhibits the ability of the arteries to constrict. Lung compliance in an older adult is decreased further, inhibiting compensatory ability.

In addition to the normal physiologic changes associated with aging, geriatric patients commonly have a history of chronic diseases. Prior heart attacks, emphysema, and diabetes are some of the common diseases that can inhibit the body's ability to compensate for hemorrhagic shock. Another important concept that must be appreciated in the elderly patient is that of relative hypotension. As a result of chronic hypertension, the bodies of elderly patients adapt to these baseline blood pressures. In these situations a blood pressure considered normal in the general population can result in a state of hypoperfusion in the elderly patient, with subsequent failure of end-organ perfusion. For example, if a patient normally has a blood pressure of 160/98 mm Hg, a blood pressure of 120/80 mm Hg may be inadequate. When faced with an elderly patient who has signs and symptoms of hypoperfusion, the paramedic must consider its presence despite an apparently normal blood pressure.

Drugs

Many of the drugs prescribed to patients to control high blood pressure will negatively affect the body's ability to compensate for shock. Beta-blockers limit the heart's ability to increase the rate and force of contraction. ACE inhibitors will stop the conversion of angiotensin I to angiotensin II. Calcium channel blockers limit the heart's ability to increase the heart rate and the force of contractility as well as limit vasoconstriction. If a patient who is going into hemorrhagic shock is taking any of these medications, the initial signs of shock may be masked. Once unmasked, however, the patient will progress more quickly to decompensated shock.

Case Scenario SUMMARY

1. *What is your general impression of this patient?* Several factors in the initial assessment suggest that this patient is high priority. First, pallor often is a sign of poor perfusion and is your first sign that this patient is in shock. The patient's apparent inability to focus on you and your partner may indicate an altered mental status and is another finding that suggests he is a high-priority patient who probably is in hypovolemic shock. Although he appears to have an intact airway and adequate ventilation, further assessment is required.

2. *What additional assessment will be important in the evaluation of this patient?* The primary survey suggested that the patient is in shock and may have an altered mental status. Further evaluation of mental status, skin (for poor skin turgor, cyanosis, and diaphoresis), and vital signs will be important. Additional airway and ventilation evaluation should be done to ensure adequacy. Of course, the patient's chief complaint also should be elicited, and you should get more information about the duration and frequency of the patient's vomiting.

3. *What intervention should you initiate at this time?* The initial impression suggests that this patient is in shock. Administration of high-flow oxygen is the most important initial treatment at this time.

4. *Is this patient high priority? Why or why not?* The presence of tachycardia and dizziness, as well as the history of 3 to 4 hours of vomiting, confirm that the patient requires treatment and transport.

5. *What stage of shock is this patient in? Should you infuse IV fluids? If so, how much?* Because his blood pressure remains in the normal range, this patient is in the *compensatory* stage. However, aggressive therapy is important to prevent further deterioration and decompensation. Although IV fluid infusion remains controversial for individuals in hemorrhagic shock, it is appropriate for this patient. As a result of his vomiting, and the potential that his diabetes may be somewhat out of control, the patient is dehydrated and has the potential for hypovolemic shock. Fluid replacement with an isotonic solution such as normal saline is in order. Although local protocols vary, typical fluid replacement guidelines in a situation such as this range from 10 to 20 mL/kg of body weight. This patient typically would receive 750 to 1000 mL of normal saline.

6. *What additional treatment should be initiated?* The patient should receive high-flow oxygen and be placed in a position of comfort. His vital signs should be monitored, and he should be transported to the hospital. In some systems, medications to reduce nausea and vomiting (antiemetics) may be administered if he continues to vomit.

7. *What destination is most appropriate for this patient?* Although this patient does not appear to require specialty treatment (such as stroke care or angioplasty), he does have several factors that may influence destination. He appears to have GI bleeding, which could require infusion of blood, aggressive therapy, or even surgery (although rare). Because his diabetes could complicate his care, access to his personal physician and records of previous hospitalizations would be useful. If possible, this patient should be transported to a hospital where his physician practices and that has an emergency department and surgical capability.

8. *Given the patient's final disposition, was your treatment appropriate? Why or why not?* For patients in compensatory shock, the most important treatments include high-flow oxygen and, for nonhemorrhagic shock, fluid replacement. Your treatment was appropriate.

Chapter Summary

- The five primary types of shock are hypovolemic, cardiogenic, distributive, obstructive, and dissociative.
- Shock is a sign, not a diagnosis. If shock is not reversed, it will result in death.

- The three primary stages of shock are early (compensatory), late (progressive or decompensated), and irreversible.

- Treatment goals for a patient in shock include reperfusing tissue with oxygenated blood and repairing or stopping the cause.
- Definitive care for a patient in hypovolemic shock is not provided in the prehospital setting. These patients should be transported to the closest appropriate medical facility, such as a trauma center.

- IV fluids can increase perfusion pressures in a patient who is in shock but also can increase anemia, stop clotting, and lower body temperature.
- Age, drugs, existing medical conditions, and overall health status can affect the body's ability to compensate for shock.

REFERENCES

Alves, B., & Sheikh, A. (2001). Age specific aetiology of anaphylaxis. *Archives of Diseases in Children, 85*(4), 349.

Atkinson, P. P., & Atkinson, J. L. (1996). Spinal shock. *Mayo Clinic Proceedings, 71*(4), 384-389.

Chiu, A. M., & Kelly, K. J. (2005). Anaphylaxis: Drug allergy, insect stings, and latex. *Immunology and Allergy Clinics of North America, 25*(2), 389-405.

Debehnke, D. J. (1994). Cardiac-related acute infectious disease. In W. B. Gibler & T. P. Aufderhiede (Eds.). *Emergency cardiac care (p. 465)*. St. Louis: Mosby.

Lieberman, P. L. (2003). Anaphylaxis and anaphylactoid reactions. In N. R. Adkinson, J. W. Yunginger, W. W. Busse, B. S. Bochner, S. T. Holgate, & F. E. R. Simons (Eds.). *Middleton's allergy: Principles and practice* (p. 1499) (6th ed.). Philadelphia: Mosby.

Lilly, L. S. (2001). Ischemic heart disease. In J. Noble (Ed.). *Textbook of primary care medicine* (p. 567) (3rd ed.). St. Louis: Mosby.

Martin, G. S., Mannino, D. M., Eaton, S., & Moss, M. (2003). The epidemiology of sepsis in the United States from 1979 through 2000. *New England Journal of Medicine, 348*(16), 1546-1554. PMID: 12700374.

Munford, R. S. (2005). Severe sepsis and septic shock. In D. L. Kasper, E. Braunwald, A. S. Fauci, S. L. Hauser, D. L. Longo, J. L. Jameson, & K. J. Isselbacher (Eds.). *Harrison's principles of internal medicine* (16th ed.). New York: McGraw-Hill.

Roberts, J. R., & Hedges, J. R. (2004). *Clinical procedures in emergency medicine* (4th ed.). Philadelphia: Elsevier.

Shewmon, D. A. (1999). Spinal shock and brain death: Somatic pathophysiological equivalence and implications for the integrative-unity rationale. *Spinal Cord, 37*(5), 313-324.

Sicherer, S. H., & Simons, F. E. (2005). Quandaries in prescribing an emergency action plan and self-injectable epinephrine for first-aid management of anaphylaxis in the community. *Journal of Allergy and Clinical Immunology, 115*(3), 575-583.

Victorino, G. P., Battistella, F. D., & Wisner, D. H. (2003). Does tachycardia correlate with hypotension after trauma? *Journal of the American College of Surgeons, 196*(5), 679-684.

Zipnick, R. I., Scalea, T. M., Trooskin, S. Z., Sclafani, S. J., Emad, B., Shah, A., et al. (1993). Hemodynamic responses to penetrating spinal cord injuries. *Journal of Trauma, 35*(4), 578-583.

SUGGESTED RESOURCES

Guyton, A., & Hall, J. (2002). *Textbook of medical physiology* (2nd ed.). Philadelphia: Saunders.

Marx, J., Hockberger, R., Walls, R. (2002). *Emergency medicine: Concepts and clinical practice* (6th ed.). St. Louis: Mosby.

Hamilton, G. C., Sanders, A. B., Strange, G., Trott, A. T. (2002). *Emergency medicine: An approach to clinical problem solving*. Philadelphia: Saunders.

Chapter Quiz

1. During compensatory shock, the precapillary and postcapillary sphincters constrict. This is known as which phase of shock?
- **a.** Ischemic
- **b.** Stagnant
- **c.** Washout

2. Your patient's pulse rate is greater than 120 beats/min, his blood pressure has dropped, and his pulse pressure has narrowed. Approximately what percentage of total blood volume has been lost?
- **a.** 10%
- **b.** 20%
- **c.** 30%
- **d.** 50%

3. As arterial pressure drops, the baroreceptors are stimulated. This triggers the release of which of the following?
- **a.** Renin
- **b.** Angiotensin I
- **c.** Epinephrine
- **d.** Antidiuretic hormone

4. Your patient has internal bleeding. Which of the following will benefit your patient the most?
- **a.** High-flow oxygen
- **b.** IV isotonic fluid bolus
- **c.** PASG application
- **d.** Transport to the closest appropriate medical facility

5. As epinephrine is released during shock, it causes venous constriction. How will this affect cardiac output?
- **a.** Increase afterload
- **b.** Increase preload
- **c.** Increased heart rate
- **d.** Decreased stroke volume

6. If a patient is taking a beta-blocker, how will it affect his or her ability to compensate for shock?
- **a.** No change
- **b.** Increase cardiac contractility
- **c.** Limit tachycardia
- **d.** Cause vasodilation

Terminology

Acute respiratory distress syndrome Respiratory failure and acute noncardiac pulmonary edema caused by a direct or indirect pulmonary insult.

Afterload Pressure or resistance against which the ventricles must pump to eject blood.

Anemia Deficiency in RBCs or hemoglobin; most common form is iron-deficiency anemia.

Atrial kick Remaining 20% to 30% of blood forced into the right ventricle during atrial contraction.

Bacteremia The presence of bacteria in the blood. This condition could progress to septic shock. Fever, chills, tachycardia, and tachypnea are common manifestations of bacteremia.

Beck's triad Classic sign of cardiac tamponade that includes JVD, hypotension, and muffled heart sounds.

Cardiac output Amount of blood pumped into the aorta each minute by the heart (Heart rate × Stroke volume).

Cardiogenic shock A condition in which heart muscle function is severely impaired, leading to decreased cardiac output and inadequate tissue perfusion.

Disseminated intravascular coagulation (DIC) A complex, systemic thrombohemorrhagic disorder involving the generation of intravascular fibrin and the consumption of procoagulants and platelets.

Fick principle Describes the components needed for the oxygenation of the body's cells.

Hemolytic anemia Anemia that results from the destruction of RBCs.

Hemorrhagic anemia Anemia caused by hemorrhage.

Hypovolemic shock Inadequate tissue perfusion caused by inadequate vascular volume.

Hypoxemia Insufficient oxygenation of the blood.

Inotropic Relating to the force of cardiac contraction.

Ischemic phase Vascular response to shock when precapillary and postcapillary sphincters constrict, halting blood movement to distal tissues.

Multiple organ dysfunction syndrome Altered organ function in an acutely ill person in whom homeostasis cannot be maintained without intervention.

Perfusion Circulation of blood through an organ or a part of the body.

Preload Force exerted by the blood on the walls of the ventricles at the end of diastole.

Pulse pressure Difference between the systolic and diastolic blood pressures.

Sepsis Body-wide infection, regardless of source. Common causes include pneumonia or urinary tract infections.

Septicemia A serious medical condition characterized by vasodilation that leads to hypotension, tissue hypoxia, and eventually shock. Usually caused by gram-negative bacteria. Diagnosed by blood tests called *cultures*.

Septic shock Sepsis with hypotension, despite adequate fluid resuscitation, along with the presence of perfusion abnormalities that may include lactic acidosis, decreased urine output, and a sudden change in mental status.

Severe sepsis Sepsis associated with organ dysfunction, shock, or hypotension.

Shock Inadequate tissue perfusion that results from the failure of the cardiovascular system to deliver enough oxygen and nutrients to sustain vital organ function.

Stagnant phase Vascular response in shock when precapillary sphincters open, allowing the capillary beds to engorge with fluid; follows the ischemic phase.

Stroke volume Amount of blood ejected by either ventricle during one contraction; can be calculated as cardiac output divided by heart rate.

Systemic inflammatory response syndrome A response to infection manifested by a change in two or more of the following: temperature, heart rate, respiratory rate, and WBC count.

Turgor Normal tension of a cell or tissue.

Washout phase Vascular response in shock when postcapillary sphincters open, allowing fluid in the capillary beds to be pushed into systemic circulation; follows the stagnant phase.

Quiz Answers

CHAPTER 1

1. The components of wellness are physical, mental, and emotional well-being. Self-assessment varies by individual.

2. The ways in which paramedics promote wellness vary by locality. Some examples or possibilities for promotion of wellness include health fairs (blood pressure checks, stroke screenings, etc.) in public places; visiting schools, providing materials, giving presentations; setting good examples (exercise, weight control, fitness); providing cardiopulmonary resuscitation classes; and partnering with other healthcare entities to meet community needs.

3. Self-assessment varies by individual.

4. Cardiovascular risk factors: obesity, elevated cholesterol or triglyceride levels, hypertension, diabetes, family history, aging, smoking, elevated stress, high-fat diet, irregular or absent physical examinations or risk assessments.

5. They help identify abnormalities and therefore lead to earlier assessment and treatment. They save lives.

6. Irregular sleep patterns often lead to sleep deprivation, which can significantly affect an individual's life, both personally and professionally. It can increase stress and irritability; decrease the ability to control emotions and actions; and negatively affect decision making, motor control, and reaction time. Ways to decrease the impact of irregular sleep patterns include attempting to maintain the same wake/sleep pattern whether on or off duty, ensuring solid nutrition, decreasing or stopping caffeine intake before desired sleep time, giving yourself a break between work and sleep time to decompress as needed, eating small amounts of carbohydrates before sleep time, and creating a calm, quiet, dark sleeping area.

7. Sterilization by heat, steam, or radiation or by using a solution approved by the Environmental Protection Agency.

8. **a.** Mask for the patient as well as a mask for the paramedic. **b.** Gloves. **c.** Gloves, splash-resistant suit with a hood, air-purifying respirator.

9. Physical and mental performance is affected, as is the ability make appropriate, safe decisions.

10. *Physiologic:* Cardiac rhythm disturbances (rapid, irregular), chest tightness or pain, palpitations, dyspnea, increased respiratory rate, nausea and vomiting, gastrointestinal tract problems (e.g., diarrhea, constipation), sleep disturbances (e.g., insomnia, nightmares, excessive sleep), sweating, headaches, increased blood pressure, aching muscles and joints.

   Emotional: Panic reactions or attacks, increased startle reflex, increased irritability, quick temper, fear, denial, responses out of line with stimulus, feelings of being overwhelmed.

   Cognitive: Difficulty making decisions, critical thinking slowed or impaired, decreased level of awareness (of others, self, scene), difficulty concentrating or focusing, memory problems, strange dreams or nightmares, confusion or disorientation.

   Behavioral: Hyperactivity, withdrawn or sullen demeanor, short fuse, increased smoking, increased use of alcohol or medication, change in eating habits (not eating, excessive eating).

11. Kübler-Ross, five stages of the grieving process: anger, denial, bargaining, depression, acceptance. Variations: not all individuals go through all stages; there is no one "right" order; individuals may vacillate between two or more stages, going back and forth between them.

12. High stress levels can lead to increased incidence of disease and can negatively affect personal and professional life. It can damage relationships, shorten careers, lead to poor clinical decision-making, and affect patient care. The majority of people handle stress by themselves in a healthy manner most of the time. However, even healthy people may need assistance when they are working in extreme, bizarre, and unhealthy circumstances such as disasters, line of duty deaths, pediatric tragedies, and so forth. Individuals who have used their normal coping mechanisms for 4 to 6 weeks after an incident and still experience signs and symptoms of stress should seek additional help from a mental health provider.

13. Examples of positive coping mechanisms: exercise, spending time outdoors in nature, music, good nutrition, sufficient rest, talk with friends and co-workers, hobbies, reading. Some of these could be done while on duty; modification may be needed.

CHAPTER 2

1. The Department of Transportation was created in 1966 and began funding EMS. This funding capability went nationwide for all states in 1973.

2. The Omnibus Budget Reconciliation Act passed in 1981 and ended federal funding of EMS programs.

3. The set of acts an EMS professional is legally allowed to perform within his or her state and EMS system.

4. EMT.

5. A license to practice is provided by the state. A certificate implies passing a type of accrediting service process to perform skills and duties.

6. This is referred to as *refresher learning.* Continuing education is learning additional information or skills that expand your knowledge.

7. To stay current with new information, the paramedic must attend continuing education. Refresher education is valuable for brushing up on the material you may not have completely understood during your initial training or have since forgotten.

8. A paramedic follows protocols (standing orders) as well as online or physician direction. The paramedic also must be able to be self-directed because many patients fit under multiple protocols, and the paramedic should be able to identify which applies and when deviation from a protocol should be requested.

9. Immediately upon arrival you must size up the scene for safety for all concerned.

10. You must return to service by restocking and cleaning the unit and turning in documentation.

11. Protocols deal with treatment guidelines. Policies deal with non-patient-related issues.

12. a. Research is important for several reasons; it validates existing treatments and protocols, it provides better patient care, and it can improve the EMS system.

CHAPTER 3

1. In the United States unintentional injuries are the leading cause of death for ages 1 to 34 years.

2. True. Most injuries do have predictable and preventable components.

3. EMS providers are widely distributed among the population, reflect the composition of their communities, and may be the most medically educated individuals in a rural setting. More than 600,000 EMS providers are in the United States and are high-profile role models, considered champions of health care consumers, welcome in schools and other environments, and considered authorities on injury and prevention.

4. Injury surveillance is conducted with EMS data and is integral for developing prevention programs and campaigns. Epidemiologists and injury prevention specialists examine all the data.

5. Examples of teachable moments include a car crash victim not wearing a seat belt, parents of a child involved in a near drowning, a cyclist without a helmet involved in a bicycle crash.

6. The "five Es" of injury prevention are *e*ducation, *e*nforcement, *e*ngineering, *e*nvironment, and *E*MS.

7. Examples of grass roots campaigns include EPIC MEDICS, S.A.F.E., Safety Corridor, Kids Don't Float, or any local program.

8. e. Enforcement of bicycle helmet law for riders younger than 14 years.

9. b. Separate bike trails and road traffic with cement median, and **e.** enforcement of bicycle helmet law for riders younger than 14 years.

10. k. Education and public awareness campaign about childhood pedestrian safety.

11. g. Required window railings on upper-story windows.

12. i. Firearm and hunter safety program, and **d.** Media campaign to promote safe storage of firearms.

13. c. A low-cost child safety seat program for newborns and toddlers.

14. f. Required fencing around private pools.

15. c. A low-cost child safety seat program for newborns and toddlers.

16. a. Mandatory flame-retardant sleepwear for kids, and **h.** Stop! Drop! Roll! School education problems.

17. j. Required safety helmets during youth equestrian events.

18. d. Media campaign to promote safe storage of firearms, and **i.** Firearm and hunter safety program.

CHAPTER 4

1. An area of law in which an individual is prosecuted on behalf of society for violating laws designed to safeguard society is called *criminal law.*

2. False. A paramedic's scope of practice (not the standard of care) is the range of duties and skills a paramedic is legally allowed to perform when necessary.

3. The four elements that must be proven in a negligence case are duty, breach of duty, damages, and causation.

4. b. The Health Insurance Portability and Accountability Act (HIPAA) deals with patient privacy. It requires that all individually identifiable health information (commonly referred to as protected health information) be safeguarded and used only for purposes specifically permitted by the regulations.

5. Examples of intentional torts include assault, battery, false imprisonment, invasion of privacy, libel, and slander.

6. d. False imprisonment is the confinement or restraint of a person against his or her will or without appropriate legal justification.

7. A paramedic's standard of care may be determined by the paramedic's scope of practice, EMS protocols, applicable EMS policies or procedures, the National Standard Curriculum, literature (journals, EMS textbooks), expert witnesses, and juries.

8. True. Most insurance policies generally do not cover punitive damage awards, but will, up to the coverage limits of the policy, cover damages arising from ordinary negligence.

9. Battery is touching or contact with another person without that person's consent. Assault is a threat of imminent bodily harm to another person by someone with the apparent present ability to carry out the threat.

10. False. Expressed consent is given by a patient or his or her responsible decision maker either verbally or through some physical expression of consent. Nonverbal expressions of consent can include, for example, a nod of the head or rolling up a sleeve to allow the paramedic to start an intravenous line.

CHAPTER 5

1. The "best test" is a simple self-assessment of your decisions and actions that you can use after any call. It involves imagining yourself in front of a patient (or someone who loves the patient more than anyone in the whole world) and telling that person you did your very best for the patient.

2. *Primum non nocere* means "first do no harm." It is an ancient, minimal standard of care for all aspects of medicine.

3. A paramedic should strive to do things *for* patients instead of *to* them.

4. A code of ethics is a guide for interactions between members of a specific profession, such as physicians, and the public.

5. There are no good excuses for incompetence in a paramedic.

6. Ethics is a body of principles that people or groups of people adopt as guidelines for personal, professional, and social behavior.

7. **a** and **e.** Honor and humility.

8. The second half of the Hippocratic Oath focuses on a physician's responsibilities toward a patient.

CHAPTER 7

1. The layer of skin that contains nerve endings is the dermis.

2. Water accounts for 60% of total body weight.

3. The difference in concentration between solutions on opposite sides of a semipermeable membrane is called the *osmotic gradient.*

4. The organ system that virtually controls all body functions is the nervous system.

5. As the thoracic cavity begins to expand, the intrathoracic pressure becomes greater than atmospheric pressure.

6. Physiologically, the term *respiration* refers to the exchange of gases at the cellular level.

7. When swallowing, the structure that occludes the tracheal opening to prevent aspiration of food and liquids is the epiglottis.

8. The relative shortness of the urethra in the female and its proximity to the vaginal canal enable bacteria to enter the bladder easily.

9. The epididymis is a series of tubes located in the posterior portions of the scrotum.

10. The trachea divides into the right and left mainstem bronchi at the carina.

11. The cervical spine is the skeletal support for the head.

12. The largest portion of the brain, which provides for consciousness and higher mental functions, is the cerebrum.

13. Minute volume is best described as respiratory rate multiplied by tidal volume.

14. The skeletal muscles used for voluntary movement are controlled by the somatic nervous system.

15. The release of the neurotransmitter acetylcholine results in a negative chronotropic effect.

16. An increase in carbon dioxide production will trigger an increase in hyperventilation.

17. The structure that filters blood into a nephron is the glomerulus.

18. The anterior-most organ in the pelvis of men and women is the urinary bladder.

19. The exchange of gases between a living organism and its environment is called *respiration.*

CHAPTER 8

1. **d.** Metaplasia is the transformation of one type of mature differentiated cell into another type of mature differentiated cell.

2. **a.** Hypoxia. Hypoxic injury is the most common and probably most studied form of cellular injury.

3. **d.** Viruses are the most common cause of infection in human beings.

4. **a.** The preprogrammed death of cells is called apoptosis. This happens in response to cellular damage or injury that results in a nonfunctioning cell. This is the body's way of ridding itself of these cells. It is generally considered normal.

5. **c.** Potassium is the chief intracellular cation responsible for pH and water balance inside cells.

6. **c.** PTH is the substance needed for the body to release stored calcium into the bloodstream.

7. **c.** Normal blood pH of the human body is 7.35 to 7.45.

8. **d.** The ratio of 20:1 between bases and acids is required to maintain balance in the body.

9. **c.** Respiratory acidosis is the most likely acid-base disturbance with these laboratory values.

10. **a.** Antidiuretic hormone primarily regulates water balance in the body.

11. **d.** Sodium is the chief extracellular cation.

12. **b.** An antigen reacts with the preformed components of the immune system.

13. **b.** Hypoperfusion is the inadequate delivery of blood, oxygen, and nutrients to the cells of the body.

14. **a.** Mast cells are responsible for the release of vasoactive amines such as histamine.

15. **b.** Margination is the process of phagocytes adhering to capillary and venule walls in the early phases of inflammation.

16. **b.** Chronic inflammation. The simplest way to distinguish between acute and chronic inflammation is by the length of the response. Chronic inflammation is defined as an inflammatory response lasting longer than 2 weeks, regardless of the cause.

17. **b.** The alarm stage is the phase of the general adaptation syndrome in which the central nervous system is activated.

18. **a.** Cortisol is the primary substance released as a result of stimulation of the adrenal cortex by ACTH during stress.

CHAPTER 9

1. **b.** The term *neonate* is used to describe a child who is younger than 28 days old.

2. **c.** The head of an infant is proportionally large, constituting 25% of the baby's total weight.

3. **a.** The average weight of a newborn is approximately 3 kg.

4. **b.** All fontanelles have generally closed by 9 to 18 months of age.

5. **b.** Puberty usually begins during school age. School-age children are between the ages of 6 and 10 years. These children continue

to grow, adding approximately 3 kg of weight and 2 to 3 inches of height each year. During these years most body functions reach adult levels and body changes related to puberty begin.

6. **a.** Authoritarian parenting is a restrictive, punitive style in which the parent exhorts the child to be obedient, follow the parents' directions, and respect the parents' work and effort. Firm limits and controls are placed on the child, and little verbal exchange is allowed. This style is associated with children's low self-esteem and socially incompetent behavior.

7. **a.** Sibling rivalry refers to the natural jealousy of a child toward a brother or sister.

8. **a.** Early adolescents are at the age where they begin to develop independence and have a desire to not be seen with their parents.

9. **c.** Menopause generally occurs in women in their late 40s to early 50s.

10. **c.** Terminal drop is the drastic mental and physical decline that occurs in the few years immediately preceding death.

CHAPTER 10

1. The World Health Organization defines health as "a state of complete physical, mental, and social well-being and not merely the absence of disease or infirmity."

2. Public health works to improve the overall health of populations and communities rather than focus on providing services to a specific individual. Clinicians evaluate and treat individual patients, whereas public health professionals look at community needs and allocate resources to enhance the health of the public as a whole.

3. The structure of public health at a local level varies significantly. Public health at the local level may be a function of the state, region, county, or municipality. State and local statutes define local accountability for public health.

4. Public health activities to ensure a clean water supply and provide mass immunizations are the two advances that have had the greatest impact on public health in the last century.

5. The positive perception of local ambulance services puts them in an ideal position to approach families unwilling or unable to use private or governmental health services. Their mobility makes them ideally suited to reach people at special risk, such as the homebound, migrant populations, or those in rural areas. EMS providers generally have the requisite training to administer vaccines, and participation in vaccination programs may serve as a revenue source.

6. One study found that 60% of paramedics had no training in the formal recognition of child abuse; other studies have found similar results. Enhanced training is critical to expanding the EMS profes-

sional's capabilities to participate in screenings to identify at-risk situations and patients.

7. *All-hazards emergency preparedness* refers to a cross-cutting approach in which all forms of emergencies, including manmade and natural disasters, epidemics, and terrorist incidents, are managed from a common template that uses consistent language and structure. EMS may participate in emergency responses within an emergency services function structure, with public health officials in command of the health and medical aspects.

8. A syndromic surveillance system compares expected historic volumes of injury or illness within a community against actual, real-time rates. EMS may be able to assist public health by using dispatch data to identify potential disease outbreaks based on greater than expected numbers of cases during a given period.

9. Isolation involves the seclusion of individuals who have already contracted an illness for the duration of their contagious period to prevent transmission to others. People placed into quarantine have been exposed to a disease but do not yet have symptoms. They are secluded for the duration of the incubation period and monitored for the development of symptoms.

10. Efforts to develop a system of triage that would allow EMS providers under appropriate medical supervision to "treat and release" or transport patients to settings other than hospitals would help control healthcare costs. The use of relatively less-expensive EMS staff for primary care activities in the community setting may also significantly affect costs.

CHAPTER 11

1. **d.** The trade name is the original name assigned to a drug by the company that patents the medication. The generic name is a shortened version of the chemical name, which represents the chemical compound. The official name is listed in the *United States Pharmacopoeia*.

2. The three classification systems for drugs include the body system, class of agent, and mechanism of action.

3. **a.** Schedule I has the highest abuse potential and no therapeutic indication. Schedule V is the least controlled; drugs in this category have a current accepted medical use and the lowest potential for abuse. Schedule II, III, and IV are levels in between.

4. **c.** The autonomic system is a division of the peripheral nervous system and has two divisions of its own, the parasympathetic and sympathetic divisions. It is responsible for automatic control and is not voluntary. The somatic system is under voluntary control.

5. **d.** Enteral routes of medication administration include the sublingual, buccal, oral, rectal, and gastric routes.

6. The four main processes of pharmacokinetics are absorption, distribution, metabolism (biotransformation), and elimination/excretion.

7. **c.** Beta$_1$ receptors affect heart function. Beta$_2$ receptors act on the lungs and affect bronchodilation. Alpha$_1$ receptors are responsible for peripheral vasoconstriction. Alpha$_2$ receptors are inhibitory receptors that prevent excess release of norepinephrine.

8. **a.** The parenteral route avoids gastrointestinal absorption. Included in the parenteral routes are subcutaneous, intramuscular, intravenous, intrathecal, intralingual, intradermal, transdermal, inhalation, nasal, endotracheal, umbilical, and intraosseous.

9. **2** Endotracheal
   5 Intradermal
   1 Intravenous
   3 Intramuscular
   4 Subcutaneous

10. **d.** Metabolism alters the drug compound by the reactions of enzymes. It may render a substance more active, such as with a prodrug. It may render a chemical inactive and make it easier for elimination. It often cleaves the drug into smaller subunits called *metabolites.*

11. False. Distribution of a drug occurs more quickly to organs with higher blood flow, such as the brain, heart, liver, and kidneys, than areas with less blood flow, such as the skin, fat, and muscles.

CHAPTER 12

1. **a.** Morphine is an analgesic. Propranolol is a beta-blocker. Phenytoin is an anticonvulsant. Phenobarbital is in the barbiturate class.

2. **b.** Corrosive substances are at the extremes of the pH scale. They can be either acidic or basic. Both can cause substantial tissue damage. Ignitable chemicals have the potential to burn or explode. Reactive substances mix unfavorably with other substances. Toxic substances are harmful to the body.

3. **c.** Hydrofluoric acid is an inorganic acid used in glass etching. It is exceptionally toxic to skin and can cause deep, painful burns.

4. **d.** Crystalloid solutions are used for volume replacement. They do not contain real blood products. Ringer's lactate is a crystalloid. Packed red blood cells, whole blood, and fresh frozen plasma are examples of colloids. Other examples of crystalloids include normal saline, D$_5$W, half normal saline, and D5 $\frac{1}{2}$ NS.

5. **b.** Immunoglobulins are preformed antibodies used to treat serious infection, such as tetanus. Antibiotics are used to treat antigens, which are foreign invaders. Antidotes are used for poisons and toxins.

6. **a.** Beta-blockers or adrenergic antagonists are used to treat coronary ischemia. Sympathomimetics increase heart rate and blood pressure, which would be counterproductive in coronary ischemia. Sympathomimetics are used in respiratory problems, including asthma, chronic obstructive pulmonary disease, and anaphylaxis for their beta$_2$ agonist properties.

7. a. Atropine is a cholinergic blocking drug. It is used in advanced cardiac life support to block the effects of the parasympathetic nerves or increase heart rate. Physostigmine and pyridostigmine are cholinergic agonists. Epinephrine is a sympathomimetic.

8. b. Prolongation of the QRS complex greater than 0.10 seconds is a clinical indication of tricyclic antidepressant overdose. Other signs include prolongation of the QT interval, hypotension, and coma.

9. d. Acetaminophen (Tylenol) does not have any antiplatelet effects. Therefore it is not indicated in cardiac ischemia.

10. a. It exhibits some agonist activity. It does, however, block other agonists from acting at the site. This prevents the full agonist from having any therapeutic effect.

CHAPTER 13

1. 0.3 mL

2. 4 mL

3. 5 mL

4. 2 mL

5. 4 mL

6. 360 gtt/min (6 gtt/sec)

7. 120 gtt/min (2 gtt/sec)

8. 50 gtt/min (5 gtt/6 sec)

9. 100 gtt/min (5 gtt/3 sec)

10. 50 gtt/min (5 gtt/6 sec)

11 to 15. Remember the steps: cross out like terms, reduce the numbers above and below the line, and multiply across. Then divide the "gtt/min" by "60 sec/min." Avoid parts of a second in your answers. (DD = Dose delivered; DH = Dose on hand; * = Drug concentration)

11. 1 mg = 1000 mcg − DH: 1000 mcg/250 mL = 4 mcg/mL

$$\frac{DD: 4\,\text{mcg}/\text{min} \times 60\,\text{gtt}/\text{mL}}{DH: 4\,\text{mcg}/\text{mL}} = 60\,\text{gtt/min}$$

$$\frac{\dfrac{1}{60}\,\text{gtt}/\text{min}}{\dfrac{60}{1}\,\text{sec}/\text{min}} = 1\,\text{gtt/sec}$$

12. 1 g = 1000 mg − DH: 1000 mg/250 mL = 4 mg/mL*

$$\frac{DD: 3\,\text{mg}/\text{min} \times 60\,\text{gtt}/\text{mL}}{DH: 4\,\text{mg}/\text{mL}} = 45\,\text{gtt/min}$$

$$\frac{\dfrac{3}{45}\,\text{gtt}/\text{min}}{\dfrac{60}{4}\,\text{sec}/\text{min}} = 3\,\text{gtt/4sec}$$

13. 1 mg = 1000 mcg − DH: 1000 mcg/250 mL = 4 mcg/mL*

$$\frac{DD: \dfrac{1}{4\,\text{mcg}}\bigg/\text{min} \times 60\,\text{gtt}/\text{mL}}{DH: \dfrac{4}{1}\,\text{mcg}/\text{mL}} = 60\,\text{gtt/min}$$

$$\frac{\dfrac{1}{60}\,\text{gtt}/\text{min}}{\dfrac{60}{1}\,\text{sec}/\text{min}} = 1\,\text{gtt/sec}$$

14. 1 mg = 1000 mcg − DH: 1000 mcg/500 mL = 2 mcg/mL*

$$\frac{DD: \dfrac{1}{2\,\text{mcg}}\bigg/\text{min} \times 60\,\text{gtt}/\text{mL}}{DH: \dfrac{2\,\text{mcg}/\text{mL}}{1}} = 60\,\text{gtt/min}$$

$$\frac{\dfrac{1}{60}\,\text{gtt}/\text{min}}{\dfrac{60}{1}\,\text{sec}/\text{min}} = 1\,\text{gtt/sec}$$

15. 1 g = 1000 mg − DH: 1000 mg/500 mL = 2 mg/mL*

$$\frac{DD: \dfrac{1}{2\,\text{mg}}\bigg/\text{min} \times 60\,\text{gtt}/\text{mL}}{DH: \dfrac{2\,\text{mg}/\text{mL}}{1}} = 60\,\text{gtt/min}$$

$$\frac{\dfrac{1}{60}\,\text{gtt}/\text{min}}{\dfrac{60}{1}\,\text{sec}/\text{min}} = 1\,\text{gtt/sec}$$

16. 220 lb/2.2 lb per kg = 100 kg
Medical control tells you to add 400 mg of dopamine to a 250-mL bag of normal saline, start the drip at 3 mcg/kg/min, and continue to monitor the level of consciousness and vital signs.

17. 100 kg × 8 mcg/kg/min = 800 mcg/min (DD/min)

18. 400 mg = 400,000 mcg
400,000 mcg/250 mL = 1600 mcg/mL (DH/mL)
With a microdrip IV administration set, calculate the number of drops per second that will deliver the proper amount of drug to your patient.

19. 60 gtt/mL

20. $\dfrac{DD/\text{min}: 800\,\text{mcg}/\text{min} \times 60\,\text{gtt}/\text{mL}}{DH/\text{mL}: 1600\,\text{mcg}/\text{mL}} = $ number of gtt/min

First, cross out like terms, and zero for zero, 1:1 above and below the line:

$$\frac{DD/min:800 \ \text{mcg}/min \quad 60 \ \text{gtt}/\text{mL}}{DH/mL:1600 \ \text{mcg} \ /\text{mL}} = \text{number of gtt/min}$$

Then reduce the problem:

$$\frac{DD/min:5 \ min \times 6 \ gtt}{DH\big/mL:\dfrac{16}{1}} = \text{number of gtt/min}$$

Now multiply across:

$$\frac{DD/min:5 \ min \times 6 \ gtt}{denominator} = 30 \ gtt/min$$

21. $\dfrac{30 \ gtt/\text{min}}{60 \ sec/\text{min}} = gtt/sec$

$$\frac{1}{\dfrac{\dfrac{30 \ gtt}{60 \ sec}}{2}} = 1 \ gtt/2 \ sec$$

22. b. Intravenous or any other method that delivers the medication directly into the bloodstream, such as intraosseously, will be the fastest.

23. d. The signs and symptoms presented are the classic signs and symptoms of a transfusion reaction.

24. a. A tibial intraosseous infusion should not be used when a patient has a fracture proximal to the intraosseous site.

25. c. The vastus lateralis is the preferred site for this age group. The other sites should be avoided for this population.

CHAPTER 14

1. c. Hypoxia is an abnormal deficiency in the concentration of oxygen in arterial blood, that is, an inadequate oxygenation of the cells. Hypoventilation occurs when the volume of air that enters the alveoli and takes part in gas exchange is not adequate for the body's metabolic needs (hypoxia can be the result of this). Hypocarbia is an excess of carbon dioxide in the blood.

2. Indications for performing either needle or surgical technique include conditions in which intubation is difficult or impossible, complete upper airway obstruction (e.g., epiglottitis, acute anaphylaxis, severe inhalation injury secondary to burns), laryngeal fracture, craniofacial abnormalities, congenital laryngeal anomalies, excessive oropharyngeal hemorrhage, massive traumatic or congenital deformities, respiratory arrest or near arrest in patients who cannot be tracheally intubated, cervical spine fracture with respiratory compromise in patients who cannot be tracheally intubated, delayed or inability to ventilate the patient by any other means, and an inability to access the patient's mouth because of clenched teeth or a mass, such as a tumor.

3. c. The tongue is the most common cause of airway obstruction in an unresponsive patient. Although food, emesis, and edema can result in airway obstruction, they are not the most common causes.

4. b. Belonging to both the respiratory and gastrointestinal systems, the pharynx is responsible for helping direct food toward the esophagus during swallowing. The larynx, or voice box, and trachea are structures that belong only to the respiratory system. An anatomic landmark, the vallecula, serves no function in relation to the gastrointestinal system but is a landmark when performing endotracheal intubation with a curved laryngoscope blade.

5. Minute volume is the amount of gas moved in and out of the respiratory tract per minute. Tidal volume multiplied by ventilatory rate equals minute volume. The minute volume is the true measurement of a patient's ventilatory status and is vital in assessing pulmonary function. It ascertains the ventilatory rate as well as the depth of each inhalation.

6. a. As air passes through fluid, as with pulmonary edema, a moist crackling or popping sound is heard, referred to as *crackles* or *rales*. Wheezes are musical high-pitched sounds caused by airway constriction such as is commonly associated with asthma. Rattles (rhonchi) are a sign of congestion noted in the larger airway passages associated with conditions such as bronchitis and pneumonia. Stridor is a noise created by constriction of upper airway passages.

7. d. A Venturi mask uses interchangeable adapters at specific liter flow rates to administer precise concentrations of oxygen beneficial for patients receiving long-term supplemental oxygen and those breathing on the hypoxic drive. Nasal cannula and nonrebreather masks do not provide such precise oxygen delivery. A small-volume nebulizer is used to aerosolize inhaled beta-agonist medications with variable rates of oxygen administration.

8. During artificial ventilation gastric distention is a common complication, even when the procedure is performed correctly. Gastric distention impedes the effectiveness of ventilation and increases the risk of regurgitation. To minimize gastric distention, perform cricoid pressure, which is noninvasive and simple to perform. Apply posterior pressure over the cricoid cartilage to compress the esophagus and help prevent the flow of air into the gastrointestinal tract.

9. Endotracheal intubation is indicated in the following situations: inability of the patient to protect his or her own airway because of the absence of protective reflexes (e.g., coma, respiratory and/or cardiac arrest), inability to ventilate an unresponsive patient with less-invasive methods, present or impending airway obstruction or respiratory failure (as in inhalation injury, severe asthma, exacerbation of chronic obstructive pulmonary disease, severe pulmonary edema, severe flail chest or pulmonary contusion), and when prolonged ventilatory support is required.

10. Depending on local medical direction, common indications include a responsive patient in severe respiratory distress from suspected pulmonary edema, congestive heart failure, acute respiratory distress syndrome, drowning, chronic obstructive pulmonary disease, and pneumonia.

CHAPTER 15

1. Gathering data; establishing rapport and responding to the patient's emotions; educating and motivating patients.

2. b. The paramedic is directing the patient to address only the topic of pain.

3. c. The paramedic is confronting the patient about the headache.

4. d. The most effective and efficient method to gather information during the medical interview is to use open-ended questions. They allow patients to respond in narrative form, feel free to answer in their own way, and provide details and information that they believe to be important.

5. d. The attribution of some trait or characteristic to one person based on the interviewer's preconceived notions about a general class of people of similar characteristics is known as stereotyping.

6. b. Keeping the patient in a secure location, such as a closed bedroom, to ensure his or her safety and prevent escape is *not* a recommended method of approaching a hostile patient. Ideally, the patient should not be cornered and should have an available exit.

7. When the patient cannot answer the paramedic's questions, information may be obtained from the patient's family, medication bottles, and/or bystanders.

8. b. The best approach to dealing with your own emotions in response to a patient or situation is to continue to provide appropriate care in a nonjudgmental fashion until the encounter is over, then use appropriate outlets to discuss your emotions.

9. Three ways to communicate with a hearing-impaired patient are to use written forms of communication, use a translator proficient in sign language, or determine if the patient is able to read lips.

10. In a potentially hostile or violent patient, nonverbal cues to be alert for include clenched fists, upright or standing position, pacing, angry facial expression, and tense posture.

11. Ways of determining a patient's mental status include asking the patient simple demographic information, such as name, address, and date of birth; asking the patient if she knows who she is, where she is, what time it is, and whether she can recall what happened; asking family members on scene if the patient's behavior or affect seems appropriate.

12. c. The application of a derogatory term to a patient on the basis of an event, habit, or personality trait that may not be accurate about the underlying condition is known as *labeling*.

13. False. When appropriate, physical contact is very personal and useful, from shaking hands with the patient to even putting your arm around the patient's shoulders in a gesture of comfort or condolence.

CHAPTER 16

1. Old medical records; family members; the patient's primary care physician.

2. Family history; screening tests; immunizations.

3. b. A developmental assessment is a unique component of a pediatric history.

4. b. The best way to deal with an intoxicated person is to obtain pertinent medical history from family or caregivers. Because of alterations in mental status, the answers that an intoxicated patient provides may be incorrect.

5. b. Break patient confidentiality if the person plans to harm himself or anyone else.

CHAPTER 17

1. a. Palpating with fingertips allows the paramedic to detect fine sensations.

2. c. During the primary survey, the paramedic's goal is to identify and treat immediate life threats.

3. d. A full set of vital signs includes pulse, respirations, blood pressure, skin, AVPU, and core temperature.

4. c. The difference between pain and tenderness is the patient feels pain; you discover tenderness on palpation.

5. a. When evaluating a 6-month-old child in respiratory distress, bradycardia is an ominous sign of impending respiratory failure.

6. c. When you cannot identify a cause for a decreased level of consciousness, you need the physical examination, SAMPLE history, and vital signs to help make a differential diagnosis.

7. The skilled paramedic should be competent at auscultating lung sounds, heart tones, and blood pressure.

8. b. Sensory and motor examinations test spine and nerve integrity; CSM checks evaluate neurovascular bundle integrity in an extremity.

9. a. *Antegrade amnesia* is the term used to describe short-term memory loss of information since a head injury occurred.

10. a. *Borborygmi* is the correct term used to describe hyperactivity of bowel sounds.

CHAPTER 18

1. c. A system that allows one-at-a-time communication on the same frequency is a simplex system. You cannot interrupt the transmission because both operators use the same frequency.

2. c. A radio with a low output carried by an individual is a portable radio, also referred to as a *walkie-talkie*. These radios are carried by emergency personnel and have a lower wattage output than the mobile or base unit. To use these portable radios with a higher watt output, the units can be connected through a repeater system, which increases range.

3. **c.** A system that receives transmissions from a low output and rebroadcasts the signal at a higher output is called a *repeater system.*

4. **b.** Interoperability describes a system that allows components of different radio systems to communicate on scene. It can use specialized equipment to connect several different radio systems and components together and have them communicate with each other.

5. **a.** A radio system that allows transmitting and receiving at the same time through two different frequencies is a duplex system.

6. **d.** A radio system that uses multiple repeaters so that the computer searches for an open channel and transmits on that channel is called a *trunking system.*

7. **b.** A radio that is installed in a fixed unit that transmits at a higher wattage is a mobile radio.

8. **c.** The federal organization that regulates interstate and international communications through radio, television, wire, and satellite is the FCC. It is an independent U.S. governmental agency directly responsible to Congress and established by the Communications Act of 1934. The FCC's jurisdiction covers the 50 states, the District of Columbia, and U.S. territorial possessions.

9. **b.** The three primary modes of EMS communication are verbal, written, and electronic.

10. Good communication is important. It helps gather information needed from the caller; helps relay pertinent information to the hospital; and provides written documentation of events that happened during a call.

CHAPTER 19

1. **c.** "The patient was intoxicated" would be inappropriate to include in a PCR, which must be objective. This statement makes an assumptive leap. Slurred speech and staggered gait could be caused by several medical or traumatic conditions. The assumption that the patient is intoxicated is only an opinion.

2. Three reasons why statements such as "physical assessment unremarkable" should be avoided in a PCR: the statement does not identify what was evaluated; the statement does not identify the evaluations that were done; and the statement is open to interpretation.

3. **a.** Documenting that the father beat the child would be inappropriate in a PCR. The PCR must be objective.

4. **b.** "Patient has circumoral cyanosis" would be a pertinent positive finding. A pertinent positive finding is a sign or symptom that is significant to the working diagnosis.

5. False. All patients require a PCR.

6. False. Having that patient sign a refusal form when refusing transport will not necessarily clear the paramedic from any legal action against him or her.

7. **c.** HIPAA regulates how a paramedic must protect a patient's personal information.

8. **b.** Marking out an error with a single line and then initialing it is an appropriate way to correct an error.

9. **a.** Use only abbreviations approved for use in your agency.

10. **d.** Using the PCR to notify the patient's friend is not an accepted use of a PCR.

CHAPTER 20

1. **b.** The aqueous humor fills the anterior chamber of the eye and is similar to water. The two chambers do not exchange fluid. Aqueous humor is constantly replaced by the body.

2. **c.** Tinnitus is a constant humming in the ears.

3. **a.** Ludwig's angina is a bacterial infection of the floor of the mouth resulting from an infection in the root of the teeth, an abscessed tooth, or an injury to the mouth. Because the infection is under the tongue, swelling can push the tongue up and back, covering the airway.

4. **b.** They are highly transmittable from person to person through close contact or sharing personal grooming items. The most commonly infected group is children from 4 to 10 years of age.

5. **b.** Bell's palsy is an inflammation of the facial nerve (cranial nerve VII). It often is preceded by a viral upper respiratory tract infection. This condition can affect an individual at any age; no one segment of the population is at a higher risk.

6. **d.** Impetigo is a highly contagious skin disease caused by *Staphylococcus* or *Streptococcus* bacteria and, once diagnosed, is treated with antibiotics. It does not cause any systemic effects, which differentiates it from chickenpox.

7. Low blood pressure, nearsightedness, family history, African descent, diabetes, long-term exposure to cortisone, and previous eye injury are all risk factors for developing glaucoma.

8. **a.** Exudative retinal detachment is associated with tumors and trauma. Rhegmatogenous detachment is associated with fluids other than blood separating the retina and tractional detachment is associated with scarred tissue. Occlusive is not a type of retinal detachment.

9. **a.** Thrush is a fungal infection that typically affects infants and newborns and can cause fever, nausea, vomiting, and diarrhea.

10. b. Otitis externa is redness and irritation of the external auditory canal and is commonly associated with spending time in the water. Tinnitus is a ringing in the ear, rhinitis is a runny nose, and labyrinthitis is an infection of the labyrinth within the middle ear.

CHAPTER 21

1. Upper respiratory tract infections that require medical treatment include epiglottitis, bacterial tracheitis, and croup.

2. Reducing airway edema by cool mist, cold air, inhaled epinephrine, or nebulized saline are examples of how to treat an upper respiratory tract infection such as croup.

3. Care for a patient with a tracheostomy who called EMS for dyspnea includes ensuring oxygenation and ventilation, assisting ventilations if necessary, and IV placement and ECG monitoring followed by rapid transport.

4. Typical findings include dyspnea, tachypnea, decreased breath sounds on one side, and possibly tachycardia, low oxygen saturation level, or chest wall trauma.

5. Supportive care includes oxygen administered to maintain sufficient saturations, IV placement, ECG monitoring, and expedient transport.

6. Signs of pneumonia may include fever, chills, productive cough, dyspnea, and chest pain.

7. EMS can help patients with COPD exacerbations by using oxygen to help reduce the sensation of hypoxia, using inhaled beta-agonists such as albuterol, and possibly using IV steroids and theophylline.

8. Inhaled irritants are treated by EMS with immediate removal from the area of the offending agent and decontamination as needed. Supplemental oxygen and monitoring can also help the patient.

9. Insufficient tissue oxygenation caused by inadequate or absent respiration. Causes include COPD, status asthmaticus, pneumonia, and pulmonary edema. Various conditions can cause respiratory failure, which is insufficient tissue oxygenation.

10. Tuberculosis is a serious bacterial lung infection spread by respiratory droplets.

CHAPTER 22

1. *Coronary heart disease* refers to disease of the coronary arteries and their resulting complications, such as angina pectoris or acute myocardial infarction. Coronary artery disease affects the arteries that supply the heart muscle with blood.

2. Traits and lifestyle habits that may increase a person's chance of developing a disease are called *risk factors*.

3. The three major coronary arteries are the LAD, LCX, and RCA.

4. Stroke volume is determined by (1) the degree of ventricular filling when the heart is relaxed (preload), (2) the pressure against which the ventricle must pump (afterload), and (3) the myocardium's contractile state (contracting or relaxing).

5. Four properties of cardiac cells are automaticity, excitability (irritability), conductivity, and contractility.

6. The intrinsic rates for the heart's normal pacemaker sites are SA node (primary pacemaker), 60 to 100 beats/min; AV junction, 40 to 60 beats/min; and Purkinje fibers, 20 to 40 beats/min.

7. A rhythm that begins in the SA node has (1) a positive (upright) P wave before each QRS complex, (2) P waves that look alike, (3) a constant PR interval, and (4) regular atrial and ventricular rhythm (usually).

8. SVT includes three main types of fast rhythms: (1) atrial tachycardia, (2) atrioventricular nodal reentrant tachycardia, and (3) atrioventricular reentrant tachycardia.

9. The 5 *P*s of acute arterial occlusion are *p*ain, *p*allor, *p*ulselessness, *p*aralysis, and *p*aresthesia.

10. An aneurysm is a localized dilation or bulging of a blood vessel wall (or wall of a heart chamber). The dilated area may leak or rupture if it stretches too far.

11. Ventricular septal defect is the most common (15% to 20%) congenital heart defect.

12. Classic signs of cardiac tamponade include jugular vein distention, hypotension, and muffled heart sounds (Beck's triad), but these signs are present in less than half of all patients with cardiac tamponade.

CHAPTER 23

1. a. The central nervous system is composed of the brain and spinal cord. All remaining nervous tissue comprises the peripheral nervous system.

2. b. Neurons have three basic parts: dendrites, the cell body, and the axon.

3. d. The frontal lobe area regulates many important functions, including speech, abstract thinking, and personality.

4. c. These nerves innervate the organ systems and other related elements, such as smooth muscle and glands.

5. a. The somatic (*soma,* from the Greek for body) part of the nervous system innervates the skin and most of the skeletal muscle.

6. c. Glasgow Coma Scale: eye opening response, verbal response, motor response.

7. c. The meninges are three layered, connective tissue coverings that surround, protect, and suspend the brain and spinal cord in the cranium and spinal canal. The outermost layer is the dura mater, atop the arachnoid membrane, which is above the pia mater.

8. **b.** Hallucinations are false sensory perceptions, such as hearing voices or seeing things that are not there.

9. **d.** Delirium is *short term and temporary* mental confusion and fluctuating level of consciousness.

10. **c.** The symptoms of hemorrhagic stroke tend to occur with a higher severity and progress more rapidly than those of ischemic stroke. Patients often complain of a sudden-onset "thunderclap" headache or the "worst headache of my life." The headache is made worse by lying down or moving. At first the patient may have an abnormal meningeal examination. This quickly progresses to forceful vomiting (often without nausea); neurologic deficits; and visual disturbances such as blurry or double vision, unconsciousness, and seizures.

11. **b.** Ensure that the patient's airway remains open. Patients with an acute stroke may lose the ability to swallow if the cranial nerves are affected. They may not be able to breathe effectively if the brainstem is involved. Apply a pulse oximeter and cardiac monitor. Give oxygen as needed and per medical direction instructions. Monitor the patient's breathing effort and be prepared to assist ventilations. If inadequate breathing is present, consider intubation, particularly if the patient's GCS is less than 8. Consider the use of pharmacologically assisted intubation if necessary and approved by medical direction. Lidocaine is usually given IV approximately 90 seconds before intubation to prevent a further increase in ICP.

　　Establish IV access with a saline lock or an IV line containing normal saline or lactated Ringer's solution and run at a keep-open rate (30 mL/hr). Avoid giving large volumes of fluids unless hypotension is present. Obtain a 12-lead ECG. Do not delay transport to definitive care to perform these procedures.

12. **a.** An ischemic stroke occurs when blood flow in one of the arteries in the brain is blocked. Blockage may be caused by air, amniotic fluid, or foreign body, but a blood clot is the most common form. It occurs suddenly, with the maximal severity of the symptoms at onset without worsening or improving.

13. **b.** Status epilepticus is a single seizure lasting longer than 30 minutes or repeated seizures without full recovery of responsiveness between seizures and lasting longer than 30 minutes.

14. **c.** Syncope is a transient loss of consciousness and inability to maintain postural tone, typically resulting in a ground-level fall. Syncope is commonly known as "fainting," "passing out," "blacking out," or "falling out."

15. **d.** A migraine headache is a recurrent headache with symptom-free intervals and at least three of the following: abdominal pain, nausea or vomiting; throbbing or pulsatile character of the pain; pain located on one side of the head; associated aura (visual, sensory, motor); relief after rest or sleep; and positive family history.

16. **b.** Infectious headaches are often accompanied by fever and, depending on the pathogen, seen with a rash, neck stiffness (nuchal rigidity), confusion, altered mental status, nausea, and vomiting.

17. **c.** In shingles the patient develops extreme sensitivity and pain along a unilateral dermatome. After 1 to 3 days the pain progresses to a reddened rash with raised bumps and blisters along the same area.

18. **d.** Signs and symptoms of Alzheimer's disease vary widely as the condition progresses. In its early stages patients may have slight lapses in memory and cognition, such as trouble recognizing familiar family and friends or remembering recent events and activities. The patient may seem to have problems finding a particular word to describe something or may show difficulty performing familiar tasks. These signs often go unnoticed or are simply credited to "old age" by the patient's friends and family.

　　This decrease in mental function continues as the patient becomes unable to think clearly or solve problems and develops communication issues (problems with reading, speaking, and writing). At this stage patients begin to lose the ability to perform simple daily functions, such as bathing, grooming, dressing, preparing meals, and remembering to take scheduled medications. Even in familiar surroundings the patient becomes increasingly confused and disoriented and has a greater risk of falls and accidents.

19. **b.** This is most often caused by either a distended bladder or a distended rectum impacted with feces.

20. **a.** Hydrocephalus describes a condition of an excessive amount of cerebrospinal fluid.

21. **c.** Bell's palsy is paralysis of the facial nerve (cranial nerve VII), often caused by infection by the Herpes simplex virus.

22. **a.** Seizure activity and status epilepticus may continue after tonic and clonic movements stop. This is sometimes called *"silent" status epilepticus*. Because of the high levels of activity, the motor neurons that carry signals from the brain to the muscles have become exhausted, causing the patient to become limp while seizure activity continues in the brain.

CHAPTER 24

1. The hypothalamus releases several hormones that specifically target receptor sites in the pituitary gland, which in turn regulates body systems and maintains homeostasis.

2. TSH is released by the pituitary gland at the direction of the hypothalamus. The primary function of TSH is to increase the body's metabolic rate.

3. Alpha cells release glucagon, which is responsible for raising blood glucose levels; beta cells release insulin, which is responsible for decreasing blood glucose levels; and delta cells release somatostatin, which is responsible for buffering the effects of both insulin and glucagon.

4. Diabetes insipidus is caused by a lack of ADH from the posterior pituitary gland. It results in excess water loss in the urine and poor water absorption into the bloodstream. Signs and symptoms include polyuria, dehydration, and hypernatremia.

5. Thyrotoxicosis is caused by an overactive thyroid gland. In its extreme form this disorder is called a *thyroid storm.* Signs and symptoms of a thyroid storm include high fever, irritability, tachycardia, hypotension, vomiting, diarrhea, delirium, and coma.

6. Myxedema is caused by underactivity of the thyroid gland. It is characterized by hypothermia in the absence of cold exposure, hypoglycemia in the absence of insulin replacement therapy, and coma.

7. Patients in DKA do not have enough insulin present to allow the cells to use glucose for their metabolic needs. In response, the body breaks down fats and proteins to produce new glucose, gluconeogenesis, which has a byproduct of ketone bodies. In patients with hyperglycemic, hyperosmolar nonketotic coma, there is a significant excess of glucose in the blood but enough insulin in the system to allow for cellular metabolism without the need for gluconeogenesis.

8. Patients who are hypoglycemic have pale, cool, clammy skin; tachycardia; altered mentation; coma; and seizures. Treatment varies based on level of consciousness. If the patient is conscious and expected to be able to maintain his or her airway, he or she may be treated with oral glucose. In the absence of the ability to protect his or her own airway, the patient may be treated with IV D50 or intramuscular glucagon if the patient has poor vascular access.

9. Kwashiorkor is caused by inadequate protein caloric intake. Elderly patients with poor nutritional habits and inadequate financial resources may be at risk for this disorder.

10. Wernicke-Korsakoff syndrome is a neurologic disorder caused by an insufficiency of thiamine, or vitamin B_1. In early stages the patient may present with ataxia, nystagmus, and mental derangement. As the syndrome worsens the signs and symptoms may become permanent and include amnesia, disorientation, delirium, and hallucinations. Chronic alcoholics may have poor nutritional habits that may be complicated by liver disorders, causing hypoglycemia. Thiamine-deficient patients who are treated with D50 may develop Wernicke-Korsakoff syndrome unless they are also given thiamine simultaneously.

CHAPTER 25

1. **a.** Antibiotics only kill bacteria and generally are not effective in stopping other organisms. This is frequently misunderstood; many patients request an antibiotic thinking it will kill or stop an infection by a virus.

2. **c.** Viruses differ from all the other organisms because they are not composed of cells, the basic building block of most living things. Instead they consist of genetic material (RNA or DNA) that must use the machinery of other organisms to reproduce. Viruses cannot move on their own and need an outside mechanism to move from one host to another.

3. **a.** Anaphylaxis represents the most serious manifestation of immediate hypersensitivity. Hypersensitivity disorders manifest themselves as excessive responses to an antigen that are uncomfortable or dangerous for the patient in which they occur. They are divided into four types: type I (immediate), type II (cytotoxic), type III (immune complex mediated), and type IV (delayed).

4. Answer should include reference to the following actions: a pathogen is introduced into the body containing an *antigen,* which is recognized as foreign by *lymphocytes* during the *cognitive phase.* The lymphocytes then enlist the help of other lymphocytes, with large numbers of antigen-specific lymphocytes produced through amplification during the *activation phase.* During the activation phase and *effector phase* antibodies are produced that are specific to the pathogen's antigen and that control or kill the pathogen. Also during the effector phase many other host defenses are activated; these, along with some lymphocytes, help control the infection by *phagocytosis* (consumption and digestion) of the pathogens.

5. **b.** EMS professionals are required to have more immunizations than the general public is because of their increased exposure to communicable diseases. In addition to the standard childhood vaccinations (such as measles/mumps/rubella and polio), EMS employment generally also requires immunization against hepatitis B. Annual influenza vaccinations are usually recommended, as is maintenance of tetanus toxoid vaccination.

6. **b.** At the first sign of anaphylaxis (respiratory distress or cardiovascular compromise) epinephrine should be given per local protocol. As always, airway, breathing, and circulation take priority in assessment and treatment. Airway management is critical. Anaphylaxis represents an airway emergency in an otherwise healthy, nontraumatized patient. Any complaint of tightness of the throat or shortness of breath should be considered potential impending respiratory failure. IV access and pulse oximetry should be obtained and high-concentration oxygen administered.

   Once cardiopulmonary stability has been ensured, all interventions for less-severe allergic reactions should also be used for anaphylaxis. Aerosolized epinephrine may be given if available, permitted, and ordered by medical direction and if the patient has respiratory symptoms. Any antigenic material still in contact with the patient should be removed. If an insect stinger remains, care must be taken not to squeeze it. This can result in the release of further venom. Glucagon may be ordered by medical direction if the patient is taking a beta-blocker. Beta-agonists such as albuterol can be helpful for bronchospasm refractory to epinephrine. Glucocorticoids are available to paramedics in some EMS systems. Some patients may have already self-administered epinephrine by a prescribed EpiPen. This should be considered if further epinephrine is being given.

7. False. Physicians track histocompatibility antigens (such as ABO blood types and human leukocyte antigen) and try to match them

between donor and recipient before transplantation to prevent rejection. However, if preformed antibodies exist in the host, a hyperacute rejection can occur. Preformed antibodies can form through prior exposure to the histocompatibility antigen, such as by prior transplant, blood transfusions, or pregnancy. These antibodies are usually directed at the vascular endothelium of the transplanted organ, trigger the complement cascade, and are usually immunoglobulin G or M. This represents another example of type II (cytotoxic) hypersensitivity, although some researchers also believe components of type IV (delayed) hypersensitivity may be present in hyperacute rejection as well.

8. d. Anaphylaxis represents the most serious manifestation of immediate hypersensitivity, causing up to 1500 deaths each year.

9. b. Autoimmune diseases are present when the immune system response attacks its own tissue. Multiple sclerosis and lupus are good examples of autoimmune diseases.

10. a. Because the gastrointestinal tract, upper respiratory tract, and genitourinary tract communicate with the outside world, they are considered external barriers. Each of these body systems prevents pathogenic agents from reaching internal tissues by serving as a mechanical barrier. They also have unique features that further prevent infection.

11. c. Effector cells act to control an infection and kill or contain the pathogen causing it.

CHAPTER 26

1. a. Crohn's disease is characterized by weakness, weight loss, decrease in appetite, bloody stools, ulceration of bowel, and fistulas. The pus coming from the patient's skin is a description of a fistula that can occur in this severe inflammatory condition.

2. c. The first three questions are appropriate but can indicate one of many gastrointestinal conditions. Dark, tarry stools are typically associated with gastrointestinal bleeding.

3. b. Although all the answers are correct, the most important treatment option is to begin with the primary survey and treat all life-threatening conditions.

4. c. The most likely cause is gastroenteritis. Symptoms typically include nausea, vomiting, and diarrhea. A small-bowel obstruction would produce abdominal pain and hyperresonant sounds on percussion. Gastritis typically involves only the stomach and not the intestines. Cirrhosis usually has either jaundice or a distended and fluid-filled abdomen.

5. c. The pancreas is located in the mid-epigastric region. It can be quite painful when inflamed. The pain is typically in the middle of the abdomen and radiates to the back. Crohn's disease and ulcerative colitis are typically chronic illnesses. Hemorrhoids do not cause abdominal pain.

6. c. This patient may have a bowel obstruction. Obtaining IV access is important. Fluid replacement would be appropriate because this patient may be dehydrated from vomiting. On the basis of the patient's vital signs, placing the patient in a shock position is not necessary at this time. He should be permitted to assume a position of comfort. A nasogastric tube may be indicated, but a nasal airway is not necessary.

7. a. Appendicitis typically presents with periumbilical pain. This pain then localizes to the right lower quadrant. Rovsing's sign is present when the left side of the abdomen is palpated and the patient feels pain in the right lower quadrant. This often occurs in appendicitis. The liver is in the upper right quadrant, and hepatitis is typically painful in that location. The pancreas is in the mid-epigastric area. Gastritis also is in the mid-epigastric region.

8. b. Diverticulosis can cause painless rectal bleeding. Diverticulitis is inflammation of one of the outpouchings of the colon. Patients with diverticulosis may have painless bloody stools. Patients with diverticulitis typically present with signs of illness, including fever, shaking chills, nausea, vomiting, abdominal pain, and diarrhea. Gastritis is inflammation of the stomach and, if rectal bleeding is present, it is typically melena (dark, tarry stools). Hemorrhoids typically cause bleeding but more often small amounts of blood dripping into the toilet.

9. d. Visceral pain is common with abdominal pain. Pain that is felt in an area different from the organ of origin is called *visceral pain*.

10. a. Cholecystitis is inflammation of the gallbladder. It is common in women who are near 40 years of age. It often occurs right after eating.

11. c. This patient should receive IV fluids and medications for pain and nausea as per local protocol.

CHAPTER 27

1. Hypertension and diabetes mellitus. Many risk factors are common to both progression of kidney disease and cardiovascular complications, such as diabetes, hypertension, and high cholesterol. Diabetes mellitus and hypertension are among the strongest risk factors for chronic renal failure.

2. A condition in which the kidneys suddenly stop functioning, either partially or totally. If the cause of the acute renal failure is corrected before permanent damage occurs, the kidneys may return to normal functioning.

3. They are toxic to the nephron and can alter its ability to function. Nonsteroidal antiinflammatory drugs can be dangerous, especially in patients at risk of hypovolemia.

4. Benign prostate hypertrophy restricts the flow of urine from the urinary bladder, thus preventing the bladder from emptying.

5. Hemodialysis, peritoneal dialysis, kidney transplant. Dialysis is the process of diffusing blood across a semipermeable membrane to remove substances that the kidney would normally eliminate. Two types of dialysis treatments are available: hemodialysis and peritoneal dialysis. When the kidneys function at 10% to 15% of normal, dialysis or transplantation is the only option for the patient's survival.

6. The patient has acute renal failure caused by dehydration. Prehospital care includes rehydration and prompt transportation to the emergency department. Prehospital care for patients with acute renal failure includes airway and ventilatory support, establishing IV access, monitoring the patient's vitals signs and ECG, promptly treating for shock (hypovolemic and other types), ensuring an adequate blood pressure after a cardiac event, properly treating for ingested toxins, and promptly transporting to the emergency department.

7. Urinary tract infection (see Table 27-2).

8. Uremic frost from waste, such as urea being excreted through the skin. This is caused by fluid overload and, perhaps, an incomplete dialysis during a previous treatment. Uremic frost is dried crystals of urea excreted through the skin that appear to be a frosting on the patient's body.

9. Paraphimosis should be treated by wrapping the penis, including the glans, in a gauze dressing. The dressing should be followed by a compression bandage to reduce swelling, if permitted by medical direction. Alternatively, the penis can be wrapped in plastic followed by a cold compress. The patient should be transported promptly to the emergency department. Two of the more urgent structural conditions are phimosis or paraphimosis. These conditions are described as the inability to retract the foreskin over the glans of the penis (see Figure 27-11). Because of this, the patient may develop an infection under the foreskin and complain of a discharge. Paraphimosis is the more serious of the two conditions and occurs when the foreskin cannot be replaced over the glans after it has been retracted. The result is a tight ring around the glans that acts as a tourniquet, leading to swelling of the glans. Treatment for paraphimosis includes squeezing the glans firmly for 10 minutes or longer to reduce swelling. If approved by medical direction, wrap the glans in gauze, then apply an elastic wrap from the distal end of the penis onto the shaft to produce constant and gentle compression. An alternative treatment is to wrap the penis in plastic, then apply cold packs to reduce the swelling. Transport the patient to the emergency department when the compression dressing can be removed and the foreskin replaced over the glans. If this fails, the emergency department physician may need to incise the foreskin to alleviate the constriction. Any underlying infection must also be treated.

CHAPTER 28

1. **b.** The appendicular skeleton consists of the bones of the shoulder, hips, and limbs.

2. **a.** Abdominal pain, passage of blood with bowel movements or urination, pulsatile masses in the abdomen, or vomiting may be associated with an acute intraabdominal process such as an abdominal aortic aneurysm, for which hypotension is also a concern.

3. **b.** Pain in the lumbar back and leg resulting from irritation and impingement of the sciatic nerve, usually from a herniated disc. The pain of a herniated disc is often described as sharp, "electric," or "shooting" and radiates down the posterior aspect of one leg. The affected leg can also feel numb.

4. **b.** The treatment principles are the same for a strain or sprain: immobilization, compression of the affected joint with an elastic wrap, elevation of the affected part, application of an ice pack, and appropriate analgesia.

5. **d.** Carpal tunnel syndrome is a medical condition in which the median nerve is compressed at the wrist (within the carpal tunnel), resulting in pain and numbness of the hand.

6. **d.** Signs and symptoms of rhabdomyolysis include myalgias, stiffness, weakness, malaise, and possibly dark-brown urine. Nausea, vomiting, abdominal pain, and tachycardia can occur in severe cases. Remember that rhabdomyolysis can still be present in patients without any signs or symptoms.

7. **b.** With gout even light touch is perceived as being quite painful, such as a blanket draped over the affected toe.

8. **b.** Risk factors for septic arthritis include a history of prior joint trauma, artificial (prosthetic) joints, a history of intravenous drug abuse, sexually transmitted diseases, or a history of immunosuppression.

9. **d.** Pathologic fractures occur as a result of an underlying disease process that weakens the mechanical properties of the bone. Bone tumors are common causes of pathologic fractures, but other metabolic diseases such as osteoporosis can cause these fractures as well. Pathologic fractures may be the first presentation of a primary bone tumor in up to 10% of cases.

10. **c.** Transient synovitis, which is a nonspecific inflammation of the synovium and synovial fluid, is the most common cause of nontraumatic hip pain in children with a subsequent limp. The exact cause is not known, although it is thought to be related to recent minor trauma, recent illnesses, or a result of a medication reaction in children with allergic tendencies.

CHAPTER 29

1. Vitamin D. The skin serves as a protective barrier against the environment (e.g. heat, light, injury, infection). The skin also regulates body temperature and stores water, fat, and vitamin D.

2. Dermis. The skin is composed of three layers, with each layer performing specific protective functions. They are the epidermis, dermis, and subcutaneous fat.

3. Matching
   Bulla. **E.** A localized, fluid-filled lesion usually greater than 0.5 cm

Cyst. **F.** A walled cavity that contains fluid or purulent material

Macule. **B.** A flat, circumscribed, discolored lesion (e.g., freckle)

Nodule. **H.** An elevated, solid lesion in the deep skin or subcutaneous tissues

Papule. **J.** An elevated, solid lesion usually less than 0.5 cm

Patch. **C.** A flat, circumscribed, discolored lesion

Plaque. **I.** An elevated, solid lesion usually greater than 0.5 cm that lacks a deep component

Pustule. **D.** A lesion that contains purulent material

Vesicle. **G.** An elevated lesion that contains clear fluid; sometimes called a *water blister*

Wheal. **A.** A firm, rounded, flat-topped elevation of skin that is evanescent and pruritic

4. Matching

Crust **A.** A collection of cellular debris or dried blood; sometimes called a *scab*

Erosion **E.** A partial focal loss of epidermis that usually heals without scarring

Excoriation **D.** A linear erosion created by scratching

Fissure **G.** A vertical loss of epidermis and dermis with sharply defined walls; sometimes called a *crack*

Ulcer **C.** A full-thickness crater that involves the dermis and epidermis with loss of the surface epithelium

Scar **B.** A collection of new connective tissue

Scale **F.** A thick stratum corneum that results from hyperproliferation or increased cohesion of keratinocytes

5. **b.** Avoidance of sun. Prevention of skin cancer by avoiding sun exposure is the best approach. Parents should protect young children and teach older children about sun protection with sunscreen (at least SPF 15), appropriate clothing, hats, and avoidance of midday sun exposure. Early detection of melanoma can be life saving.

6. **a.** Melanoma recognition is enhanced by looking for asymmetry and border irregularities of any lesions.

7. True. The most important component for caretakers of a patient with decubitus ulcers (or the risk of) is to understand what causes them and make every effort with preventive methods. The prevention of pressure ulcers is one of the most important aspects of care of the immobile patient. Efforts to minimize skin pressure and stress are pivotal in the prevention of pressure ulcers.

8. True. Dermatitis literally means inflammation of the skin, but it almost always refers to a specific group of inflammatory diseases.

9. True. Contact dermatitis refers to any dermatitis arising from direct skin exposure to a substance. The cause may either be allergic or irritant induced, the latter being the most common. Contact dermatitis is caused by exposure to an allergen or by direct irritation of the skin (e.g., metals, cosmetics, soaps, tape, plants, detergents).

10. Matching

Carbuncles **D.** Interconnected erythematous nodular lesions that drain through openings in the skin

Cellulitis **A.** A red, swollen area of skin that feels hot and tender

Impetigo **B.** A combination of pustules and vesicles that, when rupture, leave a characteristic thick, golden or honey-like appearance

Folliculitis **C.** Erythematous clustered lesions with a central pustule on top of a raised lesion

Furuncles **E.** Painful nodular lesions

Psoriasis **F.** Red, discrete, flat-topped, persistent plaques and papules with thick silvery scales

11. Matching

Tinea capitis **F.** Round, scaly area on the scalp where no hair grows

Tinea corporis **A.** Annular lesions; sometimes called *ringworm*

Tinea cruris **G.** Sharply demarcated area with elevated scaling and geographic borders

Tinea manuum **C.** Dry, diffuse scaling usually seen on the palms

Tinea pedis **D.** Maceration between the toes or scaling on the soles or sides of the foot

Tinea unguium **B.** Dark debris under fingernails or toenails

Tinea versicolor **E.** Pink, tan, or white patches with fine desquamating scales

12. Matching

Herpes simplex **C.** HSV-1 or -2

Pediculosis **D.** Lice

Scabies **E.** Mites

Warts **A.** Benign lesions caused by papillomavirus

Varicella **B.** Chickenpox

13. Matching

Erythema multiforme **B.** Single or multiple wheals, sometimes geographic in appearance

Herpes zoster **C.** Vesicular eruptions that follow a dermatome

Urticaria **A.** Multiple presentations usually related to a drug reaction

CHAPTER 30

1. True. Toxicologic emergencies can pose grave dangers. The patient may be under the influence of psychoactive drugs, a victim of foul play, or a casualty of a larger hazardous materials incident.

2. Inhalation, ingestion, absorption, and injection.

3. **b.** The *Physicians' Desk Reference* contains much useful information on medications but little information on the chemical and physical properties of hazardous materials.

4. True. The regional Poison Control Center has a large database of poisons, biologic toxins, and medications that can be searched by signs and symptoms as well as by name.

5. See Table 30-1.

6. Activated charcoal. Activated charcoal has many fewer side effects and possible complications than emetics or gastric lavage.

7. **a.** Acetaminophen is involved in most accidental and intentional poisonings because of its ready availability.

8. **c.** Medications with a narrow therapeutic index are more dangerous than those with a wide therapeutic index. A narrow therapeutic index can easily lead to undermedication or an overdose. This may lead to therapeutic overdoses, accidental overdoses and, with antidepressants, suicidal behavior if patients are undermedicated.

9. False. Bases, or caustics or alkalis, have a pH *above* 7.

10. False. Hydrocarbons with a low viscosity are more likely to be aspirated and cause pulmonary complications.

11. **a.** Organophosphates inhibit the enzyme acetylcholinesterase, which is vital to nerve signaling.

12. False. Organophosphates, not nitrates and nitrites, cause SLUDGEM symptoms.

13. **c.** Cytochrome C is the enzyme vital to cellular respiration that is inhibited by the cyanide family.

14. **b.** Ethanol is a competitive inhibitor of alcohol dehydrogenase. Ethanol helps keep the protoxin methanol from being biochemically converted to formic acid.

15. True. Chelating agents effectively bind many heavy metals. Unfortunately, they also bind many metals vital to cell function and, therefore, must be closely monitored.

CHAPTER 31

1. Two: HIV-1 and -2. HIV-1 is more pathologic and HIV-2 is more restricted to West Africa.

2. Sexual contact; sharing of contaminated needles and syringes; infusion of contaminated blood and blood products.

3. Fever, anorexia, abdominal discomfort. Other symptoms include nausea, darkening of the urine, jaundiced skin color.

4. Liver.

5. Direct. Meningitis is contracted through direct contact with the patient's secretions during intubation, direct suctioning, and cardiopulmonary resuscitation with increased exposure through prolonged contact with infected persons.

6. Sickle cell disease, cardiovascular disease, anatomic or functional asplenia, diabetes mellitus, chronic renal failure or other kidney disease, HIV, organ transplantation, multiple myeloma, lymphoma, or Hodgkin's disease.

7. Skeletal.

8. Abdominal rigidity.

9. 3 to 8 weeks. Human beings are especially susceptible to tetanus when bitten by an infected animal. The incubation period is usually 3 to 8 weeks but can be 9 days (rare) or up to 7 years.

10. Integumentary. Herpes zoster is a local manifestation of reactivation of latent viral infection of dorsal root ganglia, and it is distributed along nerve fibers of the skin.

11. 12 to 25 days.

12. Immune system, integumentary, musculoskeletal, and lymph nodes.

13. Nasopharyngeal air droplets and direct contact. Period of communicability is before the prodromal period to 4 days after appearance of the rash. Immunity is acquired after illness and is permanent.

14. Before the onset of paroxysmal, violent coughing.

15. Person-to-person spread by oropharyngeal route or saliva. Kissing among adults has been implicated in the spread among adults and transmission from healthcare provider to children is common. Blood transfusions can be a mode of transmission, but resulting clinical disease is uncommon.

16. Granulomatous lesions from syphilis infection. Gummas are found on the skin and bone. Skin gummas are painless with sharp borders, whereas bone gummas cause a deep, gnawing pain.

17. Direct contact with exudates of mucous membranes, almost always from unprotected sexual intercourse.

18. Eyes, genital areas and associated organs, and the respiratory system.

19. Atrioventricular blocks, myocarditis, and left ventricular dysfunction (less common).

CHAPTER 32

1. **b.** The limbic system contains the thalamus, hypothalamus, hippocampus, and amygdale.

2. **a.** Organic means an etiology of an illness that stems from a biologic cause, such as a stroke or electrolyte imbalance.

3. **c.** Scene safety has clearly not been established in this case, so you should leave the scene until it has been secured by the police.

4. **b.** Tardive dyskinesia is a degenerative neurologic condition associated with long-term use of antipsychotic drugs marked by involuntary and repetitive movements of the mouth and face.

5. **d.** Melancholy is best described as depression, and mania (euphoria) as the opposite.

6. **d.** Posttraumatic stress disorder best fits the description. Delusions are perceiving things that are not true. Bipolar involves periods of highs and lows. She has not indicated a fear of going places.

7. **c.** Malingering is faking an illness for a tangible gain (missing work, avoiding incarceration, etc.).

8. a. Anorexia nervosa is an eating disorder characterized by a preoccupation that one is obese; drastic, intentional weight loss; and bizarre attitudes and rituals associated with food and exercise.

9. c. Of the answers listed, securing him to the backboard is the most appropriate. Three people are not sufficient. Injecting medications is not appropriate, and securing him to the stretcher will require you to untie him at the hospital. Tying his hands behind his back increases the likelihood he may have difficulty breathing or develop restraint asphyxia.

10. a. Anectine is a paralytic and requires airway and ventilatory support.

11. c. Dystonic reactions are from long-term antipsychotic medications, not alcohol.

12. d. Most deaths from MDMA (ecstasy) are related to hyperthermia and dehydration.

13. b. Chemical restraints should be given as soon as possible after the physical restraint of patients with risk factors for excited delirium. This will end struggling and hopefully prevent the possible peak of delirium that leads to sudden death.

14. b. A dissociative is a substance that causes feelings of detachment (dissociation) from one's surroundings and one's self (e.g., phencyclidine [PCP], ketamine, dextromethorphan).

15. b. In addition to the standard MONA treatment, diazepam, a benzodiazepine, is given to calm the brain, where the central nervous system stimulation is originating.

16. b. Reassurance is the most appropriate action. EMS is not in the business of teaching people a lesson or playing tricks on them. Blindfolding the patient will not decrease the hallucinations and, in fact, may increase them.

17. d. This patient is suffering from a narcotic (heroin) overdose, as shown by the depressed respiratory drive and pinpoint pupils.

18. b. Narcan will reverse the overdose and the patient will regain a gag reflex, so a nasopharyngeal airway is the best choice.

19. c. These findings and the history lead to the suspicion that GHB, the date rape drug, is the cause of the unresponsiveness.

20. c. The rash and strong chemical odor would be most consistent with inhalant usage.

CHAPTER 33

1. (1) Supply oxygen and nutrients to the cells. (2) Transport carbon dioxide and nitrogenous wastes from the tissues to the lungs and kidneys, where the wastes can be removed from the body. (3) Carry hormones from the endocrine glands to the target tissues. (4) Regulate body temperature. (5) Regulate pH through the buffering components in the blood. (6) Keep fluid and electrolytes balanced through salt and plasma proteins. (7) Regulate the immune system through white blood cell and antibody formation. (8) Form clots through the action of platelets.

2. Stem cells. Red blood cells, white blood cells, and platelets are produced from the progenitor or stem cells.

3. Without a nucleus or protein metabolic pathway, the cell has a limited life span of 100 to 120 days.

4. The average lifespan of a platelet in the blood is approximately 10 days.

5. From 42% to 52% for males and 36% to 48% for females. Hematocrit depends primarily on the number of red blood cells, but there is some effect (to a much lower extent) from the average size of the red blood cells.

6. O-negative. In general the AB-positive blood group is referred to as the *universal recipient* and O-negative blood group as the *universal donor.*

7. False. The differential for these disorders is broad and, unfortunately, unless the patient has a known diagnosis, determining the cause of the patient's symptoms in the field is impossible without sophisticated laboratory testing and, in some cases, bone marrow biopsy.

8. Tumor lysis syndrome. Patients with acute leukemias have high levels of spontaneous cell turnover, which increases after the institution of therapy. The sudden transfer of the intracellular contents and cellular breakdown products to the extravascular space can cause life-threatening elevations of uric acid, potassium, and phosphate in the tumor lysis syndrome.

CHAPTER 34

1. a. During compensatory shock, the precapillary and postcapillary sphincters constrict during the ischemic phase.

2. c. These are indications that your patient has lost 30% of his total blood volume.

3. c. As arterial pressure drops and the baroreceptors are stimulated, release of epinephrine is triggered.

4. d. Transport to the closest appropriate medical facility will help your patient the most.

5. d. Venous constriction results in increased preload.

6. c. The beta-blocker will limit tachycardia.

Abciximab (ReoPro)

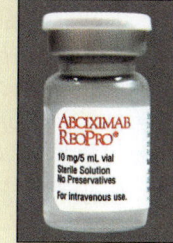

Classification: GP IIb/IIIa inhibitor

Action: Prevents the aggregation of platelets by inhibiting the integrin GP IIb/IIIa receptor.

Indications: UA/NSTEMI patients undergoing planned or emergent PCI.

Adverse Effects: Bleeding from the GI tract, internal bleeding, intracranial hemorrhage, hypotension, stroke, anaphylactic shock.

Contraindications: Bleeding from any source, severe uncontrolled hypertension, surgery or trauma within the previous 6 weeks, stroke within the previous 30 days, renal failure, thrombocytopenia, intracranial mass.

Dosage:

UA/NSTEMI with Planned PCI within 24 Hours:

- 0.25 mg/kg IV, IO (10 to 60 minutes prior to procedure), then 0.125 mcg/kg/min IV, IO infusion for 12 to 24 hours.

Percutaneous Coronary Intervention Only:

- 0.25 mg/kg IV, IO, then 10 mcg/min IV, IO infusion.

Special Considerations: Pregnancy class C

Activated Charcoal

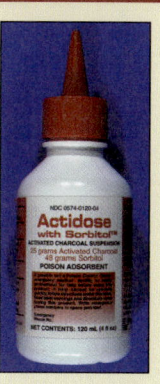

Classification: Antidote, adsorbent

Action: When certain chemicals and toxins are in proximity to the activated charcoal, the chemical will attach to the surface of the charcoal and become trapped.

Indications: Toxic ingestion

Adverse Effects: Nausea/vomiting, constipation, or diarrhea. If aspirated into the lungs, charcoal can induce a potentially fatal form of pneumonitis.

Contraindications: Ingestion of acids, alkalis, ethanol, methanol, cyanide, ferrous sulfate or other iron salts, lithium; coma; GI obstruction.

Dosage:

- **Adult:** 50 to 100 g/dose.
- **Pediatric:** 1 to 2 g/kg.

Special Considerations: Pregnancy class C

Adenosine (Adenocard)

Classification: Antiarrhythmic

Action: Slows the conduction of electrical impulses at the AV node.

Indications: Stable reentry SVT. Does not convert AF, atrial flutter, or VT.

Adverse Effects: Common adverse reactions are generally mild and short-lived: sense of impending doom, complaints of flushing, chest pressure, throat tightness, numbness. Patients will have a brief episode of asystole after administration.

Contraindications: Sick sinus syndrome, second- or third-degree heart block, or poison-/drug-induced tachycardia.

Dosage: Note: Adenosine should be delivered only by rapid IV bolus with a peripheral IV or directly into a vein, in a location as close to the heart as possible, preferably in the antecubital fossa. Administration of adenosine must be immediately followed by a saline flush, and then the extremity should be elevated.

- **Adult:** Initial dose 6 mg rapid IV, IO (over a 1- to 3-second period) immediately followed by a 20-mL rapid saline flush. If the first dose does not eliminate the rhythm in 1 to 2 minutes, 12 mg rapid IV, IO, repeat a second time if required.
- **Pediatric:**
  - **Children >50 kg:** Same as adult dosing.
  - **Children <50 kg:** Initial dose 0.1 mg/kg IV, IO (max dose: 6 mg) immediately followed by a ≥5-mL rapid saline flush; may repeat at 0.2 mg/kg (max dose: 12 mg).

Special Considerations:
- Use with caution in patients with preexisting bronchospasm and those with a history of AF.
- Elderly patients with no history of PSVT should be carefully evaluated for dehydration and rapid sinus tachycardia requiring volume fluid replacement rather than simply treated with adenosine.
- Pregnancy class C

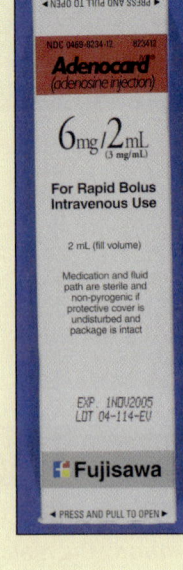

Albumin

Classification: Volume expander, colloid

Action: Increases oncotic pressure in intravascular space.

Indications: Expand intravascular volume.

Adverse Effects: Allergic reaction in some patients; an excessive volume of fluid can result in CHF and pulmonary edema in susceptible patients.

Contraindications: Severe anemia or cardiac failure in the presence of normal or increased intravascular volume, solution appears turbid or after 4 hours since opening the container, known sensitivity.

Dosage: Two preparations: 500 mL of a 5% solution and 100 mL of a 25% solution.

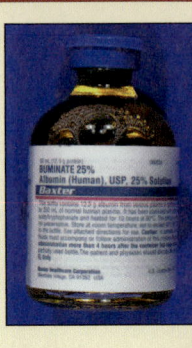 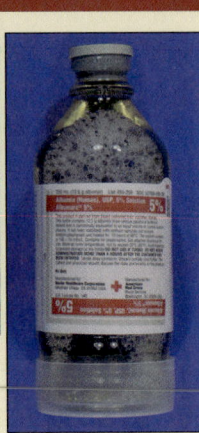

- **Adult:**
  - **5% albumin:** 500 to 1000 mL IV, IO.
  - **25% albumin:** 50 to 200 mL IV, IO.
- **Pediatric:**
  - **5% albumin:** 12 to 20 mL/kg IV; the initial dose may be repeated in 15 to 30 minutes if the clinical response is inadequate.
  - **25% albumin:** 2.5 to 5 mL/kg IV, IO.
  - Alternatively, one may administer based on grams of albumin at 0.5 to 1 g/kg/dose IV, IO. May repeat as needed (max dose: 6 g/kg/day).

Special Considerations:
- Patients with a history of CHF, cardiac disease, hypertension, and pulmonary edema should be given 5% albumin, or the 25% albumin should be diluted. Because 25% of albumin increases intravascular volume greater than the volume administered, slowly administer 25% albumin in normovolemic patients to prevent complications such as pulmonary edema.
- Pregnancy class C

Albuterol (Proventil, Ventolin)

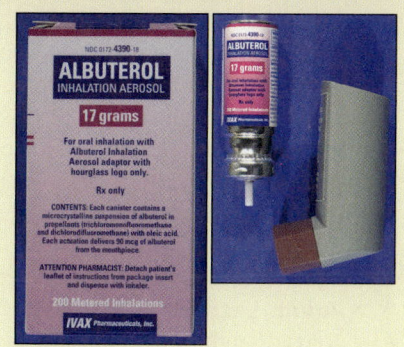

Classification: Bronchodilator, beta agonist

Action: Binds and stimulates beta$_2$ receptors, resulting in relaxation of bronchial smooth muscle.

Indications: Asthma, bronchitis with bronchospasm, and COPD.

Adverse Effects: Hyperglycemia, hypokalemia, palpitations, sinus tachycardia, anxiety, tremor, nausea/vomiting, throat irritation, dry mouth, hypertension, dyspepsia, insomnia, headache, epistaxis, paradoxical bronchospasm.

Contraindications: Angioedema, sensitivity to albuterol or levalbuterol. Use with caution in lactating patients, cardiovascular disorders, cardiac arrhythmias.

Dosage:

Acute Bronchospasm:

- **Adult:**
  - **MDI:** 4 to 8 puffs every 1 to 4 hours may be required.
  - **Nebulizer:** 2.5 to 5 mg every 20 minutes for a maximum of three doses. After the initial three doses, escalate the dose or start a continuous nebulization at 10 to 15 mg/hr.
- **Pediatric:**
  - **MDI:**
    - **4 years and older:** 2 inhalations every 4 to 6 hours; however, in some patients, 1 inhalation every 4 hours is sufficient. More frequent administration or more inhalations are not recommended.
    - **Younger than 4 years:** Administer by nebulization.
  - **Nebulizer:**
    - **Older than 12 years:** The dose for a continuous nebulization is 0.5 mg/kg/hr.
    - **Younger than 12 years:** 0.15 mg/kg every 20 minutes for a maximum of three doses. Alternatively, continuous nebulization at 0.5 mg/kg/hr can be delivered to children younger than 12 years.

Asthma in Pregnancy:

- **MDI:** Two inhalations every 4 hours. In acute exacerbation, start with 2 to 4 puffs every 20 minutes.
- **Nebulizer:** 2.5 mg (0.5 mL) by 0.5% nebulization solution. Place 0.5 mL of the albuterol solution in 2.5 mL of sterile normal saline. Flow is regulated to deliver the therapy over a 5- to 20-minute period. In refractory cases, some physicians order 10 mg nebulized over a 60-minute period.

Special Considerations: Pregnancy class C

Albuterol/Ipratropium (Combivent)

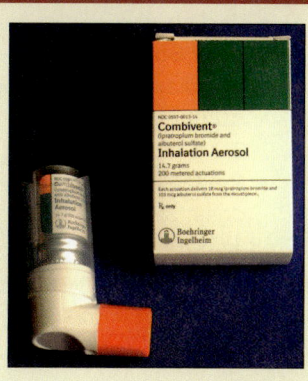

Classification: Combination bronchodilator

Action: Binds and stimulates beta$_2$ receptors, resulting in relaxation of bronchial smooth muscle, and antagonizes the acetylcholine receptor, producing bronchodilation.

Indications: Second-line treatment (if bronchodilator is ineffective) in COPD or severe acute asthma exacerbations during medical transport.

Adverse Effects: Headache, cough, nausea, arrhythmias, paradoxical acute bronchospasm.

Contraindications: Allergy to soybeans or peanuts; known sensitivity to atropine, albuterol, or their respective derivatives. Used with caution in patients with asthma, hypertension, angina, cardiac arrhythmias, tachycardia, cardiovascular disease, congenital long QT syndrome, closed-angle glaucoma.

Dosage:

- **Adult:** 2 puffs inhaled every 6 hours by MDI, with a maximum daily dose of 12 puffs/day.
- **Pediatric:** Not recommended for pediatric patients.

Special Considerations: Pregnancy class C

Aminophylline

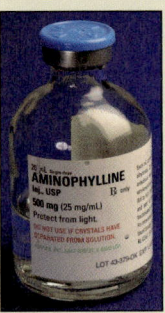

Classification: Bronchodilator

Action: Relaxes the smooth muscle of the bronchial airways and pulmonary blood vessels. May also have antiinflammatory properties.

Indications: Bronchospasm

Adverse Effects: Seizures, cardiac arrest, arrhythmias, nausea/vomiting, abdominal pain or cramping, headache, tachycardia, palpitations, anxiety, ventricular arrhythmias.

Contraindications: Known sensitivity. Use with caution in liver disease, kidney disease, seizures, cardiac arrhythmias.

Dosage: A loading dose is first administered, followed by an infusion.

- **Adult:** Load with 5 mg/kg IV, IO slowly over a 20- to 30-minute period, followed by an infusion. An infusion rate of 0.4 mg/kg/hr is effective for a nonsmoker, but a patient who smokes can require a high infusion rate at 0.8 mg/kg/hr IV, IO. When treating patients with CHF, reduce the dose to 0.2 mg/kg/hr.
- **Pediatric:** Load with 5 mg/kg slow IV, IO over a 20-minute period.
  - **Older than 12 years:** 0.4 mg/kg/hr IV, IO.
  - **10 to 12 years:** 0.7 mg/kg/hr IV, IO.
  - **1 to 9 years:** 0.8 to 1 mg/kg/hr IV, IO.
  - **6 months to 1 year:** 0.6 to 0.7 mg/kg/hr IV, IO.
  - **6 to 24 weeks:** 0.5 mg/kg/hr IV, IO.

Special Considerations: Pregnancy class C

Amiodarone (Cordarone)

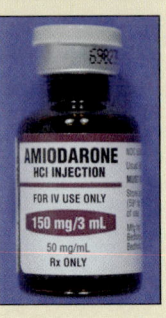

Classification: Antiarrhythmic, class III

Action: Acts directly on the myocardium to delay repolarization and increase the duration of the action potential.

Indications: Ventricular arrhythmias; second-line agent for atrial arrhythmias.

Adverse Effects: Burning at the IV site, hypotension, bradycardia.

Contraindications: Sick sinus syndrome, second- and third-degree heart block, cardiogenic shock, when episodes of bradycardia have caused syncope, sensitivity to benzyl alcohol and iodine.

Dosage:

Ventricular Fibrillation and Pulseless Ventricular Tachycardia:

- **Adult:** 300 mg IV/IO. May be followed by one dose of 150 mg in 3 to 5 minutes. After conversion, follow with a 1-mg/min infusion for 6 hours, then a 0.5-mg/min maintenance infusion over 18 hours.
- **Pediatric:** 5 mg/kg (max dose: 300 mg); may repeat 5 mg/kg IV, IO up to 15 mg/kg.

Relatively Stable Patients with Arrhythmias such as Premature Ventricular Contractions or Wide Complex Tachycardias with a Strong Pulse:

- **Adult:** 150 mg in 100 mL D₅W IV, IO over a 10-minute period; may repeat in 10 minutes up to a maximum dose of 2.2 g over 24 hours.
- **Pediatric:** 5 mg/kg very slow IV, IO (over 20 to 60 minutes); may repeat in 5-mg/kg doses up to 15 mg/kg (max dose: 300 mg).

Special Considerations: Pregnancy class D

Angiotensin-Converting Enzyme (ACE) Inhibitors: Captopril (Capoten), Enalapril (Vasotec), Lisinopril (Prinivil, Zestril), Ramipril (Altace)

Classification: Angiotensin-converting enzyme (ACE) inhibitors

Action: Blocks the enzyme responsible for the production of angiotensin II, resulting in a decrease in blood pressure.

Indications: Congestive heart failure, hypertension, post–myocardial infarction.

Adverse Effects: Headache, dizziness, fatigue, depression, chest pain, hypotension, palpitations, cough, dyspnea, upper respiratory infection, nausea/vomiting, rash, pruritus, angioedema, hypotension, renal failure.

Contraindications: Angioedema related to previous treatment with an ACE inhibitor, known sensitivity. Use with caution in aortic stenosis, bilateral renal artery stenosis, hypertrophic obstructive cardiomyopathy, pericardial tamponade, elevated serum potassium levels, acute kidney failure.

Dosage:
- **Adult:** Medication is administered orally. Dosage is individualized.
- **Pediatric:** Medication is administered orally. Dosage is individualized.

Special Considerations: Pregnancy class D

Aspirin, ASA

Classification: Antiplatelet agent, nonnarcotic analgesic, antipyretic

Action: Prevents the formation of a chemical known as thromboxane A_2, which causes platelets to clump together, or aggregate, and form plugs that cause obstruction or constriction of small coronary arteries.

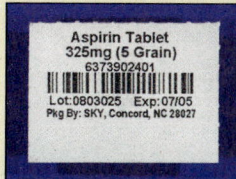

Indications: Fever, inflammation, angina, acute MI, and patients complaining of pain, pressure, squeezing, or crushing in the chest that may be cardiac in origin.

Adverse Effects: Anaphylaxis, angioedema, bronchospasm, bleeding, stomach irritation, nausea/vomiting.

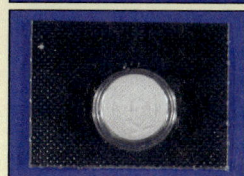

Contraindications: GI bleeding, active ulcer disease, hemorrhagic stroke, bleeding disorders, children with chickenpox or flulike symptoms, known sensitivity.

Dosage: Note: "Baby aspirin" 81 mg, standard adult aspirin dose 325 mg.

Myocardial Infarction:
- **Adult:** 160 to 325 mg PO (alternatively, four 81-mg baby aspirin are often given), 300-mg rectal suppository.
- **Pediatric:** 3 to 5 mg/kg/day to 5 to 10 mg/kg/day given as a single dose.

Pain or Fever:
- **Adult:** 325 to 650 mg PO (1 to 2 adult tablets) every 4 to 6 hours.
- **Pediatric:** 60 to 90 mg/kg/day in divided doses every 4 to 6 hours.

Special Considerations: Pregnancy class C except the last 3 months of pregnancy, when aspirin is considered pregnancy class D.

Atenolol (Tenormin)

Classification: Beta adrenergic antagonist, antianginal, antihypertensive, class II antiarrhythmic

Action: Inhibits the strength of the heart's contractions and heart rate, resulting in a decrease in cardiac oxygen consumption. Also saturates the beta receptors and inhibits dilation of bronchial smooth muscle (beta$_2$ receptor).

Indications: ACS, hypertension, SVT, atrial flutter, AF.

Adverse Effects: Bradycardia, bronchospasm, hypotension.

Contraindications: Cardiogenic shock, AV block, bradycardia, known sensitivity. Use with caution in hypotension, chronic lung disease (asthma and COPD).

Dosage: ACS:
- **Adult:** 5 mg IV, IO over a 5-minute period; repeat in 5 minutes.
- **Pediatric:** Not recommended for pediatric patients.

Special Considerations: Pregnancy class D

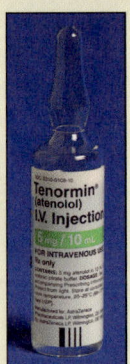

Atracurium (Tracrium)

Classification: Nondepolarizing neuromuscular blocker

Action: Antagonizes acetylcholine receptors at the motor end plate, producing muscle paralysis.

Indications: Neuromuscular blockade to facilitate ET intubation.

Adverse Effects: Flushing, edema, urticaria, pruritus, bronchospasm and/or wheezing, alterations in heart rate, decrease in blood pressure.

Contraindications: Cardiac disease, electrolyte abnormalities, dehydration, known sensitivity.

Dosage:
- **Adult:** 0.4 to 0.5 mg/kg IV, IO; repeat with 0.08 mg/kg to 0.10 mg/kg every 20 to 45 minutes as needed for prolonged paralysis.
- **Pediatric:**
  - **Older than 2 years:** Same as adult dosing.
  - **Younger than 2 years:** 0.3 to 0.4 mg/kg IV, IO.

Special Considerations:
- Do not give by IM injection.
- Pregnancy class C

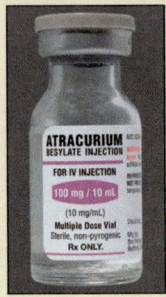

Atropine Sulfate

Classification: Anticholinergic (antimuscarinic)

Action: Competes reversibly with acetylcholine at the site of the muscarinic receptor. Receptors affected, in order from the most sensitive to the least sensitive, include salivary, bronchial, sweat glands, eye, heart, and GI tract.

Indications: Symptomatic bradycardia, asystole or PEA, nerve agent exposure, organophosphate poisoning.

Adverse Effects: Decreased secretions resulting in dry mouth and hot skin temperature, intense facial flushing, blurred vision or dilation of the pupils with subsequent photophobia, tachycardia, restlessness. Atropine may cause paradoxical bradycardia if the dose administered is too low or if the drug is administered too slowly.

Contraindications: Acute MI; myasthenia gravis; GI obstruction; closed-angle glaucoma; known sensitivity to atropine, belladonna alkaloids, or sulfites. Will not be effective for infranodal (type II) AV block and new third-degree block with wide QRS complex.

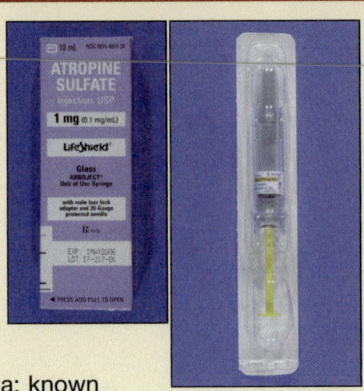

Continued

Atropine Sulfate—continued

Dosage:

Symptomatic Bradycardia:

- **Adult:** 0.5 mg IV, IO every 3 to 5 minutes to a maximum dose of 3 mg.
- **Adolescent:** 0.02 mg/kg (minimum 0.1 mg/dose; maximum 1 mg/dose) IV, IO up to a total dose of 2 mg.
- **Pediatric:** 0.02 mg/kg (minimum 0.1 mg/dose; maximum 0.5 mg/dose) IV, IO, to a total dose of 1 mg.

Asystole/Pulseless Electrical Activity:

- 1 mg IV, IO every 3 to 5 minutes, to a maximum dose of 3 mg. May be administered via ET tube at 2 to 2.5 mg diluted in 5 to 10 mL of water or normal saline.

Nerve Agent or Organophosphate Poisoning:

- **Adult:** 2 to 4 mg IV, IM; repeat if needed every 20 to 30 minutes until symptoms dissipate. In severe cases, the initial dose can be as large as 2 to 6 mg administered IV. Repeat doses of 2 to 6 mg can be administered IV, IM every 5 to 60 minutes.
- **Pediatric:** 0.05 mg/kg IV, IM every 10 to 30 minutes as needed until symptoms dissipate.
- **Infants <15 lb:** 0.05 mg/kg IV, IM every 5 to 20 minutes as needed until symptoms dissipate.

Special Considerations:

- Half-life 2.5 hours.
- Pregnancy class C; possibly unsafe in lactating mothers.

Butorphanol (Stadol)

Classification: Opioid agonist-antagonist; schedule C-IV controlled substance

Action: Produces analgesia by binding to the opioid receptor.

Indications: Moderate to severe pain.

Adverse Effects: Drowsiness, dizziness, confusion, respiratory depression, nausea/vomiting, bradycardia, hypotension.

Contraindications: Patients with active substance abuse, sensitivity to opiate agonists. Use with caution in kidney, liver, or pulmonary problems.

Dosage:

- **Adult:** 0.5 to 2 mg IV, IO every 3 to 4 hours.
- **Pediatric:** Not recommended for pediatric patients.

Special Considerations: Pregnancy class C

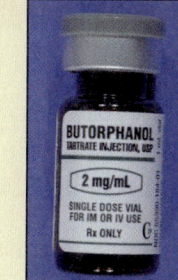

Calcium Gluconate

Classification: Electrolyte solution

Action: Counteracts the toxicity of hyperkalemia by stabilizing the membranes of the cardiac cells, reducing the likelihood of fibrillation.

Indications: Hyperkalemia, hypocalcemia, hypermagnesemia.

Adverse Effects: Soft tissue necrosis, hypotension, bradycardia (if administered too rapidly).

Contraindications: VF, digitalis toxicity, hypercalcemia.

Dosage: Supplied as 10% solution; therefore each milliliter contains 100 mg of calcium gluconate.

- **Adult:** 500 to 1000 mg IV, IO administered slowly at a rate of approximately 1 to 1.5 mL/min maximum dose 3 g IV, IO.
- **Pediatric:** 60 to 100 mg/kg IV, IO slowly over a 5- to 10-minute period; maximum dose 3 g IV, IO.

Special Considerations:

- Do not administer by IM or Sub-Q routes, which causes significant tissue necrosis.
- Pregnancy class C

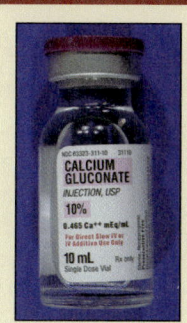

Carbamazepine (Tegretol)

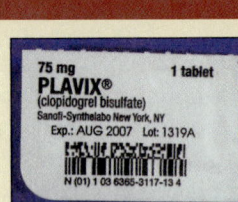

Classification: Anticonvulsant
Action: Decreases the spread of the seizure.
Indications: Partial and generalized tonic-clonic seizures.
Adverse Effects: Dizziness, drowsiness, ataxia, nausea/vomiting, blurred vision, confusion, headache, transient diplopia, visual hallucinations, life-threatening rashes.
Contraindications: AV block, bundle branch block, agranulocytosis, bone marrow suppression, MAOI therapy, hypersensitivity to carbamazepine or tricyclic antidepressants. Use with caution in petit mal, atonic, or myoclonic seizures; liver disease, patients with blood dyscrasia caused by drug therapies or blood disorders, patients with a history of cardiac disease, or patients with a history of alcoholism.
Dosage:
- **Adult:** 200 mg PO every 12 hours.
- **Pediatric:**
  - **6 to 11 years:** 100 mg PO twice daily.
  - **Younger than 6 years:** 10 to 20 mg/kg/day PO 2 or 3 times per day.

Special Considerations: Pregnancy class D

Clopidogrel (Plavix)

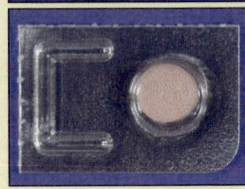

Classification: Antiplatelet
Action: Blocks platelet aggregation by antagonizing the GP IIb/IIIa receptors.
Indications: ACS, chronic coronary and vascular disease, ischemic stroke.
Adverse Effects: Nausea, abdominal pain, and hemorrhage.
Contraindications: History of intracranial hemorrhage, GI bleed or trauma, known sensitivity.
Dosage:
Unstable Angina Pectoris or Non–Q-Wave Acute Myocardial Infarction:
- **Adult:** Single loading dose of 300 mg PO followed by a daily dose of 75 mg PO.
- **Pediatric:** Not recommended for pediatric patients.

Special Considerations: Pregnancy class B

Dexamethasone (Decadron)

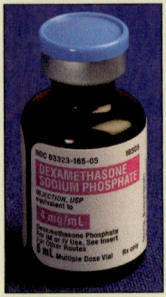

Classification: Corticosteroid
Action: Reduces inflammation and immune responses.
Indications: Various inflammatory conditions, adrenal insufficiency, nonresponsive forms of shock.
Adverse Effects: Nausea/vomiting, edema, hypertension, hyperglycemia, immunosuppression.
Contraindications: Fungal infections, known sensitivity.
Dosage:
- **Adult:** 1 to 6 mg/kg IV to a maximum dose of 40 mg.
- **Pediatric:** 0.03 to 0.3 mg/kg IV, IO divided into doses every 6 hours.

Special Considerations: Pregnancy class C

Dextrose (Dextrose 50%, Dextrose 25%, Dextrose 10%)

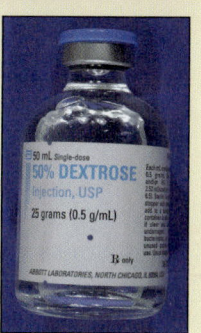

Classification: Antihypoglycemic

Action: Increases blood glucose concentrations.

Indications: Hypoglycemia

Adverse Effects: Hyperglycemia, warmth, burning from IV infusion. Concentrated solutions may cause pain and thrombosis of the peripheral veins.

Contraindications: Intracranial and intraspinal hemorrhage, delirium tremens, solution is not clear, seals are not intact.

Dosage:

Hyperkalemia:

- **Adult:** 25 g dextrose 50% IV, IO.
- **Pediatric:** 0.5 to 1 g/kg IV, IO.

Hypoglycemia:

- **Adult:** 10 to 25 g of dextrose 50% IV (20 to 50 mL of dextrose solution).
- **Pediatric:**
  - **Older than 2 years:** 2 mL/kg of dextrose 50%.
  - **Younger than 2 years:** 2 to 4 mL/kg of dextrose 10%.

Special Considerations: Pregnancy class C

Diazepam (Valium)

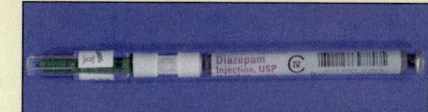

Classification: Benzodiazepine; schedule C-IV

Action: Binds to the benzodiazepine receptor and enhances the effects of GABA. Benzodiazepines act at the level of the limbic, thalamic, and hypothalamic regions of the CNS and can produce any level of CNS depression required (including sedation, skeletal muscle relaxation, and anticonvulsant activity).

Indications: Anxiety, skeletal muscle relaxation, alcohol withdrawal, seizures.

Adverse Effects: Respiratory depression, drowsiness, fatigue, headache, pain at the injection site, confusion, nausea, hypotension, oversedation.

Contraindications: Children younger than 6 months, acute-angle glaucoma, CNS depression, alcohol intoxication, known sensitivity.

Dosage:

Anxiety:

- **Adult:**
  - **Moderate:** 2 to 5 mg slow IV, IM.
  - **Severe:** 5 to 10 mg slow IV, IM (administer no faster than 5 mg/min).
  - **Low:** Low dosages are often required for elderly or debilitated patients.
- **Pediatric:** 0.04 to 0.3 mg/kg/dose IV, IM every 4 hours to a maximum dose of 0.6 mg/kg.

Delirium Tremens from Acute Alcohol Withdrawal:

- **Adult:** 10 mg IV

Seizure:

- **Adult:** 5 to 10 mg slow IV, IO every 10 to 15 minutes; maximum total dose 30 mg.
- **Pediatric:**
  - **IV, IO:**
    - **5 years and older:** 1 mg over a 3-minute period every 2 to 5 minutes to a maximum total dose of 10 mg.
    - **Older than 30 days to younger than 5 years:** 0.2 to 0.5 mg over a 3-minute period; may repeat every 2 to 5 minutes to a maximum total dose of 5 mg.
    - **Neonate:** 0.1 to 0.3 mg/kg/dose given over a 3- to 5-minute period; may repeat every 15 to 30 minutes to a maximum total dose of 2 mg. (Not a first line agent due to sodium benzoic acid in the injection.)

Continued

Diazepam (Valium)—continued

- **Rectal administration:** If vascular access is not obtained, diazepam may be administered rectally to children.
  - **12 years and older:** 0.2 mg/kg.
  - **6 to 11 years:** 0.3 mg/kg.
  - **2 to 5 years:** 0.5 mg/kg.
  - **Younger than 2 years:** Not recommended.

Special Considerations:
- Make sure that IV, IO lines are well secured. Extravasation of diazepam causes tissue necrosis.
- Diazepam is insoluble in water and must be dissolved in propylene glycol. This produces a viscous solution; give slowly to prevent pain on injection.
- Pregnancy class D

Digoxin (Lanoxin)

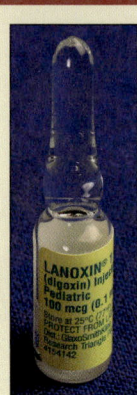

Classification: Cardiac glycoside

Action: Inhibits sodium-potassium-adenosine triphosphatase membrane pump, resulting in an increase in calcium inside the heart muscle cell, which causes an increase in the force of contraction of the heart.

Indications: CHF, to control the ventricular rate in chronic AF and atrial flutter, narrow-complex PSVT.

Adverse Effects: Headache, weakness, GI disturbances, arrhythmias, nausea/vomiting, diarrhea, vision disturbances.

Contraindications: Digitalis allergy, VT and VF, heart block, sick sinus syndrome, tachycardia without heart failure, pulse lower than 50 to 60 beats/min, MI, ischemic heart disease, patients with preexcitation AF or atrial flutter (i.e., a delta wave, characteristic of Wolff-Parkinson-White syndrome, visible during normal sinus rhythm).

Dosage: Dosage is individualized.

Special Considerations:
- Low levels of serum potassium can lead to digoxin toxicity and bradycardia. Conditions such as administration of steroids or diuretics or vomiting and diarrhea can produce low levels of potassium and subsequent digoxin toxicity.
- Pregnancy class C

Diltiazem (Cardizem)

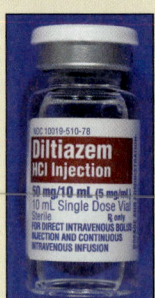

Classification: Calcium channel blocker, class IV antiarrhythmic

Action: Blocks calcium from moving into the heart muscle cell, which prolongs the conduction of electrical impulses through the AV node.

Indications: Stable narrow-QRS tachycardia caused by reentry, stable narrow-QRS tachycardia caused by automaticity, to control the ventricular rate in patients with AFib or atrial flutter (NOTE: Should *not* be given to patients with Afib or atrial flutter associated with known preexcitation [e.g., WPW syndrome]).

Adverse Effects: Flushing; headache; bradycardia; hypotension; heart block; myocardial depression; severe AV block; and, at high doses, cardiac arrest.

Contraindications: Hypotension, heart block, heart failure.

Dosage:
- **Adult:** Optimum dose is 0.25 mg/kg IV, IO over a 2-minute period; 20 mg is a reasonable dose for the average adult patient. A second, higher dose of 0.35 mg/kg IV, IO (25 mg is a typical second dose) may be administered over a 2-minute period if rate control is not obtained with the lower dose. For continued reduction in heart rate, a continuous infusion can be started at a dose range of 5 to 15 mg/hr.
- **Pediatric:** Not recommended for pediatric patients.

Special Considerations:
- Use with extreme caution in patients who are taking beta blockers because these two drug classes potentiate each other's effects and toxicities.
- Patients with a history of heart failure and heart block are at a higher risk for toxicity.
- Pregnancy class C

Diphenhydramine Hydrochloride (Benadryl)

Classification: Antihistamine

Action: Binds and blocks H_1 histamine receptors.

Indications: Anaphylactic reactions, dystonic reactions

Adverse Effects: Drowsiness, dizziness, headache, excitable state (children), wheezing, thickening of bronchial secretions, chest tightness, palpitations, hypotension, blurred vision, dry mouth, nausea/vomiting, diarrhea.

Contraindications: Acute asthma, which thickens secretions; patients with cardiac histories; known sensitivity.

Dosage:

- **Adult:** 25 to 50 mg IV, IO, IM.
- **Pediatric:** 2 to 12 years: 1 to 1.25 mg/kg IV, IO, IM.

Special Considerations: Pregnancy class B

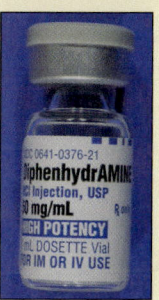

Dobutamine (Dobutrex)

Classification: Adrenergic agent

Action: Acts primarily as an agonist at $beta_1$ adrenergic receptors with minor $beta_2$ and $alpha_1$ effects. Consequently, dobutamine increases myocardial contractility and stroke volume with minor chronotropic effects, resulting in increased cardiac output.

Indications: CHF, cardiogenic shock.

Adverse Effects: Tachycardia, PVCs, hypertension, hypotension, palpitations, arrhythmias.

Contraindications: Suspected or known poisoning/drug-induced shock, systolic blood pressure <100 mm Hg with signs of shock, idiopathic hypertrophic subaortic stenosis, known sensitivity (including sulfites). Use with caution in hypertension, recent MI, arrhythmias, hypovolemia.

Dosage:

- **Adult:** 2 to 20 mcg/kg/min IV, IO. At doses >20 mcg/kg/min, increases of heart rate of >10% may induce or exacerbate myocardial ischemia.
- **Pediatric:** Same as adult dosing.

Special Considerations:

- Half-life 2 minutes
- Pregnancy class C

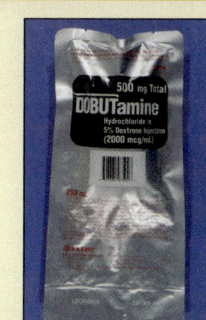

Dolasetron (Anzemet)

Classification: Antiemetic

Action: Prevents/reduces nausea/vomiting by binding and blocking a receptor for the brain chemical serotonin.

Indications: Prevent and treat nausea/vomiting.

Adverse Effects: Headache, fatigue, diarrhea, dizziness, abdominal pain, hypotension, hypertension, ECG changes (prolonged PR and QT intervals, widened QRS), bradycardia, tachycardia, syncope.

Contraindications: Known sensitivity. Use with caution in hypokalemia, hypomagnesemia, cardiac arrhythmias.

Dosage:

- **Adult:** 12.5 mg IV, IO.
- **Pediatric:** 2 to 16 years: 0.35 mg/kg IV, IO (max dose: 12.5 mg).

Special Considerations: Pregnancy class B

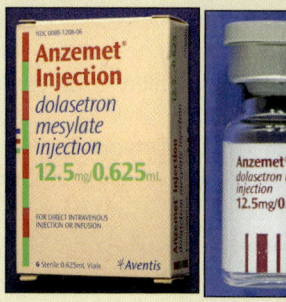

Dopamine (Intropin)

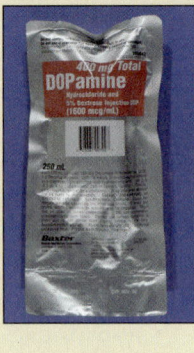

Classification: Adrenergic agonist, inotrope, vasopressor

Action: Stimulates alpha and beta adrenergic receptors. At moderate doses (2-10 mcg/kg/min), dopamine stimulates beta$_1$ receptors, resulting in inotropy and increased cardiac output while maintaining dopaminergic-induced vasodilatory effects. At high doses (>10 mcg/kg/min), alpha adrenergic agonism predominates, and increased peripheral vascular resistance and vasoconstriction result.

Indications: Hypotension and decreased cardiac output associated with cardiogenic shock and septic shock, hypotension after return of spontaneous circulation following cardiac arrest, symptomatic bradycardia unresponsive to atropine.

Adverse Effects: Tachycardia, arrhythmias, skin and soft tissue necrosis, severe hypertension from excessive vasoconstriction, angina, dyspnea, headache, nausea/vomiting.

Contraindications: Pheochromocytoma, VF, VT, or other ventricular arrhythmias, known sensitivity (including sulfites). Correct any hypovolemia with volume fluid replacement before administering dopamine.

Dosage:

- **Adult:** 2 to 20 mcg/kg/min IV, IO infusion. Starting dose 5 mcg/kg/min; may gradually increase the infusion by 5 to 10 mcg/kg/min to desired effect. Cardiac dose is usually 5 to 10 mcg/kg/min; vasopressor dose is usually 10 to 20 mcg/kg/min. Little benefit is gained beyond 20 mcg/kg/min.
- **Pediatric:** Same as adult dosing

Special Considerations:

Half-life 2 minutes

Pregnancy class C

Epinephrine

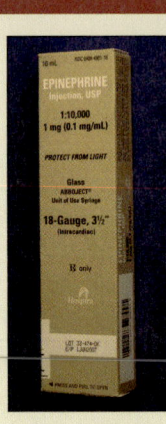 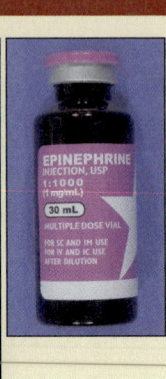

Classification: Adrenergic agent, inotrope

Action: Binds strongly with both alpha and beta receptors, producing increased blood pressure, increased heart rate, bronchodilation.

Indications: Bronchospasm, allergic and anaphylactic reactions, cardiac arrest.

Adverse Effects: Anxiety, headache, cardiac arrhythmias, hypertension, nervousness, tremors, chest pain, nausea/vomiting.

Contraindications: Arrhythmias other than pulseless VT/VF, asystole, PEA; cardiovascular disease; hypertension; cerebrovascular disease; shock secondary to causes other than anaphylactic shock; closed-angle glaucoma; diabetes; pregnant women in active labor; known sensitivity to epinephrine or sulfites.

Dosage:

Cardiac Arrest:

- **Adult:** Initial dose 1 mg (1:10,000 solution) IV, IO; may repeat every 3 to 5 minutes.
- **Pediatric:** Initial dose 0.01 mg/kg (1:10,000 solution) IV, IO; repeat every 3 to 5 minutes as needed (max dose: 1 mg).

Symptomatic Bradycardia:

- **Adult:** 1 mcg/min (1:10,000 solution) as a continuous IV infusion; usual dosage range: 2 to 10 mcg/min IV; titrate to effect.
- **Pediatric:** 0.01 mg/kg (1:10,000 solution) IV, IO; may repeat every 3 to 5 minutes (max dose: 1 mg). If giving epinephrine by ET tube, administer 0.1 mg/kg.

Asthma Attacks and Certain Allergic Reactions:

- **Adult:** 0.3 to 0.5 mg (1:1000 solution) IM or Sub-Q; may repeat every 10 to 15 minutes (max dose: 1 mg).
- **Pediatric:** 0.01 mg/kg (1:1000 solution) IM or Sub-Q (max dose: 0.5 mg).

Continued

Epinephrine—continued

Anaphylactic Shock:
- **Adult:** 0.1 mg (1:10,000 solution) IV slowly over 5 minutes, or IV infusion of 1 to 4 mcg/min, titrated to effect.
- **Pediatric:** Continuous IV infusion rate of 0.1 to 1 mcg/kg/min (1:10,000 solution); titrate to response.

Special Considerations:
- Half-life 1 minute
- Pregnancy class C

Epinephrine Autoinjectors (EpiPen, EpiPen Jr)

Classification: Adrenergic agonist, inotrope
Action: Binds strongly with both alpha and beta receptors, producing increased blood pressure, increased heart rate, bronchodilation.
Indications: Anaphylactic shock, certain allergic reactions, asthma attacks.
Adverse Effects: Headaches, nervousness, tremors, arrhythmias, hypertension, chest pain, nausea/vomiting.
Contraindications: Arrhythmias other than VF, asystole, PEA; cardiovascular disease; hypertension; cerebrovascular disease; shock secondary to causes other than anaphylactic shock; closed-angle glaucoma; diabetes; pregnant women in active labor; known sensitivity to epinephrine or sulfites.

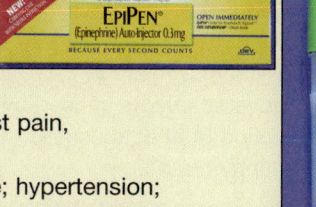

Dosage:
- **Adult:** An EpiPen contains 0.3 mg epinephrine to be administered IM into the anterolateral thigh.
- **Pediatric:** For children weighing <30 kg, an EpiPen Jr delivers 0.15 mg IM.

Special Considerations:
- Half-life 1 minute
- Pregnancy class C

Eptifibatide (Integrilin)

Classification: GP IIb/IIIa inhibitor
Action: Prevents the aggregation of platelets by binding to the GP IIb/IIIa receptor.
Indications: UA/NSTEMI—to manage medically and for those undergoing percutaneous coronary intervention.
Adverse Effects: Bleeding from the GI tract, internal bleeding, intracranial hemorrhage, hypotension, stroke, anaphylactic shock.
Contraindications: Bleeding from any source, severe uncontrolled hypertension, surgery or trauma within the previous 6 weeks, stroke within the previous 30 days, renal failure, thrombocytopenia.

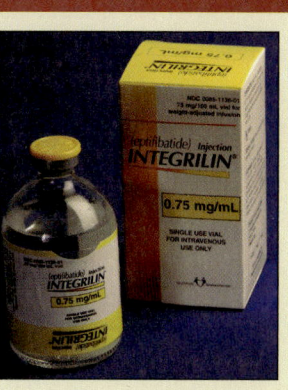

Dosage:
- **Adult:** Loading dose: 180 mcg/kg IV, IO (max dose: 22.6 mg) over 1 to 2 minutes, then 2 mcg/kg/min IV, IO infusion (max dose: 15 mg/hr).
- **Pediatric:** No current dosing recommendations exist for pediatric patients.

Special Considerations:
- Half-life approximately 90 to 120 minutes
- Pregnancy class B

Esmolol (Brevibloc)

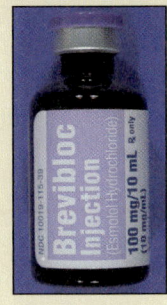

Classification: Beta adrenergic antagonist, class II antiarrhythmic

Action: Inhibits the strength of the heart's contractions, as well as heart rate, resulting in a decrease in cardiac oxygen consumption.

Indications: ACS, MI, acute hypertension, supraventricular tachyarrhythmias, thyrotoxicosis.

Adverse Effects: Hypotension, sinus bradycardia, AV block, cardiac arrest, nausea/vomiting, hypoglycemia, injection site reaction.

Contraindications: Acute bronchospasm, COPD, second- or third-degree heart block, bradycardia, cardiogenic shock, pulmonary edema, sick sinus syndrome, known sensitivity. Use with caution in patients with pheochromocytoma, Prinzmetal's angina, cerebrovascular disease, stroke, poorly controlled diabetes mellitus, hyperthyroidism, thyrotoxicosis, renal disease.

Dosage:
- **Adult:** 500 mcg/kg (0.5 mg/kg) IV, IO over a 1-minute period, followed by a 50 mcg/kg/min (0.05 mg/kg) infusion over a 4-minute period (maximum total: 200 mcg/kg). If patient response is inadequate, administer a second bolus 500 mcg/kg (0.5 mg/kg) over a 1-minute period, and then increase infusion to 100 mcg/kg/min. Maximum infusion rate: 300 mcg/kg/min.
- **Pediatric:** 500 mcg/kg (0.5 mg/kg) IV, IO over a 1-minute period, followed by an infusion at 25 to 200 mcg/kg/min.

Special Considerations:
- Half-life 5 to 9 minutes
- Any adverse effects caused by administration of esmolol are brief because of the drug's short half-life.
- Resolution of effects usually within 10 to 20 minutes.
- Pregnancy class C

Etomidate (Amidate)

Classification: Hypnotic, anesthesia induction agent

Action: Although the exact mechanism is unknown, etomidate appears to have GABA-like effects.

Indications: Induction for rapid sequence intubation and pharmacologic-assisted intubation, induction of anesthesia.

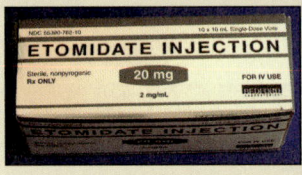
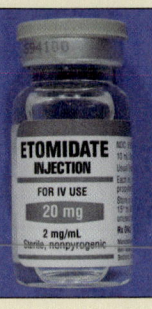

Adverse Effects: Hypotension, respiratory depression, pain at the site of injection, temporary involuntary muscle movements, frequent nausea/vomiting on emergence, adrenal insufficiency, hyperventilation, hypoventilation, apnea of short duration, hiccups, laryngospasm, snoring, tachypnea, hypertension, cardiac arrhythmias.

Contraindications: Known sensitivity. Use in pregnancy only if the potential benefits justify the potential risk to the fetus. Do not use during labor and avoid in nursing mothers.

Dosage:
- **Adult:** 0.2 to 0.6 slow mg/kg IV, IO (over 30 to 60 seconds). A typical adult intubating dose of etomidate is 20 mg slow IV. Consider less (e.g., 10 mg) in the elderly or patients with cardiac conditions.
- **Pediatrics:**
  - **Older than 10 years:** Same as adult dosing.
  - **Younger than 10 years:** Safety has not been established.

Special Considerations:
- Etomidate is used to prepare a patient for orotracheal intubation. Both personnel and equipment must be present to manage the patient's airway before administration.
- Pregnancy class C

Felbamate (Felbatol)

Classification: Anticonvulsant

Action: Although the mechanism of action is not known, it is believed that it antagonizes the effects of glycine, increases the seizure threshold in absence seizures, and prevents the spread of generalized tonic-clonic and partial seizures.

Indications: Partial seizures with and without generalization in epileptic adults; partial and generalized seizures associated with Lennox-Gastaut syndrome in children.

Adverse Effects: Nausea/vomiting, suicidal ideation and behavior, depression, insomnia, dyspepsia, upper respiratory tract infection, fatigue, headache, constipation, diarrhea, rhinitis, anxiety, aplastic anemia, photosensitivity.

Contraindications: Blood dyscrasias, hepatic disease, known sensitivity to carbomates.

Dosage: Should be individualized based on condition.

Special Considerations: Pregnancy class C

Fentanyl Citrate (Sublimaze)

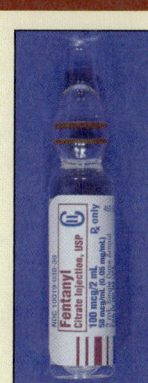

Classification: Narcotic analgesic; schedule C-II

Action: Binds to opiate receptors, producing analgesia and euphoria.

Indications: Pain

Adverse Effects: Respiratory depression, apnea, hypotension, nausea/vomiting, dizziness, sedation, euphoria, sinus bradycardia, sinus tachycardia, palpitations, hypertension, diaphoresis, syncope, pain at injection site.

Contraindications: Known sensitivity. Use with caution in traumatic brain injury, respiratory depression.

Dosage: Note: Dosage should be individualized.

- **Adult:** 50 to 100 mcg/dose (0.05 to 0.1 mg) IM or slow IV, IO (administered over 1 to 2 minutes).
- **Pediatric:** 1 to 2 mcg/kg IM or slow IV, IO (administered over 1 to 2 minutes).

Special Considerations: Pregnancy class B

Fibrinolytics: Tissue Plasminogen Activator (tPA), Streptokinase (Streptase, Kabikinase), Reteplase (Retavase), Tenecteplase (TNKase)

Classification: Fibrinolytic agent

Action: Alters plasmin in the body, which then breaks down fibrinogen and fibrin clots and reestablishes blood flow.

Indications: ST segment elevation (≥1 mm in two or more contiguous leads), new or presumed-new left bundle branch block.

Adverse Effects: Bleeding, intracranial hemorrhage, stroke, cardiac arrhythmias, hypotension, bruising.

Contraindications: ST segment depression, cardiogenic shock, recent (within 10 days) major surgery, cerebrovascular disease, recent (within 10 days) GI bleeding, recent trauma, hypertension (systolic blood pressure ≥180 mm Hg or diastolic blood pressure ≥110 mm Hg), high likelihood of left heart thrombus, acute pericarditis, subacute bacterial endocarditis, severe renal or liver failure with bleeding complications, significant liver dysfunction, diabetic hemorrhagic retinopathy, septic thrombophlebitis, advanced age (older than 75 years), patients taking warfarin (Coumadin).

Dosage: Dosing per medical direction.

Special Considerations: Pregnancy class C

Flumazenil (Romazicon)

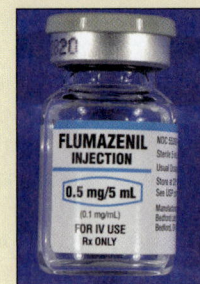

Classification: Benzodiazepine receptor antagonist, antidote

Action: Competes with benzodiazepines for binding at the benzodiazepine receptor, reverses the sedative effects of benzodiazepines.

Indication: Benzodiazepine oversedation

Adverse Effects: Resedation, seizures, dizziness, pain at injection site, nausea/vomiting, diaphoresis, headache, visual impairment.

Contraindications: Cyclic antidepressant overdose; life-threatening conditions that require treatment with benzodiazepines, such as status epilepticus and intracranial hypertension; known sensitivity to flumazenil or benzodiazepines. Use with caution where there is the possibility of unrecognized benzodiazepine dependence and in patients who have a history of substance abuse or who are known substance abusers.

Dosage:

- **Adult:** Initial dose is 0.2 mg IV, IO over a 15-second period. If the desired effect is not observed after 45 seconds, administer a second 0.2-mg dose, again over a 15-second period. Doses can be repeated a total of four times until a total dose of 1 mg has been administered.
- **Pediatric:** Children older than 1 year, 0.01 mg/kg IV, IO given over a 15-second period. May repeat in 45 seconds and then every minute to a maximum cumulative dose of 0.05 mg/kg or 1 mg, whichever is the lower dose.

Special Considerations:

- Monitor for signs of hypoventilation and hypoxia for approximately 2 hours.
- If the half-life of the benzodiazepine is longer than flumazenil, an additional dose may be needed.
- May precipitate withdrawal symptoms in patients dependent on benzodiazepines.
- Flumazenil has not been shown to benefit patients who have overdosed on multiple drugs.
- Pregnancy class C

Fosphenytoin (Cerebyx)

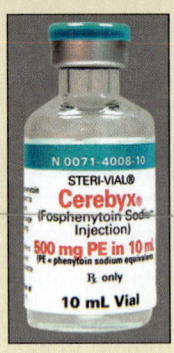

Classification: Anticonvulsant

Action: Alters the movement of sodium and calcium into nervous tissue and prevents the spread of seizure activity.

Indications: Partial and generalized seizures, status epilepticus, seizure prophylaxis.

Dosage: The dose and concentration of fosphenytoin is expressed in PE to simplify the conversion between phenytoin and fosphenytoin.

- **Adult:** The usual loading dose of fosphenytoin is 15 to 20 mg PE/kg IV, not to exceed 150 mg PE/min IV rate.
- **Pediatric:** The usual loading dose of fosphenytoin is 15 to 20 mg PE/kg IV, not to exceed 3 mg PE/kg/min (max dose: 150 mg PE/min) IV rate.

Adverse Effects: Phenytoin can cause several adverse effects often related to drug dose, including sedation, nystagmus, tremors, ataxia, dysarthria, gingival hypertrophy, hirsutism, and facial coarsening. Too-rapid administration can cause hypotension.

Contraindications:

- Bradycardia, bundle branch blocks, agranulocytosis, Adams-Stokes syndrome, hydantoin hypersensitivity
- Pregnancy class D
- Compatible with breast-feeding

Furosemide (Lasix)

Classification: Loop diuretic

Action: Inhibits the absorption of the sodium and chloride ions and water in the loop of Henle, as well as the convoluted tubule of the nephron. This results in decreased absorption of water and increased production of urine.

Indications: Pulmonary edema, CHF, hypertensive emergency.

Adverse Effects: Vertigo, dizziness, weakness, orthostatic hypotension, hypokalemia, thrombophlebitis. Patients with anuria, severe renal failure, untreated hepatic coma, increasing azotemia, and electrolyte depletion can develop life-threatening consequences.

Contraindications: Known sensitivity to sulfonamides or furosemide.

Dosage:

Congestive Heart Failure and Pulmonary Edema:

- **Adult:** The initial dose is 0.5 to 1 mg/kg IV push, given at a rate no faster than 20 mg/min.
- **Pediatric:** 1 mg/kg IV, IO or IM. If the response is not satisfactory, an additional dose of 2 mg/kg may be administered no sooner than 2 hours after the first dose.

Hypertensive Emergency:

- **Adult:** 40 to 80 mg IV, IO.
- **Pediatric:** 1 mg/kg IV or IM.

Special Considerations:

- Onset of action for IV, IO administration occurs within 5 minutes and will peak within 30 minutes.
- Furosemide is a diuretic, so the patient will likely have urinary urgency. Be prepared to help the patient void.
- Pregnancy class C

Gabapentin (Neurontin)

Classification: Anticonvulsant

Action: The exact mechanism of action has not been determined.

Indications: Seizures, neuropathic pain syndromes.

Adverse Effects: Dizziness, ataxia, sleepiness, gait disturbances, upset stomach.

Contraindications: Known sensitivity. Use with caution in elderly patients, renal impairment.

Dosage:

- **Adult:** 300 to 1800 mg PO daily.
- **Pediatric:**
  - **5 to 12 years:** 25 to 35 mg/kg/day PO divided in three divided doses daily.
  - **3 to 4 years:** 40 mg/kg/day PO divided in three divided doses daily.

Special Considerations: Pregnancy class C

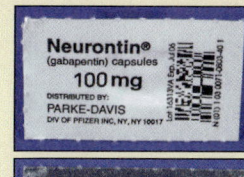
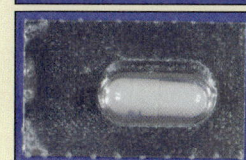

Glucagon (GlucaGen)

Classification: Hormone

Action: Converts glycogen to glucose.

Indication: Hypoglycemia, beta blocker overdose.

Adverse Effects: Nausea/vomiting, rebound hyperglycemia, hypotension, sinus tachycardia.

Contraindications: Pheochromocytoma, insulinoma, known sensitivity.

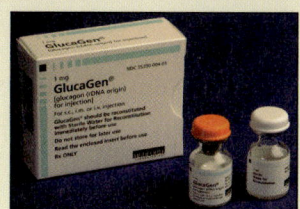

Continued

Glucagon—continued

Dosage:
Hypoglycemia:
- **Adult:** 1 mg IM, IV, IO, Sub-Q.
- **Pediatric:** (<20 kg) 0.5 mg IM, IV, IO, Sub-Q.

Beta blocker overdose:
- **Adult:** 2 to 5 mg IV, IO over a 1-minute period, followed by a second dose of 10 mg IV if the symptoms of bradycardia and hypotension recur. (Note that this dose is much higher than the dose required to treat hypoglycemia.)
- **Pediatric:** For patients weighing <20 kg, the dose is 0.5 mg.

Special Considerations: Pregnancy class B

Haloperidol (Haldol)

Classification: Antipsychotic agent
Action: Selectively blocks postsynaptic dopamine receptors.
Indications: Psychotic disorders, agitation.
Adverse Effects: Extrapyramidal symptoms, drowsiness, tardive dyskinesia, hypotension, hypertension, VT, sinus tachycardia, QT prolongation, torsades de pointes.
Contraindications: Depressed mental status, Parkinson's disease.
Dosage:
- **Adult:**
  - **Mild agitation:** 0.5 to 2 mg PO or IM.
  - **Moderate agitation:** 5 to 10 mg PO or IM.
  - **Severe agitation:** 10 mg PO or IM.
- **Pediatric:** Not recommended for pediatric patients.

Special Considerations: Pregnancy class C

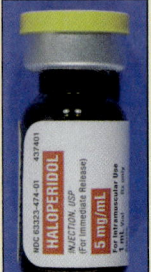

Heparin (Unfractionated Heparin)

Classification: Anticoagulant
Action: Acts on antithrombin III to reduce the ability of the blood to form clots, thus preventing clot deposition in the coronary arteries.
Indications: ACS, acute pulmonary embolism, deep venous thrombosis.
Adverse Effects: Bleeding, thrombocytopenia, allergic reactions.
Contraindications: Predisposition to bleeding, aortic aneurysm, peptic ulceration; known sensitivity or history of heparin-induced thrombocytopenia, severe thrombocytopenia, sulfite sensitivity.
Dosage:
Cardiac Indications:
- **Adult:** 60 U/kg IV (max 4000 units), followed by 12 U/kg/hr (max 1000 units). Once in the hospital, additional dosing is determined based on laboratory blood tests.
- **Pediatric:** 75 U/kg followed by 20 U/kg/hr.

Pulmonary Embolism and Deep Vein Thrombosis:
- **Adult:** 80 U/kg IV, followed by 18 U/kg/hr.
- **Pediatric:** 75 U/kg IV followed by 20 U/kg/hr.

Special Considerations:
- Half-life approximately 90 minutes
- Pregnancy class C

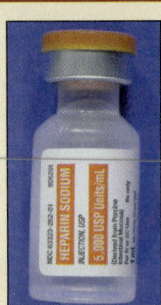

Hetastarch (Hespan)

Classification: Volume expander, colloid
Action: Causes water to move from interstitial spaces, thereby increasing the oncotic pressure within the intravascular space.
Indications: Hypovolemia when volume must be increased only in the intravascular compartment.
Adverse Effects: Anaphylactic reactions, CHF, pulmonary edema, cardiac arrhythmias, cardiac arrest, severe hypotension, pruritus, edema, platelet dysfunction, bleeding complications, dilution of the serum proteins responsible for the formation of blood clots, nausea/vomiting.
Contraindications: Bleeding disorders, intracranial bleeding, CHF, pulmonary edema, renal failure, thrombocytopenia or other coagulopathy (e.g., hemophilia), known sensitivity to hetastarch or corn.
Dosage: Note: The dosage of hetastarch required is determined by the clinical situation and the severity of the hypovolemia.
- **Adult:** 500 to 1000 mL IV, IO; more than 1500 mL of hetastarch typically is not administered because of concerns that larger doses can interfere with platelet function and promote bleeding.
- **Pediatric:** 10 mL/kg per dose IV; the total daily dosage should not exceed 20 mL/kg.

Special Considerations: Pregnancy class C

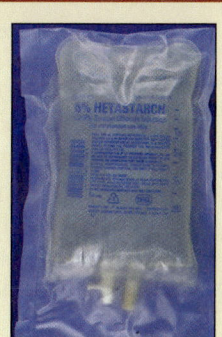

HMG Coenzyme A Statins: Atorvastatin (Lipitor), Fluvastatin (Lescol), Lovastatin (Mevacor), Pravastatin (Pravachol), Rosuvastatin (Crestor), Simvastatin (Zocor)

Classification: HMG coenzyme A statins
Action: Reduces the level of circulating total cholesterol, LDL-cholestrol, and serum triglycerides; reduces the incidence of reinfarction, recurrent angina, rehospitalization, and stroke when initiated within a few days after onset of ACS.
Indications: Acute coronary syndromes/acute myocardial infarction prophylaxis, hypercholesterolemia, hyperlipoproteinemia, hypertriglyceridemia, stroke prophylaxis.
Adverse Effects: Constipation, flatulence, dyspepsia, abdominal pain, infection, headache, flu-like symptoms, back pain, allergic reaction, asthenia, diarrhea, sinusitis, pharyngitis, rash, arthralgia, nausea/vomiting, myopathy, myasthenia, renal failure, rhabdomyolysis, chest pain, bronchitits, rhinitis, insomnia.
Contraindications: Active hepatic disease, pregnancy, breast-feeding, rhabdomyolysis
Dosage:
- **Adult:** Medication is administered orally. Dosage is individualized.
- **Pediatric:** Safe use has not been established.

Special Considerations: Pregnancy class X

Hydralazine (Apresoline)

Classification: Antihypertensive agent, vasodilator
Action: Directly dilates the peripheral blood vessels.
Indications: Hypertension associated with preeclampsia and eclampsia, hypertensive crisis.
Adverse Effects: Headache, angina, flushing, palpitations, reflex tachycardia, anorexia, nausea/vomiting, diarrhea, hypotension, syncope, peripheral vasodilation, peripheral edema, fluid retention, paresthesias.
Contraindications: Patients taking diazoxide or MAOIs, coronary artery disease, stroke, angina, dissecting aortic aneurysm, mitral valve and rheumatic heart diseases.

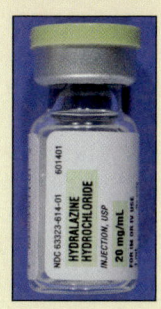

Dosage:
Preeclampsia and Eclampsia:
- **Adult:** 5 to 10 mg IV, IO. Repeat every 20 to 30 minutes until systolic blood pressure of 90 to 105 mm Hg is attained.
Acute Hypertension Not Associated with Preeclampsia:
- **Adult:** 10 to 20 mg IV, IO, or IM.
- **Pediatric:**
  - **1 month to 12 years:** 0.1 to 0.6 mg/kg IV, IO, or IM (max: 20 mg/dose).

Special Considerations: Pregnancy class C

Hydrocortisone Sodium Succinate (Cortef, Solu-Cortef)

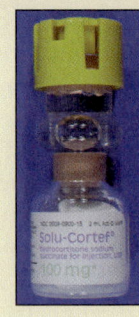

Classification: Corticosteroid

Action: Reduces inflammation by multiple mechanisms. As a steroid, it replaces the steroids that are lacking in adrenal insufficiency.

Indications: Adrenal insufficiency, allergic reactions, anaphylaxis, asthma, COPD.

Adverse Effects: Leukocytosis, hyperglycemia, increased infection, decreased wound healing, increased rate of death from sepsis.

Contraindications: Cushing's syndrome, known sensitivity to benzyl alcohol. Use with caution in diabetes, hypertension, CHF, known systemic fungal infection, renal disease, idiopathic thrombocytopenia, psychosis, seizure disorder, GI disease, glaucoma.

Dosage:

Anaphylactic Shock:
- **Adult:** 100 to 500 mg IV, IO, or IM.
- **Pediatric:** 2 to 4 mg/kg/day IV, IO, or IM (max: 500 mg).

Adrenal Insufficiency:
- **Adult:** 100 to 500 mg IV, IO, or IM.
- **Pediatric:** 1 to 2 mg/kg IV, IO, or IM.

Asthma and Chronic Obstructive Pulmonary Disease:
- **Adult:** 100 to 500 mg IV, IO, IM.
- **Pediatric:** 1 mg/kg IV, IO. The dose may be reduced for infants and children, but it is governed more by the severity of the condition and response of the patient than by age or body weight. Dose should not be less than 25 mg daily.

Special Considerations: Pregnancy class C

Hypertonic Saline (3% Saline)

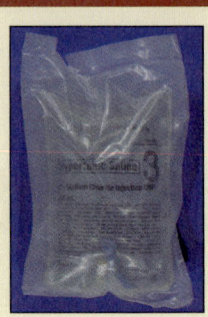

Classification: Volume expander, electrolyte solution

Action: The hyperonic nature of this fluid pulls extravascular fluid into the vascular space. Hypertonic saline may therefore be used as a volume expander in cases of hypovolemia or to reduce the edema of the swollen brain. Three percent saline has an electrolyte concentration of 514 mEq/L sodium.

Indications: Reduction of increased intracranial pressure resulting from traumatic brain injury, hypovolemic shock.

Adverse Effects: Increased rate of bleeding, alteration of blood clotting ability, osmotic demyelination syndrome.

Contraindications: Pulmonary congestion, pulmonary edema, known sensitivity. Hypertonic saline should not be administered by the IO route.

Dosage: Note: Hypertonic saline is available in several concentrations from 3% to 5%.
- **Adult:** 250-mL bag of hypertonic saline infused IV slowly over a 1-hour period.
- **Pediatric:** 6.5 to 10 mL/kg infused slowly IV over a 2-hour period.

Special Considerations:
- Hypertonic saline can cause damage to the vein in which it is administered.
- Pregnancy class C

Insulin, Regular (Humulin R, Novolin R)

Classification: Hormone

Action: Binds to a receptor on the membrane of cells and facilitates the transport of glucose into cells.

Indications: Hyperglycemia, insulin-dependent diabetes mellitus, hyperkalemia.

Adverse Effects: Hypoglycemia, tachycardia, palpitations, diaphoresis, anxiety, confusion, blurred vision, weakness, depression, seizures, coma, insulin shock, hypokalemia.

Contraindications: Hypoglycemia, known sensitivity.

Dosage:

Diabetic Ketoacidosis:

- **Adult:** 0.1 U/kg IV, IO, or Sub-Q. Because of poor perfusion of the peripheral tissues, Sub-Q administration is much less effective than the IV, IO route. IV, IO insulin has a very short half-life; therefore IV, IO insulin without an infusion is not that effective. The rate for an insulin infusion is 0.05 to 0.1 U/kg/hr IV, IO. When dosing insulin, use a U-100 insulin syringe to measure and deliver the insulin. The time from administration to action, as well as the duration of action, varies greatly among different individuals, as well as at different times in the same individual.

Hyperkalemia:

- **Adult:** 10 U IV, IO of regular insulin (Insulin R), coadministered with 50 mL of $D_{50}W$ over 5 minutes.
- **Pediatric:** 0.1 U/kg Insulin R IV, IO.

Special Considerations:

- Only regular insulin can be given IV, IO.
- Pregnancy class B

Ipratropium Bromide (Atrovent)

Classification: Bronchodilator, anticholinergic

Action: Antagonizes the acetylcholine receptor on bronchial smooth muscle, producing bronchodilation.

Indications: Asthma, bronchospasm associated with COPD.

Adverse Effects: Paradoxical acute bronchospasm, cough, throat irritation, headache, dizziness, dry mouth, palpitations.

Contraindications: Closed-angle glaucoma, bladder neck obstruction, prostatic hypertrophy, known sensitivity including peanuts or soybeans and atropine or atropine derivatives.

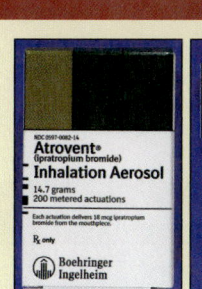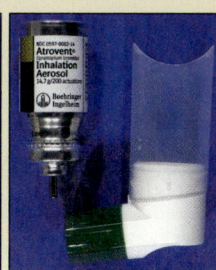

Dosage:

Nebulization:

- **Adult:** 0.5 mg every 6 to 8 hours.
- **Pediatric:** 5 to 14 years: 0.25 to 0.5 mg every 20 minutes for 3 doses as needed.

Metered-Dose Inhaler:

- **Adult:** 4 inhalations every 10 minutes, with no more than 24 inhalations per day or closer than 4 hours apart.
- **Pediatric:**
  - **Older than 12 years:** 2 to 3 puffs inhaled every 6 to 8 hours. Maximum of 12 puffs/day.
  - **5 to 12 years:** 1 to 2 puffs inhaled every 6 to 8 hours. Maximum of 8 puffs/day.

Special Considerations:

- Ipratropium bromide is not typically used as a sole medication in the treatment of acute exacerbation of asthma. Ipratropium bromide is commonly administered after a beta agonist.
- Care should be taken to not allow the aerosol spray (especially in the MDI) to come into contact with the eyes. This can cause temporary blurring of vision that resolves without intervention within 4 hours.
- Pregnancy class B

Ketamine (Ketalar)

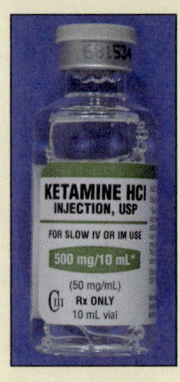

Classification: General anesthetic

Action: Produces a state of anesthesia while maintaining airway reflexes, heart rate, and blood pressure.

Indications: Pain and as anesthesia for procedures of short duration.

Adverse Effects: Emergence phenomena, hypertension and sinus tachycardia, hypotension and sinus bradycardia, other cardiac arrhythmias (rare), respiratory depression, apnea, laryngospasms and other forms of airway obstruction (rare), tonic and clonic movements, vomiting.

Contraindications: Patients in whom a significant elevation in blood pressure would be hazardous (hypertension, stroke, head trauma, increased intracranial mass or bleeding, MI). Use with caution in patients with increased ICP or increased intraocular pressure (glaucoma) and patients with hypovolemia, dehydration, or cardiac disease (especially angina and CHF).

Dosage: Administer slowly over a period of 60 seconds.

IV, IO:

- **Adult:** 1 to 4.5 mg/kg IV/IO. 1 to 2 mg/kg produces anesthesia typically within 30 seconds that typically lasts 5 to 10 minutes.
- **Pediatric:** 0.5 to 2 mg IV, IO over a 1-minute period.

IM:

- **Adult:** 6.5 to 13 mg/kg IM. 10 mg/kg IM is capable of producing anesthesia within 3 to 4 minutes with an effect typically lasting 12 to 25 minutes. In adults, concomitant administration of 5 to 15 mg of diazepam reduces the incidence of emergence phenomena.
- **Pediatric:** 3 to 7 mg IM.

Special Considerations: Pregnancy class C

Ketorolac (Toradol)

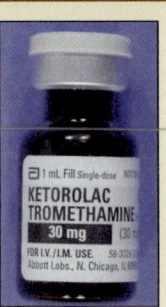

Classification: NSAID

Action: Inhibits the production of prostaglandins in inflamed tissue, which decreases the responsiveness of pain receptors.

Indications: Moderately severe acute pain.

Adverse Effects: Headache, drowsiness, dizziness, abdominal pain, dyspepsia, nausea/vomiting, diarrhea.

Contraindications: Patients with a history of peptic ulcer disease or GI bleed, patients with renal insufficiency, hypovolemic patients, pregnancy (third trimester), nursing mothers, allergy to aspirin or other NSAIDs, stroke or suspected stroke or head trauma, need for major surgery in the immediate or near future (i.e., within 7 days).

Dosage: Note: The following dosage regimen applies to single-dose administration only. IV, IO administration should occur over a period of at least 15 seconds.

- **Adult:**
  - **Younger than 65 years:** 30 mg IV, IO or 60 mg IM.
  - **Older than 65 years:** 15 mg IV, IO or 30 mg IM.
- **Pediatric:** 0.5 mg/kg IV, IO to a maximum dose of 15 mg, or 1 mg/kg IM to a maximum dose of 30 mg.

Special Considerations: Pregnancy class C; class D in third trimester

Labetalol (Normodyne, Trandate)

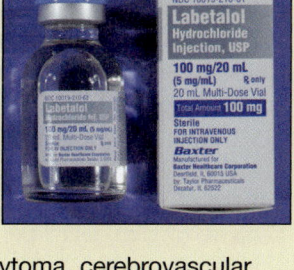

Classification: Beta adrenergic antagonist, antianginal, antihypertensive

Action: Binds with both the beta$_1$ and beta$_2$ receptors and alpha$_1$ receptors in vascular smooth muscle. Inhibits the strength of the heart's contractions, as well as heart rate. This results in a decrease in cardiac oxygen consumption.

Indications: ACS, SVT, severe hypertension.

Adverse Effects: Usually mild and transient; hypotensive symptoms, nausea/vomiting, bronchospasm, arrhythmia, bradycardia, AV block.

Contraindications: Hypotension, cardiogenic shock, acute pulmonary edema, heart failure, severe bradycardia, sick sinus syndrome, second- or third-degree heart block, asthma or acute bronchospasm, cocaine-induced ACS, known sensitivity. Use caution in pheochromocytoma, cerebrovascular disease or stroke, poorly controlled diabetes, with hepatic disease. Use with caution at lowest effective dose in chronic lung disease.

Dosage:

Cardiac Indications: Note: Monitor blood pressure and heart rate closely during administration.

Adult: 10 mg IV, IO over a 1- to 2-minute period. May repeat every 10 minutes to a maximum dose of 150 mg or give initial bolus and then follow with infusion at 2 to 8 mg/min.

Pediatric: 0.4 to 1 mg/kg/hr to a maximum dosage of 3 mg/kg/hr.

Severe Hypertension:

- **Adult:** Initial dose is 20 mg IV, IO slow infusion over a 2-minute period. After the initial dose, blood pressure should be checked every 5 minutes. Repeat doses can be given at 10-minute intervals. The second dose should be 40 mg IV, IO, and subsequent doses should be 80 mg IV, IO, to a maximum total dose of 300 mg. The effect on blood pressure typically will occur within 5 minutes from the time of administration. Alternatively, may be administered via IV infusion at 2 mg/min to a total maximum dose of 300 mg.
- **Pediatric:** 0.4 to 1 mg/kg/hr IV, IO infusion with a maximum dose of 3 mg/kg/hr.

Special Considerations: Pregnancy class C

Lamotrigine (Lamictal)

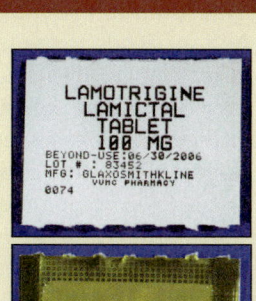
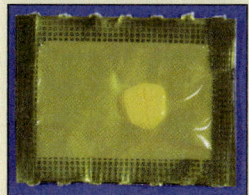

Classification: Anticonvulsant, antimanic agent

Action: The exact mechanism of action has not been determined. Studies suggest lamotrigine stabilizes neuronal membranes by acting at voltage-sensitive sodium channels, thereby decreasing presynaptic release of glutamate and aspartate, resulting in decreased seizure activity.

Indications: Seizures, bipolar disorders.

Adverse Effects: Headache, dizziness, nausea/vomiting, ataxia, diplopia.

Contraindications: Known sensitivity.

Dosage:

- **Adult:** Medication is administered orally. Dosage is individualized.
- **Pediatric:** Medication is administered orally. Dosage is individualized.

Special Considerations: Pregnancy class C

Lidocaine (Xylocaine)

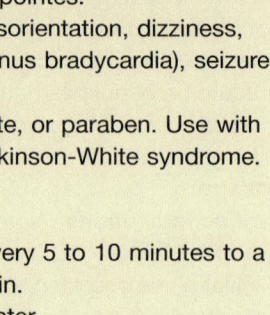

Classification: Antiarrhythmic, class IB

Action: Blocks sodium channels, increasing the recovery period after repolarization; suppresses automaticity in the His-Purkinje system and depolarization in the ventricles.

Indications: Ventricular arrhythmias, when amiodarone is not available: cardiac arrest from VF/VT, stable monomorphic VT with preserved ventricular function, stable polymorphic VT with normal baseline QT interval and preserved left ventricular function (when ischemia and electrolyte imbalance are treated), stable polymorphic VT with baseline QT-prolongation suggestive of torsades de pointes.

Adverse Effects: Toxicity (signs may include anxiety, apprehension, euphoria, nervousness, disorientation, dizziness, blurred vision, facial paresthesias, tremors, hearing disturbances, slurred speech, seizures, sinus bradycardia), seizures without warning, cardiac arrhythmias, hypotension, cardiac arrest), pain at injection site.

Contraindications: AV block; bleeding; thrombocytopenia; known sensitivity to lidocaine, sulfite, or paraben. Use with caution in bradycardia, hypovolemia, cardiogenic shock, Adams-Stokes syndrome, Wolff-Parkinson-White syndrome.

Dosage:

Pulseless Ventricular Tachycardia and Ventricular Fibrillation:

- **Adult IV, IO:** 1 to 1.5 mg/kg IV, IO; may repeat at half the original dose (0.5-0.75 mg/kg) every 5 to 10 minutes to a maximum dose of 3 mg/kg. If a maintenance infusion is warranted, the rate is 1 to 4 mg/min.
- **Adult ET tube:** 2 to 10 mg/kg ET tube, diluted in 10 mL normal saline or sterile distilled water.
- **Pediatric IV, IO:** 1 mg/kg IV, IO (maximum 100 mg). If a maintenance infusion is warranted, the rate is 20 to 50 mcg/kg/min.
- **Pediatric ET tube:** 2 to 3 mg/kg ET tube, followed by a 5-mL flush of normal saline.

Perfusing Ventricular Rhythms:

- **Adult:** 0.5 to 0.75 mg/kg IV, IO (up to 1-1.5 mg/kg may be used). Repeat 0.5 to 0.75 mg/kg every 5 to 10 minutes to a maximum total dose of 3 mg/kg. A maintenance infusion of 1 to 4 mg/min (30-50 mcg/kg/min) is acceptable.
- **Pediatric:** 1 mg/kg IV, IO. May repeat every 5 to 10 minutes to a maximum dose of 3 mg/kg. Maintenance infusion rate is 20 to 50 mcg/kg/min.

Special Considerations:

- Half-life approximately 90 minutes
- Pregnancy class B

Lorazepam (Ativan)

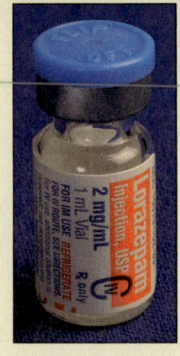

Classification: Benzodiazepine; schedule C-IV

Action: Binds to the benzodiazepine receptor and enhances the effects of the brain chemical GABA, an inhibitory transmitter, and may result in a state of sedation, hypnosis, skeletal muscle relaxation, anticonvulsant activity, coma.

Indications: Preprocedure sedation induction, anxiety, status epilepticus.

Adverse Effects: Headache, drowsiness, ataxia, dizziness, amnesia, depression, dysarthria, euphoria, syncope, fatigue, tremor, vertigo, respiratory depression, paradoxical CNS stimulation.

Contraindications: Known sensitivity to lorazepam, benzodiazepines, polyethylene glycol, propylene glycol, or benzyl alcohol; COPD; sleep apnea (except while being mechanically ventilated); shock; coma; acute closed-angle glaucoma.

Dosage: Note: IV, IO lorazepam needs to be administered slowly.

Analgesia and Sedation:

- **Adult:** 2 mg or 0.44 mg/kg IV, IO, whichever is smaller. This dose will provide adequate sedation in most patients and should not be exceeded in patients older than 50 years.
- **Pediatric:** 0.05 mg/kg IV, IO. Each dose should not exceed 2 mg IV, IO.

Continued

Lorazepam (Ativan)—continued

Seizures:

- **Adult:** 4 mg IV, IO given over 2 to 5 minutes; may repeat in 10 to 15 minutes (max total dose: 8 mg in a 12-hour period).
- **Pediatric:**
  - **Adolescents:** 0.07 mg/kg slow IV, IO given over 2 to 5 minutes (max single dose: 4 mg). May repeat in 10 to 15 minutes (max dose: 8 mg in a 12-hour period).
  - **Children and infants:** 0.1 mg/kg slow IV, IO given over 2 to 5 minutes (max single dose: 4 mg). May repeat at half the original dose in 10 to 15 minutes if seizure activity resumes.
  - **Neonates:** 0.05 mg/kg slow IV, IO given over 2 to 5 minutes. May repeat in 10 to 15 minutes.

Special Considerations:

- Be prepared to support the patient's airway and ventilation.
- Pregnancy class D

Magnesium Sulfate

Classification: Electrolyte, tocolytic, mineral

Action: Required for normal physiologic functioning. Magnesium is a cofactor in neurochemical transmission and muscular excitability. Magnesium sulfate controls seizures by blocking peripheral neuromuscular transmission. Magnesium is also a peripheral vasodilator and an inhibitor of platelet function.

Indications: Torsades de pointes, cardiac arrhythmias associated with hypomagnesemia, eclampsia and seizure prophylaxis in preeclampsia, status asthmaticus.

Adverse Effects: Magnesium toxicity (signs include flushing, diaphoresis, hypotension, muscle paralysis, weakness, hypothermia, and cardiac, CNS, or respiratory depression).

Contraindications: AV block, GI obstruction. Use with caution in renal impairment.

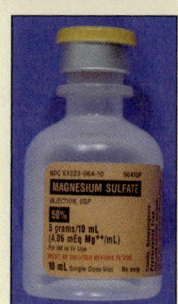

Dosage:

Ventricular Fibrillation/Pulseless Ventricular Tachycardia with Torsades De Pointes or Hypomagnesemia:

- **Adult:** 1 to 2 g in 10 mL D_5W IV, IO administered over 5 to 10 minutes.
- **Pediatric:** 25 to 50 mg/kg IV, IO over 10 to 20 minutes; may administer faster for torsades de pointes (max single dose: 2 g).

Torsades De Pointes with a Pulse or Cardiac Arrhythmias with Hypomagnesemia:

- **Adult:** 1 to 2 g in 50 to 100 mL D_5W IV, IO administered over 5 to 60 minutes. Follow with 0.5 to 1 g/hr IV, IO titrated to control torsades de pointes.
- **Pediatric:** 25 to 50 mg/kg IV, IO over 10 to 20 minutes (max single dose: 2 g).

Eclampsia and Seizure Prophylaxis in Preeclampsia:

- **Adult:** 4 to 6 g IV, IO over 20 to 30 minutes, followed by an infusion of 1 to 2 g/hr.

Status Asthmaticus:

- **Adult:** 1.2 to 2 g slow IV, IO (over 20 minutes).
- **Pediatric:** 25 to 50 mg/kg (diluted in D_5W) slow IV, IO (over 10 to 20 minutes).

Special Considerations: Pregnancy class A

Mannitol (Osmitrol)

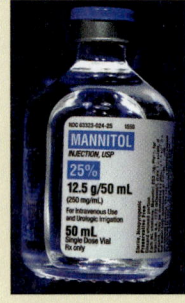

Classification: Osmotic diuretic

Action: Facilitates the flow of fluid out of tissues (including the brain) and into interstitial fluid and blood, thereby dehydrating the brain and reducing swelling. Reabsorption by the kidney is minimal, consequently increasing urine output.

Indications: Increased ICP.

Adverse Effects: Pulmonary edema, headache, blurred vision, dizziness, seizures, hypovolemia, nausea/vomiting, diarrhea, electrolyte imbalances, hypotension, hypertension, sinus tachycardia, PVCs, angina, phlebitis.

Contraindications: Active intracranial bleeding, CHF, pulmonary edema, severe dehydration. Use with caution in hypovolemia, renal failure.

Dosage:
- **Adult:** 0.5 to 2 g/kg IV, IO followed by 0.25 to 1 g/kg administered every 4 hours.
- **Pediatric:** 0.25 to 1 g/kg IV, IO followed by 0.25-0.5 g/kg every 4 hours.

Special Considerations:
- Mannitol should not be given in the same IV, IO line as blood.
- Pregnancy class C

Meperidine (Demerol)

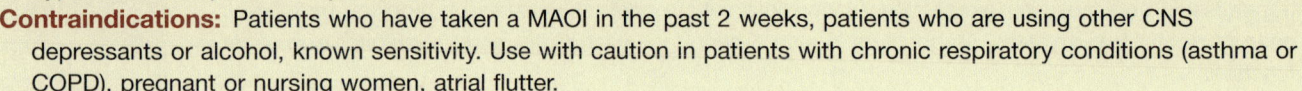

Classification: Narcotic analgesic, schedule C-II

Action: Binds to opiate receptors, producing analgesia and euphoria.

Indications: Moderate to severe pain.

Adverse Effects: Respiratory depression, nausea/vomiting, sinus bradycardia, sinus tachycardia, palpitations, hypertension, hypotension, orthostatic hypotension, diaphoresis, syncope, shock, cardiac arrest.

Contraindications: Patients who have taken a MAOI in the past 2 weeks, patients who are using other CNS depressants or alcohol, known sensitivity. Use with caution in patients with chronic respiratory conditions (asthma or COPD), pregnant or nursing women, atrial flutter.

Dosage: If given IV, IO, administer slowly.
- **Adult:** 50 to 150 mg IV, IO, IM, or Sub-Q. Elderly: 50 mg IV, IO, IM, or Sub-Q.
- **Pediatric:** 1 to 2 mg/kg IV, IO, IM, or Sub-Q.

Special Considerations:
- In adults, half-life approximately 4 hours, but its active metabolites may last 30 hours.
- Pregnancy class C; class D near term.

Methylprednisolone Sodium Succinate (Solu-Medrol)

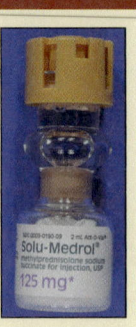

Classification: Corticosteroid

Action: Reduces inflammation by multiple mechanisms.

Indications: Anaphylaxis, asthma, COPD.

Adverse Effects: Depression, euphoria, headache, restlessness, hypertension, bradycardia, nausea/vomiting, swelling, diarrhea, weakness, fluid retention, paresthesias.

Contraindications: Cushing's syndrome, fungal infection, measles, varicella, known sensitivity (including sulfites). Use with caution in active infections, renal disease, penetrating spinal cord injury, hypertension, seizures, CHF.

Dosage:

Asthma and Chronic Obstructive Pulmonary Disease:
- **Adult:** 40 to 80 mg IV.
- **Pediatric:** 1 mg/kg (up to 60 mg) IV, IO per day in two divided doses.

Continued

Methylprednisolone Sodium Succinate (Solu-Medrol)—continued

Anaphylactic Shock:
- **Adult:** 1 to 2 mg/kg/dose, then 0.5 to 1 mg/kg every 6 hours.
- **Pediatric:** Same as adult dosing.

Blunt Spinal Cord Injury:
- **Adult:** 30 mg/kg IV, IO over a period of 1 hour, then as an infusion to run for the remaining 23 hours at a dose of 5.4 mg/kg/hr.
- **Pediatric:** Same as adult dosing.

Special Considerations:
- May mask signs and symptoms of infection.
- Pregnancy class C

Metoprolol (Lopressor, Toprol XL)

Classification: Beta adrenergic antagonist, antianginal, antihypertensive, class II antiarrhythmic

Action: Inhibits the strength of the heart's contractions as well as heart rate. This results in a decrease in cardiac oxygen consumption. Also saturates the beta receptors and inhibits dilation of bronchial smooth muscle (beta$_2$ receptor).

Indications: ACS, hypertension, SVT, atrial flutter, AF, thyrotoxicosis.

Adverse Effects: Tiredness, dizziness, diarrhea, heart block, bradycardia, bronchospasm, drop in blood pressure.

Contraindications: Cardiogenic shock, AV block, bradycardia, known sensitivity. Use with caution in hypotension, chronic lung disease (asthma and COPD).

Dosage:
Cardiac Indications:
- **Adult:** 5 mg slow IV, IO over a 5-minute period; repeat at 5-minute intervals up to a total of three infusions totaling 15 mg IV, IO.
- **Pediatric:** Not recommended for pediatric patients; no studies available.

Special Considerations:
- Blood pressure, heart rate, and ECG should be monitored carefully.
- Use with caution in patients with asthma.
- Pregnancy class C

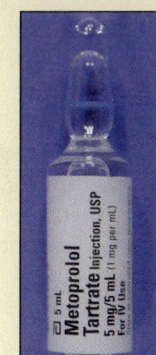

Midazolam (Versed)

Classification: Benzodiazepine, schedule C-IV

Action: Binds to the benzodiazepine receptor and enhances the effects of the brain chemical (neurotransmitter) GABA. Benzodiazepines act at the level of the limbic, thalamic, and hypothalamic regions of the CNS to produce short-acting CNS depression (including sedation, skeletal muscle relaxation, and anticonvulsant activity).

Indications: Sedation, anxiety, skeletal muscle relaxation.

Adverse Effects: Respiratory depression, respiratory arrest, hypotension, nausea/vomiting, headache, hiccups, cardiac arrest.

Contraindications: Acute-angle glaucoma, pregnancy, known sensitivity.

Dosage:
Sedation:
Note: The dose of midazolam needs to be individualized. Every dose should be administered slowly over a period of 2 minutes. Allow 2 minutes to evaluate the clinical effect of the dose given.

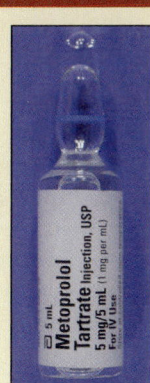

Continued

Midazolam (Versed)—continued

- **Adult:**
  - **Adult (healthy and younger than 60 years):** *Some patients require as little as 1 mg IV, IO. No more than 2.5 mg should be given over a 2-minute interval.* If additional sedation is required, continue to administer small increments over 2-minute periods (max dose: 5 mg). If the patient also has received a narcotic, he or she will typically require 30% less midazolam than the same patient not given the narcotic.
  - **Adult (60 years and older and debilitated or chronically ill patients):** This group of patients has a higher risk of hypoventilation, airway obstruction, and apnea. The peak clinical effect can take longer in these patients; therefore dose increments should be smaller, and the rate of injection should be slower. *Some patients require a dose as small as 1 mg IV, IO, and no more than 1.5 mg should be given over a 2-minute period.* If additional sedation is required, additional midazolam should be given at a rate of no more than 1 mg over a 2-minute period (max dose: 3.5 mg). If the patient also has received a narcotic, he or she will typically require 50% less midazolam than the same patient not given the narcotic.
  - **Adult—continuous infusion:** Continuous infusions can be required for prolonged transport of intubated, critically ill, and injured patients. After an initial bolus dose, the adult patient will require a maintenance infusion dose of 0.02 to 0.1 mg/kg/hr (1-7 mg/hr).
- **Pediatric (weight-based):** Pediatric patients typically require higher doses of midazolam than do adults on the basis of weight (in mg/kg). Younger pediatric patients (younger than 6 years) require higher doses (in mg/kg) than older pediatric patients. Midazolam takes approximately 3 minutes to reach peak effect; therefore wait at least 2 minutes to determine effectiveness of drug and need for additional dosing.
  - **12 to 16 years:** Same as adult dosing. Some patients in this age group require a higher dose than that used in adults, but rarely does a patient require more than 10 mg.
  - **6 to 12 years:** 0.025 to 0.05 mg/kg IV, IO up to a total dose of 0.4 mg/kg. Exceeding 10 mg as total dose usually is not necessary.
  - **6 months to 5 years:** 0.05 to 0.1 mg/kg IV, IO up to a total dose of 0.6 mg/kg. Exceeding 6 mg as total dose usually is not necessary.
- **Younger than 6 months:** Dosing recommendations for this age group is unclear. Because this age group is especially vulnerable to airway obstruction and hypoventilation, use small increments with frequent clinical evaluation. Dose: 0.05 to 0.1 mg/kg IV, IO.

Special Considerations:
- Patients receiving midazolam require frequent monitoring of vital signs and pulse oximetry. Be prepared to support patient's airway and ventilation.
- Pregnancy class D

Milrinone (Primacor)

Classification: Inotrope

Action: Milrinone is a positive inotrope and vasodilator with minimal chronotropic effect. Milrinone inhibits an enzyme, cAMP phosphodiesterase, which results in an increase in the concentration of calcium inside the cardiac cell. The result is improvement in diastolic function and myocardial contractility.

Indications: Cardiogenic shock, CHF.

Adverse Effects: Cardiac arrhythmias, nausea/vomiting, hypotension.

Contraindications: Valvular heart disease, known sensitivity.

Dosage:
- **Adult:** 50 mcg/kg IV, IO over a period of 10 minutes, followed by an infusion of 0.375 to 0.5 mcg/kg/min (max dose: 0.75 mcg/kg/min).
- **Pediatric:** Same as adult dosing.

Special Considerations: Pregnancy class C

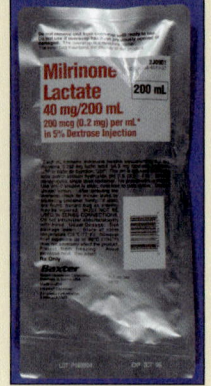

Morphine Sulfate

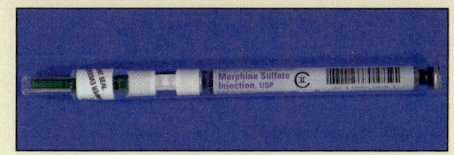

Classification: Opiate agonist, schedule C-II

Action: Binds with opioid receptors. Morphine is capable of inducing hypotension by depression of the vasomotor centers of the brain, as well as release of the chemical histamine. In the management of angina, morphine reduces stimulation of the sympathic nervous system caused by pain and anxiety. Reduction of sympathetic stimulation reduces heart rate, cardiac work, and myocardial oxygen consumption.

Indications: Moderate to severe pain, including chest pain associated with ACS, CHF, pulmonary edema.

Adverse Effects: Respiratory depression, hypotension, nausea/vomiting, dizziness, lightheadedness, sedation, diaphoresis, euphoria, dysphoria, worsening of bradycardia and heart block in some patients with acute inferior wall MI, seizures, cardiac arrest, anaphylactoid reactions.

Contraindications: Respiratory depression, shock, known sensitivity. Use with caution in hypotension, acute bronchial asthma, respiratory insufficiency, head trauma.

Dosage:

Pain:

- **Adult:** 2.5 to 15 mg IV, IO, IM, or Sub-Q administered slowly over a period of several minutes. The dose is the same whether administered IV, IO, IM, or Sub-Q.
- **Pediatric:**
  - **6 months to 12 years:** 0.05 to 0.2 mg/kg IV, IO, IM, or Sub-Q.
  - **Younger than 6 months:** 0.03 to 0.05 mg/kg IV, IO, IM, or Sub-Q.

Chest Pain Associated with Acute Coronary Syndromes, Congestive Heart Failure, and Pulmonary Edema:

Administer small doses and reevaluate the patient. Large doses may lead to respiratory depression and worsen the patient's hypoxia.

- **Adult:** 2 to 4 mg slow IV, IO over a 1- to 5-minute period with increments of 2 to 8 mg repeated every 5 to 15 minutes until patient relieved of chest pain.
- **Pediatric:** 0.1 to 0.2 mg/kg/dose IV, IO.

Special Considerations:

- Monitor vital signs and pulse oximetry closely. Be prepared to support patient's airway and ventilations.
- Overdose should be treated with naloxone.
- Pregnancy class C

Nalbuphine (Nubain)

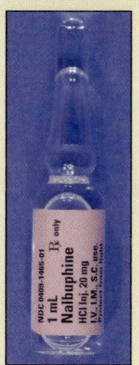

Classification: Synthetic opioid agonist-antagonist

Action: Produces analgesia by binding to the opioid receptor.

Indications: Moderate to severe pain.

Adverse Effects: Drowsiness, diaphoresis, headache, nausea/vomiting, dry mouth, respiratory depression, hypotension, bradycardia.

Contraindications: Known sensitivity.

Dosage:

- **Adult:** 10 mg IV, IO, IM, or Sub-Q.
- **Pediatric:** Not recommended for pediatric patients.

Special Considerations: Pregnancy class B

Naloxone (Narcan)

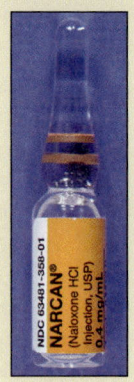

Classification: Opioid antagonist
Action: Binds the opioid receptor and blocks the effect of narcotics.
Indications: Narcotic overdoses, reversal of narcotics used for procedure-related anesthesia.
Adverse Effects: Nausea/vomiting, restlessness, diaphoresis, tachycardia, hypertension, tremulousness, seizures, cardiac arrest, narcotic withdrawal. Patients who have gone from a state of somnolence from a narcotic overdose to wide awake may become combative.
Contraindications: Known sensitivity to naloxone, nalmefene, or naltrexone. Use with caution in patients with supraventricular arrhythmias or other cardiac disease, head trauma, brain tumor.
Dosage:
- **Adult:** 0.4 to 2 mg IV, IO, ET, IM, or Sub-Q. Alternatively, administer 2 mg intranasally. Higher doses (10-20 mg) may be required for overdoses of synthetic narcotics. A repeat dose of one-third to two-thirds the original dose is often necessary.
- **Pediatric:**
  - **5 years or older or weight >20 kg:** 2 mg IV, IO, ET, IM, or Sub-Q.
  - **Younger than 5 years or weight <20 kg:** 0.1 mg/kg IV, IO, ET, IM, or Sub-Q; may repeat every 2 to 3 minutes.

Special Considerations: Pregnancy class C

Nicardipine (Cardene)

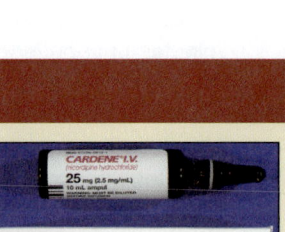

Classification: Calcium channel blocker
Action: Blocks calcium movement into the smooth muscle of the blood vessel walls, causing vasodilation.
Indications: Hypertension
Adverse Effects: Edema, headaches, flushing, sinus tachycardia, hypotension.
Contraindications: Aortic stenosis, hypotension, known sensitivity. Use with caution in heart failure, cardiac conduction abnormalities, cerebral vascular disease, depressed AV node conduction.
Dosage:
- **Adult:** 5 mg/hr IV, IO; may increase by 2.5 mg/hr every 5 to 15 minutes (max dose: 15 mg/hr). Once the patient has achieved the desired blood pressure, decrease infusion to a maintenance dose of 3 mg/hr.
- **Pediatric:** 0.5 to 1 mcg/kg/min IV, IO infusion.

Special Considerations: Pregnancy class C

Nitroglycerin (Nitrolingual, NitroQuick, NitroStat Nitro-Dur)

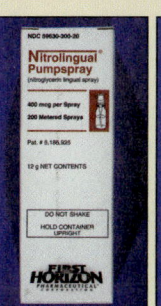
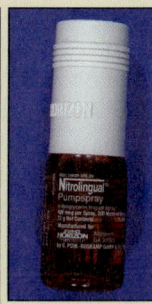

Classification: Antianginal agent

Action: Relaxes vascular smooth muscle, thereby dilating peripheral arteries and veins. This causes pooling of venous blood and decreased venous return to the heart, which decreases preload. Nitroglycerin also reduces left ventricular systolic wall tension, which decreases afterload.

Indications: Angina, ongoing ischemic chest discomfort, hypertension, myocardial ischemia associated with cocaine intoxication.

Adverse Effects: Headache, hypotension, bradycardia, lightheadedness, flushing, cardiovascular collapse, methemoglobinemia.

Contraindications: Hypotension, severe bradycardia or tachycardia, increased ICP, intracranial bleeding, patients taking any medications for erectile dysfunction (such as sildenafil [Viagra], tadalafil [Cialis], or vardenafil [Levitra]), known sensitivity to nitrates. Use with caution in anemia, closed-angle glaucoma, hypotension, postural hypotension, uncorrected hypovolemia.

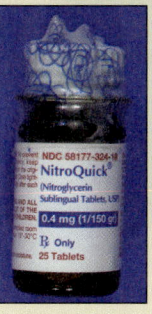
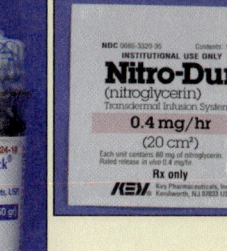

Dosage:
- **Adult:**
  - **Sublingual tablets:** 1 tablet (0.3-0.4 mg) at 5-minute intervals to a maximum of 3 doses.
  - **Translingual spray:** 1 (0.4 mg) spray at 5-minute intervals to a maximum of 3 sprays.
  - **Ointment:** 2% topical (Nitro-Bid ointment): Apply 1 to 2 inches of paste over the chest wall, cover with transparent wrap, and secure with tape.
  - **IV:**
    - **Bolus:** 12.5 to 25 mcg
    - **Infusion:** 5 mcg/min; may increase rate by 5 to 10 mcg/min every 5 to 10 minutes as needed. End points of dose titration for nitroglycerin include a drop in the blood pressure of 10%, relief of chest pain, and return of ST-segment to normal on a 12-lead ECG.
- **Pediatric IV infusion:** The initial pediatric infusion is 0.25 to 0.5 mcg/kg/min IV, IO titrated by 0.5 to 1 mcg/kg/min. Usual required dose is 1 to 3 mcg/kg/min to a maximum dose of 5 mcg/kg/min.

Special Considerations:
- Administration of nitroglycerin to a patient with right ventricular MI can result in hypotension.
- Pregnancy class C

Nitrous Oxide

Classification: Inorganic gas, inhaled anesthetic

Action: Exact mechanism is not known.

Indications: Mild to severe pain.

Adverse Effects: Delirium, hypoxia, respiratory depression, nausea/vomiting.

Contraindications: Use with caution in head trauma, increased ICP, pneumothorax, bowel obstruction, patients with COPD who require a hypoxic respiratory drive.

Dosage: Inhaled: 20% to 50% concentration mixed with oxygen.

Special Considerations:
- Ensure the safety of healthcare professionals. Only use with a scavenger gas system to ensure that unused gas is collected, or scavenged, and that providers are not exposed to significant levels of the agent.
- Pregnancy class not noted

Norepinephrine (Levophed)

Classification: Adrenergic agonist, inotrope, vasopressor

Action: Norepinephrine is an $alpha_1$, $alpha_2$, and $beta_1$ agonist. Alpha-mediated peripheral vasoconstriction is the predominant clinical result of administration, resulting in increasing blood pressure and coronary blood flow. Beta adrenergic action produces inotropic stimulation of the heart and dilates the coronary arteries.

Indications: Cardiogenic shock, septic shock, severe hypotension.

Adverse Effects: Dizziness, anxiety, cardiac arrhythmias, dyspnea, exacerbation of asthma.

Contraindications: Patients taking MAOIs, known sensitivity. Use with caution in hypovolemia.

Dosage:

- **Adult:** Add 4 mg to 250 mL of D_5W or D_5NS, but not normal saline alone. 0.5 to 1 mcg/min as IV, IO, titrated to maintain blood pressure >80 mmHg. Refractory shock may require doses as high as 30 mcg/min.
- **Pediatric:** 0.05 to 2 mcg/kg/min IV, IO infusion, to a maximum dose of 2 mcg/kg/min.

Special Considerations:

- Do not administer in same IV line as alkaline solutions.
- Half-life 1 minute
- Pregnancy class C

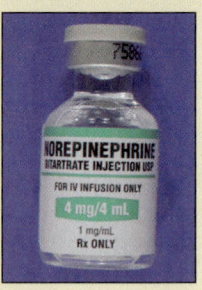

Oxygen

Classification: Elemental gas

Action: Facilitates cellular energy metabolism

Indications: Hypoxia, ischemic chest pain, respiratory distress, suspected carbon monoxide poisoning, traumatic injuries, shock, cardiac arrest.

Adverse Effects: High concentrations can cause decreased level of consciousness and respiratory depression in patients with chronic carbon dioxide retention or chronic lung disease.

Contraindications: Known paraquat poisoning.

Dosage:

Low-Concentration Oxygen:

- A dose of 1 to 4 L/min by a nasal cannula is appropriate.

High-Concentration Oxygen:

- A dose of 10 to 15 L/min via nonrebreather mask is appropriate.

Special Considerations: Pregnancy class A

Pancuronium (Pavulon)

Classification: Nondepolarizing neuromuscular blocker

Action: Antagonizes acetylcholine at the motor end plate, producing skeletal muscle paralysis.

Indications: To induce neuromuscular blockade for the facilitation of ET intubation.

Adverse Effects: Muscle paralysis, apnea, dyspnea, respiratory depression, cutaneous flushing, sinus tachycardia.

Contraindications: Known sensitivity to bromides. Use with caution in heart disease, renal disease.

Dosage:

- **Adult:** 0.04 to 0.1 mg/kg IV, IO; repeat dosing is 0.01 mg/kg every 25 to 60 minutes.
- **Pediatric:** Same as adult dosing.

Special Considerations: Pregnancy class C

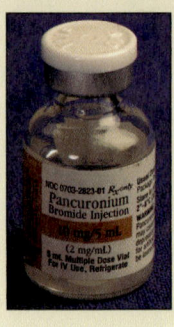

Phenobarbital (Luminal)

Classification: Anticonvulsant, barbiturate, schedule C-IV

Action: Depresses seizure activity in the cortex, thalamus, and limbic system; increases threshold for electrical stimulation of motor cortex; produces state of sedation.

Indications: Seizures

Adverse Effects: Depression, agitation, respiratory depression, accelerated metabolism of several other medications.

Contraindications: Liver dysfunction, porphyria, agranulocytosis, known sensitivity to barbiturates. Use with caution with respiratory dysfunction.

Dosage:
- **Adult:** 15 to 18 mg/kg IV, IO; infuse at a rate not faster than 60 mg/min.
- **Pediatric:** 15 to 20 mg/kg IV, IO; infuse at a rate not faster than 2 mg/kg/min.

Special Considerations:
- Be prepared to manage the patient's airway.
- Pregnancy class D

Phentolamine (Regitine)

Classification: Alpha antagonist, antihypertensive

Action: Blocks alpha adrenergic receptors, causing vasodilation.

Indications: Hypertensive emergencies and hypertension caused by pheochromocytoma, cocaine-induced vasospasm of the coronary arteries.

Adverse Effects: Sinus tachycardia, angina, dizziness, orthostatic hypotension, prolonged hypotensive episodes, nausea/vomiting, diarrhea, weakness, flushing, nasal congestion.

Contraindications: Known sensitivity. Use with caution in acute MI, angina, coronary insufficiency, evidence suggestive of coronary artery disease, peptic ulcer disease.

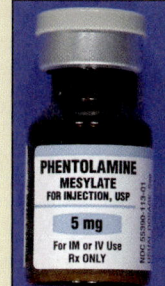

Dosage:

Hypertensive Crisis:
- **Adult:** 5 to 15 mg IV, IO or IM.
- **Pediatric:** Not recommended for pediatric patients.

Cocaine-Induced Vasospasm:
- **Adult:** 5 mg IV, IO or IM.
- **Pediatric:** Not recommended for pediatric patients.

Special Considerations: Pregnancy class C

Phenylephrine (Neo-Synephrine)

Classification: Adrenergic agonist

Action: Stimulates the alpha receptors, causing vasoconstriction, which results in increased blood pressure.

Indications: Neurogenic shock, spinal shock, cases of shock in which the patient's heart rate does not need to be increased, drug-induced hypotension.

Adverse Effects: Hypertension, VT, headache, excitability, tremor, MI, exacerbation of asthma, cardiac arrhythmias, reflex bradycardia, soft tissue necrosis.

Contraindications: Acute MI, angina, cardiac arrhythmias, severe hypertension, coronary artery disease, pheochromocytoma, narrow-angle glaucoma, cardiomyopathy, MAOI therapy, known sensitivity to phenylephrine or sulfites.

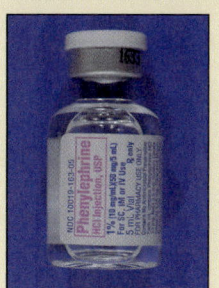

Continued

Phenylephrine (Neo-Synephrine)—continued

Dosage:

- **Adult:** 100 to 180 mcg/min IV, IO. Once the blood pressure has been stabilized, the dose can be reduced to 40 to 60 mcg/min.
- **Pediatric (2 to 12 years):** 5 to 20 mcg/kg IV, IO followed by 0.1 to 0.5 mcg/kg/min IV, IO (max dose: 3 mcg/kg/min IV, IO).

Special Considerations: Pregnancy class C

Phenytoin (Dilantin)

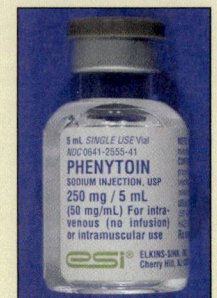

Classification: Anticonvulsant

Action: Depresses seizures by affecting the movement of sodium and calcium into neural tissue.

Indications: Generalized tonic-clonic seizures.

Adverse Effects: Nausea/vomiting, depression of cardiac conduction, sedation, nystagmus, tremors, ataxia, dysarthria, gingival hypertrophy, hirsutism, facial coarsening, hypotension.

Contraindications: Sinus bradycardia, sinoatrial block, second- and third-degree heart block, Adams-Stokes syndrome, known sensitivity to hydantoins.

Dosage:

- **Adult:** 15 to 20 mg/kg IV, IO should be administered slowly at a rate not exceeding 50 mg/min (this requires approximately 20 minutes in a 70-kg patient).
- **Pediatric:** 15 to 20 mg/kg IV, IO, administered at a rate of 1 to 3 mg/kg/min.

Special Considerations:

- Continuously monitor the ECG and blood pressure during administration.
- Pregnancy class D

Potassium Chloride

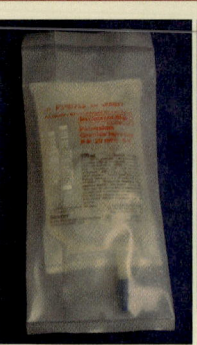
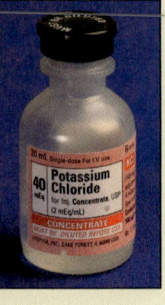

Classification: Electrolyte replacement

Action: Replaces potassium. Slight alterations in extracellular potassium levels can cause serious alterations in both cardiac and nervous function.

Indications: Hypokalemia

Adverse Effects: Hyperkalemia; AV block; cardiac arrest; GI bleeding, obstruction, or perforation; tissue necrosis if the infusion infiltrates into the soft tissues.

Contraindications: Use with caution in patients with cardiac arrhythmias, renal failure, muscle cramps, severe tissue trauma.

Dosage:

- **Adult:** Dosage must be individualized according to patient serum potassium concentration.
- **Pediatric:** Dosage must be individualized according to patient serum potassium concentration.

Special Considerations: Pregnancy class C

Pralidoxime (2-PAM)

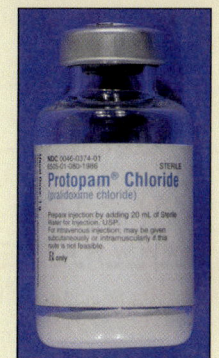

Classification: Cholinergic agonist, antidote
Action: Reactivates cholinesterase.
Indications: Toxicity from nerve agents (organophosphates) having cholinesterase activity.
Adverse Effects: Dizziness, blurred vision, hypertension, diplopia, hyperventilation, laryngospasm, nausea/vomiting, sinus tachycardia.
Contraindications: Myasthenia gravis, renal failure, inability to control the airway.
Dosage:

- **Adult:** 1 to 2 g (dilute in 100 mL normal saline) over a 15- to 30-minute period. If this is not practical or if pulmonary edema is present, the dose should be given slowly (≥5 min) by IV as a 5% solution in water.
- **Autoinjector:** Pralidoxime is also available as an autoinjector that delivers 600 mg IM. Repeat doses can be given every 15 minutes to a total of three doses (1800 mg). Pralidoxime autoinjector is not recommended for pediatric patients.
- **Pediatric:** 20 to 50 mg/kg IV, IO over a 10-minute period.

Special Considerations: Pregnancy class C

Prednisone

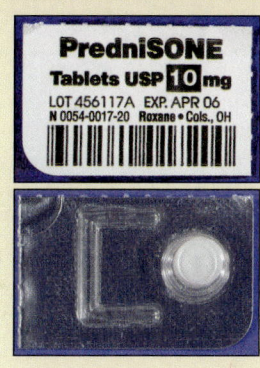

Classification: Corticosteroid
Action: Reduces inflammation
Indications: Inflammatory conditions, such as asthma with bronchospasm.
Adverse Effects: Many adverse effects of steroid use are not related to short-term use but typically are seen with long-term use and during withdrawal.
Contraindications: Cushing's syndrome, fungal infections, measles, varicella, known sensitivity.
Dosage:

- **Adult:** Dosage must be individualized.
- **Pediatric:** Dosage must be individualized.

Procainamide (Pronestyl)

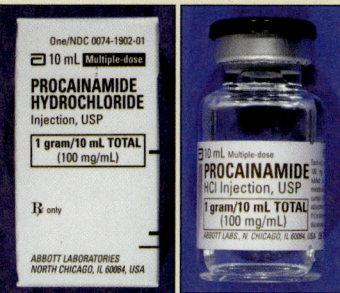

Classification: Antiarrhythmic, class IA
Action: Blocks influx of sodium through membrane pores, consequently suppresses atrial and ventricular arrhythmias by slowing conduction in myocardial tissue.
Indications: Alternative to amiodarone for stable monomorphic VT with normal QT interval and preserved ventricular function, reentry SVT if uncontrolled by adenosine and vagal maneuvers if blood pressure stable, AF with rapid rate in Wolff-Parkinson-White syndrome.
Adverse Effects: Asystole, VF, flushing, hypotension, PR prolongation, QRS widening, QT prolongation.
Contraindications: AV block, QT prolongation, torsades de pointes. Use with caution in hypotension, heart failure.
Dosage:

- **Adult:** 20 mg/min slow IV, IO (max total dose: 17 mg/kg until one of the following occurs: arrhythmia resolves, hypotension, QRS widens by >50% of original width, total dose of 17 mg/kg).

Continued

Procainamide (Pronestyl)—continued

- **Maintenance:** Infusion (after resuscitation from cardiac arrest): mix 1 g in 250 mL solution (4 mg/mL), infuse at 1 to 4 mg/min.
- **Pediatric:** 15 mg/kg slow IV, IO over 30 to 60 minutes.

Special Considerations: Pregnancy class C

Promethazine (Phenergan)

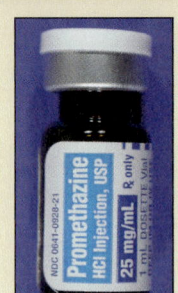

Classification: Antiemetic, antihistamine

Action: Decreases nausea and vomiting by antagonizing H_1 receptors.

Indications: Nausea/vomiting

Adverse Effects: Paradoxic excitation in children and elderly patients.

Contraindications: Altered level of consciousness, jaundice, bone marrow suppression, known sensitivity. Use with caution in seizure disorder.

Dosage:
- **Adult:** 12.5 to 25 mg IV, IO or IM.
- **Pediatric:**
  - **2 years and older:** 0.25 to 1 mg/kg IV, IO, IM (maximum rate of IV, IO administration is 25 mg/min).

Special Considerations: Pregnancy class C

Propofol (Diprivan)

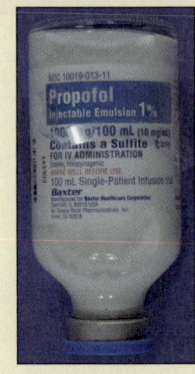

Classification: Anesthetic

Action: Produces rapid and brief state of general anesthesia.

Indications: Anesthesia induction.

Adverse Effects: Apnea, cardiac arrhythmias, asystole, hypotension, hypertension, pain at injection site.

Contraindications: Hypovolemia, known sensitivity (including soybean oil, eggs).

Dosage: A general induction dose used to produce a state of unconsciousness rapidly is 1.5 to 3 mg/kg IV, IO.

Patient Group	Dose	Rate of Administration (10 mg/mL)
Healthy adults younger than 55 years	2 to 2.5 mg/kg IV, IO	40 mg every 10 seconds
Elderly or debilitated patients	1 to 1.5 mg/kg IV, IO	20 mg every 10 seconds
Cardiac patients	0.5 to 1.5 mg/kg IV, IO	20 mg every 10 seconds
Patients with head injuries	1 to 2 mg/kg IV, IO	20 mg every 10 seconds
Pediatric (3-16 years)	2.5 to 3.5 mg/kg IV, IO	20 mg every 10 seconds

After the induction bolus, the patient must be given intermittent boluses or a maintenance infusion. For an average adult, an intermittent dose is 20 to 50 mg as needed. Alternatively, a propofol infusion may be ordered. Maintenance of anesthesia with a propofol infusion can be achieved by following the following protocols:

- **Adult patients:** 25 to 75 mcg/kg/min IV, IO
- **Elderly, debilitated, or head-injured patients:** Use approximately 80% of the normal adult dose.
- **Pediatric:** 125 to 300 mcg/kg/min IV, IO.

Continued

Propofol (Diprivan)—continued

Special Considerations:

Propofol should be administered only by personnel trained and equipped to manage the patient's airway and provide mechanical ventilation. In elderly and debilitated patients, avoid rapid administration to prevent hypotension, apnea, airway obstruction, and/or oxygen desaturation. Continue to monitor the patient's oxygenation and vital signs and try to limit use of propofol to patients who are intubated. Propofol should not be administered through the same IV catheter as blood or plasma. Pain can occur at the site of injection, which can be minimized by use of larger veins, slower rates of administration, and administration of 1 mL 1% lidocaine before propofol administration.

Propofol is listed as a pregnancy class B; however, propofol should be avoided in pregnant women because it crosses the placenta and can cause neonatal depression.

Propranolol (Inderal)

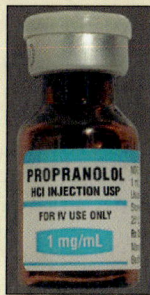

Classification: Beta adrenergic antagonist, antianginal, antihypertensive, antiarrhythmic class II

Action: Nonselective beta antagonist that binds with both the $beta_1$ and $beta_2$ receptors. Propranolol inhibits the strength of the heart's contractions, as well as heart rate. This results in a decrease in cardiac oxygen consumption.

Indications: Angina; narrow-complex tachycardias that originate from either a *reentry mechanism* (reentry SVT) or an *automatic focus* (junctional, ectopic, or multifocal tachycardia) uncontrolled by vagal maneuvers and adenosine in patients with preserved ventricular function; AF and atrial flutter in patients with preserved ventricular function; hypertension; migraine headaches.

Adverse Effects: Bradycardia, AV block, bronchospasm, hypotension.

Contraindications: Cardiogenic shock, heart failure, AV block, bradycardia, pulmonary edema, sick sinus syndrome, known sensitivity. Use with caution in chronic lung disease (asthma and COPD).

Dosage:

- **Adult:** 1 to 3 mg IV, IO at a rate of 1 mg/min; may repeat the dose 2 minutes later.
- **Pediatric:** 0.01 to 0.1 mg/kg slow IV, IO over a 10-minute period.

Special Considerations:

- Monitor blood pressure and heart rate closely during administration.
- Pregnancy class C

Courtesy Gold Standard.

Racemic Epinephrine/Racepinephrine (microNefrin, S₂)

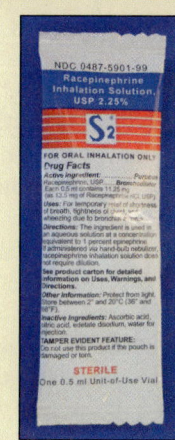

Classification: Bronchodilator, adrenergic agent

Action: Stimulates both alpha and beta receptors, causing vasoconstriction, reduced mucosal edema, and bronchodilation.

Indications: Bronchial asthma, croup.

Adverse Effects: Anxiety, dizziness, headache, tremor, palpitations, tachycardia, cardiac arrhythmias, hypertension, nausea/vomiting.

Contraindications: Glaucoma, elderly, cardiac disease, hypertension, thyroid disease, diabetes, known sensitivity to sulfites.

Dosage:

- **Adult:** Add 0.5 mL to nebulizer; for hand-bulb nebulizer, administer 1 to 3 inhalations; for jet nebulizer, add 3 mL of diluent, swirl the nebulizer and administer for 15 minutes.
- **Pediatric:**
  - **Older than 4 years:** Same as adult dosing.
  - **Younger than 4 years:** Safe and effective use has not been demonstrated.

Special Considerations:

- Monitor blood pressure, heart rate, and cardiac rhythm for changes.
- Onset of action is 1 to 5 minutes.
- Pregnancy class C

Rocuronium (Zemuron)

Classification: Neuromuscular blocker, nondepolarizing
Action: Antagonizes acetylcholine at the motor end plate, producing skeletal muscle paralysis.
Indications: To induce neuromuscular blockade for the facilitation of ET intubation.
Adverse Effects: Muscle paralysis, apnea, dyspnea, respiratory depression, sinus tachycardia, urticaria.
Contraindications: Known sensitivity to bromides. Use with caution in heart disease, liver disease.
Dosage:

- **Adult:** 0.6 to 1.2 mg/kg IV, IO.
- **Pediatric (older than 3 months):** 0.6 mg/kg IV, IO.

Special Considerations:

- Onset of action is 2 to 8 minutes.
- Duration of action is 31 minutes.
- Pregnancy class B

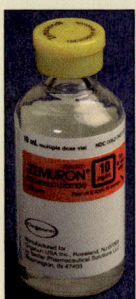

Scopolamine (Transderm Scop)

Classification: Neurologic antivertigo, antimuscarinic
Action: Antagonizes acetylcholine at muscarinic receptors.
Indications: Motion sickness
Adverse Effects: Dry mouth, drowsiness, dilated pupils and blurred vision, hallucinations, confusion.
Contraindications: Glaucoma, cardiac arrhythmias, coronary artery disease, known sensitivity.
Dosage:
Adult and children older than 12 years: 1 disc applied to skin behind ear.
Special Considerations:

- Half-life 8 hours
- Pregnancy class C

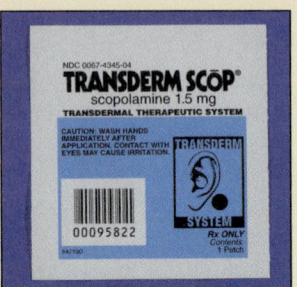

Sodium Bicarbonate

Classification: Electrolyte replacement
Action: Counteracts existing acidosis.
Indications: Acidosis, drug intoxications (e.g., barbiturates, salicylates, methyl alcohol).
Adverse Effects: Metabolic alkalosis, hypernatremia, injection site reaction, sodium and fluid retention, peripheral edema.
Contraindications: Metabolic alkalosis.
Dosage:
Metabolic Acidosis during Cardiac Arrest:

- **Adult:** 1 mEq/kg slow IV, IO; may repeat at 0.5 mEq/kg in 10 minutes.
- **Pediatric:** Same as adult dosing.

Metabolic Acidosis Not Associated with Cardiac Arrest:

- **Adult:** Dosage should be individualized.
- **Pediatric:** Dosage should be individualized.

Special Considerations:

- Do not administer into an IV, IO line in which another medication is being given.
- Because of the high concentration of sodium within each ampule of sodium bicarbonate, use with caution in patients with CHF and renal disease.
- Pregnancy class C

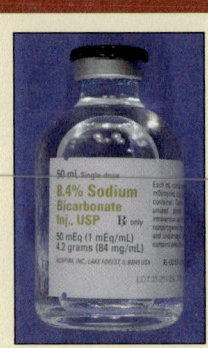

Sodium Nitroprusside (Nipride, Nitropress)

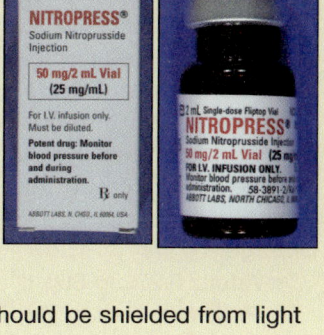

Classification: Antihypertensive agent

Action: Causes direct relaxation of both arteries and veins.

Indications: Hypertensive emergencies.

Adverse Effects: Cyanide or thiocyanate toxicity, nausea/vomiting, dizziness, headache, restlessness, abdominal pain, methemoglobinemia.

Contraindications: Hypotension, increased ICP, cerebrovascular disease, coronary artery disease, hepatic disease, renal disease, pulmonary disease.

Dosage:

- **Adult:** 0.3 to 10 mcg/kg/min IV, IO. Titrate to desired blood pressure.
- **Pediatric:** Same as adult dosing.

Special Considerations:

- Nitroprusside will break down when exposed to ultraviolet light. Therefore the infusion should be shielded from light by wrapping the bag with aluminum foil.
- Pregnancy class C

Succinylcholine (Anectine)

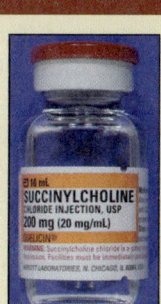

Classification: Neuromuscular blocker, depolarizing

Action: Competes with the acetylcholine receptor of the motor end plate on the muscle cell, resulting in muscle paralysis.

Indications: To induce neuromuscular blockade for the facilitation of ET intubation.

Adverse Effects: Anaphylactoid reactions, respiratory depression, apnea, bronchospasm, cardiac arrhythmias, malignant hyperthermia, hypertension, hypotension, muscle fasciculation, postprocedure muscle pain, hypersalivation, rash.

Contraindications: Malignant hyperthermia, burns, trauma. Use with caution in children, cardiac disease, hepatic disease, renal disease, peptic ulcer disease, cholinesterase-inhibitor toxicity, pseudocholinesterase deficiency, digitalis toxicity, glaucoma, hyperkalemia, hypothermia, rhabdomyolysis, myasthenia gravis.

Dosage:

- **Adult:**
  - **IV:** 0.6 mg/kg IV, IO (range 0.3-1.1 mg/kg).
  - **IM:** 3 to 4 mg/kg (max dose: 150 mg).
- **Pediatric:**
  - **IV:**
    - **Adolescents and older children:** 1 mg/kg IV, IO.
    - **Small children and infants:** 2 mg/kg IV, IO.
  - **IM:** 3 to 4 mg/kg (max dose: 150 mg).

Special Considerations:

- IV administration results in neuromuscular blockade in 0.5 to 1 minute. IM administration results in neuromuscular blockade in 2 to 3 minutes.
- IV administration in infants and children can potentially result in profound bradycardia and, in some cases, asystole. The incidence of bradycardia is greater after the second dose. The occurrence of bradycardia can be reduced with the pretreatment of atropine.
- Succinylcholine can have a significantly prolonged effect in the setting of poisoning with nerve gas agents and organophosphate pesticides.
- Pregnancy class C

Terbutaline (Brethine)

Classification: Adrenergic agonist

Action: Stimulates the beta$_2$ receptor, producing relaxation of bronchial smooth muscle and bronchodilation.

Indications: Prevention and reversal of bronchospasm.

Adverse Effects: Cardiac arrhythmias, arrhythmia exacerbation, angina, anxiety, headache, tremor, palpitations, dizziness.

Contraindications: Known sensitivity to sympathomimetics. Use with caution in hypertension, cardiac disease, cardiac arrhythmias, diabetes, elderly, MAOI therapy, pheochromocytoma, thyrotoxicosis, seizure disorder.

Dosage:

- **Adult:** 0.25 mg Sub-Q every 20 minutes for 3 doses. The usual site for the Sub-Q injection is the lateral deltoid.
- **Pediatric:** 0.01 mg/kg Sub-Q every 20 minutes for 3 doses.

Special Considerations: Pregnancy class B

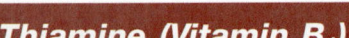

Thiamine (Vitamin B$_1$)

Classification: Vitamin B$_1$

Action: Thiamine combines with adenosine triphosphate to produce thiamine diphosphate, which acts as a coenzyme in carbohydrate metabolism.

Indication: Wernicke-Korsakoff syndrome, beriberi, nutritional supplementation.

Adverse Effects: Itching, rash, pain at injection site.

Contraindications: Known sensitivity.

Dosage:

Wernicke-Korsakoff Syndrome:

- **Adult:** 100 mg IV, IO.
- **Pediatric:** Not recommended for pediatric patients.

Special Considerations: Pregnancy class A

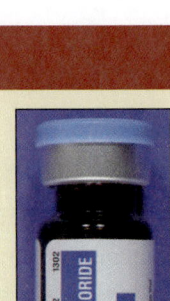
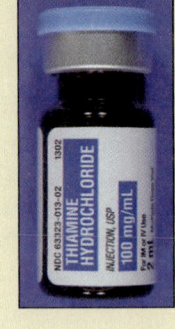

Tirofiban (Aggrastat)

Classification: GP IIb/IIIa inhibitor

Action: Prevents the aggregation of platelets by binding to the GP IIb/IIIa receptor.

Indications: UA/NSTEMI—to manage medically and for those undergoing PCI.

Adverse Effects: Bleeding from the GI tract, internal bleeding, intracranial hemorrhage, hypotension, stroke, anaphylactic shock.

Contraindications: Bleeding from any source, severe uncontrolled hypertension, surgery or trauma within the previous 6 weeks, stroke within the previous 30 days, renal failure, thrombocytopenia.

Dosage: 0.4 mcg/kg/min IV, IO for 30 minutes, then 0.1 mcg/kg/min IV, IO infusion for 48 to 96 hours.

Special Considerations:

- Half-life approximately 2 hours
- Pregnancy class B

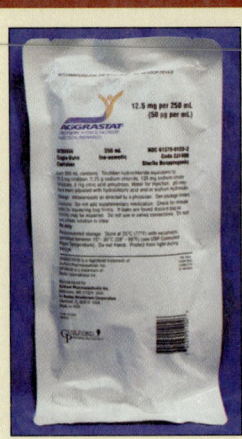

Valproic Acid (Depakote)

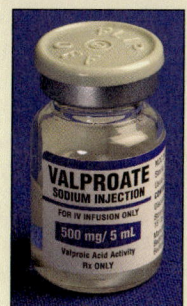

Classification: Anticonvulsant, antimanic

Action: Although the exact mechanism of action is unknown, it is suggested that valproic acid increases brain concentrations of GABA.

Indications: Seizures, mood disorders.

Adverse Effects: Tremor, transient hair loss, weight gain, weight loss.

Contraindications: Liver disease.

Dosage: Dosing is individualized.

Special Considerations:

- Although generally well tolerated, valproic acid does require regular monitoring of blood levels to ensure maintenance of therapeutic levels while minimizing adverse drug reactions.
- Pregnancy class D

Vasopressin

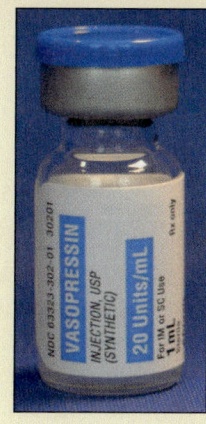

Classification: Nonadrenergic vasoconstrictor

Action: Vasopressin causes vasoconstriction independent of adrenergic receptors or neural innervation.

Indications: Adult shock-refractory VF or pulseless VT, asystole, PEA, vasodilatory shock.

Adverse Effects: Cardiac ischemia, angina

Contraindications: Responsive patients with cardiac disease

Dosage:

- **Adult:** 40 U IV/IO may replace either the first or second dose of epinephrine.
- May be given ET but the optimal dose is not known.

Special Considerations: Pregnancy class C

Vecuronium (Norcuron)

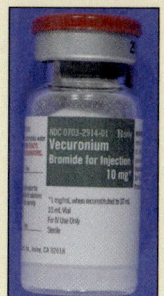

Classification: Neuromuscular blocker, nondepolarizing

Action: Antagonizes acetylcholine at the motor end plate, producing skeletal muscle paralysis.

Indications: To induce neuromuscular blockade for the facilitation of ET intubation.

Adverse Effects: Muscle paralysis, apnea, dyspnea, respiratory depression, sinus tachycardia, urticaria.

Contraindications: Known sensitivity to bromides. Use with caution in heart disease, liver disease.

Dosage:

- **Adult:** 0.08-0.1 mg/kg IV, IO.
- **Pediatric:** Dosage is individualized.

Special Considerations: Pregnancy class C

Verapamil (Isoptin)

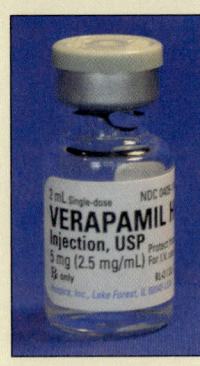

Classification: Calcium-channel blocker; class IV antiarrhythmic

Action: Blocks calcium from moving into the heart muscle cell, which prolongs the conduction of electrical impulses through the AV node. Also dilates arteries.

Indications: Atrial fibrillation, hypertension, PSVT, PSVT prophylaxis.

Adverse Effects: Sinus bradycardia; first-, second-, or third-degree AV block; congestive heart failure; reflex sinus tachycardia; transient asystole; AV block; hypotension.

Contraindications: Second- or third- degree AV block (except in patients with a functioning artificial pacemaker; hypotension (systolic pressure <90 mm Hg) or cardiogenic shock; sick sinus syndrome (except in patients with a functioning artificial pacemaker); Wolff-Parkinson-White syndrome; Lown-Ganong-Levine syndrome; severe left ventricular dysfunction; known sensitivity to verapamil or any component of the formulation; atrial flutter or fibrillation and an accessory bypass tract (WPW, Lown-Ganong-Levine syndrome); in infants <1 yr.

Dosage:

- **Adult:** 2.5 to 5 mg IV, IO over 2 minutes (3 minutes in elderly patients). May repeat at 5 to 10 mg every 15-30 minutes to a maximum dose of 30 mg.
- **Pediatric:**
  - **Children 1-16 yrs:** 0.1 mg/kg IV, IO (maximum 5 mg/dose) over 2 minutes. May repeat in 30 minutes to a maximum dose of 10 mg.
  - **Infants <1 year:** Not recommended.

Special Considerations: Pregnancy class C

Warfarin (Coumadin)

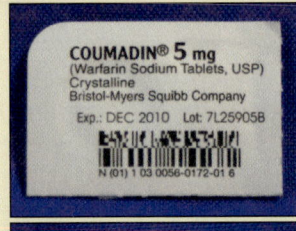

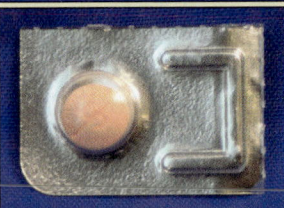

Classification: Anticoagulant

Action: Inhibit the synthesis of vitamin K dependent clotting factors.

Indications: Treatment and/or prophylaxis of thrombosis related to acute coronary syndromes, stroke, deep venous thrombosis, pulmonary embolism, atrial fibrillation, cardiac valve replacement.

Adverse Effects: Bleeding, angina, edema, rash, abdominal cramps, gastrointestinal bleeding, vomiting, hematuria, retroperitoneal hematoma, anaphylactoid reactions, skin necrosis.

Contraindications: Bleeding tendencies, recent or potential surgery of the eye or CNS, major regional lumbar block anesthesia or surgery resulting in large, open surfaces, patient who has a history of falls or is a significant fall risk, unsupervised senile or psychotic patient, eclampsia/preeclampsia, threatened abortion, pregnancy.

Dosage: Dosage is individualized.

Special Considerations: Pregnancy class X

Herbal Supplements

Herbal Product	Uses	Important Facts
Alfalfa	Digestive disorders, arthritis, to increase blood clotting, as a diuretic, cystitis	Should not be used during pregnancy, in patients who have lupus erythematosus; seeds should not be eaten; may increase prothrombin time and prolong bleeding when taken with anticoagulants; may potentiate hypoglycemic action; avoid concurrent use with estrogen and oral contraceptives; may cause hypotension, photosensitivity
Aloe	Minor burns, sunburns, cuts, abrasions, bed sores, diabetic ulcers, acne, stomatitis	Should not be used internally during pregnancy; should not be given to children <12 years; should not be used by persons with kidney disease, cardiac disease, or bowel obstruction; should not be used topically by persons hypersensitive to aloe, garlic, onions, or tulips; may cause GI spasms, intestinal mucosa damage, hemorrhagic diarrhea, red-colored urine, nephrotoxicity, contact dermatitis, delayed healing of deep wounds, hypokalemia, uterine contractions causing spontaneous abortion, premature labor; aloe products taken internally may increase the effects of antiarrhythmics, cardiac glycosides, antidiabetics, loop diuretics, potassium-wasting drugs, systemic steroids, and thiazides; if taken internally, avoid concurrent use with licorice—may cause hypokalemia; aloe may lower serum potassium levels with long-term use
Arginine	Congestive heart failure, erectile dysfunction, peripheral vascular disease, angina, interstitial cystitis, chronic renal failure	Safety in pregnancy and children not established; should not be used by persons with severe hepatic disease; may cause nausea, vomiting, anorexia, increased BUN, hyperkalemia; ACE inhibitors taken with arginine (IV) may lead to fatal hypokalemia; concurrent use of alcohol, NSAIDs, platelet inhibitors, and salicylates may cause gastric irritation
Astragalus	Bronchitis, COPD, colds, flu, GI conditions, weakness, fatigue, chronic hepatitis, ulcers, hypertension, viral myocarditis	Should not be used during pregnancy and lactation; should not be used by persons with acute infections, in the presence of fever, or inflammation; may cause allergic reactions; may decrease or increase action of antihypertensives, avoid concurrent use

Herbal Product	Uses	Important Facts
Belladonna	Irritable bowel syndrome, nervous system disorders, headache, menopausal symptoms, premenstrual syndrome, radiation burns, muscle and bone aches	Should not be used during pregnancy and lactation; should not be used in children; may cause dilated pupils, flushed skin, dry mouth, tachycardia, confusion, nervousness, hallucinations, allergic rashes; should not be used in persons who are sensitive to anticholinergic drugs or who are allergic to members of the nightshade family, such as bell peppers, potatoes, and eggplant; atropine is an ingredient in belladonna, therefore drugs that interact with atropine will interact with belladonna
Betel nut	CNS stimulation, schizophrenia, anemia	Should not be used during pregnancy and lactation; should not be used in children; may cause skin color changes, dilated pupils, blurred vision, difficulty breathing, increased salivation, incontinence, diaphoresis, fever, confusion, psychosis, amnesia, feeling of euphoria; may cause tremors, stiffness in persons also taking antipsychotic medications; chewing betel nuts may cause nausea, vomiting, stomach cramps, diarrhea, chest pain, arrhythmias; do not use concurrently with alcohol, antiglaucoma agents, beta-blockers, calcium channel blockers, cardiac glycosides, MAOIs, neuroleptics
Bilberry	Improve night vision; prevent cataracts, macular degeneration, and glaucoma; treat varicose veins and hemorrhoids; prevent hemorrhage after surgery; prevent and treat diabetic retinopathy and myopia; decrease diarrhea, dyspepsia; control insulin levels	Safety in pregnancy not established; may cause constipation; use caution if taking concurrently with anticoagulants, antiplatelets, aspirin, insulin, iron (avoid concurrent use), NSAIDs, oral antidiabetics
Black Cohosh	Menopausal symptoms, arthritis	Use during pregnancy may cause uterine stimulation; should not be used during lactation; should only be given to children under supervision of a qualified herbalist; should not be used in patients with a history of estrogen receptor–positive breast cancer; may cause hypotension, bradycardia, uterine stimulation, spontaneous abortion, nausea, vomiting, anorexia; avoid concurrent use with antihypertensives, oral contraceptives, sedatives/hypnotics; use cautiously with hormone replacement therapy
Blessed Thistle	Anorexia, GI discomfort, to improve memory, for liver disorders such as jaundice, hepatitis, myrroghia, and dyspepsia; to stimulate lactation	Should not be used during pregnancy; may cause nausea, vomiting, anorexia, contact dermatitis

Herbal Product	Uses	Important Facts
Burdock	Arthritis, diabetes, some skin disorders (e.g., psoriasis, eczema, poison ivy)	May cause hypotension, hypoglycemia; use with caution in persons with diabetes or cardiac disorders; avoid concurrent use with antidiabetics, antihypertensives, calcium channel blockers
Chondroitin	Joint conditions (in combination with glucosamine), coronary artery disease, interstitial cystitis, hyperlipidemia	Safety in pregnancy and children not established; should not be used in persons with bleeding disorders or renal failure; may cause headache, restlessness, euphoria, nausea, vomiting, anorexia, bleeding; do not use concurrently with anticoagulants, NSAIDs, or salicylates
Coenzyme Q10	Ischemic heart disease, CHF, angina pectoris, hypertension, arrhythmias, diabetes mellitus, breast cancer, deafness, Bell's palsy, decreased immunity, mitral valve prolapse, periodontal disease, infertility	Should not be used at excessive levels during pregnancy and lactation; safety in children not established; may cause nausea, vomiting, anorexia, diarrhea, epigastric pain; avoid concurrent use with anticoagulants, beta-blockers, HMG-CoA reductase inhibitors, oral antidiabetics, phenothiazines, or tricyclic antidepressants
Cranberry	Urinary tract disorders; susceptibility to kidney stones	Should not be used by persons with oliguria, anuria; may cause diarrhea (large doses), hypersensitivity reactions
Creatine	Enhance athletic performance	Safety in pregnancy and children not established; may cause nausea, vomiting, anorexia, bloating, weight gain, diarrhea, dehydration, cramping (high doses)
Dandelion	As a laxative, antihypertensive, diuretic	Should not be used during pregnancy and lactation; safety in children not established; should be used with caution in persons with diabetes mellitus or fluid and electrolyte imbalances; avoid use in persons with irritable bowel syndrome, digestive diseases, bile duct obstruction, intestinal obstruction, latex allergy; may cause nausea, vomiting, anorexia, cholelithiasis, gallbladder inflammation, contact dermatitis; avoid concurrent use with antihypertensives, diuretics, insulin, lithium, oral antidiabetics
Devil's Claw	Anorexia, joint pain and inflammation, allergies, headache, heartburn, dysmenorrhea, GI upset, malaria, gout, nicotine poisoning	Should not be used during pregnancy and lactation; should not be given to children; avoid use in persons with peptic or duodenal ulcer disease, cholecystitis; may cause nausea, vomiting, anorexia; use cautiously with antiarrhythmics
DHEA	Atherosclerosis, hyperglycemia, cancer, to improve memory and cognitive functioning	Safety in pregnancy and children not established; avoid use in persons with estrogen-sensitive tumors, prostate cancer, or benign prostatic hypertrophy; may cause arrhythmias (high doses), insomnia, restlessness, irritability, anxiety, increased mood, aggressiveness, acne; avoid concurrent use with hormone replacement therapy

Herbal Product	Uses	Important Facts
Dong Quai	Menopausal symptoms, menstrual irregularities (e.g., dysmenorrhea, PMS, menorrhagia), headache, neuralgia, herpes infections, malaria	Safety in pregnancy and children not established; avoid use in persons with bleeding disorders, excessive menstrual flow, or acute illness; may cause nausea, vomiting, diarrhea, anorexia, increased menstrual flow, hypersensitivity reactions, photosensitivity, fever, bleeding; use cautiously with antiplatelets, oral anticoagulants, chamomile, dandelion, horse chestnut, red clover, St. John's wort
Echinacea	Prevention and treatment of infection (especially a cold or the flu); impaired immune status	Should not be used during pregnancy and lactation; should not be given to children <2 years; avoid use in persons with autoimmune diseases; may cause hepatotoxicity, hypersensitivity reactions, acute asthma attack, angioedema
Ephedra*	Asthma, bronchitis, headache, pulmonary congestion, joint pain and inflammation, to promote weight loss	May cause palpitations, tachycardia, hypertension, chest pain, arrhythmias, stroke, MI, cardiac arrest, anxiety, nervousness, insomnia, hallucinations, headache, dizziness, poor concentration, tremors, confusion, seizures, psychosis, nausea, vomiting, anorexia, constipation or diarrhea, hepatotoxicity, dysuria, urinary retention, hypersensitivity reactions, exfoliative dermatitis, uterine contractions, dyspnea; should not be used during pregnancy and lactation; should not be given to children; should not be used by persons with hypersensitivity to sympathomimetics, narrow-angle glaucoma, seizure disorders, hyperthyroidism, diabetes mellitus, prostatic hypertrophy, arrhythmias, heart blocks, hypertension, psychosis, tachycardia, angina pectoris; avoid concurrent use with anesthetics, antidiabetics, beta-blockers, MAOIs, oxytocics, phenothiazines, sympathomimetics, tricyclic antidepressants, xanthines
Evening Primrose Oil	Premenstrual syndrome; hot flashes; inflammatory disorders; migraine headache	May cause uterine contraction in pregnant women; may lower seizure threshold in seizure disorders or individuals taking phenothiazines; do not use concurrently with phenothiazines
Garlic	Improve circulation; lower blood lipid levels; HTN; inflammatory/menstrual disorders; earaches; diarrhea; cold and flu symptoms; many others	May increase bleeding time—should not be used before or immediately after surgery or with drugs or herbs that affect clotting; should not be used medicinally during pregnancy and lactation—may stimulate labor and cause colic in infants; should not be used by persons with hypothyroidism, stomach inflammation, gastritis; may cause dizziness, headache, irritability, nausea, vomiting, anorexia, hypothyroidism, hypersensitivity reactions, contact dermatitis, diaphoresis, garlic odor, irritation of the oral cavity, decreased red blood cells; do not use concurrently with anticoagulants

*On February 6, 2004, the Food and Drug Administration issued a final rule prohibiting the sale of dietary supplements containing ephedra.

Herbal Product	Uses	Important Facts
Ginger	Nausea, indigestion, sore throat; motion and morning sickness; inflammation; migraine headaches	Safety in pregnancy not established; should not be used by persons with cholelithiasis; may cause nausea, vomiting, anorexia, hypersensitivity reactions; may increase the risk of bleeding when used concurrently with anticoagulants or antiplatelets
Ginkgo	Decrease disturbances of cerebral functioning and peripheral vascular insufficiency in persons with Alzheimer disease or other types of age-related dementia, as an antioxidant, to improve peripheral artery disease, enhance circulation throughout the body, depressive mood disorders, sexual dysfunction, asthma, glaucoma, menopausal symptoms, multiple sclerosis, headaches, tinnitus, dizziness, arthritis, altitude sickness, intermittent claudication	Safety in pregnancy and children not established; should not be used in persons with coagulation or platelet disorders, hemophilia; may cause transient headache, anxiety, restlessness, nausea, vomiting, anorexia, diarrhea, hypersensitivity reactions, rash; avoid concurrent use with anticonvulsants, anticoagulants, MAOIs, platelet inhibitors
Ginseng	Physical/mental exhaustion; stress; viral infection; diabetes; headache	Safety in pregnancy and children not established; should not be used by persons with hypertension, cardiac disorders; may cause decreased diastolic BP, increased QT interval, hypertension, chest pain, palpitations, edema, insomnia, hypertonia, anxiety, restlessness (high doses), headache, nausea, vomiting, anorexia, diarrhea (high doses), hypersensitivity reactions, rash; avoid concurrent use with immunosuppressants, insulin, MAOIs, oral antidiabetics, stimulants
Glucosamine	Joint conditions (in combination with chondroitin)	Should not be used during pregnancy and lactation, should not be given to children; may cause drowsiness, headache, nausea, vomiting, anorexia, constipation or diarrhea, heartburn, epigastric pain, cramps, indigestion, hypersensitivity reactions, rash (rare); may increase the effects of antidiabetics
Goldenseal	Gastritis, GI ulceration, peptic ulcer disease, mouth ulcer, bladder infection, sore throat, postpartum hemorrhage, skin disorders (e.g., pruritus, boils, hemorrhoids, anal fissures, eczema), cancer, TB, may promote wound healing and reduce inflammation	Should not be used during pregnancy because it is a uterine stimulant; safety during lactation and in children not established; should not be used by persons with cardiovascular conditions such as heart block, arrhythmias, hypertension; should not be used locally by persons with purulent ear discharge or by those with ruptured eardrum; may cause bradycardia, asystole, heart block, CNS depression, seizures, paralysis (increased doses), paresthesia, dyspnea (prolonged use), restlessness, nervousness, irritability, cardiovascular collapse, coma, death,

Herbal Product	Uses	Important Facts
		hallucinations, delirium (prolonged use), nausea, vomiting, anorexia, diarrhea or constipation, abdominal cramping, mouth ulcers, hypersensitivity reactions, rash, contact dermatitis, phototoxicity (topical); do not use concurrently with alcohol, antiarrhythmics, anticoagulants, antihypertensives, azole antifungals, benzodiazepines, beta-blockers, calcium channel blockers, cardiac glycosides, CNS depressants, statins, vitamin B
Gotu Kola	Internally: Hypertension, cancer, hepatic disorders, leprosy, varicose veins, chronic interstitial cystitis, cellulite, periodontal disease, to increase fertility; Externally: To promote wound healing, to treat skin disorders (e.g., psoriasis, eczema, keloids)	Safety in pregnancy and children not established; may cause sedation, hypersensitivity reactions (e.g., burning [topical use], contact dermatitis, rash, pruritus), increased blood glucose, increased cholesterol levels; do not use concurrently with antidiabetics, antilipidemics
Grapeseed	Antioxidant, disease prevention, leg cramps, inflammation, vision problems	Safety in pregnancy and children not established; may cause dizziness, nausea, anorexia, hepatotoxicity, rash
Green Tea	Used as a general antioxidant, anticancer agent, diuretic, antibacterial, antilipidemic, and antiatherosclerotic	Should not be used by persons with kidney inflammation, GI ulcers, insomnia, cardiovascular disease, increased intraocular pressure; contains caffeine; may cause hypertension, palpitations, arrhythmia (high doses), anxiety, nervousness, insomnia (high does), nausea, heartburn, increased stomach acid (high doses), hypersensitivity reactions; antacids may decrease the therapeutic effects of green tea; large amounts may increase the action of xanthines and some bronchodilators; do not use concurrently with MAOIs
Hawthorn	Cardiovascular disorders (e.g., hypertension, arrhythmias, arteriosclerosis, CHF, Buerger disease, stable angina pectoris)	Safety in pregnancy and children not established; may cause hypotension, arrhythmias, fatigue, sedation, nausea, vomiting, anorexia, hypersensitivity reactions; avoid concurrent use with antihypertensives, CNS depressants; carefully monitor concurrent use with cardiac glycosides
Horse Chestnut	Fever, phlebitis, hemorrhoids, prostate enlargement, edema, inflammation, diarrhea, varicose veins	Safety in pregnancy and children not established; may cause nephropathy, nephrotoxicity, hepatotoxicity, severe bleeding, shock, nausea, vomiting, anorexia, pruritus, hypersensitivity, rash, urticaria, muscle spasms; do not use concurrently with anticoagulants, aspirin, and other salicylates; may increase the hypoglycemic effects of diabetic medications

Herbal Product	Uses	Important Facts
Horsetail	Internally: Oral diuretic for treatment of edema, osteoporosis; Externally: To promote wound healing	Safety in pregnancy and children not established; may cause weakness, dizziness, fever, weight loss, cold feeling in extremities (very large quantities), nausea, vomiting, anorexia, hypersensitivity reactions, thiamine deficiency; avoid use by persons with edema, cardiac disease, renal disease, nicotine sensitivity; contains nicotine and should not be used for prolonged periods; the active chemicals in this herb are absorbed through the skin and can cause death; avoid concurrent use with cardiac glycosides, cerebral stimulants, diuretics, lithium, xanthines
Kava	Anxiety, depression, insomnia, stress, to promote wound healing	Safety in pregnancy not established; should not be used in children <12 years; should not be used by persons with major depressive disorder or Parkinson disease; most side effects and adverse reactions occur when high doses are taken for a long period; may include pulmonary hypertension, liver damage, increased reflexes, blurred vision, red eyes, nausea, vomiting, anorexia, weight loss, hematuria; decreased platelets, lymphocytes, bilirubin, protein, and albumin; increased red blood cell volume, hypersensitivity reactions, skin yellowing and scaling (high doses), dyspnea; do not use concurrently with antiparkinsonian, benzodiazepines, CNS depressants; antipsychotics taken with kava may result in neuroleptic movement disorders; concurrent use with barbiturates may result in increased sedation
Lavender	Anxiety, insomnia	Safety in pregnancy and children not established; may cause CNS depression, headache, drowsiness, dizziness, euphoria, nausea, vomiting, increased appetite, constipation, hypersensitivity reactions, contact dermatitis; avoid concurrent use with alcohol, antihistamines, opioids, and sedatives/hypnotics
Licorice	Constipation, asthma, malaria, hepatitis, abdominal pain, GI disorders, infections, eczema, chronic fatigue syndrome, insomnia	Safety in pregnancy and children not established; should not be used by persons with liver disease, renal disease, hypokalemia, hypertension, arrhythmias, CHF; may cause cardiac arrest, hypokalemia, hypertension, edema, headache, weakness, nausea, vomiting, anorexia, hypersensitivity reactions; do not use concurrently with antiarrhythmics, antihypertensives, azole antifungals, cardiac glycosides, corticosteroids, diuretics
Lycopene	Cancer prevention	Safety of supplements in pregnancy and children not established; may cause nausea, anorexia

Herbal Product	Uses	Important Facts
Marshmallow	Cough, sore throat, gastric disorders (e.g., IBS, gastritis, constipation), minor skin disorders	Safety in pregnancy and children not established; may cause nausea, vomiting, anorexia, hypersensitivity reactions; may reduce the absorption of oral medications—do not use concurrently
Melatonin	Insomnia, to inhibit cataract formation, to increase longevity, treat jet lag, prevent weight loss in cancer patients	Safety in pregnancy and children not established; may cause tachycardia, headache, change in sleep patterns, confusion, hypothermia, sedation; nausea, vomiting, anorexia; hypersensitivity reactions (rash, pruritus); decreased progesterone, estradiol, LH levels; use cautiously with benzodiazepines; avoid concurrent use with cerebral stimulants, DHEA, magnesium, succinylcholine, zinc
Milk Thistle	Hepatotoxicity caused by poisonous mushrooms, cirrhosis of the liver, chronic candidiasis, hepatitis C, exposure to toxic chemicals, liver transplantation	Safety in pregnancy and children not established; may cause nausea, vomiting, anorexia, diarrhea, menstrual changes, hypersensitivity reactions; should not be used with drugs metabolized by the P-450 enzyme
Passion Flower	Anxiety, sleep disorders, neuralgia, nervous tachycardia, restlessness, opiate withdrawal	Safety in pregnancy and children not established; may cause CNS depression (high doses), severe nausea, vomiting, drowsiness, prolonged QT interval, nonsustained ventricular tachycardia, liver toxicity, hypersensitivity reactions, anorexia; avoid concurrent use with CNS depressants and MAOIs
Propolis	Inflammation, to promote wound healing	Safety in pregnancy and children not established; may cause nausea, anorexia, oral mucositis, stomatitis, hypersensitivity reactions, dermatitis, eczema
Pycnogenol (bark of maritime pine tree) (Horphag Research, Geneva, Switzerland)	Hypoxia in cardiac or cerebral infarction, inflammation; also used as an antioxidant and an antitumor	Safety in pregnancy and children not established; may cause reduced blood platelet aggregation
Pygeum	Urinary tract infections, benign prostatic hypertrophy, to increase prostatic secretions that may cause sterility	Safety in pregnancy and children not established; may cause nausea, vomiting, anorexia, GI irritation; avoid concurrent use with anticoagulants, antiplatelets, hormones, immunostimulants, NSAIDs
Saw Palmetto	Benign prostatic hypertrophy; urinary problems; chronic and subacute cystitis; to increase breast size, sperm count, and sexual potency	Should not be used during pregnancy; safety during lactation and in children not established; may cause headache, nausea, vomiting, anorexia, constipation or diarrhea, abdominal pain and cramping, dysuria, urine retention, impotence, hypersensitivity reactions, back pain
Slippery Elm	Internally: Cough, GI conditions; Externally: For smoothing skin and as a poultice to treat skin inflammation, wounds, burns	May cause spontaneous abortion if used during pregnancy; safety during lactation and in children not established; may cause nausea, vomiting, anorexia

Herbal Product	Uses	Important Facts
Soy	To lower cholesterol, treat hyperactivity, fever, headache, anorexia, chronic hepatitis, menopausal symptoms, osteoporosis, various cancers	No absolute contraindications are known; may cause hypersensitivity reactions, nausea, bloating, diarrhea, abdominal pain; avoid concurrent use with thyroid agents
Spirulina	To promote weight gain in malnourished clients malnutrition, promote weight loss, and for oral leukoplakia	Safety in pregnancy and children not established; may cause nausea, vomiting, anorexia, hypersensitivity reactions; avoid concurrent use with thyroid hormones
St. John's Wort	Anxiety, depression, sleep disorders, viral infection, hemorrhoids, vitiligo, burns	Safety in pregnancy and children not established; may cause dizziness, insomnia, restlessness, fatigue (PO), constipation, abdominal cramps (PO), photosensitivity, rash, hypersensitivity reactions; avoid concurrent use with ACE inhibitors, loop diuretics, thiazide diuretics, alcohol (inconclusive research), immunosuppressants, MAOIs (inconclusive research), NSAIDs, oral contraceptives, SSRIs, sulfonamides, sulfonylureas, tetracyclines; concurrent use of amphetamines, antidepressants, tricyclic antidepressants, trazodone may cause serotonin syndrome; taken PO in combination with indinavir may decrease the antiretroviral action of this drug
Valerian Root	Anxiety, stress, depression, insomnia	Safety in pregnancy and children not established; may cause insomnia, headache, restlessness, nausea, vomiting, anorexia, hepatotoxicity (overdose), hypersensitivity reactions, vision changes, palpitations; may enhance effects of alcohol or sedating substances; avoid if taking antidepressants, pain medications, tranquilizers, antihistamines, anticholinergic drugs, or kava; may increase effects of anesthetics; avoid before surgery; avoid concurrent use with CNS depressants, MAOIs, phenytoin, warfarin

Data from Skidmore-Roth, L. (2004). *Mosby's handbook of herbs and natural supplements* (3rd ed.). St. Louis: Mosby.

GI, Gastrointestinal; *BUN,* blood urea nitrogen; *ACE,* angiotensin-converting enzyme; *IV,* intravenous; *NSAIDs,* nonsteroidal antiinflammatory drugs; *COPD,* chronic obstructive pulmonary disease; *CNS,* central nervous system; *MAOI,* monoamine oxidase inhibitor; *CHF,* congestive heart failure; *HMG-CoA,* 3-hydroxy-3-methylglutaryl coenzyme A; *DHEA,* dehydroepiandrosterone; *PMS,* premenstrual syndrome; *MI,* myocardial infarction; *HTN,* hypertension; *BP,* blood pressure; *TB,* tuberculosis; *IBS,* irritable bowel syndrome; *LH,* luteinizing hormone; *PO,* by mouth; *SSRI,* selective serotonin reuptake inhibitor.

Glossary

800 MHz A type of radio signal in the ultra-high-frequency range that allows splitting a frequency into individual talk groups used as communication links with other system users.

9-1-1/E9-1-1 A set of three numbers that automatically sends the call to the emergency dispatch center. E9-1-1 is enhanced 9-1-1, which gives the dispatcher the ability to determine the caller's location by routing the call through several CAD systems.

Abandonment Terminating care when it is still needed and desired by the patient and without ensuring that appropriate care continues to be provided by another qualified healthcare professional.

Abbreviation A shorter way of writing something.

Abdominal compartment syndrome Syndrome caused by diffuse intestinal edema, a result of fluid accumulation in the bowel wall. It may be caused by overresuscitation with crystalloids and results in shock and renal failure.

Abdominal evisceration An injury in which a severe laceration or incision of the abdomen breaches through all layers of muscle to allow abdominal contents, most often the intestines, to protrude above the surface of the skin.

Aberrant Abnormal.

Abortion The ending of a pregnancy for any reason before 20 weeks' gestation; the lay term miscarriage is referred to as a *spontaneous abortion.*

Abruptio placentae Separation of the placenta from the uterine wall after the twentieth week of gestation.

Abscess A collection of pus.

Absence seizure A generalized seizure characterized by a blank stare and an alteration of consciousness.

Absolute refractory period Corresponds with the onset of the QRS complex to approximately the peak of the T wave; cardiac cells cannot be stimulated to conduct an electrical impulse, no matter how strong the stimulus.

Absorption Movement of small organic molecules, electrolytes, vitamins, and water across the digestive tract and into the circulatory system. Also the movement of a drug from the site of input into the circulation.

Abuse Use of a substance for other than its approved, accepted purpose or in a greater amount than prescribed.

Acalculus cholecystitis Inflammation of the gallbladder in the absence of gallstones.

Acceptance A grief stage in which the individual has come to terms with the reality of his or her (or a loved one's) imminent death.

Accessory muscles Muscles of the neck, chest, and abdomen that become active during labored breathing.

Accessory pathway An extra bundle of working myocardial tissue that forms a connection between the atria and ventricles outside the normal conduction system.

Accreditation Recognition given to an EMD center by an independent auditing agency for achieving a consistently high level of performance based on industry best practice standards.

Acetylation A mechanism in which a drug is processed by enzymes.

Acetylcholinesterase A body chemical that stops the action of acetylcholine (a neurotransmitter involved in the stimulation of nerves).

Acid Fluid produced in the stomach; breaks down the food material within the stomach into chyme.

Acid-base balance Delicate balance between the body's acidity and alkalinity.

Acidic pH less than 7.0.

Acids Materials that have a pH value less than 7.0 (e.g., hydrochloric acid, sulfuric acid).

Acquired immunity Specific immunity directed at a particular pathogen that develops after the body has been exposed to it once (e.g., immunity to chickenpox after first exposure).

Acquired immunodeficiency syndrome (AIDS) An acquired immunodeficiency disease that can develop after infection with HIV.

Acrocyanosis Cyanosis of the extremities.

Action potential A five-phase cycle that reflects the difference in the concentration of charged particles across the cell membrane at any given time.

Activated charcoal An adsorbent made from charred wood that effectively binds many poisons in the stomach; most effective when administered within 1 hour of intake.

Activation phase In phases of immunity, the stage at which a single lymphocyte activates many other lymphocytes and significantly expands the scope of immune response in a process known as amplification.

Active immunity Induced immunity in which the body can continue to mount specific immune response when exposed to the agent (e.g., vaccination).

Active listening Listening to the words that the patient is saying as well as paying attention to the significance of those words to the patient.

Active range of motion The degree of movement at a joint as determined by the patient's own voluntary movements.

Active transport A process used to move substances against the concentration gradient or toward the side that has a higher concentration; requires the use of energy by the cell but is faster than diffusion.

Acute arterial occlusion A sudden blockage of arterial blood flow that occurs because of a thrombus, embolus, tumor, direct trauma to an artery, or an unknown cause.

Acute care Short-term medical treatment usually provided in a hospital for patients who have an illness or injury or who are recovering from surgery.

Acute coronary syndrome (ACS) A term used to refer to patients presenting with ischemic chest discomfort. Acute coronary syndromes consist of three major syndromes: unstable angina, non–ST-segment elevation myocardial infarction, and ST-segment elevation myocardial infarction.

Acute exposure An exposure that occurs over a short timeframe (less than 24 hours); usually occurs at a spill or release.

Acute renal failure (ARF) When the kidneys suddenly stop functioning, either partially or completely, but eventually recover full or nearly full functioning over time.

Acute respiratory distress syndrome (ARDS) Collection of fluid in the alveoli of the lung, usually as a result of trauma or serious illness.

Addiction The involvement in a repetitive behavior (gambling, substance abuse, etc.). In physical addiction the individual has become dependent on an external substance and develops physical withdrawal symptoms if the substance is unavailable.

Additive effect The combined effect of two drugs given at the same time that have similar effects.

Adenosine triphosphate (ATP) Formed from metabolism of nutrients in the cell; serves as an energy source throughout the body.

Adipocyte A fat cell; a connective tissue cell that has differentiated and become specialized in the synthesis (manufacture) and storage of fat.

Adipose (fat) connective tissue Tissue that stores lipids; acts as an insulator and protector of the organs of the body.

Administrative law A branch of law that deals with rules, regulations, orders, and decisions created by governmental agencies.

Adrenergic Having the characteristics of the sympathetic division of the autonomic nervous system.

Adrenocortical steroids Hormones released by the adrenal cortex essential for life; assist in the regulation of blood glucose levels, promote peripheral use of lipids, stimulate the kidneys to reabsorb sodium, and have antiinflammatory effects.

Adsorb To gather or stick to a surface in a condensed layer.

Adult respiratory distress syndrome (ARDS) A life-threatening condition that causes lung swelling and fluid buildup in the air sacs.

Advance directive A document in which a competent person gives instructions to be followed regarding his or her healthcare in the event the person later becomes incapacitated and unable to make or communicate those decisions to others.

Advanced emergency medical technician (AEMT) An EMS professional who provides basic and limited advanced skills to patients who access the EMS system.

Adverse effect (reaction) An unintentional, undesirable, and often unpredictable effect of a drug used at therapeutic doses to prevent, diagnose, or treat disease.

Advocate A person who assists another person in carrying out desired wishes; a paramedic should function as a patient's advocate in all aspects of prehospital care.

Aerosol A collection of particles dispersed in a gas.

Affect Description of the patient's visible emotional state.

Afferent division Nerve fibers that send impulses from the periphery to the central nervous system.

Affinity The intensity or strength of the attraction between a drug and its receptor.

Afterload Pressure or resistance against which the ventricles must pump to eject blood.

Ageism Stereotypical and often negative bias against older adults.

Agonal respirations Slow, shallow, irregular respirations resulting from anoxic brain injury.

Agonist A drug that causes a physiologic response in the receptor to which it binds.

Agonist-antagonist A drug that blocks a receptor. It may provide a partial agonist activity, but it also prevents an agonist from exerting its full effects.

Agoraphobia Consistent anxiety and avoidance of places and situations where escape during a panic attack would be difficult or embarrassing.

Air emboli Bubble of air that has entered the vasculature. Emboli can result in damage similar to a clot in the vasculature, typically resulting in brain injury or pulmonary emboli when neck vessels are damaged.

Air embolism Introduction of air into venous circulation, which can ultimately enter the right ventricle, closing off circulation to the pulmonary artery and leading to death.

Air trapping A respiratory pattern associated with an obstruction in the pulmonary tree; the breathing rate increases to overcome resistance in getting air out, the respiratory effort becomes more shallow, the volume of trapped air increases, and the lungs inflate.

Airbag identification The various shapes, sizes, colors, and styles of visual identification labels indicating that an airbag is present.

Airbags Inflatable nylon bags designed to supplement the protection of occupants during crashes; one of the most common new technology items confronting responders at crash scenes; also known as *supplemental restraint systems.*

Air-reactive materials Materials that react with atmospheric moisture and rapidly decompose.

Alarm reaction The body's autonomic, sympathetic nervous system response to stimuli designed to prepare the individual to fight or flee.

Alcoholic ketoacidosis (AKA) Condition found in patients who chronically abuse alcohol accompanied by vomiting, a build-up of ketones in the blood, and little or no food intake.

Alcoholism Addiction and dependence on ethanol; often develops over many years.

Aldosterone A hormone responsible for the reabsorption of sodium and water from the kidney tubules.

Alkali A substance with a pH above 7.0; also known as a *base* or *caustic.*

Alkaline pH greater than 7.0.

Alkaloids A group of plant-based substances containing nitrogen and found in nature.

Allergen A substance that can provoke an allergic reaction.

Allergic reaction An abnormal immune response, mediated by immunoglobulin E antibodies, to an allergen that should not cause such a response and to which the patient has already been exposed; usually involves excessive release of immune agents, especially histamines.

All-hazards emergency preparedness A cross-cutting approach in which all forms of emergencies, including manmade and natural disasters, epidemics, and physical or biologic terrorism, are managed from a common template that uses consistent language and structure.

Allografting Transplanting organs or tissues from genetically nonidentical members of the same species.

All-terrain vehicle (ATV) Any of a number of models of small open motorized vehicles designed for off-road and wilderness use; three-wheeled (all-terrain cycles) and four-wheeled (quads) versions are most often used for personnel insertion; six- and eight-wheeled models exist for specialized applications.

Alpha particle A positively charged particle emitted by certain radioactive materials.

Altered mental status Disruption of a person's emotional and intellectual functioning.

Altitude illness A syndrome associated with the relatively low partial pressure of oxygen in the atmosphere at altitudes encountered during mountain climbing or travel in unpressurized aircraft.

Alveolar air volume In contrast to dead air space, alveolar volume is the amount of air that does reach the alveoli for gas exchange (approximately 350 mL in the adult male). It is the difference between tidal volume and dead-space volume.

Alveoli Functional units of the respiratory system; area in the lungs where the majority of gas exchange takes place; singular form is *alveolus.*

Alzheimer's disease Progressive dementia seen mostly in the elderly and marked by decline of memory and cognitive function.

Amniotic sac (bag of waters) The fluid-filled protective sac that surrounds the fetus inside the uterus.

Amplitude Height (voltage) of a waveform on the ECG.

Ampule A sealed sterile container that holds a single dose of liquid or powdered medication.

Amygdala Almond-shaped structure at the end of each hippocampus that attaches emotional significance to incoming stimuli; has a large role in the fear response; plural form is *amygdale.*

Amylase Enzyme in pancreatic juice.

Amyotrophic lateral sclerosis (ALS) Autoimmune disorder affecting the motor roots of the spinal nerves, causing progressive muscle weakness and eventually paralysis.

Anal canal Area between the rectum and the anus.

Analgesia A state in which pain is controlled or not perceived.

Anaphylactic reaction An unusual or exaggerated allergic reaction to a foreign substance.

Anaphylactoid reaction Reaction that clinically mimics an allergic reaction but is not mediated by immunoglobulin E antibodies, so it is not a true allergic reaction.

Anaphylaxis Life-threatening allergic reaction.

Anasarca Massive generalized body edema.

Anatomic plane The relation of internal body structures to the surface of the body; imaginary straight line divisions of the body.

Anatomic position The position of a person standing erect with his or her feet and palms facing the examiner.

Anatomy Study of the body's structure and organization.

Anchor point A single secure connection for an anchor.

Anchors The means of securing the ropes and other elements of the high-angle system.

Anemia Deficiency in red blood cells or hemoglobin; most common form is iron-deficiency anemia.

Anesthesia A process in which pain is prevented during a procedure.

Aneurysm Localized dilation or bulging of a blood vessel wall or wall of a heart chamber.

Anger A stage in the grieving process in which the individual is upset by the stated future loss of life.

Angina pectoris Chest discomfort or other related symptoms of sudden onset that may occur because the increased oxygen demand of the heart temporarily exceeds the blood supply.

Anginal equivalents Symptoms of myocardial ischemia other than chest pain or discomfort.

Angioedema Swelling of the tissues, including the dermal layer; often found in and around the mouth, tongue, and lips.

Angle of Louis An angulation of the sternum that indicates the point where the second rib joins the sternum; also called the *manubriosternal junction.*

Anhedonia Lack of enjoyment in activities one used to find pleasurable.

Anion A negatively charged ion.

Anorexia nervosa Eating disorder characterized by a preoccupation that one is obese; drastic, intentional weight loss; and bizarre attitudes and rituals associated with food and exercise.

Anoxia A total lack of oxygen availability to the tissues.

Antagonist A drug that does not cause a physiologic response when it binds with a receptor.

Antegrade amnesia The inability to remember short-term memory information after an event during which the head was struck.

Antepartum The period before childbirth.

Anterior The front, or ventral, surface.

Anterior cord syndrome Collection of symptoms seen after the compression, death, or transection of the anterior portion of the spinal cord.

Anthrax An acute bacterial infection caused by inhalation, contact, or ingestion of *Bacillus anthracis* organisms. Three forms of anthrax disease may occur depending on the route of exposure. Inhalational anthrax disease occurs after the inhalation of anthrax spores. Cutaneous anthrax disease is the most common form and occurs after the exposure of compromised skin to anthrax spores. Gastrointestinal anthrax disease occurs after the ingestion of live *B. anthracis* in contaminated meat.

Antiarrhythmic Medications used to correct irregular heartbeats and slow hearts that beat too fast.

Antibacterial Medication that kills or limits bacteria.

Antibiotic In common medical terms, a drug that kills bacteria.

Antibody Agents produced by B lymphocytes that bind to antigens, thus killing or controlling them and slowing or stopping an infection; also called *immunoglobulin.*

Antidiuretic hormone (ADH) A hormone released in response to detected loss of body water; prevents further loss of water through the urinary tract by promoting the reabsorption of water into the blood.

Antidote A substance that can reverse the adverse effects of a poison.

Antifungal Agent that kills fungi.

Antigen A marker on a cell that identifies the cell as "self" or "not self"; antigens are used by antibodies to identify cells that should be attacked as not self.

Antihistamine Medication that reduces the effects of histamine.

Antiinflammatory mediators Protein entities, often produced in the liver, that act as modulators of the immune response to the proinflammatory response to injury; also called *cytokines.*

Antipyretic medication A medication that reduces or eliminates a fever.

Antisepsis Prevention of sepsis by preventing or inhibiting the growth of causative microorganisms; in the field, the process used to cleanse local skin areas before needle puncture with products that are alcohol or iodine based.

Antivenin A substance that can reverse the adverse effects of a venom by binding to it and inactivating it.

Antiviral An agent that kills or impedes a virus.

Antonym A root word, prefix, or suffix that has the *opposite* meaning of another word.

Anucleated Cells of the body that do not have a central nucleus, such as those in cardiac muscle.

Anus The end of the anal canal.

Anxiety The sometimes vague feeling of apprehension, uneasiness, dread, or worry that often occurs without a specific source or cause identified. It is also a normal response to a perceived threat.

Aorta Delivers blood from the left ventricle of the heart to the body.

Aortic valve Semilunar valve on the left of the heart; separates the left ventricle from the aorta.

Apex Tip.

Apex of the heart Lower portion of the heart, tip of the ventricles (approximately the level of the fifth left intercostal space); points leftward, downward, and forward.

Apgar score A scoring system applied to an infant after delivery; key components include appearance, pulse, grimace, activity, and respiration.

Aphasia Loss of speech.

Apnea Respiratory arrest.

Apnea monitor A technologic aid used to warn of cessation of breathing in a premature infant; also may warn of bradycardia and tachycardia.

Apocrine glands Sweat glands that open into hair follicles, including in and around the genitalia, axillae, and anus; secrete an organic substance (which is odorless until acted upon by surface bacteria) into the hair follicles.

Appendicitis Inflammation of the appendix.

Appendicular region Area that includes the extremities (e.g., arms, pelvis, and legs).

Appendicular skeleton Consists of all the bones not within the axial skeleton: upper and lower extremities, the girdles, and their attachments.

Appendix Accessory structure of the cecum.

Application of principles The step at which the paramedic applies critical thinking in a clinical sense and arrives at a field impression or a working diagnosis.

Aqueous humor Fluid that fills the anterior chamber of the eye; maintains intraocular pressure.

Arachnoid mater Second layer of the meninges.

Arachnoid membrane Weblike middle layer of the meninges.

Areolar connective tissue A loose tissue found in most organs of the body; consists of weblike collagen, reticulum, and elastin fibers.

Arnold-Chiari malformation A complication of spina bifida in which the brainstem and cerebellum extend down through the foramen magnum into the cervical portion of the vertebrae.

Arrector pili Smooth muscle that surrounds each follicle; responsible for "goose bumps," which pull the hair upwards.

Arrhythmia Term often used interchangeably with dysrhythmia; any disturbance or abnormality in a normal rhythmic pattern; any cardiac rhythm other than a sinus rhythm.

Arterial puncture Accidental puncture into an artery instead of a vein.

Arterioles Small arterial vessels; supply oxygenated blood to the capillaries.

Arteriosclerosis A chronic disease of the arterial system characterized by abnormal thickening and hardening of the vessel walls.

Arthritis Inflammation of a joint that results in pain, stiffness, swelling, and redness.

Artifact Distortion of an ECG tracing by electrical activity that is noncardiac in origin (e.g., electrical interference, poor electrical conduction, patient movement).

Artificial anchors The use of specially designed hardware to create anchors where good natural anchors do not exist.

Arytenoid cartilages Six paired cartilages stacked on top of each other in the larynx.

Ascending colon Part of the large intestine.

Ascites Marked abdominal swelling from a buildup of fluid in the peritoneal cavity.

Asepsis Sterile; free from germs, infection, and any form of life.

Asphyxiants Chemicals that impair the body's ability to either get or use oxygen.

Aspiration Inhalation of foreign contents into the lungs.

Aspiration pneumonitis Inflammation of the bronchi and alveoli caused by inhaled foreign objects, usually acids such as stomach acid.

Assault A threat of imminent bodily harm to another person by someone with the obvious ability to carry out the threat.

Assay A test of a substance to determine its components.

Assessment-based management Taking the information you obtain from your assessment and using it to treat the patient.

Asthma A reversible obstructive airway disease characterized by chronic inflammation, hyperreactive airways, and episodes of bronchospasm.

Asynchronous pacemaker Fixed-rate pacemaker that continuously discharges at a preset rate regardless of the patient's intrinsic activity.

Asystole A total absence of ventricular electrical activity.

Ataxia Inability to control voluntary muscle movements; unsteady movements and staggering gait.

Atelectasis An abnormal condition characterized by the collapse of alveoli, preventing the respiratory exchange of carbon dioxide and oxygen in a part of the lungs.

Atherosclerosis A form of arteriosclerosis in which the thickening and hardening of the vessel walls are caused by a buildup of fatty deposits in the inner lining of large and middle-sized muscular arteries (from *athero*, meaning gruel or paste, and *sclerosis*, meaning hardness).

Atlas First cervical vertebra.

Atopic A genetic disposition to an allergic reaction that is different from developing an allergy after one or more exposures to a drug or substance.

Atresia Absence of a normal opening.

Atria Two receiving chambers of the heart; singular form is *atrium*.

Atrial kick Remaining 20% to 30% of blood forced into the right ventricle during atrial contraction.

Atrioventricular junction The atrioventricular node and the nonbranching portion of the bundle of His.

Atrioventricular node A group of cells that conduct an electrical impulse through the heart; located in the floor of the right atrium immediately behind the tricuspid valve and near the opening of the coronary sinus.

Atrioventricular sequential pacemaker Type of dual-chamber pacemaker that stimulates first the atrium, then the ventricle, mimicking normal cardiac physiology.

Atrioventricular valve Valve located between each atrium and ventricle; the tricuspid separates the right atrium from the right ventricle, and the mitral (bicuspid) separates the left atrium from the left ventricle.

Atrophy Decrease in cell size that negatively affects function.

Attenuated vaccine A vaccine prepared from a live virus or bacteria that has been physically or chemically weakened to produce an immune response without causing the severe effects of the disease.

Attributes Qualities or characteristics of a person.

Auditory ossicles Three small bones (malleus, incus, and stapes) that articulate with each other to transmit sounds waves to the cochlea.

Augmented limb lead Leads aVR, aVL, and aVF; these leads record the difference in electrical potential at one location relative to zero potential rather than relative to the electrical potential of another extremity, as in the bipolar leads.

Aura Sensory disturbances caused by a partial seizure; may precede a generalized seizure.

Auricle Outer ear; also called the *pinna*.

Auscultation The process of listening to body noises with a stethoscope.

Authority having jurisdiction The local agency having legal authority for the type of rescue and the location at which it occurs.

Autoantibodies Antibodies produced by B cells that mistakenly attack and destroy "self" cells belonging to the patient; autoantibodies are the pathophysiologic agent of most autoimmune disorders.

Autografting Transplanting organs or tissues within the same person.

Autoignition point The temperature at which a material ignites and burns without an ignition source.

Autologous skin grafting The transplantation of skin of one patient from its original location to that of a wound on the same patient, such as a burn. Autologous means "derived from the same individual."

Automatic location identification Telephone technology used to identify the location of a caller immediately.

Automatic number identification Telephone technology that provides immediate identification of the caller's 10-digit telephone number.

Automaticity Ability of cardiac pacemaker cells to initiate an electrical impulse spontaneously without being stimulated from another source (such as a nerve).

Autonomic dysreflexia Massive sympathetic stimulation unbalanced by the parasympathetic nervous system because of spinal cord injury, usually at or above T6.

Autonomic dysreflexia syndrome A condition characterized by hypertension superior to an SCI site

caused by overstimulation of the sympathetic nervous system.

Autonomic nervous system Division of the peripheral nervous system that regulates many involuntary processes.

AVPU Mnemonic for *a*wake, *v*erbal, *p*ain, *u*nresponsive; used to evaluate a patient's mental status.

Axial compression (loading) The application of a force of energy along the axis of the spine, often resulting in compression fractures of the vertebrae.

Axial loading Application of excessive pressure or weight along the vertical axis of the spine.

Axial region Area that includes the head, neck, thorax, and abdomen.

Axial skeleton Part of the skeleton composed of the skull, hyoid bone, vertebral column, and thoracic cage.

Axis Imaginary line joining the positive and negative electrodes of a lead; also the second cervical vertebra.

Axon Branching extensions of the neuron where impulses exit the cell.

Azotemia The increase in nitrogen-containing waste products in the blood secondary to renal failure.

B lymphocytes Cells present in the lymphatic system that mediate humoral immunity (also known as *B cells*).

B pillar The structural roof support member on a vehicle located at the rear edge of the front door; also referred to as the *B post*.

Babinski's sign An abnormal finding indicated by the presence of great toe extension with the fanning of all other toes on stimulation of the sole of the foot when it is stroked with a semi-sharp object from the heel to the ball of the foot.

Bacillus anthracis A gram-positive, spore-forming bacterium that causes anthrax disease in human beings and animals.

Bacteremia The presence of bacteria in the blood. This condition could progress to septic shock. Fever, chills, tachycardia, and tachypnea are common manifestations of bacteremia.

Bacteria Prokaryotic microorganisms capable of infecting and injuring patients; however, some bacteria, as part of the normal flora, assist in the processes of the human body.

Bacterial tracheitis A potentially serious bacterial infection of the trachea.

Band A range of radio frequencies.

Bargaining A stage of the grieving process. The individual may attempt to "cut a deal" with a higher power to accomplish a specific goal or task.

Bariatric ambulance Ambulance designed to transport morbidly obese patients.

Barotrauma An injury resulting from rapid or extreme changes in pressure.

Barrier device A thin film of material placed on the patient's face used to prevent direct contact with the patient's mouth during positive-pressure ventilation.

Base of the heart Top of the heart; located at approximately the level of the second intercostal space.

Baseline Straight line recorded on ECG graph paper when no electrical activity is detected.

Bases Materials with a pH value greater than 7.0; also known as *caustic.*

Basilar skull fracture Loss of integrity to the bony structures of the base of the skull.

Basophils Type of granulocyte (white blood cell or leukocyte) that releases histamine.

Battery Touching or contact with another person without that person's consent.

Battle's sign Significant bruising around the mastoid process (behind the ears).

Beck's triad Classic signs of cardiac tamponade that include jugular venous distention, hypotension, and muffled heart sounds.

Behavior The conduct and activity of a person that is observable by others.

Behavioral emergency Actions or ideations by the patient that are harmful or potentially harmful to the patient or others.

Belay A safety technique used to safeguard personnel exposed to the risk of falling; the belayer is the person responsible for operation of the belay.

Bell's palsy An inflammation of the facial nerve (cranial nerve VII) that is thought to be caused by herpes simplex virus.

Benchmarking Comparison of operating policies, procedures, protocols, and performance with those of other agencies in an effort to improve results.

Benzodiazepine Any of a group of minor tranquilizers with a common molecular structure and similar pharmacologic activity, including antianxiety, sedative, hypnotic, amnestic, anticonvulsant, and muscle-relaxing effects.

Beriberi Disease caused by a deficiency of thiamine and characterized by neurologic symptoms, cardiovascular abnormalities, and edema.

Beta particle A negatively charged particle emitted by certain radioactive materials.

Bevel The slanted tip at the end of the needle.

Bicuspid valve Left atrioventricular valve in the heart; also called the *mitral valve.*

Bile salts Manufactured in the liver; composed of electrolytes and iron recovered from red blood cells when they die.

Bilevel positive airway pressure (BiPAP) A form of noninvasive, mechanical ventilation in which two (bi) levels of positive-pressure ventilation; one during inspiration (to keep the airway open as the patient inhales) and the other (lower) pressure during expiration to reduce the work of exhalation.

Bilevel positive airway pressure (BiPAP) device Breathing device that can be set at one pressure for inhaling and a different pressure for exhaling.

Bioassay A test that determines the effects of a substance on an organism and compares the result with some agreed standard.

Bioavailability The speed with which and how much of a drug reaches its intended site of action.

Bioburden Accumulation of bacteria in a wound; does not necessarily imply an infection is present.

Biologic agent A disease-causing pathogen or a toxin that may be used as a weapon to cause disease or injury to people.

Biot respirations Irregular respirations varying in rate and depth and interrupted by periods of apnea; associated with increased intracranial pressure, brain damage at the level of the medulla, and respiratory compromise from drug poisoning.

Biphasic Waveform that is partly positive and partly negative.

Bipolar disorder An illness of extremes of mood, alternating between periods of depression and episodes of mania (type I) or hypomania (type II).

Bipolar limb lead ECG lead consisting of a positive and negative electrode; a pacing lead with two electrical poles that are external from the pulse generator; the negative pole is located at the extreme distal tip of the pacing lead, and the positive pole is located several millimeters proximal to the negative electrode. The stimulating pulse is delivered through the negative electrode.

Birth canal Part of the female reproductive tract through which the fetus is delivered; includes the lower part of the uterus, the cervix, and the vagina.

Blast lung syndrome Injuries to the body from an explosion, characterized by anatomic and physiologic changes from the force generated by the blast wave hitting the body's surface and affecting primarily gas-containing structures (lungs, gastrointestinal tract, and ears).

Bleeding Escape of blood from a blood vessel.

Blister agent A chemical used as a weapon designed specifically to injure the body tissue internally and externally of those exposed to its vapors or liquid; the method of injury is to cause painful skin blisters or tissue destruction of the exposed surface area (e.g., mustard, lewisite).

Blocked premature atrial complex Premature atrial contraction not followed by a QRS complex.

Blocking A position that places the emergency vehicle at an angle to the approaching traffic, across several lanes of traffic if necessary; this position begins to shield the work area and protects the crash scene from some of the approaching traffic.

Blood Liquid connective tissue; allows transport of nutrients, oxygen, and waste products.

Blood agents Chemicals absorbed into the body through the action of breathing, skin absorption, or ingestion (e.g., hydrogen cyanide, cyanogen chloride).

Blood alcohol content Milligrams of ethanol per deciliter of blood divided by 100; a fairly standard measure of how intoxicated a person is.

Blood-brain barrier A layer of tightly adhered cells that protects the brain and spinal cord from exposure to medications, toxins, and infectious particles.

Blood pressure Force exerted by the blood against the walls of the arteries as the ventricles of the heart contract and relax.

Bloody show Passage of the protective blood and mucus plug from the cervix; often is an early sign of labor.

Body mass index A calculation strongly associated with subcutaneous and total body fat and with skinfold thickness measurements.

Body surface area (BSA) Area of the body covered by skin; measured in square meters.

Boiling liquid expanding vapor explosion An explosion that can occur when a vessel containing a pressurized liquid ruptures.

Boiling point The temperature at which the vapor pressure of the material being heated equals atmospheric pressure (760 mm Hg); water boils to steam at 100°C (212°F).

Bone Hard connective tissue; consists of living cells and a matrix made of minerals.

Borborygmi Hyperactivity of bowel sounds.

Borderline personality disorder Cluster B disorder marked by unstable emotions, relationships, and attitudes.

Botulism A severe neurologic illness caused by a potent toxin produced by *Clostridium botulinum* organisms; the three forms are food borne, wound, and infant (also called intestinal) botulism.

Bowel sounds The noises made by the intestinal smooth muscles as they squeeze fluids and food products through the digestive tract.

Bowman's capsule Located in the renal corpuscle.

Boyle's law Gas law that demonstrates that as pressure increases, volume decreases; explains the pain that can occur in flight in the teeth and ears and barotrauma in the gastrointestinal tract.

Bradycardia Heart rate slower than 60 beats/min (from *brady*, meaning "slow").

Bradykinesia Abnormal slowness of muscular movement.

Bradypnea A respiratory rate that is persistently slower than normal for age; in adults, a rate slower than 12 breaths/min.

Brain injury A traumatic insult to the brain capable of producing physical, intellectual, emotional, social, and vocational changes.

Brainstem Part of the brain that connects it to the spinal cord; responsible for many of the autonomic functions the body requires to survive (also called *vegetative functions*).

Brake bar rack A descending device consisting of a U-shaped metal bar to which several metal bars are attached that create friction on the rope. Some racks are limited to use in personal rappelling, whereas others also may be used for lowering rescue loads.

Braxton-Hicks contractions (false labor) Benign and painless contractions that usually occur after the third month of pregnancy.

Breach of duty Violation by the defendant of the standard of care applicable to the circumstances.

Breech presentation Presentation of the buttocks or feet of the fetus as the first part of the infant's body to enter the birth canal.

Bronchioles Smallest of the air passages.

Bronchiolitis An acute, infectious, inflammatory disease of the upper and lower respiratory tracts that results in obstruction of the small airways.

Bronchitis Inflammation of the lower airways, usually with mucus production. Often chronic and related to tobacco abuse.

Bronchopulmonary dysplasia (BPD) Respiratory condition in infants usually arising from preterm birth.

Bronchospasm Wheezing.

Brown-Séquard syndrome Group of symptoms that develop after the herniation or transection of half of the spinal cord manifested with unilateral damage.

Bruit The blowing or swishing sound created by the turbulence within a blood vessel.

Bubonic Relating to an inflamed, enlarged lymph gland.

Buccal An administration route in which medication is placed in the mouth between the gum and the mucous membrane of the cheek and absorbed into the bloodstream.

Buffer systems Compensatory mechanisms that act together to control pH.

Bulbourethral glands Pair of small glands that manufacture a mucous-type secretion that unites with the prostate fluid and spermatozoa to form sperm.

Bulimia nervosa Eating disorder consisting of a pattern of eating large amounts of food in one sitting (binging) and then forcing oneself to regurgitate (purging), with associated guilt and depression.

Bulk containers Large containers and tanks used to transport large quantities of hazardous materials.

Bulla A localized, fluid-filled lesion usually greater than 0.5 cm.

Bundle branch block (BBB) Abnormal conduction of an electrical impulse through either the right or left bundle branches.

Bundle of His Fibers located in the upper portion of the interventricular septum that conduct an electrical impulse through the heart.

Burnout Exhaustion to the point of not being able to perform one's job effectively.

Bursitis Chronic or acute inflammation of the small synovial sacs known as bursa.

Burst Three or more sequential ectopic beats; also referred to as a *salvo* or *run*.

Cadaveric transplantation Transplantation of organs from an already deceased person to a living person.

Calibration Regulation of an ECG machine's stylus sensitivity so that a 1-mV electrical signal will produce a deflection measuring exactly 10 mm.

Call processing time The elapsed time from the moment a call is received by the communications center to the time the responding unit is alerted.

Cancer A group of diseases that allow unrestrained growth of cells in one or more of the body organs or tissues.

Capacitance vessels Venules that have the capability of holding large amounts of volume.

Capillaries Tiny vessels that connect arterioles to venules; deliver blood to each cell in the body.

Capillary leak Loss of intravascular fluid (plasma, water) from a loss of capillary integrity or an opening of gap junctions between the cells of the capillaries. May be caused by thermal injury to capillaries or the intense inflammatory reaction to burn injury, infection, or physical trauma.

Caplet A tablet with an oblong shape and a film-coated covering.

Capnograph A device that provides a numerical reading of exhaled CO_2 concentrations and a waveform (tracing).

Capnography Continuous analysis and recording of CO_2 concentrations in respiratory gases.

Capnometer A device used to measure the concentration of CO_2 at the end of exhalation.

Capnometry A numeric reading of exhaled CO_2 concentrations without a continuous written record or waveform.

Capsid Layer of protein enveloping the genome of a virion; composed of structural units called the capsomeres.

Capsule A membranous shell surrounding certain microorganisms, such as the pneumococcus bacterium; also a small gelatin shell in which a powdered or granulated form of medication is placed.

Capture Ability of a pacing stimulus to depolarize successfully the cardiac chamber being paced; with one-to-one capture, each pacing stimulus results in depolarization of the appropriate chamber.

Carbamate A pesticide that inhibits acetylcholinesterase.

Carbon dioxide narcosis Condition mostly seen in patients with chronic obstructive pulmonary disease, in whom carbon dioxide is excessively retained, causing mental status changes and decreased respirations.

Carboys Glass or plastic bottles commonly used to transport corrosive products.

Carbuncle A series of abscesses in the subcutaneous tissues that drain through hair follicles.

Cardiac arrest Absence of cardiac mechanical activity confirmed by the absence of a detectable pulse, unresponsiveness, and apnea or agonal, gasping respirations.

Cardiac cycle Period from the beginning of one heartbeat to the beginning of the next; normally consisting of PQRST waves, complexes, and intervals.

Cardiac output Amount of blood pumped into the aorta each minute by the heart.

Cardiac rupture An acute traumatic perforation of the ventricles or atria.

Cardiac sphincter Circular muscle that controls the movement of material into the stomach.

Cardiogenic shock A condition in which heart muscle function is severely impaired, leading to decreased cardiac output and inadequate tissue perfusion.

Cardiomyopathy A disease of the heart muscle.

Cardiovascular disorders A collection of diseases and conditions that involve the heart (cardio) and blood vessels (vascular).

Carina Area in the bronchial tree that separates into the right and left mainstem bronchi.

Carotid bruit The noise made when blood in the carotid arteries passes over plaque buildups.

Carpal tunnel syndrome A medical condition in which the median nerve is compressed at the wrist (within the carpal tunnel), resulting in pain and numbness of the hand.

Carpopedal spasm Cramping of the extremities secondary to hyperventilation-induced hypocalcemia.

Cartilage Connective tissue composed of chondrocytes; exact makeup depends on the location and function in the body.

Cartilaginous joint Unites two bones with hyaline cartilage or fibrocartilage.

Case law Interpretations of constitutional, statutory, or administrative law made by the courts; also known as *common law* or *judge-made law*.

Catabolic Refers to the metabolic breakdown of proteins, lipids, and carbohydrates by the body to produce energy.

Catabolism Process of breaking down complex substances into more simple ones.

Catalepsy Abnormal state characterized by a trancelike level of consciousness and postural rigidity; occurs in hypnosis and in certain organic and psychological disorders such as schizophrenia, epilepsy, and hysteria.

Cataract A partial or complete opacity on or in the lens or lens capsule of the eye, especially one impairing vision or causing blindness.

Catatonia A state of psychologically induced immobility with muscular rigidity, at times interrupted by agitation.

Catatonic schizophrenia A form of schizophrenia characterized by alternating periods of extreme withdrawal and extreme excitement. During the withdrawal stage stupor, waxy flexibility, muscular rigidity, mutism, blocking, negativism, and catalepsy may be seen; during the period of excitement, purposeless and impulsive activity may range from mild agitation to violence. See *Catatonia.*

Cathartics Substances that decrease the time a poison spends in the gastrointestinal tract by increasing bowel motility.

Catheter shear/catheter fragment embolism Breaking off the tip of the intravenous catheter inside the vein, which then travels through the venous system; it can lodge in pulmonary circulation as a pulmonary embolism.

Cation A positively charged ion.

Cauda equina Peripheral nerve bundles descending through the spinal column distal to the conus medullaris. Cauda equina are not spinal nerves.

Cauda equina syndrome A group of symptoms associated with the compression of the peripheral nerves still within the spinal canal below the level of the first lumbar vertebra, characterized by lumbar back pain, motor and sensory deficits, and bowel or bladder incontinence.

Caudal A position toward the distal end of the body; usually inferior.

Causation In a negligence case, the negligence of the defendant must have caused or created the harm sustained by the plaintiff; also referred to as *proximate cause.*

Caustic A substance with a pH above 7.0; also known as a *base* or *alkali.*

Cecum First segment of the large intestine; the appendix is its accessory structure.

Cell body Portion of the neuron containing the organelles, where essential cellular functions are performed.

Cell-mediated immunity Form of acquired immunity; results from activation of T lymphocytes that were previously sensitized to a specific antigen.

Cellular swelling Swelling of cellular tissues, usually from injury.

Cellulitis An inflammation of the skin.

Cementum A layer of tough tissue that anchors the root of a tooth to the periodontal membrane/ligament.

Central cord syndrome Collection of symptoms seen after the death of the central portion of the spinal cord.

Central nervous system (CNS) The brain and spinal cord.

Central neurogenic hyperventilation Similar to Kussmaul respirations; characterized as deep, rapid breathing; associated with increased intracranial pressure.

Central retinal artery occlusion (CRAO) A condition in which the blood supply to the retina is blocked because of a clot or embolus in the central retinal artery or one of its branches.

Central vein A major vein of the chest, neck, or abdomen.

Central venous catheter A catheter through a vein to end in the superior vena cava or right atrium of the heart for medication or fluid administration.

Centrioles Paired, rodlike structures that exist in a specialized area of the cytoplasm known as the centrosome.

Centrosome Specialized area of the cytoplasm; plays an important role in the process of cell division.

Cephalic A position toward the head; usually superior.

Cerebellum Area of the brain involved in fine and gross coordination; responsible for interpretation of actual movement and correction of any movements that interfere with coordination and the body's position.

Cerebral contusion A brain injury in which brain tissue is bruised in a local area but does not puncture the pia mater.

Cerebral palsy Neuromuscular condition in which the patient has difficulty controlling the voluntary muscles because of damage to a portion of the brain.

Cerebral perfusion pressure (CPP) Pressure inside the cerebral arteries and an indicator of brain perfusion; calculated by subtracting intracranial pressure from mean arterial pressure (CPP = MAP − ICP).

Cerebrospinal fluid (CSF) Fluid that bathes, protects, and nourishes the central nervous system.

Cerebrovascular accident (CVA) Blockage or hemorrhage of the blood vessels in the brain, usually causing focal neurologic deficits; also known as a *stroke.*

Cerebrum Largest part of the brain, divided into right and left hemispheres.

Certification An external verification of the competencies that an individual has achieved and typically involves an examination process; in healthcare these processes are typically designed to verify that an individual has achieved minimal competency to ensure safe and effective patient care.

Certified Flight Paramedic (FP-C) A certification obtained by paramedics on successful completion of the Flight Paramedic Examination.

Certified Flight Registered Nurse (CFRN) A nurse who has completed education, training, and certification beyond a registered nurse with a focus on air medical transport of potentially critically ill or injured patients.

Cerumen Earwax.

Ceruminous glands Glands lining the external auditory canal; produce cerumen or earwax.

Cervical spondylosis Degeneration of two or more cervical vertebrae, usually resulting in a narrowing of the space between the vertebrae.

Cervical vertebrae First seven vertebrae in descending order from the base of the skull.

Cervix Inferior portion of the uterus.

Chalazion A small bump on the eyelid caused by a blocked oil gland.

Charles' law Law stating that oxygen cylinders can have variations in pressure readings in different ambient temperatures.

Chelating agent A substance that can bind metals; used as an antidote to many heavy metal poisonings.

Chemical Abstracts Services (CAS) number Unique identification number of chemicals, much like a person's Social Security number.

Chemical asphyxiants Chemicals that prevent the transportation of oxygen to the cells or the use of oxygen at the cellular level.

Chemical name A precise description of a drug's chemical composition and molecular structure.

Chemical restraints Agents such as sedatives that can suppress a patient's neurologic and/or motor capabilities and reduce the threat to the paramedic; also known as *pharmacologic restraints*.

Cheyne-Stokes respirations A pattern of gradually increasing rate and depth of breathing that tapers to slower and shallower breathing with a period of apnea before the cycle repeats itself; often described as a crescendo-decrescendo pattern or periodic breathing.

Chief complaint The reason the patient has sought medical attention.

Child maltreatment An all-encompassing term for all types of child abuse and neglect, including physical abuse, emotional abuse, sexual abuse, and neglect.

Chloracetophenone Tear gas; commercially known as *Mace*.

Choanal atresia Narrowing or blockage of one or both nares by membranous or bony tissue.

Choking agent An industrial chemical used as a weapon to kill those who inhale the vapors or gases; the method of injury is asphyxiation resulting from lung damage from hydrochloric acid burns (e.g., chlorine, phosgene); also known as a pulmonary agent.

Cholangitis Inflammation of the bile duct.

Cholecystitis Inflammation of the gallbladder.

Choledocholithiasis The presence of gallstones in the common bile duct.

Cholelithiasis The presence of stones in the gallbladder.

Cholinergic Having the characteristics of the parasympathetic division of the autonomic nervous system.

Cholinesterase inhibitor A chemical that blocks the action of acetylcholinesterase; thus the neurotransmitter acetylcholine is allowed to send its signals continuously to innervate nerve endings.

Chordae tendineae Fibrous bands of tissue in the valves that attach to each part or cusp of the valve.

Chorioamnionitis Infection of the amniotic sac and its contents.

Choroid Vascular layer of the eyeball.

Choroid plexus Group of specialized cells in the ventricles of the brain; filters blood through cerebral capillaries to create the cerebrospinal fluid.

Chromatin Material within a cell nucleus from which the chromosomes are formed.

Chromosomes Any of the threadlike structures in the nucleus of a cell that function in the transmission of genetic information; each consists of a double strand of DNA attached to proteins called histones.

Chronic Long, drawn out; applied to a disease that is not acute.

Chronic exposure An exposure to low concentrations over a long period.

Chronic obstructive pulmonary disease (COPD) A progressive and irreversible condition characterized by diminished inspiratory and expiratory capacity of the lungs.

Chronic renal failure The gradual, long-term deterioration of kidney function.

Chronology The arrangement of events in time.

Chronotropism A change in heart rate.

Chute time The time required to get a unit en route to a call from dispatch.

Chyme Semifluid mass of partly digested food expelled by the stomach into the duodenum.

Ciliary body Consists of muscles that change the shape of the lens in the eye; includes a network of capillaries that produce aqueous humor.

Circadian A daily rhythmic activity cycle based on 24-hour intervals or events that occur at approximately 24-hour intervals, such as certain physiologic occurrences.

Circadian rhythm The 24-hour cycle that relates to work and rest time.

Circumflex artery Division of the left coronary artery.

Circumoral paresthesia A feeling of tingling around the lips and mouth caused by hyperventilation.

Circumstantial thinking Adding detours and extra details to conversations but eventually returning to the main topic.

Cirrhosis A chronic degenerative disease of the liver.

Civil law A branch of law that deals with torts (civil wrongs) committed by one individual, organization, or group against another.

Clarification Using a phrase or question in an attempt to clarify any ambiguous statements or words.

Classic heat stroke Heat stroke caused by environmental exposure that results in core hyperthermia greater than 40°C (104°F).

Clean To wash with soap and water.

Cleft lip Incomplete closure of the upper lip.

Cleft palate Incomplete closure of the hard and/or soft palate of the mouth.

Clinical performance indicator A definable, measurable, skilled task completed by the dispatcher that has a significant impact on the delivery of patient care.

Clitoris Small, erectile structure superior to the entrance to the vagina.

Closed-ended questions A form of interview question that limits a patient's response to simple, brief words or phrases (e.g., "yes or no," "sharp or dull").

Closed fracture Fracture of the bone tissue that has not broken the skin tissue.

Clostridium botulinum A bacterium that produces a powerful toxin that causes botulism disease in human beings, waterfowl, and cattle.

Cluster A personality disorders Odd and eccentric type of personality disorders, including paranoid, schizoid, and schizotypal; characterized by social isolation and odd thought processes.

Cluster B personality disorders Emotional and dramatic type of personality disorders, including histrionic, borderline, antisocial, and narcissistic; characterized by impulsive, unpredictable behavior, and manipulation of others.

Cluster C personality disorders Anxious and fearful type of personality disorders, including avoidant, dependent, and compulsive; marked by anxiety, shyness, and avoidance of conflict.

Cluster headache A migraine-like condition characterized by attacks of intense unilateral pain. The pain occurs most often over the eye and forehead and is accompanied by flushing and watering of the eyes and nose. The attacks occur in groups, with a duration of several hours.

CNS-PAD An acronym for *c*entral *n*ervous *s*ystem padding: *p*ia mater, *a*rachnid mater, *d*ura mater.

Coagulation Formation of blood clots with the associated increase in blood viscosity.

Coagulation cascade A set of interactions of the circulating clotting factors.

Coagulation necrosis Dead or dying tissue that forms a scar or eschar.

Cocaine hydrochloride Fine, white powdered form of cocaine, a powerful central nervous system stimulant; typically snorted intranasally.

Coccyx (coccygeal vertebrae) Terminal end of the spinal column; a tail-like bone composed of three to five vertebra. No nerve roots travel through the coccyx.

Cochlea Bony structure in the inner ear resembling a tiny snail shell.

Code of ethics A guide for interactions between members of a specific profession (such as physicians) and the public.

Codependence A psychological concept defined as exhibiting too much and often inappropriate caring behavior.

Cognition Operation of the mind by which one becomes aware of objects of thought or perception; includes all aspects of perceiving, thinking, and remembering.

Cognitive disability An impairment that affects an individual's awareness and memory as well as his or her ability to learn, process information, communicate, and make decisions.

Cognitive phase In the phases of immune response, the stage at which a foreign antigen is recognized to be present.

Cold diuresis The occurrence of increased urine production on exposure to cold.

Cold protective response The mechanism associated with cold water in which individuals can survive extended periods of submersion.

Cold zone A safe area isolated from the area of contamination; also called the *support zone*. This zone has safe and easy access. It contains the command post and staging areas for personnel, vehicles, and equipment. EMS personnel are stationed in the cold zone.

Collagen A fibrous protein that provides elasticity and strength to skin and the body's connective tissue.

Collapsed lung See *Pneumothorax*.

Colostomy Incision in the colon for the purpose of making a temporary or permanent opening between the bowel and the abdominal wall.

Combination deployment Using a mix of geographic coverage and demand posts to best serve the community given the number of ambulances available at any one time.

Combining form A word root followed by a vowel.

Combining vowel A vowel that is added to a word root before a suffix.

Comfort care Medical care intended to provide relief from pain and discomfort, such as the control of pain with medications.

Command post The location from which incident operations are directed.

Comminuted skull fracture Breakage of a bone or bones of the skull into multiple fragments.

Communicable period The period after infection during which the diease may be transmitted to another host.

Communication The exchange of thoughts, messages, and information.

Compartment syndrome (CS) A condition in which compartment pressures increase in an injured extremity to the point that capillary circulation is stopped; often only correctable through surgical opening of the compartment.

Compensatory pause Pause for which the normal beat after a premature complex occurs when expected; also called a *complete pause*.

Complete abortion Passage of all fetal tissue before 20 weeks of gestation.

Complex Several waveforms.

Complex partial seizure A seizure affecting only one part of the brain that does alter consciousness.

Compliance The resistance of the patient's lung tissue to ventilation.

Compound presentation Presentation of an extremity beside the major presenting fetal part.

Compound skull fracture Open skull fracture.

Compound word Word that contains more than one root.

Computer-aided dispatch (CAD) A computer-aided system that automates dispatching by enhanced data collection, rapid recall of information, dispatch mapping, as well as unit tracking and the ability to track and dispatch resources.

Concealment To hide or put out of site; provides no ballistic protection.

Concept formation The initial formation of an overall concept of care for a particular patient begins when the paramedic arrives on location of the incident.

Conception The act or process of fertilization; beginning of pregnancy.

Concurrent medical direction Consultation with a physician or other advanced healthcare professional by telephone, radio, or other electronic means, permitting the physician and paramedic to decide together on the best course of action in the delivery of patient care.

Concussion A brain injury with a transient impairment of consciousness followed by a rapid recovery to baseline neurologic activity.

Conducting arteries Large arteries of the body (e.g., aorta and the pulmonary trunk); have more elastic tissue and less smooth muscle; stretch under great pressures and then quickly return back to their original shapes.

Conduction system A system of pathways in the heart composed of specialized electrical (pacemaker) cells.

Conductive hearing loss Type of deafness that occurs where there is a problem with the transfer of sound from the outer to the inner ear.

Conductivity Ability of a cardiac cell to receive an electrical stimulus and conduct that impulse to an adjacent cardiac cell.

Confidentiality Protection of patient information in any form and the disclosure of that information only as needed for patient care or as otherwise permitted by law.

Confined space By Occupational Safety and Health Administration (OSHA) definition, a space large enough and configured so that an employee can enter and perform assigned work but has limited or restricted means for entry or exit (e.g., tanks, vessels, silos, storage bins, hoppers, vaults, and pits are spaces that may have limited means of entry); not designed for continuous employee occupancy.

Confrontation Focusing on a particular point made during the interview.

Congenital Present at or before birth.

Conjunctiva Thin, transparent mucous membrane that covers the inner surface of the eyelids and the outer surface of the sclera.

Conjunctivitis Inflammation of the conjunctiva.

Connective tissue Most abundant type of tissue in the body; composed of cells that are separated by a matrix.

Conscious sedation A medication or combination of medications that allows a patient to undergo what could be an unpleasant experience by producing an altered level of consciousness but not complete anesthesia. The goal is for the patient to breathe spontaneously and maintain his or her own airway.

Consensus formula Formula used to calculate the volume of fluid needed to properly resuscitate a burn patient. The formula is 2 to 4 mL/kg/% total body surface area burned. This is the formula currently regarded by the American Burn Association as the standard of care in adult burn patients. Several other, similar formulas exist that also may be used.

Consent Permission.

Constricted affect Emotion shown in degrees less than expected.

Contamination The deposition or absorption of chemical, biologic, or radiologic materials onto personnel or other materials.

Contamination reduction zone See *Warm zone.*

Continuing education (CE) Lifelong learning.

Continuous positive airway pressure (CPAP) The delivery of slight positive pressure throughout the respiratory cycle to prevent airway collapse, reduce the work of breathing, and improve alveolar ventilation.

Continuous positive airway pressure (CPAP) device Breathing device that allows delivery of slight positive pressure to prevent airway collapse and improve oxygenation and ventilation in spontaneously breathing patients.

Continuous quality improvement (CQI) Programs designed to improve the level of care; commonly driven by quality assurance.

Contractility Ability of cardiac cells to shorten, causing cardiac muscle contraction in response to an electrical stimulus.

Contraction Rhythmic tightening of the muscular uterine wall that occurs during normal labor and leads to expulsion of the fetus and placenta from the uterus.

Contraction interval The time from the beginning of one contraction to the beginning of the next contraction.

Contraction time The time from the beginning to the end of a single uterine contraction.

Contraindication Use of a drug for a condition when it is not advisable.

Contrecoup injury An injury at another site, usually opposite the point of impact.

Contributory negligence An injured plaintiff's failure to exercise due care that, along with the defendant's negligence, contributed to the injury.

Conus medullaris Terminal end of the spinal cord.

Conus medullaris syndrome Complications resulting from injury to the conus medullaris.

Conventional silo A vertical structure used to store ensiled plant material in a aerobic environment.

Cor pulmonale Right-sided heart failure caused by pulmonary disease.

Core body temperature The measured body temperature within the core of the body; generally measured with an esophageal probe; normal is 98.6° F.

Cornea Avascular, transparent structure that permits light through to the interior of the eye.

Coronary artery disease Disease of the arteries that supply the heart muscle with blood.

Coronary heart disease Disease of the coronary arteries and their resulting complications, such as angina pectoris or acute myocardial infarction.

Coronary sinus Venous drain for the coronary circulation into the right atrium.

Corrosive A substance able to corrode tissue or metal (e.g., acids and bases).

Corticosteroids See *Adrenocortical steroids*.

Cosmesis Of or referring to the improvement of physical appearance.

Costal angle The angle formed by the margins of the ribs at the sternum.

Costochondritis Inflammation of the cartilage in the anterior chest that causes chest pain.

Coughing A protective mechanism usually induced by mucosal irritation; the forceful, spastic expiration experienced during coughing aids in the clearance of the bronchi and bronchioles.

Coup contrecoup An injury most often associated with a blow to the skull in which the force of the impact is transmitted through the skull bones to the opposite side of the head, where the bruise, fracture, or other sign of injury appears.

Coup injury An injury directly below the point of impact.

Couplet Two consecutive premature complexes.

Cover A type of concealment that hides the body and offers ballistic protection.

Crack cocaine Solid, brownish-white crystal form of cocaine, a powerful central nervous system stimulant; typically smoked.

Crackles (rales) As the name implies, when fluid accumulates in the smaller airway passages, air passing through the fluid creates a moist crackling or popping sound heard on inspiration.

Cranial nerve Twelve pairs of nerves that exit the brain and innervate the head and face; some also are part of the visceral portion of the peripheral nervous system.

Cranium The vaultlike portion of the skull, behind and above the face.

Creatinine End product of creatine metabolism; released during anaerobic metabolism. Elevated levels of creatinine are common in advanced stages of renal failure.

Creatine kinase An enzyme in skeletal and cardiac muscles that is released into circulation as a result of tissue damage. Can be used as a laboratory indicator of muscle damage.

Credentialing A local process by which an individual is permitted by a specific entity (e.g., medical director) to practice in a specific setting (e.g., EMS agency).

Crepitation A crackling sound indicative of bone ends grinding together.

Crepitus The grating, crackling, or popping sounds and sensations experienced under skin and joints.

Cricoid cartilage Most inferior cartilage of the larynx; only complete ring in the larynx.

Cricothyroid membrane A fibrous membrane located between the cricoid and thyroid cartilages.

Cricothyrotomy An emergency procedure performed to allow rapid entrance to the airway (by the cricothyroid membrane) for temporary oxygenation and ventilation.

Crime scene A location where any part of a criminal act has occurred or where evidence relating to a crime may be found.

Criminal law A branch of law in which the federal, state, or local government prosecutes individuals on behalf of society for violating laws designed to safeguard society.

Cross tolerance Decreasing responsiveness to the effects of a drug in a drug classification (such as narcotics) and the likelihood of development of decreased responsiveness to another drug in that classification.

Crossmatch The process by which blood compatibility is determined by mixing blood samples from the donor and recipient.

Croup A viral infection of the upper airway; respiratory distress caused by narrowing below the glottis and characterized by hoarseness, inspiratory stridor, and a barking cough.

Crown The visible part of a tooth.

Crowning The appearance of the first part of the infant at the vaginal opening during delivery.

Crush points Formed when two objects are moving toward each other or when one object is moving toward a stationary object and the gap between the two is decreasing.

Crush syndrome Renal failure and shock after crush injuries.

Crust A collection of cellular debris or dried blood; often called a *scab*.

Cryogenic Pertaining to extremely low temperatures.

CSM *C*irculation, *s*ensation, and *m*ovement.

Cullen's sign Yellow-blue ecchymosis surrounding the umbilicus.

Cultural beliefs Values and perspectives common to a racial, religious, or social group of people.

Cultural imposition The tendency to impose your beliefs, values, and patterns of behavior on an individual from another culture.

Cumulative action Increased intensity of drug action evident after administration of several doses.

Current Flow of electrical charge from one point to another.

Current health status Focus on the environmental and personal habits of the patient that may influence the patient's general state of health.

Cushing syndrome Disorder caused by the overproduction of corticosteroids; characterized by a "moon face," obesity, fat accumulation on the upper back, increased facial hair, acne, diabetes, and hypertension.

Cushing's triad Characteristic pattern of vital signs during rising intracranial pressure, presenting as rising hypertension, bradycardia, and abnormal respirations.

Customs A practice or set of practices followed by a group of people.

Cyanogen chloride A highly toxic blood agent.

Cyanosis A bluish coloration of the skin as a result of hypoxemia, or deoxygenation of hemoglobin.

Cyclohexyl methyl phosphonofluoridate G nerve agent. The G agents tend to be nonpersistent, volatile agents.

Cyclothymia A less-severe form of bipolar disorder marked by more frequently alternating periods of a dysphoric mood that does not meet the criteria for depression and hypomania.

Cylinders Nonbulk containers that normally contain liquefied gases, nonliquified gases, or mixtures under pressure; cylinders also may contain liquids or solids.

Cyst A walled cavity that contains fluid or purulent material.

Cystic fibrosis (CF) Genetic disease marked by hypersecretion of glands, including mucus glands in the lungs.

Cystic medial degeneration A connective tissue disease in which the elastic tissue and smooth muscle fibers of the middle arterial layer degenerate.

Cystitis Infection isolated in the bladder.

Cytokines Protein molecules produced by white blood cells that act as chemical messengers between cells; released in response to injury.

Cytoplasm Fluid-like material in which the organelles are suspended; lies between the plasma membrane and the nucleus.

Cytoplasmic membrane Encloses the cytoplasm and its organelles; forms the outer border of the cell.

Cytosol Liquid medium of the cytoplasm.

Dalton's law (law of partial pressure) Law relating to the partial pressure of oxygen during transport; defines that it is more difficult for oxygen to transfer from air to blood at lower pressures.

Damages Compensable harm or other losses incurred by an injured party (plaintiff) because of the negligence of the defendant.

Data interpretation The step that uses all the data gathered in the concept formation stage with the paramedic's knowledge of anatomy, physiology, and pathophysiology to continue the decision-making process.

Daughter cells Two cells that result from mitosis.

Dead air space Not all the air inspired during a breath participates in gas exchange and can be further classified as anatomic or physiologic dead space. In the average adult male this equates to approximately 150 mL. Anatomic dead space includes airway passages such as the trachea and bronchi, which are incapable of participating in gas exchange. Alveoli that have the potential to participate in gas exchange but do not because of disease or obstruction, as in chronic obstructive pulmonary disease (COPD) or atelectasis, are referred to as physiologic dead space.

Deafness A complete or partial inability to hear.

Debridement Removal of foreign material or dead tissue from a wound (pronounced *da brēd'*).

Decannulation Removal of a tracheostomy tube.

Decompensated shock A clinical state of tissue perfusion that is inadequate to meet the body's metabolic demands; accompanied by hypotension; also called *progressive* or *late shock.*

Decompression sickness An illness occurring during or after a diving ascent that results when nitrogen in compressed air converts back from solution to gas, forming bubbles in tissues and blood.

Decontamination The process of removing dangerous substances from the patient; may involve removing substances from the skin (external decontamination) and/or removing substances from the gastrointestinal tract (internal decontamination).

Deep fascia Fibrous, nonelastic connective tissue that forms the boundaries of muscle compartments.

Deep partial-thickness burn A burn in which the mid- or deeper dermis is injured. Results in injury to the deeper hair follicle, glandular, nerve, and blood vessel structures.

Deep venous thrombosis (DVT) A blood clot that forms in the deep venous system of the pelvis or legs; may progress to a pulmonary embolism.

Defamation The publication of false information about a person that tends to blacken the person's character or injure his or her reputation.

Defendant The person or institution being sued; also called the *respondent.*

Defibrillation Therapeutic use of electric current to terminate lethal cardiac dysrhythmias.

Degenerative joint disease See *Osteoarthritis.*

Dehydration A state in which the body has an excessive water loss from the tissues.

Delayed reaction A delay between exposure and onset of action.

Delirium Short-term and temporary mental confusion and fluctuating level of consciousness, often caused by intoxication from various substances, hypoglycemia, or acute psychiatric episodes.

Delirium tremens (DT) The most severe form of ethanol withdrawal, including hallucinations, delusions, confusion, and seizures.

Delta wave Slurring of the beginning portion of the QRS complex caused by preexcitation.

Delusion False perception and interpretation of situations and events that a person believes to be true no matter how convincing evidence is to the contrary.

Delusions of reference A belief that ordinary events have a special, often dangerous, meaning to the self.

Demand pacemaker Synchronous pacemaker that discharges only when the patient's heart rate drops below the preset rate for the pacemaker.

Dementia Long-term decline in mental faculties such as memory, concentration, and judgment; often seen with degenerative neurologic disorders such as Alzheimer's disease.

Dendrite Branchlike projections from a neuron that receive impulses or sensory information.

Denial A common defense mechanism that presents with feelings of disbelief, such as "no, that can't be right" when a life-threatening or terminal diagnosis is received; one of the stages of the grief response.

Denominator The number or mathematic expression below the line in a fraction; the denominator is the sum of the parts.

Dentin A hard but porous tissue found under the enamel and cementum of a tooth.

Deoxyribonucleic acid (DNA) Specialized structure within the cell that carries genetic material for reproduction.

Depersonalization A sudden sense of the loss of one's identity.

Deployment Matching production capacity of an ambulance system to the changing patterns of call demand.

Depolarization Movement of ions across a cell membrane, causing the inside of the cell to become more positive; an electrical event expected to result in contraction.

Depressed skull fracture A fracture of the skull with inward displacement of bone fragments.

Depression Sorrow and lack of interest in the things that previously produced pleasure.

Derealization A sudden feeling that one's surroundings are not real, as if one is watching a movie or television, not reality.

Dermatomes Areas of the body innervated by specific sensory spinal nerves; also a device used to remove healthy skin from somewhere on the body of the burn patient for the purpose of transplanting (grafting) at another site, such as an excised burn wound or other open wound.

Dermis Located below the epidermis and consists mainly of connective tissue containing both collagen and elastin fibers; contains specialized nervous tissue that provides sensory information, pain, pressure, touch, and temperature, to the central nervous system; also contains hair follicles, sweat and sebaceous glands, and a large network of blood vessels.

Descending colon Part of the large intestine.

Desired action The intended beneficial effect of a drug.

Developmental disabilities Disabilities that involve some degree of impaired adaptation in learning, social adjustment, or maturation.

Diabetes insipidus (DI) Disorder caused by insufficient production of ADH in the posterior pituitary gland, causing a larger than normal increase in the secretion of free water in the urine and poor absorption of water into the bloodstream.

Diabetic ketoacidosis (DKA) Condition found in diabetic patients caused by the lack or absence of insulin, leading to an increase of ketone bodies and acidosis in the blood.

Dialysis The process of diffusing blood across a semipermeable membrane to remove substances that the kidney would normally eliminate.

Dialysis shunt Shunt composed of two plastic tubes (one inserted into an artery, the other into a vein) that stick out of the skin to allow easy access and attachment to a dialysis machine for filtering waste products from the blood.

Diapedesis Migration of phagocytes through the endothelial wall of the vasculature into surrounding tissues.

Diaphragm Muscle that separates the thoracic cavity from the abdominal cavity.

Diaphragmatic hernia Protrusion of the abdominal contents into the chest cavity through an opening in the diaphragm.

Diaphysis Shaft of the bone where marrow is found that forms red and white blood cells.

Diastole Phase of the cardiac cycle in which the atria and ventricles relax between contractions and blood enters these chambers; when the term is used without reference to a specific chamber of the heart, the term implies ventricular diastole.

Diastolic blood pressure The pressure exerted against the walls of the large arteries during ventricular relaxation.

Diencephalon Portion of the brain between the brainstem and cerebrum; contains the thalamus and hypothalamus and the temperature regulatory centers for the body.

Differential diagnosis The list of problems that could produce the patient's chief complaint.

Differentiation Process of cell maturation; the cell becomes specialized for a specific purpose, such as a cardiac cell versus a bone cell.

Diffuse axonal injury (DAI) A type of brain injury caused by shearing forces that occur between different parts of the brain as a result of rotational acceleration.

Diffusion Spreading out of molecules from an area of higher concentration to an area of lower concentration.

Digestion Chemical breakdown of food material into smaller fragments that can be absorbed into the circulatory system.

Digestive tract Series of muscular tubes designed to move food and liquid.

Digoxin A medication derived from digitalis that acts by increasing the force of myocardial contraction and the refractory period and decreasing the conduction rate of the atrioventricular node; used to treat heart failure, most supraventricular tachycardias, and cardiogenic shock.

Dilation Spontaneous opening of the cervix that occurs as part of labor.

Diplomacy Tact and skill in dealing with people.

Direct (closed-ended) questions Questions that can be answered with short responses such as "yes" or "no."

Direct communication Method of intercellular communication in which one cell communicates with the cell adjacent to it by using minerals and ions.

Dirty bomb A conventional explosive device used as a radiologic agent dispersal device.

Disaster An incident involving 100 or more persons.

Disaster Medical Assistance Team (DMAT) Field-deployable hospital teams that include physicians, nurses, emergency medical technicians, and other medical and nonmedical support personnel.

Disaster Mortuary Operations Teams Teams composed of forensic and mortuary professionals trained to deal with human remains after disaster situations.

Discrimination Treatment or consideration based on class or category rather than individual merit.

Disease period The interval between the first appearance of symptoms and resolution.

Disinfect To clean with an agent that should kill many of, or most, surface organisms.

Disinfection Process of cleaning the ambulance, the cot, and equipment; disinfectant substances are toxic to body tissues.

Disorganized schizophrenia A subtype of schizophrenia characterized by an earlier age of onset, usually at puberty, and a more severe disintegration of personality than occurs in other forms of the disease; symptoms include incoherence, loose associations, gross disorganization or behavior, and flat or inappropriate affect.

Dispatch A central location that receives information and collects, disseminates, and transmits the information to the proper resources.

Dispatch factors Training and education of communications personnel, rapid call taking, call prioritization (selecting the most appropriate resources to respond), managing out-of-chute times (getting crews on the road quickly), and providing crews with route selection assistance.

Dispatch life support The provision of clinically approved, scripted instructions by telephone by a trained and certified emergency medical dispatcher.

Disseminated intravascular coagulation (DIC) A complex, systemic, thrombohemorrhagic disorder involving the generation of intravascular fibrin and the consumption of procoagulants and platelets.

Dissociatives Substances that cause feelings of detachment (dissociation) from one's surroundings and self; includes PCP, ketamine, and dextromethorphan.

Distal A position farthest away from the attachment of a limb to the trunk.

Distracting injury An injury that occupies the patient's attention and focus. The injury causes significant enough pain that the patient may not feel pain from other injuries, particularly spine injuries.

Distraction A self-defense measure that creates diversion in a person's attention.

Distress Stress that is perceived as negative; it may be seen as physical or mental pain or suffering.

Distributing arteries Blood vessels that have well-defined adventitia layers and larger amounts of smooth muscle; capable of altering blood flow.

Distribution The movement of drugs from the bloodstream to target organs.

Distributive shock Inadequate tissue perfusion as a result of fluid shifts between body compartments. Burn shock is a distributive shock in which plasma and water are lost from the vascular tree into the surrounding tissues. This shock also is seen in the setting of sepsis, in which a similar fluid redistribution occurs.

Diuretic An agent that promotes the excretion of urine.

Diversity Differences of any kind such as race, class, religion, gender, sexual preference, personal habitat, and physical ability.

Diverticulitis Inflammation of a diverticulum, especially of the small pockets in the wall of the colon that fill with stagnant fecal material and become inflamed.

Diverticulosis A condition of the colon in which outpouches develop.

Documentation Written information to support actions that lead to conclusive information; written evidence.

Donor skin site A site on the body from which healthy skin is removed for the purpose of grafting a burn or other open wound.

Do not resuscitate (DNR) orders Orders limiting cardiopulmonary resuscitation or advanced life support treatment in the case of a cardiac arrest. These orders may be individualized in that they may allow for differing levels of interventions. When individualized, they usually grant or deny permission for chest compressions, intubation or ventilation, and life-saving medications.

Dorsal Referring to the back of the body; posterior.

Dosage The amount of medication that can be safely given for the average person for a specified condition. Also the administration of a therapeutic agent in prescribed amounts.

Dose The exact amount of medication to be given or taken at one time.

Down syndrome A genetic syndrome characterized by varying degrees of mental retardation and multiple physical defects.

Downregulation The process by which a cell decreases the number of receptors exposed to a given substance to reduce its sensitivity to that substance.

Dromotropism The speed of conduction through the atrioventricular junction.

Drop (or drip) factor The number of drops per milliliter that an intravenous administration set delivers.

Drowning A process resulting in primary respiratory impairment from submersion or immersion in a liquid medium.

Drug Any substance (other than a food or device) intended for use in the diagnosis, cure, relief, treatment, or prevention of disease or intended to affect the structure or function of the body of human beings or animals.

Drug allergy The reaction to a medication with an adverse outcome.

Drug antagonism The interaction between two drugs in which one partially or completely inhibits the effects of the other.

Drug dependence A physical need or adaptation to the drug without the psychological need to take the drug.

Drug interaction The manner in which one drug and a second drug (or food) act on each other.

Drug overdose Internalization of more than the safe amount of a medication or drug; often associated with illegal drugs when a user administers too great an amount of substance; may be used to commit suicide.

Drug-food interaction Changes in a drug's effects caused by food or beverages ingested during the same period.

Dual-chamber pacemaker Pacemaker that stimulates the atrium and ventricle.

Dual-stage airbags An airbag with two inflation charges inside; only one of the two charges may deploy during the initial crash, causing the bag to inflate; the second charge of the dual-stage airbag may remain.

Ductus arteriosus Blood vessel that connects the pulmonary trunk to the aorta in a fetus.

Ductus deferens Also known as *vas deferens;* tubes that extend from the end of the epididymis and through the seminal vesicles.

Ductus venosus Fetal blood vessel that conects the umbilical vein and the inferior vena cava.

Due process The constitutional guarantee that laws and legal proceedings must be fair regarding an individual's legal rights.

Due regard Principle used when driving an emergency vehicle of ensuring that all other vehicles and citizens in the area see and grant the emergency vehicle the right of way.

Duodenum First part of the small intestine; has important accessory structures that help digest various types of nutrients.

Duplex A radio system that allows transmitting and receiving at the same time through two different frequencies.

Dura mater Toughest layer of the meninges; top layer.

Durable power of attorney for healthcare A type of advanced directive that allows an individual to appoint someone to make healthcare decisions for him or her if the person's ability to make these decisions or communicate wishes is lost.

Duty to act A legal obligation (created by statute, contract, or voluntarily) to provide services.

Dysarthria An articulation disorder in which the patient is not able to produce speech sounds.

Dyspareunia Pain during sexual intercourse.

Dyspepsia Epigastric discomfort often occurring after meals.

Dysphagia Difficulty swallowing.

Dysphoric mood (dysphoria) An unpleasant emotional state characterized by sadness, irritability, or depression.

Dysplasia Abnormal cell growth; cells take on an abnormal size, shape, and organization as a result of ongoing irritation or inflammation.

Dyspnea An uncomfortable awareness of one's breathing that may be associated with a change in the breathing rate, effort, or pattern.

Dysrhythmia An abnormal heart rhythm.

Dysthymia A constant, chronic, low-grade form of depression.

Dystonia Impairment of muscle tone, particularly involuntary muscle contractions of the face, neck, and tongue; often caused by a reaction to certain antipsychotic medications.

Ebola A viral hemorrhagic fever illness caused by the Ebola virus (Filovirus family); seen mostly in Africa; transmitted by person-to-person contact with body fluids of infected individuals; no specific treatment is available, and it often is fatal within several days.

Ecchymosis Collection of blood within the skin that appears blue-black, eventually fading to a greenish-brown and yellow. Commonly called a *bruise.*

Eclampsia A life-threatening condition of pregnancy and the postpartum period characterized by hypertension, edema, and seizures.

Economic abuse Preventing others from having or keeping a job; forcing control of another's paycheck; restricting access or forcing conditions on others to receive an allowance; stealing money; not allowing others to know about or have access to economic assets.

Ecstasy (MDMA) A synthetic, hallucinogenic stimulant drug similar to both methamphetamine and mescaline.

Ectopic Impulse(s) originating from a source other than the sinoatrial node.

Ectopic pregnancy A pregnancy that implants outside the uterus, usually in the fallopian tube.

Eczema A disorder of the skin characterized by inflammation, itching, blisters, and scales.

Edema A collection of water in the interstitial space.

Effector The muscle, gland, or organ on which the autonomic nervous system exerts an effect; target organ.

Effector phase In phases of immunity, the stage at which the infection is eradicated.

Efferent division Nerve fibers that send impulses from the central nervous system to the periphery.

Efficacy The ability of a drug to produce a physiologic response after attaching to a receptor.

Efflux Flowing out of.

Ejection fraction Fraction (expressed as a percentage) of blood ejected from the ventricle of the heart with each contraction. Generally at least 60% of the blood entering the ventricle should be forced to the lungs or systemic circulation.

Elasticity Ability of muscle to rebound toward its original length after contraction.

Electrical alternans A beat-to-beat change in waveform amplitude on the ECG.

Electrodes Adhesive pads that contain a conductive gel and are applied at specific locations on the patient's chest wall and extremities and connected by cables to an ECG machine.

Electrolytes Elements or compounds that break into charged particles (ions) when melted or dissolved in water or another solvent.

Elevated mood (euphoria) Exaggerated sense of happiness and joy; a feeling of being on top of the world.

Elimination The process of removing a drug from the body.

Elixir A clear, oral solution that contains the drug, water, and some alcohol.

Emancipated minor A self-supporting minor. This status often depends on the minor receiving an actual court order of emancipation.

Embryo The developing egg from fertilization until approximately 8 weeks of pregnancy.

Emergency decontamination The process of decontaminating people exposed to and potentially contaminated with hazardous materials by rapidly removing most of the contamination to reduce exposure and save lives, with secondary regard for completeness of decontamination.

Emergency medical dispatching (EMD) The science and skills associated with the tasks of an emergency medical dispatcher.

Emergency medical responder (EMR) An EMS professional who provides initial basic life-support care to patients who access the EMS system; formerly called *first responder.*

Emergency Medical Treatment and Active Labor Act (EMTALA) A federal law that requires a hospital to provide a medical screening examination to anyone who comes to that hospital and to provide stabilizing treatment to anyone with an emergency medical condition without considering the patient's ability to pay.

Emergency operations center A gathering point for strategic policymakers during an emergency incident.

Emergency service function (ESF) A grouping of government and certain private sector capabilities into an organizational structure to provide the support, resources, program implementation, and services most likely to be needed to save lives, protect property and the environment, restore essential services and critical infrastructure, and help victims and communities return to normal, when feasible, after domestic incidents.

Emesis Vomiting.

Emotional/mental impairment Impaired intellectual functioning (such as mental retardation), which results in an inability to cope with normal responsibilities of life.

Empathy Identification with and understanding of another's situation, feelings, and motives.

Emphysema Lung disease in which destruction of the alveoli creates dyspnea; often associated with tobacco abuse.

Empyema A collection of pus in the pleural cavity.

EMS Emergency medical services.

EMS system A network of resources that provides emergency care and transportation to victims of sudden illness or injury.

Emulsification The breakdown of fats on the skin surface by alkaloids, creating a soapy substance; penetrates deeply.

Emulsion A water and oil mixture containing medication.

Enabling behavior Behavior that allows another individual to continue to stay ill.

Enamel Hard, white outer surface of a tooth.

Encephalitis Inflammation and usually infection of brain tissue.

Encephalopathy A condition of disturbances of consciousness and possible progression to coma.

Endocardium Innermost layer of the heart that lines the inside of the myocardium and covers the heart valves.

Endocrine communication Method of intercellular communication in which one cell communicates with target cells throughout the body by using hormones.

Endocrine gland Where hormones are manufactured.

Endogenous Produced within the organism.

Endolymph Fluid that fills the labyrinth.

Endometriosis Growth of endometrial tissue outside the uterus, often causing pain.

Endometritis Infection of the endometrium.

Endometrium Innermost tissue lining of the uterus that is shed during menstruation.

Endoplasmic reticulum (ER) Chain of canals or sacs that wind through the cytoplasm.

Endorphins Neurotransmitters that function in the transmission of signals within the nervous system.

Endothelial cells A thin layer of flat epithelial cells that lines serous cavities, lymph vessels, and blood vessels.

Endotoxin A substance contained in the cell wall of gram-negative bacteria, generally released during the destruction of the bacteria by either the host organism's defense mechanisms or by treatment with medications.

Endotracheal (ET) Within or through the trachea.

Endotracheal intubation An advanced airway procedure in which a tube is placed directly into the trachea.

End-stage renal disease (ESRD) When the kidneys function at 10% to 15% of normal and dialysis or transplantation is the only option for the patient's survival.

Enlargement Implies the presence of dilation or hypertrophy or both.

Enteral A drug given for its systemic effects that passes through the digestive tract.

Enteric-coated tablets Tablets that have a special coating so they break down in the intestines instead of the stomach.

Enteral drug One that is given and passed through any portion of the digestive tract.

Entrapment A state of being pinned or entrapped.

Envenomation The process of injecting venom into a wound; venomous animals include snakes, insects, and marine creatures.

Environmental emergency A medical condition caused or exacerbated by weather, terrain, atmospheric pressure, or other local environmental factors.

Environmental hazards Hazards related to the weather and time of day, including extremes of heat, cold, wetness, dryness, and darkness, that increase risks to crews and patients.

Enzyme A large molecule (protein) that performs a biochemical reaction in the cell.

Eosinophils Type of granulocyte (white blood cell, or leukocyte) involved in immune response to parasites as well as in allergic responses.

Epicardium Also known as the *visceral pericardium;* the external layer of the heart wall that covers the heart muscle.

Epidemiologist Medical professional who studies the causes, distribution, and control of disease in populations.

Epidemiology The study of the causes, patterns, prevalence, and control of disease in groups of people.

Epidermis The outermost layer of the skin; made of tightly packed epithelial cells.

Epididymis Convoluted series of tubes located in the posterior portion of the scrotum; final maturation of sperm occurs here.

Epidural hematoma A collection of blood between the skull and dura mater.

Epidural space Potential area above the dura mater; contains arterial vessels.

Epiglottitis An inflammation of the epiglottis.

Epilepsy Group of neurologic disorders characterized by recurrent seizures, often of unknown cause.

Epiphyseal plate Found in children who are still generating bone growth; also known as the *growth plate.*

Epiphysis Either end of the bone where bone growth occurs during the developmental years.

Epistaxis Bloody nose.

Epithelial tissue Covers most of the internal and external surfaces of the body.

Epithelialization Migration of basal cells across a wound and the growth of skin over a wound.

Eponym A word that derives its name from the specific person (or place or thing) for whom (or which) it is named.

Erosion A partial focal loss of epidermis. This lesion is depressed, moist, and does not bleed; usually heals without scarring.

Erythema multiforme An internal (immunologic) reaction in the skin characterized by a variety of lesions.

Erythrocytes Red blood cells.

Erythropoiesis The development and differentiation of red blood cells; typically occurs in the bone marrow.

Erythropoietin A hormone that stimulates peripheral stem cells in the bone marrow to produce red blood cells.

Escape Term used when the sinus node slows or fails to initiate depolarization and a lower pacemaker site spontaneously produces electrical impulses, assuming responsibility for pacing the heart.

Eschar A thick wound covering that consists of necrotic or otherwise devitalized tissue or cellular components. In a burn wound, this is the burned tissue or skin of the wound.

Esophageal atresia (EA) A condition in which the section of the esophagus from the mouth and the section of the esophagus from the stomach end as a blind pouch without connecting to each other.

Esophagitis Inflammation of the esophagus.

Esophagoduodenoscopy Medical procedure in which an endoscope is used to look at the esophagus, stomach, and duodenum.

Esophagus Tube surrounded by smooth muscle that propels material into the stomach.

Essential hypertension High blood pressure for which no cause is identifiable; also called *primary hypertension.*

Estimated date of confinement The due date of the fetus.

Estrogen A female hormone produced mainly by the ovaries from puberty to menopause that is responsible for the development of secondary sexual characteristics and cyclic changes in the thickness of the uterine lining during the first half of the menstrual cycle.

Ethanol (ETOH) Colorless, odorless alcohol found in alcoholic beverages such as beer, wine, and liquor.

Ethics Societal principles of conduct that people or groups of people adopt as guidelines for personal behavior.

Ethnocentrism Viewing your life as the most desirable, acceptable, or best and acting a manner conveying superiority to another culture's way of life.

Eukaryotes One of the two major classes of cells found in higher life forms (more complex in structure).

Eustachian tube A small tube connecting the middle ear to the posterior nasopharynx; allows the ear to adjust to atmospheric pressure.

Eustress Stress that occurs from events, people, or influences that are perceived as good or positive. Eustress can increase productivity and performance.

Euthymic mood A normal, baseline emotional state.

Evaluation of treatment A reassessment of the patient overall and specifically the body system(s) affected by that treatment to answer two critical questions: Did the treatment work as intended? What is the clinical condition of the patient after the treatment?

Evasive tactic A self-defense measure in which the moves and actions of an aggressor are anticipated and unconventional pathways are used during retreat for personal safety.

Excision In reference to burn surgery, this is the sharp, surgical removal of burned tissue that will never regain function. Excision is carried out before skin grafting.

Excitability Ability to respond to a stimulus.

Excited delirium Acute and sudden agitation, paranoia, aggression, hyperthermia, dramatically increased strength, and decreased sensitivity to pain related to long-term use of stimulant drugs; often ends in sudden death.

Excoriation A linear erosion created by scratching. It is a hollowed out area that is sometimes crusted.

Excretion Removal of waste products from the body.

Exertional heat stroke A condition primarily affecting younger, active persons characterized by rapid onset (developing in hours) and frequently associated with high core temperatures.

Exhaled CO_2 detector A capnometer that provides a noninvasive estimate of alveolar ventilation, the concentration of exhaled CO_2 from the lungs, and arterial carbon dioxide content; also called an *end-tidal CO_2 detector.*

Exhaustion The last stage of the stress response and the body's inability to respond appropriately to subsequent stressors.

Exhaustion stage Occurs when the body's resistance to a stressor (decreased reaction to the stress, tolerance) and the ability to adapt fail; the ability to respond appropriately to other stressors may then fail; the immune system can be affected, and the individual may be at risk physically or emotionally.

Exogenous Produced outside the organism.

Exotoxin Proteins released during the growth phase of the bacteria that may cause systemic effects.

Expiratory reserve volume Amount of gas that can be forcefully expired at the end of a normal expiration.

Explanation Sharing objective information related to a message.

Explosive Any chemical compound, mixture, or device, the primary or common purpose of which is to function by detonation or rapid combustion (i.e., with substantial instantaneous release of gas and heat); found in liquid or solid forms (e.g., dynamite, TNT, black powder, fireworks, ammunition).

Exposure When blood or body fluids come in contact with eyes, mucous membranes, nonintact skin, or through a needlestick; it also can occur through inhalation and ingestion.

Expressed consent Permission given by a patient or his or her responsible decision maker either verbally or through some physical expression of consent.

Exsanguinate Near complete loss of blood; not conducive with life.

Exsanguination Bleeding to death.

Extensibility Ability to continue to contract over a range of lengths.

Extension posturing (decerebrate) Occurs as a result of an injury to the brainstem; presents as the patient's arms at the side with wrists turned outward.

External anal sphincter Muscle under voluntary control that allows a controlled bowel movement.

External auditory canal Tube from the external ear to the middle ear; lined with hair and ceruminous glands.

External bleeding Observable blood loss.

External ear Includes the auricle and external auditory canal.

External respiration The exchange of gases between the alveoli of the lungs and the blood cells traveling through the pulmonary capillaries.

External urinary sphincter Ring of smooth muscle in the urethra under voluntary control.

Extracellular Outside the cell or cytoplasmic membrane.

Extracellular fluid (ECF) The fluid found outside of the cells.

Extubation Removal of an endotracheal tube from the trachea.

Exudate Drainage from a vesicle or pustule.

Eyebrows Protect the eyes by providing shade and preventing foreign material (sweat, dust, etc.) from entering the eyes from above.

Eyelids Protect the eyes from foreign objects.

Facilitated diffusion Movement of substances across a membrane by binding to a helper protein integrated into the cell wall and highly selective about the chemicals allowed to cross the membrane.

Facilitated transport The transport of substances through a protein channel carrier with no energy input.

Facilitation Encouraging the patient to provide more information.

Factitious disorder Condition in which patients intentionally produce signs and symptoms of illness to assume the sick role.

Fainting (syncope) A brief loss of consciousness caused by a temporary decrease in blood flow to the brain.

Fallopian tube Paired structures extending from each side of the uterus to each ovary; they provide a way for the egg to reach the uterus.

False imprisonment Confinement or restraint of a person against his or her will or without appropriate legal justification.

False motion Abnormal movement of a bone or joint typically associated with a fracture or dislocation.

Fascia Anatomically, the tough connective tissue covering of the muscles of the body. Fascia contains the muscles within a compartment.

Fascicle Small bundle of nerve fibers.

Fasciotomy A surgical incision into the muscle fascia to relieve intracompartmental pressures; the emergency treatment for compartment syndrome.

Fear Physical and emotional reaction to a real or perceived threat.

Febrile seizure Seizure caused by too rapid of a rise in body temperature; rarely seen after age 2 years.

Fecalith A hard impacted mass of feces in the colon.

Feces Undigested food material that has been processed in the colon.

Federal Communication Commission (FCC) An independent U.S. government agency, directly responsible to Congress, established by the Communications Act of 1934; it regulates interstate and international communications by radio, television, wire, satellite, and cable. The FCC's jurisdiction covers the 50 states, the District of Columbia, and U.S. possessions.

Fetus The term used for an infant from approximately 8 weeks of pregnancy until birth.

Fibrin A threadlike protein formed during the clotting process that crisscrosses the wound opening and forms a matrix that traps blood cells and platelets, thereby creating a clot. Fibrin is formed by the action of thrombin and fibrinogen.

Fibrinolysis The breakdown of fibrin, the main component of blood clots.

Fibrinolytic agent Clot-busting drug; used in very early treatment of acute myocardial infarction, stroke, deep vein thrombosis, pulmonary embolism, and peripheral arterial occlusion.

Fibroblasts A cell that gives rise to connective tissue.

Fibrous connective tissue Composed of bundles of strong, white collagenous fibers (protein) in parallel rows; tendons and ligaments are composed of this type of tissue; relatively strong and inelastic.

Fibrous joints Two bones united by fibrous tissue that have little or no movement.

Fibrous tunic Layer of the eye that contains the sclera and the cornea.

Fick principle Describes the components needed for the oxygenation of the body's cells.

Finance officer The person responsible for providing a cost analysis of an incident.

Fine ventricular fibrillation Ventricular fibrillation with fibrillatory waves less than 3 mm in height.

FiO$_2$ Fraction of inspired oxygen.

"First on the Scene" program An educational program that teaches people what to do and what not to do when they come upon an injury emergency.

First-degree burn Superficial burn involving only the epidermis, such as a minor sunburn.

First-pass effect The breakdown of a drug in the liver and walls of the intestines before it reaches the systemic circulation.

First responder unit The closest trained persons and vehicle assigned to respond to a call; often the closest available fire department vehicle.

Fissure A vertical loss of epidermis and dermis with sharply defined walls (sometimes called a *crack*).

Fistula An abnormal tunnel that has formed from within the body to the skin.

Fixed positioning Establishing a single location in a central point to station an emergency vehicle, such as a fire station.

Fixed-rate pacemaker Asynchronous pacemaker that continuously discharges at a preset rate regardless of the patient's heart rate.

Fixed-station deployment Deployment method of using only geographically based stations.

Fixed-wing aircraft Airplanes used for longer distance medical flights; they can travel higher and faster than rotor-wing aircraft.

Flail segment A free-floating section of the chest wall that results when two or more adjacent ribs are fractured in two or more places or when the sternum is detached.

Flammable The capacity of a substance to ignite.

Flammable gases Any compressed gas that meets requirements for lower flammability limit, flammability limit range, flame projection, or flame propagation as specified in CFR Title 49, Sec. 173.300(b) (e.g., acetylene, butane, hydrogen, propane).

Flammable range The concentration of fuel and air between the lower flammable limit or lower explosive limit and the upper flammable limit or upper explosive limit; the mixture of fuel and air in the flammable range supports combustion.

Flammable solid A solid material other than an explosive that is liable to cause fires through friction or retained heat from manufacturing or processing or that can be ignited readily; when ignited, it burns so vigorously and persistently that it creates a serious transportation hazard (e.g., phosphorus, lithium, magnesium, titanium, calcium resinate).

Flash electrical burn A burn resulting from indirect contact with an electrical explosion.

Flashpoint The minimal temperature at which a substance evaporates fast enough to form an ignitable mixture with air near the surface of the substance.

Flat affect A complete or near-complete lack of emotion.

Flat bones Specialized bones that protect vital anatomic structures (e.g., ribs and bones of the skull).

Flexible deployment See *System status management.*

Flexion posturing (decorticate) Occurs from an injury to the cerebrum; presents as a bending of the arms at the elbow, the patient's arms pulled upwards to the chest, and the hands turned downward at the wrists.

Flight of ideas Moving quickly from topic to topic during conversation but without any connection or transition.

Flow rate The number of drops per minute an intravenous administration set will deliver.

Fluctuance A wavelike motion felt between two fingertips when palpating a fluid-filled structure such as a subcutaneous abscess.

Fluctuant nodule A movable and compressible mass; typically a pocket of pus or fluid within the dermis.

Focal atrial tachycardia Atrial tachycardia that begins in a small area (focus) within the heart.

Focal deficit Alteration or lack of strength or sensation in the body caused by a neurologic problem.

Focal injury An injury limited to a particular area of the brain.

Follicle Small, tubelike structure in which hair grows; contains a small cluster of cells known as the hair papilla.

Follicles Vesicles within the cortex of the ovary.

Folliculitis Inflammation of the follicle; localized to hair follicles and is more common in immunocompromised patients; are usually multiple and measure 5 mm or less in diameter; erythematous, pruritic, and frequently have a central pustule on top of a raised lesion, often with a central hair.

Fontanelles Membranous spaces at the juncture of an infant's cranial bones that later ossify.

Foramen Open passage.

Foramen magnum Opening in the floor of the cranium where the spinal cord exits the skull.

Foramen ovale The opening in the interatrial septum in a fetal heart.

Foreign body Any object or substance found in a organ or tissue where it does not belong under normal circumstances.

Form of thought Ability to compose thoughts in a logical manner.

Formed elements Located in the bloodstream; erythrocytes, leukocytes, and thrombocytes, or platelets.

Formulary A book that contains a list of medicinal substances with their formulas, uses, and methods of preparation.

Fractile response time Method used to determine the time at which 90% of all requests for service receive a response; considered a more definitive measure of performance than averages.

Francisella tularensis A hardy, slow-growing, highly infectious, aerobic organism; human infection may result in tularemia, also known as *rabbit fever* or *deer fly fever.*

Free nerve endings Most common type of dermal nerve ending; responsible for sensing pain, temperature, and pressure.

Free radical A molecule containing an extra electron, which allows it to form potentially harmful bonds with other molecules.

Frontal lobe Section of cerebrum important in voluntary motor function and the emotions of aggression, motivation, and mood.

Frontal plane Imaginary straight line that divides the body into anterior (ventral) and posterior (dorsal) sections.

Frostbite A condition in which the skin and underlying tissue freeze.

Frostnip Reversible freezing of superficial skin layer marked by numbness and whiteness of the skin.

Fully deployed Assigning ambulances to a street corner post.

Fulminant Sudden, intense occurrence.

Functional reserve capacity At the end of a normal expiration, the volume of air remaining in the lungs.

Fundus Superior aspect of the uterus.

Fungi Plantlike organisms that do not contain chlorophyll; the two classes of fungi are yeasts and molds.

Furuncles Inflammatory nodules that involve the hair follicle (e.g., boils).

Gag reflex A normal neural reflex elicited by touching the soft palate or posterior pharynx; the responses are symmetric elevation of the palate, retraction of the tongue, and contraction of the pharyngeal muscles.

Gagging A reflex caused by irritation of the posterior pharynx that can result in vomiting.

Gamma A type of electromagnetic radiation.

Gamma-hydroxybutyrate (GHB) A drug structurally related to the neurotransmitter gamma-aminobutyric acid, usually dissolved in liquid, that causes profound central nervous system depression.

Gamma rays A type of electromagnetic radiation that can travel great distances; can be stopped by heavy shielding, such as lead.

Gamow bag Portable hyperbaric chamber that can help with altitude sickness emergencies.

Ganglion The junction between the preganglionic and postganglionic nerves.

Gangrenous necrosis Tissue death over a large area.

Gases Substances inhaled and absorbed through the respiratory tract.

Gasoline and electric hybrid vehicle Vehicle designed to produce low emissions by combining a smaller than normal internal combustion gasoline engine with a special electric motor to power the vehicle.

Gasping Inhaling and exhaling with quick, difficult breaths.

Gastric The route used when a tube is placed into the digestive tract, such as a nasogastric, orogastric, or gastrostomy tube.

Gastric distention Swelling of the abdomen caused by an influx of air or fluid.

Gastric lavage A method of internal decontamination that involves emptying the stomach contents through an orogastric or nasogastric tube.

Gastritis Inflammation of the stomach.

Gastroenteritis Inflammation of the stomach and the intestines.

Gastrostomy tube A tube placed in a person's stomach that allows continuous feeding for an extended time.

Gay-Lussac's law A gas law sometimes combined with Charles' law that deals with the relation between pressure and temperature; in an oxygen cylinder, as the ambient temperature decreases, so does the pressure reading.

Gel cap Soft gelatin shell filled with liquid medication.

Gene The biologic unit of inheritance, consisting of a particular nucleotide sequence within a DNA molecule that occupies a precise locus on a chromosome and codes for a specific polypeptide chain.

Generalized anxiety disorder Condition characterized by excessive worries about everyday life.

Generalized seizure Excessive electrical activity in both hemispheres of the brain at the same time.

Generic name The name proposed by the first manufacturer when a drug is submitted to the FDA for approval; often an abbreviated form of the drug's chemical name, structure, or formula.

Geospatial demand analysis Understanding the different locations of demand within a community.

Germ theory Controversial theory developed in the 1600s in which microorganisms were first identified as the possible cause of some disease processes.

Germinativum Basal layer of the epidermis where the epidermal cells are formed.

Gestation or gestational age The number of completed weeks of pregnancy from the last menstrual period.

Glasgow Coma Scale (GCS) Neurologic assessment of a patient's best verbal response, eye opening, and motor function.

Glaucoma Increased intraocular pressure caused by a disruption in the normal production and drainage of aqueous humor; causes often are unknown.

Global positioning system (GPS) A satellite-based geographic locating system often placed on an ambulance to track its exact location.

Glomerulus Network of capillaries in the renal corpuscle.

Glottis The true vocal cords and the space between them.

Gluconeogenesis Creation of new glucose in the body by using noncarbohydrate sources such as fats and proteins.

Glycogenolysis Breakdown of glycogen to glucose in the liver.

Glycolysis Process by which glucose and other sugars are broken down to yield lactic acid (anaerobic glycolysis) or pyruvic acid (aerobic glycolysis). The breakdown releases energy in the form of adenosine triphosphate.

Glycoside A compound that yields a sugar and one or more other products when its parts are separated.

Golgi apparatus Substance that concentrates and packages material for secretion out of the cell.

Gomphoses Joint in which a peg fits into a socket.

Gout A metabolic disease in which uric acid crystals are deposited onto the cartilaginous surfaces of a joint, resulting in pain, swelling, and inflammation.

Graft Connection by a surgeon of a piece of the patient's saphenous vein to an artery and vein; in lieu of using the patient's own blood vessel, a cow's artery or a synthetic graft may be used.

Graham's law Law stating that gases move from a higher pressure or concentration to an area of lower pressure or concentration; takes into consideration the effect of simple diffusion at a cellular level.

Gram-negative bacteria Bacteria that do not retain the crystal violet stain used in Gram's stain and that take the color of the red counterstain.

Gram-positive bacteria Bacteria that retain the crystal violet stain used in Gram's stain.

Grandiose delusions Dramatically inflated perceptions of one's own worth, power, or knowledge.

Granulocyte A form of leukocyte that attacks foreign material in the wound.

Gravida Number of pregnancies.

Gravidity The number of times a patient has been pregnant.

Great vessels Large vessels that carry blood to and from the heart; superior and inferior venae cavae, pulmonary veins, aorta, and pulmonary trunk.

Greenstick fracture The incomplete fracturing of an immature bone.

Grey-Turner's sign Bruising along the flanks that may indicate pancreatitis or intraabdominal hemorrhage.

Ground effect The cushion of air created by downdraft when a helicopter is in a low hover. Ground effect benefits the helicopter flight because it increases lift capacity, meaning less power is required for the helicopter to hover. When the helicopter has ground effect, it is said to be in ground effect. If a helicopter does not have ground effect, it is said to be operating out of ground effect.

Ground electrode Third ECG electrode (the first and second are the positive and negative electrodes), which minimizes electrical activity from other sources.

Grunting A short, low-pitched sound heard at the end of exhalation that represents an attempt to generate positive end-expiratory pressure by exhaling against a closed glottis, prolonging the period of oxygen and carbon dioxide exchange across the alveolar-capillary membrane; a compensatory mechanism to help maintain patency of small airways and prevent atelectasis.

Guarding The contraction of abdominal muscles in the anticipation of a painful stimulus.

Guidelines For emergency medical dispatchers, an unstructured, subjective, unscripted method of telephone assessment and treatment; a less-effective process than protocols.

Guillain-Barré syndrome Autoimmune neurologic disorder marked by weakness and paresthesia that usually travel up the legs.

Gum Plant residue used for medicinal or recreational purposes.

Gurgling Abnormal respiratory sound associated with collection of liquid or semisolid material in the patient's upper airway.

Gurney Stretcher or cot used to transport patients.

Gustation Sense of taste.

Hair papilla Small cluster of cells within a follicle; growth of hair starts in this cluster of cells, which is hidden in the follicle.

Half Duplex A radio system that use two frequencies: one to transmit and one to receive; however, like a simplex system, only one person can transmit at a time.

Half-life The time required to eliminate half of a substance from the body.

Hallucination False sensory perceptions originating inside the brain.

Hallucinogen Substance that causes hallucinations and intense distortions and perceptions of reality; includes LSD, psilocybin mushrooms, peyote, and mescaline.

Hamman's sign A crunching sound occasionally heard on auscultation of the heart when air is in the mediastinum.

Hangman's fracture A fracture of the axis, the second cervical vertebra. This may occur with or without axis dislocation.

Hazard Communication Standard (HAZCOM) Occupational Safety and Health Administration standard regarding worker protection when handling chemicals.

Hazardous materials A substance (solid, liquid, or gas) capable of posing an unreasonable risk to health, safety, environment, or property.

Hazardous Waste Operations and Emergency Response (HAZWOPER) Occupational Safety and Health Administration and Environmental Protection Agency regulations regarding worker safety when responding to hazardous materials emergencies.

Head bobbing Indicator of increased work of breathing in infants; the head falls forward with exhalation and comes up with expansion of the chest on inhalation.

Head injury A traumatic insult to the head that may result in injury to the soft tissue or bony structures of the head and/or brain injury.

Headache A pain in the head from any cause.

Health A state of complete physical, mental, and social well-being, not merely the absence of disease or infirmity.

Health Insurance Portability and Accountability Act (HIPAA) Rules governing the protection of a patient's identifiable information.

Healthcare professional An individual who has special skills and knowledge in medicine and adheres to the standards of conduct and performance of that medical profession.

Healthcare A business associated with the provision of medical care to individuals.

Heart disease A broad term referring to conditions affecting the heart.

Heart failure A condition in which the heart is unable to pump enough blood to meet the metabolic needs of the body.

Heartbeat Organized mechanical action of the heart.

Heat emergencies Conditions in which the body's thermoregulation mechanisms begin to fail in response to ambient heat, causing illness.

Hematemesis Vomiting of bright red blood.

Hematochezia Bright red blood in the stool.

Hematocrit A measure of the relative percentage of blood cells (mainly erythrocytes) in a given volume of whole blood; also called *volume of packed red cells* or *packed cell volume.*

Hematoma Collection of blood beneath the skin or within a body compartment.

Hematuria Blood found in the urine.

Hemiparesis Muscle weakness of one half of the body.

Hemiplegia Paralysis of one side of the body.

Hemoglobin A protein found on red blood cells that is rich in iron.

Hemolytic anemia Anemia that results from the destruction of red blood cells.

Hemopoietic tissue Connective tissue found in the marrow cavities of bones (mainly long bones).

Hemoptysis The coughing up of blood.

Hemorrhage Heavy bleeding.

Hemorrhagic anemia Anemia caused by hemorrhage.

Hemorrhagic stroke Rupture of a blood vessel in the brain causing decreased perfusion and potentially leading to rising intracranial pressure.

Hemorrhoids Swollen, distended veins in the anorectal area.

Hemostasis Stopping a hemorrhage.

Hemothorax Blood within the thoracic cavity, a potentially life-threatening injury.

Henry's law Law associated with decompression sickness that deals with the solubility of gases in liquids at equilibrium.

Hepatic artery The artery that supplies the liver with blood and nutrients from the circulatory system.

Hepatic duct Connects the gallbladder to the liver; secretes bile into the gallbladder.

Hepatitis Inflammation of the liver.

Hering-Breuer reflex A reflex that limits inspiration to prevent overinflation of the lungs in a conscious, spontaneously breathing person; also called the *inhibito-inspiratory reflex.*

Hernia Protrusion of any organ through an abdominal opening in the muscle wall of the cavity that surrounds it.

Herniated disc A condition in which an intervertebral disc weakens and protrudes out of position, often affecting adjacent nerve roots.

Herniation Protrusion of the brain through an abnormal opening, often the foramen magnum.

Heroin (diacetylmorphine) The most popular, powerful, and addictive member of the opioids.

Herpes simplex A skin eruption caused by the herpes simplex virus, divided into two types; HSV-1 causes oral infection and HSV-2 causes genital infections.

Herpes zoster A skin eruption that follows a particular nerve distribution (dermatome); caused by the varicella zoster virus in persons who have had varicella sometime in their lives (also called *shingles*).

Hiatus A gap or a cleft.

Hiccup (hiccoughing) Intermittent spasm of the diaphragm resulting in sudden inspiration with spastic closure of the glottis; usually annoying and serves no known physiologic purpose.

High angle An environment in which the load is predominantly supported by the rope rescue system.

High voltage Greater than 1000 V.

High-altitude cerebral edema The most severe high-altitude illness, characterized by increased intracranial pressure.

High-altitude pulmonary edema A high-altitude illness characterized by increased pulmonary artery pressure and edema, leading to cough and fluid in the lungs (pulmonary edema).

High-angle terrain (vertical terrain) A steep environment such as a cliff or building side where hands must be used for balance when ascending.

Hilum Point of entry for bronchial vessels, bronchi, and nerves in each lung.

Hilus Indentation through which the renal artery, vein, lymphatic vessels, and nerves enter and leave the kidney.

Hippocampi Structures within the limbic system that filter incoming information, determine what stimuli is important, and commit the experiences to memory.

His-Purkinje system Portion of the conduction system consisting of the bundle of His, bundle branches, and Purkinje fibers.

Histamine A substance released by mast cells that promotes inflammation.

History of present illness A narrative detail of the symptoms the patient is experiencing.

Hollow organ An organ (a part of the body or group of tissues that performs a specific function) that contains a channel or cavity within it, such as the large and small intestines.

Homan's sign Pain and tenderness in the calf muscle on dorsiflexion of the foot.

Home care The provision of health services by formal and informal caregivers in the home to promote, restore, and maintain a person's maximal level of comfort, function, and health, including care toward a dignified death.

Homeostasis A state of equilibrium in the body with respect to functions and composition of fluids and tissues.

Homeotherm Organism with a stable independent body temperature; an organism whose stable body temperature is generally independent of the surrounding environment.

Homonyms Terms that sound alike but are spelled differently and have different meanings.

Honeymoon phase A period of remorse by the abuser characterized by the abuser's denial and apologies.

Hordeolum A common acute infection of the glands of the eyelids.

Hormones Chemicals within the body that reach every cell through the circulatory system.

Hospice A care program that provides for the dying and their special needs.

Hospital Incident Command System An emergency management system that uses a logical management structure, defined responsibilities, clear reporting channels, and a common nomenclature to help unify hospitals with other emergency responders.

Hospital off-load time The time necessary for a crew to become available once they arrive at a hospital.

Hot load Loading a patient into a helicopter while the rotors are spinning.

Hot zone The primary danger zone around a crash scene that typically extends approximately 50 feet in all directions from the wreckage.

Hover The condition in which a helicopter remains fairly stationary over a given point, moving neither vertically nor horizontally.

Hub The plastic piece that houses a needle and fits onto a syringe.

Human immunodeficiency virus (HIV) The virus that can cause AIDS.

Human leukocyte antigen Leukocyte antigen that transplant surgeons attempt to match to prevent incompatibility.

Humoral immunity Immunity from antibodies in the blood.

Humoral Pertaining to elements in the blood or other body fluids.

Huntington's disease Programmed cell death of certain neurons in the brain, leading to behavioral abnormalities, movement disorders, and a decline in cognitive function.

Hydration Process of taking in fluids with the normal daily output.

Hydraulic A water hazard caused when water moves over a uniform obstruction to flow.

Hydraulic injection injuries High-pressure fluid that leaks from hydraulic hoses and is injected into the body.

Hydrocarbon A member of a large class of chemicals belonging to the petroleum derivative family; they have a variety of uses, such as solvents, oils, reagents, and fuels; the psychoactive ingredient in many abused inhalants.

Hydrocele Collection of fluid in the scrotum or along the spermatic cord.

Hydrocephalus An excessive amount of cerebrospinal fluid.

Hydrogen cyanide A highly toxic blood agent.

Hydrogen ion concentration Concentration of hydrogen ions in a given solution, such as water or blood; used to calculate the pH of a substance.

Hydrogen sulfide A hazardous gas produced by the decomposition of organic material prevalent when manure is stored in a liquid form for an extended period.

Hydrophilic Attracts water molecules.

Hydrophobic Repels water molecules.

Hydrostatic pressure Pressure exerted by a fluid from its weight.

Hydroxylysine An amino acid found in collagen.

Hymen Thin of layer of tissue that may cover the vaginal orifice in women who have not had sexual intercourse.

Hypercalcemia A state in which the body has an abnormally high level of calcium.

Hypercapnia An increased amount of carbon dioxide in the blood; may be a result of hypoventilation.

Hypercarbia An excess of CO_2 in the blood.

Hyperdynamic Excessively forceful or energetic. Term is used to describe shock states in which the heart is pumping aggressively to make up for fluid losses, such as in burn or septic shock.

Hyperextension Extension beyond a joint's normal range of motion.

Hyperflexion Flexion beyond a joint's normal range of motion.

Hyperkalemia A state in which the body has an abnormally elevated potassium level.

Hypermagnesemia A state in which the body has an abnormally elevated concentration of magnesium in the blood.

Hypermetabolic A state or condition of the body characterized by excessive production and utilization of energy molecules such as protein.

Hyperopia Farsightedness; difficulty seeing objects close to the person.

Hyperosmolar hyperglycemic nonketotic coma (HHNC) Condition caused by a relative insulin insufficiency that leads to extremely high blood sugar levels while still allowing for normal glucose metabolism and an absence of ketone bodies.

Hyperplasia Abnormal cell division that increases the number of a specific type of cell.

Hyperpnea Increased respiratory rate or deeper than normal breathing; also called *hyperventilation.*

Hyperresonant A high-pitched sound.

Hypersensitivity disorder A disorder in which the immune system responds inappropriately and excessively to an antigen (in this response, known as allergens).

Hypersensitivity pneumonitis Inflammation in and around the tiny air sacs (alveoli) and smallest airways (bronchioles) of the lung caused by an allergic reaction to inhaled organic dusts or, less commonly, chemicals; also called *extrinsic allergic alveolitis, allergic interstitial pneumonitis,* or *organic dust pneumoconiosis.*

Hypersensitivity reaction An immune response that is excessive beyond the bounds of normalcy to a point that it leads to damage (as with endotoxins) or is potentially damaging to the individual.

Hypersensitivity An altered reactivity to a medication that occurs after prior sensitization; response is independent of the dose.

Hypertension Elevated blood pressure.

Hypertensive emergencies Situations that require rapid (within 1 hour) lowering of blood pressure to prevent or limit organ damage.

Hypertensive urgencies Significant elevations in blood pressure with nonspecific symptoms that should be corrected within 24 hours.

Hyperthermia A core body temperature greater than 98.6°F.

Hypertonic In a membrane, the side with the higher concentration in an imbalance in the ionic concentration from one side to the other.

Hypertrophic scar Scar that forms with excessive amounts of scar tissue. The scar remains contained by the wound boundaries but may be slightly raised and can impair function.

Hypertrophy Enlargement or increase in the size of a cell(s) or tissue.

Hyperventilation Blowing off too much carbon dioxide.

Hyphema Blood in the anterior chamber of the eye.

Hypocalcemia A state in which the body has an abnormally low calcium level.

Hypocarbia An inadequate amount of carbon dioxide in the blood.

Hypokalemia A state in which the level of potassium in the serum falls below 3.5 mEq/L.

Hypomagnesemia A state in which the body has an abnormally low serum concentration of magnesium.

Hypomania An episode of a lesser form of mania that may transition into mania or alternate with depression.

Hypoperfusion The inadequate circulation of blood through an organ or a part of the body; shock.

Hypotension Low blood pressure significant enough to cause inadequate perfusion.

Hypothalamus Interface between the brain and the endocrine system; provides control for many autonomic functions.

Hypothermia A core body temperature below 95°F (35°C).

Hypotonic In a membrane, the side with the lower concentration when an imbalance exists in the ionic concentration from one side to the other.

Hypoventilation Occurs when the volume of air that enters the alveoli and takes part in gas exchange is not adequate for the body's metabolic needs.

Hypovolemic shock Inadequate tissue perfusion caused by inadequate vascular volume.

Hypoxemia An abnormal deficiency in the concentration of oxygen in arterial blood.

Hypoxia Inadequate oxygenation of the cells.

Iatrogenic drug response An unintentional disease or drug effect produced by a physician's prescribed therapy; *iatros* means "physician," and *-genic* is a word root meaning "produce."

Icterus Jaundice.

Idiosyncrasy The unexpected and usually individual (genetic) adverse response to a drug.

Ileostomy Surgical creation of a passage through the abdominal wall into the ileum.

Ileum Last segment of the small intestine; area of decreased absorption where chyme is prepared for entry into the large intestine.

Ileus Decreased peristaltic movement of the colon.

Immediately dangerous to life or health concentrations (IDLHs) Maximal environmental air concentration of a substance from which a person could escape within 30 minutes without symptoms of impairment or irreversible health effects.

Immersion To be covered in water or other fluid.

Immunity Protection from legal liability in accordance with applicable laws; also the body's ability to resist a particular disease.

Immunodeficiency Deficit in the immune system and its response to infection or injury.

Immunoglobulin See *Antibody.*

Impetigo A highly contagious infection caused by staphylococcal or streptococcal bacteria. A superficial vesicopustular skin infection that primarily occurs on exposed areas of the face and extremities from scratching infected lesions; usually begins at a traumatized region of the skin, where a combination of vesicles and pustules develops; the pustules rupture and crust, leaving a characteristic thick, golden or honeylike appearance.

Implied consent The presumption that a patient who is ill or injured and unable to give consent for any reason would agree to the delivery of emergency health care necessitated by his or her condition.

Incarcerated hernia Hernia of intestine that cannot be returned or reduced by manipulation; it may or may not become strangulated.

Incendiary device A device designed to ignite a fire.

Incidence The rate at which a certain event occurs, such as the number of new cases of a specific disease occurring during a certain period in a population at risk.

Incidence rate The rate of contraction of a disease versus how many are currently sick with the disease.

Incident commander The person responsible for the overall management of an emergency scene.

Incident scene hazards Hazards directly related to the specific incident scene, including control of crowds, traffic, the danger of downed electrical wires, the presence of hazardous materials, and the location of an emergency.

Incomplete abortion An abortion in which the uterus retains part of the products of the pregnancy.

Incomplete cord transection A partial cutting (severing) of the spinal cord in which some cord function remains distal to the injury site.

Incontinence Inability to control excretory functions; usually refers to the involuntary passage of urinary or fecal matter.

Incubation period The time between exposure to a disease pathogen and the appearance of the first signs or symptoms.

Incus The anvil-shaped bone located between the malleus and stapes in the middle ear.

Index of suspicion The expectation that certain injuries or patterns of injuries have resulted to a body part, organ, or system based on the mechanism of injury and the force of impact to the patient.

Indication The appropriate use of a drug when treating a disease or condition.

Indicative change ECG changes seen in leads looking directly at the wall of the heart in an infarction.

Induration Hardened mass within the tissue typically associated with inflammation.

Infarction Death of tissue because of an inadequate blood supply.

Inferior Toward the feet; below a point of reference in the anatomic position.

Inferior vena cava Vessels that return venous blood from the lower part of the body to the right atrium.

Infiltration Complication of intravenous therapy when the catheter tip is outside the vein and the intravenous solution is dispersed into the surrounding tissues.

Inflammation A tissue reaction in an injury, infection, or insult.

Influx Flowing into.

Ingestion Process of bringing food into the digestive tract.

Inhalants Substances such as aerosols, fuels, paints, and other chemicals that produce fumes at room temperature; they are breathed in, producing a high.

Inhalation A route in which the medication is aerosolized and delivered directly to the lung tissue.

Injury Intentional or unintentional damage to a person resulting from acute exposure to thermal, mechanical, electrical, or chemical energy or from the absence of such essentials as heat or oxygen.

Injury risk A real or potential hazardous situation that puts individuals at risk for sustaining an injury.

Injury surveillance An ongoing systematic collection, analysis, and interpretation of injury data essential to the planning, implementation, and evaluation of public health practice, closely integrated with the timely dissemination of the data to those who need to know.

Inner ear Holds the sensory organs for hearing and balance.

Inotropic Relating to the force of cardiac contraction.

Inotropism A change in myocardial contractility.

Inspiratory reserve volume Amount of gas that can be forcefully inspired in addition to a normal breath's tidal volume.

Integrity Doing the right thing even when no one is looking.

Integumentary system The largest organ system in the body, consisting of the skin and accessory structures (e.g., hair, nails, glands).

Intense affect Heated and passionate emotional responses.

Intentional injury Injuries and deaths self-inflicted or perpetrated by another person, usually involving some type of violence.

Intentional tort A wrong in which the defendant meant to cause the harmful action.

Interatrial septum Septum dividing the atria in the heart.

Intercalated discs The cell-to-cell connection with gap junctions between cardiac muscle cells.

Interference The ability of one drug to limit the physiologic function of another drug.

Intermittent claudication Pain, cramping, muscle tightness, fatigue, or weakness of the legs when walking or during exercise.

Internal anal sphincter Muscle under autonomic control; has stretch receptors that provide the sensation of the need to defecate.

Internal bleeding Escape of blood from blood vessels into tissues and spaces within the body.

Internal respiration The exchange of gases between blood cells and tissues.

Internal urinary sphincter Ring of smooth muscle in the urethra that is under autonomic control.

International medical surgical response teams Specialty surgical teams that can respond both in the United States and internationally.

Interoperability Describes a radio system that can use the components of several different systems; it can use specialized equipment to connect several different radio systems and components together and have them communicate with each other.

Interpretation Stating the conclusions you have drawn from the information.

Interstitial compartment Area consisting of fluid outside cells and outside the circulatory system.

Interstitium Extravascular and extracellular milieu; also known as the *third space.*

Interval Waveform and a segment; in pacing, the period, measured in milliseconds, between any two designated cardiac events.

Interventricular septum Septum dividing the ventricles in the heart.

Intimal In reference to blood vessels, the innermost lining of an artery; composed of a single layer of cells.

Intimate partner violence and abuse (IPVA) Formerly called *domestic violence,* this is a learned pattern of assaultive and controlling behavior, including physical, sexual, and psychological attacks as well as economic control, which adults or adolescents use against their intimate partners to gain power and control.

Intimate space The area within 1.5 feet of a person.

Intoxication Being under the effect of a toxin or drug; common terminology (nonmedical) refers to intoxication as being under the effect of alcohol or illegal drugs.

Intracardiac The injection of a drug directly into the heart.

Intracellular Inside of the cell or cytoplasmic membrane.

Intracellular fluid (ICF) Fluid found within cells.

Intracerebral hematoma Bleeding within the brain tissue itself.

Intracerebral hemorrhage Bleeding within the brain tissue, often from smaller blood vessels.

Intracranial pressure (ICP) Pressure inside the brain cavity; should be very low, usually less than 15 mm Hg.

Intradermal Route of the injection of medication between the dermal layers of skin.

Intralingual Direct injection into the underside of the tongue with a small volume of medication.

Intramuscular (IM) An injection of medication directly into the muscle.

Intranasal The route that offers direct delivery of medications into the nasal passages and sinuses.

Intraosseous An administration route used in emergency situations when peripheral venous access is not established; a needle is passed through the cortex of the bone and the medication is infused into the capillary network within the bone matrix.

Intraosseous infusion The process of infusing medications, fluids, and blood products into the bone marrow cavity for subsequent delivery to the venous circulation.

Intraperitoneal Abdominopelvic organs surrounded by the peritoneum.

Intrathecal The direct deposition of medication into the spinal canal.

Intravascular compartment Area consisting of fluid outside cells but inside the circulatory system; the majority of intravascular fluid is plasma, which is the fluid component of blood.

Intravenous (IV) Administration route offering instantaneous and nearly complete absorption through peripheral or central venous access.

Intravenous (IV) bolus The delivery of a drug directly into an infusion port on the administration set using a syringe.

Intravenous cannulation Placement of a catheter into a vein to gain access to the body's venous circulation.

Intravenous therapy Administration of a fluid into a vein.

Intrinsic rate Rate at which a pacemaker of the heart normally generates impulses.

Intussusception Invagination of a part of the colon into another part of the colon; also referred to as *telescoping.*

Invasion of privacy Disclosure or publication of personal or private facts about a person to a person or persons not authorized to receive such information.

Invasive wound infection An infection involving the deeper tissues of a wound that may be destructive to blood vessels and other structures of the skin and soft tissues.

Investigational drug A drug not yet approved by the Food and Drug Administration.

Involuntary consent The rendering of care to a person under specific legal authority, even if the patient does not consent to the care.

Ion Electrically charged particle.

Ionizing radiation Particles or pure energy that produces changes in matter by creating ion pairs.

Iris Colored part of the eye; ring of smooth muscle that surrounds the pupil; controls the size (diameter) of the pupil.

Irregular bones Unique bones with specialized functions not easily classified into the other types of bone (e.g., vertebrae).

Ischemia Decreased supply of oxygenated blood to a body part or organ.

Ischemic phase Vascular response to shock when precapillary and postcapillary sphincters constrict, halting blood to distal tissues.

Ischemic stroke Lack of perfusion to an area of brain tissue; caused by a blood clot, air, amniotic fluid, or a foreign body.

Islets of Langerhans Groups of cells located in the pancreas that produce insulin, glucagon, somatostatin, and pancreatic polypeptide.

Isoelectric line Absence of electrical activity; observed on the ECG as a straight line.

Isografting Transplanting tissue from a genetically identical person (i.e., identical twin).

Isolation The seclusion of individuals with an illness to prevent transmission to others.

Isotonic A balance in the ionic concentration from one side of the membrane to the other.

Jacking the dash Making cuts into the front pillar and A pillar and lifting the dash, instrument panel, steering wheel, column, and even the pedals off a trapped driver or front seat passenger.

Jejunum Second part of the small intestine; major site of nutrient absorption.

Joint dislocation Disruption of articulating bones from their normal location.

Joints Point where two or more bones make contact to allow movement and provide mechanical support.

J-point Point where the QRS complex and ST segment meet.

Jugular venous distension (JVD) The presence of visually enlarged external jugular neck veins.

Jump kit A hard- or soft-sided bag used by paramedics to carry supplies and medications to the patient's side.

Junctional bradycardia A rhythm that begins in the atrioventricular junction with a rate of less than 40 beats/min.

Jurisprudence The theory and philosophy of law.

Kehr's sign Acute left shoulder pain caused by the presence of blood or other irritants in the peritoneal cavity.

Keloid An excessive accumulation of scar tissue that extends beyond the original wound margins.

Keratinized Accumulation of the protein keratin within the cytoplasm of skin cells. These cells comprise the epidermis of the skin. These dead cells function as the first defense against invaders and minor trauma.

Keratinocytes Epidermal cells.

Keratitis Inflammation and swelling of the cornea.

Kernicterus Excessive fetal bilirubin; associated with hemolytic disease.

Ketonemia The presence of ketones in the blood.

Kinetic energy M [mass] × ½ V [velocity]²; also called the *energy of motion.*

Knee bags Airbags mounted low on the instrument panel designed to deploy against the driver's and front seat passenger's knees in a frontal collision.

Korotkoff sounds The noise made by blood under pressure tumbling through the arteries.

Kussmaul respirations An abnormal respiratory pattern characterized by deep, gasping respirations that may be slow or rapid.

Kwashiorkor A form of malnutrition caused by inadequate protein intake compared with the total needed or required calorie intake.

Kyphosis Abnormally increased convexity in the curvature of the thoracic spine as viewed from the side; also called *hunchback.*

Labeling The application of a derogatory term to a patient on the basis of an event, habit, or personality trait that may not be accurate about the underlying condition.

Labia majora Rounded folds of external adipose tissue of the external female genitalia.

Labia minora Thinner, pinkish folds of skin that extend anteriorly to form the prepuce of the external female genitalia.

Labile Affect that changes frequently and rapidly.

Labor The process by which the fetus and placenta are expelled from the uterus. Usually divided into three stages, starting with the first contraction and ending with delivery of the placenta.

Labyrinth Series of bony tunnels inside the inner ear.

Labyrinthitis An inflammation of the structures in the inner ear.

Lacrimal ducts Small openings at the medial edge of the eye; drain holes for water from the surface of the eye.

Lacrimal fluid Watery, slightly alkaline secretion that consists of tears and saline that moisten the conjunctiva.

Lacrimal gland One of a pair of glands situated superior and lateral to the eye bulb; secretes lacrimal fluid.

Lacrimation Tearing of the eyes.

Lactic acid Byproduct of anaerobic metabolism.

Landing zone An area used to land a helicopter that is 100 feet × 100 feet and free of overhead wires.

Large intestine Organ where a large amount of water and electrolytes is absorbed and where undigested food is concentrated into feces.

Laryngoscope An instrument used to examine the interior of the larynx; during endotracheal intubation the device is used to visualize the glottic opening.

Laryngotracheobronchitis Croup.

Larynx Lies between the pharynx and the lungs; outer case of nine cartilages that protect and support the vocal cords.

Lassa fever A viral hemorrhagic fever illness caused by the Lassa virus (Arenavirus family).

Latent period Period during and after infection in which the disease is no longer transmissable.

Lateral A position away from the midline of the body.

Lateral recumbent Lying on either the right or left side.

Lead Electrical connection attached to the body to record electrical activity.

Left A position toward the left side of the body.

Left coronary artery Vessel that supplies oxygenated blood to the left side of the heart muscle.

Legally blind Less than 20/200 vision in at least one eye or a extremely limited field of vision (such as 20 degrees at its widest point).

Lens Transparent, biconvex elastic disc suspended by ligaments.

Leptomeningitis Inflammation of the inner brain coverings.

Lesions A wound, injury, or pathologic change in body tissue; any visible, local abnormality of the tissues of the skin, such as a wound, sore, rash, or boil.

Lethal concentration 50% (LC50) The air concentration of a substance that kills 50% of the exposed animal population; also commonly noted as LCt50; this denotes the concentration and the length of exposure time that results in 50% fatality in the exposed animal population.

Lethal dose 50% (LD50) The oral or dermal exposure dose that kills 50% of the exposed animal population in 2 weeks.

Leukocytes White blood cells.

Leukocytosis An increase in the number of white blood cells in the blood; typically results from infection, hemorrhage, fever, inflammation, or other factors.

Leukopenia A decrease in the total number of white blood cells in the blood.

Liability The legal responsibility of a party for the consequences of his or her acts or omissions.

Libel False statements about a person made in writing that blacken the person's character or injure his or her reputation.

Lice Wingless insects that live in human hair.

Licensure Permission granted to an individual by a governmental authority, such as a state, to perform certain restricted activities.

Life-threatening conditions A problem to the circulatory, respiratory, or nervous system that will kill a patient within minutes if not properly managed.

Ligaments Fibrous connective tissue that connects bones to bones, forming joint capsules.

Limbic system The part of the brain involved in mood, emotions, and the sensation of pain and pleasure.

Linear laceration Laceration that generally has smooth margins, although not as precise as those of an incision.

Linear skull fracture A line crack in the skull.

Lipid accumulation Accumulation of lipids in cells, usually as a result of the failure or inadequate performance of the enzyme that metabolizes fats.

Lipid peroxidation Process of cellular membrane destruction from exposure of the membrane to oxygen free radicals.

Lipophilic Substances that tend to seek out and bind to fatty substances.

Liquefaction necrosis Dead or dying tissue in which the necrotic material becomes softened and liquefied.

Liver Largest internal organ in the body; serves as a major detoxifier in the body.

Living will A type of advanced directive with written and signed specific instructions to healthcare providers about the individual's wishes regarding what types of healthcare measures or treatments should be undertaken to prolong life.

Loaded airbag An airbag that has not deployed during the initial crash.

Local damage Damage present at the point of chemical contact.

Local effect The effects of a drug at the site where the drug is applied or in the surrounding tissues.

Lock out, tag out An industrial workplace safety term describing actions taken to shut off power to a device, appliance, machine, or vehicle and to ensure that power remains off until work is completed.

Logistics officer The person responsible for assembling supplies used during an incident.

Long bones Bones that are longer than they are wide, have attachments for muscles to allow movement, and are found in limbs (e.g., the femur).

Looseness of associations (LOA) Going off track during conversation to varying degrees.

Low-angle terrain An environment in flat or mildly sloping areas in which rescuers primarily support themselves with their feet on the terrain surface.

Low vision Level of visual impairment in which an individual is unable to read a newspaper at the usual viewing distance even if wearing glasses or contact lenses. It is not limited to distance vision and can be a severe visual impairment.

Low voltage Less than 1000 V.

Lower airway Portion of the respiratory tract below the glottis.

Lower airway inhalation injury Injury to the anatomic portion of the respiratory tree below the level of the glottis. Generally caused by the inhalation of the toxic byproducts of combustion.

Lower flammable limit The minimal concentration of fuel in the air that will ignite; below this point too much oxygen and not enough fuel are present to burn (too lean); also called the *lower explosive limit.*

Ludwig's angina A bacterial infection of the floor of the mouth resulting from an infection in the root of the teeth, an abscessed tooth, or an injury to the mouth.

Lumbar vertebrae Vertebrae of the lower back that do not attach to any ribs and are superior to the pelvis.

Lumen An opening in the bevel of a needle.

Lungs Organs that allow the mechanical movement of air to and from the respiratory membrane.

Lymph Fluid that flows through the lymphatic ducts and aids in immune response and debris removal.

Lymph nodes Filter out foreign materials and collect infection-fighting cells that kill pathogens.

Lymphadenopathy Swelling of lymph nodes.

Lymphatic system The network of vessels, ducts, nodes, valves, and organs involved in protecting and maintaining the internal fluid environment of the body; part of the circulatory system.

Lymphatic vessels Unidirectional tubes that carry fluid or lymph within the lymphatic system.

Lymphedema Edema that follows when lymphatic pathways are blocked and fluid accumulates in the interstitial space.

Lymphocyte A form of leukocyte.

Lyse To destroy a cell.

Lysergic acid diethylamide (LSD) A powerful synthetic hallucinogen, often called *acid* and found on small squares of blotter paper.

Lysosomes Membrane-walled structures that contain enzymes.

Macrophages A monocyte that has matured and localized in one particular type of tissue; active in the immune system by activating agents that kill pathogens, absorbing foreign materials, and slowing infections and infectious agents.

Macule A flat, circumscribed, discolored lesion (e.g., freckle) measuring less that 1 cm.

Mainstem bronchi Each of two main breathing tubes that lead from the trachea into the lungs. There is one right mainstem bronchus and one left mainstem bronchus.

Malaise General feeling of illness without any specific symptoms.

Malfeasance Performing a wrongful act.

Malignant Highly dangerous or virulent; often used to describe a deadly form of cancer or a spreading of cancer.

Malignant hypertension Severe hypertension with signs of acute and progressive damage to end organs such as the heart, brain, and kidneys.

Malingering Faking illness for a tangible gain (missing work, avoiding incarceration, etc.).

Malleus Hammer-shaped bone located at the front of the middle ear; receives vibrations from the tympanic membrane.

Malocclusion The condition in which the teeth of the upper and lower jaws do not line up.

Mammary glands Female organs of milk production; located within the breast tissue.

Mania An excessively intense enthusiasm, interest, or desire; a craze.

Manure gas A name used for several different gases formed by decomposition of manure (methane, carbon dioxide, ammonia, hydrogen sulfide, and hydrogen disulfide); in certain concentrations all are toxic to animals and human beings.

Marasmus A form of nutritional deficiency from an overall lack of calories that results in wasting.

Marburg A viral hemorrhagic fever illness caused by the Marburg virus (Filovirus family).

Margination Process of phagocytes adhering to capillary and venule walls in the early phases of inflammation.

Marijuana Dried mixture of shredded leaves, stems, and seeds of the hemp plant that are usually smoked and contain many psychoactive compounds, most notably tetrahydrocannabinol (THC).

Mark 1 antidote kit Self-injected nerve agent antidote kit consisting of atropine and 2-pralidoxime (2-PAM).

Mast cells Connective tissue cell that contains histamine; important in initiating the inflammatory response.

Material safety data sheet (MSDS) A document that contains information about the specific identity of a hazardous chemical; information includes exact name and synonyms, health effects, first aid, chemical and physical properties, and emergency telephone numbers.

Matrix Nonliving material that separates cells in the connective tissue.

Mechanical processing Physical manipulation and breakdown of food.

Mechanism of action The manner in which a drug works to produce its intended effect.

Mechanism of injury The way an injury occurs on the body.

Meconium A dark green substance that represents the infant's first bowel movement.

Medial A position toward the midline of the body.

Median lethal dose The dose that kills 50% of the drug-tested population.

Mediastinitis Infection of the mediastinum; a serious medical condition.

Mediastinoscopy Surgical procedure of looking into the mediastinum with an endoscope.

Mediastinum Area that includes the trachea, esophagus, thymus gland, heart, and great vessels.

Medical asepsis Medically clean, not sterile; the goal in prehospital care because complete asepsis is not always possible.

Medical direction Physician oversight of paramedic practice; also called *medical control*.

Medical director A physician responsible for the oversight of the EMS system and the actions of the paramedics; also known as a *physician advisor*.

Medical ethics A field of study that evaluates the decisions, conduct, policies, and social concerns of medical activities.

Medical practice act Legislation that governs the practice of medicine; may prescribe how and to what extent a physician may delegate authority to a paramedic to perform medical acts; varies from state to state.

Medical terminology Greek- and Latin-based words (typically) that function as a common language for the medical community.

Medically clean Disinfected.

Medulla Most inferior part of the brainstem; responsible for some vegetative functions.

Medulla oblongata Lowest portion of brain tissue and the interface between the brain and the spinal cord; responsible for maintenance of basic life functions such as heart rate and respirations.

Meissner corpuscle Encapsulated nerve endings in the superficial dermis responsible for sensing vibrations and light touch.

Melancholy An episode of dysphoric mood with disruptions of homeostasis, including alterations in appetite, activities, and sleep patterns; also called *major* or *severe depression*.

Melena Foul-smelling, dark, and tarry stools stained with blood pigments or with digested blood, often indicating gastrointestinal bleeding.

Melting point The temperature at which a solid changes to a liquid (e.g., ice melting to water at 0°C (32°F).

Membrane potential Difference in electrical charge across the cell membrane.

Menarche The onset of the menstrual cycle.

Meninges Covering of the brain and spinal cord; layers include the dura mater, arachnoid, and pia mater.

Meningitis Irritation of the connective tissue covering the central nervous system, often from infection or hemorrhage.

Meningocele A type of spina bifida in which the spinal cord develops normally but a saclike cyst that contains the meninges and cerebrospinal fluid protrudes from an opening in the spine, usually in the lumbosacral area.

Meningomyelocele The severest form of spina bifida in which the meninges, cerebrospinal fluid, and a portion of the spinal cord protrude from an opening in the spine and are encased in a sac covered by a thin membrane; also called *myelomeningocele.*

Menopause Cessation of menstruation in the human female.

Menstruation Cyclical shedding of endometrial lining.

Mental illness Any form of psychiatric disorder.

Mental retardation Developmental disability characterized by a lower than normal IQ.

Merocrine glands Sweat glands that open directly to the surface of the body; produce a fluid (mainly water) when the temperature rises that allows the body to dispel large amounts of heat through the evaporation process.

Mesentery Layers of connective tissue found in the peritoneal cavity.

Metabolism Sum of all physical and chemical changes that occur within an organism.

Metabolites The smaller molecules from the breakdown that occurs during metabolism.

Metaplasia The transformation of one type of mature differentiated cell into another type of mature differentiated cell.

Metastatic Spread of cancerous cells to a distant site.

Metered-dose inhaler (MDI) A handheld device that disperses a measured dose of medication in the form of a fine spray directly into the airway.

Methamphetamine A powerful, highly addictive central nervous system stimulant found in either a white powder form or a clear crystal form ("crystal meth").

Methemoglobinemia The oxidation of hemoglobin from the ferrous iron to the ferric iron state.

Methicillin-resistant Staphylococcus aureus Any of several bacterial strains of *S. aureus* resistant to methicillin (a penicillin) and related drugs; typically acquired in the hospital.

Micturition Urination.

Midbrain Lies below the diencephalon and above the pons; works with the pons to route information from higher within the brain to the spinal cord and vice versa.

Middle ear Air-filled chamber within the temporal bone; contains the auditory ossicles.

Migraine headache A recurring vascular headache characterized by unilateral onset, severe pain, sensitivity to light, and autonomic disturbances during the acute phase, which may last for hours or days.

Milliampere (mA) Unit of measure of electrical current needed to elicit depolarization of the myocardium.

Millivolt (mV) Difference in electrical charge between two points in a circuit.

Minor In most states, a person younger than 18 years.

Minute volume Amount of gas moved in and out of the respiratory tract per minute. Tidal volume multiplied by ventilatory rate equals minute volume. The minute volume is the true measurement of a patient's ventilatory status and is vital in assessing pulmonary function. It ascertains the ventilatory rate and the depth of each inhalation.

Miosis Pinpoint pupils.

Miscarriage (spontaneous abortion) Loss of the products of conception before the fetus can survive on its own.

Misfeasance Performing a legal act in a harmful manner.

Mitochondria Power plant of the cell and body; site of aerobic oxidation.

Mitosis Process of division and multiplication in which one cell divides into two cells.

Mitral valve Left atrioventricular valve in the heart; also called the *bicuspid valve.*

Mittelschmerz Pain occurring at time of ovulation.

Mixed episode A period of manic-like energy and agitation coupled with the pessimism and dysphoria of severe depression.

Mobile data computer A device used in an ambulance or first responder vehicle to retrieve and send call information; has its own memory storage and processing capability.

Mobile data terminal A device used like a mobile data computer but without its own memory storage and processing capability.

Mobile radio A radio installed in an emergency vehicle; usually transmits by higher wattage than a portable radio.

Modern deployment Deployment that considers workload and how available resources can achieve a balance among coverage, response times, and crew satisfaction.

Mold A multicellular type of fungus that grows hyphae.

Monoblasts Immature monocytes.

Monocytes Type of white blood cell (leukocyte) designed to consume foreign material and fight pathogens; generally become macrophages within a few days after release into the bloodstream.

Monomorphic Having the same shape.

Mons pubis A hair-covered fat pad overlying the symphysis pubis.

Mood The dominant and sustained emotional state of a patient; the emotional lens through which a patient views the world.

Morals Values that help a person define right (what a person ought to do) versus wrong (what a person ought not to do).

Morbid obesity Having a body mass index of 40 or more; equates to approximately 100 lb more than ideal weight.

Morbidity Nonfatal injury rates; state of being diseased; propensity to cause disease or illness.

Mortality Death rate.

Mortality rate The number of patients who have died from a disease in a given period.

Motor cortex Area of brain tissue on the frontal lobe that controls voluntary movements.

Mucosa Layer of cells lining body cavities or organs (e.g., the lining of the mouth and digestive tract); generally implies a moist surface.

Multiformed atrial rhythm Cardiac dysrhythmia that occurs because of impulses originating from various sites, including the sinoatrial node, the atria, and/or the atrioventricular junction; requires at least three different P waves seen in the same lead for proper diagnosis.

Multipara A woman who has given birth multiple times.

Multiple-casualty incident An incident involving 26 to 99 persons.

Multiple organ dysfunction syndrome Altered organ function in an acutely ill person in whom homeostasis cannot be maintained without intervention.

Multiple-patient incident An incident involving two to 25 persons.

Multiple sclerosis (MS) Autoimmune disorder in which the immune system attacks the myelin sheath surrounding neurons, causing widespread motor problems and pain.

Multiplex A system that allows the crew to transmit voice and data at the same time, enabling the crew to call in a patient report while transmitting an ECG strip to the hospital.

Murphy's sign An inspiratory pause when the right upper quadrant is palpated.

Muscle tissue Contractile tissue that is the basis of movement.

Muscular dystrophy (MD) Hereditary condition causing malformation of muscle tissue and leading to malformation of the musculoskeletal system and physical disability.

Mutate To change in an unusual way.

Mutism A condition in which a person will not speak.

Myasthenia gravis Autoimmune disorder affecting acetylcholine receptors throughout the body, causing widespread muscle weakness.

Mycoses Diseases caused by fungi.

Mydriasis Dilation of the pupils.

Myelomeningocele Developmental anomaly of the central nervous system in which a hernial sac containing a portion of the spinal cord, the meninges, and cerebrospinal fluid protrudes through a congenital cleft in the vertebral column; occurs in approximately two of every 1000 live births, is readily apparent, and is easily diagnosed at birth.

Myocardial cells Working cells of the myocardium that contain contractile filaments and form the muscular layer of the atrial walls and the thicker muscular layer of the ventricular walls.

Myocardial depressant factor An inflammatory mediator (cytokine) produced as a result of significant burn injury; known to affect the contractile function of the cardiac ventricles.

Myocardial infarction (MI) Necrosis of some mass of the heart muscle caused by an inadequate blood supply.

Myocarditis Inflammation of the middle and thickest layer of the heart, the myocardium.

Myocardium Middle and thickest layer of the heart; contains the cardiac muscle fibers that cause contraction of the heart as well as the conduction system and blood supply.

Myoglobin A protein within muscle that functions as an oxygen carrier. When released in large quantities into the bloodstream, these proteins block the small vessels of the kidneys.

Myoglobinuria Presence of myoglobin in the urine; almost always a result of a pathologic (disease) state such as widespread muscle injury.

Myometrium Muscular region of the uterus.

Myopia Nearsightedness; difficulty seeing objects at a distance.

Myositis A rare muscle disease in which the body's immune system is activated, resulting in inflammation and pain of muscle tissue.

Myotomes Areas of the body controlled by specific motor spinal nerves.

Myxedema Severe form of hypothyroidism characterized by hypothermia and unresponsiveness.

N-95 particulate mask (medical) A facial mask worn over the nose and mouth that removes particulates from the inspired and expired air.

Nasal flaring Widening of the nostrils on inhalation; an attempt to increase the size of the airway and increase the amount of available oxygen.

Nasal polyps Small, saclike growths consisting of inflamed nasal mucosa.

Nasogastric (NG) The administration route used when a nasogastric tube is in place; bypasses the voluntary swallowing reflex.

Nasogastric tube A tube placed by way of the nose into the stomach.

Nasolacrimal duct Opening at the medial corner of the eye that drains excess fluid into the nasal cavity.

Natal Connected with birth.

National Disaster Medical System An organized response to an event that includes field units, coordination of patient transportation, and provision of hospital beds. The field component is composed of many volunteer teams of medical professionals.

National Fire Protection Association (NFPA) International voluntary membership organization that promotes improved fire protection and prevention and establishes safeguards against loss of life and property by fire; writes and publishes national voluntary consensus standards.

National Flight Paramedics Association (NFPA) Association established in 1984 to differentiate the critical care paramedic from the flight paramedic; has developed a position statement recommending the training considered necessary to perform the duties of a flight paramedic.

National Highway Traffic Safety Administration (NHTSA) An agency within the U.S. Department of Transportation that was first given the authority to develop EMS systems, including the development of curriculum.

National Medical Response Team Quick response specialty teams trained and equipped to provide mass casualty decontamination and patient care after the release of a chemical, biologic, or radiologic agent.

National Registry of EMTs (NREMT) A national organization developed to ensure that graduates of EMS training programs have met minimal standards by measuring competency through a uniform testing process.

National Standard Curriculum (NSC) Document providing information or course planning and structure, objectives, and detailed lesson plans. It also suggests hours of instruction for the EMT-A.

Natural immunity Nonspecific immunity that mounts a generalized response to any foreign material or pathogen (e.g., inflammation).

Natural killer cells Specialized lymphocytes capable of killing infected or malignant cells.

Nebulizer A machine that turns liquid medication into fine droplets in aerosol or mist form.

Necrosis Death of an area of tissue.

Necrotizing Causing the death (necrosis) of tissue.

Negative battery cable An electrical power cable that allows the vehicle's electrical system to be grounded or neutral as an electrical circuit.

Negative pressure Pressure that acts as a vacuum, pulling more fluid from the vascular space at a faster rate than before, further depleting the intravascular volume; also known as *inhibition pressure*.

Neglect Failure to provide the basic needs of an individual can be physical, educational, or emotional.

Negligence The failure to act as a reasonably prudent and careful person would under similar circumstances.

Negligence per se Conduct that may be declared and treated as negligent without having to prove what would be reasonable and prudent under similar circumstances, usually because the conduct violates a law or regulation.

Nematocyst The stinging cells many marine creatures use to envenomate and immobilize prey.

Neonatal abstinence syndrome Withdrawal symptoms that occur in newborns born to opioid-addicted mothers.

Neonate An infant from birth to 1 month of age.

Neoplasm Cancerous growth; a tumor that may be malignant or benign.

Neovascularization New blood vessel growth to support healing tissue.

Nephron Functional unit of the kidney.

Nephrotoxic Chemicals, medications, or other substances that can be toxic to the kidneys.

Nerve Neurons and blood vessels wrapped together with connective tissue; the body's information highways.

Nervous tissue Tissue that can conduct electrical impulses.

Neural tube defects Congenital anomalies that involve incomplete development of the brain, spinal cord, and/or their protective coverings.

Neuralgia Pain caused by chronic nerve damage.

Neuroeffector junction Interface between a neuron and its target tissue.

Neurogenic shock Shock with hypotension caused by a sudden loss of control over the sympathetic nervous system. Loss can be caused by a variety of mechanisms from traumatic injury to disease and infection.

Neuroglia Supporting cells of nervous tissue; functions include nourishment, protection, and insulation.

Neurons Conducting cells of nervous tissue; composed of a cell body, dendrites, and axon.

Neuropeptide A protein that may interact with a receptor after circulation through the blood.

Neuroses Mental diseases related to upbringing and personality in which the person remains "in touch" with reality.

Neurotransmitters A chemical released from one nerve that crosses the synaptic cleft to reach a receptor.

Neutralizing agent A substance that counteracts the effects of acids or bases; brings the pH of a solution back to 7.0.

Neutron radiation Penetrating radiation that can result in whole-body irradiation.

Neutrophils A form of granulocyte that is short lived but often first to arrive at the site of injury; capable of phagocytosis.

Newborn asphyxia The inability of a newborn to begin and continue breathing at birth.

Newly born An infant in the first minutes to hours after birth; also called *newborn.*

Nodule An elevated, solid lesion in the deep skin or subcutaneous tissues.

Noncardiogenic pulmonary edema (NCPE) Fluid collection in the alveoli of the lung that does not result from heart failure.

Nonfeasance Failure to perform a required act or duty.

Nonproprietary name Generic name.

Nonsteroidal antiinflammatory drug (NSAID) Medications used primarily to treat inflammation, mild to moderate pain, and fever.

Nonverbal cues Expressions, motions, gestures, and body language that may be used to communicate other than with words.

Normal flora Nonthreatening bacteria found naturally in the human body that, in some cases, are necessary for normal function.

Nuclear envelope The outer boundary between the nucleus and the rest of the cell to the endoplasmic reticulum for protein synthesis.

Nuclear membrane Membrane in the cell that surrounds the nucleus.

Nucleoplasm Protoplasm of the nucleus as contrasted with that of the cell.

Nucleus Area within a cell where the genetic material is stored.

Nullipara A woman who has not borne a child.

Numerator The number or mathematic expression written above the line in a fraction; the numerator is a portion of the denominator.

Nystagmus Involuntary rapid movement of the eyes in the horizontal, vertical, or rotary planes of the eyeball.

Obesity An excessively high amount of body fat or adipose tissue in relation to lean body mass.

Objective information Verifiable findings, such as information seen, felt, or heard by the paramedic.

Obsessive-compulsive disorder (OCD) An anxiety disorder marked by frequent, intrusive, unwanted, and bothersome thoughts (obsessions) and repetitive rituals (compulsions).

Obstructed lane +1 Blocking with an emergency vehicle to stop the flow of traffic in the lane in which the damaged vehicle is positioned plus one additional lane or the shoulder of the roadway.

Occipital lobe Most rearward portion of the cerebrum; mainly responsible for processing the sense of sight.

Occupational Safety and Health Administration (OSHA) A unit of the U.S. Department of Labor that establishes protective standards, enforces those standards, and reaches out to employers and employees through technical assistance and consultation programs.

Official name A drug's name as listed in the *United States Pharmacopoeia.*

Offline medical direction Prospective and retrospective medical direction (e.g., protocols and standard operating procedures).

Oils In medicine, substances extracted from flowers, leaves, stems, roots, seeds, or bark for use as therapeutic treatments.

Olfactory Sense of smell.

Olfactory fatigue Desensitization of the sense of smell.

Olfactory tissue Located within the nasopharynx; contains receptors that enable the ability of smell (olfaction).

Omphalocele Protrusion of abdominal organs into the umbilical cord.

Oncotic pressure The net effect of opposing osmotic pressures in the capillary beds.

Online medical direction Direct voice communication by a medical director (or designee) to a prehospital professional while he or she is attending to the patient; also called *direct medical direction.*

Oocyte The female gamete; product of the female reproductive system.

Oogenesis Egg production.

Open-ended questions A form of interview question that allows patients to respond in narrative form so that they may feel free to answer in their own way and provide details and information that they believe to be important.

Open fracture Fracture of the bone tissue that breaks the skin and may or may not still be exposed.

Open pneumothorax Injury to the thoracic cavity in which the cavity is breached, allowing air into the space between the lung and the chest wall.

Operations Carries out the tactical objectives of the incident commander.

Ophthalmic Route of administration in which medications are applied to the eye, such as antibiotic eye drops.

Ophthalmoscope An instrument used to examine the inner parts of the eye; consists of an adjustable light and multiple magnification lenses.

Opioids Powerful pain-relieving drugs derived from the seed pods of the poppy plant or drugs that are similar in molecular structure.

Oral A route of administration in which the medication is placed in the mouth and swallowed; the drug is absorbed through the gastrointestinal tract.

Oral cavity First part of the gastrointestinal tract; includes salivary glands, teeth, and tongue.

Organ A structure composed of two or more kinds of tissues organized to perform a more complex function than any one tissue alone can.

Organ of Corti Organ of hearing located in the cochlea.

Organ systems The coordination of several organs working together.

Organelles Structures within the cell that perform specialized functions.

Organic An etiology of an illness that stems from a biologic cause, such as a stroke or electrolyte imbalance.

Organism An entity composed of cells and capable of carrying on life functions.

Organophosphate A pesticide that inhibits acetylcholinesterase.

Orogastric (OG) tube A tube placed by way of the mouth into the stomach.

Oropharynx Starts at the uvula; back of the oral cavity that extends down to the epiglottis.

Orphan drugs Products developed for the diagnosis and/or treatment of rare diseases or conditions, such as sickle cell anemia and cystic fibrosis.

Orthopnea Dyspnea relieved by a change in position (either sitting upright or standing).

Orthostatic vital signs Serial measurements of the patient's pulse and blood pressure taken with the patient recumbent, sitting, and standing. Results are used to assess possible volume depletion; also called the *tilt test* or *postural vital signs.*

Osmolarity The number, or concentration, of solute per liter of water.

Osmosis The passive movement of water from a higher to a lower concentration.

Osmotic gradient The difference in the concentration from one side of a membrane to the other in the presence of an imbalance in the ionic concentration.

Osmotic pressure The pressure exerted by the concentration of the solutes in a given space.

Osteoarthritis A disorder in which the cartilaginous covering of the joint surface starts to wear away, resulting in pain and inflammation of a joint; also known as *degenerative joint disease.*

Osteomyelitis An infection of bone.

Osteoporosis Reduction in the amount of bone mass, which leads to fractures after minimal trauma.

Ostomy Hole; usually refers to a surgically made hole in some part of the body (e.g., tracheostomy, gastrostomy, colostomy).

Otic Route of administration in which medications are applied to the ear, such as antibiotic drops.

Otitis externa A condition manifested by redness and irritation of the external auditory canal; also called *swimmer's ear.*

Otosclerosis Abnormal growth of bone that prevents structures in the ear from working properly; thought to be a hereditary disease.

Otoscope An instrument used to examine the inner ear; consists of a light source and magnifying lens; the tip is covered with a disposable cone.

Oval window A membranous structure that separates the middle ear from the inner ear.

Ovarian follicle The ovum and its surrounding cells.

Ovarian medulla Inner portion of the ovary.

Ovarian torsion Twisting of an ovary on its axis such that the venous flow to the ovary is interrupted.

Ovaries Site of egg production in females.

Overdose The accidental or intentional ingestion of an excess of a substance with the potential for toxicity.

Over-the-counter (OTC) Drugs that can be purchased without a prescription.

Overweight State of increased body weight in relation to height.

Ovulation Mid-cycle release of an ovum during the menstrual cycle.

Ovum (oocyte) Human egg that, when fertilized, implants in the lining of the uterus and results in pregnancy.

Oxidation A normal chemical process in the body caused by the release of oxygen atoms created during normal cell metabolism.

Oxidation ability The ability of a substance to readily release oxygen to stimulate combustion.

Oxygen-limiting silo A vertical structure used to store ensiled plant material in an anaerobic environment.

Oxyhemoglobin Hemoglobin that has oxygen molecules bound to it.

P wave First wave in the cardiac cycle; represents atrial depolarization and the spread of the electrical impulse throughout the right and left atria.

Pacemaker Artificial pulse generator that delivers an electrical current to the heart to stimulate depolarization.

Pacemaker cells Specialized cells of the heart's electrical conduction system capable of spontaneously generating and conducting electrical impulses.

Packaging Placing the injured or ill patient in a litter and securing him or her for evacuation.

Painful stimulus Any stimulus that causes discomfort to the patient, triggering some sort of response.

Palliative care Provision of comfort measures (physical, social, psychological, and spiritual) to terminally ill patients.

Pallor Pale, washed-out coloration of skin. Often a result of extreme anemia or chronic illness. A patient with pallor can be referred to as pallid.

Palpation The process of applying pressure against the body with the intent of gathering information.

Palpitations An unpleasant awareness of one's heartbeat.

Pancreatitis Inflammation of the pancreas.

Pandemic A disease that affects the majority of the population of a single region or that is epidemic at the same time in many different regions.

Panic attack A sudden, paralyzing anxiety reaction characterized by an overwhelming sense of fear, anxiety, and impending doom, often with physical symptoms such as chest pain and difficulty breathing.

Papillary dermis Section of the dermis composed of loose connective tissue that contains vasculature that feeds the epidermis.

Papillary muscles Muscles attached to the chordae tendineae of the heart valves and the ventricular muscle of the heart.

Papule An elevated, solid lesion usually less than 0.5 centimeters in diameter; may arise from the epidermis, dermis, or both.

Para The number of pregnancies carried to 20 weeks or more.

Paracrine communication Method of intercellular communication in which cells communicate with cells in close proximity through the release of paracrine factors, or cytokines.

Paradoxic motion (of a segment of the chest wall) Part of the chest moves in an opposite direction from the rest during respiration.

Paranoid delusions False perceptions of persecution and the feeling that one is being hunted or conspired against; this is the most common type of delusion.

Paranoid schizophrenia A form of schizophrenia characterized by persistent preoccupation with illogical, absurd, and changeable delusions, usually of a persecutory, grandiose, or jealous nature, accompanied by related hallucinations.

Paraphimosis Tight, constricting band caused by the foreskin when it is retracted behind the glans penis.

Paraplegia Paralysis of the lower extremities. The injury can be either complete (a complete loss of muscle control and sensation below the injury site) or incomplete (a partial loss of muscle control or sensation below the injury site).

Parasites An organism that lives within or on another organism (the host) but does not contribute to the host's survival.

Parasympathetic division A division of the autonomic nervous system; responsible for the relaxed state of the body known as "feed and breed."

Parasympathetic nervous system The subdivision of the autonomic nervous system usually involved in activating vegetative functions, such as digestion, defecation, and urination.

Parasympatholytics Drugs that block or inhibit the function of the parasympathetic receptors.

Parasympathomimetics Drugs that mimic the parasympathetic division of the autonomic nervous system.

Parenteral Administration route used for systemic effects and given by a route other than the digestive tract.

Paresthesia Abnormal sensation described as numbness, tingling, or pins and needles.

Parietal lobe Section of the cerebrum responsible for the integration of most sensory information from the body.

Parietal pleura Lining of the pleural cavity attached tightly to the interior of the chest cage.

Parity The number of pregnancies that have resulted in birth.

Parkinson's disease Progressive movement disorder caused by dysfunction in the cerebellum; rigidity, tremor, bradykinesia, and postural instability are characteristic.

Parkmedic A National Park Service ranger who has undergone additional wilderness medical training and who operates in certain parks under the medical direction of emergency physicians from University of Southern California–Fresno; scope of practice lies between a traditional EMT-Intermediate and EMT-Paramedic, with additional wilderness medical training.

Paroxysmal atrial tachycardia Atrial tachycardia that starts or ends suddenly.

Paroxysmal nocturnal dyspnea (PND) A sudden onset of difficulty breathing that awakens the patient from sleep.

Paroxysmal supraventricular tachycardia (PSVT) A regular, narrow QRS tachycardia that starts or ends suddenly.

Partial agonist A drug that when bound to a receptor may elicit a physiologic response, but it is less than that of an agonist; may also may block the response of a competing agonist.

Partial pressure The pressure exerted by an individual gas in a mixture.

Partial seizure A seizure confined to one area of the brain.

Partial-thickness burn Burns that involve any layer of the dermis. The depth of these burns varies and depends on location, so they are further subcategorized as superficial partial-thickness or deep partial-thickness burns. Also called *second-degree burns.*

Partially sighted Level of vision in persons who have some type of visual problem and may need assistance.

Passive immunity Induced immunity that only lasts as long as the injected immune agents are alive and active (e.g., immunoglobulin injection).

Passive range of motion Degree of movement at a joint determined when the examiner causes the movement with the patient at rest.

Passive transport The ability of a substance to traverse a barrier without any energy input; generally occurs from a higher to a lower concentration.

Past medical history A summary of all past health-related events.

Patch A flat, circumscribed, discolored lesion measuring greater than 1 cm.

Pathologic fracture Fractures that occur as a result of an underlying disease process that weakens the mechanical properties of the bone.

Pathophysiology Functional changes that accompany a particular syndrome or disease.

Patients with terminal illness Patients with advanced stage of illness or disease with an unfavorable prognosis and no known cure.

Pattern recognition Gathering patient information, relating it to the healthcare professional's knowledge of pathophysiology and the signs and symptoms of illnesses and injuries, and determining whether the patient's presentation fits a particular pattern.

Pattern response Anticipating the equipment and emergency care interventions needed on the basis of the patient's history and physical examination findings.

Patterned injuries Those that leave a distinctive mark, indicating that an object was used in the assault (e.g., cigarette burns, electrical cord whipping, human bites, glove injuries, attempted strangulation, and slaps).

Peak expiratory flow The greatest rate of airflow that can be achieved during forced expiration beginning with the lungs fully inflated.

Peak flow meter A device used to assess the severity of respiratory distress.

Pediculosis Human infestation with lice.

Pelvic inflammatory disease (PID) An infection of a woman's reproductive organs, usually from a bacterial infection, that spreads from the vagina to the upper parts of the reproductive tract.

Penetrating trauma Any mechanism of injury that causes a cut or piercing of skin.

Penis Male sex organ with three columns of erectile tissue; transfers sperm during copulation.

Percussion A diagnostic technique that uses tapping on the body to differentiate air, solids, and fluids.

Performance-based response system A contractual agreement between the EMS provider and the government authority to provide ambulance response to a particular municipality or region with time requirements for each response and total responses on a monthly basis.

Perfusion Circulation of blood through an organ or a part of the body.

Pericardial cavity The potential space between the two layers of the pericardium.

Pericardial effusion An increase in the volume and/or character of pericardial fluid that surrounds the heart.

Pericardial tamponade Life-threatening injury in which blood collects within the pericardium until the increasing pressure prevents the heart from filling with blood, causing death.

Pericardiocentesis A procedure in which a needle is inserted into the pericardial space and the excess fluid is drawn out (aspirated) through the needle.

Pericarditis Inflammation of the double-walled sac (pericardium) that encloses the heart.

Pericardium Two-layer serous membrane lining the pericardial cavity.

Perinatal From the twenty-eighth week of gestation through the first 7 days after delivery.

Perineal body See *Perineum.*

Perineum The tissue between the mother's vaginal and rectal openings; may be torn during delivery.

Periodontal membrane/ligament Ligamentous attachment between the root of a tooth and the socket of the bone within which it sits.

Periosteum Fibrous connective tissue rich in nerve endings that envelops bone.

Peripheral nervous system All the nerves outside the central nervous system.

Peripheral vein A vein outside the chest or abdomen, such as the veins of the upper and lower extremities.

Peripherally inserted central catheter (PICC) line A thin tube inserted into a peripheral vein (usually the arm) and threaded into the superior vena cava to allow fluid or medication administration.

Peristalsis The wavelike contraction of the smooth muscle of the gastrointestinal tract.

Peritoneal cavity The space between the parietal and visceral peritoneum; also called the *peritoneal space.*

Peritoneum Double-layered serous membrane that lines the abdominal cavity and covers the organs located in the abdominopelvic cavity.

Peritonitis Inflammation of the peritoneum, typically caused by infection or in response to contact with blood or digestive fluids.

Peritonsillar abscess (PTA) An infection of tissue between the tonsil and pharynx, usually the result of a significant infection in the tonsils.

Permeability Ability of a membrane channel to allow passage of electrolytes once it is open.

Permissible exposure limit Allowable air concentration of a substance in the workplace as established by the Occupational Safety and Health Administration; these values are legally enforceable.

Permit-required confined space A confined space with one or more of the following characteristics: (1) contains or has a potential to contain a hazardous atmosphere; (2) contains a material with the potential for engulfing an entrant; (3) has an internal configuration such that an entrant could be trapped or asphyxiated by inwardly converging walls or by a floor that slopes downward and tapers to a smaller cross-section; or (4) contains any other recognized serious safety or health hazard.

Personal protective equipment (PPE) Equipment used to protect personnel; includes items such as gloves, eyewear, masks, respirators, and gowns.

Personal space The area around an individual that the person perceives as an extension of himself or herself. In the United States, personal distance is 1.5 to 4 feet.

Personality disorders Patterns of interacting with others and the world that are rigid and harmful, causing social and occupational problems.

Pertinent negative In a patient assessment, the signs and symptoms found not to be present that support a working diagnosis.

Pertinent positive In a patient assessment, the signs and symptoms found to be present that support a working diagnosis.

Pesticide A chemical material used to control a pest (insect, weed, etc.).

Petechiae A tiny pinpoint rash on the upper area of the neck and the face; may indicate near strangulation or suffocation; caused by an occlusion of venous return from the head while arterial pressure remains normal; may be present in mothers after childbirth.

pH A numeric assignment used to define the hydrogen ion concentration of a given chemical. The lower the pH, the higher the hydrogen ion concentration and the more acidic the solution.

Phagocyte Cells that are part of the body's immune system that play a predominant role in the destruction of invading microorganisms.

Phagocytosis Ingestion and digestion of foreign materials by phagocytes (cells, such as macrophages, designed to perform this function).

Pharmaceutics The science of preparing and dispensing drugs.

Pharmacogenetics The study of inherited differences (variation) in drug metabolism and response.

Pharmacokinetics The process by which a drug is absorbed, distributed, metabolized, and eliminated by the body.

Pharmacologic restraints Agents such as sedatives that can suppress a patient's neurologic and/or motor capabilities so that the threat to the paramedic is reduced; also known as *chemical restraints*.

Pharmacology The study of drugs, including their actions and effects on the host.

Pharmacopoeia A book describing drugs, chemicals, and medicinal preparations in a country or specific geographic area, including a description of the drug, its formula, and dosage.

Phases of rescue The training and organizational concept that groups all the activities that take place at a typical vehicle crash with entrapment into four categories, with each known as a phase of rescue.

Phlebitis Inflammation of a vein.

Phobia An intense fear of a particular object or situation.

Phosphate A salt of phosphoric acid that is important in the maintenance of the acid-base balance of the blood.

Phospholipid bilayer A double layer composed of three types of lipid molecules that comprise the plasma membrane.

Photoreceptor cells Rods and cones contained in the sensory part of the retina; they relay impulses to the optic nerve.

Photosensitivity A condition in which the patient's eyes are sensitive or feel pain when exposed to bright light.

Physical abuse Inflicting a nonaccidental physical injury on another person such as punching, kicking, hitting, or biting.

Physical disabilities Disabilities that involve limitation of mobility.

Physical restraints Straps, splints, and other devices that prevent movement of all or part of the patient's body.

Physician advisor A physician responsible for the oversight of the EMS system and the actions of the paramedics; also known as a *medical director*.

Physiology Study of how the body functions.

Pia mater Last meningeal layer; adheres to the central nervous system.

Pierre Robin sequence A congenital anomaly characterized by a very small lower jaw (micrognathia), a tongue that tends to fall back and downward (glossoptosis), and cleft palate.

Pill Dried powder forms of medication in the form of a small pellet; the term "pill" has been replaced with tablet and capsule.

Pinch points A machinery entanglement hazard formed when two machine parts move together and at least one of the parts moves in a circle.

Pinocytosis Absorption or ingestion of nutrients, debris, and fluids by a cell.

Placards Diamond-shaped signs placed on the sides and ends of bulk transport containers (e.g., truck, tank car, freight container) that carry hazardous materials.

Placenta (afterbirth) The organ inside the uterus that exchanges nutrition and waste between mother and fetus.

Placenta previa Placement of the placenta such that it partially or completely covers the cervix.

Placental abruption (abruptio placenta) Separation of part of the placenta away from the wall of the uterus.

Placental barrier Many layers of cells that form between maternal and fetal circulation that protect the fetus from toxins.

Plague An acute infectious disease caused by the anaerobic, gram-negative bacterium *Yersinia pestis;* transmitted naturally from rodents to human beings through flea bites; three common syndromes are bubonic (most likely form of the disease to be seen from naturally occurring infections), pneumonic (most likely form of the disease to result from an act of terrorism), and septicemic plague.

Plaintiff The person who initiates a lawsuit by filing a complaint; also known as a *claimant, petitioner,* or *applicant.*

Planning Supplies past, present, and future information about the incident.

Plaque An elevated, solid lesion usually greater than 0.5 cm in diameter that lacks any deep component.

Plasma Pale, yellow material in the blood; made of approximately 92% water and 8% dissolved molecules.

Plasma level profile The measurement of blood level of a medication versus the dosage administered.

Plasma membrane The outer covering of a cell that contains the cellular cytoplasm; also known as the *cell membrane.*

Platelets One of three formed elements in the blood; also called *thrombocytes.*

Pleura Serous membrane that lines the pleural cavity.

Pleural cavities Areas that contain the lungs.

Pleural effusion Collection of fluid in the pleural space, usually fluid that has seeped through the lung or chest wall tissue.

Pleural friction rub Noise made when the visceral and parietal pleura rub together.

Pleurisy Painful rubbing of the pleural lining.

Plural Amount that refers to more than one person, place, or thing.

Pluripotent Cell line that has the ability to differentiate into multiple different cell lines based on the right physiologic stimulus.

Pneumomediastinum Air entrapped within the mediastinum; a serious medical condition.

Pneumonia An inflammation and infection of the lower airway and lungs caused by a viral, bacterial, parasitic, or fungal organism.

Pneumonia Infection of the lungs.

Pneumothorax A collection of air in the pleural space, usually from either a hole in the lung or a hole in the chest wall.

Pocket mask A clear, semirigid mask designed for mouth-to-mask ventilation of a nonbreathing adult, child, or infant.

Poikilothermic An organism whose temperature matches the ambient temperature.

Point of maximum impulse (PMI) The apical impulse; the site where the heartbeat is most strongly felt.

Poison Any substance that can harm the human body; also known as a *toxin.*

Poisoning Exposure to a substance that is harmful in any dosage.

Poisonous Describes gases, liquids, or other substances of such nature that exposure to a very small amount is dangerous to life or is a hazard to health; also known as *toxic* (e.g., cyanide, arsenic, phosgene, aniline, methyl bromide, insecticides, pesticides).

Polarized state Period after repolarization of a myocardial cell (also called the *resting state*) when the outside of the cell is positive and the interior of the cell is negative.

Poliomyelitis Viral infection that tends to attack the motor roots of the spinal nerves, often leading to physical disability and even paralysis of the diaphragm.

Polydipsia Excessive thirst.

Polymorphic Varying in shape.

Polyphagia Excessive eating.

Polypharmacy The concurrent use of several medications.

Polyuria Excessive urination.

Pons Area of the brainstem that contains the sleep and respiratory centers for the body, which along with the medulla control breathing.

Portable radio Also referred to as a *walkie-talkie.* These radios are carried by emergency personnel and have a lower wattage output than the mobile or base unit. To use these portable radios with a higher watt output, the units can be connected through a repeater system to increase their output, which increases range.

Portal hypertension Increased venous pressure in the portal circulation.

Portal vein A vein composed of a group of vessels that originate from the digestive system.

Positive battery cable Also known as the *hot cable,* this electrical power cable allows a vehicle's electrical system to carry the current or electrical energy from the battery to the electrically powered appliances throughout the vehicle.

Positive end-expiratory pressure (PEEP) The amount of pressure above atmospheric pressure present in the airway at the end of the expiratory cycle. When forcing air into the lungs (positive-pressure ventilation), airway pressure is maintained above atmospheric pressure at the end of exhalation by means of a mechanical device, such as a PEEP valve.

Positive-pressure ventilation Forcing air into the lungs.

Postconcussion syndrome Symptoms of a concussion that persist for weeks to 1 year after an initial injury to the head.

Posterior The back, or dorsal, surface.

Postganglionic neuron The nerve that travels from the ganglia to the desired organ or tissue.

Postictal State that begins at the termination of seizure activity in the brain and ends with the patient returning to a level of normal behavior.

Postnatal The period immediately following the birth of a child and lasting for approximately 6 weeks.

Postpartum Pertaining to the mother after delivery.

Posttraumatic stress disorder (PTSD) An anxiety disorder that occurs after a traumatic, often life-threatening event.

Posture A patient's overall attitude and frame of mind.

Potassium The main intracellular ion (electrolyte), with the chemical designation K+.

Potential difference Difference in electrical charge between two points in a circuit; expressed in volts or millivolts.

Potentiating To augment or increase the action of.

Potentiation A prolongation or increase in the effect of a drug by another drug.

Pounds per square inch (psi) The amount of pressure on an area that is 1 inch square.

Poverty of speech A disorder of thought form characterized by very little spontaneous, voluntary speech and short answers to questions.

Powder Medication ground into a fine substance.

Power take-off Element that connects a tractor to an implement; also called a *driveshaft*.

Prearrival instructions Clinically approved instructions provided by telephone by a trained and certified emergency medical dispatcher.

Precapillary sphincters Smooth muscle located at the entrances to the capillaries; responsive to local tissue needs.

Preeclampsia A complication of pregnancy that includes hypertension, swelling of the extremities and, in its most severe form, seizures (see *Eclampsia*).

Preexcitation Term used to describe rhythms that originate from above the ventricles but in which the impulse travels by a pathway other than the atrioventricular node and bundle of His; thus the supraventricular impulse excites the ventricles earlier than normal.

Prefix A sequence of letters that comes before the word root and often describes a variation of the norm.

Preganglionic neuron The nerve that extends from the spinal cord (central nervous system) to the ganglion.

Prehospital care report (PCR) The report written by the paramedic after the call has been completed. The report becomes part of the patient's permanent medical record.

Preload Force exerted by the blood on the walls of the ventricles at the end of diastole.

Premature birth Delivery between the twentieth and thirty-seventh weeks of pregnancy.

Premature complex Early beat occurring before the next expected beat; can be atrial, junctional, or ventricular.

Premature or preterm infant Infant born before 37 weeks of gestation.

Prenatal Preceding birth.

Preoccupation A topic or theme that consistently recurs in a person's thought process and conversations.

Prepuce A fold formed by the union of the labia minora over the clitoris.

Presbycusis Age-related hearing loss.

Presbyopia Loss of function of the lens to adjust to close reading; usual onset in middle age.

Presenting part The first part of the infant to appear at the vaginal opening, usually the head.

Pressured speech Rapid, loud, and intense speech that often results from racing thoughts and is frequently seen during manic episodes.

Preterm birth Birth before 37 weeks of gestation.

Preterm delivery Delivery between the twentieth and thirty-seventh weeks of pregnancy.

Prevalence rate The fraction of the population that currently has a certain disease.

Priapism A prolonged and painful erection.

Primary apnea The newly born's initial response to hypoxemia consisting of initial tachypnea, then apnea, bradycardia, and a slight increase in blood pressure; if stimulated, responds with resumption of breathing.

Primary blast injury Injuries caused by an explosive's pressure wave.

Primary cord injury A spinal cord injury caused by a direct traumatic blow.

Primary hypertension High blood pressure for which no cause is identifiable; also called *essential hypertension*.

Primary injury prevention Keeping an injury from occurring.

Primary skin lesion A lesion that has not been altered by scratching, rubbing, scrubbing, or other types of trauma.

Primary triage The initial sorting of patients to determine which are most injured and in need of immediate care.

Primary tumor A collection of cells that grow out of control, far in excess of normal rates. A primary tumor is a tumor that develops in one tissue only (e.g., a liver primary tumor originates in the liver).

Primigravida A woman who is pregnant for the first time.

Primipara A woman who has given birth to her first child.

Primum non nocere Latin for "first, do no harm."

Prions Infectious agents composed of only proteins.

Prodromal An early symptom of a disease.

Prodrome A symptom indicating the onset of a disease.

Prodrug A substance that is inactive when it is given and is converted to an active form within the body.

Profession A group of similar jobs or fields of interest that involve a responsibility to serve the public and require mastery of specific knowledge and specialized skills.

Professional A person who has special knowledge and skills and conforms to high standards of conduct and performance.

Professional malpractice A type of tort case addressing whether a professional person failed to act as a reasonably prudent and careful person with similar training would act under similar circumstances.

Professionalism Following the standards of conduct and performance for a profession.

Progesterone A female hormone secreted after ovulation has occurred that causes changes in the lining of the uterus necessary for successful implantation of a fertilized egg.

Prokaryotes One of the kingdoms of cells; simpler in structure and found in lower life forms such as bacteria.

Proliferative phase Portion of the menstrual cycle in which the endometrial lining grows under the influence of estrogen.

Prone Position in which the patient is lying on his or her stomach (face down).

Proprioception Ability to sense the orientation, location, and movement of the body's parts relative to other body parts.

Prospective medical direction Physician participation in the development of EMS protocols and procedures, and participation in the education and testing of EMS professionals; a type of offline medical direction.

Prostaglandins A class of fatty acids that has many of the properties of hormones.

Prostate Glandular tissue that produces prostatic fluid and muscular portion that contracts during ejaculation to prevent urine flow; dorsal to the symphysis pubis and the base of the urinary bladder.

Protein Any one of a number of large molecules composed of amino acids that form the structural components of cells or carry out biochemical functions.

Protocols A set of treatment guidelines written for the paramedic to follow. A written form of medical direction.

Protoxin A substance converted to a toxin through a biochemical process in the body; would be harmless if they were not converted (e.g., methanol and ethylene glycol).

Proximal A position nearer to the attachment of a limb to the trunk.

Pruritus Itching of the skin.

Psoriasis A common chronic skin disorder characterized by erythematous papules and plaques with a silver scale.

Psychological abuse The verbal or psychological misuse of another person, including threatening, name calling, ignoring, shaming unfairly, shouting, and cursing; mind games are another form of psychological abuse.

Psychomotor Pertaining to motor effects of cerebral or psychic activity.

Psychomotor agitation Excessive motor activity that is usually nonproductive and tedious, resulting from inner tensions (pacing, fidgeting, hand wringing, etc.)

Psychoses A group of mental disorders in which the individual loses contact with reality; psychosis is thought to be related to complex biochemical disease that disorders brain function. Examples include schizophrenia, bipolar disease (also known as *manic-depressive illness*), and organic brain disease.

Psychosis An abnormal state of widespread brain dysfunction characterized by bizarre thought content, typically delusions and hallucinations.

Psychosocial development The social and psychological changes human beings undergo as they grow and age.

Psychosocial factors Life events that affect a person's emotional state, such as marriage, divorce, or death of a loved one.

Public health The discipline that studies the overall health of populations and intervenes on behalf of those populations rather than on behalf of individuals.

Public Safety Answering Point (PSAP) A dispatch center set up to receive and dispatch 9-1-1 calls.

Pull-in point Machinery entanglement hazard created when an operator attempts to remove material being pulled into a machine.

Pulmonary abscess A collection of pus within the lung itself.

Pulmonary arteries Left and right pulmonary arteries supplying the lungs.

Pulmonary bleb Cavity in the lung much like a balloon; may rupture to create a pneumothorax.

Pulmonary circulation Blood from the right ventricle is pumped directly to the lungs for oxygenation through the pulmonary trunk; blood becomes oxygenated and is then delivered through the pulmonary arteries for the left atrium.

Pulmonary edema A buildup of fluid in the lungs, usually a complication of left ventricular fibrillation.

Pulmonary embolism Movement of a clot into the pulmonary circulation.

Pulmonary embolus A blood clot that has lodged in the pulmonary artery, causing shortness of breath and hypoxia.

Pulmonary trunk Vessels that deliver blood from the right ventricle of the heart to the lungs for oxygenation.

Pulmonary veins Vessels that return blood to the left atrium of the heart.

Pulmonic valve Right semilunar valve; separates the right ventricle and the pulmonary trunk.

Pulp Center of a tooth that contains nerves, blood vessels, and connective tissue.

Pulse deficit A difference between the apical pulse and the peripheral pulse rates.

Pulse generator Power source that houses the battery and controls for regulating a pacemaker.

Pulse oximetry A noninvasive method of measuring the percentage of oxygen-bound hemoglobin.

Pulse pressure The difference between the systolic and diastolic blood pressures.

Pulseless electrical activity (PEA) Organized electrical activity observed on a cardiac monitor (other than ventricular tachycardia) without the patient having a palpable pulse.

Pulsus alternans A beat-to-beat difference in the strength of a pulse (also called *mechanical alternans*).

Pulsus paradoxus A fall in systolic blood pressure of more than 10 mm Hg during inspiration (also called *paradoxic pulse*).

Pupil Central opening in the iris.

Purkinje fibers Fibers found in both ventricles that conduct an electrical impulse through the heart.

Purpura Reddish-purple nonblanchable discolorations greater than 0.5 cm in diameter; large purpura are called ecchymoses.

Pustule A lesion that contains purulent material.

Pyelonephritis Infection of the kidney.

Pyrogens Substances, such as endotoxins from certain bacteria, that stimulate the body to produce a fever.

Pyrophorics Substances that form self-ignitable flammable vapors when in contact with air.

QRS complex Several waveforms (Q wave, R wave, and S wave) that represent the spread of an electrical impulse through the ventricles (ventricular depolarization).

Quadriplegia Paralysis affecting all four extremities.

Quality assurance Programs designed to achieve a desired level of care.

Quality improvement Programs designed to improve the level of care; commonly driven by quality assurance.

Quality improvement unit (QIU) Trained and certified quality specialists who have the knowledge and skills to measure dispatcher performance against established standards accurately and consistently.

Quarantine The seclusion of groups of exposed but asymptomatic individuals for monitoring.

Quick response unit A type of responder with paramedic-level skills but no transport capability.

R wave On an EGG, the first positive deflection in the QRS complex, representing ventricular depolarization.

Raccoon eyes Bruising around the orbits of the eyes.

Racing thoughts The subjective feeling that one's thoughts are moving so fast that one cannot keep up; often seen during manic episodes.

Radio frequency Channel that allows communication from one specific user to another. For simple communication, both users must be on the same frequency or channel.

Radioactive The ability to emit ionizing radioactive energy.

Radioactive substances Any material or combination of materials that spontaneously emit ionizing radiation and have a specific activity greater than 0.002 mcCi/g (e.g., plutonium, cobalt, uranium 235, radioactive waste).

Radioactivity The spontaneous disintegration of unstable nuclei accompanied by the emission of nuclear radiation.

Range of motion The full and natural range of a joint's movement.

Rapid medical assessment A quick head-to-toe assessment of a medical patient who is unresponsive or has an altered mental status.

Rapid sequence intubation (RSI) The use of medications to sedate and paralyze a patient to achieve endotracheal intubation rapidly.

Rapid trauma assessment A quick head-to-toe assessment of a trauma patient with a significant mechanism of injury.

Rattles (rhonchi) Attributable to inflammation and mucus or fluid in the larger airway passages; descriptive of airway congestion heard on inspiration. Rhonchi are commonly associated with bronchitis or pneumonia.

Red blood cell count The number of red blood cells per liter of blood.

Rebound tenderness Discomfort experienced by the patient that occurs when the pressure from palpation is released.

Receptor A molecule, such as a protein, found inside or on the surface of a cell that binds to a specific substance (such as hormones, antigens, drugs, or neurotransmitters) and causes a specific physiologic effect in the cell.

Reciprocal change Mirror image ECG changes seen in the wall of the heart opposite the location of an infarction.

Reciprocity The ability for an EMS professional to use his or her certification or license to be able to practice in a different state.

Recompression A method used to treat divers with certain diving disorders, such as decompression sickness.

Rectal The drug administration route for suppositories; the drug is placed into the rectum (colon) and is absorbed into the venous circulation.

Rectum End of the sigmoid colon; feces are further compacted into waste here.

Reentry Spread of an impulse through tissue already stimulated by that same impulse.

Referred pain Pain felt at a site distant to the organ of origin.

Reflection Echoing the patient's message using your own words.

Reflection on actions A final step that may involve a personal reflection or a run critique; in certain instances this may be done formally, but in most instances it is accomplished informally.

Refractoriness Period of recovery that cells need after being discharged before they are able to respond to a stimulus.

Refresher education The process of refreshing information and skills previously learned.

Registration The process of entering an individual's name and essential information into a record as a means of verifying initial certification and monitoring recertification.

Regurgitation Backward flow of blood through a valve during ventricular contraction of the heart.

Rejection In terms of organ transplantation, the process by which the body uses its immune system to identify a transplanted organ and kill it; the medical management of posttransplant patients is largely directed at preventing rejection.

Relative refractory period Corresponds with the downslope of the T wave; cardiac cells can be stimulated to depolarize if the stimulus is strong enough.

Relief medic Emergency medical technician who has obtained additional training and certification in disaster and relief medical operations.

Rem Roentgen equivalent man.

Renal calculi Kidney stones formed by substances such as calcium, uric acid, or cystine.

Renal corpuscle Large terminal end of the nephron.

Renal insufficiency A decrease in renal function to approximately 25% of normal.

Renal pyramids Number of divisions in the kidney.

Repeater A system that receives transmissions from a low-wattage radio and rebroadcasts the signal at a higher wattage to the dispatch center.

Reperfusion phenomenon Series of events that result from the reperfusion of tissue damaged in a crush injury or tissue that is profoundly hypoxic; can lead to crush syndrome (rhabdomyolysis).

Repolarization Movement of ions across a cell membrane in which the inside of the cell is restored to its negative charge.

Res ipsa loquitur Latin phrase meaning "the thing speaks for itself." In negligence cases, this doctrine can be imposed when the plaintiff cannot prove all four components of negligence, but the injury itself would not have occurred without negligence (e.g., a sponge left in a patient after surgery).

Rescue The act of delivery from danger or entrapment.

Residual volume After a maximal forced exhalation, the amount of air remaining in the lungs and airway passages not able to be expelled.

Resistance The amount of weight moved or lifted during isotonic exercise. Also the ability of the body to defend itself against disease-causing microorganisms.

Resistance stage The stage of the stress response in which the specific stimulus no longer elicits an alarm reaction.

Respiration The exchange of gases between a living organism and its environment.

Respiratory arrest Absence of breathing.

Respiratory distress Increased work of breathing (respiratory effort).

Respiratory failure A clinical condition in which there is inadequate blood oxygenation and/or ventilation to meet the metabolic demands of the body tissues.

Respiratory membrane Where gas exchange takes place; oxygen is picked up in the bloodstream and carbon dioxide is eliminated through the lungs.

Respiratory syncytial virus A virus linked to bronchiolitis in infants and children.

Respiratory tract Passages to move air to and from the exchange surfaces.

Respondeat superior Latin phrase meaning "let the master answer." Under this legal doctrine, an employer is liable for the acts of employees within their scope of employment.

Response area The geographic area assigned to an emergency vehicle for responding to the sick and injured.

Response assignment plan An approved, consistent plan for responding to each call type.

Response mode A type of response, either with or without lights and sirens use.

Response time The time from when the call is received until the paramedics arrive at the scene.

Restraint Any mechanism that physically restricts an individual's freedom of movement, physical activity, or normal access to his or her body.

Restraint asphyxia Suffocation of a patient stemming from an inability to expand the chest cavity during inspiration because of restraint and immobilization.

Reticular activating system Group of specialized neurons in the brainstem; involved in sleep and wake cycles; maintains consciousness.

Reticular cells The cells forming the reticular fibers of connective tissue; those forming the framework of lymph nodes, bone marrow, and spleen are part of the reticuloendothelial system and under appropriate stimulation may differentiate into macrophages.

Reticular dermis Section of the dermis composed of larger and denser collagen fibers; provides most of the skin's elasticity and strength. This layer contains most of the skin structures located within the dermis.

Reticular formation A cloud of neurons in the brainstem and midbrain responsible for maintaining consciousness.

Retina Outer pigmented area and inner sensory layer that responds to light.

Retinal detachment A condition in which the retina is lifted or pulled from its normal position, resulting in a loss of vision.

Retractions Use of accessory muscles of respiration to assist in ventilation during times of distress; sinking in of the soft tissues above the sternum or clavicle or between or below the ribs during inhalation.

Retreat Leaving the scene when danger is observed or when violence or indicators of violence are displayed; requires immediate and decisive action.

Retrograde Moving backward or moving in the opposite direction to that which is considered normal.

Retrograde amnesia The inability to remember events or recall memories from before an event in which the head was struck.

Retroperitoneal Abdominopelvic organs found behind the peritoneum.

Retrospective medical direction Physician review of prehospital care reports and participation in the quality improvement process; a type of offline medical direction.

Reuptake Absorption of neurotransmitters from the synapse into the presynaptic neuron to be reused or destroyed.

Review of systems A review of symptoms for each organ system.

Rhabdomyolysis Complex series of events that occur in patients with severe muscle injury (e.g., crush injuries); destruction of the muscle tissues results in a release of cellular material and acidosis that can lead to acute renal failure.

Rheumatoid arthritis (RA) A painful, disabling disease in which the body's immune system attacks the joints.

Rhinitis Inflammation of the mucous membranes of the nose, usually accompanied by swelling of the mucosa and a nasal discharge.

Rhinorrhea Persistent discharge of fluid (such as blood or cerebrospinal fluid) from the nose.

Rhonchi Rattling or rumbling in the lungs.

Ribonucleic acid (RNA) Specialized structures within the cell that carry genetic material for reproduction.

Ribosome Substance in organelle where new protein is synthesized; forms the framework for the genetic blueprint.

Right A position toward the right side of the body.

Right block or left block Terms describing a responding vehicle arriving on scene and turning at a right or left angle. In this block position, the emergency vehicle acts as a physical barrier between the crash scene work area and approaching traffic.

Right coronary artery Blood vessel that provides oxygenated blood to the right side of the heart muscle.

Risk factors Traits and lifestyle habits that may increase a person's chance of developing a disease.

Risus sardonicus Distorted grinning expression caused by involuntary contraction of the facial muscles.

Roentgens Denote ionizing radiation passing through air.

Rolling the dash Rescue tasks involving strategic cuts to the firewall structure followed by pushing, spreading, or even pulling equipment to move the dash, firewall, steering wheel, column, and pedals away from front seat occupants.

Rollover protective structure A structure mounted on a tractor designed to support the weight of the tractor if an overturn occurs; if a tractor has this structure and the operator wears a seat belt, the operator will stay in the safety zone if the tractor overturns.

Root word In medical terminology, the part of the word that gives the primary meaning.

Rotor-wing aircraft Helicopter that can be used for hospital-to-hospital and scene-to-hospital transports; usually travels a shorter distance and is used in the prehospital setting for certain types of transport.

Routes of administration Various methods of giving drugs, including oral, enteral, parenteral, and inhalational.

Rovsing's sign Pain in the right lower quadrant elicited by palpation of the abdomen in the left lower quadrant.

S1 The sound of the tricuspid and mitral valves closing.

S2 The sound of the closing of the pulmonary and aortic valves.

Sacrum (sacral vertebrae) A heavy, large bone at the base of the spinal cord between the lumbar vertebrae and the coccyx. Roughly triangular in shape, it comprises the back of the pelvis and is made of the five sacral vertebrae fused together.

Safety officer The person responsible for ensuring that no unsafe acts occur during the emergency incident.

Sagittal plane Imaginary straight line that runs vertically through the middle of the body, creating right and left halves.

Saliva Mucus that lubricates material like food that is placed in it; enzymes begin the digestive process of starchy material.

Salivary glands Located in the oral cavity; produce saliva.

Saponification A form of necrosis in which fatty acids combine with certain electrolytes to form soaps.

Sarin A nerve agent.

Saturation of peripheral oxygen The percentage of hemoglobin saturated with oxygen (SpO_2).

Scabies A contagious skin disease of the epidermis marked by itching and small raised red spots caused by the itch mite *(Sarcoptes scabiei)*.

Scale Thick stratum corneum that results from hyperproliferation or increased cohesion of keratinocytes (can include eczema or psoriasis).

Scar A collection of new connective tissue; may be hypertrophic or atrophic and implies dermoepidermal damage.

Schizophrenia A group of disorders characterized by psychotic symptoms, thought disorder, and negative symptoms (social isolation and withdrawal); types include paranoid, disorganized, and catatonic.

Sciatica Pain in the lumbar back and leg caused by irritation and impingement of the sciatic nerve, usually from a herniated disc.

Sclera Firm, opaque, white outer layer of the eye; helps maintain the shape of the eye.

Scope of practice A predefined set of skills, interventions, or other activities that the paramedic is legally authorized to perform when necessary; usually set by state law or regulation and local medical direction.

Scrotum Loose layer of connective tissue that support the testes.

Sebaceous glands Found in the dermis; secrete oil (sebum) in the shaft of the hair follicle and the skin.

Sebum Oil secreted by the sebaceous glands in the shaft of the hair follicle and the skin; prevents excessive drying of the skin and hair; also protects from some forms of bacteria.

Second messenger A molecule that relays signals from a receptor on the surface of a cell to target molecules in the cell's nucleus or internal fluid where a physiologic action is to take place; also called a *biochemical messenger*.

Secondary apnea When asphyxia is prolonged, a period of deep, gasping respirations with a simultaneous fall in blood pressure and heart rate; gasping becomes weaker and slower and then ceases.

Secondary blast injury Injuries caused by shrapnel from the fragments of an explosive device and from things that have been attached to it.

Secondary contamination The risk of another person or healthcare provider becoming contaminated with a hazardous material by contact with a contaminated victim.

Secondary cord injury A spinal cord injury that develops over time after a traumatic injury to the spinal column or the blood vessels that supply the spinal cord with blood. Generally caused by ischemia, swelling, or compression.

Secondary device An explosive, chemical, or biologic device hidden at the scene of an emergency and set to detonate or release its agent after emergency response personnel are on scene.

Secondary hypertension High blood pressure that has an identifiable cause, such as medications or an underlying disease or condition.

Secondary injury prevention Preventing further injury from an event that has already occurred.

Secondary skin lesion Any lesion that has been altered by scratching, scrubbing, or other types of trauma.

Secondary triage Conducted after the primary search; determines the order of treatment and transport of the remaining patients.

Secondary tumor A tumor that has spread from its original location (e.g., lung tumor that spreads to brain); also called *metastasis*.

Secretion Release of water, acids, enzymes, and buffers that aid in the breakdown and digestion of food in the digestive tract.

Secretory phase Portion of the menstrual cycle in which the corpus luteum secretes progesterone to maintain the endometrial lining in case of fertilization.

Sedative-hypnotics Prescription central nervous system depressant drugs that cause powerful relaxation and euphoria when abused; typically barbiturates and benzodiazepines.

Segment Line between waveforms; named by the waveform that precedes and follows it.

Seizure A temporary alteration in behavior or consciousness caused by abnormal electrical activity of one or more groups of neurons in the brain.

Self-injury An unhealthy coping mechanism involving intentionally injuring one's own body, often through cutting or burning oneself to relieve emotional tension; also known as *self-mutilation*.

Sellick maneuver Technique used to compress the cricoid cartilage against the cervical vertebrae, causing occlusion of the esophagus, thereby reducing the risk of aspiration; cricoid pressure.

Semicircular canals Three bony fluid-filled loops in the internal ear; involved in balance of the body.

Semilunar (SL) valves Valves shaped like half moons that separate the ventricles from the aorta and pulmonary artery.

Seminal fluid Liquid produced in the seminal vesicles.

Seminal vesicles Ducts that produce seminal fluids.

Sensing Ability of a pacemaker to recognize and respond to intrinsic electrical activity.

Sensorineural hearing loss A type of deafness that occurs when the tiny hair cells in the cochlea are damaged or destroyed. In addition, damage to the auditory nerve prevents sounds from being transmitted from the cochlea to the brain.

Sensory cortex Area of brain tissue on the frontal lobe responsible for receiving sensory information from different parts of the body.

Sepsis Pathologic state, usually accompanied by fever, resulting from the presence of microorganisms or their poisonous products in the bloodstream; commonly called *blood poisoning.*

Septic abortion An abortion associated with intrauterine infection.

Septic arthritis Invasion of microorganisms into a joint space, causing infection of the joint.

Septic shock Sepsis with hypotension, despite adequate fluid resuscitation, along with the presence of perfusion abnormalities that may include lactic acidosis, decreased urine output, and a sudden change in mental status.

Septicemia A serious medical condition characterized by vasodilation that leads to hypotension, tissue hypoxia, and eventually shock; usually caused by gram-negative bacteria; diagnosed by blood tests called cultures.

Septum Tough piece of tissue that divides the left and right halves of the heart.

Serious apnea Cessation of breathing for longer than 20 seconds or any duration if accompanied by cyanosis and sinus bradycardia.

Serosanguineous discharge Blood and fluid discharged from the body.

Serous membrane Membrane that lines the thoracic, abdominal, and pelvic cavities; composed of the parietal membrane, which adheres to the cavity wall, and the visceral membrane, which adheres to the organ.

Serum base deficit Implies that the blood buffer, bicarbonate, is being used to combat a metabolic acidosis. Metabolic acidosis occurs in the setting of numerous shock states, such as burn shock. This number is reported on a standard blood gas assay and is detected in an arterial or venous blood sample.

Serum lactate Measure in the blood; a byproduct of anaerobic metabolism. As such, it is a good measure of end organ and cellular perfusion in shock states. Elevated serum lactate levels, or lactic acidemia, implies that cells, tissues, or organs are not receiving adequate oxygen to carry out their metabolic activities.

Sesamoid bones Specialized bones found within tendons where they cross a joint; designed to protect the joint (e.g., the patella [kneecap]).

Severe sepsis Sepsis associated with organ dysfunction, shock, or hypotension.

Sexual abuse Forced and/or coerced sex, violent sexual acts against the victim's will (rape), or withholding sex from the victim; includes fondling, intercourse, incest, rape, sodomy, exhibitionism, sexual exploitation, or exposure to pornography. According to the National Center on Child Abuse and Neglect, to be considered child abuse these acts must be committed by a person responsible for the care of a child (e.g., a babysitter, parent, or daycare provider) or related to the child. If a stranger commits these acts, it is considered sexual assault and handled solely by the police and criminal courts.

Sexual assault Sexually explicit conduct used as an expression of interpersonal violence against another individual; nonconsenting sexual acts achieved through power and control.

Shaft The length of a needle; the needle shaft connects to the hub. Also called the *cannula.*

Shear points Hazardous machinery locations created when the edges of two objects are moved toward or next to one another closely enough to cut a relatively soft material.

Shingles Infection of a nerve, often by the herpes zoster virus, causing severe pain and a rash along a unilateral dermatome.

Shock Inadequate systemic perfusion that results from the failure of the cardiovascular system to deliver sufficient oxygen and nutrients to sustain vital organ function.

Short bones Specialized bones of the skeleton designed for compactness and strength, often with limited movement (e.g., bones of the wrist [carpals])

Short haul The transport of one or more people externally suspended below a helicopter.

Shoulder dystocia Impaction of a newborn's anterior shoulder underneath the mother's pubic bone, slowing or preventing delivery.

Shunt Insertion of catheters into an artery and a vein from outside the body. Most shunts are located on the forearm. When not in use to dialyze a patient, the catheters are connected to each other with clear tubing, allowing the continuous flow of blood from artery to vein, then covered with self-adhering roller gauze for protection.

Side effect An effect of a drug other than the one for which it was given; may or may not be harmful.

Side impact airbags Deployable airbags located inside any or all vehicle doors, front and rear outboard seatbacks, as well as along all or a portion of the roof line.

Sighing Involuntary and periodic slow, deep breath followed by a prolonged expiratory phase. Occurring approximately once per minute, the act of sighing is thought to open atelectatic (collapsed) alveoli.

Sigmoid colon Part of the large intestine.

Signs and symptoms Signs are a medical or trauma condition of the patient that can be seen, heard, smelled, measured, or felt during an examination. Symptoms are conditions described by the patient, such as shortness of breath, or pieces of information bystanders tell you about the patient's chief complaint.

Silo gas The gases produced from the fermentation of plant material inside a silo.

Simple asphyxiants Inert gases and vapors that displace oxygen in inspired air (e.g., carbon dioxide, nitrogen).

Simple partial seizure A seizure affecting only one part of the brain without an alteration in consciousness.

Simple pneumothorax Injury to the thoracic cavity in which a lung is ruptured, allowing air into the space between the chest wall and the lungs.

Simplex A system that allows only one-at-a-time communication. The transmission cannot be interrupted; both operators use the same frequency.

Singular command Command type involving one agency.

Sinoatrial node Pacemaker site of the heart; where impulse formation begins in the heart.

Sinus block (barosinusitis) A condition of acute or chronic inflammation of one or more of the paranasal sinuses; produced by a negative pressure difference between the air in the sinuses and the surrounding atmospheric air.

Sinus rhythm A normal heart rhythm.

Sinuses Cavities within the bones of the skull that connect to the nasal cavity.

Situational awareness The state of being aware of everything occurring in the surrounding environment and the relative importance of all these events.

Size-up The art of assessing conditions that exist or can potentially exist at an incident scene.

Skeletal muscles Muscles that affect movement of the skeleton, usually by voluntary contractions.

Skin grafting Transplantation of skin, either from the same person or from a cadaver, to the site of a wound, such as a burn.

Skin turgor The elasticity of the skin; good skin turgor returns the skin's natural shape within 2 seconds.

Slander False statements spoken about a person that blacken the person's character or injure his or her reputation.

Slipped capital femoral epiphysis A disease in which a posterior displacement of the growth plate of the femur occurs (the epiphysis).

SLUDGEM Mnemonic for *s*alivation, *l*acrimation, *u*rination, *d*efecation, *g*astrointestinal pain, *e*mesis, and *m*iosis.

Smallpox A disease caused by variola viruses, which are members of the Orthopoxvirus family; eradicated in the 1970s but still remains a threat as a bioterrorism agent.

Sneezing Occurs from nasal irritation and allows clearance of the nose.

Sniffing position Neck flexion at the fifth and sixth cervical vertebrae, with the head extended at the first and second cervical vertebrae. This position aligns the axes of the mouth, pharynx, and trachea, opening the airway and increasing airflow.

Snoring Noisy breathing through the mouth and nose during sleep; caused by air passing through a narrowed upper airway.

Social distance The acceptable distance between strangers used for impersonal business transactions. In the United States, social distance is 4 to 12 feet.

Sodium bicarbonate Neutralizes hydrochloric acid from the stomach.

Solid organ An organ (a part of the body or group of tissues that performs a specific function) without any channel or cavity within it; examples include the kidneys, pancreas, liver, and spleen.

Solubility Pertaining to the ease with which a drug can dissolve.

Solution A medication dissolved in a liquid, often water.

Soman A G nerve agent. The G agents tend to be nonpersistent, volatile agents.

Somatic Portion of the peripheral nervous system that carries impulses to and from the skin and musculature; responsible for voluntary muscle control.

Somatic delusions False perceptions of the appearance or functioning of one's own body.

Somatic nervous system Division of the peripheral nervous system whose motor nerves control movement of voluntary muscles.

Somatic pain Pain that arises from either the cutaneous tissues of the body's surface or deep tissues of the body, such as musculoskeletal tissue or the parietal peritoneum.

Somatoform disorders A group of disorders characterized by the manifestation of psychological problems as physical symptoms; this includes conversion disorder, hypochondriasis, somatization disorder, and body dysmorphic disorder.

Sore throat Any inflammation of the larynx, pharynx, or tonsils.

Space blanket A blanket resembling aluminum foil used to help the patient maintain body temperature.

Space-occupying lesion A mass, such as a tumor or blood collection, within a contained body space, such as the skull.

Spacer A hollow plastic tube that attaches to the metered-dose inhaler on one end and has a mouthpiece on the other; sometimes called a *holding chamber*.

Span of control The amount of resources that one person can effectively manage.

Special needs Conditions with the potential to interfere with usual growth and development;

may involve physical disabilities, developmental disabilities, chronic illnesses, and forms of technologic support.

Specialty center A hospital that has met criteria to offer special care as a burn center, level I trauma center, stroke center, or pediatric center.

Specific gravity The ratio of a liquid's weight compared with an equal volume of water (which has a constant value of 1); materials with a specific gravity of less than 1.0 float on water and materials with a specific gravity greater than 1.0 sink.

Sperm Mucus-type secretion made of prostatic fluid and spermatozoa.

Spermatic cord Nerves, blood vessels, and smooth muscle that surround the vas (ductus) deferens.

Spermatocele Benign accumulation of sperm at the epididymis presenting as a firm mass.

Spermatogenesis Spermatozoa formation.

Spermatozoa Product of the male reproductive system.

Sphincters Smooth muscles that regulate flow through the capillary beds.

Spina bifida (SB) A neural tube defect that affects the back portion of the vertebrae, which fail to close, usually in the area of the lower back; meninges, the spinal cord, or both may protrude through this opening.

Spina bifida occulta Mildest form of spina bifida in which the spinal cord is intact but one or more vertebrae fail to close in the lumbosacral area.

Spinal cord Long stalk of nerve tissue that is the interface between the brain and the body; extends from the foramen magnum to the lumbar spine and contains the main reflex centers of the body.

Spinal cord injury (SCI) An injury to the spinal cord that results from trauma; usually a permanent injury.

Spinal cord injury without radiological abnormality A spinal cord injury not detected on a standard radiograph.

Spinal nerves Paired nerves that originate from the spinal cord and exit the spine on either side between vertebrae; each has a sensory root and a motor root.

Spinal shock Shock with hypotension caused by an injury to the spinal cord.

Spirit A medication that contains volatile aromatic substances.

Split-thickness skin graft A skin graft in which only a fraction of the thickness of the natural dermis is taken.

Spontaneous abortion See *Miscarriage*.

Spontaneous bacterial peritonitis (SBP) Infection of cirrhotic fluid in the abdominal cavity.

Spontaneous pneumothorax Pneumothorax occurring without trauma, usually by rupture of a pulmonary bleb.

Sprain An injury to a ligament that results when the ligament is overstretched, leading to tearing or complete disruption of the ligament.

Stagnant phase Vascular response in shock when precapillary sphincters open, allowing the capillary beds to engorge with fluid; follows the ischemic phase.

Stair chair A collapsible, portable chair with handles on the front and back used to carry patients in sitting position down stairs.

Standard of care Conduct exercising the degree of care, skill, and judgment that would be expected under like or similar circumstances by a similarly trained, reasonable paramedic in the same scenario.

Standard operating procedures (SOPs) An organized set of guidelines distributed across the organization.

Standing orders Written instructions that authorize EMS personnel to perform certain medical interventions before establishing direct communication with a physician.

Standard precautions Infection control practices in healthcare designed to be observed with every patient and procedure and prevent the exposure to bloodborne pathogens.

Stapes The stirrup-shaped bone that links the middle ear to the inner ear; connects to the malleus and incus.

Status asthmaticus Condition of severe asthma that is minimally responsive to therapy; a serious condition.

Status epilepticus A single seizure lasting longer than 30 minutes or repeated seizures without full recovery of responsiveness between seizures and lasting longer than 30 minutes.

Statute A law passed by a legislature.

Statute of limitations A law that sets the time limits within which parties must take action to enforce their rights.

Statutory law Statutes and ordinances enacted by Congress, state legislatures, and city councils.

Steady state An evenly distributed concentration of a drug in the plasma.

Stellate laceration A laceration with jagged margins.

Stem cells Formative cells whose daughter cells may give rise to other cell types.

Stenosis Abnormal constriction or narrowing of a structure.

Stereotyping The attribution of some trait or characteristic to one person on the basis of the interviewer's preconceived notions about a general class of people of similar characteristics.

Sterile Free of any living organism.

Sterilization Process that makes an object free of all forms of life (e.g., bacteria) by using extreme heat or certain chemicals.

Sterilize To kill all microorganisms.

Stimuli Anything that excites or incites an organism or part to function, become active, or respond.

Stomach Organ located at the inferior end of the esophagus; large storage vessel surrounded by multiple layers of smooth muscle; cells within it produce acid.

Stored energy Any energy (mechanical, electrical, hydraulic, compressed air, etc.) that has the potential of being released either intentionally or inadvertently, causing further injury or problems.

Strain An injury to a muscle that results when the muscle is overstretched, leading to tearing of the individual muscle fibers.

Strainer A water hazard formed by an object or structure in the current that allows water to flow but that strains out large objects, such as boats and people.

Strangulation Compression of the vessels that carry blood, leading to ischemia.

Stratum corneum Outer layer of the epidermis where skin cells are shed.

Stress Mental, emotional, or physical pressure, strain, or tension resulting from stimuli.

Stressor A stimulus that produces stress.

Stricture A specific form of narrowing, usually from scar tissue formation.

Stridor A harsh, high-pitched sound heard on inspiration associated with upper airway obstruction; often described as a high-pitched crowing or "seal-bark" sound.

Stroke volume Amount of blood ejected by either ventricle during one contraction; can be calculated as cardiac output divided by heart rate.

Struck-by A situation in which a responder, working in or near moving traffic, is struck, injured, or killed by traffic passing the incident scene.

Stye An external hordeolum.

Stylet A relatively stiff but flexible metal rod covered by plastic and inserted into an endotracheal tube; used for maintaining the shape of the relatively pliant tube and "steering" it into position.

Subarachnoid hemorrhage Bleeding from the arteries between the arachnoid membrane and the pia mater that occurs suddenly and often is fatal.

Subcutaneous (Sub-Q) Injection of medication in a liquid form underneath the skin into the subcutaneous tissue.

Subcutaneous emphysema Air entrapped beneath the skin, typically caused by rupture of a structure containing air; feels like crackling when palpated.

Subcutaneous tissue Thick layer of connective tissue found between the layers of the skin; composed of adipose tissue and areolar tissue; insulates, protects, and stores energy (in the form of fat).

Subdural hematoma A collection of blood in the subdural space, which is between the dura mater and arachnoid layer of the meninges.

Subdural space Area below the dura mater; contains large venous vessels, drains, and a small amount of serous fluid.

Subjective information Information told to the paramedic.

Sublingual Medication placed under the tongue.

Sucking chest wound Open thoracic injury characterized by air being pulled into and pushed out of the wound during respiration.

Sudden cardiac death (SCD) An unexpected death from a cardiac cause that either occurs immediately or within 1 hour of the onset of symptoms.

Suffix Added to the end of a root word to change the meaning; usually identifies the condition of the root word.

Suicide The act of ending one's own life.

Sulfur mustard The most well known and commonly used of the vesicants.

Summarization Briefly reviewing the interview and your conclusions.

Summation The combined effects of two or more drugs equaling the sum of each of their effects.

Superficial burn A burn with a pink appearance that does not exhibit blister formation; painful both with and without tactile stimulation (e.g., sunburn); also known as a *first-degree burn.*

Superficial fascia Connective tissue that contains the subcutaneous fat cells.

Superficial partial-thickness burn Burns involving the more superficial dermis. These burns have a moist, pink appearance, and when lightly touched, are painful and sensate. Blood vessels, hair shafts, nerves, and glands may be injured, but not to the extent that regeneration cannot take place.

Superior Situated above or higher than a point of reference in the anatomic position; top.

Superior vena cava Vessel that returns venous blood from the upper part of the body to the right atrium of the heart.

Supernormal period Period during the cardiac cycle when a weaker than normal stimulus can cause cardiac cells to depolarize; extends from the end of phase 3 to the beginning of phase 4 of the cardiac action potential.

Supine Position in which the patient is lying on his or her back (face up).

Supine hypotensive syndrome A fall in the pregnant patient's blood pressure when she is placed supine; caused by the developing fetus and uterus pressing against the inferior vena cava.

Suppository Medications combined to make them a solid at room temperature; when placed in a body opening such as the rectum, vagina, or urethra, they dissolve because of the increase in body temperature and are absorbed through the surrounding mucosa.

Supraglottic Any airway structure above the vocal cords (e.g., the epiglottis).

Suprasternal notch A depression easily felt at the base of the anterior aspect of the neck, just above the angle of Louis.

Supraventricular Originating from a site above the bifurcation of the bundle of His, such as the sinoatrial node, atria, or atrioventricular junction.

Supraventricular dysrhythmias Rhythms that begin in the sinoatrial node, atrial tissue, or the atrioventricular junction.

Surfactant Specialized cells within each alveolus that keep it from collapsing when little or no air is inside.

Surge capacity The ability to expand care based on a sudden mass casualty incident; developed in the emergency management plan.

Susceptibility Vulnerability or weakness; the opposite of resistance.

Suspension Medication suspended in a liquid, such as an oral antibiotic.

Sutures Seams between flat bones.

Sweat glands Odor-forming glands in the body; two types are merocrine and apocrine.

Swimmer's ear See *Otitis externa*.

Sympathetic division of the autonomic nervous system Division of the autonomic nervous system that, when stimulated, provides a fight-or-flight response, including increased heart rate, pupil dilation, bronchodilation, and the shunting of blood to the muscles.

Sympathetic nervous system Division of the autonomic nervous system that prepares the body for stress or the classic fight-or-flight response.

Sympatholytics Drugs that block or inhibit adrenergic receptors.

Sympathomimetics Drugs that mimic the sympathetic division of the autonomic nervous system.

Sympathy Sharing the patient's feelings or emotional state in relation to an illness.

Symphysis Cartilaginous joint; unites two bones by means of fibrocartilage.

Synapse Microscopic space at the neuroeffector junction that neurotransmitters cross to stimulate target tissues.

Synaptic communication Method of intercellular communication in which neural cells communicate to adjacent neural cells by using neurotransmitters.

Synaptic junction The open space in which neurotransmitters traverse to reach a receptor.

Synchondroses Cartilaginous joint; unites the bones by means of hyaline cartilage.

Synchronized intermittent mandatory ventilation (SIMV) A ventilator setting that generally allows the patient to inspire at will and to the depth that he or she desires.

Syncope A transient loss of consciousness and inability to maintain postural tone, typically resulting in a ground-level fall; also know as *passing out* or *fainting*.

Syndesmosis Joint in which the bones are united by fibrous, connective tissue forming an intraosseous membrane or ligament.

Synergism The interaction of drugs such that the total effect is greater than the sum of the individual effects.

Synonym A root word, prefix, or suffix that has the same or almost the same meaning as another word, prefix, or suffix.

Synovial fluid Fluid located within the joint capsules of synovial joints; provides lubrication and cushioning during manipulation of the joint.

Synovial joint Freely movable; enclosed by a capsule and synovial membrane.

Synovium Soft tissue that lines the noncartilaginous surfaces of a joint.

Synthetic drugs Drugs chemically developed in a laboratory; also called *manufactured drugs*.

Syrup A medication dissolved in water with sugar or a sugar substitute to disguise taste.

System At least two kinds of organs organized to perform a more complex task than can a single organ.

System Status Management The dynamic process of staffing, stationing, and moving ambulances based on projected call volumes; also called *flexible deployment*.

Systemic damage Damage remote to the site of exposure or absorption.

Systemic effect Drug action throughout the body.

Systemic inflammatory response syndrome A response to infection manifested by a change in two or more of the following: temperature, heart rate, respiratory rate, and white blood cell count.

Systole Contraction of the heart (usually referring to ventricular contraction) during which blood is propelled into the pulmonary artery and aorta; when the term is used without reference to a specific chamber of the heart, the term implies ventricular systole.

Systolic blood pressure The pressure exerted against the walls of the large arteries at the peak of ventricular contraction.

T lymphocytes Cells present in the lymphatic system that mediate cell-mediated immunity (also known as *T cells*).

Tablets Medications that have been pressed into a small form that is easy to swallow. They are a specific shape, color, and may have engraving for identification.

Tachycardia A heart rate grater than 100 beats/min.

Tachyphylaxis The rapidly decreasing response to a drug or physiologically active agent after administration of a few doses; rapid cross-tolerance.

Tachypnea An increased respiratory rate, usually greater than 30 breaths/min.

Tactical EMS EMS personnel specially trained and equipped to provide prehospital emergency care in tactical environments.

Tactical patient care Patient care activities that occur inside the scene perimeter or hot zone.

Tangential thinking A progression of thoughts related to each other but that become less and less related to the original topic.

Tardive dyskinesia A neurologic syndrome caused by the long-term or high-dose use of dopamine agonists, usually antipsychotic medications; characterized by repetitive, involuntary, and purposeless movements such as grimacing, rapid movements of the face, lip smacking, and eye blinking. Symptoms may last for a significant period after removal of the offending agent.

Teachable moment The time just after an injury has occurred when the patient and observers remain acutely aware of what has happened and may be more receptive to learning how the event or illness could have been prevented.

Teamwork The ability to work with others to achieve a common goal.

Teeth Provide mastication of food products in preparation for entry into the stomach.

Telematic A system set up as mayday call reporting, such as On-Star and Tele-aid. This system can send information from an automobile that has been involved in an accident directly to an emergency dispatch center with the exact location and the amount of damage that may have occurred.

Telephone aid Ad-libbed instructions most often used in emergency dispatch centers by dispatchers who have had previous training as paramedics, EMTs, or cardiopulmonary resuscitation providers; strictly relies on the dispatcher's experience and prior knowledge of a particular situation or medical condition and is considered an ineffective form of telephone treatment.

Telson Venom-containing portion of a scorpion's abdomen that is capable of venomous injection into human beings.

Temporal demand Measurement of call demand by hour of the day.

Temporal lobe Cerebrum beneath the temporal bone; area where processing of hearing and language occurs.

Temporal modeling Predicting the times when calls occur.

Tendonitis Inflammation of a tendon, often caused by overuse.

Tendons Tough, fibrous bands of connective tissue that connect muscle to muscle and muscle to bones.

Tension-building phase Period when tension in the relationship is high and heightened anger, blaming, and arguing may occur between the victim and the abuser.

Tension pneumothorax Life-threatening injury in which air enters the space between the lungs and the chest wall but cannot exit. With each breath, the pressure increases until it prevents ventilation and causes death.

Teratogen A drug or agent that is harmful to the development of an embryo or fetus.

Term gestation A gestation equal to or longer than 37 weeks.

Terminal drop A theory that holds that mental and physical functioning decline drastically only in the few years immediately preceding death.

Terminal illness Advanced stage of illness or disease with an unfavorable prognosis and no known cure.

Tertiary blast injury Injuries caused by the patient being thrown like a projectile.

Testes Male reproductive organs suspended within the scrotum.

Testicular torsion Twisting of the spermatic cord inside the scrotum that cuts off the blood supply to the testis.

Testosterone Male hormone secreted within the testes.

Tetany Repeated, prolonged contraction of muscles, especially of the face and limbs.

Tetraplegia Paralysis to all four extremities as a result of a spinal cord injury high in the spine. The injury can either be complete (a complete loss of muscle control and sensation below the injury site) or incomplete (a partial loss of muscle control or sensation below the injury site).

Thalamus Structure located within the limbic system that is the switchboard of the brain, through which almost all signals travel on their way in or out of the brain.

Therapeutic abortion Planned surgical or medical evacuation of the uterus.

Therapeutic dose The dose required to produce a beneficial effect in 50% of the drug-tested population; also called *effective dose*.

Therapeutic index The ratio between the amount of drug required to produce to produce a therapeutic dose and a lethal dose of the same drug. A narrow therapeutic index is dangerous because the possibility of underdosing or overdosing is higher.

Therapeutic threshold The level of a drug that elicits a beneficial physiologic response.

Thermogenesis The process of heat generation.

Thermolysis A chemical process by which heat is dissipated from the body; sometimes results in chemical decomposition.

Thermoreceptor A sensory receptor that responds to heat and cold.

Third space Extravascular and extracellular milieu; also known as the *interstitium*.

Thirst mechanism Sensation activated by cells in the hypothalamus when cells called osmoreceptors detect an imbalance in body water; as the body is replenished by drinking fluid, the osmoreceptors sense a return to baseline and turn off this mechanism.

Thoracic vertebrae A group of 12 vertebrae in the middle of the spinal column that connect to ribs.

Thought blocking A symptom of thought disorder in which a patient is speaking and then stops mid-sentence, unable to remember what he or she was saying and unable to continue.

Thought content The dominant themes and ideas of a patient; may include delusions, hallucinations, and preoccupations.

Threatened abortion Vaginal bleeding or uterine cramping during the first half of pregnancy without cervical dilation.

Threshold limit value The airborne concentrations of a substance; represents conditions under which nearly all workers are believed to be repeatedly exposed day after day without adverse effects.

Thrombocytes One of three formed elements in the blood; also known as *platelets.*

Thrombocytopenia A lower than normal number of platelets circulating in the blood.

Thromboembolism Movement of a clot within the vascular system.

Thrombophlebitis Development of a clot in a vein in which inflammation is present.

Thromboplastin Blood coagulation factor.

Thrombus Blood clot.

Thrush A fungal infection of the mouth.

Thyroid storm Severe form of hyperthyroidism characterized by tachypnea, tachycardia, shock, hyperthermia, and delirium.

Thyrotoxicosis A condition in which the thyroid gland produces excess thyroid hormone; also called *hyperthyroidism* or *Graves' disease.*

Tidal volume The volume of air moved into or out of the lungs during a normal breath; can be indirectly evaluated by observing the rise and fall of the patient's chest and abdomen.

Time on task The average time a unit is committed to manage an incident.

Tincture A medicine consisting of an extract in an alcohol solution (e.g., tincture of iodine, tincture of mercurochrome).

Tinea capitis Located on the head and scalp; appears as a round, scaly area where no hair is growing; diffuse scaling.

Tinea corporis Located on the body; appears annular (e.g. ringworm).

Tinea cruris Located on the groin and genitalia; appears as a sharply demarcated area with elevated scaling, geographic borders.

Tinea manuum Located on the hands; appears as dry, diffuse scaling, usually on the palm.

Tinea pedis Located on the feet; appears as maceration between the toes, scaling on soles or sides of the foot, sometimes vesicles and/or pustules.

Tinea unguium Located on or under fingernails or toenails; appears as dark debris under the nails.

Tinea versicolor Located on the trunk; appears as pink, tan, or white patches with fine, desquamating scale.

Tinnitus A ringing, roaring sound or hissing in the ears that is usually caused by certain medicines or exposure to loud noise.

Tissue A group of cells that are similar in structure and function.

Tocolytic A medication used to slow uterine contractions.

Tolerance Decreasing responsiveness to the effects of a drug; increasingly larger doses are necessary to achieve the effect originally obtained by a smaller dose.

Tongue Muscular organ that provides for the sensation of taste; also directs food material toward the esophagus.

Tonic-clonic seizure Form of generalized seizure with a tonic phase (muscle rigidity) and a clonic phase (muscle tremors).

Topical Medication administered by applying it directly to the skin or mucous membrane.

Tort A wrong committed on the person or property of another.

Total body surface area burned (TBSAB) Used to describe the amount of the body injured by a burn and expressed as a percentage of the entire body surface area.

Total body water (TBW) The total amount of fluid in the body at any given time.

Totally blind Description of someone who has no vision and uses nonvisual media or reads Braille.

Toxic organic dust syndrome A flulike illness caused by the inhalation of grain dust, with symptoms including fever, chest tightness, cough, and muscle aches; inhalation may occur in an agricultural setting or from covering a floor with straw.

Toxicology The study of poisons.

Toxidrome A classification system of toxic syndromes by signs and symptoms.

Toxin A poisonous substance of plant or animal origin.

TP segment Interval on the ECG between two successive PQRST complexes during which electrical activity of the heart is absent; begins with the end of the T wave through the onset of the following P wave and represents the period from the end of ventricular repolarization to the onset of atrial depolarization.

Trachea Air passage that connects the larynx to the lungs.

Tracheal stoma A surgical opening in the anterior neck that extends from the skin surface into the trachea, opening the trachea to the atmosphere.

Tracheitis Inflammation of the mucous membranes of the trachea.

Tracheostomy A surgically created hole in the anterior trachea for breathing.

Tracheoesophageal fistula (TEF) An abnormal opening between the trachea and the esophagus.

Trade name The name given a chemical compound by the company that makes it; also called the *brand name* or *proprietary name.*

Transcellular compartment Compartment classified as extracellular but distinct because it is formed from the transport activities of cells; cerebrospinal fluid, bladder urine, the aqueous humor, and the synovial fluid of the joints are considered transcellular.

Transdermal Through the skin.

Transection A complete cutting (severing) across the spinal cord.

Transient ischemic attack (TIA) Neurologic dysfunction caused by a temporary blockage in blood flow; by definition the symptoms resolve within 24 hours but usually within 1 or 2 hours.

Transient synovitis A nonspecific inflammation of a joint, usually the hip, that affects the synovium and synovial fluid in children.

Transverse colon Part of the large intestine.

Transverse plane Imaginary straight line that divides the body into top (superior) and bottom (inferior) sections; also known as the *horizontal plane*.

Traumatic asphyxia Life-threatening injury in which the thorax is severely crushed, preventing ventilation; typically results in death.

Traumatic iritis An inflammation of the iris caused by blunt trauma to the eye.

Triage Classifying patients based on the severity of illness or injury.

Tricuspid valve Right atrioventricular valve of the heart.

Trigeminal neuralgia Irritation of the seventh cranial nerve (trigeminal nerve), causing episodes of severe, stabbing pain in the face.

Trip audit The review of a prehospital care report written by a paramedic to a peer or a third party.

Tripod position Position used to maintain an open airway that involves sitting upright and leaning forward with the neck slightly extended, chin projected, and mouth open and supported by the arms.

Trismus Spasm of the muscles used for chewing, resulting in limited movement of the mouth because of pain.

Trunking system A system that uses multiple repeaters (five or more) so that the computer can search for an open channel to transmit by.

Tube trailers Trailers that carry multiple cylinders of pressurized gases.

Tuberculosis (TB) A highly contagious bacterial infection known for causing pneumonia and infecting other parts of the body.

Tularemia A disease resulting from infection of *Francisella tularensis*; normally transmitted through handling infected small mammals such as rabbits or rodents or through the bites of ticks, deerflies, or mosquitoes that have fed on infected animals; also known as *rabbit fever* or *deer fly fever*.

Tumor, benign An abnormal growth of cells that is not malignant (i.e., is not known for spreading and growing aggressively).

Tumor, malignant An abnormal growth of cells that is known for being aggressive and spreading to other parts of the body.

Tumor necrosis factor-alpha An inflammatory cytokine released in response to a variety of physical trauma, including burns. In burn injuries, massive quantities are produced by the liver; has been implicated as the causative agent in myocardial depression seen in burns.

Tumor, primary A tumor in the location where it originates (e.g., a primary lung tumor is in the lung).

Tumor, secondary A tumor that has spread from its original location (e.g., lung tumor that spreads to the brain); also called *metastasis*.

Tunica adventitia Outermost layer of the blood vessel; made of mainly elastic connective tissue; allows the vessel to expand to great pressure or volume.

Tunica intima Innermost layer of the blood vessel; composed of a single layer of epithelial cells; provides almost no resistance to blood flow.

Tunica media Middle layer of the blood vessel; mainly composed of smooth muscle; functions to alter the diameter of the lumen of the vessel and is under autonomic control, which enables the body to adjust blood flow quickly to meet immediate needs.

Tunics Layers of an elastic tissue and smooth muscle in the blood vessels.

Tunnel vision Focusing on or considering only one aspect of a situation without first taking into account all possibilities.

Turbinates Large folds found in the nasal cavity; highly vascular area in the nose that warms and humidifies inhaled air.

Turgor Normal tension of a cell or tissue.

Tympanic membrane A thin, translucent, pearly gray oval disk that protects the middle and conducts sound vibrations; eardrum.

Type and crossmatch Mixing a sample of a recipient's and donor's blood to evaluate for incompatibility.

Type I ambulance Regular truck cab and frame with a modular ambulance box mounted on the back.

Type II ambulance Van-style ambulance.

Type III ambulance A van chassis with a modified modular back.

Type IV (quaternary) blast injuries All other miscellaneous injuries caused by an explosive device.

Ulcer A full-thickness crater that involves the dermis and epidermis, with loss of the surface epithelium; this lesion is depressed and may bleed; it usually heals with scarring.

Umbilical An administration route that may be used on a newborn infant; because the umbilical cord was the primary source of nutrient and waste exchange, it provides an immediate source of drug exchange.

Umbilical cord The cord, containing two arteries and a vein, that connects the fetus to the placenta.

Umbilical cord prolapse Appearance of the umbilical cord in front of the presenting part, usually with compression of the cord and interruption of blood supply to the fetus.

Umbilical vein route Route of administration that achieves access through the one umbilical vein set between the two umbilical arteries.

Unethical Conduct that does not conform to moral standards of social or professional behavior.

Unified command Command type involving multiple agencies.

Unintentional injury Injuries and deaths not self-inflicted or perpetrated by another person (accidents).

Unintentional tort A wrong that the defendant did not mean to commit; a case in which a bad outcome occurred because of the failure to exercise reasonable care.

Unipolar lead Lead that consists of a single positive electrode and a reference point; a pacing lead with a single electrical pole at the distal tip of the pacing lead (negative pole) through which the stimulating pulse is delivered. In a permanent pacemaker with a unipolar lead, the positive pole is the pulse generator case.

Unit hour utilization (UhU) A measure of ambulance service productivity and staff workload.

United Nations (UN) number The four-digit number assigned to chemicals during transit by the U.S. Department of Transportation; the *2008 Emergency Guidebook* lists useful information about these chemicals.

Upper airway Portion of the respiratory tract above the glottis.

Upper flammable limit The concentration of fuel in the air above which the vapors cannot be ignited; above this point too much fuel and not enough oxygen are present to burn (too rich); also called the *upper explosive limit.*

Upper respiratory tract infection (URI) Viral syndrome causing nasal congestion, coughing, fever, and runny nose.

Upregulation The process by which a cell increases the number of receptors exposed to a given substance to improve its sensitivity to that substance.

Upstream A term describing the approaching traffic side of the damaged vehicles and the crash scene.

Uremia A term used to describe the signs and symptoms that accompany chronic renal failure.

Uremic frost Dried crystals of urea excreted through the skin that appear to be a frosting on the patient's body.

Ureter A thin-walled pair of tubes that drain urine from each kidney to the bladder.

Urethra Passageway for both urine and male reproductive fluids; opening at the end of the bladder.

Urethral meatus Opening of the urethra between the clitoris and vagina.

Urinary bladder A muscular sac responsible for storing urine before it is eliminated from the body.

Urinary retention The inability to empty the bladder or completely empty the bladder when urinating.

Urinary system Eliminates dissolved organic waste products by urine production and elimination.

Urticaria Also known as *hives;* a skin condition in uhich a wheal on the skin forms from edema; often caused by a reaction to a drug or through contact with substances (skin contact or even inhaled), causing hypersensitivity in the patient.

Uterine cavity Innermost region of the uterus.

Uterine prolapse Protrusion of part or all of the uterus out of the vagina.

Uterine tubes Tubular structures that extend from each side of the superior end of the body of the uterus to the lateral pelvic wall; they pick up the egg released by the ovary and transport it to the uterus; also known as *fallopian tubes.*

Uterus Muscular organ approximately the size of a pear; grows with the developing fetus.

Uvula Fleshy tissue resembling a grape that hangs down from the soft palate.

Vagina Female organ of copulation, the lower part of the birth canal, extending from the uterus to the outside of the body; extends from the cervix to the outside of the body.

Vaginal orifice Opening of the vagina.

Vaginitis An inflammation of the vaginal tissues.

Vallecula The depression or pocket between the base of the tongue and the epiglottis.

Vancomycin-resistant *Enterococcus* Bacteria resistant to vancomycin (a potent antibiotic); commonly acquired by patients in the hospital or patients who have indwelling catheters.

Vapor density The weight of a volume of pure gas compared with the weight of an equal volume of pure dry air (which has a constant value of 1); materials with a vapor density less than 1.0 are lighter than air and rise when released; materials with a vapor density greater than 1.0 are heavier than air and sink when released.

Vapor pressure The pressure exerted by a vapor against the sides of a closed container; a measure of volatility—high vapor pressure means it is a volatile substance.

Varicella An acute contagious vesicular skin eruption caused by the varicella zoster virus (chickenpox).

Varices Distended veins.

Varicocele Dilation of the venous plexus and internal spermatic vein, presenting as a lump in the scrotum.

Variola major A member of the *orthopoxvirus* family that causes the most common form of smallpox; the most likely form of the organism to be used as a weapon.

Vas deferens Tubes that extend from the end of the epididymis and through the seminal vesicles; also known as the *ductus deferens*.

Vascular access device Type of intravenous device used to deliver fluids, medications, blood, or nutritional therapy; usually inserted in patients who require long-term intravenous therapy.

Vascular headaches Headaches that involve changes in the diameter or size and chemistry of blood vessels that supply the brain.

Vascular resistance Amount of opposition that the blood vessels give to the flow of blood.

Vascular tunic Layer of the eye that contains most of the vasculature of the eye.

Vector A mode of transmission of a disease, typically from an insect or animal.

Vegetative functions Autonomic functions the body requires to survive.

Vehicle hazards Hazards directly related to the vehicle itself, including undeployed airbags; fuel system concerns; electrical system and battery electricity; stability of the vehicle; sharp glass and metal; leaking hot antifreeze; and engine oil, transmission oil, or antifreeze spills. Even the contents inside a vehicle's trunk or cargo area are typical vehicle hazards that can be encountered.

Vehicle stabilization Immediate action taken to prevent any unwanted movement of a crash-damaged vehicle.

Vena cava One of two large veins returning blood from the peripheral circulation to the right atrium of the heart.

Venipuncture Piercing of a vein.

Venom The poison injected by venomous animals such as snakes, insects, and marine creatures.

Venous return Amount of blood flowing into the right atrium each minute from the systemic circulation.

Ventilation The mechanical process of moving air into and out of the lungs.

Ventral Referring to the front of the body; anterior.

Ventricles Either of the two lower chambers in the heart.

Ventricular fibrillation Disorganized electrical activity of the ventricular conduction system of the heart, resulting in inefficient contractile force. This is the main cause of sudden cardiac death in electrical injuries.

Venules Small venous vessels that return blood to the capillaries.

Verbal apraxia Speech disorder in which the person has difficulty saying what he or she wants to say in a correct and consistent manner.

Verbal stimulus Any noise that elicits some sort of response from the patient.

Vertebrae Specialized bones comprising the spinal column.

Vertebral foramen Open space in the middle of vertebra.

Vertigo An out-of-control spinning sensation not relieved by lying down that may get worse when the eyes are closed.

Very high frequency A type of radio signal used to make two-way radio contact between the communications center and the responders. Now considered old technology compared with more contemporary 800-MHz radio systems.

Vesicants Agents named from the most obvious injury they inflict on a person; will burn and blister the skin or any other part of the body they touch; also known as *blister agents* or *mustard agents*.

Vesicles The "shipping containers" of the cell. They are simple in structure, consisting of a single membrane filled with liquid; they transport a wide variety of substances both inside and outside the cell.

Vestibule Space or cavity that serves as the entrance to the inner ear.

Veterinary medical assistance team Teams designed to provide animal care and assistance during disasters.

Vials Glass containers with rubber stoppers at the top.

Viral hemorrhagic fevers A group of viral diseases of diverse etiology (arenaviruses, filoviruses, bunyaviruses, and flaviviruses) having many similar characteristics, including increased capillary permeability, leukopenia, and thrombocytopenia, resulting in a severe multisystem syndrome.

Viral shedding Release of viruses from an infected host through some vector (e.g., sneezing, coughing, bleeding).

Virions Small particles of viruses.

Virulence A term to refer to the relative pathogenicity or the relative ability to do damage to the host of an infectious agent.

Virus Microorganism that invades cells and uses their machinery to live and replicate; cannot survive without a host, does not have a cell wall of its own, and consists of a strand of DNA or RNA surrounded by a capsid.

Visceral Portion of the peripheral nervous system that processes motor and sensory information from the internal organs; includes the autonomic nervous system.

Visceral pain Deep pain that arises from internal areas of the body that are enclosed within a cavity.

Visceral pleura Lining of the pleural cavity that adheres tightly to the lung surface.

Viscosity The thickness of a liquid; a high-viscosity liquid does not flow easily (e.g., oils and tar); a low-viscosity liquid flows easily (e.g., gasoline) and poses a greater risk for aspiration and consequent pulmonary damage.

Visual acuity card A standardized board used to test vision.

Vitreous chamber The most posterior chamber of the eyeball.

Vitreous humor Thick, jellylike substance that fills the vitreous chamber of the eyeball.

Voice over Internet protocol Telephone technology that gives Internet users the ability to make voice telephone calls.

Volatility A measure of how quickly a material passes into the vapor or gas state; the greater the volatility, the greater its rate of evaporation.

Volkmann contracture A deformity of the hand, fingers, and wrist caused by injury to the muscles of the forearm; also known as *ischemic contracture.*

Voltage Difference in electrical charge between two points.

Volume of packed red cells A measure of the relative percentage of blood cells (mainly erythrocytes) in a given volume of whole blood; also called *hematocrit* or *packed cell volume.*

Voluntary guarding Conscious contraction of the abdominal muscles in an attempt to prevent painful palpation.

Volvulus Intestinal obstruction caused by a knotting and twisting of the bowel.

Vomiting Forceful ejection of stomach contents through the mouth.

Vowel The letters *a, e, i, o, u,* and sometimes *y.*

Vulva The region of the external genital organs of the female, including the labia majora, labia minora, mons publis, clitoris, and vagina.

Vulvovaginitis Inflammation of the external female genitalia and vagina.

VX Most toxic of the nerve agent class of military warfare agents.

Warm zone Area surrounding the hot zone that functions as a safety buffer area, decontamination area, and as an access and egress point to and from the hot zone; also called the *contamination reduction zone.*

Warts Benign lesions caused by the papillomavirus.

Washout phase Vascular response in shock when postcapillary sphincters open, allowing fluid in the capillary beds to be pushed into systemic circulation; follows the stagnant phase.

Water solubility The degree to which a material or its vapors are soluble in water.

Water-reactive materials Materials that violently decompose and/or burn vigorously when they come in contact with moisture.

Waveform Movement away from the baseline in either a positive or negative direction.

Wernicke-Korsakoff syndrome Neurologic disorder caused by a thiamine deficiency; most often seen in chronic alcoholics; characterized by ataxia, nystagmus, weakness, and mental derangement in the early stages. In later stages, the condition is much more likely to become permanent and is characterized by amnesia, disorientation, delirium, and hallucinations.

Wheal A firm, rounded, flat-topped elevation of skin that is evanescent and pruritic (itches); also known as a *hive.*

Wheeze A musical, whistling sound heard on inspiration and/or expiration resulting from constriction or obstruction of the pharynx, trachea, or bronchi. Wheezing is commonly associated with asthma.

Wilderness command physician A physician who has received additional training by a Wilderness Emergency Medical Services Institute–endorsed course in wilderness medical care and medical direction of wilderness EMS providers and operations.

Wilderness emergency medical technician An emergency medical technician who has obtained EMT certification by Department of Transportation criteria and has completed additional modules in wilderness care; sometimes abbreviated as WEMT, W-EMT, or EMT-W.

Wilderness EMS An individual or group that preplans to administer care in an austere environment and then is called on to perform these duties when needed.

Wilderness EMS system A formally structured organization integrated into or part of the standard EMS system and configured to provide wilderness medical care to a discrete region.

Wilderness first aid A level of certification indicating a provider has been trained in traditional first aid with added training in wilderness care and first aid administration in austere environments.

Wilderness first responder A first responder who has obtained certification by Department of Transportation criteria and has completed additional modules in wilderness care.

Wilderness medicine Medical management in situations where care and prevention are limited by environmental considerations, prolonged extrication, or resource availability.

Window phase The period after infection during which the antigen is present but no antibody is detectable.

Withdrawal Physical and/or psychological signs and symptoms that result from discontinuing regular administration of a drug; effects are usually the opposite of the effects of the drug itself because the body has changed itself to maintain homeostasis.

Wolff-Parkinson-White syndrome Type of preexcitation syndrome characterized by a slurred upstroke of the QRS complex (delta wave) and wide QRS.

Word root The foundation of a word; establishes the basic meaning of a word.

Word salad The most severe form of looseness of associations in which the topic shifts so rapidly that it interrupts the flow of sentences themselves, producing a jumble of words.

Workload management Planning resources and support services around demand.

Wrap point A machinery entanglement hazard formed when any machine component rotates.

Xenografting Transplanting tissue from a member of a different species (e.g., porcine heart valves harvested from pigs).

Years of potential life lost (YPLL) A method that assumes that, on average, most people will live a productive life until the age of 65 years.

Yeast A unicellular type of fungus that reproduces by budding.

Yersinia pestis The anaerobic, gram-negative bacterium that causes plague disease in human beings and rodents.

Zone of coagulation In a full-thickness burn wound, the central area of the burn devoid of blood flow. This tissue is not salvageable and becomes visibly necrotic days after the injury.

Zone of stasis or ischemia Outside the zone of coagulation, where blood supply is tenuous. The capillaries may be damaged but oxygenated blood can still pass through them to perfuse the surrounding tissues.

Illustration Credits

Chapter 1

Figure 1-2. Courtesy U.S. Department of Agriculture, Center for Nutrition Policy and Promotion, Alexandria, VA.

Chapter 2

Figure 2-5. Chapleau, W., & Pons, P. (2007). *Emergency medical technician: Making the difference.* St. Louis: Mosby/JEMS.

Chapter 3

Figures 3-1, 3-5, 3-7, 3-12, 3-13. Courtesy Josh Krimston.

Figure 3-2. Centers for Disease Control and Prevention. (2003). *10 Leading causes of death by age group, United States, 2003.* Atlanta, GA: National Center for Health Statistics, National Vital Statistics System.

Figures 3-3, 3-4, 3-6. Courtesy Paul Maxwell.

Figure 3-14. Courtesy Alaska State Injury Prevention and Emergency Medical System.

Figure 3-15. Courtesy San Diego Medical Services Enterprise; photo courtesy John Creel.

Chapter 4

Figure 4-2. EMS Data Systems Inc. Phoenix, AZ.

Figures 4-3. Courtesy State of Wisconsin Department of Health and Human Services.

Figure 4-4. Courtesy Missouri Department of Health, Bureau of Emergency Medical Services, Jefferson City, MO.

Figure 4-5. Stoy, W., Platt, T., & Lejeune, D. A. (2007). *Mosby's EMT-Basic textbook* (2nd ed.). St. Louis: Mosby.

Chapter 7

Figures 7-22, 7-25, 7-27, 7-28, 7-29, 7-30, 7-31, 7-36, 7-39, 7-43, 7-44, 7-46, 7-47, 7-54, 7-57, 7-58, 7-60, 7-61, 7-63, 7-64, 7-65, 7-66, 7-67, 7-68, 7-69, 7-72, 7-73, 7-74. Drake, R., Vogl, W., & Mitchell, A. (2005). *Gray's anatomy for students.* New York: Churchill Livingstone.

Figure 7-5. Modified from Drake, R., Vogl, W., & Mitchell, A. (2005). *Gray's anatomy for students.* New York: Churchill Livingstone.

Figures 7-8; 7-10; 7-17, B and C; 7-35; 7-37; 7-38; 7-42; 7-45; 7-50; 7-53; 7-56; 7-70; 7-71; 7-75. Herlihy, B. (2007). *The human body in health and illness* (3rd ed.). Philadelphia: Saunders.

Figure 7-9. McCance, K. L., & Heuther, S. (2006). *Pathophysiology: The biologic basis for disease in adults and children* (5th ed.). St. Louis: Mosby.

Figure 7-16. Modified from Thibodeau, G., & Patton, K. (2005). *The human body in health and disease* (4th ed.). St. Louis: Mosby.

Figure 7-48. Aehlert, B. (2007). *ECGs made easy* (3rd ed.). St. Louis: Mosby/JEMS.

Figure 7-49. Huszar, R. (2007). *Basic dysrhythmias: Interpretation and management* (3rd ed.). St. Louis: Mosby.

Figures 7-51, 7-52. Thibodeau, G. A., & Patton, K. (2003). *Anatomy and physiology* (5th ed.). St. Louis: Mosby.

Chapter 8

Figure 8-1. Lewis, S. M., Heitkemper, M. M., Dirksen, S. R., et al. (2000). *Medical-surgical nursing: Assessment and management of clinical problems* (5th ed.). St. Louis, Mosby.

Figures 8-2, 8-3. Herlihy, B. (2007). *The human body in health and illness* (3rd ed.). Philadelphia: Saunders.

Figures 8-4; 8-7; 8-8; 8-9; 8-10; 8-11; 8-13, A and B; 8-14, 8-15, 8-16, 8-17, 8-18, 8-19, 8-20, 8-21, 8-22, 8-24. McCance, K. L., & Heuther, S (2006). *Pathophysiology: the biologic basis for disease in adults and children* (5th ed.). St Louis: Mosby.

Figure 8-5. Jorde, L. B., Carey, J. C., Bamshad, M. J., et al. (2006). *Medical genetics* (3rd ed.). St. Louis: Mosby.

Figure 8-13, C. Mudge-Grout, C. (1992). *Immunologic disorders.* St. Louis: Mosby–Year Book.

Figure 8-23. Cotran, R. S., Kumar, V., & Collins, T. (1999). *Robbins pathologic basis of disease* (6th ed.). Philadelphia: W. B. Saunders.

Chapter 11

Figure 11-3. Gould, B. E. (2006). *Pathophysiology for the health professions* (3rd ed.). Philadelphia: Saunders.

Figure 11-4. Lehne, R. A. (2007). *Pharmacology for nursing care* (6th ed.). Philadelphia: Saunders.

Figure 11-6, B. Aehlert, B. (2005). *PALS pediatric advanced life support study guide.* St. Louis: Mosby/JEMS.

Chapter 12

Figure 12-1. Fulcher, E. M., Soto, C. D., & Fulcher, R. M. (2003). *Pharmacology: Principles & applications: A worktext for allied health professionals.* Philadelphia: Saunders.

Drug photos. Gold Standard (2008). *Clinical pharmacology.* Tampa Bay, FL: Elsevier; Chapleau, W. (2007). *Emergency first responder: Making the difference.* St. Louis: Mosby; Guy, J. (2008). *Pharmacology for the prehospital professional.* St. Louis: Mosby/JEMS.

Chapter 13

Figures 13-9, 13-15, 13-16, 13-17, 13-18, 13-19, 13-21, 13-22, 13-23. deWit, S. (2005). *Fundamental concepts and skills for nursing* (2nd ed.). Philadelphia: Saunders.

Figure 13-10. Henry, M., & Stapleton, E. (2007). *EMT prehospital care* (3rd ed.). St. Louis: Mosby/JEMS.

Figure 13-13. Hockenberry, M., & Wilson, D. (2007). *Wong's nursing care of infants and children* (8th ed.). St. Louis: Mosby.

Figure 13-14. Photo courtesy Wolfe Tory Medical, Salt Lake City, UT.

Figures 13-25, 13-32, 13-33, 13-34, 13-35, 13-36, 13-37. Drake, R., Vogl, W., & Mitchell, A. (2005). *Gray's anatomy for students.* New York: Churchill Livingstone.

Figures 13-29, 13-30, 13-31. McKenry, L., Tessier, E., & Hogan, M. A. (2006). *Mosby's pharmacology in nursing* (22nd ed.). St. Louis: Mosby.

Figure 13-44. Courtesy Pyng Corporation, Richmond, BC, Canada.

Figure 13-45. Courtesy Vidacare Corporation, San Antonio, TX.

Chapter 14

Figures 14-2, 14-3, 14-5, 14-6. Heuther, S., & McCance, K. (2008). *Understanding pathophysiology* (4th ed.). St. Louis: Mosby/JEMS.

Figures 14-4, 14-8, 14-9. Seidel, H., Ball, J., Dains, J., et al. (2002). *Mosby's guide to physical examination* (5th ed.). St. Louis: Mosby.

Figure 14-7. Thompson, J., Wilson, S. (1996). *Health assessment for nursing practice.* St. Louis: Mosby.

Figures 14-11; 14-20; Skill 14-3, Step 5; Skill 14-4; Skill 14-6, Step 1. Chapleau, C., & Pons, P. (2007). *Emergency medical technician: Making the difference.* St. Louis: Mosby/JEMS.

Figures 14-13, 14-21, 14-22, 14-23, 14-31, 14-36, 14-37, 14-38, 14-44. Shade, B., Rothenberg, M., Wertz, E., et al. (2002). *Mosby's EMT-intermediate textbook* (2nd ed.). St Louis: Mosby.

Figure 14-14. Sorrentino, S., & Gorek, B. (2007). *Mosby's textbook of long-term care nursing assistants* (5th ed.). St. Louis: Mosby.

Figure 14-16. Henry, M., & Stapleton, E. (2004). *EMT prehospital care* (3rd ed.). St. Louis: Mosby.

Figure 14-20. Herlihy, B., & Maebius, N. (2003). *The human body in health and illness* (2nd ed.). Philadelphia: Saunders.

Figure 14-24. Cummins, R. (1996). *ACLS scenarios: Core concepts for case-based learning.* St. Louis: Mosby-Year book.

Figure 14-26. A, Courtesy Allied Healthcare Products. **B,** Courtesy O Two Medical Technologies.

Figure 14-27. Hockenberry, M., Wilson, D., Winklestein, et al. (2003). *Wong's nursing care of infants and children* (7th ed.). St. Louis, Mosby.

Figures 14-28, 14-30. Courtesy Nellcor.

Figures 14-29, 14-41. Roberts, J., & Hedges, J. (1998). *Clinical procedures in emergency medicine* (3rd ed.). Philadelphia: WB Saunders.

Figure 14-42. Benumof, B. (1996). *Airway management: Principles and practice.* St. Louis: Mosby-Year Book.

Chapter 17

Figures 17-4, 17-29, 17-30, 17-34, 17-39, 17-40, 17-42, 17-43, 17-44, 17-48. Seidel, H., Ball, J., Dains, J., et al. (2006). *Mosby's guide to physical examination* (6th ed.). St. Louis: Mosby.

Figures 17-6, 17-30, 17-31, 17-32. Bonewit-West, K. (2008). *Clinical procedures for medical assistants* (7th ed.). Philadelphia: Saunders.

Figures 17-13, 17-14, 17-18. Courtesy Wilderness Medical Associates, Portland, ME.

Figure 17-38. Swartz, M. (1989). *Textbook of physical diagnosis, history, and examination.* Philadelphia: Saunders.

Chapter 18

Figure 18-1. Chapleau, W. (2007). *Emergency first responder: Making the difference.* St. Louis: Mosby.

Figures 18-2, 18-3. Chapleau, W., & Pons, P. (2007). *Emergency medical technician: making the difference.* St. Louis: Mosby/JEMS.

Chapter 19

Figure 19-1. Reprinted with permission from Mountain Valley EMS Agency, Modesto, CA.

Figure 19-6. Courtesy Greater Community Hospital Ambulance, Creston, IA.

Figure 19-7. Courtesy Mettag, Draper, UT.

Chapter 20

Figure 20-1. Mandell, G., Bennett, J., & Dolin, R. (2005). *Principles and practice of infectious disease.* (6th ed., Vol. 2). New York: Churchill-Livingstone.

Figures 20-2, 20-3, 20-5, 20-6, 20-7, 20-9. Zitelli, B., & Davis, H. (2002). *Atlas of pediatric physical diagnosis* (4th ed.). St. Louis: Mosby.

Figure 20-4. Sanders, M. (2007). *Mosby's paramedic textbook* (3rd ed.). St. Louis: Mosby/JEMS.

Chapter 21

Figures 21-2, 21-8, A; 21-11; 21-33. Marx, J., Hockberger, R., & Walls, R. (2006). *Rosen's emergency medicine: Concepts and clinical practice.* (6th ed., Vol. 2). St. Louis: Mosby

Figure 21-3. Modified from Herlihy, B. (2007). *The human body in health and illness* (3rd ed.). Philadelphia: Saunders.

Figure 21-4. Chapleau, W. (2007). *Emergency first responder: Making the difference.* St. Louis: Mosby.

Figures 21-5, 21-6. Modified from Drake, R., Vogl, W., & Mitchell, A. (2005). *Gray's anatomy for students.* New York: Churchill Livingstone.

Figure 21-8, C. Rakel, R. E. *Textbook of family medicine* (6th ed.). Philadelphia: Saunders.

Figure 21-9. Cummings, C. W., Haughey, B. H., Thomas, J. R., et al. (2005). *Cummings otolaryngology, head and neck surgery* (4th ed.). St. Louis: Mosby.

Figure 21-10. Modified from Long, S. S., Pickering, L. K., & Prober, C. G. (2003). *Principles and practice of pediatric infectious diseases* (2nd ed.). New York: Churchill Livingstone.

Figure 21-13. Khatri, V. P., & Asensio, J. A. (2003). *Operative surgery manual.* Philadelphia: Saunders.

Figures 21-14, 21-15, 21-16, 21-17, 21-18, 21-35. Drake, R., Vogl, W., & Mitchell, A. (2005). *Gray's anatomy for students.* New York: Churchill Livingstone.

Figure 21-21. Thibodeau, G. A., & Patton, K. T. (2004). *Structure and function of the body* (12th ed.). St. Louis: Mosby.

Figure 21-22. Modified from Mason, R. J., Broaddus, C., Murray, J. F., et al. (2005). *Murray and Nadel's textbook of respiratory medicine* (4th ed.). Philadelphia: Saunders.

Figure 21-23. Modified from Townsend, C. M., Beauchamp, D., Evers, M., et al. (2004). *Sabiston textbook of surgery: The biological basis of modern surgical practice* (17th ed.). Philadelphia: Saunders.

Figure 21-24. Ford, M. D., Delaney, K. A., Ling, L., et al. (2000). *Clinical toxicology.* Philadelphia: Saunders.

Figures 21-27, 21-28. McCance, K. L., & Heuther, S. (2006). *Pathophysiology: the biologic basis for disease in adults and children* (5th ed.). St. Louis: Mosby.

Figure 21-29. Kumar, V. K., Abbas, A. K., & Fausto, N. (2005). *Robbins and Cotran pathologic basis of disease* (7th ed.). Philadelphia: Saunders.

Figure 21-30. Mason, R. J., Broaddus, C., Murray, J. F., et al. (2005). *Murray and Nadel's textbook of respiratory medicine* (4th ed.). Philadelphia: Saunders.

Figure 21-31. Mandell, G. L., Bennett, J., & Dolin, R. (2005). *Principles and practice of infectious diseases* (6th ed.). New York: Churchill Livingstone.

Figure 21-32. Modified from Mandell, G. L., Bennett, J., & Dolin, R. (2005). *Principles and practice of infectious diseases* (6th ed.). New York: Churchill Livingstone.

Figure 21-34. Zipes, D. P., Libby, P., Bonow, R., et al. (2005). *Braunwald's heart disease: A textbook of cardiovascular medicine* (7th ed.). Philadelphia: Saunders.

Chapter 22

Figures 22-1, 22-2, 22-3, 22-100. Drake, R., Vogl, W., & Mitchell, A. (2005). *Gray's anatomy for students.* New York: Churchill Livingstone.

Figures 22-4, 22-5, 22-6, 22-13. Herlihy, B. (2007). *The human body in health and illness* (3rd ed.). Philadelphia: Saunders.

Figure 22-7. Sanders, M. (2007). *Mosby's paramedic textbook* (3rd ed.). St. Louis: Mosby/JEMS.

Figures 22-8, 22-9, 22-10. Canobbio, M. (1990). *Cardiovascular disorders.* St. Louis: Mosby–Year Book.

Figures 22-15, 22-17, 22-28, 22-30. Urden, L. D., Stacy, K. M., & Lough, M. E. (2006). *Thelan's critical care nursing* (5th ed.). St. Louis: Mosby.

Figures 22-11, 22-12, 22-14, 22-31, 22-47, 22-62. Crawford, M., & Spence, M. (1994). *Common sense approach to coronary care* (6th ed.). St. Louis: Mosby–Year Book.

Figure 22-16. Methodist Hospital. (1986). *Basic electrocardiography: A modular approach.* St. Louis: Mosby–Year Book.

Figures 22-18, 22-22, 22-85, 22-86, 22-87, 22-88, 22-89, 22-90, 22-91, 22-92, 22-93, 22-94, 22-95, 22-96, 22-113. Phalen, T., & Aehlert, B. (2006). *The 12-lead ECG in acute coronary syndromes* (2nd ed.). St. Louis: Mosby/JEMS.

Figure 22-19. Closhesy, J., et al. (1996). *Critical care nursing* (2nd ed.). Philadelphia: W. B. Saunders.

Figure 22-20; Skill 22-8, Step 1. Lounsbury, P., & Frye, S. (1992). *Cardiac rhythm disorders: A nursing process approach* (2nd ed.). St. Louis: Mosby–Year Book.

Figures 22-21, 22-24, 22-25, 22-29, 22-34, 22-35, 22-37, 22-39, 22-44, 22-45, 22-52, 22-53, 22-54, 22-57, 22-58, 22-60, 22-61, 22-63, 22-65, 22-66, 22-67, 22-69, 22-70, 22-72, 22-75, 22-77, 22-78, 22-79, 22-80, 22-81, 22-82. Aehlert, B. (2007). *ECGs made easy* (3rd ed.). St. Louis: Mosby/JEMS.

Figures 22-23, 22-40, 22-42, 22-97. Goldberger, A. (2006). *Clinical electrocardiography: A simplified approach* (7th ed.). St. Louis: Mosby.

Figures 22-26, 22-48, 22-59, 22-83. Chou, T. (1996). *Electrocardiography in clinical practice: Adult and pediatric* (4th ed.). Philadelphia: Saunders.

Figure 22-27. Thibodeau, G. A., & Patton, K. (2003). *Anatomy and physiology* (5th ed.). St. Louis: Mosby.

Figures 22-32, 22-43, 22-49, 22-51, 22-55, 22-73, 22-74, 22-76. Shade, B., Collins, T., Wertz, E., et al. (2007). *Mosby's EMT-Intermediate textbook for the 1999 National Standard Curriculum* (3rd ed.). St. Louis: Mosby/JEMS.

Figures 22-33, 22-46, 22-50, 22-64, 22-68, 22-71, 22-106. Aehlert, B. (2007). *ACLS study guide* (3rd ed.). St. Louis: Mosby.

Figure 22-38. Kinney, M. (1995). *Andreoli's comprehensive cardiac care* (8th ed.). St. Louis: Mosby–Year Book.

Figure 22-41. Zipes, D. P., Libby, P., Bonow, R., et al. (2005). *Braunwald's heart disease: A textbook of cardiovascular medicine* (7th ed.). Philadelphia: Saunders.

Figures 22-56, 22-84. Grauer, K. (1998). *A practical guide to ECG interpretation* (2nd ed.). St. Louis: Mosby–Year Book.

Figures 22-98; 22-99, A; 22-102; 22-126. Seidel, H., Ball, J., Dains, J., et al. (2006). *Mosby's guide to physical examination* (6th ed.). St. Louis: Mosby.

Figure 22-99, B. Zatouroff, M. (1996). *Physical signs in general medicine* (2nd ed.). London: Mosby-Wolff.

Figures 22-103, 22-109, 22-110, 22-111, 22-112, 22-125. Kumar, V. K., Abbas, A. K., & Fausto, N. (2005). *Robbins and Cotran pathologic basis of disease* (7th ed.). Philadelphia: Saunders.

Figure 22-104. E. Braunwald & R. M. Califf (Eds.) (1996). *Atlas of heart diseases: Acute myocardial infarction and other acute ischemic syndromes* (Vol. 3). Singapore: Current Medicine.

Figure 22-105. Huether, S., & McCance, K. (2004). *Understanding pathophysiology* (3rd ed.). St. Louis: Mosby.

Figures 22-107, 22-108, 22-114. Gould, B. E. (2006). *Pathophysiology for the health professions* (3rd ed.). Philadelphia: Saunders.

Figures 22-115, 22-116, 22-117, 22-118, 22-119, 22-120, 22-121, 22-122, 22-123. Hockenberry, M., & Wilson, D. (2007). *Wong's nursing care of infants and children* (8th ed.). St. Louis: Mosby.

Figure 22-124. Zitelli, B., & David, H. (2002). *Atlas of pediatric physical diagnosis* (4th ed.). St. Louis: Mosby.

Chapter 23

Figure 23-1. Black, J. M., & Hokanson Hawks, J. (2005). *Medical-surgical nursing: Clinical management for positive outcomes* (7th ed.). Philadelphia: Saunders.

Figures 23-2, 23-3, 23-4, 23-5, 23-7, 23-8. Drake, R., Vogl, W., & Mitchell, A. (2005). *Gray's anatomy for students.* New York: Churchill Livingstone.

Figure 23-20. Kidwell, C. S., Starkman, S., Eckstein, M., et al. (2000). Identifying stroke in the field. Prospective validation of the Los Angeles Prehospital Stroke Screen (LAPSS). *Stroke, 31,* 71-76.

Figures 23-21, 23-22. Cohen, J., & Powderly, W. G. (2004). *Infectious diseases* (2nd ed.). St. Louis: Mosby.

Chapter 24

Figure 24-2. Thibodeau, G., & Patton, K. (2005). *The human body in health and disease* (4th ed.). St. Louis: Mosby.

Figure 24-3. Kumar, V. K., Abbas, A. K., & Fausto, N. (2005). *Robbins and Cotran pathologic basis of disease* (7th ed.). Philadelphia: Saunders.

Chapter 25

Figures 25-1, 25-2, 25-3. Cohen, J., & Powderly, W. G. (2004). *Infectious diseases* (2nd ed.). London: Mosby.

Figures 25-4, 25-5. Drake, R., Vogl, W., & Mitchell, A. (2005). *Gray's anatomy for students.* New York: Churchill Livingstone.

Figure 25-6. Kumar, V. K., Abbas, A. K., & Fausto, N. (2005). *Robbins and Cotran pathologic basis of disease* (7th ed.). Philadelphia: Saunders.

Figures 25-7, 25-8, 25-9. Harris, E., Budd, R. C., Firestein, G. S., et al. (2005). *Kelley's textbook of rheumatology* (7th ed.). Philadelphia: Saunders.

Chapter 26

Figure 26-1. Chapleau, W. & Pons, P. (2007). *Emergency first responder: Making the difference*. St. Louis: Mosby/JEMS.

Figures 26-2 to 26-8, 26-18, 26-27, 26-28, 26-29. Drake, R., Vogl, W., & Mitchell, A. (2005). *Gray's anatomy for students*. New York: Churchill Livingstone.

Figures 26-9, 26-10. Feldman, M., Friendman, L. S., & Brandt, L. *Sleisenger and Fordtran's gastrointestinal and liver disease* (8th ed.). Philadelphia: Saunders.

Figure 26-11. Harris, E., Budd, R. C., Firestein, G. D., Genovese, M., & Sergent, J. (2005). *Kelley's textbook of rheumatology* (7th ed.). Philadelphia: Saunders.

Figure 26-12. Stoy, W. A., Platt, T. E., Lejeune, D. A. (2005). *Mosby's EMT-Basic textbook* (2nd ed.) St. Louis: Mosby.

Figures 26-13, 26-20, 26-21, 26-26, 26-27. McCance, K. L., & Huether, S. (2006). *Pathophysiology: The biologic basis for disease in adults and children* (5th ed.). St. Louis: Mosby.

Figure 26-14. Cumming, C. W., Haughey, B. H., Thomas, J. R., Harker, L., Flint, P., Robbins, K. et al. (2005). *Cummings otolaryngology, head and neck surger* (4th ed.). St. Louis: Mosby.

Figures 26-16, 26-17. Damajanov, I., Linder, J. (1996). *Anderson's pathology* (10th ed.). St. Louis: Mosby.

Figure 26-19. Phipps, W. P., Sands, J. K., Marek, J. F. (1999). *Medical-surgical nursing: Concepts and clinical practice* (6th ed.). St. Louis: Mosby.

Figures 26-23, 26-24, 26-25, 26-31. Stevens, A., Lowe, J. (2000). *Pathology* (2nd ed.). London: Mosby.

Figures 26-26, 26-30. Damjanov, I., Linder, J., editors. (1996). *Anderson's pathology* (10th ed., Vol. 2). St. Louis: Mosby.

Chapter 27

Figures 27-1, 27-5. Herlihy, B. (2007). *The human body in health and illness* (3rd ed.). Philadelphia: Saunders.

Figures 27-2, 27-3, 27-7. Gould, B. E. (2006). *Pathophysiology for the health professions* (3rd ed.). Philadelphia: Saunders.

Figures 27-4, 27-8, 27-9, 27-11, 27-12. Drake, R., Vogl, W., & Mitchell, A. (2005). *Gray's anatomy for students*. New York: Churchill Livingstone.

Figure 27-6. Brenner, B. *The kidney* (7th ed., Vol. 1). Philadelphia: Saunders.

Chapter 28

Figure 28-1. Branch, W. T. (2006). Office practice of medicine. In J. Marx, R. Hockberger, & R. Walls (Eds.) (2006). *Rosen's emergency medicine: Concepts and clinical practice* (6th ed.). St. Louis: Mosby.

Figures 28-3, 28-6. Black, J. M., & Hokanson Hawks, J. (2005). *Medical-surgical nursing: Clinical management for positive outcomes* (7th ed.). Philadelphia: Saunders.

Figure 28-5. Noble, J. (2001). *Textbook of primary care medicine* (3rd ed.). St. Louis: Mosby.

Chapter 29

Figures 29-1, 29-2, 29-3, 29-5, 29-6, 29-7, 29-9, 29-11, 29-12, 29-13, 29-14, 29-15, 29-16, 29-17, 29-18, 29-19, 29-21, 29-22, 29-23, 29-24, 29-25, 29-26, 29-27, 29-28, 29-29, 29-30, 29-31, 29-32, 29-33, 29-34, 29-35, 29-38, 29-39, 29-40, 29-41, 29-42. Habif,

T. P., Campbell, J. I., Chapman, S., et al. (2005). *Skin disease: Diagnosis and treatment* (2nd ed.). St. Louis: Mosby.

Figures 29-4, 29-10. Weston, W. L., Lane, A. T., & Morelli, J. G. (1996). *Color textbook of pediatric dermatology* (2nd ed.). St. Louis: Mosby–Year Book.

Figure 29-20. Black, J. M., & Hokanson Hawks, J. (2005). *Medical-surgical nursing: Clinical management for positive outcomes* (7th ed.). Philadelphia: Saunders.

Chapter 30

Figure 30-1. Auerbach, P. (2007). *Wilderness medicine* (5th ed.). St. Louis: Mosby. **A,** Courtesy Michael Cardwell & Associates. **B,** Courtesy Indiana University Medical Center. **C,** Courtesy Paul Auerbach and Riley Rees (brown recluse bite after 6 hours) and Paul Auerbach (brown recluse bite after 24 hours). **D,** Courtesy Richard M. Houseman, Department of Entomology, University of Missouri–Columbia (striped scorpion) and R. David Gaban (giant hairy scorpion).

Figure 30-2. A, Auerbach, P. (2007). *Wilderness medicine* (5th ed.). St. Louis: Mosby. **B,** Courtesy Sherman Minton. **C,** Courtesy Michael Cardwell and Carl Barden, Medtoxin Venom Laboratory, DeLand, FL. **D,** Courtesy Charles Alfaro.

Figure 30-3. Auerbach, P. (2007). *Wilderness medicine* (5th ed.). St. Louis: Mosby. **A,** Courtesy Larry Madin, Woods Hole Oceanographic Institution, MA. **B,** Part 1, photo courtesy Howard Hall; part 4, photo courtesy Robert D. Hayes. **C,** Courtesy John Williamson.

Chapter 31

Figure 31-1. Courtesy Centers for Disease Control and Prevention, Sol Silverman, Jr.

Figure 31-2. Courtesy Centers for Disease Control and Prevention, Patricia Walker, Regions Hospital, MN.

Figures 31-3, 31-7, 31-9, 31-10, 31-12, 31-15. Courtesy Centers for Disease Control and Prevention.

Figure 31-4. Courtesy Centers for Disease Control and Prevention, Edwin P. Ewing, Jr.

Figure 31-5. Courtesy Centers for Disease Control and Prevention, Thomas Hooten.

Figure 31-6. Courtesy Centers for Disease Control and Prevention, Barbara Andrews.

Figure 31-8. Courtesy Centers for Disease Control and Prevention, National Immunization Program, Barbara Rice.

Figure 31-11. Courtesy Centers for Disease Control and Prevention, Thomas F. Sellers, Emory University, Atlanta, GA.

Figure 31-13. Courtesy Centers for Disease Control and Prevention, Lourdes Fraw, Jim Pledger.

Figure 31-14. Courtesy Centers for Disease Control and Prevention, Reed & Carnrick Pharmaceuticals, Monheim, Germany.

Chapter 32

Figure 32-1. Thibodeau, G. A., & Patton, K. (2003). *Anatomy and physiology* (5th ed.). St. Louis: Mosby.

Chapter 33

Figures 33-1, 33-2, 33-4, 33-5. Applegate, E. (2006). *The anatomy and physiology learning system* (3rd ed.). Philadelphia: Saunders.

Figure 33-3. Marx, J., Hockberger, R., & Walls, R. (2006). *Rosen's emergency medicine: Concepts and clin2ical practice* (6th ed., Vol. 2). St. Louis: Mosby.

Chapter 34

Figure 34-5. Guyton, A., & Hall, J. (2006). *Textbook of medical physiology* (11th ed.). Philadelphia: Saunders.

Figure 34-6, 34-9, 34-10, 34-11, 34-12, 34-13. Gould, B. E. (2006). *Pathophysiology for the health professions* (3rd ed.). Philadelphia: Saunders.

Figure 34-8. Chapleau, W., & Pons, P. (2007). *Emergency medical technician: Making the difference.* St. Louis: Mosby/ JEMS.

Index

Page numbers followed by *f, t,* or *b* indicate figures, tables, or boxed material, respectively. Numbers in **boldface** indicate volume number.